TRAUMA MANAGEMENT

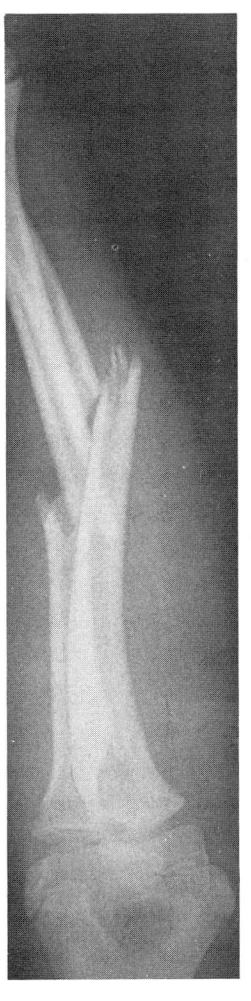

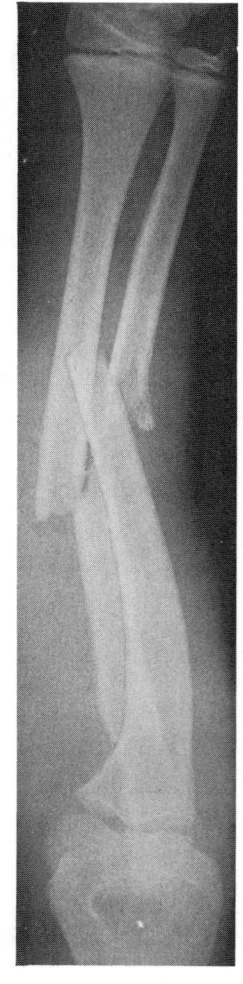
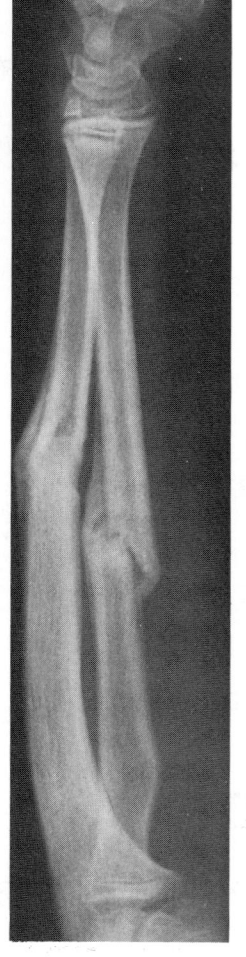
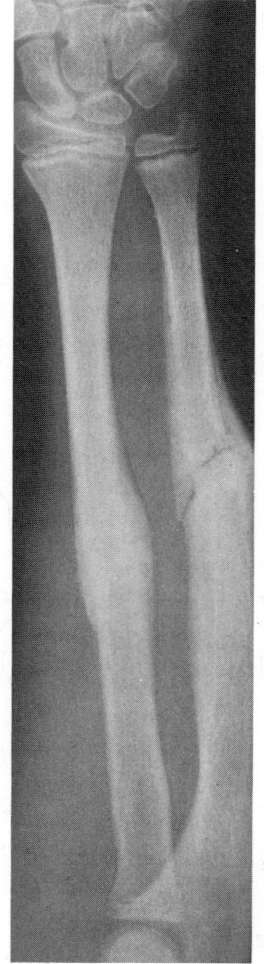
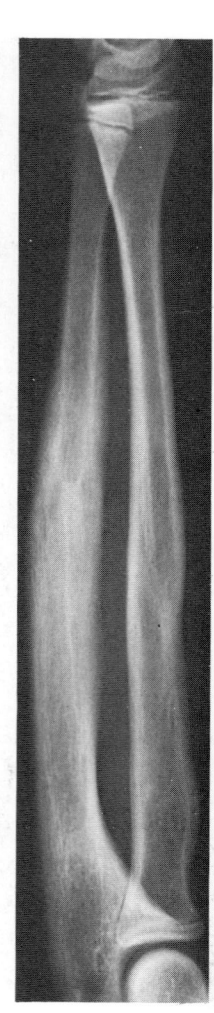

TRAUMA MANAGEMENT

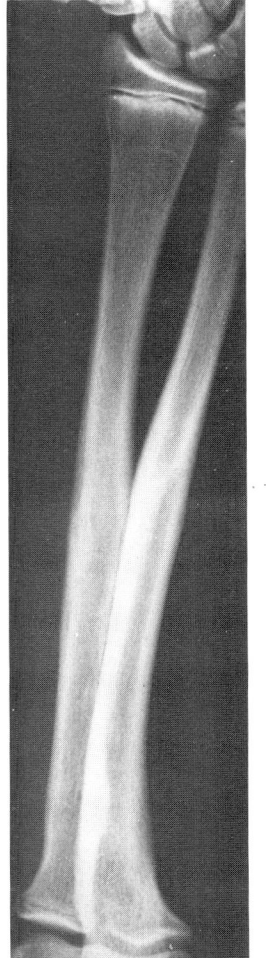

EDWIN F. CAVE
Member, Board of Consultation,
Massachusetts General Hospital

JOHN F. BURKE
Visiting Surgeon, Massachusetts General Hospital;
Associate Professor of Surgery, Harvard Medical
School; Chief of Staff, Shriners Burns Institute

ROBERT J. BOYD
Assistant Orthopedic Surgeon, Massachusetts
General Hospital; Clinical Instructor in Orthopedic
Surgery, Harvard Medical School

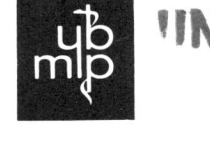

YEAR BOOK MEDICAL PUBLISHERS, INC.
35 East Wacker Drive / Chicago

Copyright © 1974 by Year Book Medical Publishers, Inc.

All rights reserved. No part of this publication may be reproduced, stored in a retrieval system, or transmitted, in any form or by any means, electronic, mechanical, photocopying, recording, or otherwise, without prior written permission from the publisher.

Printed in the United States of America.

Library of Congress Catalog Card Number: 74-78365

International Standard Book Number: 0-8151-1454-0

This volume is dedicated to our Senior Editor,

DR. EDWIN F. CAVE

whose inspired leadership, enthusiasm, personal persuasiveness and extensive clinical experience have made possible the completion of this revision. He continued an active role on the Editorial Board, despite devastating personal illness, which necessitated his retirement from practice. His courage and determination have been an inspiration to us all, and we gratefully acknowledge his invaluable guidance and assistance.

Preface

WHEN THE EDITORIAL BOARD was formed to revise *Fractures and Other Injuries*, it was determined that the more general subject of trauma would be emphasized. We have thus enlarged our volume, attempting to encompass more fully the surgical aspects of injury, pertinent to the general field of trauma.

Advances in surgery, particularly of cardiac, chest, vascular and abdominal trauma, have been rapid and account for the expansion of our text in these areas. Although new devices have become available for fracture fixation, joint replacement and external stabilization of the spine, and are described in this edition, the basic approach to fracture management has changed relatively little. Perhaps the greatest single advance in fracture treatment in the past ten years has been the increased number and availability of well-trained orthopedic surgeons, allowing wider application of known principles. We hope that this book will help to increase further the number of surgeons well prepared to deal with trauma, an ever increasing problem. Accidental injury and death have reached staggering proportions, becoming a national emergency, and show no sign of abating.

The original edition of this book, *Experience in the Management of Fractures and Dislocations*, edited by Dr. P. D. Wilson, became the basis for *Fractures and Other Injuries*, edited by Dr. E. F. Cave, which has led to our present text and which provides a sound foundation. We believe that there is a need for such a text and hope that this book will prove to be of value to all those concerned with the management of trauma.

The authors have been selected from the members and former members of the Massachusetts General Hospital Staff with special interest and competence in the subjects assigned. The opinions expressed in the various chapters represent primarily the thoughts of the individual authors, but these opinions are substantiated in the main by the members of the Editorial Board, consisting of Dr. E. F. Cave, Dr. J. F. Burke and Dr. R. J. Boyd.

The drawings were made in the Medical Art Department of Massachusetts General Hospital by Mrs. Edith Tagrin and Mr. Paul Andriesse and by Mr. Sidney Rosenthal of Arrco Medical Art and Design, Inc. Photographs were made under the direction of Mr. Stanley Bennett of our hospital. Their fine efforts made our task easier, and they deserve a large share of credit for whatever success the book may have. Bibliographical references to pertinent material appear at the end of the chapters. All of the authors, we are sure, are grateful to the many patients who have taught us so much about their injuries, and to them we owe an everlasting debt. The Year Book Medical Publishers have been of enormous help from the beginning of our endeavor, both in editing the manuscript and in arranging the illustrations.

Great appreciation is expressed by the Editorial Board to all the individual authors who are responsible for the thoughts contained in the following pages. We thank Mrs. Judith Wood for her assistance in typing the manuscripts.

Special thanks are due Miss Marion Buchanan, who devoted countless hours to the Editorial Board duties and almost single handedly managed the extensive secretarial chores. Without her intelligent and loyal devotion to the job at hand, the present volume could not have been prepared.

JOHN F. BURKE

ROBERT J. BOYD

July 1, 1974

List of Contributors

ATHANASOULAS, CHRISTOS A.: Assistant Radiologist, Massachusetts General Hospital; Assistant Professor of Radiology at the Massachusetts General Hospital, Harvard Medical School

AUFRANC, OTTO E.: Visiting Orthopedic Surgeon, Massachusetts General Hospital; Lecturer on Orthopedic Surgery, Harvard Medical School; Chief of Orthopedic Surgery Division, New England Baptist Hospital (Retired)

AUSTEN, W. GERALD: Chief of General Surgical Services, Massachusetts General Hospital; Professor of Surgery, Harvard Medical School

BAKER, EDWARD P., JR.: Assistant in Neurosurgery, Massachusetts General Hospital; Clinical Assistant in Surgery, Harvard Medical School

BARNES, BENJAMIN A.: Senior Surgeon and Chief of the Transplant Service, Department of Surgery, New England Medical Center Hospital; Professor, Department of Surgery, Tufts University School of Medicine

BARR, JOSEPH S., JR.: Assistant Orthopedic Surgeon, Massachusetts General Hospital; Clinical Instructor in Orthopedic Surgery, Harvard Medical School

BAUM, STANLEY: Radiologist and Chief of Cardiovascular Radiology, Massachusetts General Hospital; Professor of Radiology at the Massachusetts General Hospital, Harvard Medical School

BEHRINGER, GLENN E.: Associate Visiting Surgeon, Massachusetts General Hospital; Associate Clinical Professor of Surgery, Harvard Medical School

BENDIXEN, HENRIK H.: Chief of Anesthesia, Columbia University College of Physicians and Surgeons; formerly Anesthetist, Massachusetts General Hospital.

BOYD, ROBERT J.: Assistant Orthopedic Surgeon, Massachusetts General Hospital; Clinical Instructor in Orthopedic Surgery, Harvard Medical School

BROWN, THORNTON: Visiting Orthopedic Surgeon, Massachusetts General Hospital; Associate Clinical Professor of Orthopedic Surgery, Harvard Medical School

BUCKLEY, MORTIMER J.: Associate Visiting Surgeon, Massachusetts General Hospital; Associate Professor of Surgery, Harvard Medical School

BURKE, JOHN F.: Visiting Surgeon, Massachusetts General Hospital; Associate Professor of Surgery, Harvard Medical School; Chief of Staff, Shriners Burns Institute

CANNON, BRADFORD: Visiting Surgeon, Massachusetts General Hospital; Associate Clinical Professor of Surgery, Harvard Medical School

CAVE, EDWIN F.: Member of the Board of Consultation, Massachusetts General Hospital

CHANDLER, HUGH P.: Assistant Orthopedic Surgeon, Massachusetts General Hospital; Clinical Instructor in Orthopedic Surgery, Harvard Medical School

COHEN, JONATHAN: Consultant of Orthopedic Surgery, Kennedy Memorial Hospital; Professor of Orthopedic Surgery, Tufts University School of Medicine

X / LIST OF CONTRIBUTORS

CONSTABLE, JOHN D.: Associate Visiting Surgeon, Massachusetts General Hospital; Assistant Clinical Professor of Surgery, Harvard Medical School

DAGGETT, WILLARD M.: Associate Visiting Surgeon, Massachusetts General Hospital; Associate Professor of Surgery, Harvard Medical School; Established Investigator of the American Heart Association Award Number 70-131

DARLING, R. CLEMENT: Associate Visiting Surgeon and Chief, Peripheral Vascular Clinic, Massachusetts General Hospital; Assistant Clinical Professor of Surgery, Harvard Medical School

EGBERT, LAWRENCE D.: Division of Anesthesiology, Johns Hopkins Hospital; formerly Associate Anesthetist, Massachusetts General Hospital

GEFFIN, BENNIE: Associate Anesthetist, Massachusetts General Hospital; Staff Anesthesiologist, Lynn Hospital; Assistant Professor of Anesthesia at the Massachusetts General Hospital, Harvard Medical School

HARRIS, WILLIAM H.: Visiting Orthopedic Surgeon, Massachusetts General Hospital; Associate Clinical Professor of Orthopedic Surgery, Harvard Medical School

HERNDON, JAMES H.: Orthopedic Surgeon, Blodgett Memorial Hospital and Mary Free Bed Hospital, Grand Rapids, Michigan; Assistant Clinical Professor, Michigan State University; formerly Chief Resident in Orthopedic Surgery, Massachusetts General Hospital

HUDDLESTON, JAMES I.: Assistant Orthopedic Surgeon, Massachusetts General Hospital; Clinical Instructor in Orthopedic Surgery, Harvard Medical School

JONES, WILLIAM N.: Associate Orthopedic Surgeon, Massachusetts General Hospital; Clinical Instructor in Orthopedic Surgery, Harvard Medical School

JOPLIN, ROBERT J.: Member Department of Orthopedic Surgery, Placid Memorial Hospital, Lake Placid, New York; formerly Member Senior Consulting Staff, Massachusetts General Hospital

KENZORA, JOHN E.: Assistant in Orthopedic Surgery, Children's Hospital Medical Center; Orthopedic Staff Member, Peter Bent Brigham Hospital; Instructor in Orthopedic Surgery, Harvard Medical School

KERR, WALTER S., JR.: Visiting Urologist, Massachusetts General Hospital; Assistant Clinical Professor of Surgery, Harvard Medical School

KJELLBERG, RAYMOND N.: Visiting Neurosurgeon, Massachusetts General Hospital; Associate Clinical Professor of Surgery, Harvard Medical School

LOWELL, J. DRENNAN: Senior Assistant in Orthopedic Surgery, Peter Bent Brigham Hospital; Visiting Assistant in Orthopedic Surgery, Children's Hospital Medical Center; Member of the Board of Consultation, Massachusetts General Hospital; Assistant Professor of Orthopedic Surgery, Harvard Medical School

MACAUSLAND, WILLIAM R., JR.: Assistant Orthopedic Surgeon, Massachusetts General Hospital; Associate Clinical Professor of Orthopedic Surgery, Harvard Medical School

MALT, RONALD A.: Visiting Surgeon and Chief of Gastroenterological Surgery, Massachusetts General Hospital; Associate Professor of Surgery, Harvard Medical School

MILLENDER, LEWIS H.: Attending Hand Service, Department of Orthopedic Surgery, Robert Breck Brigham Hospital; Clinical Instructor in Orthopedic Surgery, Harvard Medical School

MONCURE, ASHBY C.: Associate Visiting Surgeon, Massachusetts General Hospital; Assistant Professor of Surgery at the Massachusetts General Hospital, Harvard Medical School

MUNDTH, ELDRED D.: Associate Visiting Surgeon, Massachusetts General Hospital; Associate Professor of Surgery, Harvard Medical School

NALEBUFF, EDWARD A.: Chief of Hand Surgery, Robert Breck Brigham Hospital; Assistant Clinical Professor of Orthopedic Surgery, Harvard Medical School

NORTON, PAUL L.: Member of the Board of Consultation, Massachusetts General Hospital

OJEMANN, ROBERT G.: Associate Visiting Neurosurgeon, Massachusetts General Hospital; Associate Clinical Professor of Surgery, Harvard Medical School

OTTINGER, LESLIE W.: Assistant Surgeon and Coordinator of the Internship and Residency Training Program, Massachusetts General Hospital; Associate Professor of Surgery at the Massachusetts General Hospital, Harvard Medical School

OTTO, WILLIAM J.: Clinical Assistant in Radiology, Massachusetts General Hospital; Visiting Radiologist, Beverly Hospital

PATEL, DINESH: Assistant in Orthopedic Surgery, Massachusetts General Hospital; Clinical Instructor in Orthopedic Surgery, Harvard Medical School

PIERCE, DONALD S.: Associate Orthopedic Surgeon, Massachusetts General Hospital; Clinical Associate in Orthopedic Surgery, Harvard Medical School

QUINBY, WILLIAM C., JR.: Associate Surgeon, Massachusetts General Hospital; Assistant Clinical Professor of Surgery, Harvard Medical School

REMENSNYDER, JOHN P.: Assistant Surgeon and Chief of Plastic Surgery, Massachusetts General Hospital; Assistant Clinical Professor of Surgery, Harvard Medical School

RISEBOROUGH, EDWARD J.: Senior Associate in Orthopedic Surgery, Children's Hospital Medical Center; Assistant Clinical Professor of Orthopedic Surgery, Harvard Medical School

RODKEY, GRANT V.: Visiting Surgeon, Massachusetts General Hospital; Associate Clinical Professor of Surgery, Harvard Medical School

ROWE, CARTER R.: Visiting Orthopedic Surgeon, Massachusetts General Hospital; Associate Clinical Professor of Orthopedic Surgery, Harvard Medical School

RUSSELL, PAUL S.: Visiting Surgeon, Massachusetts General Hospital; John Homans Professor of Surgery, Harvard Medical School

SCANNELL, J. GORDON: Visiting Surgeon, Massachusetts General Hospital; Clinical Professor of Surgery, Harvard Medical School

SLEDGE, CLEMENT B.: Surgeon in Chief, Robert Breck Brigham Hospital; Chief of Orthopedic Surgery, Peter Bent Brigham Hospital; Member of the Board of Consultation, Massachusetts General Hospital; Professor of Orthopedic Surgery, Harvard Medical School

TRAVIS, KENNETH W.: Assistant in Anesthesiology, Children's Hospital Medical Center; Clinical Assistant in Anesthesiology, Harvard Medical School

VANDER SALM, THOMAS J.: U. S. Navy, Virginia Beach, Virginia; formerly Chief Resident in Surgery, Massachusetts General Hospital

WALTMAN, ARTHUR C.: Assistant Radiologist, Massachusetts General Hospital; Assistant Professor of Radiology at the Massachusetts General Hospital, Harvard Medical School

WELCH, CLAUDE E.: Senior Consultant in Surgery, Massachusetts General Hospital; Clinical Professor of Surgery *Emeritus*, Harvard Medical School

WEPSIC, JAMES G.: Assisting Visiting Neurosurgeon, Massachusetts General Hospital; Clinical Instructor in Surgery, Harvard Medical School

WHEELOCK, FRANK C., JR.: Visiting Surgeon, Massachusetts General Hospital; Assistant Clinical Professor of Surgery, Harvard Medical School

WHITE, JAMES C.: Senior Consulting Staff, Massachusetts General Hospital; Professor of Surgery at Massachusetts General Hospital, Harvard Medical School (Emeritus)

WYMAN, EDWIN T., JR.: Assistant Orthopedic Surgeon, Massachusetts General Hospital; Clinical Instructor in Orthopedic Surgery, Harvard Medical School

Table of Contents

1. History of the Fracture Clinic of the M. G. H., *Edwin F. Cave and Robert J. Boyd* 1
2. Measurement and Recording of Joint Motion, *Edwin F. Cave and Robert J. Boyd* 9
3. Metabolic Response to Trauma, *Benjamin A. Barnes and Paul S. Russell* 39
   Introduction, 39 / Acute Response to Trauma, 40 / Variations Due to Complications or to Therapy, 50 / Convalescence, 56 / Summary, 64.
4. Repair of Bone and Fracture Healing, *John E. Kenzora* 71
   Repair of Bone, 73 / Remodeling, 82 / Healing of Necrotic Compact Bone, 83 / Healing of a Small Hole in Bone, 87 / Healing of a Fractured Diaphysis Treated by External Cast Immbolization, 91 / Healing of a Complete Osteotomy Treated by Intramedullary Fixation, 98 / Healing of a Fractured Diaphysis Without Any Form of Immobilization, 101 / Primary Bone Healing Fracture Healing and the Compression Plate, 104 / Other Features of Fracture Healing, 106.
5. Delayed Union, Nonunion and Malunion of Long Bones; Nonunion with Infection, *Edwin F. Cave and Robert J. Boyd* 115
   Nonunion of Femoral Shaft Fractures, 123 / Nonunion of Closed Fractures of Tibia and Fibula, 127 / Nonunion of the Tibia and Fibula Secondary to Open Fractures, 128 / Nonunion of Forearm Fractures, 128 / Nonunion of Humeral Shaft Fractures, 129 / Nonunion of Clavicle, 130 / Malunion, 130 / Nonunion and Infection, 135.
6. Technique of Bone Grafting, *Edwin F. Cave and Robert J. Boyd* 159
   Onlay Graft, 159 / Inlay Graft, 162 / Subperiosteal Iliac Graft, 162 / "Neighborhood Graft," 163 / Dowel Graft, 163 / Slotted Graft, 163 / Bank Bone, 163 / Rejection of Bone Grafts, 163.
7. Pathologic Fractures, *Edwin T. Wyman, Jr.* 167
   Treatment, 170 / Metastatic Fractures, 171.
8. Early Examination and Treatment of the Injured Patient, *Glenn E. Behringer* 177
   The Airway, 178 / Control of External Hemorrhage, 180 / Control of Major Internal Hemorrhage, 181 / Shock, 181 / Cardiac Arrest, 183 / Splinting of Fractures, 183 / Examination of the Patient, 184 / Immediate Therapy, 187 / Priority of General Surgery, 188.

9. Use and Abuse of X-Ray in Trauma, *William J. Otto* 191
   Historical Background, 191 / Legal Problems, 191 /
   Radiation Hazards, 192 / Proper Use of Fluoroscopy, 193 /
   General Principles in Traumatic Radiology, 194.
10. Angiography of Trauma, *Christos A. Athanasoulis,
    Arthur C. Waltman and Stanley Baum* 197
    Method, 197 / Trauma to the Chest and Great Vessels, 198 /
    Abdominal Trauma, 198 / Trauma of the Extremities, 206 /
    Trauma Following Disk and Hip Surgery, 206 / Pelvic
    Fractures with Hemorrhage, 210 / Multiple Trauma, 210.
11. Shock, *Mortimer J. Buckley and W. Gerald Austen* 213
    Treatment of Shock States, 218.
12. Trauma and the Anesthetist, *Lawrence D. Egbert* 235
    Resuscitation, 235 / Evaluation of the Patient, 236 / Specific
    Anesthetic Problems, 237 / The Unstable Cardiovascular
    System, 238 / Induction of Anesthesia, 238 / The Full
    Stomach, 239 / Neurologic Trauma, 239 / Eye, Ear and
    Maxillofacial Trauma, 240 / Psychologic Problems, 241 /
    Treatment of Pain in the Traumatized Patient, 242 /
    Conclusions, 242.
13. Facial Injuries, *Bradford Cannon and John D. Constable* 243
    Emergency Care and Transportation, 243 / Examination of the
    Patient, 244 / General Considerations in Treatment, 248 /
    Management of Fractures, 249 / Management of Soft
    Tissues, 264 / Dressings, 267 / Postoperative Care, 267.
14. Diagnosis and Treatment of Head Injuries, *Edward P. Baker, Jr.* . . . 269
    First Aid and Transportation, 270 / Evaluation of Head
    Injuries, 272 / Intrinsic Brain Injuries, 279 / Other Conditions
    That May Complicate the Diagnosis of Head Trauma, 283 /
    Injuries to the Coverings of the Brain, 286 / Complications of
    Skull Fractures, 291 / Intracranial Hematomas, 295 /
    Nonsurgical Adjuncts to Management, 308 / Irreversible
    Coma and Brain Death, 313 / Organ Transplantation, 314.
15. Injuries to the Spinal Cord and Cauda Equina, *James
    G. Wepsic* 317
    Anatomy, 317 / Basic Evaluation, 324 / Immobilization, 330 /
    Fractures and Dislocations, 333 / Neurologic Syndromes
    Associated with Cord Injury, 336 / Indications for
    Operation, 336 / Spinal Cord Hypothermia, 339 / Late
    Surgical Considerations, 339 / Medical and Nursing Care, 339.
16. Injuries to the Spine: Neurologic Considerations; Fractures
    and Dislocations, *Donald S. Pierce and Robert G. Ojemann* 343
    Cord Injury, 343 / The Cervical Spine, 345 / The Thoracic Spine
    (Upper 10 Thoracic Vertebrae), 381 / The Lumbar Spine
    (Including T11 and T12), 384 / Fractures of the Transverse
    Processes, 391 / Urinary Tract, 393 / The Bowels, 395 /
    Physical Therapy, 395 / The Spinal Injury Team, 396.
17. Shoulder Girdle Injuries, *Carter R. Rowe* 399
    Anatomy and Function, 399 / Clinical Examination, 403 / The
    Clavicle: Anatomic Considerations, 404 / Acromioclavicular
    Injuries, 404 / Sternoclavicular Dislocations, 409 / Fractures
    of the Clavicle, 411 / Fractures of the Scapula, 416 / Dislocations
    of the Shoulder, 417 / Fractures of Head and Neck of the
    Humerus, 441 / Injuries to the Rotator Cuff, 446 / Surgical

Approaches to Shoulder Joint, 450 / Shoulder Exercises, 450.

18. Humeral Shaft Fractures, *Robert J. Boyd* 455
Anatomic Considerations, 455 / Physical Examination, 457 / Etiology and Types of Fractures, 457 / Treatment, 457 / Complications, 464.

19. Fractures and Dislocations of the Elbow, *William R. MacAusland, Jr.* 469
Dislocations, 469 / Fracture-Dislocations, 474 / Fractures of the Elbow, 478 / Epiphyseal Injuries, 493.

20. Fractures of the Forearm, *William N. Jones and Joseph S. Barr, Jr.* 497
Anatomy, 497 / Incidence: Age and Sex Distribution, 499 / Mechanism of Injury, 499 / X-Ray Examination, 499 / Treatment, 500 / Open Fractures of Forearm, 506.

21. Fractures of the Distal End of the Radius, *Joseph S. Barr, Jr. and Edwin T. Wyman, Jr.* 513
Anatomy, 513 / Mechanism of Injury, 513 / Associated Injuries, 516 / X-Ray Examination, 516 / Treatment, 516 / Prognosis, 521 / Complications, 522 / Smith's and Barton's Fractures, 525.

22. Injuries to the Carpal Bones, *Edwin F. Cave and Robert J. Boyd* 527
Development of the Carpus, 527 / Anatomy, 528 / Diagnosis by X-Ray Examination, 529 / Treatment, 531.

23. Soft Tissue Injuries of the Hand, *John P. Remensnyder* 555
Nature of Hand Injuries, 555 / Principles of Repair, 556 / Specific Injuries, 564.

24. Skeletal and Ligamentous Injuries of the Hand, *Edward A. Nalebuff and Lewis H. Millender* 583
Ligamentous Injury, 583 / Fractures, 594.

25. Fractures of the Pelvis, *William N. Jones and Walter S. Kerr, Jr.* 605
Pelvic Fractures Associated with Other Injuries, 605 / Anatomy of the Pelvis, 607 / Mechanism of Injury, 608 / Treatment, 609.

26. Fractures of the Hip: Head, Neck and Trochanter, *Otto E. Aufranc, J. Drennan Lowell, Hugh P. Chandler and Paul L. Norton* 619
Historical Considerations, 620 / Materials and Design of Fixation Devices, 623 / Epidemiology, 624 / Intracapsular Fractures, 625 / Extracapsular (Trochanteric) Fractures, 654 / Clinical Complications in Fractures of the Hip, 673 / Pathologic Fractures, 675 / Hip Fractures in Children, 675 / Summary, 677.

27. Dislocations of the Hip and Fractures of the Acetabulum, *Carter R. Rowe* 681
Dislocations of the Hip, 681 / Fractures of the Acetabulum, 692 / Surgical Approaches to the Hip, 704.

28. Reconstructive Surgery of the Hip Following Trauma, *William H. Harris* 711
Early Reconstructions, 711 / Late Reconstruction, 712.

29. Fractures of the Femoral Shaft, *Dinesh Patel and Thornton Brown* 719
Anatomic Considerations, 719 / Signs and Symptoms, 722 /

Treatment, 722 / Complications, 747.

30. Injuries Involving the Knee, *William R. MacAusland, Jr* 753
    General Considerations, 753 / Soft Tissue Injuries of the Knee, 755 / Injuries of the Ligaments of the Knee, 756 / Injuries of the Semilunar Cartilage, 762 / Combined Lesions of Medial Meniscus and Internal Collateral and Anterior Cruciate Ligaments, 764 / Lesions of the Knee Extensor Apparatus, 765 / Traumatic Dislocation of the Patella, 767 / Fractures of the Patella, 768 / Traumatic Separation of Distal Femoral Epiphysis, 774 / Fractures of the Lower End of the Femur (Supracondylar), 776 / Dislocation of the Knee, 784 / Fractures of the Proximal Fibula, 786 / Dislocation of the Proximal Fibula, 786 / Fractures of the Proximal Tibia, 786.

31. Fractures of the Tibia and Fibula, *Edwin T. Wyman, Jr. and Joseph S. Barr, Jr.* 793
    Mechanism and Type, 793 / Initial Evaluation and X-Ray Examination, 793 / Healing Times, 795 / Treatment, 796.

32. Ankle Injuries, *Edward J. Riseborough and Otto E. Aufranc* 809
    Causes and Mechanism of Ankle Fractures, 809 / Emergency Treatment, 809 / X-Ray Examination, 811 / Anatomic Points of Clinical Significance Around the Ankle, 813 / Important Ligaments of the Ankle, 815 / Muscles and Tendons Around the Ankle, 815 / Motions of the Ankle, 817 / Ligamentous Injuries, 820 / Bone Injuries, 823.

33. Injuries of the Foot, *Robert J. Joplin* 837
    Soft Tissue Injuries, 837 / Fractures of the Os Calcis, 839 / Fractures and Dislocations of the Talus, 848 / Fractures of the Tarsal Navicular, 850 / Metatarsal Fractures, 851 / Metatarsal Fractures with Tarsometatarsal Dislocations, 853 / Phalangeal Fractures, 856 / Treatment of Injuries of Some Lesser Bones of the Foot, 860.

34. Epiphyseal Injuries, *Clement B. Sledge* 869
    Historical Note, 869 / Epidemiology, 869 / Anatomy and Physiology of the Epiphyseal Plate, 870 / Blood Supply to the Epiphysis, 873 / Course of the Fracture Line, 873 / General Notes on Epiphyseal Separations, 876 / Management of Injuries, 876.

35. Operative Treatment of Fractures, *Edwin F. Cave, Robert J. Boyd and James I. Huddleston* 887
    Training of the Fracture Surgeon, 888 / Preparation of the Patient, 890 / Operative Techniques, 892.

36. Use and Abuse of Metal Implants, *Jonathan Cohen and Thornton Brown* 913
    Metallurgy, 913 / Failure, 923 / Mechanical and Biologic Interactions of Host and Implant, 928.

37. Treatment of Open Fractures, *Thomas Vander Salm and Edwin F. Cave* 935
    General Principles in the Approach to the Patient, 935 / Principles of Fracture Handling, 935 / Complications and Treatment, 940 / Summary, 942.

38. Sepsis Following Trauma: Prevention and Control, *John F. Burke* 943

General Principles, 943 / Measures Important in Preventing Sepsis, 943 / Control of Established Infection, 949.

39. Injuries to Major Tendons, *Edwin F. Cave and Robert J. Boyd* 957
Anatomy, 957 / Mechanism of Injury, 957 / Pathologic Process, 957 / Symptoms and Signs, 958 / Treatment, 958.

40. Soft Tissue Repairs, *Bradford Cannon and John Remensnyder, Jr.* 969
Methods of Wound Closure, 971 / Care of the Open Wound, 978 / Delayed Primary Closure, 979 / Skin Grafting, 979 / Indications For and Uses of Flaps, 982 / Summary, 991.

41. Chest Injuries: Chest Wall, Lung, Esophagus and Pleural Spaces, *Ashby C. Moncure and J. Gordon Scannell* 993
Resuscitation, 993 / Control of Bleeding, 995 / Stabilization of the Chest Wall, 996 / Maintenance of a Clear Airway, 998 / Management of Blood and Air in the Pleural Space, 999 / Management of the External Wound, 1001 / Special Considerations, 1002 / Summary, 1002.

42. Cardiac Trauma: Heart and Great Vessels, *Willard M. Daggett, Eldred D. Mundth, Mortimer J. Buckley and W. Gerald Austen* 1005
Management of the Patient in the Emergency Room in Relation to Cardiovascular Trauma, 1005 / Blunt Trauma to the Heart and Great Vessels, 1006 / Penetrating Trauma to the Heart and Great Vessels, 1011.

43. Management of Respiratory Failure Associated with Chest Trauma, *Kenneth W. Travis, Henrik H. Bendixen and Bennie Geffin* 1015
What is Traumatized, 1015 / Associated Injuries, 1016 / Early Manifestations, 1016 / Diagnosis, 1016 / Functional Disturbance, 1016 / Pathophysiology, 1020 / Wet Lung Syndrome, 1021 / Early Treatment, 1022 / Maintenance of Respiratory Care, 1022 / General Care, 1025 / Physiologic Assessment of Respiratory Functions, 1027 / Complications of Mechanical Ventilation, 1027 / Stabilization of the Flail Chest, 1028 / Weaning from the Ventilator, 1029 / Extubation, 1029 / Conclusion, 1030 / Equations, 1030.

44. Management of Abdominal Injuries, *Grant V. Rodkey and Claude E. Welch* 1033
General Considerations, 1033 / Diagnosis of Abdominal Visceral Injury, 1033 / General Treatment, 1035 / Treatment of Specific Injuries, 1039 / Postoperative Care, 1050 / Mortality, 1052.

45. Liver and Extrahepatic Biliary System, *Ronald A. Malt* 1057
Liver, 1057 / Extrahepatic Biliary System, 1068.

46. Injuries to the Genitourinary Tract, *Walter S. Kerr, Jr.* 1071
Kidney, 1071 / Ureter, 1076 / Bladder, 1078 / Urethra, 1080 / Penis, 1085 / Scrotum and Testes, 1086.

47. Peripheral Nerve Injuries, *Raymond N. Kjellberg and James C. White* 1087
Anatomic Structure, 1087 / Metabolic Determinants in Nerve Repair, 1088 / Degrees of Injury, 1093 / Types of Injury, 1096 / Diagnosis of Injury, 1097 / Nerve Repair, 1101 / Postoperative

XVIII / TABLE OF CONTENTS

Care, 1108 / Recovery After Nerve Suture, 1108 / Orthopedic Measures to Correct Presistent Paralysis, 1112 / Painful Syndromes After Nerve Injury, 1113.

48. Peripheral Vascular Injuries, *Ashby C. Moncure and R. Clement Darling* 1115
Arterial Injury, 1115 / Venous Injury, 1125.

49. Volkmann's Contracture, *William C. Quinby, Jr.* 1129
Nature of the Process, 1129 / Mechanisms of Ischemia, 1130 / Recognition of Impending Volkmann's Contracture, 1131 / Management of Impending Contracture, 1133 / Management of Established Muscle Ischemia, 1134 / Summary, 1135.

50. Treatment of Burns, *William C. Quinby, Jr. and John F. Burke* 1137
Burn Shock, 1137 / Infection, 1142 / Burn Wound, 1147 / Function of Systems and Organs, 1154.

51. Injuries Due to Cold, *Frank C. Wheelock, Jr. and Leslie W. Ottinger* 1163
Historical Considerations, 1163 / Definitions and Factors Producing Injury Due to Cold, 1163 / Pathology and Physiology, 1164 / Clinical Findings, 1165 / Early Treatment, 1165 / Late Treatment, 1166 / Other Forms of Cold Injury, 1166.

52. Rehabilitation Medicine, *Donald S. Pierce* 1169
Crutch Walking, 1171 / Exercise, 1173 / Heat, 1175 / Massage, 1178 / Electrodiagnosis, 1178 / Electrotherapy, 1178 / Instruction of Patient in Home Care, 1179 / Problems in Rehabilitation, 1180.

53. Replanting Amputated Arms, *Ronald A. Malt and William H. Harris* 1183
Emergency Care, 1183 / Judgment, 1185 / Operation, 1186 / Postoperative Care, 1191.

54. Fat Embolism, *James H. Herndon* 1195
Pathogenesis, 1195 / Pathophysiology, 1195 / Clinical Manifestations, 1196 / Diagnosis, 1196 / Treatment, 1197.

Index 1199

1 | History of the Fracture Clinic of the M.G.H.

EDWIN F. CAVE and ROBERT J. BOYD

THE FRACTURE CLINIC of the Massachusetts General Hospital was established in 1917 by Charles L. Scudder and was the first such clinic in the United States. Dr. Scudder was the first Chief of the Clinic, and assigned with him were Henry C. Marble, George A. Leland, Torr W. Harmer and Richard H. Miller, from the East and West Surgical Services. After World War I, great impetus was given to the study of the treatment of fractures throughout the United States, and in 1919 the Fracture Clinic began to function as a separate unit of the Surgical Services. Postgraduate teaching of fracture treatment was initiated by Dr. Scudder, who was assisted by the above-named general surgeons and by Robert B. Osgood, Chief of the Orthopedic Service, Zabdiel B. Adams and Philip D. Wilson, also from the Department of Orthopedic Surgery.

In 1920, Dr. Scudder retired from hospital service and was succeeded as Chief of the Clinic by Daniel F. Jones of the Surgical Service and in 1924 by Nathaniel Allison of the Orthopedic Service as Associate Chief. During the period of service of Drs. Jones and Allison, the Fracture Clinic reached its full stride in providing the best of care for patients suffering from injury and as a teaching service. Although end-result studies of fractures were begun largely at the instigation of Dr. Osgood in 1919, the value of these studies was not evident until the late 1920s, when (in 1928) sufficient knowledge of the treatment of fractures had accumulated to permit giving the first postgraduate course in the management of fractures and dislocations. Dr. Jones retired in 1929; he was replaced as

CHARLES L. SCUDDER
1917–1920

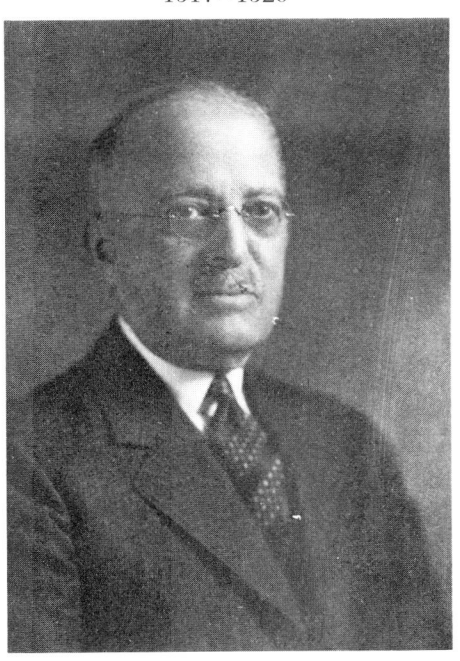

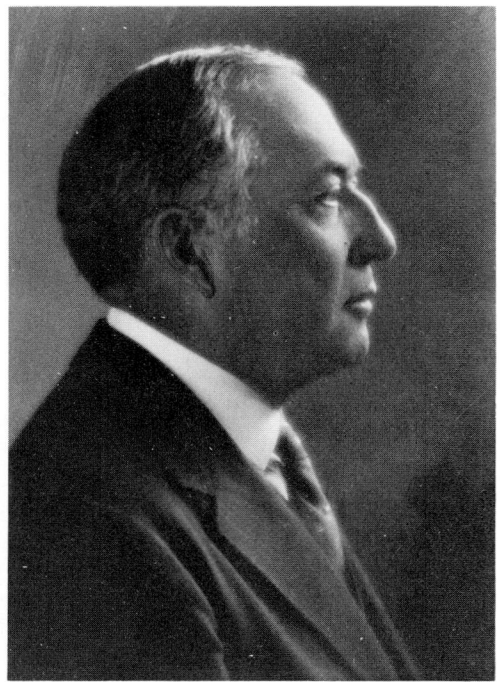

DANIEL F. JONES
1920–1929

involving the skull have been admitted to the Orthopedic Service unless there were major complicating injuries involving the central nervous system, abdomen or urologic organs, in which case the patient has been admitted to the appropriate section and any fractures associated with these injuries have been cared for by the fracture surgeons.

The Massachusetts General Hospital Fracture Clinic has experienced many changes in fracture management since its beginning in 1917. Then, with few exceptions, all fractures and dislocations were treated by manipulation and splinting. Many of the splints were ill-fitting, and plaster-of-Paris bandages often were of poor quality. "Setting" of the plaster was always a problem, and catalyzing agents (such as salt) were added to speed the process. Patients with fractured hips were immobilized in large double spicas, which soon became loose and did not provide stability to the fracture. The re-

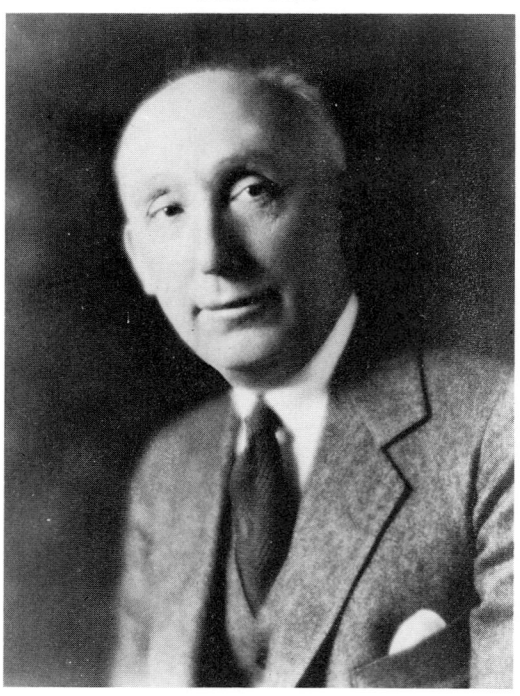

NATHANIEL ALLISON
1924–1930

Chief by Henry Marble. Dr. Allison relinquished his duties at the Massachusetts General Hospital in 1930; he was succeeded by Philip D. Wilson as Associate Chief. George W. Van Gorder was made Associate Chief when Dr. Wilson moved to New York in 1934. Drs. Marble and Van Gorder were replaced by Arthur W. Allen as Chief and M. N. Smith-Petersen as Associate Chief in 1940. They served until 1947. Edwin F. Cave was Chief from 1947 to 1957.

Dr. Otto E. Aufranc was appointed Chief of the Fracture Clinic in 1957. With his knowledge and sound judgment concerning skeletal injury, he has directed the Clinic in a way comparable to that which had existed for many years.

Before World War II, fracture admissions to the wards were rotated, in order, to the East and West Surgical Services and the Orthopedic Service. Since 1947, all patients with fractures other than those

Chapter 1: HISTORY OF THE FRACTURE CLINIC OF THE M.G.H. / 3

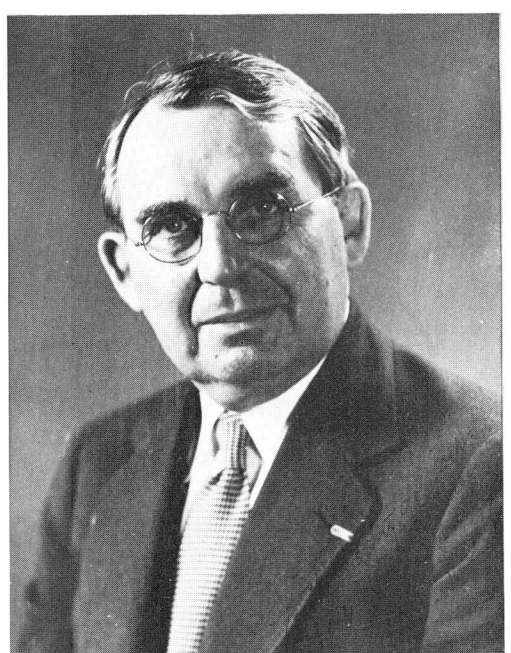

HENRY C. MARBLE
1929–1940

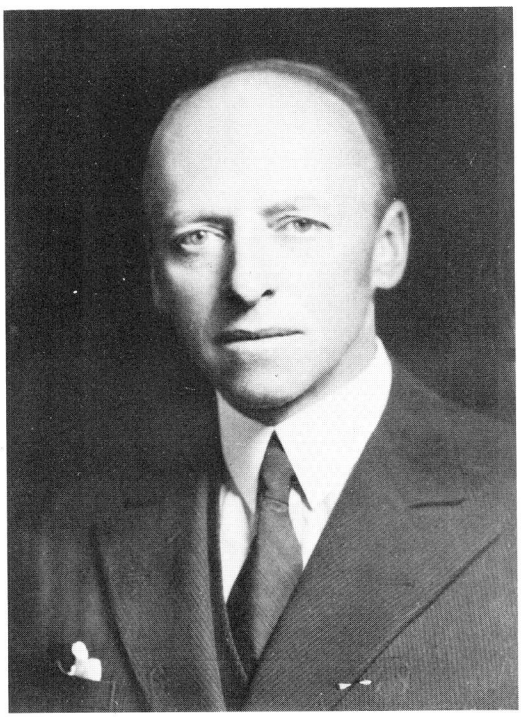

PHILIP D. WILSON
1930–1934

culty, however, lay in the fact that the plates and screws he employed corroded in tissue, caused reaction, broke and frequently had to be removed. Lane himself believed that when this occurred, it was due to "dirty surgery."

In America, fracture management continued along "conservative" lines until about 1915, when William O'Neill Sherman, surgeon to the Carnegie Steel Company, Pittsburgh, accumulated a vast experience from openly reducing, and securing with steel, long-bone fractures, particularly those of the femur. Sherman was an able surgeon and a master of technique in applying plates and screws. He was dexterous and quick, and since he was dealing with relatively young persons (steelworkers) and since his operations were done soon after injury, a high percentage of his patients did well, soon were out of bed and returned to work at a relatively early date. The quality of metsult was a high mortality; for those patients who did survive, there remained joint stiffness, muscle weakness and often leg shortening—all of which contributed to permanent invalidism. Nevertheless, we have, as have most fracture clinics, continued to treat the vast majority of long-bone fractures by traction or closed manipulation and external splinting. This practice will, of course, continue; but, as surgical techniques in general have improved, the operative management of fractures has developed, and with considerable justification. Some of these developments have occurred in our own Clinic. The operative management of fractures had been advocated sporadically, only to be abandoned for many generations, but it was more firmly established early in the century by Sir Arbuthnot Lane of Guy's Hospital, London. Lane believed that the "no-touch technique" was a major factor in a successful open reduction. His chief diffi-

al, however, still was a problem, and, as in the case of Lane, many of the plates and screws advocated by Sherman, and employed by others, broke, infection supervened and the metal had to be removed. Not infrequently, osteomyelitis and nonunion of bone followed. The no-touch technique was not the answer, although it was continuously practiced in some clinics in the United States and abroad.

Some members of the present Massachusetts General Hospital Fracture Clinic will remember Sherman as rotund, ruddy complexioned and having a strong personality. He spoke fluently and did not fail to state his opinion with force. He dressed like a "Broadway actor" and obviously was fond of his food. It was always an exciting day when he visited Wards E and A at our Hospital, along with other fracture "greats," such as William E. ("Bill") Darrach, Bancroft, Blake, Cotton, Gallie, Estes, Murray and others, in company with Drs. Scudder, Jones, Allison, Smith-Petersen, Marble, Wilson and the other Clinic members. These visits usually took place at the time of the combined meeting of the Philadelphia, New York, Brooklyn and New England Fracture committees. The meeting was always followed by a fine dinner, where drink and food were not deficient, and where, as a result, many lively arguments took place as to the best methods of fracture management.

The establishment of the Fracture Committee of the American College of Surgeons in 1922 by Dr. Scudder did much to improve the care of the injured patient throughout the country. Other representatives on this committee from Massachusetts General Hospital have been Drs. Allison, Osgood, Wilson, Marble, Leland, Reggio and Cave.

Regional subcommittees were established in various sections of the United States and Canada. Representatives from

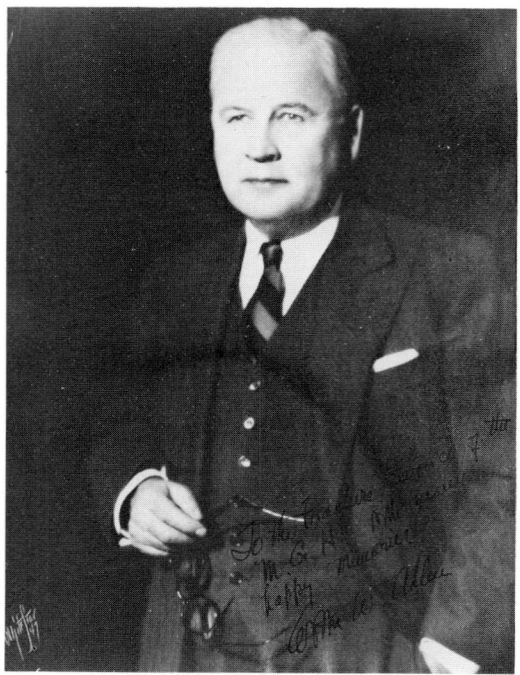

ARTHUR W. ALLEN
1940–1947

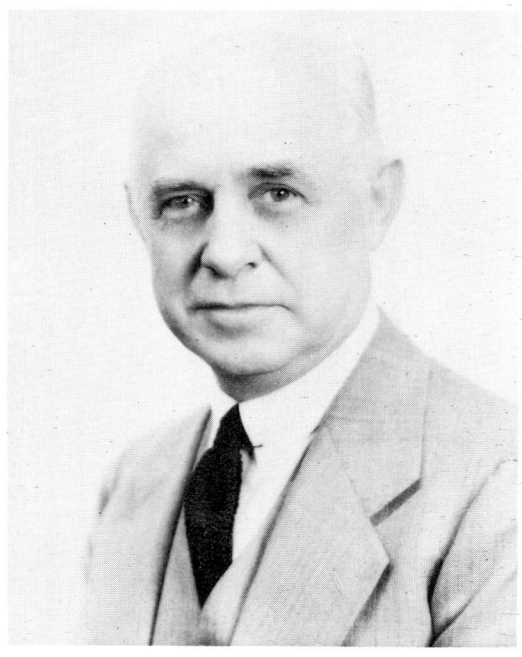

GEORGE W. VAN GORDER
1934–1940

these groups have done much to stimulate interest in the early care of the injured and the methods of transportation.

In 1949, the "Fracture Committee" of the College of Surgeons became the "Committee on Trauma," which emphasized the fact that when bone is broken there always is soft-tissue damage of varying degree; also that, owing to mechanized industry and the high-speed automobile, the patient with multiple injuries appears more and more frequently in the emergency ward. Thoracic wounds and abdominal or pelvic wounds often are associated with injuries to the extremities.

Since 1929, when Venable and Stuck brought out Vitallium, to be followed a few years later by the standardization of steel manufacture, open treatment of fractures has been more and more widely accepted.

The thin, flanged nail for femoral-neck fractures, conceived by Smith-Petersen of the Massachusetts General Hospital Fracture Clinic in 1925, caused reaction in tissue in the early cases. Some nails broke or extruded themselves as corrosion occurred around the nail. Now, however, such an occurrence is rare, and the Smith-Petersen nail still is an excellent means of securing femoral-neck fractures. With improvement in metal construction has come also improved surgical technique. Proper choice of a case for operation; attention to the fact that soft tissues must be in good condition before they can be incised; adequate, carefully placed incisions; gentleness in handling tissue; sufficient but not unnecessary periosteal reflection; careful reduction and firm fixation of the fracture; careful wound closure without tension; postoperative elevation of the extremity—all have contributed to the use of open treatment of fractures, when necessary, to restore normal anatomy and permit shorter hospitalization.

Nevertheless, the fundamental principles for promoting bone healing remain unchanged. These principles we should never fail to teach. Let us remember that

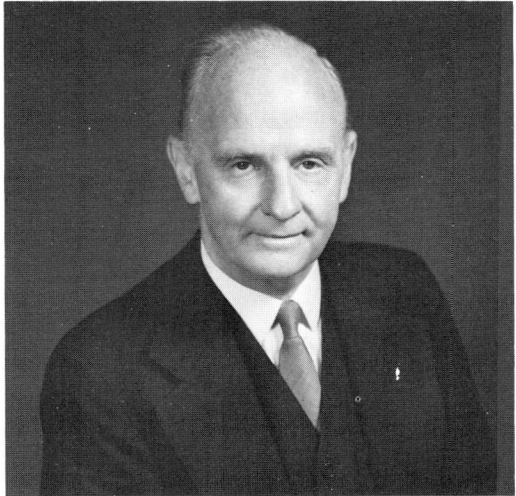

EDWIN F. CAVE
1947–1957

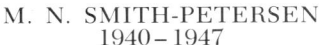

M. N. SMITH-PETERSEN
1940–1947

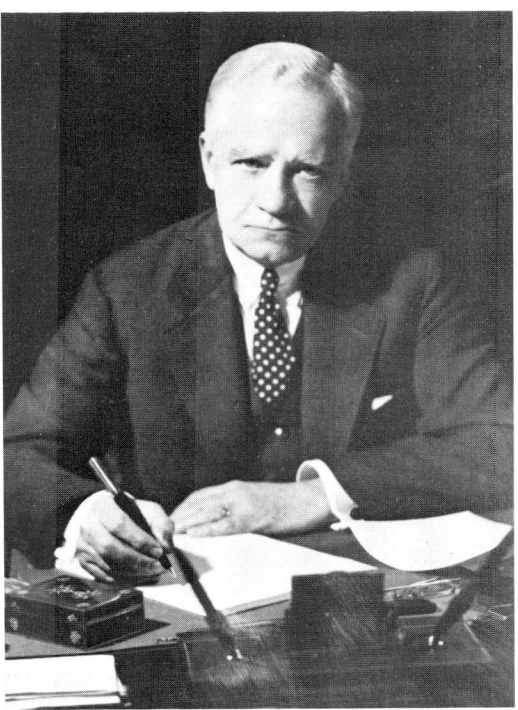

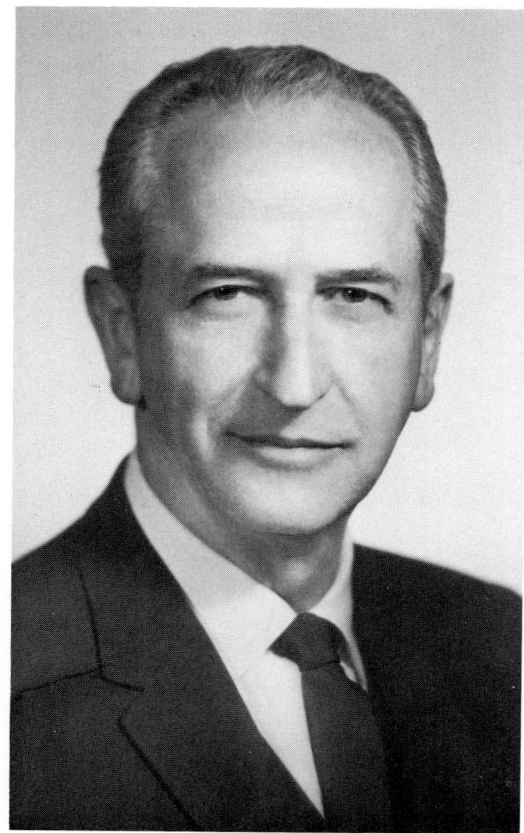

OTTO E. AUFRANC
1957–1973

open treatment of fractures still is high on the list of causes of nonunion of bone, largely because of poor surgery. The members of our Clinic strive to keep these thoughts uppermost in our minds and to preach what we practice.

Medullary nailing, looked on with disfavor when our wounded soldiers first returned from German prison camps after World War II, carrying great long steel rods in their femurs, now is an accepted form of treatment of long-bone fractures. Some will wonder why it was not thought of long ago. It was tried by Nicolaysen in 1897, by Delbet in 1906, by Lambotte in 1909, by Hey Groves in 1961 and by others, but it had to be abandoned because of poor quality of metal. Now medullary nailing is here to stay, and many fracture surgeons believe that it has been the greatest advance in fracture management since the Smith-Petersen nail. Our Clinic members have seen all of these new mechanical devices in their development. We have tried many of them.

Even more important, however, has been our increase in knowledge as to the methods of handling the whole patient: the management of the entire patient at the scene of the accident, careful and simple splinting, gentle and rapid transportation, early evaluation of all possible injuries, blood transfusion and judicious use of drugs to combat possible infection. The importance of skin coverage for any bone after injury did not become fully appreciated until World War II. Now, our Plastic Service is an extremely important part of the Fracture Clinic. These advances and others have, over the years, been appreciated and tried by members of our Clinic. We, as a group, may be regarded by some as too surgically minded and as "an operating clinic." However, the fundamental ideas of patient care, wound management and splinting of a fracture remain the same, and we shall continue to keep them uppermost in our minds in caring for the injured and in teaching our students.

In 1967, the Fracture Ward Service essentially ceased to exist as a separate unit and gradually was absorbed into the Orthopedic Service. Therefore, all patients with major skeletal injury were cared for in the orthopedic wards and in the Outpatient Orthopedic Clinic, except those whose major injury was abdominal or urologic or was related to the head or chest. These, of course, were admitted to the appropriate sections of the Surgical Service.

Recently, the question of a separate "Trauma Service" has been raised. It appears that such a service would have considerable merit in that all forms of injury could be handled in a separate unit. A major difficulty is finding the proper surgeon to direct the Clinic. There always is rivalry between the various divisions in the departments of surgery. Consequently, in most hospitals it has been difficult to have a separate trauma service, because it is extremely rare that one surgeon would have sufficient knowledge of all forms of trauma to justify his appointment as Chief. In certain clinics, especially in the Montreal General Hospital, the Trauma Service has been directed cooperatively by a plastic surgeon and an orthopedic surgeon. Nevertheless, it is not realistic to think that "two heads are better than one" in directing any unit. There must be *one* "commanding officer." However, the real advantages of a separate trauma service remain to be convincingly demonstrated in a hospital such as ours, where cooperation between surgeons and services is the rule, and where there appears to be little to gain from the administrative or physical standpoint in establishing such a service.

The Massachusetts General Hospital Fracture Clinic continues to function and remains a vital part of our teaching and research programs. We are investigating newer methods of data recording and retrieval, and the members of our Clinic continue with primary responsibility for the ongoing review of our fracture experience, the teaching of the principles of fracture care and the supervision of our residents' fracture cases.

BIBLIOGRAPHY

Delbet, P.: Osteosynthesis, Policlinico 24:332, 1917.

Groves, E. W. H.: *On Modern Methods of Treating Fractures* (Bristol, England: John Wright & Sons, Ltd., 1916).

Lambotte, M. A.: Technique et indications de la prothèse perdue dans le traitement des fractures, Presse méd. 17:321, 1909.

Lane, Sir Arbuthnot: *The Operative Treatment of Fractures* (London: Medical Publishing Co., 1914).

Lane, Sir Arbuthnot: The operative treatment of simple fractures, Surg. Gynecol. Obstet. 8:344, 1909.

Murray, C. R.: Primary operative fixation of long bone fractures in adults, Am. J. Surg. 51:739, 1941.

Nicolaysen, J.: Lidt om Diagnosen og Behandlingen af. Fr. colli femoris, Nord. Med. Ark. 8:n:r 16:1 (Med 2 Taffer Festband tillegn. Axel Key, 1897).

Sherman, W. O'N.: The bone plating problems—report of 200 cases, Int. J. Surg. 29:2, 1916.

Venable, C. S., and Stuck, W. G.: *The Internal Fixation of Fractures* (Springfield, Ill.: Charles C Thomas, Publisher, 1947), pp. 210 and 211.

2 | Measurement and Recording of Joint Motion

EDWIN F. CAVE and ROBERT J. BOYD

THE STANDARDIZATION of joint motion based on the principles of the Neutral Zero Method as described by Cave and Roberts in 1936 was updated by the Committee for the Study of Joint Motion, American Academy of Orthopaedic Surgeons. The results of the Committee's study were published by the A.A.O.S. in 1965 in a pamphlet entitled *Joint Motion—Method of Measuring and Recording*. The illustrations appearing at the end of this chapter have been reproduced in part from the above publication with the kind permission of the American Academy of Orthopaedic Surgeons.

The general principles of this system of joint motion measurement, which has been widely adopted and presently is in use, are as follows*:

1. All motions of a joint are measured from defined Zero Starting Positions. Thus, the degrees of motion of a joint are added in the direction the joint moves from the Zero Starting Position.

2. The extended "anatomical position" of an extremity is, therefore, accepted as zero degrees, rather than 180 degrees.

3. This method will eliminate the confusion that has existed in the past of measuring joint motions from various starting positions.

*From *Joint Motion—Method of Measuring and Recording*, American Academy of Orthopaedic Surgeons, 1965.

4. The motion of the extremity being examined should be compared to that of the opposite extremity. The difference may be expressed in degrees of motion as compared to the opposite extremity, or in percentages of loss of motion in comparison with the opposite extremity.

5. If the opposite extremity is not present, the motion should be compared to the average motion of an individual of similar age and physical build. Likewise, motions of the spine may be compared to individuals of similar age and physique.

6. Motions are described as active or passive.

7. A distinction is made between the terms "extension" and "hyperextension." Extension is used when the motion opposite to flexion, at the Zero Starting Position, is a natural motion. This is present in the wrists and shoulder joints. If, however, the motion opposite to flexion at the Zero Starting Position is an unnatural one, such as that of the elbow or knees, it is referred to as hyperextension.

8. The motion of a joint may be painful. Every effort should be made by the examiner to be gentle. A more accurate estimate of motion may be obtained if the extremity is examined in the position of greatest comfort to the patient.

9. Ankylosis is accepted as the complete loss of motion of a joint.

10. The use of a goniometer is optional, and it should be used according to the surgeon's discretion.

11. The recording of joint motion should be accurately and clearly tabulated by the examiner.

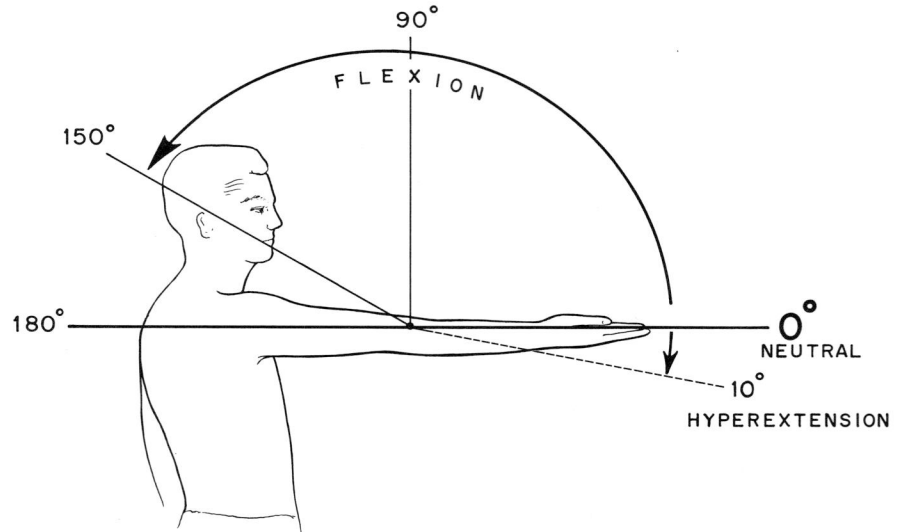

Fig. 2-1. — Motion of elbow. *Zero Starting Position:* The extended straight arm (Zero degrees). Natural motion is present in FLEXION. The opposite motion to FLEXION, to the Zero Starting Position, is EXTENSION. As the motion beyond the Zero Starting Position is an unnatural one, it is referred to as HYPEREXTENSION.

Motions are measured as follows:

FLEXION: Zero to 150 degrees.

EXTENSION: 150 degrees to Zero (from the angle of greatest flexion to the Zero Starting Position).

HYPEREXTENSION: This is measured in degrees beyond the Zero Starting Position. This motion is not present in all individuals. When it is present, it may vary from 5 to 15 degrees.

Chapter 2: MEASUREMENT AND RECORDING OF JOINT MOTION / 11

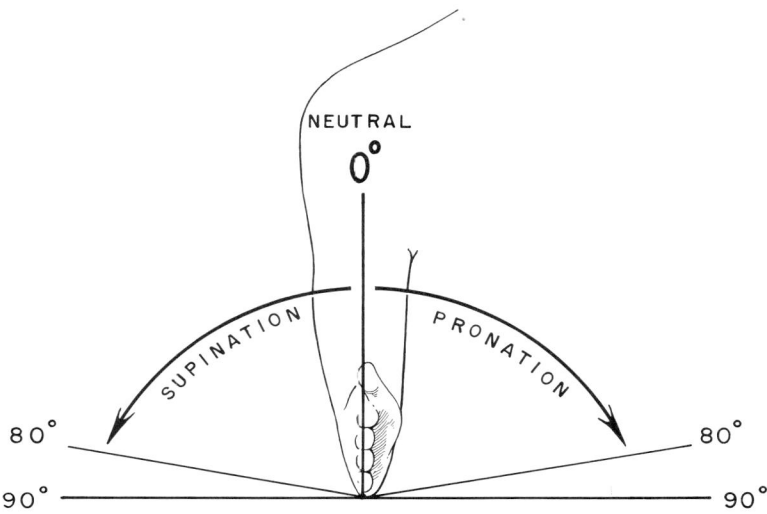

Fig. 2-2.—Motion of forearm. *Zero Starting Position:* The vertical upright position or "thumbs up" position, with the forearms at the side of the body and the elbow flexed 90 degrees.
Motions are measured as follows:
Pronation and Supination:
PRONATION: Zero to 80–90 degrees.
SUPINATION: Zero to 80–90 degrees.
TOTAL FOREARM MOTION: 160–180 degrees.
Individuals may vary in the range of supination and pronation. Some individuals may reach the 90 degrees arc, whereas others may have only 70 degrees plus.

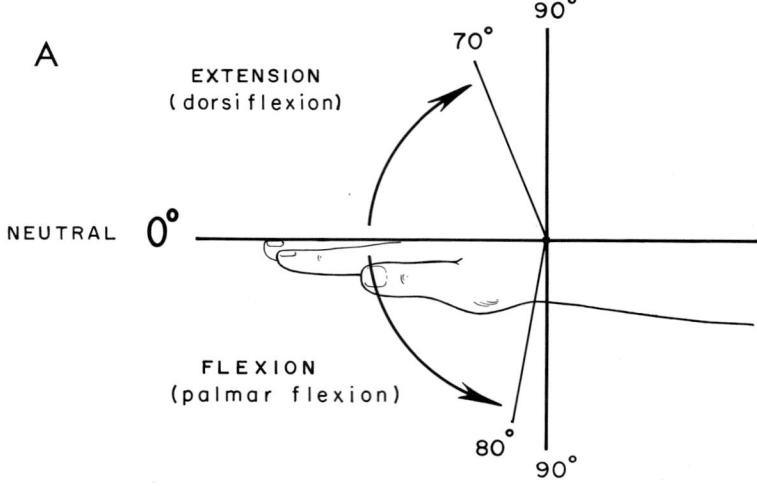
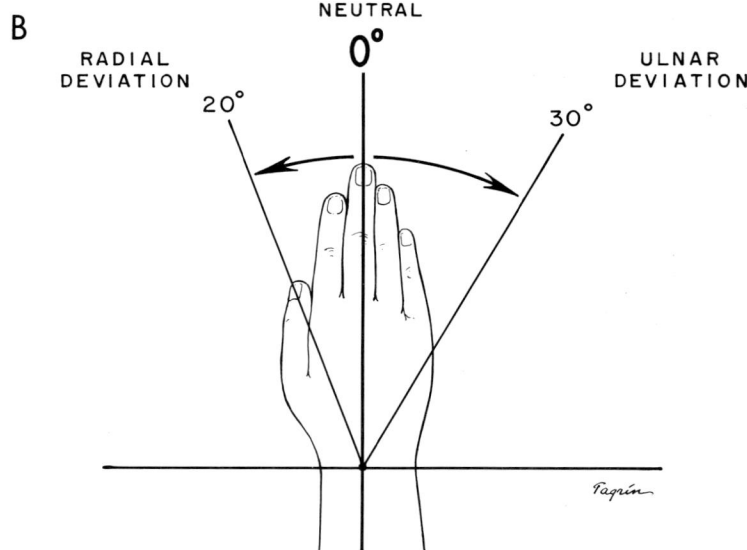

Fig. 2-3. — Motion of wrist. *Zero Starting Position:* The extended wrist in line with the forearm. The wrist has natural motion in FLEXION, EXTENSION, and ULNAR and RADIAL DEVIATION from the Zero Starting Position. There is some degree of rotatory circumduction at the wrist, which cannot be measured accurately.

   A. *Flexion and Extension:*
FLEXION (palmar flexion): Zero to 80 degrees ±.
EXTENSION (dorsiflexion): Zero to 70 degrees ±.
B. *Radial and Ulnar Deviation:*
RADIAL DEVIATION: Zero to 20 degrees.
ULNAR DEVIATION: Zero to 30 degrees.

   Ulnar deviation usually is measured with the wrist in pronation. When measured in supination, there is some increase in ulnar deviation.

Chapter 2: MEASUREMENT AND RECORDING OF JOINT MOTION / 13

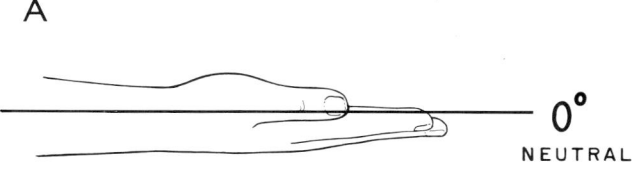

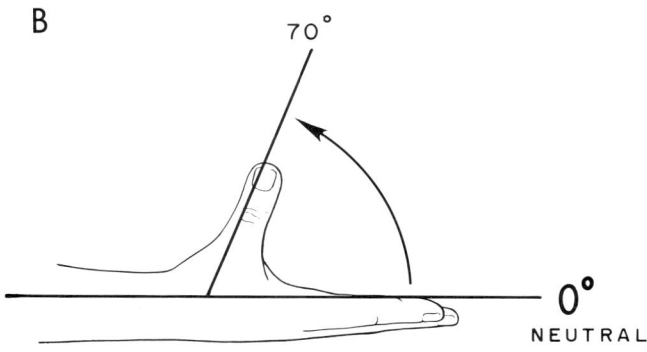

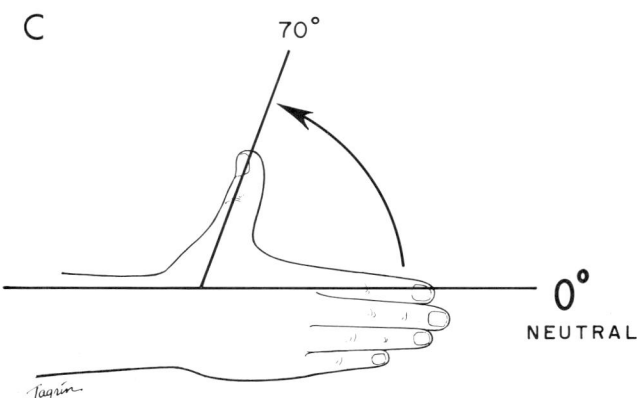

Fig. 2-4. — Motion of thumb. The motions of the thumb are complex. All definitions are necessarily somewhat arbitrary. The principal motions are: ABDUCTION, ADDUCTION, FLEXION, EXTENSION and OPPOSITION (circumduction).

A, ABDUCTION and ADDUCTION: *Zero Starting Position:* The extended thumb alongside the index finger, which is in line with the radius. ABDUCTION is defined as the angle created between the metacarpal bones of the thumb and the index finger. This motion may take place in two planes.

B illustrates ABDUCTION at a right angle to the plane of the palm. With the hand in supination, the thumb will point to the ceiling (ABDUCTION-CIRCUMDUCTION).

C illustrates ABDUCTION parallel to the plane of the palm (ABDUCTION-EXTENSION).

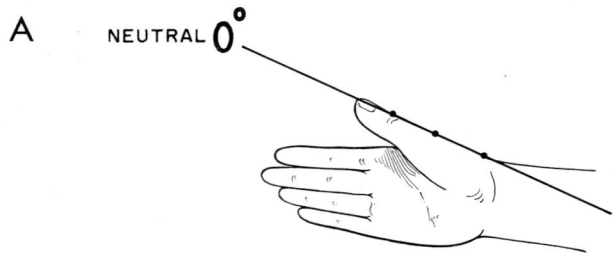
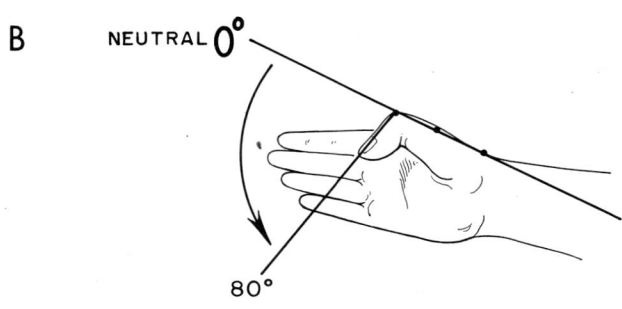
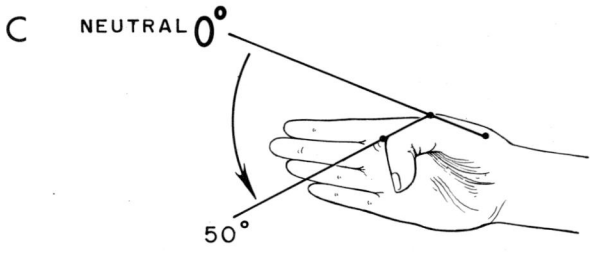
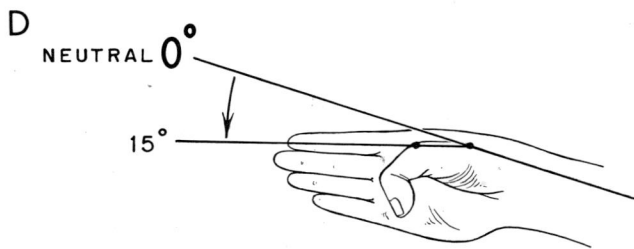

Fig. 2-5.—Motion of thumb (flexion).
  A. Zero Starting Position: The extended thumb.
  B. Flexion of interphalangeal joint: Zero to 80 degrees ±.
  C. Flexion of metacarpophalangeal joint: Zero to 50 degrees ±.
  D. Flexion of carpometacarpal joint: Zero to 15 degrees ±.

Chapter 2: MEASUREMENT AND RECORDING OF JOINT MOTION / 15

ZERO STARTING POSITION

① ②

③

OR

FLEXION TO TIP OF
LITTLE FINGER

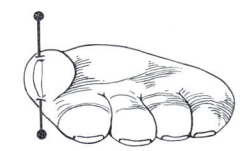

FLEXION TO BASE OF
LITTLE FINGER

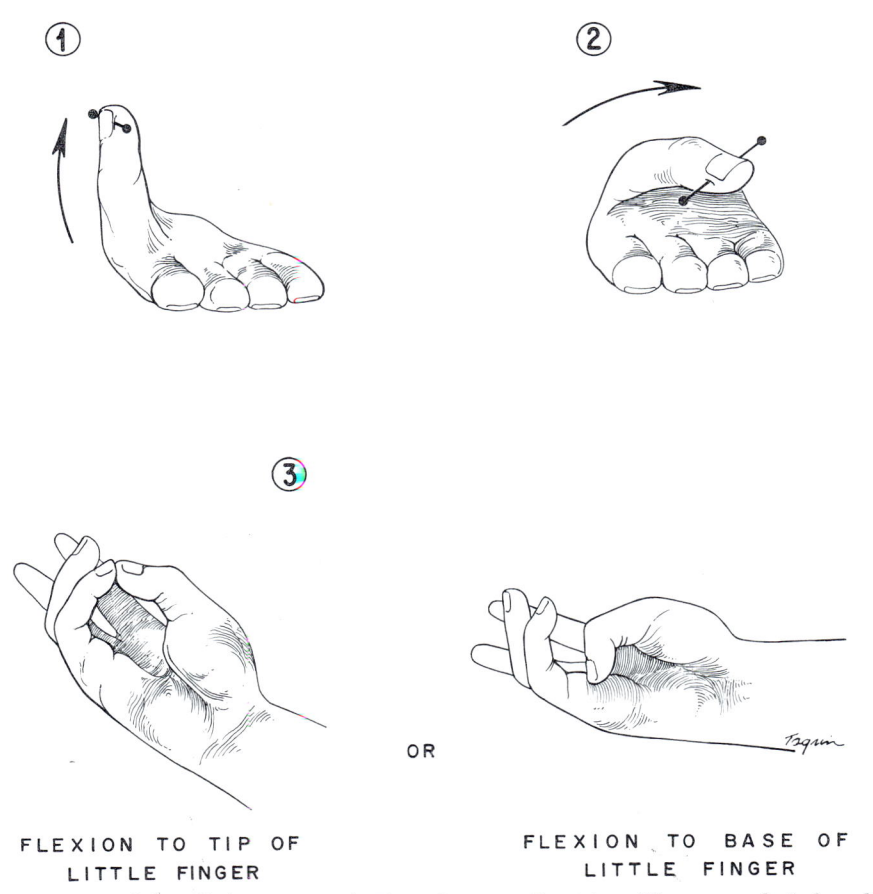

Fig. 2-6.—Motion of thumb (opposition). *Zero Starting Position:* The extended thumb in line with the index finger. The motion of opposition is a complete motion, consisting of three elements:
 1. ABDUCTION (ABDUCTION-CIRCUMDUCTION).
 2. ROTATION.
 3. FLEXION. This motion usually is considered complete when the tip, or pulp, of the thumb touches the tip of the little finger. Some surgeons, however, consider the arc of opposition complete when the tip of the thumb touches the base of the little finger. Both methods are illustrated.

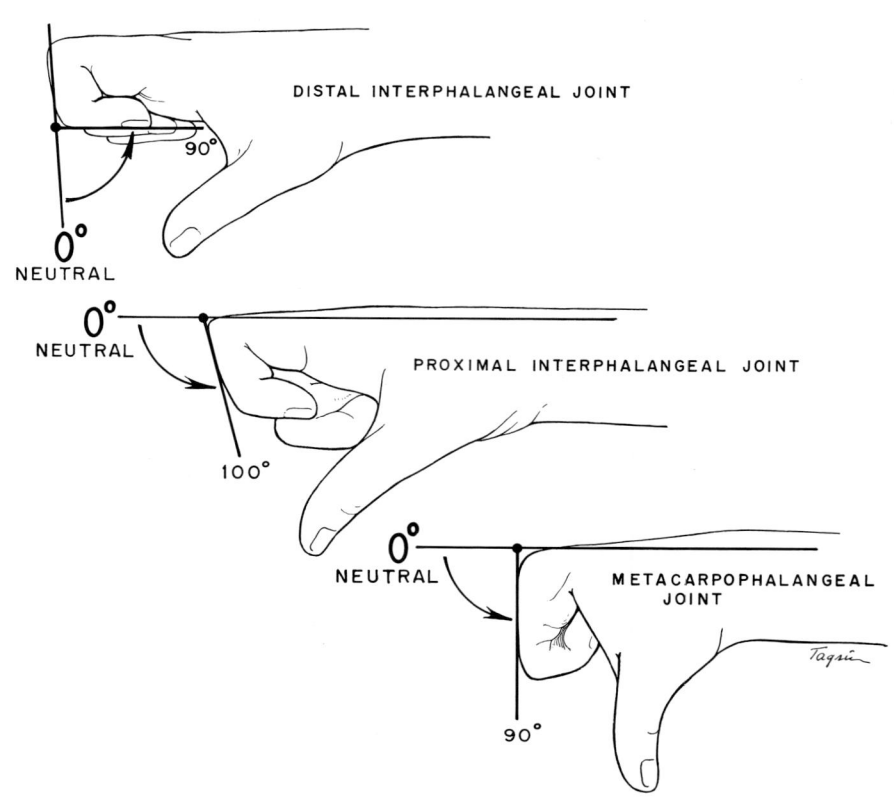

Fig. 2-7.—Motion of fingers (flexion). *Zero Starting Position:* The extended fingers parallel to one another and in line with the plane of the dorsum of the hand and wrist. FLEXION: This motion can be estimated in degrees or in centimeters. FLEXION is a natural motion in all joints of the fingers.

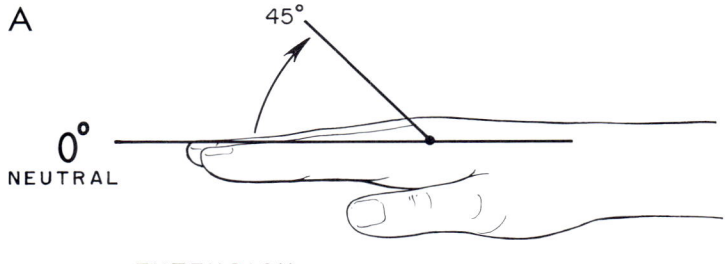

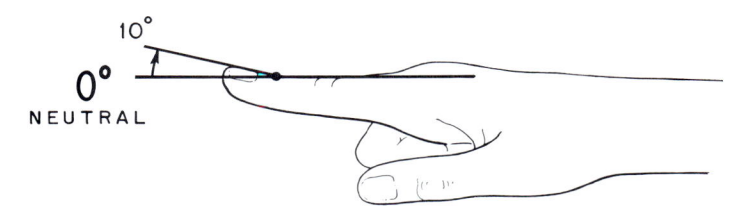

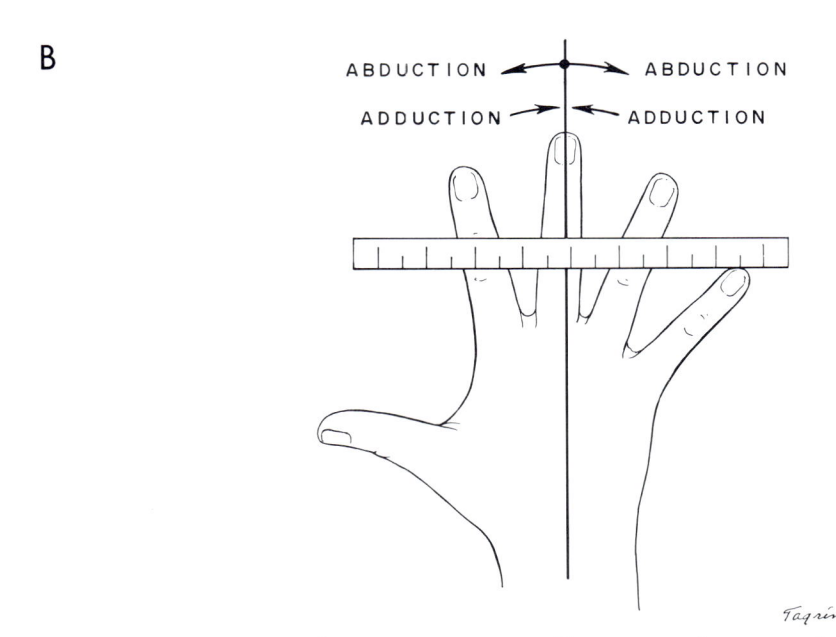

Fig. 2-8. — Fingers. **A,** EXTENSION and HYPEREXTENSION. EXTENSION is a natural motion at the metacarpophalangeal joint but an unnatural one in the proximal interphalangeal joint and the distal interphalangeal joint. **B,** ABDUCTION AND ADDUCTION (finger spread). This motion takes place in the plane of the palm away from, and to, the long or middle finger of the hand. This can be indicated in centimeters or inches. Spread of the fingers can be measured from the tip of the index finger to the tip of the little finger. Individual fingers spread from tip to tip of indicated fingers.

18 / *Edwin F. Cave and Robert J. Boyd*

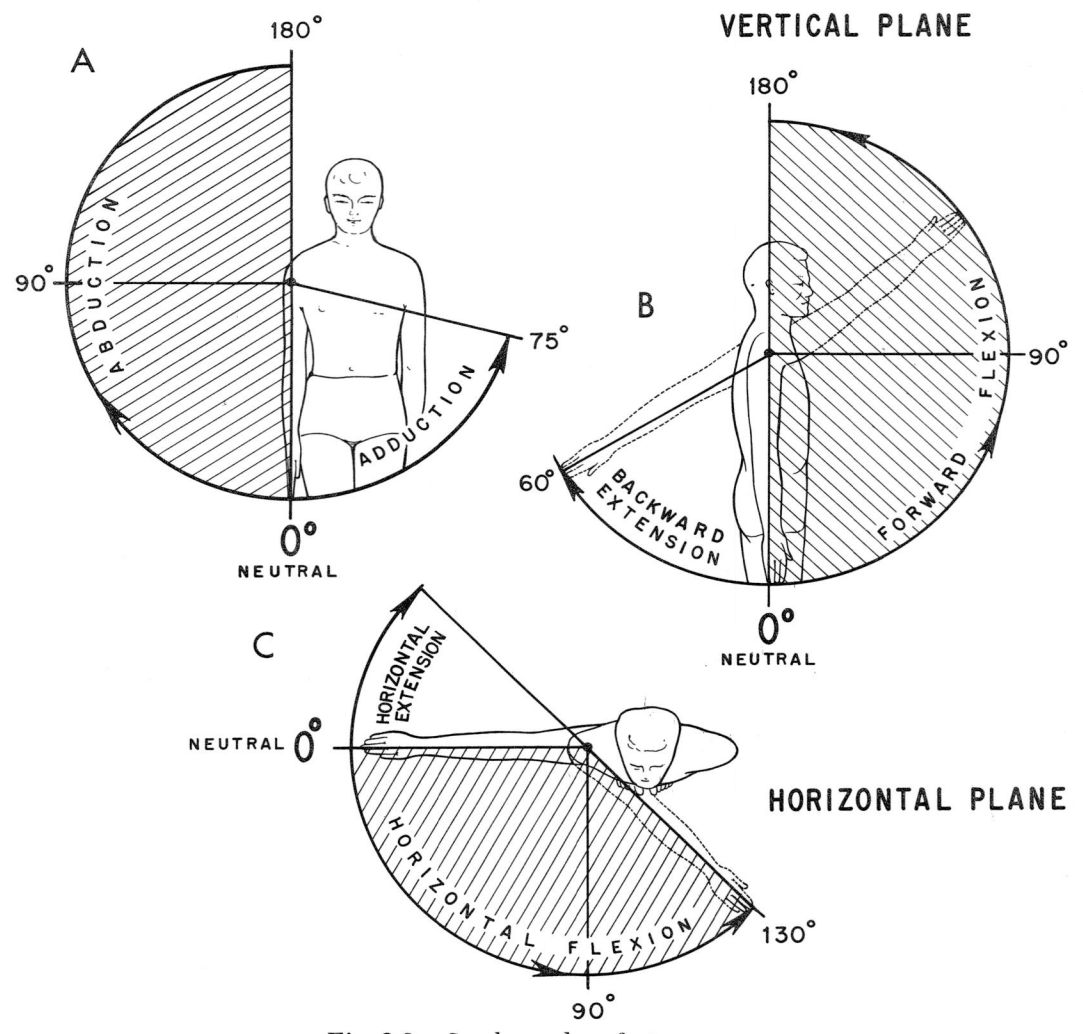

Fig. 2-9.—See legend on facing page.

Chapter 2: MEASUREMENT AND RECORDING OF JOINT MOTION / 19

←
Fig. 2-9.—Motion of shoulder. It is important to differentiate true glenohumeral motion in relation to scapulothoracic motion. The total upward motion of the arm at the shoulder from Zero degrees to 180 degrees is a smooth, rhythmic combination of true glenohumeral motion, plus the upward and forward rotation of the scapula on the chest wall, or scapulothoracic motion. As the shoulder has an almost 360-degree range of motion, the patient should be examined in the standing position. (If the shoulder is examined with the patient lying down, only 180 degrees of motion are available.)

Zero Starting Position: The patient standing erect, with the arm at the side of the body.

I.—*Vertical or Upward Motion of the Shoulder*

A, ABDUCTION and ADDUCTION. ABDUCTION is the upward motion of the arm away from the side of the body in the coronal plane, from Zero degrees to 180 degrees. ADDUCTION is the opposite motion of the arm toward the midline of the body, or beyond it in an upward plane.

B, FORWARD FLEXION (or forward elevation) and BACKWARD EXTENSION. FORWARD FLEXION is the forward, upward motion of the arm in the anterior sagittal plane of the body, from Zero to 180 degrees. The opposite motion to the Zero position may be termed "depression" of the arm. BACKWARD EXTENSION is the upward motion of the arm in the posterior sagittal plane of the body from Zero degrees to approximately 60 degrees.

II.—*Horizontal Motion of the Shoulder*

C, HORIZONTAL FLEXION. *Horizontal flexion* is the motion of the arm in the horizontal plane anterior to the coronal plane across the body. This motion is measured from Zero degrees to approximately 130–135 degrees. *Horizontal extension* is the horizontal motion posterior to the coronal plane of the body.

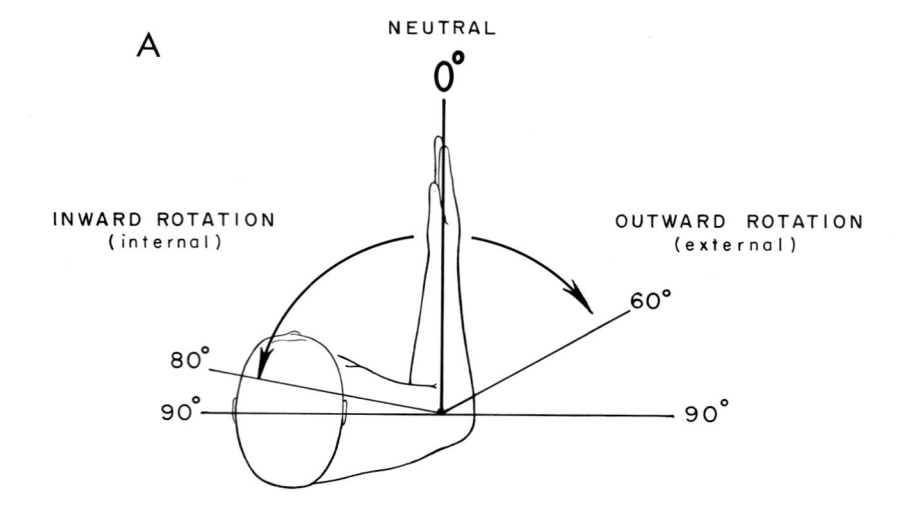

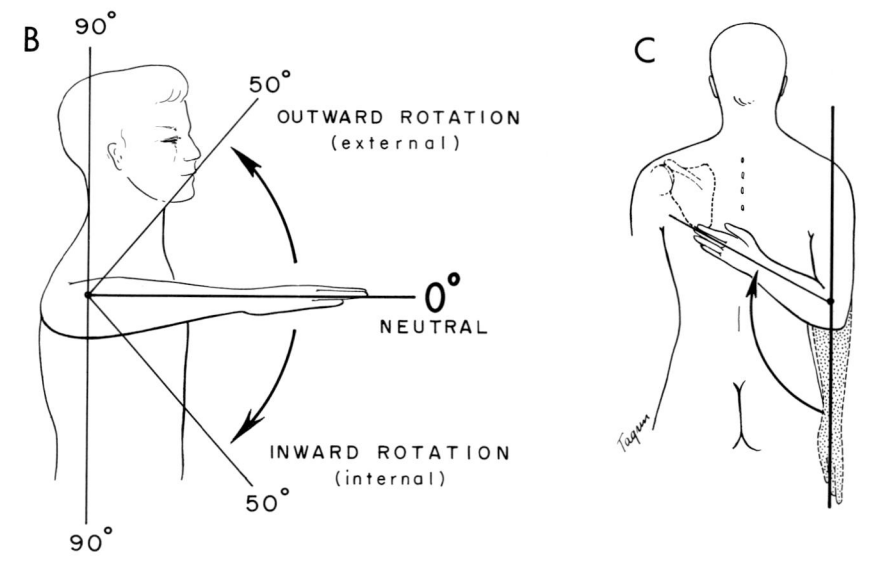

Fig. 2-10.—Motion of shoulder (rotation). *Neutral Position:* It is customary to measure rotation of the shoulder in two positions—one with the arm at the side of the body, the second in 90 degrees of abduction. Rotation can also be measured in any position where vertical and horizontal planes or coordinates cross.

A, ROTATION WITH ARM AT SIDE OF BODY: Inward and outward motion is recorded in degrees of motion from the neutral starting point.

B, ROTATION IN ABDUCTION: Rotation in this position is less than with the arm at the side of the body. It is recorded in degrees of motion from the Zero Starting Position.

C, INTERNAL ROTATION POSTERIORLY: A clinical method of estimating function is the distance the finger tips reach in relation to the scapula or the base of the neck.

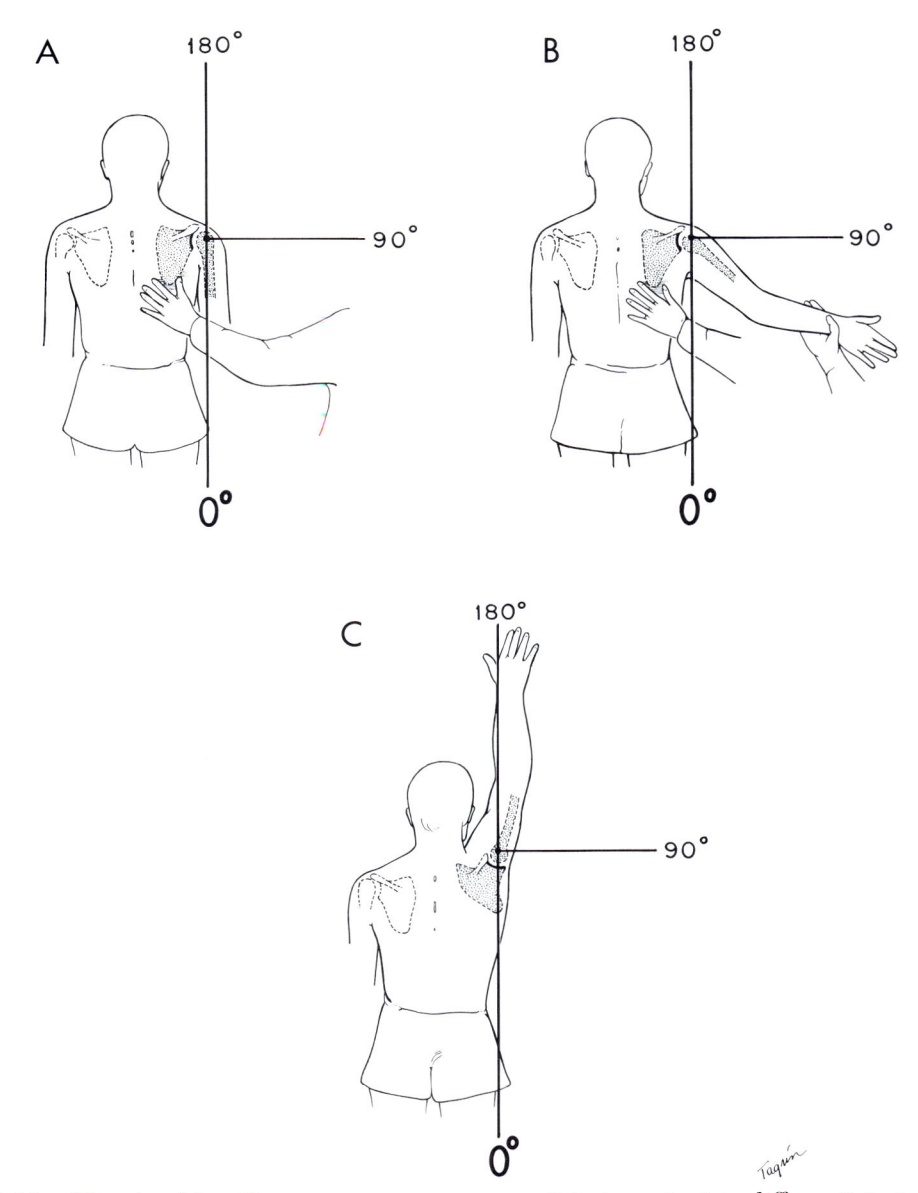

Fig. 2-11.—The shoulder. GLENOHUMERAL MOTION. It is important to differentiate true glenohumeral motion in relation to scapulothoracic motion. The total upward motion of the arm at the shoulder from Zero degrees to 180 degrees is a smooth, rhythmic combination of true glenohumeral motion, plus the upward and forward rotation of the scapula on the chest wall, or scapulothoracic motion. **A,** THE NEUTRAL STARTING POSITION with the arm at the side of the body. **B,** TRUE GLENOHUMERAL MOTION is estimated by fixing the scapula with the hand and elevating the arm passively with the other hand. **C,** "COMBINED" GLENOHUMERAL WITH SCAPULOTHORACIC MOTION. The rotation of the scapula upward and forward over the chest wall allows the arm to reach farther upward. Normally, the range is 180 degrees.

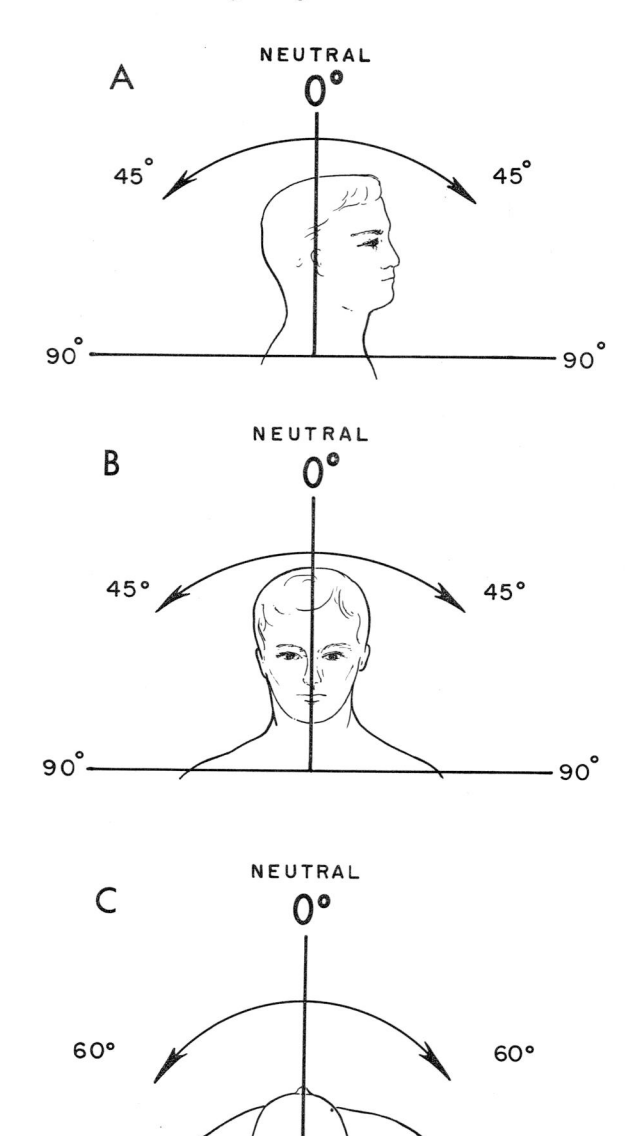

Fig. 2-12.—Motion of cervical spine. *Zero Starting Position:* The correct standing or sitting position.

A, FLEXION and EXTENSION: These motions usually are designated in degrees; however, the examiner may indicate the number of inches the chin lacks from touching the chest.

B, LATERAL BEND: This motion also is measured in degrees, but can be indicated by the number of inches the ear lacks from reaching the shoulder.

C, ROTATION: This is estimated in degrees from the neutral position, or in percentages of motion, as compared to individuals of similar age and physical build.

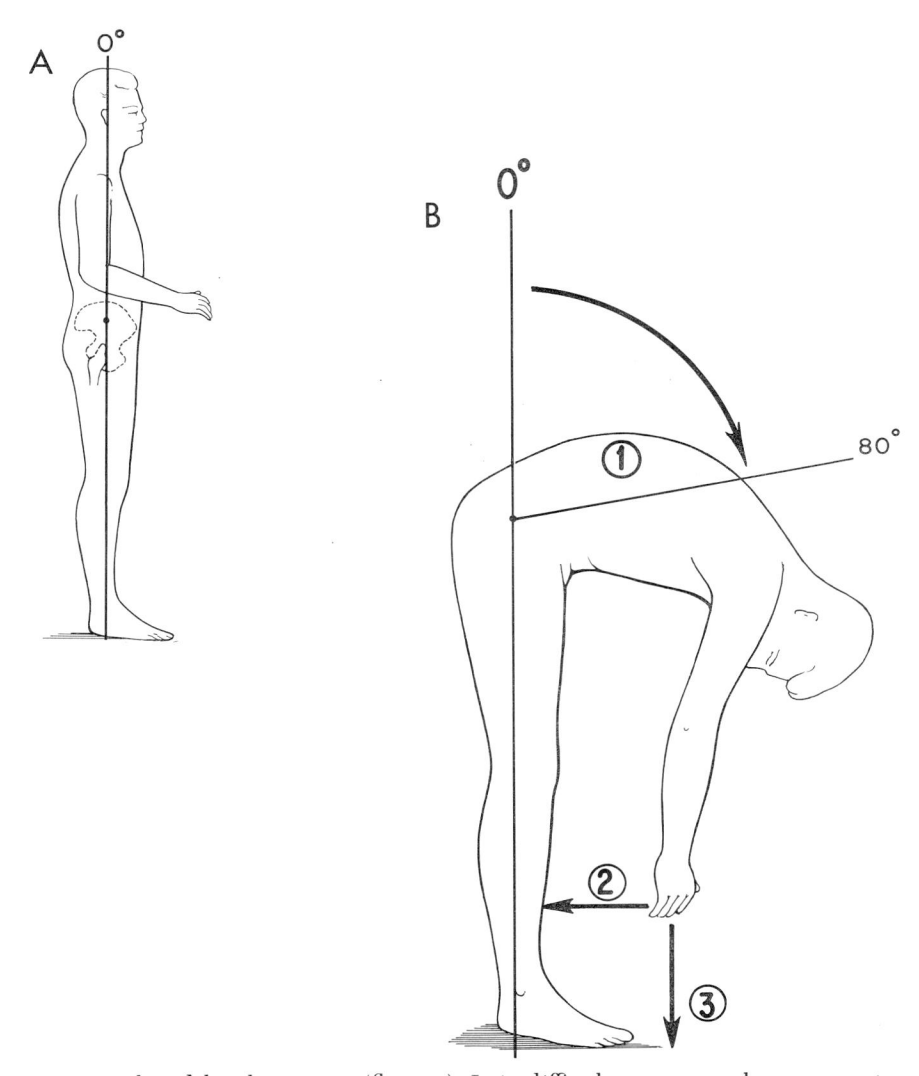

Fig. 2-13.—Dorsal and lumbar spine (flexion). It is difficult to accurately measure true spine motion by physical examination. This is due to soft tissue coverage of the spine, the normal curves of the spine, variations of motion in different sections of the spine and the presence of hip motion. In fact, one may bend forward 90 degrees, with the motion taking place entirely in the hips and not in the spine. It has been found that the use of the steel or plastic tape measure (see Fig. 2-14) is the most accurate method of estimating true spine motion in flexion.

A, *Zero Starting Position:* The correct standing position.

B, FLEXION: Four clinical methods of estimating the range of spinal flexion are:

1. By measuring the degrees of forward inclination of the trunk in relation to the longitudinal axis of the body. The examiner should "fix" the pelvis with his hands. The loss (or not) of lordosis should also be noted.

2. By indicating the level the finger tips reach along the patient's leg. For instance, finger tips to the patella or finger tips to midtibia.

3. By measuring the distance in inches or centimeters between the finger tips and the floor.

4. By the steel or plastic tape measure method (see Fig. 2-14).

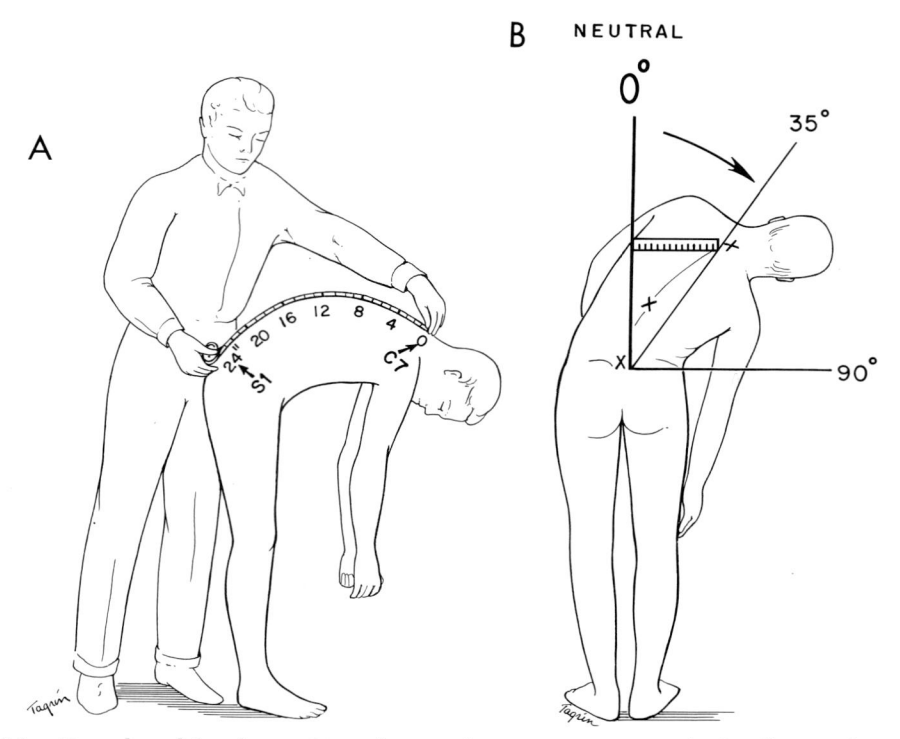

Fig. 2-14.—Dorsal and lumbar spine—the steel tape measure method. This perhaps is the most accurate clinical method of measuring true motion of the spine in flexion. The flexible steel or plastic tape adjusts very accurately to the dorsal and lumbar contours of the spine. With the patient standing, the 1-inch marker of the tape is held over the spinous process of C7 and the distal tape is held over the spinous process of S1.

A, as the patient bends forward, if the lumbar curve reverses and the spinous processes spread, this will be indicated by lengthening of the tape measure. In the normal healthy adult, there is, on the average, an increase of 4 inches in forward flexion. If the patient bends forward with his back straight (as in rheumatoid spondylitis), the tape will not record motion. One is able to record motion of the dorsal spine per se by taping from the spinous process of C7 to D12. Likewise, motion of the lumbar spine can be measured from the spinous process of D12 to S1. Usually, if the total spine in flexion is 4 inches, the examiner will find that 1 inch occurs in the dorsal spine and 3 inches occurs in the lumbar spine.

B, lateral bending. The vertical steel tape, if held firmly and straight, may also aid in measuring the motion of lateral bending. This can be estimated as follows:

1. In the degrees of lateral inclination of the trunk, or
2. By noting the position of the spinous process of C-7 with relation to the pelvis.
3. Note the level of the lumbar spine reflecting the base of lateral motion. This level may be lumbosacral or higher and may vary from right to left in the same patient.
4. The knee joint may be used as a fixed point. Record the distance of the finger tips from the knee joint on lateral bending.

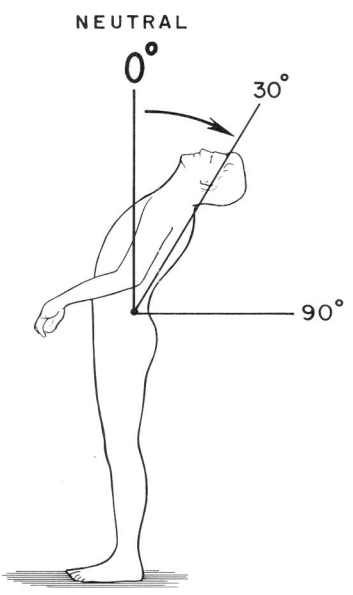

Chapter 2: MEASUREMENT AND RECORDING OF JOINT MOTION / 25

Fig. 2-15.—Motion of spine. Extension may be recorded with the patient standing or lying prone on a firm surface. The range of extension is recorded in degrees.

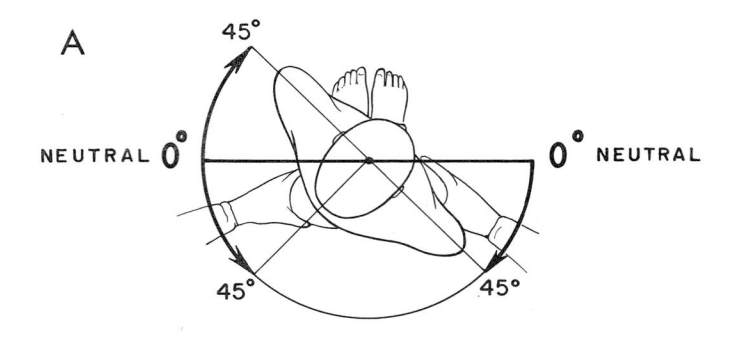

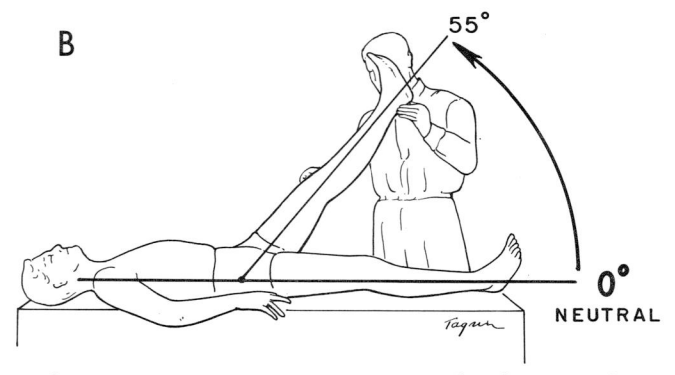

Fig. 2-16.—Motion of spine. **A,** ROTATION: To estimate the degrees of rotation of the spine, the pelvis must be held firmly by the examiner's hands and the patient is instructed to rotate to the right or the left. This motion is recorded in degrees, or in percentages of motion, as compared to individuals of similar age and physical build. **B,** STRAIGHT LEG RAISING TEST: Although this is not a record of spine motion, it is included here because of its use in examinations of the back. The test is carried out with the patient supine on a firm, level examining table. The upward motion of the straight leg is a passive motion and is measured in degrees from the Zero Starting Position. This range of motion varies considerably in individuals of different physical builds. The motion of one leg should be compared to the opposite leg. Rotation of the pelvis occurs after a point is reached and may provide an "error" in the actual straight leg raising present. (This is a passive test with the patient completely relaxed. It may also be performed actively, but the level of rise is likely to be inaccurate.)

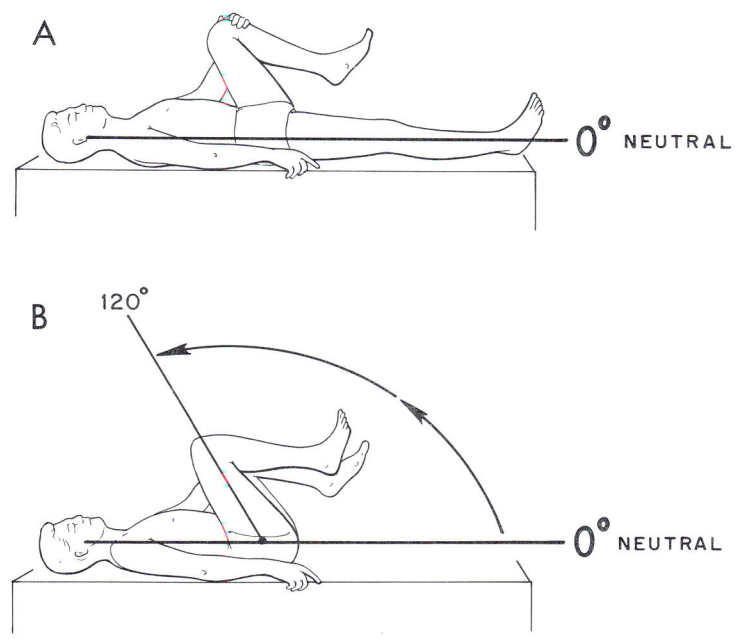

Chapter 2: MEASUREMENT AND RECORDING OF JOINT MOTION / 27

Fig. 2-17.—Motion of hip. The hip is a "ball-and-socket" joint. Due to its deeper socket, the range of motion is less than that of the shoulder. Motions of the hip are measured with the patient lying either supine or prone. This simplifies terminology, as compared to the shoulder, as only one hemisphere of motion is measured at a time. Errors in hip motion occur when pelvis rotation is not noticed. FLEXION: **A,** *Zero Starting Position* of the right hip: The patient lies supine on a firm, flat surface with the opposite hip held in full flexion. This flattens the lumbar spine and demonstrates a flexion deformity of the hip if it is present. **B,** the motion of flexion is recorded from Zero to 110 or 120 degrees. The examiner should place one hand on the iliac crest to note the point at which the pelvis begins to rotate.

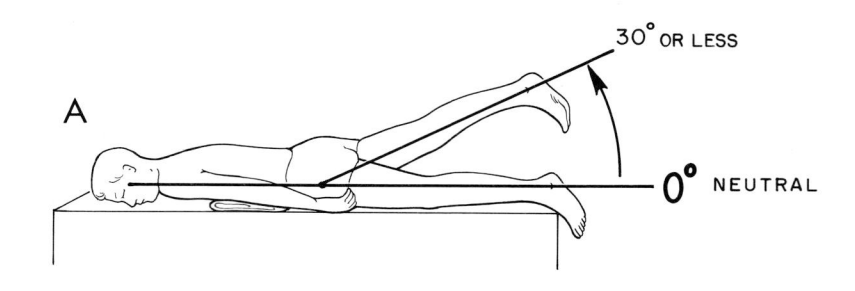

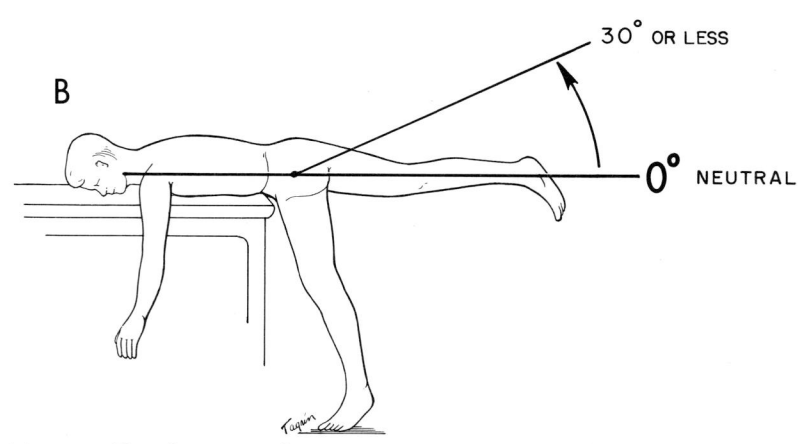

Fig. 2-18.—Motion of hip (extension). *Zero Starting Position:* The patient lies prone on a firm, level surface. The upward motion of the hip is measured in degrees from the Zero Starting Position. Two methods are commonly used: **A**, with the patient face down and a small pillow under the abdomen, the leg is extended with the knee straight or flexed. **B**, with the opposite extremity flexed over the end of the examining table. From this position the hip is extended. This method is a more accurate method of measuring extension. There is an anatomic question whether extension is present in the hip at all. Extension as seen from examination is that deviation of the extremity past the Zero Starting Position and reflects some back motion.

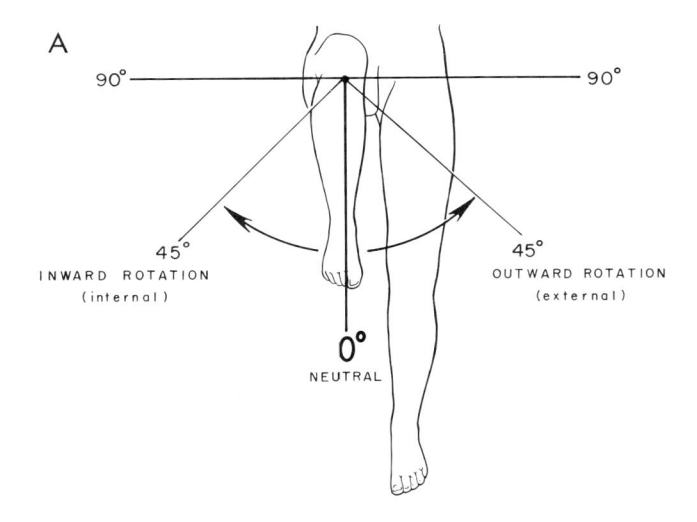

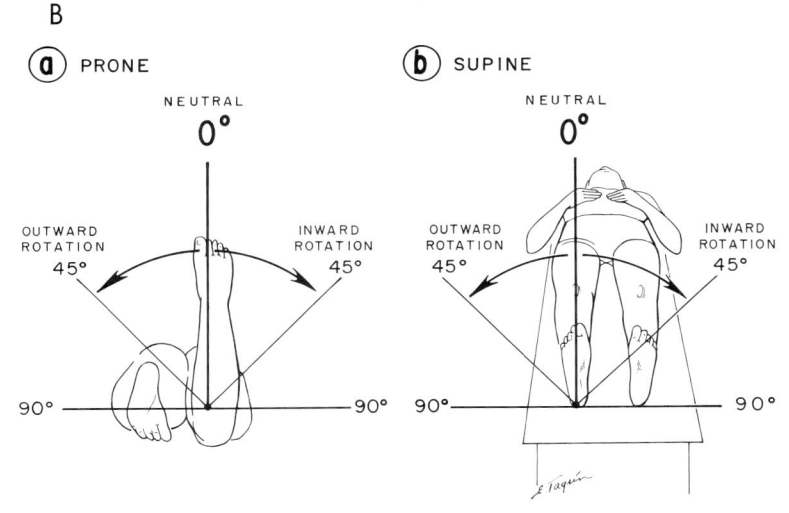

Chapter 2: MEASUREMENT AND RECORDING OF JOINT MOTION / 29

Fig. 2-19.—Motion of hip (rotation). Rotation of the hip is measured in flexion and in extension.
   A, ROTATION IN FLEXION: *Zero Starting Position:* With the patient lying supine, the hip and knee are flexed to 90 degrees each, with the thigh perpendicular to the transverse line across the anterior superior spines of the pelvis. INWARD ROTATION (internal): This is measured by rotating the leg away from the midline of the trunk with the thigh as the axis of rotation, thus producing inward rotation of the hip. OUTWARD ROTATION (external): This is measured by rotating the leg toward the midline of the trunk with the thigh as the axis of rotation, thus producing outward rotation of the hip.
   B, ROTATION IN EXTENSION: *Zero Starting Position:* With the patient lying face down, the knee is flexed to 90 degrees and is perpendicular to the transverse line across the anterior superior spines of the pelvis.
   (a) INWARD ROTATION is measured by rotating the leg outward. OUTWARD ROTATION is measured by rotating the leg inward.
   (b) Rotation in extension can also be measured with the patient supine.

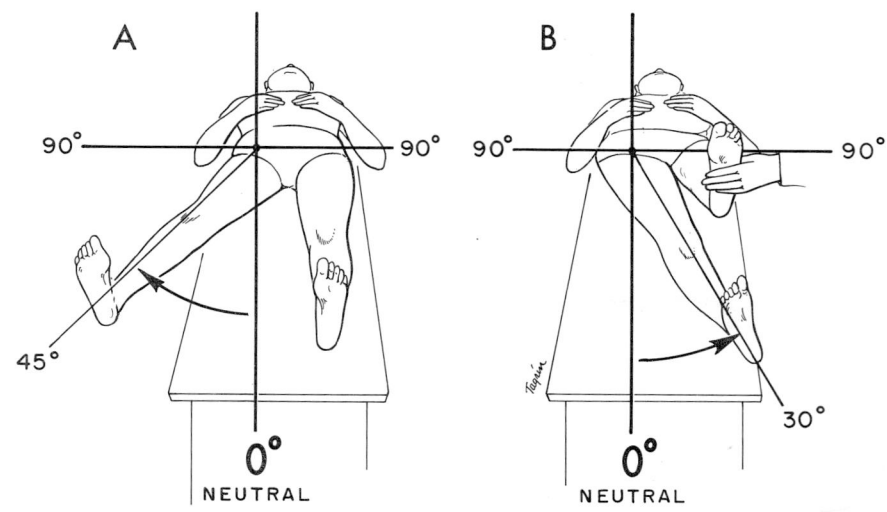

Fig. 2-20.—Motion of hip: ABDUCTION and ADDUCTION. *Zero Starting Position:* The patient lies supine with the legs extended at a right angle to a transverse line across the anterior superior spines of the pelvis. **A,** ABDUCTION: The outward motion of the extremity is measured in degrees from the Zero Starting Position. ABDUCTION IN FLEXION: See Figure 2-21. **B,** ADDUCTION: In measuring adduction, the examiner should elevate the opposite extremity a few degrees to allow the leg to pass under it.

Fig. 2-21.—Motion of hip: ABDUCTION IN FLEXION. Abduction can be measured in degrees at any level of flexion. Usually this is carried out in 90 degrees of flexion.

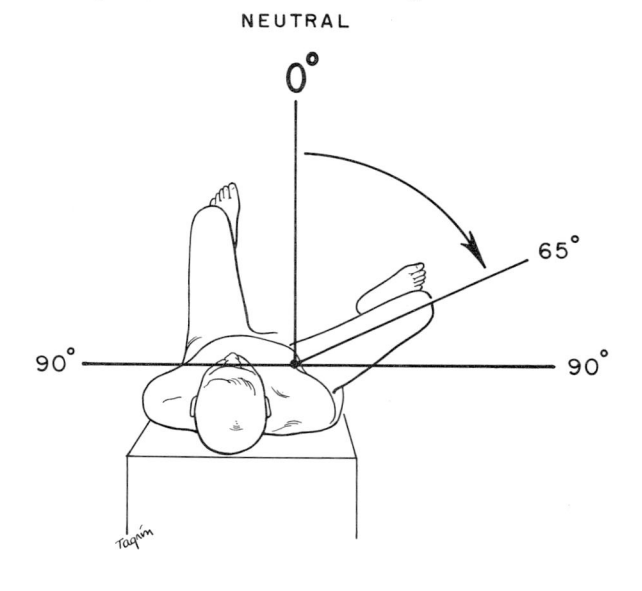

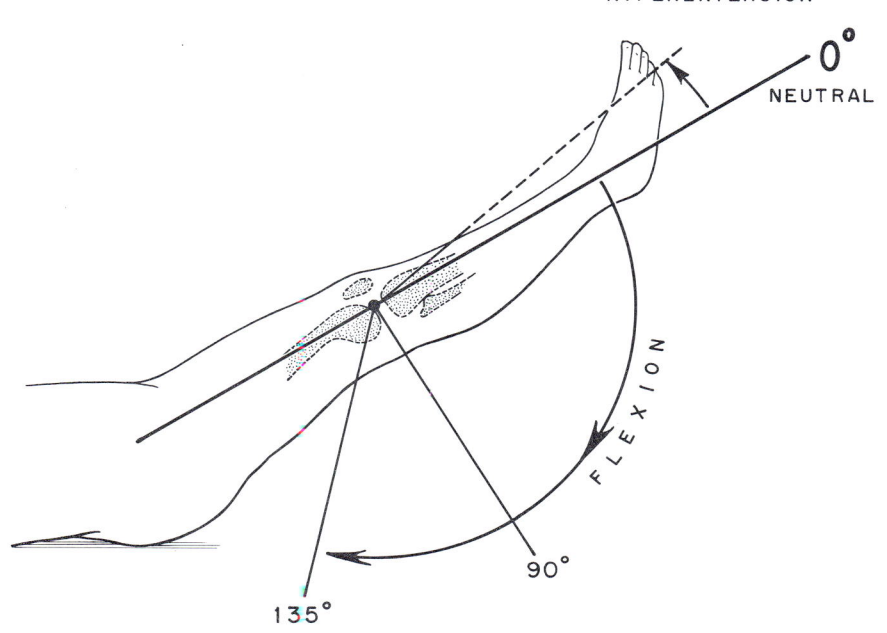

Chapter 2: MEASUREMENT AND RECORDING OF JOINT MOTION / 31

Fig. 2-22. — Motion of knee. The knee is considered to be a modified hinge joint, with its primary motion in flexion. The motion opposite to FLEXION, to the Zero Starting Position, is EXTENSION. As the motion beyond the Zero Starting Position is an unnatural one, it is referred to as HYPEREXTENSION. There is a small degree of natural rotation of the tibia on the femoral condyle in FLEXION and EXTENSION. This cannot be measured accurately. Abnormal lateral motion may be estimated in degrees.

FLEXION: *Zero Starting Position:* The extended straight knee with the patient either supine or prone. FLEXION is measured in degrees from the Zero Starting Position. HYPEREXTENSION is measured in degrees opposite to flexion at the Zero Starting Position.

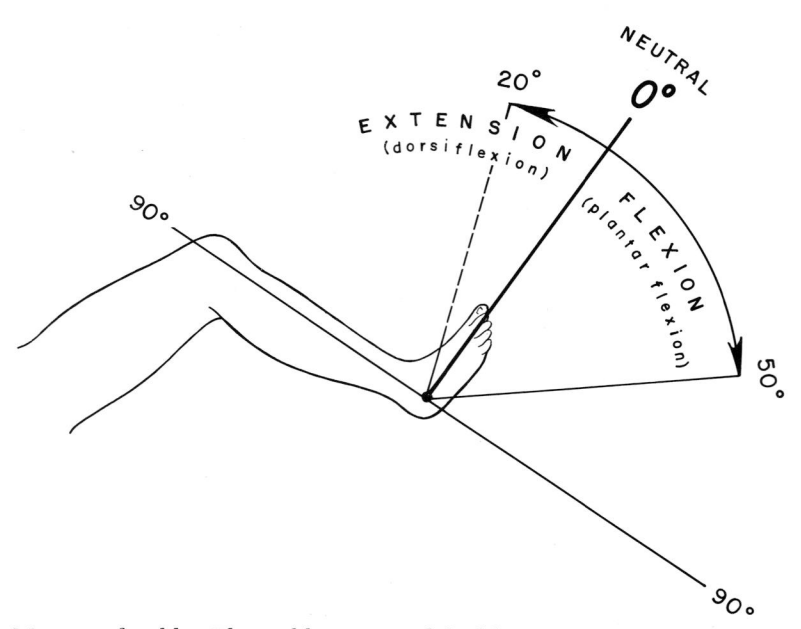

Fig. 2-23.—Motion of ankle. The ankle is a modified hinge joint, with its primary motion of **FLEXION** and **EXTENSION** at the tibiotalar joint. There is a slight degree of lateral motion present with the ankle in plantar flexion. This cannot be estimated accurately. Motions of the ankles should be measured with the knee in flexion in order to relax the heel cord.

Zero Starting Position: With the leg at a right angle to the thigh and the foot at a right angle to the leg. EXTENSION (dorsiflexion) and FLEXION (plantar flexion): These motions are measured in degrees from the right angle neutral position, or in percentages of motion, as compared to the opposite ankle.

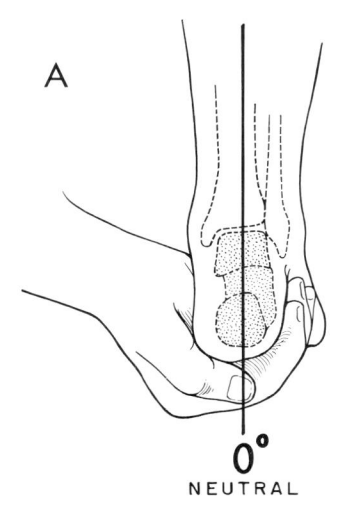

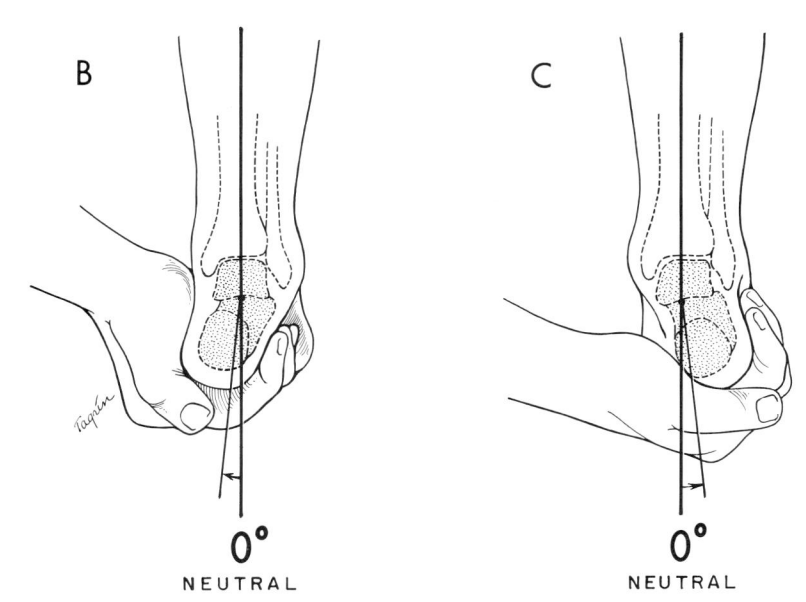

Chapter 2: MEASUREMENT AND RECORDING OF JOINT MOTION / 33

Fig. 2-24. — Hind part of foot (passive motion). Motion of the foot is compound but can be broken down as (1) the hind part of the foot (the subtalar joint) and (2) the fore part of the foot (midtarsal joints).

Motions of the hind part of the foot (passive motion): **A,** *Zero Starting Position:* The heel is aligned with the midline of the tibia. **B, INVERSION**: The heel is grasped firmly in the cup of the examiner's hand. Passive motion is estimated in degrees, or percentages of motion, by turning the heel inward. **C, EVERSION**: This motion is estimated by turning the heel outward.

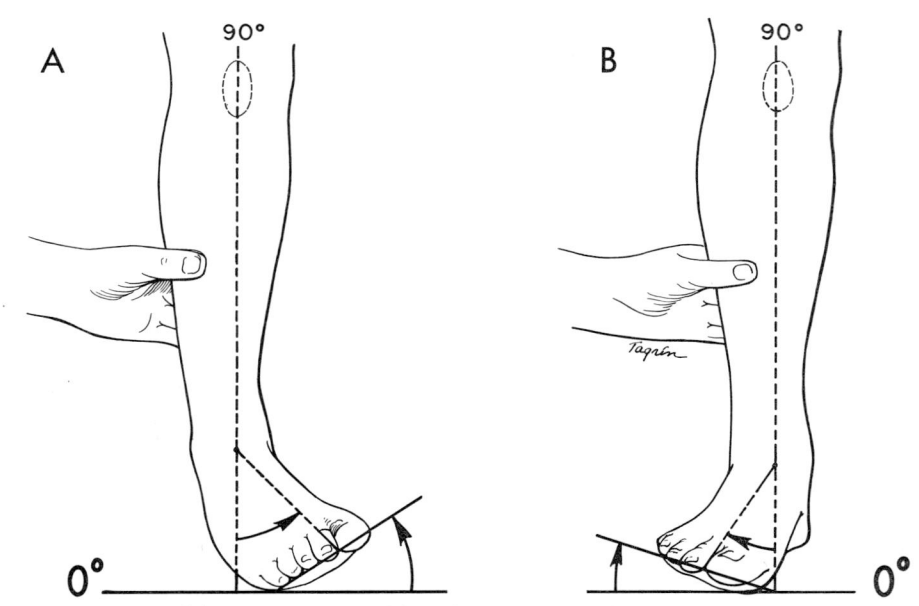

Fig. 2-25.—Motion of foot. Fore part of foot (active motion). *Zero Starting Position:* The axis of the foot is the second toe. The foot is aligned with the tibia in the long axis from the ankle to the knee. **A, ACTIVE INVERSION**: The foot is directed medially. This motion includes supination, adduction and some degree of plantar flexion. This motion can be estimated in degrees, or expressed in percentages, as compared to the opposite foot. **B, ACTIVE EVERSION**: The sole of the foot is turned to face laterally. This motion includes pronation, abduction and dorsiflexion.

NOTE: Problems exist when the foot motions are divided in fore and hind foot descriptions. Care must be made to record motions pertaining to that part of the foot described or the whole foot, as the case may be.

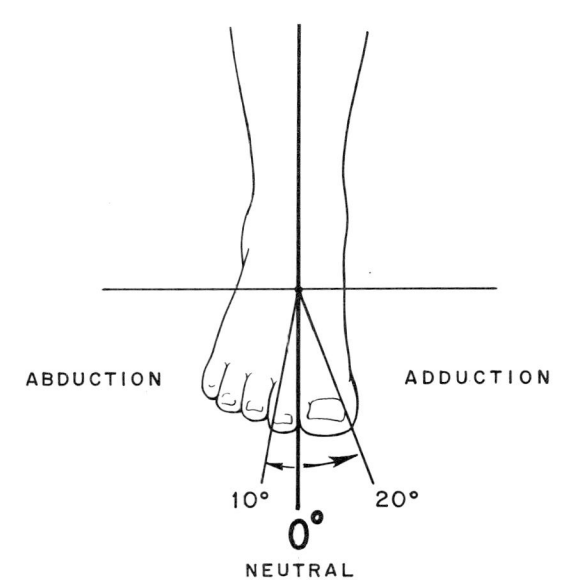

Fig. 2-26.—Motion of foot. Fore part of foot (passive motion). ADDUCTION and ABDUCTION: These passive motions are obtained by grasping the heel and moving the fore part of the foot inward or outward. This motion must take place in the plane of the sole of the foot.

36 / *Edwin F. Cave and Robert J. Boyd*

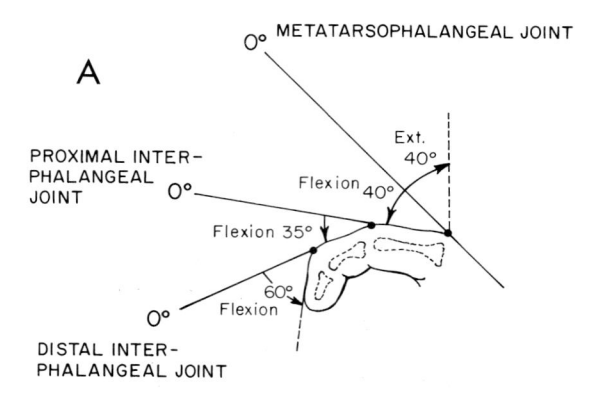

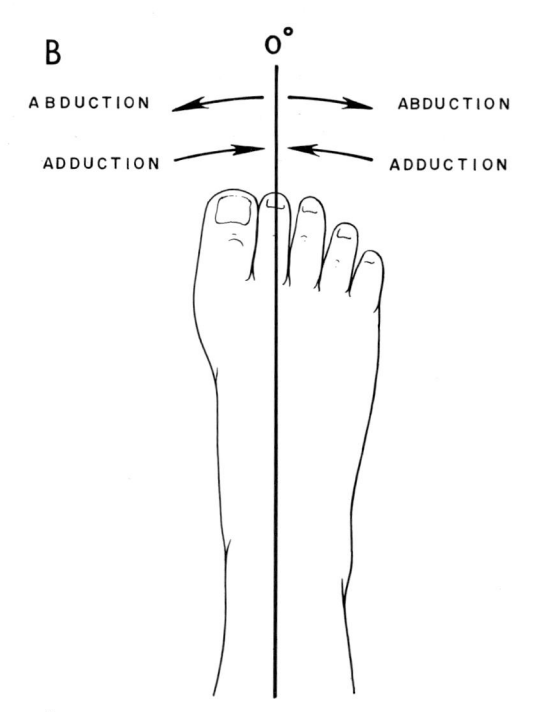

Fig. 2-27.—Motion of toes. **A,** motion in FLEXION is present in the interphalangeal and metatarsophalangeal joints of the toes. EXTENSION is present at the metatarsophalangeal joint. These motions can be simply expressed in degrees. **B,** ABDUCTION AND ADDUCTION (toe spread): This can be measured in relation to the second toe, which is the midline axis of the foot.

BIBLIOGRAPHY

American Society for Surgery of The Hand, Personal Consultations, 1960–1962.

Cave, E. F. (ed.): *Fractures and Other Injuries* (Chicago: Year Book Medical Publishers, Inc., 1958).

Cave, E. F., and Roberts, S. M.: A method of measuring and recording joint function, J. Bone Joint Surg. 18:455, 1936.

Clark, W. A.: A system of joint measurements, J. Orth. Surg., Vol. 2, No. 12, 1920.

Codman, E. A.: *The Shoulder* (Boston: T. Todd, 1934).

Combined Meeting, Orthopaedic Associations of the English Speaking World, Vancouver, B. C., June, 1964.

Evaluation of Industrial Disability (Comm. of California Medical Assn. & The Industrial Acc. Comm. of the State of California) (Oxford University Press, 1960).

Executive Committee of American Academy of Orthopaedic Surgeons, September 12, 1959 (Executive Committee Meeting).

Executive Committee of American Orthopaedic Association, January, 1960 (Executive Committee Meeting).

Gardner, E., Gray, D. J., and O'Rahilly, R.: *Anatomy* (Philadelphia: W. B. Saunders Company, 1960).

Glimcher, M. J., and Brown, T.: Department of Biophysics, Massachusetts Institute of Technology, 1959.

Harris, R. I.: A memorandum of movements of joints, 1918.

Joint Motion – Method of Measuring and Recording, American Academy of Orthopaedic Surgeons, 1965.

Journal American Medical Association: A guide to the evaluation of permanent impairment of the extremities & back. Special edition, February 15, 1958.

McBride, E. D.: *Disability Evaluation: Principles of Treatment of Compensable Injuries* (5th ed.; Philadelphia: J. B. Lippincott Company, 1953).

Outline of Treatment of Fractures: American College of Surgeons, 7th ed., 1960.

Solomon, L.: Personal communication, Johannesburg, South Africa.

The United States Armed Forces Medical Journal, Vol 6, No. 3, March, 1955; The Joint Motion Measurements – Dept. of the Army & The Air Force. T. M. 8-640:A.F.P. 160-14-1 March, 1956.

Workman's Compensation Board, Toronto, Canada, Forms 43 & 149.

3 | Metabolic Response to Trauma

BENJAMIN A. BARNES and PAUL S. RUSSELL

There is a circumstance attending accidental injury which does not belong to disease, viz., that the injury done has, in all cases, a tendency to produce both the disposition and the means of cure.—
JOHN HUNTER[67]

INTRODUCTION

IT IS APPROPRIATE at the outset of a volume on trauma to consider those responses following injury that are systemic, not localized to the injured part and observed after a wide variety of traumatic insults to the body. The remainder of this volume presents specific examples of trauma in various anatomic sites together with their clinical implications and treatment. Nevertheless, all major trauma evokes a far-embracing biologic response similar in all patients to a considerable extent. This response, known to antiquity as the *vis medicatrix naturae*, is the subject of this introductory chapter. In other chapters, complementary topics are presented on fracture healing, management of shock and respiratory insufficiency, anesthesia and treatment of burns. As the above quotation attests, John Hunter recognized the response in the eighteenth century, and definition and analysis have intrigued many since. In the 1920s, Cannon evolved his brilliant interpretation of the integrating mechanism in mammals responding to pain, hunger, fear and rage. He was principally concerned with the functional anatomy of the nervous system and with the hormones of the adrenal medulla, which could be detected then by exquisitely sensitive biologic assays. He wrote, "The most significant feature of these bodily reactions in pain and in the presence of emotion-provoking objects is that they are of the nature of reflexes. . . . The pattern of the reaction . . . is deeply inwrought in the workings of the nervous system."[18] His early demonstrations of the physiologic basis for part of the response to injury were followed by increasingly complex interpretations more deeply inwrought in every organ system as successive physicians applied more penetrating techniques in metabolic research. In 1936, Selye[109] emphasized the sweeping scope of the response, which he later called the "general adaptation syndrome," ushered in by an "alarm reaction" defined as "the sum of all nonspecific phenomena elicited by sudden exposure to stimuli to which the organism is quantitatively or qualitatively not adapted." His endocrine and morphologic data added a comprehensive interpretation to the novel biochemical studies by Cuthbertson[24] on the reaction to injury, the results of which appeared in 1930. World War II and subsequent wars have occasioned many additional observations, among which the contributions of J. E. Howard, O. Cope and F. D. Moore have been notable, so that in recent years our understanding has been extended considerably.

A presentation of the metabolic response to injury apart from the variations brought about by complications and by therapy would be artificial. Therefore, as in clinical situations, the response of the patient to injury and to certain complications and therapy will be considered together. The responses observed vary from trivial to major ones, as when the body contends with near-lethal injury and its complications. The response following excessively complicated injuries with visceral damage calls into play more varied changes specific to the structures involved. For illustrative purposes, we will accordingly concentrate on the response following an intermediate type of injury, such as traumatic fracture of the femur or pelvis without visceral damage in an otherwise healthy young adult. Observations on the response to surgical procedures, which can be viewed as a highly controlled type of trauma, have been most instructive and will be discussed also.

ACUTE RESPONSE TO TRAUMA

SUPPORT OF THE CIRCULATION.—Commonly, trauma leads to pain and anxiety, to external and internal blood loss immediately following injury, to an accumulation of edema fluid at the site of injury, starting at once and extending over the next 12–36 hours, and to a decrease in blood volume, causing cardiovascular insufficiency with inadequate perfusion of the tissues. Experimentally, it has been shown that the insult of 30 minutes of ischemia will produce alterations in muscle, readily identified by light microscopy, consisting of edema fluid, hyaline and granular degeneration and vacuolization associated with focal necrosis.[29] Viscera may be functionally impaired by only a few minutes of total ischemia. Cardiac volume receptors and arterial baroreceptors initiate the integrated response to a decrease in blood volume by neural and humoral mechanisms. Cardiac rate increases promptly, and systemic arterial vasoconstriction distributes the waning cardiac output to essential organs.

Epinephrine and norepinephrine secretion is the familiar response of the sympathetic nervous system to trauma, pain, anxiety and diminished blood volume. The adrenal medulla, other paraspinal collections of chromaffin tissue and postganglionic sympathetic nerve endings share in the secretion, and the relative proportion of epinephrine to norepinephrine released by the medulla is about 2 to 1.[66] Following an uncomplicated major operation, 16 µg of epinephrine are excreted in the urine per 24 hours (normal 5 µg per 24 hours) and 60 µg of norepinephrine in the urine per 24 hours (normal 25 µg per 24 hours). Extensive trauma may lead to maximal excretion of 60 µg of epinephrine and 500 µg of norepinephrine per 24 hours. These excretion rates correspond to about 1–5% of the hormones secreted because of rapid in vivo oxidation to inactive metabolites. In the absence of complications, they return to normal in a week or less.[48, 57, 66] Epinephrine augments the cardiac output by a positive inotropic and chronotropic action. Venous return to the heart is improved by a rise in peripheral venous pressure as vasoconstriction reduces the capacity of the veins, normally containing 50% of the total blood volume. Epinephrine, altering the relative distribution of blood throughout the body, favors flow to cardiac and skeletal muscle and causes a reduction in the circulation to skin and abdominal viscera. Perspiration, mydriasis, rise in plasma nonesterified fatty acids, increase in basal metabolic rate, and hyperglycemia, with a possible secondary glycosuria, are associated phenomena. On the other hand, norepinephrine, which is also the substance involved in neurohumoral transmission between postganglionic adrenergic nerve fibers and effector cells, supports the blood supply and function of many viscera. The balance of these hormones and their contingent actions following stress remain to be fully clarified.

Clinical corollary: The pressor response to acute hypovolemia is generally consistent and predictable, with the optimal response being obtained from endogenous hormones. Only occasionally, as set forth in the chapter on shock (Chapter 12), are pressor drugs needed to restore the patient's normal blood pressure and circulation if whole blood and plasma are given promptly to maintain the central venous pressure between 10 and 15 cm water, urine volume greater than 25 ml per hour and hematocrit between 35 and 45%. Where a cardiac stimulant and vasodilator to improve tissue perfusion is needed, 2 mg of isoproterenol in 1,000 ml 5% dextrose in water may be given intravenously at a rate determined by the clinical situation.

Antidiuretic hormone (ADH) secretion is evoked by stimuli traversing the hypothalamiconeurohypophyseal tract to the posterior pituitary gland. The hypothalamus, in turn, is stimulated by pain and by afferent stimuli coming from the cardiac volume receptors located in the wall of the left atrium and possibly at other intrathoracic sites. The existence of intravascular volume receptors was suspected early by Leaf[81] following studies of the diuretic response seen in subjects depleted of extracellular fluid electrolyte and with simultaneous expansion of extracellular fluid volume. Experimental evidence for their intrathoracic location was suggested by the doubling of urine volume achieved in dogs when constrained to breathe against a constant negative pressure of −10 cm of water. The ensuing increase in intrathoracic blood volume presumably initiated afferent impulses to the hypothalamus originating from volume receptors in the walls of the great veins or in the atria of the heart.[50] Morphine, anesthetic agents and other stimuli characteristic of the postoperative period also increase ADH activity.[42] The retention of water and sodium chloride by this hormone's potent action on the distal renal tubules reduces urine formation at a critical moment. This conservation of body fluids aids the defense of vascular and extracellular spaces depleted by blood loss and sequestration of extracellular fluid at the site of primary injury. ADH release may be activated in a few minutes and has been shown in normal volunteers to occur after acute hemorrhage of 500–1,000 ml.[49, 89, 130] This promptness and sensitivity are noteworthy.

Aldosterone is secreted by the adrenal cortex in response to adrenocorticotropic hormone (ACTH) and more strikingly in response to elevations in plasma angiotensin, which is produced from precursors in the blood through the action of renin, a hormone originating in the juxtaglomerular cells of the renal cortex. These cells produce renin when pressure in their circulation falls or when sodium concentration in the distal tubule declines, as invariably occurs with the decrease in renal blood flow following major hemorrhage.[126] The existence of a volume receptor controlling renin release, as established for ADH, appears unlikely at present. Further activation of aldosterone secretion by hyperkalemia, another proved stimulus, is not part of the early response to trauma unless substantial muscle damage has caused this complication. The sensitivity of the aldosterone response has been studied in normal volunteers sustaining a hemorrhage of approximately 15% of their blood volume.[115] During the 24-hour period following this minimal stress, aldosterone excretion in the urine rose from the prehemorrhage value of 180 μg to 600 μg per 24 hours. Sodium excretion in the urine fell right off within 15 minutes, during which time only 250 ml of blood had been removed. In Figure 3-1, adapted from Skillman et al.,[115] are seen the dramatic promptness and magnitude of this response. Plasma cortisol levels were not increased by the controlled hemorrhage, and this is evidence against a significant

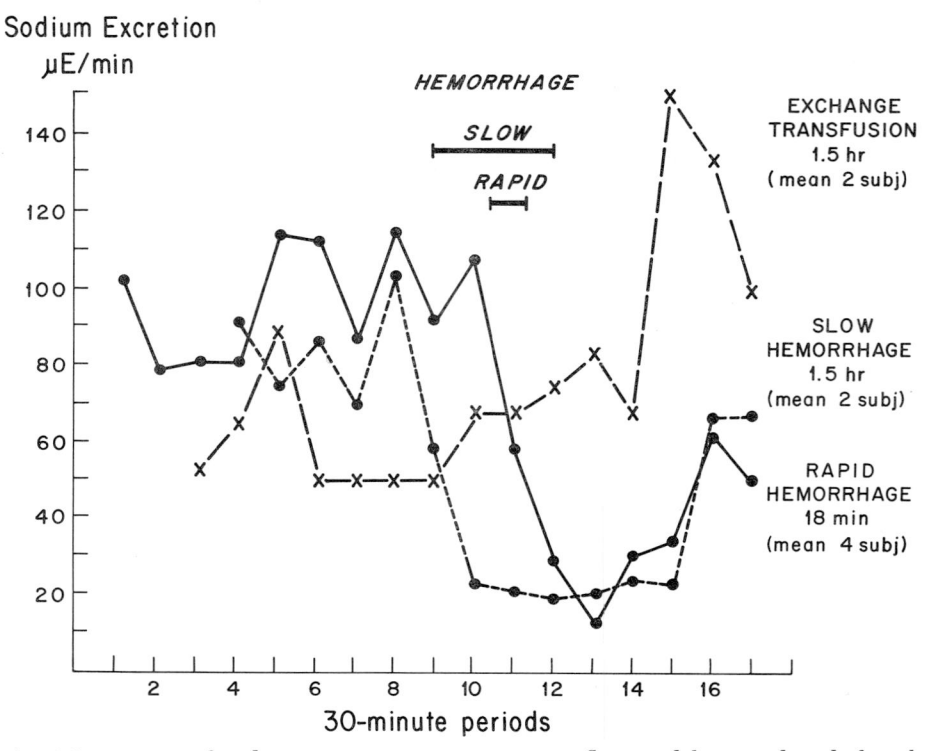

Fig. 3-1.—Mean rates of sodium excretion in urine as influenced by rapid and slow hemorrhage and by exchange transfusion.

secretion of ACTH and in favor of the initiation of aldosterone secretion by the renin mechanism. The resorption of sodium chloride and water from the renal tubules and loss of potassium effected by aldosterone is a response admirably designed to defend the composition and volume of the extracellular space after trauma when dehydration and hyperkalemia may be threatening survival. Furthermore, the effectiveness of aldosterone secretion is potentiated when caused by blood loss sufficient to alter perfusion of the liver. This organ, the principal site for the metabolism of aldosterone, clears the blood of 90–100% by conjugation in a single pass.[136] The normal half-life of aldosterone in the blood, 30 minutes, is almost doubled following a hemorrhage of 3% of the body weight, which diminishes hepatic blood flow.[32] Thus, the secretion of aldosterone may, where liver perfusion is altered, be reinforced by a decrease in the rate of conjugation of aldosterone. As with sodium and water, stress from hemorrhage activates mechanisms that conserve a vital hormone.

These responses supporting the circulation are summarized in Figure 3-2, adapted from Gauer and Henry.[49] These authors emphasize that ADH release and constriction of the resistance vessels (systemic arteries) are early compensations and that aldosterone release and constriction of the capacity vessels (systemic veins) occur later. These mechanisms and the net shift of fluid from the interstitial to the vascular space compensate for acute blood loss of a liter or less without the hemoglobin concentration in the blood being depressed to a point at which oxygen transport is seriously ham-

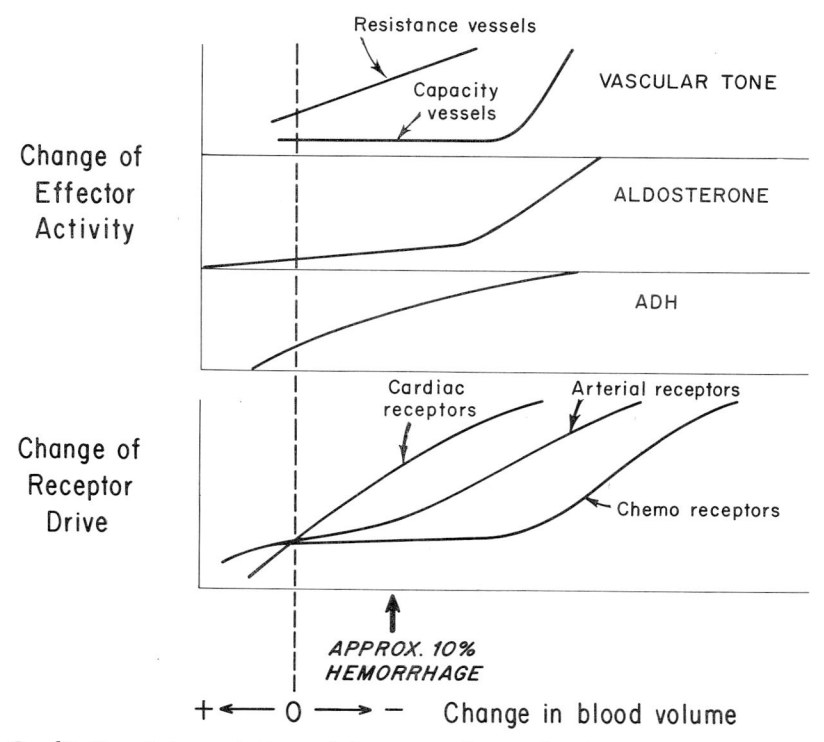

Fig. 3-2.—Qualitative interpretation of homeostatic mechanisms supporting circulation as blood volume varies. Below are receptor drives of cardiac (volume), arterial (pressure) and chemo (oxygen tension) receptors. Above are resultant effector activities.

pered. In Figure 3-3, adapted from Skillman et al.,[115] observations in a normal volunteer following hemorrhage are displayed. The gradual increase in plasma volume over 24 hours is complete compensation for the volume lost. Note the departures of the calculated plasma volume above the dashed line, revealing that transcapillary filling starts during the blood loss. The initial and most rapid rate of transcapillary filling at the termination of a liter of hemorrhage is 1.5–2.0 ml/min, gradually decreasing as the average capillary pressure is restored concurrently with the blood volume to normal. The protein transfers associated with injury are considered in a subsequent section.

Clinical corollary: The combined effects of ADH and aldosterone minimizing water and sodium chloride losses by the kidneys demand caution in fluid therapy to avoid excess salt loading and overhydration in the period immediately following operation or injury. The guiding principle is to limit prescribed fluids to those needed to compensate for proved or suspected requirements and deficits. When fluid intake must be curtailed, 5% dextrose in water is the preferred vehicle by which antibiotics and other medications are given intravenously, since about 500 ml of water may be removed each 24 hours by insensible loss from the lungs and skin without imposing any excretory load on the kidneys.

CORTISOL SECRETION.—Following trauma, cortisol increases in the serum from a normal level of 15 μg/100 ml to a peak value of 50–75 μg/100 ml within 6–12 hours.[48, 108, 118] To produce this rise, the

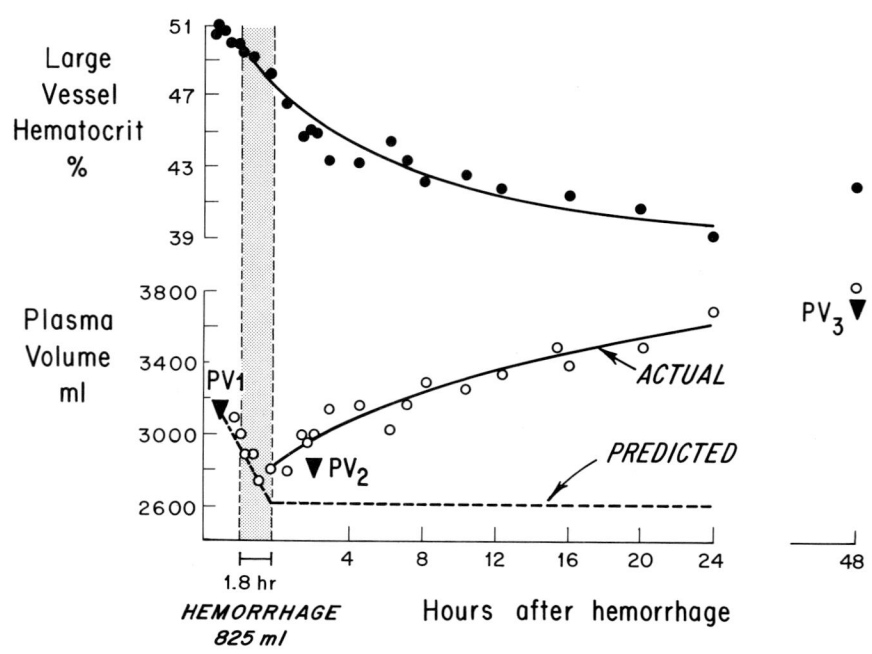

Fig. 3-3.—Large vessel hematocrit and plasma volume changes following 825-ml hemorrhage. Dashed line represents predicted plasma volume in absence of compensatory transcapillary filling. Open circles are plasma volumes, PV, calculated from hematocrit, Hct, assuming constancy of red cell mass, RCM, according to the relationship

$$PV = RCM \left(\frac{1}{Hct} - 1\right)$$

PV_1, PV_2 and PV_3 are determinations of plasma volume by independent tracer dilution methods.

concentration of cortisol in adrenal vein blood may increase tenfold.[66] The urinary excretion is elevated for a longer period, indicating continuing hypersecretion by the adrenal cortex, but the concentration in the serum returns in many instances to normal within 48 hours, well before many of the metabolic changes to be described have taken place. Emotion, pain, anxiety and alterations in pH and temperature are effective stimuli for cortisol secretion.[20, 40, 44, 62, 108] Although stimulation of the adrenal cortex directly by efferent nerves and other humoral substances is possible, adrenocorticotropic hormone (ACTH) is the common mediator. The amount of cortisol secreted varies with the extent of trauma and also with the development of complications in the post-injury or postsurgical period.[22, 44, 48, 108] Common anesthetic agents, however, do not increase cortisol excretion in the urine when given apart from operation. Spinal anesthesia has been observed to delay the onset of cortisol secretion until anesthesia has subsided, suggesting that sensory nerves, or possibly other afferent nerves, are required for the normal, prompt response.[58, 90]

Some of these interrelations are clearly seen in Figure 3-4, adapted from Hume et al.[66] Operations of intermediate severity were performed in 3 patients, of whom 2 were paraplegics with sensory deficits below T12 and T4. The top chart shows the normal secretory response of 17-hy-

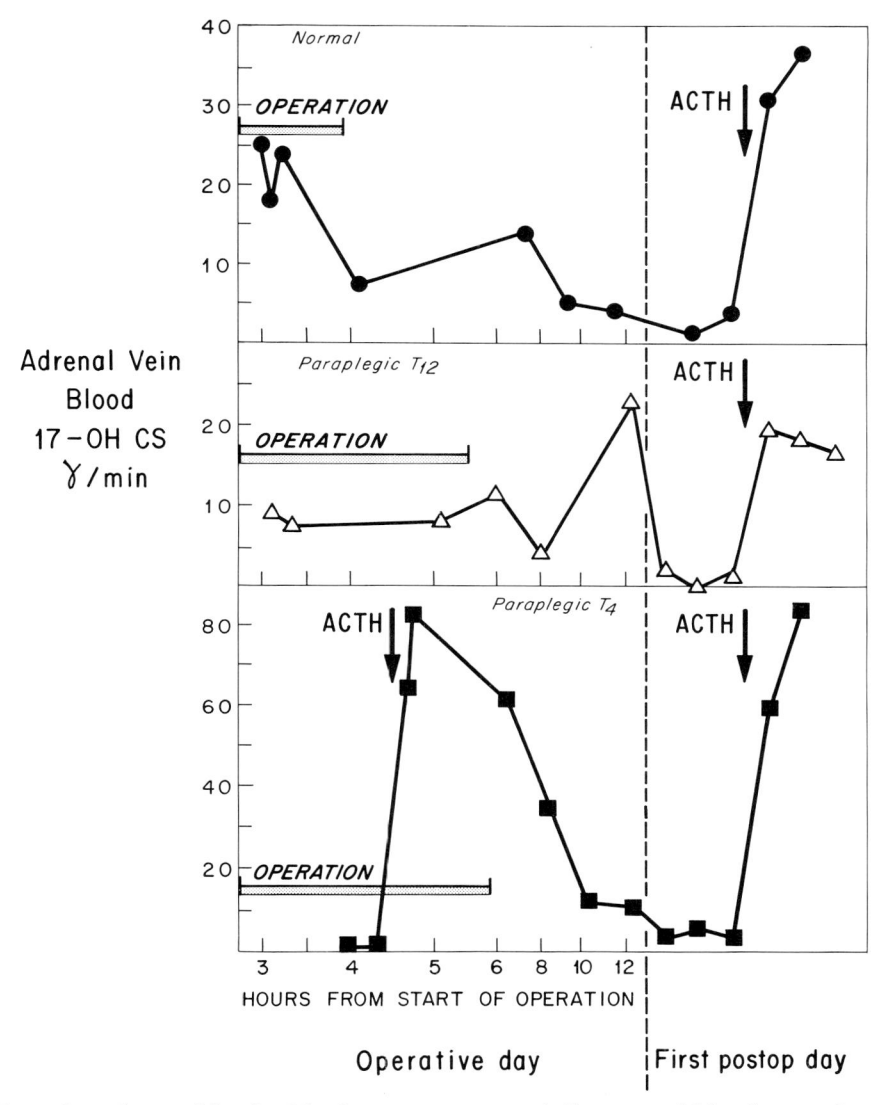

Fig. 3-4.—Adrenal vein blood 17-hydroxycorticosteroid (fraction of blood steroids including cortisol and certain congeners) secretion rates in nonparalyzed and paraplegic patients in relation to operation and ACTH administration.

droxycorticosteroids (including cortisol), with a rise of 24 μg/min. The first paraplegic patient had a muted response during the operation but a normal response postoperatively. The second paraplegic, with the sensory loss at a higher level, had no response during the operation until given ACTH. On the first postoperative day, all patients responded to ACTH, establishing that the adrenal glands were responsive, although operative stress could not stimulate the glands in the 2 patients with lesions of the spinal cord.

Cortisol facilitates gluconeogenesis, in which glucose is produced from protein. During fasting, this sustains an adequate level of blood glucose, which serves as the chief substrate for the energy metabolism of the central nervous system. Cortisol also facilitates the mobilization and degradation of protein, mainly from skeletal muscle, possibly to provide essential amino acids for protein synthesis by the liver or by the injured tissues during repair. Other known actions of cortisol, such as effects on fat metabolism, capillary permeability, muscle function, the psyche and lymphoid tissues, may be enhanced by the increased secretion of this hormone, but the evidence is, in general, against a direct effect simply proportional to the level of cortisol secretion. A conditioning or permissive role of cortisol governing certain responses, as originally defined by Ingle et al.,[68] is more consistent with recent evidence summarized by Cuthbertson.[26]

1. The time of maximal levels of steroids in the plasma within 48 hours is earlier than the time of maximal loss of nitrogen in the urine occurring between 2 and 6 days postinjury. The variable interval following different types of trauma between these maxima and the lack of correlation between total urinary corticosteroids and nitrogen excretion argue against a catabolic response proportional to *increased* production of corticosteroids.

2. The net loss of nitrogen after trauma is significantly decreased by prior protein depletion in man and animals. However, since the increased levels of corticosteroids in the plasma are not altered by this protein depletion, the nitrogen losses under these circumstances also do not appear to be directly related to increase in adrenal secretion.

3. Adrenalectomized animals surviving on sodium chloride therapy have no catabolic response after injury and adrenalectomized animals maintained on *constant* doses of steroids have a normal response. Observations on adrenalectomized patients undergoing surgical procedures and also on patients undergoing adrenalectomy, who are maintained on *constant* doses of steroid therapy, confirm that *increased* exogenous steroids are not required to permit responses after trauma identical to those seen in individuals with intact adrenal function.[70, 86, 103]

The above facts, consistent with an essentially normal catabolic response occurring after trauma in subjects surviving solely on constant exogenous steroid therapy, do not, however, establish that corticosteroid levels in the plasma are unaltered. As with aldosterone, the balance of production, excretion, utilization and destruction or inactivation in the liver must be considered jointly. Liver function may be impaired by trauma and related events, since arterial hypoxemia with contents in the range of 6–9 ml/100 ml or circulatory insufficiency causes centrilobular liver cell necrosis, a release of hepatic enzymes including glutamic oxalocetic and pyruvic transaminases and reduced excretion indicated by elevation of serum bilirubin and alkaline phosphatase.[74, 102] Also, operative stress has been shown to decrease hepatic conjugation of steroids, perhaps related to transient hypoxia or hepatic circulatory insufficiency, and this decrease is roughly correlated with a reduction in Bromsulphalein clearance.[125] A related phenomenon has been observed in the immediate postoperative period, in which the increase in plasma cortisol levels following a test dose of 50 mg intravenously was noted in 3 of 5 patients to be greater than in control observations made prior to operation.[108] Also, ACTH proved to be more potent in raising plasma cortisol in the postoperative period, and major surgery resulted in higher plasma cortisol levels than can be attained by ACTH therapy in the preoperative period.[118] An example, adapted from Moore,[90] is displayed in Figure 3-5. Thus, in addition to production, excretion and destruction of adrenocorticosteroids there are significant variables in any formulation covering the function of these hormones. Since little is understood concerning cellular

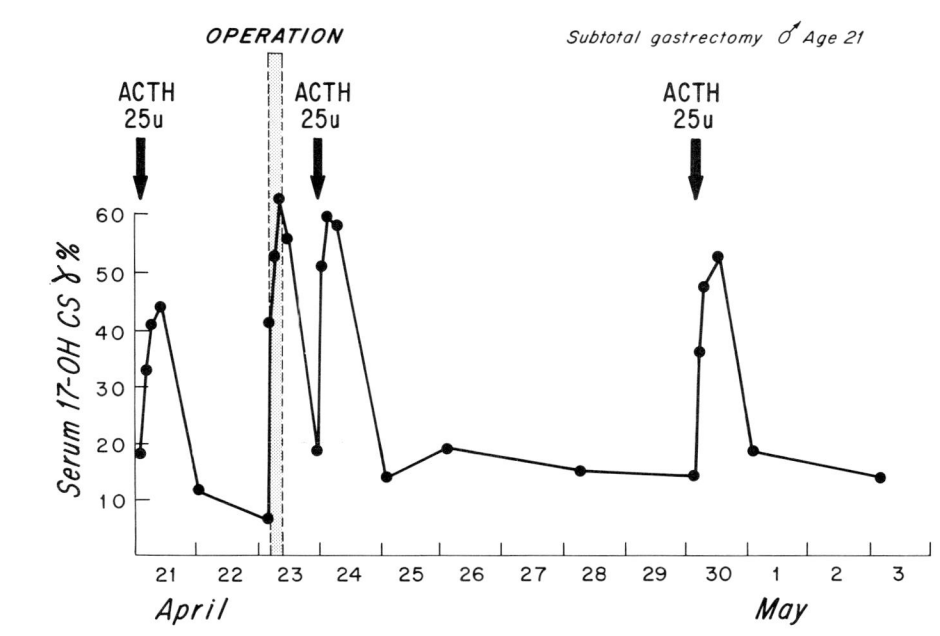

Fig. 3-5.—Serum 17-hydroxycorticosteroids (fraction of blood steroids including cortisol and certain congeners) in response to ACTH preoperatively and postoperatively and in response to operation.

mechanisms of utilization, unraveling the action at the cellular level will be a major advance.

Clinical corollary: The possibility of an inadequate or absent response of the adrenal glands to stress exists whenever a patient has been on steroid therapy within 6 months prior to trauma, has a neurologic lesion interrupting normal afferent pathways from the injured area or has had adrenal gland disease or surgery. In these circumstances, to prevent adrenal insufficiency, which could be fatal, 200 mg of cortisol (hydrocortisone) is given intravenously as soon as possible after the injury or immediately preoperatively when an elective procedure is planned. The postoperative steroid therapy is adjusted for each patient, continuing parenteral or oral therapy every 6 hours with due consideration being given to subsequent complications, which demand continuing high doses. In the absence of complications, the total daily dose is reduced stepwise to 10–20 mg of prednisone orally, or prednisolone parenterally, within the first 5 days following an isolated stress. Prednisone and prednisolone have a sodium-retaining effect, but if hyponatremia develops secondary to natriuresis and not secondary to inadequate intake, 10 mg of desoxycorticosterone acetate intramuscularly may be added every 6 hours as required.

CARBOHYDRATE METABOLISM.—Hyperglycemia and, occasionally, glycosuria occur after trauma and persist for a few days unless complications prolong the original stress. A diabetic type of response in a glucose tolerance test and diminished sensitivity to a test dose of insulin are common following severe fractures.[64, 106] These changes in carbohydrate metabolism are proportional to the injury and are ascribed to the action of cortisol stimulating gluconeogenesis and of catecholamines inhibiting secretion of insulin. As a rule, these transient changes in carbohydrate metabolism require no specific therapy, but they are part of the superbly designed response to trauma that safeguards a supply of glucose for nerve tissue and enhances the utilization of fat as the chief source of energy in the body as a whole.

The intravenous infusion of epinephrine in humans at a rate of 6 μ/min suppresses insulin secretion while causing a sustained hyperglycemia in the range of 200–300 mg/100 ml.[101] This rate of administration is approximately 20 times the basal secretory rate of epinephrine in man and far less than the secretory rate during stress or the rate of administration for a maximal pressor effect on the circulation. Since insulin is not required for the utilization of glucose by the central nervous system but is required for its peripheral utilization by heart, kidney cortex and skeletal muscle, the action of epinephrine is remarkably suited to support blood glucose, which is the specific energy substrate essential for the central nervous system in acute fasting.[13] The conversion of glycogen to glucose is also enhanced by catecholamines, but this is a minor source of energy, since stores of muscle and liver glycogen total about 150 and 75 gm respectively in normal adult man. Contrariwise, gluconeogenesis from protein sources taps a large caloric reserve equivalent to 24,000 Cal in a normal adult. Not all these calories are available, since conversion into glucose catabolizes lean tissue, and when one-third to one-half of the lean tissue mass is lost in this process, a profound cachexia ensues, with the loss of ventilatory ability and the consequent development of sepsis in the vulnerable lower respiratory tract. As noted above, cortisol facilitates this process occurring in the liver, where glucogenic amino acids, particularly alanine, are converted into glucose. This energy-requiring process oxidizes fatty acids as a fuel and is accompanied by the discharge into the blood of acetoacetate and β-hydroxybutyrate. These keto acids appearing in blood and urine are part of the ketosis of fasting, which, in most circumstances, develops simultaneously with gluconeogenesis and produces a metabolic acidosis. Other aspects of glucose metabolism are considered in the sections on hypoxia and on energy requirements and expenditures.

FAT METABOLISM. – The normal serum nonesterified fatty acid or free fatty acid (FFA) level of 0.3–0.6 mEq/L is increased following trauma to 1.5–2.0 mEq/L. Insulin (0.1 U/kg) causes an abrupt fall and epinephrine (0.5 mg) an abrupt rise in FFA levels.[34] The calorigenic action of catecholamines is causally related to this mobilization of fatty acids.[120] The serum free fatty acids, due to utilization in tissues and due to rapid exchange with acids in the fat depots, have a half-life in the serum of about 2 minutes, which is indicative of the dynamic state of this major energy source. Mobilization of depot fat by epinephrine occurs in less than 10 minutes, and the response provides all tissues with their principal supply of energy except for the glycolytic tissues, such as nerve, erythrocytes, leukocytes, kidney medulla and bone marrow.[60, 119, 128] Cortisol exerts a permissive influence on this mobilization.[119] In summary, the preceding section and this one indicate that the mobilization of fat and suppression of insulin are controlled by the catecholamines, which joint action favors fat over carbohydrate as a fuel source for the majority of tissues.

During convalescence, the amount of fat mobilized and oxidized depends on the net balance between the caloric needs of the body and the available exogenous and endogenous sources of energy other than body fat. Where calories from oral or intravenous feedings and from protein or carbohydrate stores are sufficient, the demand on fat depots disappears. On the other hand, when a patient contends with the tremendous energy requirements associated with septic fevers and complications or with the evaporation of liters of water from the body's surface, as occurs in extensively burned patients, substantial amounts of fat are oxidized. Oxidation of 600 gm of fat per day in a patient with generalized septic peritonitis has been reported providing more than 5,000 Cal of energy.[91] The mobilization of fat during a prolonged convalescence generally exceeds the catabolism of protein, so that the decrease in body weight fortunately is not a balanced loss of all tissues but represents proportionately a greater loss of fat.

SERUM PROTEINS. — An acute response potentially of great clinical significance is the changes in concentration of serum proteins following trauma. Present data are merely descriptive, but helpful correlations with clinical conditions undoubtedly will be made. Serum albumin decreases about 20%, reaching a minimum between 4 and 10 days, and serum fibrinogen increases twofold or more, reaching a maximum between 5 and 18 days following trauma.[23, 98, 131] Proteins altered immediately after trauma are collectively designated "acute phase reactive proteins," and they do not include most of the gamma globulins, which rise later after injury and commonly in relation to septic complications.

Experimental studies of protein turnover show that ^{14}C-labeled glycine is incorporated in newly synthesized serum glycoprotein by the liver at an accelerated rate within hours of injury.[19] Two independent studies[95, 121] confirm that the half-life of serum albumin after operations of intermediate extent is reduced about 30% due to the loss of albumin in the operative area. The normal ratio of extravascular to intravascular albumin mass is approximately 1.0, and the sequestration of albumin-rich fluid at a fracture site increases the ratio to values of 1.3–2.7. In severe burns, the ratio may rise to 3.6.[30] In humans, albumin has a normal turnover rate of about 0.2 gm/kg/day or 5% of the total albumin pool per day, equivalent to the synthesis of 14 gm/day in 70 kg min. The effects of trauma, such as those associated with gastrectomy or bilateral adrenalectomy, double this turnover rate, revealing the hepatic potential of synthesizing more than 30 gm of albumin per day.[6, 30] The turnover of gamma globulins is also increased following major fractures, even in the absence of infection.[31]

COAGULATION OF BLOOD. — Tendencies to hemorrhage and also to thrombosis occur following trauma. The interpretation in individual cases is complicated by pre-existing disease, such as cirrhosis of the liver, by the effects of multiple transfusions and by the functional failure of organs during cardiovascular insufficiency that normally maintain the coagulation mechanism.[107] Changes in the coagulability of the blood following trauma often appear biphasic, with an initial shortening of the conventional bleeding time and an increase in platelet concentration. This phase, obviously of value in controlling hemorrhage, rarely causes complications unless accompanied by cardiovascular collapse and poor tissue perfusion. These may usher in a second phase dominated by disseminated intravascular coagulation, thought to occur throughout the vascular tree and causing obstruction of the microcirculation and exhaustion of the finite supply of clotting factors. This phenomenon, a consumption coagulopathy, has been investigated intensively.[7, 8, 59, 87, 99]

Simmons and associates[112] measured prothrombin time, partial thromboplastin time, recalcification time, platelet count, fibrinogen and fibrinolysin in 240 severely injured combat casualties seen within 1–2 hours following wounding. The only therapy received prior to the above determinations was morphine and surgical dressing. In comparison with control values, the means of these determinations were not changed significantly, but the variance was significantly greater, indicating that the tendency to hypercoagulation and hypocoagulation was present shortly after injury in this group of soldiers. An even greater range would be expected in injured civilians, with age and pre-existing liver disease adding further variability. The soldiers studied did not, in a single instance, have clinical evidence of a hemorrhagic diathesis at the time of the initial examination, but the changes in clotting factors predisposing to hemorrhage in some soldiers were interpreted as laboratory evidence for the early stages of disseminated intravascular coagulation. Subsequently, a few developed a hemorrhagic diathesis as the pathologic intravascular coagulation depleted the clotting factors and as multiple transfusions attenuated the clotting mechanism further, as described below in the section on transfusions. The severity of cardiovascular insufficiency was roughly quantitated by grouping the soldiers on the basis of pH, serum lactic acid and blood pressure. Of the clotting factors measured, only the increases in prothrombin time and partial thromboplastin time could be correlated with the severity of shock, and it is possible that cessation of hepatic production of factors V and VII, which are characterized by half-lives of a few hours, may be responsible. An important clinical indication for platelet transfusions prior to debridement emerged from the study, since soldiers with platelet counts of less than 120,000 per mm³ generally had excessive bleeding if an extensive debridement was attempted. All those receiving multiple transfusions tended to converge on common values in the clotting studies performed (e.g., four banked blood transfusions generally resulted in a platelet count of 100,000 and rarely less than 75,000 per mm³) and, therefore, the infrequent appearance of a hemorrhagic diathesis after multiple transfusions could not be correlated with the test results. The diathesis presumably represented abnormalities peculiar to an individual yet to be recognized by suitable tests. Since an incompatible transfusion may cause generalized bleeding in an injured part or an operative field, the possibility of a transfusion reaction being responsible always must be considered. In general, the tendency to hemorrhage occurs in the first few days after trauma, and intravascular thrombosis leading to pulmonary embolism is a later complication of disordered blood coagulation compounded by immobilization of the patient.

Clinical corollary: In patients with a history of prolonged or severe cardiovascular insufficiency following trauma, clotting factors must be checked prior to an operation and deficiencies treated by fresh whole blood transfusions, platelet transfusions or specific clotting factors, as available. In each patient after injury or operation it is mandatory to exclude the possibility of continuing hemorrhage from vessels that can be controlled only by direct surgery. In this circumstance, the procrastination occasioned by attempts to adjust the clotting factors could lead to fatality.

VARIATIONS DUE TO COMPLICATIONS OR TO THERAPY

HYPOXIA.—The pathogenesis of hypoxia during cardiovascular insufficiency following trauma has received new attention with recent experiences in Vietnam. Pulmonary congestion and insufficiency in the absence of trauma to the lungs have been observed repeatedly in severely injured casualties.[41, 84, 85, 113, 114, 129] Examples and instructive interpretations of the pulmonary disability are available for reference.[3, 54] Cardiac output is affected adversely by reduced oxygenation of the blood at a critical moment after trauma, when intrapulmonary shunting of blood often is rising due to a progressive atelectasis. This frequently is a consequence of inadequate ventilation secondary to pain, sedation, anesthesia, reduced compliance of chest wall or lung, pulmonary edema, oxygen therapy, abdominal distention and elevated diaphragm. Since, in the presence of intrapulmonary shunting, systemic arterial oxygen content is dependent on cardiac output as well as on the size of the intrapulmonary shunt, a progressive spiral of cardiac insufficiency may develop, with declining arterial oxygen contents (and oxygen tensions) in turn further depressing myocardial function. A theoretic treatment for this important aspect of hypoxia has been developed.[75]*

The degree of hypoxia in the tissues is difficult to assess during cardiopulmonary insufficiency because no convenient measure of it exists. It is not directly related to arterial or venous oxygen tension, saturation or content. Consumption of oxygen by a particular tissue is determined by blood flow, hemoglobin concentration in the blood and the arteriovenous (A-V) saturation difference of the tissue as expressed in the following equation:

$$\text{Oxygen consumption} = \dot{Q}t \times \text{Hgb} \times (S_A - S_V) \times 1.34 \times 10^{-4} \text{ tissue in ml per min}$$

where $\dot{Q}t$ equals tissue blood flow in ml per min, Hgb equals concentration of hemoglobin in gm/100 ml binding 1.34 ml oxygen per gm, S_A equals per cent saturation of hemoglobin in arterial blood, S_V equals per cent saturation of mixed venous blood from tissue and where the trivial contribution of oxygen carried in solution at normal oxygen tensions is ignored. Although systemic artery oxygen tensions are helpful in following pulmonary function because of their sensitivity to intrapulmonary shunting, they do not measure the factors in the equation relevant to oxygen consumption by the tissues throughout the body. However, oxygen tensions are informative in estimating S_A, as, for example, the per cent saturation of normal hemoglobin is greater than 90 when the oxygen tension is 70 mm Hg or higher. At the bedside, in addition to a hemoglobin determination and an estimate of S_A by arterial oxygen tensions or by noting the presence and severity of cyanosis, tissue perfusion ($\dot{Q}t$) is evaluated by clinical criteria to permit an opinion as to the degree of hypoxia, if any. Although tissue perfusion is intuitively evaluated by considering vital signs, the peripheral circulation, urine volume and state of consciousness among other prognostics, serial cardiac outputs provide for the critically ill patient a much-needed quantitative measure.*

Figure 3-6, adapted from Smith, illustrates the relationship between cardiac output, maximal oxygen capacity of blood and maximal oxygen available to the tissues (equivalent to the oxygen content of venous blood being negligible) as the hematocrit varies.[116] One curve shows the fall in cardiac output as the viscosity of the blood increases with rising hematocrit. A second shows the rise in maximal oxygen capacity of the arterial blood as the hemoglobin content increases with rising hematocrit. The product of these two functions yields the third curve depicting the maximal oxygen available from arterial blood reaching a maximum when the hematocrit is about 40%. This figure emphasizes the critical role of a

---

*Decrease in oxygen content of arterial blood =

$$\frac{\dot{V}O_2}{(\dot{Q}_T - \dot{Q}_S)} \times \frac{\dot{Q}s}{\dot{Q}_T} \times 100$$

due to intrapulmonary shunting in ml per cent. Where $\dot{V}O_2$ is oxygen consumption in ml per min, $\dot{Q}s$ blood flow in shunt in ml per min and $\dot{Q}_T$ cardiac output in ml per min. $\dot{Q}_T$ is the most important physiologic variable affecting oxygen content and tension in arterial blood in the presence of a relatively fixed shunt.

*Repeated cardiac outputs are determined by indicator dilution methods where a bolus of indicator of known mass, m (dye or radioisotopically labeled substance), is injected into a central vein. The rise and fall over time of the concentration of the indicator, C(t), is measured for less than a minute in samples of blood drawn from a peripheral artery. Ignoring a correction for the effects of recirculation of the indicator cardiac output, C.O., is computed from the relation:

$$\text{C.O} = \frac{m}{\int C(t)\, dt}$$

In practice, a correction for the effects of recirculation is made by a simple graphic method.

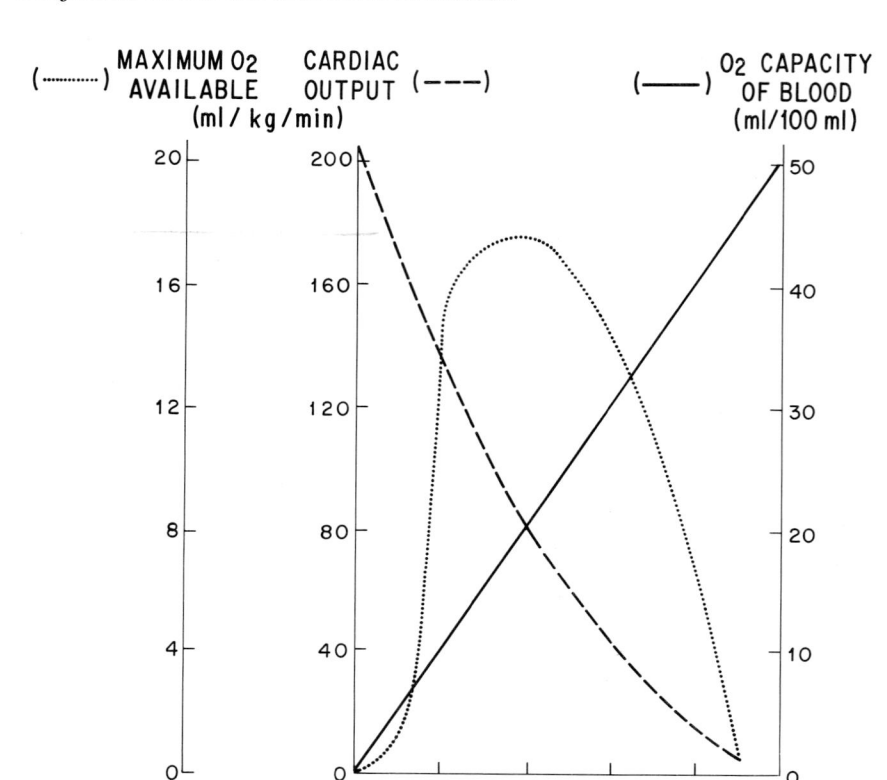

Fig. 3-6.—Availability of oxygen to tissues in relation to cardiac output and hematocrit.

normal hematocrit for optimal oxygen transport. From this figure and the above equation it may be appreciated that, in addition to adequate ventilation, a cardiac output and hematocrit approaching normal are essential for correcting hypoxia.

In tissues receiving oxygen in normal amounts, glucose, fatty acids and amino acids are oxidized to provide energy by the stepwise formation of high-energy phosphate bonds in a series of oxidation reductions under enzymatic control. In the absence of adequate amounts of oxygen, the chain of respiratory enzymes cannot remove the hydrogen atoms or electrons generated by the Krebs or citric acid cycle and their contribution to the energy needs of the cells is sharply limited. The decreasing operation of the Krebs cycle results in pyruvate accumulating in the cells, threatening, in turn, the remaining source of energy derived from the Embden-Meyerhof pathway of glucose oxidation, which also generates pyruvate. The anaerobic removal of pyruvate by reduction to lactate is the metabolic adjustment that permits continued, but inefficient, cell respiration, utilizing glucose as an energy source. Nicotinamide adenine dinucleotide, normally oxidized by the respiratory enzymes, is oxidized in the conversion of pyruvate to lactate, and this latter normal metabolite accumulating in pathologic amounts causes a metabolic acidosis, to be discussed, commonly seen in cardiovascular collapse.[65] Mortality rates following trauma and hemorrhagic shock are correlated with lactic acid elevations.[9, 100] Elevations of lactic acid resulting from hemorrhagic shock in man greater than 6 mEq/L (about 50 mg/100 ml) have been associated with a 50% mortality, and when lactic acid exceeds 14 mEq/L (about 120 mg/100 ml), the mortality approaches 100%.[37]

ACID-BASE DISORDERS.—These complications, although well defined by the usual determinations of arterial blood pH, PCO_2 and bicarbonate, may be confusing, because alterations in acid-base balance invariably are an accompanying manifestation of one or more primary disorders. These must be recognized to identify the etiology of a particular alteration and to design appropriate therapy. Acid-base disorders can be divided into those characterized by a pathologic accumulation or loss of carbonic acid from the body and the remainder characterized by an accumulation or loss of all other anions or cations. The former are named respiratory disturbances because of the control of carbonic acid concentration in the body exerted by pulmonary function. The lungs, responsible for the excretion of about 15,000 mEq of carbonic acid per day, cause a profound acidosis or alkalosis by decreasing or increasing this excretory rate by 2 or 3%. The latter are named metabolic disturbances, connoting a number of sources and excretory pathways for acids and bases.

Acidosis is the most common disorder in acid-base balance seen early in the severely injured. First, lactic acid accumulates because of poor tissue perfusion, hypoxia and anaerobic metabolism, as described above in the section on hypoxia. Second, bank blood preserved with an acid-citrate-dextrose solution (ACD blood) initially produces an acidosis, as noted in the discussion on transfusions below. Third, acidosis is promoted by the accumulation of carbonic acid in the body due to inadequate ventilation. Although the early acid-base disorders frequently represent this mixture of metabolic acidosis and respiratory acidosis, a patient may develop respiratory alkalosis secondary to hyperventilation stimulated by pain, anxiety and chronic hypoxia. This hypoxia, compensatory hyperventilation and associated moderate respiratory alkalosis are familiar early signs of impending respiratory insufficiency, requiring assisted ventilation with oxygen for treatment.

A metabolic alkalosis may develop insidiously after 18–36 hours following trauma by several mechanisms.[83] First, the gradual oxidation of sodium citrate received with ACD blood transfusions causes alkalosis following the initial acidosis mentioned above. Second, nasogastric suction for treatment of abdominal trauma, paralytic ileus and persistent nausea and vomiting cause a preferential loss of hydrogen and chloride ions. Third, normal compensatory renal mechanisms frequently are impaired because of poor perfusion, prior disease and limited excretion of sodium due to the persistent effects of ADH and aldosterone.

The above acid-base disorders lead to compensatory responses in the buffer systems of the body and in pulmonary and renal function, but these may not suffice to restore the pH to normal. Experimental acidosis in animals with a serum pH less than 6.8 has been associated with cardiac dysfunction and impaired inotropic response to norepinephrine and with changes in pulmonary artery pressure and resistance.[35] Clinical studies confirm that minimal alterations occur in cardiac output and in response to epinephrine when the serum pH is greater than 6.9, but a progressive increase in pulmonary blood pressure has been striking at lower pH values.[2] Earlier work established that, in some patients, severe acidosis depresses responses to pressor agents[17] and leads to heart block and cardiac arrest if not treated promptly with sodium bicarbonate.[122, 123] Also, in experimental acidosis, the mobilization of FFA caused by norepinephrine is depressed, and the available oxidizable substrates for tissue energy requirements likewise are decreased.[97]

With extremes in acidosis and alkalosis there is a concomitant shift in the oxyhemoglobin dissociation curve. Acidosis diminishes the affinity of hemoglobin for oxygen, i.e., a shift in the curve to the right, and this interferes with normal saturation of blood in the pulmonary capillaries unless the patient is breathing oxygen-enriched air. However, with a low pH, at any given tissue oxygen tension, proportionately more oxygen will be released from the hemoglobin molecule if the per cent saturation achieved in the lungs is normal. Since the undesirable effects of a shift to the right may be compensated by oxygen therapy, such a shift need not be a serious disadvantage to the patient. Contrariwise, a shift to the left seen with alkalosis results in a tighter binding of the oxygen by hemoglobin, and the only available compensatory mechanisms to maintain oxygen transport are the reduction of tissue oxygen tensions, thus increasing the A-V difference, an increase in cardiac output or an elevation in circulating hemoglobin to abnormal levels by transfusion. The fact that each of these mechanisms has obvious disadvantages explains the urgency of correcting an alkalosis. Temporary relief may be obtained by 100% oxygen therapy, which, by increasing the oxygen in solution in the blood, may contribute 25–30% of the total oxygen transport required. The depletion of the normal erythrocyte component, 2,3-diphosphoglycerate (2,3-DPG), in bank blood, described below, and the state of hypothermia also shift the oxyhemoglobin dissociation curve to the left, acting in a synergistic manner with alkalosis.

Clinical corollary: The lactic acidosis of cardiovascular insufficiency accompanied by cardiac arrhythmias and arrest is an emergency requiring, in addition to other supportive measures, immediate sodium bicarbonate therapy, 100–200 mEq intravenously over a 5–15-minute period and repeated as required to raise serum pH to the 7.30–7.45 range. Other types of metabolic acidosis are corrected gradually, guided by frequent monitoring of pH, serum bicarbonate and arterial PCO_2.

Most types of metabolic alkaloses respond to 150–300 mEq of sodium chloride intravenously, provided that renal function is capable of responding by a natriuresis. In the presence of good hepatic function, 75–150 mEq of ammonium chloride intravenously may be prescribed for an intractable alkalosis. In the presence of acute renal failure, peritoneal dialysis or hemodialysis will be required until life-sustaining renal function returns.

Respiratory acidosis as part of deteriorating pulmonary function with arterial PCO_2 greater than 60 mm Hg requires positive-pressure ventilation by cuffed endotracheal or tracheostomy tube to improve ventilation and pulmonary excretion of carbonic acid.

MULTIPLE BLOOD TRANSFUSIONS.—The effects of more than four to six 500-ml blood transfusions include an initial metabolic acidosis, a tendency to lower ionized blood calcium, depression of the coagulation mechanism chiefly due to thrombocytopenia, hyperkalemia and, as we have seen, a late metabolic alkalosis. An immediate effect is the microembolization, to a greater or lesser degree, of the pulmonary capillary circulation by aggregates of platelets and leukocytes observed in some patients.[69] The initial acidosis is a direct consequence of ACD bank blood having a pH between 6 and 7 due to the citric acid added for optimal preservation.[11, 82] Since sodium citrate is also added to buffer the pH in this range, the ultimate oxidation of the citrate favors a metabolic alkalosis. About 17 mEq of sodium citrate are in each unit of ACD bank blood. Eight or ten units provide 136–170 mEq of sodium, an amount sufficient to cause a moderate metabolic alkalosis, particularly in the presence of impaired renal function.[82] Because of the limited viability of platelets in bank blood, the absence of reserve platelet stores in the patient and the slow rate of thrombocytopoiesis, platelet depletion is the most common cause of defective coagulation occasioned by multiple transfusions. To a lesser degree, the coagulation mechanism is altered by the absence in bank blood of certain labile components, factor V (Ac-globulin) and factor VIII (antihemophilic factor) in particular.[53] Binding ionized calcium in the patient's blood by excess citrate in ACD bank blood usually is not a problem, since there are sufficient reserves in the extracellular fluid and skeleton. However, when the circulation is sluggish and the exchange with extracellular fluid is poor, it may be prudent to give 1 gm of calcium gluconate intravenously every second or third transfusion and ensure that every third or fourth transfusion is given no more than a few hours after its collection.[11, 53] This is a necessary precaution, particularly in patients with associated liver disease.

After a few days of storage, bank blood has a significant depletion of 2,3-DPG, and this causes hemoglobin to bind oxygen more firmly, creating a serious impediment to oxygen transport.[4, 5] In clinical aseptic shock, 2,3-DPG in the erythrocytes may be half normal, and experimentally it has been shown that reductions in 2,3-DPG are associated with diminished oxygen consumption and cardiovascular collapse even when blood volume and hemoglobin concentrations are maintained near normal values.[88] The oxygen tension at which 50% of erythrocyte hemoglobin is saturated normally is 25 mm Hg. In critical depletions of 2,3-DPG, this may be 15 mm Hg or less.

Clinical corollary: Freshly collected whole blood transfusion is the most widely applicable therapy for the hemorrhagic diathesis associated with multiple transfusions. Providing freshly collected blood for every fourth transfusion, when 10 or more may be required, has prophylactic value against deterioration of the clotting mechanism.

When a patient has received multiple transfusions of bank blood or is contending with advanced sepsis, impaired oxygen transport due to a deficiency of 2,3-DPG may exist. The oxygen tension at which 50% of the erythrocyte hemoglobin is saturated should be determined. A value in the range of 15–20 mm Hg or less is treated by exchange transfusions of freshly collected whole blood or frozen blood, which preserves erythrocyte 2,3-DPG.

TRAUMATIZED MUSCLE.—Trauma and ischemia of soft tissues, principally skeletal muscle, lead to increased permeability of the cell membrane and to the release of potassium, enzymes and myoglobin from within cells. Quantitation of muscle destruction by measuring the serum concentration of released intracellular enzymes is in a primitive stage, although the evaluation of myocardial infarction by serial serum enzyme determinations already has been useful. Myokinase and creatine phosphokinase probably are the most representative enzymes for skeletal muscle destruction.[124, 127] Contusion of muscle elevates serum creatine phosphokinase levels whereas a surgical incision across muscle does not. The escape of potassium from injured cells raises this ion in the extracellular space. Because of the normal concentration of potassium within the cells of 150 mEq/L and outside the cells of 4 mEq/L, only a very modest change in cell membrane permeability may elevate the extracellular potassium to 7 or 8 mEq/L, at which level cardiac irregularities appear. The normal, impressive capacity of the kidney to excrete excess potassium after trauma may be limited because of inadequate renal perfusion or pre-existing renal disease.

Myoglobin released from damaged muscle may precipitate in renal tubules, but the well-recognized renal dysfunction that follows ischemia is secondary to the hypotension and marginal renal perfusion that often complicate severe injuries. This striking clinical entity probably would be better termed "renal ischemic syndrome" rather than "acute tubular necrosis," as it is, since all renal structures are concerned to a varying degree. It is characterized by a prompt and dramatic fall in urine volume and by a rapid rise in blood urea nitrogen products, often leading to all the manifestations of uremia. It was first described in association with extensive crushing injuries incurred during the bombing of London in World War II and was termed the "crush syndrome."[10, 12] Acute tubular necrosis is not prevented by amputation of a crushed extremity, however, since the renal disability is secondary to diminished renal perfusion initiated by the primary trauma and not, apparently, to any circulating toxic factors derived from injured tissues. It may vary in severity from a mild and transient period of renal insufficiency to severe and even irreversible renal failure. This "crush syndrome" renal failure should be suspected after extensive trauma in the presence of progressive oliguria and myoglobin in the urine or serum.

GASTROINTESTINAL ULCERATION.—The gastrointestinal tract may respond to stress and to injury in other parts of the body by the development of acute ulcerations. Epigastric distress, gnawing pain, interference with nutrition, hemorrhage and perforation caused by these ulcerations contribute significantly to post-trauma morbidity and mortality.[47, 51] Patients with severe burns appear to be somewhat more prone to gastrointestinal ulcerations than do those with other types of trauma. In a study of 291 autopsies on patients with fatal burns, 8.9% had duodenal ulcers and 14.4% had gastric ulcers.[110] When present, duodenal ulcers usually are single or, rarely, double, and gastric ulcers commonly are multiple, superficial erosions. The explanation for these gastrointestinal ulcerations is not known, but since ACTH and exogenous steroid medication can be associated with gastrointestinal ulcerations and increased loss of pepsin of gastric origin in the urine,[39, 55] the endogenous adrenal secretions are at least implicated as possibly contributing to this interesting and mysterious condition.

Clinical corollary: Throughout convalescence, presence of upper gastrointestinal symptoms and of positive stool guaiac tests should be checked to alert the responsible physician to potential gastrointestinal ulcerations. Ulcer diets and medications may be required and should be instituted on a prophylactic basis if the patient is receiving steroid therapy.

CONVALESCENCE

ENERGY REQUIREMENTS AND EXPENDITURES.—Altered energy requirements and expenditures associated with trauma and recovery have been investigated in patients by means of indirect calorimetry. By this technique, oxygen consumption is measured directly, and since the quantity of energy liberated in the body averages approximately 4.8 Cal per liter of oxygen, consumption of oxygen may be converted to a caloric equivalent. Oxygen consumption has been determined postoperatively at intervals following common surgical procedures, in large part gastrectomies.[79] Total consumption was determined by interpolation and there was no correlation between the temperature of the patient and the energy expenditure calculated from oxygen consumption. Elevations in temperature not associated with a commensurate increase in oxygen consumption were interpreted as the result of defective control of body temperature in the presence of normal or slightly elevated energy expenditures. Injury and surgical operations raise the basal metabolic rate (BMR) less than 20% for 5–10 days unless major septic complications develop, which may cause increases of 30–40%.[21, 77] It has been observed experimentally that 7% of the elevation in BMR may be accounted for by the additional oxygen required to degrade the protein necessary to provide the observed nitrogen losses in the feces and urine.[14] Calculations of data derived from patients establish that the nitrogen losses observed would require a similar elevation in the BMR of approximately 10%.[14, 76]

Under basal conditions, the heat of vaporization of insensible water loss from the surface of the body and lungs amounts to 30–35% of the total caloric expenditure. Major second-degree and third-degree burns commonly increase the BMR over 40% because of the energy required to evaporate water from burned and denuded areas, which has been estimated as ranging between 5 and 10 L per day.[15, 104] The heat of vaporization at skin temperatures is about 580 Cal/L, and for an insensible water loss of 3 L from the surface of the body, the total heat of vaporization would be 1,740 Cal. It is instructive to consider the additional physiologic burden caused by this obligatory caloric expenditure, which must be satisfied to avoid an intolerable decrease in body temperature. To estimate the oxygen required to produce this amount of heat, we assume that only carbohydrate and fat are being oxidized by a patient in a ratio of 2 to 3, corresponding to a respiratory quotient of 0.8 and also to a caloric equivalent of 4.8 Cal/L oxygen as determined by standard physiologic tables. In fact, protein and often more fat than assumed here are oxidized for energy, and such alterations would decrease the caloric equivalent of oxygen and increase the oxygen required. The oxygen equivalent of 1,740 Cal amounts of 363 L (1,740/4.8), and if this additional consumption of oxygen per day is distributed over all ventilations at a frequency of 20 per minute, 12.6 ml of extra oxygen will need to be transferred to the blood with each breath (363 × 10³/20 × 60 × 24). Since, at rest or at maximal exercise, the ratio of minute ventilatory volume to minute oxygen consumption is about 18, the ventilatory load per breath is augmented 227 ml (12.6 × 18). The oxygen consumption must be increased 252 ml/min (12.6 × 20), and, assuming a normal A-V oxygen content difference of 5 ml/100 ml of blood, cardiac output must increase 5 L/min or about threefold to transport the extra oxygen (252/5 × 10). This conservative estimate does not include the oxygen requirement for the additional ventilatory and cardiac work entailed, and it reveals the imposing extra demands on pulmonary and cardiac function inexorably following increased caloric expenditures for any cause.

The energy balance in a typical patient undergoing a major surgical procedure followed by 12 days of uncomplicated convalescence is displayed in Figure 3-7, adapted from Kinney.[76] The "calories in" from the day of operation through the seventh day are less than the "calories out," and the accumulated difference over the day of operation and through the first 7 postoperative days is 8,900 Cal. Calculations revealing the source of these calories are instructive. The horizontal dashed line indicates the caloric equivalent of endogenous *and* exogenous protein degraded per day. This averages 400 Cal per day or a total of 3,200 Cal from protein (8 × 400). The remaining 5,700 Cal over 8 days is derived largely from fat depots and, to a negligible extent, from limited reserves of glycogen. Because the total protein intake on days 3 through 7 is equivalent to 800 Cal, only 2,400 Cal are derived from body protoplasm (3,200 −800). The patient's weight, assuming no significant change in state of hydration, falls 3.63 kg, of which 3.0 kg represents loss of hydrated tissue protein (0.8 Cal per gm of hydrated tissue protein) and of which 0.63 kg represents loss of fat (9 Cal per gm of fat). In this example, the protein expended to produce an average of 400 Cal per day would result in 15 gm of nitrogen being excreted by the kidney per day (26.5 Cal per gm of urinary nitrogen). The contribution of 2,400 Cal from body protoplasm represents only 27% of the total caloric requirement over the 8 days (2,400 × 100/8,900). This characteristic limited caloric contribution of protein conserves

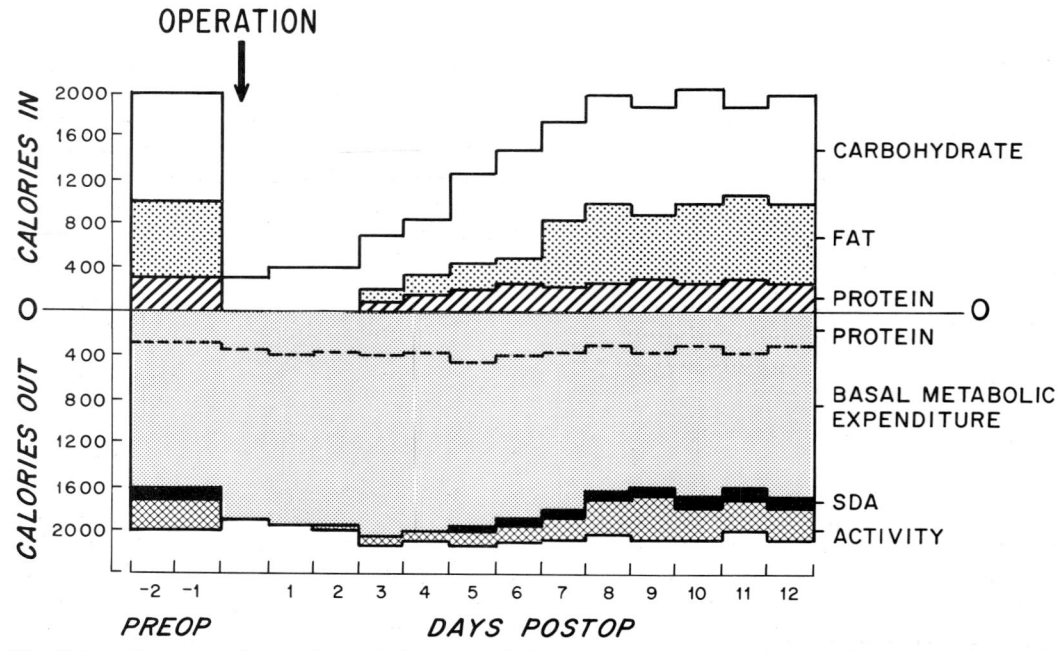

Fig. 3-7.—Energy balance in model patient following major surgical procedure. SDA (specific dynamic action) indicates calories required to oxidize endogenous and exogenous protein. Cross-hatched area designated as "activity" indicates calories expended for activity beyond those covering basal activity (cardiac muscle, ventilatory muscles, synthetic and other thermodynamic work of tissues, and heat production).

specialized and reactive tissues, notably a poor source of energy, and contradicts the often repeated concept that increased nitrogen excretion is an essential part of the adjustment, providing a major share of required calories during fasting.[38]

Clinical corollary: A warm environment and attention to minimizing energy losses occasioned by evaporation from weeping surfaces or from wet dressings conserves calorie stores in the patient and relieves the cardiorespiratory system of extra obligations for oxygen transport.

When a patient cannot take foods of sufficient caloric value orally, fat and protein depots make up the deficit of energy expenditure over intake. Over a few weeks, this loss of normal tissue is not a serious disadvantage unless nutrition prior to injury has been inadequate.

LEAN TISSUE.—The metabolic response of lean tissue to trauma has been studied extensively following the original investigations by Cuthbertson starting in 1928. In his studies, fractures in animals precipitated losses of nitrogen, phosphorus and sulfur in the urine, reaching a maximal value between the second and sixth days and gradually returning to normal over 1–2 months.[24] These excretions are reproducible and the ratios of the elements lost are consistent with their origin from skeletal muscle. The loss of nitrogen is a consequence of the mobilization of protein from lean tissue generally and not merely from the site of injury, but certain protein sources are spared. For example, part of the serum proteins and liver do not suffer net losses and, furthermore, the nutritional state prior to injury modifies the loss of nitrogen and associated minerals, since nutritionally depleted animals have a shorter and less severe period of negative balance.[28, 46, 96]

The relationship observed in man of

nitrogen excretion to the degree of trauma assigned a value of 1 to 10 on an arbitrary scale is displayed in Figure 3-8, adapted from Kinney.[78] This model chart has three upwardly concave lines representing the relation of maximal daily nitrogen excretion to magnitude of trauma in patients under three circumstances: depletion of protein stores prior to trauma, normal nutrition on zero nitrogen intake post-trauma and on 12 gm per day post-trauma. Figure 3-8 emphasizes the smaller losses following trauma sustained by depleted patients and also the increasing ineffectiveness of protein or nitrogen intake to cover obligatory losses as the extent of trauma increases. Note that the two upper curves are not parallel and that points at A, B and C are increasingly separated, demonstrating that less of the protein or nitrogen intake is being utilized as the magnitude of the trauma increases. Evidently, massive protein intake in the early days following trauma accomplishes little and has the certain disadvantage of increasing the excretory load for the kidney.

The maximal net loss of nitrogen per day in man occurs between the fourth and eighth days and may attain, following extensive trauma, a value of 10–30 gm, equivalent to 300–900 gm of hydrated, lean tissue.[25, 27] This rate of loss, if continued by the persistence of unresolved complications, can be tolerated for only a few weeks before serious secondary consequences, particularly intercurrent respiratory tract infections, start an inexorable downward spiral toward death. Following trauma in patients, the respiratory tract often proves to be their Achilles heel because, beyond a certain degree of muscle wasting, the capacity to ventilate and to protect the lungs from bacterial

Fig. 3-8.—Magnitude of trauma and maximal nitrogen excretion in depleted individuals and in normal individuals on 0 gm and 12 gm nitrogen intake per day. Shaded area represents normal range of nitrogen excretion by individual in balance on protein intake of 70 gm per day.

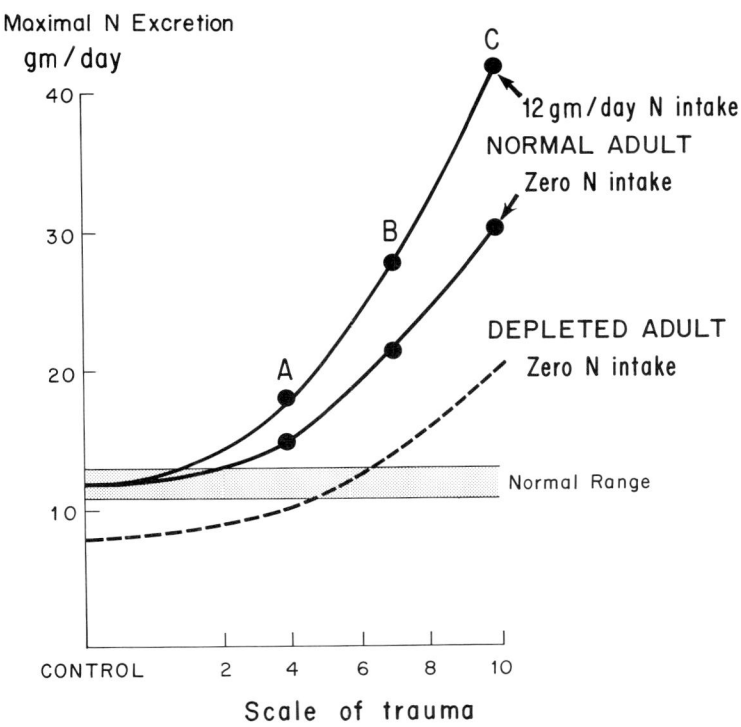

infection by vigorous coughing is reduced to a point at which disseminated pneumonia and irreversible pulmonary insufficiency exact their toll. Fortunately, following most severe trauma, the wasting of lean tissue subsides after the first week unless complications intervene. Wasting of lean tissue is accentuated by steroid medication, which evokes an artificial and continuing response unlike that occasioned by the normal, brief elevation of endogenous steroids. In patients with chronic disease, a trial of steroid therapy, 30 mg of prednisone or 150 mg of hydrocortisone per day, increased the degradation of serum albumin from 14 gm to 18 gm per day.[105] The anabolic rate was not increased proportionately, resulting in a net depletion of albumin stores. Larger doses have a more profound effect, and skeletal muscle also is affected adversely; however, detailed studies concerning dose relationships and other tissues are yet to be completed in man. Moore et al.[93] have published a compositional study of a patient who became "cushingoid" while receiving chronic ACTH medication. The patient had been given ACTH initially because of peritoneal adhesions and other complications following a sigmoid resection for rectal prolapse. ACTH had been continued for 9 weeks at the time of the compositional studies, and they provide disquieting evidence. In comparison to normal predicted values, the blood volume was increased 18%, the intracellular water and potassium were decreased 30–35%, the total body fat was increased 78% and extracellular sodium, chloride and water were unchanged. The preferential diminution of the intracellular phase, as indicated by the reduction in intracellular potassium and water, is attributed to the endogenous steroid secretion stimulated by ACTH and is consistent with muscle atrophy complicating chronic steroid medication.

IMMOBILIZATION. — Of particular interest to physicians treating fractures is the metabolic response to immobilization, which has been studied extensively in volunteers, quadriplegics with poliomyelitis and patients following trauma. Normal volunteers placed in plaster casts from the umbilicus to the toes sustained urinary losses of 14–18 gm per day of nitrogen in contrast to control subjects on the same diet, who lost 12 gm per day.[33] The nitrogen loss reached a maximum at about 10 days after immobilization and thus is later than that seen following fever or injury. Urinary calcium increased on the second or third day following casting and reached a maximum in the fifth week, with an average loss of 340 mg per day and a maximal loss of 590 mg per day. These observations have been confirmed and extended in a study of patients with extensive acute poliomyelitis resulting in quadriplegia.[132-134] Such patients have the response to an acute infection and to acute motor neuron paralysis added to that of immobilization. Urinary nitrogen losses peaked during the third week of illness in the range of 18–39 gm per day. The maximal negative nitrogen balance averaged 12 gm per day, equivalent to 360 gm of lean tissue. The maximal urinary calcium excretion averaged slightly more than 500 gm per day, with a total loss over 6 months of about 50 gm. This represents a negligible part of the total skeletal calcium, amounting to about 1.2 kg in an adult, but may lead to complications in the urinary tract. A maximal excretion of 670 mg per day has been reported during immobilization in the treatment of lower-extremity fractures.[63] In a series of 14 cases selected because of the development of urinary tract complications following immobilization, the onset of urinary tract symptoms due to hypercalciuria occurred as early as the eighth day and as late as 6 months following injury.[80] The nephrocalcinosis and pelvic or ureteral calculi noted were unilateral in 60% of the cases. In adolescent patients, immobilization of a large part of the skeleton may result not only in hypercalciuria and related complications but also in hypercalcemia as the osteoporosis of disuse progresses at a pace greater than that generally seen in adults. Hypercalcemia as high as 9 mEq/L and hypophosphatemia have been reported, which mimic the findings of hyperparathyroidism, leading to unnecessary explorations of the parathyroid glands.[1]

Techniques employing bone-seeking radioisotopes have settled the relative importance of decrease in bone formation or increase in bone resorption as the cause of disuse osteoporosis. Comparative studies of normal individuals and of patients extensively paralyzed with poliomyelitis demonstrate that the rate of bone formation in the immobilized patient is 0.4–0.5 gm per M² per day, a value higher than normal. Bone resorption proceeds at the rate of 0.6–0.7 gm per M² per day, a value 2 to 3 times the normal rate.[61] Thus, the proportionately greater increase in bone resorption accounts for the development of disuse osteoporosis. When the daily calcium balance becomes essentially zero after several months of immobilization, the formation and resorption of bone are equal at normal or slightly less than normal rates. Therefore, in contrast to earlier interpretations, the absence of skeletal stress does not necessarily result in continuing high calcium excretion. In these subjects, the observations of decreased intestinal absorption of calcium, increased serum calcium *and* serum phosphorus and hypercalciuria out of proportion to the hypercalcemia are, taken together, evidence against a role for the parathyroid glands in the development of disuse osteoporosis.[61]

Clinical corollary: Urinary tract infections and hypercalciuria secondary to immobilization are best prevented by daily urine volumes greater than 2,500 ml. Medication to decrease urinary pH generally increases calcium mobilization from the skeleton and has not proved helpful in the treatment of hypercalciuria. Early passive and active exercises decrease urinary calcium losses and muscle wasting secondary to disuse.

COMPOSITIONAL CHANGES.—Considering the body as a whole, Moore *et al.* have collected extensive clinical data employing isotope dilution techniques to define compositional changes in surgical disease.[92, 93] Following trauma there is no sudden or surprising change in composition within a few hours other than a relative increase in the volume of the extracellular space due to the edema of injury and a tendency for a slight decrease in the concentration of its components. The cell mass, as represented largely by skeletal muscle, starts to decrease gradually over a period of days but in the process guards its intracellular composition. The freed components of the decreasing cell mass are transmitted via the extracellular space to tissues requiring them for energy, synthetic functions or repair and to the kidneys for excretion, with the result that restricted renal reserve may be unmasked by observed increases in blood urea nitrogen and potassium. The nature of the trauma in large part controls the magnitude and duration of the edema and cell destruction before repair halts the catabolic trend. In uncomplicated trauma, this point is reached in a few days to 2 weeks at most, with immobilization prolonging the interval to the turning point.

The local edema fluid due to trauma may reach a maximum of 2–6 L or more, with a greater or lesser accumulation of red cells, depending on capillary and small vessel injury. The total cell mass may reach its minimum of 75–80% of the preinjury mass days or weeks after the edema fluid has been removed by restoration of normal lymphatic and capillary function. The fat depots contributing to the energy requirements may lose 5–10 kg or more, an amount that may represent almost all or only a small proportion of the body fat, depending on the total fat content of the patient prior to injury.

These generalities are modified in countless ways by variations in severity of the original trauma and by complications that usually favor a repeated expan-

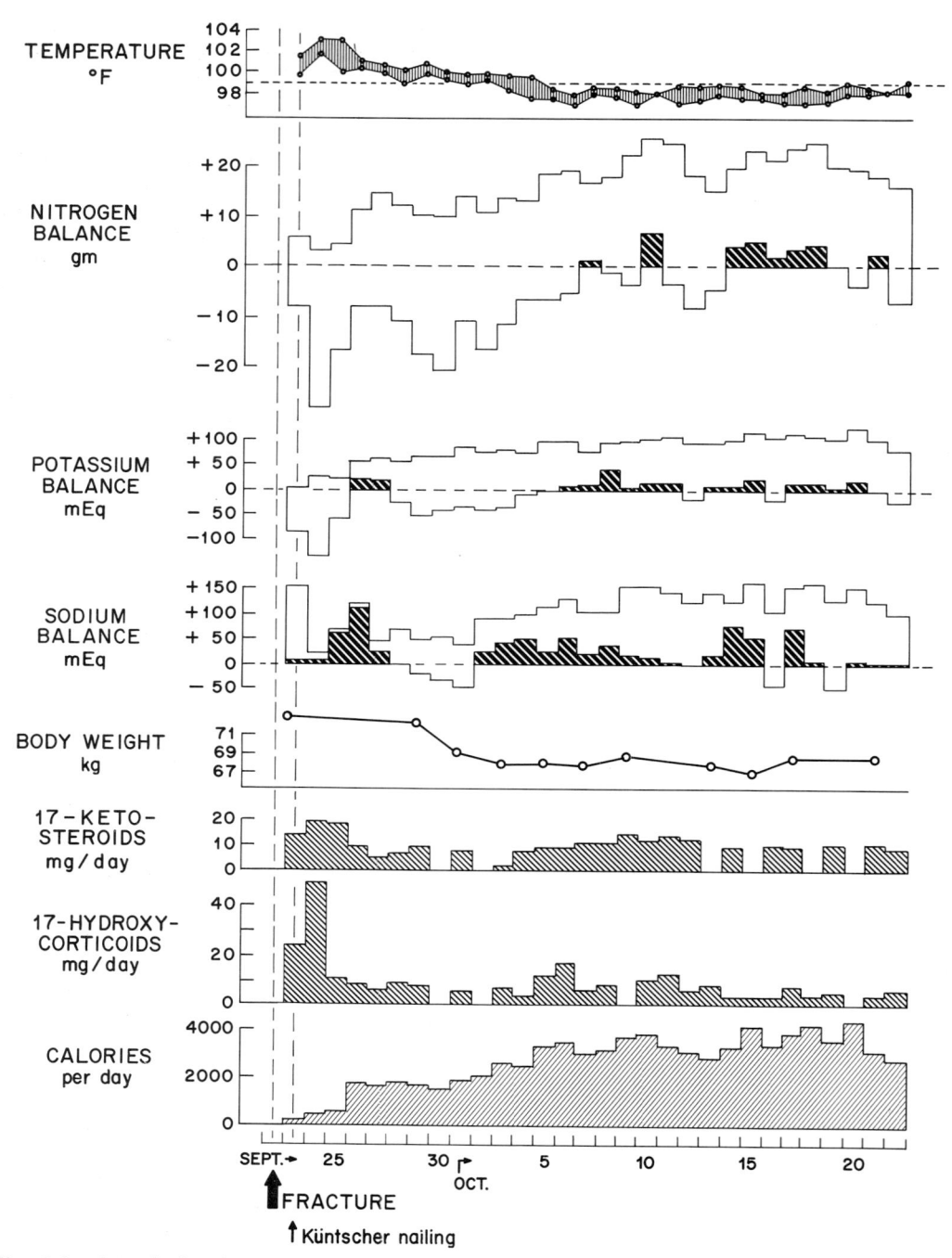

Fig. 3-9.—Metabolic data following fracture of femur. Nitrogen, potassium and sodium balance are plotted with intake measured up from zero line and output measured down from top of intake column. Shaded area above or below zero line represents the positive or negative balance. 17-ketosteroids include androgens; 17-hydroxycorticoids include cortisol.

sion of the extracellular space, as in the late development of peritonitis following abdominal or pelvic trauma. A further loss of cell mass and fat thus may occur as the body responds to a second stress and wave of endogenous steroids as it meets the demands for additional energy sources as well as it is then able to do. As an example of typical changes in body composition following a major fracture, Figures 3-9 and 3-10, adapted from Moore et al.,[94] present metabolic balance data and certain data on body composition. Careful inspection will reveal illustrations of many of the features of convalescence already described in this chapter.

Clinical corollary: No striking compositional changes are seen immediately following trauma to a normal person that demand replacement therapy for any component of the intercellular or extra-

Fig. 3-10.—Compositional data following fracture of femur. Fluid balance charted as balance data in Figure 3-9.

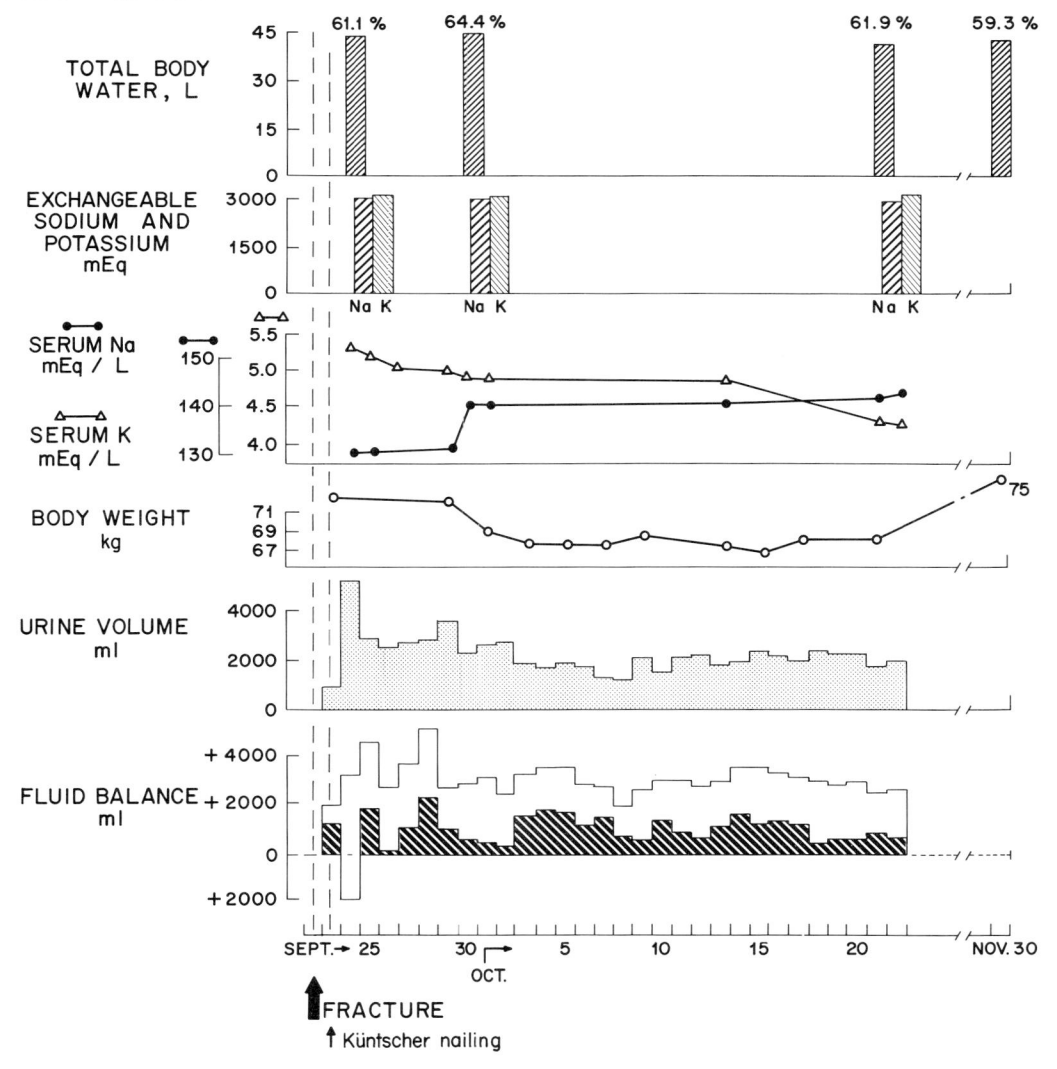

cellular space. Volume changes due to blood loss or fluid sequestration commonly require therapy. Specific replacement therapy for sodium, potassium and other components may be indicated because of depletions existing prior to injury or due to a complication developing after injury.

OTHER ENDOCRINE FUNCTIONS.—Apart from the secretion of ACTH, other hormones normally secreted by the anterior pituitary presumably play a permissive role and do not exert any significant, specific influence, as suggested by convalescence following hypophysectomy or following injury to patients who previously had their hypophysis removed. Although growth hormone is stimulated by emotional stress,[56] its function during convalescence has not been established. The secretion of gonadotropins has been reported to be increased in 8 of 18 patients studied during the first week following an operation, but no correlation of the urinary gonadotropin titers was observed with anesthesia, age, sex or extent of trauma.[117] During convalescence from extensive trauma, gonadotropins probably are suppressed, as suggested by the frequent temporary loss of libido and regular menses. Changes in thyroid gland function measured by iodine uptake and serum concentrations of triiodothyronine and protein-bound iodine after operations have been inconsistent,[43, 71, 111] and the minor changes reported are scarcely sufficient to account for the temporary rise in BMR observed after trauma discussed previously. The function of the parathyroid glands also has no recognized specific relation to the metabolic response following trauma. These and other endocrine functions following trauma have been the subject of an informative review by Johnston.[72]

SUMMARY

The perfection of the metabolic response to injury is appreciated with increasing respect as the interrelations of one adjustment to another are unfolded by medical research. The synoptic view presented in this chapter may serve as an introduction to our future understanding of the response to injury and to a consideration in following chapters of many injuries that have their unique local characteristics.

The major features of the generalized metabolic response are:

1. An immediate response supporting the circulation by actions of nerve reflexes, epinephrine, norepinephrine, antidiuretic hormone, aldosterone and fluid shifts.

2. An immediate increase in cortisol secretion affecting gluconeogenesis, protein catabolism, fat mobilization and cellular metabolism broadly.

3. An alteration in energy sources and utilization with glucose being preferentially conserved for the glycolytic tissues, particularly nerve, and with fat being the major energy substrate for other tissues.

4. An early tendency to hypercoagulability of the blood, followed in rare instances by disseminated intravascular coagulation, leading to a hemorrhagic diathesis occasionally compounded with the adverse effects of multiple transfusions.

5. A variable early respiratory insufficiency commonly leading to respiratory acidosis and metabolic acidosis secondary to anaerobic respiration and lactate accumulation.

6. A variable negative caloric balance with wasting of hydrated lean tissue at a maximal rate of 300–900 gm per day and of fat at a maximal rate of 400–600 gm per day until parenteral intake returns to normal.

7. A variable calciuria secondary to immobilization at a maximal rate of 400–600 mg per day.

8. An infinite number of variations on these metabolic themes are observed as a consequence of complications related to previously existing disease, to sepsis and to associated visceral injury.

APPENDIX
CALORIC AND NUTRITIONAL BALANCE BY INTRAVENOUS FEEDING

Parenteral and oral regimens for optimal nutrition in a patient following trauma no longer are a matter of great debate. High protein and high caloric diets or intravenous feedings modify, but do not prevent, the loss of protein after injury or operation.[25, 73] Observations on the nitrogen-sparing effect achieved by nonprotein calories during a fast have been reviewed and provide ample justification for the common use of 5% dextrose solutions.[16] The provision of a minimum of 700 calories by dextrose mitigates the ketosis of fasting, conserves lean tissue and consequently reduces fluid requirements for renal excretion. For example, the excretion of 1 gm of nitrogen as urea requires 40–60 ml of water if the kidney is concentrating maximally (> 1,000 mOsm/L); when a patient is excreting upward of 20 gm of nitrogen a day there is an obligatory loss of water of about 1,000 ml. Additional amounts are needed to cover the renal excretion of intracellular minerals associated with the nitrogen. The minimum of 700 calories needed to achieve maximal nitrogen sparing during a fast requires 175 gm of dextrose, which, if given intravenously, should be administered slowly enough to avoid hyperglycemia and glycosuria. At times, 5–10 U of regular insulin given intravenously with each 50 gm of dextrose may prevent wasteful glycosuria. Intensive intravenous infusions of amino acids and dextrose should be confined to debilitated patients unable to eat or to those facing a protracted catabolic phase, as seen in extensively burned patients or in patients contending with prolonged septic complications or with chronic intrinsic gastrointestinal disease or fistulas causing malabsorption.[52] Under such circumstances, it is very desirable to provide calories and essential foods by the intravenous route. A method of nutrition known as "hyperalimentation," championed by Rhoads and his colleagues, has made this possible by the use of centrally placed catheters that are directed through a superficial vein in the upper extremity or the neck into the superior vena cava.[36, 45, 135] Hypertonic, potentially sclerosing solutions enter the superior vena cava, where rapid dilution prevents, in most cases, damage to the vessel wall or to formed elements in the blood. The constituents of a typical solution for this therapy are presented in Table 3-1. Normal growth rates in neonatal infants achieved by this solution attest to its nutritional efficacy. However, careful precautions must be taken to ensure sterility of the central catheter and of solutions containing amino acids, to avoid the complication of air embolism when using a constant infusion pump and to minimize glycosuria during and rebound hypoglycemia following the infusion. A typical regimen for an adult patient prescribes 2.5 L over a 12-hour period. This provides more than 80 gm of protein and 2,300 calories. Vitamin and trace mineral supplements are given either in the infusate or by the addition of fresh plasma or whole blood.

TABLE 3-1.—NUTRIENTS AND MINERALS IN INFUSATE FOR HYPERALIMENTATION[45]

CONSTITUENT	CONTENT /L
Protein (as amino acids)	33 gm
Glucose	200 gm
Sodium°	5 mEq
Potassium°	16 mEq
Chloride°	11.7 mEq
Calcium	183 mg (9.2 mEq)
Magnesium	30.6 mg (2.6 mEq)
Phosphorus	67 mg (2.2 mM)

°Adjusted further at bedside, generally bringing Na, K and Cl to about 40, 40 and 70 mEq/L, respectively, as indicated by the patient's serum electrolyte concentrations. At pH >6.5, almost all amino acids are anions and provide almost half of the anions in the above solution.

BIBLIOGRAPHY

1. Albright, F., Burnett, C. H., Cope, O., and Parson, W.: Acute atrophy of bone (osteo-

porosis) simulating hyperparathyroidism, J. Clin. Endocrinol. 1:711, 1941.
2. Andersen, M. N., Border, J. R., and Mouritzen, C. V.: Acidosis, catecholamines and cardiovascular dynamics: When does acidosis require correction?, Ann. Surg. 166:344, 1967.
3. Bendixen, H. H., and Laver, M. B.: Hypoxia in anesthesia; a review, Clin. Pharmacol. Ther. 6:510, 1965.
4. Benesch, R., and Benesch, R. E.: The effect of organic phosphates from the human erythrocyte on the allosteric properties of hemoglobin, Biochem. Biophys. Res. Commun. 26:162, 1967.
5. Benesch, R., and Benesch, R. E.: Intracellular organic phosphates as regulators of oxygen release by haemoglobin, Nature, London 221: 618, 1969.
6. Birke, G., Liljedahl, S. O., Plantin, L. O., et al.: Albumin catabolism in burns and following surgical procedures, Acta Chir. Scand. 118: 353, 1959.
7. Borowiecki, B., and Sharp, A. A.: Trauma and fibrinolysis, J. Trauma 9:522, 1969.
8. Brinkhous, K. M., and Scarborough, D. E.: Some mechanisms of thrombus formation and hemorrhage following trauma, J. Trauma 9:684, 1969.
9. Broder, G.: Excess lactate: An index of reversibility of shock in human patients, Science 143:1457, 1964.
10. Bull, G. M., Joekes, A. M., and Lowe, K. G.: Renal function studies in acute tubular necrosis, Clin. Sci. 9:379, 1950.
11. Bunker, J. P.: Metabolic effects of blood transfusion, Anesthesiology 27:446, 1966.
12. Bywaters, E. G. L., and Beall, D.: Crush injuries with impairment of renal function, Br. Med. J. 1:427, 1941.
13. Cahill, G. F., Jr.: Starvation in man, N. Engl. J. Med. 282:668, 1970.
14. Cairnie, A. B., Campbell, R. M., Pullar, J. D., et al.: The heat production consequent on injury, Br. J. Exp. Pathol. 38:504, 1957.
15. Caldwell, F. T., Osterholm, J. L., Sower, N. D., et al.: Metabolic response to thermal trauma of normal and thyroprivic rates at three environmental temperatures, Ann. Surg. 150: 976, 1959.
16. Calloway, D. H., and Spector, H.: Nitrogen balance as related to caloric and protein intake in active young men, Am. J. Clin. Nutr. 2:405, 1954.
17. Campbell, G. S., Houle, D. B., Crisp, N. W., et al.: Depressed response to intravenous symphathicomimetic agents in humans during acidosis, Dis. Chest 33:18, 1958.
18. Cannon, W. B.: Bodily Changes in Pain, Hunger, Fear and Rage (New York: D. Appleton and Company, 1929).
19. Chandler, A. M., and Neuhaus, O. W.: Synthesis of serum glycoproteins in response to injury, Am. J. Physiol. 206:169, 1964.
20. Cooper, C. E., and Nelson, D. H.: ACTH levels in plasma in preoperative and surgically stressed patients, J. Clin. Invest. 41:1599, 1962.
21. Cope, O., Nardi, G. L., Quijano, M., et al.: Metabolic rate and thyroid function following acute thermal trauma in man, Ann. Surg. 137: 165, 1953.
22. Cope, O., Nathanson, I. T., Rourke, G. M., et al.: Metabolic observations, Ann. Surg. 117: 937, 1943.
23. Crockson, R. A., Payne, C. J., Ratcliff, A. P., et al.: Time sequence of acute phase reactive proteins following surgical trauma, Clin. Chim. Acta 14:435, 1966.
24. Cuthbertson, D. P.: The disturbance of metabolism produced by bony and non-bony injury, with notes on certain abnormal conditions of bone, Biochem. J. 24:1244, 1930.
25. Cuthbertson, D. P.: Further observations on the disturbance of metabolism caused by injury, with particular reference to the dietary requirements of fracture cases, Br. J. Surg. 23: 505, 1935.
26. Cuthbertson, D. P.: Physical Injury and Its Effects on Protein Metabolism, in Munro, H. N., and Allison, J. B. (eds.), Mammalian Protein Metabolism (New York: Academic Press, 1964), Vol. 2.
27. Cuthbertson, D. P.: Post-shock metabolic response, Lancet 1:433, 1942.
28. Cuthbertson, D. P., and Robertson, J. S.: The metabolic response to injury, J. Physiol. 89: 53P, 1937.
29. Dahlback, L. O., and Rais, O.: Morphologic changes in striated muscle following ischemia. Immediate postischemic phase, Acta Chir. Scand. 131:430, 1966.
30. Davies, J. W. L., Ricketts, C. R., and Bull, J. P.: Studies of plasma protein metabolism. Part I. Albumin in burned and injured patients, Clin. Sci. 23:411, 1962.
31. Davies, J. W. L., Ricketts, C. R., and Bull, J. P.: Studies of plasma protein metabolism. Part II. Pooled v-globulin in burned and injured patients, Clin. Sci. 24:371, 1963.
32. Davis, J. O., Olichrey, M. J., Brown, T. C., et al.: Metabolism of aldosterone in several experimental situations with altered aldosterone secretion, J. Clin. Invest. 44:1433, 1965.
33. Deitrick, J. E., Whedon, G. D., and Shorr, E.: Effects of immobilization upon various metabolic and physiologic functions of normal men, Am. J. Med. 4:3, 1948.
34. Dole, V. P.: Relation between non-esterified fatty acids in plasma and metabolism of glucose, J. Clin. Invest. 35:150, 1956.
35. Downing, S. E., Talner, N. S., and Gardner, T. H.: Cardiovascular responses to metabolic acidosis, Am. J. Physiol. 208:237, 1965.
36. Dudrick, S. J., Wilmore, D. W., Vars, H. M., et al.: Long-term total parenteral nutrition with growth, development, and positive nitrogen balance, Surgery 64:134, 1968.
37. Duff, J. H., Scott, H. M., and Peretz, D. I.: The diagnosis and treatment of shock in man based on hemodynamic and metabolic measurements, J. Trauma 6:145, 1966.
38. Duke, J. H., Jr., Jorgensen, S. B., Long, C. L., et al.: Contribution of protein to the caloric expenditure following injury. Presented at the 31st Annual Meeting of The Society of University Surgeons, Pittsburgh, February 12–14, 1970.

39. Eastcott, H. H. G., Fawcett, J. K., and Rob, C. G.: Some factors affecting uropepsinogen excretion in man, Lancet 1:1068, 1953.
40. Egdahl, R. H.: Pituitary-adrenal response following trauma to the isolated leg, Surgery 46:9, 1959.
41. Eiseman, B., and Ashbough, D. G. (eds.): Pulmonary effects of nonthoracic trauma, in Proceedings of Conference conducted by Committee on Trauma, Division of Medical Services, National Academy of Sciences, National Research Council, J. Trauma 8:649, 1968.
42. Eisen, V. D., and Lewis, A. A. G.: Antidiuretic activity of human urine after surgical operations, Lancet 2:361, 1954.
43. Engstrom, W. W., and Markardt, B.: The effects of serious illness and surgical stress on the circulating thyroid hormone, J. Clin. Endocrinol. 15:953, 1955.
44. Espiner, E. A.: Urinary cortisol excretion in stress situations and in patients with Cushing's syndrome, J. Endocrinol. 35:29, 1966.
45. Filler, R. M., Eraklis, A. J., Rubin, V. G., et al.: Long-term total parenteral nutrition in infants, N. Engl. J. Med. 281:589, 1969.
46. Fleck, A., and Munro, H. N.: Protein metabolism after injury, Metabolism 12:783, 1963.
47. Fogelman, J. M., and Garvey, J. M.: Acute gastroduodenal ulceration incident to surgery and disease, Am. J. Surg. 112:651, 1966.
48. Franksson, C., Gemzeli, C. A., and von Euler, V. S.: Cortical and medullary adrenal activity in surgical and allied conditions, J. Clin. Endocrinol. 14:608, 1954.
49. Gauer, O. H., and Henry, J. P.: Circulatory basis of fluid volume control, Physiol. Rev. 43:423, 1963.
50. Gauer, O. H., Henry, J. P., Sieker, H. O., et al.: Effect of negative pressure breathing on urine flow, J. Clin. Invest. 33:287, 1954.
51. Gear, M. W. L.: Perforated duodenal ulcer following injury or operation, Br. J. Surg. 55:585, 1968.
52. Gilder, H., Moody, F. G., Cornell, G. N., et al.: Components of body weight loss in surgical patients, Metabolism 10:134, 1961.
53. Goldstein, R., Bunker, J. P., and McGovern, J. J.: The effects of storage on whole blood and anticoagulants upon certain coagulation factors, Ann. N. Y. Acad. Sci. 115:422, 1964.
54. Gomez, A. C.: Pulmonary insufficiency in nonthoracic trauma, J. Trauma 8:656, 1968.
55. Gray, S. J., and Ramsey, C. G.: Adrenal influences upon the stomach and the gastric responses to stress, Recent Prog. Horm. Res. 13:583, 1967.
56. Greenwood, F. C., and Landon, J.: Growth hormone secretion in response to stress in man, Nature, London 210:540, 1966.
57. Halme, A., Pekkarinen, A., and Turunen, M.: On the excretion of noradrenaline, adrenaline, 17-hydroxycorticosteroids and 17-ketosteroids during the postoperative stage, Acta Endocrinol. (Supp. 32) 24:1, 1957.
58. Hammond, W. G., Vandam, L. D., Davis, J. M., et al.: Studies in surgical endocrinology. IV. Anesthetic agents as stimuli to change in corticosteroids and metabolism, Ann. Surg. 148:199, 1958.
59. Hardaway, R. M.: Disseminated intravascular coagulation in experimental and clinical shock, Am. J. Cardiol. 20:161, 1967.
60. Harvel, R. J.: The autonomic nervous system and intermediary carbohydrate and fat metabolism, Anesthesiology 29:702, 1968.
61. Heaney, R. P.: Radiocalcium metabolism in disuse osteoporosis in man, Am. J. Med. 33:188, 1962.
62. Hodges, J. R., Jones, M. T., and Stockham, M. A.: Effect of emotion on blood corticotrophin and cortisol concentrations in man, Nature, London 193:1187, 1962.
63. Howard, J. E., Parson, W., and Bigham, R. S., Jr.: Studies on patients convalescent from fracture; urinary excretion of calcium and phosphorus, Bull. Johns Hopkins Hosp. 77:291, 1945.
64. Howard, J. M.: Studies of the absorption and metabolism of glucose following injury, Ann. Surg. 141:321, 1955.
65. Huckabee, W. E.: Relationships of pyruvate and lactate during anaerobic metabolism, J. Clin. Invest. 37:244, 1958.
66. Hume, D. M., Cooper, B. C., and Bartter, F.: Direct measurement of adrenal secretion during operative trauma and convalescence, Surgery 52:174, 1962.
67. Hunter, J.: *The Surgical Works of John Hunter, F.R.S.*, Palmer, J. F. (ed.) (London: Longman Rees, Orme Brown, Green & Longman, 1837), Vol. III, p. 239.
68. Ingle, D. J., Ward, E. O., and Kuizenga, M. H.: Relationship of adrenal glands to changes in urinary non-protein nitrogen following multiple fractures in force-fed rat, Am. J. Physiol. 149:510, 1947.
69. Jenevein, E. P., Jr., and Weiss, D. L.: Platelet microemboli associated with massive blood transfusion, Am. J. Pathol. 45:313, 1964.
70. Jepson, R. P., Jordan, A., Levell, M. J., et al.: Metabolic response to adrenalectomy, Ann. Surg. 145:1, 1957.
71. Johnston, I. D. A.: Endocrine aspects of the metabolic response to surgical operation, Ann. R. Coll. Surg. Engl. 35:270, 1964.
72. Johnston, I. D. A.: *The Endocrine Response to Trauma.* (Br. Postgrad. Med. Fed.) (The scientific basis of medicine annual reviews.) (London: The Athlone Press, 1968).
73. Johnston, I. D. A., Marino, J. D., and Stevens, J. Z.: The effects of intravenous feeding on the balances of nitrogen, sodium, and potassium after operation, Br. J. Surg. 53:885, 1966.
74. Kantrowitz, P. A., Greenberger, N. J., et al.: Severe postoperative hyperbilirubinemia simulating obstructive jaundice, N. Engl. J. Med. 276:590, 1967.
75. Kelman, G. R., Nunn, J. F., Prys-Robert, C., et al.: The influence of cardiac output on arterial oxygenation: A theoretical study, Br. J. Anaesth. 39:450, 1967.
76. Kinney, J. M.: A consideration of energy exchange in human trauma, Bull. N. Y. Acad. Med. 36:617, 1960.
77. Kinney, J. M.: The effect of injury on

metabolism, Br. J. Surg. 54 (supp.): 435, 1967.
78. Kinney, J. M.: Protein Metabolism in Human Pathological States. The Effect of Injury upon Human Protein Metabolism, in *Protein Metabolism, Influence of Growth Hormone, Anabolic Steroids, and Nutrition in Health and Disease.* An international symposium. Sponsored by Ciba. Edited by F. Gross (Berlin: Springer-Verlag, 1962).
79. Kinney, J. M., and Francis, R. C.: Caloric equivalent of fever. I. Patterns of postoperative response, Trans. Am. Surg. Assoc. 80:282, 1962.
80. Leadbetter, W. F., and Engster, H. C.: The problem of renal lithiasis in convalescent patients, J. Urol. 53:269, 1945.
81. Leaf, A.: Antidiuretic mechanism not regulated by extracellular fluid tonicity, J. Clin. Invest. 31:60, 1952.
82. Litwin, M. S., Smith, L. L., and Moore, F. D.: Metabolic alkalosis following massive transfusion, Surgery 45:805, 1959.
83. Lyons, J. H., and Moore, F. D.: Post-traumatic alkalosis; incidence and pathophysiology of alkalosis in surgery, Surgery 60:93, 1966.
84. Martin, A. M., Simmons, R. L., and Heister, K. C. A.: Respiratory insufficiency in combat casualties. I. Pathologic changes in the lungs of patients dying of wounds, Ann. Surg. 170:30, 1969.
85. Martin, A. M., Soloway, H. B., and Simmons, R. L.: Pathologic anatomy of the lungs following shock and trauma, J. Trauma 8:687, 1968.
86. Mason, A. S.: Metabolic response to total adrenalectomy and hypophysectomy, Lancet 2:632, 1955.
87. Merskey, C., Johnson, A. J., Kleiner, G. J., et al.: The defibrination syndrome: Clinical features and laboratory diagnosis, Br. J. Haematol. 13:528, 1967.
88. Miller, L. D., Oski, F. A., Diaco, J. F., et al.: The affinity of hemoglobin for oxygen; its control and in vivo significance. Presented at the 31st Annual Meeting of the Society of University Surgeons, Pittsburgh, February 12–14, 1970.
89. Moore, F. D.: The effect of hemorrhage on body composition, N. Engl. J. Med. 273:567, 1965.
90. Moore, F. D.: Endocrine changes after anesthesia, surgery, and unanesthetized trauma in man, Recent Prog. Horm. Res. 13:511, 1967.
91. Moore, F. D., Haley, H. B., Bering, E. A., Jr., et al.: Further observations on total body water. II. Changes of body composition in disease, Surg. Gynecol. Obstet. 95:155, 1952.
92. Moore, F. D., McMurrey, J. D., and Parker, H. V.: Body composition; total body water and electrolytes, intravascular and extravascular phase volumes, Metabolism 5:447, 1956.
93. Moore, F. D., Olesen, K. H., McMurrey, J. D., et al.: *The Body Cell Mass and Its Supporting Environment. Body Composition in Health and Disease* (Philadelphia: W. B. Saunders Company, 1963).
94. Moore, F. D., Steenburg, R. W., Ball, M. R., et al.: Studies in surgical endocrinology; urinary excretion of 17-hydroxycorticoids, and associated metabolic changes in cases of soft tissue trauma of varying severity and in bone trauma, Ann. Surg. 141:145, 1955.
95. Mouridsen, H. T.: Turnover of human serum albumin before and after operations, Clin. Sci. 33:345, 1967.
96. Munro, H. N., and Chalmers, M. I.: Fracture metabolism at different levels of protein intake, Br. J. Exp. Pathol. 26:396, 1945.
97. Nahas, G. G., and Poyart, C.: Effect of arterial pH alterations on metabolic activity of norepinephrine, Am. J. Physiol. 212:765, 1967.
98. Owen, J. A.: Effect of injury on plasma proteins, Adv. Clin. Chem. 9:1, 1967.
99. Penick, G. D., and Roberts, H. R.: Intravascular clotting; focal and systemic, Int. Rev. Exp. Pathol. 3:269, 1964.
100. Peretz, D. I., Scott, H. M., Duff, J., et al.: The significance of lacticacidemia in the shock syndrome, Ann. N. Y. Acad. Sci. 119:1133, 1965.
101. Porte, D., Jr., Graber, A. L., Kuzuya, T., et al.: The effect of epinephrine on immunoreactive insulin levels in man, J. Clin. Invest. 45:228, 1966.
102. Refsum, H. E.: Arterial hypoxaemia serum activities of GO-T, GP-T and LDH, and centrilobular liver cell necrosis in pulmonary insufficiency, Clin. Sci. 25:369, 1963.
103. Robson, J. M., Horn, D. B., Dudley, H. A., et al.: Metabolic response to adrenalectomy, Lancet 2:325, 1955.
104. Roe, C. F., and Kinney, J. M.: The caloric equivalent of fever. II. Influence of major trauma, Ann. Surg. 161:140, 1965.
105. Rothchild, M. A., Schreiber, S. S., Oratz, M., et al.: The effects of adrenocortical hormones on albumin metabolism studied with albumin-I^{131}, J. Clin. Invest. 37:1229, 1958.
106. Sachar, L., Walker, W., and Whittico, J.: Carbohydrate tolerance, blood ketone levels and nitrogen balance after human trauma, Arch. Surg. 60:837, 1950.
107. Salzman, E. W.: Does intravascular coagulation occur in hemorrhagic shock in man?, J. Trauma 8:867, 1968.
108. Sandberg, A. A., Eik-Nes, K., Samuels, L. T., et al.: Effect of surgery on blood levels and metabolism of 17-hydroxycorticosteroids in man, J. Clin. Invest. 33:1509, 1954.
109. Selye, H.: The general adaptation syndrome and the diseases of adaptation, J. Clin. Endocrinol. 6:117, 1946.
110. Sevitt, S.: Duodenal and gastric ulceration after burning, Br. J. Surg. 54:32, 1967.
111. Shipley, R. A., and MacIntyre, F. H.: Effect of stress, TSH and ACTH on the level of hormonal I^{131} of serum, J. Clin. Endocrinol. 14:309, 1954.
112. Simmons, R. L., Heisterkamp, C. A., Collins, J. A., et al.: Coagulation disorders in combat casualties. I. Acute changes after wounding. II. Effects of massive transfusion. III. Postresuscitative changes, Ann. Surg. 169:455, 1969.
113. Simmons, R. L., Heisterkamp, C. A., Collins, J. A., et al.: Respiratory insufficiency in combat casualties. III. Arterial hypoxemia after wounding, Ann. Surg. 170:45, 1969.
114. Simmons, R. L., Heisterkamp, C. A., Collins,

J. A., et al.: Respiratory insufficiency in combat casualties. IV. Hypoxia during convalescence, Ann. Surg. 170:53, 1969.
115. Skillman, J. J., Lauler, D. P., Hickler, R. D., et al.: Hemorrhage in normal man: Effect on renin, cortisol, aldosterone, and urine composition, Ann. Surg. 166:865, 1967.
116. Smith, E. E., and Crowell, J. W.: Influence of hematocrit ratio on survival of unacclimatized dogs at simulated high altitude, Am. J. Physiol. 205:1172, 1963.
117. Sohval, A. R., Weiner, I., and Soffer, L. J.: The effect of surgical procedures on urinary gonadotropin excretion, J. Clin. Endocrinol. 12:1053, 1952.
118. Steenburg, R. W., Lennihan, R., and Moore, F. D.: Studies in surgical endocrinology; free blood 17-hydroxycorticoids in surgical patients; their relation to urine steroids, metabolism and convalescence, Ann. Surg. 143:180, 1956.
119. Steinberg, D.: Catecholamine stimulation of fat mobilization and its metabolic consequences, Pharmacol. Rev. 18:217, 1966.
120. Steinberg, D., Nestel, P. H., Buskirk, E. R., et al.: Calorigenic effect of norepinephrine correlated with plasma free fatty acid turnover and oxidation, J. Clin. Invest. 43:167, 1964.
121. Sterling, K., Lipsky, S. R., and Freedman, L. J.: Disappearance curve of intravenously administered I[131] tagged albumin in the postoperative injury reaction, Metabolism 4:343, 1955.
122. Stewart, J. S. S.: Management of cardiac arrest, with special reference to metabolic acidosis, Br. Med. J. 1:476, 1964.
123. Stewart, J. S. S., Stewart, W. K., Morgan, H. G., et al.: A clinical and experimental study of the electrocardiographic changes in extreme acidosis and cardiac arrest, Br. Heart J. 27:490, 1965.
124. Swaiman, K. F., and Bradley, W. E.: Creatine phosphokinase in detection of visceral muscle injury, Proc. Soc. Exp. Biol. Med. 130:612, 1969.
125. Tyler, F. H., Schmidt, C. D., Eik-Nes, K., et al.: Role of liver and adrenal in producing elevated plasma 17-hydroxycorticosteroid levels in surgery, J. Clin. Invest. 33:1517, 1954.
126. Vander, A. J.: Control of renin release, Physiol. Rev. 47:359, 1967.
127. Vassella, F., Richterick, R., and Rossi, E.: The diagnostic value of serum creatine kinase in neuromuscular and muscular disease, Pediatrics 35:322, 1965.
128. Warner, W. A.: Release of free fatty acids following trauma, J. Trauma 9:692, 1969.
129. Webb, W. R.: Pulmonary complications of non-thoracic trauma: Summary of the National Research Council Conference, J. Trauma 9:700, 1969.
130. Weinstein, H., Berne, R. M., and Sachs, H.: Vasopressin in blood: Effect of hemorrhage, Endocrinology 66:712, 1960.
131. Werner, M., and Cohnen, G.: Changes in serum proteins in the immediate postoperative period, Clin. Sci. 36:173, 1969.
132. Whedon, G. D.: Osteoporosis: Atrophy of Disuse, in Rodahl, K., Nicholson, J. T., and Brown, E. M. (eds.), *Bone as a Tissue* (New York: McGraw-Hill Book Company, 1960).
133. Whedon, G. D., and Shorr, E.: Metabolic studies in paralytic acute anterior poliomyelitis. I. Alterations in nitrogen and creatine metabolism, J. Clin. Invest. 36:942, 1957.
134. Whedon, G. D., and Shorr, E.: Metabolic studies in paralytic acute anterior poliomyelitis. II. Alterations in calcium and phosphorus metabolism, J. Clin. Invest. 36:966, 1957.
135. Wilmore, D. W., and Dudrick, S. J.: Growth and development of an infant receiving all nutrients exclusively by vein, JAMA 203:860, 1968.
136. Yates, F. E., and Urquhart, J.: Control of plasma concentrations of adrenocortical hormones, Physiol. Rev. 42:359, 1962.

4 | Repair of Bone and Fracture Healing

JOHN E. KENZORA*

BONE is one of the more specialized connective tissues, specifically adapted to mechanical, protective and locomotive functions. Like most connective tissues, bone consists of a population of different cells and an extracellular matrix. One of the most distinguishing characteristics of bone is the fact that a solid mineral phase of calcium and phosphorus is deposited in an extracellular matrix of collagen. In addition, the matrix has a specific microscopic architecture much different from other collagenous tissues, such as tendon and skin.

All connective tissues respond to certain external, chemical and physical stimuli by changes in the rates at which extracellular matrix is produced and resorbed as well as by changes in the microscopic organization of the tissue. Bone, as one of the connective tissues, likewise will respond to these stimuli. The *repair of bone* is a specific biologic response to the stimulus of bone injury or death in that the bone responds by replacing the injured areas with new living bone. Because the gross and microscopic appearance of coarse cancellous bone differs markedly from that of compact bone, the cellular mechanisms required for the replacement of injured or dead areas are different. The repair of injured spongy bone, therefore, will be studied separately from that of injured compact bone. *Fracture healing* is a very specialized form of bone repair in which there is a discontinuity of tissue. This will produce a further different cellular response.

The understanding and descriptions of the sequence of biologic events that occur in injured spongy and compact bone have important further clinical implications. The comprehension of the principles of bone grafting, avascular necrosis and healing of certain defects of bone is made easier once the fundamentals of bone repair are evident.

It must be pointed out that bone repair differs from repair in most connective tissues because bone is one of the few tissues capable of perfect healing. By definition, bone healing means that injured areas of bone will be replaced with new living bone and, specifically, that a fracture will heal by filling in the discontinuity with new living bone. Most other connective tissues heal injured areas with scar tissue. It must be stressed that the repair of bone is a cell-mediated phenomenon. Therefore, for repair to occur there must be a large enough pool of undifferentiated cells that are capable of further proliferation and modulation to cells of osteogenic lineage; that is, to osteoblasts, osteocytes and osteoclasts. Adequate new bone production requires that sufficient numbers of undifferentiated

---

*Assistant in Orthopedic Surgery, Children's Hospital Medical Center; Instructor in Orthopedic Surgery, Harvard Medical School; Junior Associate in Orthopedic Surgery, Peter Bent Brigham Hospital.

cells modulate to osteoblasts, which then must secrete enough new bone matrix. New bone must also form in the proper areas. Osteoclasts are also cells of osteogenic lineage and are essential during certain phases of bone repair. Bone resorption can occur as the result of primary cell modulation to osteoclasts or by dedifferentiation of osteocytes to uninuclear cells with organelles similar to classic osteoclasts. This process, when it occurs, is called osteocytic osteolysis. By definition, any cell that participates in resorption of bone is an osteoclast, regardless of the number of nuclei present, and thus mononuclear osteoclasts may participate in the repair of bone.

The undifferentiated cells within bone are really partly differentiated, as there are only a specific number of allowable modulations. For example, they cannot form the specialized cells of liver, brain, kidney, etc. Fracture healing, however, does include certain additional modulations to those already described, which depend on the local cell environment. Under certain local conditions, chondroblasts, chondrocytes and cartilage tissue may form, whereas, under other local conditions, fibroblasts, fibrocytes and fibrous connective tissue form. Synovioblasts, synoviocytes and synovial fluid may even be produced if the local environment is appropriate. Regardless of the tissues produced or resorbed, living cells are responsible for their production and removal.

In summary, for bone repair or fracture healing to go on to completion, adequate *numbers* of osteoblasts must be present and produce sufficient *quantities* of new bone of proper internal architecture (*quality*) and *distribution;* that is, the injured area or fracture site will be replaced with normal living bone.

Just as important as the healing of the fracture site is the repair of bone as an organ and the restoration of a functional unit. A fracture that has gross axial displacement and angulation not only deforms the bone but it also malaligns the joints above and below the fracture. The fracture site may heal perfectly, but if displacement and angulation are not corrected, a *functionally* poor result will occur. To prevent a clinically poor functional result, displacement and alignment must be properly assessed and corrected. Only a certain amount of geometric deformity can be corrected by external remodeling. External remodeling refers to the control of size, shape and distribution of over-all mass possessed by the organ bone. In regard to fracture healing, it is the ability of a bone to maintain or return to an appropriate size and shape. Young growing bones have greater potential for controlling these parameters than do adult bones. In addition, only young growing bones have epiphyseal plates. As will be pointed out later, this feature confers a limited ability to correct malalignment of the bone ends, because asymmetric rates of growth are possible within epiphyseal plates.

In contrast, internal remodeling is the change in the internal microscopic architecture that occurs at the fracture site. Included are all the changes in the callus between the earliest fine cancellous randomly oriented bone and the final restoration to compact osteonal bone. These changes occur with fractures in both growing and adult bone, but the rate will be greater in the growing bone. In a particular case, if the bone is young enough and the angulation and displacement are not severe, complete correction of the shaft may occur. In this case, external remodeling is complete. The adult bone, on the other hand, can correct neither displacement nor angulation. Internal remodeling occurs at the fracture site, but the only external remodeling that can occur will be the local resorption of the sharp convexities and the partial filling in of concavities with new bone. In addition, the marrow cavity may be restored. Details of remodeling phenomena will be presented at the end of this chapter.

These remodeling potentials have important clinical implications. In the adult fracture, minimal angular deformity is permissible, depending on the bone and the site within the bone, particularly in planes coronal to adjacent joint planes. Some displacement is permissible, provided that the local deformity produced is acceptable and the involved joints are aligned. In growing bones, a certain amount of angulation and displacement is allowable, provided that neither exceeds the biologic potential of the bone to remodel with further growth. In addition, metaphyseal deformity will correct more completely and quickly than diaphyseal deformity because of the proximity to the epiphyseal plate and to the metaphyseal cutback zone, where funnelization occurs. The healing of the fracture site and remodeling occur simultaneously but, for purposes of clarity, they will be discussed individually.

A discussion of the general repair of dead cancellous and compact bone follows. In each case, this is the cellular response to the death of bone cells. In both the spongy and cortical bone, the structural integrity of the organ is intact and cell death is induced by exogenous techniques. Because the bone is intact, the variables of motion, gap size and alignment are eliminated and the bone repair will become evident. Later, when fracture healing is presented, these same variables become part of the local environment, and the cellular response will change accordingly.

REPAIR OF BONE

General Considerations

Before the sequence of cellular events is presented, two general phenomena must be mentioned. These are the *source* of cells and the *types* of cells that are available for tissue repair.

A fracture cannot heal without the presence of living cells. For healing to proceed, sufficient *numbers* of cells must *differentiate* to osteoblasts, which then must produce sufficient quantities of bone matrix of adequate *quality* in the proper *distribution* to bridge the fracture gap. Which cells are primarily responsible for healing and where do they come from?

Cells of the osteogenic lineage, i.e., osteoblasts, osteocytes, osteoclasts, chondroblasts and fibroblasts may all contribute to fracture healing to varying degrees under particular circumstances.[7, 8, 10, 14, 27, 29, 30, 35, 40, 42, 50, 51, 57, 62, 65, 79, 81, 86, 92, 93] These specialized cells are all descended from less-differentiated cells, which themselves derive from pluripotential or mesenchymal cells. The undifferentiated cells themselves come from various sources. The deep or cambium cell layer of the periosteum and the endosteum are two potential cell sources.[6, 9, 43, 59, 83-85] The endosteum, which is a single cell layer, is considered a minor source of undifferentiated cells. Blood vessels, marrow, osteons and fascial planes near the fracture site contain undifferentiated cells, which, on appropriate stimulation, may differentiate into osteogenic cells. This is the largest pool of available cells that may be called on to assist in healing.[95] The monocyte, a white blood cell found in the blood and in marrow, may be capable of transformation or dedifferentiation to an osteoclast,[2, 11, 37, 91] which then may participate in bone repair phenomena. Most cells that participate in fracture healing are undifferentiated and come from marrow and periosteal sources.

Repair of Dead Coarse Cancellous Bone (FIGS. 4-1–4-9)

Experimentally, one can induce cell necrosis of a sizable piece of bone in situ and observe the healing at any or all stages. The cell death is produced in situ; that is, with the bone structure intact. The sequence of events that follow the injury will now be presented.

NECROSIS[45, 48].—The initial biologic response to severe bone injury is cell necrosis. When living cells are cut off from

74 / *John E. Kenzora*

A
---- Live bone ---- → ← -- Zone of Cell Necrosis -- → ← ---- Live bone ----

Living blood vessel

Marrow with inflammatory response

Normal trabeculae with osteocytes in lacunae, and lined by some osteoblasts

Trabeculum with empty lacunae and absent osteoblasts

Marrow contains only cell ghosts. Fat cells may appear normal. Live vessels absent

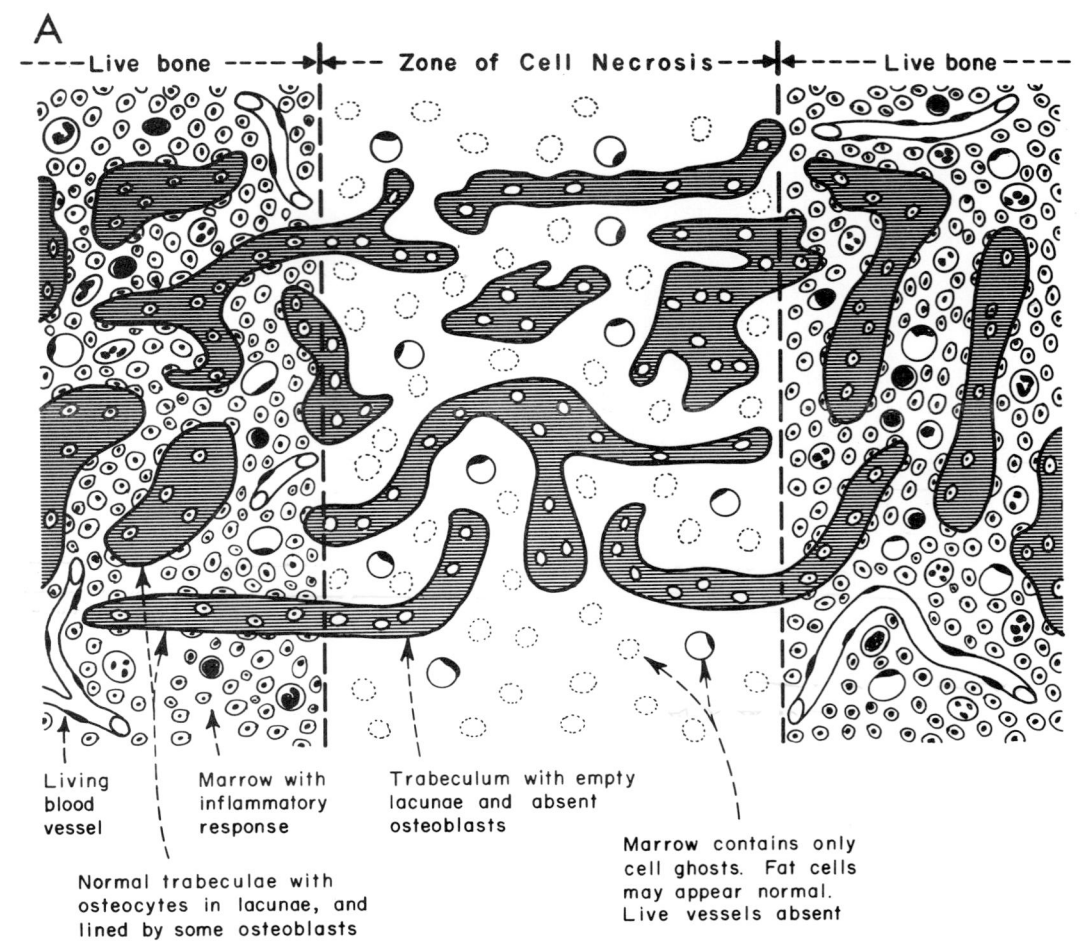

Fig. 4-1.—Healing of dead coarse cancellous bone. **A,** 4 days after cell necrosis. The diagram is a medium-power representation of mature spongy bone. The zone between the vertical dashed lines lost its blood supply 4 days previously. The major biologic feature in this zone is cell necrosis. Most osteocyte lacunae are empty. Osteoblasts and endothelial cells were lost several days ago. The marrow contains cell ghosts, except for signet-shaped fat cells, which remain for long periods. The bone on each side of the necrotic zone is alive with intact osteoblasts and osteocytes. The marrow contains live vessels and has undergone a major cell modulation to chronic inflammatory cells. **(Continued.)**

their sources of nutrition and respiration, they will die. With infarcted spongy bone, the first cells to die are those of hematopoietic lineage and the osteoblasts. Endothelial cells are next to show evidence of necrosis. Although osteocytes begin to die within a few hours, half still are functional 12 hours after total loss of systemic blood supply. Virtually all osteocytes are dead within 4 days.[47] Although all dying cells undergo pyknosis, karyolysis, nuclear clumping and eventual total dissolution, many osteocyte lacunae retain what appears histologically to be live osteocytes for many months. The marrow spaces eventually contain only ghosts of fat cells and amorphous debris.

Hematopoietic marrow replaced by rapidly dividing mesenchymal cells and new blood vessels

Revascularization and invasion of empty marrow spaces by mesenchymal cells. Cells in the trabeculae are necrotic but the trabeculae remain mechanically intact

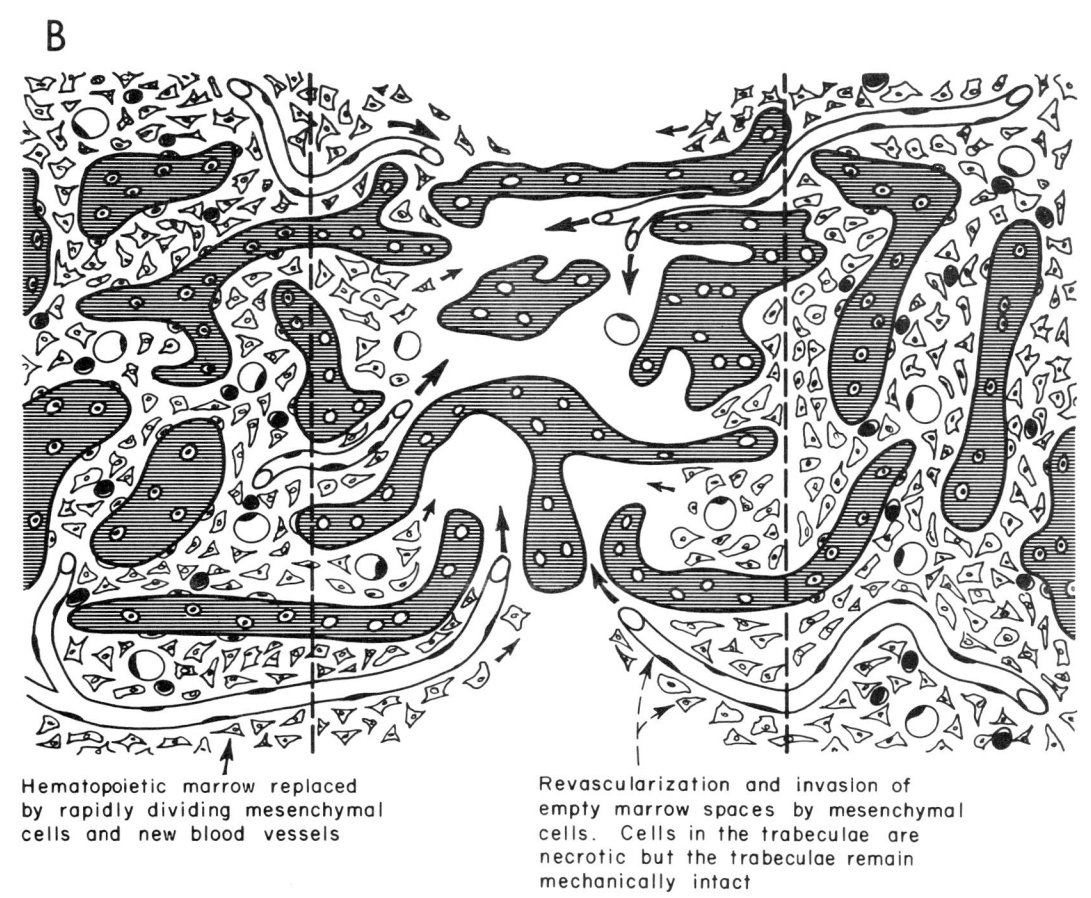

Fig. 4-1 (cont.). — **B,** 7–10 days after cell necrosis. The major biologic response is inflammatory. The chronic inflammatory tissue has gradually been replaced by sheets of mesenchymal cells. These undifferentiated cells, along with new blood vessels, begin to invade the empty marrow spaces of the necrotic bone. **(Continued.)**

The bone matrix during this phase remains unchanged mechanically, architecturally and radiographically. What remains is the normal mineralized matrix of the coarse cancellous framework devoid of living cells and blood supply.

INFLAMMATORY RESPONSE.—The live marrow of coarse cancellous bone adjacent to the dead marrow is replaced rapidly by reactive tissues. Initially there is a preponderance of acute inflammatory cells, i.e., polymorphonuclear leukocytes, but within a day or so these cells are replaced by a chronic type of inflammatory cells, i.e., lymphocytes, plasma cells, monocytes and macrophages. Some of the phagic type of cells can be observed after they have entered the infarcted areas, presumably removing necrotic marrow debris. Within 1 week of infarction, the inflammatory tissue has again changed its make-up. At this time, the vast majority of cells present are mesenchymal cells and vascular sprouts. These latter cells are proliferating rapidly and soon form a syncytium, which expands into necrotic marrow spaces be-

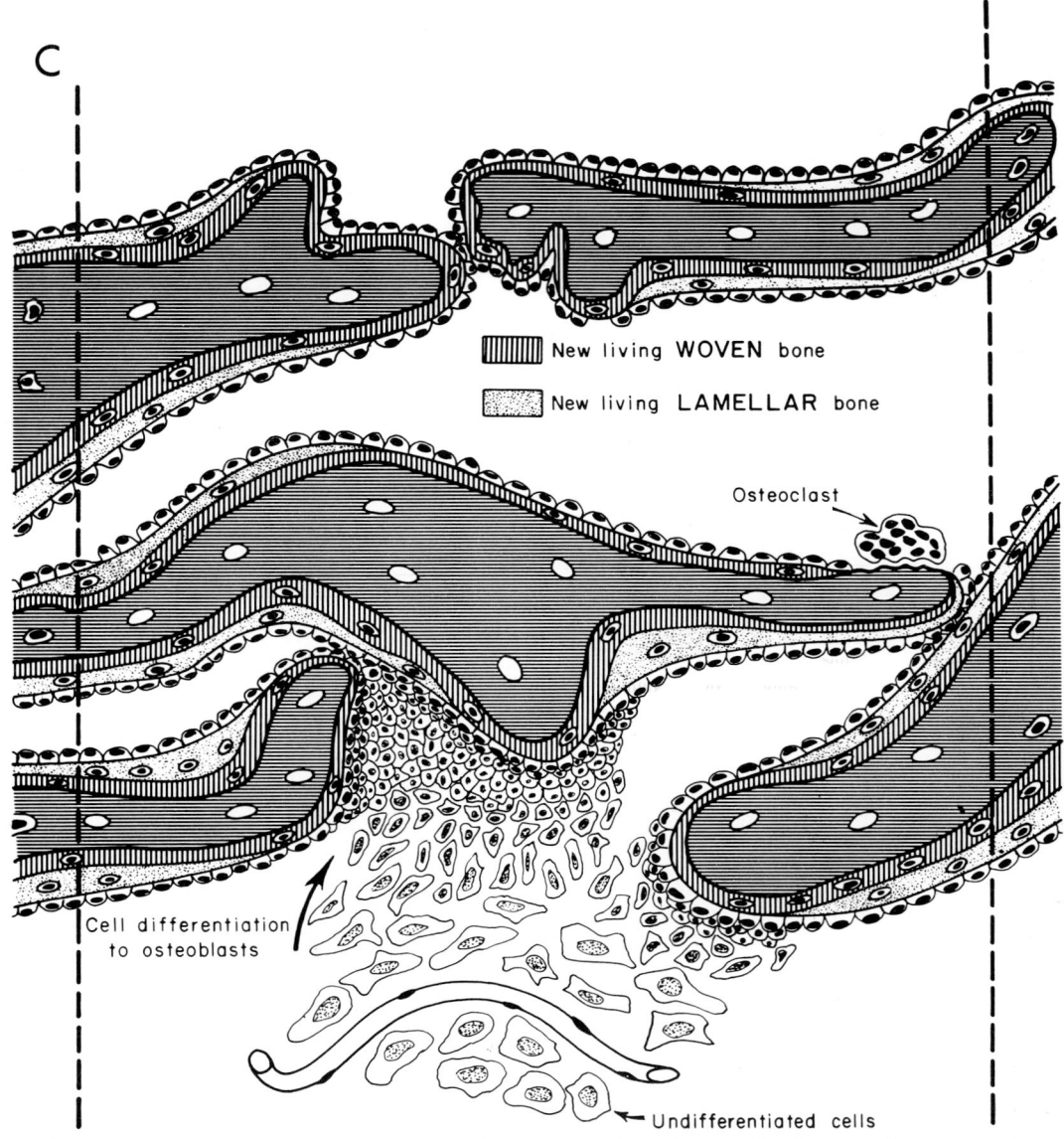

Fig. 4-1 (cont.).—C, 2–3 weeks after cell necrosis. This phase of healing is characterized by cytodifferentiation and matrix synthesis. The empty marrow spaces rapidly filled with a syncytium of mesenchyme. Somewhat behind the revascularizing tissue in space and time is cell differentiation. In some areas, the mesenchyme polarizes to certain dead trabecular bone surfaces. Here, there is a morphologic cellular transition from undifferentiated cells to cells that seem fibroblastic, to cells that resemble the basophilic polyhedric osteoblast. Early, small amounts of osteoid are secreted onto the surfaces of the dead trabeculae. Later, large amounts of new bone containing live osteocytes are added. Initially, the bone is woven by nature; later it is lamellar. Here and there a rare osteoclast may be seen apparently removing necrotic debris. **(Continued.)**

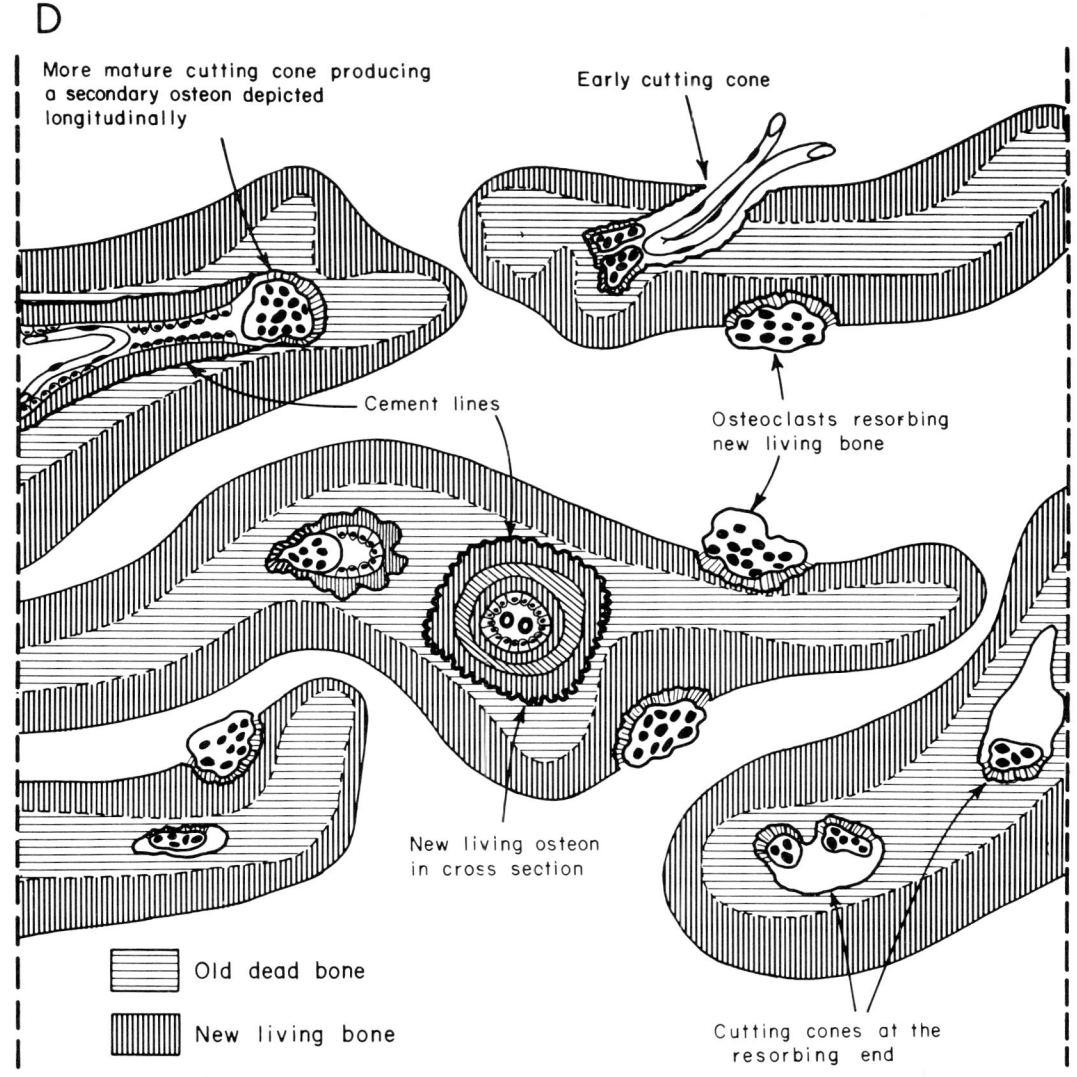

Fig. 4-1 (cont.).—D, many weeks after cell necrosis. Large volumes of new living bone have been added to the surfaces of the dead trabeculae. This increases both the physical and radiologic density of the tissue. Internal remodeling has begun. Osteoclasts are seen on the surfaces of the trabeculae and at the head of cutting cone mechanisms and functions are threefold. The first is to remove as much of the old dead bone as possible. The second is to replace the removed necrotic bone with new living bone. The third is to reduce the over-all size of the enlarged trabeculae to normal. Early and mature cutting cones are depicted in longitudinal and in cross section. Large volumes of dead bone remain. A single osteon is shown. Osteons are seen only where trabeculae are thick and therefore are found in only a few trabeculae. **(Continued.)**

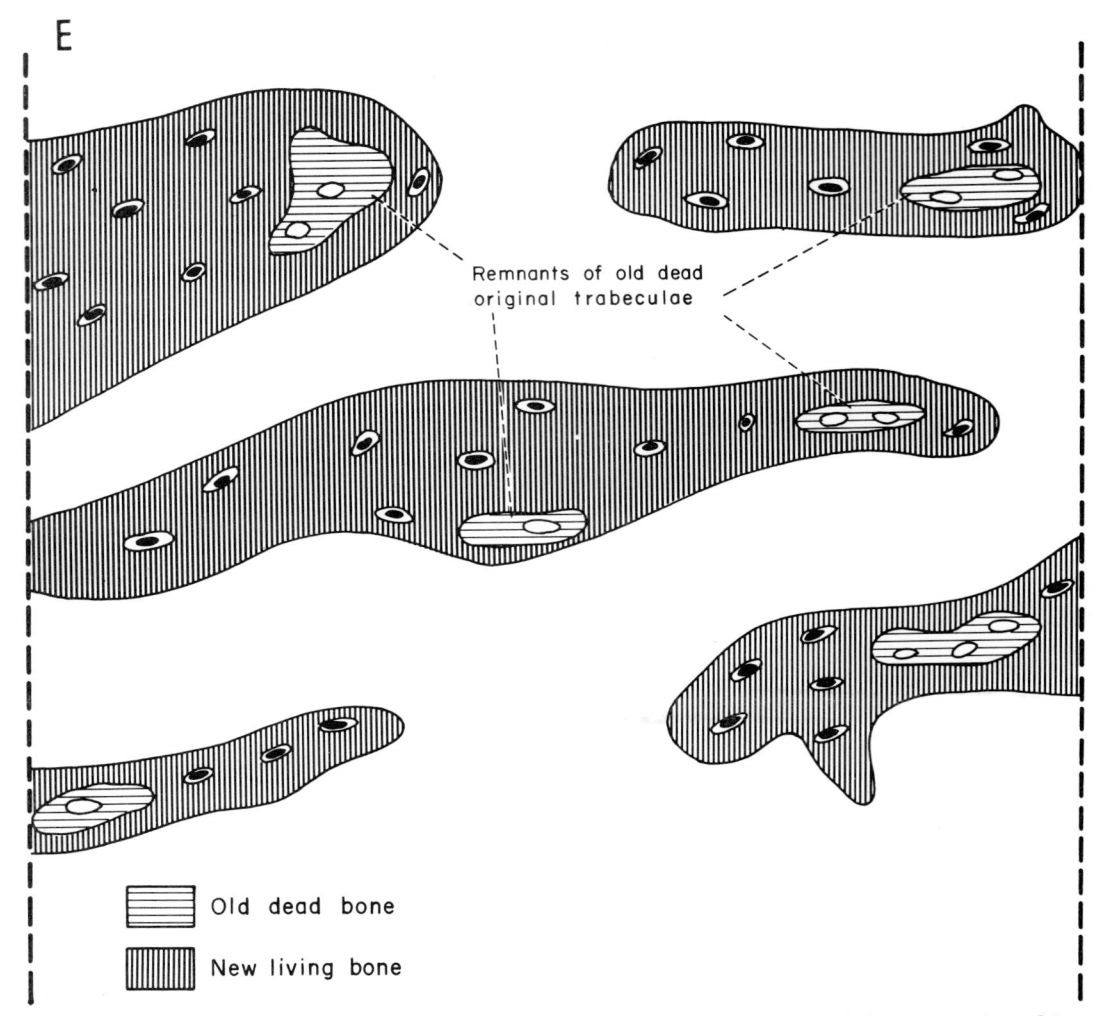

Fig. 4-1 (cont.). — **E,** months to years after cell necrosis. End-stage remodeling, manifested by slow resorption and replacement, may occur for many years. Indeed, small areas of necrotic trabeculae may be seen indefinitely.

tween necrotic bone trabeculae. This has been called granulation tissue because it resembles the revascularizing tissues in all other organs that have sustained injury.

REVASCULARIZATION. — The undifferentiated cells and vascular tuft cells continue to divide at a rapid rate without differentiation for some time, and they spread in a mass of cells into the interstices of the dead spongy bone. As there is no bony barrier to their migration, there is little need for any extensive modulation to osteoclasts at this time. The live cells merely have to move into and occupy pre-existing spaces. Bone resorption is not a prerequisite for revascularization. The syncytium of cells continues to fill the empty intertrabecular spaces until the revascularization process is complete or is interrupted by some other event.

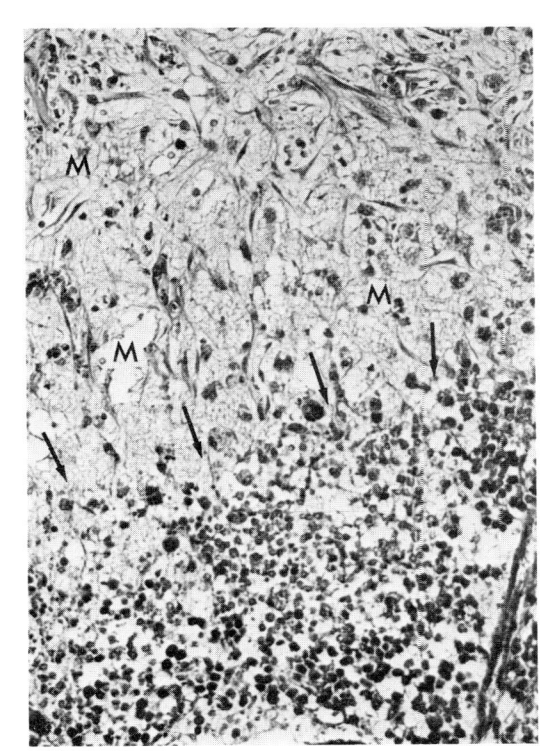

Chapter 4: REPAIR OF BONE AND FRACTURE HEALING / 79

Fig. 4-2.—The healing of dead coarse cancellous bone. Four days after cell necrosis. This medium-power photomicrograph is taken from the marrow at the junction of living and dead tissue. The tissue in the inferior third or so of the picture is necrotic marrow. The cells in this zone are dead and show various phases of cell necrosis, including pyknosis, nuclear clumping, karyolysis and total fragmentation. The tissue in the upper half of the photograph, labeled *M*, is mesenchyme. It is made up of undifferentiated cells and new blood vessels.

CYTODIFFERENTIATION.—At the same time that undifferentiated cells are spreading into empty spaces, some of the cells in more proximal spaces that have been revascularized are modulating to cells of osteogenic lineage. Some pluripotential cells become oriented and polarize their cell processes toward dead bone surfaces. The most superficial of these cells can be seen to assume a fibroblastic appearance. Appropriate histochemical stains demonstrate small amounts of collagenous matrix around these fibroblastic cells. Closer to the bone surface, the cytoplasm and cell membranes assume a polyhedric appearance, with affinity for hematoxylin, i.e., basophilia. Cytoplasmic basophilia is due to the large content of RNA and rough-surfaced endoplasmic reticulum. The nucleus becomes large and basophilic and polarizes to the side of the cell farthest away from the bone surface. A large Golgi apparatus can be seen adjacent to the nucleus and between it and the bone surface. These intracellular changes are indicative of a "blastic" cell—a cell actively secreting an extracellular material. Connective tissue stains reveal that these cells appear to have secreted a collagenous matrix against the dead bone surface. Some of the cells become com-

Fig. 4-3.—This is a high-power view from the mesenchyme of Figure 4-2. The undifferentiated cells are large cells with fairly large pole nuclei and indistinct cell membranes. The cytoplasm appears loose and may assume a spindle or stellate shape.

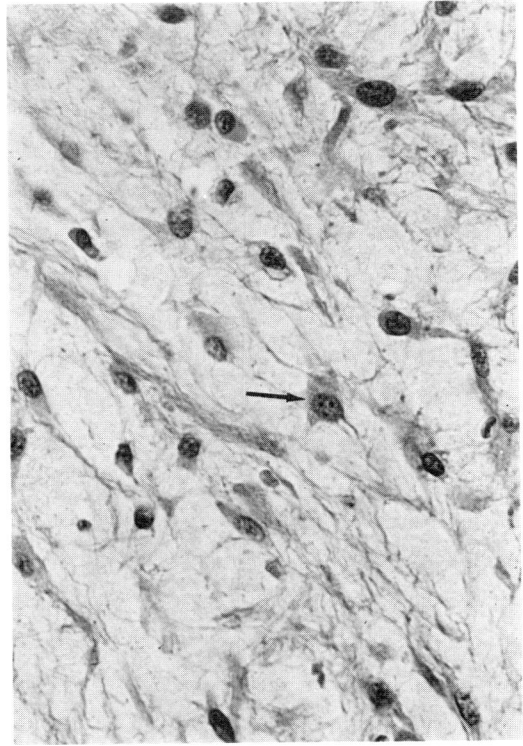

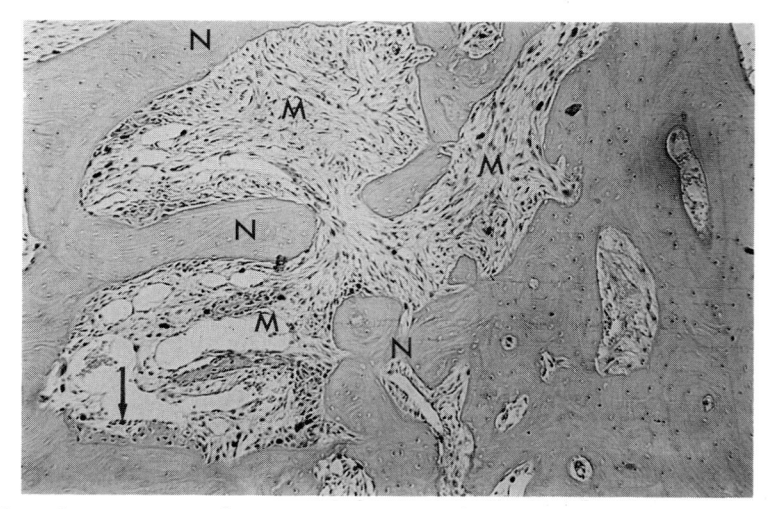

Fig. 4-4.—This photomicrograph represents revascularization. The mesenchymal tissue, M, has completely filled the intertrabecular spaces bounded by necrotic trabeculae, N. In one small area, under the arrow, there is some differentiation to osteoblasts and early new bone formation. Note that the spaces fill with loose connective tissue prior to new bone formation, both spatially and temporally.

pletely surrounded by a matrix that becomes mineralized; i.e., new bone tissue containing live osteocytes is being produced. Many of the dead trabeculae become completely surrounded by a cocoon of new live bone. Some necrotic trabeculae undergo partial resorption by osteoclasts prior to the addition of new bone;

Fig. 4-5.—Modulation and synthesis. This photograph shows mesenchymal tissue, M, streaming toward necrotic trabecular surfaces. N. As cells approach the bone surface, they undergo a modulation first toward a fibroblastic cell and then to preosteoblasts (*upper arrows*) and finally to osteoblasts. Initially, in the healing sequence, living woven bone is produced. The woven bone is obvious by the randomly scattered fat osteocytes present in large numbers and the absence of lamellation.

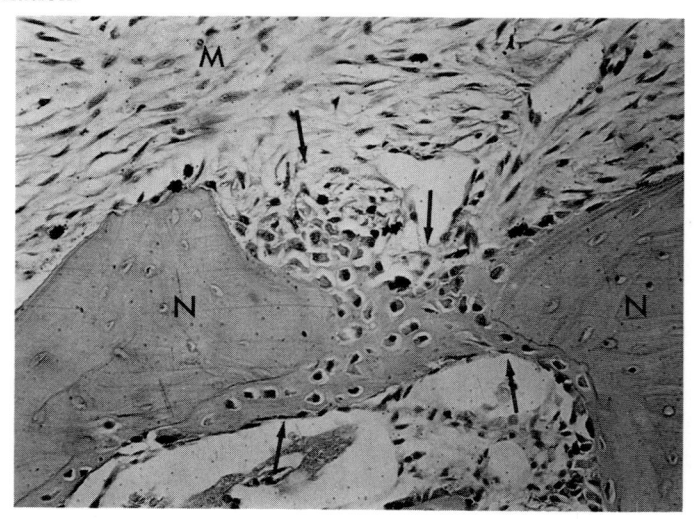

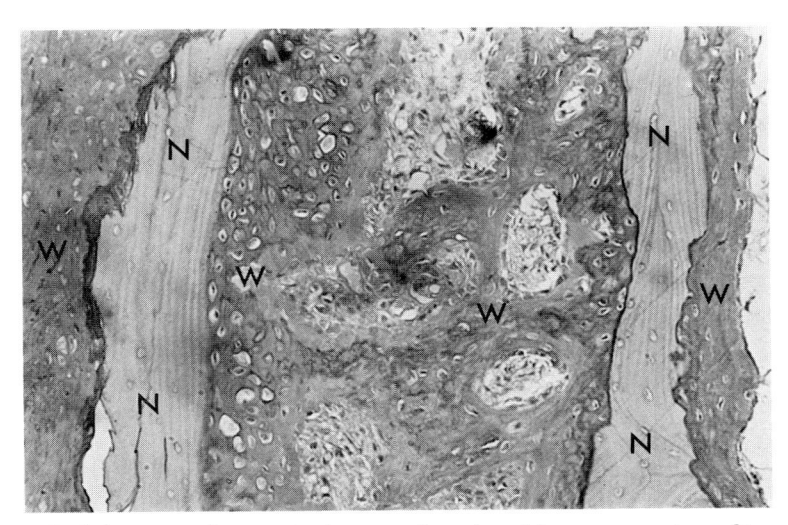

Fig. 4-6.—Two lightly stained necrotic bone trabeculae, N, are seen at medium power. The necrotic bone is lamellar in nature. Large amounts of living woven bone (W) occupy virtually the entire intertrabecular spaces. X-rays taken now would reveal an increased radiodensity in this area.

however, the majority undergo little or no preliminary resorption. As more new bone is added to pre-existing dead bone, the total mass of bone per unit volume increases and so does the radiodensity. If differentiation to osteoblasts and bone synthesis are not interrupted, all of the dead trabeculae will become coated with new living bone and the previously dead area will become more radiodense.

Fig. 4-7.—Slightly later in the healing, the nature of the new bone switches from live woven to live lamellar bone. This medium-power photomicrograph demonstrates a large central necrotic trabeculum (N) surrounded by a layer of darker-staining live woven bone (W). The woven bone, in turn, is surrounded by live lamellar bone (L). Note that there is no evidence of extensive resorption at this time.

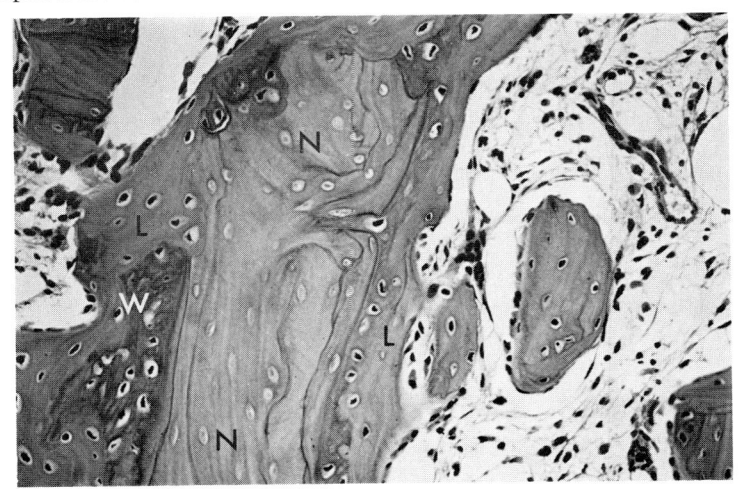

82 / John E. Kenzora

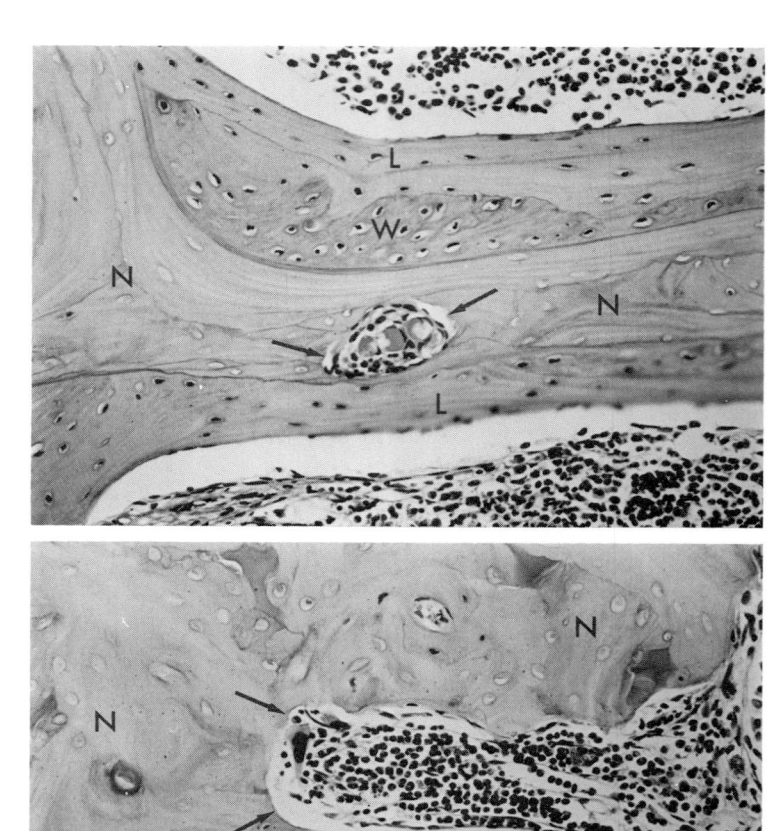

Fig. 4-8 (top).—Early remodeling. This photograph shows the same features as Figure 4-7 except that early remodeling has commenced. In the center of the necrotic bone (N), a cutting cone has resorbed the area of bone indicated by the arrows.

Fig. 4-9 (bottom).—A high-power view of a cutting cone eroding necrotic bone. The cutting cone is visualized longitudinally. The resorbing end is indicated by arrows. Here, several osteoclasts can be seen. Just behind the osteoclasts, new lamellar bone has been produced (L).

REMODELING

Appropriate cells at this terminal phase of healing recognize that large volumes of dead bone are present and that this dead bone must be removed. Locally, there is cytodifferentiation to osteoclasts and cutting cones and resorption areas now can be recognized here and there, especially in the central dead areas of the trabeculae. Dead bone is resorbed and replaced by live bone. The size of individual trabeculae is reduced to normal. Theoretically, this process continues until no dead bone remains and all trabeculae are of normal size and shape. Resorption of all necrotic bone may be complete in children and laboratory animals but only approaches completeness to varying degrees in adults.

HEALING OF NECROTIC COMPACT BONE (FIGS. 4-10–4-14)

Compact bone is located primarily in the diaphyses of long bones. The most simple form of healing, that is, healing influenced by as few variables as possible, can be studied by inducing necrosis in a diaphysis in situ, without cutting or fracturing the bone. This can be done by various means experimentally, but one method of creating necrosis is to freeze a segment of diaphysis in situ.[32, 45] Healing then may be observed over a period of time by various means, including x-ray, microradiography, histology and radioautography.

NECROSIS.—If a segment of diaphysis is frozen for an adequate period using appropriate cryosurgical apparatus, the frozen segment of bone undergoes necrosis. All cells in the exposed zone are dead by the time thawing is complete. This includes periosteum, osteocytes, osteoblasts, marrow and fat cells. All these cells undergo pyknosis, with eventual lysis. Initially, the bone will appear normal grossly, but biologically an entire cross-sectional segment of bone is necrotic. The necrotic cortical bone, at this time, is normal mechanically, radiographically and architecturally. Histologically, all cells are dead but the matrix is normal. Within a few days, most of the osteocyte lacunae will appear empty, as will the contents of haversian canals.

INFLAMMATORY RESPONSE.—Just as in the case of coarse cancellous bone, the live marrow adjacent to the dead marrow is replaced, first by acute inflammatory cells, then by chronic inflammatory cells and at 1 week by a granulomatous tissue made up primarily of undifferentiated cells and new blood vessels. Almost immediately these cells proceed to invade areas of dead marrow as a mass of new cells. On the periosteal surface, living cambial cells on each side of the necrotic periosteum undergo a hyperplastic response and build up a shoulder of undifferentiated cells. Subperiosteally, at the junction of living and dead bone, a small amount of new woven bone may be produced. The amount of new bone produced is small and the duration of response is short. This new bone never extends beyond the junction of living and dead cortex and its function remains unclear. As cell division continues, the masses of new cells on each side of the necrotic zone approach one another, thereby filling in the periosteal defect. There is some contribution to the healing periosteum from surrounding connective tissues.

Intracortically, cells in living osteons adjacent to necrotic osteons also proliferate in preparation for revascularization.

REVASCULARIZATION AND DIFFERENTIATION.—Undifferentiated cells from the three sources just described, i.e., periosteal, endosteal and osteonal, undergo a primary modulation to cutting cones or, in other words, to osteoclasts and osteoblasts. In order for healing to occur in the mass of solid cortical bone there must be space in which the healing can take place. Space is provided by the osteoclasts, which begin to core out channels in the dead bone. The channeling process begins at the junction of live and dead bone and continues into the dead bone. The live–dead junction may occur at any point along the longitudinal axis of a particular osteon. The osteoclasts proceed from periosteal, endosteal and osteonal live areas and advance by resorbing bone in front of them. In doing so, a core of dead bone is removed, providing a potentially empty channel or space in which healing may occur. As the resorption continues, more and more of the dead bone is resorbed and the cortex actually becomes osteoporotic. X-rays will show a decreased radiodensity from 2 to 4 months after the initial necrosis.[24, 32, 45]

84 / John E. Kenzora

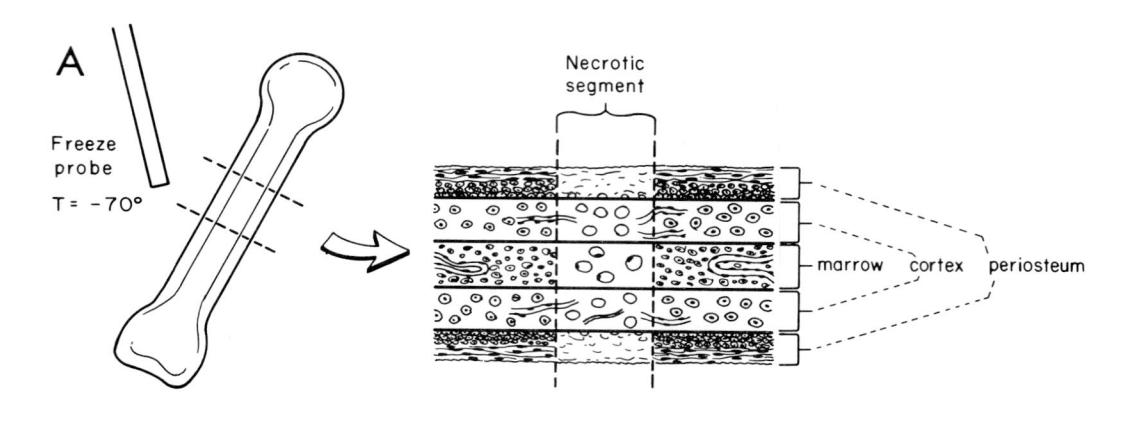

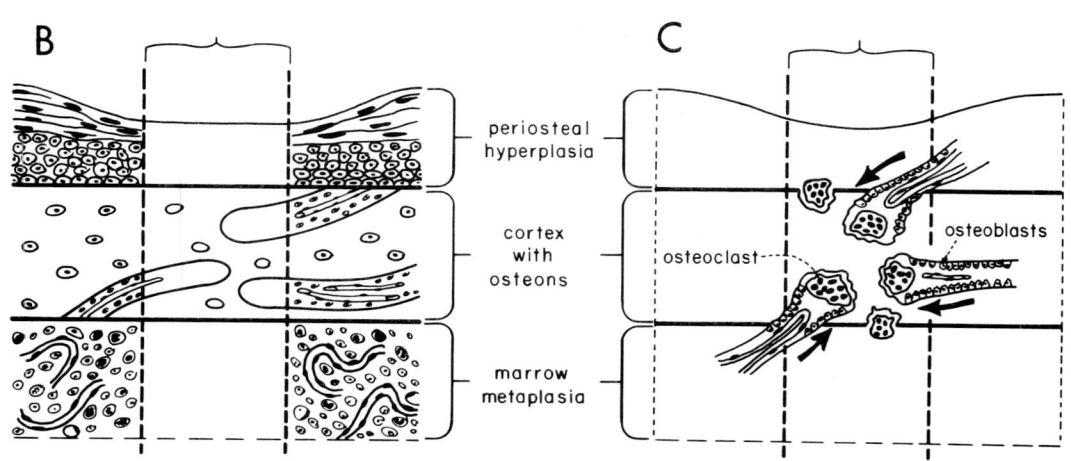

Fig. 4-10.—Healing of dead compact (diaphyseal) bone. **A**, cell necrosis. The mid-diaphyseal portion of a mature long bone is killed, using a cryosurgical probe. This permits study of bone healing without the variables encountered by a fracture gap and by motion. The diagram to the right is a low-power representation of the mid-diaphysis. Both cortices are shown. The initial biologic event is necrosis. This manifests by complete cell necrosis of the zone within the vertical dashed lines; the necrosis includes cells of the periosteum, cortex and marrow. **B**, 1 week after cell necrosis. This diagram is magnified about twice that of **A**. Only one periosteal surface and one cortex are seen. The zone within the vertical dashed lines still is necrotic. The periosteum on each side of the dead zone is hyperplastic. Undifferentiated cells within haversian canals and the marrow rapidly increase in number. **C**, 3 weeks after cell necrosis. Cutting cone mechanisms have formed from the periosteal surface, from within adjacent living osteons and from the marrow. Active resorption of the necrotic zone has begun. (**Continued.**)

During this stage, the bone resorption is so extensive that the bone may undergo a pathologic fracture. Throughout this early phase of revascularization, resorption is prominent, but there is also, to a lesser degree, concomitant bone formation.

FURTHER DIFFERENTIATION WITH SYNTHESIS.—Immediately behind the osteoclasts, both temporally and spatially, other cells modulate to osteoblasts. The osteoclasts have just cored out a large volume of bone and now undifferentiated cells from various sources stream toward

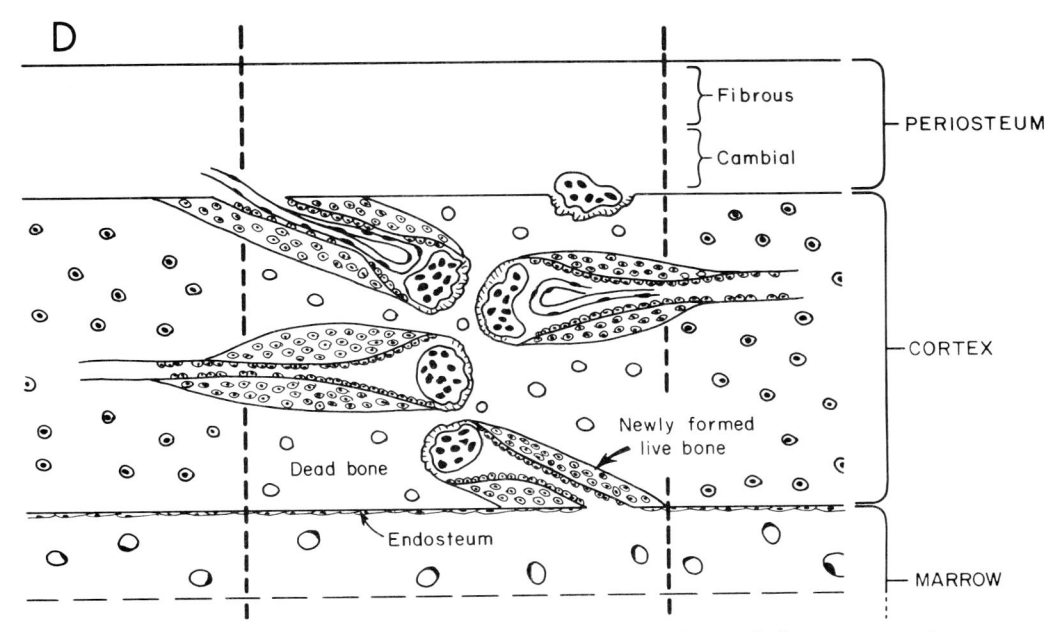

Fig. 4-10 (cont.).—D, several months after cell necrosis. This and the next two diagrams are slightly magnified from those shown in **A–C**. There has been extensive resorption in the necrotic cortex and some new bone formation. Large volumes of dead bone remain to be resorbed. The overlying previously dead periosteum has been repopulated with living cells. No new periosteal or endosteal bone has been produced. (**Continued.**)

Fig. 4-10 (cont.).—E, 4–6 months after cell necrosis. Large numbers of newly formed osteons have been produced. The necrotic segment is less porotic than in **D**. Resorption continues at a less marked level, as large volumes of dead bone still remain to be resorbed. (**Continued.**)

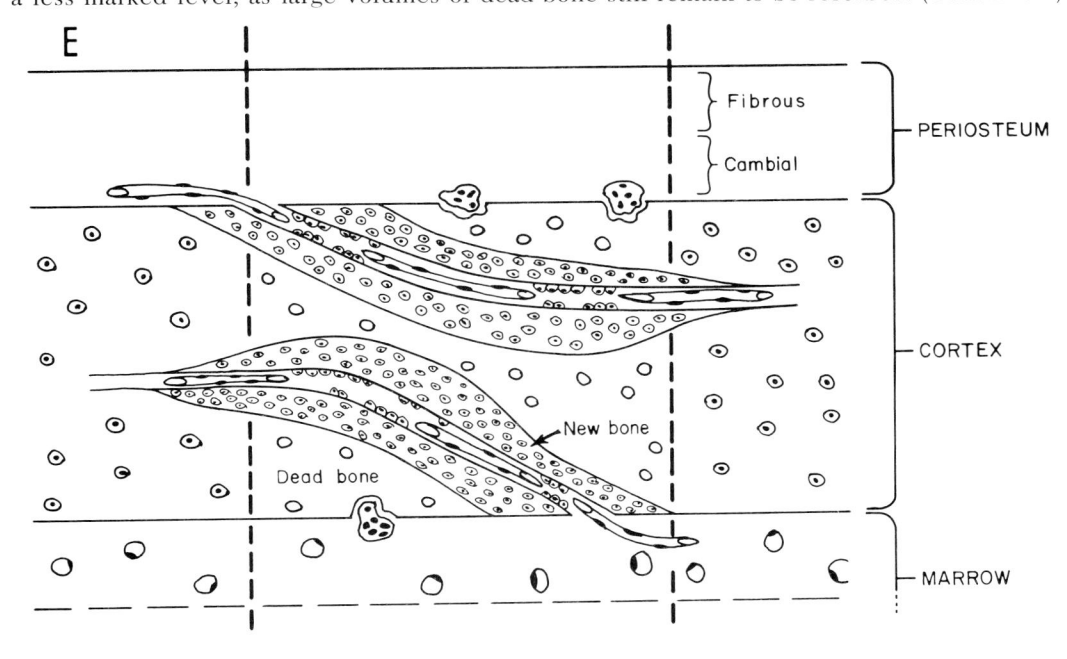

```
                    F
```

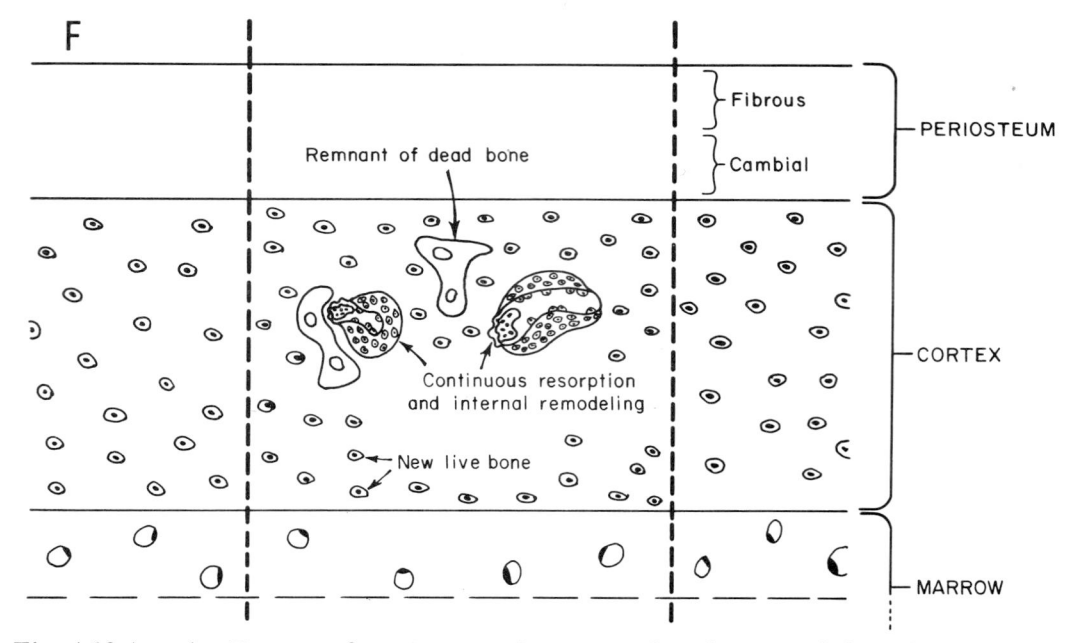

Diagram labels:
- Remnant of dead bone
- Fibrous } Cambial } PERIOSTEUM
- Continuous resorption and internal remodeling
- New live bone
- CORTEX
- MARROW

Fig. 4-10 (cont.). — F, years after necrosis. The zone within the vertical dashed lines now is mostly living osteonal bone, but small amounts of dead bone may persist forever. Internal remodeling may occur at a markedly decreased level indefinitely.

the dead bone surfaces of the hollow canal and modulate to osteoblasts, which immediately begin to synthesize new living bone on the dead bone surface and, in so doing, produce a phosphate-rich junction called a cement line. The cellular entity made up of osteoclasts eroding a core of dead bone with osteoblasts and blood vessels immediately behind is called a cutting cone.[31, 44] As described in the preceding paragraph, initially the major function of the cutting cone is resorption with minimal new bone production, whereas, in the later phases, new bone production is the major function and resorption is minimal. As new bone begins filling in the newly created channels, the osteoporosity is gradually decreased.

Cutting cones from one side of the necrotic bone continue to core out dead bone, at least until they have met cutting cones coming from the other side of the necrotic bone. The channels gradually fill in with new bone and the radiodensity gradually returns to normal.

REMODELING. — At the time living cutting cones from one side have met those from the other, large volumes of dead cortical bone still exist. This stage occurs at about 4 months experimentally. Some new cutting cones are produced continuously and indefinitely as they mimic their predecessors by removing dead bone and replacing it with live bone. The extent of this reaction, or, in other words, the amount of dead bone remaining, will be limited by a number of factors, which include age and the volume of initial necrosis. In the adult animal, about half of the dead bone has been replaced by the end of the first year and large amounts of dead bone may persist indefinitely. In the immature animal, all the dead bone may be replaced without evidence of any previous injury. Of course, in the young, this will be accomplished mainly by the ex-

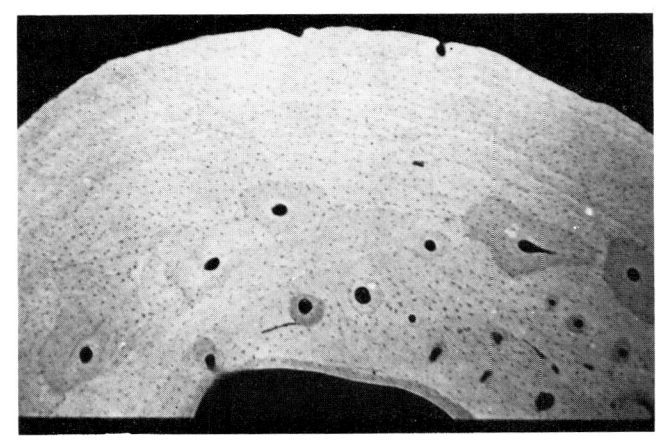

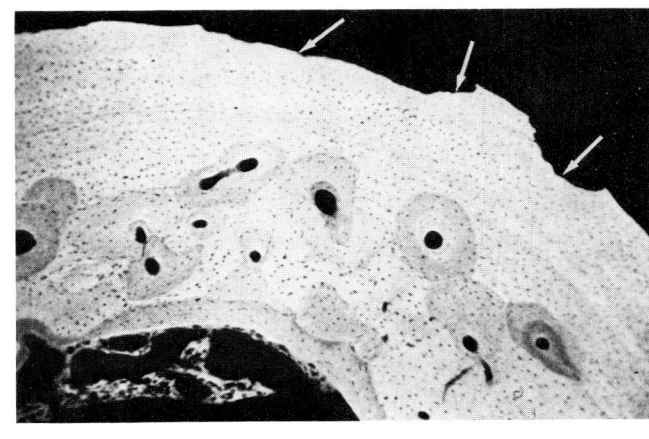

Chapter 4: REPAIR OF BONE AND FRACTURE HEALING / 87

Fig. 4-11 (top). — Healing of dead compact bone. Figures 4-11–4-14 come from the research work of Dr. Fumio Kato while at the Orthopedic Research Laboratories of the Children's Hospital Medical Center, Harvard Medical School. Figure 4-11 is a microradiograph of a control adult monkey ulna. Note the relatively smooth periosteal and endosteal surfaces. The majority of the haversian systems are mature, as indicated by the radiodensity surrounding the canals. A few osteons appear somewhat darker, indicating incomplete mineralization.

Fig. 4-12 (bottom). — Three to 4 weeks after a segment of ulnar diaphysis was killed, the present situation is seen near the junction of living and dead cortex. There is extensive periosteal resorption, as indicated by the arrows. Cutting cone mechanisms from adjacent living osteons and from the marrow cavity are not yet apparent.

ternal remodeling potential of cylinderization, whereby the entire cortex may be resorbed endosteally and replaced subperiosteally. This process will be elucidated later.

HEALING OF A SMALL HOLE IN BONE (FIGS. 4-15–4-19)

Bone healing to this point has been discussed without the variables of motion and size of the fracture gap. These variables now will be introduced.[4, 69, 72] Experimentally, a small drill hole is made in the diaphysis of adult rabbits and the healing studied at various intervals. There is virtually no motion; only a small gap must be filled in. The pattern of events will be followed in the same sequence as that already outlined. The injury caused by drilling a small hole in bone is not extensive. The periosteum is necrosed at the site of penetration, as is all the bone and marrow for a millimeter or two around the hole. Blood rapidly fills the gap and clots. Within hours, large numbers of polymorphs are seen within the clot in the fracture gap and in the marrow; by 24 hours, many lymphocytes, plasma cells and macrophages are seen. The normal marrow in the vicinity of the drill hole is replaced by granulation tissue made up primarily of undifferentiated cells. The nature of the periosteal "inflammatory response" is somewhat different. Even with this relatively small injury, the periosteum responds 360 degrees around the bone and for extensive

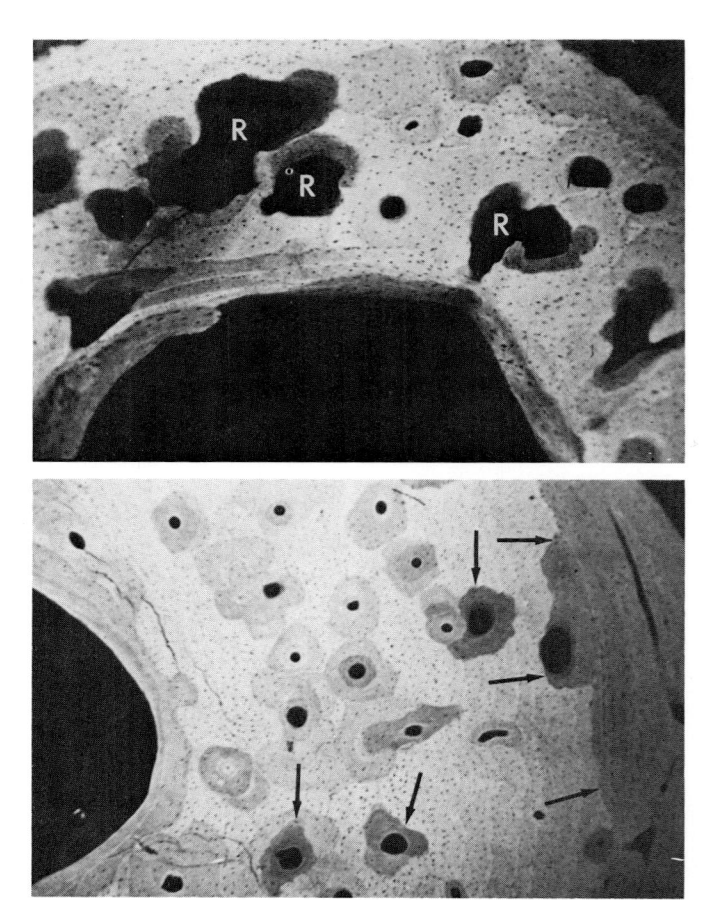

Fig. 4-13 (top).—Between 8 and 16 weeks, the cortex appears markedly porotic. During this time, the bone is mechanically weak. The porosity is produced by cutting cones from adjacent living osteons intracortically and from newly formed cutting cones from the periosteum and endosteum. R indicates resorption cavities. There is some minimal new bone formation demonstrated by dark gray areas around portions of the circumference of the resorption canals.

Fig. 4-14 (bottom).—Between 6 and 12 months after necrosis, new bone formation predominates. Newly formed bone is incompletely mineralized and appears darker by microradiography. The darker the bands surrounding the canals the more immature the bone with regard to mineralization. Full mineralization may require many months. The horizontal arrows indicate new periosteal bone, the vertical arrows newly formed osteons. At the end of 1 year, about 50% of the bone has been replaced with live bone; the other 50% is the original necrotic bone. Further resorption and replacement continue indefinitely at a much slower rate.

distances up and down the length of the bone. The cambium, or deep cell layer of periosteum, becomes many times thicker, primarily due to division of the undifferentiated cells located here. The fibrous periosteum nearest the small hole is lifted from the bone surface by a nubbin of underlying hyperplastic cells, which, in effect, forms an elevated ring around the hole. These same cells, with further multiplication, begin to cross the fracture gap through the clot and approach the opposite side. When the cells meet over the gap, they continue dividing, forming a mound of cells resembling a blastema. The endosteum responds in

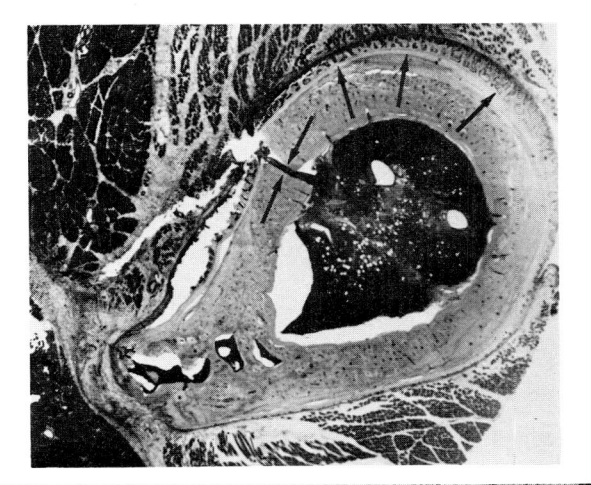

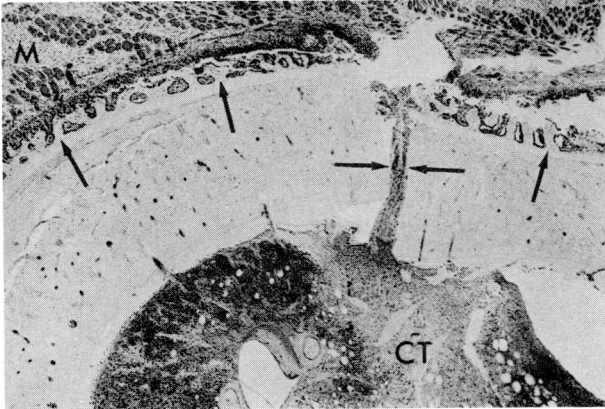

Chapter 4: REPAIR OF BONE AND FRACTURE HEALING / 89

Fig. 4-15 (top). — Figures 4-15–4-19 depict the healing of a small drill hole in bone. Figure 4-15 is a very low-power cross section of an adult rabbit femur. A small defect, seen between the arrows, was made 1 week before. A hematoma may be seen in the gap and adjacent marrow. Already the periosteum has reacted by forming new woven bone around most of the bone circumference.

Fig. 4-16 (bottom). — The defect at 2 weeks is between the horizontal arrows. The hematoma no longer is in evidence. In its place, in the gap, periosteally and endosteally, sheets of undifferentiated connective tissue (*CT*) are seen. Undifferentiated cells are also seen in large numbers between muscle bundles (*M*). The vertical arrows point out newly formed periosteal woven bone. Several small trabeculae of new bone have formed within the fracture gap.

the same manner, but this layer of cells is much thinner than the periosteum and the reaction therefore is less extensive. Blood vessels from the marrow cavity and periosteal surface enter the gap and introduce undifferentiated cells into the gap. By 3 days, some of the cells have modulated to osteoblasts and new woven bone trabeculae can be seen subperiosteally and subendosteally adjacent to the gap and occasionally in the gap itself. The subperiosteal and endosteal new bone is appositional whereas that in the midst of the marrow and gap, away from the bone surfaces, is purely intramembranous by formation (formed from mesenchyme and without a bony template). By 1 week, the periosteum and endosteum again are intact layers and a few underlying woven bone trabeculae have bridged the gap. Simultaneously, new bone has been produced around the entire circumference of bone and up and down the shaft for long distances. Woven bone trabeculae continue to form until the gap is filled and a small mound of new bone exists subperiosteally and endosteally. The majority of these trabeculae are oriented at right angles to the bone shaft.

Over the next 2–3 weeks, the trabecular bone becomes compacted with the addition of more new bone on the sides of the original trabeculae. The bone trabeculae originally filling the gap were woven in nature and oriented perpendicular to the shaft. Then, primary lamellar

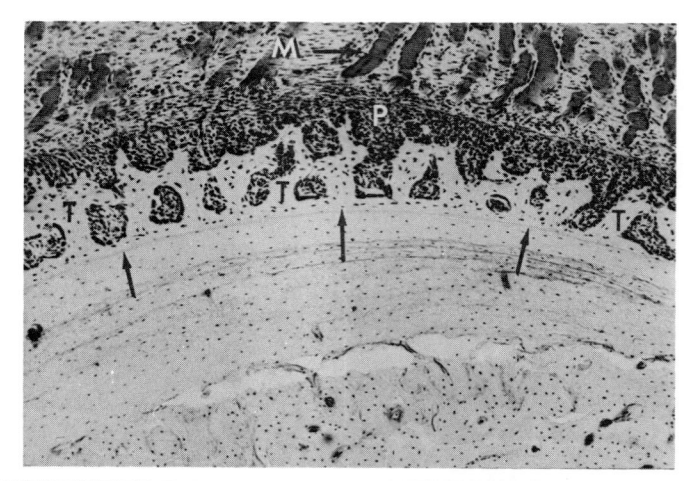

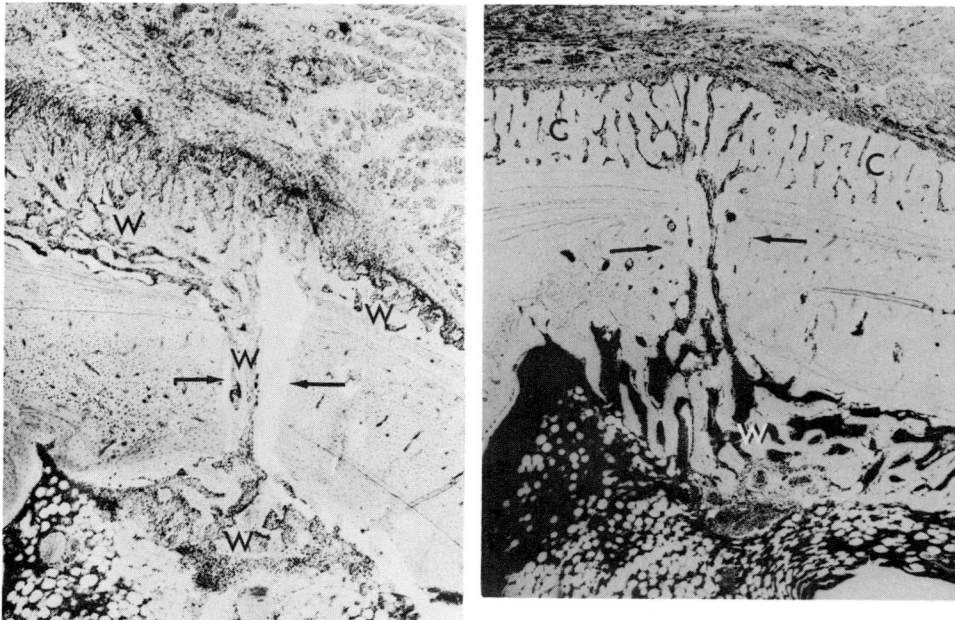

Fig. 4-17 (top).—This is a medium-power photomicrograph of the periosteal reaction at 2 weeks. The vertical arrows point to the line that represents the bone surface prior to the injury. Newly formed woven bone trabeculae (*T*) are seen, with their major orientation at right angles to the bone surface. The cambial layer of periosteum (*P*) is several times thicker than normal and tends to blend with proliferating cells between muscle fibers (*M*).

Fig. 4-18 (bottom left).—This was taken several days after the Figure 4-17. Arrows demarcate the defect. Now, large amounts of woven bone (*W*) can be seen covering the gap on the periosteal and endosteal surfaces. Within the gap a small amount of woven bone is seen.

Fig. 4-19 (bottom right).—Between 3 and 4 weeks, the gap is completely filled with woven trabecular bone. The periosteal new bone is now compacted (*C*), whereas the endosteal new bone (*W*) remains spongy. At this stage, the gap is completely filled with new bone but this new bone still is woven in nature and oriented at 90 degrees to the normal.

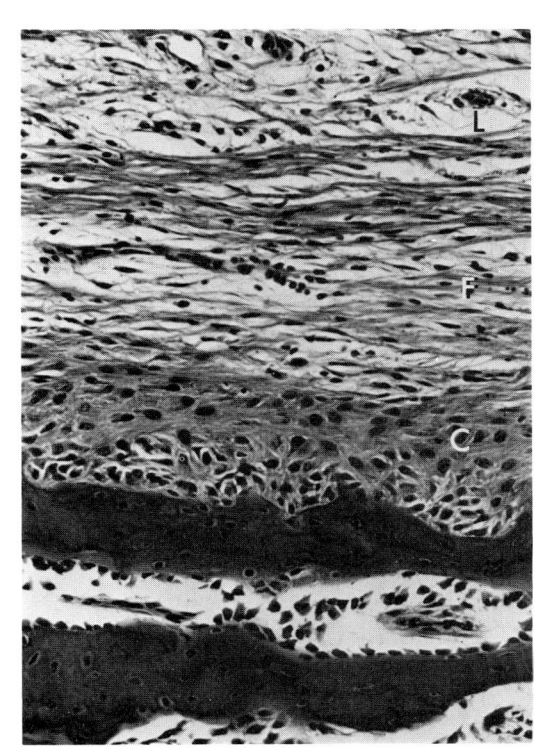

Fig. 4-20. — A high-power view of normal periosteum from a growing rabbit long bone. The periosteum is made up of two distinct layers. The cambium (C) is the deeper layer and in a growing animal may be many cell layers thick, as seen here. The deepest cells of this layer are osteoblasts, the superficial cells are undifferentiated. Between are the preosteoblasts. The other, more superficial, layer of periosteum is the fibrous (F) layer. This layer is made up of fibroblasts and collagen fibers that run parallel to the bone surface. Loose areolar connective tissue (L) surrounds the periosteum and extends into all the fascial planes.

bone was added to the woven trabecular surfaces and the large intertrabecular spaces gradually filled in.

The callus that bridges the gap at about 3 weeks thus is a mixture of woven and lamellar bone. No cartilage has been produced. There has been virtually no contribution to healing from the bone ends themselves.

Over the next few months, however, cutting cones from endosteum, periosteum and diaphyseal osteons slowly resorb the reactive bone in the fracture gap and replace it with bone of the same nature and fiber orientation as that in the rest of the shaft. Excess bone in the periosteal and endosteal callus mass is resorbed. The defect is healed when there is no evidence that there ever was a bone defect. The total time to heal this defect is much longer than one might think.

HEALING OF A FRACTURED DIAPHYSIS TREATED BY EXTERNAL CAST IMMOBILIZATION
(FIGS. 4-21 – 4-26)

A situation analogous to the common midshaft fracture treated by closed reduction and cast application is discussed here. The most simple experimental fracture of this nature to study is the midshaft transverse fracture. The most consistent way to produce and reproduce the injury is to break the shaft and periosteum transversely, using an osteotome or power saw. Moreover, soft tissue interposition is minimized by this technique. Attempts to break the shaft manually produce wide variations in the nature of the fracture and in the extent of soft tissue injury; therefore, this method is not used. An external cast is applied and the fracture studied at various time intervals after sacrificing the animal.

The initial situation is dissimilar to that in the preceding section because the defect is a complete fracture and the plaster cast permits gross motion at the fracture site. That is, there will be rotary motion and, in addition, there will be shear, bending and tractional forces to contend with. End-to-end fragment alignment and apposition will not be as good.

Immediately following the osteotomy, an extensive hematoma forms (Fig. 4-21, A). Hemorrhage will be much greater than in previous situations because the relatively poor apposition and increased motion create a larger dead space and potential for some continual trauma. As

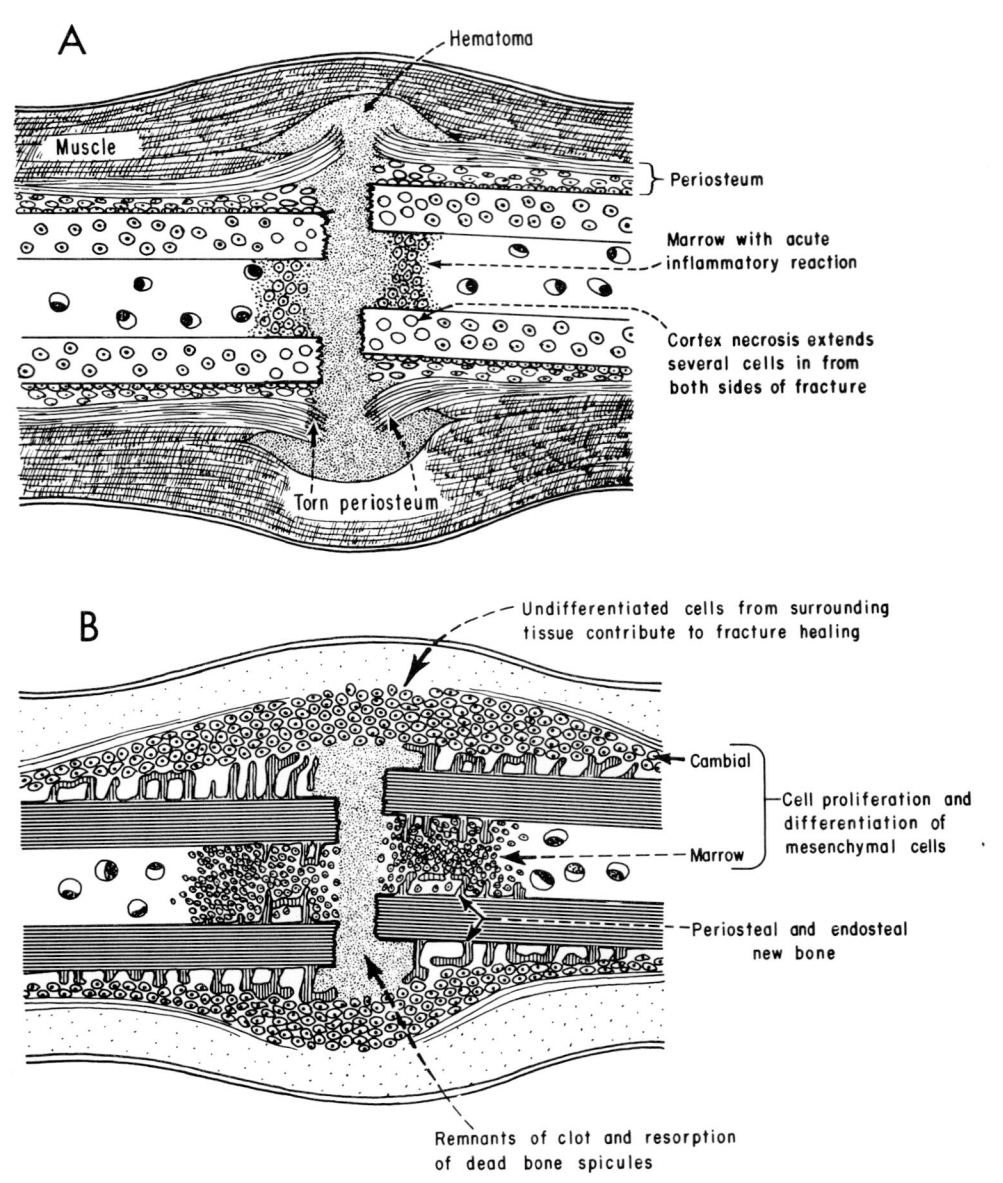

Fig. 4-21.—Fracture healing. Figure 4-21, **A–E** illustrates the biology of fracture healing in the situation in which a diaphyseal fracture is immobilized in a cast. The bone depicted is adult. **A,** 24 hours after fracture. At this time, an extensive hematoma has formed between the fracture fragments. There is necrosis of all cell types, for a millimeter or so, on both sides of the fracture gap. Soft tissues are swollen and inflamed. Histologically, an acute inflammatory response is noted in the marrow on each side of the necrotic zone.—**B,** 1 week after fracture. The periosteum is hyperplastic along the entire diaphysis, with the cambial layer becoming several times thicker than normal. The periosteum over the fracture gap is thicker than anywhere else. The cells that make up this virtual blastema come from the live cambial cells from each side of the fracture gap and from undifferentiated cells in surrounding connective tissue. New woven bone trabeculae have formed appositionally on each side of the fracture and soon will form along the entire diaphysis. The marrow cavity has transformed into a massive syncytium of mesenchyme except in the fracture gap itself. Here, significant clot still remains. (**Continued.**)

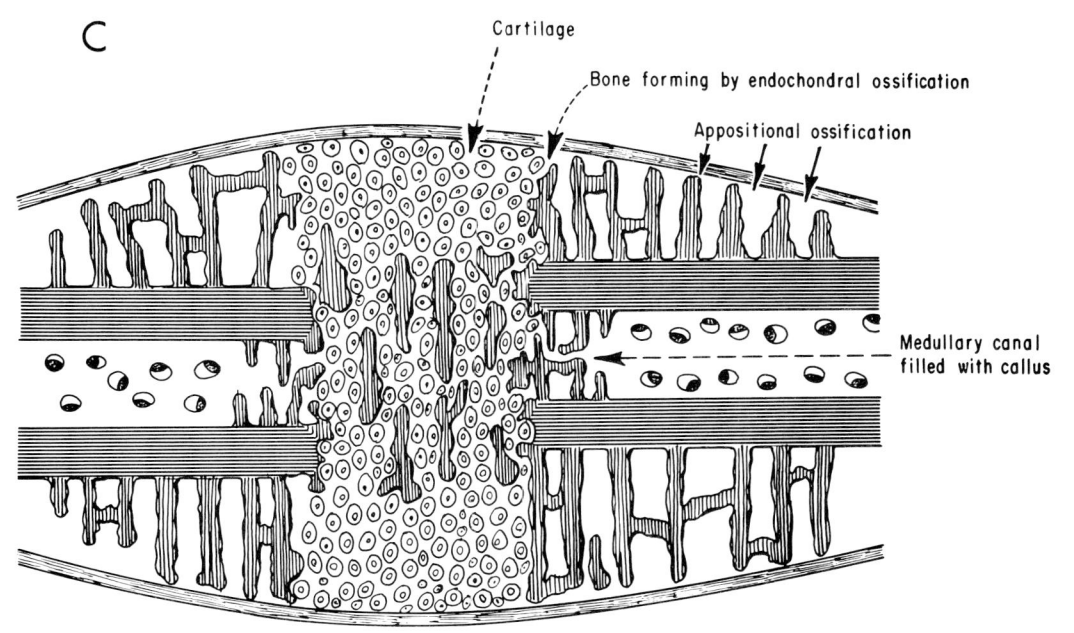

Fig. 4-21 (cont.).—**C**, 3 weeks after fracture: fragments weakly joined. By now, large volumes of woven trabecular bone have formed along the diaphysis periosteally, more forming near the fracture than distally. Similar bone forms in the marrow cavity near the fracture site. This type of bone is called "fine cancellous" because of its gross appearance. Depending on local environment, various amounts of hyaline cartilage are produced. The bone trabeculae that form along the edges of the cartilage do so by an endochondral ossification sequence, whereas the remainder of the trabeculae form appositionally. The cartilage is continuously resorbed as more and more trabeculae form by the endochondral sequence. The fracture is well stuck together, as depicted diagrammatically, but there is no bony union. Even so, this early callus acts as an internal splint that resists motion and produces a more beneficial environment for bone formation. (**Continued.**)

in all the other injuries, there is complete cell necrosis on each side of the fracture surface for several millimeters periosteally, endosteally and intraosteally. Within hours, an acute inflammatory response is evident in the live marrow adjacent to dead marrow and in the soft tissues around the periosteum. Over the next few days, this is replaced by a chronic inflammatory response with large numbers of macrophages, which appear to remove necrotic debris. The entire periosteum undergoes a hyperplastic response and begins growing around and through the hematoma. Subperiosteal bone is produced almost immediately, more forming close to the fracture site than at more distal locations (Fig. 4-21, B).

A limited modulation to osteoclasts occurs between the fracture fragments. These cells are seen resorbing bits of dead bone matrix debris in the blood clot and may resorb small amounts of dead bone on the end of each fragment. This is not a major cellular response but it may be sufficient to be manifested radiologically by an apparent increase in the size of the fracture gap.

Endosteally, the marrow changes its cellular make-up for large distances on each side of the fracture. Undifferentiated cells and newly forming blood vessels rapidly replace the hematopoietic elements and soon begin to invade the necrotic marrow and hematoma between the fracture ends.

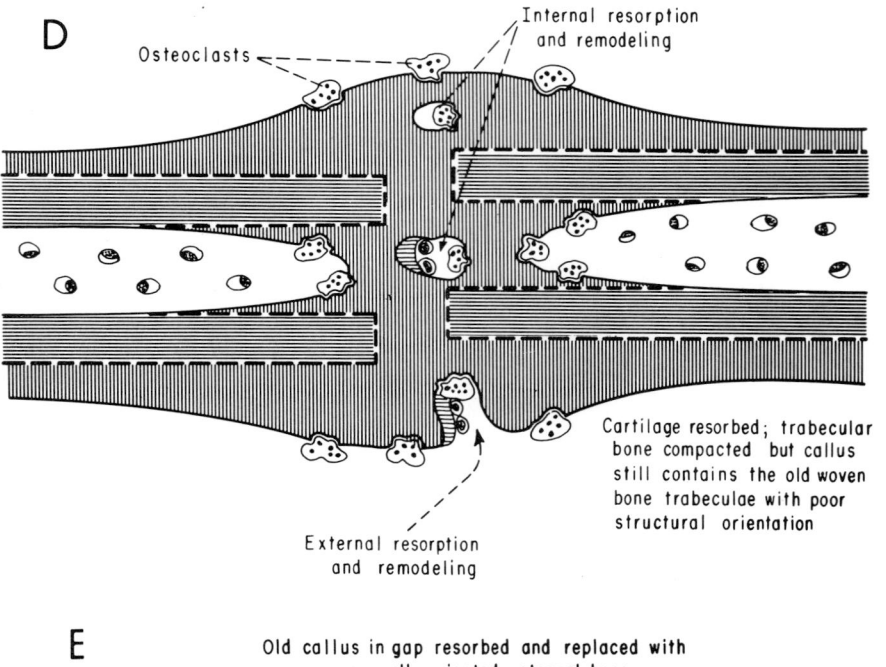

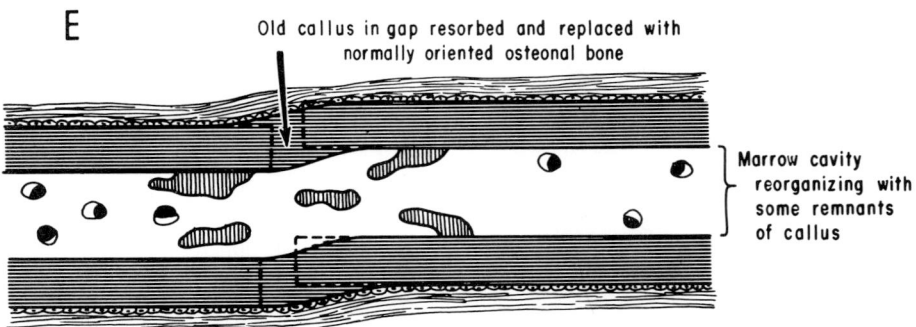

Fig. 4-21 (cont.).—D, 6–12 weeks after fracture. When most of the cartilage has been resorbed there is early bone union. This diagram demonstrates bony union. During this time interval, the fine cancellous bone, which made up the earlier bony callus, becomes compacted. Compaction occurs as additional living lamellar bone is added to the surfaces of the fine cancellous trabeculae. As more and more bone is added, the intertrabecular spaces decrease in size and the physical and radiologic densities increase. The marrow cavity remains plugged with this compact bone. The organization and architecture of the callus, however, are poor. This is illustrated by changes in lamination, which are shown at 90 degrees to one another. External and internal remodeling has started. E, years after the fracture. All excess callus has been resorbed. The poorly oriented bone of the preceding phase has been replaced by high-quality osteonal bone in normal orientation. The dashed lines indicate the position of the original fragments. The marrow cavity has been restored as a result of long-term endosteal resorption; however, some remnants of the original callus may persist indefinitely, as indicated. Because the bone is adult, the potential for external remodeling is minimal and displacement has not been corrected.

Experimental studies by Rhinelander[70, 71] revealed that the endosteal vessels, which are ramifications of the nutrient artery, are primarily responsible for vascularizing the callus. Once revascularization of the fracture gap and hematoma is completed, a pool of undifferentiated cells exists, which may modu-

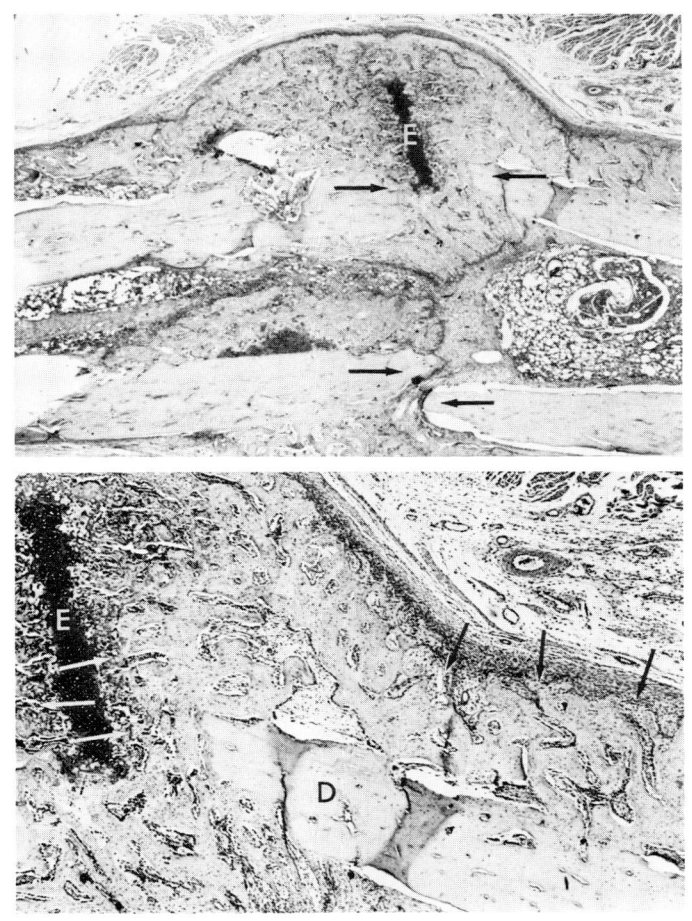

Fig. 4-22. (top).—This photograph illustrates an adult long bone fracture, reduced without significant angulation or displacement and immobilized with a tight-fitting plaster cast. Six weeks after fracture there is early bony union. Arrows depict the fracture sites of both cortices. A large mound of callus is seen over the cortex. The dark vertical band marked E is cartilage. Bone immediately on each side is forming by endochondral ossification. Farther away, on each side of the fracture, the bone of the callus has formed appositionally from the periosteum.

Fig. 4-23 (bottom).—A medium-power view of Figure 4-22. The cortical bone near the fracture is dead (D). The reactive bone forming above the cortex (*vertical arrows*) is appositional, having been formed from periosteum. Horizontal arrows indicate bone forming by endochondral ossification (E).

late under appropriate local environmental stimuli. For a week or so, these cells maintain a mesenchymal appearance. Trueta also has studied the vascularity during fracture healing and believes that the periosteal blood supply is more significant because fractures healed better when the endosteal blood vessels were destroyed than when the periosteal vessels were interrupted.[15, 86] In any case, it seems that a fracture will heal satisfactorily if either source is intact and that both contribute vessels and cells to the callus. Cells from the hyperplastic periosteum, meanwhile, grow around and through the hematoma, between the bone ends, to meet similar cells from the other side. The fibrous nature of the periosteum initially is lost as dividing cells traverse the fracture gap and hematoma; indeed, the cambial cells blend in with connective tissue cells of overlying muscle and fascia (Fig. 4-21, B). The surrounding soft tissue connective tissues supply both undifferentiated cells and blood vessels to the external forming callus. As just described, the most abundant blood supply to the callus is found endosteally and periosteally near the fracture edges and this is also where most of the new woven bone is laid down initially (Fig. 4-21, B and C and Figs. 4-22–4-26). The physiologic fact that living bone must have a blood supply whereas cartilage is nourished by diffusion bears repeating at this time. Cytodifferentiation to osteoblasts

Fig. 4-24 (top).—A high-power view of callus bone forming by endochondral ossification. Primary trabeculae (i.e., trabeculae with cartilage cores) are seen along each side of the central mass of cartilage (*C*).

Fig. 4-25 (bottom).—This pattern probably is a more typical picture of cast immobilization fracture healing. With more and more motion, large amounts of cartilage (*C*) are produced. Cartilage is seen extruding from well above the periosteal surface (*oblique arrows*) down between the fragments (*horizontal arrows*) and through the entire marrow cavity. Large volumes of fine cancellous woven bone (*W*) are seen on each side of the cartilage. The entire marrow cavity is stuffed full of callus. Bony union will occur as soon as bone trabeculae replace the central cartilage areas and meet trabeculae from the opposite side. The fracture depicted here clinically would be stuck together, but rather weakly.

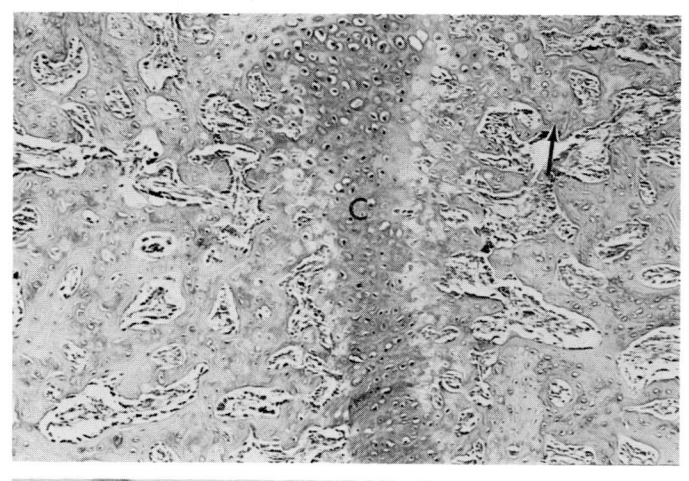

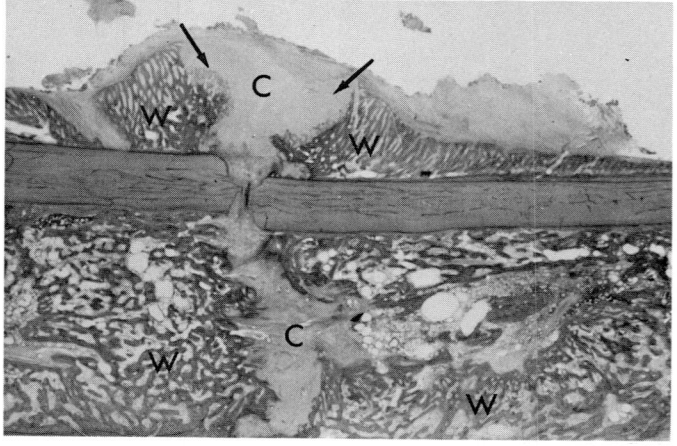

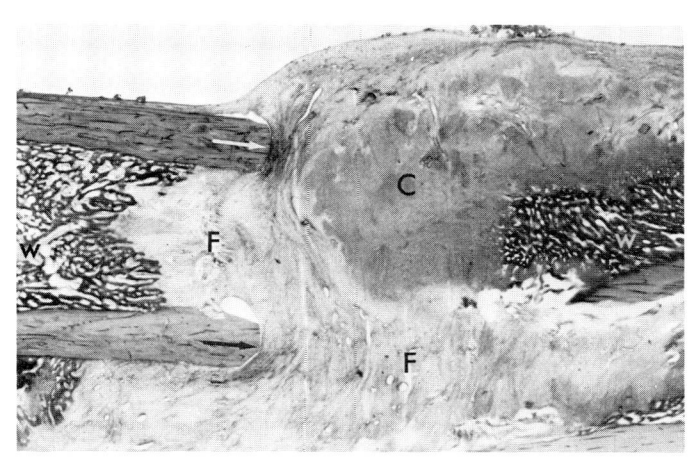

Fig. 4-26.—Loose case immobilization. With gross motion occurring at the fracture site, large volumes of cartilage (C) and fibrous tissue (F) are produced. Large amounts of woven bone form in addition, but at some distance from the fracture site. As long as motion persists, the fracture will not unite by bone and a fibrocartilaginous delayed union or nonunion will result.

occurs in these highly vascularized locations and for short distances into the fracture gap also. These cells produce new, fine cancellous woven bone trabeculae, which are oriented perpendicular to the bone surface. More centrally in the fracture defect, undifferentiated cells appear to infiltrate the hematoma at a greater rate than new blood vessels. The resulting paucity of blood vessels indicative of relative anoxia, together with continual motion in the fracture gap, produces an environment conducive to cell modulation to chondrocytes, and consequently large amounts of cartilage are produced between, above and below the bone ends (Figs. 4-21, C and 4-26). The bone ends now are held together by a weak callus that will tend to resist further gross motion. Callus is the aggregate of all the reactive tissues produced in response to the fracture. At this stage of the healing, this includes bone, cartilage and fibrous connective tissues, together with their accompanying cells.[20, 21, 41, 81] In addition, mast cells are seen throughout the healing stages but are present in largest numbers during the early stages. These cells contain vasoactive materials and heparin and they may play significant roles in the inflammatory response and in controlling cytodifferentiation and remodeling.[26, 53, 73] Heparin is known to inhibit new bone production in tissue culture and thus the mast cell could help regulate fracture healing by shutting off or allowing bone production.

The cartilaginous component of the callus is progressively removed by cells surrounding blood vessels and by chondroclasts and is replaced by osteoblasts, which secrete new bone onto freshly cored cartilage surfaces. In other words, an active endochondral ossification sequence is established similar in appearance and function to an epiphyseal plate. The majority of cartilage is located subperiosteally, but significant amounts may be seen in the endosteal callus close to the fracture gap and between the bone ends themselves. Endochondral new bone formation continues to replace the cartilage until most of the cartilage is gone. When this is completed, the fracture is united by a bony bridge for the first time. Fine cancellous woven bone trabeculae will comprise the bulk of the fracture callus, but trabeculae with cartilage cores (primary trabeculae) are found where cartilage was located previously. The over-all orientation of the trabeculae is perpendicular to the shaft, in a sunburst pattern. Now, motion at the fracture site has been eliminated and the large spaces between the trabeculae begin to fill in with additional bone, but this is primary lamellar bone in nature. This new lamellar bone is secreted onto the surfaces of the woven bone trabeculae in a centripetal manner, gradually eliminating the spaces of the fine cancellous network.

The cancellous bone undergoes a progressive compaction, which ceases when the callus is converted to compact bone. The callus of the marrow cavity, fracture gap and periosteum now comprise a solid mass of new bone of greater than adequate quantity but of poor mechanical quality and distribution (Fig. 4-21, D).

Remodeling processes begin to remove the excess endosteal and periosteal bone callus primarily by osteoclastic resorption. Cutting cones from endosteal, periosteal and osteonal sources then enter the callus bone in the fracture gap and replace the poor-quality bone with osteonal bone.

Not only does the quality of bone improve from a mixture of woven and primary lamellar bone to one of pure haversian bone but the orientation of the osteons becomes normal and the distribution of material ideal.

Osteoclasts eventually remove all the endosteal and periosteal callus, thereby restoring the medullary canal and normal external geometry of the bone. Hematopoietic elements replace the endosteal callus. When all callus in the fracture gap has been replaced by osteonal bone and there is little or no histologic evidence of the initial bone injury, the fracture is biologically healed. Complete biologic healing can be expected in growing children. In the adult, remodeling may never be complete and histologic and radiographic evidence of the original injury may persist until death (Fig. 4-21, E).

In summary, the healing depicted here, which is essentially that which occurs with most long bone fractures treated in a cast, differs from other situations in that motion occurs at the fracture site, apposition is not as good and there may be some malalignment. These mechanical differences are expressed in healing qualitatively by increased cytodifferentiation to cartilage with endochondral ossification and quantitatively by increases in total amounts of callus formed. The callus is distributed over large areas of the bone internally and externally and initially is poorly organized as fine cancellous bone.[13, 25, 38, 94]

Hematoma in Fracture Healing

The significance of the fracture hematoma is not clear. One theory states that hematoma inhibits fracture healing whereas another theory states that fractures cannot heal without hematoma. There probably is some truth in both theories. A large hematoma between and around the fracture fragments produces a large dead space filled with clotted blood and few if any undifferentiated cells. Extensive hematoma makes excellent reduction and immobilization difficult. This could lead to excessive motion and, together with the massive dead clot, could produce extensive anoxia. Anoxia is not favorable to cellular modulation to osteoblasts.[62, 79] On the other hand, if clot is continually removed from the fracture gap, healing will not occur. In essence, removing the clot implies the removal of undifferentiated cells. Without these cells, new bone cannot form.

It seems that some clot is necessary to produce a jelly-like bridge between the fragments. The fibrin strands that form serve as a lattice on which immigrating undifferentiated cells can climb.

HEALING OF A COMPLETE OSTEOTOMY TREATED BY INTRAMEDULLARY FIXATION (FIGS. 4-27 – 4-29)

The next fracture situation to be considered is the complete fracture with a relatively small defect, in which there will be an element of twisting motion but no shear or bending motion. A complete mid-diaphyseal transverse osteotomy is surgically created and the fragments are reduced and held together internally by an intramedullary device. The number of variables is minimal. The osteotomy is equivalent to a complete transverse midshaft fracture except that soft tissue trauma is less. The use of an intramedullary device seriously impairs any contribution from endosteal sources of blood supply and cells. Indeed, if a Küntscher rod is used, it eliminates altogether the endosteal blood supply and infarcts at least the inner half of the entire cortex.[17, 18, 46, 54, 70, 71, 89] Because the osteotomy is transverse and the fracture is reduced surgically, apposition is good and the gap to be healed is small. The intramedullary device virtually eliminates bending or shear motion. Some gap motion occurs as a result of torque forces but this motion is minimal.

When this situation is produced in animals, the healing sequence can be followed accurately.

Necrosis of all cells will occur for several millimeters on both sides of the osteotomy. The entire diaphyseal marrow and endosteum die and are unable to contribute to fracture repair indefinitely, if ever. Hemorrhage and a subsequent clot forms between the bone ends and in the vicinity of the cut periosteum and overlying soft tissues. The inflammatory response is seen primarily in the periosteum and overlying soft tissues. As with all healing, this cell response rapidly progresses through acute and chronic white cell stages during the first 4 or 5 days and then enters a granulomatous phase. By this time, periosteum has reacted throughout its length, width and depth. The cambium or deep cell layer becomes many cells thicker than normal; the closer to the osteotomy the more extensive the hyperplasia. The granulomatous reaction is seen in the soft tissues around the torn periosteum, manifested as extensive new vascular and mesenchymal cells within tissue fascial planes. The intermuscular cleavage planes become obscured and mesenchymal cells seem to blend into and perhaps arise from epiphyseal and perimysial connective tissues. The cut ends of periosteum were lifted from the bone surface by blood clot. The periosteal defect soon becomes filled by cells contributed from adjacent living cambial cells and from cells that seem to arise from the intermuscular fascial planes. A thick layer of undifferentiated cells now surrounds the osteotomy site and many of these cells eventually will grow through the hematoma and enter the fracture site itself. The combination of hematoma, bone debris, rotary motion and the torn periosteum prevents the periosteum from growing directly and straight across the gap to meet the opposite cut edge of periosteum. Instead, the periosteum grows over the gap and around and through the hematoma at some distance from the actual bone and gap surfaces. By 1 week, extensive appositional new woven bone is being produced by the periosteum onto the surfaces of the bone fragments. More bone forms near the gap than at a distance from it and, in doing so, creates a circumferential shoulder of woven trabecular bone on each side of the gap. Most trabeculae that form are perpendicular to the bone surface, as are the blood vessels that nourish the new bone. As the proliferating cambium layer covers the gap area, trabeculae are produced at the edges of the gap and continue to grow into the gap. The periosteum directly above the gap may produce a small amount of cartilage, while off to each side new bone is produced. Slight motion and hematoma produce areas of relative anoxia and this may be the local environmental factor that causes cell modulation to cartilage instead of bone. Only small amounts of cartilage are produced unless more extensive motion occurs. Indeed, in some instances in which the internal fixation may have almost eliminated motion, virtually no cartilage is seen (Figs. 4-27 and 4-28). Now, the two fragments are stuck together by callus that is made up from one bone surface to the other by woven bone

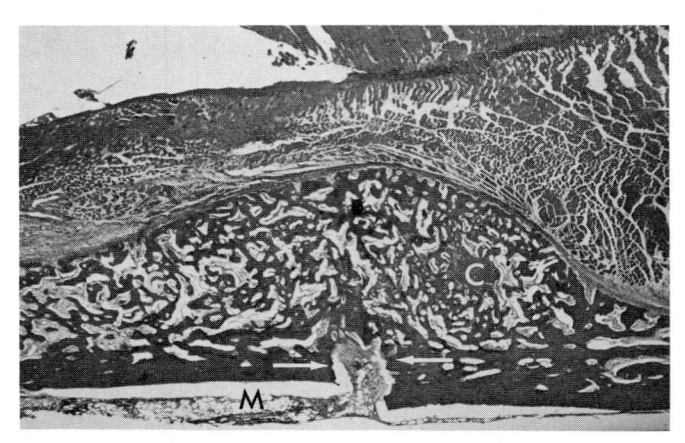

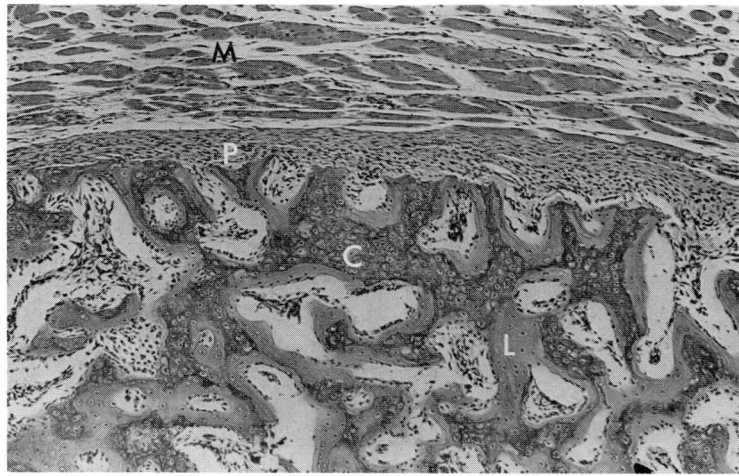

Fig. 4-27 (top). — Figures 4-27–4-29 illustrate the type of healing that occurs with intramedullary fixation. The long bone in Figure 4-22 was osteotomized, anatomically reduced and immobilized with an intramedullary device. Only minimal rotary motion was permitted. Within 6–8 weeks, the fracture was united by a fairly large fine cancellous woven bony callus (C). The fracture site is demarcated by arrows and contains only connective tissue. There has been no contribution to fracture healing from the marrow cavity (M), which was infarcted when the intramedullary device was inserted. No cartilage is evident and this probably reflects lack of motion at the fracture site.

Fig. 4-28 (bottom). — This is a medium-power view of the periosteal callus shown in Figure 4-27. The callus can be seen to be made up of two types of bone. The first bone seen forms rapidly with significant amounts of mucoproteins. It somewhat resembles cartilage and has been called "chondro-osteoid" (C) by some. Later, this bone is covered by a more mature lamellar type of bone (L). This latter bone continues to form on bony surfaces, changing the gross appearance of the callus from spongy to compact. The periosteum here is indicated by (P) and the surrounding muscle by (M).

to cartilage to woven bone. As mentioned above, the callus may consist entirely of bone tissue but this is the less common finding, as small amounts of cartilage usually are found. This early callus acts as a temporary bond that resists further motion.

Blood vessels from the adjacent bony

callus and from the periosteum penetrate and resorb the cartilage. New bone is produced in this area of callus by an endochondral ossification mechanism. Soon almost no cartilage remains and the entire callus is made up of dense trabecular woven bone. This same type of bone makes up the bone shafts of human embryos and is called "fine cancellous" woven bone. Virtually no motion occurs beyond this stage. The next step in the biology is compaction; that is, more new bone is added to the trabecular surfaces of the callus and the bone assumes a true compact nature. This latter bone is laid down as primary lamellar bone containing no mature osteons. The callus at this stage is a mixture of woven and lamellar bone. Now the osteotomy is united by new compact bone. There is, however, a small mass of callus that surrounds the osteotomy site, and this callus is bone with poor architectural and mechanical properties. By clinical criteria, the fracture site may be "healed," because there is bony union without local pain, tenderness or motion. Extensive local remodeling, however, still must occur before the fracture can be considered "biologically" healed. Subperiosteal resorption must occur to remove this excessive bump of callus. In addition, cutting cones must resorb the poor-quality bone filling the gap and replace it with normal-appearing osteonal bone. When biologic healing is complete there will be no histologic or mechanical proof that an injury ever occurred. In growing animals and children, this process may go on to completion within months or a few years. In clinical practice, though, children's fractures rarely are fixed by intramedullary means. In an adult, the process of biologic healing may never become complete and, indeed, some excess original fracture callus may remain forever. The infarcted inner half or so of the diaphyseal cortex will be partly resorbed and replaced as described above under Healing of Necrotic Compact Bone.

HEALING OF A FRACTURED DIAPHYSIS WITHOUT ANY FORM OF IMMOBILIZATION

The poorest local conditions for fracture healing occur when no attempt is made to treat the fracture. One method that can be used to study this situation is to osteotomize a long bone including per-

Fig. 4-29.—When the intramedullary device is loose, permitting some motion, cartilage (C) is produced over the gap (*arrows*). Woven bone (W) is also produced, but this is at some distance from the gap. The callus in this case is made up of cartilage, bone and fibrous tissue.

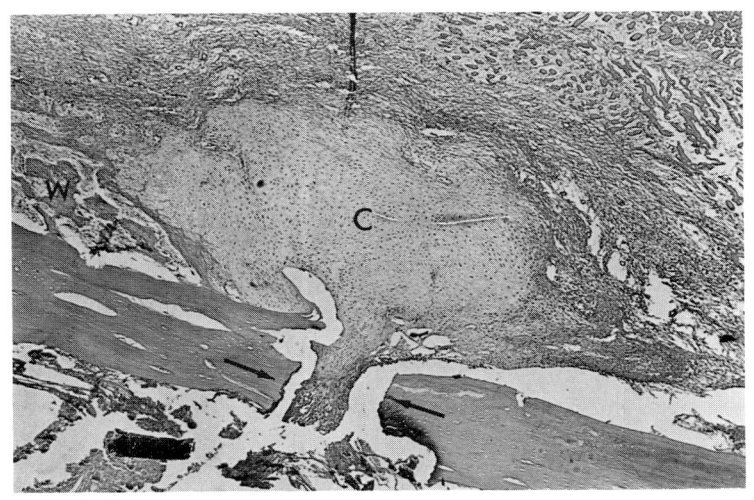

iosteum, to repair only overlying subcutaneous soft tissues and skin and to observe the healing at various periods following surgery. No attempt is made to immobilize the fracture fragments. This would ensure gross motion of the fracture fragments and would guarantee poor alignment and poor apposition.

The initial phase of necrosis will be about the same as in the cast immobilization fracture in extent and location. The hematoma that forms is large in extent because the moving bone ends will continue to remove early clots from lacerated vessels and, in addition, these moving sharp fragments will traumatize more soft tissues.

Bleeding may continue for much longer periods than when the fracture is immobilized. The inflammatory response in the marrow and soft tissues around the fracture will be the same as with cast immobilization up to the point of cytodifferentiation. The periosteum also responds as with any fracture by a hyperplasia of the cambium layer and soon with early bone formation. More bone will be produced subperiosteally near the fracture site than more distally. The endosteum and marrow likewise undergo tissue replacement to granulation tissue.

The endosteal granulation tissues then begin to revascularize and fill in the fracture gap by penetrating the blood clot nearest them. The undifferentiated cells can penetrate the hematoma only a limited distance. The gross motion centrally appears to inhibit new cells from crossing the fracture gap to meet similar cells from the opposite surface. Instead, these undifferentiated cells continue to divide and, together with some new vessels, grow around the bone ends closely adherent to the fractured dead bone surface.

The periosteum, with cell contributions from the overlying soft tissues, grows through and/or around the hematoma and joins up with the periosteal sleeve from the opposite side. Some cells from the cambium layer may extend along the periosteal surface and around the fracture ends to join those cells of endosteal origin. These cells, too, are unable to cross the hematoma.

Under some circumstances, cells may be able to cross the hematoma to meet their similar members from the other side despite motion. Under the most favorable circumstances, these cells modulate to cartilage and fibrous connective tissue throughout the central areas of hematoma. A fibrocartilage union is produced and this will limit gross motion. If a favorable cell environment persists, the cartilage will slowly be converted to fine cancellous woven bone by endochondral ossification and will slowly heal in a manner similar to that of cast immobilization. Because of the large amount of cartilage, the healing time will be prolonged by all criteria and there may be delayed union. With a slightly less favorable local environment, the undifferentiated cells in the center of the fracture gap may modulate to fibroblasts and fibrocytes and produce dense, irregular fibrous connective tissue, i.e., scar. As long as motion persists, blood vessels are incapable of reaching the central areas and this may be a factor influencing cell modulation. If local circumstances do not change, the scar tissue remains as such and a fibrous nonunion will result. If the local environment can be beneficially altered at this time, by cast immobilization, bone graft or both, the fracture may go on to heal. Vessels will penetrate the scar and repopulate the area with undifferentiated cells. Under these improved conditions, a graft may produce or induce a humoral agent that stimulates new bone formation, contribute living donor osteogenic cells and provide a bony framework. If all these variables are operable, sufficient new bone can be produced to achieve bony consolidation.

Under the worst circumstances, undifferentiated cells and new vessels are permanently unable to penetrate the hematoma. They grow around the bone ends and the fracture surface in a layer. On the fracture ends there is a modulation to cartilage cells and fibrocartilage (Fig. 4-30). Endosteally, on each side of the gap, new bone, cartilage and fibrous tissue will be produced in sufficient quantity to close off the entire marrow cavity. Thus, the entire bone end will become solid. Likewise, a shoulder of new subperiosteal bone may be built up at the edge of the fragments, making the bone ends broader. This periosteal reac-

Fig. 4-30.—If gross motion continues indefinitely, a pseudarthrosis will occur. This photograph is taken from the end of the marrow cavity of one of the fracture fragments. New bone has filled the entire marrow space (i.e., all the bone in the picture). Fibrocartilage (C) has formed over the ends of the fragments, (arrows) including the bony cap in the marrow cavity. A potential space is seen above the cartilage and this is filled with fluid. When seen at low power, this resembles a synovial joint, thus the term pseudarthrosis.

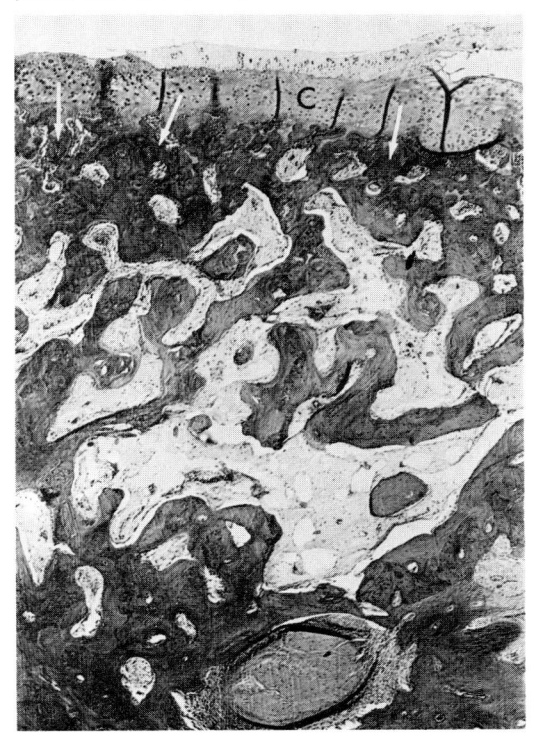

tive bone does not extend across the gap either. With time, it becomes compacted, sclerotic and relatively ischemic. The entire fracture surface eventually is coated with fibrocartilage, which can appear very similar to hyaline cartilage if sufficient cartilage matrix is secreted. The fibrocartilaginous cap adds to the local ischemia. Radiologically, the gross appearance of the fracture under these conditions has been compared to an "elephant's foot." The periosteum, which has surrounded the hematoma and is an intact layer, also undergoes cell change. The superficial layer, the fibrous zone, hypertrophies. The cambial zone, which was hyperplastic and consisted mainly of mesenchymal cells, modulates to a thin layer of flat cells without a basement membrane. With time, the hematoma is slowly resorbed and replaced by a fluid similar to synovial fluid. The fracture ends now are capped with fibrocartilage, rub against one another and are separated from one another by a fluid. The bone ends remain within a fibrous pseudocapsule, which is lined by a synovial-like layer of cells that secrete a synovial fluid. This anatomic and poorly functional entity is called a *pseudarthrosis* and, in fact, appears very similar to a synovial joint. Without some further extensive form of treatment, the pseudarthrosis will remain indefinitely.

In clinical practice, an occasional pseudarthrosis is found that by x-ray does not appear like an "elephant's foot." In this situation, the fragments become sclerotic and assume a long, thin, tapered appearance. It is difficult to demonstrate the pathophysiology in these rare cases, but when they occur there appears to be a local defect in cell modulation to osteoblasts. Biopsies usually reveal dense fibrous connective tissue containing only fibrocytes and a few blood vessels. In some conditions, such as congenital pseudarthrosis, there may be an inherited local periosteal defect in cell modulation. When a pseudarthrosis follows trauma, the injury has been severe enough to permanently damage local soft tissues and periosteum. Open fractures and infections are additional features of soft tissue injury[22, 29] that may have adverse effects on local cell responses and inhibit bone repair.

PRIMARY BONE HEALING: FRACTURE HEALING AND THE COMPRESSION PLATE[1, 3, 5, 16, 19, 28, 36, 52, 55, 56, 60, 68, 75-77, 78, 87]

All the fracture healing situations to this point have healed by what is called "secondary bone healing." That is to say, the major contribution to healing has come from cells derived from endosteum, periosteum and overlying soft tissues. Osteonal contributions have been minimal, if at all, until very late, when remodeling is occurring.

"Primary bone healing" implies that the bone ends initially unite with bone that is osteonal and of normal orientation. The healing cells are derived from cells within surviving osteons and Volkmann's canals. Neither periosteum nor endosteum contributes osteogenic cells in this type of healing. The process may be studied experimentally. Animals with good haversian bone should be used — for example, dogs, cats or goats. A complete mid-diaphyseal osteotomy is made and an appropriate AO compression plate is inserted without undue periosteal stripping, using the accepted AO techniques.[58, 66]

This open technique, barring complications, results in a number of highly desirable features. Open reduction and internal fixation in this situation produce almost perfect alignment without displacement and virtually eliminate motion. There is some question presently as to whether compression is maintained across the fracture site for more than a very short time. Everyone agrees, however, that this technique can provide maximal apposition with minimal motion between the cortices under the plate. The fracture cortices diametrically opposite the plate are also close together but frequently are forced open slightly as compression is applied.

The cortices adjacent to the plate undergo primary bone healing, whereas those opposite the plate usually undergo secondary healing as described above under Healing of a Small Hole in Bone.

The osteotomy creates a zone of necrosis on each side of the defect just like any of the previous osteotomies. A hematoma forms endosteally and periosteally in the soft tissues but not in between the bone ends, because there is no room for a hematoma. The periosteum reacts by undergoing a limited hyperplasia in the vicinity of the fracture but virtually no new bone is produced. The minimal cell response seems to occur to enable the periosteum to heal itself. A short-lived acute inflammation occurs in the soft tissues around the periosteum and in the marrow endosteally. Within 2–3 days, chronic inflammatory cells and macrophages are present and participate in the removal of necrotic debris. Some new blood vessels and undifferentiated cells in the same areas appear but do not enter the fracture gap. Undifferentiated cells that accompany the blood vessels within haversian systems and Volkmann's canals begin to multiply. This cell activity occurs at some distance from the fracture site, at the junction of living and dead bone and throughout the remainder of the osteon.

New cutting cone mechanisms are produced at the junction of live and dead bone. The cutting cones, headed by a few osteoclasts, move toward the fracture site along the empty haversian canal, resorbing the matrix of the surrounding necrotic osteon plus or minus a little more necrotic bone. The cutting cones reach the fracture site, cross this very narrow space and either enter another empty haversian canal or begin to cut directly into the necrotic bone on the opposite

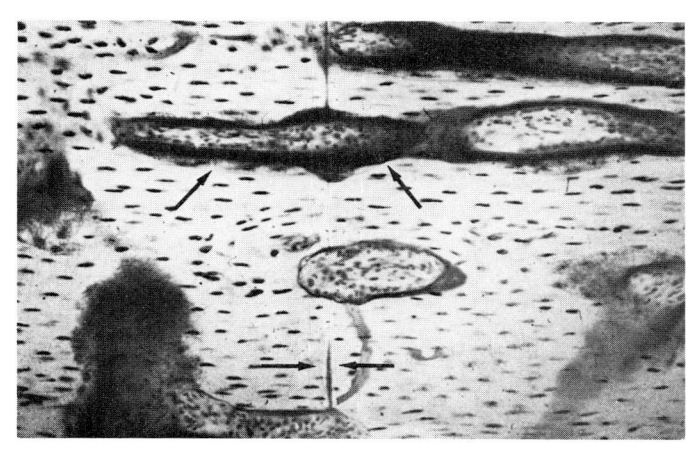

Fig. 4-31. — Primary bone healing in a dog. A medium-power photograph from the fracture gap under a compression plate. Note how small the gap is (*horizontal arrows*), i.e., virtually absent. At this phase of healing, cutting cones with new bone formation can be seen crossing the fracture site at several levels. Two oblique arrows point out a cutting cone, which extends well beyond both sides of the fracture site. This photograph is from the experimental work of Dr. M. Allgöwer, who pioneered the development and use of compression plate internal fixation for fractures.

side of the fracture. Implied by the very nature of the cutting cone is the fact that a new living osteon is made immediately behind the resorbing osteoclasts, and this osteon will not need to be remodeled. The same process occurs until all the dead segments of osteons have been resorbed and replaced by new living osteons, though fewer cutting cones remain operable as time goes on. Initially, resorption will be the major response and new bone formation the minor response, just as described above under Healing of Necrotic Compact Bone. X-rays during this early phase, which may last for 2 or 3 months, may show a decreased radiodensity on each side of the fracture. As the zone of necrosis is fairly narrow, the resorption is manifested by an apparent widening of the fracture site 8–10 weeks postoperatively. Later, as more and more osteons mature, resorption will be minimal and matrix formation maximal. As mineralization of the new matrix becomes complete, radiodensity approaches normal. In more than 60% of Segmüller's cases,[78] the fracture lines no longer were visible at 14–16 weeks. A stage is finally reached at which the fracture line has been crossed by many new osteons and the fracture is clinically healed. The timing of this event is difficult to assess, but most compression plates are left in situ about 2 years before they are removed and normal weight bearing is permitted. The 2-year time is an empirical judgment, as the incidence of refracture varies inversely with the length of time the plate remains in place. Some dead bone still remains at this phase and will slowly be resorbed and replaced by new generations of osteons. This latter phase of healing may never be complete. The total length of time required for biologic healing is not known, but, again, in the adult, it may require many months to years and indeed may really take as long as fractures treated with cast immobilization.

The advantages of compression plates for fracture treatment are clinical, in that external immobilization may not be required at all or may be discontinued early and in that adjacent joints may be mobilized very soon after surgery, if not immediately.

OTHER FEATURES OF FRACTURE HEALING

DISUSE OR IMMOBILIZATION OSTEOPOROSIS. — Clinical fracture healing often is further complicated by other biologic responses. Fractures that require cast immobilization for more than a few weeks frequently show secondary changes throughout the remainder of the bone.

Although the biologic changes described for the healing of coarse cancellous and compact bone hold for fractures through metaphyses[79] and diaphyses respectively, extensive osteoporosis may be found a short distance from the fracture line if a cast is required for more than 4–6 weeks. This is a normal response also. If muscular and weight-bearing stresses are removed from a bone, the bone will respond to its new circumstances, in compliance with Wolff's law, by undergoing resorption. The bone cortices thin, mainly by endosteal resorption; individual trabeculae become smaller and those that were small to begin with may disappear completely. No matter what the forces on the bone as a whole, however, the cell responses at the fracture site and for some distance on each side of the fracture are in accordance with the discussions in this chapter.

VARIATION FROM BONE TO BONE AND IN THE NATURE OF THE FRACTURE. — Certain features of healing are seen in clinical practice that cannot be duplicated experimentally. For example, fracture of the middle tibia and humerus behave differently than fractures of the femur. Clinically, the effects of gravity and variations of blood supply are among the reasons proffered to explain these differences. The extent of soft tissue injury — and this includes skin, muscle fascia, periosteum and blood vessels to and from bone — that surrounds a fracture is extremely important in clinical fractures.[22, 39] The amount of soft tissue injury will vary with the nature of the injury, the area over which the force was applied and whether the fracture was open or closed. Early and/or late sepsis also plays a role. All these variables probably express themselves in the same way at the biologic level; that is, they decrease the number of undifferentiated cells that are available to participate in fracture healing and they may influence the modulation of those cells that can participate.

REMODELING. — Discussion to this point has been concerned with the cellular events at the fracture site. Just as important as the healing of the fracture, per se, is what happens to the bone as a whole. For example, how does a displaced fracture correct in childhood and in adulthood? What about an angulated and displaced fracture?

In general, the deformities of displacement and angulation are said to be corrected by "remodeling phenomena." Remodeling is of two broad types: internal and external. Internal remodeling refers to changes in the nature of the bone *tissue* at microscopic levels. The initial callus that forms with most fractures is a mixture of relatively randomly oriented woven bone trabeculae and cartilage. The cartilage is gradually resorbed and replaced with primary woven bone trabeculae through an endochondral ossification mechanism so that the callus now is almost entirely made up of woven bone. The major orientation of these trabeculae is at right angles to the surface of the bone, but many trabeculae are randomly formed. This type of bone is called fine cancellous woven bone because of its resemblance to embryonic cortical bone; that is, it appears to be cortical bone grossly, but if it is examined closely or by a low-power magnifying glass, it really is spongy or cancellous. At this time, the large spaces between the woven bone trabeculae are occupied by blood vessels and mesenchymal cells. Some of these cells modulate to osteoblasts and secrete new bone matrix onto the surfaces of the woven bone trabeculae. This most recent bone is laid down as primary lamellar bone. It continues to be produced in a centripetal fashion until there is only room enough centrally for blood vessels and some associated cells. This process is called *compaction,* for now the callus is as solid or compact as regular cortical bone. The callus now is a mass of primary lamellar bone with central cores of woven bone. This same callus has been a bulbous mass around the fracture site for some time. Subperiosteal and endosteal osteoclasts remove excess callus from the periosteal and endosteal surfaces respectively. This is a feature of external remodeling. The bone between the fracture fragments likewise is a mixture of lamellar and woven bone. Now the distribution and quantity of the new bone are adequate, but the quality and orientation are not yet ideal. The final stage of internal remodeling is the resorption of the lamellar bone from between the fragments and the concomitant replacement with properly oriented osteonal bone. All of these events comprise *internal* remodeling. It is of interest to note that normal diaphyseal bone undergoes identical changes between the embryonic and the adult stages of growth and development.

External remodeling refers to changes in the size and shape of the *organ* bone. Extensive external remodeling can occur only in young growing bones. In these young bones, the bone increases its length by endochondral ossification mechanisms located primarily in the epiphyseal plate and to a lesser extent in the base of the growing articular cartilages. The ends of bones increase in size and change shape by the process called hemispherization. The diaphyseal cortex grows thicker and changes shape and distribution of mass as a result of the balance between periosteal new bone formation and endosteal resorption. This process is called cylinderization. As the bone grows in length and width, it maintains a fairly constant over-all shape at the metaphyses due to a process called funnelization. This is due to a balance between formation and resorption at the ring of Ranvier and the cutback zone respectively.[23, 74] Longitudinal growth, hemispherization and funnelization cease at maturity. However, periosteal new bone formation and endosteal resorption continue at an extremely slow rate indefinitely. Thus, in the adult, there is some, albeit minimal, potential for external remodeling.

What, in essence, is being stressed is that the external remodeling phenomena that are invoked to correct shaft deformities are in actuality the identical cellular mechanisms that permit the bone shaft to grow longer, wider and thicker and at the same time control shape; that is, the delicate balance between bone resorption and bone formation. The total remodeling permitted is absolutely delimited by the amount of normal growth potential remaining at the time of injury. Deformities in metaphyses have advantages over those in diaphyses. This is due to the fact that resorption rates in the cutback zone and formation rates at the ring of Ranvier are very high. In addition, the epiphyseal plate is capable of asymmetric growth. Thus, the rates of normal and fracture remodeling are much greater in metaphyses than elsewhere.

DISPLACED FRACTURES (FIG. 4-32).—A growing animal will be able to completely correct displacement if enough growth remains. If the total width of the two displaced fragments is less than the width of the mature bone, the normal cell phenomena of cylinderization can completely correct the deformity. In effect, what happens is that endosteal osteoclasts completely resorb the deformed bone from within, whereas periosteal osteoblasts produce an entire new cortex from without. The adult animal is unable to correct *any* displacement. A bayonet fracture will heal with the fragments maintained in this position. As pointed out,

108 / *John E. Kenzora*

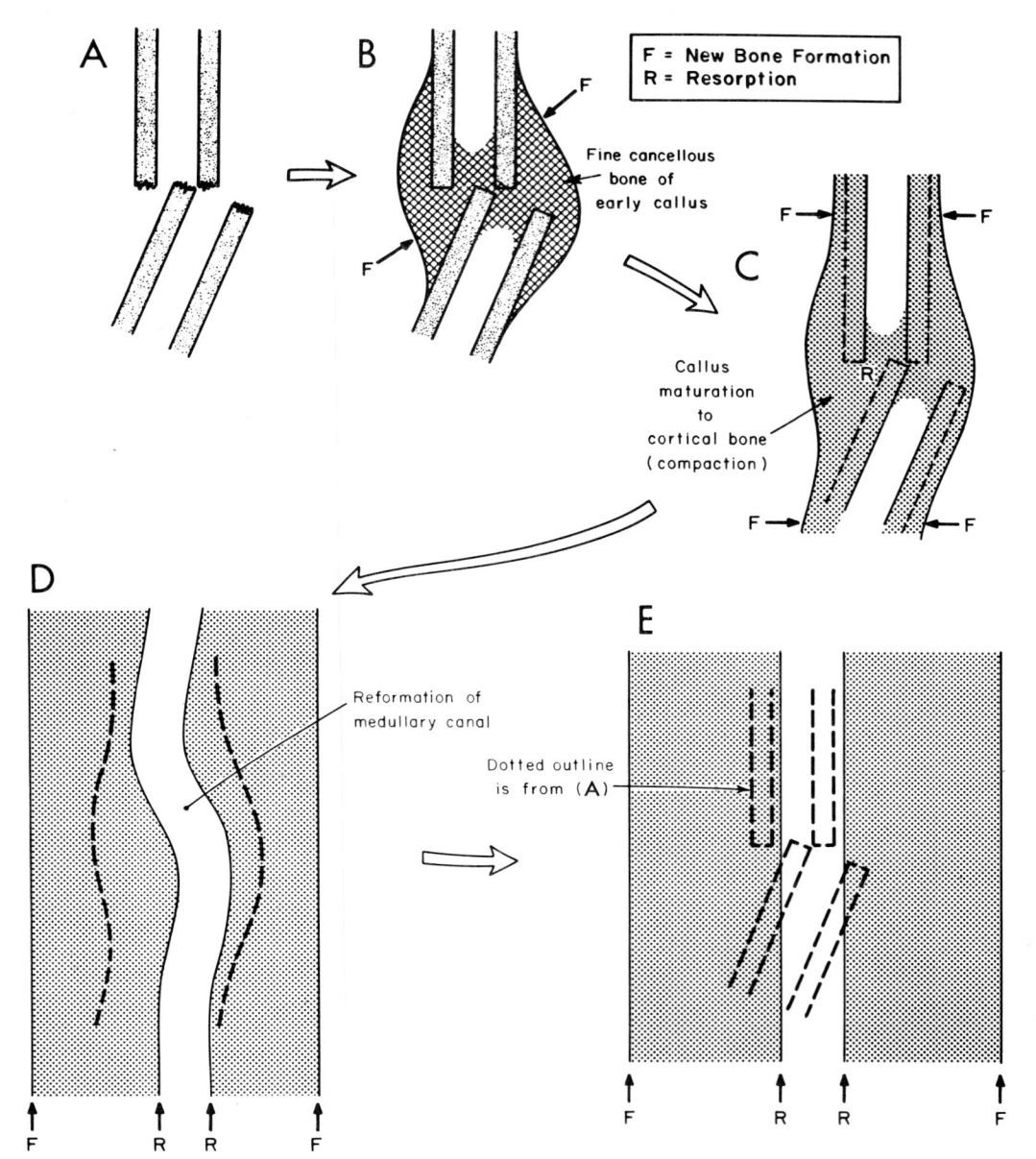

Fig. 4-32.—Remodeling: the correction of diaphyseal angulation and displacement in a growing bone. In general, if the total width of the displaced and angulated shaft fragments is less than the width of the shaft at termination of growth, both the angulation and displacement of the shaft will correct. This comes about via the normal biologic growth patterns inherent in the term *cylinderization*. Appropriate periosteal new bone formation and endosteal resorption can correct the diaphyseal deformities as illustrated. The malalignment of the joints above and below an angulated fracture, however, cannot correct by cylinderization.

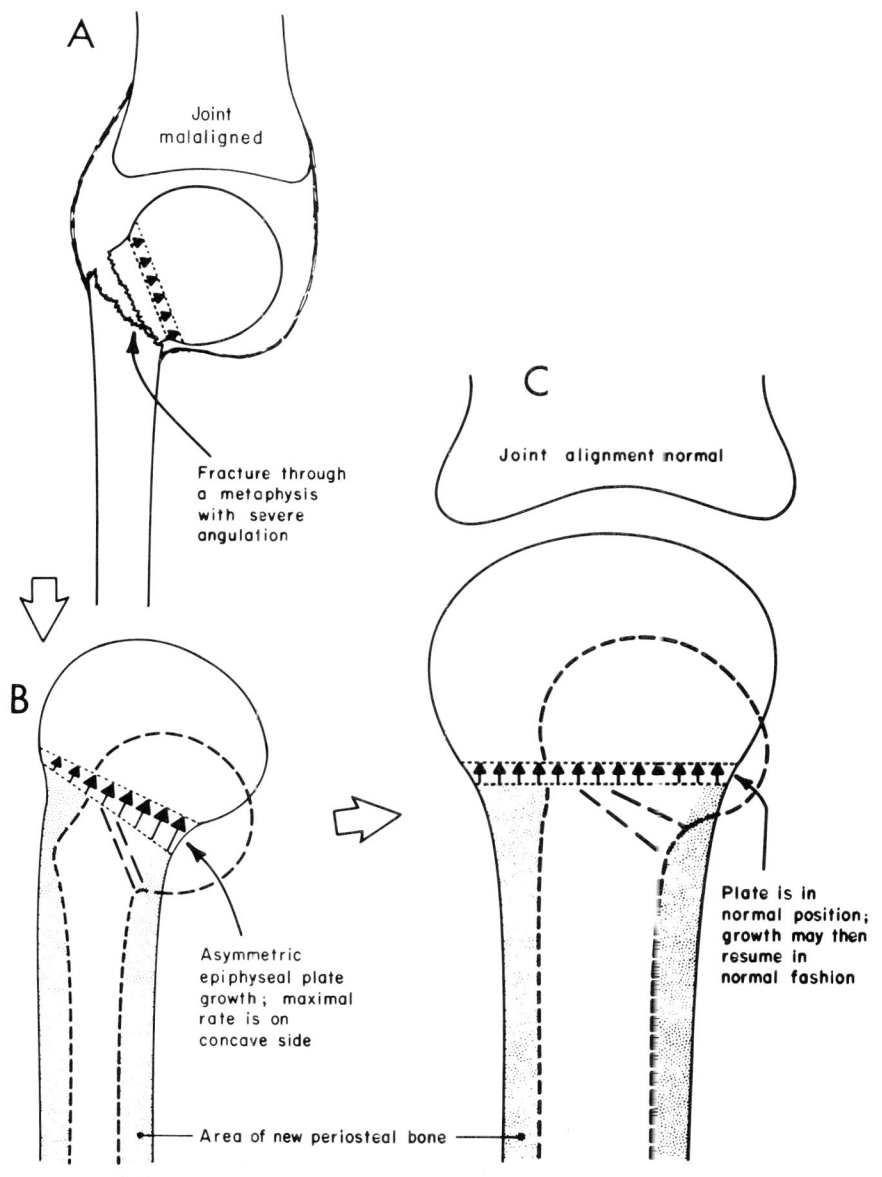

Fig. 4-33.—Remodeling: the correction of joint malalignment and epiphyseal plate angulation in a growing bone. This deformity can occur secondary to angulated fractures in diaphyses or metaphyses. In general, the closer to the epiphyseal plate the quicker the correction. The joint surface and plate angulation can correct only by asymmetric epiphyseal plate growth. The relative rate of growth on the side of the concavity of the fracture is greater than that on the convexity. This increased rate is depicted by an increased thickness of the plate and by vertical arrows. In actuality, the plate probably is no thicker on the concavity. The cutback zone on the concavity very likely remains fairly inactive, relative to that of the opposite side, until the bone end straightens.

some very limited external remodeling potential exists. The sharp corners will be rounded off and the medullary canal restored by osteoclastic resorption, but displacement will persist.

ANGULATION (FIG. 4-33).—Angulated fractures present at least two problems. The first is that the shaft of the long bone is bent. The second and most important is that the joints above and below an angulated fracture are malaligned relative to each other. These alterations introduce serious cosmetic and functional handicaps. A growing animal may remodel *shaft* angulation entirely, by the normal cellular processes of cylinderization, provided that sufficient growth remains. As is the case in displacement, endosteal osteoclasts completely resorb the angulated cortices from within. They may also resorb some subperiosteal bone at the convexity of the angulation. Concomitantly, subperiosteal osteoblasts make an entirely new cortex. This process will completely straighten out the shaft but cannot alter the angulation of the bone ends. The angulation at the bone ends and joint surfaces can be corrected only by asymmetric growth at the epiphyseal plates. The concave side of the plate grows at a relatively greater rate than the convex side; that is, there is a gradation in rate of growth from one side of the epiphyseal plate to the other. An adult can neither correct the shaft angulation nor the joint malalignment. Once the fracture site heals, angulation and displacement are permanent. Thus, angulation of more than a few degrees in adult fractures in planes other than those of the joint is unacceptable. The major reason for active intervention in the treatment of displaced and/or angulated fractures is the maintenance of normal function. Most adult fractures heal, but because the remodeling potential is so low, angulation in planes other than those of the joint cannot be permitted, since the joints would be malaligned and a poor functional result would ensue.

ROTATION.—On grounds purely empirical, it is generally believed that neither a growing bone nor a mature bone can correct rotary defects. Although it may be theoretically possible to explain a mechanism to correct rotation, there are few data to show that it ever occurs.

More exacting details of the cellular processes of remodeling and how they affect the correction of displaced and angulated fractures will be presented in a forthcoming text. The in-depth study of these problems is not within the clinically oriented scope of the present volume.

ACKNOWLEDGMENTS

The general format of this chapter, in which fracture healing is presented as a special case of the more general response of bone repair and healing, was developed at Harvard Medical School by Dr. Melvin J. Glimcher for both undergraduate and graduate teaching courses in the biology of bone. I am indebted to Professor Glimcher for advice on many of the illustrations, for use of the teaching syllabi utilized in these courses and for his help in preparing the manuscript. Concepts have been developed to explain the correction of various deformities and displacements of bone, based on normal bone growth and development. Remodeling phenomena have been defined using these criteria. To my knowledge, the roles of asymmetric epiphyseal plate growth and cylinderization in the correction of angular and axial displacements of fractures have never been presented in this fashion before.

I would like to thank Dr. Fumio Kato for permission to use data and scientific illustrations from his forthcoming articles with Dr. Glimcher on the Role of the Internal Architecture of Bone in the Sequence of Bone Repair.

In addition, I should like to give special credit to Myrtelina Shamsi, our excellent histology technician, for the tissue sections which were used for some of the photographs.

BIBLIOGRAPHY

1. Allgöwer, M.: Healing of Clinical Fractures of the Tibia with Rigid Internal Fixation, in Robinson, R. A. (ed.), *The Healing of Osseous Tissue* (Washington, D. C.: National Academy of Sciences – National Research Council, 1967), p. 81.
2. Allgöwer, M.: Studies on the Acquired Ability of Circulating Monocytes to Synthesize Collagen under Certain Experimental Conditions and the Implications in Wound Healing, in Robinson, R. A. (ed.), *The Healing of Osseous Tissue* (Washington, D. C.: National Academy of Sciences – National Research Council, 1967), p. 121.
3. Anderson, L. D.: The treatment of ununited fracture of the long bones; compression plate fixation and the effect of different types of internal fixation on fracture healing, J. Bone Joint Surg. 47-A:191, 1965.
4. Anderson, L. D.: Healing of Standard Discontinuities of Long Bones as Observed Roentgenographically, Grossly, and Histologically in the Adult Dog, in *The Healing of Osseous Tissue – A Workshop* (Washington, D. C.: National Academy of Sciences – National Research Council, 1965), p. 41.
5. Bagby, G. W., and Janes, J. M.: The effect of compression on the rate of fracture healing using a special plate, Am. J. Surg. 95:761, 1958.
6. Bassett, C. A.: Current concepts of bone formation, J. Bone Joint Surg. 44-A:1217, 1962.
7. Bassett, C. A.: Biophysical Principles Affecting Bone Structure, in Bourne, G. H. (ed.), *The Biochemistry and Physiology of Bone*, Vol. 3, *Development and Growth* (2d ed.; New York: Academic Press, 1971), Chap. 1.
8. Bassett, C. A.: Bioelectric responses and bone formation, J. Bone Joint Surg. 53-A:1655, 1971.
9. Bassett, C. A., Creighton, D. K., and Stinchfield, F. E.: Contributions of endosteum, cortex and soft tissues to osteogenesis, Surg. Gynecol. Obstet. 112:145, 1961.
10. Becker, R. O., and Murray, D. G.: A method for producing cellular dedifferentiation by means of very small electrical currents, Trans. N. Y. Acad. Sci. 29:606, 1967.
11. Bloom, W., and Fawcett, D. W.: *A Textbook of Histology* (9th ed.; Philadelphia: W. B. Saunders Company, 1968).
12. Blount, W. P.: *Fractures in Children* (Baltimore: The Williams & Wilkins Company, 1954).
13. Bourgois, R., and Burny, F.: Measurement of the stiffness of fracture callus in vivo, a theoretical study, J. Biomech. 5:85, 1972.
14. Brooke, S. M., and Helal, B.: Primary osteoarthritis, venous engorgement and osteogenesis, J. Bone Joint Surg. 50-A:493, 1968.
15. Cavadias, A. X., and Trueta, J.: An experimental study of the vascular contribution to the callus of fracture, Surg. Gynecol. Obstet. 120:731, 1965.
16. Charnley, J., and Baker, S. L.: Compression arthrodesis of the knee, J. Bone Joint Surg. 34-B:187, 1952.
17. Danckwardt-Lilliestrom, G.: Reaming of the medullary cavity and its effects on diaphyseal bone. A fluorochromic, microangiographic and histologic study on the rabbit tibia and dog femur, Acta Scand., Supp. 128, 1969.
18. Danckwardt-Lilliestrom, G., Lorenzi, G. L., and Olerud, S.: Intramedullary nailing after reaming. An investigation on the healing process in osteotomized rabbit tibias, Acta Scand., Supp. 134, 1970.
19. Dingwall, J. S., Duncan, D. B., and Horney, F. D.: Compression plating in large animal orthopedics, J. Am. Vet. Med. Assoc. 158:1651, 1971.
20. Duthie, R. B.: The Possible Role of Mast Cells in Tissue Injury and Their Presence in Fracture Sites, in Robinson, R. A. (ed.), *The Healing of Osseous Tissue – A Workshop* (Washington, D. C.: National Academy of Sciences – National Research Council, 1965), p. 195.
21. Duthie, R. B., and Barker, A. N.: Histochemistry of the preosseous stage of bone repair studied by autoradiography; effects of cortisone, J. Bone Joint Surg. 37-B:691, 1955.
22. Edwards, P.: Fractures of the shaft of the tibia: 492 consecutive cases in adults, importance of soft tissue injury, Acta Scand. Orthop., Supp. 76, 1965.
23. Enlow, D. H.: *Principles of Bone Remodeling* (Springfield, Ill.: Charles C Thomas, Publisher, 1963).
24. Enneking, W. F.: The repair of bone transplants. Presentation at the Boston Orthopaedic Club, November, 1972.
25. Falkenberg, J.: An experimental study of the rate of fracture healing as assessed from the tensile strength and Sr 85 activity of the callus with special reference to the effect of intramedullary nailing, Acta. Scand., Supp. 50, 1961.
26. Flatmark, A. L.: Fracture union in the presence of delayed blood coagulation. A clinicoexperimental investigation, Acta Chir. Scand., Supp. 344:1, 1964.
27. Földes, I., Olah, E. H., and Tasnady, L.: Studies on respiration during regenerative chondral bone formation (formation of callus), Acta Biol. Acad. Sci. Hung. 15:1, 1964.
28. Friedenberg, Z. B., and French, G.: The effects of known compression forces on fracture healing, Surg. Gynecol. Obstet. 94:743, 1952.
29. Friedenberg, Z. B., Harlow, M. C., and Brighton, C. T.: Healing of nonunion of the medial malleolus by means of direct current: A case report, J. Trauma 11:883, 1971.
30. Friedenberg, Z. B., Roberts, J. R., Didizian, N. H., and Brighton, C. T.: Stimulation of fracture healing by direct current in the rabbit fibula, J. Bone Joint Surg. 53-A:1400, 1971.
31. Frost, H. M.: *The Laws of Bone Structure* Springfield, Ill.: Charles C. Thomas, Publisher, 1964).
32. Gage, A. A., Greene, G. W., Jr., Neiders, M., and Emmings, F. G.: Freezing bone without excision; an experimental study of bone-cell destruction and manner of regrowth in dogs, JAMA 196:770, 1906.
33. Ham, A. W., and Leeson, T. S.: *Histology* (4th ed.; J. B. Lippincott Company, 1961).
34. Ham, A. W., and Harris, W. R.: Repair and Transplantation of Bone, in Bourne, G. H. (ed.),

The Biochemistry and Physiology of Bone, Vol. 3, *Development and Growth* (2d ed.; New York: Academic Press, 1971), p. 337.
35. Hancox, N. M.: *Biology of Bone* (London: Cambridge University Press, 1972).
36. Harris, W. H., Coutts, R. D., Davis, L., and MacKenzie, A.: Experimental analysis of the role of compression vs. the role of stabilization in skeletal responses, J. Bone Joint Surg. 54-A: 1800, 1972.
37. Hay, E. D.: Origin of Osteoblasts from Mononuclear Leukocytes in Regenerating Newt Limbs, in Robinson, R. A. (ed.), *The Healing of Osseous Tissue* (Washington, D. C.: National Academy of Sciences – National Research Council, 1967), p. 129.
38. Henry, A. N., Freeman, M. A. R., and Swanson, S. A. U.: Studies on the mechanical properties of healing experimental fractures, Proc. R. Soc. Med. 61:40, 1968.
39. Holden, C. E. A.: The role of blood supply to soft tissue in the healing of diaphyseal fractures, J. Bone Joint Surg. 54-A:993, 1972.
40. Holtrop, M.: The Origin of Bone Cells in Endochondral Ossification, in Proceedings, Third European Symposium on Calcified Tissues, Davos, 1965 (Berlin: Springer-Verlag, 1966).
41. Hulth, A., and Olerud, S.: Early fracture callus in normal and cortisone treated rats. A study by a combination of tetracycline labelling, microangiography and microradiography, Acta Orthop. Scand. 34:1, 1964.
42. Jarry, L., and Uhthoff, H. K.: Post traumatic sclerosis of bone, J. Bone Joint Surg. 50-B:2, 1968.
43. Jarry, L., and Uhthoff, H. K.: Pluripotency of periosteum and endosteum in fracture healing J. Bone Joint Surg. 57-B:387, 1969.
44. Johnson, L. C.: The Kinetics of Skeletal Remodelling, Structural Organization of the Skeleton, *Birth Defects, Original Article Series*, Vol. II, No. 1, p. 67, 1966.
45. Kato, F. and Glimcher, M. J.: The relationship between cellular modulation and architectural structures in bone healing. To be published.
46. Kelly, P. J.: Anatomy, physiology and pathology of the blood supply of bones, J. Bone Joint Surg. 50-A:766, 1968.
47. Kenzora, J. E.: The osteocytic, living, dying and dead; a histologic functional study, J. Bone Joint Surg. 54-A:1126, 1972.
48. Kenzora, J. E., Uosipovich, Z., Steel, R., and Warshawsky, H.: Tissue biology following experimental infarction of femoral heads. Part I, J. Bone Joint Surg. 51-A:1021, 1969.
49. Key, J. A., and Conwell, A. E.: The Management of Fractures, Dislocations and Sprains in *Repair of Fractures* (6th ed.; St. Louis: The C. V. Mosby Company, 1956), Chap. 2.
50. Laurnen, E. L., and Kelly, P. J.: Blood flow, oxygen consumption, carbon dioxide production and blood-calcium and pH changes in tibial fractures in dogs, J. Bone Joint Surg. 51-A:298, 1969.
51. Lavine, L. S., Lustrin, O., Shamos, M. H., Rinaldt, R. A., and Liboff, A. R.: Electric enhancement of bone healing, Science 175: 1118, 1972.
52. Lettin, A. W.: The effects of axial compression on the healing of experimental fractures of the rat tibia, Proc. R. Soc. Med. 58:882, 1965.
53. Lindholm, R., Lindholm, S., Liukko, P., Paasimäki, J., Osikääntä, S., Rossi, R., Autio, E., and Tamminent, E.: The mast cell as a component of callus in healing fractures, J. Bone Joint Surg. 51-B: 148, 1969.
54. MacNab, I.: The blood supply of tubular and cancellous bone, J. Bone Joint Surg. 40-A: 1433, 1958.
55. Miller, L. S.: Charnley compression clamp in treatment of nonunion of the tibia, South. Med. J. 61:606, 1968.
56. Milner, J. C., and Rhinelander, F. W.: Compression fixation and primary bone healing, Surg. Forum 19:453, 1968.
57. Mindell, E. R., Rodbard, S., and Kwasman, B. G.: Chondrogenesis in bone repair. A study of the healing fracture callus in the rat, Clin. Orthop. 79:187, 1971.
58. Müller, M. E., Allgöwer, M., and Willenegger, H.: *Technique of Internal Fixation of Fractures*, G. Segmüller (ed.) (Berlin and New York: Springer-Verlag, 1965).
59. Murakami, H., and Emergy, M. A.: The role of elastic fibres in the periosteum in fracture healing in guinea pigs. Histologic studies of the elastic fibres in the periosteum and the possible relationship between the osteogenic cells and the cells that form elastic fibres, Can. J. Surg. 10:359, 1967.
60. Olerud, S., and Danckwardt-Lilliestrom, G.: Fracture healing in compression osteosynthesis in the dog, J. Bone Joint Surg. 50-B:844, 1968.
61. Peacock, E. E., and Van Winkle, W., Jr.: *Surgery and Biology of Wound Repair* (Philadelphia: W. B. Saunders Company, 1970), Chap. XI.
62. Prasad, G. C., and Reynolds, J. J.: Effect of environmental factors on the repair of bone in vitro, J. Bone Joint Surg. 50-B:401, 1968.
63. Pritchard, J. J.: General Histology of Bone (Chap. 1) and The Osteoblast (Chap. 2), in Bourne, G. H. (ed.), *The Biochemistry and Physiology of Bone* (New York: Academic Press, 1971), Vol. 1.
64. Pritchard, J. J.: Bone Healing, in *The Scientific Basis of Medicine, Annual Reviews 1963*, Univ. of London, The Athlone Press, 1963. Chap. XVIII, p. 286.
65. Pritchard, J. J., and Ruzicka, A. J.: Comparison of fracture repair in the frog, lizard and rat, J. Anat. 84:236, 1950.
66. Pugh, P. D.: An early impression of techniques employed by the Association for the Study of Osteosynthesis, Proc. R. Soc. Med. 61:982, 1968.
67. Rabhan, W. N., and Haas, L. M.: The role of fracture hematoma in the union of long bones, J. Bone Joint Surg. 51-A:1036, 1969.
68. Rahn, B. A., Gallinaro, R., Baltensperger, A., and Perren, S. M.: Primary bone healing, an experimental study in the rabbit, J. Bone Joint Surg. 53-A:783, 1971.
69. Reynolds, F. C., and Key, J. A.: Fracture healing after fixation with standard plates, contact splints and medullary nails. An experimental study, J. Bone Joint Surg. 36-A: 577, 1954.

70. Rhinelander, F. W.: The normal microcirculation of diaphyseal cortex and its response to fracture, J. Bone Joint Surg. 50-A: 784, 1968.
71. Rhinelander, F. W., and Baragry, R. A.: Microangiography in bone healing. I. Undisplaced closed fractures, J. Bone Joint Surg. 44-A:1273, 1962.
72. Robinson, R. A. (ed.): *The Healing of Osseous Tissue—A Workshop*, October 23–25, 1965, (Washington, D.C.: National Academy of Sciences—National Research Council, 1967).
73. Rokkanen, P., and Slätes, P.: The repair of experimental fractures during long term anticoagulant treatment. An experimental study on rats, Acta Orthop. Scand. 35:21, 1964.
74. Rubin, P.: *Dynamic Classification of Bone Dysplasias* (Chicago: Year Book Medical Publishers, Inc., 1964).
75. Schenk, R., and Willenegger, H.: Morphologic findings in primary fracture healing, Symp. Biol. Hung. 7:75, 1967.
76. Schenk, R., and Willenegger, H.: Zum histologischen Bild der sogenannten Primärheilung der Knochenkompakta nach experimentellen Osteotomien am Hund, Experientia 19:593, 1963.
77. Schenk, R., and Willenegger, H.: Zur Histologie der primären Knochenheilung, Langenbeck Arch. Klin. Chir. 308:440, 1964.
78. Segmüller, G.: Bone repair and internal fixation, Prog. Surg. 5:87, 1966.
79. Sevitt, S.: The healing of fractures of the lower end of the radius, J. Bone Joint Surg. 53-B:519, 1971.
80. Shaw, J. L., and Bassett, C. A.: The effects of varying oxygen concentrations on osteogenesis and embryonic cartilage in vitro, J. Bone Joint Surg. 49-A:1, 1967.
81. Slatis, P., et al.: The normal repair of experimental fractures. A histoquantitative study of rats, Acta Orthop. Scand. 36:221, 1965.
82. Sledge, C. B., and Asher, M.: The effect of inorganic orthophosphate on the rates of collagen formation and degradation in bone and cartilage, J. Bone Joint Surg. 54-A:1122, 1972.
83. Tonna, E. A.: The Source of Osteoblasts in Healing Fractures in Animals of Different Ages, in Robinson, R. A. (ed.), *The Healing of Osseous Tissue* (Washington, D. C.: National Academy of Sciences—National Research Council, 1967), p. 93.
84. Tonna, E. A., and Cronkite, E. P.: Cellular response to fracture studied with tritiated thymidine, J. Bone Joint Surg. 43-A:352, 1961.
85. Tonna, E. A., and Cronkite, E. P.: Changes in the skeletal cell proliferative response to trauma concomitant with aging, J. Bone Joint Surg. 44-A:1557, 1962.
86. Trueta, J.: *Studies of the Development and Decay of the Human Frame* (Philadelphia: W. B. Saunders Company, 1968), Chaps. 24–26.
87. Uhthoff, H. K., Lavigne, P., and Dubuc, F.: The importance of compression and rigidity of the plate and the structural changes in bone—the late bony changes beneath the plate, J. Bone Joint Surg. 54-B:763, 1972.
88. Urist, M. R., Wallace, T. H., and Adams, T.: The function of fibrocartilaginous fracture callus. Observations on transplants labelled with tritiated thymidine, J. Bone Joint Surg. 47-B:304, 1965.
89. Varma, B. P., et al.: Fracture healing with intramedullary nail fixation of the long bones. An experimental study, Acta Orthop. Scand. 38:419, 1967.
90. Vaughn, L. C.: The repair of fractures in pigs, Vet. Rec. 79:2, 1966.
91. Walker, D. G.: Reversal of osteopetrosis by the serial transfer of osteolytic stem cells. A paper read at the twentieth annual meeting of the Orthopaedic Research Society, Dallas, Texas, January 17, 1974.
92. Weiss, R., et al.: The influence of cortisone on the healing of experimental fractures in rats, Acta Anat. (Basel) 59:163, 1964.
93. Wray, J. B.: Studies of metabolic activity in the healing of fractures, J. Bone Joint Surg. 51-A:1694, 1969.
94. Yamagishi, M., and Yoshiyuki, Y.: The biomechanics of fracture healing, J. Bone Joint Surg. 37-A:1035, 1955.
95. Young, R. W.: The Control of Cell Specialization in Bone, in Robinson, R. A. (ed.), *The Healing of Osseous Tissue* (Washington, D.C.: National Academy of Sciences—National Research Council, 1967), p. 111.

5 Delayed Union, Nonunion and Malunion of Long Bones; Nonunion with Infection

EDWIN F. CAVE and ROBERT J. BOYD

THE FUNDAMENTAL PRINCIPLES of bone healing do not change, but methods of management of a broken bone have varied from generation to generation, from decade to decade and often from year to year. Hippocrates wrote, "Put the bone ends together and hold them still enough and long enough." This fundamental idea still prevails, but during the latter part of the nineteenth and early part of the twentieth centuries, the operative treatment of fractures came into vogue and this was especially true in the early 1930s, when the quality of metals was improved and the reaction to metal in tissue was diminished or practically eliminated. Then, many surgeons treating fractures used a more radical approach and carried out open reductions on the closed fractures. Unfortunately, they began to "treat the x-ray" and not the extremity as a whole. Thus, the operative treatment has caused many disasters when used by those lacking in fundamental knowledge of bone healing and with improper operative techniques and inadequate follow-up care of the patient. This is not to condemn open reduction of fractures, but it is to remind the reader that the fundamental principles of bone healing still prevail as it is realized that the majority of long bone fractures will heal if reduced adequately and held sufficiently long with external fixation.

During the present century, the management of a long bone fracture actually has improved in many ways. Accurate diagnoses have been possible; proper x-ray techniques and methods of external splinting have been perfected; surgical procedures have been improved; metals used for internal fixation have been standardized and the care of the whole patient has been enhanced; but, as these advances have been made, nonunion of bone actually has been on the increase, and this increased incidence of nonunion after fracture must be laid largely at the door of the surgeon. In many instances, harm is done by the use of inadequate or improper incisions, poor internal fixation and improper postoperative care, any one of which may lead to delayed union and nonunion of bone. When such errors in judgment and poor results occur, the surgeon must be held responsible.

In general, the common causes of nonunion are: lack of adequate reduction of the fracture and faulty immobilization. And when bone fails to heal after fracture, the cause in an extremely high percentage of cases is a local one. Generalized body disturbance does not cause nonunion of bone, except in cases of extreme malnutrition, extreme vitamin deficiency or intrinsic bone disease.

Fractures of certain long bones, namely, those of the femoral neck, the femoral shaft, the lower shaft of the tibia and, at times, the humeral shaft, may require a longer period of time to unite than do fractures of certain other bones. The slowness of union of fractures in the areas listed is generally attributed to lack of adequate blood supply to the part, because, in these instances, the fracture usually occurs at the level of or beyond the entrance of the nutrient artery to bone, and circulation to the fracture surfaces is cut off. Therefore, unless prompt and accurate reduction of the fracture is carried out, healing of bone may be delayed and nonunion may result.

The local causes of delayed union or nonunion are:

1. Inadequate reduction of the fracture.
2. Inadequate external fixation.
3. Trauma to soft parts, which interferes with circulation to bone fragments.
4. Improper operative interference, causing trauma to bone ends and interference with blood supply.
5. Inadequate internal fixation.
6. Too much "hardware" (plates, screws, bands, medullary nails, etc.).
7. Improper application of metal for internal fixation.
8. Distraction of bone fragments, due to improperly applied traction.
9. Too early motion of the injured part.
10. Too early weight bearing on an injured lower extremity.
11. Sacrifice of bone fragments in open fractures.
12. Infection.

The larger the bone the longer the time required for healing in most instances. The fractured phalanx will be stabilized, and the finger can be used in a few days, without fear of delayed healing, but a fracture of the femur must be protected

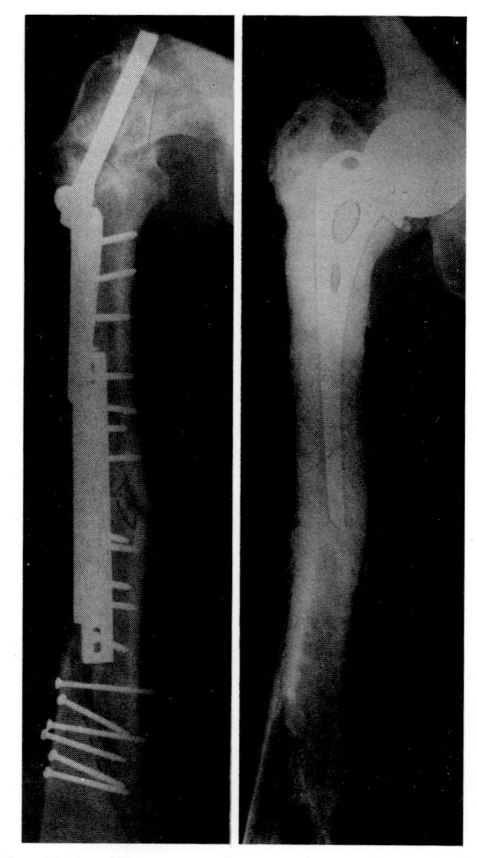

Fig. 5-1.—How much metal can bone tolerate? The original fractures, sustained in an automobile accident, were located at the base of the femoral neck, the upper third of the femur and the midshaft of the femur. The third fracture developed in the lower third of the femur from minor trauma to porotic bone during convalescence from the original injury. **Left,** the result of treatment: nonunion of the base of the femoral neck and a refracture of the distal portion of the shaft. A sterile abscess developed over the plates in the lateral aspect of the femur. Eventually the sterile abscess was evacuated, hardware removed and the wound closed. The fractures united except for the one at the base of the femoral neck. **Right,** 2 years after union of the femoral shaft and insertion of a Vitallium prosthesis for the ununited femoral neck fracture. The patient, now ambulatory and walking with a cane, was perfectly able to carry out his duties as a hotel executive.

Chapter 5: DELAYED UNION, NONUNION AND MALUNION OF LONG BONES

for months because of the size of the bone, its weight-bearing function and very large muscle attachments, which exert pull on the fractured fragments.

There is no rule as to how long a fracture of a particular bone must be immobilized, but the arbitrary periods shown in the list below can be accepted for a working formula, particularly if internal fixation is not applied.

1. Phalanges — A few days to 2 weeks
2. Metacarpals — 2–3 weeks
3. Carpal bones, other than the navicular — 3–6 weeks
4. Carpal navicular — 10–16 weeks
5. Forearm bones:
    a) Children — 6–8 weeks
    b) Adults — 8–14 weeks
6. Humeral shaft — 8–12 weeks
7. Clavicle:
    a) Children — 3 weeks
    b) Adults — 4–6 weeks
8. Metatarsal bones — 3–4 weeks
9. Tarsal bones — 6–8 weeks
10. Tibia:
    a) Without fracture of the fibula:
        (1) Young children — 6 weeks
        (2) Older children and adults — 8–16 weeks
    b) With fracture of the fibula:
        (1) Young children — 6–8 weeks
        (2) Older children and adults — 12–20 weeks
11. Femur:
    a) Children — 6–8 weeks
    b) Older children and adults — 12–24 weeks

Nonunion (clinical) of fractures does not occur in the following:
1. The vertebral body.
2. The skull.
3. The scapula.
4. The ribs.

The time factor in the healing of fractures may be the most important phase of all fracture management, and courage on the part of the surgeon and cooperation by the patient are required to continue with immobilization until bone heals. Unless traction is required, immobilization must be complete, and plaster of Paris is the most effective means of providing such fixation. Braces that are worn part time do not give uninterrupted fixation and often give the patient a false sense of security.

No two fractures are alike as to cause the resultant deformity, and the management of no one fracture can be exactly comparable to that of another. This statement can be applied to an even greater degree in regard to nonunion of bone. The causes of nonunion listed below are the common ones, but, in certain cases, a combination of factors may exist. Soft tissue scar bone loss and infection all play a part in the delayed healing of many open fractures. In recent years, as operative treatment of fractures has become more frequent, improper operations have become a major cause. In an analysis of 120 closed fractures that eventually resulted in operation for correction of longstanding nonunion, the causes were listed as follows:

Improper operative interference	44
Inadequate external fixation	12
Inadequate closed reduction	12
Interposed soft tissue	11
Distraction	11
Infection	7
Too early weight bearing	7
Improper operative technique	3
Failure of reduction	3
Abnormal metabolic bone change	3 (1 malnutrition)
Infection and improper operative technique	2
Inadequate closed reduction and fixation	2
Too early weight bearing and broken medullary nail	1

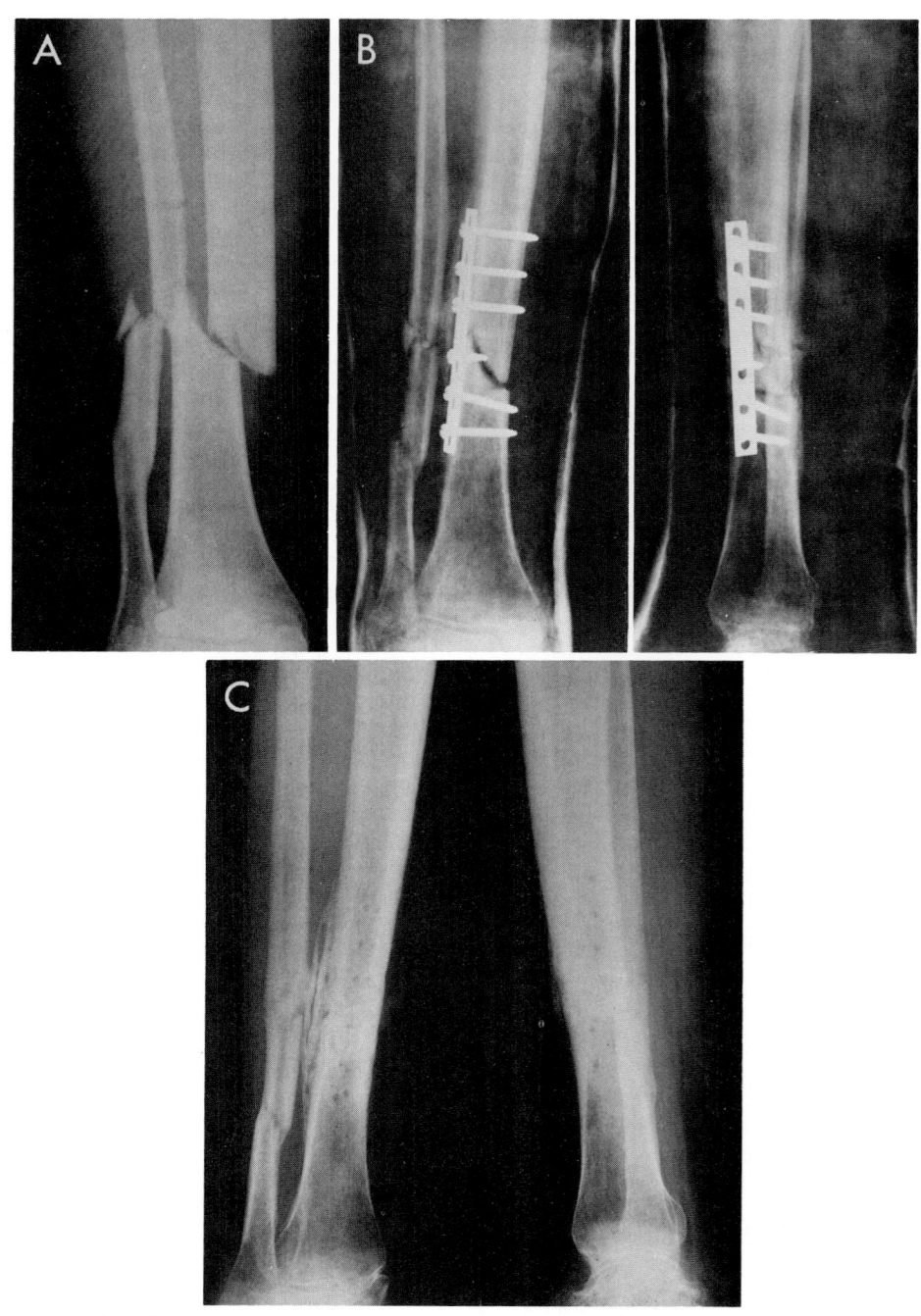

Fig. 5-2.—Delayed union of bone due to improperly applied slotted plate. **A,** the fresh fracture. **B,** anteroposterior and lateral views showing screws placed so that the fracture cannot impact. Removal of metal and subperiosteal application of iliac bone promoted union in 4 additional months. **C,** anteroposterior and lateral views revealing bone union.

Metal interference
   and distraction   1
Intentional operative
   procedure to
   improve motion   1

In 81 open fractures, the causes of nonunion were listed as follows:

Improper operative
   interference   20
Infection   13
Inadequate external
   fixation   12
Bone loss   10
Distraction   7
Soft tissue trauma   6
Inadequate reduction   3
Too early weight
   bearing   3
Interposed soft tissue   2
Faulty operative
   technique   2
Soft tissue loss and
   improper operative
   interference   1
Infection and
   improper operative
   technique   1
Bone loss and
   infection   1

It is discouraging to note that improper operative interference was the principal cause of nonunion in both closed and open fractures.

At times, it may be difficult to determine whether one is dealing with delayed union, and occasionally one cannot be sure that nonunion actually exists.

The presence of *delayed* union must be determined almost entirely from the x-ray film. Certain bones give evidence of healing in more or less prescribed periods of time. The best evidence of bone healing is callus formation, as shown by the film. Calcification of periosteum is not true callus formation. The more accurately a fracture is aligned the less demand there will be for callus. In such a case, a gradual obliteration of the fracture line, without loss of position, and the absence of unusual bone atrophy, or excessive sclerosis at the fracture site, are the best evidences of progressive bone healing.

There is no reliable clinical test for delayed union. As a fracture is healing, manual tests for motion should not be

Fig. 5-3.—Callus requirement is increased with malposition. **A,** anatomic reduction. **B,** large callus requirement; slow union.

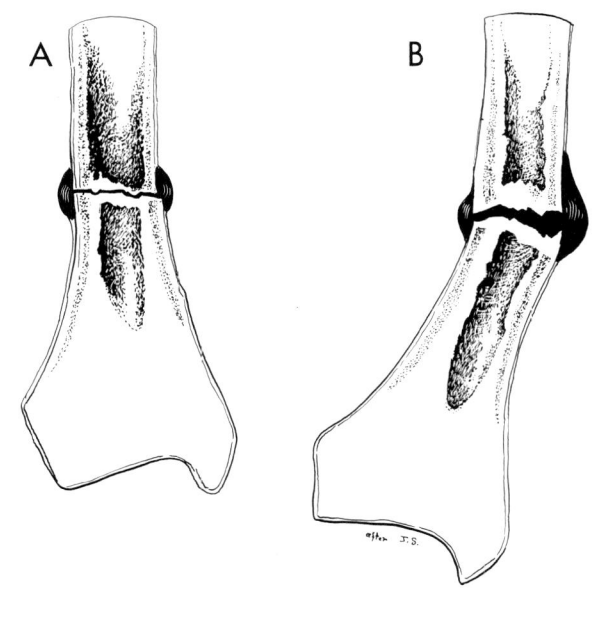

made at the fracture site because any movement may interrupt the new bone bridge that is uniting the fracture.

Nonunion of bone occurs when the repair process has stopped completely, and it is suggested by the following clinical findings:

1. Pain on use of the extremity.
2. Progressive bowing of the extremity.
3. Edema of the extremity.
4. Increased surface temperature at the fracture site.

By roentgenogram, the following should be looked for to determine the presence of nonunion:

1. Excess (false) callus production at the fracture site.
2. Gradual bowing at the fracture site.
3. Unusual sclerosis at the fracture site.

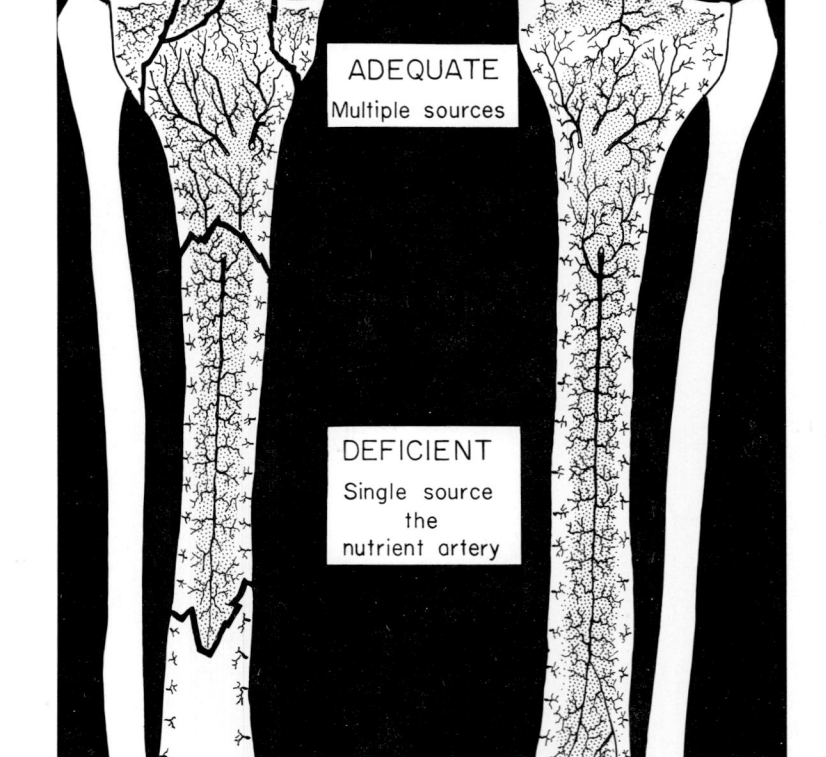

Fig. 5-4.—The tibial blood supply.

Chapter 5: DELAYED UNION, NONUNION AND MALUNION OF LONG BONES / 121

4. Unusual bone atrophy below and above the fracture site.

Although definite rules cannot be put down as to the exact technique of management of any group of cases of nonunion of bone, certain considerations always are necessary and certain principles must be adhered to. When confronted with an ununited fracture, the surgeon must ask himself the following questions:

1. *Which bone and what part of the bone are involved?*

The trochanteric area and the supracondylar area of the femur will unite more promptly than will the shaft of the femur because cancellous bone heals more promptly than cortical bone and because the blood supply is more abundant in the former areas. The same applies to the upper and lower ends of the other long bones. The femoral neck and the carpal navicular are notoriously slow in uniting.

2. *How long has nonunion existed?*

The longer nonunion has existed the greater the sclerosis of bone ends and atrophy of the soft tissue and of the shaft, especially beyond the fracture line. Sclerosed bone will require a long time to revascularize even if it is covered by "fresh" bone and nourished by a good muscular covering.

3. *What is the condition of the soft parts?*

Scar in skin, subcutaneous tissue and muscle will preclude good circulation to the fracture and to the bone graft. Therefore, the graft must be inserted through an incision over the most viable soft tissue.

4. *What is the condition of the joints above and below the site of fracture?*

Immobile joints will add strain to the fracture site. Therefore, after the graft is applied, the fracture must be protected until there is solid union. Medullary fixa-

Fig. 5-5. — Sclerosis of bone in a manufacturer, aged 52. **A,** 2 years after open fracture; complete nonunion of tibia. **B,** 1 year after grafting and 3 years after injury; complete healing. The onlay graft was removed from the proximal fragment. Iliac bone slabs were also packed around the fracture site.

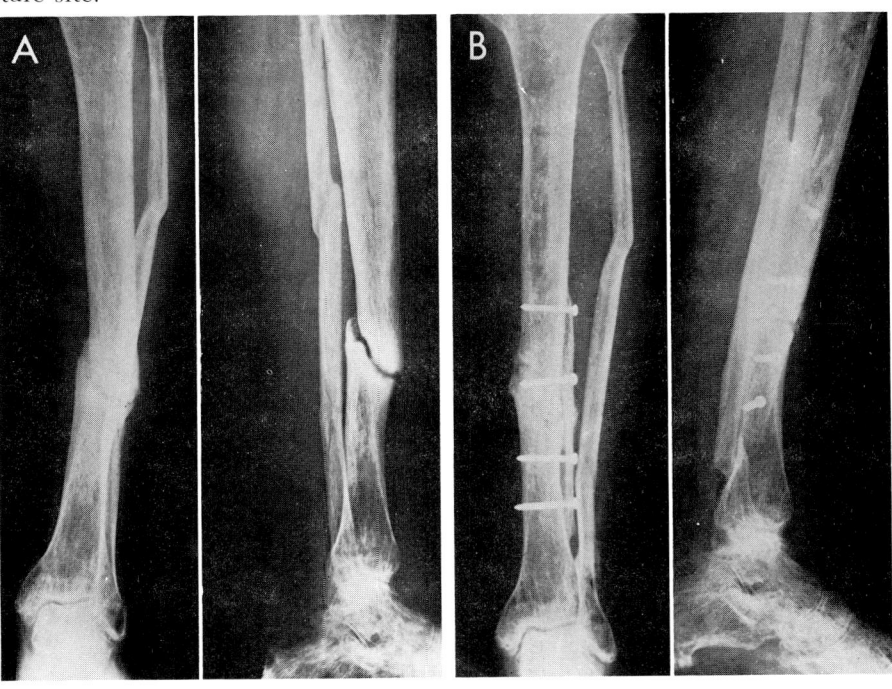

tion has allowed much earlier joint motion after operations for nonunion.

5. *Is the fracture in satisfactory alignment?*

An ununited fracture in good alignment should not be mobilized by excising scar at the fracture site. Fibrous union gives some stability, and subperiosteal iliac bone may be all that is required to promote union.

6. *To what degree is there sclerosis of bone ends at the fracture site?*

Sclerosed bone, with excessive callus formation, need not necessarily be excised completely, but the shaft should be reshaped by trimming down the excess sclerotic area before applying the graft. Such reshaping will enhance the local circulation, allow the introduction of bone and result in easier wound closure.

7. *To what degree is there osteoporosis of bone below and/or above the fracture site?*

Osteoporosis calls for as early use of the extremity as is consistent with healing of the ununited fracture. Until joint motion can be initiated or weight is borne, muscle-setting exercises are of benefit.

8. *To what degree is there bone loss?*

Bone loss is, at times, the most severe deterrent to bone healing, and it frequently follows gunshot wounds or ill-advised debridement where bone is sacrificed. To promote union, bone must be replaced by grafting or the shaft must be shortened at the fracture site.

9. *To what degree is there shortening of the injured bone?*

Bone lengthening has been largely

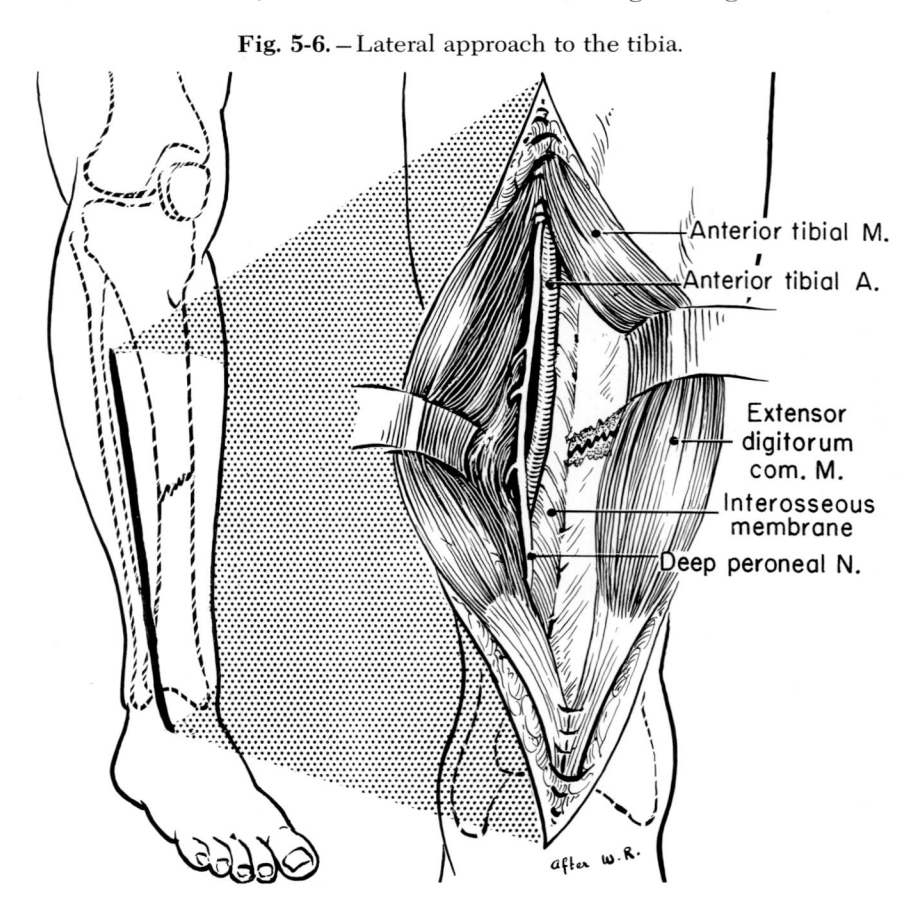

Fig. 5-6.—Lateral approach to the tibia.

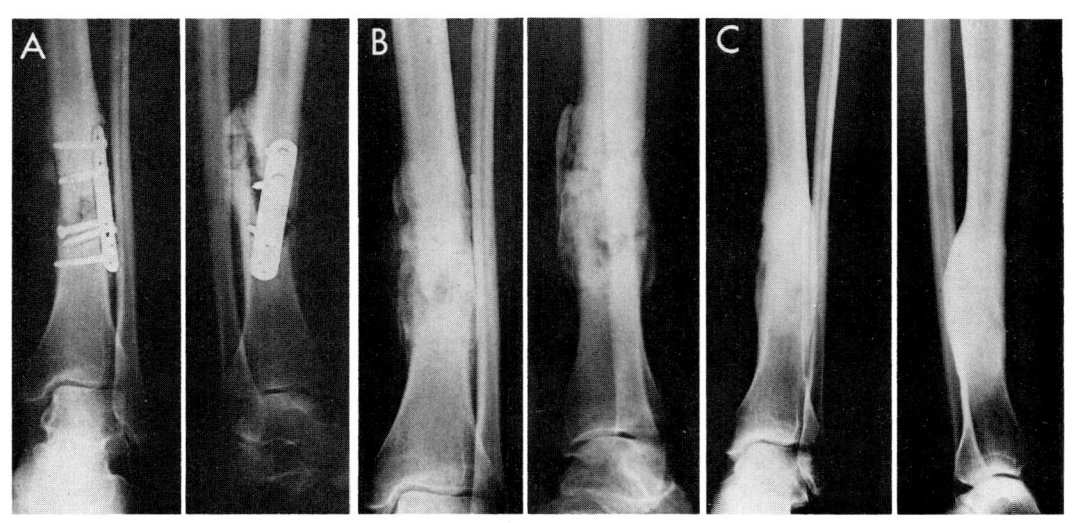

Fig. 5-7.—Nonunion of 6 months' duration following faulty application of plate and screws in the tibia of a housewife, aged 26. **A,** 6 months after injury and operation. **B,** 4 months after removal of plate and screws and subperiosteal application of iliac slabs of bone posteriorly, mesially and laterally; bone has healed. **C,** 7 years after bone graft; complete recovery.

abandoned as an operative procedure, since it is better to obtain union even though a considerable degree of shortening must be accepted. Shortening of the upper extremity can be accepted; shortening of the lower extremity can be compensated for by a lift on the shoe. If the shortening is too great, amputation can be done at the point of election and a prosthesis used.

10. *If union can be established, will the patient have a useful extremity?*

If, despite bone union, there is severe, painful limitation of joint motion with marked shortening, with a painful, relatively useless hand or foot, amputation may be the procedure of choice.

NONUNION OF FEMORAL SHAFT FRACTURES

Nonunion in fractures of the femoral shaft occurs second in frequency only to that of the tibia. In 46 cases of nonunion of the femur, the causes were as follows:

Improper operative interference	8
Inadequate external fixation	8
Distraction	7
Infection	5
Interposed soft tissue	4
Bone loss	4
Abnormal metabolic bone change	3
Inadequate closed reduction	3
Infection and improper operative technique	1
Too early weight bearing	1
Too early weight bearing and broken medullary nail	1
Intentional operative procedure to improve motion	1

TREATMENT OF NONUNION OF CLOSED FEMORAL FRACTURES.—Since the introduction of medullary nailing, nonunion of the femur has been less frequent, when it has occurred, it has been corrected more easily by intramedullary fixation. Before the use of the medullary nail, the onlay bone graft or the subperiosteal application of iliac bone was used. The onlay bone graft frequently was followed by failure. The subperiosteal application of iliac bone succeeded in some cases in which the onlay graft failed, but it required prolonged external immobilization of the extremity afterward.

If the soft tissues will permit, a high

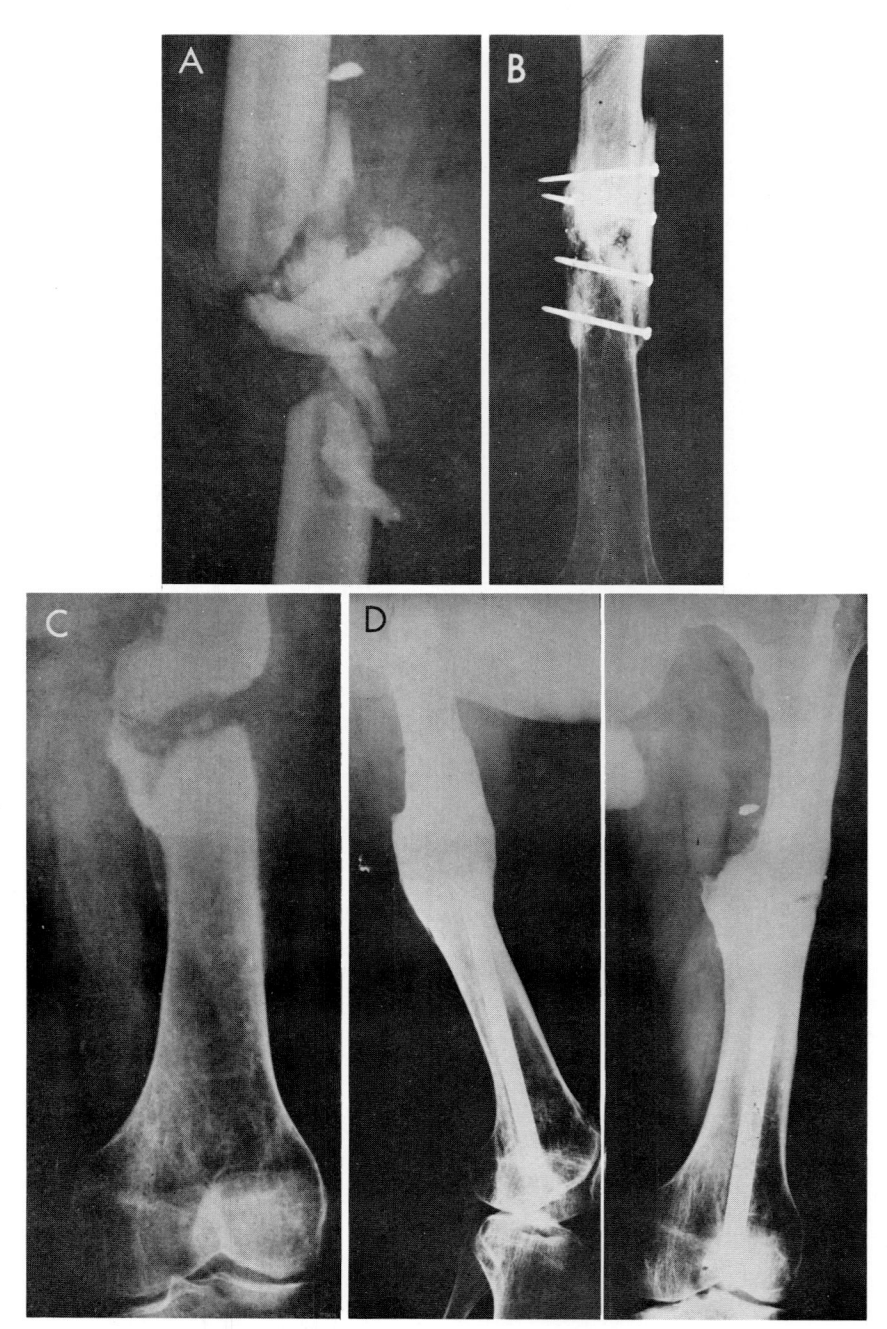

Fig. 5-8.—Use of medullary nail in old ununited infected fracture of femur and extreme bone loss, extreme bone sclerosis and 3-inch shortening, secondary to gunshot wound in a soldier, aged 29. **A,** wound shortly after injury. **B,** 4 years later, after several attempts at bone grafting. **C,** 5 years after wound, following removal of screws and graft. **D,** bone union without infection following medullary nailing 8 years after injury.

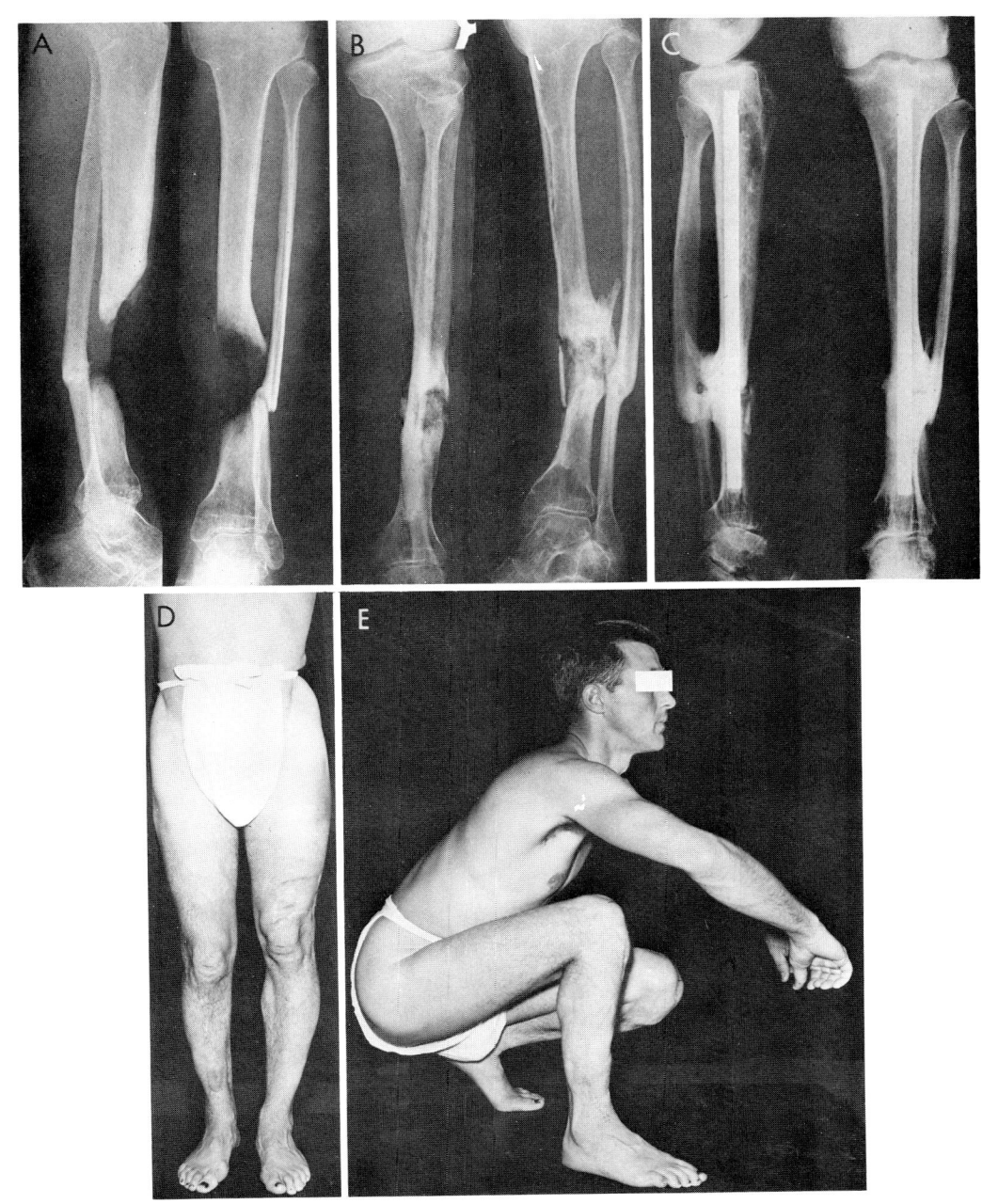

Chapter 5: DELAYED UNION, NONUNION AND MALUNION OF LONG BONES / **125**

Fig. 5-9. — Nonunion of the right tibia with deformity in soldier, aged 23. **A,** extensive bone loss of tibia following open fracture; union of fibula of 2 years' duration. **B,** 1 year after attempted bone graft. **C,** 5 years after injury and 1 year after medullary nailing and graft; bone union. **D** and **E,** end result: bone union; 1-inch shortening; good knee function.

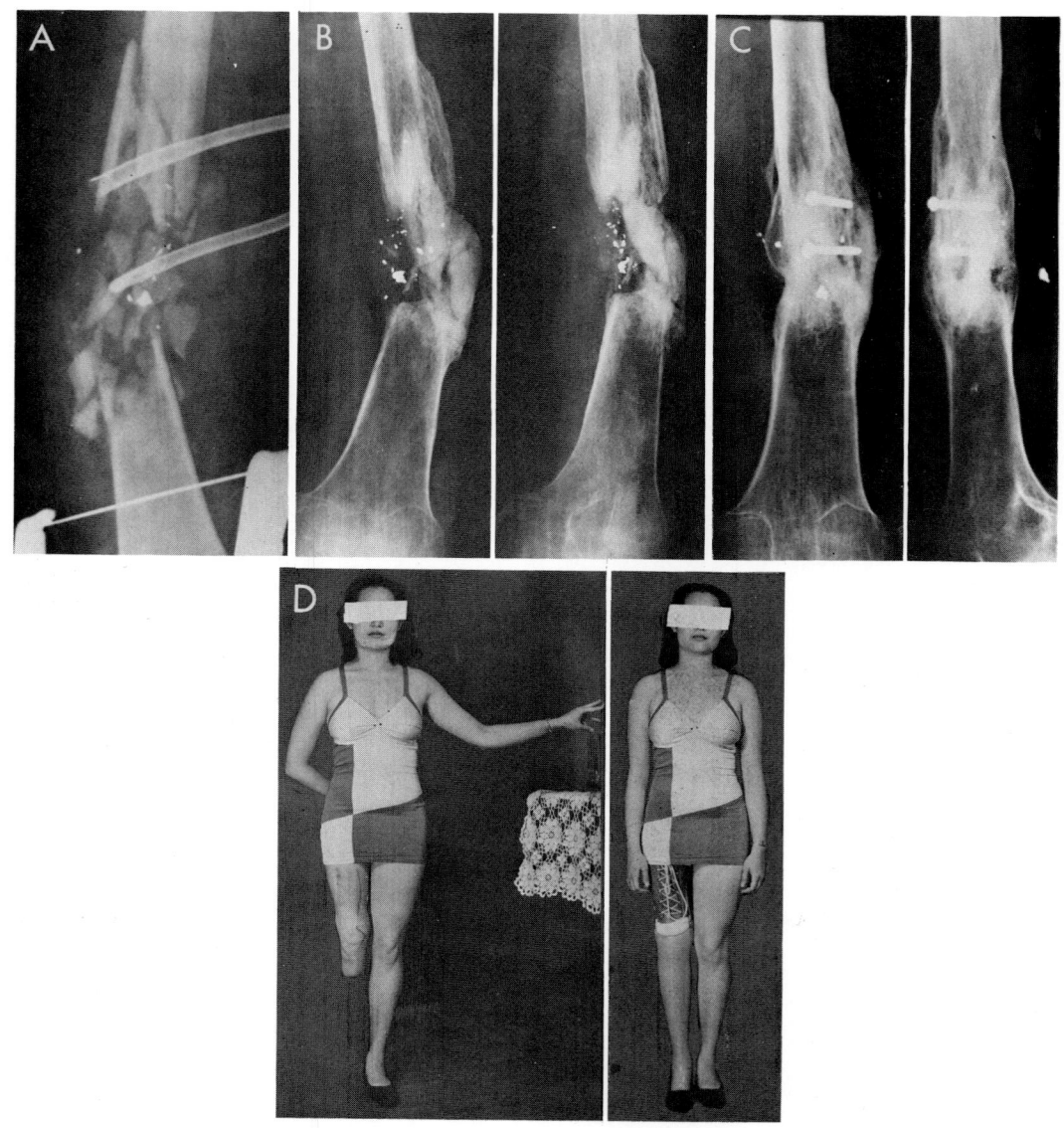

Fig. 5-10. — Producing union by bone shortening. **A**, gunshot wound of femur (woman, aged 17, in the home), resulting in gangrene of foot and distal leg and followed by amputation; bone loss and nonunion of femur. **B**, 1 year later; draining sinus; nonunion of femur. **C**, 2 years after injury (femur had been shortened and secured with 2 screws); union obtained. **D**, 5 years after injury; union of the shortened femur and a mobile knee; prosthesis worn satisfactorily.

percentage of cases of nonunion of the femoral shaft can be treated successfully by the medullary nail and the addition of subperiosteal iliac bone.

The compression plate has been advocated by some.[18] Postoperative care will depend greatly on the condition of the soft tissues, the quality of the bone to be stabilized, the mobility of the joints above and below the fracture and the return of strength to the quadriceps and the hamstring muscles. If stability is ob-

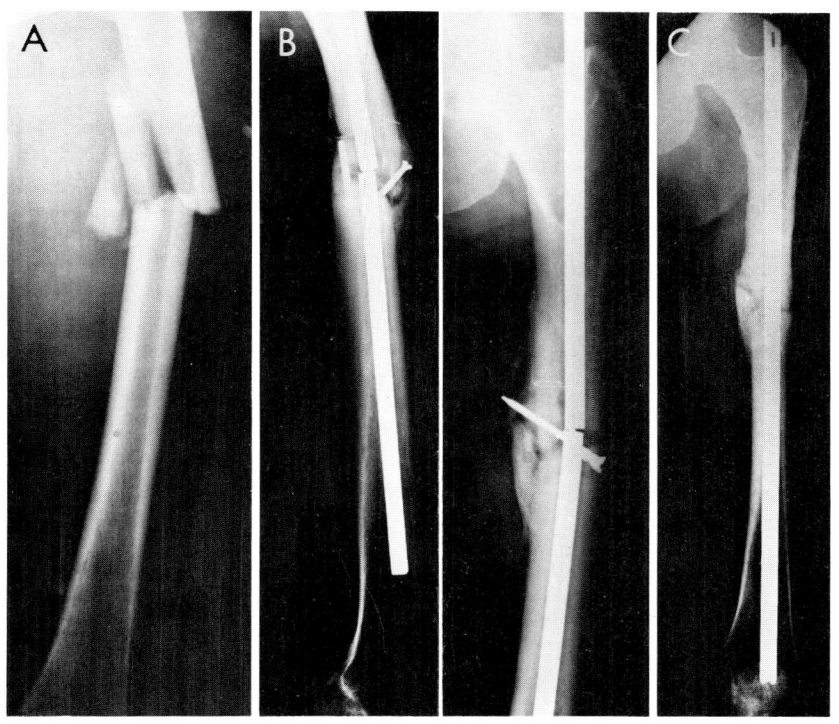

Chapter 5: DELAYED UNION, NONUNION AND MALUNION OF LONG BONES / **127**

Fig. 5-11.—Comminuted fracture of the upper shaft of the femur (housewife, aged 34); nonunion resulted. **A,** the original fracture. **B,** 2 years after insertion of medullary nail, which broke 18 months after it was inserted because it was of too small diameter and was not inserted far enough down the shaft; nonunion. **C,** after removal of screws and broken nail and the insertion of a larger (12-mm) nail, which reached to the level of the adductor tubercle, and of bone grafts.

tained by the nail and muscle control is satisfactory, partial weight bearing with crutches can be allowed within a few days. When stability of the fracture is in doubt, the medullary nail may be supplemented by a walking plaster spica.

Crutches should be continued until bone union is established. The time will vary from 4 months to 1 year, or longer.

TREATMENT OF NONUNION OF OPEN FEMORAL FRACTURES.—Ununited open fractures of the femoral shaft offer a serious problem because usually there has been extensive damage to the soft tissues, resultant scar formation, possibly latent bone infection and, not infrequently, bone loss.

The medullary nail is by far the best means of handling such problems. Before inserting the nail it usually is wise to eliminate all sinuses and sequestra, insofar as possible. If drainage persists despite what was considered to be adequate debridement, the surgeon may be justified in introducing the medullary nail, because often stability of a fracture will not only encourage healing of bone but will also diminish the reaction to infection, and it may even encourage closure of a draining sinus. Bone grafts may be added through a separate incision.

NONUNION OF CLOSED FRACTURES OF TIBIA AND FIBULA

If the ununited tibia is in alignment and the soft tissue in good condition, it is probable that subperiosteal iliac bone will work successfully in promoting union. If the fibula is united in malposi-

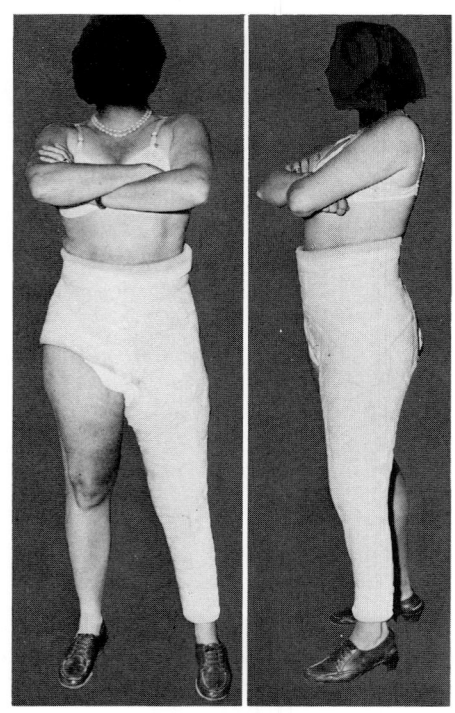

Fig. 5-12.—A "walking" plaster spica supplementing medullary fixation for an ununited fracture of the femoral shaft of 2 years' duration. Spica was applied in a standing position and was worn for 6 months without difficulty by a housewife, aged 34.

tion and prevents proper alignment of the tibial fracture, it should be osteotomized, realigned and, possibly, stabilized with a Rush pin.

If the fracture of the tibia is maligned, the surgeon will, of necessity, osteotomize the fibula, usually through a separate incision, and expose, mobilize and realign the tibia. Iliac bone should be placed around the tibia, especially posteriorly and laterally. In any case, prolonged external fixation by means of plaster is necessary until union is firm.

NONUNION OF THE TIBIA AND FIBULA SECONDARY TO OPEN FRACTURES

In the management of the ununited open fracture of the tibia and fibula, much depends on the condition of the skin, subcutaneous tissue and surrounding muscle. Very often, scarring will be so extensive anteriorly over the tibia that a direct incision in this area will be impossible and the approach must be posterior.

A full-thickness skin graft over the scarred tibia may increase nutrition to the area, but it is doubtful that the routine anterior approach to the ununited tibial fracture can be used in many cases, even after a skin graft. There is considerable doubt as to whether a full-thickness skin graft actually nourishes the bone, as does normal skin and subcutaneous tissue.

NONUNION OF FOREARM FRACTURES

Nonunion of the forearm bones occurs third in frequency, following nonunion of the tibia and the femur. Seventeen cases in a series of 201 occurring in all long bones involved the radius and/or ulna. Of the 17 cases, 5 were open fractures and 12 were closed. In 13 cases, the soft tissues were in excellent condition at the time of operation.

Of the 12 closed fractures, 2 were treated by onlay tibial grafts to the radius and ulna and 10 were stabilized by the use of onlay iliac bone; 8 of the 10 were secured by screws. All united solidly.

Of the 5 patients with open fractures, 1 was an 8-year-old boy who had had the upper two-thirds of his radial shaft avulsed in an automobile accident. This fracture was treated by transplantation of a 6-inch section of the fibula. The result, 7 years later, was continued growth of the distal radial epiphysis with reasonably good length to the forearm but marked limitation of supination. However, there was good return of function of the entire extremity except for limited rotation.

The second case was that of a 52-year-old woman whose forearm had been badly mangled in an automobile accident 1 year previously. She sustained a severe open fracture of both bones of the forearm. The radius was plated and the ulna

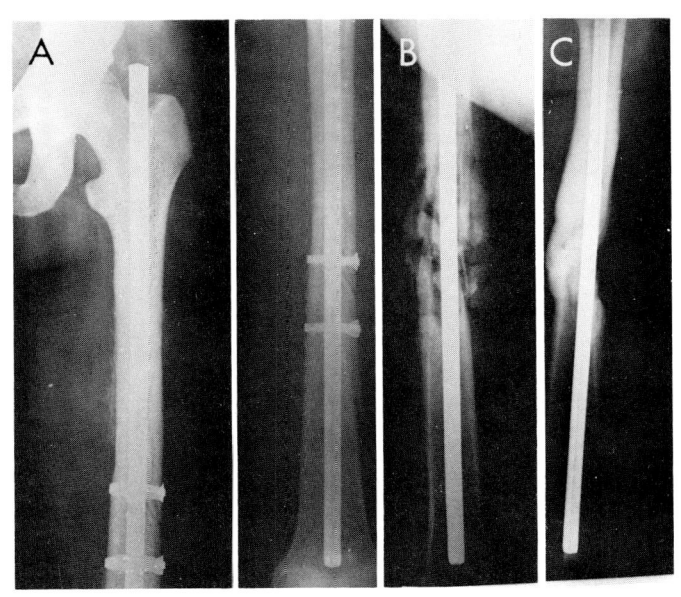

Fig. 5-13.—Infection following medullary nailing. **A,** anteroposterior and lateral views, showing successful reduction of fracture, medullary nailing and application of Parham bands to appose the long oblique fracture. **B** reveals sequestration associated with draining sinuses and development of infection. Parham bands were removed. Medullary nail was left in place. Further sequestration. **C** shows union of fracture. No longer any infection. Nail left in place.

wired shortly after the accident. Primary healing of the wounds occurred, but the bones developed nonunion at one point in the ulna and in two areas of the segmental fracture in the radius. Treatment consisted in open reduction through separate incisions, internal fixation of the ulna with a Rush pin and the addition of iliac bone. The middle fragment of the radius was removed, freshened at the bone ends, replaced and stabilized with a tibial onlay graft. Iliac bone was supplemented. The result 1 year after removal of the Rush pin was firm union and a useful extremity but marked limitation of supination.

NONUNION OF HUMERAL SHAFT FRACTURES

Fractures of the humeral shaft are comparable in many ways to those of the femur. Nonunion of the humerus is less common, however, because gravity tends to realign the humerus, as the patient is ambulatory. Consequently, one of the major causes of nonunion in the lower extremity, distraction, is not present in the humerus. Furthermore, operative treatment, a common cause of nonunion, has been used less frequently in the humerus than in the femur and tibia. As with the femur, the medullary nail has been the savior for some ununited humeri. By its use, stability is increased and joint motion can be initiated earlier.

To date, the Küntscher or Lottes nail has been the most satisfactory type of medullary fixation for the humeral shaft. It is inserted either from above through the greater tuberosity or from below through the condyles. If it is put in from above, one of the larger femoral or tibial nails can be used, if needed. From below, it is better to apply the smaller Küntscher or Lottes nail, introducing it through the lateral humeral condyle or posteriorly, beginning above the olecranon fossa.

The preferred grafts are those from the

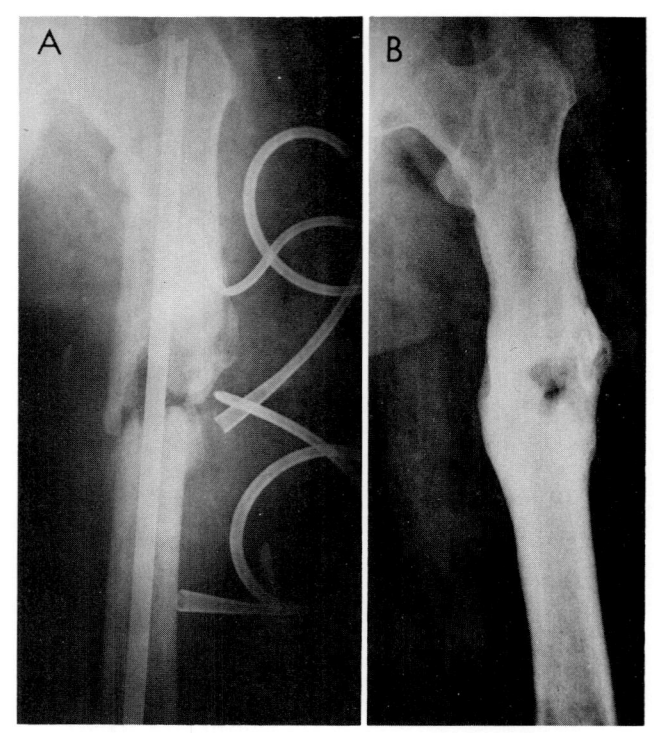

Fig. 5-14.—Infection of femoral shaft fracture following introduction of a medullary nail. Admitted to Massachusetts General Hospital 7 months after injury and operation. Extensive drainage of the thigh (*Staphylococcus aureus*), necessitating debridement and wound irrigation. *The medullary nail was left in position. This is important.* Union finally was accomplished. Drainage ceased. When union was firm, the nail was removed.

ilium, and they can be added in large quantity.

In the humerus, external fixation in the form of plaster may also have to be utilized in conjunction with the medullary nail.

Any humeral shaft fracture is easily and safely exposed through Henry's incision. This incision follows the course of the cephalic vein, and the entire shaft can be exposed without danger to any nerves or vessels (see Fig. 18-5, A in Chapter 18, Humeral Shaft Fractures).

NONUNION OF CLAVICLE

Although rare, nonunion of the clavicle usually is symptomatic, and internal fixation with bone grafting is indicated. Figure 5-30 illustrates the problem and successful healing following intramedullary fixation with autogenous iliac graft added.

Figure 5-31 shows a similar problem treated by fixation, utilizing the compression plating technique.

MALUNION

Malunion of long bone fractures is defined as significant alteration of normal bone configuration, length and alignment following fracture.

Some malunion problems require correction of the deformity to improve function of an extremity but rarely to regain length. Most often, as is shown in Figure 5-32, malunion needs no specific

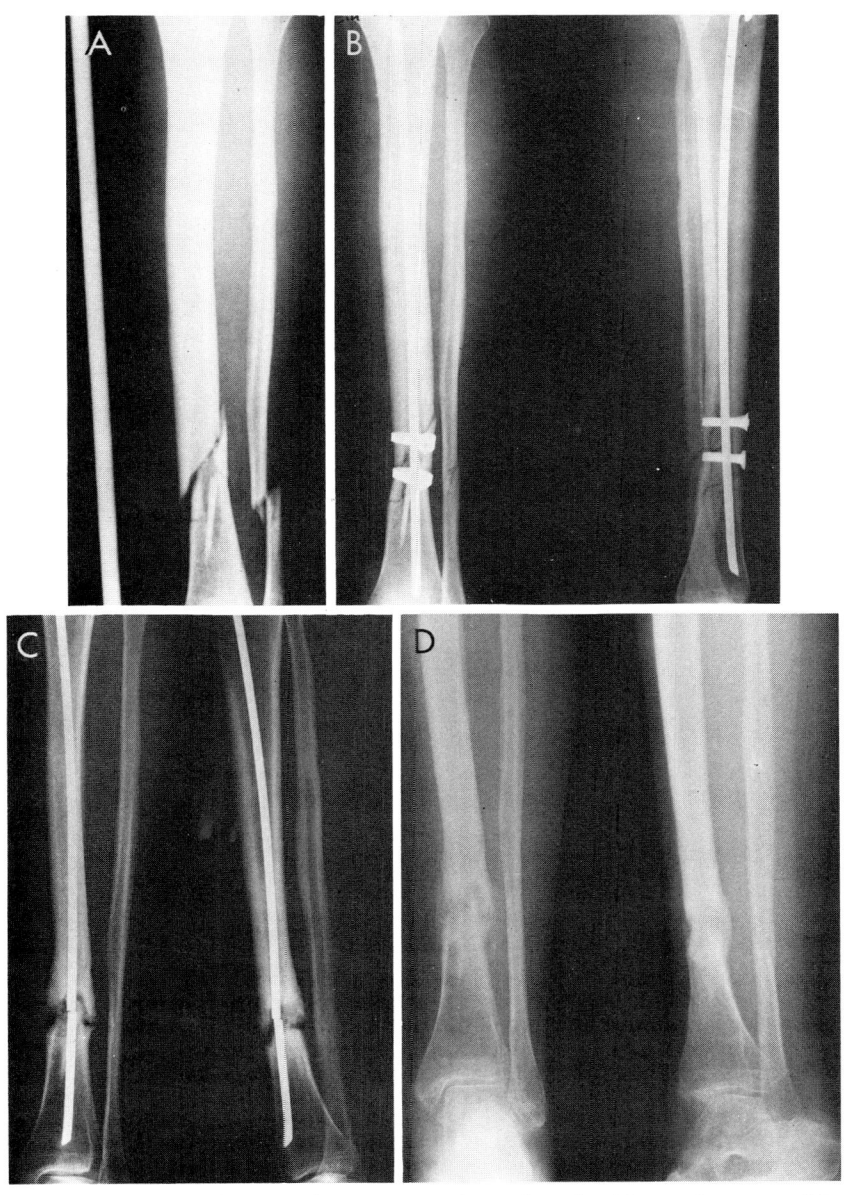

Chapter 5: DELAYED UNION, NONUNION AND MALUNION OF LONG BONES / 131

Fig. 5-15. — Unnecessary and harmful use of metal. **A,** closed, oblique fracture of distal end of tibia and fibula. It should have been treated adequately with long leg plaster for a period of 4 or 6 months. Operative treatment was elected. **B,** anteroposterior and lateral views, showing the result of having introduced a Rush pin and Parham bands. Nonunion resulted. Bands were removed later. **C** reveals nonunion with a broken Rush pin. Eleven months postinjury, following removal of the broken rod, bone grafting was required. A Phemister-type graft was applied, followed by plaster fixation for 7 months. **D,** bone union.

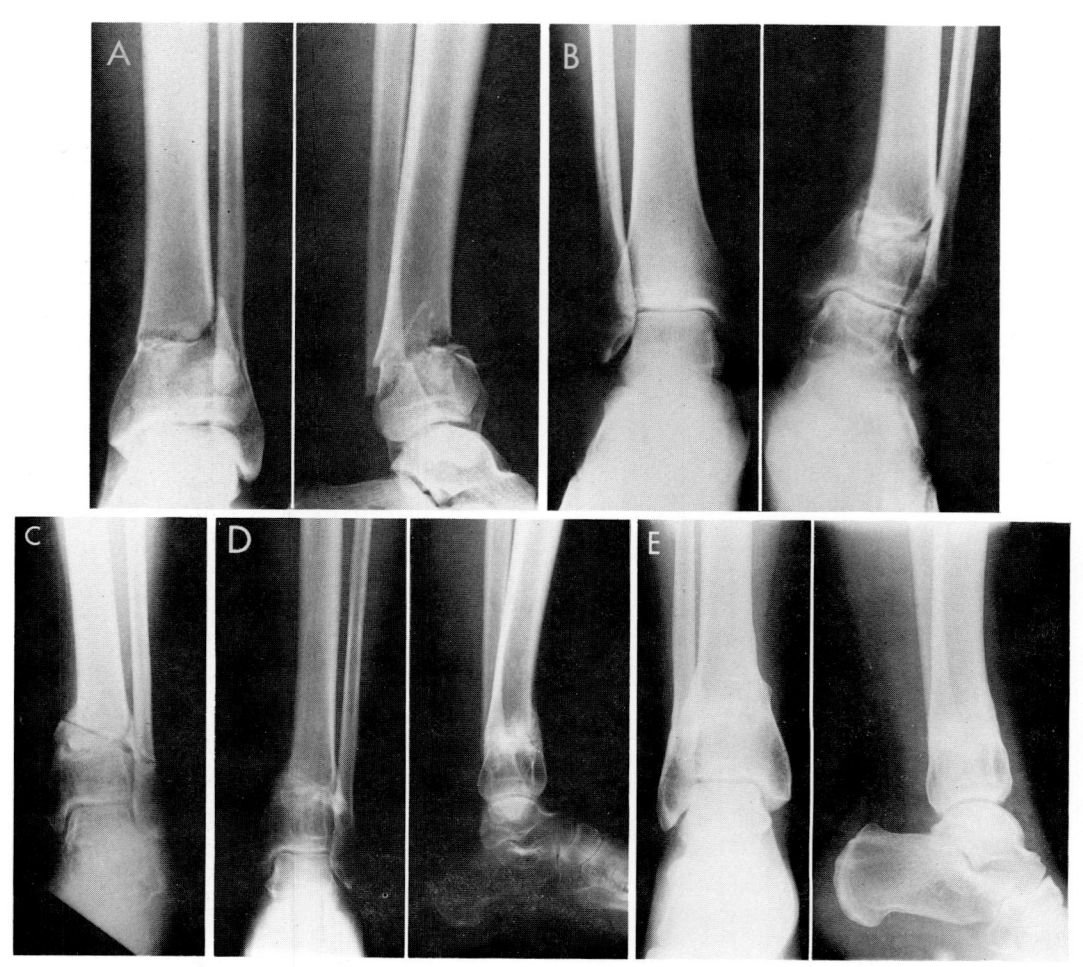

Fig. 5-16. — "Boot-top" fractures frequently are slow in healing, but they will heal satisfactorily if aligned properly and held sufficiently long with plaster fixation. **A,** anteroposterior and lateral views, revealing a comminuted fracture of the distal ends of the tibia and fibula with posterior bow. The ideal form of treatment would have been to correct the deformity by applying pressure on the leg posteriorly, just above the ankle, and, if necessary, accepting a temporary position of equinus of the foot. Plaster fixation must be prolonged until union is firm. Operation is not indicated. **B,** anteroposterior views of uninjured and injured extremities, revealing inversion deformity and delay in healing of the fracture 4 months after injury. Weight bearing was allowed too early. **C,** anteroposterior view after osteotomy of the distal end of the fibula in order to mobilize the tibia; re-creation of the tibial fracture and insertion of a wedge of iliac bone mesially at the fracture site to realign the ankle. **D,** anteroposterior and lateral views, showing complete correction of the deformity, normal alignment of the ankle and union of the fracture. **E,** end result.

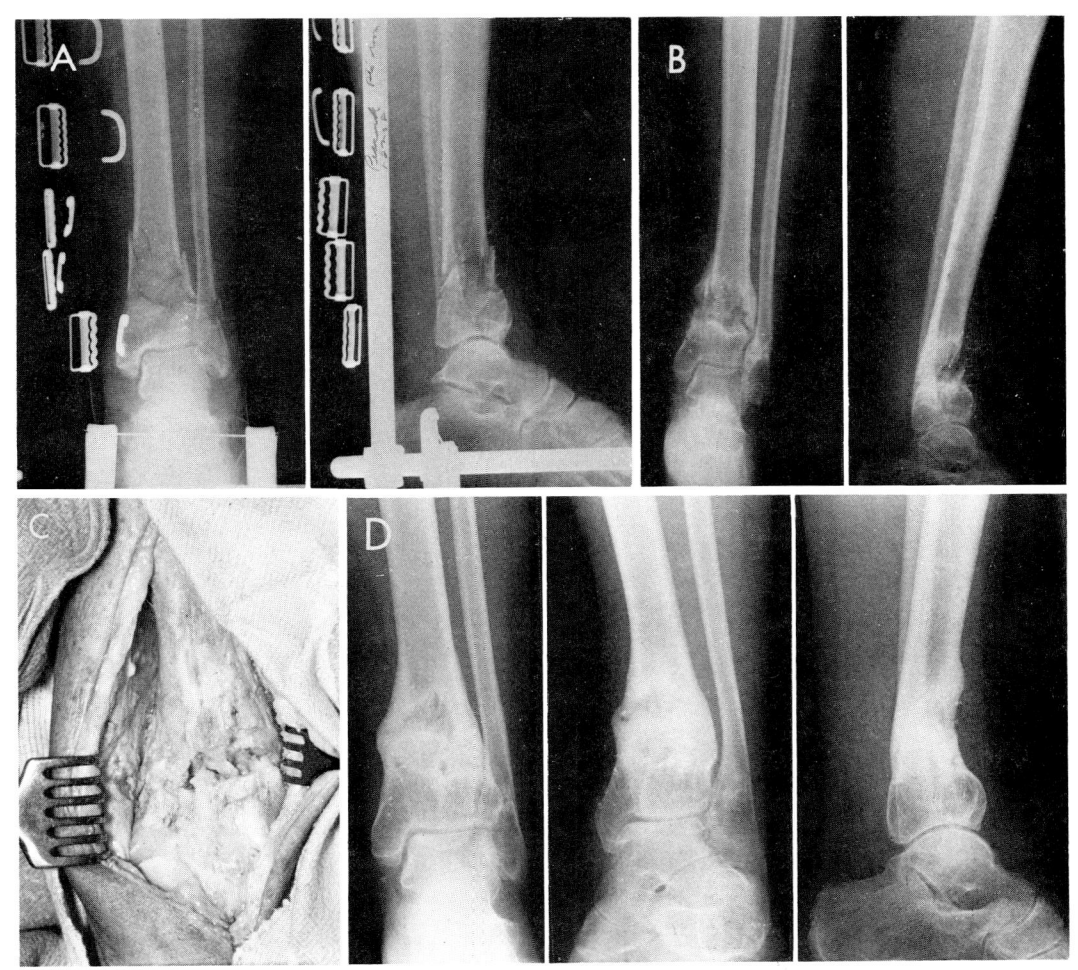

Chapter 5: DELAYED UNION, NONUNION AND MALUNION OF LONG BONES / 133

Fig. 5-17.—Nonunion from a "boot-top" fracture, due to unnecessary operation. **A,** anteroposterior and lateral views of comminuted fracture of the distal tibia and fibula in excellent alignment. Long leg plaster immobilization with the foot in a few degrees of equinus probably would have brought about a good result in 4 or 6 months. The surgeon in charge elected to "operate upon the fracture and put the fragments in better position." This failed and resulted in nonunion. **B,** anteroposterior and lateral views 11 months after injury. **C,** appearance of ununited tibia at time of operation. Bone graft was required. Bone was introduced from the ilium to fill the defect in the distal end of the tibia. This was followed by 6 months of plaster immobilization, which brought about bone union and an excellent result (**D**).

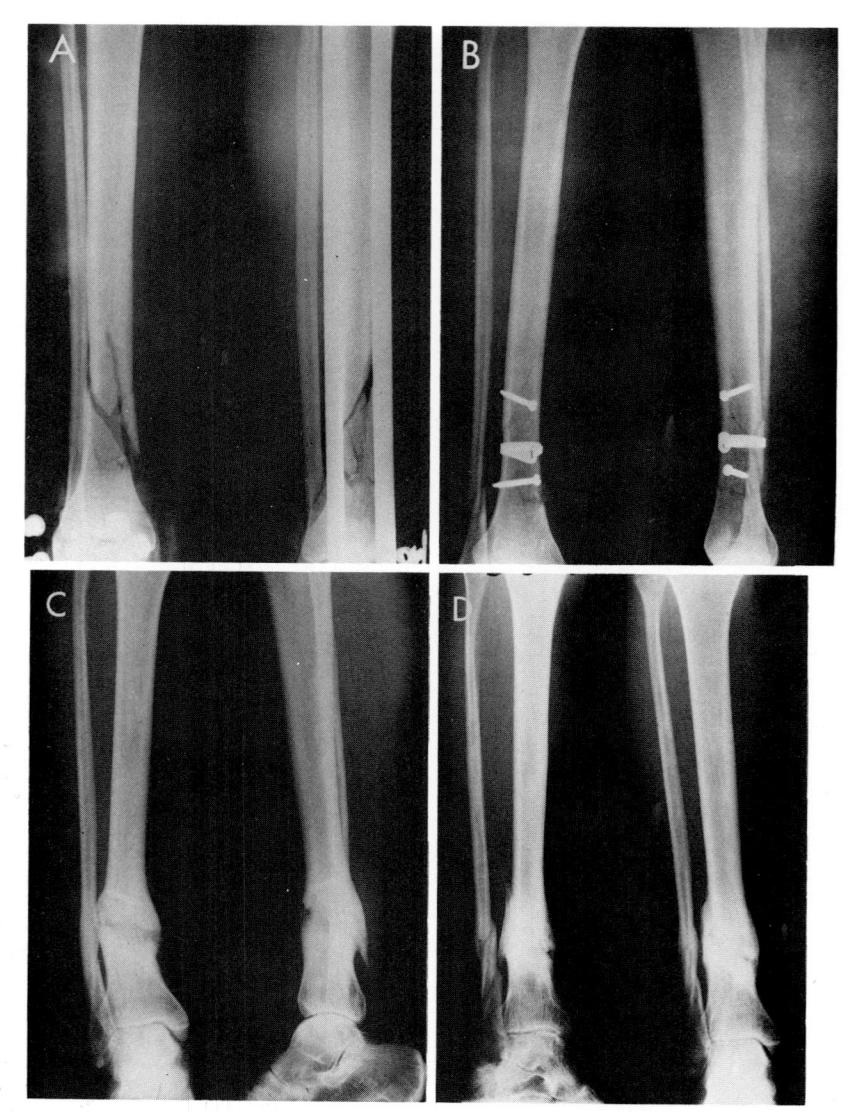

Fig. 5-18.—This illustrates the result from unnecessary operation, too much faith in "hardware" and too early weight bearing, superimposed on delayed union. **A** shows oblique, comminuted fracture of the distal end of the tibia and fibula in excellent position. Plaster fixation would have brought about a successful result. **B,** introduction of 2 screws and a Parham band. **C,** situation after removal of hardware. Weight bearing was allowed, with resultant deformity, excess callus production and nonunion of the tibia. The fibula had united. **D,** to correct the deformity, the fibula was osteotomized and the tibia was reshaped and realigned without excision of the fibrous union. Iliac bone grafts were introduced, followed by plaster immobilization for 5 months, when union was firm. (From Cave, E. F.: Healing of fractures and nonunion of bone. The 7th Murray S. Danforth Oration, Rhode Island Med. J. 48:77, 1965.)

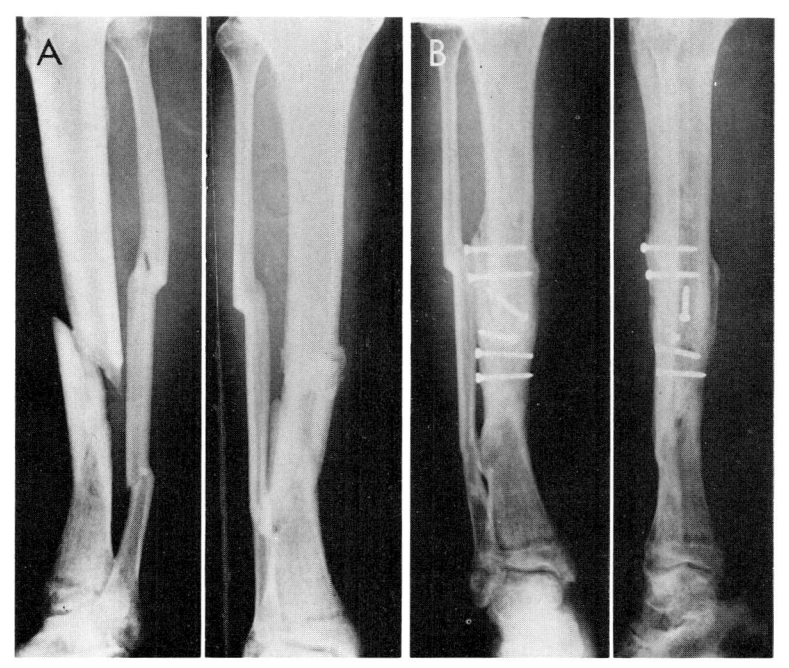

Fig. 5-19.—Segmental fractures of the tibia and fibula following extensive open injury to bone and soft tissue 2 years previously, in a man (a teacher), aged 59. **A,** nonunion of the malaligned upper tibial fracture. **B,** 3 years after injury and 1 year after onlay tibial graft (removed from proximal fragment) and iliac bone. To correct the deformity, the fibula was osteotomized at the distal fracture.

treatment. However, as noted in Figure 5-33, the pronounced degree of femoral bowing, which limited knee and lower-extremity function, required operative correction, with resultant problems from the surgery, illustrating the hazards involved.

Internal rotation deformity at the femoral shaft fracture site treated in traction may occur if the distal fragment rotation is not aligned properly. Failure to achieve satisfactory alignment may impede walking and running if the deformity is excessive.

In Figure 5-34, malrotation occurred in the midfemoral shaft fracture site, resulting in internal rotation of the foot in walking of approximately 60 degrees and hip pain on attempting to walk with the toes straight ahead. Rotational osteotomy with compression plate fixation was carried out above the fracture site.

NONUNION AND INFECTION

When a surgeon is faced with the management of a long bone fracture that is ununited and infected, and with or without severe deformity, certain principles must be observed in management, in order to clear the infection, promote union and restore function to the extremity.

Since this problem is encountered more frequently in both bones of the leg, we shall first direct our remarks toward this area and believe that the principles laid down can be followed in the management of the ununited, infected fractures of other long bones.

So often the question arises as to whether the extremity can and should be saved. There are important considerations: (1) the age of the patient; i.e., the younger the patient the greater the effort that should be made to save the arm or

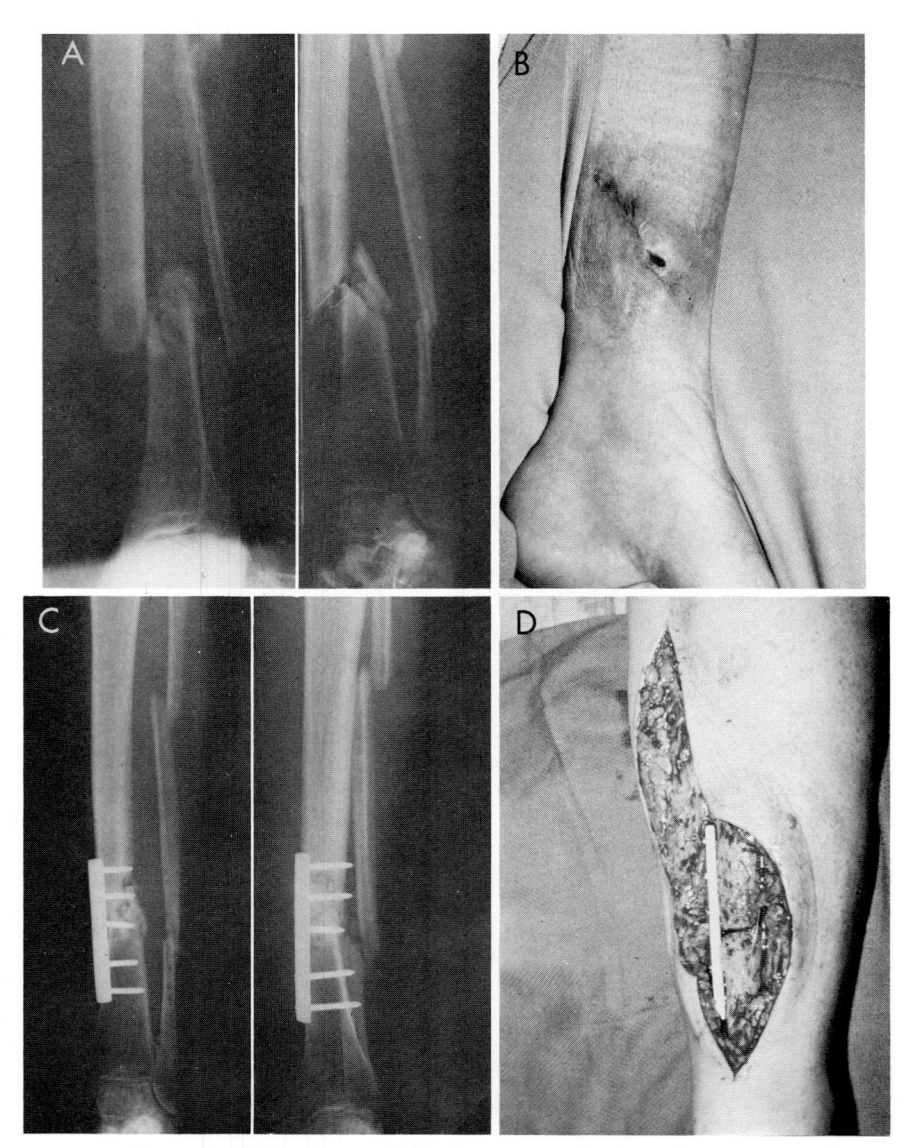

Fig. 5-20. — Open fracture of the tibia and fibula sustained when skiing. Treated primarily by open reduction and wire fixation. The patient was immobilized in a long leg plaster of Paris cast for 6 months after injury, at the end of which time a short plaster was applied. Fracture became infected. Patient was allowed to bear weight too early. Nonunion resulted. **A,** anteroposterior and oblique views, showing ununited fractures of tibia and fibula. **B,** appearance of skin; draining sinus anteromesially. **C,** osteotomy of fibula at distal fracture site. Through a lateral incision, re-creation of distal fibular fracture. Through anteromesial incision, reduction of tibial fracture and application of plate. **D,** anteromesial incision with plate applied. (**Continued.**)

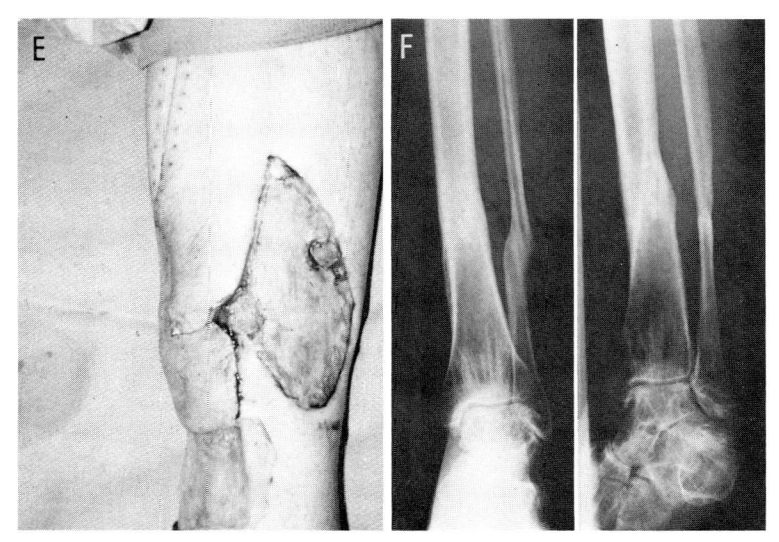

Chapter 5: DELAYED UNION, NONUNION AND MALUNION OF LONG BONES / 137

Fig. 5-20 (cont.).—**E,** skin coverage of fracture and plate and split-skin graft to replace flap. Removal of plate was necessary because of sterile abscess. **F,** anteroposterior and lateral views, revealing bone union. All tissue healed.

leg. (2) How extensive is the infection and will so much bone have to be sacrificed that an unacceptable degree of shortening will result? This is especially true in the lower extremity. (3) How good is the foot or hand? A painful, stiff, essentially useless hand or foot when present with infection and nonunion of the long bones would hardly call for an effort to clear infection and promote bone union; therefore, amputation may be the treatment of choice.

In most of the infected, ununited fractures of the tibia in our series there has been a good foot. Such fractures have been primarily in young individuals who have sustained severe injury by automobile accident or in sports and, other than a fractured leg, are healthy, productive citizens. Therefore, during recent years, we have been making more and more of an effort to save such an extremity, and with considerable justification.

The surgeon should first direct his effort to clearing the infection of the bone. This means thorough debridement, sequestrectomy and removal of all dead, infected bone, no matter how much is required to accomplish this purpose. In the ununited, infected fracture of the leg, usually the fibula has united, perhaps with some shortening and deformity, but if it is in reasonably good alignment, it should be left so and effort directed to removing the infected bone from the tibia. This procedure is done through an anterior approach, because more often than not the leg has been operated on previously or has suffered from an open fracture and there already is a scar anteriorly, and the stabilizing-grafting procedure will be done posteriorly.

Once the surgeon is convinced that all dead, infected bone has been removed, it is justifiable to temporarily pack the wound with fine-mesh gauze and within a few days do a split-skin graft over the defect anteriorly.

Next, bone grafts are introduced, preferably through a posterior incision. It is desirable to have the infection cleared entirely, but in a few cases we have introduced bone grafts posteriorly when there has been persistent, although relatively slight, drainage anteriorly.

The advantage of the posterior incision

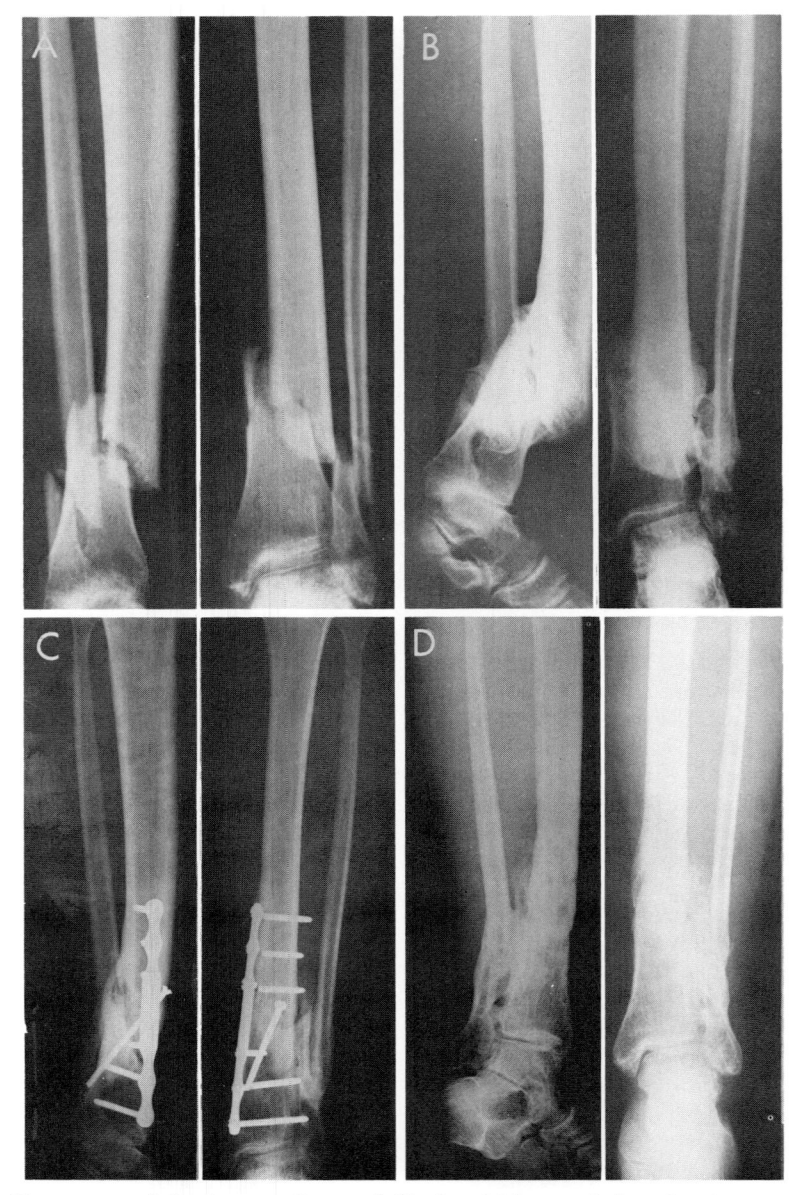

Fig. 5-21.—Nonunion of the lower tibia and fibula of 16 years' duration in a nurse, aged 33. **A,** the original open fracture, sustained at age 17, 16 years before admission. **B,** condition of bone and ankle joint at time of admission: complete pseudarthrosis of both tibia and fibula, deformity and traumatic arthritis of the ankle joint. **C,** 13 months after osteotomies at fracture sites, application of plate and screws to tibia and of iliac bone around both tibia and fibula. Note that screws in proximal fragment have broken, indicating failure of bone to heal. **D,** 8 months after removal of plate and screws and application of iliac bone around fracture sites of tibia and fibula and continuous plaster fixation; union established. The ankle joint realigned, but traumatic arthritis persisted, although patient was symptom-free and had a good range of ankle motion.

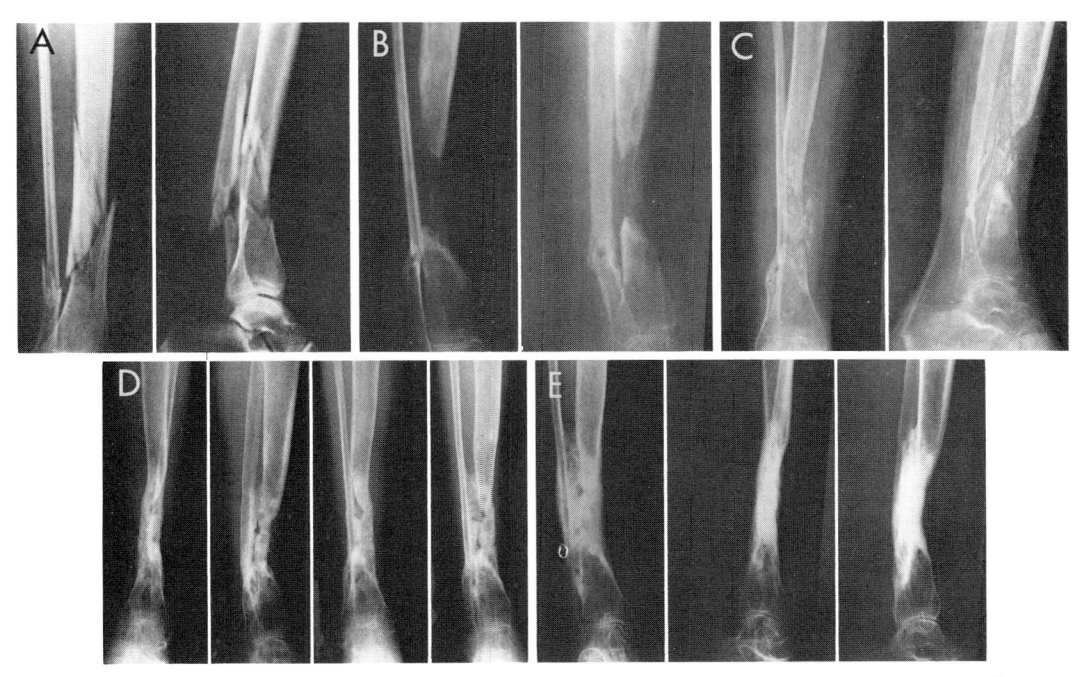

Chapter 5: DELAYED UNION, NONUNION AND MALUNION OF LONG BONES / 139

Fig. 5-22.—These illustrations indicate disaster subsequent to unnecessary open reduction and internal fixation of a comminuted fracture of the tibia and fibula. **A,** anteroposterior and lateral views, showing original injury. This fracture would have healed perfectly well with plaster immobilization. Early operation was carried out, but infection developed, necessitating debridement and extensive sequestrectomy, with approximately 2 inches of bone loss of the tibia. This required months of hospital care, followed by a full-thickness skin graft to the anterior aspect of the tibia. The patient arrived in our clinic with massive bone loss of the tibia (**B**). **C** represents introduction of iliac bone through a posterior approach (see Fig. 5-37), bone grafts bridging the gap in the tibia and creating synostosis between the healed fibula and the upper and lower fragments of the tibia. **D** illustrates successful bone graft, promoting union of the tibial fragments and synostosis between the tibia and fibula. **E,** solid union of the tibia and fibula 6 years after injury and 4 years after bone graft. A successful result—but only after many years of hospitalization and repeated operations, which could have been avoided by "conservative" management.

is that bone grafts can be introduced through sound tissue and without penetrating the interosseous membrane, thus avoiding communication with the infected area anteriorly. The posterior aspect of the ilium furnishes a more fruitful source of bone than does the anterior aspect, and with the patient in the prone position, the approach to the posterior ilium is relatively easy. The grafts should be taken before the tibia is exposed. Usually 6 or 8 grafts, approximately 3 or 3½ inches in length, using both tables of the ilium, and ⅛ inch thick, are desirable (see Fig. 6-5,

right, in Chapter 6, Technique of Bone Grafting). These are preserved. The iliac wound is closed in layers. The posterior approach to the tibia then is made.

The operation is done with a pneumatic tourniquet inflated.

The object of the bone graft is to create synostosis between the intact fibula and the defective tibia. A large amount of bone can be utilized for this purpose.

Prior to introducing the grafts, the surfaces of the tibia and fibula should be scarified with osteotomes and the grafts placed subperiosteally and in contact

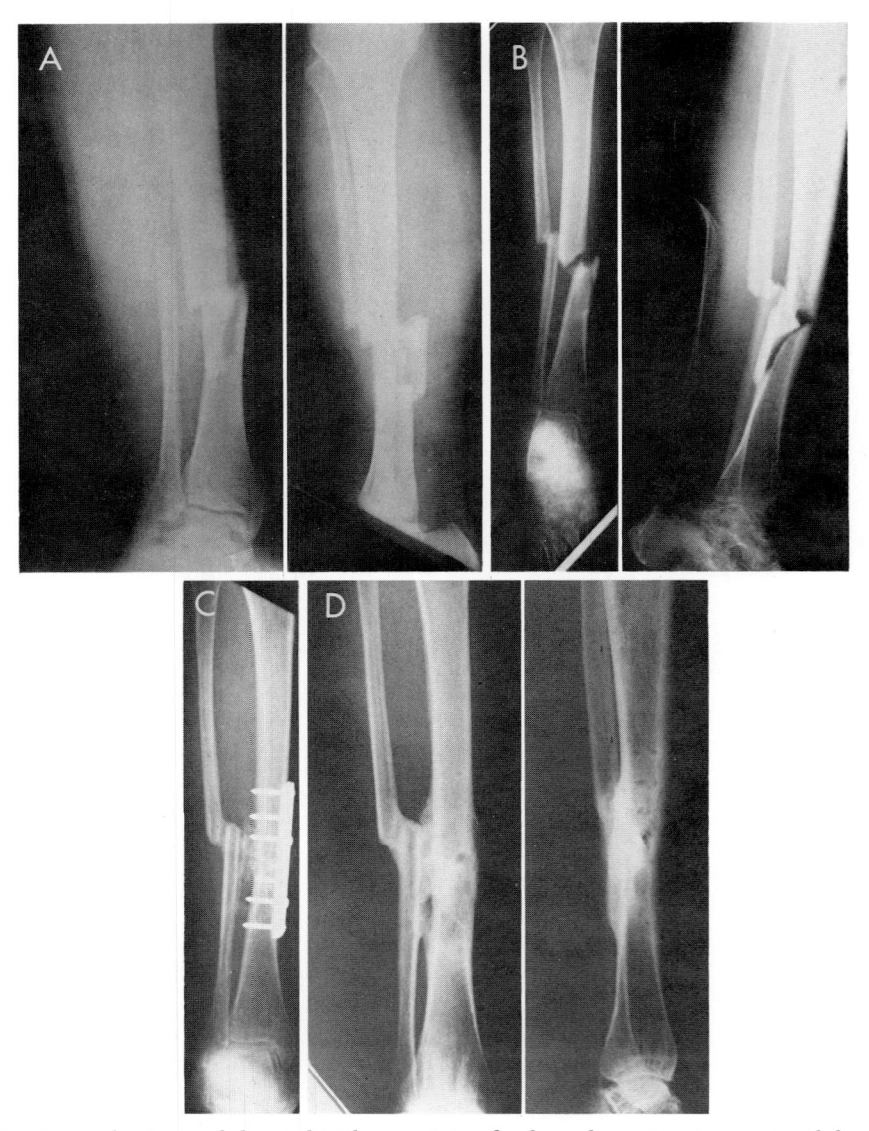

Fig. 5-23.—Open fracture of the right tibia sustained when the patient was struck by an automobile that got out of control and came onto the sidewalk. **A,** anteroposterior and lateral views of original injury. Treated with closed reduction and long leg plaster of Paris cast. Reduction was lost. A second closed reduction was performed and transverse wires through the proximal and distal tibia were incorporated in the plaster, which was removed after 5 weeks. Patient was in long leg cast up to time of admission to Massachusetts General Hospital 9 months later. **B** shows frank nonunion 9 months after injury and plaster immobilization. **C,** following fibular osteotomy and open reduction of tibial fracture, application of "compression" plate and iliac bone grafts. **D,** after plate was removed because of "sterile" abscess. Bone union resulted.

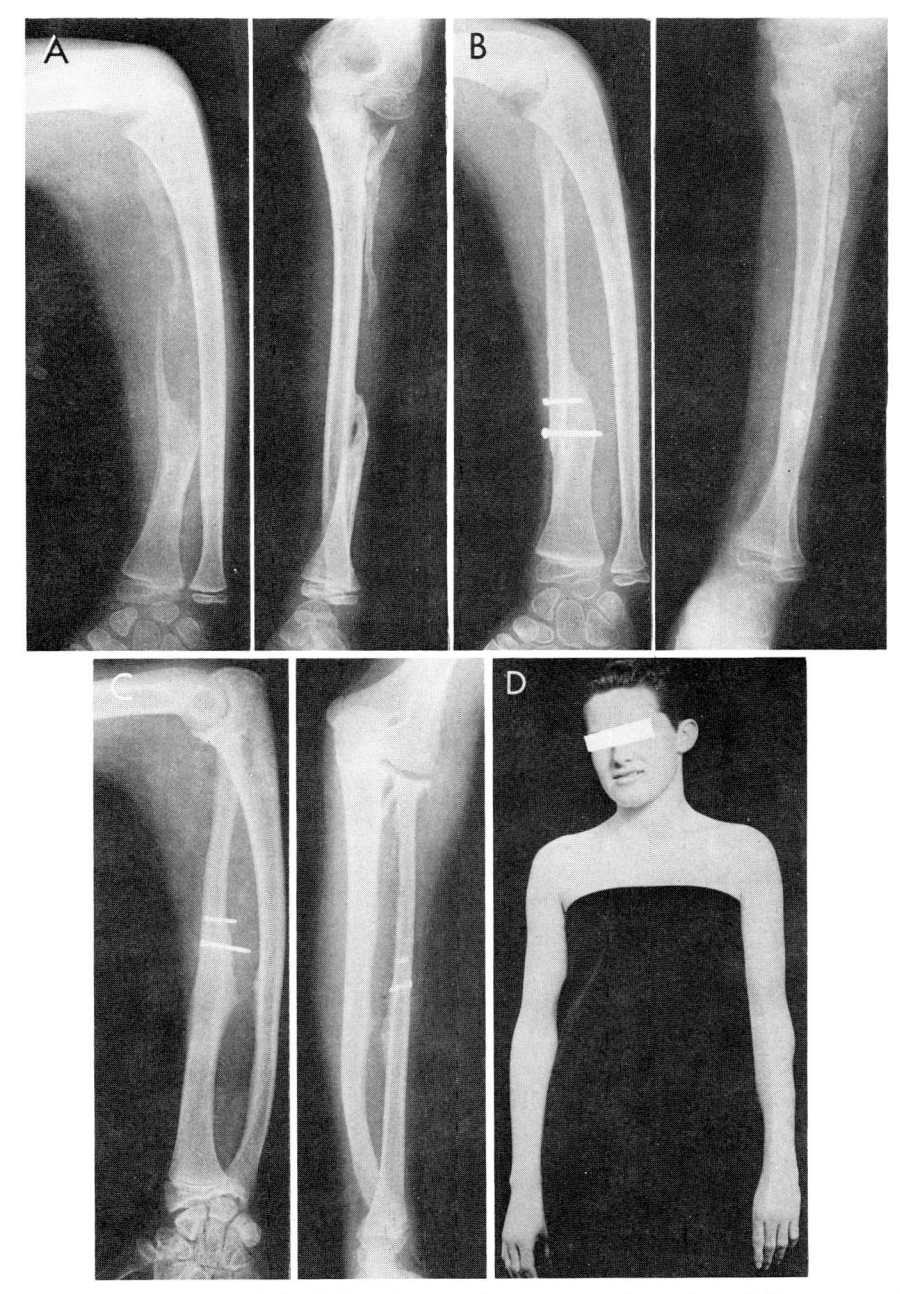

Chapter 5: DELAYED UNION, NONUNION AND MALUNION OF LONG BONES / 141

Fig. 5-24.—Open fracture of the left radius with extensive bone loss following avulsion of upper two-thirds of radius in an 8-year-old boy injured in an automobile accident. **A,** x-ray on admission 4 months after injury. (See text regarding operation.) **B,** fibula transplant 6 months after operation. **C,** 7 years after operation: continued growth of radius from distal epiphysis; some angulation of ulna. **D,** 7 years after injury: general alignment satisfactory; hand function excellent, but no supination of forearm, although pronation to 60 degrees.

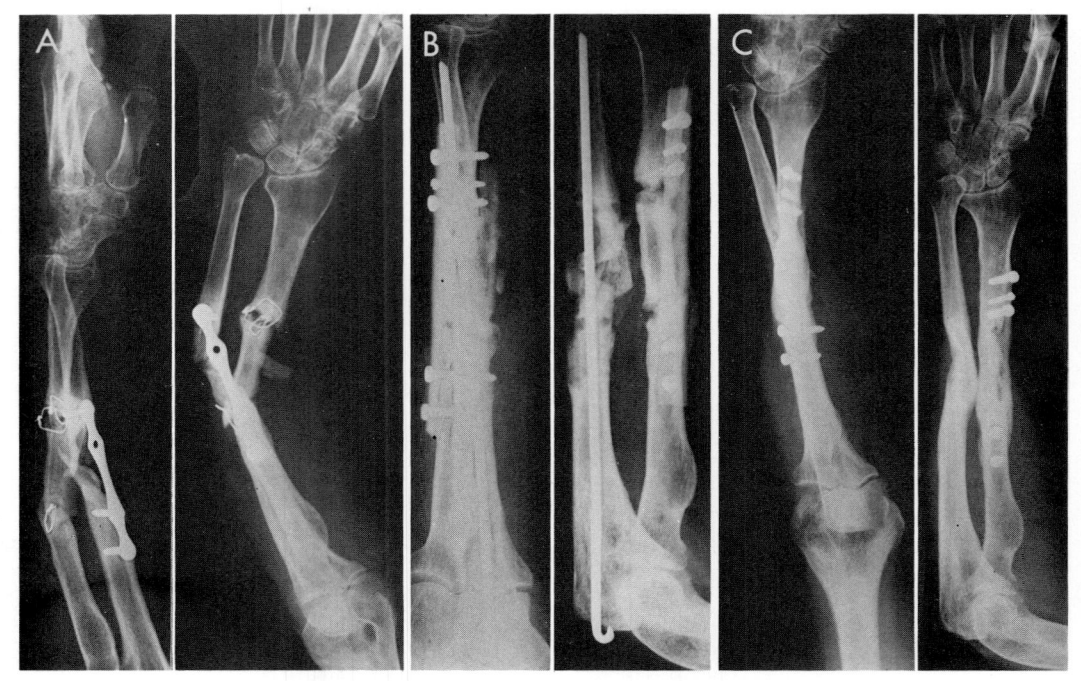

Fig. 5-25.—Nonunion of an old open fracture of the radius and ulna in a woman aged 52.

with the two bones. In addition, they bridge the gap in the tibia. The tourniquet then is released and the wound is easily closed with suture material of the surgeon's choice, which will approximate the muscle structures, the subcutaneous tissue and skin. A long plaster is applied, with the knee in approximately 30 degrees of flexion and the foot in a neutral position.

THE UNUNITED, INFECTED FRACTURE OF THE FEMUR.—The septic femur, which is ununited, presents a very difficult problem because of the necessity of preserving a reasonable length to the extremity. In the upper extremity, shortening can be accepted, but in the lower extremity shortening of more than 1½ or 2 inches may cause permanent disability and require the wearing of an elevated shoe. Therefore, every effort should be made to preserve the length of the femur. The infection must be cleared by sequestrectomy and debridement. A similar procedure of skin grafting or secondary wound closure can be carried out and the bone graft can be done through an incision remote from the original one. The posterior approach to the femur is recommended. The surgeon may elect to use intramedullary fixation in the form of a Küntscher nail, which we believe is preferable to the application of a plate and screws.

Barrel-staved grafts from the ilium, which are placed subperiosteally, following the principles of Phemister,[20] should be satisfactory for the bone-grafting procedure. These grafts are removed in the routine fashion and according to the technique described above. Immobilization of the femur is desirable. External fixation in the form of plaster should be avoided if possible, but a plaster spica may be necessary if it is not possible to employ internal fixation.

THE UNUNITED, INFECTED FRACTURE OF THE HUMERAL SHAFT.—Shortening can

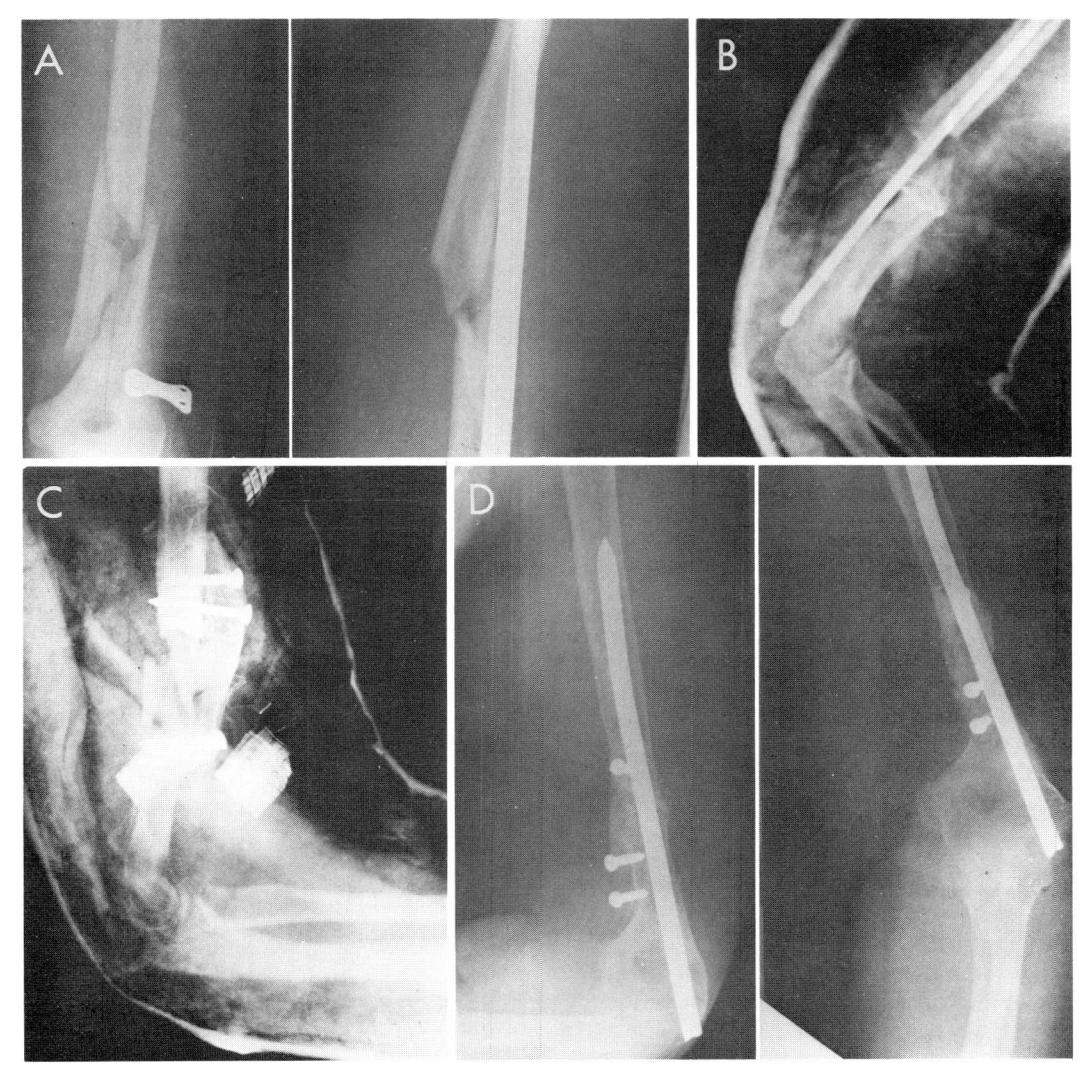

Chapter 5: DELAYED UNION, NONUNION AND MALUNION OF LONG BONES / 143

Fig. 5-26. — **A**, anteroposterior and lateral views of closed, comminuted fracture of the distal right humerus. External immobilization would have produced union. Operation was unwisely attempted on two occasions. Nonunion resulted. **B**, lateral view, showing misuse of medullary nail, which did not engage distal fragment. **C**, another attempt was made to stabilize the fracture with onlay iliac bone graft. Both procedures failed. **D**, union was established by open reduction and internal fixation with a cut-down Lottes nail, introduced from below through the lateral humeral condyle, supplemented by application of iliac bone and held with 3 screws, 36 months after injury.

be accepted in the humerus if necessary to appose bone ends in order to gain union, but, again, the principle of sequestrectomy and wound debridement should be followed with secondary closure if possible; if not, skin grafting, followed by the application of barrel-staved grafts should be done. The use of internal fixation in the form of an intramedullary nail sometimes is a reasonable thing to do.

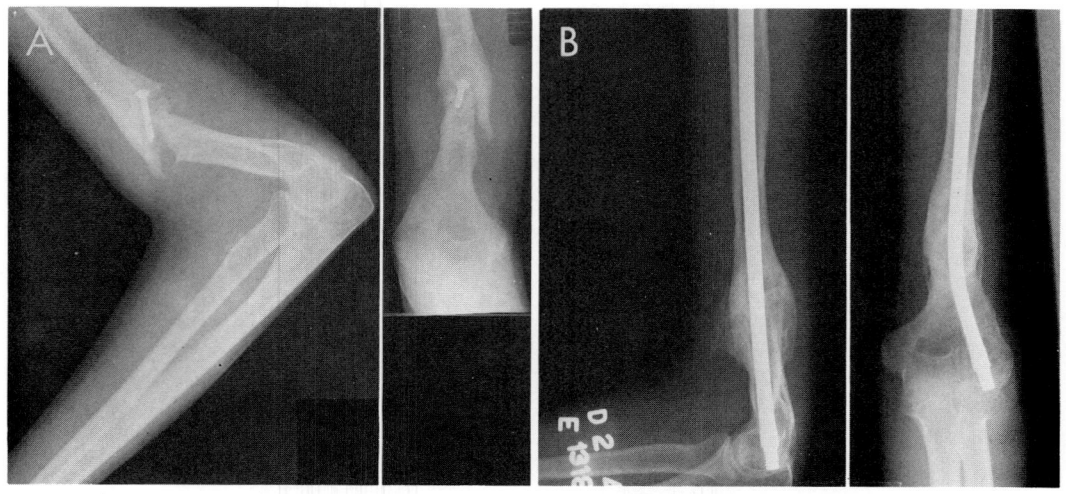

Fig. 5-27.—Nonunion, postoperative, old fracture of the distal shaft of the humerus, secondary to an automobile accident. **A,** nonunion of humerus, the nonunion secondary to inadequate internal fixation. Treatment: Exposure of the fracture with Henry's incision, removal of screw, debridement and realignment of fracture, retrograde insertion of Lottes nail, followed by light plaster spica to prevent tendency to rotation for 4 months. **B,** end result: bone union but limited elbow motion. Flexion to 50 degrees; further flexion to 125 degrees. Normal pronation and supination. Carrying on full-time work as a secretary.

The use of a compression plate may be possible; however, if a bone is too porotic, the principle of compression can be applied with Kirschner wires inserted through the bone above and below the fracture. At best, however, this is an awkward form of fixation.

THE UNUNITED, INFECTED FRACTURE OF BOTH BONES OF THE FOREARM.—Infection and nonunion in combination is relatively rare in the radius and ulna, certainly in civilian practice. In the military it is more common.

The same principles should be followed; namely, sequestrectomy, debridement and acceptance of some shortening to bring about apposition of bone. Or, if one bone is intact and length is preserved, iliac bone can be introduced to occupy the defective space in the affected bone.

The physician treating fractures must keep the following points uppermost in mind:

1. The vast majority of fractures will heal if reduced and held sufficiently long by uninterrupted external fixation.

2. Improperly executed operations on long bone fractures account for the increasing number of cases of nonunion of bone.

3. The existence of delayed union is determined entirely by the x-ray film. Testing for motion at the fracture site during the healing stage is contraindicated. Immobilization must be continued.

4. Nonunion of bone may be determined by local physical examination as well as by the x-ray film.

5. When nonunion is established, it should be corrected surgically.

6. The infected fracture with nonunion should be treated by debridement and removal of all avascular infected tissue, skin graft, as a rule, and appropriate bone graft, usually with a remote approach through sound and clean soft tissue.

7. Each case of an ununited fracture is a problem unto itself, and the operation must be planned accordingly, considering the bone involved, the soft tissue around the fracture, the entire extremity and the patient as a whole.

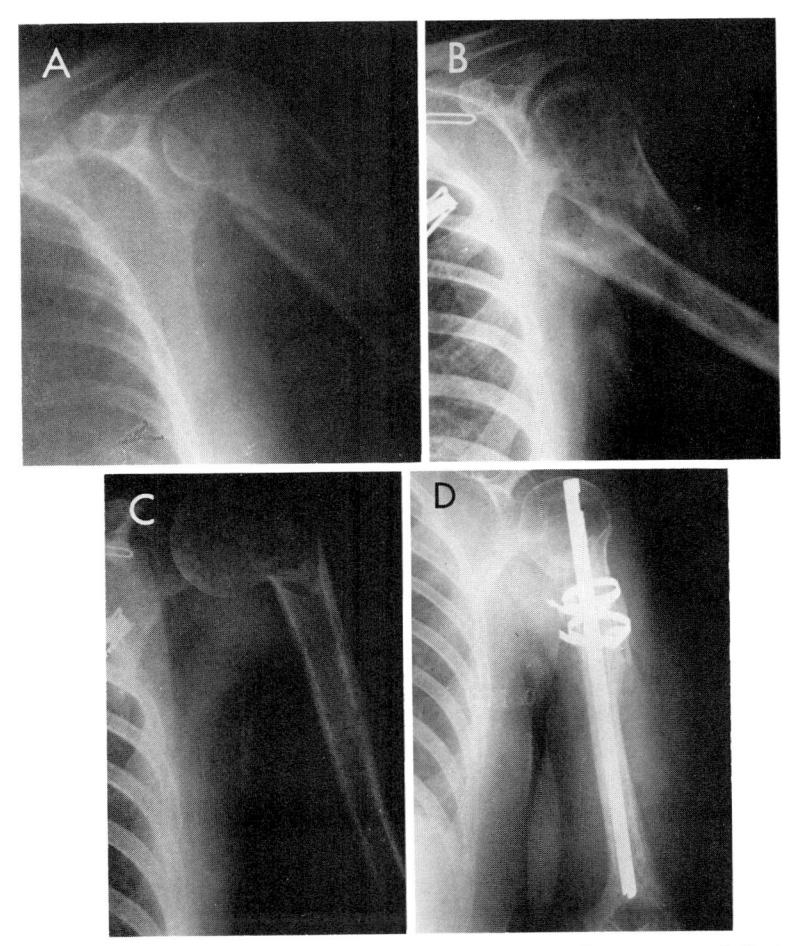

Chapter 5: DELAYED UNION, NONUNION AND MALUNION OF LONG BONES / **145**

Fig. 5-28.—**A,** fracture of the upper shaft of the left humerus when patient fell. A hanging cast was applied. Nonunion resulted (**B** and **C**). Treatment: Open reduction through anterior incision, following course of cephalic vein, and retrograde introduction of cloverleaf medullary nail. Parham bands were used to appose oblique fracture (**D**). Result: bone union with good return of function.

146 / *Edwin F. Cave and Robert J. Boyd*

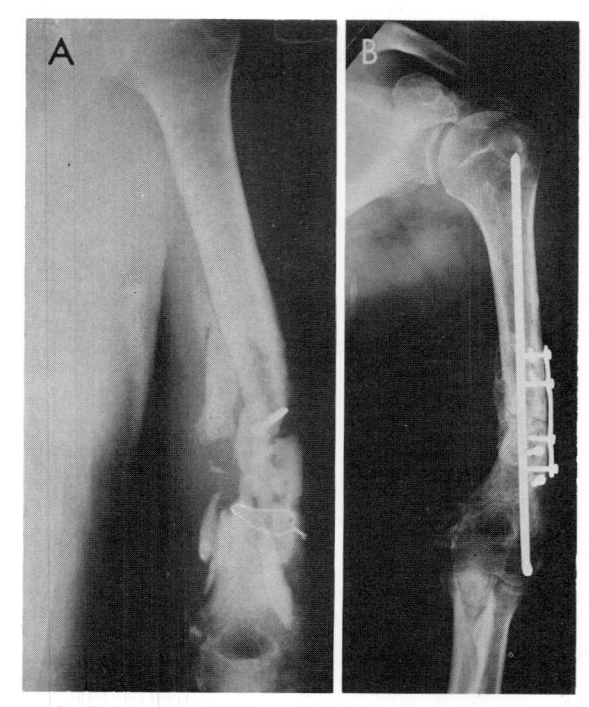

Fig. 5-29.—**A,** open, markedly comminuted fracture of the left humerus (man, aged 57) secondary to bullet (.45 cal.) wound 2 years before admission. Open reduction had been attempted, but nonunion had resulted. **B,** 6 months after operation to promote union, bone healing was accomplished by bone shortening (¾ inch), by stabilization with a Rush pin to prevent angulation and by a plate and screws to prevent rotation at the fracture site. In addition, a tibial onlay graft was secured with 4 screws and iliac bone chips were added.

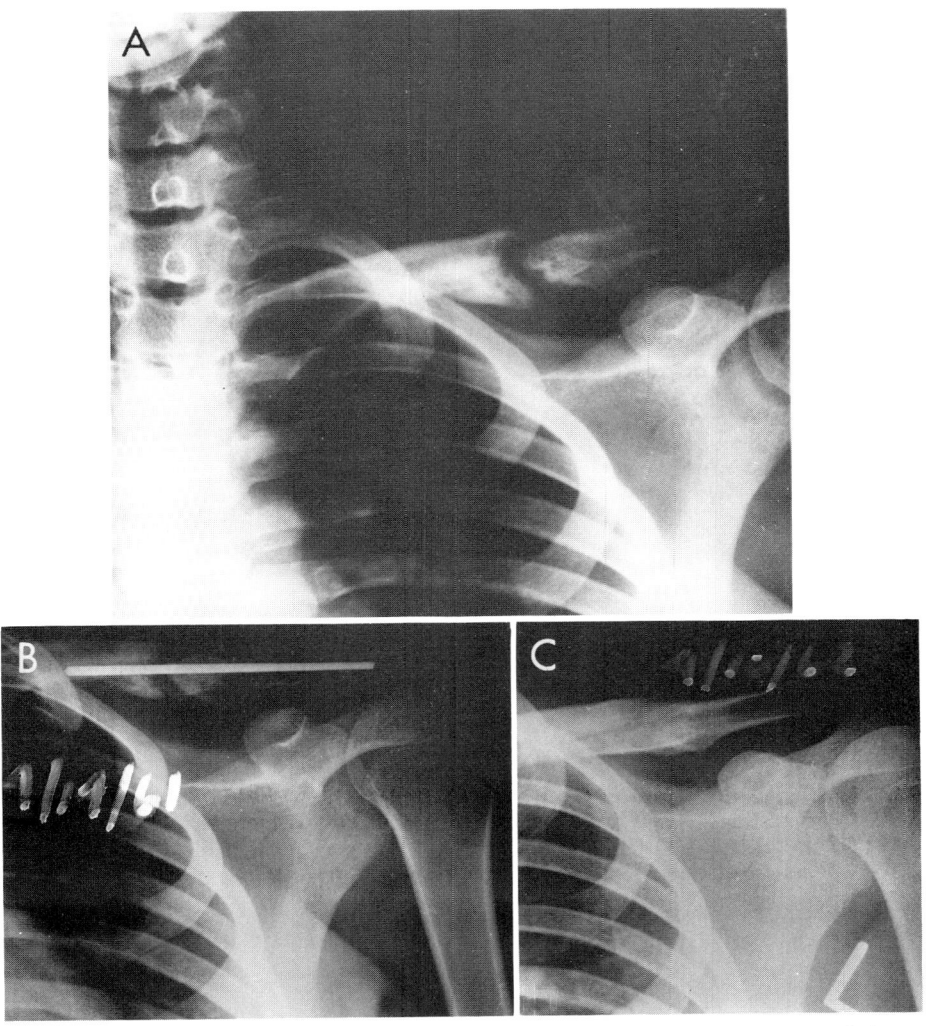

Chapter 5: DELAYED UNION, NONUNION AND MALUNION OF LONG BONES / **147**

Fig. 5-30.—Nonunion of the clavicle, result of an injury sustained in an automobile accident 9 months prior to admission. Treated with a brace for 3 weeks, followed by open reduction. **A,** anteroposterior view, revealing complete nonunion and absorption of bone at the fracture site. **B,** following open reduction, introduction of threaded Kirschner wire and bone graft from ilium. **C,** complete union, after which wire was removed. Excellent return of function.

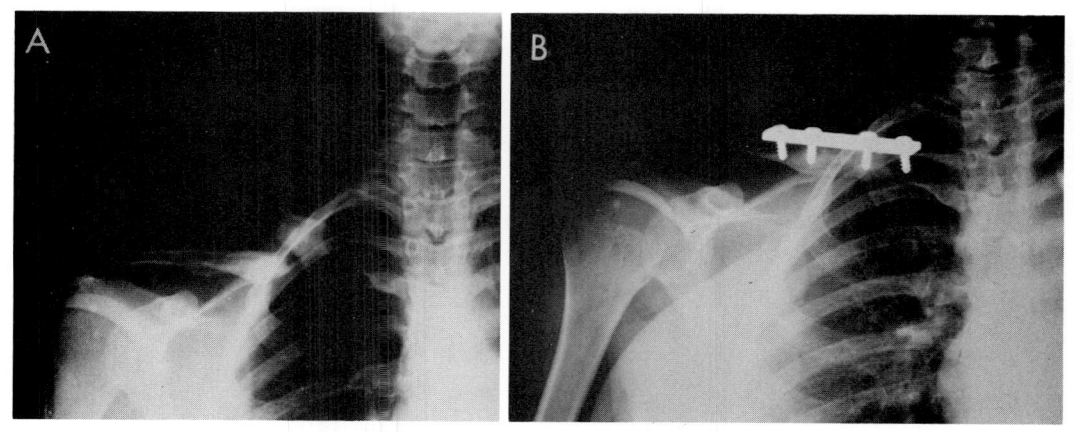

Fig. 5-31.—**A,** 23-year-old secretary with painful nonunion of the right clavicle 14 months following injury, who also had elbow pain and paresthesias of the hand. Symptoms cleared after fixation, using a compression plate (**B**). The plate was removed 1½ years later after solid union had occurred, because of prominence and mild tenderness over the plate.

Fig. 5-32.—**A,** displaced fracture of the tibia and fibula, which could not be reduced perfectly (one-third contact of tibia in left-hand view). This position was accepted. Union was firm after 8 months and the leg is straight without shortening (**B**).

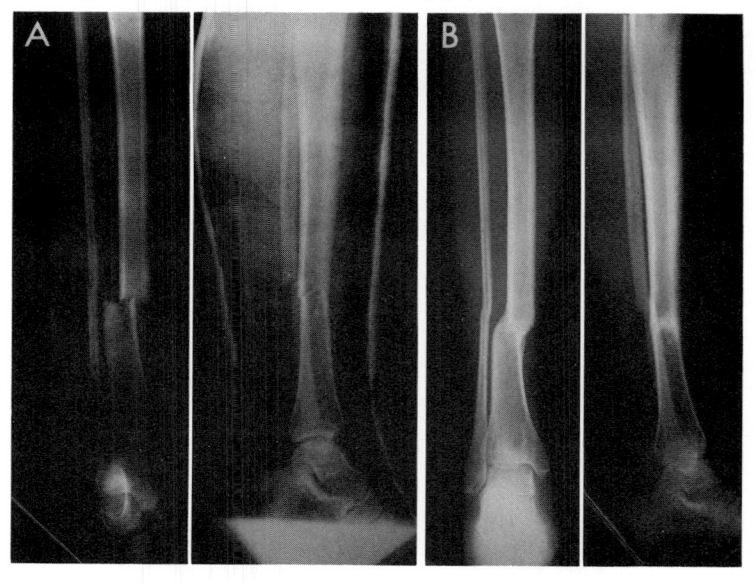

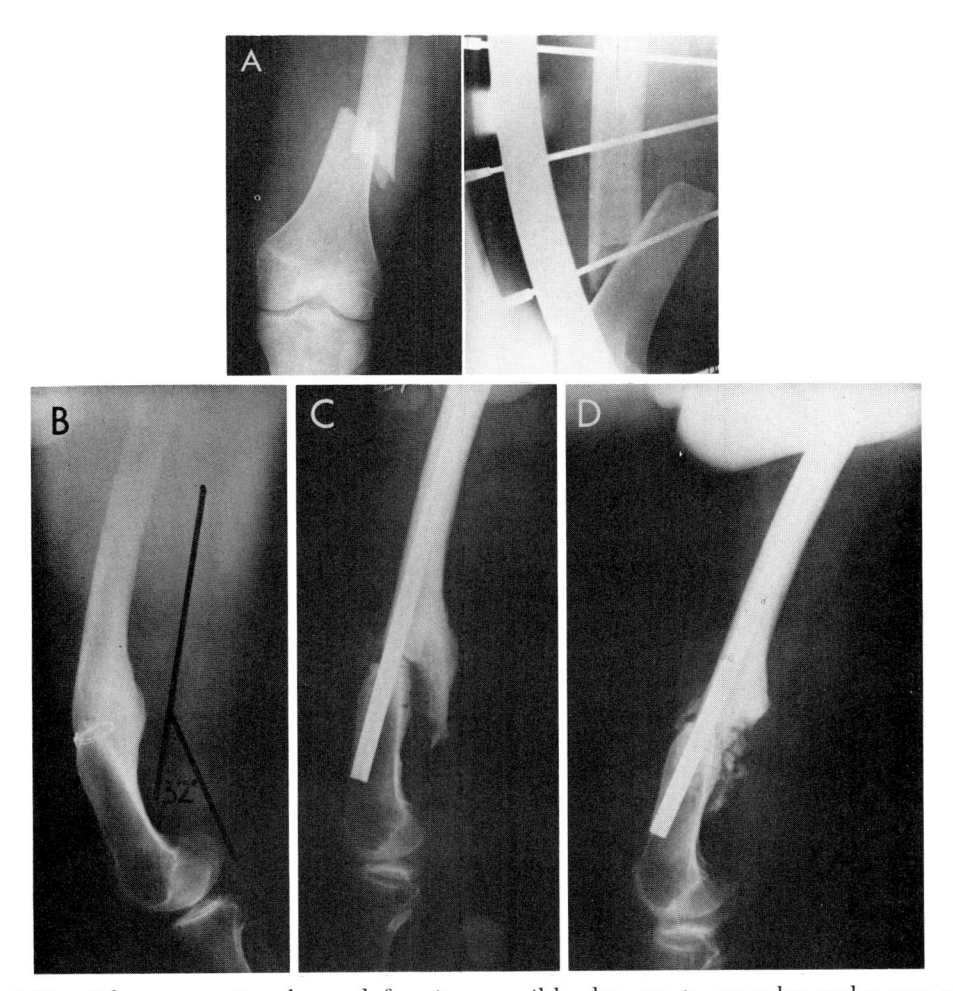

Chapter 5: DELAYED UNION, NONUNION AND MALUNION OF LONG BONES / 149

Fig. 5-33.—When correcting bony deformity, possible damage to vascular and nerve structures must constantly be kept in mind. **A,** anteroposterior and lateral views of closed, displaced fracture of distal femur. **B,** fracture healed with marked anterior bow (32 degrees). **C,** at time of osteotomy, anterior bow was corrected and femur stabilized with a medullary nail, but the projecting fragment of the proximal fragment of the femur interfered with vascular and nerve structures above the popliteal space. This required immediate resection of the large bone fragment. **D,** symptoms and signs of partial Volkmann's contracture persisted, requiring eventual lengthening of the Achilles tendon.

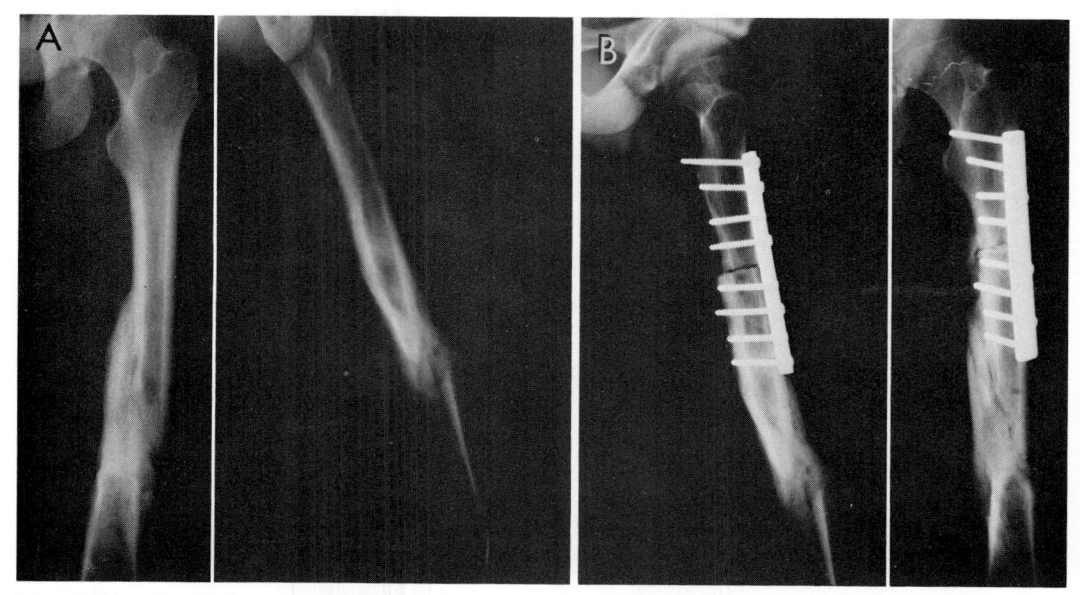

Fig. 5-34.—**A,** 60-degree rotatory malunion with marked internal rotation of the left femur distal to the fracture site because of failure to appreciate the degree of external rotation of the proximal femur in traction. Patient walked awkwardly, with the foot in 20–30 degrees of internal rotation, and had hip pain on attempting to walk with the toes ahead. **B,** excellent correction with compression plate, uneventful healing and marked improvement in gait.

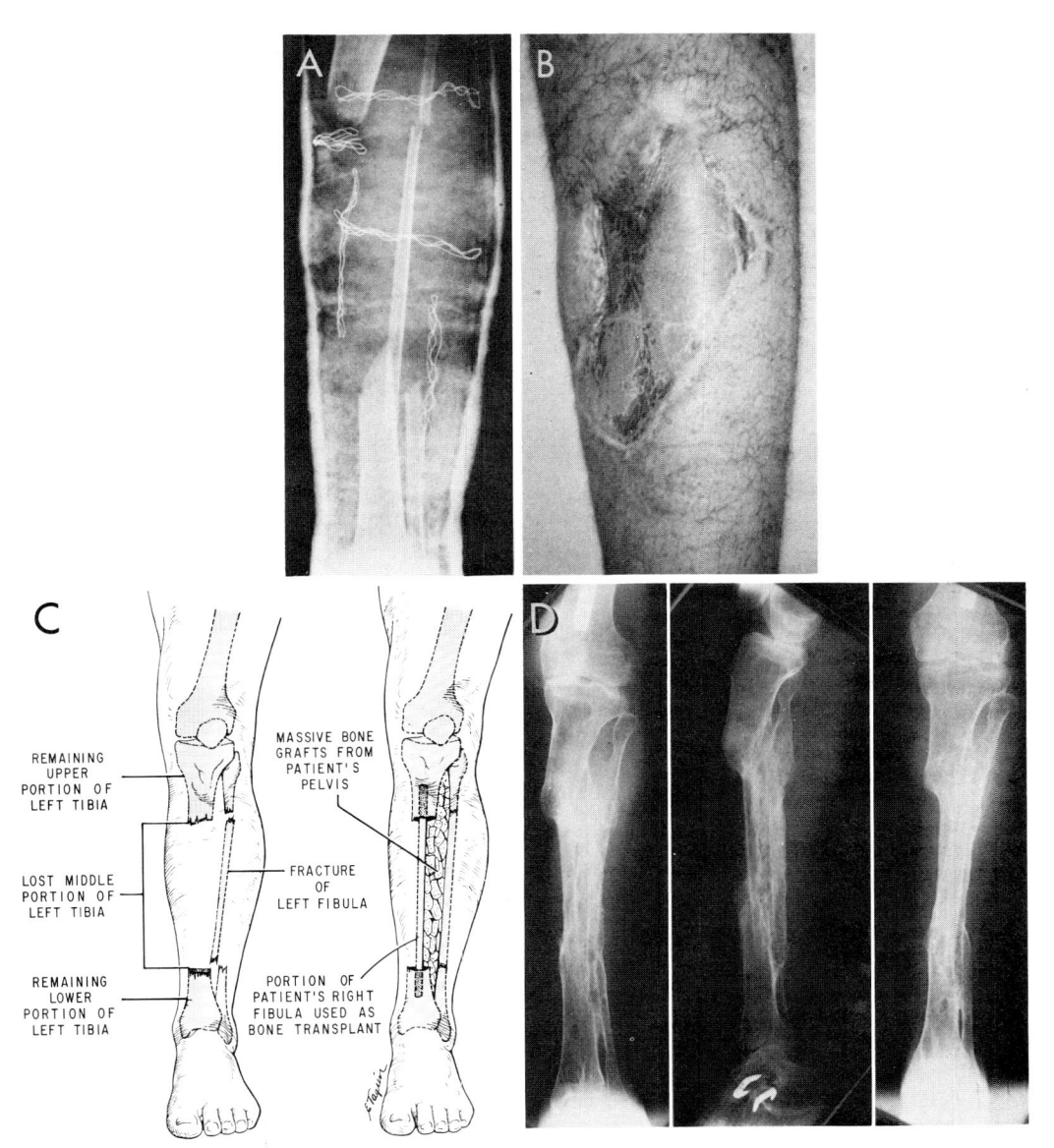

Chapter 5: DELAYED UNION, NONUNION AND MALUNION OF LONG BONES / 151

Fig. 5-35.—**A,** open fracture of the right tibia and fibula with extensive bone loss (8 inches) of tibia, secondary to automobile accident. Treated primarily by plaster fixation and skin grafting. **B,** appearance of anterior aspect of leg prior to bone grafting. **C,** technique of promoting union: transplantation of 10 inches of opposite fibula to defect in tibia. Operation was done in two stages, both through a posterior approach to tibia and fibula, and supplemented by massive iliac bone. Union firm after 12 months. Because of deformity of foot, secondary to peroneal injury, foot stabilization with staples was carried out. **D,** end result, 5 years: bone union. (Courtesy of Aufranc, O. E., Jones, W. N., and Turner, R. H.: Fracture of the Month No. 70, Nonunion of the tibial fracture with bone defect, JAMA 196:4, 1966.)

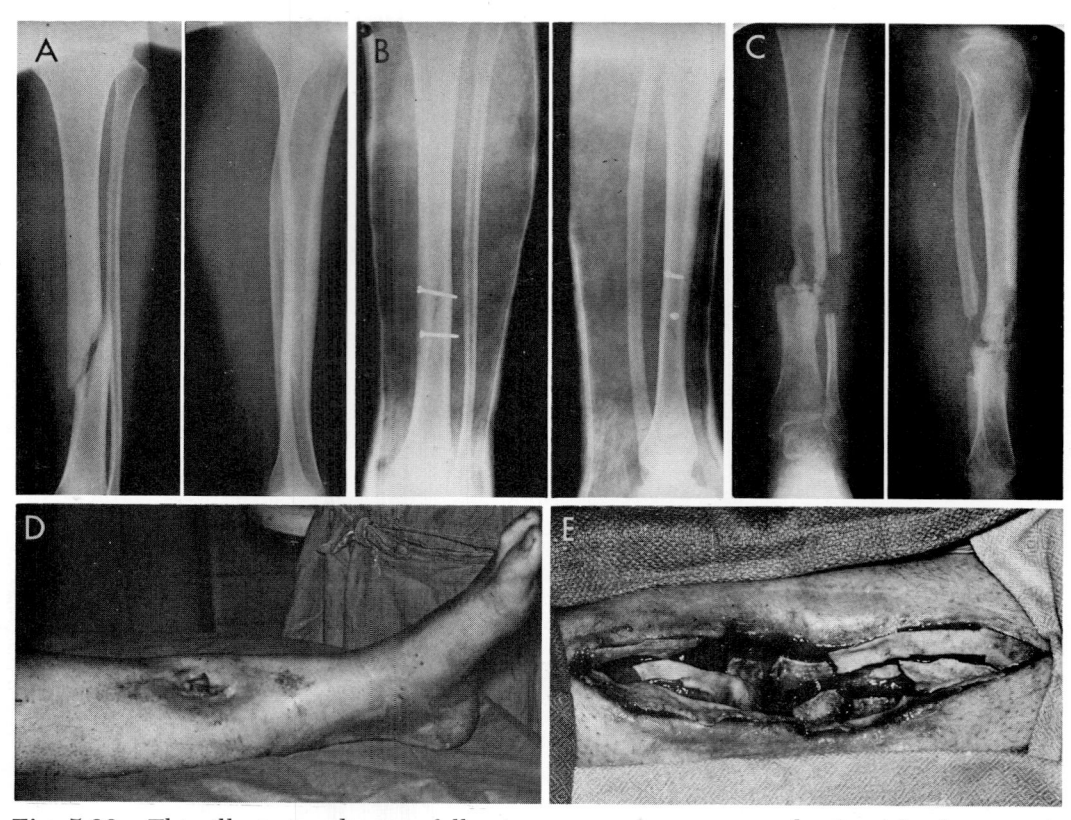

Fig. 5-36.—This illustrates disaster following unnecessary open reduction of a fracture. **A**, a slightly displaced, oblique fracture of the tibia with an intact fibula. This fracture would have healed with external fixation. **B**, following open reduction with adequate application of 2 screws and plaster of Paris. **C**, the result after infection and nonunion had developed and after the nearby fibula had been used for bone graft. **D**, appearance of the leg at time of admission for corrective surgery. **E**, following debridement and sequestrectomy and application of split-skin grafts. (**Continued.**)

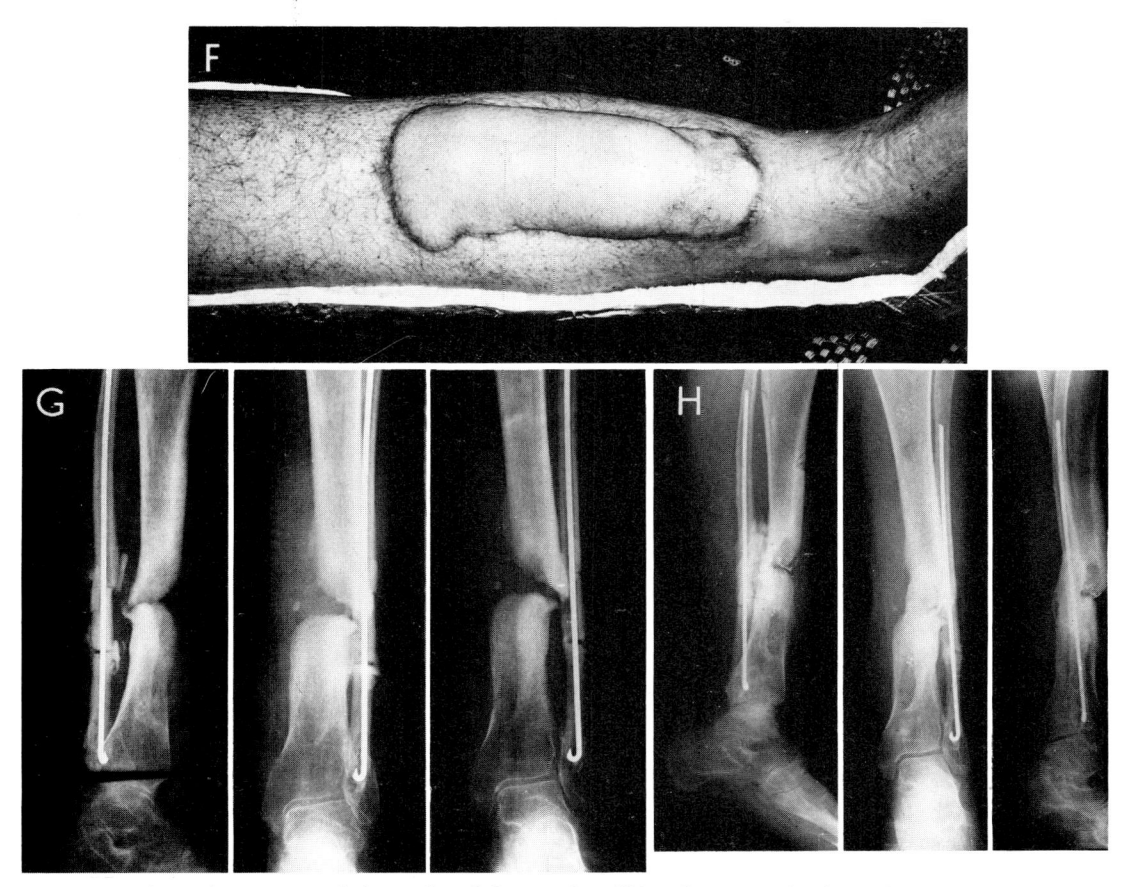

Chapter 5: DELAYED UNION, NONUNION AND MALUNION OF LONG BONES / 153

Fig. 5-36 (cont.).—**F,** a graft from the abdominal wall has been applied. **G,** through a posterior approach, the missing section of the fibula was replaced by a portion of the fibula from the opposite leg and stabilized with a Rush pin. **H,** after the 2d stage operation, again through the posterior approach. A massive amount of iliac bone has created synostosis between the tibia and fibula and union of the tibia has occurred. (From Cave, E. F.: Healing of fractures and nonunion of bone. The 7th Murray S. Danforth Oration, Rhode Island Med. J. 48:77, 1965.)

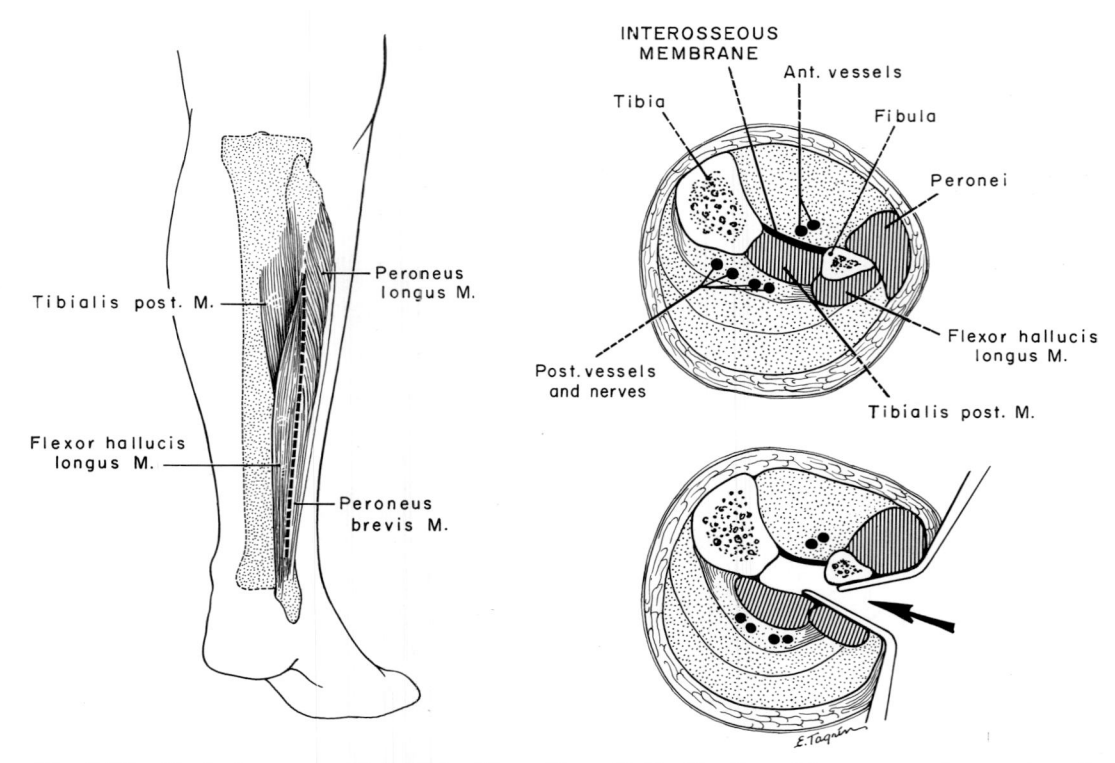

Fig. 5-37.—Posterior approach to tibia. (From Cave, E. F.: Healing of fractures and nonunion of bone. The 7th Murray S. Danforth Oration, Rhode Island Med. J. 48:77, 1965.)

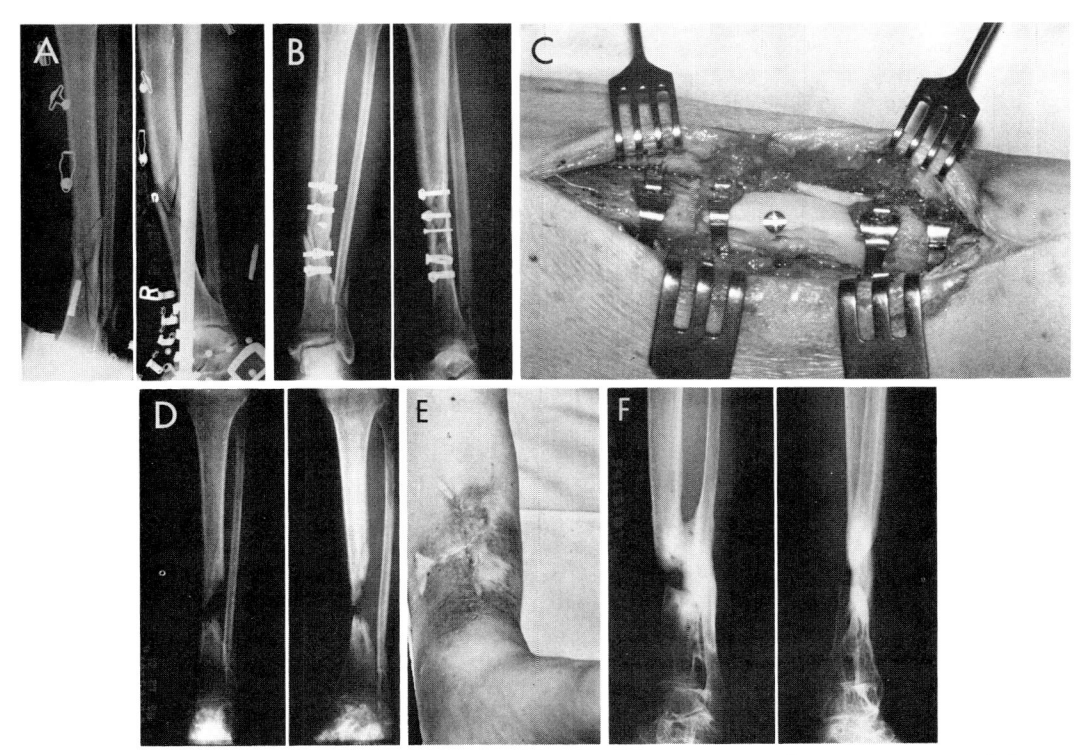

Chapter 5: DELAYED UNION, NONUNION AND MALUNION OF LONG BONES / 155

Fig. 5-38.—This case illustrates how the fibula can hypertrophy and assume responsibility of the tibia. **A,** anteroposterior and lateral views of closed, comminuted fracture of the tibia and fibula as a result of skiing. Ideal case for immobilization with plaster fixation. **B,** shows application of screws and Parham bands. Infection developed. Screws and Parham bands were removed. **C,** appearance at time of admission. "Dead" fragment of tibia. Metal was removed, along with sequestra, resulting in bone loss of the tibia, as shown in anterior and lateral views (**D**). Because of scar anteriorly (**E**), posterior bone graft was carried out. Infection recurred, but eventually union was accomplished. **F,** 10 years after injury. Although there is a large gap in the tibia, bone graft has caused synostosis between the intact fibula and fragments of the tibia. Despite the fact that the patient has 1 inch of shortening, he has a useful leg and has returned to his full time occupation as an optometrist. (From Cave, E. F.: Healing of fractures and nonunion of bone. The 7th Murray S. Danforth Oration, Rhode Island Med. J. 48:77, 1965.)

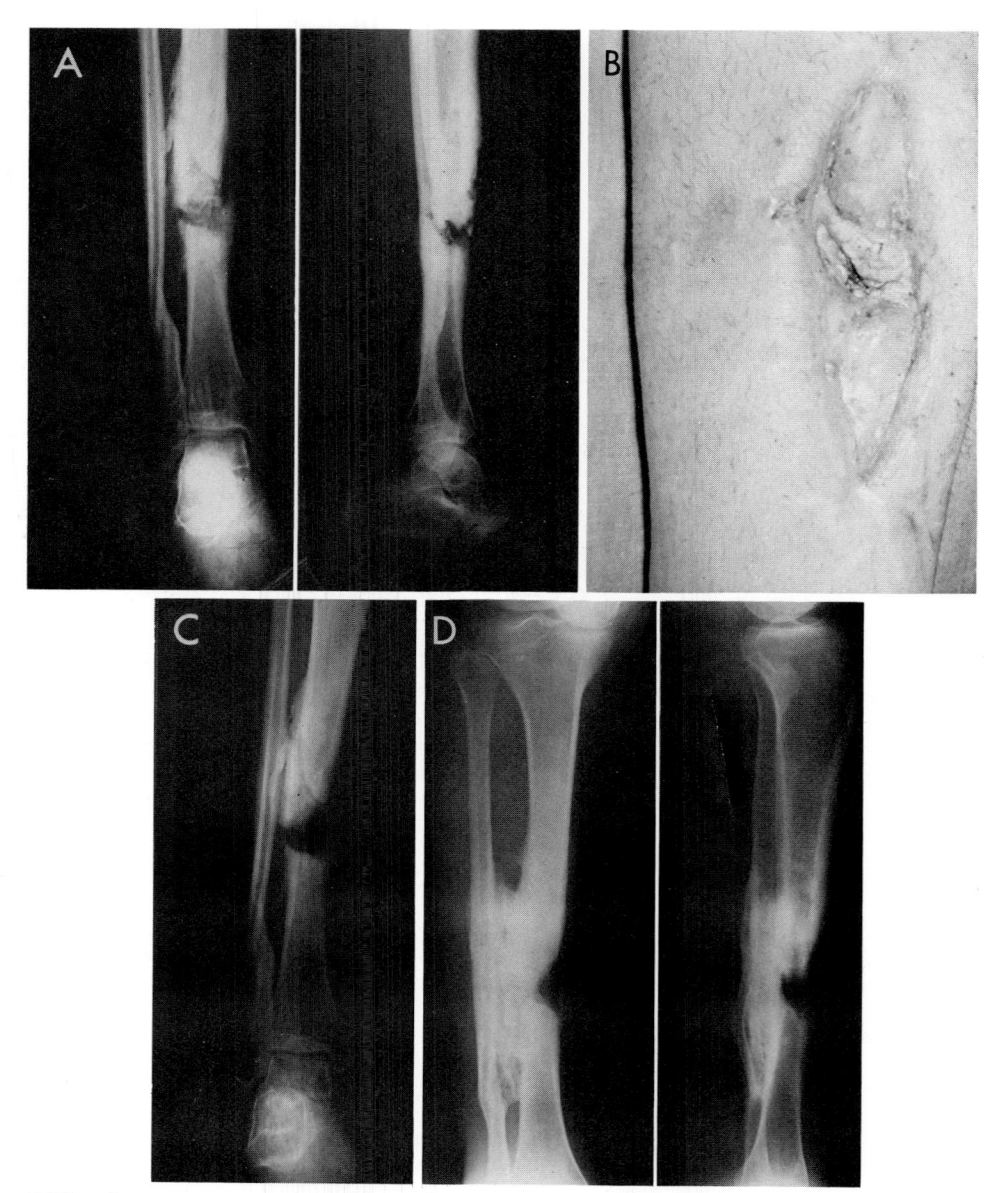

Fig. 5-39.—**A,** anteroposterior and lateral views showing nonunion of the tibia following open fracture of both bones of the right leg, sustained when the leg was struck by a falling, heavy object. Primary treatment consisted in closed reduction and a plaster of Paris cast; 6 days later, the application of a plate. **B,** appearance of anterior aspect of leg at time of admission with infection and nonunion. **C,** following sequestrectomy for removal of dead, infected bone from tibia, done through an anterior incision. **D,** anteroposterior and lateral views, showing bone graft to tibia and fibula with union. Patient ambulatory without support.

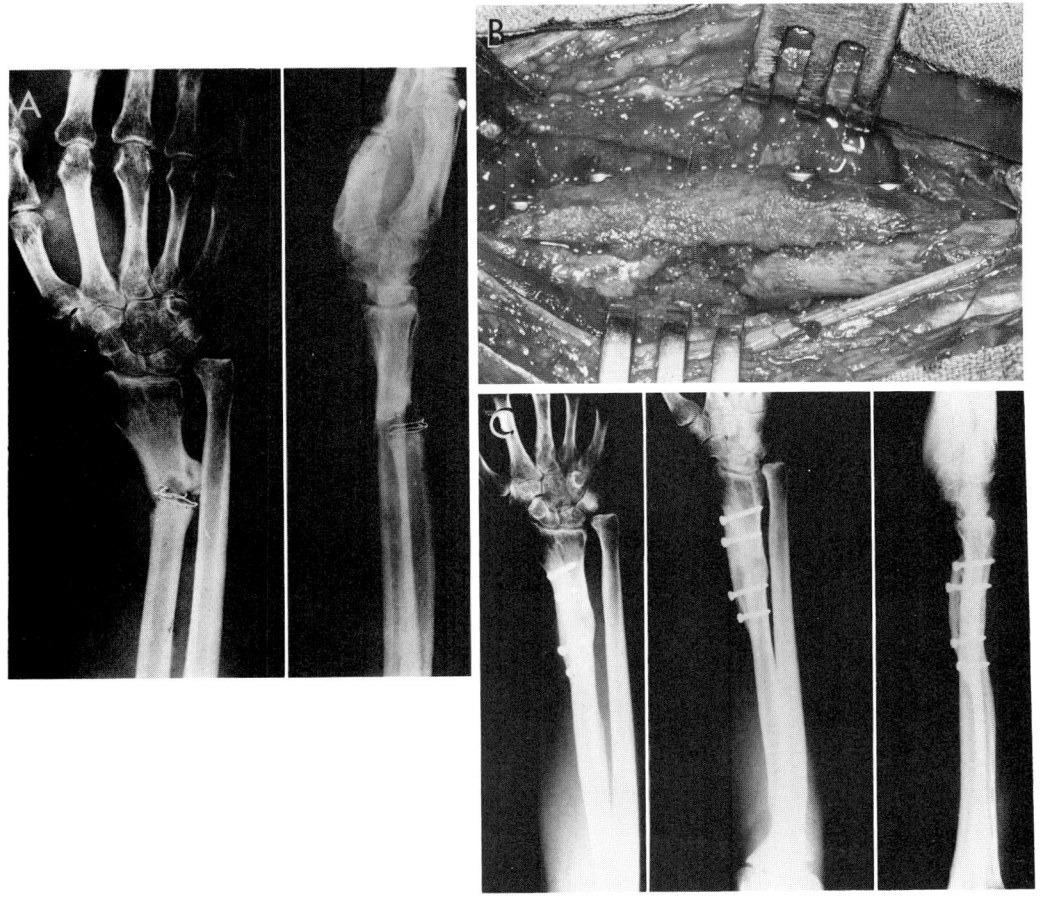

Chapter 5: DELAYED UNION, NONUNION AND MALUNION OF LONG BONES / 157

Fig. 5-40.—**A,** anteroposterior and lateral views illustrating nonunion of the distal portion of the right radius, inadequately treated with "wire loop." Operation was required to promote union and restore length to radius. **B,** application of bone graft (iliac crest) as length of radius is restored. Defect between main radial fragments packed with iliac bone chips. **C,** anteroposterior, oblique and lateral views. Bone union with restoration of radial length. Excellent function.

BIBLIOGRAPHY

1. Abbott, L. C., Schottstaedt, E. R., Saunders, J. B. deC. M., and Bost, F. C.: The evaluation of cortical and cancellous bone as grafting material: A clinical and experimental study, J. Bone Joint Surg. 29:381, 1947.
2. Bennett, G. A.: Fracture healing, in Lectures on Reconstruction Surgery of the Extremities, Am. Acad. Orthop. Surgeons Lect., p. 461, Course No. XIII, 1944.
3. Bennett, G. A., and Bauer, W.: The Healing of Fractures, in Scudder, C. (ed.), *The Treatment of Fractures* (Philadelphia: W. B. Saunders Company, 1939), Chap. XI.
4. Bishop, W. A., Stauffer, R. C., and Swenson, A. L.: Bone grafts: An end-result study of the healing time, J. Bone Joint Surg. 29:961, 1947.
5. Brav, E.: Personal communication, June, 1956.
6. Bush, L. F.: The use of homogenous bone grafts, J. Bone Joint Surg. 29:620, 1947.
7. Bush, L. F., and Garber, C. Z.: Bone bank, JAMA 137:588, 1948.
8. Campbell, W. C.: In Speed, J. S., and Knight, R. A. (eds.), *Operative Orthopedics* (3d ed.; St. Louis: The C. V. Mosby Company, 1956), Vol. 1, Chap. XI, p. 795.
9. Campbell, W. C.: Ununited fractures, Arch. Surg. 24:990, 1932.
10. Chandler, F. A., and Fox, T. A.: Amputation for discrepancy of limb length, J. Bone Joint Surg. 31-A:420, 1948.
11. Cubbins, W. R., Callahan, B. S., and Scuderi, C. S.: The causes of non-union. Bone growth and regeneration, Surg. Gynecol. Obstet. 62:427, 1936.
12. d'Aubigné, R. M.: Surgical treatment of non-union of long bones, J. Bone Joint Surg. 31-A:256, 1948.
13. Funsten, R. V., and Lee, R. W.: Healing time in fractures of the shafts of the tibia and femur, J. Bone Joint Surg. 27:395, 1945.
14. Harmon, P. H.: A simplified surgical approach to the posterior tibia for bone-grafting and fibular transference, J. Bone Joint Surg. 27:496, 1945.
15. Jores, L.: Experimentelle Untersuchungen über die Einwirkung mechanischen Druckes auf den Knochen, Beitr. Pathol. Anat. 66:433, 1920.
16. Key J. A.: The choice of operations for delayed and nonunion of long bones, Ann. Surg. 118:665, 1943.
17. McLaughlin, H. L., Gaston S. R., and Neer, C. S.: Open reduction and internal fixation of fractures of the long bones, J. Bone Joint Surg. 31-A:94, 1949.
18. Murray, W. R., Lucas, D. B., and Inman, V. T.: Treatment of nonunion of fractures of the long bones by the two-plate method, J. Bone Joint Surg. 46-A:1027, 1964.
19. Phemister, D. B.: Biologic principles in the healing of fractures and their bearing on treatment, Ann. Surg. 133:433, 1951.
20. Phemister, D. B.: Treatment of ununited fractures by onlay bone grafts without screw or tie fixation and without breaking down of the fibrous union, J. Bone Joint Surg. 29:946, 1947.
21. Ray, R. D., LaViolette, D., Buckley, H. D., and Mosiman, R. S.: Studies of bone metabolism: I. A comparison of the metabolism of strontium in living and dead bone, J. Bone Joint Surg. 37-A:143, 1955.
22. Reynolds, F. C., and Oliver, D. R.: Clinical evaluation of merthiolate bone bank: Preliminary report, J. Bone Joint Surg. 31-A:792, 1949.
23. Senn, N.: *Principles of Surgery* (Philadelphia: F. A. Davis Company, 1890).
24. Starr, K. W.: *The Causation and Treatment of Delayed Union in Fractures of the Long Bones* (London: Butterworth & Co., Ltd., 1947).
25. Urist, M. R.: The pathogenesis and treatment of delayed union and nonunion: A survey of 85 ununited fractures of the shaft of the tibia and 100 control cases with similar injuries, J. Bone Joint Surg. 36–A:931, 1954.
26. Urist, M. R.: The physiologic basis of bone-graft surgery, with special reference to the theory of induction, Clin. Orthop. 1:207, 1953.
27. Urist, M. R., and Johnson, R. W., Jr.: Calcification and ossification: IV. Healing of fractures in man under clinical conditions, J. Bone Joint Surg. 25:375, 1943.
28. Urist, M. R., and McLean, F. C.: The local physiology of bone repair: With particular reference to the process of new bone formation by induction, Am. J. Surg. 85:444, 1953.
29. Watson-Jones, R., and Coltart, W. D.: Slow union of fractures: With a study of 804 fractures of the shafts of the tibia and femur, Br. J. Surg. 30:260, 1943.
30. Weaver, J. B.: Experience in use of homogenous (bone bank) bone, J. Bone Joint Surg. 31-A:778, 1949.
31. Wilson, P. D.: Experience with the bone bank, Ann. Surg. 126:932, 1947.
32. Young, H. G., and Blaisdell, J. S.: A comparative study of several methods of treatment of fractures of the shaft of the tibia, Surg. Clin. North Am. 23:967, 1943.

6 | Technique of Bone Grafting

EDWIN F. CAVE and ROBERT J. BOYD

THE TECHNIQUE OF BONE GRAFTING has been improved as our knowledge of bone repair has increased. Added to the technical advances in bone transplants has been improvement in the design of instruments, particularly the thin, sharp osteotomes devised by Smith-Petersen and the motor-driven saws and drills of Albee, Luck and Stryker. The type of graft to be employed not only depends on the local situation to be dealt with, but also is a matter of preference of the individual surgeon. Some surgeons still use the massive inlay graft for an ununited tibia, whereas other surgeons condemn it completely and use only the onlay graft.

Since the introduction of the massive inlay tibial graft (Fig. 6-1) by Albee[2] in 1915, other types of transplants have been developed—the multiple bone chips of Hibbs,[13] the onlay grafts of Henderson[12] and Campbell[6] and the subperiosteal application of bone slabs advocated by Phemister. The dowel graft has frequently been employed for nonunion of the carpal navicular, for malleolar or condylar fractures and, at times, for nonunion of the femoral neck. Massive autogenous bone fragments or bank bone is used to fill large defects secondary to bone loss from injury or after resection of tumors.

The usual sources for bone grafts are the tibia and the ilium. In recent years, bank bone has been used to some extent.

Onlay Graft

The onlay graft may be used for any fracture of any of the long bones when bone loss is not great. The common source of bone for the graft is the tibia. The graft may be taken from the proximal, or at times the distal, fragment of the

Fig. 6-1.—The sliding inlay graft is cut with a double-blade circular saw. The distal portion of the graft is cut through and replaced in the slot in the upper end of the tibia after the graft is moved downward.

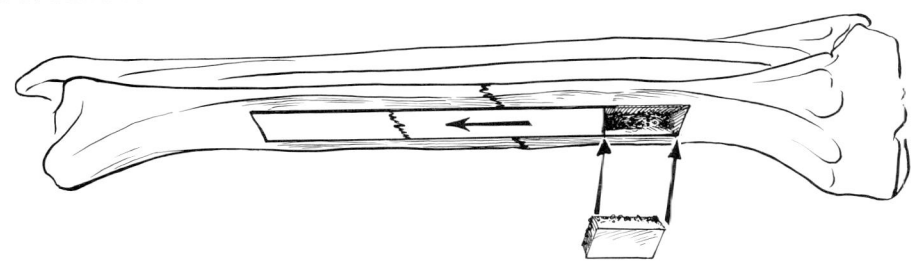

fractured bone, depending on the site of the fracture; or it may be removed from the opposite tibia. It should be cut with a motor drill and a motor saw (Fig. 6-2). The tibia is exposed with a long, curving incision that is carried down to periosteum. The periosteum is incised and gently reflected from the tibia sufficiently to obtain a graft without damaging periosteum and other soft tissue. Improvement in the design of motor drills and saws has simplified the taking of grafts. The usual onlay tibial graft should be from 3 to 4 in. long and from $3/8$ to $1/2$ in. wide. The entire cortex is removed. When possible, it is better to take the graft from the upper part of the tibia. A single-blade saw is used to outline the graft, and a small drill

Fig. 6-2. — The onlay graft is removed with a single-blade motor saw. The graft is beveled slightly toward the center. Drill holes at the 4 corners eliminate the possibility of fracture of the tibia. Drill holes to accommodate screws for securing the graft may be made with the graft in situ. They are staggered to prevent splitting of the graft. The graft is fitted accurately to the lateral aspect of recipient bone.

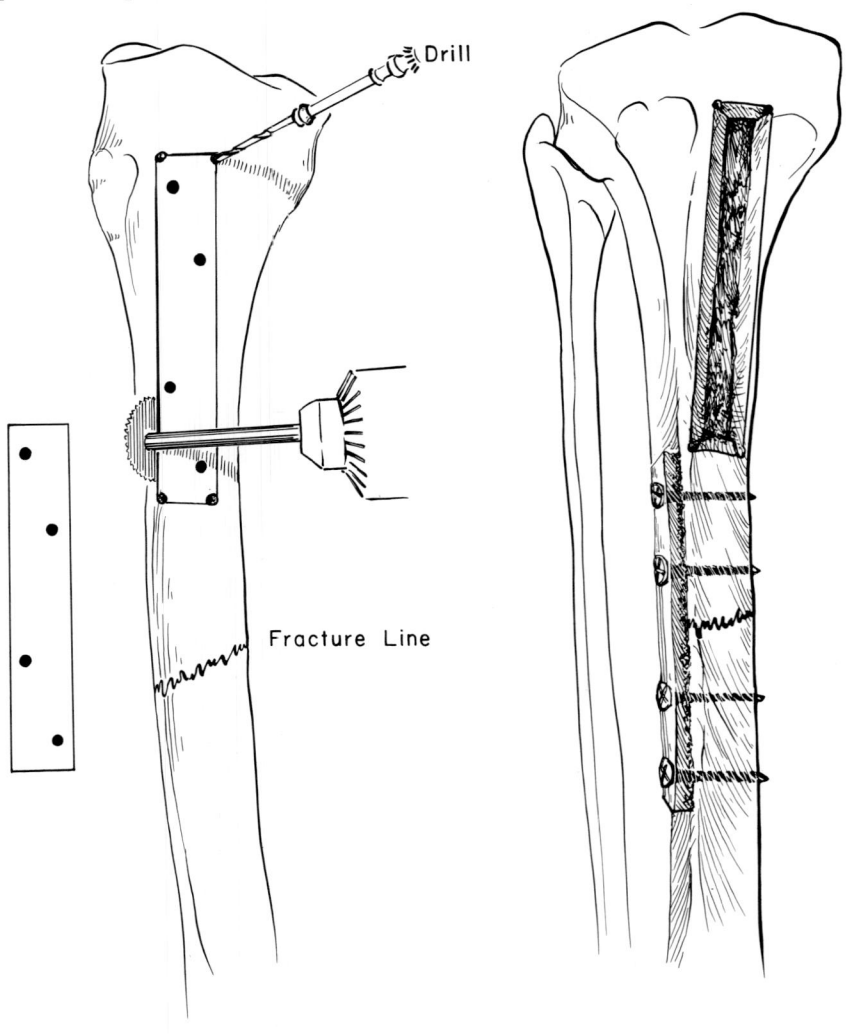

is employed to mobilize the graft's 4 corners in order to avoid fracture of the shaft of the bone. The motor saw should be used at low speed, so as not to burn bone. It is angulated slightly toward the central portion of the bone in order to bevel the graft slightly; this also helps to avoid fracture of the shaft of the tibia. After the graft is cut and while it is still in its bed, it is possible to make drill holes in the graft which will accommodate screws.

The recipient bone is leveled on 1 side with osteotomes to permit accurate fitting of the graft. The graft is secured to an area of bone that has the best blood supply from surrounding muscles. In the tibia, it is well to apply the graft to the lateral aspect of the bone (Fig. 6-2). Usually the graft is secured by screws, which are staggered to prevent splitting of the graft; the screws traverse the graft as well as both cortices of the bone to which it is applied. It must fit accurately but must not be placed under stress, because stress, if present, may eventually produce fracture of the graft.

Onlay grafts may also be taken from the iliac crest. These grafts are particularly useful for application to the radius or ulna (see Chapter 20). The graft is removed by exposing the anterior and mesial iliac crest subperiosteally on both the inner and outer aspects for a length of about 4 in. and a depth of about 2 in. With a single-blade motor saw or with sharp, straight and curved osteotomes, the graft is cut obliquely (Fig. 6-3). The soft, cancellous bone is gouged out, leaving the strong cortex, which will fit the curving contour of the radius or ulna. Four screws are needed to secure the graft to the recipient bone. This type of graft is also applicable to the humeral shaft. Boyd[3] has advocated the use of a double, or "twin," onlay graft (Fig. 6-4), particularly in congenital pseudarthrosis of the tibia. This type of graft is also applicable for use in any long bone when there is considerable bone loss and when it is desirable to maintain length. The graft is usually removed from the opposite tibia, although bank bone may be used.

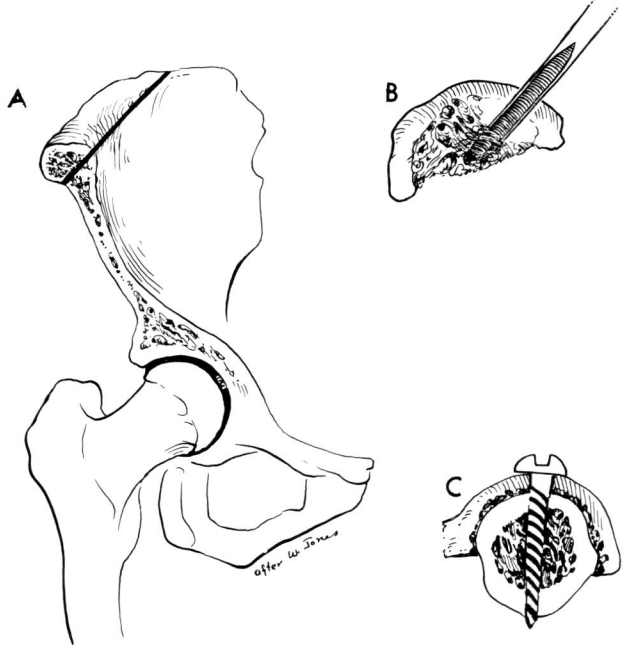

Fig. 6-3. — Massive graft from ilium. **A**, the graft is cut in an oblique manner. **B**, cancellous bone is partially removed. **C**, the curving iliac crest fits the contour of the bone.

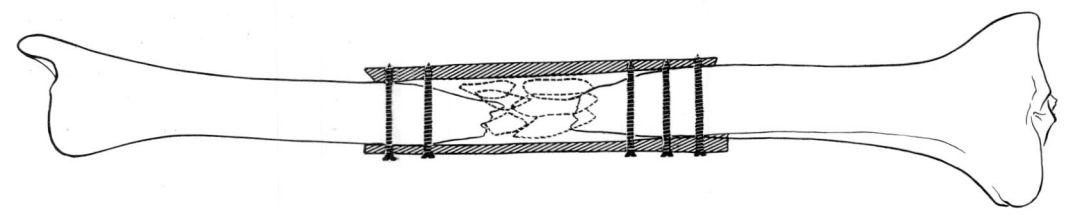

Fig. 6-4.—Double, or "twin," onlay graft.

It is well to supplement the double onlay graft with iliac bone chips interposed between the 2 grafts and the ends of the fragments.

Inlay Graft

The inlay tibial graft has been employed in our clinic very rarely during the past 25 years. In our experience, it is less effective than the onlay graft, although it is still in favor in some clinics. It may be removed from the proximal or distal fragment, above or below the fracture site. The inlay graft may also be removed from the opposite tibia. It is cut with a double-blade motor saw, which is also used to make a slot across the fracture line, into which the graft is placed (Fig. 6-1). Generally, internal fixation is not used with this type of graft.

Subperiosteal Iliac Graft

The subperiosteal iliac graft has been found most useful, and it is being employed with increasing favor, particularly when the fracture is in reasonably good alignment and mobilization of the area of nonunion or repositioning of bone frag-

Fig. 6-5.—Technique of removing iliac grafts. **A,** making use of only the outer table of the ilium. **B,** "horizontal" grafts, utilizing both tables of the ilium.

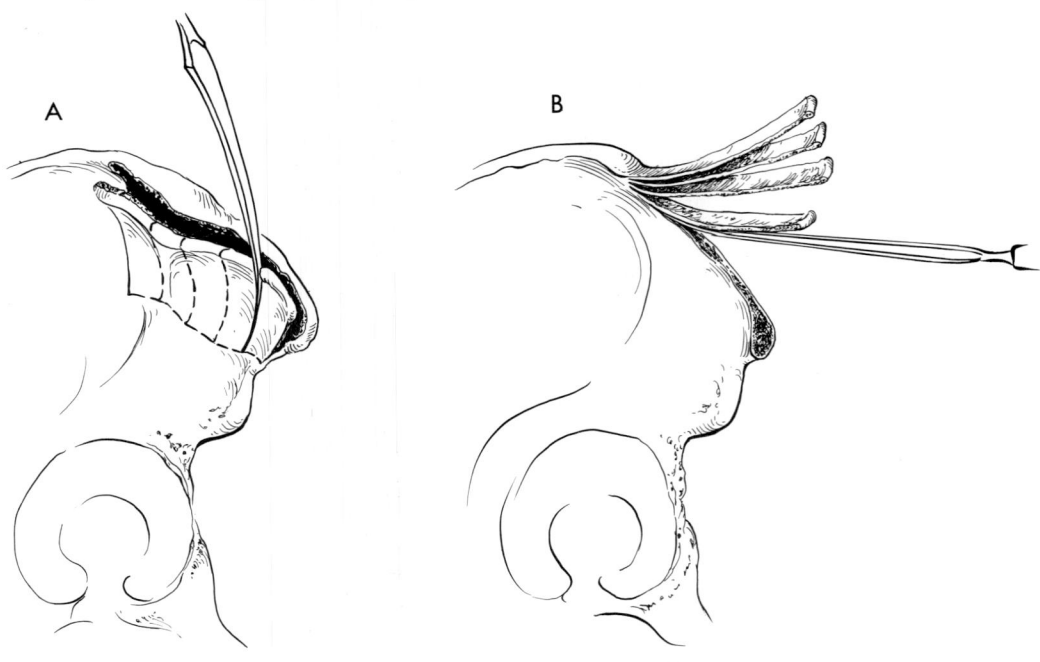

ments is not necessary. If realignment is necessary, a plate and screws are used to stabilize the bone before inserting the subperiosteal iliac bone around the shaft under the periosteum. For application of this type of graft, the bone is exposed subperiosteally with an adequate incision. The grafts are removed from the ilium, as shown in Figure 6-5, and are applied to the area of the bone that is most effectively covered by muscle. These grafts do not need to be long or very thick, and they are placed in a barrel-stave fashion about the fracture site.

"Neighborhood" Graft

The osteoperiosteal "neighborhood" graft may serve the same purpose as the subperiosteal iliac graft. It is usually removed from the proximal fragment of the shaft, and it is made up of periosteum and a layer of cortical bone thin enough to bend but thick enough to be of value as a source of new bone. It is taken, as wide as possible, from the upper fragment of the bone and is placed about the fracture site under periosteum (Fig. 6-6). As a rule, this graft is used in conjunction with some form of internal fixation. It may be employed in fresh fractures or in fractures in which operation has, of necessity, been delayed.

Dowel Graft

The dowel graft is used most often in the ununited navicular fracture of, or for delayed union in fractures of, the femoral neck. For the navicular fracture, the graft is usually removed from the tibia with the motor saw. For grafting an ununited femoral neck, a longitudinal section of the fibula or the entire fibula may be employed. In each case the graft is shaped in cylindrical fashion with a rasp. When the dowel graft is used in the femoral neck, it may be supplemented by internal fixation in the form of a flanged nail (Fig. 6-7) or a combination of nail and plate. In the carpal navicular bone, the dowel graft gives stability and is supplemented by external plaster fixation.

Slotted Graft

The slotted graft has had a limited use in our clinic. This method of bone grafting has been effective for the ununited internal malleolus (Figs. 6-8 and 6-9), and some surgeons prefer it for the carpal navicular bone.

Bank Bone

The use of bank bone has met with moderate enthusiasm since it was introduced some years ago, and is particularly useful when large defects are to be filled. However, it is generally agreed that heterogenous bone from the bone bank does not act as effectively for grafting as does autogenous bone and that the hazard of infection is greater.

Bone grafts are used primarily as a source of bone to promote healing of a fracture. Albee[2] maintained that the massive bone transplant lives in its new location. Opposing this view were others—Leriche and Policard, Groves, Gallie, Phemister and Ghormley—who believed that the graft dies, leaving only the matrix surviving to act as support for newly proliferating osteoblasts, which in time completely replace the bone graft. The massive grafts have considerable value as stabilizing elements, but in practically every case they must be supplemented by external fixation in the form of plaster. Notable exceptions are the subperiosteal, iliac and tibial grafts used in conjunction with medullary fixation.

Rejection of Bone Grafts

Fresh autogenous bone graft has long been recognized as clinically superior to homogenous bone graft. This may be related to the survival of periosteal cells in the autografts and the formation of new bone of donor origin. It has been demonstrated experimentally that homogenous and heterogenous bone grafts are not as effective in producing osteogenesis as is autogenous bone. Much experimental evidence suggests that this is probably on an immunologic basis. Although homog-

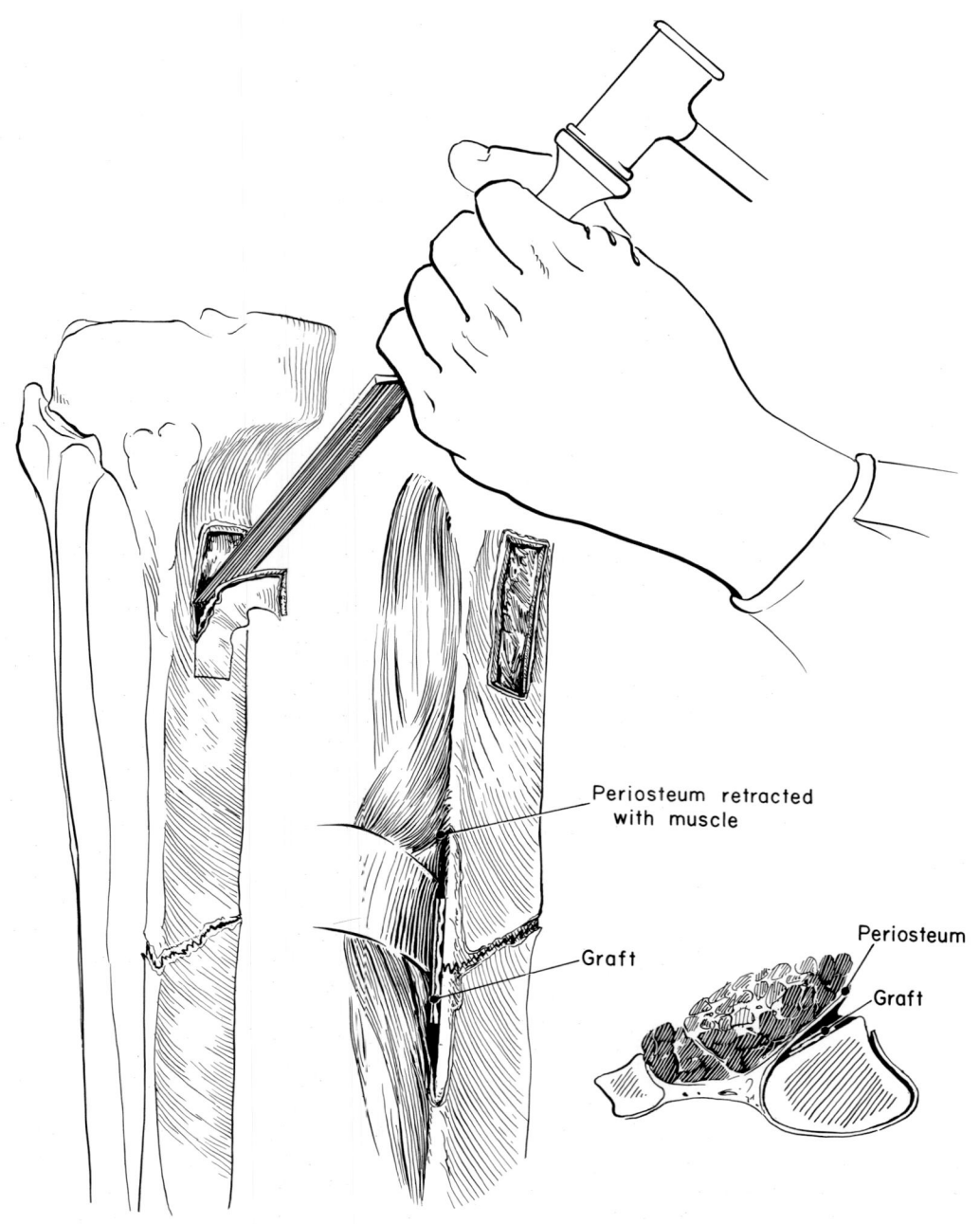

Fig. 6-6.—Osteoperiosteal "neighborhood" graft.

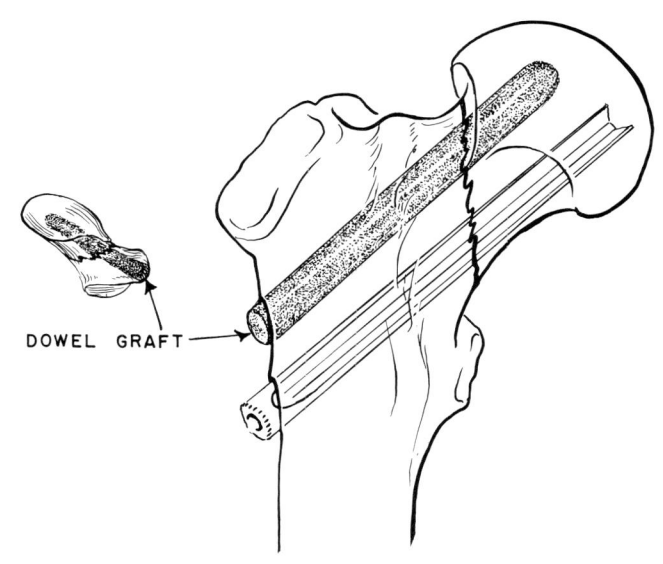

Fig. 6-7.—Dowel graft.

enous bone grafts show immunologic rejection at about 1 week, they do not slough and they act as a support and framework for newly proliferating osteoblasts, which replace the bone graft in time.

Heterogenous bone is definitely antigenic, producing circulating antibodies. Homogenous bone graft antigenicity has been demonstrated, although it is not clear whether circulating antibodies are produced. Fresh bone homograft appears to have antigens in common with skin antigens, as noted by Chalmers[7] and others. Freezing and freeze drying of bone homografts appear to inactivate the antigens they have in common with skin. Decalcification, deproteinization, and deproteinization and freezing of bone homograft appear to leave sufficient

Fig. 6-8.—Slotted grafts are cut with a motor saw, turned on themselves and replaced into the slots.

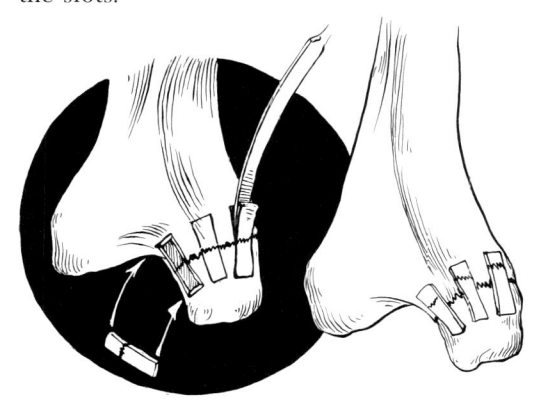

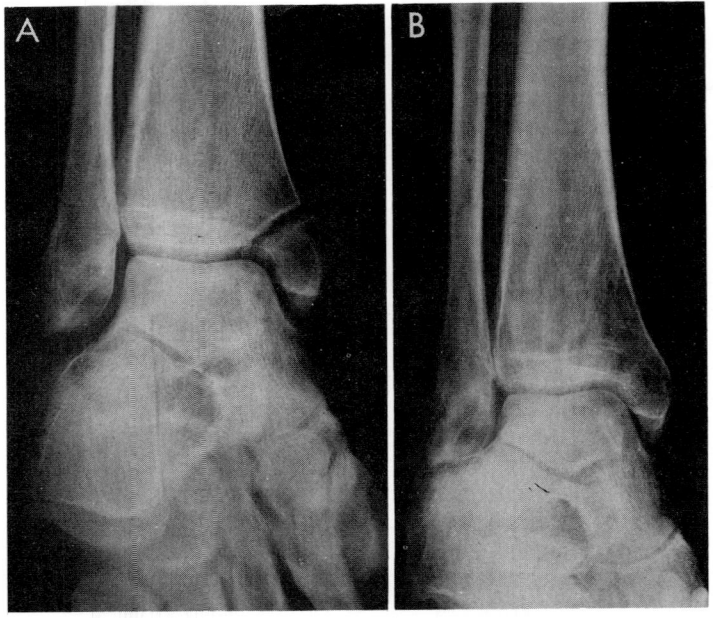

Fig. 6-9.—**A**, ununited fracture of internal malleolus in 41-year-old guard. **B**, bone union that resulted from use of the slotted graft.

common antigen to cause acceleration of skin rejection, as noted by Chalmers[7] as well as by Brooks et al.[4]

The ultimate importance of bone antigens to the effectiveness of bone homograft material remains uncertain.

Fresh autogenous bone graft is recommended for use preferentially, with freeze-dried homogenous bone the next most desirable material. The latter is particularly useful when large defects are to be filled.

BIBLIOGRAPHY

1. Abbott, L. C.: The use of iliac bone in the treatment of ununited fractures, Am. Acad. Orthop. Surgeons Lectures on Reconstruction Surgery of the Extremities. Course No. I, p. 13, 1944.
2. Albee, F. H.: *Bone Graft Surgery* (Philadelphia: W. B. Saunders Company, 1915).
3. Boyd, H. B.: The treatment of difficult and unusual nonunion, with special reference to the bridging of defects, J. Bone Joint Surg. 25:535, 1943.
4. Brooks, D. B., Heiple, K. G., Herndon, C. H., and Powell, A. E.: Immunological factors in homogenous bone transplantation: IV. The effect of various methods of preparation and irradiation on antigenicity, J. Bone Joint Surg. 45-A:1617, 1963.
5. Burwell, R. G., and Gowland, G.: Studies in the transplantation of bone: I. Assessment of antigenicity; serological studies, J. Bone Joint Surg. 43-B:814, 1961.
6. Campbell, W. C.: in Speed, J. S., and Knight, R. A. (eds.), *Operative Orthopedics* (3d ed.; St. Louis: C. V. Mosby Company, 1956), Vol. 1, Chap. IV, p. 174.
7. Chalmers, J.: Transplantation immunity in bone homografting, J. Bone Joint Surg. 41-B:160, 1959.
8. Gallie, W. D.: The transplantation of bone, Br. Med. J. 2:840, 1931.
9. Ghormley, R. K.: Choice of bone graft methods in bone and joint surgery, Ann. Surg. 115:247, 1942.
10. Groves, E. W. H.: Ununited fractures, with special reference to gunshot injuries and the use of bone grafting, Br. J. Surg. 6:203, 1918.
11. Heiple, K. G., Chase, S. W., and Herndon, C. H.: A comparative study of the healing process following different types of bone transplantation, J. Bone Joint Surg. 45-A: 1593, 1963.
12. Henderson, M. S.: The massive bone grafts, JAMA 107:1104, 1936.
13. Hibbs, R. A.: Operative orthopedics, Ann. Surg. 55:682, 1912.
14. Orell, S.: Interposition of os purum in osteosynthesis after osteotomy, resections of bone and joints (interposition-osteosynthesis), Surg. Gynecol. Obstet. 59:638, 1934.

7 | Pathologic Fractures

EDWIN T. WYMAN, JR.

A PATHOLOGIC FRACTURE can be said to be that fracture which occurs through abnormal bone. The bone is weakened and will give way with little stress, at times only that placed on it by normal function. These fractures are often called "spontaneous," but that should not imply that no force is required to produce the fracture.

Certain types of pathologic fractures (by strict definition) rightfully are not really considered or treated as such. An example is the metatarsal stress fracture through bones with disuse atrophy; this occurs during weight-bearing rehabilitation after cast immobilization for a tibial fracture. The vertebral compression fracture (Fig. 7-1) through osteoporotic bone in the postmenopausal woman is another example. The subcapital femoral neck fracture occurring during a weight-bearing turn (without a precipitating fall) in the osteoporotic aged patient is a third. It is important in treatment of these fractures to realize that the fracture has not occurred through "normal" bone.

CLASSIFICATION.—Since pathologic fractures occur only through bone that is diseased, a classification would actually be a list of all bone pathology. No attempt will be made here to list all these conditions. Suffice it to say that fractures will occur most frequently in those bones under the most biomechanical stress (i.e., weight bearing) in those conditions which give the most replacement of normal osseous tissue by diseased tissue. The disease can be generalized as in rickets or syringomyelia, congenital as in osteogenesis imperfecta (Fig. 7-2), or iatrogenic as in long-term, high-level steroid therapy (Fig. 7-3). On the other hand, the condition underlying the fracture can be localized, as in primary or metastatic bone tumors, benign bone cysts or osteomyelitis.

HEALING TIMES.—A generalization cannot be stated concerning the length of healing time of pathologic fractures since so much depends on the underlying condition. Fractures through the delicate bone of osteogenesis imperfecta heal more rapidly than normal, but with bone of the same poor quality. Fractures through bone in the area of a benign bone cyst heal in about the same time as would be required if the cyst did not exist (Fig. 7-4). Fractures through bone containing Paget's disease (Fig. 7-5) or areas of old, healed osteomyelitis take much longer to heal. Indeed, femoral neck fractures in bone afflicted with Charcot's disease rarely, if ever, heal at all.

TYPES OF FRACTURES.—Although pathologic fractures can occur in all the same forms as nonpathologic fractures, they usually occur with less force and so tend to be less comminuted and displaced. They may be considerably angulated. The bone often will appear to have simply crumbled, and the patient may give a history of some pain for days or weeks before acute fracture (probably from small microfractures).

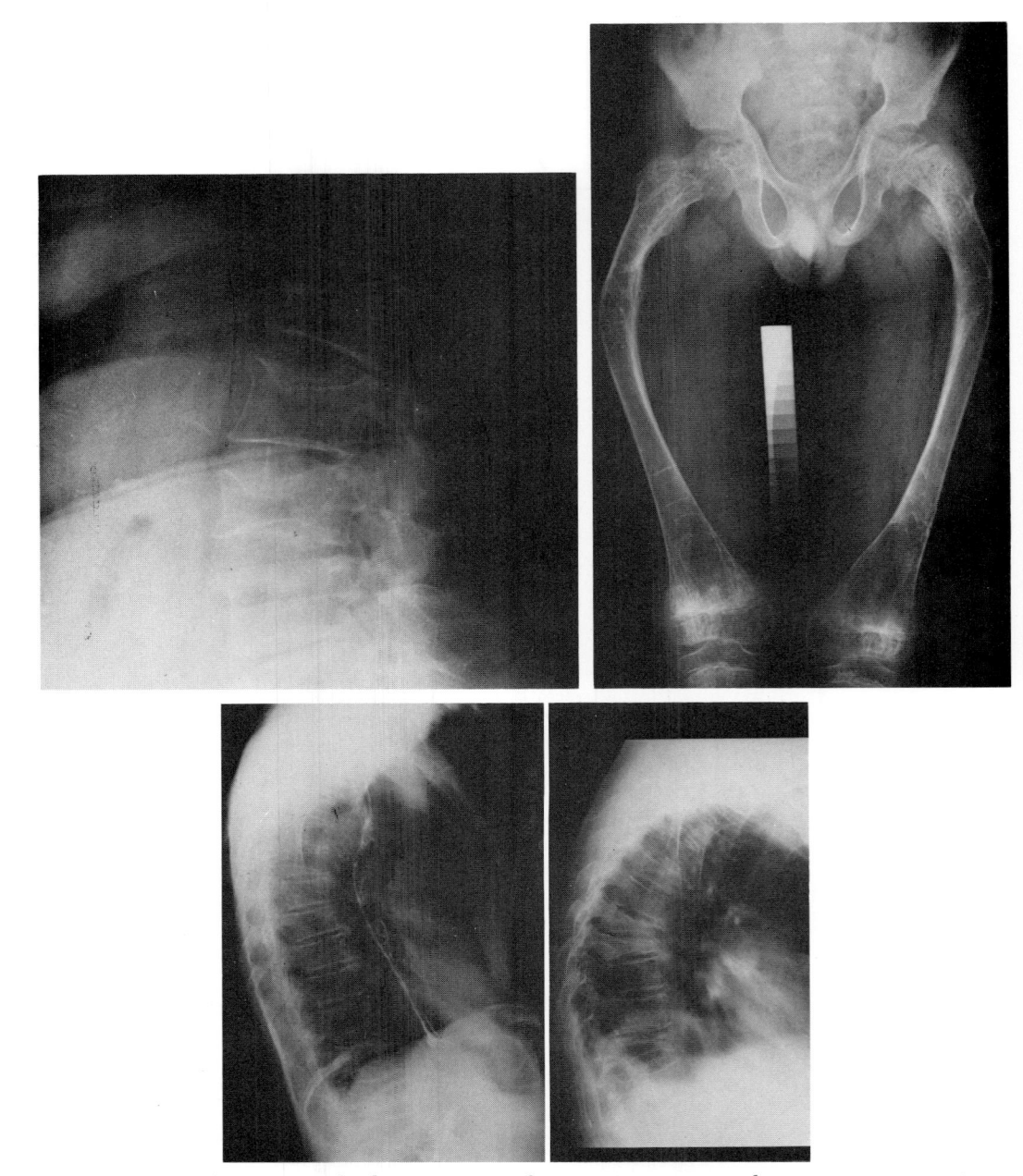

Fig. 7-1 (top left).—Vertebral compression fracture in patient with severe osteoporosis.
Fig. 7-2 (top right).—Osteogenesis imperfecta in a 9-year-old child. Decalcification of disease and femoral deformity resulting from 16 fractures are shown.
Fig. 7-3 (bottom).—Multiple compression fractures of dorsal spine (views taken 4 months apart) in patient on high doses of steroids for pemphigus.

Chapter 7: PATHOLOGIC FRACTURES / 169

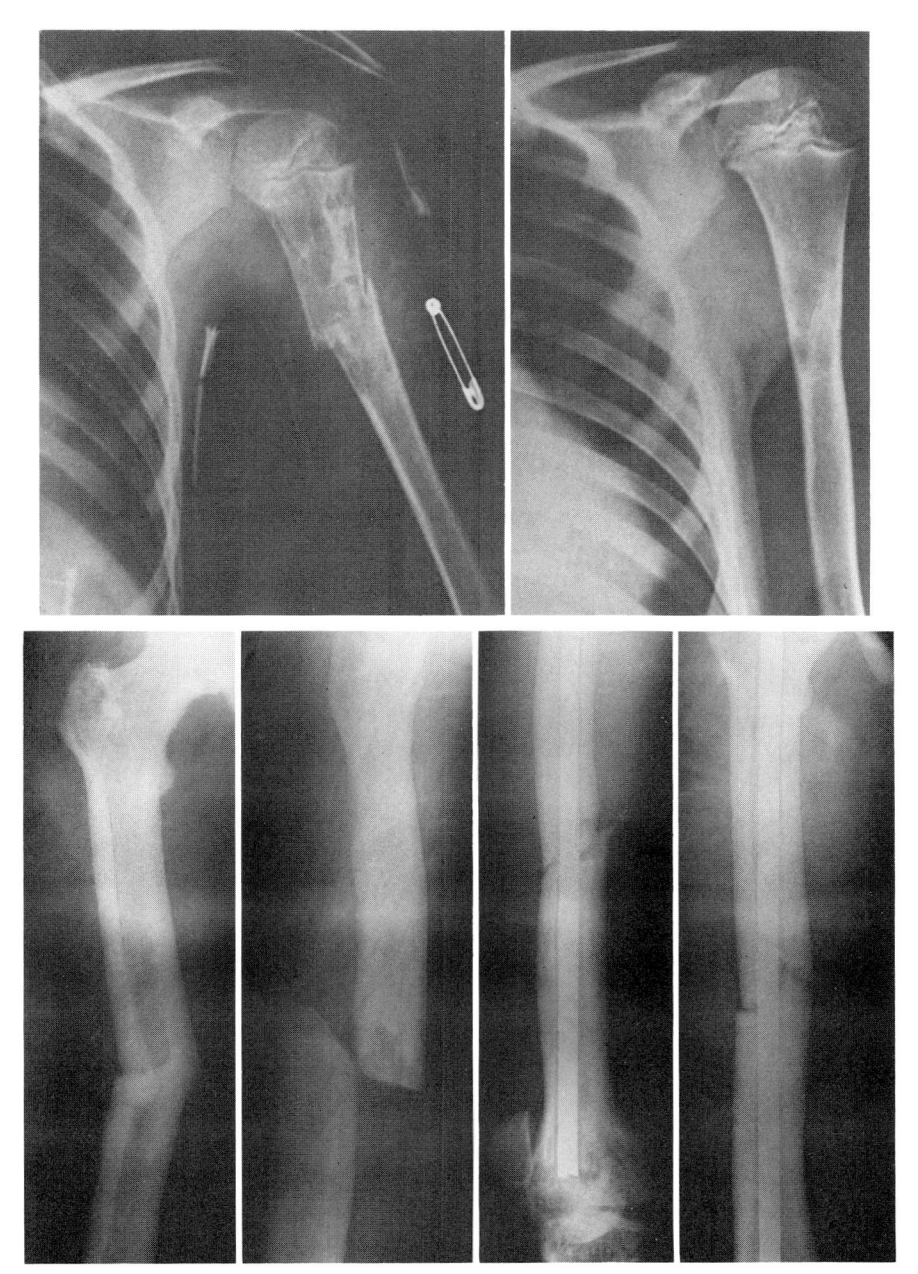

Fig. 7-4 (top).—Multilocular bone cyst. Left, pathologic fracture of proximal third of humerus in a child, treated in plaster shoulder spica. Right, 3 years later; obliteration of cystic lesion and healed fracture.
Fig. 7-5 (bottom).—Pathologic fracture in woman with Paget's disease occurred while she was walking. Fixation with Küntscher nail allowed early ambulation (right) although healing was delayed.

Pathologic dislocations also occur and should be mentioned. These usually are a result of acute sepsis. Treatment of the sepsis is so intimately involved with treatment of the dislocation as to be inseparable from it. Diagnosis as to the cause of the dislocation should not be a problem except in the rare case of chronic infection with an organism such as the treponema of syphilis.

TREATMENT

Treatment is focused in 2 directions: the treatment of the underlying condition and the treatment of the fracture.

TREATMENT OF THE UNDERLYING CONDITION.—The first important step is to make the diagnosis. This may be obvious, as in the patient with a prior, well-documented osteomyelitis. A fracture through a benign nonossifying fibroma in a child may make further diagnostic steps, e.g., biopsy, undesirable. However, if the diagnosis is not reasonably certain, and if biopsy is the method of choice to obtain the diagnosis, the procedure should be done either before the changes of fracture healing confuse the microscopic picture or after fracture healing is complete. The microscopic picture of a healing fracture can look deceptively malignant. At times, as in a pathologic fracture through a primary malignant bone tumor without metastases, the definitive surgical treatment of the tumor, i.e., amputation, eliminates all need for treatment of the fracture. In some cases, as in fractures through areas of prior heavy irradiation, no treatment is available for the underlying condition.

Therapy of the underlying condition should be started immediately and made to mesh with the treatment of the fracture. Often one will fit nicely with the other, such as curettage and bone grafting of a unicameral bone cyst after fracture (Fig. 7-6), since both conditions will require immobilization of the limb.

TREATMENT OF THE FRACTURE.—As noted in the foregoing discussion, the treatment of the fracture depends some-

Fig. 7-6.—Pathologic fracture occurred during light lifting in giant-cell tumor of proximal humerus. Simultaneous treatment of the cyst by curettage and bone grafting and of the fracture by immobilization allowed complete healing.

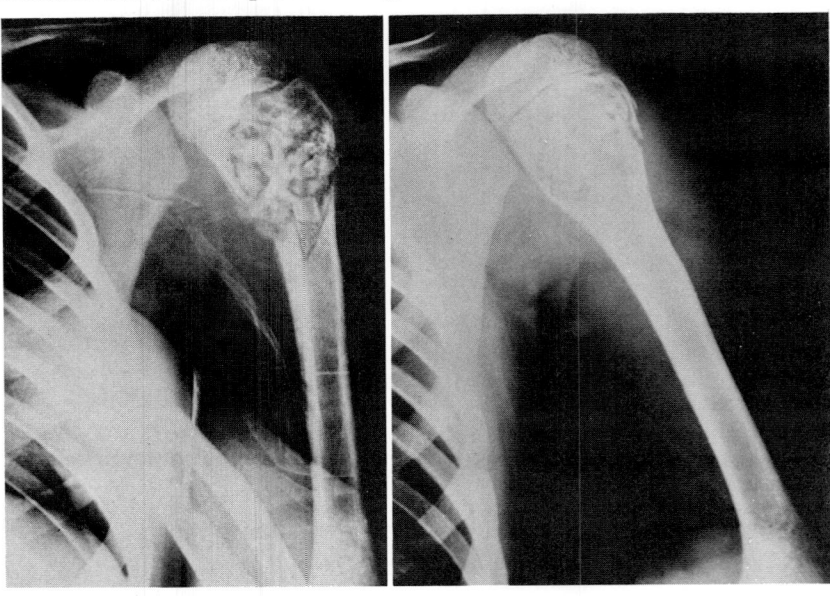

what on the treatment of the underlying pathologic condition. Treatment usually is conservative, with some exceptions. Fixation of a fracture usually treated by closed methods may be carried out at the time of biopsy. Fixation of a fracture through a deformed area of fibrous dysplasia to attain the corrective effects of an osteotomy may be attempted. Amputation may be selected as the best therapeutic approach in a fracture which is unlikely to heal through an area of chronically recurrent osteomyelitis when the limb distal to the break is borderline in function.

The treatment of pathologic fractures, then, involves the meshing of therapy of both underlying condition and fracture into the therapy most beneficial to the patient. Although the fracture treatment is often no different from the treatment of the same fracture under nonpathologic conditions, this bifid approach can yield unusual and stimulating therapeutic programs which require the best of the physician's clinical skill and judgment.

METASTATIC FRACTURES

The treatment of pathologic fractures through areas of bone containing metastases follows the principles just stated. However, in these patients, life expectancy is limited and the primary goals should be to return the patient to as high a level of general function as possible, as soon as possible, to eliminate pain and to reduce to a minimum the hospitalization needed for fracture treatment.

Of all the pathologic fractures treated in general orthopedic practice, except for those occurring because of osteoporosis, metastatic fractures are the most common and challenging. With better radiotherapeutic and chemotherapeutic techniques, patients with metastatic disease are living longer and the incidence of metastatic fracture is therefore increasing.

Diagnosis is seldom a problem. The patient, the family and the physician treating the patient up to the point of fracture are only too aware of the diagnosis. The fracture is viewed as a terminal event and greeted by all with despair. But all too often the fracture does not precede the patient's death by a few days or weeks, but by months or even years. The patient then should not be treated passively, since this may lead to increased hospital time, increased pain and malunion of the fracture in a position allowing little or no function (Fig. 7-7).

Tumors commonly metastasizing to bone originate in the breast, prostate, kidney, thyroid, lung and lymph structures. Metastases from renal and thyroid malignancies may be particularly bloody at operation, a factor to be carefully planned for if operation is elected.

Therapy should be initiated to convince patient, family and other involved physicians of the desirability of an aggressive program to attain the goals of greater comfort, improved function and prompt return of the patient to home. This may be relatively simple, as in a patient with a metastatic forearm fracture who can be made comfortable and the arm made functional with a simple cast. In children, healing times of fractures are so short that, even in fractures of long bones, operative fixation is seldom necessary. Many metastatic fractures, such as those in vertebral bodies, are not amenable to any surgical stability procedures, and therapy must depend solely on elimination of gravity, external support, and chemotherapeutic and radiotherapeutic measures.

The orthopedic goals of therapy of metastatic fractures are to provide firm fixation and stability to the area by the quickest possible method, in conjunction with x-ray and chemotherapy. Often, and particularly in weight-bearing long bones, this means open fixation (Fig. 7-8). Although general alignment of the fracture is important, minor degrees of displacement, malalignment and shortening should be accepted to gain stability. Because of the tendency for other metastatic areas to appear in the same bone, as well

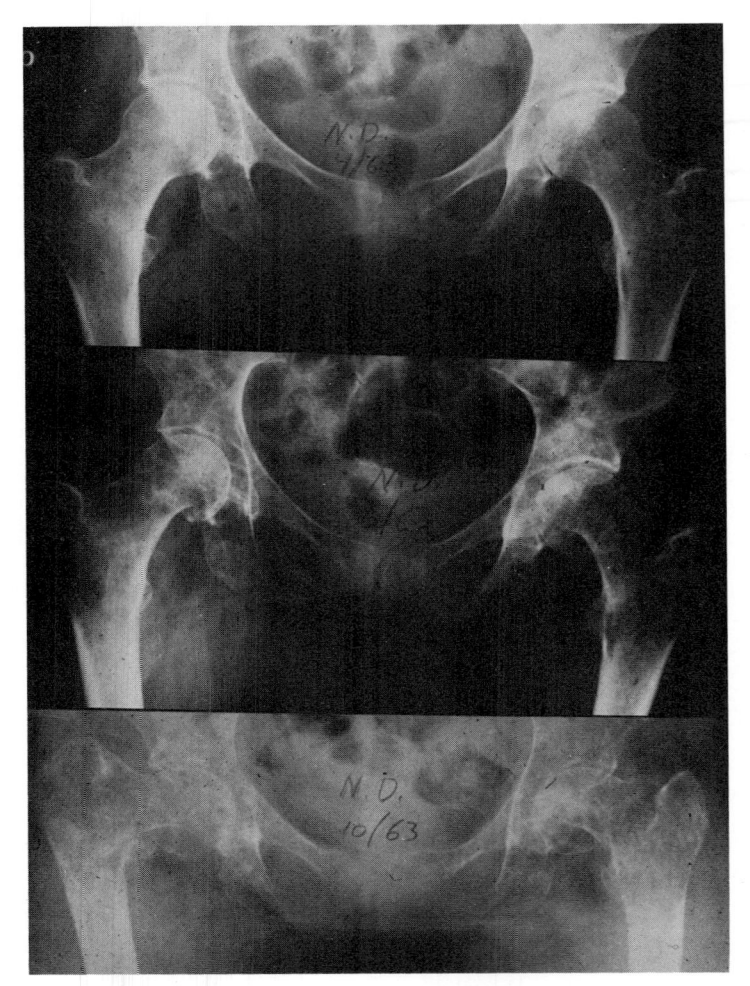

Fig. 7-7.—**Top,** metastatic breast carcinoma in both upper femora in 38-year-old woman bedridden from spinal metastases. Bilateral femoral neck fractures (**center**), though not treated, healed (**bottom**), but were followed by bilateral intertrochanteric fractures. The patient was in constant pain, had large decubiti and posed a difficult nursing problem until her death 6 months later. Fixation of the fractures at the time of initial symptoms of fracture would have eased pain and nursing difficulties.

as further dissolution of the bone by tumor in the area of fracture, intramedullary fixation is the method of choice; Küntscher and Rush rods are most often used. Postoperatively the patient is mobilized as quickly and to as great a level of function as possible, since the patient tends to deteriorate rapidly if kept in bed for a long period. The usual high priority for protection and immobilization to gain bone union is foregone in this instance. Fractures often tend to heal rapidly in any case, both because there is less cortical bone and greater blood supply in the area and because, at best, the patient does not place normal functional stresses on the area. Postoperative pain relief is often remarkable, and patient morale significantly improved.

The use of methylmethacrylate cement

Chapter 7: PATHOLOGIC FRACTURES / 173

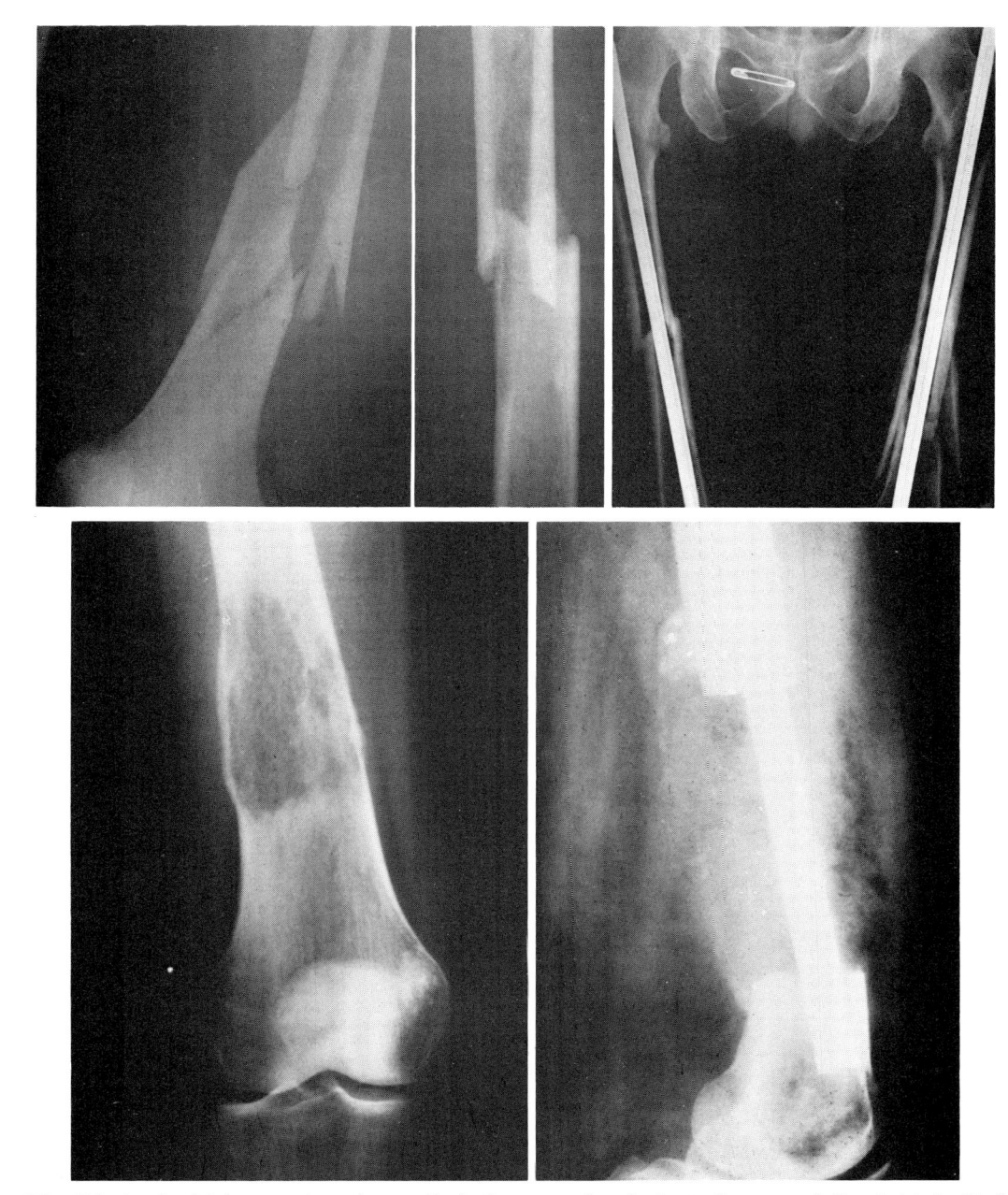

Fig. 7-8. (top) — Malignant lymphoma. **Left**, 2 views of pathologic fracture of distal third of left femur and midshaft of right femur through metastatic areas. **Right**, anteroposterior view after open reduction and retrograde insertion of Küntscher nails. Patient subsequently was comfortable until death, 6 months later.
Fig. 7-9. (bottom) — **Left**, symptomatic lesion of multiple myeloma (microfractures) treated by excision and rod (**right**) with methylmethacrylate reinforcement. Patient was comfortable for 2 years.

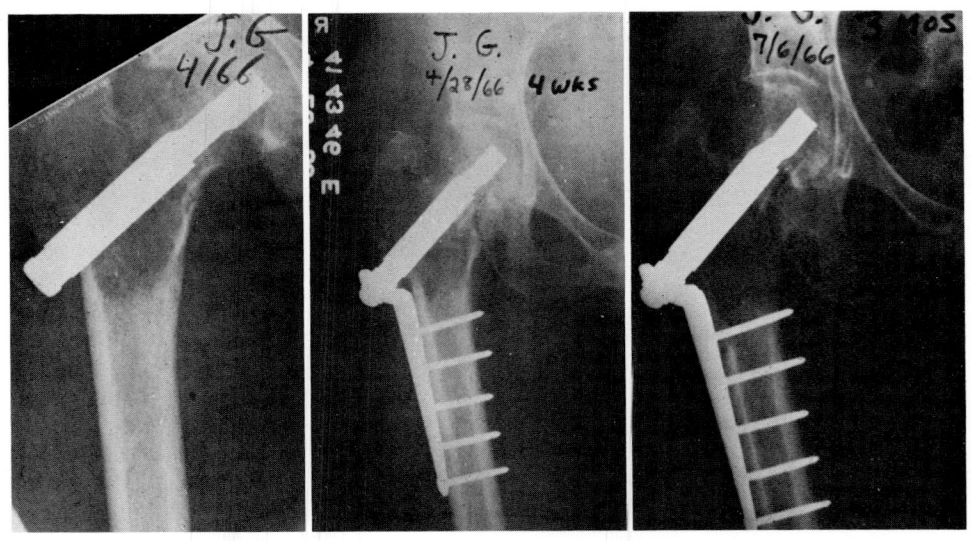

Fig. 7-10.—Metastatic carcinoma of breast. Femoral neck fracture occurred while patient was standing, without a fall. Fixation with sliding nail allowed settling of metastasis without displacement of the femoral head or protrusion of the nail into the acetabulum. Patient was ambulatory and comfortable for 5 months.

to provide stability, perhaps with excision of an entire area of metastasis, can be extremely useful (Fig. 7-9). The sliding-nail concept in metastatic femoral neck fractures is the method of choice for fixation, since its ability to collapse as the tumor further erodes the bone prevents protrusion of the nail into the acetabulum (Fig. 7-10).

PROPHYLACTIC FIXATION.—Prior to acute fracture, patients will often pass through a period of weeks when a previously known asymptomatic metastatic area will become painful. The reason proposed for this is that small cortical cracks appear in the weakened metastatic area. These microfractures cannot be seen on x-ray and continue until the bone suddenly gives way completely, often on such minimal stress as a normal step or a turn to the side. In this symptomatic period before complete fracture occurs, prophylactic fixation should be carried out if feasible (Fig. 7-11). At this time the patient's general condition is better than

Fig. 7-11.—Multiple lesions in femora before actual fracture of the bones. Küntscher nails were inserted, from above, through the trochanters without exposing the femoral shafts.

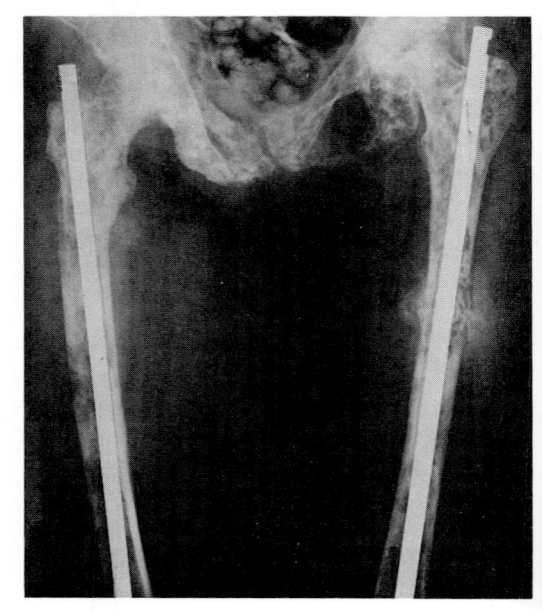

after complete fracture, and the fracture may be fixed without completely opening the fracture area (i.e., by closed nailing). In addition to these advantages, prophylactic nailing seems to retard further anatomic collapse of the area despite further tumor replacement of bone in the area.

BIBLIOGRAPHY

1. Barry, H. C.: Fractures of the femur in Paget's disease in bone in Australia, J. Bone Joint Surg. 49-A:1359, 1967.
2. Coron, A. G., Banks, H. H., Aliapoulios, M. A., et al.: The management of pathological fractures in patients; the metastatic carcinoma of the breast, Surg. Gynecol. Obstet. 127:1225, 1968.
3. Ebrenhaft, J. L., and Tedrich, R. T.: Intramedullary bone fixation in pathologic fractures, Surg. Gynecol. Obstet. 88:519, 1949.
4. Fitts, W. T., Jr.: Fractures in metastatic carcinoma, Am. J. Surg. 85:282, 1953.

8 | Early Examination and Treatment of the Injured Patient

GLENN E. BEHRINGER

THIS CHAPTER will be concerned with the care of the injured patient from the time he is admitted to the hospital until the time he is sent to the wards for further observation or to the operating room for definitive therapy. In the emergency ward, examination and treatment must proceed simultaneously (Table 8-1). The purposes of the patient's stay in the emergency ward are to control abnormalities that might be fatal immediately, to prepare the patient as adequately as possible for early surgery and to obtain, by means of a thorough physical examination, an accurate estimate of the injuries as a base line from which changes in his condition can be measured. Historical material, if available, is important in management, and the examiner should inquire about pre-existing cardiovascular, pulmonary, renal or endocrine disease.

It is obvious that these same principles apply anywhere an injured person is encountered, be it in the street, at home or on the battlefield. In these areas, however, only a necessary minimal amount of care should be given before removal to a hospital. The essential measures that might be lifesaving include the maintenance of an airway, the control of hemorrhage, closed cardiac massage and the emergency splinting of fractures.

When the patient arrives in the hospital he is undressed completely (the clothes cut off if necessary) and placed on a Bradford frame or litter, by which he can be transported easily. The frame is put on an operating table or truck in the emergency ward. The surgeon then begins the examination and treatment. This will not be a routine, leisurely head-to-toe, system-by-system observation; it must be rapid and arranged to give pre-

TABLE 8.1.—PROGRAM FOR INITIAL EXAMINATION AND TREATMENT

1. Establish an airway; consider laryngeal obstruction and tension pneumothorax; close sucking chest wounds.
2. Control active hemorrhage.
3. Treat shock. Give blood for oligemic shock. Suspect cardiac tamponade or tension pneumothorax with chest injuries. Be prepared for cardiac arrest; institute electrocardiographic monitoring early.
4. Splint fractures.
5. Examine the patient completely. Obtain history. Do a neurologic examination as indicated.
6. Carry out special laboratory examinations. Most important are blood, urine and x-ray examinations.
7. Administer necessary medication, including analgesics, antibiotics, tetanus toxoid or antitoxin and oxygen. Apply dressings to open wounds. Patients with serious injuries must have the stomach emptied and be put on constant urinary drainage.
8. Establish priority of individual wounds for therapy.

cedence to the establishment of proper respiratory function, the control of hemorrhage and the treatment of shock. Thereafter, fractures are splinted, the history and physical examinations are completed and medication and therapy are administered. These procedures will now be considered in detail.

THE AIRWAY

A sudden interference in respiration may be due to any one of several causes. The most important (Fig. 8-1) are: (1) pharyngeal obstruction caused by excessive secretions or by a relaxed tongue or jaw; (2) laryngeal obstruction from a foreign body or inflammatory exudate; (3) tracheal obstruction; (4) reduction in pulmonary volume due to a traumatic or spontaneous tension pneumothorax or to lungs filling with water. In addition to disordered respiration from mechanical causes, the observer must recognize such disturbances of rhythm as Cheyne-Stokes respiration, the Kussmaul breathing of diabetic acidosis and the characteristically slow, labored respirations typical of increased intracranial pressure.

When secretions are profuse, the use of a suction catheter is necessary. A no. 14 rubber catheter is passed through the nares and the pharynx is cleared out. Often the aspirator can be made to enter the trachea by advancing it through the larynx as the patient inspires. Even if this maneuver should fail, it may produce a vigorous cough which will open the lower respiratory tree. Insertion of an oropharyngeal airway will hold the tongue anteriorly, although the mandible must be held forward to keep the pharynx open.

Every emergency ward should be

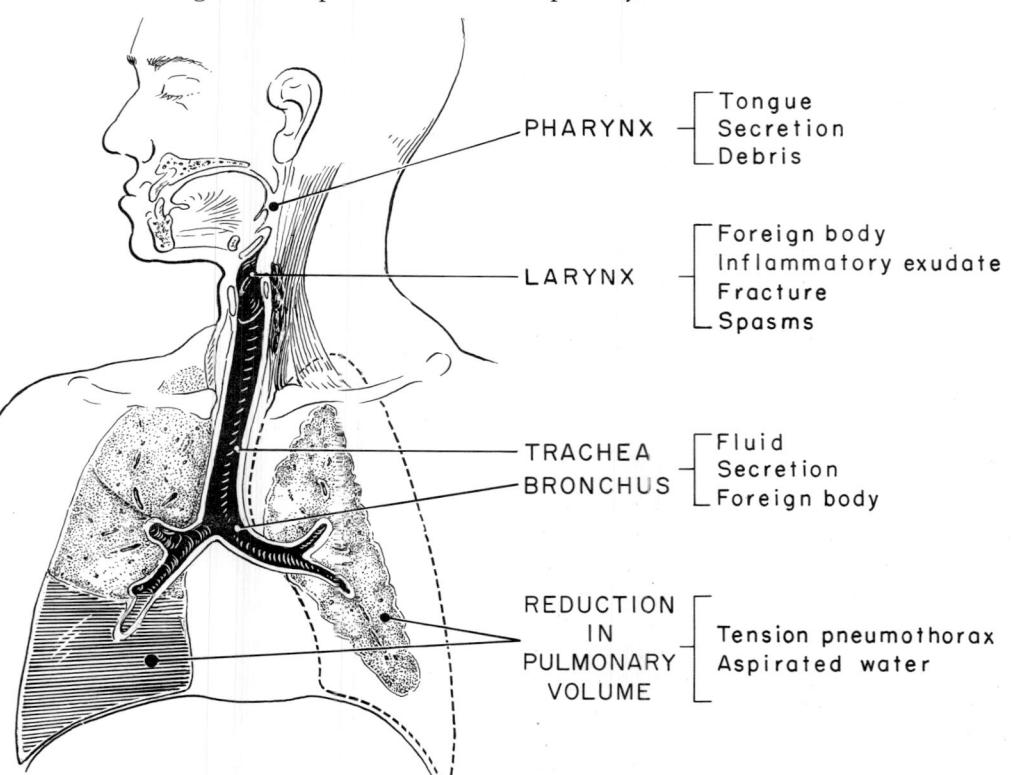

Fig. 8-1.—Important causes of respiratory embarrassment.

Chapter 8: EARLY EXAMINATION AND TREATMENT OF THE INJURED PATIENT / 179

equipped with proper aspirating equipment, instruments for direct laryngoscopy and an assortment of endotracheal tubes. Direct laryngoscopy is the only method by which the larynx can be inspected well, and it is the best method to clear the airway. The laryngoscopy is most important when the patient is comatose and the cough reflex is lost.

If there are no profuse secretions or if aspiration does not succeed in clearing the respiratory tract, a lower obstruction is present. The larynx is the most common site because of the narrow aperture between the vocal cords. The patient with such an obstruction is cyanotic; retraction is visible in the supraclavicular areas and often in the intercostal spaces on every attempt at inspiration. When the stethoscope is used, no breath sounds are heard in either lung. In a child this is usually due to a foreign body although diphtheritic membranes may be the cause. The foreign body may, at times, be dislodged by up-ending the child and delivering a forceful slap to the posterior thorax. If this fails and direct laryngoscopy cannot be carried out rapidly and skillfully, a tracheostomy is necessary.

Tracheostomy is done through the second tracheal ring (Fig. 8-2). The neck is slightly hyperextended. In emergency,

Fig. 8-2.—Emergency tracheostomy. **A**, position of patient with neck hyperextended. **B**, vertical skin incision is likely to produce less bleeding than horizontal. **C**, site of tracheal incision. **D**, insertion of special 3-pronged retractor and tracheostomy tube. **E**, final appearance.

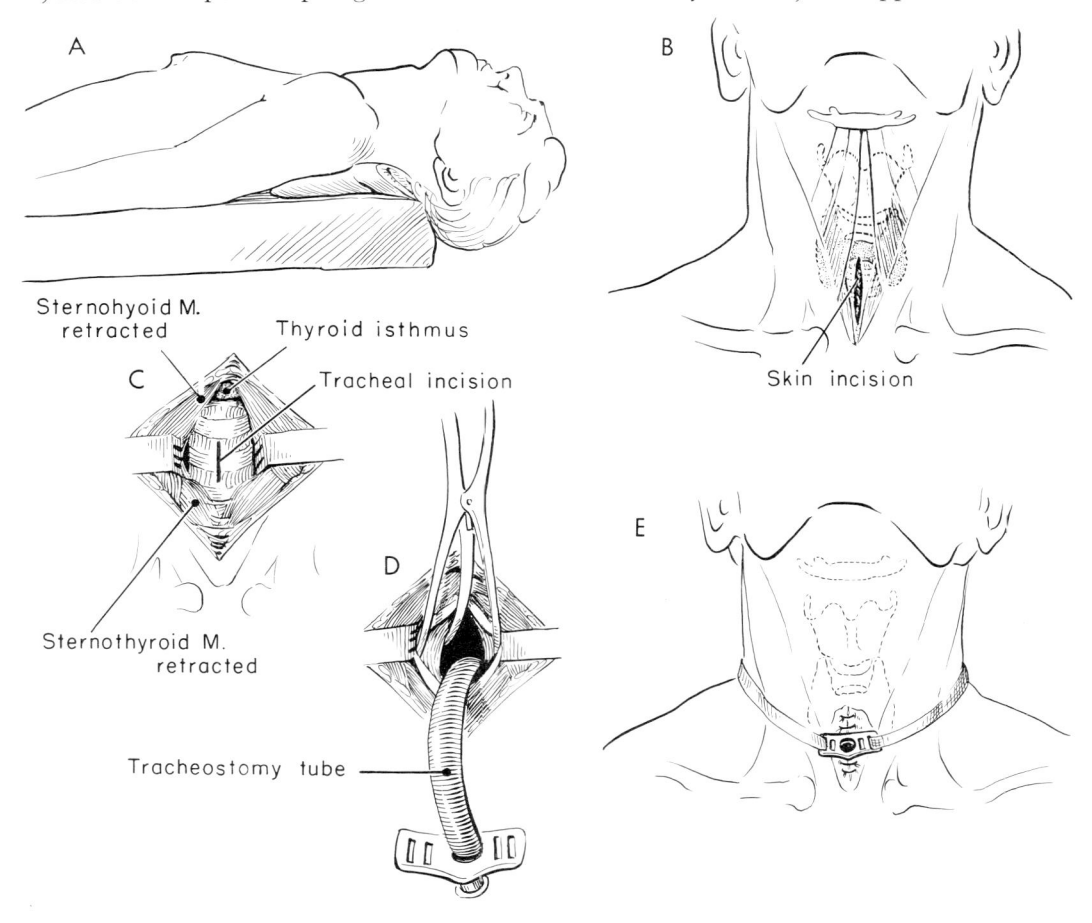

no anesthesia need be given, although in less pressing instances procaine is used. A vertical incision is made, since troublesome bleeding is less likely to occur than with an incision on the horizontal plane. The incision is carried down immediately to the second tracheal cartilage. This is opened adequately. A tracheostomy tube is then inserted. This procedure will be aided by use of a 3-pronged retractor to hold the trachea open as the tube is slipped in place.

Tracheal or bronchial obstruction is rarely encountered. If present, it is nearly always due to secretions, since foreign bodies small enough to pass between the vocal cords will descend to one of the smaller bronchi.

In a patient who has an obvious reason for poor pulmonary ventilation on admission to the emergency ward, a cuffed endotracheal tube should be immediately inserted and the patient placed on assisted ventilation with a mechanical respirator. These conditions include unconsciousness, hemorrhagic shock, chest injury or pre-existing chronic pulmonary disease. The establishment of proper ventilation and pulmonary gas exchange is monitored in such conditions by serial determinations of arterial blood gases and pH.

A tension pneumothorax is an important cause of dyspnea. It must be recognized and treated rapidly or death may occur. It must be suspected in the presence of any chest injury and particularly in injuries that have caused fractured ribs or subcutaneous emphysema. Spontaneous pneumothorax may occur from ruptured blebs or from unknown causes in young adults. Whenever tension is increased above the normal intrapleural pressure, the opposite lung is compressed. The trachea is deviated away from the side of the pneumothorax; breath sounds are absent, and the percussion note is tympanitic on the affected side. If this lesion is suspected, the chest must be tapped immediately before x-rays are taken.

The chest tap is performed with an ordinary no. 18 needle in the second interspace anteriorly. If air is present under tension it will escape rapidly. If a tension pneumothorax is thus found, the unphysiologic effects of this condition will be immediately relieved. However, this type of decompression is not adequate to reinflate the lung, especially if a large air leak is present. A no. 16 Foley catheter with a 5-ml bag should be introduced in the second interspace anteriorly, with the head of the bed elevated. This can be done, after proper skin preparation, through a small incision under local anesthesia, using a chest trocar or Kelly clamp. The tube is then placed on closed-chest suction drainage with a negative pressure of 10 cm of water.

Another major emergency that produces a dangerous pneumothorax is the open wound of the chest. When the laceration extends into the free pleural cavity, air is sucked into the chest with every inspiration. Unless the incision can be closed by suture immediately, an occlusive pressure dressing is applied and maintained until a definitive operation can be carried out. Chest tube suction and positive-pressure respiratory assistance through a cuffed endotracheal tube may be required to maintain proper ventilatory exchange.

CONTROL OF EXTERNAL HEMORRHAGE

Hemorrhage is most often venous in type, but it may be purely arterial or combined arterial and venous. If the vessels involved are relatively small or superficial, they may be grasped with hemostats and ligated. If this is not feasible and the hemorrhage is from an extremity, the extremity is elevated well above the level of the heart and a pressure dressing applied. If profuse bleeding continues, it is better to apply a tourniquet than to grope blindly with hemostats for the involved artery, since such action may damage a major vessel, making subsequent repair more difficult. When dealing with major arterial hemorrhage in areas where the use of a tourniquet is not possible, such as the neck or the supraclavicular, axillary or inguinal areas, the simplest, most delicate and effective maneuver is to obturate the hole in the vessel with the index finger, maintaining the "finger in the dike" until the vessel has been exposed surgically and controlled proximally and distally.

If a tourniquet is applied, no time must be wasted in preparing the patient for immediate operation. The patient should be in the operating room and anesthetized in preparation for removal of the tourniquet no later than 1 hour after it was applied.

CONTROL OF MAJOR INTERNAL HEMORRHAGE

Major internal hemorrhage must be recognized promptly. There are 3 important types: intra-abdominal, intrapleural and intrapericardial. Each produces a characteristic set of symptoms. Intra-abdominal hemorrhage will be considered in detail in Chapter 44. In brief, it may be noted here that such hemorrhage may occur with penetrating trauma or with blunt trauma when the abdominal wall has not been broken. It should be suspected particularly when the lower ribs have been fractured, producing lacerations of either liver or spleen. Falling blood pressure, rising pulse, increasing abdominal or shoulder pain and vomiting are danger signals.

Intrapleural hemorrhage is rarely severe enough to endanger life. Major bleeding follows laceration of intercostal arteries associated with multiple rib fractures. It is suspected in the presence of a dull percussion note and absent breath sounds over the affected area and is confirmed by x-ray examination of the chest and thoracentesis. This type of hemorrhage usually subsides spontaneously, and only rarely is an emergency thoracotomy necessary.

Intrapericardial hemorrhage, on the other hand, may be fatal if only a small amount of blood has been lost, since, if the pericardium is intact, cardiac tamponade will occur. It should be suspected whenever there has been penetrating or blunt trauma to the chest. The patient's pulse pressure diminishes. Venous pressure becomes high, and a paradoxical pulse is noted. A paradoxical pulse can be detected by inflating the blood pressure tourniquet to the upper level at which the cardiac sounds can just be heard; on every inspiration the sounds will disappear.

The diagnosis is established by pericardicentesis. A no. 18 needle is inserted through the left costoxiphoid angle and deviated upward and medially at an angle of 45 degrees to the abdomen and midline. If blood is found, it is aspirated until the motion of the heart can be felt against the needle. If the blood should reaccumulate rapidly, a thoracotomy may be necessary.

SHOCK

Shock requires immediate treatment. "Shock" is a clinical, descriptive term referring to a syndrome of hypotension, rapid pulse, sweating and prostration, with diminution in sensorium or loss of consciousness. This condition is most often caused by blood loss (oligemic shock), due to either internal or external bleeding. The same syndrome may be produced by intracranial hemorrhage secondary to cerebral trauma. It is also seen with severe crushing injuries. The possibility of a superimposed myocardial infarction must not be overlooked.

Whatever the cause of shock, emergency treatment should be instituted at once. The blood pressure and pulse rate are taken *and recorded,* to be followed with similar observations every 15–30 minutes as required. Venous blood is drawn for immediate typing and cross match. Intravenous routes for infusion are established. Usually a large-bore intravenous catheter is placed in an arm vein for rapid fluid administration. A smaller catheter is introduced into the superior vena cava, through either the subclavian or jugular vein, for monitoring the central venous pressure and also for fluid administration if necessary. When massive, rapid volume replacement is required, both forearms may be used, as well as the inferior vena cava cannulated through the femoral veins in the groin. The primary treatment of oligemic shock is the administration of blood. However, there is a necessary delay in this procedure due to the necessity for cross matching. During this time the patient's circulating fluid volume may be restored with rapid infusion of Ringer's lactate solution and colloid in the form of human plasma protein fraction, Albumisol or Plasmanate. Oxygen is administered by mask if the patient's respiratory ability is adequate or by mechanical respirator through a cuffed endotracheal tube if it is not. The practice in the Emergency Ward at the Massachusetts General Hospital is to replace blood loss with cross-matched blood. Only in the most dire emergencies is cross matching not carried out. In such situations type-specific blood is used. "Universal donor" or neutralized blood is no longer employed.

Volume replacement and proper oxygenation should result in prompt improvement of the patient. This is monitored by rise of the arterial blood pressure, the central venous pressure and the urine output. If adequate volume replacement has been carried out and there has been no response to therapy, the surgeon must re-examine the patient to decide which of the usual causes is present. The usual causes are:

1. Continuing hemorrhage. Internal hemorrhage from an intra-abdominal injury is the commonest cause of continued shock.

2. An associated cerebral injury or damage to the spinal cord.

3. A tension pneumothorax or hemopericardium.

4. Massive intraperitoneal contamination from extensive abdominal injuries. This produces a shocklike state that is not responsive to blood replacement and becomes progressively worse as time passes. The colon, intestine or stomach is the most common site of injury, but extensive extravasation of urine or pancreatic enzymes can cause the same picture.

The route of administration of fluids has been mentioned, but several technical points with regard to insertion of indwelling intravenous catheters should be noted. These catheters should be inserted under the best of aseptic conditions possible under the circumstances attendant on the injury, since sepsis extending from the skin into a major venous channel can lead to serious or fatal septicemia. The catheters should be firmly secured with a sterile, occlusive dressing, with an antibiotic ointment applied at the puncture site.

Puncture of the jugular or femoral veins does not present a difficult technical problem, but subclavian vein catheterization may be complicated by hemorrhage from a lacerated vessel wall or by pneumothorax from penetration of the pleura and lung. To avoid these complications, the patient should be placed in the Trendelenburg position with the shoulders hyperextended over a roll beneath the vertebral column and the head rotated to the side opposite that selected for the puncture. Use of aseptic technique with sterile gloves and instruments is important. After suitable shaving and preparation of the area, local anesthetic is infiltrated into the skin and subcutaneous tissues at the inferior borders of the midpoint of the clavicle. A commercially available 8-in. no. 16 needle-catheter combination is inserted through the wheal and advanced beneath the inferior border of the clavicle, with the needle point directed at a finger tip pressed firmly into the suprasternal notch. With the needle parallel to the frontal plane of the patient, the needle enters the anterior wall of the subclavian vein and blood returns through the needle. The needle is advanced a few millimeters after the blood is observed to insure the intraluminal position of the beveled tip. The catheter is then advanced to its full length and the needle withdrawn. This should position the tip of the catheter in the superior vena cava in an adult. The needle hub is then connected to a central venous pressure apparatus that is set with 0 at the level of the right auricle with a spirit level. The position of this catheter should be checked with a chest x-ray as soon as possible. It is incumbent on anyone who is involved in the emergency care of patients to practice this technique in the postmortem room until he gains confidence and facility in the technique.

In the initial phases of the treatment of shock, the central venous pressure will be low, perhaps 0, indicating low circulating fluid volume and poor venous return to the right side of the heart. However, with rapid infusion of adequate amounts of blood, colloid and crystalloid solutions, the pressure will rise to normal levels of 10–15 cm of water. A rise to the range of 20 cm or above indicates impending overload of the right side of the heart and necessitates slowing the infusion rate lest pulmonary edema develop.

CARDIAC ARREST

Cardiac arrest occurring during the initial treatment of trauma and shock must be detected and treated immediately to restore cardiac function and prevent irreversible central nervous system damage. The most common causes of arrest in the situations under discussion are poor coronary blood flow and myocardial oxygenation. It thus becomes apparent why proper respiratory exchange and blood pressure should be established as rapidly as possible in the emergency room and why electrocardiographic monitoring should be established early in the treatment of shock. Cardiac function may effectively cease either because of asystole or because of fibrillation. The detailed management of these problems will be discussed in Chapter 11.

The treatment of cardiac arrest, whether it is detected clinically or electrocardiographically, is the immediate institution of closed-chest cardiac massage. This method of assisting the circulation is quickly begun, simple and effective. A rigid support is placed beneath the patient's chest, since the ordinary hospital bed is too yielding to permit good cardiac compression. The operator then kneels at the patient's side. The heel of 1 hand, with the other on top of it, is placed over the lower sternum, and the chest is firmly and sharply compressed about 60 times a minute. This movement of the lower thoracic wall squeezes the heart between the sternum and the vertebral column, causing ejection of blood; the relaxation allows cardiac filling. Pulmonary ventilation is meanwhile carried out by the mechanical ventilator. The compression of the chest in closed-chest massage is not sufficient to induce respiratory exchange. Frequent assessment of the carotid pulse is important to make sure effective circulation is being produced, as proved by a palpable peripheral arterial pulse wave. Care should be exercised in carrying out this procedure since overzealous massage may produce rib fractures, damage to liver, spleen and pancreas and to the heart itself.

A heart in asystole may often be restarted by continuous massage, or circulation may often be maintained while instruments are obtained to open the chest. In ventricular fibrillation, shown by the electrocardiographic recording, defibrillation may be successfully carried out by the use of an external defibrillator (see Chapter 42).

SPLINTING OF FRACTURES

During the early examination and treatment period, all obvious fractures are splinted. The methods for splinting various fractures will be discussed individually in later chapters.

EXAMINATION OF THE PATIENT

When the emergency therapy has been completed, the surgeon can proceed with a more leisurely and complete examination. This will include the history, the physical examination and indicated laboratory studies.

The History

As full a history should be obtained as possible. The exact manner in which a patient fell may give the diagnosis of a fracture almost as accurately as does the x-ray examination. The position in which a person was hit with a bullet or stabbed with a knife will aid in establishing the tract of the missile or weapon and may indicate whether or not a surgical exploration may be necessary. Other accurate notations of the time, position and principal features of the accident must be obtained as medicolegal details. The patient's conduct since the accident is important. If he lost consciousness after a lucid interval, a subdural hematoma is suggested. If he complained of pain or vomited or voided blood since the injury, diagnostic leads may be presented.

The Physical Examination

The physical examination should follow an expeditious routine that will include the following essential points.

THE IMPORTANT VITAL SIGNS.—These include the level of consciousness, the blood pressure, the pulse and the respiratory rate. These data should be recorded and a chart started.

EXTERNAL SIGNS.—Indications of violence, cutaneous signs of drug use or the odor of ethanol on the breath should be noted and described, if present.

THE EXTREMITIES.—If the patient is conscious he should be asked to move each extremity in turn. Peripheral sensation should be carefully checked. Unless this is done, particularly when the hand is injured, nerve lacerations will be neglected completely. Tests of motion and sensation must cover the entire extremity, including the fingers and toes, with individual tests of each digital nerve when indicated. Any abnormality of reflexes should be noted.

The peripheral arteries should be palpated. The radial and ulnar arterial pulsations at the wrist are particularly important in fracture of the elbow in children.

In the foot, the posterior tibial and dorsalis pedis arteries must be palpated when there is a fracture of the femur or about the knee. A cold, white extremity means injury of the major arteries, arterial compression from hematoma or, rarely, severe vasospasm.

Fractures should be diagnosed or at least suspected at this time. Dislocation should be obvious on inspection. Deformity, local tenderness and impairment of function are the classic signs of fracture. If a fracture is suspected, the entire length of the bone should be examined carefully, and x-ray examination should include the entire bone.

At this time, if any fractures are open, sterile dressings are placed on the wounds. All fractured extremities are then splinted, preferably with splints of radiolucent materials, so that no further damage will occur before definite treatment is carried out.

THE HEAD AND NECK.—Inspection of the face will suggest most of the common fractures. Fractures of the nasal bones are accompanied by epistaxis, swelling and often by lateral displacement. Crepitus may be elicited. Depressed fractures of the zygoma are demonstrated by comparison of the characteristic depression of the malar eminence with the opposite side. Fractures of the mandible show varying degrees of deformity, usually with malocclusion of the teeth.

Drainage from the nose or ears must be noted. Rhinorrhea is diagnostic of a fracture of the skull into 1 of the frontal or sphenoidal sinuses. Bleeding from the external auditory meatus after trauma to the head indicates a fracture of the temporal bone into the auditory canal.

It is necessary to obtain a rapid estimate of the damage sustained by the brain. The examiner has already noted the vital signs (level of consciousness, blood pressure, pulse and character of respirations). A semi- or unconscious state, an elevated blood pressure, a slow and full pulse or slow and deep respirations indicate major cerebral injuries. Inequality or dilatation and fixation of the pupils are serious signs.

The cranial nerves must then be tested in order. These tests are summarized in Chapter 14.

It cannot be emphasized too strongly that this general neurologic evaluation must be a part of the initial survey and not deferred for the neurosurgeon. It is only in this way that changes in neurologic status that may indicate immediate surgical intervention can be appreciated.

A history of "striking bottom" when diving must make the examiner suspect fracture of the cervical spine. Extreme care must be displayed in the handling of such patients in order to avoid spinal cord injury. A firm collar or head traction should be applied as soon as possible before further motion is carried out. Other serious neck injuries are uncommon, except for lacerations sustained in suicide attempts; in these, major blood vessels may be injured, and control of hemorrhage then becomes important.

THE CHEST. — Major injuries that require the most urgent treatment have already been noted: the open sucking chest wound, the tension pneumothorax and cardiac tamponade. Other abnormalities of the chest which must be watched for on the original examination will just be noted here, since they will be discussed fully in Chapter 41.

Inspection of the patient may show restricted motion of 1 side of the chest. Subcutaneous emphysema, indicative of pulmonary damage, may be visible or may be demonstrated by light palpation. Percussion and auscultation must always be carried out to determine the presence or absence of pneumothorax or hemothorax. Gentle palpation and localized pain on respiration may indicate rib fractures. In doubtful cases, the patient's chest should be compressed between the hands of the surgeon. The clavicle and sternum also must be palpated carefully. In addition to fracture of these bones, luxation of the sternoclavicular joint or costochondral junction may be found. In all these fractures, careful physical examination is particularly important because the early x-ray picture may be equivocal or negative.

THE ABDOMEN. — Careful observation of the abdomen is especially important in the early appraisal of the patient because, in the great majority of cases, the diagnosis of visceral injury is not possible immediately after the trauma and becomes apparent only after a few hours. Here a base line must be established immediately by questioning the patient about abdominal pain, vomiting, voiding and defecating after the injury. The presence of blood in any of these discharges is especially important. The abdomen should be inspected carefully to note any distention. The character of the peristalsis should be noted. Percussion may suggest fluid, presumably blood, in either lateral gutter. Palpation will show any local areas of tenderness. The rectal examination must not be neglected. The examiner should be concerned particularly with the presence of blood on the glove.

THE PELVIS AND BACK. — It must not be forgotten that the patient has a back side as well as a front. It is a mistake to spend several hours repairing an obvious, extensive abdominal wound and then to turn the patient over, for the first time, to discover irreparable damage to the buttocks, rectum and urethra.

Injuries of the spinal cord often cause abdominal pain or are associated with visceral injury. It is particularly important, in patients with these injuries, to test for any disturbance of mobility or sensation or reflex changes in the legs.

Fractures of the pelvis are usually diagnosed by bimanual compression of the pelvic girdle either laterally or in an anteroposterior direction. If a pelvic fracture is present, the surgeon should anticipate the onset of hypovolemic shock since these injuries are associated with slow but massive blood loss into the pelvic retroperitoneum either from the fracture sites themselves or from laceration of major pelvic blood vessels.

In these fractures the possibility of urethral trauma should be suspected. Evidence of urinary extravasation in the perineum or inability to pass a urethral catheter associated with the appearance of blood on the catheter is confirmatory evidence.

Laboratory Examinations

In nearly every case, special examinations must be carried out before definite treatment can be accomplished. These procedures will be discussed briefly.

BLOOD. — The hematocrit is an essential part of the blood examination. Immediately after a severe hemorrhage the hematocrit stays at essentially normal levels and remains so until hemodilution takes place. Unless blood volume studies are carried out, the magnitude of blood loss cannot be quantitated. Hence the early hematocrit reading serves chiefly to establish a base line. Electrolyte determinations on venous blood should also be done to serve as baseline values to aid in future management, since considerable volumes of crystalloid solution may be administered in the immediate resuscitative management of shock.

If any degree of respiratory embarrassment is present on admission, or is anticipated, arterial blood should be drawn for gas determinations and pH.

URINE. — Urine must be obtained — by catheter if necessary. In severely injured patients it is easier to insert a Foley catheter at once so that renal output can be measured accurately and recorded. Inability to pass a catheter, particularly in the presence of a pelvic injury, is strong evidence of urethral laceration. The urine sediment must be examined for gross and microscopic blood and tested for sugar, since a suspected cerebral injury may actually be diabetic coma. The instillation of 60 ml of sterile saline into the bladder is often carried out at the time of catheterization. If the examiner does not obtain a quantitative return of the injected fluid, a laceration of the bladder is probable.

DIAGNOSTIC PARACENTESIS. — The examiner may secure a confirmation of a diagnosis by tapping the appropriate body cavity. Thoracentesis to establish the presence of air or blood in the pleural cavity is a most important diagnostic and therapeutic procedure. Pericardicentesis is occasionally necessary as an emergency procedure. Abdominal tap, in 4 quadrants, may establish the presence of intraperitoneal bleeding. It should be emphasized that this procedure is of value only if results are positive, i.e., if blood is aspirated. A negative tap, however, does not rule out intraperitoneal hemorrhage.

LUMBAR PUNCTURE. — Lumbar puncture may be necessary as an immediate diagnostic or therapeutic measure. It is contraindicated when increased intracranial pressure is suspected.

SIGMOIDOSCOPY. — This procedure is valuable when wounds of the rectum are suspected and it will establish a definite diagnosis.

GASTRIC ASPIRATION. — Blood will occasionally be found in the stomach on passage of a Levin tube, indicating injury to that organ.

X-RAY EXAMINATION.—X-ray films will be necessary in nearly every injury. The examiner should order the proper examinations at the outset, so that repeated trips of the patient to the radiology department will not be necessary. There are numerous principles to remember, among which the following are the most important:

1. X-rays for fractures of the long bones should include the entire involved bone. Anteroposterior and lateral views are essential. Oblique views are often indicated. In children, where the epiphyseal lines are confusing, the opposite normal bone should be examined for comparison.

2. The demonstration of skull fractures requires a fairly cooperative patient because of special positions and long exposure. It is possible to delineate major defects on a limited examination consisting of anteroposterior and lateral views.

3. Fractures, particularly of the ribs, may be present but not appear on the x-ray film initially. Therefore, if a fracture is suspected clinically, a repeat study should be carried out in 7–10 days when the fracture line may be visible due to resorption of bone at the site of injury.

4. With chest injuries, provision should be made for fluoroscopy at the time of the original examination.

5. When an abdominal injury is suspected, plates should be made with the patient both lying and sitting, since only in the latter position can free air under the diaphragm be seen. When looking for free air in the peritoneal cavity, an upright or lateral position should be maintained for 5–10 minutes before a film is taken.

6. When penetrating wounds from metallic fragments or other foreign bodies are encountered, all clothing should be removed and the litter should be clean before any x-rays are taken. A laparotomy for a shell fragment that is lying loose on the litter has been done more than once. Furthermore, when penetrating wounds are encountered, it is essential to examine the whole anatomic area involved. The bullet may be located in subcutaneous tissue just off the film.

IMMEDIATE THERAPY

The therapeutics of control of hemorrhage and oligemic shock and of obstruction of the airway have been considered, but other therapy must be carried out simultaneously with the physical examination or immediately afterward. This will include:

1. Splinting of fractures as they are encountered.

2. Administration of analgesics. Morphine, or 1 of its derivatives, is usually given to allay apprehension and to relieve pain. However, there are several contraindications to its routine use. If there is a cerebral injury, morphine must not be given since it may produce profound depression, coma and death. If necessary to control restlessness, pentobarbital sodium or Valium is safer. When abdominal injuries are suspected, morphine would dull the patient's appreciation of increasing pain and cloud the diagnosis. Morphine should be given only to allay severe pain and should be given intravenously rather than subcutaneously to patients who demonstrate shock. If given subcutaneously, it will be absorbed poorly. After repeated doses a cumulative effect will be noted as circulation improves and this will lead to severe respiratory depression. Intravenous Talwin will provide analgesia with less respiratory depression.

The intravenous use of mannitol or Lasix in shock patients may be helpful in maintaining renal blood flow and promoting glomerular filtration, thus preventing the later development of acute renal failure.

3. Administration of antibiotics. Anti-

biotics should be given immediately to all patients with open wounds and to those with suspected abdominal or chest injuries. In general, penicillin and Keflin are used for soft-tissue injuries while penicillin and kanamycin are given to patients with possible abdominal or chest injuries. Later, a shift to a more appropriate drug may be made on the basis of information obtained from culture and sensitivity tests. Dosage schedules will be discussed in Chapter 38.

4. Administration of tetanus antitoxin or toxoid. Fortunately a high proportion of the population has been immunized against tetanus and will have had their immunity maintained by periodic booster doses. If such is the case, another injection is given. If immunization has never been carried out, tetanus antitoxin must be given. Human tetanus immune globulin is used to avoid the anaphylactic reactions formerly seen with material prepared from horse serum. The prophylactic dose is 250 units. Larger doses of 400–500 units are recommended for patients with tetanus-prone wounds or when more than 24 hours has elapsed between the time of injury and treatment.

5. Administration of oxygen. Oxygen must be given to patients in shock and to those with poor pulmonary ventilation due to chest or cerebral injuries. Depending on the patient's ventilatory ability, oxygen may be administered by nasal catheter, by face mask or by a mechanical respirator via a cuffed endotracheal tube. The efficiency of the patient's respiration is monitored by frequent determinations of arterial blood gas values and pH.

6. Application of temporary dressings to all wounds. No attempt should be made to change dressings until the time has come for definite surgery.

7. Use of urinary catheter. An inlying catheter is essential to the treatment of any serious injury. Only in this way can total urinary output be checked accurately and oliguria or anuria be recognized and treated at an early stage.

8. Preoperative orders. Frequently the patient goes directly from the accident room to the surgical theater. Before general anesthesia is given the patient's stomach must be emptied. This can usually be accomplished by a Levin tube. If the patient has eaten immediately before the accident, vomiting must be induced or the stomach lavaged with a large gastric tube. If the latter situation cannot be accomplished because of an uncooperative patient, the anesthesiologist must be made aware of the problem so that anesthesia induction can be carried out in a manner to prevent vomiting and aspiration. Aspiration of gastric contents can be immediately fatal and aspiration pneumonia has a very serious prognosis.

The aspiration of gastric contents is usually inexcusable because it is nearly always due to a lack of awareness on the part of the surgeon or anesthetist. Every surgeon of experience has heard of such a catastrophe. It is particularly likely to happen in children, since they retain digested food in the stomach for many hours. Therefore, the only safe procedure is to be sure that the stomach has been emptied mechanically.

Preoperative medication is also necessary. Atropine is essential, particularly if Pentothal Sodium is to be used. Sedatives or analgesics should be used sparingly and only in amounts necessary to make the patient comfortable and controllable.

PRIORITY OF GENERAL SURGERY

Finally, an order of priority for surgical procedures must be established. The following considerations will apply to the individual patient with multiple wounds or to a group of casualties with different types of injuries. In general, the routine to be followed must consider: (1) major arterial hemorrhage and (2) severe interference with the airway (these conditions have the highest priority; sucking chest wounds are closed at once); (3) abdominal injuries; (4) major arterial injuries, in which restoration of the circulation is feasible by suture or graft; (5) open fractures; (6) chest injuries; (7) head injuries. When the chest and abdomen are injured simultaneously, as by a missile that penetrates the diaphragm, it is best to explore the chest first, so that the diaphragm can be sutured and the pulmonary function stabilized.

When the initial diagnosis and therapy are completed, the patient is sent either to the operating room for definitive surgery or to the ward for further observation. In either case, a complete record of the initial history, examination, laboratory studies and procedures carried out must accompany him.

9 | Use and Abuse of X-Ray in Trauma

WILLIAM J. OTTO

HISTORICAL BACKGROUND

ON NOVEMBER 8, 1895, Wilhelm Konrad Röntgen, working alone in his Würzburg laboratory, was experimenting with a Crookes-Hittorf tube. When he activated the tube, he noticed that some platinocyanate crystals on a nearby table were glowing, even though the tube was completely covered with paper. He immediately grasped the significance of this observation: "a new kind of ray" was being produced, which could penetrate matter. A few intensive weeks of investigation defined the properties of the new "x-rays," including the vital fact that they darkened a photographic plate.

Röntgen's first paper, published in December 1895, was a marvel of brevity and lucidity. Scientists and laymen alike were excited by the paper and its illustrations, including an x-ray photograph of Frau Röntgen's hand, the bones clearly visible. The medical application was obvious. No other scientific discovery has ever been promulgated, refined and exploited so quickly. Over 1,000 papers on the medical uses of the roentgen ray were published in 1896 and multiple diagnostic possibilities were quickly established. But the impact of Frau Röntgen's metacarpals has never been superseded. The diagnosis of trauma, particularly fracture detection, and the x-ray are forever linked in the public mind. This has led to the exciting field of traumatic radiology; it has also led to some problems for physicians and patients alike.

LEGAL PROBLEMS

The sensitized physician often equates the term "medical-legal" with "malpractice." Fortunately, the physician will encounter legal authority most often as an expert witness in accident cases, workmen's compensation claims and so forth. The majority of medicolegal cases involve accidental trauma; the specialist most often involved is the orthopedic surgeon; the medical exhibit most often introduced is the radiograph. The courts view the radiograph as objective and unbiased evidence. Knowing this, the physician treating a patient with a potential medicolegal case is under pressure to document his clinical findings with radiographs.

Even greater pressure is exerted by the looming threat of malpractice. One of the oldest and most vexing malpractice problems involves the need for x-ray examination in cases of suspected fracture. The prevailing opinion remains that radiographs are not required, but the physician who relies on his clinical judgment alone and errs has placed himself at risk. The physician therefore feels compelled to verify his clinical impressions with x-ray examination, even when the results will not change the therapeutic approach. The same reasoning applies to follow-up studies after fracture reduction and to diagnostic evaluation of head trauma.

Recent studies have shown that routine skull films in children with head trauma are of little help in the diagnosis and management of the patient. Further work of this type stressing clinical evaluation may give the practitioner some relief. For the present, however, most physicians will continue to obtain radiographs for the record, both to protect themselves and to satisfy patients who insist on the procedure.

The result is overutilization of x-ray facilities, increased medical costs and unnecessary radiation exposure. This may ultimately lead to a national policy on standards of care and malpractice. Until then, every practitioner must deal with this problem in the light of his own practice situation and the needs of individual patients.

RADIATION HAZARDS

The radiation dose to an adult patient from properly performed diagnostic studies should never approach a level where somatic injury need be feared. In the energy range of diagnostic x-rays, an acute dose of perhaps 200 rad could be delivered to a body part without any detectable sequelae. Radiographs of the spine, abdomen or hips may result in a skin dose of 1-2 rad per film. The safety margin is therefore quite large. A properly adjusted modern fluoroscope should deliver 1-3 rad/minute at the tabletop. However, an older or improperly operated fluoroscope may deliver 10 rad/minute or more, emphasizing the relative risk of fluoroscopy.

The somatic risk to the fetus is much higher than to the adult, particularly in the first trimester. Doses in the range of 25-50 rad, perhaps less, may be damaging in the first weeks after conception. The need for radiographs of a pregnant patient must be weighed against this risk, particularly when the abdomen cannot be shielded. Usually in cases of trauma the need is clear-cut; but a careful history may detect early pregnancy and modification of the procedure may be possible to reduce fetal dose.

The epiphyses of a growing child are also susceptible to radiation damage, but the dose required is higher than that received in proper diagnostic studies. Of more concern are the effects of chronic exposure to small doses of radiation. This is primarily a hazard to the physician rather than to the patient. Many pioneer radiologists died of leukemia, other blood dyscrasias and skin tumors probably induced by their long exposure to relatively large doses of radiation. Smaller, chronic doses may result in premature aging and a shortening of the life span. This is extremely controversial but the wise physician will insure that his personal radiation exposure is as low as possible. Film badge or other monitoring systems will record the doses recieved and may disclose breaks in technique leading to higher than needed exposure.

The genetic effects of ionizing radiation are more insidious and potentially more dangerous. At risk is the entire gene pool of the population rather than of any one individual. There is probably no threshold dose for genetic damage and radiation effects appear to be cumulative throughout reproductive life. The health needs of an individual will often require radiologic study involving gonadal radiation exposure. The physician can do no more than minimize this exposure, but should do not less. Because of atomic testing, controversial nuclear power plants and other widely publicized issues, the public is informed and concerned about this problem. In counseling anxious patients, the physician can emphasize that the basic danger of genetic radiation lies in its ability to increase the frequency of mutations in the gene pool of the population as a whole. At the dose

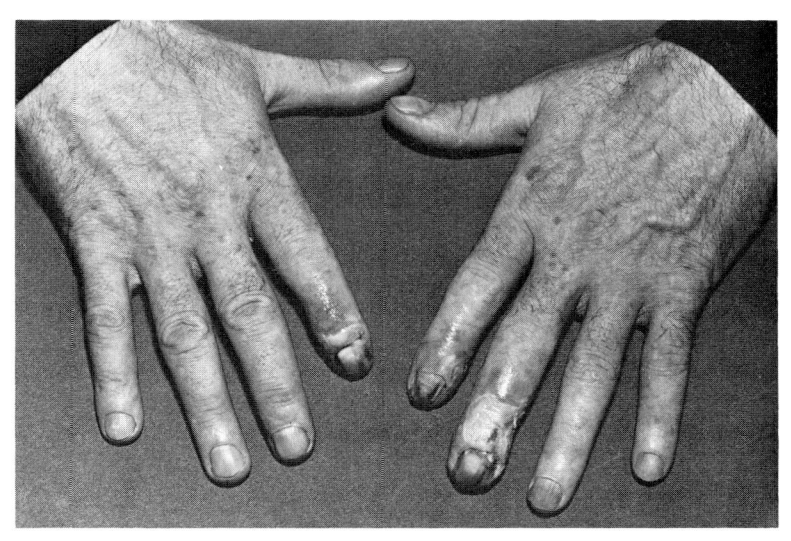

Fig. 9-1.—Radiation necrosis and dermatitis. Hands of a hospital technician who served as an orderly for 10 years, helping to reduce fractures under fluoroscopic observation. Multiple operations, with removal of several fingers, were ultimately required. (Courtesy of Dr. E. M. Daland.)

levels of diagnostic x-ray, the risk to an individual's immediate offspring is statistically nil.

Reduction of a patient's radiation exposure dose can be accomplished by rigorous attention to basic procedures. X-ray tubes should have adequate filtration, at least 2 mm of aluminum and preferably more. Accurate columniation should define the beam to the area of interest; at no time should the beam dimensions be larger than the film. The fastest possible screen–film combination consistent with acceptable detail should be used. When possible, the gonads should be shielded. Darkroom facilities must be adequate to yield radiographs of excellent quality. Well-trained technicians and modern exposure-control devices will minimize the need for repeat films.

Reduction of radiation exposure of medical personnel is also possible. Technicians and nurses should leave the room before an exposure is made; they should not hold or position the patient. Fluoroscopy entails the greatest risk. Protective garments should always be worn. The hands, even with lead gloves, must never enter the direct beam (Fig. 9-1).

In perspective, the risks of diagnostic radiology are very low in comparison to the benefits. Good practice and common sense will minimize the hazards. Whether the clinician refers his patients to a radiologist or obtains his own radiographs he should constantly be vigilant and demand high standards of radiation safety. He should take care that his own example does not lead his assistants into unsafe practices.

PROPER USE OF FLUOROSCOPY

The widespread introduction of image intensifiers with a bright television display, visible in a lighted room, has increased the ease of fluoroscopic fracture reduction but has done little to reduce the hazards to patient and personnel. Fluoroscopic reduction of routine fracture is unacceptable practice. In rare, selected instances a fracture reduction may be improved by the use of fluoroscopy, with benefit to the patient. Fluoroscopy is useful in foreign body localization and can shorten the time needed for operative internal fixation. In all cases, the physician must use the best available equipment, minimize the fluoroscopic time and avoid exposure of himself and his assistants. He should realize that the radiologist's lead gloves and apron are designed for scattered radiation and do not offer sufficient protection in the direct beam. Alternative methods, such as Polaroid film or a 90-second processor close at hand, can reduce the need for fluoroscopy. The instrument is designed to study dynamic function; it is a misuse to fluoroscope a static situation. Film is far superior, provides a permanent record, and the radiation dose is much less.

GENERAL PRINCIPLES IN TRAUMATIC RADIOLOGY

The basic goal is to obtain radiographs of the highest quality and diagnostic import with the least possible discomfort or danger to the injured patient. No patient demands more of equipment and technical skill than the victim of severe trauma. Some patients may require studies for which personnel and equipment are not available. Although decisions regarding transfer to a larger center are usually made on clinical grounds, proper weight must be given to the immediate and future needs for x-ray examination. Poor quality radiographs may be worse than no study at all, particularly in areas of complex anatomy such as the cervical spine. Too often a report of "no fracture seen on poor films" becomes "the x-rays are negative." When possible, x-ray examination can be delayed until the patient's condition stabilizes. Poor quality films should be regarded as a screening study and repeated when conditions permit.

The clinician interested in the field of trauma should keep abreast of new equipment that will facilitate radiography in his patients. High output generators permit shorter exposure times. Radiotransparent litters fit over the x-ray tables; the patient need not be shifted back and forth. Some x-ray tables have removable light-weight tops that themselves become litters. Upright and angling Bucky cassette holders, free-floating tabletops that move in all directions, ceiling mounted tubes and other ingenious devices can increase the speed and ease of the examination.

Sophisticated radiologic procedures may greatly enhance diagnostic capability. Many of these have extended the traditional bounds of radiology. For example, ultrasonic echo studies can detect traumatic pericardial effusion, thermography can identify poor vascular perfusion, and radionucleides can localize subdural hematomas.

Angioradiology is a growing subspecialty that has considerable interest in the diagnosis of trauma (Fig. 9-2). The ability to visualize injured vessels directly and to diagnose laceration and hematoma in organs such as liver, kidney and spleen can be of enormous help to the surgeon. The need for regional coopera-

Fig. 9-2.—Angiographic diagnosis of splenic trauma. Subcapsular hematoma displaces the visualized splenic tissue. Angiography has greatly increased the radiologist's ability to diagnose injury to internal organs. (Courtesy of Dr. D. J. Fleischli.)

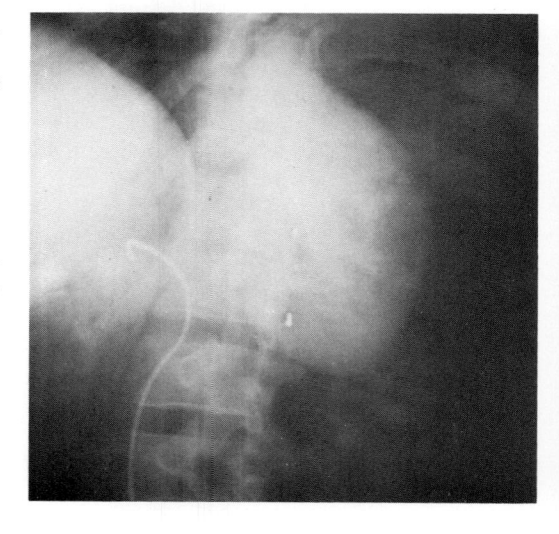

tion is evident, so that as many patients as possible can have access to the skills and equipment needed for these special procedures.

Fortunately, most patients require only the standard x-ray examinations familiar to all. The most important requirements for good practice are cooperation and continued communication among the clinician, technicians and radiologists. Without these, the most elaborate technical facilities and sophisticated procedures will fall short of their potential contribution.

BIBLIOGRAPHY

1. Camps, F. E.: *Gradwohl's Legal Medicine* (Baltimore: The Williams & Wilkins Company, 1968).
2. Curran, W. J.: *Tracy's the Doctor as a Witness* (2d ed.; Philadelphia: W. B. Saunders Company, 1965).
3. Medical Research Council: *The Hazards to Man in Nuclear and Allied Radiation* (London: Her Majesty's Stationery Office, 1956).
4. Moritz, A. R., and Helberg, D. S.: *Trauma and Disease – Selections from the Recent Literature* (Brooklyn: Central Book Co., 1959).
5. Stetler, C. J., and Moritz, A. R.: *Doctor and Patient and the Law* (St. Louis: C. V. Mosby Company, 1962).

10 | Angiography of Trauma

CHRISTOS A. ATHANASOULIS,
ARTHUR C. WALTMAN and STANLEY BAUM

TRAUMA IN OUR highly mechanized, highly automated society has become a great environmental health problem. Accidental injury is the leading cause of death among persons 1–37 years of age and is the fourth leading cause of death in all ages.[4]

Early recognition of the site and the extent of injury is of paramount importance for successful management. Delay in diagnosis may occur in patients with multiple injuries, since occult, life-threatening, great vessel or visceral injuries may be obscured by multiple musculoskeletal trauma. Hence, the value of angiography in the evaluation of the injured patient becomes apparent. Not only may angiography confirm the site or extent of an injury that is clinically suspected, but it may also disclose serious but clinically unrecognized injuries. In light of the angiographic findings then, the clinical problems can be reassessed and priorities set before surgical treatment is undertaken.

It is not suggested that all injured patients be transferred directly to the angiography suite on arrival at the emergency ward. Each patient presents a different problem. On the other hand, the argument that angiography is time-consuming for an often critically injured patient is not correct either. It is important to realize that angiography can be safely and expediently performed while general supportive measures are taken and, often, while the operating theater is being prepared to receive the patient.

This use of angiography presents a challenge to the radiologist who performs the vascular procedures: to keep abreast of recent developments in angiography, to be available and able to mobilize rapidly his team around the clock, and to be able to function in harmony with the "trauma team" in order to provide the best care for the injured patient.

METHOD

All angiographic procedures are performed according to the Seldinger[38] and Odman[39] techniques for percutaneous catheterization of the aortic branches. In the majority of patients the approach is through either femoral artery. If the femoral pulses are absent, or if they cannot be palpated due to the presence of edema or large hematomas in the groin, an axillary artery, usually the left, is catheterized.

The catheter is placed in the appropriate position, using image-intensified fluoroscopy and television monitoring. Iodinated contrast medium is injected through the catheter with a pressure injector, and serial radiographs are exposed. Capability for simultaneous biplane radiography is desirable when studying injured patients, since precise information is sought in the minimal possible time.

TRAUMA TO THE CHEST AND GREAT VESSELS

The importance of prompt definitive diagnosis of aortic or great vessel rupture assumes its proper perspective when one considers that rupture of the aorta or a great vessel is present in 16% of fatal automobile accidents.[26] About 20% of patients with aortic rupture survive for more than 1 hour if there are no associated cardiac injuries,[53] but if aortic rupture is undiagnosed and untreated 60% die within 2 weeks.[41]

The clinical findings of trauma to the aorta and great vessels are frequently minimal and obscured by other injuries.[24, 28] The presence of hemothorax or of a widening mediastinum on serial chest roentgenograms should alert one to the possibility of a ruptured aorta. Aortography permits a definitive diagnosis[13, 24, 28, 33, 37] and makes possible life-saving surgical correction.[16]

Intravenous aortography is not recommended since it does not provide adequate concentration of contrast and often fails to demonstrate the vascular "tear."

Percutaneous catheterization of the thoracic aorta permits optimal opacification and pinpoints the site of the traumatic tear or laceration. Some controversy exists as to whether forward arteriography via a right axillary artery approach is preferable to retrograde femoral aortography.[24, 28, 37] We prefer the retrograde femoral technique, which when cautiously performed is a safe procedure, even in cases of aortic transection. This method also permits evaluation of associated rupture of abdominal viscera in patients with multiple injuries.

The angiographic appearance may vary from irregularity of the aortic wall to a large false saccular aneurysm.[24, 28] An intimal tear with or without dissection is readily demonstrable (Figs. 10-1 and 10-2). The most common site of rupture is the isthmus (45% in autopsy series), followed by the supravalvar area.[28, 41]

In other instances, laceration or transection of aortic branches, the innominate, the subclavian, the internal mammary or an intercostal artery may be precisely demonstrated by thoracic aortography[13, 49] (Fig. 10-3).

ABDOMINAL TRAUMA

Abdominal trauma constitutes only 7% of injuries caused by automobile accidents, yet the resultant morbidity is notably high.[32] Angiography provides an excellent means for early diagnosis.[6, 22, 23, 32] The main indication for angiographic evaluation of the abdominal viscera is suspected injury to the liver, spleen, kidney, pancreas or the retroperitoneum.[22, 32]

Liver

Injury to the liver is not as common as injury to the kidney or spleen, yet it is the most significant in terms of mortality.[1, 54] Although the massive hemorrhage and shock associated with rupture of the liver constitute a surgical emergency, in most patients in whom liver injury is suspected there is ample time for angiographic evaluation. In deciding whether or not angiography is needed, it is important to keep in mind that very often the clinical picture is inconclusive and that the exact site and extent of liver injury may be difficult to assess even at surgery.

The indications, therefore, for angiography in liver injury are:[10]

1. To diagnose hepatic damage and to localize and evaluate its extent.
2. To follow the course of an angiographically demonstrated lesion, if operation is not performed.
3. To evaluate for complications of liver trauma (aneurysms, hemobilia) following conservative or surgical management, even if angiography was not originally performed.

The angiographic finding in hepatic trauma may include any of the following.[1, 10, 19, 42, 44, 46]

Chapter 10: ANGIOGRAPHY OF TRAUMA / 199

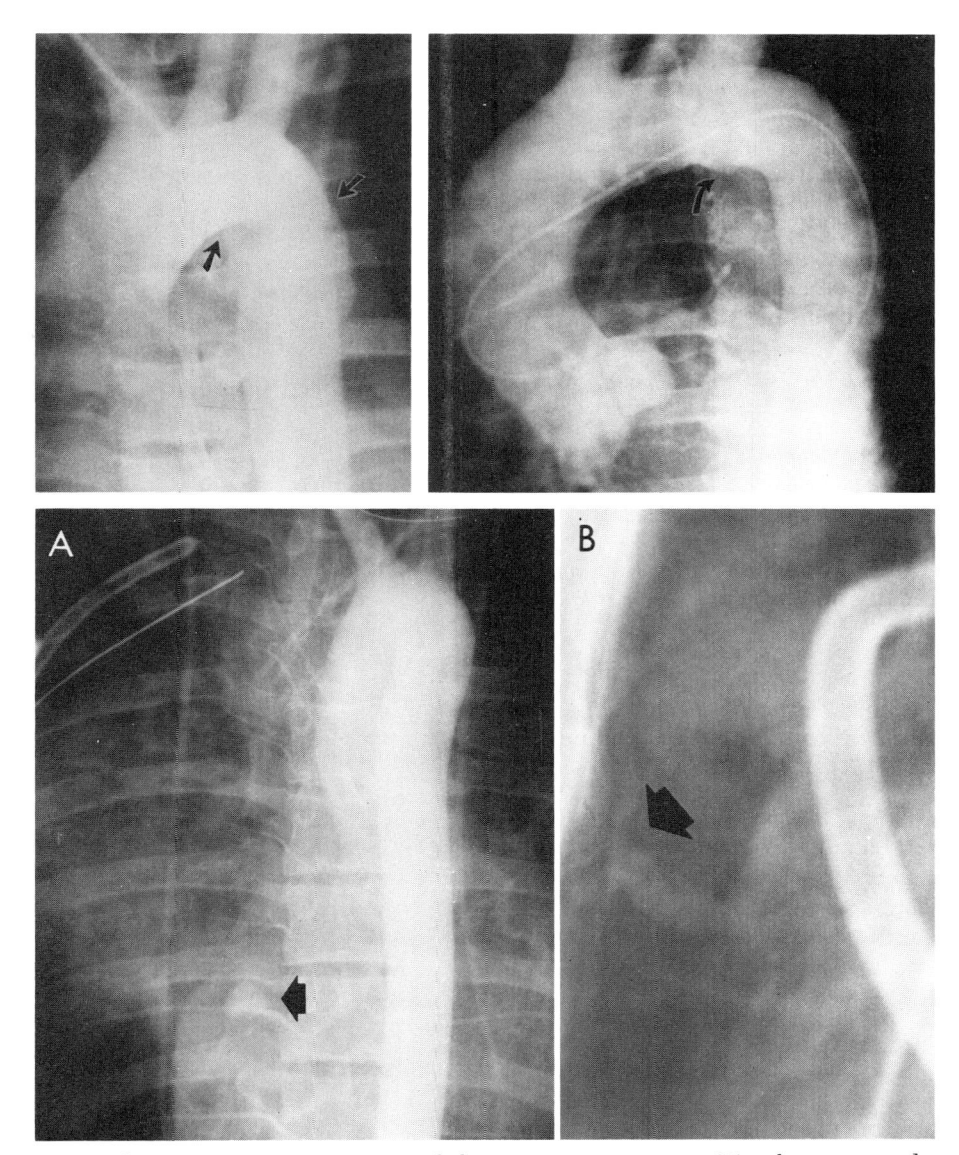

Fig. 10-1 (top left).—Traumatic rupture of thoracic aorta in man, 25, who sustained a chest injury in an automobile accident. Right transaxillary thoracic aortogram demonstrates rupture of the aorta at the isthmus, with discontinuity of the aortic wall *(arrows)* and false saccular aneurysm formation.

Fig. 10-2 (top right).—Intimal tear of thoracic aorta in man, 50, with chest injury from an automobile accident. Retrograde aortogram in the right posterior oblique projection shows minor discontinuity of the aortic wall *(arrow)* due to intimal tear.

Fig. 10-3 (bottom).—Mediastinal hemorrhage from internal mammary artery in patient who sustained trauma to the chest in an automobile accident. Radiograph showed a large right pleural effusion and a widened mediastinum. **A,** retrograde thoracic aortogram, anteroposterior projection, shows extravasation of contrast along the right border of the thoracic spine. **B,** lateral projection shows the extravasation to originate from the internal mammary artery in the anterior mediastinum. This was confirmed at surgery.

1. Hepatic contusion
    a Straightening and elongation of arterial branches
    b Delayed flow
    c Multiple small areas of contrast accumulation in the affected area
2. Hepatic laceration (Fig. 10-4)
    a Arterial occlusion
    b Contrast extravasation
    c Pseudoaneurysm formation
    d Arterioportal fistula
    e Arteriobiliary fistula
3. Intrahepatic or subcapsular hematoma
    a Arterial displacement
    b Liver displacement
    c Contrast extravasation

Small peripheral liver contusions will not be demonstrated by selective hepatic arteriography; however, these are probably clinically insignificant.

Spleen

The spleen is the organ most commonly injured in blunt abdominal trauma.[3, 52] Whereas physical signs, laboratory studies and simple radiography may suggest the diagnosis, only a splenic angiogram confirms or excludes the presence of splenic rupture. If negative, the splenic angiogram may make an exploration unnecessary; if positive, it will prevent the sequences of a delayed rupture.

The angiographic findings of splenic rupture have been extensively described.[3, 6, 31, 34, 42, 44] The inadequacy of midstream abdominal aortography alone to provide the diagnosis must be emphasized. Celiac axis or selective splenic artery catheterization is mandatory if one is to avoid false-negative or false-positive interpretation.

The definitive criteria for an angiographic diagnosis of spleen rupture are:

1. Gross or multifocal small points of contrast extravasation in the arterial phase of the angiogram, persisting into the capillary and venous phase (Fig. 10-5).
2. Direct intrasplenic arteriovenous communication.
3. Subcapsular hematoma, readily demonstrable in the capillary phase with

Fig. 10-4.—Liver rupture in man, 22, who had intraperitoneal hemorrhage following blunt abdominal trauma in an automobile accident. At exploration a ruptured spleen was removed and a laceration of the dome of the liver was oversewn. **A,** selective hepatic arteriogram following surgery shows continuing hemorrhage and contrast extravasation within the liver. **B,** subselective middle hepatic artery injection localizes the site of bleeding to a branch of the middle hepatic artery.

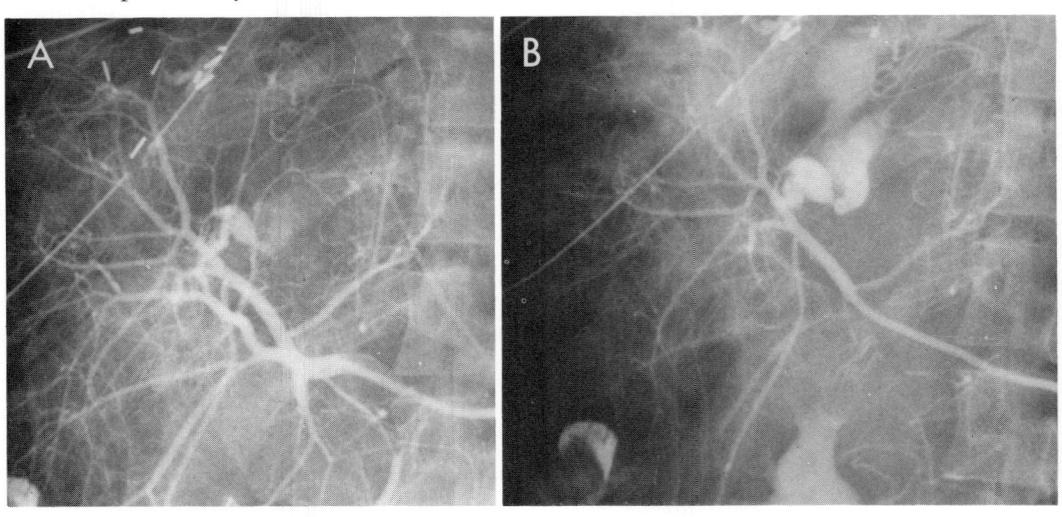

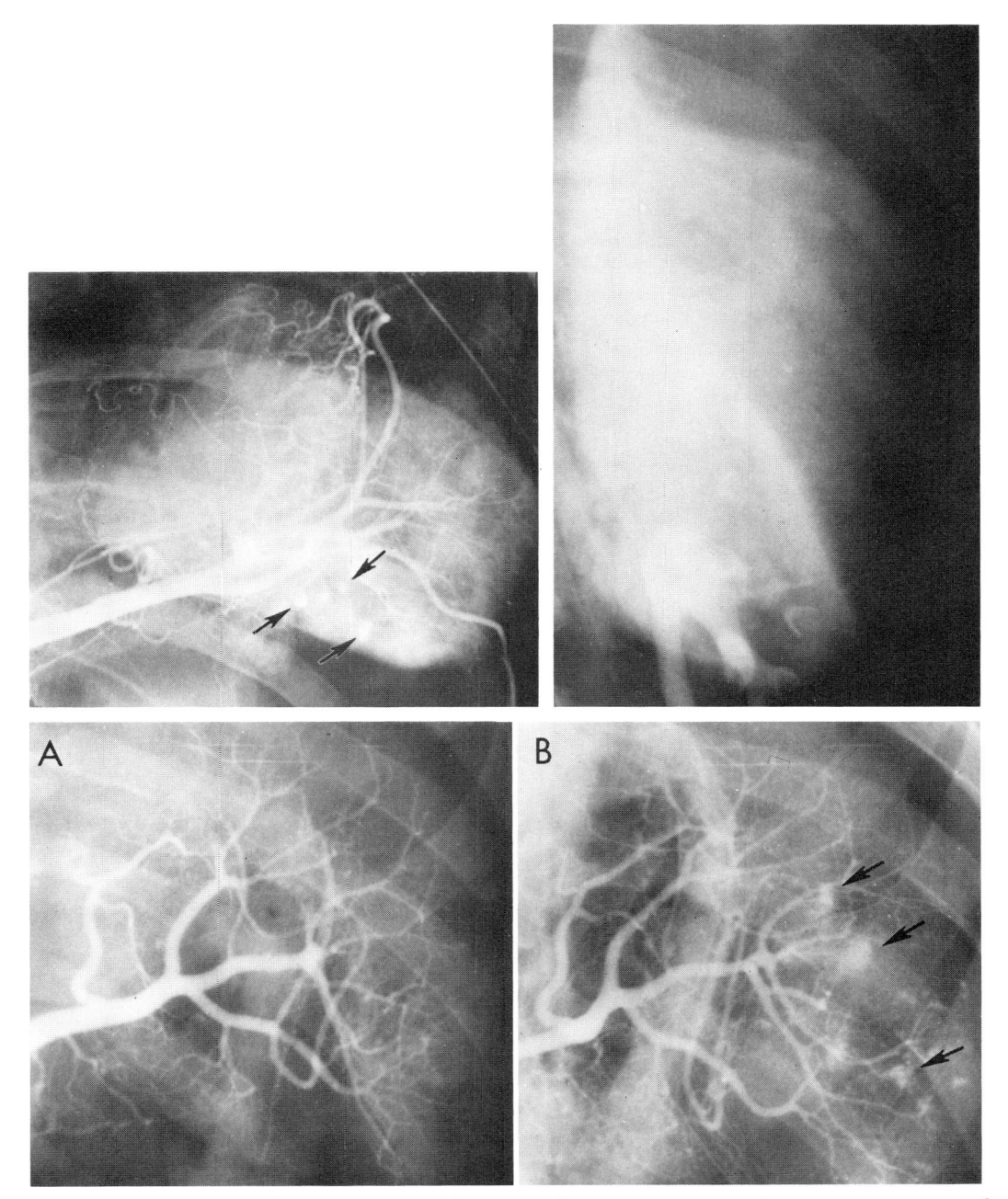

Fig. 10-5 (top left).—Splenic rupture. Selective splenic arteriogram shows extravasation of contrast along the inferior and medial aspects of the spleen. At surgery a tear of the capsule with hematoma was found.

Fig. 10-6 (top right).—Splenic subcapsular hematoma. Left upper quadrant pain and fullness followed injury to the left lower chest. Late phase of a selective splenic arteriogram demonstrates a large subcapsular hematoma along the lateral aspect of the spleen. The spleen was surgically removed.

Fig. 10-7 (bottom).—Splenic rupture. **A,** selective splenic arteriogram, arterial phase, reveals no definite evidence of rupture. Because of strong clinical suspicion, the splenic arteriogram was repeated after intra-arterial injection of 10 µg epinephrine. **B,** multiple foci of contrast extravasation are now clearly demonstrated *(arrows)*, indicating splenic rupture.

or without contrast extravasation (Fig. 10-6).

4. Definite wedge-shaped defect during the capillary phase, with arterial displacement in the involved areas, due to a tear with hematoma.

The so-called "indirect" signs of spleen rupture, such as "mottled" splenogram, questionable stretching of splenic artery branches and displacement of the opacified spleen away from the diaphragm or the lateral thoracic wall, are totally unreliable and should not be considered in the interpretation of the angiogram.

In several instances the angiographic findings may be subtle. Splenic arteriography in more than 1 projection (anteroposterior and right posterior oblique) may then be needed. Also, repeat angiography after the injection of epinephrine into the splenic artery may enhance contrast extravasation[51] (Fig. 10-7).

Pancreas

Traumatic pancreatic pseudocysts present no clinical diagnostic problem. Only when they present as a delayed manifestation of trauma, or when a left upper quadrant mass may be clinically attributed to the pancreas or a splenic delayed hematoma, is angiography utilized to clarify the nature and the location of the mass lesion.

Depending on the part of the pancreas it is connected with, a pseudocyst may or may not produce displacement of arteries, displacement of adjacent opacified viscera and displacement or thrombosis of veins, usually the splenic[9] (Fig. 10-8).

Kidney

In blunt or penetrating abdominal trauma, which by location may have involved the kidney, the extent of the renal damage needs to be precisely evaluated. A normal excretory urogram does not exclude renal vascular or parenchymal injury.[30] Unrecognized or untreated renal

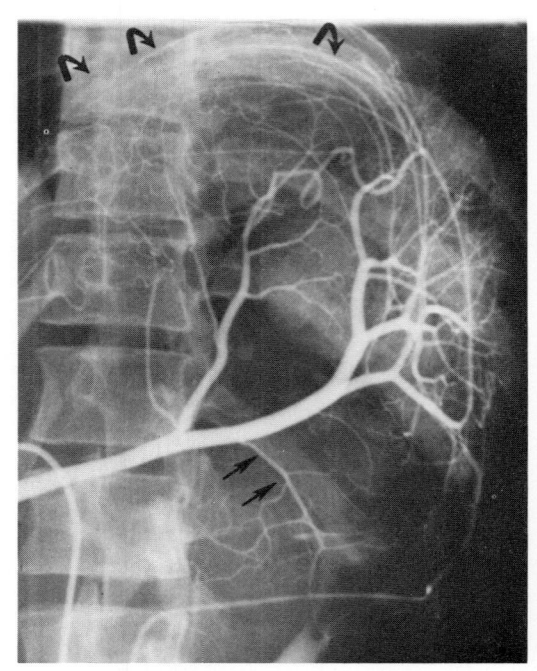

Fig. 10-8.—Traumatic pancreatic pseudocyst. Woman, 22, was seen with a large left upper quadrant mass 2 weeks following abdominal trauma in an automobile accident. Selective splenic arteriogram, arterial phase, shows no evidence of splenic rupture. However, there is splaying of the short gastric arteries *(curved arrows)* and stretching of the pancreatica magna artery *(straight arrows)*, indicating a mass lesion in the region of the body and tail of the pancreas. At surgery this proved to be a pancreatic pseudocyst.

trauma on the other hand may result in renal infarction, hypertension or hydronephrosis;[2, 5, 29, 30] hence, the need for precise angiographic evaluation in all patients suspected of having major renal injury.[14]

The angiographic findings of renal trauma may include any of the following.[18, 27, 29, 30, 40, 44]

1. Renal artery occlusion, secondary to shearing forces sustained during severe trauma or fall. Midstream abdominal aortography can adequately demonstrate the occlusion and must be performed immediately if the kidney is to be salvaged.[12, 20]

2. Contrast extravasation during the

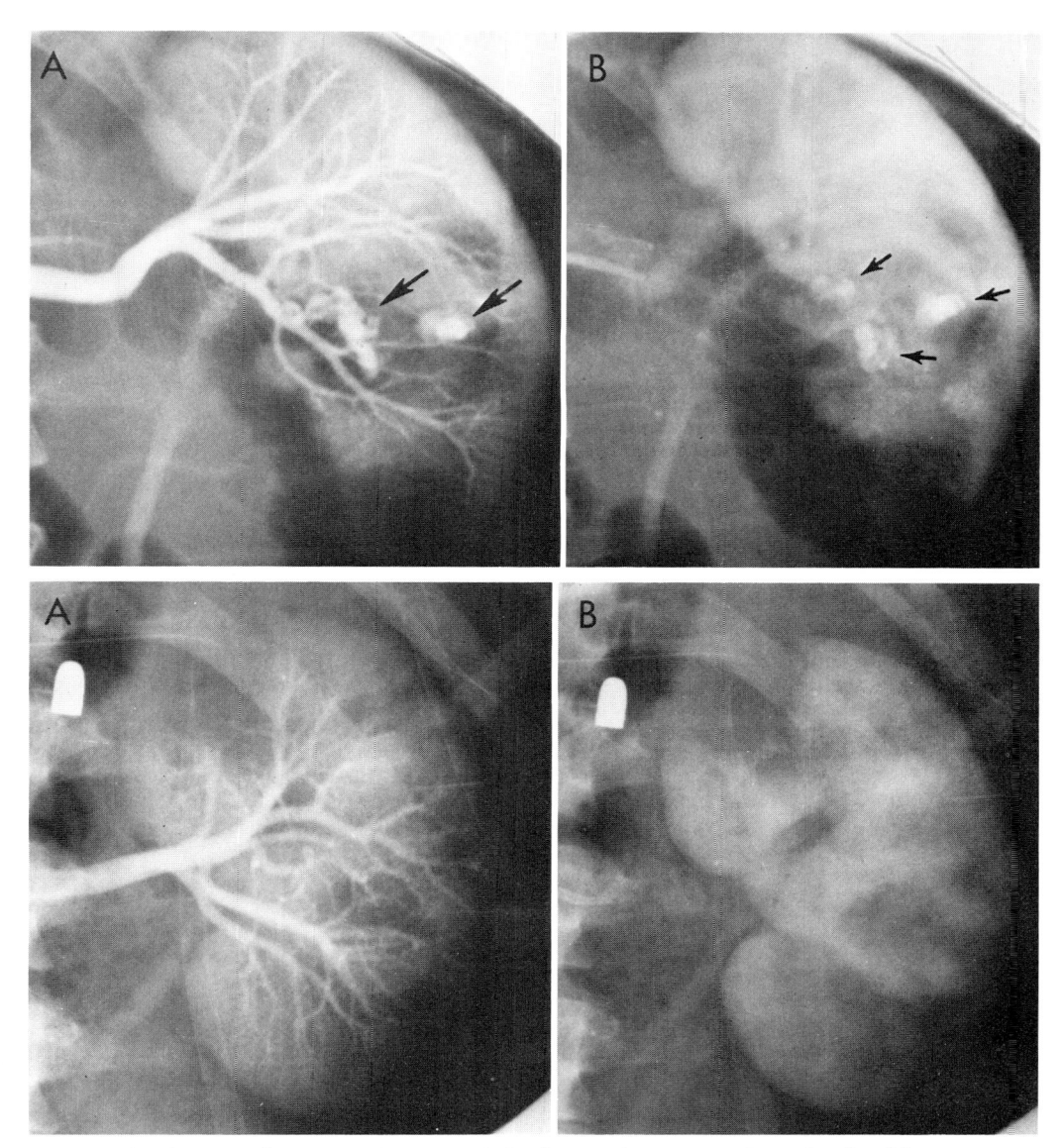

Fig. 10-9 (top).—Renal trauma. Patient, 19, had gross hematuria 1 week after blunt trauma to the abdomen. **A,** selective left renal arteriogram, arterial phase, shows multiple areas of contrast extravasation, which persisted into the late nephrographic phase, **B**. At surgery a large intrarenal hematoma was found.

Fig. 10-10 (bottom).—Renal hematoma. Patient had hematuria following bullet injury of the left flank. **A,** selective left renal arteriogram, arterial phase, shows lack of opacification of the most peripheral arterial branches to the upper pole of the kidney. **B,** in the late nephrographic phase there is a wedge-shaped defect in the upper pole due to a renal hematoma. A wedge resection was performed.

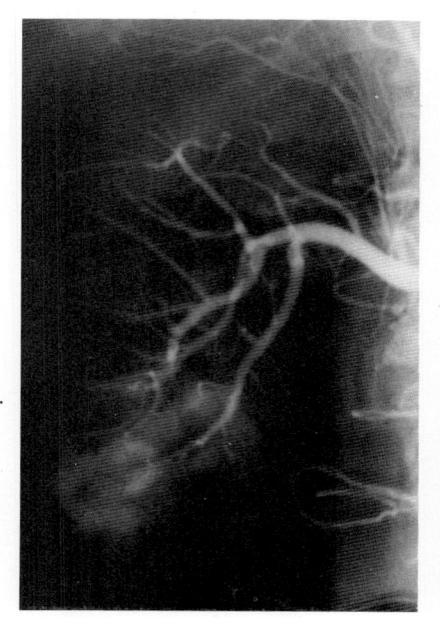

Fig. 10-11.—Renal hematoma. Patient had gross hematuria following bullet injury to the right flank. Selective right renal arteriogram, arterial phase, shows incomplete filling and displacement of the renal artery branches in the midportion of the kidney, due to intrarenal hematoma. A second renal artery accounts for the defect in the inferior pole of this kidney.

Fig. 10-12.—Renal rupture. Patient had hematuria following blunt trauma to the left abdomen in an automobile accident. **A,** selective left renal arteriogram shows no contrast extravasation. The defect in the inferior pole is due to the presence of a second renal artery supplying this area. **B,** during the nephrographic phase following midstream aortography, a defect is clearly demonstrated *(arrows)*, indicating renal rupture. **C,** a radiograph obtained at the end of this study, when the collecting system was opacified, shows contrast extravasation in the area of the renal rupture due to injury of the collecting system.

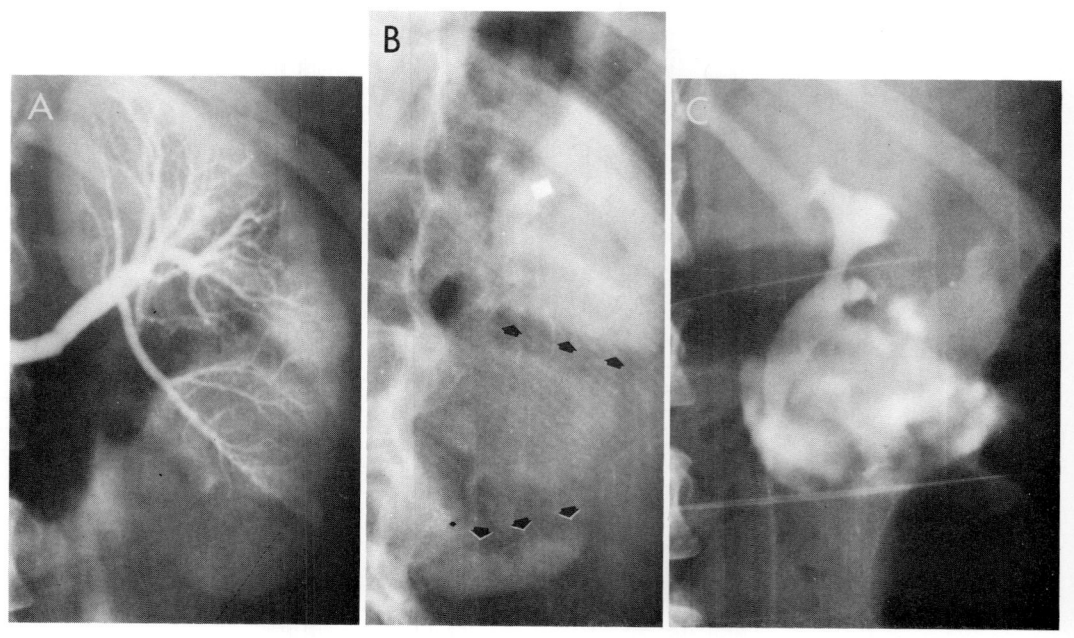

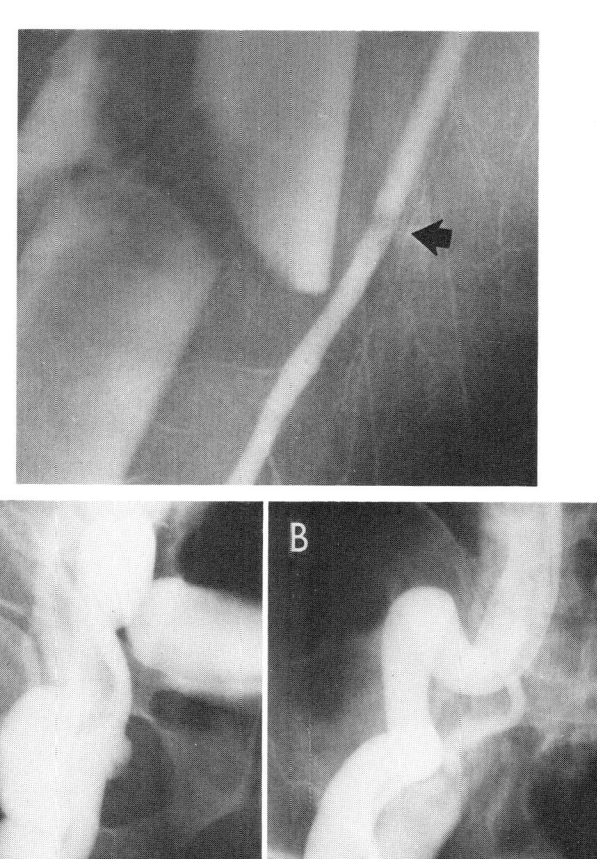

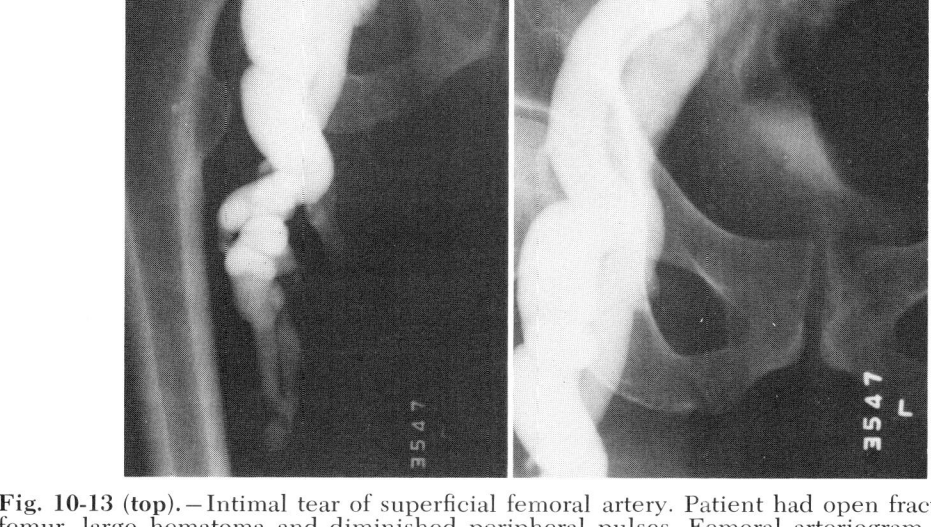

Fig. 10-13 (top).—Intimal tear of superficial femoral artery. Patient had open fracture of the femur, large hematoma and diminished peripheral pulses. Femoral arteriogram shows the presence of a filling defect in the superficial femoral artery adjacent to the fracture site, due to intimal tear (surgically proved).

Fig. 10-14 (bottom).—Traumatic arteriovenous fistula in man, 65, who presented with congestive heart failure 29 years after bullet injury of the right groin. A bruit and thrill were audible over the area of the right groin. Femoral arteriogram shows an arteriovenous fistula involving branches of the profunda artery and vein (**A**) with intense opacification of the common femoral and iliac veins (**B**).

arterial phase, or pseudoaneurysm formation (Fig. 10-9).

3. Arteriovenous fistula due to perforating injury,[29] or percutaneous needle biopsy.[7] In this instance, the angiographic demonstration of "siphoning effect," causing ischemia of a segment of the kidney, is of great importance before surgical correction.[29]

4. Arterial displacement due to intrarenal, perirenal or diffuse retroperitoneal hematoma (Figs. 10-10 and 10-11).

5. Parenchymal tear or complete renal transection, best appreciated during the nephrographic phase. Selective renal arteriography may be useful in establishing viability of the parenchymal margins on the basis of their homogenous or nonhemogenous opacification[29] (Fig. 10-12).

6. Renal vein thrombosis. Enlarged kidney and delayed arterial flow may suggest the possibility. Selective renal venography will confirm the diagnosis.

7. Underlying renal pathology, such as hydronephrosis or tumor.

TRAUMA OF THE EXTREMITIES

As the emphasis increases on primary repair of an injured vessel rather than ligation,[17, 38] angiography in trauma of the extremities is assuming increasing importance in the evaluation of the site and extent of vascular injury prior to reconstruction.[11, 33]

Arteriography is not always indicated when the site of injury is clinically obvious and the pulses distal to the injury are absent. It is in cases in which arterial injury is suspected, and the distal pulse is intact, that arteriography is most valuable. In such instances early recognition and repair of an incomplete laceration, an intimal tear or arterial contusion may prevent delayed arterial occlusion, ischemia and gangrene.[11, 15]

The indications for angiography in peripheral trauma are therefore:[11, 25]

1. Pulse deficit, if the site of obstruction is not clinically apparent.

2. No pulse deficit, but clinically suspected vascular injury (Fig. 10-13).

3. Suspected arterial aneurysm or arteriovenous fistula (Fig. 10-14).

4. Large or enlarging soft tissue swelling.

5. Postoperative control of vascular reconstruction.

When large soft-tissue hematomas are present and peripheral arteriography excludes arterial injury, peripheral venography may be considered to evaluate for large vein transection, which may be amenable to immediate surgical repair.

TRAUMA FOLLOWING DISK AND HIP SURGERY

Although rare, the development of an arteriovenous fistula following lumbar disk surgery has been reported.[8] This is 1

Fig. 10-15.—Following lumbar disk surgery, patient had congestive heart failure and abdominal bruit. Pelvic arteriogram shows an arteriovenous fistula between the right common iliac artery and vein.

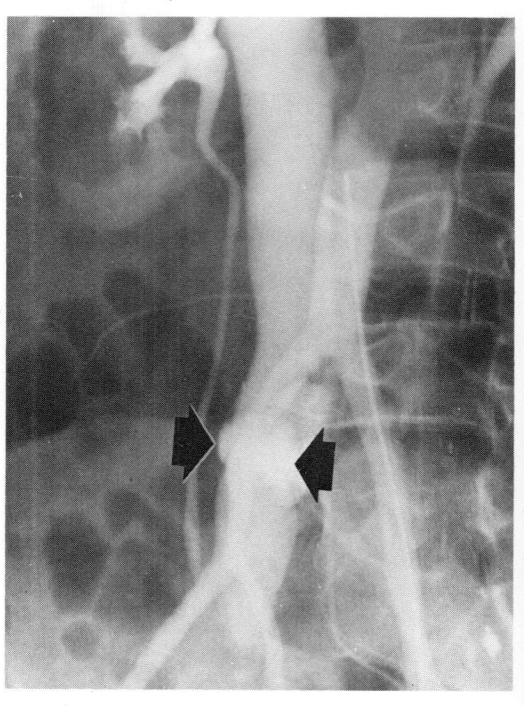

Chapter 10: ANGIOGRAPHY OF TRAUMA / **207**

more instance in which angiography can precisely localize the fistula and define the vessels involved, thus facilitating surgical repair[47] (Fig. 10-15).

Major hip surgery, a cup prosthesis or total hip replacement may also be associated with vascular injury and massive hemorrhage. Pelvic arteriography applied in 2 such patients demonstrated contrast extravasation from branches of the superior gluteal artery in 1 instance in which a graft had been obtained from the iliac bone, and from a branch of the inferior gluteal artery in another.

Following angiographic demonstration of the bleeding artery and selective placement of the catheter in the superior or the inferior gluteal artery, autologous clot may be introduced with angiographic and clinical control of hemorrhage

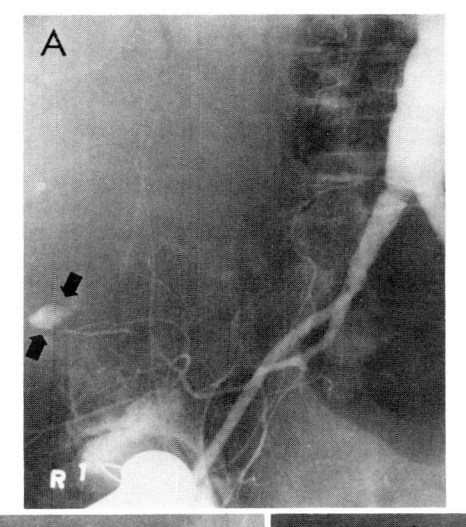

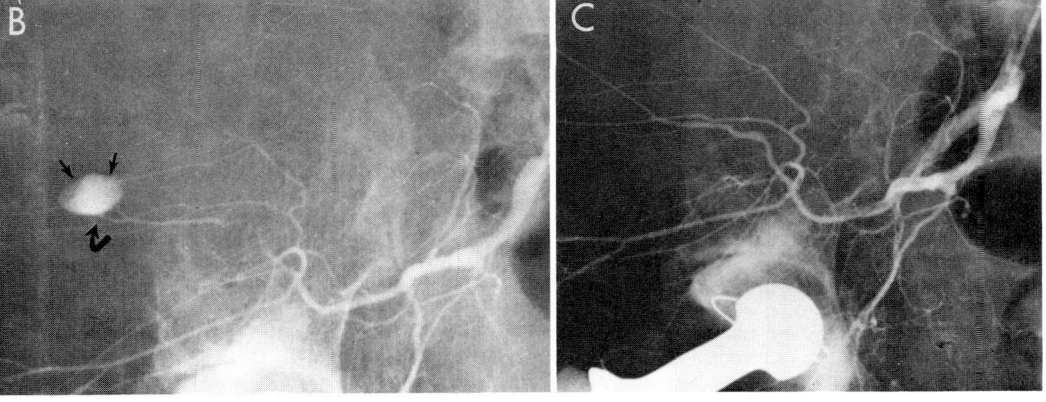

Fig. 10-16.—Angiographic localization and control of massive pelvic and retroperitoneal hemorrhage following total hip replacement. At surgery a graft was obtained from the right iliac bone. **A,** pelvic arteriogram shows extravasation from branches of the right hypogastric artery. **B,** selective right hypogastric arteriogram demonstrates to better advantage the extravasation *(straight arrows).* The bleeding artery is a branch of the superior gluteal artery *(curved arrow).* **C,** right hypogastric arteriogram following introduction of autologous clot through the angiographic catheter shows no extravasation. After this procedure the patient required no further blood replacement.

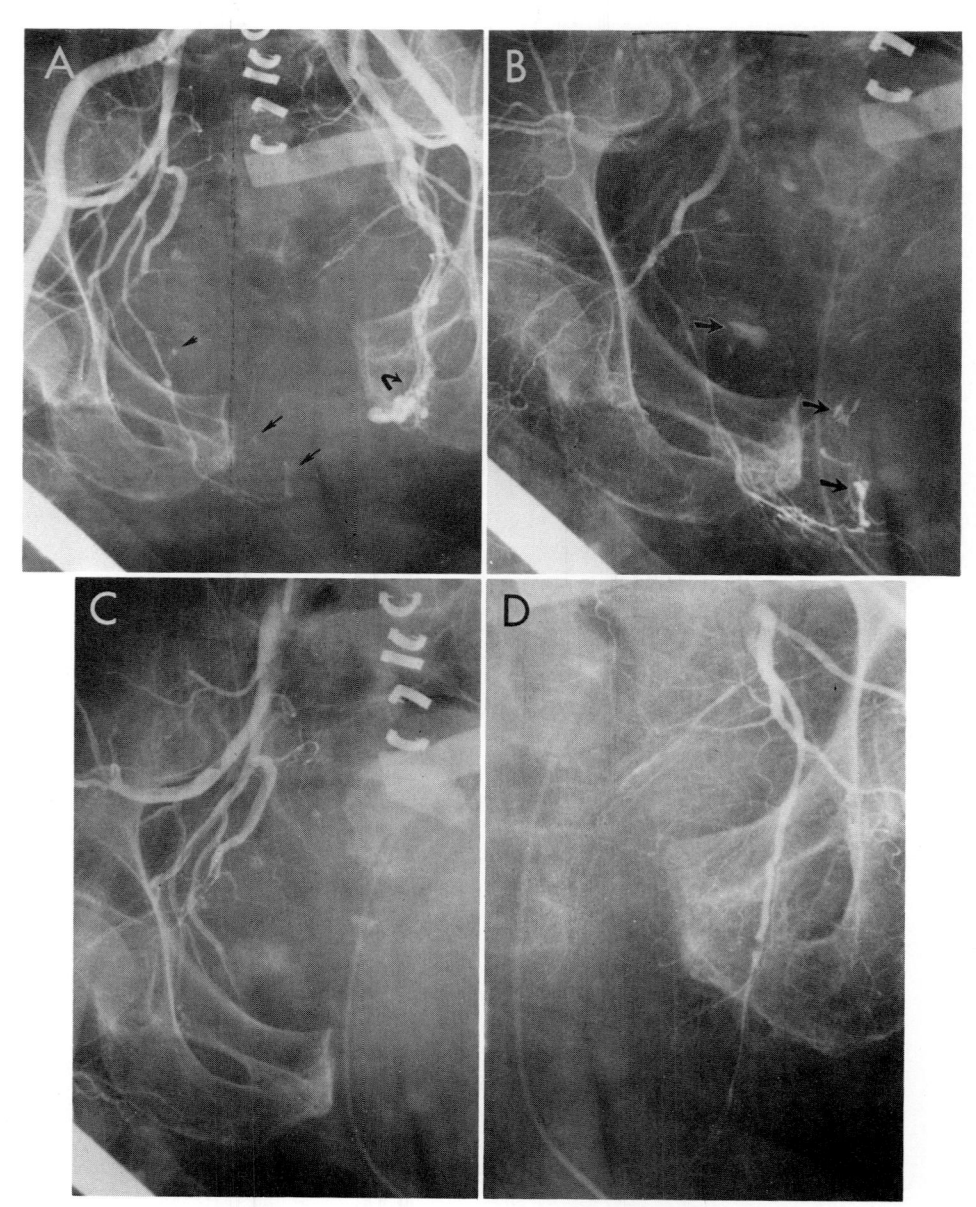

Fig. 10-17.—Angiographic localization and control of bleeding in a patient with multiple pelvic injuries from an automobile accident. **A,** pelvic arteriogram shows multiple bleeding sites *(straight arrows)* from branches of the right internal pudendal artery. A traumatic arteriovenous malformation is on the left side *(curved arrow).* **B,** selective right hypogastric arteriogram confirms the extravasation from bleeding sites in the right pelvis. **C,** right hypogastric arteriogram following introduction of autologous clot through the angiographic catheter shows complete control of the bleeding angiographically. The same procedure was repeated after selective catheterization of the left hypogastric artery and introduction of autologous clot. Arteriogram (**D**) shows occlusion of the arterial branch leading to the arteriovenous malformation. The patient required no further blood transfusions.

Chapter 10: ANGIOGRAPHY OF TRAUMA / 209

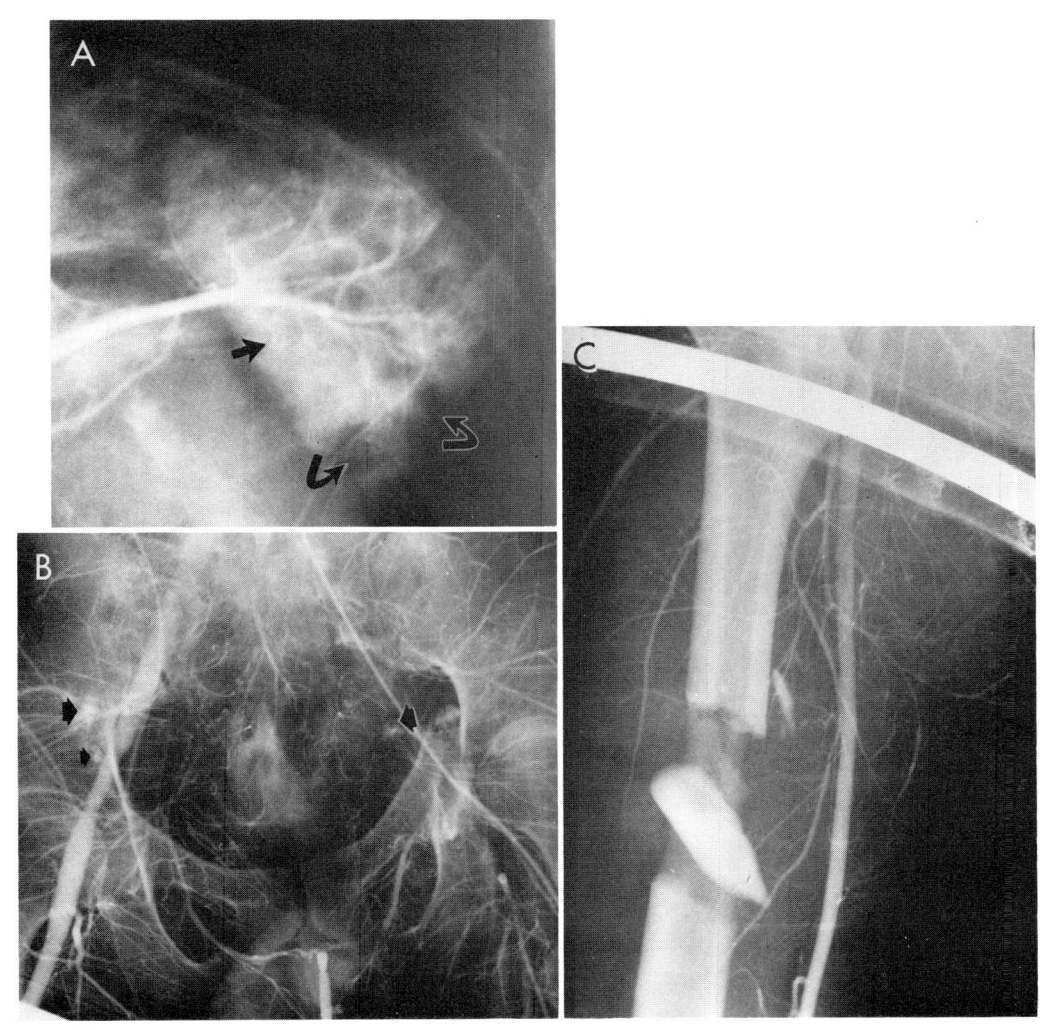

Fig. 10-18.—Angiography in multiple trauma. A 20-year-old man sustained multiple abdominal, pelvic and peripheral injuries following a fall from a third-story window. **A,** selective splenic arteriogram shows contrast extravasation *(straight arrow)* and a defect in the splenogram *(curved arrows)*, indicating splenic rupture. **B,** pelvic arteriogram shows multiple sites of arterial bleeding from branches of the hypogastric artery bilaterally. **C,** right femoral arteriogram excludes arterial injury at the site of the comminuted femoral fracture associated with large soft-tissue hematoma.

(Fig. 10-16). This seems to be a promising way to control massive hemorrhage following hip surgery.

PELVIC FRACTURES WITH HEMORRHAGE

The value of arteriography in the management of massive hemorrhage associated with fractures of the bony pelvis was recently reported.[52] Since then, 3 more patients with pelvic fractures and hemorrhage have been studied. In all 3, percutaneous arteriography of the pelvic arteries demonstrated points of extravasation from branches of either or both hypogastric arteries. Following localization of the bleeding vessel, selective catheterization of the hypogastric artery or 1 of the branches can be undertaken, and the bleeding artery may be occluded with autologous blood clot or by a Fogarty catheter introduced through the angiographic catheter. The hemorrhage was angiographically and clinically controlled in 2 patients (Fig. 10-17).

If pelvic arteriography fails to demonstrate the bleeding site, venography of the femoral and iliac veins may be performed to rule out large vein transection or laceration amenable to surgical repair.[45]

Since assessment of the type of pelvic vascular damage is important for management, and since surgical or conservative management is often unsatisfactory,[43] arteriographic methods for localization and control of hemorrhage from pelvic fractures seem to be extremely promising.

MULTIPLE TRAUMA

It is indeed convenient to group the indications for angiography, together with the corresponding findings, according to the organ or the area involved. Unfortunately, injuries do not follow textbook rules. Very often, a person falling from a height or involved in a rapid deceleration accident sustains multiple injuries. The physical findings are confusing or are perhaps totally lacking if there is associated head injury.[32]

Before surgical intervention, these patients are generally observed in the emergency ward and general supportive measures undertaken. It is during this period that angiography may be performed to evaluate the site and extent of injuries (Fig. 10-18). Given the appropriate clinical setting, "total body angiography" is no more unrealistic than total body radiography in the evaluation of the severely injured patient.[21, 32]

BIBLIOGRAPHY

1. Aakhus, T., and Enge, I.: Angiography in rupture of the liver, Acta Radiol. [Diagn.] 11: 353, 1971.
2. Abrams, H. L.: Renal Arteriography in Hypertension, in Abrams, H. L. (ed.), *Angiography*, (2d ed.; Boston: Little, Brown & Company, 1971), Vol. 2, p. 877.
3. Abrams, H. L.: Splenic Arteriography, in Abrams, H. L. (ed.), *Angiography* (2d ed.; Boston: Little, Brown & Company, 1971), Vol. 2, p. 1003.
4. Artz, C. P.: Presidential address: Make your commitment, J. Trauma 12:99, 1972.
5. Banowsky, L. H., Wolfel, D. A., and Lackner, L. H.: Consideration in diagnosis and management of renal trauma, J. Trauma 10:587, 1970.
6. Baum, S., Roy, R., Finkelstein, A. K., and Blakemore, W. S.: Clinical application of selective celiac and superior mesenteric arteriography, Radiology 84:279, 1965.
7. Bennett, A. R., and Wiener, S. N.: Intrarenal arteriovenous fistula and aneurysm: A complication of percutaneous renal biopsy, Am. J. Roentgenol. 95:372, 1965.
8. Birkeland, I. W., and Taylor, T. K.: Major vascular injuries in lumbar disc surgery, J. Bone Joint Surg. 51-B:4, 1969.
9. Boijsen, E.: Pancreatic Angiography, in Abrams, H. L. (ed.), *Angiography* (2d ed.; Boston: Little, Brown & Company, 1971), Vol. 2, p. 953.
10. Boijsen, E., Kaude, J., and Tylén, U.: Angiography in hepatic rupture, Acta Radiol. [Diagn.] 11:363, 1971.
11. Bron, M. K.: Femoral Arteriography, in Abrams, H. L. (ed.), *Angiography* (2d ed.; Boston: Little, Brown & Company, 1971), Vol. 2, p. 1221.
12. Cornell, S. H., Reasa, D. A., and Culp, D. A.: Occlusion of the renal artery secondary to acute or remote trauma, JAMA 219:1754, 1972.
13. Davies, E. R., and Roylance, J.: Aortography in the investigation of traumatic mediastinal hematoma, Clin. Radiol. 21:297, 1970.
14. Del Villar, R. G., Ireland, G. W., and Cass, A. S.: Management of renal injury in conjunction with the immediate surgical treatment of acute severe trauma patient, J. Urol. 107:208, 1972.

15. Dillard, B. M., Nelson, D. L., and Norman, H. G., Jr.: Review of 85 major traumatic arterial injuries, Surgery 63:391, 1968.
16. Dobbell, A. R. C., MacNaughton, E. A., and Crutchlow, E. T.: Successful early treatment of subadventitial rupture of the thoracic aorta, N. Engl. J. Med. 270:410, 1964.
17. Doty, D. B., Treiman, R. L., Rothschild, P. D., and Gaspar, M. R.: Prevention of gangrene due to fracture, Surg. Gynecol. Obstet. 125:284, 1967.
18. Elkin, M., Meng, C. H., and de Paredes, R. G.: Roentgenologic evaluation of renal trauma with emphasis on renal angiography, Am. J. Roentgenol. 98:1, 1966.
19. Enge, I., Knutrud, O., and Normann, T.: Central rupture of the liver with traumatic haemobilia: A pre- and post-operative angiography study, Br. J. Radiol. 41:789, 1968.
20. Evans, A., and Mogg, R. A.: Renal artery thrombosis due to closed trauma, J. Urol. 105:330, 1971.
21. Freeark, R. J.: Role of angiography in the management of multiple injuries, Surg. Gynecol. Obstet. 128:761, 1969.
22. Freeark, R. J., Love, L., and Baker, R. J.: An active diagnostic approach to blunt abdominal trauma, Surg. Clin. North Am. 48:97, 1968.
23. Freeark, R. J., Shoemaker, W. C., and Baker, R. J.: Aortography in blunt abdominal trauma, Arch. Surg. 96:705, 1968.
24. Freed, T. A., Neal, M. P., Jr., and Vinik, M.: Roentgenographic findings in extracardiac injury secondary to blunt chest automobile trauma, Am. J. Roentgenol. 104:424, 1968.
25. Girl, J.: Arteriography in arterial gunshot wounds, Acta Radiol. [Diagn.] 11:78, 1971.
26. Greendyke, R. M.: Traumatic rupture of aorta: Special reference to automobile accidents, JAMA 195:527, 1966.
27. Halpern, M.: Angiography in renal trauma, Surg. Clin. North Am. 48:1221, 1968.
28. Heitzman, E. R., and McAfee, J. G.: Aneurysms of the Thoracic Aorta and Its Branches, in Abrams, H. L. (ed.), *Angiography* (2d ed.; Boston: Little, Brown & Company, 1971), Vol. 2.
29. Lang, E. K., Trichel, B. E., Turner, R. W., Fontenot, R. A., Johnson, B., and St. Martin, E. C.: Renal arteriography in the assessment of renal trauma, Radiology 98:103, 1971.
30. Lecky, J. W.: Renal Angiography, in Robbins, L. L. (ed.), *Golden's Diagnostic Radiology* (Baltimore: Williams & Wilkins Company, 1971), Section 18, p. 309.
31. Lepasoon, J., and Olin. T.: Angiographic diagnosis of splenic lesions following blunt abdominal trauma, Acta Radiol. [Diagn.] 11:257, 1971.
32. Lim, R. C., Jr., Glickman, M. G., and Hunt, T. K.: Angiography in patients with blunt trauma to the chest and abdomen, Surg. Clin. North Am. 52:551, 1972.
33. Love, L.: Arterial trauma. Semin. Roentgenol. 5:267, 1970.
34. Love, L., Greenfield, G. B., Braun, T. W., Moncada, R., Freeark, R. J., and Baker, R. J.: Arteriography of splenic trauma, Radiology 91:96, 1968.
35. Margolies, M. N., Ring, E. J., Waltman, A. C., Kerr, W. S., Jr., and Baum, S.: Arteriography to manage hemorrhage from pelvic fractures, N. Engl. J. Med. 287:317, 1972.
36. Mills, R. H. B.: The problems of closed liver injuries, Acta Chir. Scand. 2:267, 1961.
37. Molnar, W., and Page, W. G.: Traumatic rupture of the thoracic aorta, Radiol. Clin. North Am. 4:403, 1966.
38. Morris, G. C., Jr., Beall, A. C., Jr, Roof, W. R., and DeBakey, M. E.: Surgical experience with 220 acute arterial injuries in civilian practice, Am. J. Surg. 99:775, 1960.
39. Odman, P.: Percutaneous selective angiography of the main branches of the aorta, Acta Radiol. 45:1, 1956.
40. Olsson, O., and Lunderquist, A.: Angiography in renal trauma, Acta Radiol. (Diagn.) 1:1, 1963.
41. Parmley, L. F., Mattingly, T. W., Manion, W. C., and Jahnke, E. J., Jr.: Non-penetrating traumatic injury of aorta, Circulation 17:1086, 1958.
42. Pollard, J. J., and Nebesar, R. A.: Abdominal angiography, N. Engl. J. Med. 279:1035, 1968.
43. Quimby, W. C., Jr.: Pelvic fractures with hemorrhage. Editorial, N. Engl. J. Med. 284:668, 1971
44. Redman, H. C., Reuter, S. R., and Bookstein, J. J.: Angiography in abdominal trauma, Ann. Surg. 169:57, 1969.
45. Reynolds, B. M., and Balsano, N. A.: Venography in pelvic fractures: A clinical evaluation, Ann. Surg. 173:104, 1971.
46. Rösch, J., and Steckel, R. J.: Selective Angiography of the Abdominal Viscera, in Robbins, L. L. (ed.), *Golden's Diagnostic Radiology* (Baltimore: Williams & Wilkins Company, 1972), Section 18, p. 17.
47. Saldino, R. M., White, A. A., and Palubinskas, A. J.: Arteriovenous fistula, a complication of lumbar disc surgery, Radiology 98:565, 1971.
48. Seldinger, S. L.: Catheter replacement of needle in percutaneous arteriography: A new technique, Acta Radiol. 39:368, 1953.
49. Siegelman, S. S., Rosenberg, R. F., and Furman, S.: Angiographic evaluation of injury to the great vessels, Arch. Surg. 100:565, 1970.
50. Solheim, K.: Closed abdominal injuries, Acta Chir. Scand. 126: 574, 1963.
51. Stein, H. L.: The diagnosis of traumatic laceration of the spleen by selective arteriography, direct serial magnification angiography and intra-arterial epinephrine, Radiology 93:367, 1969.
52. Stivelman, R. L., Glaubitz, J. P., and Crampton, R. S.: Laceration of the spleen due to nonpenetrating trauma: One hundred cases, Am. J. Surg. 106:889, 1963.
53. Strassman, G.: Traumatic rupture of aorta, Am. Heart J. 33:508, 1947.
54. Williams, L. F., Jr., and Byrne, J. J.: Trauma to the liver at the Boston City Hospital from 1955 to 1965, Am. J. Surg. 112:368, 1966.

11 | Shock

MORTIMER J. BUCKLEY and
W. GERALD AUSTEN

SHOCK has been historically described in many different fashions, passing through a long evolution of definition. Periods of severe trauma, usually occurring in wartime, have greatly accelerated the process of delineation. One of the outstanding treatises concerning the investigative evaluation of the shock processes is *Traumatic Shock*, written by Cannon.[19] This monograph, which reviewed the experiences of the Allied shock teams in World War I, gave one of the first quantitative evaluations of shock and described well the inter-reaction of heart, vasomotor tone, blood volume and oxygenation. The conclusions, which related the progress of shock to a build-up of fixed acids and which suggested that a deficit in alkali reserve was a secondary effect of impaired oxygen transport, still hold today. Subsequent studies carried out by Keith (see Ref. 78), Blalock[13] and Parsons and Phemister[64] in the 1920s and 1930s further delineated much of the physiologic and anatomic defects associated with wounds. Again, in World War II, the battlefield studies of the physiologic changes produced by low perfusion enhanced our understanding of the shock state. A shock study team headed by Beecher[7] in the Mediterranean operation during that war first used a biochemical laboratory near the battlefield and its members were able to show that the predominant cause of traumatic shock was the loss of blood and other fluids. This loss frequently led to inadequate tissue perfusion and acidosis. More recently, shock units in Korea and Vietnam[20, 42] have been able to further define the effects of the hypotensive and hypoperfused state on renal and pulmonary function. Simultaneous with these efforts has been the development of multiple shock units throughout the United States. The evaluation and finally the therapy of the shock patient have slowly changed from the pragmatic application of multiple therapeutics based on evident clinical changes readily discerned at the bedside. With the advent of more invasive procedures, a more specific definition of the shock state has become possible and, in many circumstances, more definitive therapy of the injured systems can be achieved before irreversible damage has occurred.

To discuss shock, we first need a clear definition. Hypotension, weak pulse, pallid facies and cyanosis of the nail beds and lips have been constant findings in all forms of shock. Although the clinical description still is applicable, a more definitive physiologic definition would be helpful. Shock can be described as the clinical state that follows cellular hypoxia and damage caused by inadequate flow of blood to critical organs. As extensive investigations have been made into the clinical shock state,[24] the deficits at the cellular level have become evident, and it is clear that the therapy of shock must be directed not only to the evident clinical changes, such as hypotension and lowered cardiac output, but to the basic deficits producing the derangement in cellular metabolism as well.

Shock, then, may be initiated by failure of any one of many systems. A severe disruption in the normal interaction between the energy source (the heart), the responsiveness of the arterial system (arterial resistance), the capacity of the venous bed (venous tone), the volume and characteristics of the flowing fluid (blood) and the effectiveness of ventilation (oxygenation), and the manner in which these systems interact to deliver oxygen and metabolites to the cell, may result in a progressive deterioration ending in the shock state. Shock may be categorized according to the systems that have failed and, thus, we have basically divided the shock state into (1) cardiogenic, (2) hypoxic, (3) hypovolemic, (4) bacteremic and (5) neurogenic.

PATHOLOGIC PHYSIOLOGY. — Although the shock state may be initiated by the failure of one of the basic interacting systems described previously, the end point often is similar. One of the most difficult problems at present is to recognize the shock state in its earliest initiation, and much investigation now is being directed to that point. Once the shock state has been allowed to progress to the point that severe obtundation, hypotension, anuria and acidosis have occurred, the reversibility of this state is less likely.

Multiple tests have been designed to follow changes in the organ systems and to detect early evidence of deterioration of normal homeostasis. Cardiac activity has been followed for years by simple intermittent measurement of blood pressure and pulse. In the very ill or severely traumatized patient, these signs may deteriorate only when the shock process is quite far advanced. Constant monitoring of the changes in arterial pressure and frequent determination of the cardiac output give a better understanding of the compensatory mechanisms that are functioning before severe hypotension occurs. Similarly, the filling pressures of the heart may be of greater significance in determining evidence of cardiac failure than the systemic pressure produced. Blood pressure may be maintained at normal levels in the presence of a falling cardiac output. This is accomplished by a rise in peripheral resistance. The increase in peripheral resistance is variable in different organ systems and usually results in reduced flow to the skin, kidneys and intestines, with preferential maintenance of flow to the heart and brain. Similarly, increased cardiac output can compensate for decreased peripheral resistance, as seen in some septic states. However, these compensatory mechanisms are only transient and, once exhausted, usually result in a severe, resistant hypotensive state.

In the quiet, controlled situation, pulse rate may be a valid indication of changes in circulating blood volume and cardiac output. However, in the severely traumatized patient or in the patient who is actively bleeding, pulse rate may vary widely and may be only an indication of pain and apprehension. Again, the mechanism of rate increase can compensate for only relatively short periods of time before secondary effects on the myocardium and the periphery will occur.

Changes in filling pressure of the heart may also produce changes in the pulse rate, and only through an effective measurement of this filling pressure can cardiac activity be monitored closely. The filling pressure of the right heart, as measured by central venous pressure, does not always reflect the effective filling of the left ventricle.[22] Recent studies of shock states have shown the critical need for measurement of the left atrial filling pressure and, if possible, measurement of left ventricular pressure, especially in shock states resulting from acute myocardial infarction.[67] Severe left ventricular failure may exist even in the presence of normal or low filling pressures in the right heart. Central venous pressures are only a measure of the filling pressure of the right ventricular system, and they relate primarily to the pulmonary circulation.[25] Left atrial filling pressures can be measured accurately, in the clinical situation, only by either direct left atrial catheterization or intermittent pulmonary wedge pressure measurement.[77] In some circumstances, a measure of the end-diastolic pressure in the main pulmonary artery may relate to mean left atrial pressure.[53] With this data available, cardiac function can be more readily measured and related to peripheral resistance and cardiac output to determine over-all cardiovascular compensation.

Shifts in body fluids often produce rapid changes in hematocrit that result in either hemodilution or hemoconcentration, depending on the form of shock. Hypovolemia resulting from blood loss is slowly compensated by dilution of the hematocrit and restoration of circulating blood volume by a shift of fluid from the extravascular space. However, in the presence of severe hypotension, the shift occurs slowly because of the loss of effective pressure in the capillary circulation.[59] Intravascular fluid shifts to the extravascular and intracellular spaces may occur rapidly, with an associated elevated hematocrit, as seen in those conditions associated with plasma and other fluid loss; for example, burns, peritonitis, septicemia and fistulas.[60] These shifts may occur at a rapid rate, but the compensation as evidenced by an elevated hematocrit may lag well behind the disease process. Thus, the measurement of blood hematocrit alone does not relate immediately to the ongoing compensatory mechanisms. A more definitive measurement of blood volume, plasma volume and body water is most helpful in determining these shifts and the rapidity with which they occur, in order to initiate compensatory therapy. The shift of extravascular fluid into the intravascular space during hemorrhagic shock is thought to be related to changes in capillary hydrostatic pressure and oncotic pressure.[28] However, sequestration of red blood cells in poorly perfused areas or in an injured capillary bed may also be a cause for a falling hematocrit in a patient in severe shock.[30] Red cell mass may also be diminished acutely with diffuse intravascular coagulation initiated with the shock state.[43] Plasma loss during all forms of severe low-output shock states, particularly with endotoxin shock, has been attributed to capillary injury, with a rapid loss of fluid and protein into the extravascular space.[55] The compensatory mobilization of fluid from other extravascular sites to maintain adequate circulating blood volume can occur for an extended period before severe hemoconcentration, hypovolemia and hypotension occur. These rapid shifts that can occur in intravascular and extravascular volumes show that simple indicators, such as blood hemoglobin or hematocrit, are not adequate tests of changes in blood volume. Blood volume determinations, useful in the research setting, often are impractical in the management of patients with shock,[29, 76] when usually we must rely on three basic measurements of circulatory compensatory activity—arterial pressure, cardiac output and cardiac filling pressures.

Ventilatory mechanics generally are evaluated by measuring the respiratory rate and tidal volume of the patient. These measurements may be an indication of the adequacy of ventilation, but many other events may affect these parameters. Apprehension, severe pain, as well as metabolic processes, such as septicemia and fever, will markedly change these responses and make them poor indicators of the adequacy of oxygen delivery.[9] The most adequate method to determine the efficiency of oxygen transport to the cell has been the measurement of arterial blood gases, pH and the blood levels of pyruvate and lactate. Even in the presence of seemingly adequate ventilatory exchange, the cellular needs for oxygen may be so pronounced, as in some septic states, that cellular acidosis may occur and anaerobic metabolism with the production of lactate acidemia may ensue.[18]

Subsequent to the initiation of the shock state, the pituitary adrenal axis becomes more active with the release of antidiuretic hormone from the pituitary. The release of adrenocorticotropic hormone increases corticosteroid secretion from the adrenal gland, which is also able to release higher levels of epinephrine from the medulla. These hormonal responses result in protein breakdown, water and electrolyte retention, elevated blood sugar and increased cardiovascular activity. These factors in the presence of decreased perfusion and oxygenation of the cell result in anaerobic metabolism, with a rising level of lactic acid in the cells and blood, and progressive metabolic acidosis.[58] Recent studies have shown that as this cellular damage progresses, breakdown products may be released from the cell, which results in progression of the shock state. These breakdown products may be very important and may be critical in the propagation of the shock state so often described as irreversible and associated with severe hypotension, poor peripheral perfusion, obtundation, oliguria and acidosis.[49] In addition to the release of catecholamines, histamine and serotonin, vasoactive polypeptides are released into the circulation during periods of severe shock. Bradykinin, a vasoactive agent released by proteases working on bradykininogen, has been found to be released in hemorrhagic shock. This agent is active on the smooth muscle and small blood vessels. Multiple other vasoactive materials have been found in the research laboratory but their clinical importance has not been established.[83] Similarly, depressant factors, such as a myocardial depressant factor released in the shock state, have been found in the research animal but have not been totally identified in the clinical shock state.[79]

MONITORING SYSTEMS. — Most of the shock states, despite their manner of initiation, have in common a similar physiology. Numerous measurements must be used to determine the form and efficacy of the therapy selected. Needless to say, adequate care for shock patients requires a well-equipped intensive care unit, staffed by specially trained nurses, supported by available deeply interested physicians and backed by well-trained technicians. In such a physical setting, the following needs may be met.

Cardiac activity must be monitored closely. Pulse rate and blood pressure must be recorded, if possible, constantly. This is especially true in the severely hypotensive patient. An electrocardiogram monitor may be used to observe rate and to check for cardiac arrhythmias. The measurement of peripheral blood pressure alternately with a sphygmomanometric system may be useful in the mildly ill patient, but this system requires constant supervision and work. One that is more reasonable and more functional measures arterial pressure directly by means of a catheter placed either in the radial artery or in some other suitable peripheral arterial trunk, which, when connected to a transducer and an oscilloscope, gives a constant read-out of blood pressure and its pulse form. As computer techniques become more available, further interpretation of the pulse contour may yield added information concerning the contractile state of the myocardium, cardiac output and peripheral vasomotor tone. At present, this recording is mainly helpful in evidencing early changes in systemic arterial pressure. The catheter inserted for measurement of arterial pressure is also a ready source of arterial blood for the determination of pH, P_{CO_2} and P_{O_2} as well as a sampling site for blood electrolytes and hematocrit. The value of these measurements will be discussed subsequently. Ideally, cardiac output should be measured in these patients; when related to arterial pressure, this measurement is helpful in determining the type of pressor agent that might be needed. Patients who are hypotensive and who have a high cardiac output and a low peripheral resistance would not be candidates for treatment with such agents as isoproterenol. Conversely, patients with a normal blood pressure and a marked increase in peripheral resistance should be treated with agents that will reduce peripheral resistance and maintain cardiac output or return cardiac output to normal levels. These determinations of cardiac output generally can be accomplished by a dye-dilution technique, since the radial artery catheter, already in place, may be used for sampling and since another catheter, usually in place for the measurement of central filling pressures, is available for injection. Alternatively, a Fick determination of cardiac output may be carried out. There are drawbacks to this method, however, as it requires a long period of sampling in order to determine oxygen consumption and it is cumbersome in an intensive care unit. Repeat measurements of cardiac output are helpful in determining the effectiveness of individual forms of therapy, frequently before clinical evidence of this improvement is available.

The effective circulating blood volume can be measured in a number of ways. It is important to have an estimate of this value in order to determine adequate fluid, electrolyte and blood replacement. The systems available to measure blood volume, however, because of the rapid variations in the patient in shock or because of excessive time required for determination, have proved cumbersome and have produced variable results. Some shock units with specially trained technical help have found the determination of blood volume, plasma volume and extracellular fluid volume helpful from an analytic viewpoint and, in some circumstances, from a therapeutic viewpoint in the evaluation of patients in shock.[72, 84] In practice, however, the effective circulating blood volume may best be determined by measuring the filling pressures of the left heart.[38] Direct transseptal measurement of the left atrial pressure has been useful to some investigators, but sometimes it is difficult to do safely. Recently, however, the Swan-Ganz catheter has been used to measure pulmonary capillary wedge pressures intermittently and pulmonary artery pressures constantly in order to determine left heart filling pressures.[53] This catheter, easily placed by the flow direction technique, is quite safe.[77] The measurement of these pressures has greatly facilitated volume replacement in patients who have had variable cardiac function. Measurement of left-sided filling pressure as well as changes in arterial PO_2 may be used to determine maximal tolerable volume expansion. If this is not possible, central venous pressure may be used as a measurement of critical filling pressure as long as the physician realizes that this is a measurement of right heart filling pressure and that a normal or low central venous pressure may be present in association with a severely elevated left atrial pressure and vice versa. It should be emphasized that the measurement of central venous pressure is a very adequate system when dealing with patients who do not evidence left ventricular disease.[3, 44] This would apply to a majority of people seen in the younger age group subsequent to trauma or with sepsis, etc. It is important, however, that whenever a patient does not respond favorably to venous volume filling guided by central venous pressure measurements, a more direct measurement of left ventricular filling should be carried out before large amounts of volume are added to attempt to correct the patient's clinical course.

Adequate peripheral organ perfusion may be reflected by the temperature and color of the patient's extremities. Certainly these are not quantitative measurements of effective peripheral organ flow. Indirect evaluation of peripheral blood flow may be obtained by monitoring urinary output. The volume and specific gravity of the urine produced must be recorded carefully. This is done most accurately with indwelling catheter drainage of the bladder. Ideally, the osmolarity and sodium and potassium concentration of the urine should be evaluated frequently. Fixed osmolarity and an elevated level of sodium may point to intrinsic renal injury associated with hypoxia or hypotension. Rising osmolarity and normal urinary concentrations of sodium in the presence of a falling urinary output certainly suggest decreased renal blood flow and may be related to a decreased cardiac output.

Evidence of organ hypoperfusion may be demonstrated by the development of a metabolic acidosis; therefore, frequent measurement of blood pH should be made.

TREATMENT OF SHOCK STATES

The individual treatment of the shock patient must take into recognition multiple processes that are ongoing. In order to get a clearer definition of the pathophysiology occurring when individual organ systems fail, the following presentation will outline the intervention that may be carried out to correct this specific organ failure. The physician, however, must realize that each shock patient may have variable inter-reactions of the different organ systems and that what is said about one form of shock, such as cardiogenic shock and its treatment, may also apply to the patient who has hypovolemic shock or septic shock. The inter-reactions of these organ systems are evident and therefore the treatment must follow from these inter-reactions.

CARDIOGENIC SHOCK. — Cardiogenic shock is that condition resulting from extensive loss of functioning myocardial tissue. This usually is secondary to acute myocardial infarction causing a decreased cardiac output and a loss of compliance of the ventricular wall. It usually is marked by a cardiac index less than 2 L/min/M^2 and by mean left atrial pressure more than 15 mm Hg, and, in most circumstances, more than 20 mm Hg. Cardiogenic shock, then, is a low perfusion state resulting from loss of pump function by the left ventricle. It must be clearly distinguished from cardiogenic shock secondary to mechanical problems, such as tamponade, constrictive pericarditis, valvar heart disease and congenital anomalies. It must also be distinguished from low peripheral resistance states with normal or increased cardiac outputs, which can give the same clinical picture of hypotension. Through the use of cardiac output determinations and direct catheterization of the left heart, or indirect measurement of left atrial filling pressure, the true cardiogenic shock state has been defined more clearly.

Shock resulting from myocardial failure attributable to acute infarction, or to diffuse myocardial disease either of a chronic nature or associated with acute cardiomyopathies, provides a difficult therapeutic problem in the presence of adequate ventilation and normal or elevated blood volumes. Severe peripheral cyanosis, rapid weak pulse, hypotension and decreased urinary output are the usual signs. If the state is not corrected, severe metabolic acidosis ensues. The modalities of therapy are many, and all are only moderately helpful.

INOTROPIC AGENTS. — Certainly the residual, normal myocardial muscle in the shock state needs maximal efficiency to compensate for the nonfunctioning and poorly functioning myocardium. Pathologic studies have shown that usually 40% or more of ventricular musculature has been involved either by acute or chronic infarction in the process leading to shock.[63] Agents employed under these circumstances, therefore, rely on the compensatory power of the residual muscle. Isoproterenol has become one of the most commonly used agents because of its strong inotropic effect on the heart and its vasodilator activity in the periphery. This drug is given by intravenous drip with a concentration of 1–2 mg/250 ml of intravenous solution. The rate of infusion usually is between 1 and 4 µg/min. The level of drug used is determined by the resultant increase in both peripheral organ flow and arterial pressure. The secondary chronotropic effect of isoproterenol may, in some circumstances, limit its effectiveness because of the frequent presence of irritability associated with infarcted myocardium. When isoproterenol cannot be tolerated, epinephrine may be used. Epinephrine has inotropic functions similar to isoproterenol and may be given in similar concentrations of 1–2 mg of epinephrine in 250 ml of intravenous solution and at rates between 1 and 4 µg/min. Both of these agents, in rare circumstances, may be given at much higher doses. Again, epinephrine may be restricted by its chronotropic effect, which is not as evident as that seen with isoproterenol. Its major drawback, however, is its mixed peripheral vasoactivity, which may critically reduce circulation to underperfused peripheral organs when given in high doses. In many patients, neither of these agents is totally effective in the therapy of cardiogenic shock. In some circumstances, to maintain systemic pressure, norepinephrine[39] may have to be employed. Infusion usually is at a rate of 2–20 µg/min. When norepinephrine is used there is a marked peripheral vasoconstrictive effect, but the over-all increase in mean aortic pressure resulting from its infusion may allow more efficient coronary flow through diseased coronary arteries. Norepinephrine has been found to be most effective in those patients with normal or increased cardiac outputs who have reduced peripheral resistance. When norepinephrine is used, it should be infused for short periods; attempts should be made to wean the patient from this agent by increasing circulating blood volume if possible and replacing it, when tolerated, with other inotropic agents.

In some patients in cardiogenic shock, the combined use of agents such as isoproterenol and epinephrine or isoproterenol and norepinephrine may be salutary. The vasodilator effect of isoproterenol may counteract some of the peripheral constrictor effects seen with the other catecholamines. Together, they may give the maximal inotropic effect that is sought and thereby increase cardiac output without a massive increase in peripheral resistance. This form of treatment has to be individualized and closely monitored as to the changes in both cardiac output and heart rate, but also to be sure that peripheral vasoconstriction is being relieved by the added isoproterenol.

Many have suggested digitalization in the treatment of low cardiac output subsequent to acute myocardial infarction.[47] In the acutely ill patient, this may be difficult because of associated reduced urinary output and frequent changes in potassium ion concentration. Therefore, we would advocate the use of other inotropic agents until the patient has become more stabilized; we would favor digitalization as a means of more chronic inotropic therapy, particularly after weaning from isoproterenol, from epinephrine or a combination of the two. Even in the presence of severe pulmonary edema, the use of such short-acting inotropic agents as epinephrine or isoproterenol may be more effective. If, however, the pulmonary edema is clinically tolerable and the patient can undergo safely a period of time for digitalization, we would advocate digitalization. Digoxin is the most readily managed agent and should be given in doses up to 1–1.5 mg for the necessary inotropic effect. The dose usually is divided and given over 24–48 hours and maintained with an effective daily supplementary dose.

VOLUME EXPANSION.—Recent studies of the treatment of cardiogenic shock have shown that in the presence of markedly elevated left atrial pressures, volume expansion has little, if any, benefit. In general, in most patients in cardiogenic shock, intravascular volume should be maintained so that left atrial pressure will be at a level of approximately 15 mm Hg. Frequently this measurement is associated with normal or even low central venous pressure. If an increase in cardiac output is achieved by volume expansion and is not associated with a critical decrease in arterial PO_2, volume may be increased. This may be continued as long as it is accompanied by a rise in cardiac output. As volume is added, there is, of course, the risk of pulmonary edema. This form of therapy in association with the use of inotropic agents may allow the achievement of a more efficient state of ventricular contraction and the resolution of cardiogenic shock. The material used for volume expansion ideally should include oncotic and osmotic agents. Most of the patients in chronic failure with severe myocardial disease already will have an increased sodium and fluid load in the body, and further volume might best be handled by administering salt-poor albumin solutions. However, the patient in acute cardiogenic shock may be treated early with plasma, salt-poor albumin or albumin and Ringer's lactate. In some circumstances, whole blood or packed blood cells may be indicated. If the patient being treated for an acute problem has evidence of mitral regurgitation, higher filling pressures may be required to gain satisfactory peripheral perfusion. Over-all, however, increases beyond 20 mm Hg filling pressure in the left heart generally have not been helpful.

TREATMENT OF METABOLIC ACIDOSIS.— If metabolic acidosis is present, the use of sodium bicarbonate should be considered. The deficiency is not in the blood itself but in the capillary perfusion system, with resultant hypoxia of the cells. Sodium bicarbonate may be used in transiently correcting metabolic acidosis, thereby rendering the prescribed pressor agents more effective and myocardial contractility and oxygen transport more normal. However, unless capillary perfusion and transport of oxygen to the individual cells can be restored, the progression of metabolic acidosis will not be corrected. The use of two or three ampules of sodium bicarbonate (14–132 mEq) to correct metabolic acidosis is reasonable. However, large infusions of sodium bicarbonate solutions add a moderately severe amount of sodium to the circulation, which eventually may lead to pulmonary edema and hypernatremia. Again, Cannon[19] stated in his monograph on traumatic shock: "In the treatment of low alkali content of the blood, therefore, the important matter is not to increase the sodium bicarbonate of the blood in the late stages of shock, but to restore early the essential lack—the needed oxygen—by a better blood supply, or, preferably, to prevent reduction of alkali reserve by providing adequate oxygen through early improvement of the circulation."

CONTROL OF HEART RATE.—The development of severe bradyarrhythmias may require mechanical intervention to control the heart rate during shock states. As already mentioned, drugs such as isoproterenol are very effective in increasing heart rate. However, when bradycardia is present in association with ventricular irritability, it may be dangerous to use an agent such as isoproterenol. The use of vagolytic agents such as atropine (dose 1–2 mg intravenously) will help to resolve those arrhythmias related to increased vagal tone.[35] The use of flow-directed transvenous pacing wires,[50] which can be inserted percutaneously through a large needle, has made possible rapid and easy control of many bradyarrhythmias and also control of ventricular rates in the presence of heart block. Once the catheter has been placed either in the atrium or the ventricle of the right heart, electrical pacing can be utilized. (If heart block is present, ventricular pacing is required.) In some circumstances, the placing of a catheter in the right atrium and in the right ventricle and sequential pacing from these sites in order to obtain a more ideal P–R interval has produced an even greater increase in cardiac output than simple atrial or ventricular pacing alone.[21] These wires, once in place within the heart, can be used as monitoring devices to determine the origin of severe tachyarrhythmias.[85] The over-all beneficial result from sequential pacing, however, has not been evident in increased survival.

Because tachyarrhythmias frequently occur in the patient with an acute myocardial infarction, many physicians are justifiably reluctant to use digitalis prophylactically. If these arrhythmias appear, however, and if they are supraventricular in origin, digitalis generally is the ideal agent for their control.[47] Some supraventricular arrhythmias, however, are either poorly responsive or totally unresponsive to digitalization and may require quinidine or beta blocking agents for their suppression. Electrical cardioversion may be required.

Tachyarrhythmias originating from the ventricle are particularly life-threatening and need rapid intervention. These may be precursed by the appearance of ventricular premature contractions. Rare premature ventricular contractions from a single focus generally are not of concern, especially if they are of a chronic nature. However, the appearance of new premature contractions occurring three or more times per minute, or premature contractions occurring from multiple foci, should have careful evaluation and therapy. Early therapy may include the use of lidocaine as an intravenous bolus (1–2 mg/kg), or the use of agents such as procainamide (100–300 mg IV), quinidine (100–200 mg IV) or, in special circumstances, Dilantin (50–200 mg IV). Ventricular tachycardia or persistent ventricular irritability may require the use of intravenous lidocaine either as a bolus or as a constant infusion of 1–4 mg/min. Quinidine, procainamide, bretylium and occasionally Dilantin, alone or in combination, may be necessary to control resistant arrhythmias. Finally, persistent ventricular tachycardia and, in all circumstances, ventricular fibrillation must be treated with electrical defibrillation. Occasionally, when all agents fail to control arrhythmias, circulatory assistance and acute surgical intervention may be indicated.

OXYGEN THERAPY.—The adequacy of oxygenation should be determined; if desaturation has occurred, it should be corrected either by oxygen mask or, in severely obtunded patients, with intubation and respiratory assistance. In many circumstances, positive-pressure resistance may be required throughout expiration in order to overcome the alveolar effects of left atrial hypertension.[9] The acute condition of the cardiac patient may be managed most easily with an endotracheal tube and assisted ventilation utilizing humidified oxygen in concentrations high enough to maintain an arterial PO_2 of 100–150 mm Hg. This treatment also avoids the decreased ventilation associated with pain from areas of trauma. As the patient becomes more awake, he may be sedated with morphine in order to make the endotracheal tube tolerable, or the tube may be removed if his arterial gases show that he is capable of adequate ventilation while breathing unassisted. As the patient is considered for weaning from assisted ventilation, blood arterial gases must be followed closely so that the patient is able to maintain an arterial PO_2 of greater than 80 mm Hg for long periods without CO_2 retention. Once this has been established and the patient has been shown to have a satisfactory vital capacity and tidal volume, he may be extubated and allowed to resume normal breathing. An increased inspired oxygen content may be helpful after extubation for a period of hours to days in order to be sure of the patient's adequate oxygenation. If the endotracheal tube must remain for longer than 48–72 hours, a nasotracheal tube may be substituted. When the period of ventilatory assist may be expected to be greater than 5 days, a tracheostomy should be carried out. (Also see Treatment of Hypoxic Shock, below.)

DIURETICS.—Renal function is dependent on adequate perfusion. When adequate blood volume has been established and maximal myocardial response has been obtained, diuretics may be useful therapy if evidence exists of abnormal renal retention of water in the presence of adequate renal perfusion. Mannitol, an osmotic diuretic (average dose of 12.5–25 gm administered intravenously), has been described as having a specific effect on intrarenal blood flow, thus giving some protection during low perfusion states.[37] Ethacrynic acid and furosemide are two efficient diuretic agents that have been helpful in the treatment of patients in severe cardiogenic shock and pulmonary edema. Because of the ototoxicity associated with ethacrynic acid,[65] furosemide may be preferable as a primary agent. The dose generally is in the range of 20–100 mg; in rare circumstances, up to 1 gm of the drug may be used. However, if patients are not responsive to doses of up to 100 mg, they usually are suffering from either acute tubular necrosis or renal perfusion so low that further diuretic administration will not be useful. Again, it must be emphasized that the measurement of urinary electrolytes and osmolarity, as well as urinary volume, should be carried out frequently. Baseline studies are ideal in this circumstance and would reveal the normal retention of sodium in the patient who either is hyponatremic or has an underperfused kidney with a reduced serum sodium. When the urine volume is low and the patient apparently has adequate intervascular volume, the differential between decreased kidney perfusion with high urine osmolarity and frequently low sodium content can be distinguished from the fixed specific gravity and high sodium and potassium content seen subsequent to acute tubular injury. Diuretics, however, may cloud this picture, and the best time to determine the baseline values is either prior to administration of diuretics or at intervals when a lack of response to those diuretics is evident. In some instances, such as in blunt abdominal trauma or aortic injury, arteriography should be carried out in the oliguric patient to evaluate the patency of the renal vessels and the possibility of direct renal trauma.

ASSISTED CIRCULATION.—Low-output cardiogenic shock associated with loss of compliance of the left ventricle generally is associated with a mortality ranging from 85% to 100%.[71] This is especially true if the previously outlined therapy of volume replacement, pressors, etc. has failed to reverse the shock state within 4–6 hours. Because of this evident high mortality, many groups have been anxious to apply forms of assisted circulation to treat resistant cardiogenic shock.

The most widely used form of assisted circulation is that of external cardiac massage. A vigorous attempt at resuscitation should be made for patients who have arrested secondary to acute myocardial infarction if the arrest has occurred within the preceding few minutes and if evidence exists that cerebral function still may be present. Resuscitation should be carried out, with maintenance of an airway either by mouth-to-mouth breathing or by intubation and positive-pressure breathing. External massage is applied by direct compression over the middle and lower thirds of the sternum at rates sufficient to maintain a peripheral circulation and to keep the pupils of the eyes from dilating. The compression most likely to produce satisfactory peripheral flow is about 80–100 beats per minute. The sternum must be compressed forcibly enough to produce a peripheral arterial pulse but not so forceful as to fracture the ribs and injure abdominal organs. This form of assisted circulation allows time to apply the previously mentioned drug therapy, defibrillation and volume expansion. These interventions may allow the patient to achieve a reasonable level of cardiac function.

The shock state, however, that requires assisted circulation over prolonged periods generally is one of progressive hypotension associated with increasing left atrial pressures, pulmonary edema, hypoxia and progressive acidosis. A number of cardiac assist devices have been applied to patients in this state in an attempt to correct the shock process and, it is hoped, to increase survival. The physiologic principles that these assist devices are based on are as follows: decreased preload, reduced afterload and direct cardiac compression (similar to the effect of external massage). Cardiopulmonary bypass units are the devices used most commonly to decrease cardiac preload. Difficulties with prolonged heparinization and blood element destruction in the required oxygenator of total bypass units has limited their long-term use for shock patients. Recent advances with membrane lung units have made prolonged use more feasible.[14,51,52] Left atrial bypass units (pumping blood from the left atrium to the systemic artery), such as the transseptal left atrial shunt of Dennis[32] or the directly anastomosed pump of De Bakey,[31] have been able to avoid the use of an oxygenator by pumping oxygenated blood from the left atrium, but have had limited clinical use because of persistent problems with clotting and hemolysis. In some circumstances, these units have had physiologic problems similar to those seen with venoarterial pumping (cardiopulmonary bypass). The severely injured left ventricle that is not greatly improved by decreased filling (preload) may be unable to eject against the elevated arterial pressure (afterload) produced by the artificial pump. As long as the mitral valve remains competent, intraventricular pressure then may increase and produce higher O_2 requirements. Because of this problem, direct left ventricular-arterial bypass units have been designed. The closed-chest left ventricle-to-aorta technique[86] has had some clinical application. At present, the direct, implanted left ventricle-to-aorta bypass pump[11] has not been tried clinically but shows promise.

Counterpulsation is another method of partial circulatory assistance. This technique is designed to reduce cardiac afterload. Its application to patients was first reported by Clauss et al.,[23] who used an external pumping system (arterio-arterial), with withdrawal of blood during systole and reinfusion during diastole. Thus, the term "counterpulsation." The theory of counterpulsation is based on the fact that this form of pumping reduces aortic systolic pressure (afterload), thereby lowering peak left ventricular pressure, and delivers more oxygenated blood to the myocardium by increasing diastolic aortic pressure.

Because of difficulties with hemolysis and pressure wave propagation, the application of counterpulsation by arterio-arterial pumping has been greatly limited. During the past 5 years, another form of counterpulsation, intra-aortic balloon pumping, has become widely used.[10,16,48] By the rapid deflation of the balloon within the aorta, just prior to systole, reduction in peak systolic pressure of the left ventricle can be obtained. When the balloon is inflated rapidly at the end of diastole, diastolic augmentation is accomplished and coronary flow can be increased. It is in this circumstance that simultaneously left ventricular oxygen requirements can be reduced and myocardial oxygen delivery increased.

External, synchronous, regional pressure variation (external counterpulsation) has also been developed to treat patients in cardiogenic shock. Soroff et al.[74] have designed a unit that encases the legs in a water jacket, which, when pumped in cycle with the ECG, can produce effective counterpulsation waves in the arterial pressure trace. Encouraging results have been reported employing this technique in a limited number of patients. Since the pump system is noninvasive, early application might be accomplished more readily than with any of the other assist devices.

To evaluate the effectiveness of intra-aortic balloon assist for cardiogenic shock secondary to acute myocardial infarction, we have studied a series of patients in cardiogenic shock secondary to acute myocardial infarction. These patients were managed with pressor agents, electrical pacing, volume expansion, digitalis, diuretics, respiratory assistance and sedation. Patients who failed to respond to this medical regimen had an over-all mortality rate of 100%. Thirty-two similar patients who did not respond to medical treatment were treated with intra-aortic balloon assist. Cardiac index was increased 30%, mean arterial pressure was increased 10% and left atrial pressure was reduced 20%. The over-all survival of these patients was approximately 20%.

Subsequent to this series, a number of patients have undergone cardiac catheterization[54] and surgical procedures that have appeared to significantly increase the over-all survival from refractory cardiogenic shock secondary to acute myocardial infarction.[17, 61, 62] Patients who have failed to improve with balloon assist have undergone cineangiographic evaluation of the coronary circulation and left ventricular contraction. In most cases, the patients then have undergone surgery involving coronary artery bypass grafts, infarct resection, valve replacement or frequently a combination of these procedures.[17] This has produced an approximate 35% survival in this group of patients who have failed to respond to medical therapy and mechanical assist alone.

Detailed study of the patients who have undergone balloon assist have shown that there is a need for early institution of balloon pumping. Prolonged utilization of medical therapy in the patient remaining in shock has led to increased myocardial damage and reduced success of the assist and operative procedures. At present, we believe that the indication for balloon assist is the presence of persistent cardiogenic shock secondary to acute myocardial infarction. To determine this shock state properly, left-sided filling pressures and cardiac outputs must be recorded. A short period of pressor support and volume expansion, where indicated, should be attempted, but if no response has occurred in 2 hours, the balloon assist should be initiated.

The balloon can be easily placed under local anesthesia as long as the patient has adequate femoral vessels. In more than 100 patients in whom the balloon has been tried, only 4 were failures because of inability to pass the balloon catheter retrograde from the femoral artery to the thoracic aorta. Most patients have been anticoagulated with heparin, and this has been supplemented by dextran (25 ml/hr) in order to reduce platelet aggregation. Postoperatively, patients have not required heparin, since dextran alone has been adequate to prevent thrombosis and emboli. Balloon assist has been carried out for periods of up to 14 days, with an average duration of 4 days. At present, only two small emboli have been documented in postmortem studies in these balloon-assist patients. No aortic ruptures have occurred in our series, and no severe trauma to the aorta has occurred. Three instances of elevation of aortic plaques have been found at the time of autopsy. At no time have these dissections been deleterious to the patient. No balloon ruptures have occurred in our patients.

Further application of balloon assist has been made for the patient who is unable to be weaned from cardiopulmonary bypass following heart surgery. We have utilized balloon assist to wean patients who have not responded to long periods of pressor support and partial cardiopulmonary bypass. In those patients who evidence at least regular cardiac contraction and some left ventricular ejection, we have been able to gain over 40% long-term survival.

Thus, intra-aortic balloon assist has become a successful form of therapy for cardiogenic shock. When used alone for acute myocardial infarction, success is limited, but when combined with surgical treatment of the cardiac defect, the rate of success has been reasonably good. Finally, this form of assist can improve the patient's chance of survival after undergoing complex cardiac procedures that have led to poor cardiac function at the time the patient is to come off cardiopulmonary bypass.

TREATMENT OF HYPOXIC SHOCK. — Hypoxia probably is the most common cause of diminished blood pressure in the immediate postoperative period, especially if relaxant anesthetics have been used. Similarly, hypoxia may be a cause of shock in the post-traumatic period, when pain or trauma to the chest cage may restrict normal respiratory exchange. Therapy of this condition entails the same steps that are required in other situations that produce inadequate ventilation: obstructed airway, trauma to the lungs or chest wall, collapse of part or all of one lung, obstruction to pulmonary blood flow and depression of the central respiratory center.

The airway should be maintained by the clearing of secretions and, in the obtunded patient, by an oropharyngeal airway or an endotracheal tube. Adequate chest wall and diaphragmatic force must be proved either by measurement of vital capacity or measurement of inspiratory force. An inspiratory force of 20–25 cm of H_2O should be present in order to maintain adequate exchange. Vital capacity should be at least three times the patient's tidal volume in order to have adequate respiratory reserve.[9] The stability of the chest wall must be maintained; where disrupted, it should be stented internally by direct surgery or a positive-pressure respirator, or externally by sandbags or traction.[70] Usually, positive-pressure respiratory support is preferred. Atelectasis is the most common pulmonary problem seen post-trauma and can lead to marked intrapulmonary shunting and hypoxia.[8] Pulmonary physiotherapy in the cooperative patient or pulmonary physiotherapy and varied positive-pressure respiration in the obtunded patient are most helpful in attempting to expand the collapsed segments. Collapse of the lung from pneumothorax should be corrected by aspiration, tube thoracotomy or both.

Depression of the respiratory center, observed in connection with drug ingestion, anesthetic agents, increased intracranial pressure and hypoxia, requires the use of assisted ventilation. Frequent use of varied increased positive-pressure respirations is a necessary adjunct in order to avoid rapid changes in compliance seen with constant-pressure or constant-volume respirators.[34] Every 30–60 minutes, the patient should be maximally ventilated either manually or with increased volume from the respirator.

The adequacy of ventilation can be estimated by measuring tidal volume and comparing it to the estimated needs from a nomogram.[6, 66] A more exact measure is given by determining arterial blood gases. An arterial Po_2 of 75 mm Hg has been used as a point of satisfactory oxygenation in patients breathing room air. In the absence of intracardiac defects, this level indicates moderate intrapulmonary shunting. Close observation of the arterial Po_2 is most helpful in determining the need for changes in respiratory management. The partial pressure of CO_2 in the arterial blood should be below 45 mm Hg in order to prevent respiratory acidosis and possible narcosis.[9] CO_2 retention usually is not a problem in patients who maintain a satisfactory arterial Po_2 unless the patient has intrapulmonary disease.

Once a patient has been maintained for a prolonged period on a respirator, return to normal respirations must be gradually established by a program of weaning from the respirator. As soon as the change is tolerable, the inspired O_2 concentration should be lowered to levels that will maintain an arterial Po_2 of 100–150 mm Hg; this is desirable in order to avoid changes in the lung associated with prolonged high levels of inspired oxygen partial pressures.[1] Usually a patient should not be tried off assisted respiration if the arterial Po_2 is below 75 mm Hg while the patient is breathing 100% oxygen on the respirator or if his vital capacity is less than 10 ml/kg body weight (approximately twice the patient's predicted tidal volume). If the above criteria have been met and as soon as a stable respiratory situation has been obtained, the patient should be tried off the respirator for short periods—for about 5 minutes once an hour in order for the physician to assess the patient's ventilatory capacities. While off the respirator, the patient should inspire 100% oxygen with high humidification. Again, arterial gas studies should be repeated and unassisted respiratory periods should be prolonged if proper gas exchange is maintained. With rare exception, no patient should be kept off assisted respirations if he is unable to maintain an arterial Po_2 of 60 mm Hg or if acidosis develops.

Great care during this period must be taken to distinguish the inadequate ventilation seen in the apprehensive patient who has become dependent on his respirator from inadequacy that stems from organic problems. The use of mild sedation and much reassurance often can help the apprehensive patient, both by reducing metabolic need associated with agitation and by helping the patient to make more effective respiratory movements.

The tracheostomized patient or the patient with an endotracheal tube needing assisted ventilation requires careful, meticulous care of his respiratory tree. All aspirating equipment should be kept sterile. The occluding cuff on the tube should be deflated at least once an hour, and when inflated again, the pressure used should be just occlusive. There may be some correlation between prolonged cuff inflation (especially during hypotensive periods) and subsequent tracheal stenosis. Newly designed tracheostomy tubes have sought to avoid this with soft occluding balloons.[40] (Further discussion concerning respiratory insufficiency is undertaken in Chapter 43.)

There are some cases of severe pulmonary trauma, or occasions after periods of prolonged respiratory assistance necessitated by the combination of chest and lung trauma, in which recovery with conventional therapy is impossible. These patients may need the application of membrane lung oxygenation. At present, this form of therapy has limited success. The units available clinically have layers of silastic dividers either flat[14, 52] or in the coil[51] that separate the oxygen from the blood. Problems with boundary phenomena and areas of stagnation still reduce the efficiency of the membranes and necessitate large surface units. A greater clinical success probably will be obtained when better forms of membranes are available and when earlier applications of this technique are carried out. Basically, the technique involves using an extracorporeal circuit utilizing a pump head that allows bypass of the pulmonary circuit and oxygenation of the blood through a membrane oxygenator. Such oxygenators are useful because they allow prolonged periods of respiratory support without excessive blood element and blood protein trauma associated with the disk or bubble oxygenator systems. Heparinization of the patient is necessary in this technique, a process that makes its use quite dangerous in the severely traumatized patient who has multiple areas for potential hemorrhage.

TREATMENT OF HYPOVOLEMIC SHOCK.— Hypovolemia is one of the most common problems encountered in traumatized patients. The evident loss of whole blood from open wounds or from the GI tract is readily evident. Hidden losses occurring with ruptured internal organs, such as liver or spleen, and with severe fractures, particularly of the long bones, such as the femur, may be harder to define. Losses of fluid rich in colloid and protein, as seen with external burns and pancreatitis, may not be recorded easily. Such deficits may be anticipated in the burn patient from the extent of the burn. Similarly, the loss of water and electrolytes in the febrile patient can only be estimated. Thus, the traumatized patient may present with severe hypovolemia, which is the interreaction of multiple processes. Correction of this deficit in its simplest form is the replacement of the fluid that is lost. This is most evident in the way a patient's condition can be corrected after the acute loss of 3–4 units of blood, if he receives a very early replacement of a similar volume of whole blood. However, the secondary events occurring soon after the onset of hypovolemia make the therapeutic condition less straightforward to deal with. We can say, then, that the therapy of hypovolemic shock relies on replacing the loss that has occurred, correcting the secondary events that have resulted and controlling the basic process that produced the volume loss.

It is quite evident that the site of hemorrhage should be controlled. External bleeding points should be clamped immediately, or where this is not possible, external compression should be applied to control blood loss. Blood loss into traumatized tissue associated with long bone fractures should be controlled with external splinting of the fracture in order to reduce trauma and bleeding further. When bleeding is progressive and severe, surgical exploration should be performed and the source controlled. The recent advent of specific arteriographic[57] evaluation of bleeding points from the spleen, liver and fracture sites in the pelvis has made it possible to localize moderately active bleeding points and to control these points surgically with greater accuracy than has been seen previously.

In some circumstances, the injection of vasoconstrictor agents or clot[57,69] into small, discrete bleeding arteries may control the bleeding or greatly reduce its rate.

Plasma loss should be contained by applying pressure to the traumatized area, splinting fractures, covering burns and controlling the disease process. Specific water loss may be diminished by controlling the disease process where possible; for example, treating bacterial enteritis with antibiotics and antispasmodics, bowel obstruction with surgical correction or pyrexia with aspirin and external cooling.

VOLUME REPLACEMENT — Whole fresh blood still is the ideal agent for replacing loss in hemorrhagic shock. Properly typed and cross-matched blood is not always available immediately and it may be necessary to use other substances. Type O Rh negative blood with low anti-A titer can be administered until type-specific blood is available. Recent experience has shown the usefulness of frozen blood.[46] When available, frozen blood can be given, with low risk of transfusion reaction and minimal depression of clotting factors. At present, this blood is not widely available and does require a 1–2 hour period of preparation. Even more readily used have been lactated Ringer's solution, dextran, albumin and type-specific plasma.[4]

The rapid infusion of 1–2 liters of lactated Ringer's solution has been found to be an effective measure in determining the amount and rapidity of blood loss.[73] Blood pressure and pulse may stabilize and urine output increase in patients in whom blood loss has not been severe. As the infused fluid diffuses from the intravascular space, hypotension may ensue if blood loss was severe or is continuing. Typed and cross-matched blood, when available, then may be given, since a period of time has been gained for accurate typing and cross matching. Ringer's lactate in combination with albumin or plasma under ideal circumstances may be used to a greater extent than previously has been believed safe. Experience in the battlefields of Vietnam[20] and again in the patient undergoing open heart surgery[15] has shown that low hematocrits in the range of 15–20% will be tolerated readily by patients who can compensate for their decreased circulating oxygen volumes with an increase in cardiac output. Thus, while type-specific blood is being obtained for the young patient who has been severely traumatized and needs rapid replacement of his intravascular volume, he may be maintained easily with a large volume of Ringer's lactate infusion and albumin, reducing the chance of blood reaction and hemolysis that might occur if an improper or poorly cross-matched unit were to be used. However, the severely traumatized older patient may tolerate severe hemodilution poorly if his cardiac compensation already is compromised and he cannot increase his cardiac output sufficiently to compensate for the decreased circulating red cell mass and O_2 capacity reduction.

In some circumstances, a satisfactory volume expansion may be seen with the infusion of high molecular weight dextran (average molecular weight 75,000). The attendant difficulties with clotting when greater than 1 liter is given make this substitute limited in its usefulness.[45] There is disputed evidence as to any added value of low molecular weight (average molecular weight 45,000) dextran in low volume, high hematocrit states. The decreased cellular agglutination observed after its administration may be only a function of its increasing intravascular volume rather than a direct effect on cellular properties.[12, 41] The increase in hematocrit secondary to untreated hemorrhage or plasma loss results in increased blood viscosity. When corrections are made for the reduction in viscosity secondary to plasma volume expansion obtained with dextran infusion, there is little evidence that dextran decreases viscosity specifically.[68]

Stored, type-specific plasma is the ideal replacement fluid for plasma deficits. Its use is associated with a low incidence of hepatitis and allergic and pyrogenic reactions. Limited supply, however, usually makes this an impractical agent where massive replacement is needed. Pooled plasma is more readily available, but the increased risk of hepatitis makes this a somewhat hazardous agent. Albumin has the lowest incidence of associated risks, but its supply is limited and it is expensive.

RENAL PROTECTION. — Rapid volume replacement with restoration of renal circulation is the most effective means of preserving renal function in hypovolemic shock.

When accessible, local renal hypothermia may have a protective effect on renal function.[73] This is a process that is applicable only in special circumstances and as yet is unproved clinically. Experimentally, mannitol infusions have had a protective effect on renal function in kidneys subjected to decreased arterial flow.[37]

STEROIDS. — In simple hemorrhagic shock there had been no proved usefulness of steroids. Occasionally, with prolonged shock secondary to ruptured abdominal aneurysms or other causes, adrenal vein thrombosis may occur with secondary adrenal infarction.[4] This has occurred without any evident associated sepsis. Such a circumstance may be an indication for steroid therapy. In the presence of severe hypovolemic shock, Lillehei et al.[56] and others[27] have reported the usefulness of large doses of steroids (1–2 gm in one dose of methylprednisolone). This thesis is hard to prove but is based on the fact that microcirculatory instability may occur with prolonged shock and steroids act to restore normal capillary permeability and release the severe constriction that has occurred in the pre- and postcapillary bed. At present, opinions concerning the effectiveness of steroids in producing this change are varied. Lillehei also believes that there is a positive inotropic effect of the steroids on the myocardium.[56]

VASOPRESSORS.—Pressor drugs have little usefulness in hypovolemic shock. Generally, patients already are severely vasoconstricted and circulating catechols are elevated during the early shock state. However, in the presence of severe hypovolemic shock, a critical level of perfusion of the brain and heart must be maintained and pressors such as epinephrine or norepinephrine may be used transiently, until circulating blood volume is restored. Also, isoproterenol may be helpful if there is evidence of myocardial depression such as would occur in an older person with coronary disease or in most patients after prolonged hypovolemic shock.

BLOCKING AGENTS.—Restoration of peripheral flow in many instances cannot be accomplished by volume replacement alone. Chlorpromazine[26] and morphine[33] experimentally and clinically have been shown to produce peripheral vasodilatation and increased organ flow. Experimental models have shown increased animal survival following hemorrhagic shock if the animals have been treated with phenoxybenzamine, an adrenergic blocking agent.[5, 80] These vasodilating agents reduce the vasoconstriction that has occurred in the microcirculation—especially in the postcapillary bed. Reduced capillary hydrostatic pressure results and a more normal peripheral circulation and better cellular perfusion are produced.

It must be emphasized that as shock is prolonged there may be secondary effects on all organs. The comments made previously regarding the heart and lungs should be re-emphasized. Evidence of cardiac or respiratory insufficiency persisting after seemingly adequate volume replacement must be evaluated and the problems treated in the manner outlined previously. This rapid deterioration of other organ systems is especially frequent in the older patient with coronary artery disease and chronic pulmonary disease.

TREATMENT OF BACTEREMIC SHOCK.—The treatment of bacteremic shock depends in considerable degree on the infective agent and the site of the infection. Infections, by their injurious effects locally, may lead to shock. Bacterial cholangitis may have the effect of acutely reducing liver excretory function. Bacterial pyelonephritis may have a similar detrimental effect on renal function. Bacterial meningitis may produce cerebrospinal pathology that will lead to coma. These specific deficits, however, are not the usual cause of the events that produce bacteremic shock.

Marked changes in peripheral circulation occur with the release of toxins from bacterial sources. The early response to these toxins is a hyperkinetic state with decreased peripheral resistance.[75, 81] Early therapeutic intervention may arrest this condition. Frequently, however, the process progresses and shock ensues. This state usually is marked by reduced cardiac output, increased peripheral resistance and metabolic acidosis. The pathophysiology depends on the infecting organism. Certain species of gram-positive bacteria, that is, staphylococci and clostridia, produce exotoxins that act directly on the smooth muscles of vessels, resulting in severe vasoconstriction and ischemia. Many gram-negative bacteria, such as *Escherichia coli, Aerobacter aerogenes* and pyocyaneus, produce an endotoxin that, together with plasma factors, results in vasoconstriction directly and possibly also through the release of other vasoactive substances, probably catecholamines. Prolonged vasoconstriction results in peripheral pooling and stagnation of blood, with decreased venous return. Further blood volume loss occurs as a result of increased capillary loss of plasma into the interstitial space. The increased fluid loss across the capillary is thought to be related to increased hydrostatic pressure across the capillary bed. This increased hydrostatic pressure may be related to a difference in response between the pre- and postcapillary sphincters.[55] Loss may also occur due to a direct toxic effect on the capillary wall.

Therapy then must be directed to control of the source of the bacterial organism and toxin and restoration of adequate circulation. When possible, drainage of sepsis with identification of the bacteria is ideal. In many situations, either the condition of the patient will not allow immediate drainage or such drainage is impossible, as in the case of pyelonephritis or bacterial endocarditis.

ANTIBIOTIC THERAPY. — The nature and source of the infection generally determine the type of antibiotic treatment used. Before therapy is initiated, cultures must be taken of blood, urine, sputum and, when possible, of any other suspected areas. Suspected gram-positive infection requires coverage with large doses of penicillin (10–20 million units per day) unless resistant staphylococcal infection is suspected. In that case, oxacillin (6–12 gm per day) or sodium cephalothin is indicated. When gram-negative organisms are suspected, chloromycetin (1–2 gm per day), tetracycline (1–2 gm per day), colistin (1.5–5 mg per kg per day IM only) kanamycin or gentamicin (15 mg per kg per day) are used, depending on the bacterial agent, the age of the patient, the source of the infection or a combination of these factors.[36, 82] Although, ideally, treatment should be for a culture-proved organism, quite frequently time cannot be taken to gain culture identification of an infecting organism. Thus, the infant with severe trauma may warrant coverage of a respiratory infection with an agent that will suppress gram-negative bacteria, whereas an adult may require suppression for a gram-positive infecting agent.

VOLUME THERAPY. — Circulating blood volume should be restored with either Ringer's lactate solution or, in certain conditions in which plasma protein is deficient, with plasma, albumin or a combination of both. Whole blood is not indicated unless there is actual bleeding or pre-existing anemia. Volume therapy should be monitored by measuring urinary output and central venous pressure as well as blood pressure, pulse and respirations. Again, note must be taken of the fact that even in the presence of active infection, indwelling pressure monitoring is necessary. Arterial sampling sites are useful to determine not only blood pressure but serial measurements of pH, PCO_2 and PO_2. Similarly, the Swan-Ganz catheter may be of great benefit, since shock secondary to bacterial agents is seen frequently in the older age groups. It is difficult to carry out proper volume replacement in these patients without knowing the function of their left ventricle. The disease process may be initiated with bacteremia and secondary hypotension due to an infected urinary tract in the older man with prostatism, but his shock state will be determined mainly by myocardial insufficiency secondary to his coronary artery disease. Therefore, in order to be fully cognizant of these factors, filling pressures of the left side of the heart are necessary. Such ventricular failure can occur even in the presence of adequate oxygenation when the challenge of early infection requires a greatly increased cardiac output.

GENERAL MEASURES. — Throughout the period of patient care for problems related to bacteremic shock, careful observation must be made to note aggravating problems that might increase the patient's metabolic requirements. Fever with its accompanying tachycardia may greatly increase the oxygen requirements to a point that might overstrain the patient's ability to oxygenate the arterial blood. Fever can be controlled to some degree by the use of rectal aspirin and exposure of the patient's body surface; if the temperature persists at a level > 103°

F rectally, active cooling with alcohol sponging or a cooling blanket may be indicated. In order to safely carry this out in some patients, they may have to be sedated to prevent severe reactions with shivering, which would obviate the effect of the cooling.

TREATMENT OF NEUROGENIC SHOCK.—Neurogenic shock results from a failure of the proper homeostatic reaction between the central nervous system and the cardiovascular system. This reaction is seen not only in the traumatized patient reacting to his pain and his fears but also in the observer of the accident. A slowed heart rate associated with vagal reflexes may be seen resulting in hypotension and syncope. Usually this condition reverses itself, but when it occurs in the patient who is undergoing treatment for severe trauma, intravenous atropine (1–2 mg) may be necessary to prevent severe prolonged hypotension and hypoxia.

At times, associated with severe trauma to the spinal cord, and observed more frequently with the use of spinal anesthesia, is the paralysis of the sympathetic nervous system to the lower half of the body. This results in a loss of proper vasomotor tone and gradual, and at times severe hypotension. When this becomes prolonged, it should be reversed with the intravenous use of pressor agents, ideally phenylephrine (10 mg per 500 ml) or another peripheral vasoconstrictor,[2] which will act to restore a more physiologic peripheral resistance. Volume replacement may be required during this state because of the pooling of circulating blood volume in the intestinal vasculature and the peripheral veins. The use of volume alone in the correction of this defect may be dangerous, for a volume overload may ensue as normal vasomotor tone returns. This is especially true in the patients who have diminished cardiac function. Such a patient may readily go into pulmonary edema because he cannot easily excrete the free water overload through the kidneys.

A special awareness of loss of peripheral vasomotor tone and vasomotor response should be noted in patients who have been on prolonged drug treatment prior to the time of their trauma. Such drugs as reserpine[2] may deplete the normal stores of catecholamine and blunt a patient's response to a severe stress situation. Similarly, these patients will show a lack of response to drugs such as Aramine, which require endogenous catecholamines as their major intermediary. Therefore, if patients are found to be severely hypotensive, and by history are known to have been on drugs that will affect their peripheral vasomotor tone, early therapy with norepinephrine given intravenously should be carried out to correct any hypotensive state. Again, they must have careful monitoring of their volume replacement during these periods, ideally by a pulmonary wedge pressure or, in most circumstances, by close observation of the central venous pressure. Excessive use of a vasoconstrictor must be avoided to prevent reduced flow to peripheral organs, and this may become evident if urinary flow is decreased despite seemingly adequate volume replacement.

Again, the previously outlined steps in the management of cardiac function, hypoxia and volume replacement may apply to the treatment of neurogenic shock in order to stabilize all organs that are involved.

BIBLIOGRAPHY

1. Ahlsson, W. T. L.: A study on oxygen toxicity at atmospheric pressure, Acta Med. Scand. (supp.) 190:1, 1947.
2. Alper, M. H., Flache, W., and Krayer, O.: Pharmacology of reserpine and its implications for anesthesia, Anesthesiology 24:524, 1963.
3. Artz, C. P.: Volume replacement in shock, Surg. Gynecol. Obstet. 122:112, 1966.
4. Austen, W. G., and Buckley, M. J.: Treatment of various forms of surgical shock, Prog. Cardiovasc. Dis. 10:97, 1967.
5. Aviado, D. M.: Pharmacologic approach to the treatment of shock, Ann. Intern. Med. 62:1050, 1965.
6. Baldwin, E. deF., Cournand, A., and Richards, D. W., Jr.: Pulmonary insufficiency. I. Physiologic classification, clinical methods of

analysis, standard values in normal subjects, Medicine 27:243, 1948.
7. Beecher, H. K. (ed.): *Surgery in World War II: The Physiologic Effects of Wounds* (Washington, D. C.: Office of The Surgeon General, Department of the Army, 1952).
8. Bendixen, H. H.: Atelectasis and shunting, Anesthesiology 25:595, 1964.
9. Bendixen, H. H., Egbert, L. D., Hedley-White, J., Laver, M. B., and Pontoppidan, H.: *Respiratory Care* (St. Louis: The C. V. Mosby Company, 1965).
10. Bergman, D., Kripke, D. C., Cohen, M. N., Laniado, S., and Goetz, R. H.: Clinical experience with the unidirectional dual-chambered intra-aortic balloon assist, Circulation 43(Supp. I):1-82, 1971.
11. Bernhard, W. F., LaFarge, C. G., Kritrilakis, S., and Robinson, T.: Development and evaluation of a left ventricular-aortic assist device. (Artificial Heart Program Conference: Proceedings, Washington, D. C., June 9–13, 1969.) (Washington, D. C.: Government Printing Office, 1969), p. 559.
12. Bernstein, E. F., Emmings, F. G., Mackey, G. C., Castaneda, A., and Varco, R. L.: Effect of low molecular weight dextran on red blood cell change during extracorporeal circulation, Trans. Am. Soc. Artif. Intern. Organs 8:23, 1963.
13. Blalock, A.: Experimental shock: Cause of low blood pressure produced by muscle injury, Arch. Surg. 22:959, 1930.
14. Bramson, M. L., Hill, J. D., Osborn, J. J., and Gerbode, F.: Partial veno-arterial perfusion with membrane oxygenation and diastolic augmentation, Trans. Am. Soc. Artif. Intern. Organs 15:412, 1969.
15. Buckley, M. J., Austen, W. G., Goldblatt, A., and Laver, M. B.: Severe hemodilution and autotransfusion for surgery of congenital heart disease, Surg. Forum 22:160, 1971.
16. Buckley, M. J., Leinback, R. C., Kastor, J. A., Laird, J. D., Kantrowitz, A. R., Madras, P. N., Sanders, C. A., and Austen, W. G.: Hemodynamic evaluation of intra-aortic balloon pumping in man, Circulation 41(Supp. II):II-130, 1970.
17. Buckley, M. J., Mundth, E. D., Daggett, W. M., DeSanctis, R. W., Sanders, C. A., and Austen, W. G.: Surgical therapy for early complications of myocardial infarction, Surgery 70:814, 1971.
18. Burke, J. F., Pontoppidan, H., and Welch, C. E.: High output respiratory failure: An important cause of death ascribed to peritonitis or ileus, Ann. Surg. 158:581, 1963.
19. Cannon, W. B.: *Traumatic Shock* (New York: D. Appleton & Co., 1923).
20. Carey, L. C., Lowery, B. D., and Cloutier, C. T.: Hemorrhagic Shock, in *Current Problems in Surgery* (Chicago: Year Book Medical Publishers, Inc., January, 1971).
21. Chamberlain, D. A., Leinbach, R. C., Vassaux, C. E., Kastor, J. A., DeSanctis, R. W., and Sanders, C. A.: Sequential atrioventricular pacing in heart block complicating acute myocardial infarction, N. Engl. J. Med. 282:577, 1970.
22. Civetta, J. M., Gabel, J. C., and Laver, M. B.: Disparate ventricular function in surgical patients, Surg. Forum 22:136, 1971.
23. Clauss, R. H., Birtwell, W. C., Albertal, G., Lunzer, S., Taylor, W. J., Fosberg, A. M., and Harken, D. E.: Assisted circulation: I. Arterial counterpulsator, J. Thorac. Cardiovasc. Surg. 41:447, 1961.
24. Cloutier, C. T., Lowery, B. D., and Carey, L. C.: Acid-base disturbances in hemorrhagic shock, Arch. Surg. 98:551, 1969.
25. Cohn, J. N., Tristani, F. E., and Khatri, I. M.: Studies in clinical shock and hypotension. VI. Relationship between left and right ventricular function, J. Clin. Invest. 48:2008, 1969.
26. Collins, V. J., Jaffee, R., and Zahony, I.: Shock: A different approach to therapy, Illinois Med. J. 122:350, 1962.
27. Connolly, J. E.: The use of adrenal cortical compounds in hemorrhagic shock, Lancet 79: 460, 1959.
28. Cope, E., and Litwin, S. B.: Contribution of the lymphatic system to the replenishment of the plasma volume following a hemorrhage, Ann. Surg. 156:655, 1962.
29. Dagher, F. J., Lyons, J. H., Finlayson, D. C., Shamsai, J., and Moore, F. D.: Blood Volume Management: A Critical Study, in Welch, C. E. (ed.), *Advances in Surgery* (Chicago, Year Book Medical Publishers, Inc., 1965), Vol. 1, p. 69.
30. Deavers, S., Smith, E. L., and Huggins, R. A.: Critical role of arterial pressure during hemorrhage in the dog on the release of fluid in the circulation and trapping of red cells, Am. J. Physiol. 195:73, 1958.
31. De Bakey, M. E., Liotta, D., and Hall, C. W.: Left Heart Bypass Using an Implantable Blood Pump, in *Mechanical Devices to Assist the Failing Heart* (Washington, D. C.: National Academy of Sciences, 1966), p. 223.
32. Dennis, C., Hall, D. P., Moreno, J. R., and Senning, A.: Left atrial cannulation without thoracotomy for total left heart bypass, Acta Chir. Scand. 123:267, 1962.
33. Eckenhoff, J. E., and Oech, S. R.: The effects of narcotics and antagonists upon respiration and circulation in man, Clin. Pharmacol. Ther. 1: 483, 1960.
34. Egbert, L. D., Laver, M. B., and Bendixen, H. H.: Intermittent deep breaths and compliance during anesthesia in man, Anesthesiology 24: 57, 1963.
35. Eger, E. I.: Atropine, scopolamine and related compounds, Anesthesiology 23:365, 1962.
36. Feingold, D. S.: Antimicrobial chemotherapeutic agents: The nature of their action and selective toxicity, N. Engl. J. Med. 269:900, 957, 1963.
37. Flores, J., DiBona, D. R., Beck, C. H., and Leaf, A.: The role of cell swelling in ischemic renal damage and the protective effect of hypertonic solute, J. Clin. Invest. 51:118, 1972.
38. Forrester, J. S., Diamond, G., McHugh, T. J., and Swan, H. J. C.: Filling pressures in the right and left sides of the heart in acute myocardial infarction, N. Engl. J. Med. 285:190, 1971.
39. Friedberg, C. K.: *Diseases of the Heart* (3d ed.; Philadelphia: W. B. Saunders Company, 1966), p. 459.
40. Geffin, B., Grillo, H. C., Cooper, J. D., and Pontoppidan, H.: Stenosis following trache-

ostomy for respiratory care, JAMA 216:1984, 1971.
41. Gelin, L. E.: Disturbance of flow properties of blood and its counter-action in surgery, Acta Chir. Scand. 122:287, 1961.
42. Hardaway, R. M.: Clinical management of shock, Milit. Med. 134:643, 1969.
43. Hardaway, R. M., Brune, W. H., Greever, E. F., Burns, J. W., and Mock, H. P.: Studies on the role of intravascular coagulation in irreversible hemorrhagic shock, Ann. Surg. 155:241, 1962.
44. Harkin. H. N.: Hypovolemic Shock, in Moyer, C. A., et al. (eds.), *Surgery, Principles and Practice* (3d ed.; Philadelphia: J. B. Lippincott Company, 1965) p. 124.
45. Howard, J. M., et al.: Studies of dextrans of various molecular sizes, Ann. Surg. 143:369, 1956.
46. Huggins, C. E.: Frozen blood. Ann. Surg. 160:643, 1964.
47. Hurst, J. W., and Logue, R. B.: *The Heart* (2d ed.; New York: McGraw-Hill Book Company, 1970), p. 548.
48. Kantrowitz, A., Tjonneland, S., Ereed, P. S., Phillips, S. J., Butner, A. N., and Sherman, J. L, Jr.: Initial clinical experience with intra-aortic balloon pumping in cardiogenic shock, JAMA 203:113, 1968.
49. Kellermeyer, R. W., and Grahan, R. C., Jr.: Kinins—possible physiologic and pathologic roles in man, N. Engl. J. Med. 279:754, 1968.
50. Kimball, J., and Killip, T.: A simple bedside method for transvenous intracardiac pacing, Am. Heart J. 70:35, 1965.
51. Kolobow, T., Zapol, W. M., Sigman, R. L., and Pierce, J.: Partial cardiopulmonary bypass lasting up to seven days in alert lambs with membrane lung blood oxygenation, J. Thorac. Cardiovasc. Surg. 60:781, 1970.
52. Lande, A. J., Fillmore, S. J., Subramanian, V., Tiedemann, R. N., Carlson, R. G., Block, J. A., and Lillehei, C. W.: Twenty-four hour venous arterial perfusions of awake dogs with a simple membrane oxygenator, Trans. Am. Soc. Artif. Intern. Organs 15:181, 1969.
53. Lappas, D., Lell, W. A., Gabel, J. C., Civetta, J. M., and Lowenstein, E.: Indirect measurement of left atrial pressure in surgical patients: A comparison of pulmonary capillary wedge and pulmonary artery diastolic to left atrial pressure, Anesthesiology, 38:294, 1973.
54. Leinbach, R. C., Mundth, E. D., Dinsmore, R. E., Harthorne, J. W., Buckley, M. J., Kantrowitz, A., Austen, W. G., and Sanders, C. A.: Selective coronary and left ventricular cineangiography during intra-aortic balloon assist for cardiogenic shock, Am. J. Cardiol. 26:644, 1970.
55. Lewis, D. H., and Mellander, S.: Competitive effects of sympathetic control and tissue metabolites on resistance and capacitance vessels and capillary filtration in skeletal muscle, Acta Physiol. Scand. 56:162, 1962.
56. Lillehei, R. C., Langerbeam, J. K., and Rosenberg, J. C.: The Nature of Irreversible Shock, in Bock, K. D. (ed.), *Shock. Pathogenesis and Therapy. An International Symposium* (Berlin: Springer-Verlag, 1962), p. 106.
57. Margolies, M. N., Ring, E. J., Waltman, A. C., Kerr, W. S., Jr., and Baum, S.: Arteriography to manage hemorrhage from pelvic fractures, N. Engl. J. Med. 287:317, 1972.
58. Migone, L.: Metabolic Aspects of Shock, in Bock, K. D. (ed.), *Shock. Pathogenesis and Therapy. An International Symposium* (Berlin: Springer-Verlag, 1962) p. 76.
59. Moore, F. D.: *Metabolic Care of the Surgical Patient* (Philadelphia: W. B. Saunders Company, 1959), p. 154.
60. Moyer, C. A.: *Surgery, Principles and Practice* (Philadelphia: J. B. Lippincott Company, 1961) p. 301.
61. Mundth, E. D., Buckley, M. J., Leinbach, R. C., DeSanctis, R. W., Sanders, C. A., Kantrowitz, A., and Austen, W. G.: Myocardial revascularization for the treatment of cardiogenic shock complicating acute myocardial infarction, Surgery 70:78, 1971.
62. Mundth, E. D., Yurchak, P. M., Buckley, M. J., Leinbach, R. C., Kantrowitz, A. R., and Austen, W. G.: Circulatory assistance and emergency direct coronary artery surgery for shock complicating acute myocardial infarction, N. Engl. J. Med. 283:1382, 1970.
63. Page, D. L., Caulfield, J. B., Kastor, J. A., et al.: Myocardial changes associated with cardiogenic shock, N. Engl. J. Med. 285:133, 1971.
64. Parsons, E., and Phemister, D. B.: Haemorrhage and "shock" in traumatized limbs. Experimental study, Surg. Gynecol. Obstet. 51:196, 1930.
65. Pillay, V. K. G., Schwartz, F. D., Aimi, K., and Kark, R. M.: Transient and permanent deafness following treatment with ethacrynic acid in renal failure, Lancet 1:77, 1969.
66. Radford, E. P., Jr.: Ventilation standards for use in artificial respiration, J. Appl. Physiol. 7:451, 1955.
67. Rahimtoola, S. H., Loeb, H. S., Ehsani, A., Sinno, M. Z., Chuquimia, R., Lal, R., Rosen, K. M., and Gunnar, R. M.: Relationship of pulmonary artery to left ventricular diastolic pressures in acute myocardial infarction, Circulation 46:283, 1972.
68. Replogle, R. L., Kundler, H., and Gross, R. E.: Studies on the hemodynamic importance of blood viscosity, J. Thorac. Cardiovasc. Surg. 50:658, 1965.
69. Rosch, J., Dotter, C. T., and Brown, M. J.: Selective arterial embolization: A new method for control of acute gastrointestinal bleeding, Radiology 102:303, 1972.
70. Scannell, J. G.: Chest Wall, Lungs and Mediastinum, in Warren, R. (ed.), *Surgery* (Philadelphia: W. B. Saunders Company, 1963), p. 598.
71. Scheidt, S., Aschein, R., and Killip, T.: Shock after acute myocardial infarction: A clinical and hemodynamic profile, Am. J. Cardiol. 26:556, 1970.
72. Shires, T., and Carrico, C. J.: Current Status of the Shock Problem, in *Current Problems in Surgery* (Chicago: Year Book Medical Publishers, Inc., March, 1966).
73. *Ibid.*, p. 3.
74. Soroff, H. S., Giron, F., Fuiz, U., Birtwell, W. C., Hirsch, L. J., and Deterling, R. A., Jr.: Physiologic support of heart action, N. Engl. J. Med. 280:693, 1969.
75. Spink, W. W.: Pathogenesis and Therapy of Shock due to Infection: Experimental and

Clinical Studies, in Bock, K. D. (ed.), *Shock. Pathogenesis and Therapy. An International Symposium* (Berlin: Springer-Verlag, 1962), p. 225.
76. Suzuki, F., Baker, R. J., and Shoemaker, W. C.: Red cell and plasma volume alterations after hemorrhage and trauma, Ann. Surg. 160:263, 1964.
77. Swan, H. J. C., Ganz, W., Forrester, J., Marcus, H., Diamond, G, and Chonette, D.: Catheterization of the heart in man with use of a flow-directed balloon-tipped catheter, N. Engl. J. Med. 283:447, 1970.
78. Thal, A. P., Brown, E. B., Jr., Hermreck, A. S., and Bell, H. H.: *Shock* (Chicago: Year Book Medical Publishers, Inc., 1971).
79. Thal, A. P., Wilson, R. F., Kalfuss, L., and Andre, J.: The Role of Metabolic and Humoral Factors in Irreversible Shock, in Mills, L. C., and Moyer, J. H. (eds.), *Shock and Hypotension: Pathogenesis and Treatment* (New York: Grune & Stratton, Inc., 1965).
80. Vick, J. A., Ciuckta, H. P., and Menckel, J. H.: Vasodilator therapy in acute hemorrhagic shock, Circ. Res. 16:58, 1965.
81. Weil, M. H., and Spink, W. W.: Shock syndrome associated with bacteremia due to gram negative bacilli, Arch. Intern. Med. 101:184, 1958.
82. Weinstein, L.: Antibiotics, in Goodman, L. S., and Gilman, A. (eds), *The Pharmacological Basis of Therapeutics* (3d ed.; New York: The Macmillan Company, 1965).
83. Werle, E.: *Kallikrein, Kallidin and Related Substances: Polypeptides which Affect Smooth Muscles and Blood Vessels* New York: Pergamon Press, 1960).
84. Williams, J. A., Grable, E., Howard, F. A., and Fine, J.: Blood losses and plasma volume shifts during and following major surgical operations, Ann. Surg. 156:648, 1962.
85. Yurchak, P. M.: Personal communication.
86. Zwart, H. H. J., Kralios, A., Kwan-Gett, C. S., Backman, D. K., Fotte, J. L., Andrade, J. D., Carlton, F. M., Schoonmaker, F., and Kolff, W. J.: First clinical application of transarterial closed-chest left ventricular (TaCLV) bypass, Trans. Am. Soc. Artif. Intern. Organs 16:386, 1970.

12 | Trauma and the Anesthetist

LAWRENCE D. EGBERT

THE INJURED PATIENT often presents an unstable, rapidly changing, unpredictable situation. Anesthetists spend most of their time creating or adjusting unstable physiologic systems and can be most useful in a major emergency. Two textbooks have been written in the past decade about trauma and emergency surgery,[1,2] and we will not spend this chapter paraphrasing them. Instead, some ways will be suggested in which an anesthetist can join in the care of the severely injured patient. For the severely injured patient, perhaps unconscious or with a crushed chest or in shock, the assistance of an anesthetist should be requested early.

RESUSCITATION

Immediate evaluation of the airway is essential. Chest movements do not mean that the airway is patent, nor that air is moving into and out of the lungs. Put your hand or your face over the patient's mouth or your ear on his chest. If you do not feel any air moving or do not hear the sound of air moving, assume that no air is being ventilated. If the patient moves his respiratory muscles but no air, he is obstructed. Pull the mandible forward to open the airway. Suction out the mucus, blood or vomitus or any teeth or foreign materials. If there is no suction machine immediately available, turn the patient on his side, tilt the head down and manually remove any obstructing substances. The patient's airway must be opened so that ventilation can occur. Providing an open airway and alveolar ventilation has priority over all diagnostic and therapeutic procedures.

The patient may be obstructed or may be both apneic and obstructed. For the apneic patient, ventilation must be provided. This is done by machine, bag and mask, mouth to mask, mouth to mouth or mouth to nose. Do whichever is fastest. After some ventilation is provided, the urgency is less and further evaluation is possible.

Ventilation must be provided before cardiac massage, since the patient gains little from hypoxic blood being circulated.

Diagnosis of the presence or absence of circulation is made quickly by palpating the carotid or femoral artery or auscultating the chest. If circulation is inadequate, cardiac massage should be instituted immediately after ventilation has been started. Inadequate circulation is present if the brain is not receiving enough oxygenated blood. Thus, the patient who is exsanguinated must be treated as rapidly as the patient who has been electrocuted. Success in restoring adequate circulation is confirmed when the patient awakens.

Mouth-to-mouth resuscitation and external cardiac massage techniques have been well described, but many physicians are grossly lacking in these skills. It is essential to develop such skills, and practice is required. Skills in resuscitation and cardiac massage should be reviewed and practiced at least every few months. The American Heart Association recommends practice at cardiopulmonary resuscitation at least once a year.

After resuscitation has been started, continued evaluation is essential. Is the airway free and ventilation easy? Is the tidal volume adequate? Estimate this by listening to his chest, by watching the chest move with artificial ventilation, by measuring the exhaled volume of gas with a meter or by measurement of arterial P_{CO_2}. As the situation becomes more stable, more accurate measurements can be made. If resuscitation has been adequate and the injury not too severe, it may be possible to have the treatment completed before ever having the opportunity to insert an intravenous needle, but we should be prepared to insert an arterial needle.

You will note the delay in mentioning tracheal intubation. After ventilation and cardiac massage are started, intubation may be performed. Resuscitation usually forces large amounts of air into the stomach, which inhibits adequate ventilation and increases the likelihood of regurgitation later; intubation, therefore, is extremely important. Intubation must be done as soon as possible *after* starting ventilation and cardiac message.

Other problems then must be considered. Does the patient have a pneumothorax, a hemothorax or a tension pneumothorax? If percussion reveals a pneumothorax, a needle and, later, a catheter will remove the air. A tension pneumothorax is rapidly aggravated by positive-pressure ventilation. If there is an open chest wound, positive-pressure ventilation, preferably through an endotracheal tube, is essential. How stable is the chest wall? The positive-pressure ventilation will help stabilize broken ribs (see Chapter 43).

In the severely injured patient, a large-bore intravenous needle is mandatory. Most people prefer plastic catheters to ordinary steel needles, since plastic needles are much less likely to become dislodged. A large needle will permit rapid administration of fluids and restoration of blood volume. As resuscitation proceeds, proper fluids should be administered, but, in the emergency ward, saline, then plasma may be given immediately to restore circulation.

EVALUATION OF THE PATIENT

We need certain information concerning the patient who is to have an emergency operation. We need to know the patient's ability to cope with a circulatory challenge from anesthesia, from surgical manipulations, from changes in position and from further losses of blood. To depend on heart rate and arterial blood pressure to guide us in estimating blood volume is hazardous. Patients are notorious for having a normal blood pressure and then collapsing when anesthesia is induced. Inserting a long plastic catheter into the superior vena cava via the antecubital or external jugular vein to measure the central venous pressure increases one's ability to estimate the capabilities of the circulatory system. This is done by connecting the long catheter to a meter, most simply a column of heparinized saline with an end open to atmospheric pressure. A ruler is placed behind the column of saline with the zero point at the level of the right atrium. If the stopcock is turned to open the flow of saline from the tubing in front of the ruler and blocking flow from the reservoir bottle, flow will stop when the column of saline balances the pressure in the superior vena cava. The central venous pressure is read in centimeters of water from the level of the saline. As blood and fluid are replaced, the CVP gives valuable information that one is or is not overloading the circulation.

Hematocrit is useful after the patient

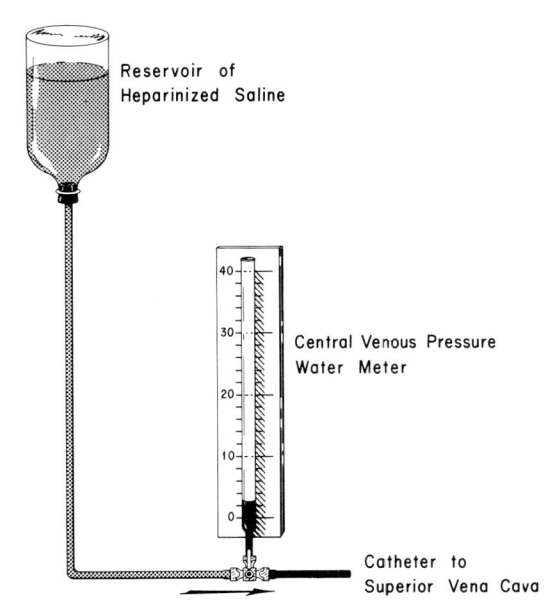

Fig. 12-1.—Central venous pressure.

has stabilized but is virtually useless as an estimate of blood volume when active bleeding is occurring. Actual measurement of the blood volume may be helpful but is time consuming, difficult and not easily available for the emergency room patient.

It is important for the anesthetist to know if the patient still is bleeding. The central venous pressure, the heart rate, the arterial blood pressure and the hematocrit, if he has not been bleeding for several hours, should be known. Finally, an estimate should be made of the possibilities for further bleeding.

Attempts should be made to determine past history, so that pertinent problems can be treated before operation. The closer one can arrive at an elective situation the better. However, when this is not possible, the anesthetist should be involved in the decision to compromise the "ideal" situation. If operation is so urgent that it is not possible to obtain the central venous pressure, hematocrit and other important information, the anesthetist should share the sense of urgency. Rushing to operate when careful consideration of other medical lesions would be to the patient's benefit is, of course, inadvisable. Too often the anesthetist appears to be obstructing the progress of care because he has not been involved early enough and does not share the surgeon's sense of the urgent need to operate.

In Chapter 43 are discussed the tests useful to evaluate the respiratory system. It should be stressed that a static measurement, for example, tidal volume or arterial PCO_2, may not give much information concerning what will happen the next moment, whereas a capacity measurement, such as vital capacity or the 1-second timed expiratory capacity or inspiratory force pressure, all rather easily measured, will give an idea of the patient's ability to cope with his environment and therefore help more in predicting what the blood gases will be an hour from now. Anything that helps predict what will occur next is useful in the emergency situation.

Whenever possible, *emergency operations should be made to look like elective operations.*

SPECIFIC ANESTHETIC PROBLEMS

Emergency operations present several special problems for the anesthetist. The circulatory system often is unstable. Food or blood often is in the stomach. The patient is terrified. Other diseases may be present that we are unaware of. Diseases that are likely to create anesthetic complications include most heart diseases, but especially coronary artery disease, aortic valvar disease, ventricular arrhythmias, congestive failure and hypertension. Respiratory diseases, such as asthma, upper respiratory tract infections, chronic bronchitis or emphysema, are common and complicate anesthetic management. Anemia, diabetes and many endocrine diseases often complicate anesthesia. The anesthetist should treat the emergency patient with the utmost respect and try to be prepared for any contingency.

THE UNSTABLE CARDIOVASCULAR SYSTEM

Rapid bleeding may make replacement difficult, and may continue so that so much blood is required, the risk of repeated transfusion may offset the risk of operating under less than optimal conditions. Hematocrit must be monitored repeatedly, as well as heart rate, arterial blood pressure, central venous pressure and urine output. Blood and plasma should be available during induction of anesthesia. An assistant to monitor and help transfuse the patient during this dangerous time is essential. Many of these patients are acidotic (pH of bank blood is 6.75–6.80; PCO_2 of bank blood is approximately 140 mm Hg). Tissue perfusion, including liver and kidney, is poor. It has been shown that when transfusion has to proceed at the rate faster than 100 ml per minute, the mortality rate is very high and usually is higher than we would anticipate from the injury alone.[1]

The person in shock reduces his circulation to all less-vital organs. The percentage of circulation that goes to the brain and the heart may be considerably higher than in the same person when he has a normal blood volume. The sympathetic nervous system is stimulated by the lower pressure in the baroreceptors and is producing large amounts of norepinephrine. Blood pressure thus is maintained to perfuse the brain and the heart. Two points emerge in preparing this type of patient for anesthesia. First, most of the anesthetic agent will go to the brain and the heart whereas in the patient with a normal blood volume, dilution occurs, so that the concentration of drug that enters the coronary and cerebral vessels is much less than in the shocked patient. Thus, anesthetic doses should be reduced in the patient in shock.

In shock, drugs that reduce sympathetic tone should be administered only with great caution, if at all. Anesthesia with thiopental, halothane or spinal block may depress sympathetic reflexes so that the precarious balance of the circulation changes and the patient's condition deteriorates *rapidly*. However, the administration of cyclopropane, which stimulates the sympathetic nervous system, often will permit the further loss of blood without much change in the vital signs that the anesthetist is using to estimate the state of the circulation. At the end of the operation, when cyclopropane is discontinued, the circulation may collapse.

INDUCTION OF ANESTHESIA

The speed of induction of anesthesia is important. Rapid induction reduces the patient's ability to cope with the changes imposed by anesthesia. For the shocked patient, most anesthetists use a slow induction of anesthesia with an anesthetic agent that is rapidly reversible. If this is cyclopropane, after the anesthetic is stabilized with an endotracheal tube inserted and the various measuring devices attached and functioning, an agent that dilates the vascular bed may be used if simultaneously the rate of transfusion is increased. Monitoring the central venous pressure reduces the hazard of this change. Anesthetics that dilate the vascular bed are halothane, barbiturates and morphine, with or without curare. Morphine has a real advantage in dilating the vascular space, since it does not depress the myocardium. Extreme care should be used if spinal anesthesia is planned, because of the dilatation of the peripheral vascular bed with precipitous shock if blood volume is low.

The slow induction of anesthesia recommended for the shocked patient is hazardous in the patient with a full stomach. If general anesthesia is necessary in the shocked patient who also has a full stomach, we need to balance the risk of the shock with the risk of vomiting and aspirating. We need to consider the risk of a rapid induction of anesthesia on the circulatory system with the sudden sympathetic nervous system effects and either raising or lowering blood pressure excessively.

THE FULL STOMACH

The vast majority of patients who have been injured have food in their stomachs. Normally, an adult empties his stomach in 2½–6 hours. When he is in pain or is frightened or has received a narcotic, the emptying time is greatly prolonged. We prefer that the patient not be operated on until 4 hours after he has eaten. Since exceptions are common, this principle is a guide only. Many patients undergo rapid anesthetic induction despite a markedly unstable circulatory system, simply because of a concern that the patient will vomit and aspirate. There is no simple rule here. If the patient needs an operation immediately, the risks are real but must be accepted. Nevertheless, we must remind ourselves not to hurry into operations that could be delayed until the patient is made comfortable, shock is treated with adequate blood replacement, the general condition has stabilized, and he has emptied his stomach.

The stomach can be emptied artificially. Insertion of a gastric tube may empty the stomach but cannot be relied on to do so. Even if the insertion of the tube has made the patient vomit, we cannot be certain that the stomach is emptied. Likewise, administration of apomorphine does not guarantee complete emptying.

Pressure applied on the cricoid cartilage to keep the gastric contents in the esophagus while the endotracheal tube is being inserted may help prevent regurgitation and aspiration. However, rupture of the esophagus is a possible result of this maneuver. Some anesthetists prefer to sit the patient up, which will require more pressure to move the stomach contents toward the pharynx, whereas others lower the head so that if the stomach contents enter the pharynx, they do not fall into the trachea. Most anesthetists attempt to insert an endotracheal tube rapidly, which often can be done before the patient can vomit. The cuff on the tube then must be inflated immediately.

However, the safest technique remains regional anesthesia. For general anesthesia, endotracheal intubation while the patient is awake is least likely to allow aspiration. Although this may be a painful and unpleasant experience for the patient, it is well worth the discomfort in many emergency situations.

If there is vomiting during the induction of general anesthesia, a powerful and carefully tested suction machine used promptly and properly will make actual drowning rare. After vomiting, severe laryngospasm usually is seen if gas induction is employed. Postoperative tracheitis, bronchitis and pneumonitis often result, especially if the patient is undergoing abdominal or thoracic operations, where his ability to cough and breathe deeply is limited (see Chapter 43).

In such a patient requiring general anesthesia, we are forced to accept the real hazard of aspiration of gastric contents. In the traumatized patient, who may be totally uncooperative and who cannot be operated on under regional anesthesia, endotracheal intubation while he is awake may be necessary.

NEUROLOGIC TRAUMA

If the unconscious patient is not breathing adequately, he must be assisted. The airway must be cleared. The vigor of the patient's reflexes should be tested. The cough reflex can be evaluated by catheterizing the patient's trachea. The patient's ability to clear his airway can be measured by the use of the inspiratory force meter. This is done simply by briefly obstructing the airway and measuring the negative pressure that the patient creates. The airway should be obstructed for this test just after the patient finishes exhalation. Do not obstruct him for more than 1 minute. The lowest pressure that the patient creates out of 5 consecutive attempted breaths while

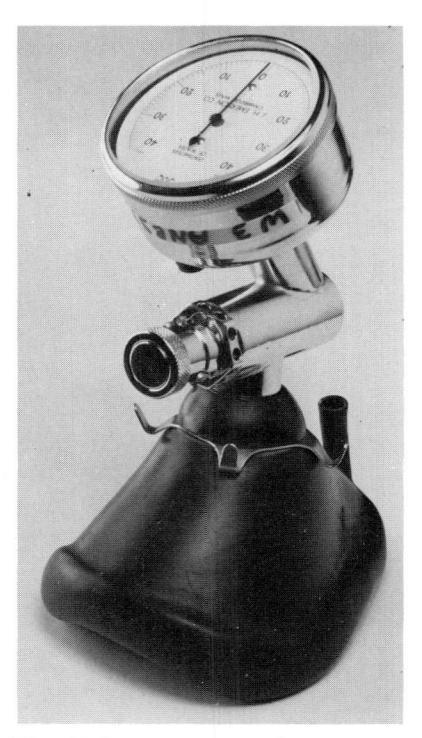

Fig. 12-2. — Inspiratory force meter.

totally obstructed is used. Patients may have a tidal volume sufficient to maintain normal blood gases, but only be strong enough to create 5 cm of H_2O negative pressure when obstructed. Needless to say, the patient who can neither cough well nor take large inspirations is quite likely to become hypoxic in a short period, and will need assisted respirations, added oxygen and careful maintenance of a clear airway by aspiration of foreign material and secretions at regular intervals. A patient, although unconscious but with an inspiratory force of more than 20 or 30 cm H_2O, will need less care of his upper airway.

Anesthetic care of the neurologic patient is complex. If the patient is unconscious, the administration of succinylcholine and intubation, using a coiled-wire endotracheal tube, will permit operation. Local anesthetic may be sufficient for the first part of an operation for subdural hematoma, but the anesthetist must be prepared in the event the patient wakes up in the middle of the procedure. General anesthesia should be with agents that permit use of the cautery, although many emergency neurosurgical procedures can be carried out without cautery if necessary. If cyclopropane is required in shock from blood loss, the cautery may not be used. Halothane now is being utilized for many intracranial problems requiring emergency operation. It has the advantage of relatively rapid reversibility by hyperventilation. However, increased cerebral blood flow with this agent can result in increased cerebral edema. Methohexital and nitrous oxide allow ready reversibility but maintenance of anesthesia is more complicated. The anesthetic is more likely to be marred by coughing and straining. Narcotics have the well-known disadvantage of depression of respiration, removing what may be a crucial sign of changing intracranial pressure.

At the end of any neurosurgical operation, the circulatory and respiratory systems must be carefully evaluated as to ability to cope with the vicissitudes of the postoperative state. Will the patient need constant respiratory care, occasional checking or is he able to take care of his respiratory needs himself?

EYE, EAR AND MAXILLOFACIAL TRAUMA

Eye or ear trauma unaccompanied by other lesions can be handled by the anesthetist in a manner similar to the management of elective operations.

With facial injuries, several problems appear. Most surprising is the amount of bleeding that can occur and not be appreciated. The patient may have swallowed large quantities of blood, gone into shock and been treated for this, then vomit and aspirate the blood during the induction of anesthesia. Facial edema may be massive. The combination of face and neck swelling, plus facial fractures, may obstruct the patient's airway. These patients often are hypoxic. Great effort is required for breathing and the airway must be improved immediately. Inserting the airway may be very difficult. This should not require general anesthesia; local is much safer. The anesthetist must maintain his skill at blind nasotracheal intubation, which is required frequently in the patient with facial injuries.

If the trachea has been lacerated, the airway will be obstructed partially by blood. The trachea and bronchi need to be cleared. A coiled-wire endotracheal tube should be inserted, similar to a tracheostomy, while the neck is prepared for operation. Later, for repair of the trachea, a fresh coiled-wire tube may be inserted through the larynx into the wound, so that the surgeon then can direct it farther into the distal portion of the trachea. The trachea then may be repaired over the tube.

After initial evaluation in the emergency ward, we need to check and recheck the patient's condition. The frequency of checking depends on the rate at which the patient is changing. If the patient is very unstable, he will need continual reevaluation. Also, if he is unstable, postoperative care will be different. (Refer to the section on Resuscitation at the beginning of this chapter and to Chapter 43.)

Often we can make predictions about what will happen in the hours and days postoperatively. We can predict, for example, that many patients who have a ruptured bowel will need respiratory assistance during the postoperative period, despite normal lungs preoperatively. Knowing this, large doses of morphine and curare may be used during the anesthesia, because later control of ventilation will be facilitated. However, if it is determined that the patient will be breathing normally postoperatively, an anesthetic agent should be used that does not last as long and which can be removed more easily. Measurement of inspiratory force, tidal volume and vital capacity and testing of reflex activity will help us to decide when the patient is recovered from the anesthetic and whether he is able to take care of his own respiration or requires respiratory assistance. In the elderly patient or the patient in shock, those severely injured will be more likely to require postoperative respiratory support. Postoperatively, periodic testing of Pa_{CO_2}, Pa_{O_2} and pH, measured with the patient breathing spontaneously but with the endotracheal tube still in place, will help decide when to remove the tube and when to allow the patient to breathe spontaneously. Normal Pa_{CO_2} is from 38 to 42 mm Hg; pH ranges from 7.36 to 7.44. Estimates of physiologic shunting, using Pa_{CO_2}, are extremely useful in evaluating the recovery of the respiratory system.

PSYCHOLOGIC PROBLEMS

Anesthesia is administered to allow the patient to avoid the pain and shock of surgical manipulations. Each physician should recognize the severe emotional stress that the trauma imposes. One moment the patient is active and healthy and the next he is helpless and in agony, dependent on strangers for his life, stunned by the unknown and possibly devastating outcome of his injury. Most patients consider major traumatic experiences in the same way they consider facing death; they *are* facing death.

A major difference between emergency and elective operations is that patients who are awaiting elective operations have had some time to organize their thoughts. They can choose a physician they trust. They can select the hospital and arrange their affairs. They have the opportunity to do the necessary work of worrying. The emergency patient has little or no opportunity to do any of this. He is far more likely to be left with psychic scars than the elective patient. The emergency patient is confronted with frantic activity of many unknown people. He sees and feels the concern and the doubts of his attendants.

Whenever possible, we should realize that the emergency patient usually will benefit by spending some time at this work of worrying. He will profit by knowing what is going on, by finding out where he is, who is taking care of him, what he should be doing to help, what will hurt and what will not and what predictions are being attempted about what may happen over the next few hours or days.

If possible, we might even consider delaying the operation for a short time so that the patient can get information and make decisions concerning his affairs and his family, thus giving him a few moments to adjust psychologically in this time of crisis.

TREATMENT OF PAIN IN THE TRAUMATIZED PATIENT

The amount of narcotics required depends on the nature of the lesion, on the nature of the patient and on the physician-patient relationship. The patient in shock will have a poor perfusion of skeletal muscle, and intramuscular injection of morphine might not be effective. When the shock is improved suddenly, the patient may have a massive effect from the morphine, which has been administered over the past several hours. Intravenous injections of small doses of narcotics are far better, and a therapeutic dose can be achieved gradually.

Before a restless patient is given morphine, it should be determined that the restlessness is not due to hypoxia, CNS injury, shock or syncope. In each of these situations, the restlessness will become less, but at the risk of aggravating the underlying problem. Oxygen may be used to reduce the confusion of the hypoxic patient. Local infiltration may reduce pain. Axillary block for the upper extremity, epidural or femoral-sciatic nerve block for the lower extremity and intercostal nerve blocks for trunk pain often are effective. If this is possible, real benefit will result, as these methods are far less likely to cause respiratory and circulatory depression than are narcotics.

CONCLUSIONS

In the care of the severely traumatized patient, conditions often are unstable and unpredictable. These patients present a real challenge, and we must be prepared to cope with a rapidly changing situation. Often immediate operation is required to correct the basic lesion, and we are forced to operate with less than complete knowledge and preparation of the patient. The incidence of operative and postoperative anesthetic complications is high. To give us the best chance of providing safe and effective anesthesia at minimal risk, the anesthetist must be involved in the care of the patient at the earliest possible opportunity—in the emergency ward.

BIBLIOGRAPHY

1. Greene, N. M. (ed.): *Anesthesia for Emergency Surgery* (Philadelphia: F. A. Davis Co., 1963).
2. Wolfson, L. J.: *Anaesthesia for the Injured* (Philadelphia: F. A. Davis Co., 1962).
3. Milstein, B. B.: *Cardiac Arrest and Resuscitation* (London: Lloyd-Luke Ltd., 1963).
4. Janis, I. L. (ed.): *Personality: Dynamics, Development & Assessment* (New York: Harcourt, Brace & World, Inc., 1969).

13 | Facial Injuries
BRADFORD CANNON and JOHN D. CONSTABLE

INJURIES TO THE FACE are a not infrequent accompaniment of injuries elsewhere in the body. A severe blow to the face may produce extensive lacerations of the soft tissues without fracture or may cause multiple fractures with only soft tissue contusion. Usually there are injuries to both the soft tissue and the bony structures. A fracture must not be overlooked because of the severity of the lacerations or of the edema of the facial tissues. Both should be treated promptly and definitively if the patient's general condition warrants.

In few injuries is the final outcome so directly dependent on early proper care as in the treatment of a severe facial injury. The bony and cartilaginous framework of the face supports the soft tissues and teeth and provides attachment to the muscles of expression and mastication. The character of the face and the emotional expression, as well as the functions of chewing and eating and the maintenance of binocular vision, depend on a normal anatomic and functional relationship between these structures. Failure to restore the displaced bone to its normal position or failure to resolve the puzzle of a jagged laceration of the eyelid, nose or mouth may result in disfigurements that will permanently alter the appearance and function of the face. Only by early reduction of all fractures and adequate splinting of the fragments before fixation of the bones has occurred can the normal contours of the face be restored, and only by accurate layer closure of the soft tissues will function be re-established and scarring minimized.

The surgeon caring for these injuries will be awed by the maze of techniques, appliances, prejudices and conflicting opinions that have found their way into the surgical literature in recent decades. It is not our purpose to review all the methods that have been used in treating facial injuries but merely to report those that have proved most simple and effective and to emphasize that these make use of simple equipment almost universally available.

EMERGENCY CARE AND TRANSPORTATION

In the emergency care and transportation of patients with severe facial injuries three problems are of concern to the surgeon. The arrest of hemorrhage and the establishment and maintenance of an adequate airway are both lifesaving, and the support and protection of the damaged tissues influence the eventual outcome.

Local pressure or packing of the wound or wounds with sterile gauze usually is sufficient to control hemorrhage, but clamping of a lacerated large blood vessel sometimes is necessary. The clamp may be left in place or the bleeding vessel ligated if feasible. In all these manipulations, interference with respiration or the respiratory passage is to be avoided. Prompt blood replacement should be instituted in conjunction with the control of hemorrhage.

The normal airway may be obstructed either by backward displacement of the tongue and floor of the mouth or by hemorrhage. A collapse of the mandibular arch or a backward and downward displacement of the roof of the mouth will crowd the tongue against the pharynx. Traction on the tongue with a suture or even with a safety pin or towel clip inserted through the tip, or traction on the displaced bone, should relieve the obstruction effectively. The insertion of an endopharyngeal tube or an endotracheal tube may be desirable. In the insertion of either, additional damage to the soft tissues must be avoided. Although many surgeons enthusiastically recommend tracheostomy for the patient with severe facial trauma, rarely is it needed or desirable if the patient can be observed adequately (see Fig. 13-24). An endotracheal tube often will suffice to ensure an adequate airway until definitive reduction of facial fractures has been obtained, after which it rarely will be necessary.

Although often dramatic, facial injuries rarely are of top priority once an airway has been established. Support and protection of the damaged tissues by application of a well-padded bandage beneath the chin and around the head and face will reduce the possibility of further contamination, slow the development of local edema and reduce the patient's local discomfort. Under no circumstances should any but the most urgent manipulation be done until after a careful general evaluation of the patient can be made and he is in the operating room, prepared for definitive treatment.

For transporting the conscious patient, the upright position has proved best. He is able to cough effectively and can rid the mouth of obstructing blood or secretion by leaning forward. The unconscious patient should be transported in a face-down position. The displaced tissue of the mouth will fall forward away from the pharynx, and the aspiration of blood or vomitus will be reduced to a minimum.

EXAMINATION OF THE PATIENT

External lacerations or abrasions of the face will be obvious, but the detailed pattern of laceration, important in carrying out the repair, may be obscured by dried blood or a dressing. In particular, actual losses of skin or soft tissue usually will be found to be much less extensive than estimated on original examination. Gross displacement in fractures will also be obvious but other fractures may be difficult to identify, so that any patient who has received a blow to the face should be considered as having a fracture until it is ruled out. This calls for a systematic examination of every such patient. On inspection, any loss of symmetry of the structures of the face should be apparent unless masked by swelling of the soft tissues. Also, malocclusion of the teeth, partial or complete paralysis of the seventh nerve, abnormal or restricted motions of the upper or lower jaw and any limitation of normal range of motion and vision of the eyes should be noted. Drainage of cerebrospinal fluid from the ear or nose may indicate fractures with laceration of the dura. Nasal bleeding indicates torn mucosa. Membranes of the tongue, palate or alveolar processes may be cut by the sharp edges of fractured bones or torn if the bones to which they are attached are displaced.

Fractures of the nasal bones and cartilage, the most common fracture of the facial bones, usually can be identified best by inquiring of the patient as to any cosmetic change and by direct palpation of any displacement. In children, minor displacements may occur and should be sought for even without the corroborating evidence of bleeding from the nose. Within the nasal cavity, swelling of the septum may indicate a septal fracture and the formation of a hematoma. Laceration of the mucosa following a blow is the most positive evidence of a fracture. X-ray examination often fails to show a nasal fracture, especially if the injury involves the cartilaginous framework. A negative film should not preclude treatment of a clinically displaced nasal fracture (see Fig. 13-8).

The next most common fracture of the facial bones is that of the zygoma, which usually results from a direct blow. The three major suture lines attaching the zygoma to the maxilla, frontal and temporal bones are the common sites of fracture or separation. Displacement often is downward and backward. Fracture of the substance of the massive zygoma seldom occurs except by a penetrating object, such as a missile. The irregular fracture line or asymmetry may be discovered by palpation of the infraorbital rims at the zygomaticomaxillary suture line or of the external orbital rim at the zygomaticofrontal suture line or of the zygomatic arch. Anesthesia often is found in the distribution of the infraorbital nerve, since the fracture line crosses its canal and the nerve is either crushed or severed. A shattering of the maxillary antral walls accompanies fractures of the zygoma. Palpation in the upper buccal fornix may reveal bony irregularities. X-ray examination will reveal details of these fractures. Unless the injury is severe, fractures of the zygoma are not associated with malocclusion, but the backward displacement of the bone or the inward displacement of the zygomatic arch may interfere with the forward excursion of the coronoid process and limit opening of the mouth (see Fig. 13-10).

Fractures of the orbit can be identified by palpation of the orbital rims. There may be lateral displacement of the medial wall of the orbit to which the inner canthus is attached. Diplopia, partial or complete loss of vision, impaired extraocular movements, corneal abrasions and damage to the globe must all be checked and recorded before any definitive treatment is undertaken.

Fracture of the orbital rim or wall accompanies many if not most of the fractures of the middle third of the face. Serious fractures of the root of the nose may be associated with lateral displacement of the medial wall of the orbit and a variety of fractures occur on the orbital rim. The pure orbital floor fracture is described by the beguiling term "blowout." By "blowout" is implied a fracture of the thin membranous bone of the orbital floor. The fracture results from a sudden increase in intraorbital pressure due to a direct blow on the orbital contents, with the eyeball transmitting the force of the blow, which breaks through the thin floor of the orbit into the relatively compressible air-filled maxillary antrum. The orbital rim remains intact, a feature that makes it easy to overlook this fracture. The soft tissue contents of the floor of the orbit may or may not be displaced into the antrum. If displaced, there will be enophthalmos and diplopia, with limited movement of the inferior rectus and inferior oblique muscles. Upward rotation of the eye, both actively and passively, will be restricted. X-ray of the maxillary sinus often will demonstrate the herniated orbital contents. Laminagrams may be of great value in doubtful cases (see Fig. 13-14).

The most serious injuries to the facial bones are those crossing the face transversely at the level of the orbits or at the level of the floor of the antrum. These are characterized by complete separation of the facial bony structures from the skull, with downward and backward and occasionally rotational displacement. By grasping the upper jaw and immobilizing the head, abnormal mobility usually can be demonstrated. Malocclusion always is present in these fractures, usually with premature contact of the molars and an open bite (see Fig. 13-15).

At the turn of the century, Le Fort studied areas of structural weakness between the maxillae and adjacent bones and proposed a classification of midfacial fractures that recently has gained wide popularity. Three types are described (see Fig. 13-15): Le Fort I is a transverse

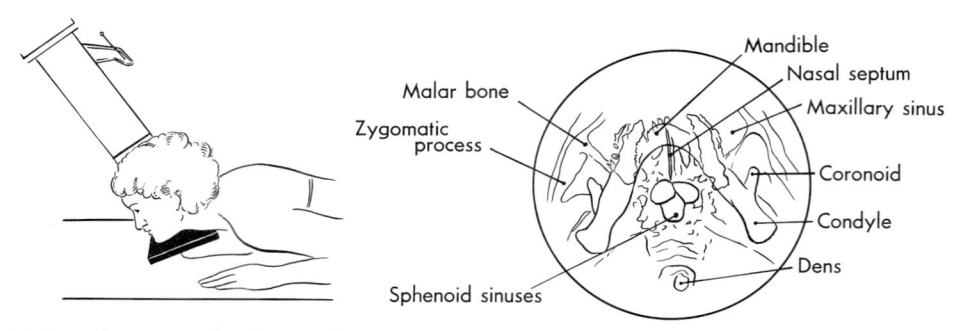

Fig. 13-1.—The vertical submental position, showing the pose and the bony landmarks that are useful in interpreting the x-ray film.

fracture above the apices of the teeth that may include the alveolar processes, palatal bone and pterygoid processes. It is essentially a detachment of the hard palate and maxillary teeth. Le Fort II is a pyramidal fracture involving the frontal processes of the maxillae, the lacrimal bones, the orbital floor, zygomaticomaxillary suture lines, the lateral antral walls and the pterygoid plates. This fracture adds the entire nasal skeleton and the remainder of the maxillae to a Le Fort I. Le Fort III is a transverse fracture with craniofacial separation at the orbital level, involving the zygomaticofrontal sutures and the nasofrontal sutures and crossing the orbital floor. This fracture adds the zygomas to a Le Fort II. Displacements in each of these fractures result in dental malocclusion, often with significant posterior displacement of the detached bones. The posterior displacement may be the result of the trauma itself and the downward displacement the result of gravity.

Although it is easy to label a Le Fort numbered fracture, detailed identification of the structures involved must not be disregarded. Combinations of this strict classification can and often do occur; for example, a Le Fort II on one side and a Le Fort III on the opposite side. Unfortunately, the Le Fort classification does not include vertical fractures or pure alveolar fractures, nor does it include the displaced zygomatic fractures with their associated injuries of adjacent bones.

Mandibular fractures alone of facial fractures are subject to significant muscle displacement—in this case, by the muscles of mastication. They usually are palpable, except those of the condyle, and usually result in malocclusion.

X-ray studies of the facial and jaw bones are important for confirmation of

Fig. 13-2.—The Waters position, showing the pose and the bony landmarks that are useful in interpreting the x-ray film.

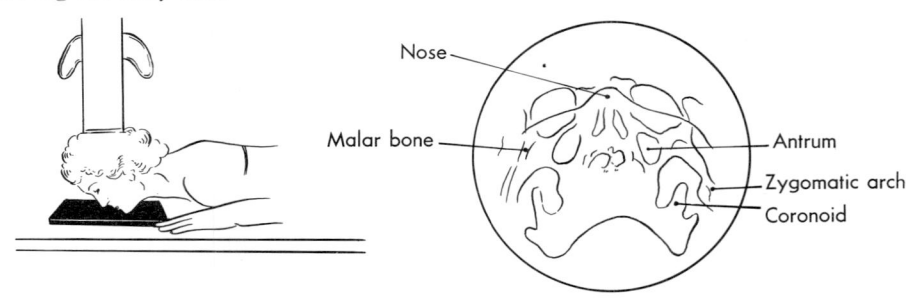

Chapter 13: FACIAL INJURIES / **247**

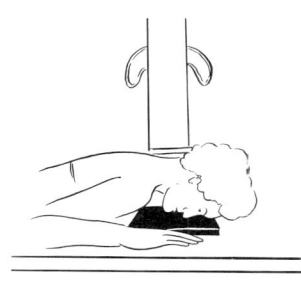

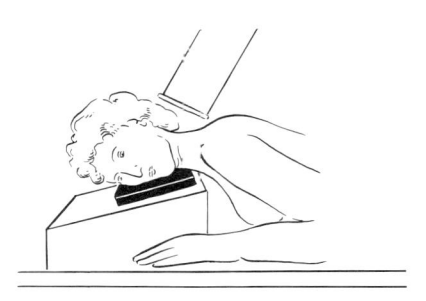

Fig. 13-3.—Positions for x-rays of the mandible: **left**, posteroanterior; **right**, lateral.

Fig. 13-4.—Sites of fractures of the mandible, showing types of displacement resulting from the action of the muscles attached to the fragments: *a*, direction of pull of temporal muscle; *b*, attachment of external pterygoid muscle; *c*, direction of pull of internal pterygoid and masseter muscles; *d*, direction of pull of geniohyoid and genioglossus muscles; *1*, common site of fracture of neck of condyle; *2*, site and direction of fracture of angle of mandible without tooth in posterior fragment, in which overriding of the posterior fragment can be expected, as shown in sketch at right; *3*, site and direction of fracture of mandible with tooth in posterior fragment and in which overriding does not occur; *4*, common site of fracture in the region of the mental foramen, with types of fracture and displacements illustrated below.

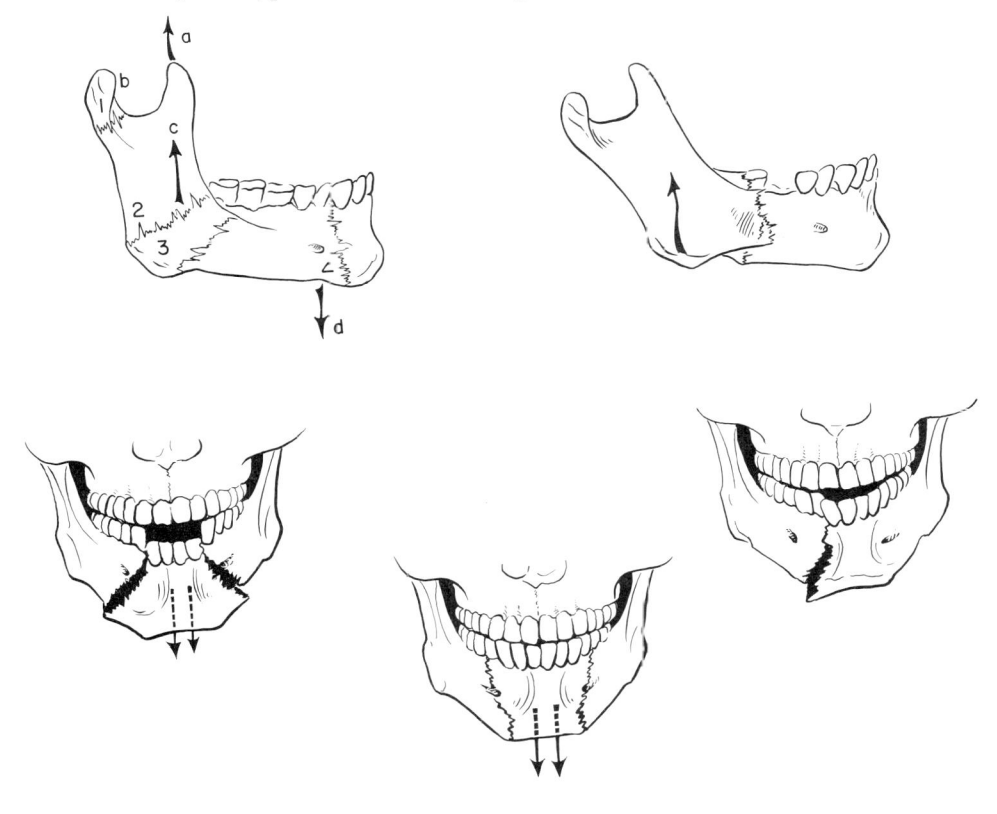

the clinical findings and as part of the patient's record. Proper posing of the head is essential for informative films. By posing in both the vertical submental and Waters positions, fracture and displacement of the rims of the orbits, the zygomatic arches, the lateral and medial walls of the antrums, the bony structure of the nose, the alveolar arches and the palate will be visualized. Detailed visualization of the nose requires a soft lateral view and an anteroposterior downward view with a small film held against the roof of the mouth. Mandibular x-ray studies should include views of each side of the jaw, the symphysis and both condyles. The direction of the mandibular fracture lines, the amount of displacement, the degree of overriding of the posterior fragment and the condition of the teeth adjacent to the fracture line may all influence the method of treatment chosen.

GENERAL CONSIDERATIONS IN TREATMENT

Critical injuries of the brain, chest and abdomen and major fractures often must take priority in treatment over facial injuries. Examination of the cervical spine should not be overlooked, since the force of a blow to the face may be transmitted to that area. The definitive care of the facial injury should be postponed until the patient has recovered consciousness or until other, more severe injuries have been attended to. The lacerated edges of skin can be drawn together with adhesive strips or loose suturing, and the displaced bony structures of the face or jaw supported by a bandage. In the presence of other injuries, minimal manipulation is permissible to lessen the patient's discomfort and to simplify later repair.

If circumstances permit, lacerations of the face and nasal fractures should receive definitive treatment as soon as possible before swelling has become prominent and before organization of blood clots or infection develops. Except for those of the nose, reduction of facial fractures within the first 12–24 hours after injury is optimal, but treatment can be delayed for a week or even longer without excessively compromising the end result, if the condition of the patient makes this necessary. Delays of more than about 10 days in the replacement of bone fragments may make realignment impossible because of their rapid fusion and fixation. Lacerations in a child often are treated best by adhesive strips (Steri-Strips) alone. A dread of hospitals, anesthesia, sutures and so forth need never be kindled in the child's mind.

Anesthesia

Local anesthesia is desirable in the definitive repair of most facial lacerations and minor fractures. Local infiltration with procaine or Xylocaine is satisfactory for most skin lacerations, but nerve block (infraorbital, mental or other) may be preferable to avoid distortion of the soft tissues. Nerve block may also be desirable if maintenance of an adequate airway is difficult and if, at the same time, complete anesthesia of the face is needed. Complete anesthesia can be obtained by block of the second and third divisions of the fifth cranial nerve and infiltration of the cervical nerves that extend upward across the body of the mandible. In children, general anesthesia may be essential for repair of facial lacerations. For manipulation of nasal fractures, excellent anesthesia can be obtained with cocaine to the mucosa and external block with procaine. In complex injuries of the face and jaws, endotracheal anesthesia is preferable because of the length of the procedure and the desirability of a tube in the trachea during and after the operation. Nasal intubation is optimal but, if too difficult to perform in the presence of severe fractures, an oral endotracheal tube may be used, with intramaxillary fixation being delayed until the patient is awake and the tube is removed. Occasionally, tracheostomy must be resorted to despite its complications. In such cases, the tube should be removed as soon as possible. The use of an endotracheal tube, even for as long as 3 or 4 days, will eliminate many unnecessary tracheostomies. The postoperative dangers of aspiration of secretions and the hazards of immediate fixation of the teeth in occlusion must be kept in mind when general anesthesia is used. Postoperatively, the endotracheal tube should be kept in place until the patient is virtually fully conscious.

Preparation of the Wound

Thorough cleansing of all facial wounds is an essential preliminary to definitive treatment. A local anesthetic may be injected before the wound preparation or, better, after the preliminary washing. Final preparation should include irrigation and gentle scrubbing, mild detergent soap being used. If dirt or oil has been ground into the skin, vigorous scrubbing with a brush is necessary. Visible pigment that cannot be removed in this way should be surgically debrided. Despite the trauma of such a procedure, it is time well spent and may eliminate the need for a later and less satisfactory operation to correct traumatic tattoos. Loose dirt, hair, glass and other foreign bodies and totally detached chips of bone should be sought for and removed. A detailed history of the nature of the trauma producing the injury may furnish helpful clues as to what may be found in the tissues.

Debridement of the tissues of the face should be minimal, in contrast to the complete wound excision recommended elsewhere in the body. An ill-advised debridement of skin around the eyelids or mouth or the failure to replace skin lost from them may result in a significant deformity. "It is better to save tissue which may die than to sacrifice any which may survive."

A piece of skin partially or even completely detached often survives as a free transplant if replaced in its normal position, sutured loosely with minimal tension and protected by a firm dressing. Fragments of bone with attached periosteum are similarly often salvageable and of great importance.

Antibiotics

Although different views are widely held, it is our belief that facial lacerations and facial fractures, however extensive and complex, seldom require the use of systemic antibiotics either before or after treatment, except in unusual circumstances. The principal exception is the patient with cerebrospinal rhinorrhea, in which routine prophylactic treatment against meningitis is indicated. Tetanus prophylaxis, however, must not be overlooked.

MANAGEMENT OF FRACTURES

Fractures of the facial bones differ from most fractures because the displacement is produced by the trauma itself and not by the pull of attached muscles. Consequently, in the reduction of fractures of the face, the displaced bones must be replaced in their original position and held in place only against the minimal elasticity of the soft tissues and the force of gravity. The disconnected bones in a mandibular fracture, on the other hand, are displaced by the action of the very powerful muscles of mastication. In the reduction and fixation of these fractures, appropriate splinting must be employed to control the pull of these muscles.

The two most useful aids in the diagnosis of fractures, malocclusion of the teeth and palpable deformity of the bony prominences of the face, are equally valuable in determining the accuracy of the reduction of fractures of the jaw or face. Such simple indicators should be an inducement to utilize definitive surgical methods in their treatment. The opportunity to reduce the displaced facial bone through the unsutured overlying laceration should not be overlooked. Many combinations of fracture and laceration can be used in this way to ensure an accurate reduction without the need for any new cuts in the skin. In other areas of the body, the skin over a compound open fracture would not be closed without reduction of the bone—the face should be no exception. The final reduction thus can be achieved promptly, the patient will be relieved of the discomfort of unstable fragments and the constant adjustment of complicated appliances will be unnecessary. These principles are in keeping with the current trend toward prompt reduction and positive fixation of fractures elsewhere in the body. The morbidity and duration of hospitalization will be reduced by employing definitive and accurate techniques.

Fractures of Nasal Structures

The nasal bones form the forward and lateral sides of the upper third of the nose. They are thin and convex in their lower half, yet are solid in their upper third. They are held as if in a vise by the ascending processes of the superior maxilla and rest on a shelf, the nasal spine of the frontal bone.

It is imperative that septal fractures and dislocations of the nose be realigned and held in place soon after an injury. Rapid organization of the injured parts in malposition occurs and makes reduction and realignment impossible after a few days. An intact septum that is realigned or a fractured or dislocated septum reduced and held in place will hold the

Fig. 13-5.—Types of nasal fractures frequently encountered.

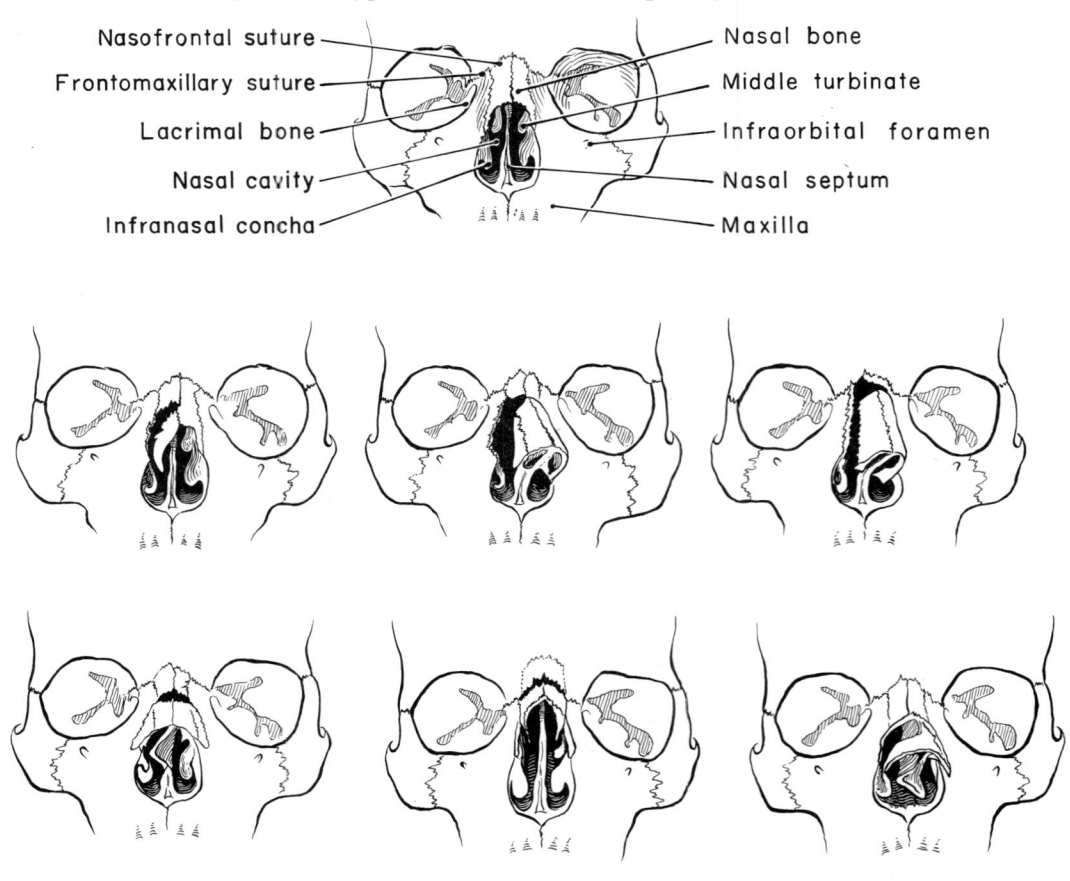

nasal bones and the cartilaginous dorsum in their normal contour. Without septal support, the nasal bones and cartilaginous dorsum will collapse after reduction. Fixation of the septum may be accomplished by gentle, intranasal packing, using either petrolatum-impregnated or dry fine-mesh gauze strips. Most nasal fractures are of the lower one-half of the nasal skeleton where the bone is thin. Frequently they include the thin portion of the ascending process of the superior maxilla. Fractures of the upper one-half, where the bone is thick and quite solid, are less frequent. Rarely are the nasal bones disarticulated in their upper third because they are held firmly in a facet created by the frontal bone and the ascending processes of the superior maxilla. A fracture there usually results from a crushing blow that separates the ascending processes, driving the bone either into the nasal passage or laterally beneath the soft tissue of the cheek. A depressed fracture in this area often involves the perpendicular plate of the ethmoid in the region of the cribriform plate and may be associated with cerebrospinal rhinorrhea. Cerebrospinal rhinorrhea is not a contraindication to reduction. Instead, reduction should be carried out as soon as the condition of the patient permits. Reduction and immobilization of the bone hastens the sealing of the dural leaks and reduces the likelihood of invasive infection of the meninges. Cerebrospinal rhinorrhea is an indication for prophylactic antibiotics.

Fig. 13-6. — One method of reducing a nasal fracture—using a blunt instrument within the nose. Palpating fingers check the reduction externally.

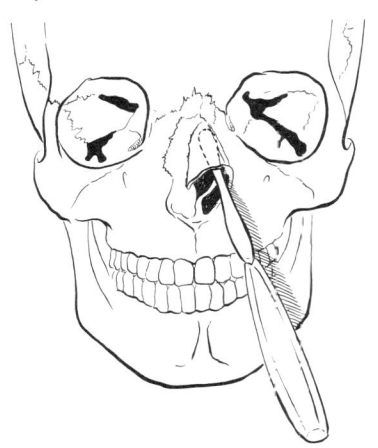

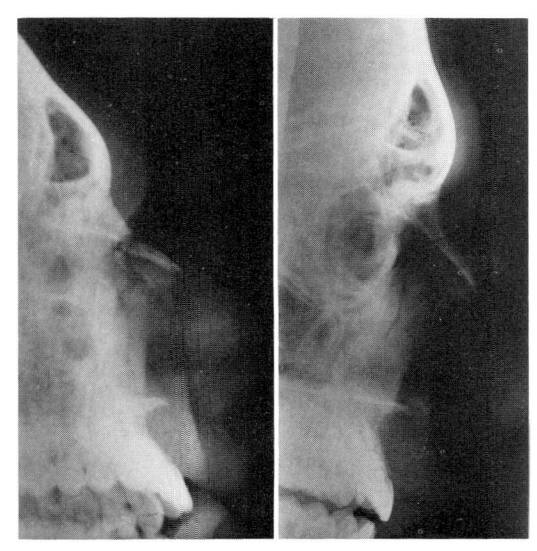

Fig. 13-7. — Fracture of the nose, obvious from both clinical and x-ray (**left**) examination. Fracture was reduced (**right**) under local anesthesia by inserting a blunt instrument into the nose and elevating the fragment into position; elaborate splinting was not necessary. X-ray studies will not always be so helpful. The surgeon often must rely on clinical examination to make a diagnosis of fracture of the nasal bones or nasal cartilages.

The majority of nasal fractures, except in children, may be reduced under local anesthesia, using topical anesthesia (cocaine) within the nose and infiltration of procaine or its equivalent subcutaneously over the bones. Most nasal fractures can be reduced by elevation, using a blunt instrument within the nose. The fragments can be manipulated and the reduction controlled and checked for accuracy by external digital pressure. In badly comminuted fractures it may be necessary to use a special forceps to grasp fragments of bone and bring them into accurate position. Most nasal fractures may need nothing more than an adhesive or metal or dental composition splint.

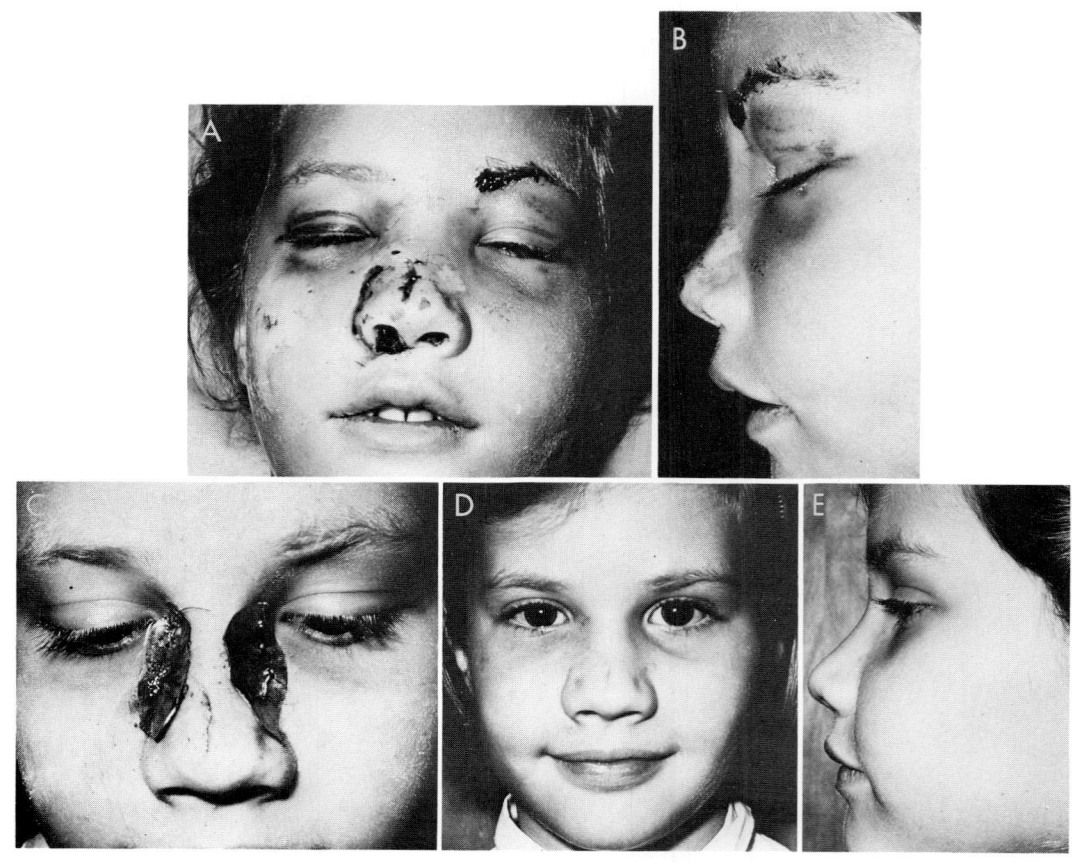

Fig. 13-8.—Nasal fracture reduction maintained with metal splints. **A** and **B**, a child seen 1 week after injury of the nose with lacerations and considerable displacement. **C**, after reduction of the fractures, with the position maintained by metal splints and wires through the nose. **D** and **E**, result at 2 months. X-ray films showed no definite evidence of fracture in this largely cartilaginous injury.

Those that have lost the support of the septum require additional splinting. To accomplish the splinting, the technique of through-and-through wires passed between and below the comminuted fragments and fastened to pieces of soft metal molded to the side of the nose has proved simple and effective. Complex fractures involving the root of the nose with displacement of the medial wall of the orbit and/or the frontal sinus often require open reduction and direct wiring of the fragments.

A common mistake in attempting to reduce a nasal fracture is passing the elevator too high within the nose so that it rests either beneath the unbroken nasal bones or beneath the nasal process of the frontal bone. Care should be taken, therefore, that the elevator lies beneath the displaced fragments only.

Fractures of the Zygoma

The zygoma is a rather flat bone with three main articulations. These are with the frontal bone, the superior maxilla and the zygomatic process of the temporal bone. The largest and firmest articulation is with the superior maxilla. Separation at this articulation usually involves the maxillary antrum. The zygomatic bone itself rarely is fractured but is displaced in the direction of the force of the blow. The displacement may be posterior, medial or both and with an upward or downward rotation. The lateral posterior surface of the zygoma, which forms the anterior wall of the temporal fossa, is in close contact with the coronoid process of the mandible. Backward or medial displacement may limit motion of the coronoid process and hence of the mandible. The outer third of the floor of the orbit is formed by the zygoma so that displacement downward, inward or upward will cause a change in the volume of the orbit. This, in turn, may produce diplopia by pushing the globe forward when the orbital contents are compressed or by inward and downward displacement of the globe if the orbit is enlarged. Diplopia may result without volume change in the orbit by interference with normal movement of the extraocular muscles. The lateral palpebral ligament is attached to the frontal process of the zygoma so that the eye is rotated when the zygomaticofrontal suture is separated and the zygo-

Fig. 13-9.—Depressed fracture of the zygomatic arch, which impinged on the coronoid process of the mandible. The chief complaint was limitation of motion of the mandible. The temporal approach was used for reduction. A blunt instrument, passed beneath the temporal fascia and the zygomatic arch, was used to pry the fracture outward. No splinting was necessary.

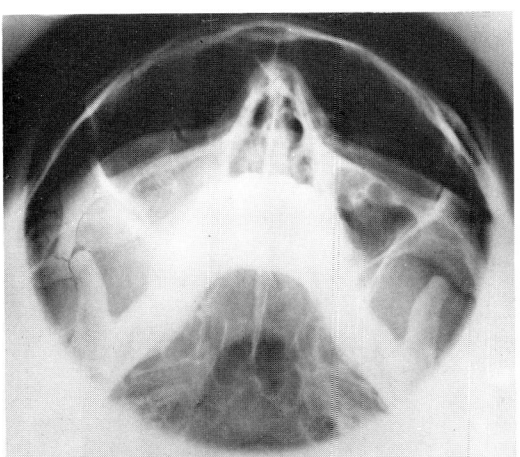

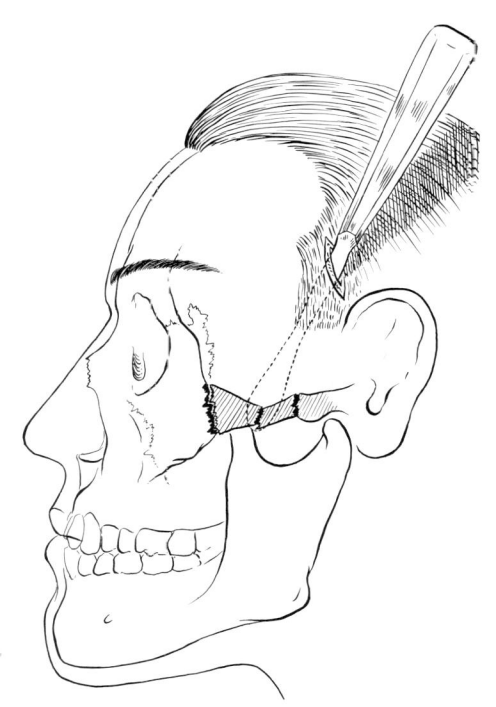

Fig. 13-10.—The Gillies method for elevation of depressed fractures of the zygomatic arch. An incision made within the hairline permits access to the temporal fossa by an instrument passed beneath the temporal fascia.

ma displaced downward. This anatomic fact makes precise reduction at this site very important.

The direction of displacement of the zygomatic bone, which usually can be determined accurately from examination and by x-rays, will influence the selection of the method of treatment. There are several methods of reduction of fractures involving the zygomatic bone, each of which has special indications. When the zygomatic arch alone has been fractured or when the zygoma has been rotated posteriorly toward the temporal fossa, reduction by the temporal approach of Gillies is indicated. An incision is made parallel to the temporal artery within the hairline about 3 cm anterior to the ear. The temporal fascia, which inserts on the arch, is exposed and incised and a blunt-tipped elevator is inserted beneath this

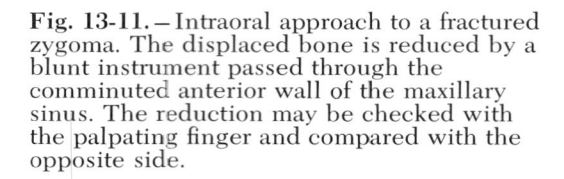

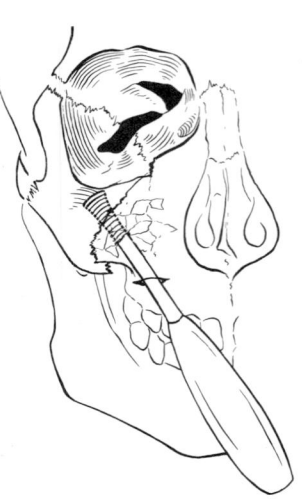

Fig. 13-11.—Intraoral approach to a fractured zygoma. The displaced bone is reduced by a blunt instrument passed through the comminuted anterior wall of the maxillary sinus. The reduction may be checked with the palpating finger and compared with the opposite side.

Fig. 13-12.—**Top,** compound injury of the lateral orbital wall caused by a hook that avulsed the bone and overlying soft tissue. **Bottom left,** x-ray film revealed fracture of zygomatic arch and lateral displacement of zygoma. The zygoma was exposed through the open wound and wired to the frontal and maxillary bones. **Bottom right,** after wiring. The soft tissue wound and the bone healed without complications.

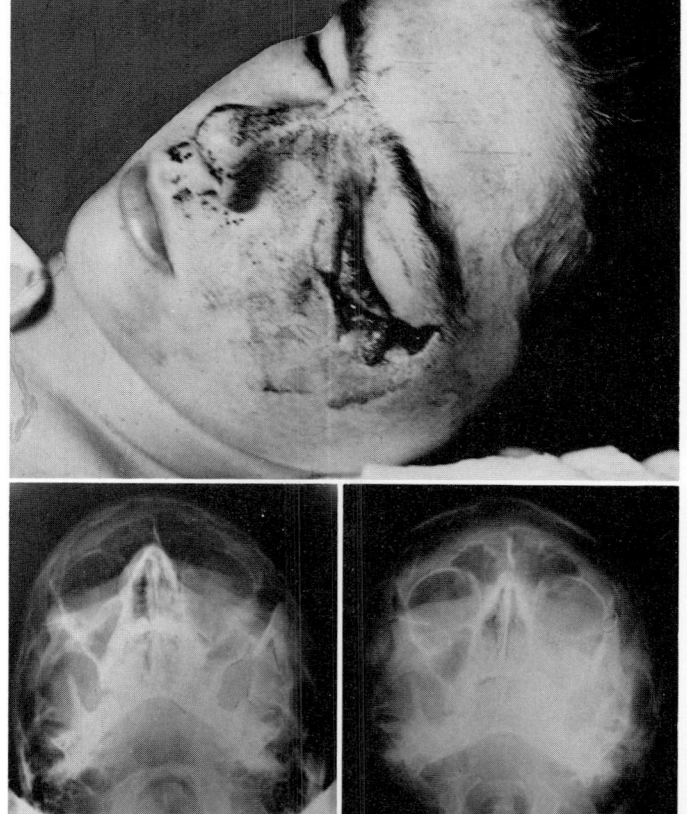

Chapter 13: FACIAL INJURIES / 255

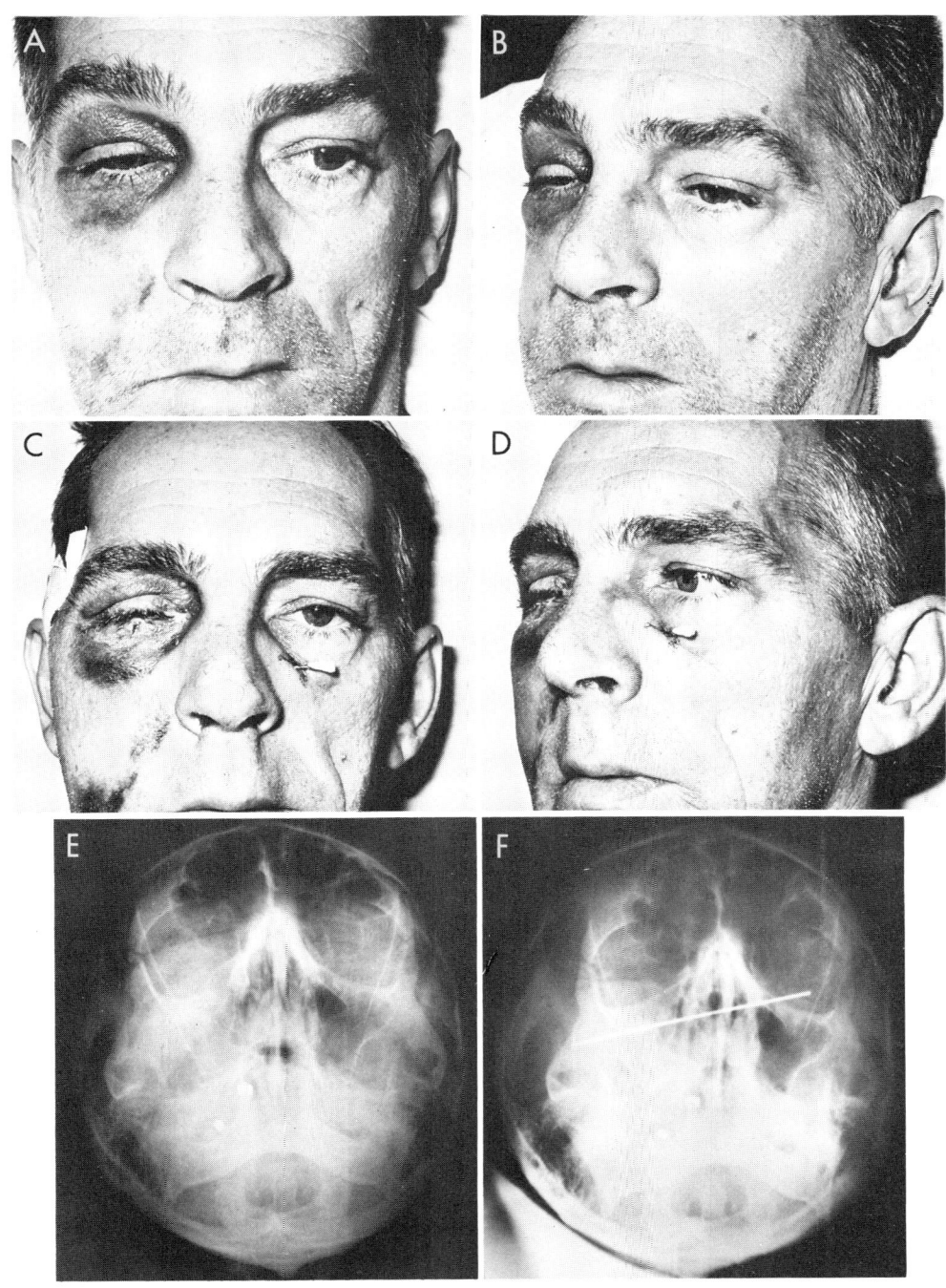

Fig. 13-13.—Unstable fracture of the zygoma with a Kirschner wire after reduction. **A** and **B**, preoperative, showing lack of malar prominence on lateral view. **C** and **D**, after reduction and fixation with a wire from the normal side. Malar prominence restored. **E** and **F**, pre- and postoperative x-ray films, with the wire still in place in F.

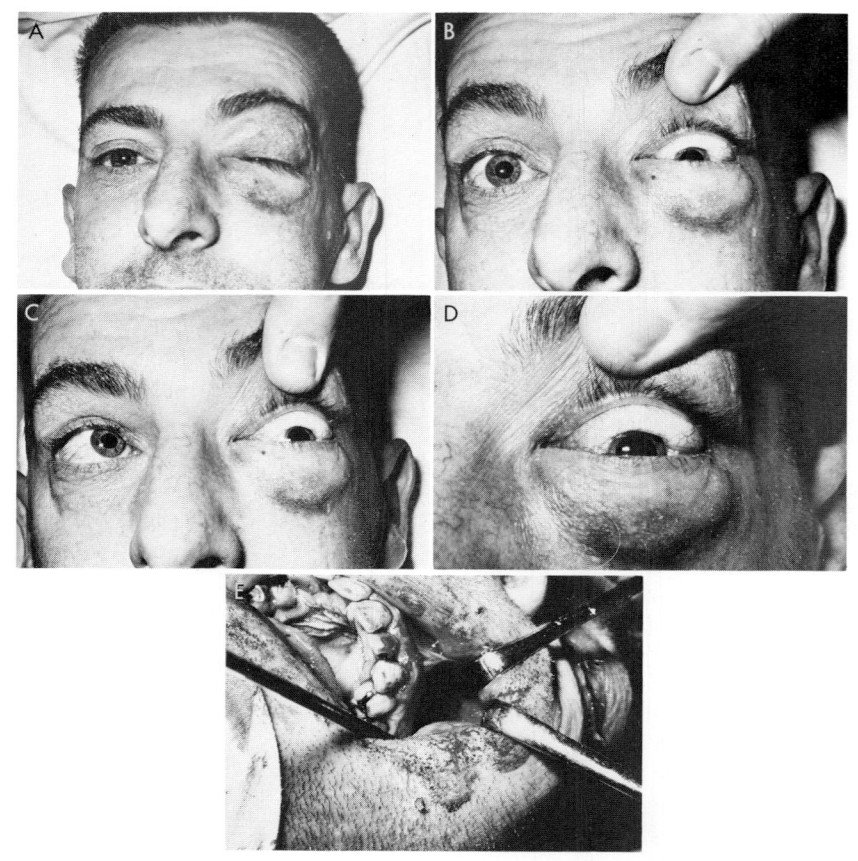

Fig. 13-14.—"Blowout" fracture of the orbit. **A–D,** preoperative views demonstrating expanded pupil (**B**), inability to raise the left eye on upward gaze (**C**) and subconjunctival air (**D**). **E,** operative approach through the antrum, showing prolapsed orbital fat. *(Continued.)*

fascia, which guides the instrument under the temporal arch. Using the instrument as a lever, the bones can be sprung back into position. If considerable force is necessary, a folded gauze pad may be placed beneath the handle of the instrument as a fulcrum. The temporal fossa can also be approached intraorally and reduction carried out from below. Through an incision made in the buccal mucosa just above the last molar tooth, a blunt elevator is passed upward parallel to the anterior border of the ramus and into the temporal fossa. Here, it lies behind the displaced zygoma, which then can be moved laterally or anteriorly.

The most ubiquitous approach for the reduction of zygomatic fracture is through the antrum, because the blow in most fractures is in front and the bone is driven backward and downward into the antrum. The antrum is entered through an incision in the buccal fornix above the bicuspid teeth. A blunt instrument passed between the fracture lines of the anterior wall of the antrum is used to engage and elevate the bone. The accuracy of reduction may be checked by comparison with the uninjured side. Usually, the reduced fragments lock themselves in place, but if there is much comminution, splinting may be necessary. A pack in the antrum provides good support for the loose fragments of the antral wall and

Chapter 13: FACIAL INJURIES / **257**

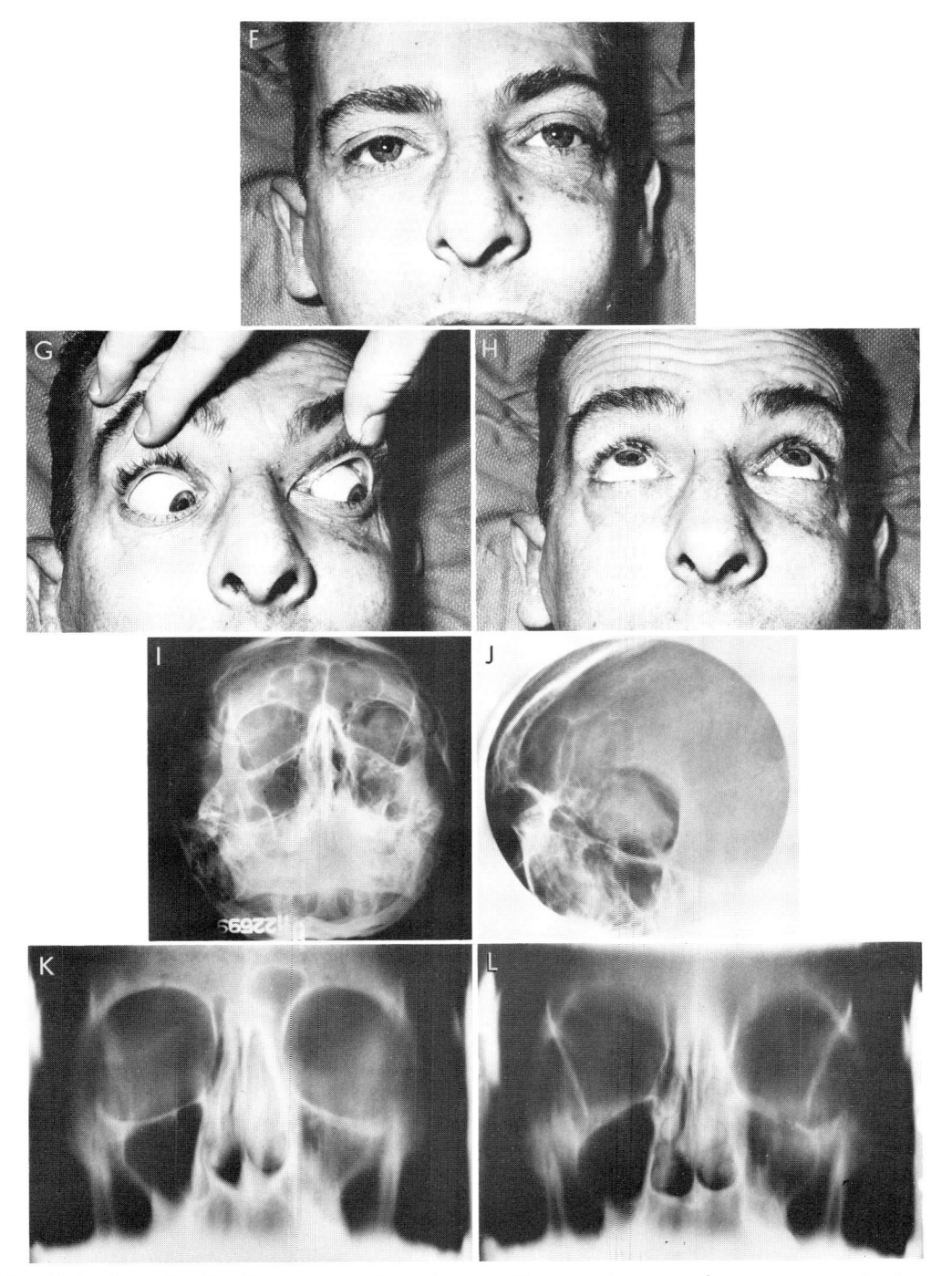

Fig. 13-14 (cont.).—**F–H,** postoperative views, with normal range of eye movements. **I,** preoperative x-ray film (Waters view), showing soft tissue in the antrum and free air in the orbit. **J,** air in the orbit. **K** and **L,** laminagrams, demonstrating intact rim of the orbit but an orbital floor defect at 1.5 cm from the orbital rim (**L**).

floor of the orbit but may be uncomfortable for the patient. Packing usually is inadequate to support the body of the zygoma, so wire skeletal fixation becomes essential. This type of fixation often is necessary when there are comminutions or a wide separation of the zygoma from adjacent bones. In the area of the frontozygomatic suture line, a fracture may be exposed by incision through the overlying skin. Two drill holes, one in the frontal bone and the other in the zygoma, permit wiring the two bones together with stainless steel. One point of open reduction and fixation normally will be sufficient but occasionally wiring of the intraorbital fracture will also prove necessary.

A variety of other methods of splinting the unstable zygoma and facial bones may be needed. These depend on fixation to adjacent or contralateral undisplaced and unfractured structures. Threaded or unthreaded Kirschner wires, available in every modern operating room, have proved singularly useful. The loose bone may be impaled on the wire and after accurate positioning of the bone, the wire is "drilled" across the face to engage solid bony structures on the opposite side. Often preferably a threaded wire may be inserted on the normal or stable side and advanced across the face until it engages on the inferior surface of the fractured zygoma on the opposite side. In this way, the fractured bone does not need to be transfixed, only supported. The wire is removed in 2–3 weeks.

Fig. 13-15.—Varieties of upper and lower transverse fractures of the maxilla and associated facial bones. **A,** unilateral alveolar fracture, with extension into the antrum and palatal process. **B,** low transverse fracture across the floor of the antrum—Le Fort I. **C,** higher transverse fracture through the complex suture lines of the nasal, malar, lacrimal and ethmoid bones but without detaching the zygomata—Le Fort II. **D,** high transverse fracture through the orbits, with multiple bony separations in the lacrimal-ethmoid region and detachment of the zygomata together with the maxillae—Le Fort III. **E,** low transverse fracture showing backward displacement of the upper arch and resultant open-bite malocclusion.

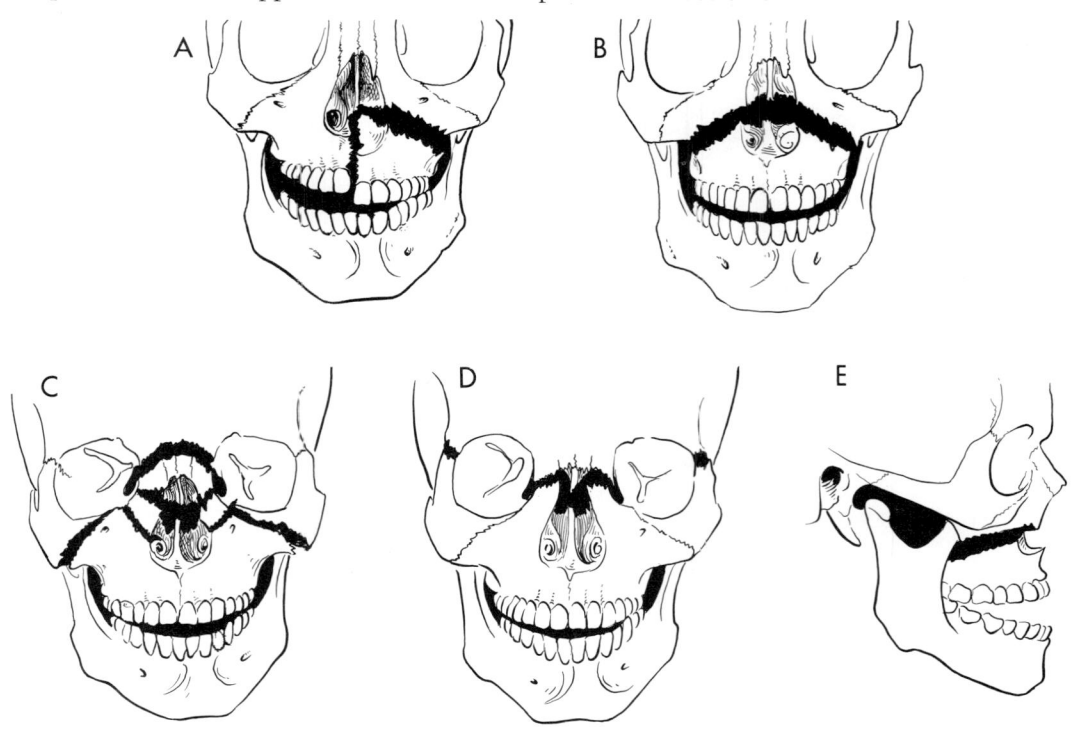

Transversing the antrum and nasal passages does not seem to lead to complications. On occasion, a 30-ml Foley catheter with the bag fully distended in the antrum may be a useful method of support. The "blowout" fracture of the orbital floor may be approached by one of two routes. Exposure through the antrum will avoid an external incision yet permit visualization of the displaced orbital contents and the fractured membranous bones. Reduction of the soft tissue and bone and support with an antral pack will suffice. The more popular approach is through an external eyelid incision. The herniated soft tissues are returned to the orbit and the floor reconstructed with a patch of silastic, cartilage or bone if the bony fragments are sufficient.

Fractures of the Maxilla

The maxilla is attached to the skull by several buttresses, chief among them being the ascending process of the maxilla, the lateral and posterior walls of the maxillary antrum and the palatal bone. The nasal, malar, lacrimal, ethmoid and other facial bones, any or all of which may be involved in severe fractures of the maxilla, are considered part of the maxillary complex. All degrees of fractures of the maxilla are encountered, from a crack through one or two of these buttresses to a complete separation of the attachments to the skull. These transverse fractures of the upper jaw cross the face either at the level of the floor of the antrum with separation of the alveolar process from its attachment to the facial bony structure (Le Fort I) or at the level of the orbit with separation of the maxillary complex from the skull (Le Fort II and III). The most significant deformity in each of these transverse fractures is elongation of the face caused by the separation of the fractured bone from the skull. There is malocclusion of the teeth as a result of the downward and often backward displacement of the maxillary teeth.

Methods of treatment of these complex transverse fractures of the face fortunately have kept pace with the universal trend toward prompt and direct reduction and fixation of all fractures. Appliances that require special preparation and repeated and painful adjustment and that consequently fail to achieve the immediate and definitive result can be avoided. Internal fixation of the displaced fragments to the stable portions of the skull—

Fig. 13-16.—Direct wiring of the floating maxilla to the orbital rim. **Left,** the wire is fixed below the zygomaticofrontal suture line if the zygoma is stable. **Right,** if the zygoma is unstable, the wire for fixation must be attached to the stable zygomatic processes of the frontal bones in the upper lateral orbital rim. The wires are passed through the soft tissues of the face either anteriorly over to the malar prominence or posteriorly through the temporal fossa. In addition, interdental fixation of the mandible to the maxilla (not shown) will be necessary to restore normal occlusion.

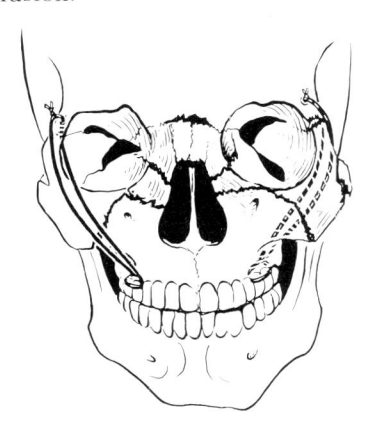

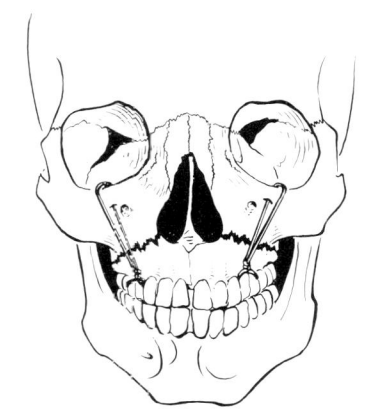

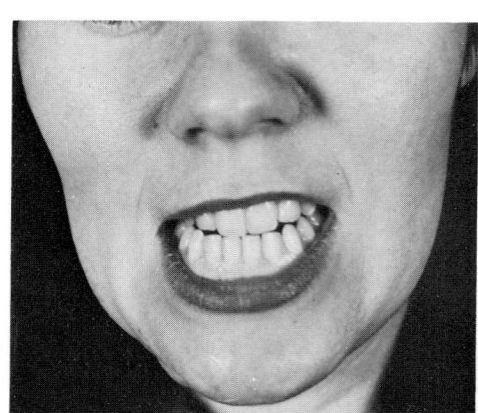

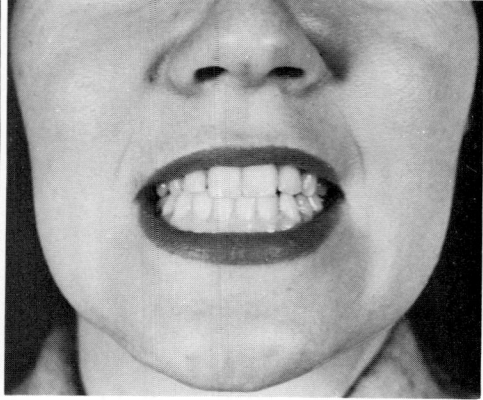

Fig. 13-17.—**Left,** malocclusion of the teeth associated with a transverse fracture of the middle third of the face. The malocclusion was overlooked. **Right,** restoration of occlusion, which required refracture of the maxilla through the floor of the nose and antrum, support of the alveolar arch with wires through the face anchored to the orbital rim and wiring of the upper and lower teeth in occlusion for about 6 weeks.

Fig. 13-18.—Methods of direct fixation of the teeth in occlusion. The normal relationship is established and stabilized by elastic traction to wire hooks or buttons (**A**), by direct wiring between opposing pairs of teeth (**B**) or by using arch bars attached to multiple teeth and held to each other with wire or elastic bands (**C**).

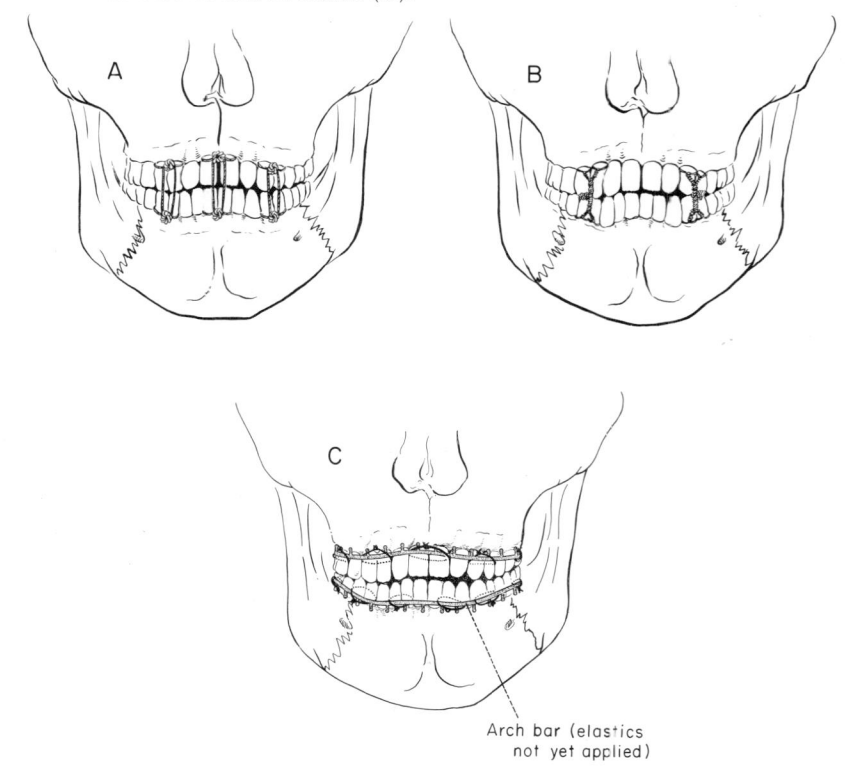

Arch bar (elastics not yet applied)

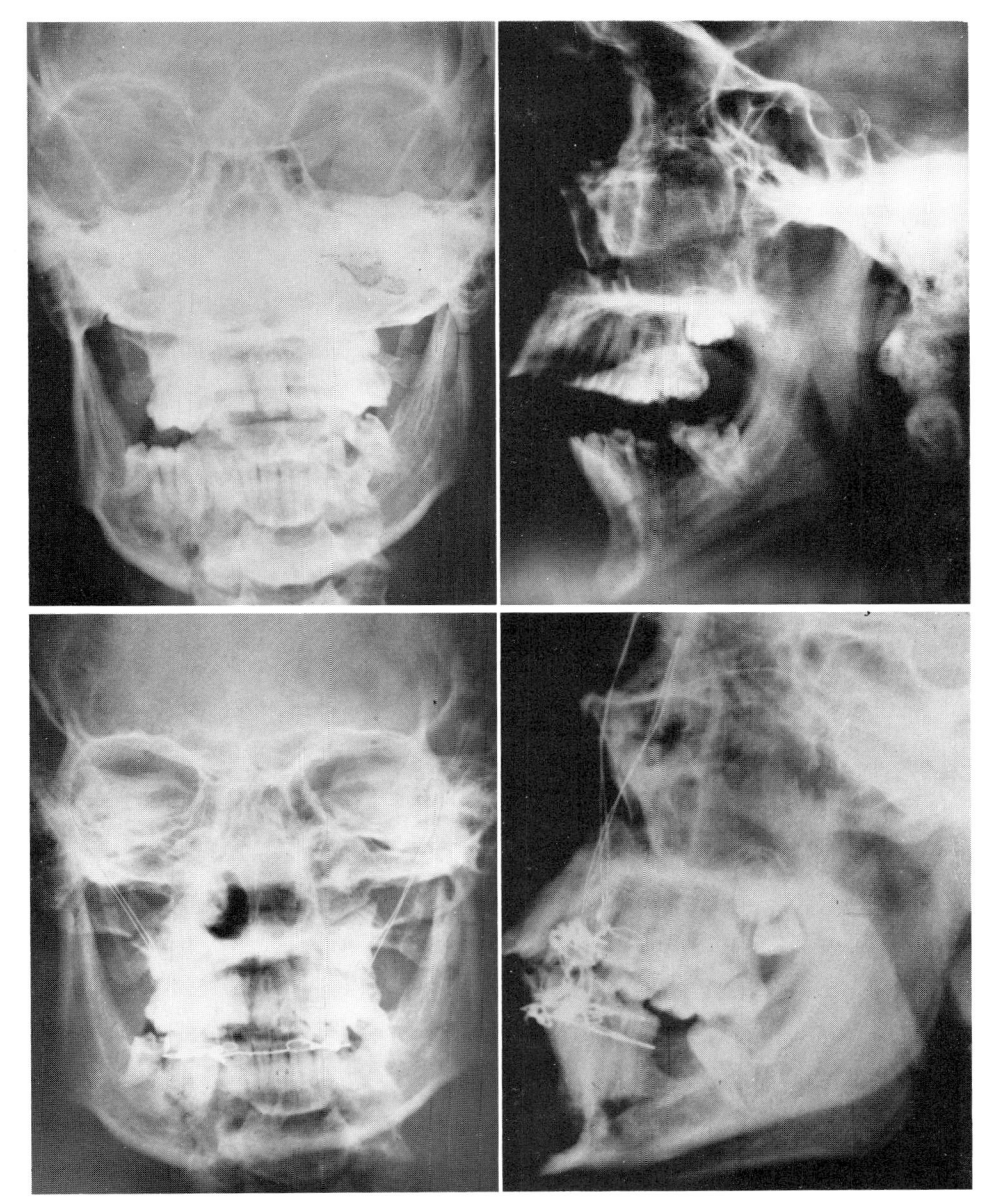

Fig. 13-19.—Severe fracture of the face and jaw from an automobile accident. **Top views,** the fracture of the face traverses the antrum, with complete separation of the floor and alveolar processes, which are displaced downward and backward. The right malar bone is also displaced downward and backward, and there is a fracture of the mandible at the right mental foramen. **Bottom views,** the facial fracture was reduced and supported by wires passed through the facial tissues, looped through holes in the zygomatic process of the frontal bone and anchored to molar teeth in the upper alveolar arch. The displaced malar bone was elevated and then held in place with a gauze pack in the antrum. Finally, the malocclusion, due both to the displaced fracture of the face and to the mandibular fracture, was reduced and fixed by wiring the upper and lower teeth together.

to the orbital rims or the zygomatic arches or the frontal bones, depending on the level of the fracture—by wires that pass directly through the soft tissues of the face is a most practical addition to the methods applicable to the treatment of facial fractures.

The goal of treatment is to support the face and to restore normal occlusion. The bones of the face must be mobilized and obvious displacements of the zygoma, lacrimal and other facial bones corrected. Occasionally, these bones may need to be fixed by open reduction before the occlusion is re-established and the total face restored to normal position. If the mandible is fractured and displaced, it is desirable to reduce and fix it first, because it serves as a valuable guide in repositioning the fractured maxillary complex. The use of internal wire fixation for support of the upper alveolar process and the sagging framework of the face has meant that materials available in every well-organized operating room have replaced all manner of complex splints, inefficient head caps and unstable and consequently painful guy wires. After application of an arch bar, the intact dental arch is anchored directly to the stable orbital rims, zygomatic arches or frontal bones by the wires passed through the substance of the cheeks. Small incisions will suffice for exposure of the sites of suspension and for making the needed small drill hole. If the upper jaw is edentulous, the wire may be attached to an intact dental plate or directly to the bony alveolus. When this method is used, immediate and accurate reduction and fixation are possible, occlusion can be re-established promptly and no other splinting will be required. Support for the upper jaw and splinting of the teeth in occlusion by intramaxillary elastics must be continued for 6–8 weeks. The wires

Fig. 13-20.—**Left view,** bilateral fracture of the mandible at the angles. A molar tooth retained in the posterior fragment on the left side of the face prevents overriding by the ramus. Open reduction and wiring were necessary on the right side only **(right view).** The jaw was immobilized for 8 weeks by fixing the teeth in occlusion.

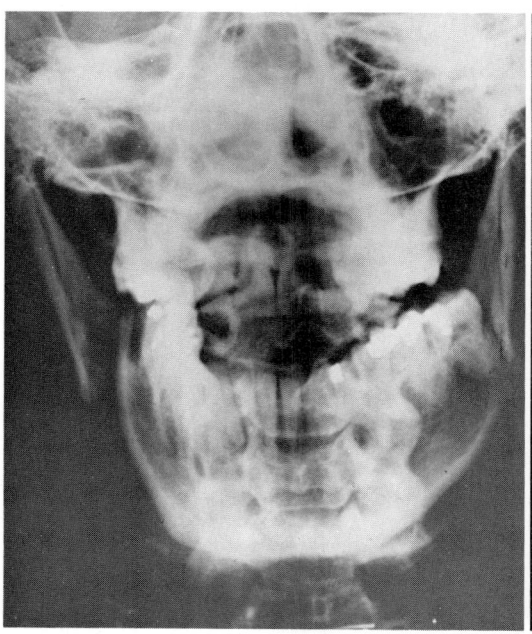

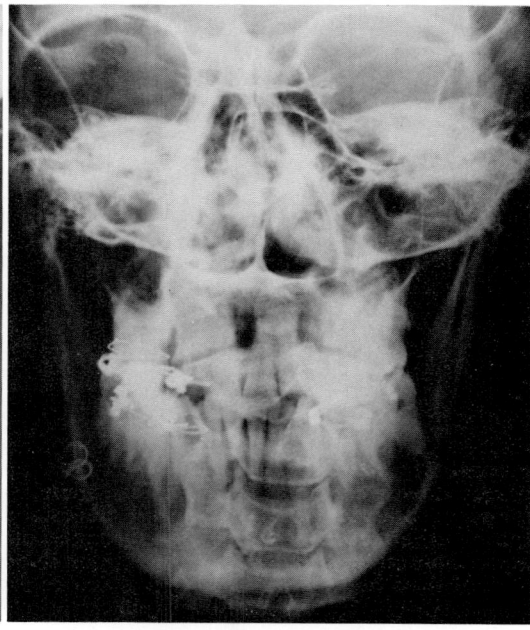

passing through the cheek are removed at that time*; other wires used for reduction may be left in place indefinitely.

Fracture of the alveolar process may involve any segment of the alveolar arch. Fixation by wiring to the adjacent undisplaced teeth or interdental fixation may be employed. Rarely is the displacement so severe that the blood supply to the bones and retained teeth is destroyed.

Fractures of the Mandible

Most mandibular fractures can be reduced and fixed in position by wiring of the upper and lower teeth in occlusion. Wires around two pairs of opposing molar teeth on each side of the upper and lower jaws may be twisted together to form four buttons to which elastic bands can be attached, or the wires on the opposing teeth are attached to each other to furnish more absolute fixation. The latter is undesirable if a general anesthetic has been used, because the mouth cannot be easily emptied of vomitus, thus increasing the chance of aspiration. Intermaxillary fixation is obtained more easily by the use of dental arch bars with interdental elastic bands. Attachment of the bars to the teeth is a little more complex, but more teeth are involved in the fixation and greater stability is obtained. Final fixation of the teeth in occlusion may have to be delayed until the patient is fully conscious.

When teeth are either inadequate or absent in any or all of the fragments, the problem is more complicated but still lends itself to surgical management. For example, the posterior fragment in fractures of the mandible at the angle often is edentulous because the fracture line is behind the last molar tooth. The ramus is

---

*Pullout wires of the type described by Bunnell will ease removal.

Fig. 13-21.—Left view, fracture of the neck of the mandibular condyle in a child. Although many of these fractures are best treated by splinting the jaw only, the displacement in this patient was so gross that open reduction through a small incision anterior to the ear was carried out (right view). No direct fixation of the fragment was necessary, but the teeth were wired in occlusion for several weeks.

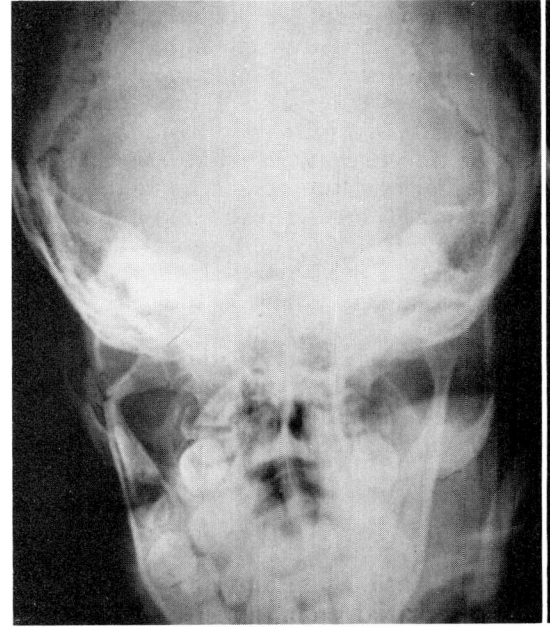

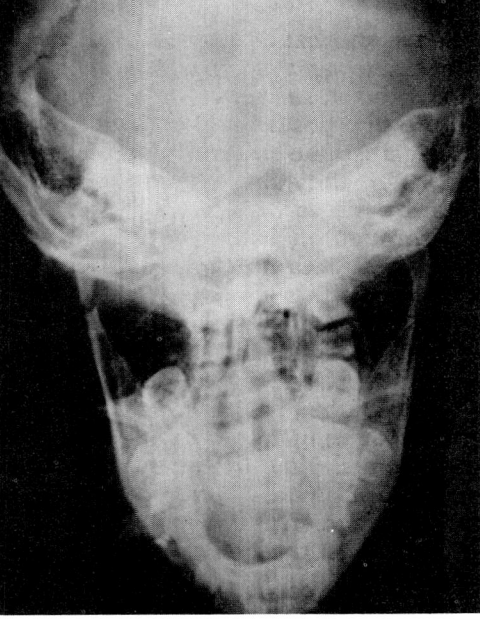

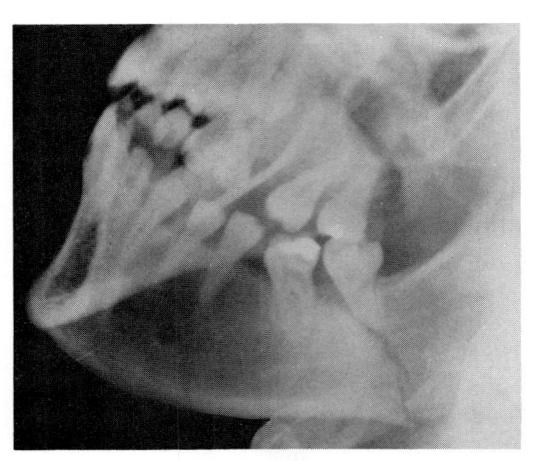

Fig. 13-22.—Fracture of the right mandible at the angle; compound into the mouth. The posterior fragment of the mandible cannot ride forward by pull of the masseter and temporal muscles because the tooth that lies in the fracture line obstructs this motion. It is safe to leave the tooth in place temporarily, until the fragments unite sufficiently to prevent overriding; then it should be extracted. Were the fracture behind the molar tooth, direct fixation of the posterior fragment probably would be necessary to prevent overriding. In either situation, wiring of the opposing upper and lower teeth in occlusion for 6–8 weeks is essential.

pulled upward and inward by the temporal, masseter and internal pterygoid muscles. If, because of the direction of the fracture, the posterior fragment does not lock against the anterior fragment (see Fig. 13-4), they must be held reduced either by direct wire fixation after exposure through an external incision or by transfixion with an internal wire-pin. Other methods, such as elastic traction to a head cap, external skeletal fixation or an intraoral dental splint, are more complex and require frequent adjustments. A totally edentulous mandible may be wired directly or may be splinted to the patient's dental plate by the passing of circumferential wires around each. The anterior fragment always must be supported against the downward pull of the geniohyoid, genioglossi, digastric and mylohyoid muscles. Occlusion will be restored if the lower plate is attached to the upper teeth or to the upper dental plate, which must be supported against the roof of the mouth by wire fixation. Fractures of the symphysis may be unstable laterally and require direct wiring of the lower border by transfixing with an internal wire-pin. The management of a fracture of one or both condyles still is a controversial matter. Some advocate open reduction of most of these fractures. Others consider this to be meddlesome surgery, because exposure and fixation of the tiny condylar fragment is difficult and may be the cause of bony ankylosis. Occasionally, excision of a single severely displaced condyle is indicated if it interferes with mandibular excursion. With rare exceptions, an excellent functional result can be expected if the mandible is splinted in normal occlusion until the condyle has united.

Fractures of the mandible with loss of bony substance require the accurate maintenance of dental occlusion. Early restoration of continuity of the bone must be planned as soon as soft tissue healing permits. Rib or iliac bone grafts may be used and will act as an effective splint for any nonimmobilized or edentulous fragments.

Since practically all mandibular fractures are compounded into the mouth, the risk of infection always is present. For this reason, nonvital loose teeth in the fracture line should be removed unless they are useful temporarily as a splint. Occasionally, external drainage of the fracture line is desirable until the mucosa is healed.

In the evaluation of the healing of mandibular fractures, the x-ray film may fail to reveal any callus. A more reliable test is clinical examination of the bony union. Fixation for 6–8 weeks is usual in uncomplicated mandibular fractures.

MANAGEMENT OF SOFT TISSUES

All fresh lacerations of the face should be repaired promptly. Only by early ac-

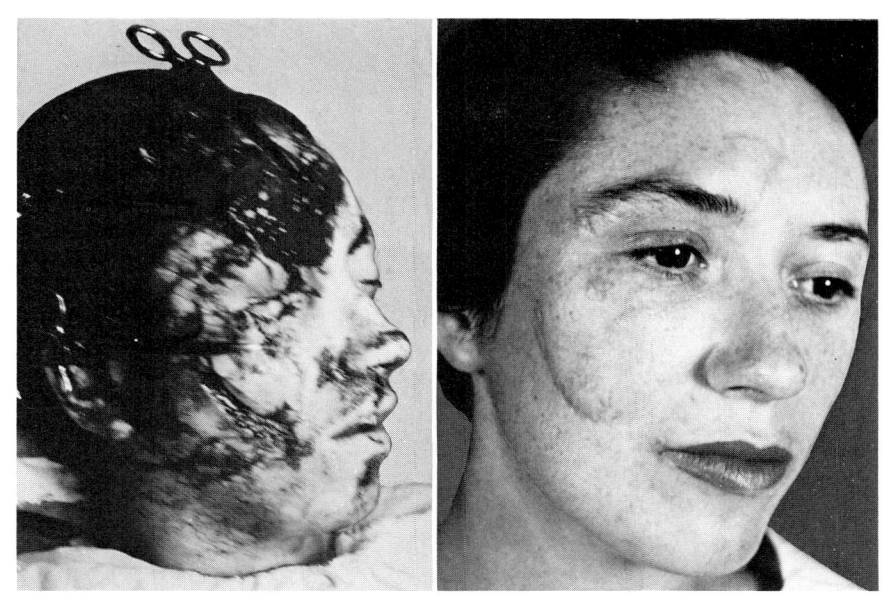

Fig. 13-23.—Left, multiple severe lacerations of face, eyelids and cheek with avulsion of portions of the scalp, the result of an automobile collision. After washing away the clotted blood, trimming the hair and removing fragments of glass from the wounds, the pattern of the lacerations became clear and primary suture was carried out. Fine (5-0) catgut was used for closure of the deep tissues and the dermis. Approximation of the skin edges was so accurate that only a minimal number of skin sutures were necessary. **Right**, final result, 1 year later.

curate closure of skin and mucous membrane can scarring and deformity be reduced. The healing power of the face is excellent and the resistance to infection high. Success depends on the observation of certain precautions, the most important of which is to do no additional damage. These include the avoidance of unnecessary debridement, the avoidance of wide sutures, which would leave stitch marks, and the avoidance of excessive tension, especially on flaps of skin with precarious blood supply. All wounds must be cleansed thoroughly, foreign material removed and hematomas evacuated. Layer closure of the subcutaneous tissues as well as the skin must be done with very fine suture material. If skin sutures are used, they should be removed within 48–72 hours. Today's trend is to use more subcutaneous sutures and substitution of a running cuticular stitch for skin sutures.

Great care and patience are necessary in identifying and replacing the jagged edges of torn and avulsed skin. If the lacerations extend through both surfaces of the eyelid, nose and mouth, with a full-thickness separation of the edges, accuracy in approximating is called for. The fitting together of obscurely misplaced flaps may require several attempts before the correct position is obtained. Obvious points of approximation, such as the vermilion border, the eyelid margin or the alar margin, are useful as starting points for suturing.

Sutures on the inner surface of the mouth, nose or eyelid should be only enough to obtain accurate apposition of the mucosa. Puncture wounds, especially of the lips, are best left unsutured. Free drainage thus is maintained and the likelihood of infection lessened. Small lacerations on the face sometimes can be approximated by adhesive support alone.

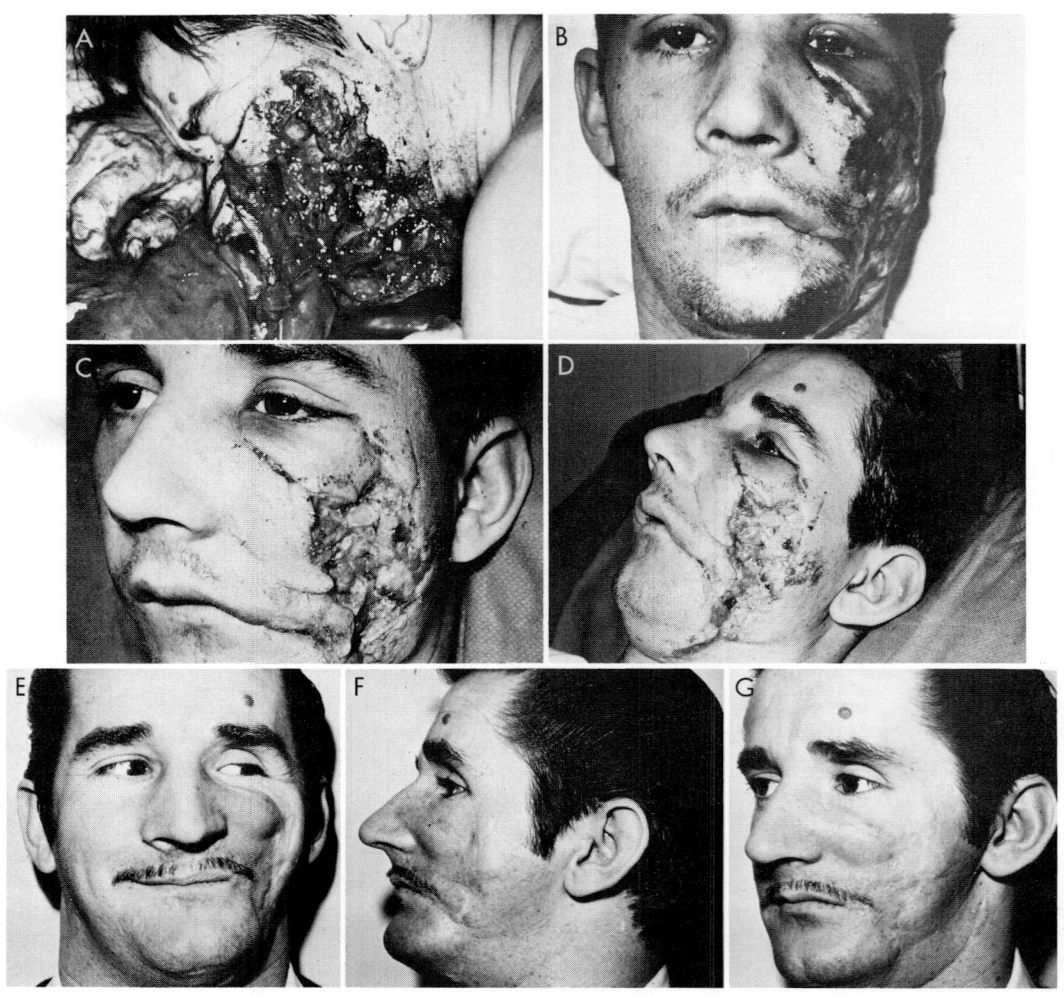

Fig. 13-24.—Severe soft tissue and bony damage to the face. **A,** patient, shortly after self-inflicted shotgun injury blowing out the left side of his face. **B,** 1 week after limited debridement, wiring of bone fragments and application of skin grafts. No tracheostomy was used. Note that the incision below the eye was not closed because of the amount of questionably viable tissue left in place. **C** and **D,** 2 weeks later. **E–G,** 2 years later after one scar revision. The incision below the eye has healed well with no additional surgery.

The method often is preferable in children because anesthesia and sutures then are unnecessary.

Skin losses, actually quite rare in these injuries, can be replaced by a skin graft if the deep tissues are not severely damaged. In extensive full-thickness losses of the cheek or nose, mucosa and skin may be approximated to close the raw surface in anticipation of later repair. This will not be indicated often in a civilian hospital except in a disaster situation with multiple casualties or under military conditions or in remote areas.

Immediate suture of divided branches of the seventh nerve in the face rarely is attainable because the fibers are tiny and identification may be impossible. If the

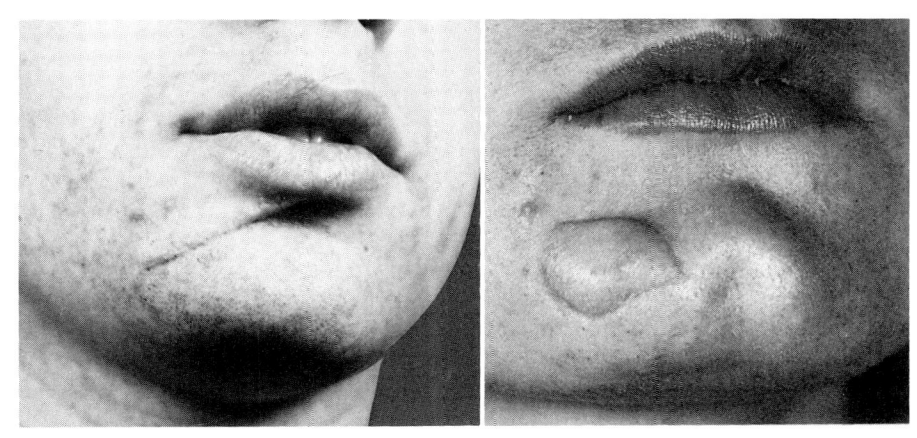

Fig. 13-25.—**Left,** thickened scar following primary suture of a laceration across a crease below the lip. Although some surgeons prefer to carry out Z-plasty or other anticipated modification of facial wounds at the time of primary closure, we usually have preferred to wait until a secondary repair can be carried out under optimal local conditions. **Right,** typical trap door flap deformity. This deformity is caused by the contraction of the scar, which, because of its U shape, constricts and thickens the skin within the circle of the scar. The deformity is correctable only by multistage thinning of the flap by opening the marginal scar.

larger trunks near the angle of the jaw can be identified, suture is indicated. Primary repair of a lacerated Stensen's duct should be considered in injuries of the cheek. A tiny probe or piece of suture material or a small silastic tube may be used as an internal splint. If the tissues of the cheek are too badly injured, repair may have to be postponed.

Among the most troublesome of all the lacerations of the face are the so-called trapdoor flaps caused by L- or U-shaped lacerations in the face. In these lacerations and in curved lacerations across the cheek, the body of the mandible or elsewhere on the nose or face, the normal contraction of the healing scar tissue produces a fullness of the skin on the concave side of the scar or thickening of the scar where it crosses normal folds. In anticipation of these deformities, some surgeons recommend primary small "zigzag" flaps to avoid straight-line suturing of such lacerations, but, in general, primary closure without the removal of normal tissue or the creation of additional scars is preferable. The amount of subsequent deformity cannot be predicted, but that secondary revision of the soft tissues may become desirable in many severe facial injuries should be anticipated in the management of the primary wound.

DRESSINGS

A firm, resilient pressure dressing is essential after the definitive primary reduction of facial fractures and after suture of facial wounds. It is also useful before treatment if there are to be unavoidable delays. Oozing of blood from the damaged tissues and the further development of edema are best controlled by such a dressing. Edema, which develops rapidly after injury and manipulation of the tissues, may persist for many weeks or months unless it is reduced to a minimum by the prompt application of a firm dressing.

POSTOPERATIVE CARE

The usual supportive measures should be continued, including fluid by vein and transfusions, until the patient is able to take sufficient fluid and food by mouth. A high-calorie, high-vitamin liquid diet must be available for all patients with interdental wiring. A home blender is of great value.

In all patients with fractures compounded into the mouth or nose, *cleanliness* is essential. Irrigations, mechanical removal of debris and mouthwashes are useful. Patients with interdental wiring may have real difficulty in keeping the mouth clean unless frequent irrigations are given. Mechanical cleansing of the teeth with a short-bristle toothbrush is desirable. An excellent method is a high-powered water jet device, such as Water Pik.

In patients with extensive fractures as well as lacerations, the dressings should be replaced after the skin sutures, if any, are removed on the second or third day. In severe injuries, the tissues need the support of a dressing for about a week. The dressing serves also as a splint for bony fragments that do not solidify before the seventh to the tenth day.

BIBLIOGRAPHY

Adams, W. M.: Internal wiring fixation of facial fractures, Surgery 12:523, 1942.

Blair, V. B., Ivy, R. H., and Brown, J. B.: *Essentials of Oral Surgery* (St. Louis: The C. V. Mosby Company, 1936).

Brown, J. B.: Deep block anesthesia of second and third divisions of fifth nerve, Surg. Gynecol. Obstet. 53:832, 1931.

Brown, J. B., and Cannon, B.: Repair of major facial injuries, Ann. Surg. 126:624, 1947.

Brown, J. B., Fryer, M. P., and McDowell, F.: Internal wire-pin stabilization for middle third facial fractures, Surg. Gynecol. Obstet. 93:676, 1951.

Cannon, B., and Murray, J. E.: Plastic surgery: Facial injuries, N. Engl. J. Med. 250:17, 1954.

Dingman, R. O.: Use of rubber bands in treatment of fractures of bones of face and jaws, J. Am. Dent. Assoc. 26:173, 1947.

Ivy, R. H., et al.: Symposium on plastic and reconstructive surgery, Clinics 2:1165, 1944.

Ivy, R. H., and Stout, R. A.: Emergency treatment of war injuries of face and jaws, Ann. Surg. 113:1001, 1941.

Kazanjian, V. H.: Primary care of injuries of face and jaws, Surg. Gynecol. Obstet. 72:431, 1941.

Additional Bibliography with Annotations

Barsky, A. J.: *Principles and Practice of Plastic Surgery* (Baltimore: The Williams & Wilkins Company, 1950).
A discussion of facial injuries with a carefully selected bibliography of the important literature on fractures of the facial bone appended.

Blair, V. P., Brown, J. B., and Byars, L. T.: Treatment of fracture of the upper jaw, Surgery 1:748, 1937.
A clear, concise presentation of the fracture patterns encountered following severe injuries to the face, with an exposition of the principles involved in their management.

Erich, J. B.: Treatment of bilateral fractures of edentulous mandible, Plast. Reconstr. Surg. 9:33, 1952.
A detailed elaboration of a specific problem of fracture splinting.

Erich, J. B., and Austin, L. T.: *Traumatic Injuries of Facial Bones* (Philadelphia: W. B. Saunders Company, 1944).
An extremely well-illustrated atlas using models of the skull to demonstrate methods of reduction and splinting of practically every type of fracture of the bones of the face and jaws.

Fry, W. K., et al.: *The Dental Treatment of Maxillofacial Injuries* (Philadelphia: J. B. Lippincott Company, 1945).
A general review of the multiple problems of facial injury, with emphasis on the important part the dental surgeon can play in the management of jaw fractures.

Kazanjian, V. H., and Converse, J. M.: *The Surgical Treatment of Facial Injuries* (Baltimore: The Williams & Wilkins Company, 1949).
An exhaustive review of many years of experience in the early and late treatment of facial injuries.

Schultz, R. C.: *Facial Injuries* (Chicago: Year Book Medical Publishers, Inc., 1970).
A very practical, well-illustrated guide to the management of facial injuries based on more than 1,000 cases treated personally by the author.

14 | Diagnosis and Treatment of Head Injuries

EDWARD P. BAKER, JR.

THE PROBLEM.—Ever since the first lethal automobile accident in the United States in 1895, the annual death toll from traffic injuries has spiraled relentlessly upward, approaching 55,000 fatalities in 1971.[1] Injuries in the home, on the job or in various miscellaneous mishaps kept apace of this increase and contributed more than half of the total of 119,000 accidental deaths. Accidents now are the most common cause of death between the ages of 1 and 44 and are the fourth most common cause of death in all age groups behind heart disease, cancer and stroke. There are more than fifty million persons injured annually in the United States and, despite the recent heightened interest in accident prevention, there are few solid grounds for optimism that this dismal epidemic will be brought under early control.

Man's earliest recorded surgical efforts were directed at the consequences of head trauma, and the importance of head injuries as a major cause of death and disability has not diminished over the intervening centuries, nor is it likely to do so in the foreseeable future. Current data indicate that head injury occurs in 70% of persons injured in traffic accidents and falls,[3] and that about the same percentage of the total killed accidentally die as a result of injury to the central nervous system. The magnitude of this medical and social problem leads one to view with alarm the growing trend in American medical schools to discontinue didactic and clinical instruction in neurosurgery for undergraduate students, and the failure of many graduate training programs in general surgery and in the various surgical specialties to provide residents with training and experience in the management of head trauma.

With more than 1,600 board-certified neurologic surgeons practicing in the United States and ample representation of the specialty in the armed forces, general surgeons seldom are required to assume primary responsibility for the management or operative treatment of severe head injuries. However, concomitant trauma to other major body systems is so common in clinical practice that general surgeons and surgical subspecialists necessarily are active participants in the care of patients with these complicated injuries, and since the presence of a serious head injury will modify treatment of other injuries (and vice versa), some familiarity with the problems encountered in the diagnosis and treatment of craniocerebral trauma is indispensable to all members of the surgical team.

This chapter is directed to trauma surgeons not specializing in neurosurgery, and attempts to outline the principles and some of the details of management of patients with head injuries, as practiced at Massachusetts General Hospital.

FIRST AID AND TRANSPORTATION

The treatment of craniocerebral injuries and the initial steps taken to prevent irreversible complications in comatose patients begin at the scene of the injury. Usually, an appreciable interval occurs between the moment of the accident and the arrival of the victim at the emergency room, and it is during these critical early minutes that the patient's chances of surviving his injuries may be irretrievably lost as a consequence of inept handling.

Ambulance attendants, police officers and firefighters in their role as rescue workers have, as their primary responsibility, the obligation to transport accident victims to an appropriate medical facility in a manner that will not compound the original injuries. In many communities, though, the level of proficiency in first aid at the accident site and in patient support while in transit to the hospital is dismally substandard because of inadequately equipped rescue vehicles, lack of community planning and, more important, poorly trained or untrained personnel. These shortcomings presently constitute a weak link in the ongoing care of trauma patients. It is more probable that major improvement in the prognosis of patients with head injuries will result from the upgrading of this phase of patient care to presently attainable levels than from advances in surgical or medical treatment in the next decade.

The steady decline in the mortality and morbidity of head injuries sustained in combat by American soldiers in the recent succession of wars is due, in large part, to the rapid evacuation of the wounded by highly trained personnel from the battlefield to well-equipped hospitals staffed by surgeons trained and prepared to provide definitive treatment. There is little doubt that the helicopter, so valuable in military medicine, will be widely used in transporting civilian casualties, but the most pressing current need concerns the first aid training of rescue workers. Formal educational programs, such as the Emergency Care Course, given annually in many centers throughout the country under the direction of the American Academy of Orthopaedic Surgeons, merit intense and active support by trauma surgeons in all specialties.

The maintenance of a patent airway is the single most important emergency measure that can be carried out in unconscious patients and this requirement always has priority over all other considerations at every phase of the patient's illness. Injury to the brain invariably results in some degree of cerebral swelling, which may be massively increased by even moderate degrees of underventilation. The resultant hypercapnia and hypoxia induce cerebral vasodilatation, which increases the brain-blood volume, leading to further brain edema and elevation of intracranial pressure to lethal levels. Airway obstruction is a common cause of death by this mechanism, and, in survivors, is a major contributor to increased neurologic disability. The deadly effects of anoxia cannot be undone by the best of care later on and must be prevented at all costs.

In the United States, the unfortunate practice of strapping the unconscious person to an ambulance litter in the supine position preparatory to a high-speed run to the nearest hospital is widely prevalent. In this position—the worst of all positions for a person in coma—the relaxed tongue and mandible fall backward, producing upper airway obstruction. This is recognizable by the "snoring" sound produced and is remedied immediately by forward pressure on the angles of the mandible and/or the insertion of a plastic oral airway. An assortment of these, together with catheters and the other equipment necessary for endotracheal suction, should be on every rescue vehicle used in transporting comatose patients. Saliva, blood from facial or oral lacerations and vomitus will gravitate into the posterior pharynx, where, unimpeded by normal cough or swallowing reflexes, they passively flow or are aspirated into the lungs. Both blood and gastric contents incite an irritative chemical pneumonitis that may be refractory to all treatment.

Patients in coma from any cause should be transported and nursed in the lateral decubitus position (the coma position) (Fig. 14-1) at all times until consciousness has been recovered. In this position, the tongue and jaw fall forward and secretions tend to flow out of the mouth rather than into the lungs, so that the hazards of aspiration are greatly reduced. Proper positioning of these patients frequently is neglected, but since attention to this detail so often represents the difference between survival and death, its importance cannot be overstressed.

It is axiomatic that every patient who is unconscious following violent trauma is to be regarded as having a cervical spine fracture until this possibility has been excluded by careful neurologic examination and satisfactory x-ray films, which must include lateral views demonstrating the odontoid and the C6–C7 interspace. Since any movement at the site of a cervical fracture may contuse or transect the spinal cord or cervical roots, the neck must be immobilized in the neutral position by means of a collar. A plastic Thomas collar is adequate for this purpose, and these devices should be standard equipment on every rescue vehicle. Special problems arise when persons must be extricated from wrecked autos or lifted from one level to another. In these instances, one person should be assigned the responsibility for maintaining the alignment of the head with the body by exerting manual traction along the axis of the spine. This topic is considered in greater detail in Chapter 15.

Bleeding from scalp lacerations may be brisk and considerable blood may be lost if the lacerations are extensive; this is controlled readily by firm pressure over a sterile dressing. Underlying depressed fractures, if present, usually are tightly impacted and are unlikely to be displaced further by the amount of pressure required to arrest the bleeding. If arterial bleeding is active on arrival at the emergency room, fine hemostats placed on the galea will evert the scalp and achieve hemostasis. Hemorrhage from exposed brain or skull should be covered lightly with a temporary dressing and dealt with in the operating room.

Not every hospital is, or should be, staffed and equipped for the complex diagnostic and operative procedures and

Fig. 14-1.—The coma position. Unconscious patients should be transported and nursed in this position to lessen the risk of aspiration. The neck is immobilized by the plastic collar and protected by careful handling until cervical spine fracture has been excluded by x-ray.

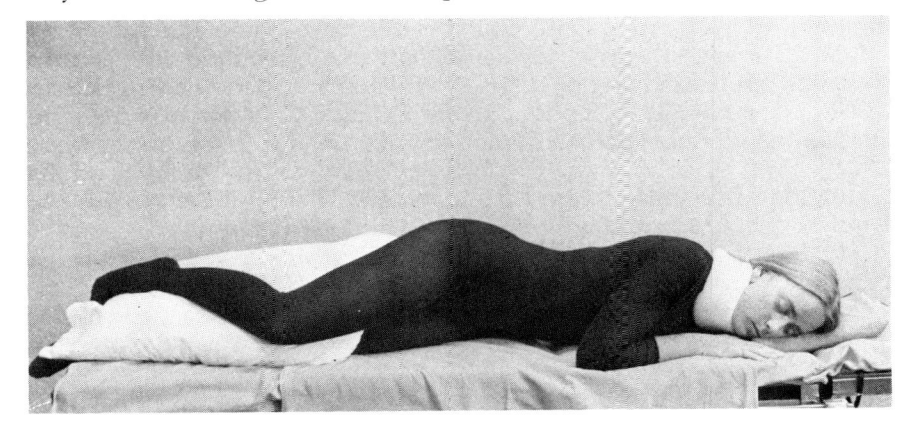

specialized postoperative care required by patients undergoing major cranial surgery. These functions are performed better in neurosurgical units, designated as such, in community hospitals or teaching centers to which patients with serious head injuries should be brought directly. Until some organization of emergency services along these lines occurs, it usually is wiser to transfer these patients immediately from the receiving hospital unaccustomed to caring for neurosurgical patients to an appropriate facility rather than to request the services of a far-away consultant. This procedure usually saves time and avoids the many serious problems that always arise when a surgeon attempts to care for these patients in a setting with inadequate facilities. Provided that shock from other injuries is not present and that coma is not progressively deepening, nonmoribund patients with head injuries can be transported safely with an intratracheal tube in place.

EVALUATION OF HEAD INJURIES

In the present era of high-velocity trauma, impact injury of the head may occur in association with every imaginable combination of body injury. The successful management of patients with such complicated multiple injuries usually requires more than one surgeon, but it is important to recognize that an assortment of surgical specialists, each acting independently to treat that portion of the patient falling within his own domain, will provide poor care unless over-all direction of management is assumed by a single person—preferably the surgeon caring for the dominant injury that threatens survival.

The evaluation of recently injured patients requires at least two examinations—the first, a quick survey to determine which body systems are involved and, later, a systematic appraisal of the individual injuries. The plan of management should be organized so that injuries posing an immediate threat to life receive attention first, and experienced surgeons, almost by reflex, begin with the respiratory system, checking for patency of the airway and adequacy of the mechanics of ventilation. Correction of airway obstruction due to secretions or fractures of facial bones or mandible by immediately inserting an endotracheal tube and aspirating the tracheobronchial tree is the first order of business, and this measure alone often results in striking improvement in the neurologic condition of obtunded patients. It is a safe rule of thumb that any unconscious person who will tolerate an endotracheal tube should have one, and certainly any comatose patient to be transported should be intubated prior to beginning his journey. The tube should be inserted without unnecessary manipulation of the neck if cervical spine fracture is a possibility, but a patent airway always has the highest priority and must be guaranteed. The profound disorders of ventilation and severe hypoxia attending chest injuries are of equally high priority, and appropriate treatment should be started before considering any of the other injuries.

If shock is present, it is not likely to be on a "central" basis as sometimes is erroneously supposed and, after first instituting corrective measures, attention should be directed toward such less fanciful causes as blood loss into the chest, abdomen or extremities. Head injuries almost never cause shock, although uncommon exceptions are encountered in infants, who may become anemic and hypovolemic from blood loss into an intracranial hematoma, in patients with massive scalp bleeding and in patients with fatal brain injuries in the few minutes before their death from failure of the medullary vital centers. Head injuries do not cause a silent abdomen, nor do they cause abdominal rigidity save as part of the pattern of generalized decerebrate rigidity. Except in the most desperate circumstances, it is unwise to begin a major neurosurgical procedure for head trauma until hypotension has been corrected by volume replacement, as such patients seldom survive.

As soon as emergency measures to provide adequate oxygenation and to restore blood volume are under way, the extent and urgency of the remaining injuries are assessed and priorities of management established. Since expanding intracranial hematomas kill quickly if not treated, surgical removal of these masses takes precedence over other injuries. Coexistent intra-abdominal hemorrhage from rupture of the liver or spleen, however, is an equally compelling indication for early surgery, and when two such life-threatening injuries demand immediate treatment and neither will await surgical correction of the other, it is necessary for two separate surgical teams to operate simultaneously—an awkward but sometimes lifesaving arrangement. With the important exception of enlarging intracranial hematomas, however, there are few cranial injuries so urgent that treatment cannot safely be postponed for the hour or two necessary for exploratory laparotomy, if this procedure is first required to arrest exsanguinating intra-abdominal hemorrhage. Delicate matters of judgment arise in the management of the patient with extremity fractures or other nonlethal injuries who is stuporous from a closed head injury not requiring cranial surgery. Lengthy operative procedures requiring anesthesia are best postponed until the patient is fully alert, but if the nature of the injury is such that early surgery is necessary, general endotracheal anesthesia should be used in preference to a spinal anesthetic. Narcotics should not be given to persons with serious head injuries, since they may depress respiration and make reliable neurologic observation difficult by altering pupillary reactions and the level of consciousness. If control of extreme agitation becomes necessary, small intravenous doses of phenothiazines can be given to titrate the patient's activity to the point of manageability.

Evaluation of the patient with a head injury should start with the history, and, if circumstances permit, the persons who brought the patient to the hospital should be interviewed before beginning a detailed examination. Trained rescue personnel and other alert observers often can provide surprisingly detailed data relative to the mechanism of injury and the patient's state of consciousness and general neurologic condition immediately thereafter; this latter information is particularly valuable, as it establishes the baseline from which subsequent improvement or deterioration is measured. Such helpful historical information is volunteered infrequently; it has to be sought actively by asking appropriate questions of the witnesses before they become unavailable. Specific inquiry should be made regarding coma and its duration, the status of limb movements, pupillary reactions, the occurrence of seizures, the extent of external blood loss and vomiting-aspiration. Relatives should be asked whether the patient is right- or left-handed to determine cerebral dominance, and questioned about the ingestion of drugs or alcohol and the existence of any prior medical or neurologic illnesses that might be related to the occurrence of the injury or to the patient's subsequent course. If the patient has recovered consciousness, he should be specifically asked if he has neck or back pain and whether limb power and sensation, vision and hearing seem normal. His replies may direct attention to the logical starting point of the physical examination. The extent of his recall of the injury and of events preceding and following the mishap is a rough index of the severity of the cerebral injury and should be recorded for medicolegal purposes.

In assessing the severity of a head injury, those with limited experience will find it helpful to consider separately the nature of the damage to the scalp, skull and brain, bearing in mind that injuries limited to the coverings of the brain usually are reparable, do not pose an immediate threat to life and can be evaluated at comparative leisure after the more pressing question of intracranial hematoma has been settled. Since enlarging intracranial hematoma is the only traumatic cranial lesion where delay of surgery for minutes or hours may spell the difference between life or death, the prime objective of the initial clinical and x-ray evaluation should be to determine whether a hematoma is present. The neurologic examination of an unconscious person is limited by the inaccessibility of all data requiring voluntary participation by the patient; however, sufficient information to arrive at a working diagnosis and to select the appropriate diagnostic studies and treatment required can be derived, within a few minutes, from the neurologic findings that are available.

The most important factors in determining the diagnosis and prognosis at any stage after head injury are the patient's state of consciousness and any changes thereof from a previously established baseline. The clinical course of patients with less severe head injuries is characterized by maximal brain dysfunction in the moments after impact, followed by steady return of consciousness toward normal. Thus, the person who is briskly alert, or who has been unconscious and is steadily awakening, is not in immediate danger and needs only close observation to ensure that his uninterrupted progress continues. Conversely, although patients with progressive brain swelling from cerebral contusions or those harboring intracranial hematomas initially may stabilize for a short period, their course is downhill as coma becomes progressively deeper and additional neurologic abnormalities appear. There are no characteristic signs that will differentiate acute subdural hematoma from cerebral contusion-laceration under those conditions, and either emergency cerebral angiography or bur-hole exploration is necessary.

A hemiparesis in an unconscious person often can be detected just by watching the patient and noting whether spontaneous limb movements are equal on the two sides. The normal response to noxious stimulation of a limb by vigorous pinching or repetitive pinprick is withdrawal, and movement can be elicited by these means if little spontaneous activity is present; alternatively tone can be assessed by elevating a limb and then dropping it onto the cot, comparing the movement to that of the contralateral extremity. The presence of a facial palsy can be determined by noting the response to digital compression of the supraorbital nerve at the orbital rim or to gentle pinprick applied to the inner nares. Failure to maintain lid closure indicates either peripheral facial palsy or profound depth of coma, with loss of all tonus. The occurrence of decorticate or decerebrate posturing on one or both sides, either spontaneously or in response to noxious stimulation, is an ominous finding that indicates injury to the upper brainstem. Decerebrate rigidity is seen more commonly after injury and is characterized by opisthotonos, forceful extension at all joints of the lower extremities and extension and internal rotation of the upper limbs (Fig. 14-2).

A dilated pupil that is unresponsive to light in a comatose patient indicates transtentorial herniation until proved otherwise and usually is due to an enlarging hematoma. Bilaterally dilated and fixed pupils are seen with injury to the midbrain, whereas constricted pupils unresponsive to light suggest a lesion of the pontomedullary region of the brainstem; either injury carries a very grave prognosis. If it can be established that either of these abnormalities was present immediately after injury, primary brainstem contusion is likely, whereas if these signs develop later, brainstem compression from an enlarging blood clot or cerebral swelling is the more probable mechanism. Roving side-to-side eye movements are observed commonly in comatose persons, and they indicate that the brainstem pathways for eye movements

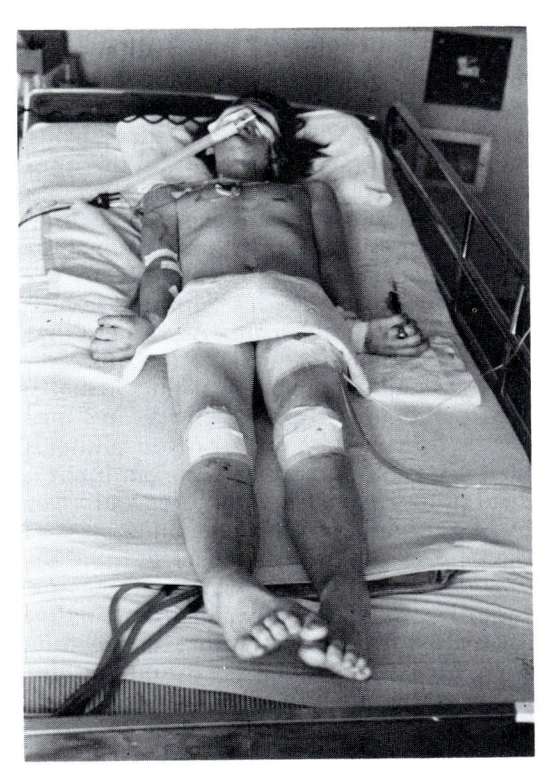

Fig. 14-2. — Decerebrate rigidity due to brainstem contusion. This patient remained decerebrate from the time of injury until death 10 days later. All limbs are rigidly extended, the arms internally rotated. Note the position of the patient's hands.

are intact. Forced conjugate deviation of the eyes to one side is due either to injury of the ipsilateral frontal eye fields for voluntary adversive gaze or to the contralateral medulla or cerebellum. These lesions can be differentiated by considering the accompanying neurologic signs and by determining whether the eyes can be brought to either side by head turning. Testing for these "doll's head" eye movements should be done only after cervical spine films have excluded fracture; their presence is normal and implies that the extensive connections between the extraocular and vestibular nuclei of the brainstem are intact.

Examination of the deep tendon reflexes takes only a few seconds and may disclose asymmetry or hyperactivity due to pyramidal tract lesions, or the reflexes may be completely absent in deep coma or in cases of cervical cord transection with spinal shock. Bilateral Babinski reflexes commonly are present in unconscious persons, and just as they often can be elicited in normal persons under general anesthesia or during sleep, they may or may not be of diagnostic importance, depending on the other findings. A unilateral extensor plantar reflex, however, always is significant and indicates a structural lesion of the contralateral cerebrum or its outflow, or of the ipsilateral spinal cord.

The vital signs alter in response to rising intracranial pressure but they do not always change according to the classic Cushing's triad of slowing of the pulse, widening of the pulse pressure with rising systolic and falling diastolic pressure and development of slow, irregular respirations. Abnormal patterns of respiration are common and if indicated by serious derangement of arterial pH and blood gases, controlled ventilation may be required.

Inspection of the head usually provides clues to the nature and force of the instrument of trauma and is useful in determining the mechanism of the brain injury. The importance of noting the location and extent of lacerations, bruises, open or depressed fractures or entry-exit sites of bullet wounds is obvious. Sometimes digital palpation of a scalp hematoma gives the false impression of an underlying depressed fracture as one feels the soft center of the hematoma; the true situation is readily clarified by x-ray. The ears and nose should be examined for evidence of bleeding or CSF leakage, and the presence of damage to the eyeballs, orbits and the facial bones determined before swelling makes such examination difficult. Ecchymosis over the tip of the mastoid (Battle's sign) or around one or both orbits (raccoon sign) in the absence of local trauma is due, respectively, to fracture of the temporal or occipital bone or to frontal fracture extending into the roof of the orbit. These signs may not appear immediately, as they depend on the diffusion of blood under the scalp to these regions of thin translucent skin.

Altered consciousness and other neurologic abnormalities after head trauma are caused by two different mechanisms, operating either singly or together in the individual patient. Brain injury is either primary, due to intrinsic damage to brain tissue (contusion-laceration) at the moment of impact or secondary to later compression of the brain by an expanding hematoma. Effective treatment plainly depends on the ability of the examiner to distinguish between these two types of injury. Some degree of primary brain injury is present in virtually every patient still unconscious on arrival at the hospital, but, although the presence or absence of an accompanying blood clot may be suggested by the clinical course and the other neurologic signs, frequently this question cannot be answered by clinical means alone, and a contrast study or surgical exploration is required. Cerebral contusion can be assumed, for the time being, to be the diagnosis in the patient with altered consciousness without other neurologic abnormalities who shows unmistakable clinical improvement during the period of the initial evaluation. If coma persists or deepens, however, or if lateralizing signs, such as a dilated pupil, hemiparesis, facial palsy or Babinski reflex, or signs of rising intracranial pressure or impending decerebration are present or appear during observation, an expanding hematoma most likely is present, and immediate cerebral angiography or bur-hole exploration is indicated.

As discussed later in this chapter, it is our practice to begin treatment of the cerebral swelling that follows brain injury by either mechanism by limiting intravenous fluids and administering parenteral steroids while the patient is in the emergency room.

X-RAY AND LABORATORY STUDIES.— Standard x-ray films of the skull supplemented if necessary by tangential or other special views, should be taken early after injury in all patients presenting with head trauma; in addition, if the injury is such that there is even a remote chance of injury to the cervical spine, frontal and lateral x-ray films demonstrating the cervical spine from C1 to C7 should be taken and examined before subjecting the neck to any movement that might damage the spinal cord. Skull x-ray films of uncooperative patients usually are technically unsatisfactory, and unless serious injury is suspected clinically, it is wiser to postpone the examination until properly positioned radiographs can be obtained. The physician in charge of the patient has the advantage of information derived from his examination, and should always view the films personally, regardless of the availability of consultants, focusing special attention on the region of the skull in relation to the external signs of injury.

Depressed fractures usually can be diagnosed from standard views of the skull, but if further information relative to the depth and extent of the depressed area is required to reach a decision on the need for surgical elevation, stereo views or an x-ray film taken with the central beam tangential to the fracture will clarify the situation. High-quality films, preferably including stereo views, demonstrating the position of indriven bone and foreign bodies are essential in planning operative treatment of penetrating brain wounds. Certain radiographic abnormalities are associated with serious complications, and their presence should prompt closer observation than otherwise might seem indicated. Thus, linear fractures crossing vascular markings of meningeal vessels or dural sinuses should alert one to the possibility of extradural hemorrhage, and the finding of intracranial air or of an air-fluid level or clouding of the paranasal sinuses indicates fracture into

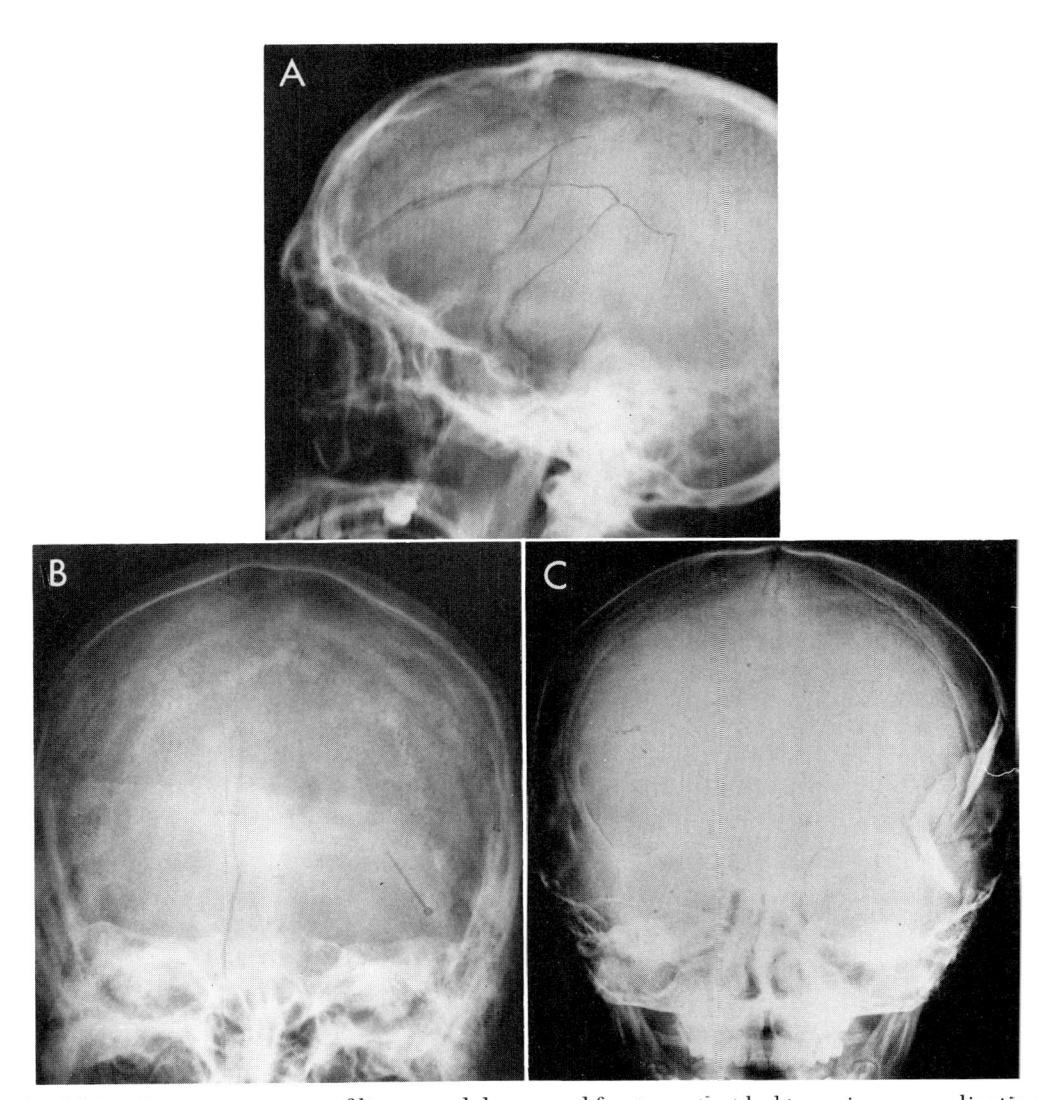

Fig. 14-3.—Roentgenograms of linear and depressed fractures that led to serious complications. **A,** linear fracture crossing groove of middle meningeal artery, which was torn, causing an extradural hematoma. **B,** linear fracture that entered ring of foramen magnum. The patient, although having extensive contrecoup injuries (see Fig. 14-6), appeared at first to have suffered only a brief concussion. On admission, she was alert and without abnormal neurologic signs but died suddenly of respiratory failure from a cerebellar pressure cone **C,** depressed temporal fracture following fall from a bicycle. (Note the characteristic lines of increased density where the edges of bone overlap.) This young girl had an immediate concussion, followed by a lucid interval and then severe convulsions. This suggested bleeding from a torn middle meningeal artery, but the artery and the dura were intact. Seizures ceased as soon as the indriven fragments of skull were elevated, and recovery was uneventful.

the sinuses and the creation of a potential pathway for bacterial contamination of the subarachnoid space. Opacification of the mastoid air cells has the same significance if old infection is excluded.

The pineal gland, which is calcified in approximately 55% of normal persons over age 20, serves as a radiographic indicator of the midline of the brain, and if it can be identified with certainty in the frontal projection, its position from the inner table on each side should be measured carefully. Displacement of more than 2 mm from the midline is presumptive evidence of a mass lesion in the hemisphere opposite the side to which the pineal is shifted; the pineal, however, may lie in a normal position if bilateral hematomas are present.

Since a high percentage of head injuries occur outside regular hospital working hours, at times when radiologic consultants are not ordinarily available, trauma surgeons must, of necessity, develop some degree of expertise in interpreting skull x-ray films. A clear account of the distinguishing features of skull fractures, and of the radiologic aspects of head trauma in general, is found in a monograph by Taveras and Wood.[48]

Cerebral angiography and bur-hole exploration share the properties of being definitive, safe and rapid methods of detecting traumatic intracranial hematomas, and one or the other is indicated in every patient suspected of having such a lesion. Direct surgical exploration has the advantage that the surface hematomas are diagnosed and treated by one procedure at the earliest possible moment, and is the preferred course for those patients deteriorating too rapidly to permit angiography. Under the most favorable of conditions, it takes almost an hour to perform a carotid angiogram, but the information derived from the study is so valuable in planning treatment that its use is advocated in all but the most urgent situations. Traumatic intracerebral hematomas are diagnosed and localized accurately by angiography, whereas they often are missed at exploration if the surgeon has no inkling of their presence beforehand. Since approximately 20% of traumatic intracranial hematomas are bilateral, the carotid circulation on both sides should be studied, either by separate injections into each cervical carotid or by attempting cross-filling with unilateral injection. This is done by injecting into one carotid artery while the opposite vessel is manually occluded in the neck. If the anterior portion of the circle of Willis is patent, contrast material will flow across the anterior cerebral arteries and opacify the vascular tree of the opposite hemisphere, usually well enough to determine whether a space-taking mass is present.

The various laboratory studies that are so helpful in the diagnosis of other diseases of the nervous system are of little value in the assessment of acute head trauma, principally because they are time-consuming and insufficiently definitive or, in the case of lumbar puncture, dangerous. Lumbar puncture should not be performed on patients with acute head injuries because of the risk of precipitating fatal transtentorial herniation or cerebellar pressure coning. Furthermore, the information obtained from the procedure is not likely to be of diagnostic specificity, since the fluid can be clear or bloody and the pressure high or low in patients with major intracranial hematomas. Radioisotope brain scanning by current techniques cannot reliably identify intracranial hematomas before 10–14 days after injury, and false positives are disturbingly frequent. The electroencephalographic abnormalities occurring soon after injury are too nonspecific for diagnosis or localization. It should be emphasized that these comments apply only to the use of these modalities in the acute situation, and any or all may be applicable to the solution of a specific diagnostic problem arising in the days or weeks following injury. The use of the ultrasonic scan to detect shifts of the midline of the brain is intellectually appeal-

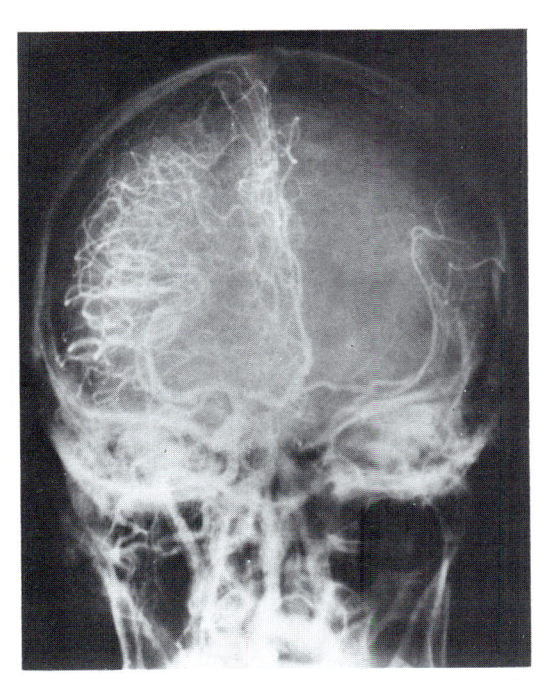

Fig. 14-4.—Acute subdural hematoma. Right carotid angiogram demonstrating separation of the terminal branches of the right middle cerebral artery from the inner table by the extracerebral collection and displacement of the pericallosal arteries to the left of their normal midline position. Manual compression of the left carotid artery in the neck during injection resulted in cross-filling of the intracranial branches of the left internal carotid artery and excluded a hematoma on this side.

ing, as it would appear to offer a quick, riskless method of screening patients with head injuries. In our hands, however, the echoencephalogram has been capricious and unreliable, and we have abandoned it in favor of other more definitive procedures. CAT scanning (Computerized Axial Tomography, EMI System) recently has become available at Massachusetts General Hospital and, because of the astonishing ability of the technique to detect tumors and to outline clearly the entire ventricular system without risk to the patient, promises to alter profoundly our current selection of procedures for the diagnosis and localization of intracranial mass lesions. This method of scanning is based on computer analysis of the differential absorption by small volumes of different tissues of a fine roentgen beam, and it is able to discriminate with great clarity between brain, blood and cerebrospinal fluid. CAT scanning for intracranial hematoma takes no more time than is required for a carotid angiogram and, although the experience with head trauma still is quite limited, it is anticipated that this technique will play a major role in the future diagnosis of the traumatic hematomas.

INTRINSIC BRAIN INJURIES

CEREBRAL CONCUSSION.—Cerebral concussion may be defined as transient post-traumatic brain dysfunction characterized clinically by unconsciousness and amnesia and pathologically by the absence of visible brain damage. Although this definition excludes macroscopic brain damage, considerable neuronal destruction has been observed in the brainstem reticular formation of animals after experimental cerebral concussion,[7] and it is probable that similar changes occur in many patients with this clinical diagnosis. Unconsciousness or coma, whether due to trauma, anesthesia or other causes, requires loss of the functional integrity of the reticular activating system of the upper brainstem, a region concerned with arousal from sleep and the maintenance of the wakeful state.[29] Lesions of the cerebral cortex alone, even if very extensive, do not result in coma.

The duration of unconsciousness after concussion is brief, and if coma persists longer than 5–10 minutes, it is likely that cerebral contusion is present. Amnesia is a constant feature of concussion, and its duration is one criterion for judging the severity of the brain injury. Both retrograde amnesia (loss of memory of events immediately preceding injury) and a somewhat longer period of anterograde amnesia (loss of memory of events after injury) may occur; the total amnesic interval tends to contract with the passage of time. Less common postconcussive phenomena, such as transient blindness or generalized seizures, may occur in children immediately after injury and are not necessarily of prognostic significance.

Patients presenting with a definite history of unconsciousness after trauma, no matter how brief, should be admitted to the hospital for 24–48 hours of observation. Those patients who were merely "dazed" or in whom the history of unconsciousness otherwise is uncertain may be discharged after careful examination, provided that a responsible relative is instructed to examine the patient periodically and to return him promptly if any abnormalities appear. An appointment for follow-up examination always should be given to such a patient. What is being observed for is the possible development of delayed intracranial hemorrhage; therefore, a complete neurologic examination is essential to establish the baseline to which any subsequent departures are compared. Since changes in the level of consciousness usually provide the earliest warning of a developing hematoma, the patient's responsiveness should be assessed hourly or even more frequently if there is unusual concern, along with speech, limb movements and vital signs. Undue reliance should not be placed on changes in the vital signs, as these are inconstant and generally occur late in the progression of a hematoma long after declining consciousness and other signs warning of the impending disaster should have been evident. In ordering observations, the physician should specify the limits of permissible variation in the vital signs and the alterations in the neurologic status of the patient that require his immediate notification.

Uncomplicated cerebral concussion requires no treatment, and prolonged bed rest or other inactivity is specifically contraindicated. If comfortable, patients should be ambulatory while hospitalized and encouraged to return to their usual activities as soon as possible after discharge, to minimize post-traumatic psychologic disturbances.

CEREBRAL CONTUSION AND LACERATION.—Cerebral contusion, or bruising of the brain, tends to be underdiagnosed clinically, relative to the great frequency with which gross structural damage of the brain occurs in closed head injury. Anatomic destruction of brain tissue to some degree probably is present in many patients diagnosed as having cerebral concussion, and certainly is present in all patients with prolonged unconsciousness or neurologic abnormalities lasting more than a few minutes. The severity of the clinical manifestations depends on the location and extent of the brain lesions, and ranges along a continuum from mild, with a picture not unlike that of a concussion except that unconsciousness lasts longer, to severe, with devastating neurologic impairment or permanent decerebration and coma. Brain contusions often occur in conjunction with skull fracture and/or intracranial hematoma, and are responsible for the failure of many patients to regain full neurologic function after successful removal of the clot. Occurring as an isolated pathologic entity, mild, moderate or severe degrees of cerebral contusion without skull fracture are very common injuries.

Bruises of the brain directly beneath the point of impact are called coup contusions and are caused by the inward deformation of the skull on impact, whereas contrecoup contusions occur on the side of the brain opposite the site of the blow and are caused by linear or rotational movement of the brain within the skull, a mechanism first demonstrated by Pudenz and Shelden[41] by high-speed cinephotography in monkeys with lucite calvarial windows. The distribution of contrecoup surface lesions is determined by the topographic features of the interior of the skull and, regardless of the point of im-

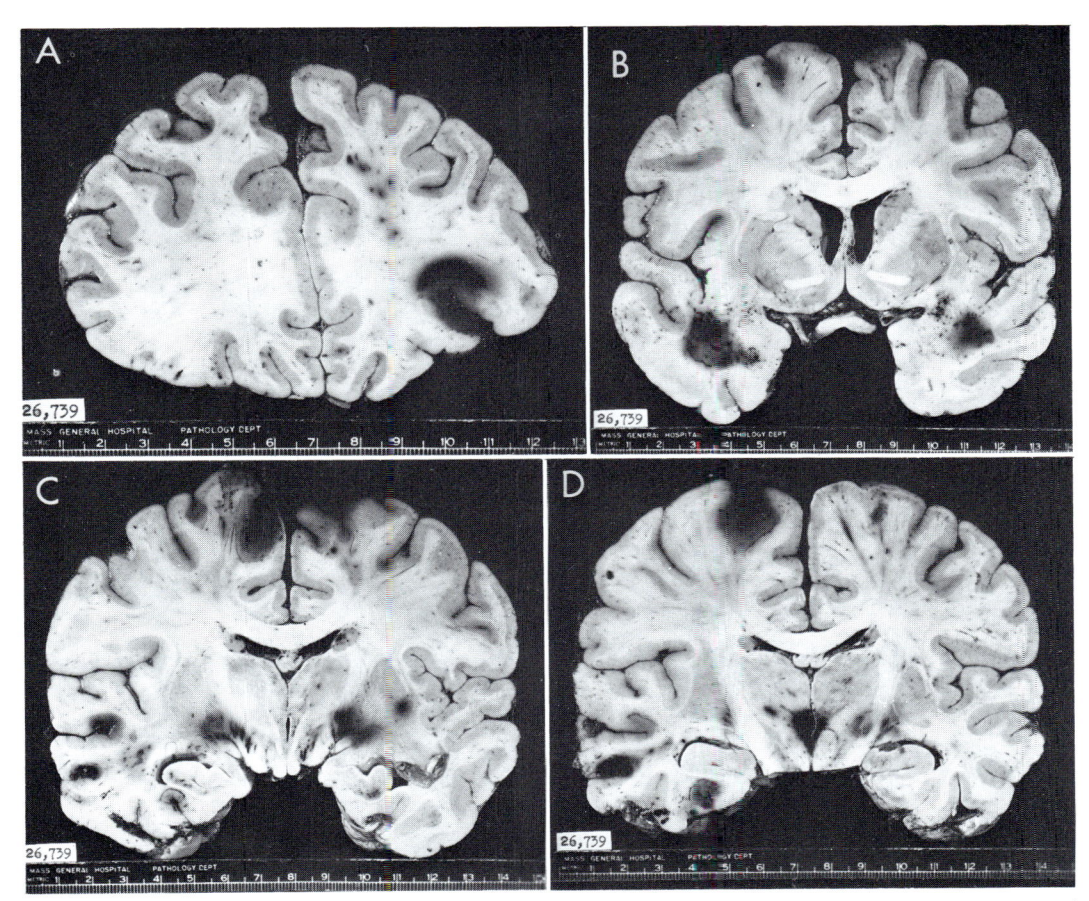

Fig. 14-5.—Primary brain injury: death 7 days after injury. Hemorrhagic lesions are scattered throughout the cerebral hemispheres and brainstem. A small subdural hematoma at the vertex has produced softening of the underlying cortex.

pact, they are found most commonly in the temporal and frontal poles and at the base of the temporal and frontal lobes, where the brain lies in relation to the sharp edge of the lesser wing of the sphenoid and the irregular surface of the floor of the anterior fossa. As the brain strikes against these bony prominences, milliseconds after impact, the cortex may be lacerated, resulting in traumatic subarachnoid hemorrhage or acute subdural hematoma. In contrast, the interior of the occipital portion of the skull is comparatively smooth and contrecoup injury of the occipital lobes after frontal trauma is uncommon. Occipital blows produce both coup and contrecoup lesions, whereas blows to the side of the head produce either coup or contrecoup injuries with approximately equal frequency.[40] Contusion of the midbrain and cerebral peduncles may result from impingement against the sharp inelastic edges of the tentorium, and is especially common after blows to the forehead or vertex.[9] Subcortical intracerebral hematomas form by coalescence of small hemorrhages within deep contusions or from shearing of a cerebral vessel, and share the predilection of contusions for the frontal and temporal poles.

In the early hours or days after injury,

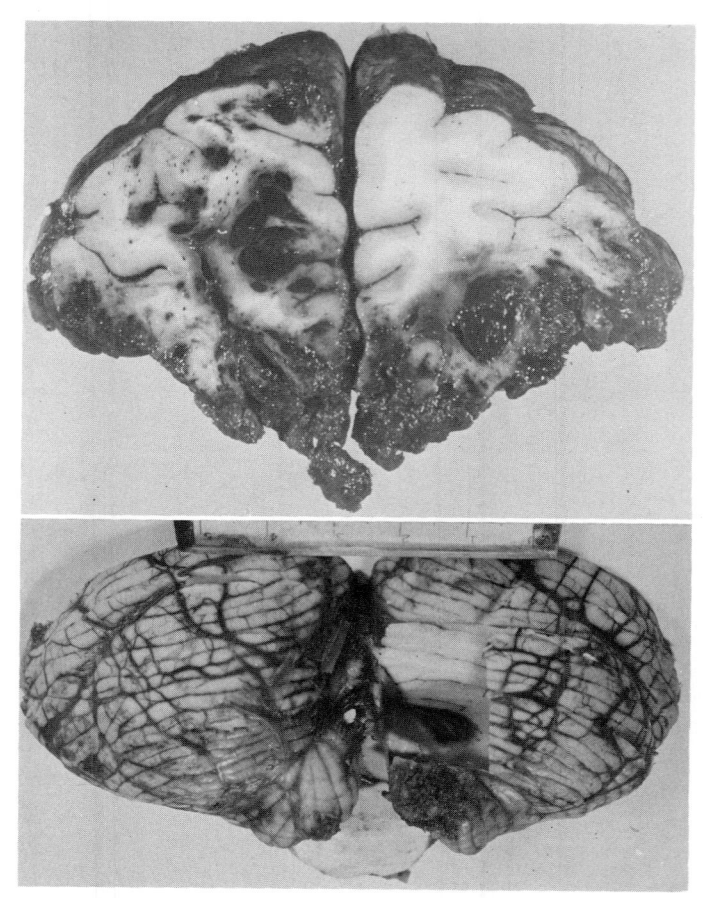

Fig. 14-6.—Contrecoup injuries in a patient who had a linear occipital fracture from an automobile accident (see Fig. 14-3, *B* for x-ray). **Top,** hemorrhage in frontal lobes. **Bottom,** herniation of tonsils with added hemorrhage in right cerebellar hemisphere. Death resulted from compression of medulla and respiratory center.

persons with milder degrees of contusion may remain drowsy, confused and restless, but if progressive improvement is not evident, the diagnosis should be reconsidered. Headache is a frequent complaint and usually is due to traumatic subarachnoid hemorrhage. Normal CSF is visually indistinguishable from water, and if lumbar puncture several days after injury yields discolored fluid, the specimen should be centrifuged promptly and the supernatant examined. The presence of xanthochromia establishes that the blood has been in the cerebrospinal fluid for more than 6–8 hours and excludes the possibility of a bloody tap. Minor amounts of blood in the CSF may be undetected unless the specimen is directly compared with a sample of water against a white background. EEG abnormalities are frequent, and an early tracing may prove useful should later seizures or other difficulties occur. As emphasized earlier, the prolonged obtundation and severe focal neurologic deficits seen in patients with more serious brain injuries are clinically identical to the syndromes produced by intracranial hematomas, and angiography is required to differentiate the two conditions.

OTHER CONDITIONS THAT MAY COMPLICATE THE DIAGNOSIS OF HEAD TRAUMA

ALCOHOL.—In 1971, drinking was a factor in approximately half of the traffic fatalities in the United States, and it is estimated that 800,000 traffic accidents result annually from the misuse of alcohol. One driver of 50 on the road at any time is dangerously inebriated. Besides the traffic accidents, the falls, assaults and other assorted mishaps to which intoxicated persons are so prone result in an extremely high incidence of severe head injuries among the drinking population.

Like other general anesthetics, alcohol depresses the reticular activating system of the brainstem, an effect that may be additive to that of trauma. Thus, an intoxicated person is rendered unconscious by a blow of lesser force than ordinarily is required to produce unconsciousness and tends to remain stuporous longer. Blood alcohol determination greatly facilitates the appraisal of the patient with head trauma who is believed to have ingested alcohol. A low level exonerates alcohol and directs attention elsewhere, whereas an elevated level permits at least an estimate of the possible role of alcohol in the symptomatology. Coma is present with blood levels of 400 mg/100 ml or greater and clinical intoxication usually is evident at 100 mg/100 ml. This latter level defines legal intoxication in Massachusetts and approximates that reached by an average-sized adult consuming 4 ounces of whiskey within a short time.

It is never safe to assume that altered consciousness in a person who appears intoxicated is due to the effects of alcohol alone if historical, physical or x-ray evidence of head trauma is present. Intracranial hematomas are very common in such persons and, if deepening stupor, lateralizing neurologic signs or other evidence of brain injury appear, appropriate diagnostic and therapeutic steps should be undertaken promptly. In cases in which the initial impression of head injury is not strong and there are no physical signs other than coma, the patient should be re-examined periodically over the course of 2 or 3 hours by the same physician. Alcohol-induced coma is of short duration and, unless progressive lightening is apparent during this brief period of observation, it is advisable to proceed with angiography to determine whether an intracranial hematoma is present.

The care of injured alcoholics may be complicated by the appearance of "rum fits" within the first 48 hours of abstinence. These seizures usually occur singly or in a flurry over several hours, but rarely the seizures may become frequent and progress to status epilepticus. Withdrawal seizures can be controlled or prevented by parenteral anticonvulsants in conventional doses and if the occurrence of seizures would seriously interfere with the treatment of other injuries, prophylactic treatment is indicated, especially if there is a history of seizures during earlier episodes of withdrawal.

OTHER DISORDERS OF THE NERVOUS SYSTEM.—Patients with pre-existing medical or neurologic diseases associated with alteration of consciousness will, at times, present in the emergency room with a bruised scalp and a nebulous history of a fall, confronting their physicians with the difficult task of determining whether the neurologic abnormalities are related to the head injury. The litany of medical diseases and intoxications modifying consciousness is vast, and usually a good bit of detective work and laboratory studies are needed before the correct diagnosis is reached. Patients with brain tumors, strokes, seizures and aneurysmal subarachnoid hemorrhage often fall, striking their heads, and, because of the complicated nature of their diseases, present thorny problems in diagnosis and early management. In most cases, a detailed history from perceptive relatives or witnesses to the fall will clarify matters but, lacking this, there are a number of neurologic clues mentioned briefly below that may help differentiate between the effects of trauma and the concomitant disorder of the nervous system.

Papilledema, if present on initial examination, is more likely due to an antecedent lesion, such as brain tumor, since it probably takes at least 12 hours for swelling of the nerve head to become manifest after an acute rise in intracranial pressure. The presence of preretinal hemorrhages favors the diagnosis of subarachnoid hemorrhage from ruptured aneurysm, although these lesions sometimes are seen with traumatic subarachnoid hemorrhage as well. Hemiparesis or other focal deficit that is disproportionately severe relative to the state of consciousness is not likely to have resulted from head injury. Although subdural hematoma over the visual cortex at the occipital pole can cause a hemianopia, this is uncommon, and the finding of a visual field defect in a patient conscious enough to participate in the examination implies an intracerebral rather than a surface lesion. The postictal coma and hemiparesis (Todd's palsy) following epileptic seizures are of short duration and, unless the seizures have been prolonged, usually clear or begin to clear within 20 or 30 minutes. The elderly provide an exception to this rule, and postictal coma may be prolonged for hours, although generally a steady trend toward improvement is soon apparent.

TRAUMATIC OCCLUSION OF THE EXTRACRANIAL CEREBRAL ARTERIES. — Acute or delayed thrombosis of the internal carotid or vertebral arteries is an uncommon sequela to either blunt trauma to the neck or penetrating cervical wounds.[44] The neurologic consequences of these major arterial occlusions depend mainly on the functional integrity of collateral flow through the circle of Willis and the presence or absence of hypotension or hypoxia due to other injuries. The diagnosis should be suspected in patients with severe neurologic deficit who nevertheless are alert and oriented and who have physical evidence of neck trauma; mandibular or clavicular fractures are seen commonly. Carotid artery occlusions in cooperative patients can be confirmed by ophthalmodynamometry, but transfemoral cerebral angiography is indicated to demonstrate the lesion and to determine the dynamic aspects of the circulation. As with other vascular occlusions, if the neurologic deficit is fixed by the time the diagnosis is made, surgical reopening of the vessel does not result in recovery of function beyond that which would be expected in the course of the normal evolution of the stroke.

CEREBRAL MANIFESTATIONS OF THE FAT EMBOLISM SYNDROME. — The diagnosis and treatment of the fat embolism syndrome are discussed in Chapter 54, and only the neurologic aspects of this interesting disorder will be considered here. Some degree of cerebral dysfunction is seen in virtually every patient with clinically significant fat embolism; in milder cases, this may appear as headache, anxiety, restlessness or irritability, whereas more severe involvement of the brain is marked by confusion, delirium, incontinence and stupor, which may progress to coma and death. Focal neurologic deficits are rare and the predominant clinical picture is one of diffuse cerebral impairment. Usually the interval between injury and the onset of symptoms is 1–3 days, but in occasional fulminating cases, severe cerebral signs may be apparent within an hour of injury. This sequence of events is reminiscent of the temporal profile of some cases of extradural hematoma in that the progressive neurologic symptoms appear after a symptom-free "lucid interval"; little confusion should exist if the fat embolism syndrome is pres-

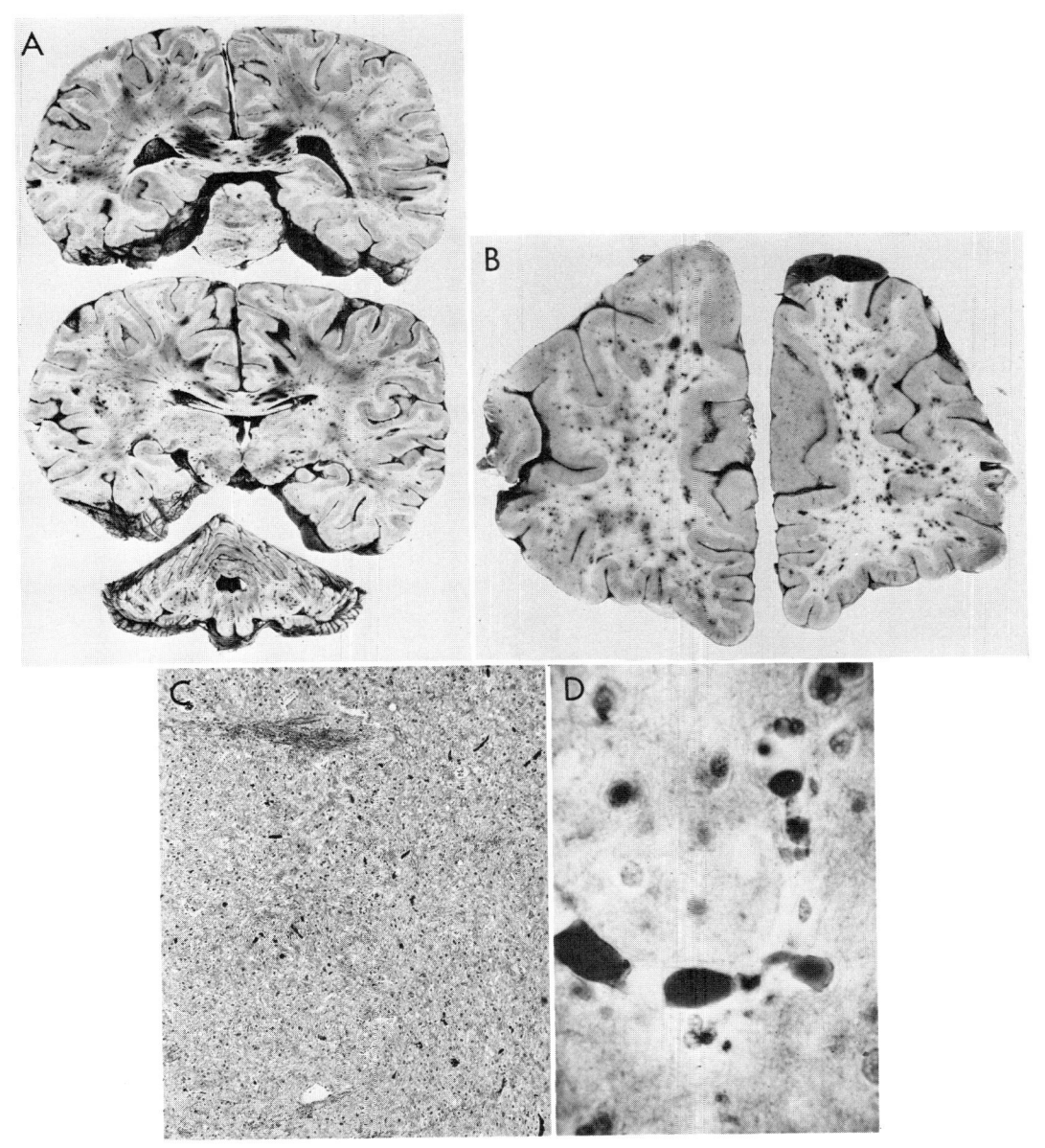

Fig. 14-7.—Cerebral fat embolism. **A** and **B**, the extensive hemorrhagic infarctions, principally within white matter, produce the characteristic picture of brain purpura. (Photos courtesy of Dr. H. R. Müller, Basel.) **C** and **D**, fat stain of the cerebrum. Many small vessels are filled with dark-staining fat emboli.

ent in fully developed form and if it is certain that the original injury spared the head. Considerable difficulty in differentiating the two conditions may arise, however, in deteriorating patients with suspected but unconfirmed fat embolism and a coexistent head injury that initially was not considered serious. In this situation, an expanding intracranial hematoma cannot be excluded on clinical grounds alone, and carotid angiography is indicated.

Two factors, hypoxia and transpulmonary embolization of fat to the brain, operating singly or together, are responsible for the cerebral manifestations of the syndrome. Arterial Po_2 of 40 or less, from any cause, results in profound cerebral dysfunction, and it is likely that the hypoxia universally present in the fat embolism syndrome explains at least the early, mild symptoms. Among the cases in Fischer et al.'s series from Massachusetts General Hospital,[8] however, neurologic signs did not improve rapidly when hypoxic patients were oxygenated to normal Po_2 and, in general, their neurologic status and the EEG abnormalities tended to lag behind other clinical indices of recovery by days. The failure of cerebral abnormalities to clear immediately with oxygenation suggests either posthypoxic brain swelling or embolization of fat to the brain. Barring paradoxic flow through a patent foramen ovale, systemic fat embolization requires passage of fat across the capillary bed of the lung, and its occurrence seems to be directly related to the amount of intravascular pulmonary fat. In fatal cases, fat emboli are found in every organ of the body, and the brain grossly appears to be sprinkled with myriads of tiny hemorrhagic lesions (Fig. 14-7, A and B), which are analogous to the evanescent skin petechiae seen so commonly. Microscopically, the lesions consist of areas of pale or hemorrhagic infarction centered around the fat-containing capillary or arteriole (Fig. 14-7, C and D).

The relative importance of hypoxia and its aftermaths and of cerebral fat embolization in producing cerebral symptoms may be difficult to determine in the individual patient, but the use of high doses of steroids, as advocated by Herndon (Chapter 54), because of the salutary effects on the lung, would also seem to be effective treatment of brain injury by either mechanism. Consideration should be given to prolonging steroid therapy beyond the recommended 3–4 days in those patients with persisting neurologic abnormalities. Fortunately, these resolve in most patients, but this is not always the case and some are left with permanent residual deficits.

INJURIES TO THE COVERINGS OF THE BRAIN

SCALP INJURIES.—Every scalp laceration, no matter how innocent in appearance, should be considered a potential penetrating wound of the brain and treatment in the emergency room not begun until x-ray films of the skull are examined. If a depressed fracture is present, it is by definition a compound depressed fracture and should be repaired in a fully equipped neurosurgical operating room. Simple linear fractures underlying scalp lacerations afford a ready avenue to the spread of infection intracranially and these wounds also preferably are debrided and sutured in the aseptic environment of the operating suite. Owing largely to the luxuriant local blood supply, properly repaired scalp lacerations usually heal rapidly. Careless treatment, though, is likely to be followed by wound infection, which may progress to subgaleal abscess formation or osteomyelitis of the skull with intracranial extension of the sepsis.

The hair should be shaved for at least 2 inches around the circumference of the wound and the surrounding scalp carefully prepped with antiseptic solution after mechanical cleansing of the skin with soap and water or ether. Satisfactory local anesthesia is obtained by injecting an agent such as 1% lidocaine with epinephrine deep to the galea. The needle should be inserted through the intact skin around the laceration rather than through the edges of the wound itself. After allowing time for the agent to take effect, the wound is irrigated with large volumes of sterile saline, taking care that all hair, dirt and other indriven foreign material is removed. After suitable draping, the wound can be explored to determine its extent and the skull palpated with gloved fingers. If an unexpected depressed fracture is discovered, the wound is closed with temporary sutures and the patient taken to the operating room for more definitive surgery.

Unless the wound was inflicted by a sharp object, there will be some contused, devitalized tissue present; this must be meticulously excised with a scalpel. It is wise to excise 2 or 3 mm of all layers of the scalp, including skin, around the entire margin of the wound. This step is particularly important if some hours have elapsed since the injury. The extent of this debridement is dictated by the amount of nonviable tissue present. Liberal use is made of saline irrigation during all phases of wound repair.

The early tensile strength of sutured scalp wounds depends almost entirely on sutures placed in the galea; a row of 3-0 silk sutures in this layer will also provide the necessary hemostasis. The galea is continuous over the forehead with the frontalis muscle, and lacerations here require a separate layer of sutures in this muscle for the reasons enumerated above and to prevent an unsightly depressed scar. The skin is closed with 4-0 silk, nylon or Dacron sutures, which can be removed in 3–5 days. If the wound is grossly contaminated, it is preferable to close with a single layer of #32 stainless steel wire placed as interrupted vertical mattress sutures. These wounds should not be drained.

The loss of scalp substance by crushing or avulsion introduces the problem of obtaining a tight closure without tension on the suture line. A great deal of scalp can be advanced to cover these defects by widely undermining in the subgaleal plane. If this maneuver proves inadequate, a relaxing incision made at a distance from the defect or a wide-based full-thickness rotational scalp flap can be employed (Fig. 14-8). These must be planned with regard to the circulation of the scalp, which is provided by three major arteries on each side—the temporal, occipital and supraorbital branches of the external carotid. Although these vessels anastomose richly with one another, the base of any proposed scalp flap should include one of the parent arteries. The donor site is closed with a split-thickness skin graft, which soon acquires a blood supply from the underlying pericranium. If available, the assistance of a plastic surgeon will be helpful in performing these latter procedures.

Birth trauma and other head injuries sustained during the early months of life may result in bleeding between scalp and skull, often producing an alarming degree of swelling and sometimes resulting in anemia. The cephalohematoma usually is located between the galea and the periosteum, and the swelling will extend over a variable sector of the skull. If the hematoma lies beneath the periosteum, its shape will conform to the outline of one of the bones of the calvarium, usually the parietal bone, since the bleeding will be limited by the dense attachments of the pericranium to the sutures of the skull. The hematoma often is associated with a fracture, and careful x-ray examination is required to determine whether any significant degree of depression is present. The temptation to aspirate the hematoma should be resisted unless it reaches truly monumental size and the scalp becomes very tightly stretched. If aspiration is required, it must be performed under the most stringent aseptic conditions to avoid contamination of the hematoma space. Left undisturbed, the collection is absorbed, and the mass feels softer within a few days and no longer is visible after several weeks. Some cephalohematomas will partially calcify to produce a hard, cosmetically unattractive mass. During this period of rapid growth of the brain and skull, remodeling usually restores normal contour within months.

LINEAR SKULL FRACTURES.—The finding on x-ray of a linear fracture of the cranial vault merely confirms that sufficient force has been applied to break the bone and, despite the connotation of "skull frac-

288 / Edward P. Baker, Jr.

SLIDING FLAP

RELAXING INCISION

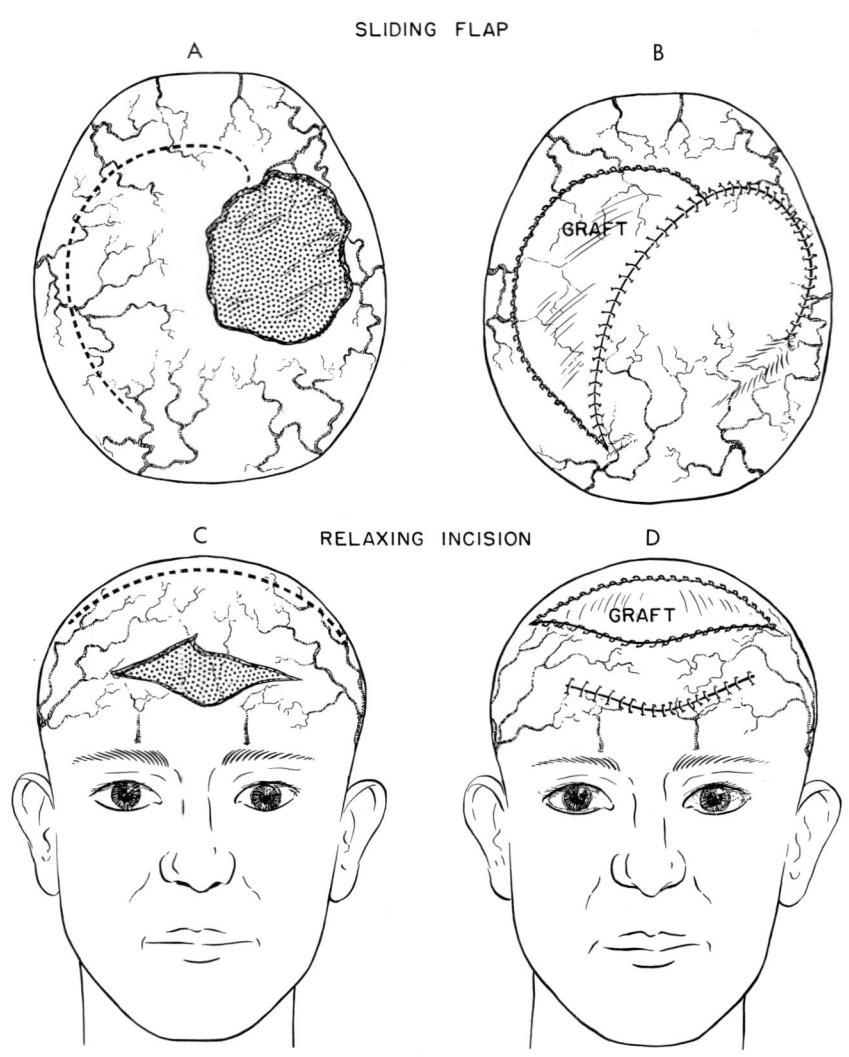

Fig. 14-8.—Repair of extensive scalp wounds to cover compound fractures in the cranial vault or areas of exposed dura mater, by sliding flap and relaxing incision. Sliding flap: **A,** extent of defect after debridement, with outline of incision designed to preserve an adequate blood supply in the pedicle. **B,** the pedicle flap has been freed and shifted to fill in the defect. The denuded area of pericranium from which the flap was taken then is covered with a split-thickness skin graft. Relaxing incision: **C,** an elliptical loss of scalp tissue can be repaired by making a longer parallel incision, leaving a well-vascularized pedicle at each end. **D,** the bridging flap has been freed, shifted forward and sutured to the anterior edge of the defect, covering the exposed healthy pericranium with a split-thickness skin graft. After suturing the grafts in place with fine silk, a snug dressing should be applied. It should be borne in mind that the scalp receives its blood supply from three principal arteries on each side (the supraorbital, temporal and occipital branches of the external carotid). There are no sizable perforating branches from the pericranium, but a sufficient capillary circulation to nourish a thin split-thickness skin graft.

ture" in the minds of the laity, does not necessarily imply injury to the brain. Skull fracture and brain injury are not synonymous terms, and it is important to keep the distinction clearly in mind. Extensive fracturing of the skull may occur and the patient remain fully alert and neurologically intact throughout; conversely, massive fatal brain injuries without demonstrable fracture are relatively common. It is not the fracture that is important but rather the effects of impact and of possible sequelae of the injury on the cranial contents. Those interested in the complex biomechanical factors involved in the formation of skull fractures should read the lucid experimental reports by Gurdjian and his colleagues.[11, 12]

The diagnosis of simple linear fracture should not be made casually, since occult compound fractures into the sinuses or middle ear may be missed unless high-quality films are examined critically and the radiographic abnormalities correlated with the neurologic findings and local signs of trauma. Simple linear fractures heal readily and the fracture itself requires no treatment. In infants and young children, the fracture line is radiographically invisible within 6–12 months, but in older persons the fracture may be visible for life, usually becoming less distinct with the passage of time.

Although the vast majority with these fractures suffer no untoward effects and recover uneventfully, delayed intracranial hemorrhage occurs in a certain percentage of patients, particularly those with fractures crossing grooves of meningeal arteries or dual venous sinuses, or extending into the foramen magnum (see Fig. 14-3). Death or crippling neurologic disability from tardy recognition and treatment of acute extradural hematomas can hardly be prevented if the patients are home in bed and the early symptoms go unnoticed; therefore, it is advisable that every patient with a skull fracture, even if asymptomatic, be hospitalized for observation over a 24–48-hour period. If comfortable and alert, the patient can be up and about and on a regular diet during his brief hospital stay. This admission policy results in hospitalizing many otherwise well patients for the sake of the few with hematomas, but the benefit to this group, we believe, justifies the cost to society.

"Growing skull fracture" is an interesting but rare complication of fractures in infants and very young children. The mechanisms responsible for enlargement of the fracture are not entirely clear, but Taveras and Ransohoff[47] postulate that an underlying cyst is formed by entrapment of cerebrospinal fluid within an arachnoidal herniation through an unrecognized dural tear, and that subsequent brain pulsations cause the bone to give way. The expansion of the original fracture into an irregularly ovoid bone defect oriented along the long axis of the fracture is evident on x-ray films taken 2–4 months after injury, and ventricular dilatation and focal brain injury under the fracture are demonstrable by pneumoencephalography. Hemiparesis, hemiatrophy and focal seizures relating to the latter findings are common.[25] Repair of the dural defect, followed by cranioplasty, should be done to prevent further loss of cerebral substance.

DEPRESSED SKULL FRACTURES. — Except in infants, whose pliable skulls react differently to deformation, depressed fractures require comminution. It is quite common for the fragments to split in the plane of the middle table and for the inner table to be more comminuted and depressed more deeply over a wider area. Equally frequent is the underestimation from preoperative x-ray films of the true degree of comminution and the extent of the depression. Nevertheless, good skull films are essential for the diagnosis of most depressed fractures, and conventional views may show gaps in the bone from which a portion of a fragment has been displaced or, more commonly, areas of increased density due either to overlapping of edges of bone or angulation of a fragment so that its density is greater than that of the surrounding skull (see Fig. 14-3, C). Tangential views directed at the point of impact are a great aid in demonstrating the depression clearly.

Depressed fractures may occur without severe brain injury, many patients remaining fully conscious throughout, but focal cerebral injury beneath the fracture is the rule, and the resultant neurologic deficit, if any, depends on the extent and location of the damage. The cortex is locally contused by minor degrees of depression, but fragments driven in beyond 5 mm are likely to lacerate both the dura and the cerebral cortex and may give rise to surface or intracerebral hematomas. Jamieson[18] found such hematomas in 30% of a large series of patients with closed or compound depressed fractures and noted a much higher incidence in the latter group. Elevation of closed fractures depressed by more than the thickness of the calvarium is indicated, particularly if the injury is near the motor strip or adjacent to the speech cortex of the dominant hemisphere. Small depressions over the cerebellum need not be elevated, and those over dural venous sinuses are best left alone for fear of precipitating major hemorrhage, unless there are progressive signs of sinus obstruction.

Compound depressed fractures, regardless of the degree of depression, should be repaired as early as possible after injury to lessen the risk of infection. The dangers of neglecting these injuries are vividly illustrated by Jennett and Miller's[21] report of 24 patients who presented with established infection due to inadequate treatment elsewhere. Fifteen had meningitis or brain abscess or both, and 4 died. Those surviving had a much higher incidence of post-traumatic epilepsy and serious neurologic residuals than did uninfected patients with similar injuries. Jennett and Miller's over-all infection rate was 4.6% and increased significantly with delay of more than 48 hours between injury and surgery.

Closed depressed fractures are best approached through a small scalp flap centered so that the incision does not lie directly over the depressed area. Generally, these fractures are tightly impacted and there may be difficulty gaining access to the extradural space. Sometimes the tip of a narrow rongeur can be inserted under an edge and a narrow channel of bone nibbled away to release the impaction; if not, a bur hole is drilled alongside the fracture and a rongeur cut is made across the depression to accomplish the same end. The depressed fragments then are carefully elevated and withdrawn so as to avoid further damage to the underlying structures, and the dura over the entire extent of the depression is exposed. Large fragments around the periphery that are only slightly canted inward can be cautiously elevated and left in situ if reduction is maintained. Intact but discolored dura may overlie a subdural hematoma and should be opened.

After thorough debridement of dural and cerebral lacerations, the dura is closed, with a graft if necessary, and the larger segments of bone wired into place. Smaller pieces of bone placed on the dura to fill in residual gaps, if protected, will be incorporated rapidly into the healing skull.

Depressed fractures in infants often are of the "ping-pong ball" variety, akin to greenstick fractures of the long bones, and occur most often incidental to delivery or from the child being accidentally dropped by a parent. These fractures do not undergo spontaneous reduction and probably all should be elevated surgically. Operative treatment consists of placing a small bur hole along one margin of the depression and then carefully inserting a suitable instrument, such as a small periosteal elevator, under the fracture, which then is gently levered outward into a normal position.

Compound depressed fractures are treated in essentially the same manner as closed fractures, with the added require-

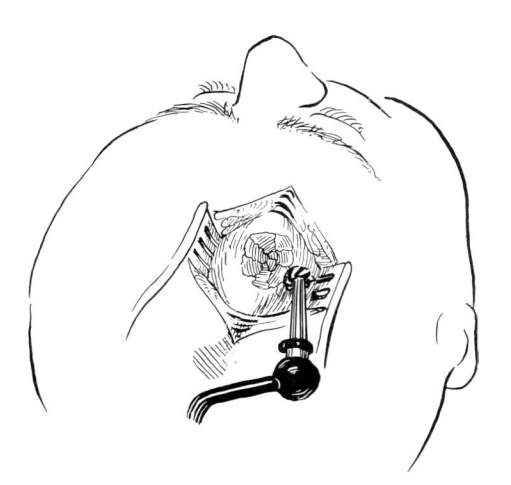

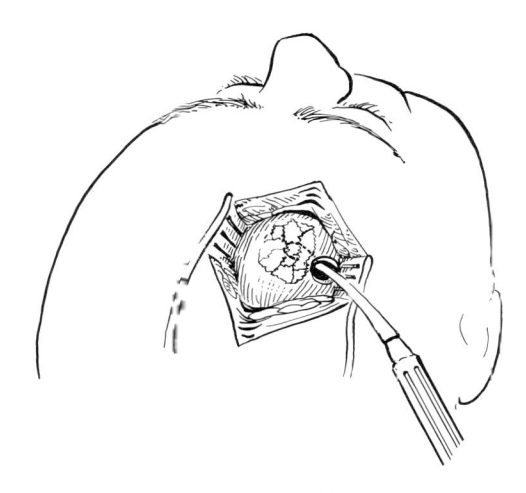

Fig. 14-9.—Elevation of a depressed fracture. Depressed fragments usually are so impacted that it is necessary to drill a bur hole alongside. The fracture then is levered outward as shown or, preferably, removed with rongeurs to permit inspection of the dura and cortex.

ment of more thorough debridement of all layers because of the element of contamination. These fractures are approached through the laceration, which first is carefully debrided layer by layer and then extended as necessary to provide adequate exposure of the fracture. Tufts of hair projecting from along tightly impacted fracture lines are a common but always striking finding; the hair is driven through the fracture at the moment of impact, when the degree of inward deformation of the skull is maximal, and then caught as the fractured area rebounds outward.

It used to be the practice to discard all bone fragments removed from compound depressed fractures and to rely on future cranioplasty to restore skull contour; this still is the best method of treatment of heavily contaminated wounds or those repaired after a delay. Kriss et al.,[23] however, reported a large series of cases in which the fragments were replaced and, provided that the dura was securely closed and repair effected within 24 hours of injury, noted normal healing of the fractures without an increase in the infection rate. These findings have been confirmed by others, and replacement of bone fragments at the time of primary repair appears to be a sound procedure under the above conditions. Bone replacement is particularly applicable to fractures of the supraorbital ridge, where later cranioplasty is notoriously difficult and often cosmetically unsatisfactory. Furthermore, the medial third of the supraorbital ridge should be preserved if at all possible, because, as Schneider[43] has emphasized, the pulley arrangement of the levator muscle attaches here, and loss of this important sector of bone results in unsightly and disabling ptosis.

COMPLICATIONS OF SKULL FRACTURES

CAROTID-CAVERNOUS FISTULA.—Carotid-cavernous fistula may occur spontaneously following rupture of an aneurysm of the intracavernous portion of the internal carotid artery, but more commonly the fistulous communication results from laceration of the carotid artery within the cavernous sinus by a basilar skull fracture or by penetrating injury. Retrograde flow of blood under arterial pressure into the orbital veins results in enormous distention and causes the pulsating exophthalmos that is a hallmark of the disease. The degree of proptosis averages 8–10 mm but may become so extreme that the lid cannot cover the globe. The patient, on recovering consciousness from his injury, is aware of an incessant rushing, roaring noise in his head synchronous with the pulse; the bruit always is easily heard by the examiner through a stethoscope placed over the orbit, forehead or temple. Conjunctival injection, chemosis, extraocular palsies and visual impairment progressing to blindness are other common signs. The intolerable bruit, ocular complications and disfigurement are compelling indications for operative relief.

Combined ligation of the cervical and intracranial internal carotid arteries together with the ophthalmic artery has failed, in a substantial percentage of cases, to obliterate the fistula, which is kept open after these ligations by the tentorial, meningeal and hypophyseal branches of the intracavernous portion of the carotid artery. Hamby[13] advocates packing the fistulous segment of the artery with muscle emboli introduced through the cervical internal carotid, after intracranial ligation of the supraclinoid carotid, and then ligating the internal, external and common carotid arteries in the neck. In our hands, this procedure has succeeded in closing the fistula in all patients in whom it has been used, but often at the price of blindness of the involved eye, due to central retinal artery occlusion.

CRANIAL NERVE INJURIES.—Certain of the cranial nerves are vulnerable to injury by fractures coursing through their foramina of exit at the base of the skull. The filaments of the olfactory nerve, the most frequently injured cranial nerve, are fixed at their points of passage through the tiny foramina of the cribriform plate, and fractures in this region may result in unilateral or bilateral anosmia, often accompanied by cerebrospinal fluid rhinorrhea. A more common mechanism of olfactory nerve injury is the avulsion of the olfactory filaments from the cribriform plate by the relative backward movement of the brain within the skull at the moment of a blow to the occiput. Anosmic patients complain bitterly of impaired taste sensation, because gustatory appreciation of flavor depends heavily on perception of aromatic substances in food by the olfactory apparatus. Unfortunately, loss of olfaction usually is permanent.

Optic nerve injuries from fractures through the optic foramen are rare, and acute blindness is due more often to direct eye trauma. Decompression of the nerve at the foramen in cases of fracture usually is futile, and since the nerve embryologically develops as a fiber tract of the brain, its axons do not have a neurilemmal sheath and regeneration after transection does not occur.

Traumatic third nerve palsies most often are due to compression of the nerve at the tentorial notch secondary to an expanding intracranial hematoma, a mechanism discussed below at greater length. These patients are deeply obtunded and, if an oculomotor palsy is present in a conscious patient, it most likely results from injury to the nerve in the orbit. With a total third nerve palsy, the lid is closed due to paralysis of the levator, the pupil is dilated and unresponsive to either direct or consensual light and the eye is deviated laterally by the unopposed lateral rectus if the abducens is intact. Partial recovery, particularly of levator function, is common. Trochlear and abducens palsies also result from injuries to the orbit or from fractures into the superior orbital fissure, and sixth nerve palsies are common, false localizing signs in the presence of raised intracranial pressure from any cause. The troublesome diplopia experienced by conscious patients with extraocular palsies is eliminated by wearing a patch over one eye; at least part of the time, the normal eye should be covered. It is wise to defer surgical correction of residual muscle paresis for at least a year to allow maximal recovery to occur, but prism glasses may be helpful in the interim.

Although the gasserian ganglion or the intracranial portion of the trigeminal nerve seldom is injured, the peripheral sensory branches of the nerve often are divided by facial lacerations or contused by fractures at their foramina of exit on the face. Anesthesia in the distribution of the supraorbital, infraorbital or mental nerves, in conjunction with signs of local trauma, is diagnostic, respectively, of frontal, maxillary or mandibular fracture. For decades, neurosurgeons have tried to produce permanent anesthesia by avulsing these nerves in patients suffering from trigeminal neuralgia, but recovery of sensation invariably occurs within 12–18 months.

The facial nerve and the auditory and vestibular portions of the acoustic nerve often are injured by fractures as they course together through the petrous pyramid of the temporal bone. Total peripheral seventh nerve palsy results in loss of all voluntary movement of the ipsilateral face and platysma and, if the injury is proximal to the geniculate ganglion, loss of taste sensation over the anterior two-thirds of the tongue and impairment of lacrimation. In contrast, central or supranuclear facial palsies caused by lesions of the motor cortex or of the projections to the facial nucleus largely spare forehead movement, since both motor cortices project to the portion of the facial nucleus concerned with innervation of the frontalis muscle. The likelihood of recovery of an immediate total peripheral facial palsy is poor, and consideration should be given to exploration of the nerve at some time after the injury if the face remains paralyzed. Delayed or "tardy" facial palsy appearing within a few days or a week after a head injury has a favorable prognosis and no treatment is required.

A clear description of the different types of temporal bone fractures and the otologic consequences of these injuries is found in Barber's[5] report. Complete deafness due to auditory nerve injury always is permanent. Partial injuries of the auditory and vestibular nerves result in tinnitus and vertigo, respectively. There is no effective treatment for tinnitus, but vertigo may be symptomatically improved by diazepam or meclizine. Patients with blood in the middle ear will have mild or moderate conductive hearing loss, which improves when the clot liquefies and drains through the eustachian canal. These patients should be examined by an otologist a month or so after the injury, as audiograms or petrous polytomography may reveal treatable hearing loss due to disruption of the middle ear ossicles.

Intracranial injuries of the ninth, tenth, eleventh and twelfth nerves are rare, and traumatic palsies of these nerves generally are caused by penetrating wounds of the neck or base of the skull.

TRAUMATIC CEREBROSPINAL FLUID RHINORRHEA AND OTORRHEA.—Traumatic cerebrospinal fluid rhinorrhea or otorrhea occurs in from 2% to 9% of patients following closed head injury[28] and is caused by basilar fractures entering the paranasal sinuses or middle ear. The fistulous pathway is created by the fracture plus mucosal and dural-arachnoidal tears, permitting communication between the sterile subarachnoid space and the contaminated environment of nasal sinuses and nasopharynx or the middle ear and external auditory canal. Traumatic pneumocephalus has the same significance, and the finding of intracranial air on skull x-rays is incontrovertible evidence of a fistula through a dural tear. Cribriform plate fractures into the ethmoid sinus, fractures through the posterior wall of the frontal sinus and fractures into the sphenoid sinus are the most common avenues of rhinorrhea, in that order, but one interesting variety, actually a form of otorrhea, occurs following fracture of the petrous pyramid, allowing escape of CSF into the middle ear, from whence it drains down the eustachian tube to the nasopharynx. Leakage from the ear requires perforation of the tympanic membrane in addition to the petrous fracture and dural tear.

The diagnosis is suggested by the appearance of thin, bloody fluid draining from the ear or nose, which forms characteristic concentric rings on the bedsheets. The nature of watery fluid in the ear never is in doubt, but later, when the fluid clears, inspection alone may be insufficient to determine whether nasal drainage consists of secretions of vasomotor rhinitis or CSF, in which case the identity of the fluid in question can be established by micro glucose and chloride determinations. Saliva and various nasal secretions have a very low glucose content, whereas CSF glucose levels approximate two-thirds those of blood and CSF chloride concentration is above 120 mEq/L. If only a drop or two of the fluid can be obtained, the presence or absence of significant glucose can be determined by the paper strips or tablets used to test diabetic urine. CSF tends to run down the back of the throat and be swallowed by supine, bedridden patients, and the diagnosis may be missed unless they are specifically questioned about this.

These patients are placed on strict bed rest, with the head of the bed elevated 45 degrees to lessen CSF flow, and instructed not to blow the nose, sneeze or sniff back the fluid, lest air and contaminated debris be driven intracranially. A loose dressing to catch the drainage and prevent constant soiling of the bedclothes is permissible, but the ear or nose must never be packed, as this will impede free drainage and increase the probability of intracranial contamination. Otorrhea generally stops within 1–3 days and operative treatment rarely is needed. Mincey[37] found that 85% of his cases of rhinorrhea closed spontaneously within a week and that the incidence of meningitis was 11%, despite prophylactic penicillin administration.

The utility of giving prophylactic antibiotics to patients with CSF leaks is controversial. MacGee et al.,[28] using data pooled from the literature, found no statistically significant difference in the incidence of meningitis among patients who received various antibiotics and those who did not. We favor withholding antibiotics unless clinical or laboratory evidence of meningitis is present, except in those patients with pre-existing otitis or sinusitis. Since the majority of the cases of meningitis associated with CSF leak are caused by pneumococcus, staphylococcus, streptococcus and hemophilus influenza in that order, antibiotics, if given, should be selected with these organisms in mind.

Surgical repair, if elected, is done after brain swelling from the original trauma has subsided and the patient is free from overt infection. Preoperatively, tomograms of the anterior fossa are essential, and many surgeons make use of intrathecal injection of various dyes or radioisotopes in efforts to localize the site of the fistula accurately. Repair of anterior fossa fistulae entails bifrontal craniotomy, intradural exploration, definition of the margins of the defect and repair with a graft of temporalis fascia or fascia lata. Antibiotic coverage is provided during the preoperative and postoperative periods. Lewin,[26] based on a series of 192 cases of CSF rhinorrhea, recommends that dural repair be considered in all cases, even when the leakage arrests spontaneously, contending that true healing of the dural tear seldom occurs, because of the interposition of brain, arachnoid or bone, and that the risk of meningitis therefore remains despite cessation of the leak. Most neurosurgeons in the United States have not had as high an incidence of late meningitis among conservatively treated patients as Lewin noted (6 of 26 patients), and, because of this factor, the risks of operation and the failure of surgical repair invariably to result in cure,[42] treat expectantly those patients in whom drainage ceases within 10–14 days. Generally accepted indications for surgical repair include persistent rhinorrhea, meningitis or the demonstration by x-ray of a wide fracture with cerebral herniation into a sinus, or of a spicule of bone penetrating into the brain.

BASILAR SKULL FRACTURE WITH HEMOTYMPANUM. — This entity deserves separate attention because of the great frequency with which it is encountered in clinical practice. Blood in the middle ear is presumptive evidence of a basilar fracture, even though the fracture frequently is not demonstrable by x-ray, and one must further assume that the potential exists for contamination of the subarachnoid space across the fracture. Seen through the otoscope, the tympanic membrane has a dark reddish purple hue, normal landmarks are obliterated and there may be splinter hemorrhages within the membrane. If the eardrum is perforated, blood appears in the external canal, in which instance, the less serious condition of laceration of the canal should be excluded by careful examination several days later, when the blood can be carefully removed. If uncomplicated by injury to the eighth nerve, there is only mild conductive hearing loss due to the presence of the blood. Aspiration of the middle-ear hematoma is meddlesome and increases the risk of sepsis. It is wise to keep these patients on bed rest for a week to allow soft tissue healing to seal the defect and to obtain follow-up otologic examination in 4–6 weeks.

INTRACRANIAL HEMATOMAS

ACUTE EXTRADURAL HEMATOMA. — In medicine, the prompt diagnosis and treatment of correctable or curable disorders always is more important than is similar acumen with diseases that, by nature, are basically untreatable. The eventual outcome of untreated extradural hematoma is death, whereas, in the early stages of evolution at least, the clot often is not accompanied by significant injury to the brain, and its prompt removal before serious brain compression has occurred will be followed by complete recovery. Since the prognosis is so dependent on early recognition and treatment, the emergency room physicians, general surgeons and pediatricians who commonly attend these patients first must be familiar with the clinical entity and be alert to its possible occurrence in patients who initially may not appear seriously injured. Compared with the mortality and morbidity of brain contusions and the other acute intracranial hematomas, the results of timely surgical evacuation of extradural hematomas are so favorable that special emphasis on the clinical features of this disorder is warranted.

The formation of a hematoma in the extradural space begins with a blow, usually to the side of the head, producing transient local deformation of the skull with stripping of dura from the inner table over a small area. Bleeding into this space ensues and further separation of dura follows as the clot expands at a rate dependent on the source of the hemorrhage. Most commonly, the hemorrhage originates from a branch of the middle meningeal artery lacerated by a fracture, and the pace of the evolution will be rapid as the clot accumulates under arterial pressure. Bleeding from middle meningeal veins, dural venous sinuses, lacerated mastoid or occipital emissary veins or from the edges of the fracture line is likely to be slower and the onset of alarming symptoms delayed for hours or even days.

Most adults with extradural hematoma (91%) have a skull fracture demonstrated by x-ray, at operation or autopsy,[10] but among children, perhaps owing to the greater elasticity of the skull and ease of dural detachment, fewer than one-half have a skull fracture.[15] Linear fractures crossing grooves of meningeal vessels or dural venous sinuses are seen most commonly and always should arouse one's suspicion regarding the possibility of extradural clot; the absence of visible fracture, however, does not exclude the diagnosis at any age.

The temporal profile of classic acute extradural hematoma is familiar to every medical student. The initiating injury, typically a low-velocity blow to the head, may produce a brief loss of consciousness, after which the patient awakens and seems comparatively well for a variable period—the so-called lucid interval, long considered a hallmark of extradural hematoma. As the hours pass, the expanding clot compresses the surface of the brain and, interfering with local cerebral circulation, gives rise to beginning cerebral edema, which, in turn, increases the over-all mass effect. Severe headache, vomiting and weakness of the contralateral limbs are present at this stage and, most important, the patient's state of consciousness begins to deteriorate. With further enlargement of the mass, the temporal lobe is displaced inward until its most medial portion, the uncus, is forced medially and downward over the free edge of the tentorium to impinge on the adjacent third nerve and brainstem. This mechanism, designated variously as uncal herniation, transtentorial herniation, tentorial pressure cone or simply "coning," is the common denominator of death from any rapidly expanding supratentorial mass lesion, whether hemorrhage, swelling, brain tumor or abscess, and it always is fatal unless the brainstem compression can be relieved quickly by one means or another. As the medial temporal lobe herniates over the tentorial edge, it displaces the oculomotor nerve, paralyzing the pupillo-constrictor fibers. The ipsilateral pupil becomes widely dilated and nonreactive to light; the patient now is in extremis. Further displacement of the uncus brings it into contact with blood vessels supplying the midbrain, impairing its circulation, and, finally, the midbrain itself is compressed and then displaced against the opposite third nerve and the unyielding contralateral tentorial edge. As these events occur, the hemiparesis becomes a hemiplegia, coma progressively deepens and the patient develops decerebrate rigidity, first on the side opposite the mass, then bilaterally (see Fig. 14-2). The opposite pupil becomes dilated and fixed to light. Midbrain hemorrhages secondary to compression and circulatory obstruction (Duret hemorrhages) extend rostrally and caudally along the axis of the brainstem, destroying centers concerned with cardiorespiratory regulation, and death follows quickly.

The diagnosis of extradural hematomas should present no difficulty when the signs and symptoms unfold in this classic sequence. There are, however, many variations of the early clinical course, particularly relating to the initial loss of consciousness and the matter of the lucid interval. Both of these phenomena are reflections of the degree of impact-produced brain injury, unrelated to the later development of the clot, and neither is an essential element of the clinical syndrome. If the fateful blow is mild, as it often is, there will be no significant brain injury and, hence, no initial loss of consciousness, a situation especially common in children.[35] Impact sufficient to cause brief unconsciousness, a concussion, results in negligible brain damage and the patient revives and remains awake until the compressive effects of the expanding hematoma become evident; this is the only clinical setting in which a pure lucid interval is present. The patient with a moderately severe brain injury may remain stuporous from its effects for hours, then begin to lighten, only to deteriorate from the later expansion of the hematoma. At the far end of the spectrum is the patient with extensive cerebral and/or brainstem injuries, comatose at the outset and worsening steadily from the superimposed brain compression. It should be emphasized that if a lucid interval is present, the patient rarely is asymptomatic during this period, and, in our experience, headache and vomiting and subtle alterations of mentation are common. Regardless of the tempo of evolution of clinical signs and symptoms up to the time of brainstem compression by the distant effects of the clot, all variants of the syndrome converge on an event—transtentorial hernia-

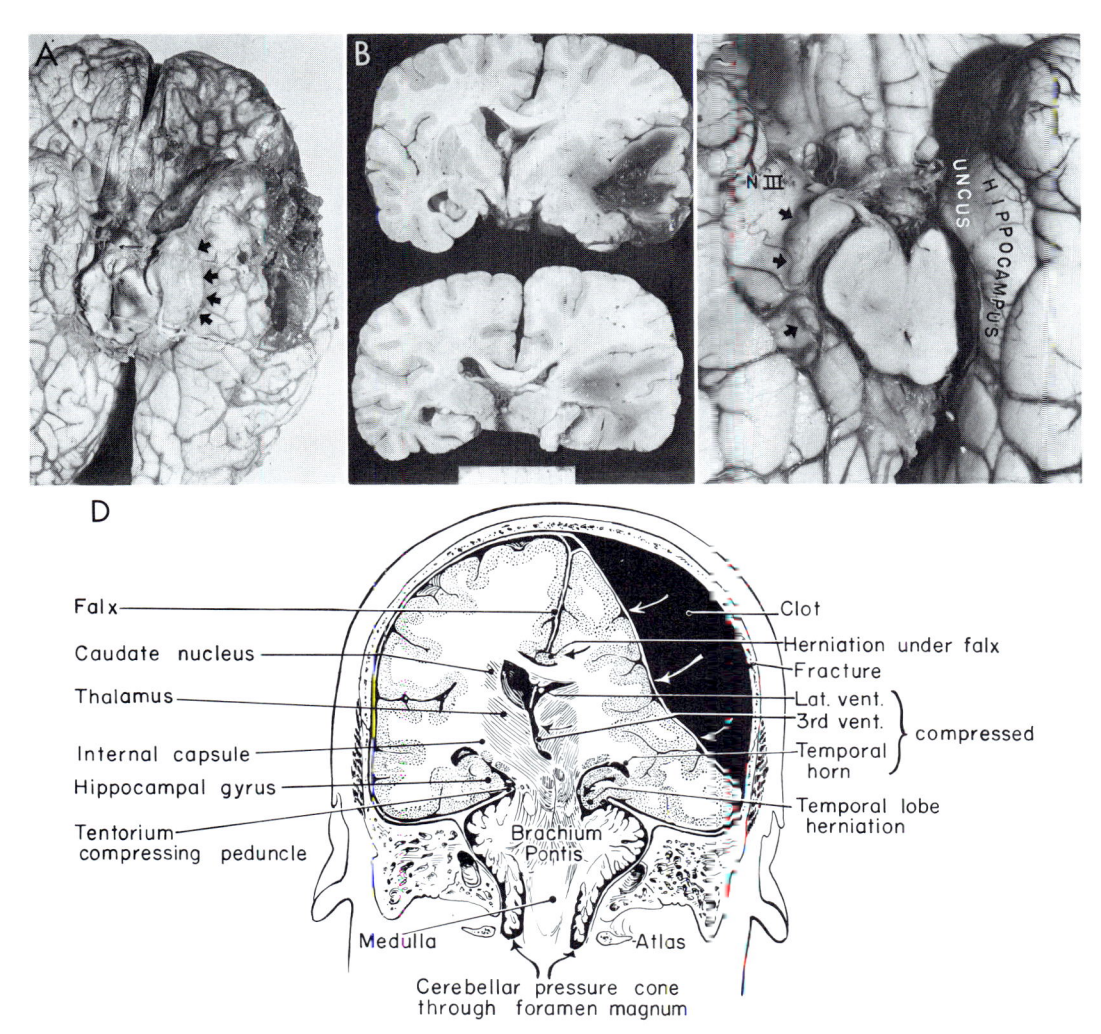

Fig. 14-10.—Mechanism of pressure-cone formation. **Top views**, lesions found at autopsy in two fatal cases. **A**, severe contusion and laceration of cortex on left side of brain following a blow on right side of head. The herniated inferior medial edge of the left temporal lobe is marked by arrows and a hemorrhage is present in the compressed midbrain. **B**, the brain cut in cross section to show extensive swelling of the left hemisphere and a large subcortical clot. **C**, right uncal herniation (at left side, marked by three arrows). The oculomotor nerve can be seen crossing under the rostral end of the hernia; its compression had caused dilatation of pupil. There is also a small hemorrhage in the compressed side of brainstem. The hippocampal gyrus and uncus on the opposite side are normal. **D**, a coronal cross section through the middle of the head illustrating herniations beneath the falx, through the tentorial notch and foramen magnum, produced by a large extradural hematoma

tion—that occurs with terrible abruptness and usually marks the last moments during which the lesion is reversible.

Removal of the hematoma early in the clinical course before transtentorial herniation has occurred clearly is the key to a favorable outcome; in a series of 167 patients with extradural hematoma, Jamieson and Yelland[19] reported a 77% mortality among patients decerebrate prior to surgery, whereas there was only one fatality among the 74 patients who were conscious at the time of operation. Although the early symptoms of headache and vomiting are not unique to extradural hematoma and are common after any head injury, the earliest tangible physical findings, lessening of consciousness from a previously established baseline or the development of any lateralizing signs, such as hyperactive reflexes, limb weakness, Babinski sign or enlarging pupil, are clear-cut danger signals that must never pass unheeded. They indicate an expanding intracranial clot until proved otherwise and call for immediate definitive action.

If the clinical signs are equivocal and nonprogressive, the diagnostic uncertainties can be clarified by carotid angiography, provided that the study is performed without delay. Extracerebral masses displace the surface of the brain, indicated angiographically by the terminal branches of the middle cerebral artery, from the inner surface of the skull, and, unless bilateral, shift the pericallosal artery and internal cerebral vein from their normal midline positions toward the opposite side. Sometimes the middle meningeal artery can be seen displaced inward with the dura, enabling one to distinguish the lesion from a subdural collection.

Patients developing clear-cut signs while under observation or those arriving at the emergency room with a clinical picture consistent with extradural hematoma should be taken directly to the operating room for exploratory bur holes without delaying for angiography or even plain skull films. It is not uncommon for these patients to die while being readied for surgery, and time-consuming tests or procedures beyond cross matching blood and endotracheal intubation are best omitted. On rare occasions, when unmistakable signs of transtentorial herniation developed during the initial emergency room examination, we have placed a temporal bur hole through the unshaven, unprepped scalp and then taken the patient to the operating suite for completion of the operation. Since the emergency release of an acute extradural hematoma in these desperate circumstances probably is the only intracranial procedure the general surgeon will ever be required to perform on his own without waiting for a neurosurgeon, the technical details of the operation as performed under more favorable conditions are presented.

The initial bur hole should be placed over the bruise or laceration, marking the point of impact, if present; otherwise, a temporal bur hole will disclose the majority of extradural clots. Access to the temporal bone and middle cranial fossa is gained through a vertical scalp incision 2 cm anterior to the ear and carried down to the zygoma. Extending the incision below the zygoma will not improve the exposure and will sever branches of the facial nerve to the frontalis muscle, paralyzing the forehead. Temporalis fascia and muscle are divided, preferably with the electrosurgical unit, and the muscle reflected from the skull and maintained with a self-retaining retractor. The fracture line frequently is seen at this stage. The bur hole is drilled and, as the clot extrudes under pressure, is enlarged with rongeurs to form a craniectomy 4 cm or larger in diameter. Removal of the entire hematoma by suction and irrigation generally can be accomplished through an opening of this size; however, experienced neurosurgeons often elect to convert this subtemporal craniectomy to a craniotomy by turning down a small osteoplastic bone flap after removing the bulk of the clot. This maneuver vastly improves the exposure, facilitates hemostasis and obviates the need for future cranioplasty. In fact, though, cranioplasty seldom is required, provided that the craniectomy is confined to the limits of the origin of the temporalis muscle and if the muscle and its overlying fascia are carefully closed as separate layers.

Removal of the clot is followed closely

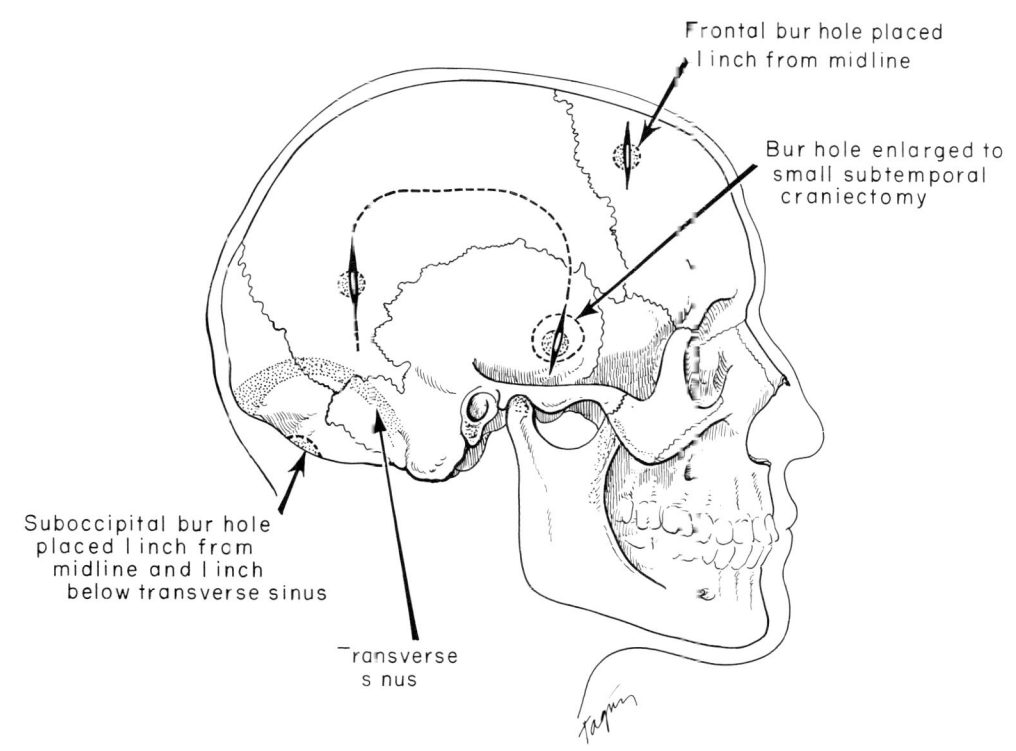

Chapter 14: DIAGNOSIS AND TREATMENT OF HEAD INJURIES / 299

Fig. 14-11.—Exploratory bur holes. Before draping, a suitable scalp flap is marked out, to be turned down in the event that solid clot is encountered. The temporal (enlarged here to a small craniectomy) and parietal bur holes can, if necessary, be incorporated into an osteoplastic bone flap. The frontal and suboccipital bur holes are placed to avoid dural venous sinuses and cranial sutures.

by re-expansion of the dura toward the inner table and sometimes, to the chagrin of the operating surgeon, by the resumption of major arterial bleeding. The origin of the hematoma may be apparent along the middle meningeal vessels, but more commonly there are multiple briskly bleeding points on the dura and the source of the hematoma cannot be determined with certainty. The risk of hypovolemic shock from this hemorrhage is particularly great in young children, who already may have lost a sizable fraction of their total blood volume into the hematoma, and these small patients always should have a blood transfusion running at the start of the operation.[32]

Hemostasis is achieved by first occluding the proximal main trunks of the middle meningeal vessels and then the major peripheral branches to prevent backbleeding within the exposed area of dura. Recalling that these vessels course in the outer of the two layers of cranial dura, they can be isolated by incising the outer layer on either side of the artery, dissecting the vessel free from the inner layer and then elevating it on a blunt dissector to be clipped or coagulated. Arterial hemorrhage beneath the temporal lobe cannot be controlled in this manner and it may be necessary to separate the dura from the floor of the middle fossa, tracing the artery back to its site of entry into the skull at the foramen spinosum, where it can be clipped, coagulated or occluded by jamming a wisp of cotton into the foramen.

Even after all visible blood vessels are secure, there is likely to be oozing from many tiny bleeding points on the dura, all of which must cease or the clot will recur. Light coagulation with the edge of the tip of a fine sucker or the application of bits of absorbably hemostatic cellulose are effective techniques for this purpose. Bone bleeding from the edges of the craniectomy is dealt with by the judicious application of bone wax, taking care not to insinuate wax under the bone edge, lest dura be stripped away and produce further bleeding. As a final step, fine silk sutures placed through the outer layer of the dura and the inner temporalis muscle are tied snugly to tent the dura against the edges of the bony defect; this maneuver controls dural oozing near the bone edge and limits the extent of any possible recurrence.

Once hemostasis is absolute, the presence of a coexistent subdural hematoma can be excluded by inspection if the dura is sufficiently thin and transparent that underlying cortical structures are clearly visible; otherwise, it is prudent to make a small dural incision. If opened, the dura is closed, followed by careful layer closure of the scalp. Drainage seldom is required, but if there is any uncertainty regarding hemostasis in the extradural space, the placement of a sialastic catheter drain led out through a separate incision and connected to low suction for 24–48 hours is advisable. If indicated by other features of the particular case at hand or if elevated intracranial pressure persists after removal of the clot, additional exploratory bur holes then are placed on the same and opposite sides in search of a second hematoma. Sites for bur holes (Fig. 14-11) should be selected with the underlying anatomic structures clearly in mind. Major dural venous sinuses and the more midline portions of the cortical veins entering the sagittal sinus are lacerated easily and these locations should be avoided. Bur holes placed directly over cranial sutures are likely to lacerate the dura, which is adherent to the underside of these joints.

ACUTE SUBDURAL HEMATOMA.—Owing to the increasing frequency of violent acceleration-deceleration injuries incurred in traffic accidents, the prevalence of this entity in the population of head-injured patients is rising steadily. In 1935, Jamieson noted a ratio of 3 extradural hematomas to 1 subdural hematoma, but by 1963 the ratio had reversed and there were 30 subdural hematomas to 1 extradural hematoma.[17] Some subdural hematomas, particularly those following a blow along the long axis of the head, develop slowly and are not associated with primary injury of the brain; the subacute clinical course then is similar to that of extradural hematomas, but over a more protracted interval. The majority of acute subdural hematomas, however, are accompanied by severe intrinsic brain injury and the expanding blood clot is only part of the problem. Traumatic intracerebral hematomas and/or contusion-lacerations of the cerebrum, which more often than not are contrecoup or bilateral, are common findings, as are impact-produced brainstem contusions. The severity of the primary brain injury usually determines the postoperative course, and patients who recover following removal of the hematoma do so gradually in a manner similar to those with contusions but without clots. The seriousness of this constellation of injuries is reflected in the 70–90% mortality reported by most investigators[34, 46] when operation is required during the first 12–24 hours after injury. In Jamieson and Yelland's series,[20] 89% of the patients with decerebrate rigidity died, and when fixed, dilated pupils were also present, the mortality rose to 95%.

More information relative to the presence of intracranial masses can be obtained by carotid angiography than by exploratory bur holes because the former procedure will disclose intracerebral clots that are easily missed at the time of exploration, even when a ventricular needle in skilled hands is passed into the frontal and temporal lobes, the usual sites of traumatic intracerebral hematomas.

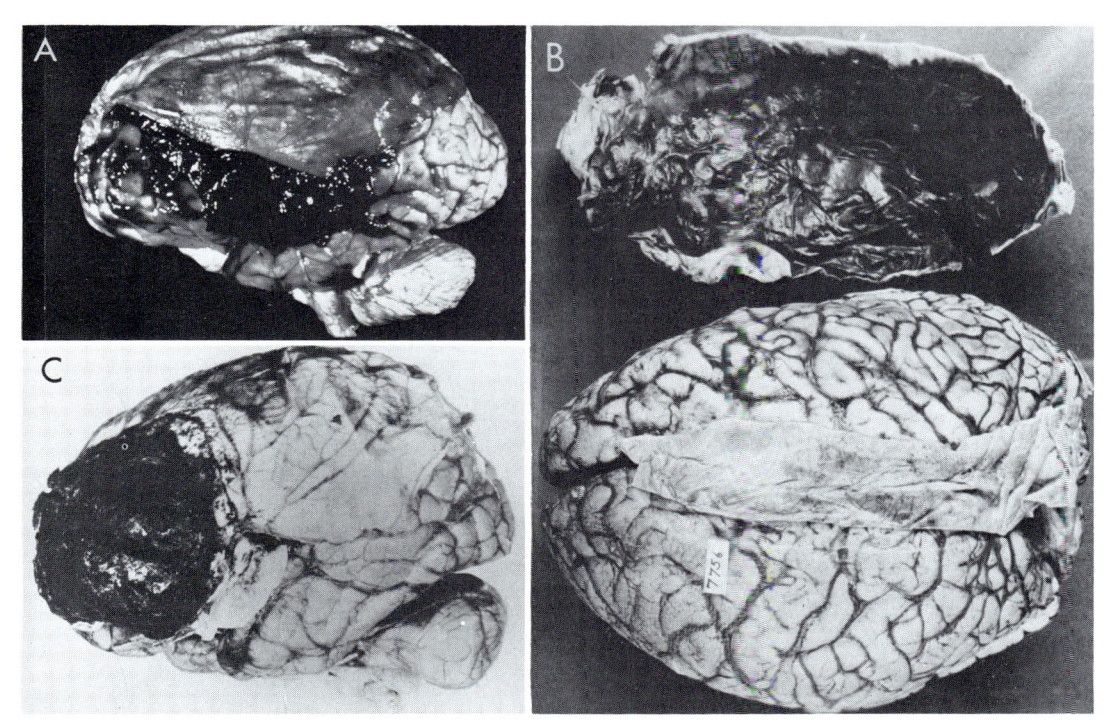

Fig. 14-12.—**A,** acute subdural hematoma. The dura is reflected to expose the hematoma and small areas of contusion of the frontal lobe. Extensive bilateral contusions were found on sectioning the brain. **B,** a more chronic hematoma. Note the degree of compression of the underlying hemisphere in this formalin-fixed specimen. **C,** acute extradural hemorrhage in a boy who was struck in the right frontal area by a pitched baseball. After a brief loss of consciousness there was a lucid interval in which he walked home and went to bed. Later, he was found in deep coma and brought to the hospital moribund. (Specimen was supplied by Dr. Timothy Leary.)

Often, though, the patient arrives in the emergency room either having coned or in the process of doing so, and time does not permit other than immediate exploration. After intubation, hyperventilation is begun, and mannitol and steroids administered as the patient is prepared for surgery, which usually is performed with the patient in the semisitting position to permit access to both sides of the head. The hematoma usually is on the side of the dilated pupil, although McKissock[33] found 9% of acute hematomas contralateral to the dilated pupil. The position of the hematoma was even less reliably predicted by a hemiparesis; 29% were ipsilateral to the hematoma, a finding probably explained by direct injury to the opposite cerebral peduncle or by compression of the peduncle contralateral to the clot against the edge of the tentorium. Because approximately 20% of acute subdural hematomas are bilateral, exploration of both sides is necessary, unless preoperative angiography has excluded this possibility. Acute hematomas are formed of solid clot and ordinarily cannot be removed through multiple bur holes or small craniectomies; usually a large osteoplastic craniotomy is required to remove the clot and control the source of bleeding. After the hematoma has been removed by suction and irrigation, areas of contusion are noted and intracerebral clots sought by passing a ventricular needle into the tips of the frontal and temporal lobes. If an intracerebral hematoma is located, a cortical incision is made in a silent area and carried down into the cavity to permit aspiration of the clot and surrounding necrotic brain. Areas of grossly pulped brain then are excised; the extent of the resection is more radical in silent areas of the brain, such as the tips of frontal or temporal lobes, and more conservative in areas close to the motor strip or the speech cortex in the dominant hemisphere.

If brain edema is severe, as it usually is, difficulty in closing the wound may be encountered as the brain rapidly expands to or beyond the plane of the dura. Little relief is gained by tapping the lateral ventricles, as they usually are compressed and scant ventricular fluid can be obtained. The dura must be closed, with a graft if necessary, or brain will herniate through the opening, compressing cortical veins around the edges of the defect and causing venous infarction of the herniated brain and further cerebral swelling. Full use of all therapeutic modalities to reduce brain swelling is in order at this point. Three possibilities confront the surgeon if the dura cannot be closed because of uncontrollable brain swelling and, unless hasty exploration of the opposite side yields a large removable hematoma, the contingencies are reduced to two. He can either perform temporal or frontal lobectomy to produce a large enough internal decompression to effect relaxation of the brain or he can convert the craniotomy to a bifrontal craniotomy as described by Kjellberg and Prieto[22] (Fig. 14-13). This is the only mechanical decompressive procedure providing more than a minor volume of increased space to patients with massive brain swelling, and it offers the additional advantage of permitting inspection of frontal, temporal and anterior parietal lobes, the subfrontal area and the space along the falx between the hemispheres, often disclosing previously unrecognized hematomas. This operation is limited in applicability to high-risk patients in desperate circumstances and has not achieved widespread use in other neurosurgical centers. The yield of the procedure has been low, but we have had a small number of high-quality survivors, some of whom were apneic, with bilaterally dilated and fixed pupils preoperatively. It would seem that controlled prospective evaluation of this and some of the other methods currently used in the management of traumatic brain injury is urgently needed.

CHRONIC SUBDURAL HEMATOMA. — No discussion of the traumatic hematomas is complete without mention of this interesting disorder, which presents weeks or months after an often minor and forgotten injury, and which so frequently mimics other conditions, such as brain tumor or stroke disease, that it has been referred to as "the great imitator" of neurologic disease. The widely held reputation for benignity enjoyed by this lesion is not warranted by the mortality rates of 20–30% reported in most series.

The bleeding most often originates from a cortical vein, which, fixed at its point of entry into the superior sagittal sinus, is lacerated by shearing forces as the brain moves slightly out of phase relative to movement of the skull at the moment of impact. This mechanism partly explains the prevalence of chronic subdural hematoma in the elderly, in whom the greater disproportion between skull volume and brain size, due to normal loss of brain substance with aging, permits a greater amplitude of displacement of the brain within its dural envelope. After bleeding is arrested, presumably by tamponade by the clot in concert with normal hemostatic processes, the blood breaks down and becomes enclosed in subdural membranes according to the timetable worked out by Munro and Merritt.[38] The inner membrane applied to the arachnoid is thin and velamentous; the outer membrane subadjacent to the dura is thick, friable and richly vascularized. By the eighteenth day after

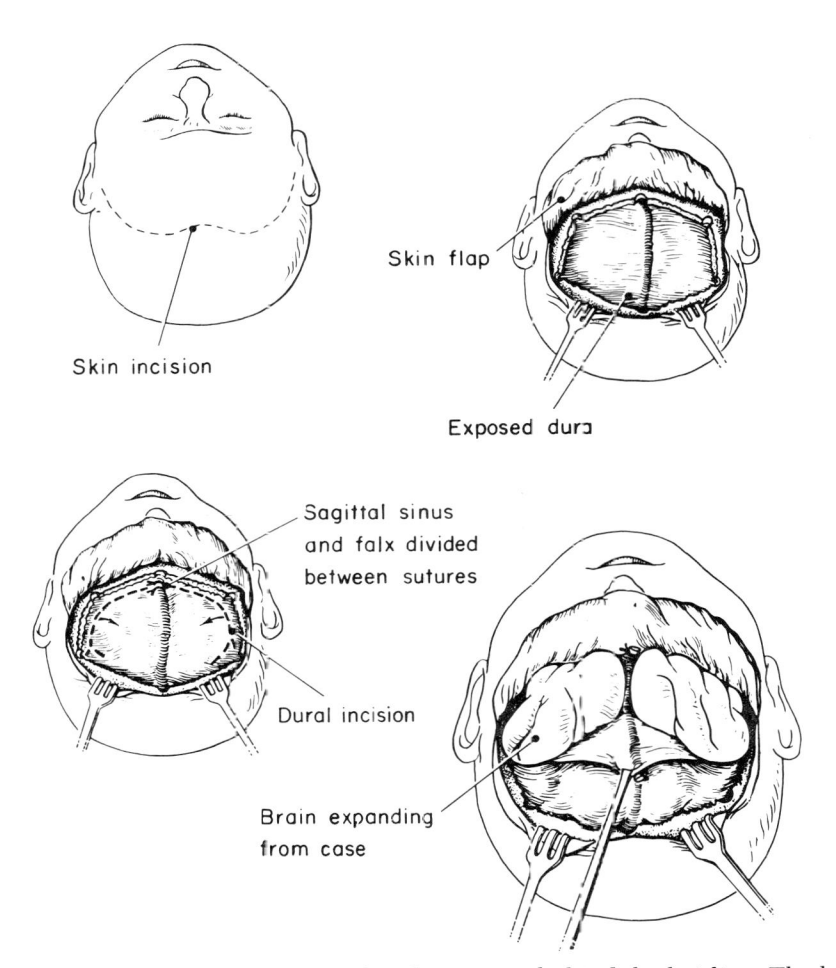

Fig. 14-13.—Bifrontal craniotomy. Coronal scalp incision behind the hairline. The bone opening extends from above the supraorbital ridge to 1 cm behind the coronal suture. The dura, sagittal sinus and falx are divided to allow anterior and lateral decompression. The dural opening is closed with a graft of pericranium or temporalis fascia.

the hemorrhage, the outer membrane is as thick as normal dura and, when seen at surgery, it usually is much thicker. Whether the mass of the enclosed hematoma increases in volume by imbibing fluid consequent to osmotic pressure generated by the breakdown products of the blood or is added to by bleeding or transudation of fluid from the vascular neomembranes remains an unsettled question.[50] The gradual enlargement of the hematoma is well tolerated by the brain at first, but eventually the compensating mechanisms begin to fail as the brain is compressed and molded by the clot, and clinical signs and symptoms become apparent.

Most patients complain of headache that often is predominantly unilateral and present for 2–4 weeks or longer before the hematoma is discovered. The most common early sign is a subtle clouding of intellectual function, frequently brought up by the patient's family ("He isn't himself"), and when seen at this stage, the patient indeed looks dull and apathetic, lacks spontaneity and performs poorly on even simple tests of cortical function. Later on, as mentation progressively worsens, hemiparesis, dysphasia, stupor, seizures and papilledema may appear. In a high percentage of cases, a pineal shift on skull films and appropriate abnormalities of the EEG and radioisotope brain scan will support the diagnosis, but we recommend carotid angiography (see Fig. 14-4) as the definitive study, except for the very elderly or those patients who are deteriorating rapidly, in which cases burhole exploration is the less risky procedure. Approximately 20% of chronic subdural hematomas are bilateral and the presence of a clot on the opposite side is determined more easily by angiography than by bilateral exploration. Preoperative assurance that the clot is unilateral enables the surgeon to operate with the patient in the more convenient lateral position and shortens anesthesia time.

The first bur hole is placed in the midtemporal region and enlarged to form a small craniectomy. The dura, darkened by the underlying hematoma, is incised to reveal the purple-brown outer subdural membrane, which, in turn, is opened to give access to the clot. If hematoma spurts out under pressure, it is important to tamponade the bur hole with a finger and allow the blood to escape very slowly over several minutes, as these fragile patients tolerate abrupt changes in intracranial dynamics poorly. At times, exploration will yield clear, yellow fluid, a subdural hygroma, which resolves with drainage. After intracranial pressure has equilibrated with the atmosphere, the subdural space is irrigated with saline and the characteristics of the hematoma examined. Completely liquid hematomas are drained by placing two or more additional bur holes and establishing through-and-through irrigation. If there is a substantial volume of old solid clot, however, removal will be inadequate unless an osteoplastic bone flap is turned down; this exposure, with proper lighting and use of brain retractors, allows access to the entire lateral aspect of the hemisphere from frontal to occipital pole. After the hematoma has been completely removed by either method, the edges of the highly vascular outer membrane are coagulated millimeter by millimeter to prevent postoperative bleeding and reaccumulation of the clot. The inner membrane is left undisturbed. The recurrence rate of chronic subdural hematomas is high, approximately 20%, and we are in agreement with Svien and Gelety[45] that no attempt should be made to strip the outer membrane beyond the limits of the exposure lest unobserved oozing results. A stainless steel clip then is placed on a tuft of arachnoid and a second clip on the opposing dura for postoperative x-ray purposes. The dura is carefully sutured if a flap has been turned or covered with small pieces of Gelfoam in the case of bur holes. Number 10 French red rubber drains are placed in the subdural space, sutured to the skin and left in place for 24–48 hours. As the dura is being closed, the subdural space is filled with Hartmann's artificial cerebrospinal fluid solution and finally the scalp is sutured with nonabsorbable material.

Failure of the brain to re-expand after removal of the compressing mass is a special problem in the management of the chronic hematomas, especially in the elderly, and predisposes to reaccumulation of the subdural collection. Nursing the patient in 20 degrees of Trendelenburg position and generous hydration are two postoperative measures to enhance brain expansion. On the morning after surgery, skull x-rays in anteroposterior, Towne and lateral projections are taken and the distance between the previously placed clips is measured to determine the width of the subdural space. Ideally, the clip on the cortex moves outward to contact the clip on the dura in a day or two, indicating full expansion of the brain, but sometimes a gap of a few millimeters as well as a residual pineal shift will persist for months, despite satisfactory clinical recovery of the patient. Re-

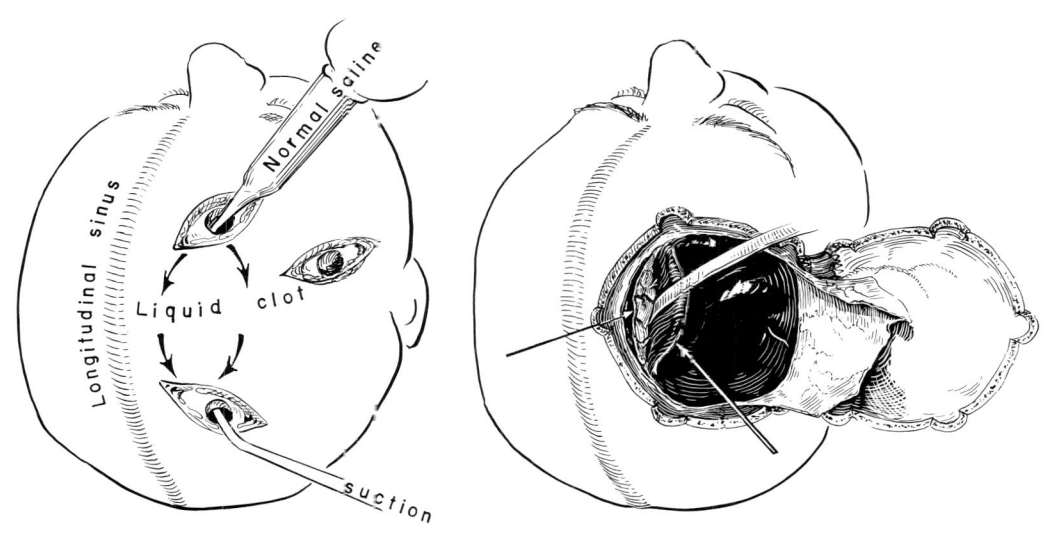

Fig. 14-14. — **Left,** removal of liquid chronic subdural hematoma by irrigating between bur holes with body-temperature saline. The cut edges of the subdural membrane then are meticulously coagulated to prevent postoperative oozing and recurrence of the clot. **Right,** removal of solid hematoma at craniotomy. The dura has been opened and the exposed hematoma is being separated from the cortex. Clot beyond the limits of the craniotomy is retrieved by suction and irrigation. The accessible portion of the outer membrane (**right arrow**) is excised and the residual cut edge (**left arrow**) carefully coagulated.

exploration, of course, is undertaken if the interval between the clips widens in conjunction with neurologic worsening.

POSTERIOR FOSSA HEMATOMAS. — Traumatic hematomas of the posterior fossa are much less common than those located above the tentorium. Wright,[53] in reviewing the experience at Massachusetts General Hospital in the decade 1955–1965, found 17 verified cases compared with 344 patients with clinically significant supratentorial hematomas treated during this same period. The extradural space was the most frequent location, a finding in keeping with other reports, and more than half of the reported cases have occurred in children. The development of signs and symptoms of an expanding extradural mass usually was delayed for hours or days after injury, suggesting that the bleeding originated from the transverse sinus or from the edges of the occipital fracture that almost universally was present. Some of the hematomas were subdural or intracerebellar in location but the true incidence of these lesions is not known, owing to the small number of reported cases.

All except one of the posterior fossa hematomas in Wright's series were caused by a direct blow to the occiput, and most of the patients in this and in other series were found to have a fracture crossing the lateral sinus or extending into the foramen magnum. Impaired consciousness, severe headache in those able to speak, sixth nerve or gaze palsies and papilledema are the most frequent findings in those not comatose at the outset. These hematomas are difficult to demonstrate radiographically, except by ventriculography or vertebral angiography, and if a subtentorial hematoma is likely on clinical grounds, exploratory suboccipital bur holes, followed by craniectomy, offers a more direct approach to diagnosis and treatment with less risk and delay. Extradural hemorrhage from a lacerated lateral sinus can spread upward and downward with equal ease, and bur holes always should be placed over the occipital lobes if a clot is found in the posterior fossa and vice versa.

In common with other posterior fossa mass lesions, hematomas obstruct the circulation of cerebrospinal fluid, and the withdrawal of CSF by lumbar puncture may result in the formation of a fatal cerebellar pressure cone. The abrupt change in intracranial dynamics created by the removal of CSF below the obstructing mass forces the cerebellar tonsils downward into the funnel-shaped foramen magnum and upper spinal canal toward the region of lower pressure. The resultant compression of the medulla by the tonsils is attended by respiratory arrest, followed shortly by cessation of heart action.

PENETRATING BRAIN WOUNDS. — The principles of management of penetrating wounds of the brain have been well established by the extensive experience of military neurosurgeons in the four major wars of this century, and it has been shown repeatedly that the mortality and morbidity from expanding hematomas and from infection of these contaminated wounds are directly related to the timing and thoroughness of the original surgical procedure. The operative mortality of penetrating cerebral wounds of 50–60% in the early years of World War I was reduced by the operative techniques of Harvey Cushing to 29% toward the end of that conflict, and was further reduced to 14% in World War II. Meirowsky[36] reported a mortality of less than 8% among soldiers reaching a neurosurgical facility during the Korean War, and in Hammon's larger series from Vietnam,[14] the operative mortality was 9.7% with extensive missile-produced brain damage, the most frequent cause of death in autopsied cases. The single most important factor responsible for improving the fate of these patients has been the recognition and application of the principle that every penetrating cerebral wound requires the earliest possible definitive debridement, with removal of all foreign material and devitalized tissue, followed by watertight closure of the dura and repair of the scalp wound without tension.

Dissipation of the energy of high-velocity military projectiles by skull and brain results in extensive tissue destruction, often at considerable distance from the missile track. At impact, the projectile may fragment and shatter bone locally, driving secondary missiles of metal and bone deep into the brain and often carrying along bits of helmet liner, skin, hair and dirt. This combination of avascular brain contaminated by diverse foreign material explains the marked propensity to deep infection of the brain if the wound is not debrided adequately in the early hours after injury.

Operation is performed with an endotracheal tube in place and the patient positioned and draped to allow wide access to the scalp. The wound of entry is excised as described above and the incision extended to expose the fracture. All contaminated bone and comminuted fragments are removed, and enough additional bone is rongeured away to provide a craniectomy adequate to expose the underlying wound of the meninges and brain. Care should be taken at this point to preserve uninjured pericranium, as it may be needed later on for use as a dural graft. Necrotic edges of the dural defect then are excised and the opening enlarged to expose the surface of the brain around the cerebral wound. Indriven bone, missile fragments, hair, etc. should be removed as encountered and submitted for bacteriologic culture. If the frontal sinuses have been entered, the sinus mucosa is totally excised and the cavity packed with antibiotic-soaked Gelfoam.

Before starting debridement of the cerebral wound, the path of the projectile and the location of radiopaque foreign bodies should be fixed clearly in the surgeon's mind by a study of the characteristics of the wound and from the preoperative skull x-ray films, which should include stereo views. Brain abscesses, due to retained fragments of bone, are common sequelae to inadequately debrided wounds, and every effort should be made to remove all bone and missile particles if they can be reached without damaging important uninjured portions of the brain. Some experienced military neurosurgeons feel so strongly about this point that they advocate reoperation a day or two later if postoperative skull films show retained bone. Residual metallic fragments apparently have a lesser tendency toward abscess formation.

Using a fine sucker tip, clot and necrotic brain are carefully aspirated under direct vision, a maneuver greatly facilitated by illumination from a fiberoptic lighted retractor. Nonviable brain sucks away without resistance, exposing bits of foreign material, which are retrieved readily. If the track is wide enough, gentle finger palpation may disclose foreign bodies that otherwise might be missed. At the conclusion of this stage of debridement, the track should remain open and the brain should pulsate; otherwise, residual hematoma and necrotic brain probably still are present. Failure to obtain these conditions after thorough debridement suggests the presence of an intracerebral or surface hematoma in the opposite hemisphere. The wound is irrigated repeatedly with sterile saline during all stages of debridement, and hemostasis must be absolute before beginning closure.

Watertight closure of the dura is an essential step that usually requires suturing a graft of locally obtained pericranium or temporalis fascia into the dural defect with a running stitch. Intact dura provides an effective barrier to infection from without, especially necessary if the paranasal sinuses have been entered, and prevents cerebrospinal fluid fistula, a particularly important consideration with transventricular wounds. The dura also prevents local cerebral herniation with subsequent infarction and greatly facilitates later cranioplasty.

The scalp is closed without drainage as a single layer with interrupted vertical mattress sutures of #32 stainless steel wire, which are left in for 2 weeks. If the defect in the scalp is so large that closure without tension cannot be accomplished, sliding or rotational scalp flaps must be advanced to cover the defect (see Fig. 14-8); the donor site is covered with thin split-thickness skin grafts placed on the pericranium.

Matson[30] has called attention to a special mechanism of hematoma formation in the hemisphere opposite the site of entry that should be suspected whenever

Fig. 14-15.—Gunshot wounds of the brain. A, characteristic small entrance and large exit wounds. B, the bullet ricocheted from the inner surface of the skull, producing tremendous cerebral damage.

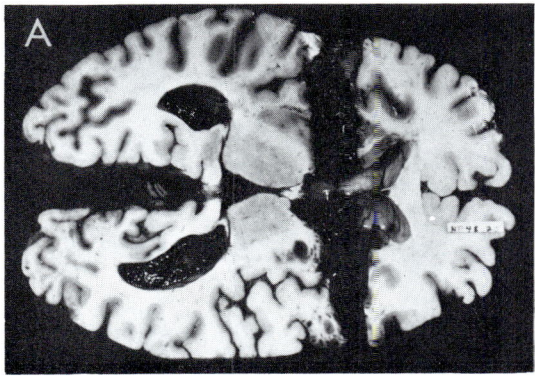

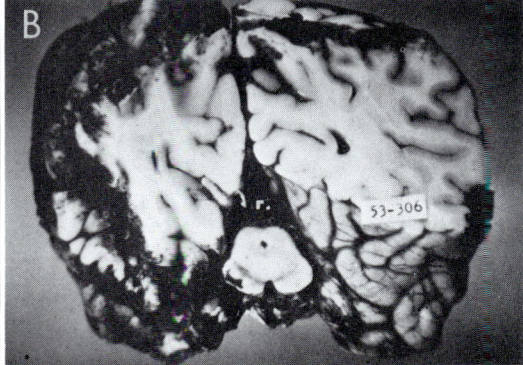

x-ray films demonstrate a metallic foreign body near the surface of the brain but distant from the site of entry. These subdural or intracerebral hematomas result from laceration of cortical vessels on the surface of the brain by a missile that has traversed the brain and strikes the opposite inner table. Its energy spent, the missile ricochets a short distance back into the brain (Fig. 14-15).

Antibiotics should be started in full therapeutic doses prior to operation and maintained throughout the postoperative period, with appropriate changes made if indicated by the results of culture and sensitivity studies. Staphylococcus is the predominant organism cultured from head wounds, but mixed infections with gram-negative organisms are frequent and should be covered by the antibiotics selected initially.

Readers interested in a more detailed discussion of projectile wounds should consult the monographs by Matson[31] and Meirowsky[36] and the reports available to date on the Vietnam experience in the *Journal of Neurosurgery* of February, 1971.

NONSURGICAL ADJUNCTS TO MANAGEMENT

CEREBRAL EDEMA AND INCREASED INTRACRANIAL PRESSURE. — A major therapeutic objective in the acute stages of head trauma is prevention and control of the cerebral edema that is such a prominent feature of the brain-injured state. The pathophysiologic processes leading to cerebral edema are complex[24, 27] and incompletely understood, but currently it is believed that brain injury results in vasoconstrictor paralysis, with congestion of the cerebrovascular bed and derangement, probably at the glial-capillary interface, of mechanisms concerned with water and electrolyte transport. The accumulation of high-protein fluid in the extracellular space, swelling of astrocytes and vascular congestion result in a net increase in cerebral volume, particularly marked in the deep hemispheral white matter. Since the brain is enclosed in a rigid skull of fixed volume already filled to capacity, an increase in volume of any of the three major intracranial components — brain tissue, blood and cerebrospinal fluid — results in an enormous rise in intracranial pressure. Initially, some compensation for an expanding mass occurs through reduction in the cerebrospinal fluid volume of the ventricles, basilar cisterns and subarachnoid space, but once the maximal amount of CSF has been displaced, small additional increases in the volume of the brain, or the mass, or of total cerebral blood, will be reflected by great rises in intracranial tension. In these circumstances, the volume of the cerebrovascular bed is determined largely by arterial Pco_2 and Po_2; hypercapnia and hypoxia are potent stimuli to further vasodilatation and, by this mechanism, disastrously enhance cerebral edema and intracranial hypertension.

HYPERVENTILATION. — Underventilation, with relative hypercapnia and hypoxia, is a common respiratory abnormality in patients with brain injuries, even though the airway may be perfectly satisfactory. The disorder is readily diagnosed by arterial blood gas analysis and should be suspected and sought for in all patients with altered consciousness or a worsening neurologic condition thought to be due to cerebral swelling. Correction of this important metabolic defect requires assisted ventilation administered via an endotracheal tube or tracheostomy. Because of the marked effect of CO_2 and O_2 on the caliber of cerebral blood vessels, cerebral swelling and increased intracranial pressure sometimes can be modified favorably by hyperventilation, provided that irreversible vasomotor paralysis has not yet occurred. Lowering arterial Pco_2 to 30 mm Hg and raising Po_2 and pH by controlled alveolar hyperventilation 25–50% above rated minute volume, with a negative pressure expiratory phase and frequent blood gas monitoring, usually produces a modest lowering of intracranial pressure that can be sustained for hours.[16]

PHARMACOLOGIC AGENTS.—In recent decades, two major classes of drugs effective in reducing cerebral edema and lowering increased intracranial pressure under certain conditions have achieved widespread use in neurosurgery. These agents, the osmotic diuretics and the adrenocortical steroids, differ widely in mode of action and in the clinical situations in which they are useful. It should be emphasized that efforts to reduce intracranial hypertension by pharmacologic means will not succeed unless any respiratory inadequacies present are corrected first.

HYPEROSMOLAR AGENTS.—The principal use of osmotic diuretics in the management of head injuries is to temporarily reverse signs of decompensation from increased intracranial pressure in crisis situations, thus gaining time for more definitive therapy. The duration of action is brief (3–6 hours) and the effect much less pronounced with repeated doses, so that these agents are not suitable for chronic intravenous administration. In uncritical hands, there is at least the theoretic possibility of masking the early focal signs of an expanding hematoma by temporarily lowering intracranial pressure.

Mannitol and urea are the most extensively used osmotic diuretics for this purpose. Following rapid intravenous administration, the molecules initially are confined to the extracellular space, creating an osmotic gradient that favors the passage of water from the brain into the bloodstream and eventual excretion by the kidneys. The expansion in circulating blood volume poses a hazard to those with fragile cardiovascular reserves, and occasional instances of congestive failure and pulmonary edema have been reported. Because of the tremendous expected diuresis, an indwelling catheter should be placed before the agent is given. The subsequent administration of excessive intravenous fluids is, of course, irrational and defeats the purpose of an osmotic diuretic.

Mannitol, the more widely used material, is a 6-carbon hexahydric alcohol that remains in the extracellular space and is cleared rapidly by the kidney. It is given intravenously as a 20% solution over 15–45 minutes; the recommended dose is 1.5 gm/kg body weight, although we have found that smaller doses (1.0 gm/kg) often produce a very satisfactory effect. Reduction in intracranial pressure usually is apparent within 20–60 minutes and lasts up to 6 hours. Wise and Chater[52] recorded pressure drops of 50–90% in a series of patients with elevated pressure due to brain tumor.

Urea, the first hyperosmolar agent to achieve extensive clinical use, now is employed less frequently because of its somewhat shorter duration of action (3–4 hours) and because of the rebound rise in pressure sometimes seen several hours after administration, when the urea concentration in brain tissue exceeds that in the extracellular space, reversing the osmotic gradient. Urea is given as a 30% solution in dosage of 0.75–1.0 gm/kg, taking great care that the material is securely infused into a large vein, since extravasation of this hypertonic fluid produces local tissue necrosis.

Glycerol, a trivalent alcohol, is absorbed from the GI tract and can be given by tube or taken orally when flavored with lemon. It is suitable for more chronic use in situations similar to those in which steroids ordinarily are employed when, because of side-effects, these latter agents are contraindicated. The usual oral dose is 1–2 gm/kg/day in six divided doses.

GLUCOCORTICOIDS.—Whereas the principal value of hyperventilation and osmotic diuretics is to provide a brief respite from increased intracranial pressure early after injury or during intervals of temporary postoperative pressure elevations, the glucocorticoids suppress elevated intracranial pressure over longer periods and commonly are used for days, weeks or, in rare instances, for months. Unlike these other modalities, the action of steroids is not rapid, and beneficial effects seldom are seen before 24 hours. The precise mechanism of action of steroids is not known, but data suggest that the effect is to decrease the abnormal cerebrovascular permeability thought to be the basic defect in vasogenic brain edema and thus retard expansion of the extracellular space and astroglial swelling.[27] Although there is ample documentation of the effectiveness of steroids in alleviating the cerebral edema and intracranial hypertension associated with primary and metastatic brain tumors, usually with striking clinical improvement, and in the reduction of experimental brain edema produced by a wide variety of means, a well-controlled study of the effects of these agents on traumatic edema of the human brain has not yet appeared. A very extensive, albeit uncontrolled, clinical experience with these drugs in the management of brain trauma has been favorable, however, and steroids are used on our service in virtually every patient with clinical evidence of structural injury of the brain.

Steroids probably are more effective in preventing the development of brain edema than in correcting it once it has occurred, and it is our practice to administer a large loading dose to seriously injured persons when they are first seen, unless compelling contraindications, such as herpetic keratitis, tuberculosis or active peptic ulcer, are present. In these cases, the risk-reward factors must be weighed carefully and a decision whether to use the drugs determined by the severity of the respective conditions. Under these liberal indications, occasional errors are made and steroids are given to patients who later prove not to be as seriously injured as was thought initially; the drug then is abruptly discontinued. Initially, dexamethasone 10 mg or methylprednisolone 40–80 mg are given intravenously to adults, with appropriate adjustments in dosage for younger patients. The usual maintenance doses of dexamethasone 4 mg (0.05 mg/kg) or methylprednisolone 40 mg (0.5 mg/kg) are given every 6 hours thereafter, or even every 4 hours for the first 24 hours in the more seriously injured patients. Duration of therapy is guided by the response of the patient to the over-all program of management, and soon after substantial neurologic improvement is established, the dosage is reduced to levels sufficient to maintain the desired effect. The best indicator of subsiding brain edema is steady improvement in the state of consciousness, but other clinical and laboratory parameters of progress must be considered also. Since exogenous steroids suppress the pituitary-adrenal axis, abrupt withdrawal of the drug after 4 or 5 days of treatment at these levels is likely to be followed by relative adrenal insufficiency, especially in elderly or debilitated patients. Slow tapering of dosage over many days will permit resumption of endogenous steroid production and avoid this problem.

Gastrointestinal bleeding is the most frequently encountered serious complication of prolonged steroid therapy, a problem compounded by other ulcerogenic variables, such as the systemic stress of injury, the specific factor of brain injury (Cushing's ulcer) and extended periods without food in the stomach. Prophylactic administration of 30 ml of an antacid preparation by Levin tube every 2–4 hours and the early institution of tube feedings will lessen the incidence of this complication. Minor GI bleeding sometimes can be controlled by titrating gastric acidity to neutrality with antacids without stopping steroids, if the need for their continued use is imperative, but generally it is wiser to discontinue the drug and attempt control with glycerol or by some other means. Delayed wound healing, increased tendency to wound infection and aggravation of diabetes or hypertension have not been major problems of this drug regimen.

FLUID REQUIREMENTS OF PATIENTS WITH INCREASED INTRACRANIAL PRESSURE.—The drastic dehydrating regimens practiced in the early days of neurosurgery in attempts to control brain swelling have long since been discarded. However, Bakay et al.[4] demonstrated that the administration of excessive amounts of 5% glucose in water to patients with cerebral edema from brain tumors resulted in a pronounced rise in intracranial pressure, and we are familiar with a number of instances of transtentorial herniation induced by the overzealous administration of hypotonic fluids in the early hours after head injury. It is preferable to keep patients with cerebral swelling on the dry side, and unless there are extraordinary water-electrolyte losses or requirements imposed by other injuries, the basic maintenance intravenous solution used on our service is 0.5 normal saline in 2.5% glucose given at 0.75 ml/kg/hr for the early days after injury. If necessitated by continuing brain edema, this mildly dehydrating regimen can be maintained for a week or longer in otherwise healthy patients, but, ordinarily, it is wise to institute tube feedings after 24–48 hours if other injuries permit.

Indications for the selection and the timing of usage of the various modalities currently available for relief from brain swelling vary widely among individual neurosurgeons, according to their experience and preferences. This factor, coupled with the heterogeneous nature of head injuries, makes the gathering of meaningful data on the relative therapeutic merits of the different regimens a difficult task, and, for obvious reasons, a controlled prospective study, for example, of the effectiveness of steroids in reducing traumatic cerebral edema, is almost impossible to design. It is anticipated that the introduction into clinical practice of subdural pressure transducers to allow continuous monitoring of intracranial pressure will permit systematic study of some of these questions and provide a rational basis for more effective use of presently available agents and of those yet to be discovered.

ANTICONVULSANT MEDICATION.—In a follow-up study of soldiers who had suffered severe head injuries during the Korean War, Caveness[6] found that 30% eventually had at least one seizure and 8% had the first seizure within 14 days of injury. Ten years later, 14 of the group still were considered to have an active seizure disorder. Factors increasing the liability of seizures included wounds adjacent to the central sulcus, especially in the parietal lobe, wounding by missile, extensive brain damage and a family history of epilepsy. Focal fits or focal fits that progressed to generalized seizures seemed to have the worst prognosis for the development of a lasting seizure disorder.

Prophylactic administration of anticonvulsant medication is advocated by many neurosurgeons, but the clinical indications for its use and the therapeutic regimens employed vary widely. In general, the use of these drugs is restricted to patients with cortical contusions, penetrating wounds of the brain and intracranial clots and to those undergoing intracranial surgery. Anticonvulsant therapy is not used prophylactically in patients with minor closed head injuries.

Diphenylhydantoin in doses of 300–400 mg/day for 70-kg adults is the most commonly used anticonvulsant, but blood levels in the therapeutic range (10–15 μg/ml) are not attained for 1–2 weeks when this drug is given by the oral or intramuscular route. Slow intravenous administration is preferred if seizures occur and control is imperative. Phenobarbital 125–250 mg/day for 70-kg adults is also widely used; the advantage of more rapidly attainable therapeutic levels, however, may be offset by the sedative properties of this drug, which may complicate neurologic evaluation.

The special problem of continuous or frequently recurring focal or generalized seizures constitutes a medical emergency, requiring urgent treatment. Large doses (1,500 mg) of parenteral diphenylhydantoin[49] and diazepam (4–10 mg) intravenously[39] have been used with success in the treatment of status epilepticus, with careful monitoring of vital signs and provisions made for coping with the cardiorespiratory problems that may attend the use of these depressant drugs.

Metabolic derangements, particularly water overload, and elevated body temperature are important factors that tend to enhance seizure activity and should be treated vigorously by water restriction, diuretics and rapid cooling of the patient, respectively. Finally, it should be kept in mind that seizures may be symptomatic of undetected intracranial clot or sepsis and appropriate investigation considered.

TEMPERATURE CONTROL.—Fever is a common accompaniment of the unconscious state and usually is due to an identifiable source, such as metabolic disturbance, atelectasis, pneumonitis or urinary tract infection. The presence of blood within the subarachnoid space may cause temperature rises to 101–102° F but this diagnosis is one of exclusion to be entertained only after a careful negative search for a treatable complication. Persistent unexplained fever in comatose patients often is erroneously attributed to the brain injury. Damage to hypothalamic thermoregulatory centers abolishes normal mechanisms of heat conservation-dissipation and results either in subnormal body temperatures without shivering or pilo-erection or in raging fever, usually unaccompanied by sweating, to 105° and beyond. Severe injuries to the hypothalamus, in addition to disordered temperature regulation, are characterized by profound coma, diabetes insipidus and failing vital signs; survival is a matter of hours.

Since fevers are poorly tolerated by patients with brain lesions and often are marked by further impairment of consciousness, heightened tendency to seizures and worsening of any focal deficits present, maintenance of normal body temperature is an important therapeutic measure. Aspirin or acetaminophen, in doses of 1.2 gm rectally in adults, is effective in lowering elevated body temperature by increasing sweating and peripheral blood flow and is used to control temperatures over 101° F. Aspirin-induced hypoprothrombinemia is a hazard with repeated doses, particularly in vitamin K-depleted patients or those with impaired liver function.

In the early 1960s, therapeutic hypothermia with maintenance of body temperature at 90–92° F for days or weeks received extensive clinical trial in the management of severe head injuries. The many serious complications and the failure of the expected benefits to materialize led to the abandonment of this modality, and the elaborate equipment developed is used rarely except to maintain normothermic temperature levels.

DIABETES INSIPIDUS.—This disorder of water metabolism, common after parasellar surgery and occurring occasionally after head injury, is due to damage to the hypothalamus and posterior pituitary and introduces unique problems of fluid-electrolyte management. Antidiuretic hormone normally is synthesized in the neurosecretory cells of the supraoptic and paraventricular nuclei of the hypothalamus and transported along the axons of these cells to the posterior lobe of the pituitary, where its release is regulated by osmoreceptors responding to changes in serum osmolarity. Secretion of this hormone into the bloodstream increases water resorption by the distal convoluted portion of the renal tubule, and its absence results in diabetes insipidus, with excretion of tremendous volumes of hypotonic urine, leading rapidly to extreme dehydration if not corrected. Post-traumatic diabetes insipidus can be temporary, intermittent or permanent and is characterized by urine volumes in excess of 200 ml/hr (often more than 1 liter/hr) of specific gravity under 1.005.

The temptation to use Pitressin at the onset of diabetes insipidus to abort the alarming polyuria is difficult to resist, but it is wiser to attempt control initially with water replacement alone, as the episode may be mild and short-lived and the use of this drug is not without risk. Conscious patients are allowed to drink ad lib or intravenous fluids are given, with each hourly volume matching the previous hour's urinary output. Most of this intravenous fluid should be glucose in water, with 1–1.5 liters/day of saline added to cover the usual daily electrolyte loss.[51] Total daily water turnover in excess of 10–12 liters becomes cumbersome and warrants the intramuscular injection of 2–3 units of Pitressin tannate in oil, which produces prompt antidiuresis lasting up to 72 hours. Once Pitressin is given, water intake must be curtailed sharply to prevent dilutional hypotonicity and water intoxication, which can occur within hours. This is the major complication of the use of antidiuretic hormone and is manifested by stupor, increased focal neurologic deficit and seizures; it is corrected by water restriction and, if severe, by cautious hypertonic saline infusion.

IRREVERSIBLE COMA AND BRAIN DEATH

The economic and medical resources of any society, no matter how affluent, are limited, and in the United States today the stresses imposed by the practice of interminably prolonging heart action and respiration by artificial means in patients having no chance of recovery have properly become a matter of public concern. To the enormous cost in dollars and the diversion of scarce hospital facilities and medical personnel into these nonproductive efforts must be added the protracted anguish of the grieving relatives of these patients. In patients with lethal head injuries producing extensive brain damage and irreversible coma, the traditional signs of death may be obscured by the use of respirators and other supportive equipment. We have been guided, in these difficult situations, by the criteria of the Ad Hoc Committee of the Harvard Medical School,[2] which define brain death and irreversible coma, and it is our practice, after consulting with the family, and unless special circumstances are present, to pronounce dead patients fulfilling all conditions and to discontinue the supportive effort. The criteria of the Ad Hoc Committee are summarized below; the original statement is quite specific and should be consulted by interested readers.

Physical findings include: a complete absence of *any* spontaneous activity, including abnormal posturing, and there is utterly no response to any external stimulation, even intense pain. Apnea is maintained during a 3-minute trial off the respirator. Both pupils are fixed to light, and no eye movements can be elicited by head turning or by ice water irrigation of the tympanic membranes. Corneal, pharyngeal, deep tendon and superficial skin reflexes are all absent. Of confirmatory value, but not essential, is the isoelectric EEG, and where facilities for obtaining reliable tracings are available, this examination should be utilized. All of the above findings must be present without change on repeated examination 24 hours later, in the view of the original Committee. The validity of the above data as indications of irreversible cerebral damage depends on the exclusion of two conditions: hypothermia (temperature below 90° F) or the presence of central nervous system depressants, such as barbiturates.

At the time of this writing, a special cooperative study involving several hospital centers is under way to determine whether these criteria for cerebral death should be less rigorous; there has been no medical evidence to date that they are insufficiently rigorous.

ORGAN TRANSPLANTATION

Transplantation of human corneas and vital organs, such as the kidney, now are clinically feasible procedures, and successful extension of these techniques to other tissues in the future can be predicted with confidence. Most transplantation centers have large populations of potential kidney recipients, each of whom must be maintained in chronic dialysis for the months of their often futile wait for a suitable donor. The number of patients needing kidney transplants stands in sad contrast to the relatively few donor organs that become available. The characteristics of the ideal donor—terminal illness of brief duration, freedom from infectious, neoplastic or degenerative diseases and youth—are met most often in patients with traumatic brain damage incompatible with survival, and virtually all organs requiring perfusion until removal are obtained from such patients at present. Surgeons attending such hopelessly injured patients should make every effort to obtain the cooperation and consent of the relatives to permit postmortem organ removal for use in these merciful endeavors, always remembering that the death of a patient is an independent event, completely separate from the requirements of potential donors, no matter how legitimate those needs may be.

BIBLIOGRAPHY

1. Accident Facts: National Safety Council, 1972 edition.
2. A Definition of Irreversible Coma: Report of the Ad Hoc Committee of the Harvard Medical School to examine the definition of brain death, JAMA 205:337, 1968.
3. A Survey of Current Head Injury Research: National Institute of Neurological Disease and Stroke, 1969.
4. Bakay, L., Crawford, J. D., and White, J. C.: The effects of intravenous fluids on cerebrospinal fluid pressure, Surg. Gynecol. Obstet. 99:48, 1954.
5. Barber, H. O.: The diagnosis and treatment of auditory and vestibular disorders after head injury, Clin. Neurosurg. 19:355, 1971.
6. Caveness, W. F.: Onset and cessation of fits following craniocerebral trauma, J. Neurosurg. 20:570, 1963.
7. Chason, J. L., Hardy, W. G., Webster, J. E., and Gurdjian, E. S.: Alterations in cell structure of the brain associated with experimental concussion, J. Neurosurg. 15:135, 1958.
8. Fischer, J. E., Turner, R. H., Herndon, J. H., and Riseborough, E. J.: Massive steroid therapy in severe fat embolism, Surg. Gynecol. Obstet. 132:667, 1971.
9. Freytag, E.: Autopsy findings in head injuries from blunt forces: Statistical evaluation of 1367 cases, Arch. Pathol. 75:402, 1963.
10. Gallagher, J. P., and Browder, E. J.: Extradural hematoma; experience with 167 patients, J. Neurosurg. 29:1, 1968.
11. Gurdjian, E. S.: Recent advances in the study of the mechanism of impact injury of the head—a summary, Clin. Neurosurg. 19:1, 1971.
12. Gurdjian, E. S., Webster, J. E., and Lissner, H. R.: The mechanism of skull fracture, J. Neurosurg. 7:106, 1950.
13. Hamby, W. B.: *Carotid-Cavernous Fistula* (Springfield, Ill.: Charles C Thomas, Publisher, 1966).
14. Hammon, W. M.: Analysis of 2,187 consecutive penetrating wounds of the brain from Vietnam, J. Neurosurg. 34:127, 1971.
15. Harwood-Nash, D. C., Hendrick, E. B., and Hudson, A. R.: The significance of skull fractures in children. A study of 1,187 patients, Radiology 101:151, 1971.
16. Hayes, G. J., and Slocum, H. L.: The achievement of optimal brain relaxation by hyperventilation techniques of anesthesia, J. Neurosurg. 19:65, 1962.
17. Jamieson, K. G.: Extradural and subdural hematomas: Changing patterns and requirements of treatment in Australia, J. Neurosurg. 33:632, 1970.
18. Jamieson, K. G.: Depressed skull fractures in Australia, J. Neurosurg. 37:150, 1972.
19. Jamieson, K. G., and Yelland, J. D. N.: Extradural hematoma: Report of 167 patients, J. Neurosurg. 29:13, 1968.
20. Jamieson, K. G., and Yelland, J. D. N.: Surgically treated traumatic subdural hematomas, J. Neurosurg. 37:137, 1972.
21. Jennett, B., and Miller, J. D.: Infection after depressed fracture of skull. Implications for management of non-missile injuries, J. Neurosurg. 36:333, 1972.
22. Kjellberg, R. N., and Prieto, A., Jr.: Bifrontal decompressive craniotomy for massive cerebral edema, J. Neurosurg. 34:488, 1971.
23. Kriss, F. C., Taren, J. A., and Kahn, E. A.: Primary repair of compound skull fractures by replacement of bone fragments, J. Neurosurg. 30:698, 1969.
24. Langfitt, T. W., Tannanbaum, H. M., and Kassell, N. F.: The etiology of acute brain swelling following experimental head injury, J. Neurosurg. 24:47, 1966.
25. Lende, R. A., and Erickson, T. C.: Growing skull fractures of childhood, J. Neurosurg. 18:479, 1961.

26. Lewin, W.: Cerebrospinal fluid rhinorrhea in nonmissile head injuries, Clin. Neurosurg. 12:237, 1964.
27. Long, D. M., Maxwell, R. E., and French, L. A.: The effects of glucosteroids on cold-induced brain edema. Ultrastructural evaluation, J. Neuropathol. Exp. Neurol. 30:680, 1971.
28. MacGee, E. E., Canthen, J. C., and Brackett, C. E.: Meningitis following acute traumatic CSF fistula, J. Neurosurg. 33:312, 1970.
29. Magoun, H. W.: *The Waking Brain* (Springfield, Ill.: Charles C Thomas, Publisher, 1958).
30. Matson, D. D.: Hematomas associated with penetrating wounds of the brain, J. Neurosurg. 3:46, 1946.
31. Matson, D. D.: *The Treatment of Acute Craniocerebral Injuries Due to Missiles* (Springfield, Ill.: Charles C Thomas, Publisher, 1948).
32. Matson, D. D.: *Neurosurgery of Infancy and Childhood* (Springfield, Ill.: Charles C Thomas, Publisher, 1969).
33. McKissock, W.: Subdural hematoma, a review of 389 cases, Lancet 1:1365, 1960.
34. McLaurin, R. L., and Tutor, F. T.: Acute subdural hematoma. Review of ninety cases, J. Neurosurg. 18:61, 1961.
35. Mealey, J. J.: Acute extradural hematoma without demonstrable skull fracture, J. Neurosurg. 17:27, 1960.
36. Meirowsky, A. M.: In *Neurological Surgery of Trauma*, Coates, J. B., Jr. (ed.) (Washington, D. C.: U.S. Government Printing Office, 1965).
37. Mincey, J. E.: Posttraumatic CSF fistula of the frontal fossa, J. Trauma 6:618, 1966.
38. Munro, D., and Merritt, H. H.: Surgical pathology of subdural hematomas based on study of 105 cases, Arch. Neurol. 35:64, 1936.
39. Nichol, C. F., Tutton, J. C., and Smith, B. H.: Parenteral diazepam in status epilepticus, Neurology 19:332, 1969.
40. Ommaya, A. K., Grubb, R. L., Jr., and Naumann, R. A.: Coup and contrecoup injury. Observations on the mechanics of visible brain injuries in the rhesus monkey, J. Neurosurg. 35:503, 1971.
41. Pudenz, R. H., and Shelden, C. H.: The lucite calvarium—a method for direct observation of the brain. I. Cranial trauma and brain movement, J. Neurosurg. 3:487, 1946.
42. Ray, B. S., and Bergland, R. M.: CSF fistula: Clinical aspects, techniques of localization and methods of closure, J. Neurosurg. 30:399, 1969.
43. Schneider, R. C.: In *Correlative Neurosurgery* (Springfield, Ill.: Charles C Thomas, Publisher, 1969).
44. Schneider, R. C., Gosch, H. H., Taren, J. A., Ferry, D. J. and Jerva, M. J.: Blood vessel trauma following head and neck injuries, Clin. Neurosurg. 19:312, 1971.
45. Svien, H. J., and Gelety, J. E.: On the surgical management of encapsulated subdural hematoma. A comparison of the results of membranectomy and simple evacuation, J. Neurosurg. 21:172, 1964.
46. Talella, A., and Morin, M. A.: Acute traumatic subdural hematoma: A review of 100 consecutive cases, J. Trauma 11:771, 1971.
47. Taveras, J. M., and Ransohoff, J.: Leptomeningeal cysts of the brain following trauma with erosion of the skull. A study of seven cases treated with surgery, J. Neurosurg. 10:233, 1953.
48. Taveras, J. M., and Wood, E. H.: *Diagnostic Neuroradiology* (Baltimore: The Williams & Wilkins Company, 1964).
49. Wallis, W., Kutt, H., and McDowell, F.: Intravenous diphenylhydantoin in treatment of acute epileptic seizures, Neurology 18:513, 1968.
50. Weir, B.: The osmolarity of subdural hematoma fluid, J. Neurosurg. 34:528, 1971.
51. Wise, B.: The management of postoperative diabetes insipidus, J. Neurosurg. 25:416, 1966.
52. Wise, B. L., and Chater, N.: The value of hypertonic mannitol solution in decreasing brain mass and lowering cerebrospinal-fluid pressure, J. Neurosurg. 19:1038, 1962.
53. Wright, R. L.: Traumatic hematomas of the posterior fossa, J. Neurosurg. 25:402, 1966.

15 | Injuries to the Spinal Cord and Cauda Equina

JAMES G. WEPSIC

SPINAL CORD INJURIES are a significant cause of serious disability or death in a youthful population. The tragic loss of neurologic function in otherwise healthy, vigorous adults, typically following diving or automobile accidents, must be dealt with carefully and systematically to ensure maximal recovery of neurologic function. This chapter deals with the major clinical and surgical considerations in early treatment of spinal cord injuries.

ANATOMY

In adults, the spinal cord extends from the foramen magnum to the L2 vertebra, suspended by the dentate ligaments, nerve roots and blood vessels within a shock-absorbing cerebrospinal fluid sac. It is covered by arachnoid and tough fibrous dura, which, in turn, are hydraulically buffered by the surrounding extradural fat and blood vessels. It further is enclosed within the bony confines of the spinal canal. This structural and buffering arrangement makes the spinal cord one of the body's most well-protected organs. Not only is there a firm bony covering around it, constructed in such a way as to allow maximal movement, but the hydraulic system within the subarachnoid space provides excellent shock absorption. The vertebral bodies, composed of a weight-bearing centrum anteriorly and protective overlapping bony arches posteriorly, are connected by two joints, the articular facets. These joints allow both flexion and extension as well as lateral motion and a small amount of rotation. Firm ligaments check this mobility from each side. The rubbery intervertebral disks separate the centra and are composed of a firm outer annular ligament restraining the softer fibrocartilage center.

The cauda equina begins at the L1–L2 interspace and extends to the sacrum. The lower part of the spinal canal with its enclosed nerve roots is less sensitive to injury than the upper portion housing the cord.

The cord receives blood supply over an extensive network of collateral vessels entering the canal over the nerve roots. These radicular arteries seem to arise from the topographic artery nearest to each particular spinal level. The degree of supply from each varies and they may number from 15 to 34, with the ventral radicular arteries usually larger than the dorsal ones. In most individuals, there usually is one ventral radicular artery, markedly larger than the rest, which originates from the aorta between T8 and L3 and provides the blood supply for most of the thoracic cord. Paraplegia can result from occlusion of this artery by traumatic or iatrogenic dissection. The arterial supply of the more superior cord is derived from the vertebral arteries. This

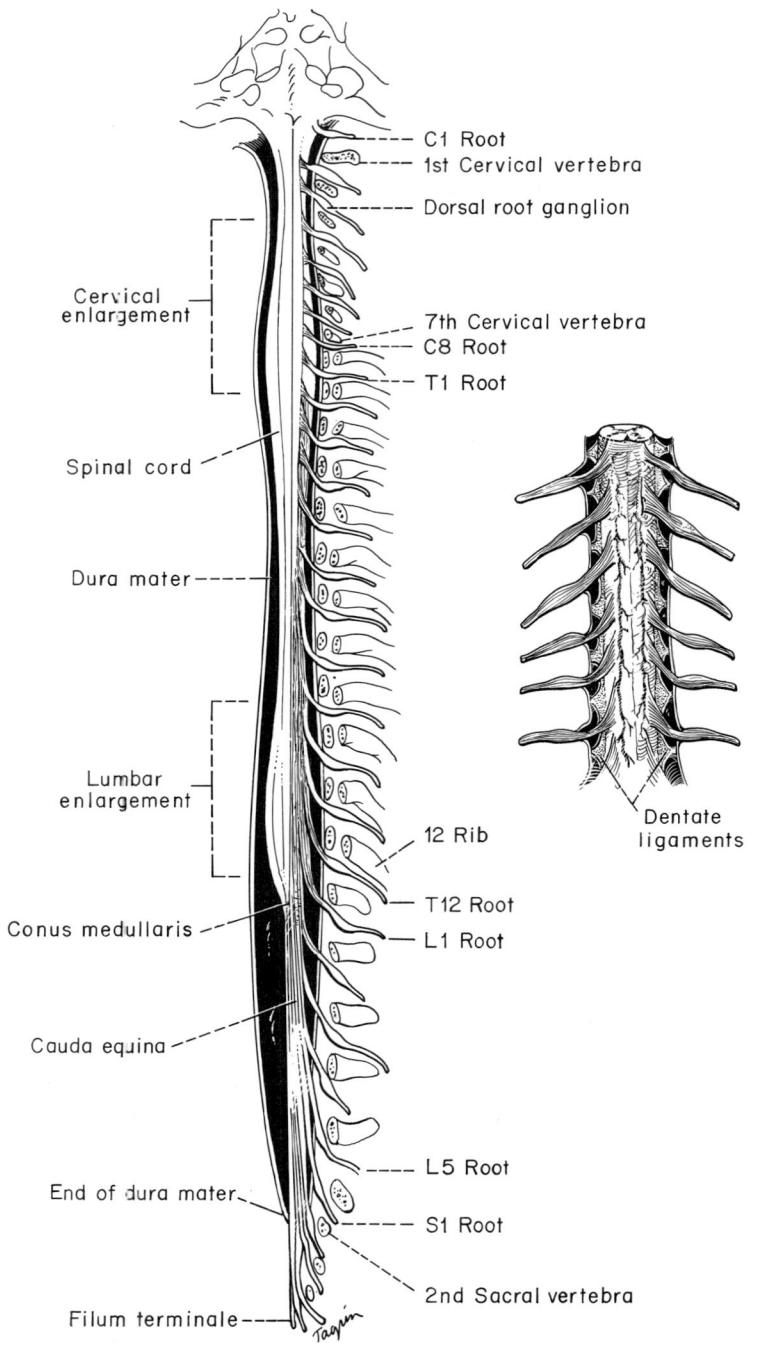

Fig. 15-1.—The spinal cord and surrounding structures. Note the position of the first, seventh and eighth cervical roots with respect to the vertebral level at which they emerge. The cervical and lumbar enlargements are depicted as well as the relationship of the dentate ligaments to the cord, posterior rootlets and dura.

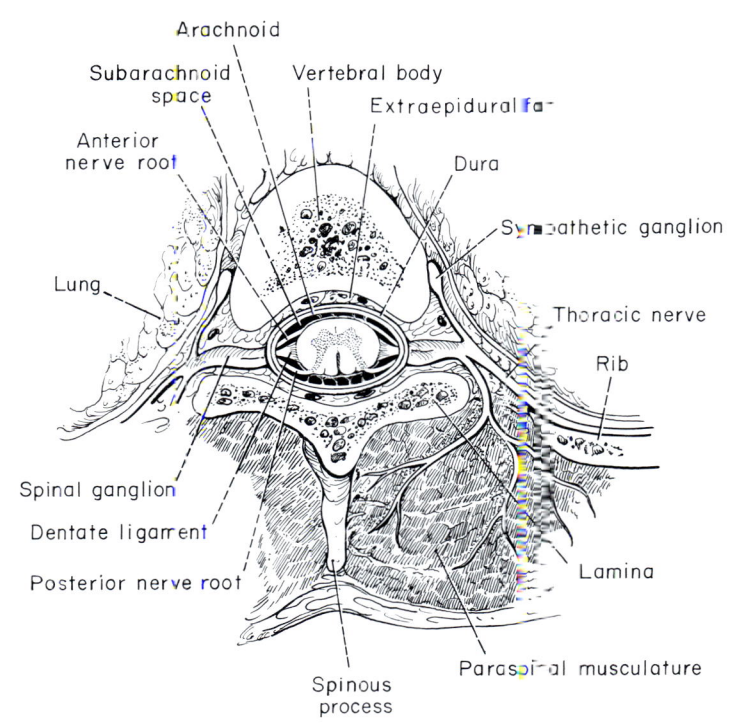

Fig. 15-2.—Transverse section through a thoracic vertebra and spinal cord. The excellent protection of the cord is apparent when the relationships of surrounding musculature, bony canal, extradural fat and spinal fluid are considered. The relationship of the dorsal root to the spinal cord is shown.

vascular architecture allows considerable turning and twisting of the cord without rupture of vessels. As the vessels terminate within the cord substance they are "end arteries," providing very little collateral circulation within the gray matter of the cord itself.

The spinal cord is almost cylindrical, with its width always greater than its dorsoventral diameter. It enlarges noticeably at the region of enervation of the upper extremities as well as at the lumbosacral region. There usually are 31 pairs of spinal nerves in man. The first pair exits from the vertebral column between C1 and the skull, with each of the remaining cervical nerves from C2 and C7 leaving *above* the vertebra of the corresponding number. Since there are 8 cervical nerves and only 7 cervical vertebrae, the eighth cervical nerve leaves the spinal column between C7 and T1. Beginning with the first thoracic nerve, all the remaining spinal nerves pass out from the vertebral column *below* the vertebra of the like number. All of the spinal nerves have dorsal root ganglia except for C1, where there may be no dorsal root.

Because of the discrepancy in length between the spinal cord and spinal canal in the adult, the intramedullary spinal segments will be higher than the numerically corresponding vertebrae. The lowermost cervical cord level (C8) lies opposite the upper part of the body of the seventh cervical vertebra. An approximate rule to determine the probable level of cord involvement after spinal column injury is to add 2 to the number of the involved vertebral spine between T10 and C2. The lumbar segments of the cord lie at approximately the level of the

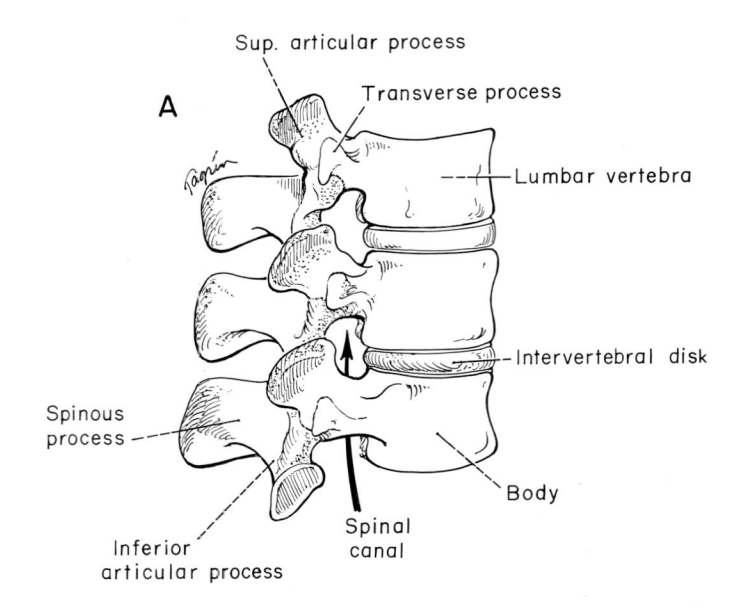

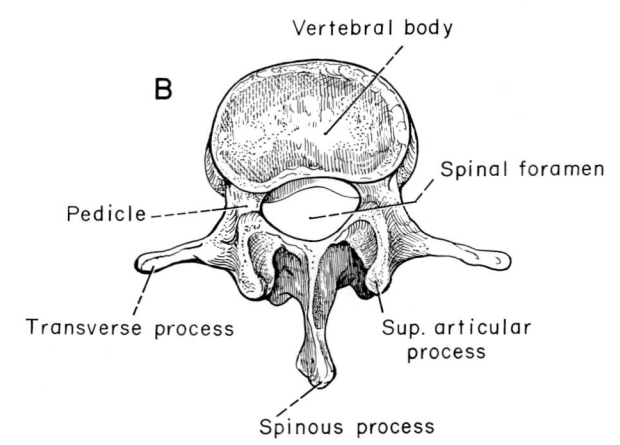

Fig. 15-3.—Bony anatomy of lumbar vertebrae.

spinous processes of T11 and T12. The sacral and coccygeal segments are at the level of the spinous process of L1.

The effects of spinal cord trauma are expressed as motor, sensory and visceral deficits distal to the site of injury. Usually, the major effect of this neural injury is to interrupt descending or ascending white matter tracts and, although gray matter lesions are of extreme importance in the midcervical region in patients with "central cord injury," the motor and sensory deficits noted on first examination are due to tract interruption.

Figure 15-6 shows a cross section of cervical spinal cord. *Motor* impulses descend in three corticospinal tracts: crossed lateral corticospinal tract, uncrossed lateral corticospinal tract and ventral corticospinal tract. These originate mainly in the precentral gyrus, descend from the cortex via the internal capsule and cerebral peduncle, crossing to the opposite side along the ventral

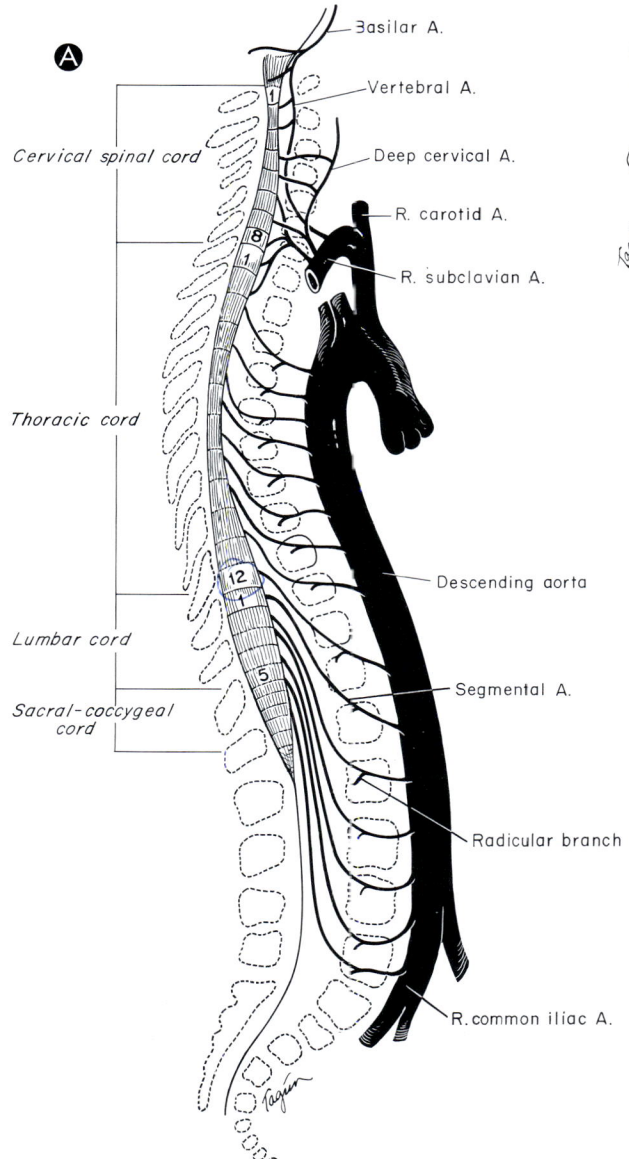

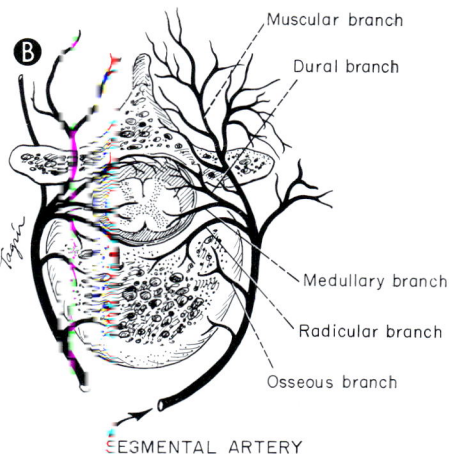

Chapter 15: INJURIES TO THE SPINAL CORD AND CAUDA EQUINA / 321

Fig. 15-4.—**A**, blood supply of the spinal cord in a human fetus arising from the subclavian artery, iliac artery and aorta. Note that the vertebral artery supplies segmental arteries in the upper cervical region whereas more direct branches from the deep cervical artery supply the mid- and lower cervical cord. The variability in this supply is great, and the most consistent feature of the detailed examination of the blood supply to the cervical cord, in particular, is its variability. The number of important large radicular branches varies, as does the level of entry or position of the vessel with respect to the anterior or posterior roots. In general, a large radicular branch arises from the aorta between T8 and L3, which provides the largest amount of blood to the thoracic cord. This is known as the artery of Adamkiewicz. **B**, the spinal anatomy of a large segmental and radicular artery is shown. Supply to the dura, muscles and bone arises from these vessels. As noted above, the entry of the medullary arteries through the intervertebral foramen is quite variable. Microscopic dissection during surgery on the posterior or anterior roots often is necessary to preserve this important blood supply.

aspect of the medulla. Although there is definite somatotropic organization above the medulla, there is no evidence for lamination in the cord. These fibers terminate on cells in posterior, intramedullary and ventral gray matter. Their interruption produces voluntary motor paralysis. Although olivospinal, rubrospinal, tectospinal and vestibulospinal tracts can be demonstrated, they are of less clinical

322 / James G. Wepsic

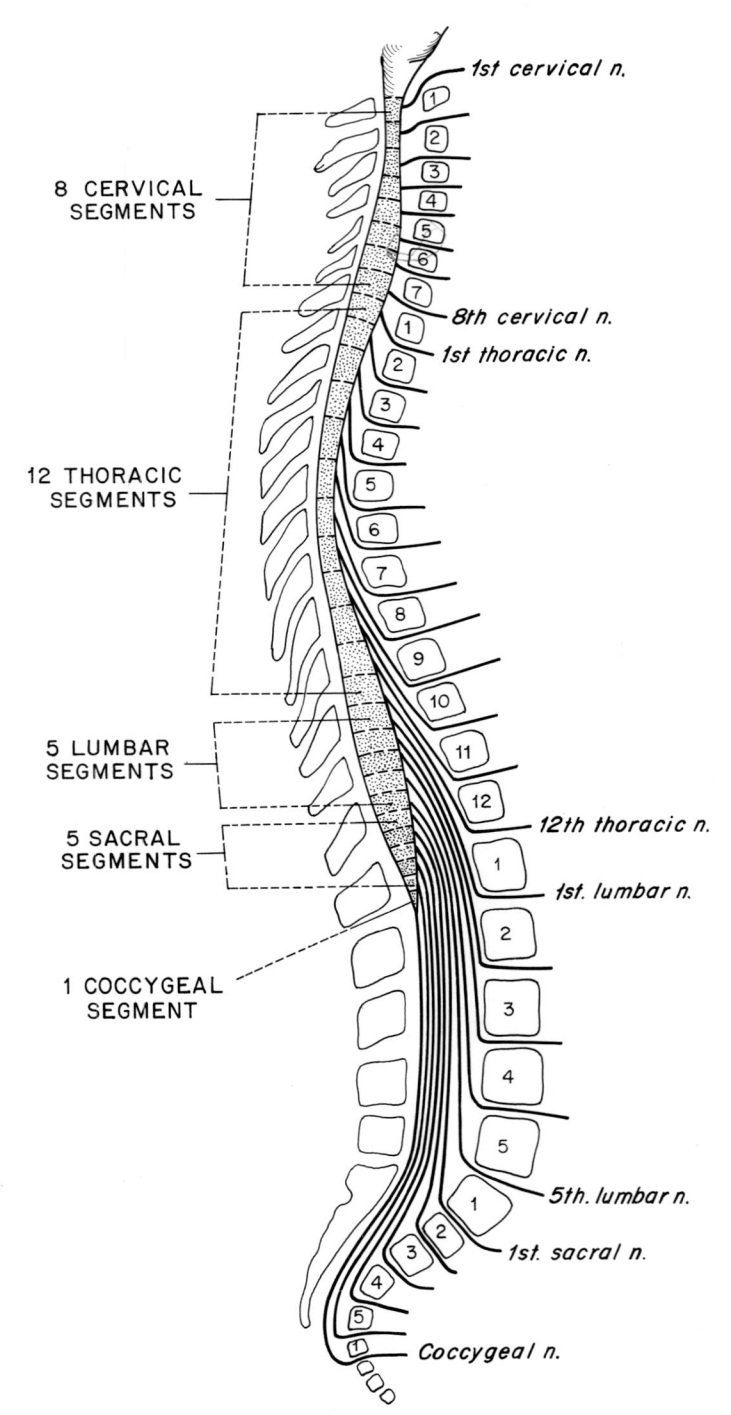

Fig. 15-5.—Relationship between spinal cord level, exiting root level and vertebral body level.

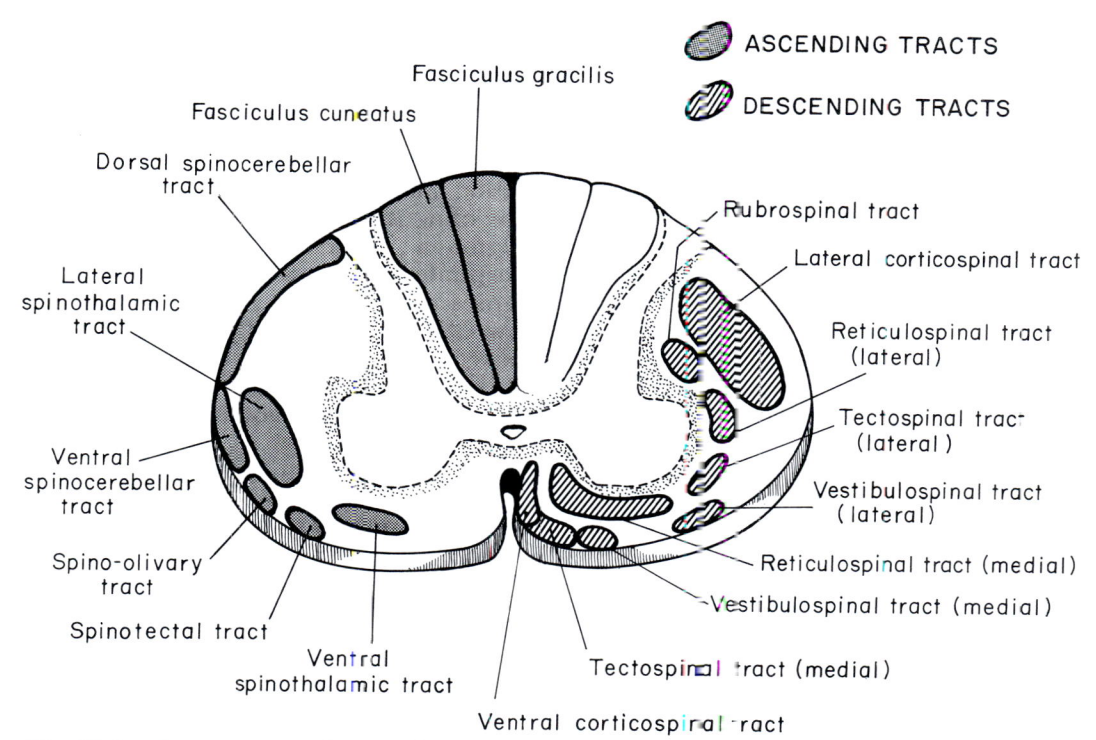

Chapter 15: INJURIES TO THE SPINAL CORD AND CAUDA EQUINA / 323

Fig. 15-6.—Cross section of cervical spinal cord depicting the long tracts. Ascending tracts are outlined at the left and descending tracts at the right. The position of the corticospinal tract, spinothalamic tract and fasciculus gracilis and cuneatus should be particularly noted, for their functions can be quickly tested to determine completeness or incompleteness of cord injury.

importance in managing the patient with cord trauma than the *reticulospinal tracts*. These originate on the pontine and medullary reticular formation. The medial tract is chiefly uncrossed and enters the anterior quadrant of the cord. The lateral tract crosses almost immediately and descends just anterior to the lateral corticospinal tract. Interruption or injury to these fibers in the cervical region will result in apnea while the patient sleeps. *Visceral activity* is modulated by these reticulospinal fibers as well as other multisynaptic chains of neurons, which terminate on both preganglionic autonomic and somatic efferent neurons. "Automatic" visceral activity usually is eventually possible in the absence of descending impulses if the relevant nerve roots and segmental cord levels are preserved in the face of a higher transection of cord.

Ascending pathways carry information concerning distal visceral and cutaneous sensibility. The spinocerebellar tracts project to vermis of cerebellum via the inferior cerebellar peduncle. The spinothalamic tracts carrying *pain and temperature sensibility* arise from cells in the dorsal gray, cross the midline via the ventral commissure and ascend in the lateral portion of the anterior quadrant to terminate chiefly in the thalamic nuclei: ventralis posterolateralis, reticularis and centra medianum. *Touch and vibration* sensibility are served by the posterior columns. The more lateral group of fibers, the fasciculus cuneatus, originates from dorsal horn cells of C1 to T6 whereas the more medial group, fasciculus gracilis, originates from cells below T6. They terminate in the nuclei cuneatus and gracilis and then project rostrally via the medial lemniscus. The afferents arising in visceral organs are conducted to higher anatomic centers mainly through short, multisynaptic chains of neurons.

BASIC EVALUATION

CLINICAL.—One should attempt to attain a thorough and detailed history of the type of injury, whether hyperextension or flexion was present and whether motor movement was impaired immediately. If paralysis was present immediately or had been present for more than 24 hours without any evidence of return of function, prognosis for significant recovery is poor. A complete general physical examination, maintaining the patient in a position of neutrality with head and spine in alignment, then should be carried out. Respiratory embarrassment often accompanies cord injuries. If the lesion is below C5, both intercostal and abdominal musculature will be flaccid, leaving only phrenically enervated diaphragmatic breathing. The cell bodies for the phren-

Fig. 15-7.—Dermatomal map of the human body. Note the position of the cervically enervated skin on the anterior chest as well as high thoracic enervation of inner aspect of arm. Reproductions of this outline should be available in areas caring for patients with spinal cord injuries so that daily charting of sensory findings can be carried out.

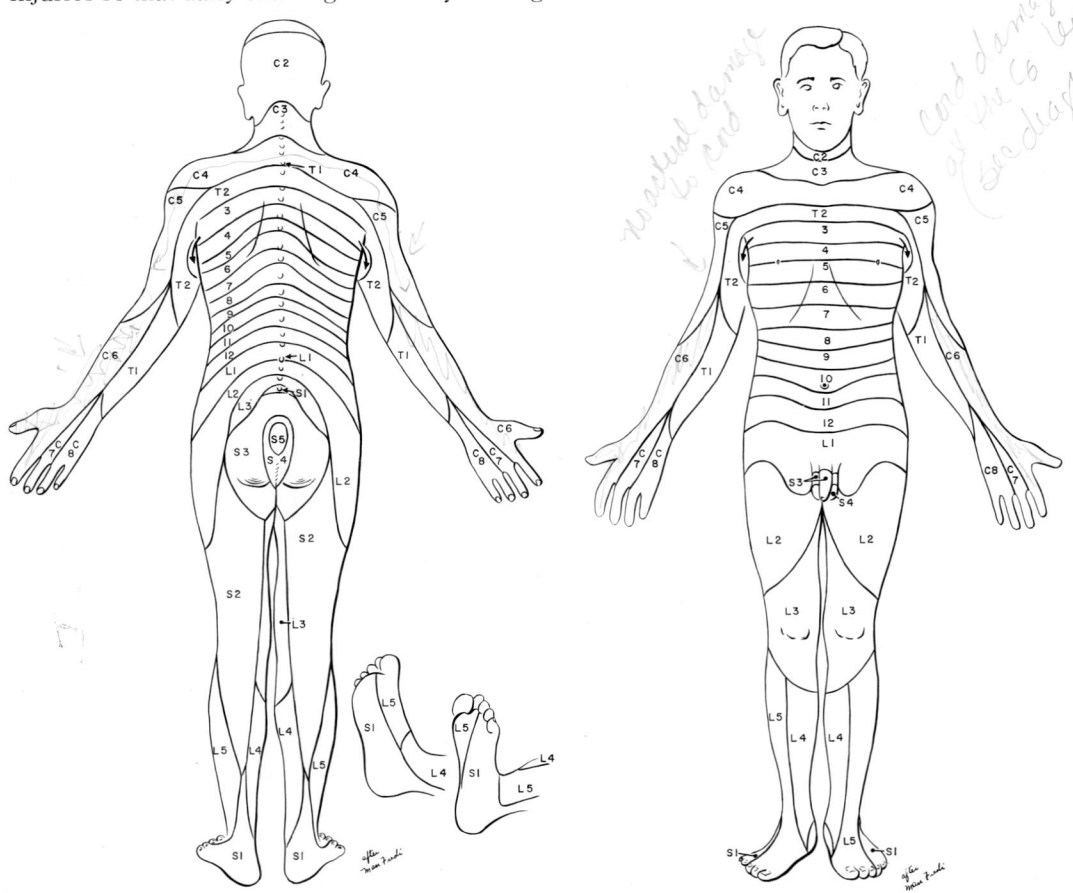

ic nerves lie at about the C4 spinal level, and cord injury at this level or above will interfere with that function as well. Measurement of arterial blood gases, tidal volume and vital capacity should be done early. If necessary, careful nasotracheal intubation may be carried out to establish assisted ventilation at a level sufficient to maintain adequate oxygenation. Care should be taken to avoid motion of the neck. If intubation is not possible, a tracheostomy may be done. Often, adequate spontaneous respiration eventually can be established once the acute effects of injury subside; therefore, it certainly is worthwhile to support a patient's ventilation early in his care. Hypotension may be seen early, due to functional sympathectomy, and may present a differential diagnostic problem in the multiply injured automobile accident victim. However, the presence of warm extremities and significant neurologic deficit should alert one to the possibility of secondary spinal cord sympathetic injury, and treatment should be instituted accordingly. Frequently, head injuries and cervical spine injuries are present together. Examination of the front and back of the head for evidence of trauma may give some clue as to the nature of spinal injury — whether it be extension or flexion.

An evaluation of the patient's motor and sensory systems should be completed. It is crucial that a thorough sensory examination, with charting of findings, be carried out as soon as possible after the injury so that documentation of progression or regression of deficit can be established. This is important in deciding on surgical treatment as well as prognosis. A rough estimate of the dermatomal level of sensory loss should be made. Muscle strength and tone should be evaluated carefully and the deep tendon reflexes noted. Reference to a motor function and reflex chart may be useful to those not routinely involved in the care of neurologic patients (Table 15-1).

Transportation of a patient who has had spinal cord injury must be carefully planned and well organized. The patient should not be moved until there are sufficient trained people to lift him as a unit, maintaining the head, neck and thorax in the position in which he was found. Jostling or motion of the neck may dislocate the fracture and produce quadriplegia or respiratory arrest. The patient who is to be transported a significant distance should be placed on a firm board or stretcher with a pillow or blanket rolls under the normal cervical and lumbar curvature. When neck injury is suspected, sandbags should be placed on either side of the head, or a Mixter 4-poster collar applied. The patient should be treated with minimal amouts of analgesics, for these may interfere with respiratory function and neurologic evaluation. If the bladder is distended, an indwelling catheter should be aseptically installed.

Medical adjuvants recently employed in trauma to the brain are useful in *immediate treatment* of trauma to the spinal cord. Patients in whom spinal cord contusion is suspected with significant spinal cord deficit now are commonly treated immediately with an osmotic diuretic, such as mannitol (2 gm/kg) as well as corticosteroid (methylprednisolone, 1 mg/kg, or dexamethasone 0.2 mg/kg). There is no experimental evidence to indicate that these agents, although proved to be of value as adjuvants to cranial neurosurgery, are effective in reducing the morbidity of spinal cord injury. However, we have noted that in patients with chronic spinal cord injury secondary to tumor or in acute trauma to the cord, an advancing neurologic deficit can be reversed with the introduction of such treatment. Therefore, it is our practice to initiate such therapy in spinal cord injury patients on arrival in the hospital.

LABORATORY STUDIES. — When a spinal cord injury is suspected, anteroposterior, lateral and open-mouth x-ray films of the neck as well as standard views of the thoracic and lumbar spine are mandatory if

TABLE 15-1.—MOTOR FUNCTION CHART*

Cord Segment	Muscles	Action to Be Tested	Nerves
Shoulder Girdle and Upper Extremity			
C1-4	Deep neck muscles (sternomastoid and trapezius also participate)	Flexion of neck Extension of neck Rotation of neck Lateral bending of neck	Cervical
C3-4	Scaleni Diaphragm	Elevation of upper thorax Inspiration	Phrenic
C5-T1	Pectoralis major and minor	Adduction of arm from behind to front	Thoracic anterior (from medial and lateral cords of plexus)
C5-7	Serratus anterior	Forward thrust of shoulder	Long thoracic
C5(3-4)	Levator scapulae	Elevation of scapula	Dorsal scapular
C4-5	Rhomboids	Medial adduction and elevation of scapula	Dorsal scapular
C5	Supraspinatus	Abduction of arm	Suprascapular
C5-6	Infraspinatus	Lateral rotation of arm	Suprascapular
C5-8	Latissimus dorsi, teres major and subscapularis	Medial rotation of arm Adduction of arm from front to back	Subscapular (from posterior cord of plexus)
C5-6	Deltoid	Abduction of arm	Axillary (from posterior cord of plexus)
C5	Teres minor	Lateral rotation of arm	Axillary (from posterior cord of plexus)
C5-6	Biceps brachii	Flexion of forearm Supination of forearm	Musculocutaneous (from lateral cord of plexus)
C6-7	Coracobrachialis	Adduction of arm Flexion of forearm	Musculocutaneous (from lateral cord of plexus)
C5-6	Brachialis	Flexion of forearm	Musculocutaneous (from lateral cord of plexus)
C6-8	Triceps brachii and anconeus	Extension of forearm	
C5-6	Brachioradialis	Flexion of forearm	
C5-7	Extensor carpi radialis	Radial extension of hand	Radial (from posterior cord of plexus)
C6-8	Extensor digitorum communis	Extension of phalanges of index finger, middle finger, ring finger, little finger	
C6-8	Extensor digitorum communis	Extension of hand	
C6-8	Extensor digiti quinti proprius	Extension of phalanges of little finger Extension of hand	
C6-8	Extensor carpi ulnaris	Ulnar extension of hand	
C5-7	Supinator	Supination of forearm	
C6-7	Abductor pollicis longus	Abduction of metacarpal of thumb Radial extension of hand	Radial (from posterior cord of plexus)

Cord Segment	Muscles	Action to Be Tested	Nerves
C6–7	Extensor pollicis brevis and longus	Extension of thumb	
C6–8	Extensor pollicis brevis and longus	Radial extension of hand	
C6–8	Extensor indicis proprius	Extension of index finger Extension of hand	
C7–T1	Flexor carpi ulnaris	Ulnar flexion of hand	
C8–T1	Flexor digitorum profundus (ulnar portion)	Flexion of terminal phalanx of ring finger, little finger	
C8–T1	Flexor digitorum profundus (ulnar portion)	Flexion of hand	
C8–T1	Adductor pollicis	Adduction of metacarpal of thumb	Ulnar (from medial cord of plexus)
C8–T1	Abductor digiti quinti	Abduction of little finger	
C8–T1	Opponens digiti quinti	Opposition of little finger	
C8–T1	Flexor digiti quinti brevis	Flexion of little finger	
C8–T1	Interossei	Flexion of proximal phalanx, extension of two distal phalanges, adduction and abduction of fingers	
C6–7	Pronator teres	Pronation of forearm	
C6–7	Flexor carpi radialis	Radial flexion of hand	
C7–T1	Palmaris longus	Flexion of hand	
C7–T1	Flexor digitorum sublimis	Flexion of middle phalanx of index finger, middle finger, ring finger, little finger	Median (C6–7 from lateral cord of plexus; C8–T1 from medial cord of plexus)
C7–T1	Flexor digitorum sublimis	Flexion of hand	
C6–7	Flexor pollicis longus	Flexion of terminal phalanx of thumb	
C7–T1	Flexor digitorum profundus (radial portion)	Flexion of terminal phalanx of index finger, middle finger	
C7–T1	Flexor digitorum profundus (radial portion)	Flexion of hand	
C6–7	Abductor pollicis brevis	Abduction of metacarpal of thumb	
C6–7	Flexor pollicis brevis	Flexion of proximal phalanx of thumb	
C6–7	Opponens pollicis	Opposition of metacarpal of thumb	Median (C6–7 from lateral cord of plexus; C8–T1 from medial cord of plexus)
C8–T1	Lumbricals (the two lateral)	Flexion of proximal phalanx and extension of the two distal phalanges of index finger, middle finger	
C8–T1	Lumbricals (the two medial)	Flexion of proximal phalanx and extension of the two distal phalanges of ring finger, little finger	

(Continued)

TABLE 15–1. (Continued)

Cord Segment	Muscles	Action to Be Tested	Nerves
		Trunk and Thorax	
	Thoracic, abdominal, and back	Elevation and depression of ribs	Thoracic and posterior lumbosacral branches
		Contraction of abdomen	
		Anteroflexion and lateral flexion of trunk	
		Hip Girdle and Lower Extremity	
T12–L3	Iliopsoas	Flexion of hip	
L2–3	Sartorius	Flexion of hip (and eversion of thigh)	Femoral
L2–4	Quadriceps femoris	Extension of knee	
L2–3	Pectineus	Adduction of thigh	
L2–3	Adductor longus	Adduction of thigh	
L2–4	Adductor brevis	Adduction of thigh	Obturator
L3–4	Adductor magnus	Adduction of thigh	
L2–4	Gracilis	Adduction of thigh	
L3–4	Obturator externus	Adduction of thigh	
L3–4	Obturator externus	Lateral rotation of thigh	
L4–5,S1	Gluteus medius and minimus	Extension of thigh	
L4–5,S1	Gluteus medius and minimus	Medial rotation of thigh	Superior gluteal
L4–5	Tensor fasciae latae	Flexion of thigh	
S1–2	Piriformis	Lateral rotation of thigh	
L4–S1	Gluteus maximus	Abduction of thigh	Inferior gluteal
L5–S2	Obturator internus	Lateral rotation of thigh	Muscular branches from sacral plexus
L4–S2	Gemelli	Lateral rotation of thigh	Muscular branches from sacral plexus
L4–S1	Quadratus femoris	Lateral rotation of thigh	Muscular branches from sacral plexus
L4–S2	Biceps femoris	Flexion of leg (assists in extension of thigh)	
L4–S1	Semitendinosus	Flexion of leg (assists in extension of thigh)	Sciatic (trunk)
L4–S1	Semimembranosus	Flexion of leg (assists in extension of thigh)	
L4–5	Tibialis anterior	Dorsal flexion of foot	
L4–5	Tibialis anterior	Supination of foot	
L4–S1	Extensor digitorum longus	Extension of toes II–V	
L4–S1	Extensor digitorum longus	Dorsal flexion of foot	Deep peroneal
L4–S1	Extensor hallucis longus	Extension of great toe	
L4–S1	Extensor hallucis longus	Dorsal flexion of foot	
L4–S1	Extensor digitorum brevis	Extension of great toe and the three medial toes	

Cord Segment	Muscles	Action to Be Tested	Nerves
L5–S1	Peronei	Plantar flexion of foot in pronation	Superficial peroneal
L5–S2	Tibialis posterior and triceps surae	Plantar flexion of foot in supination	
L5–S2	Flexor digitorum longus	Plantar flexion of foot in supination	
L5–S2	Flexor digitorum longus	Flexion of terminal phalanx, toes II–V	
L5–S2	Flexor hallucis longus	Plantar flexion of foot in supination	
L5–S2	Flexor hallucis longus	Flexion of terminal phalanx of great toe	Tibial
L5–S1	Flexor digitorum brevis	Flexion of middle phalanx, toes II–V	
L5–S2	Flexor hallucis brevis	Flexion of proximal phalanx of great toe	
S1–2	Small muscles of foot	Spreading and closing of toes	
S1–2	Small muscles of foot	Flexion of proximal phalanx of toes	
S2–4	Perineal and sphincters	Voluntary control of pelvic floor	Pudendal

*After J. C. McKinley.

the patient's life is not otherwise threatened. The patient's head and neck should be maintained in good position with manual or halter traction. Attention should be paid to obtaining good views of the lower cervical vertebrae, as these frequently are the points of fracture-dislocation and are the most difficult areas to visualize because of the superimposed radiodensity of the shoulders. Visualization of this area is facilitated by drawing down the arms and shoulders while the head is supported. Oblique or "swimmer's" views can be taken if this tactic fails to demonstrate the C7–T1 junction.

Study of the x-ray films can give information regarding fractures or dislocations of the major bone elements, presence of osteoarthritis and the presence of foreign bodies of bone within the spinal canal. The x-ray findings, although informative, never portray the total extent of clinical disruption, for, at operation, the extent of fracture and dislocation usually markedly exceeds that on the films.

The presence or absence of the *spinal subarachnoid space block* has been used as one criteria of operative intervention. If the space is compressed, due to dislocation or impingement of bony elements on the spinal cord, operative intervention has been suggested. In the past, the lumbar puncture with manometrics and application of the Queckenstedt maneuver (compression of the internal jugular veins and observation of a rise in lumbar subarachnoid pressure transmitted from distended veins around the brain) has been used to prove and disprove patency of the subarachnoid space. If there is total obstruction of spinal fluid flow, the lumbar manometer pressure will not rise on jugular compression. However, a rise in lumbar pressure with compression indicates only that a channel is present that may be as narrow as the diameter of the lumbar puncture needle. A more satisfactory method of demonstrating the subarachnoid space is *myelography*. More centers are performing emergency myelography to demonstrate the exact nature and level of a compressive lesion that may or may not be evident from clinical and plain x-ray films. When practicable, the radiopaque oil is placed in the lumbar subarachnoid space and the patient then is positioned with the upper spine dependent, allowing the dye to run in the subarachnoid space into the upper cervical region. Where this is not practicable, the spinal needle can be introduced with the patient supine, placing the needle through the C1–C2 intervertebral foramen.

Once the nature of the injury has been established, neurologic deficit defined and anatomic substrate for injury demonstrated with plain x-ray films or myelography, consideration of the patient for further therapy is in order.

IMMOBILIZATION

With any significant dislocation of the neck, it is best to immobilize the head and neck to prevent further dislocation. Several devices for skeletal traction are available. The simplest are those that can be screwed into the calvarium in a position to provide traction along the longitudinal axis of the spinal canal. Crutchfield, Barton and Vinke tongs have been used and all have specific advantages and disadvantages. Crutchfield tongs are more comfortable for the patient because they do not project into the temporal region,

Fig. 15-8.—Cervical traction with Barton tongs. **A,** location of incisions in scalp. **B,** technique of application of the tongs. On the left side (of illustration) a twist drill, protruding 4 mm, is used to make a hole in the outer table of the temporal bone. On the right side, this has been replaced by a metal pin, secured in place by the thumbscrew.

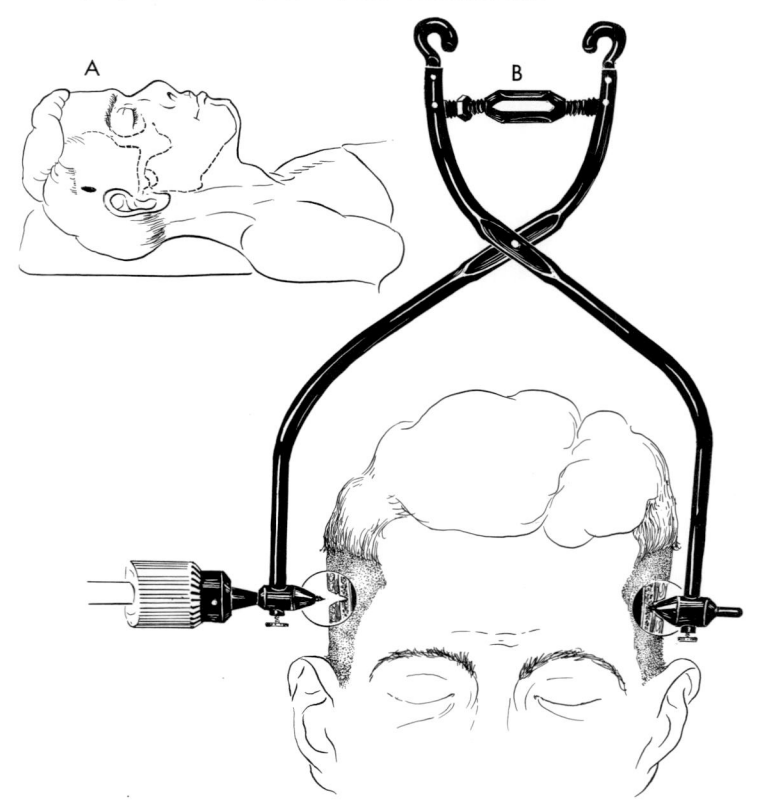

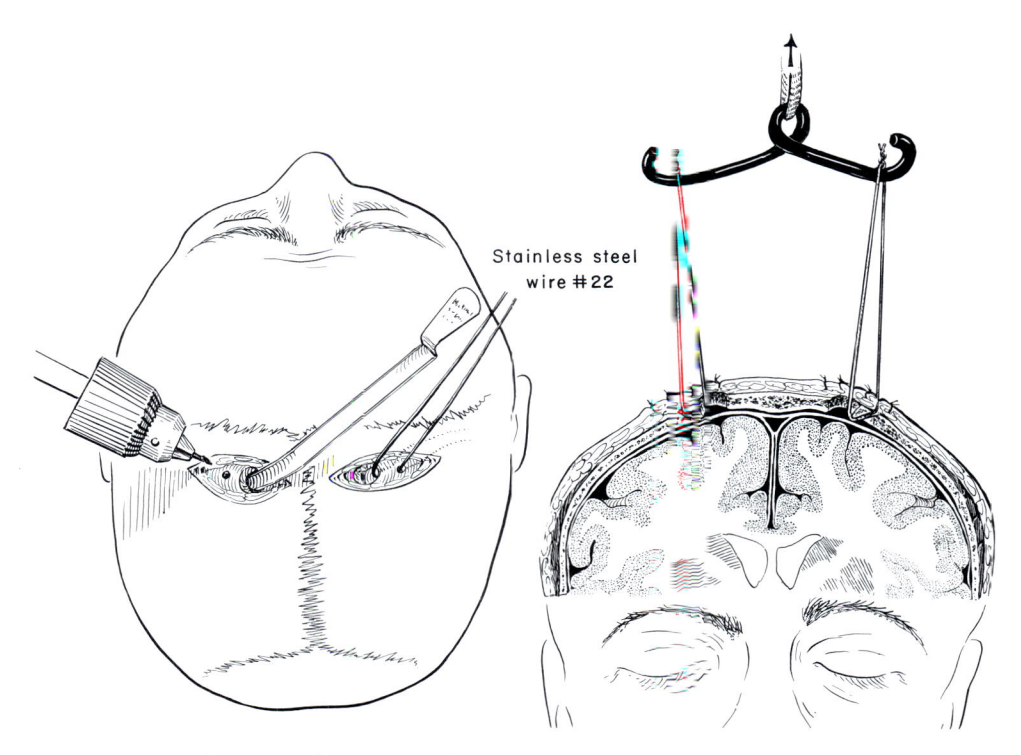

Chapter 15: INJURIES TO THE SPINAL CORD AND CAUDA EQUINA / 331

Fig. 15-9.—Cervical traction by means of cranial wires. **Left,** a 1-cm opening has been made in the bone down to the dura with a perforator bur. A metal guide is slipped into this and a second oblique hole is made with a twist drill. A stainless-steel traction wire has been passed through the two holes between bone and dura. **Right,** the traction wires are attached to a metal yoke and the incision closed with a single layer of interrupted fine-silk sutures through the galea and skin.

allowing the patient to lie on his side more easily. However, these can be distracted from the skull with greater ease and are not as stable in a patient who is restless or agitated. Barton tongs, on the other hand, rarely become dislocated but do cause some discomfort when the patient lies on his side. In children, where the calvarium is thin, or in adults with bone disorders of the skull or skull fractures, skeletal traction can be applied to the head by placing heavy wires in the extradural space and bringing them out through bur holes in the parietal area.

After x-ray films have been obtained and an airway established, skeletal traction can be placed in patients with cervical fractures or dislocations. The patient is placed supine, with a small roll beneath normal cervical lordosis, and sandbags are placed on either side of the head. The skin above the ear is shaved and prepped. Care is taken to mark off the site of tong placement so that the ends are placed symmetrically. In general, a placement directly above the pina or slightly posterior to it will allow traction to be maintained along the axis of the spine. Modest flexion or extension of the spine, if needed to accomplish realignment, can be done best by adjusting the direction of force and the level of the thorax; tong placement need not be predicated on such considerations. The Barton and Vinke tongs are placed on the temporal bone whereas Crutchfield tongs

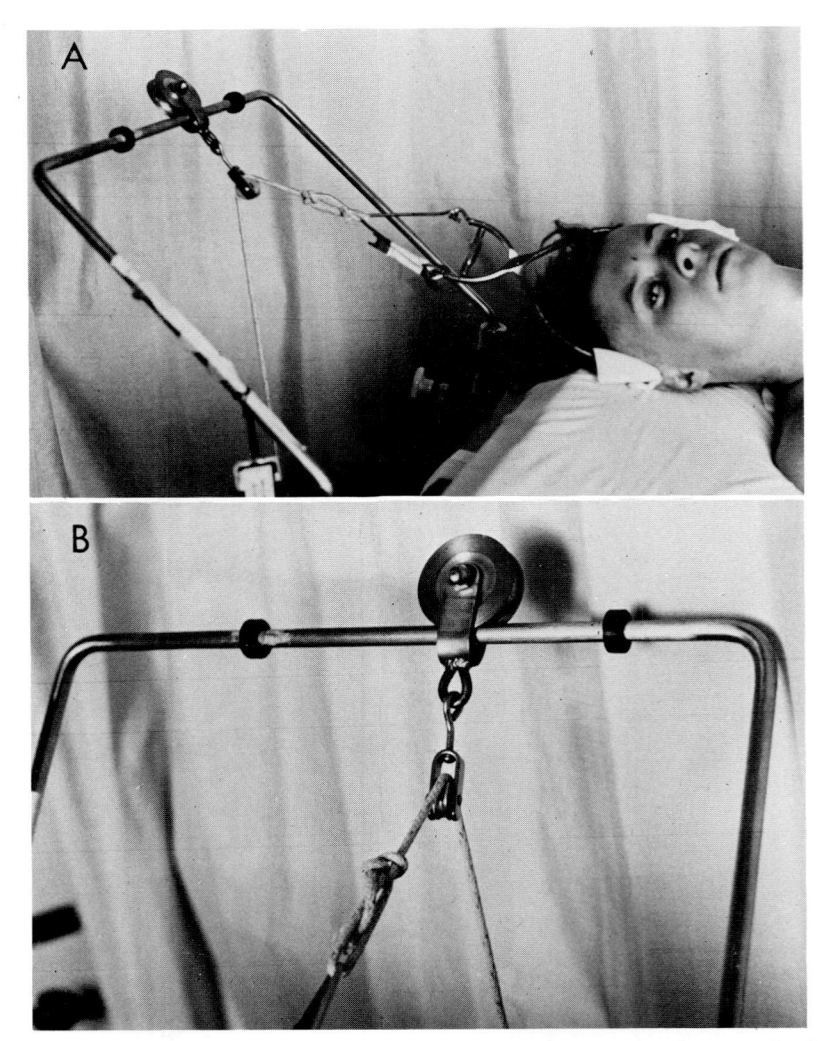

Fig. 15-10. — **A,** patient with Barton tongs in place attached to Rogers frame, which allows patient to be turned from side to side or have head elevated while maintaining the position of traction. The frame is attached to the moving portion of the bed so that it rises as the head of the bed is elevated. **B,** close-up of the double pulley arrangement, which permits traction to be applied at any position along the traverse of the frame.

are placed closer to the vertex of the skull. After infiltrating the skin over the site of installation, a small incision is made in the skin and a hole is drilled in the calvarium. The Barton tong pins can be fixed to the skull by first applying the tongs themselves to the skin incision prior to drilling the holes. The Barton tong pins then are mounted on a twist drill and used to drill the hole in the bone. Once seated in the bone, the drill can be detached and thumbscrews tightened to hold the pins to the tongs. Both Crutchfield and Vinke tongs require the twist-drill holes to be completed with a drill before the tongs are applied to these holes and tightened. Crutchfield tongs are kept in place by maintaining a tight fit of the tong tips to the skull. This requires a regular schedule of tightening to prevent distraction. The Vinke tong tips are equipped with a flange that extends between the inner and outer table of the skull and is quite effective in maintaining the tongs in proper position once they are placed.

For traction to be effective, the head of the bed must be elevated slightly so that the patient's body serves as a counterweight. Correct skeletal alignment during traction should be checked repeatedly and X-ray films obtained to be sure that the pull of the tongs is along the axis of the canal. The rope connecting the tongs to weights can be fed through the center hole of a Stryker frame or kept in place, utilizing a Rogers frame, which permits a constant angle of traction yet allows the patient to turn from side to side in a standard hospital bed. When the patient lies on his side, a small pad should be placed beneath the dependent ear and cheek to maintain a neutral lateral position of the cervical spine. Seven to 10 pounds of traction can be applied in the average adult to maintain stability. If a dislocation is present, a large amount of weight should be placed on the tongs initially to fatigue the paraspinal musculature, allowing the reduction to take place. A common error is to begin with small amounts of weight and to gradually increase the weight, hoping that realignment will take place. If it becomes apparent that the facets are locked in a dislocated position, operative reduction may be required. Closed manipulative reduction of cervical fractures carries an extreme risk and should not be done.

Care should be taken to maintain asepsis in the area of the tong points and to sedate the patient so that he will be comfortable in this traction.

Traction is not necessary in the treatment of thoracic or lumbar spine fractures, but the patient should be nursed on a frame that permits frequent changes of position without manipulation of the spine's alignment. Care to protect all bony prominences from pressure is essential.

Later immobilization is possible, utilizing a halo, a plaster body cast with attached device for skeletal fixation of the head (see Fig. 16-14, p. 355).

FRACTURES AND DISLOCATIONS

Although contusions and temporary dislocations of the spinal cord without bone abnormality may be more common, those injuries associated with bone fractures and dislocations are the most serious spinal injuries, for the majority of them cause moderate-to-severe cord damage. There are several specific types of fractures and dislocations. These will be described and illustrated before dealing with the indications and contraindications for surgical intervention. Fractures or dislocations of any type from C2 to T1 carry the most guarded prognosis. If the dislocation is between C2 and C4, the patient may die immediately or have complete quadriplegia. If respiratory function is adequate initially, it may deteriorate rapidly as intercostal and phrenic enervation muscles fail with progressive cord edema. Fractures and dislocations below C4 may produce quadriplegia with sparing of one of another group of arm muscles. In this area of cervical cord enlargment, dislocation of a few millimeters may produce a total permanent distal deficit.

Fracture-dislocations of the thoracic region may be radiographically more impressive yet spare some distal neurologic function. Those located at the thoracolumbar junction almost always are compression fractures and may result in injury to the distal cord or cauda equina. The bone deformity produced by these fractures often is pronounced enough to warrant operation to stabilize the spine. If the lesion is distal to L1, with compression of elements of the cauda equina, a more hopeful prognosis is present. Nerve root compression is more likely to recover after decompression; therefore, we believe that all traumatic lesions of the conus and cauda equina should be explored as early as possible.

Although hemorrhage within the spinal canal usually is not a major problem in spinal injury, the special case of patients with rheumatoid arthritis should be recalled. In these patients there is a higher incidence of subdural and extradural clots associated with fracture-dislo-

Fig. 15-11.—A and B, compression fracture of L3 resulting from a fall on the buttocks down an elevator shaft. Lesions of this type are more common at T12 or L1, as is shown in C. Injury occurred secondary to a fall a distance of 20 feet, with patient landing on feet, producing this fracture and open ankle fractures. Paraparesis and loss of bowel, bladder and sexual function resulted from the cord contusion. Meurig-Williams plates were placed early to help stabilize the fracture. A myelogram (D) was done, which demonstrated disk material and bone protruding into the spinal canal. This was removed and an anterior fusion performed through a retroperitoneal approach, with improvement in gait, bowel and bladder function. E, an automobile accident produced a severe compression fracture of T8, which was treated elsewhere by bed rest for 2 months. The patient's paraparesis gradually improved, then began to worsen. Tomograms then showed severe posterior dislocation of T8 into the spinal canal. This was removed through a transthoracic approach along with adjacent posteriorly displaced vertebra and a fusion was done with rib struts (F).

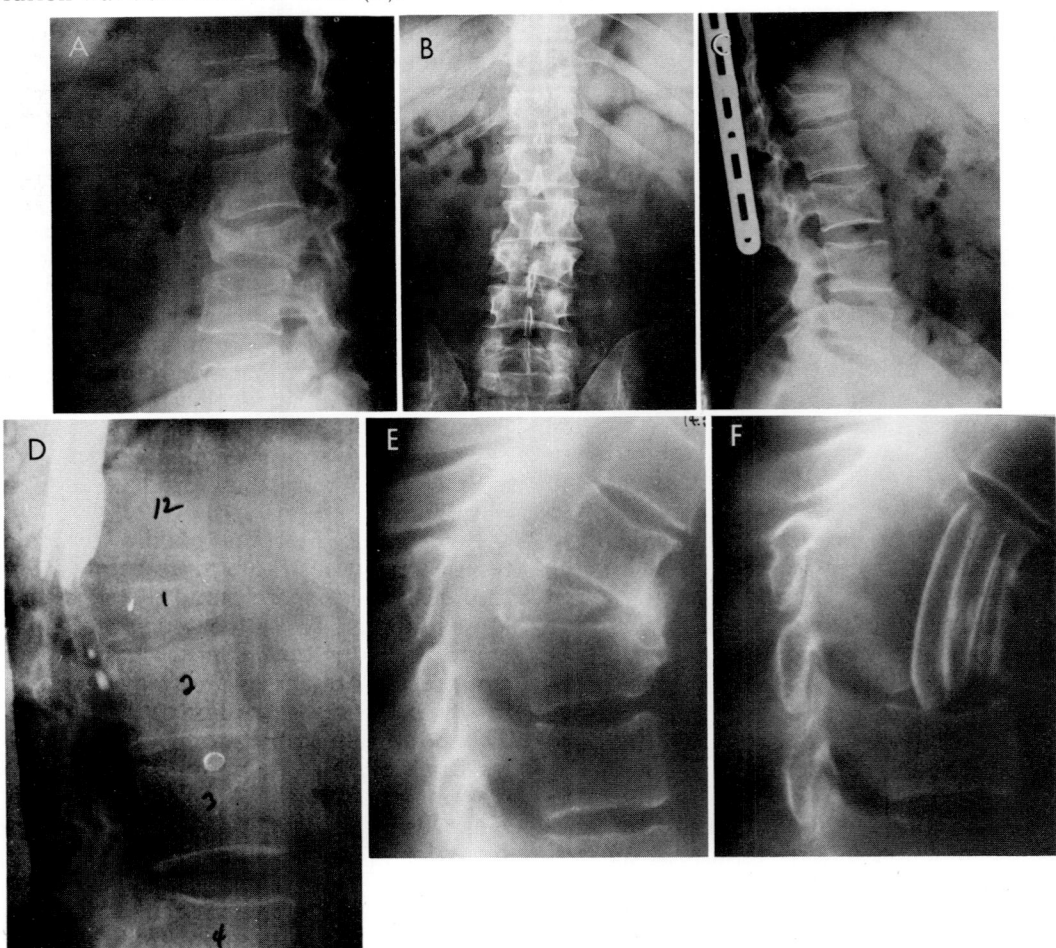

cations, thought to be due to the structural abnormalities of the bones and joints. An early exploration and clot evacuation in these patients may be fruitful.

Linear fractures, without the dislocation, are relatively mild injuries and may involve the transverse or spinous processes. If no neurologic deficit is present, they may be treated with collar immobilization and usually will produce no lasting disability.

Compression fractures usually result from *hyperflexion.* The anterior surface of the vertebra is pinched, so that the softer centrum gives way laterally or posteriorly into the spinal canal. Such fractures are common in diving accidents in the cervical region, but are seen most commonly at the thoracolumbar junction in patients with falls onto the buttocks or feet.

Atlantooccipital dislocations. These are rare and usually result in immediate death.

Atlantoaxial dislocations usually are caused by a sudden *jerking movement of the head and neck backward* and are associated with fracture of the odontoid process and rupture of the cruciate ligaments. In patients who do not die immediately, this lesion generally is not attended with neurologic deficit. When discovered, it should be treated with immobilization, and most will stabilize over a 6-week to 2-month interval. At that point, cautious fluoroscopy of the head motion should be carried out to see whether the fusion of C1 and C2 to each other and the occiput would be necessary.

Hangman's fracture. Judicial hanging produces a *bilateral avulsion fracture through the arch of the axis* without injury to the odontoid process. More recently, this type of injury has been seen in automobile accident victims. When such fracture-dislocations are seen and survival occurs, there usually is no associated neurologic deficit. This is believed to be due to increased space in the upper cervical canal as compared to the size of the cord and the fact that the patient performs his own decompression by avulsing the neural arches. These fractures usually are treated best by prolonged immobilization and will heal spontaneously.

Teardrop fractures are cervical fractures produced when *extreme flexion* causes the body of the involved vertebra to be compressed, with the anterior-inferior fragment displaced downward and forward and the posterior-inferior portion projecting into the spinal canal. This posterior portion can cause injury to the anterior portion of the spinal cord. When such a condition is present, especially in

Fig. 15-12.—**A,** teardrop fracture of C5 secondary to diving accident, with quadriplegia. **B,** fracture dislocation of C5 secondary to "head-on" football tackle quadriplegia.

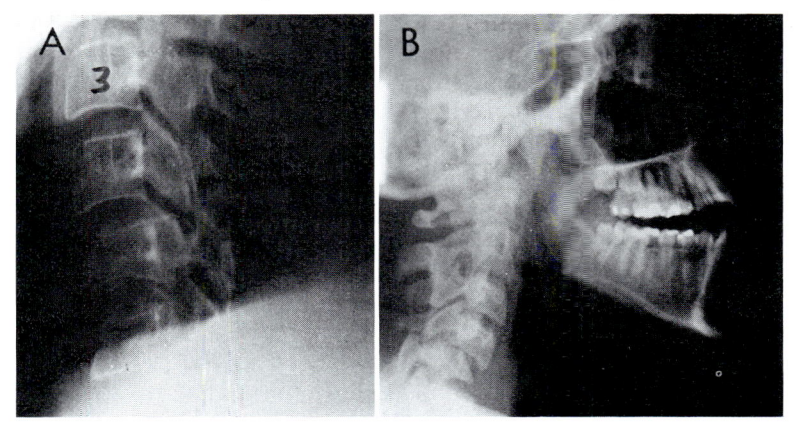

the presence of neurologic deficits and myelographic block, early operative decompression and removal of bone and herniated disk material is indicated. It usually is best to approach these lesions posteriorly, for an anterior approach, although more anatomic, has the added risk of pressing the bone fragments into the cord itself.

NEUROLOGIC SYNDROMES ASSOCIATED WITH CORD INJURY

The degree of injury to the spinal cord can vary from rapidly reversible *concussion* in which there is no neuroanatomic lesion, no blood in the spinal fluid and no subarachnoid block to complete transection of the cord, with loss of all neurologic function below this level. *Spinal cord contusion* is present when there has been bruising of the cord with subpial hemorrhage and usually blood in the CSF. Neurologic deficit always is present in contusion. The cord may be lacerated or contain a hemorrhage within it.

Anterior spinal cord injury results from acute impingement of bone or herniated disk fragments against the anterior portion of the spinal cord, resulting in immediate interruption of corticospinal and spinothalamic function, with some preservation of touch, position and vibration sense. Early operation is indicated and patients often will make an exceptional recovery if the cord has not been lacerated.

Central cervical spinal cord injury is a syndrome usually seen in *hyperextension* injuries of the cervical spine in patients with significant *cervical spondylosis*. It is characterized by marked impairment of motor movement in the upper extremities whereas motor function of the lower extremities frequently remains intact. Sensory loss and bladder dysfunction are seen as well. The mechanism of this injury remains unclear. Some believe that it is due to contusion of the cord whereas others believe that it results from relative ischemia of the central portion of the cord. Such a lesion does not require operation and frequently the patients will show a significant degree of recovery with immobilization and corticosteroids.

Brown-Séquard syndrome with loss of motor function on one side and sensory function on the other is not seen commonly in fracture-dislocations of the spine, for this state requires the presence of a unilateral cord injury sparing the opposite side. It is produced by interruption of the corticospinal tracts supplying the ipsilateral musculature and the spinothalamic tracts receiving sensibility from the contralateral side. A traumatic lateral disk herniation or extradural clot may produce such a finding and after myelography has demonstrated such a lesion, a surgical decompression may be necessary.

INDICATIONS FOR OPERATION

A progression of neurologic signs, a complete block of the subarachnoid space on manometric or myelographic tests, an open fracture, a penetrating wound of the spine, presence of foreign bodies within the spinal canal and the syndrome of acute anterior spinal cord injury are indications for immediate surgical decompression. Operations staged later in the patient's course to prevent deformity, to achieve stability and to realign dislocated fragments are important also.

Operative approach for acute neurosurgical decompression or debridement is to perform a total posterior laminectomy of the involved area, taking care not to dislocate fragments that might be broken and impinge on the spinal canal. A fusion may be performed at the initial decompression if obvious instability or dislocation is present. After all bone fragments are removed from the spinal canal, the dura is opened and the spinal cord visualized. The dentate ligaments may be sectioned if there is evidence of herniated mass anterior to the cord, but man-

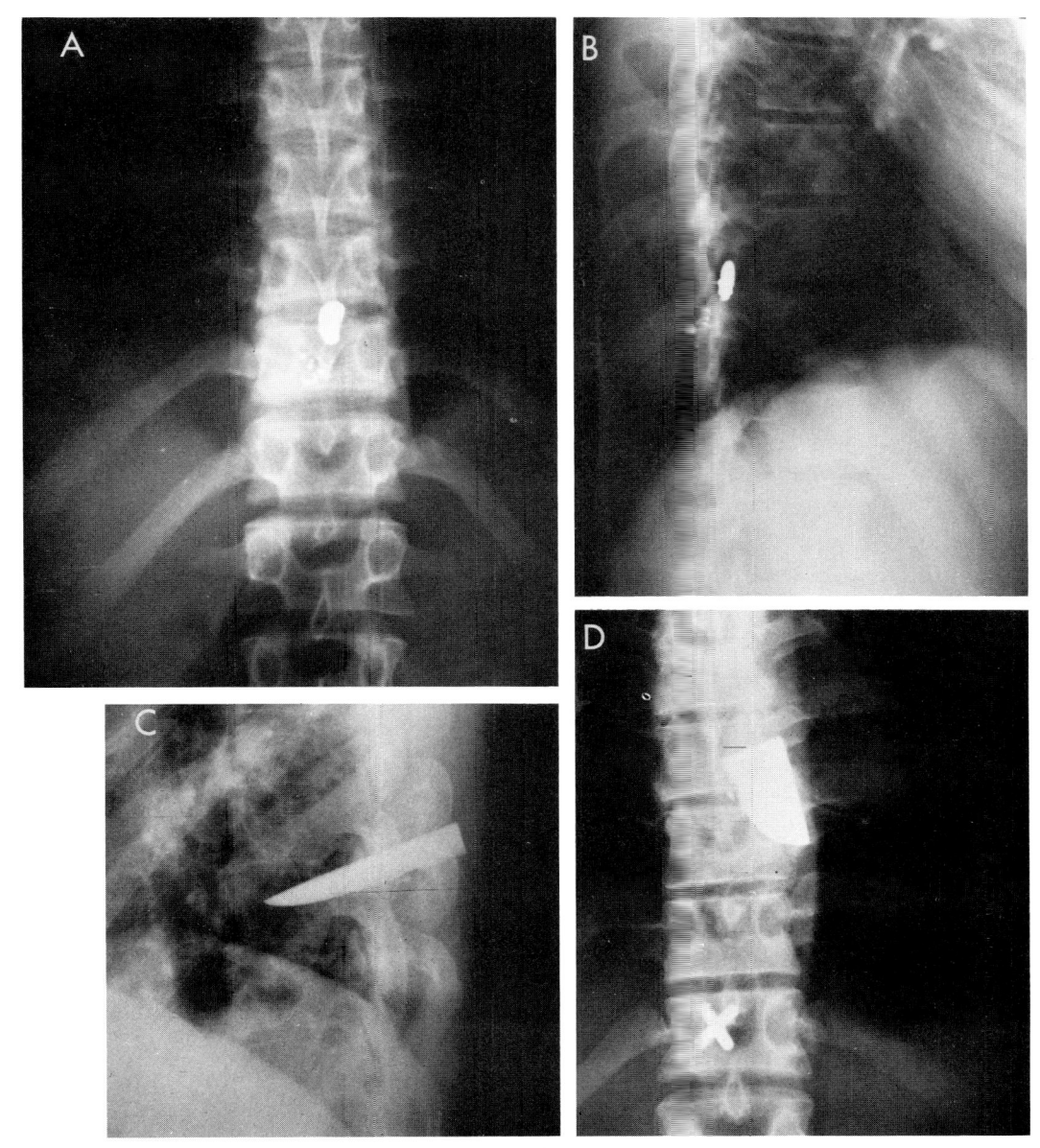

Chapter 15: INJURIES TO THE SPINAL CORD AND CAUDA EQUINA / 337

Fig. 15-13.—A and B, bullet wound of spinal cord—.32 caliber fired at short range produced immediate quadriplegia. Laminectomy 1 hour later with removal of the bullet and dural opening revealed a swollen, contused cord about 2 cm above conus. Spinal cord hypothermia with perfusion of iced Ringer's lactate at 0–5° C for 4 hours over the cord was completed. Two weeks following injury the patient ambulated with a cane. Bowel, bladder and sexual function were normal in 1 month. C and D, stab wound of spinal canal. Butcher knife stabbed into T9–10 interspace and broke off. Patient paraplegic and immediately underwent decompressive laminectomy, removal of knife blade and cooling of spinal cord. Motion returned in legs after 1 week and full ambulation in 1 month with permanent neurologic loss limited to nerve root section at T10.

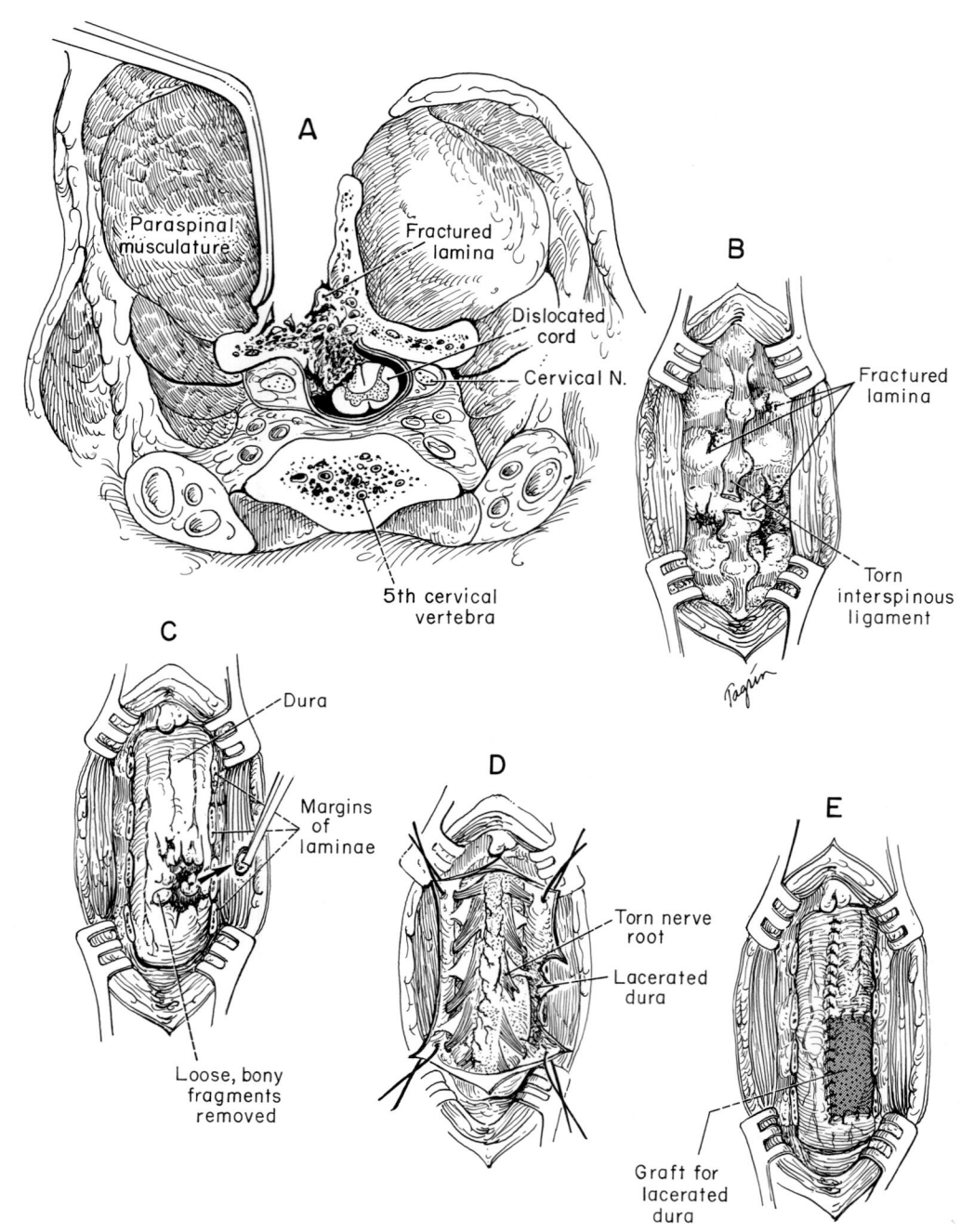

Fig. 15-14.—Technical steps in emergency decompression of C5 fracture involving lamina, dural tear and cord contusion. **A,** careful dissection of fractured, dislocated lamina. **B,** exposure of the fractured lamina and ruptured interspinous ligaments. **C,** debridement of lacerated dura. **D,** larger dural opening to evaluate cord and cool it (if the interval from injury is short and dislocation has not produced transection). **E,** dural closure with fascia lata.

ipulation of the injured spinal cord or myelotomy to decompress the swollen cord has not been rewarding.

SPINAL CORD HYPOTHERMIA

Recently, based on the experimental work of White and Alban, there has been considerable enthusiasm for acute localized perfusion of cold saline over the exposed traumatized spinal cord. They and others have demonstrated in monkeys and dogs that controlled experimental paraplegia, resulting from a measured force applied to the spinal cord, can be reversed by localized hypothermia of the cord if cooling is performed within 4–6 hours of initial trauma. Light and electron microscope studies demonstrate that the changes of spinal cord injury occur gradually and sequentially over the first 4 hours. These changes in animals receiving injury sufficient to produce *transient paraplegia* consist of early distention of venules, then extravasation of erythrocytes into the perivascular spaces, followed by small gray-matter hemorrhages and finally alterations in circulation to the cord and secondary neuronal injury. The white matter changes in these animals were less impressive and it may be the retardation of changes in these elements by cooling that makes this a worthwhile technique.

Therefore, if spinal cord injury is present and the cord, at exploration within 2–4 hours of injury, is noted to be swollen and contused, localized hypothermia should be carried out at 0–5 degrees, using a constant high-volume Ringer's lactate perfusion for at least 3 hours. Our results have been impressive, although the number of cases is small and the degree of injury cannot be quantitative, as it was in the animal experiments.

In addition to decompression and cooling the cord, a dural patch graft usually is installed to allow further cord swelling to be accommodated.

LATE SURGICAL CONSIDERATIONS

Recently we have been impressed that local root decompression and firm stabilization at the level of cervical spinal dislocation may be of value in improving local nerve root function. When skeletal immobilization or posterior fusion does not stabilize an interspace adequately, removal of a compressed dislocated vertebral body and adjacent disks, with immediate interbody fusion, may result in surprising improvement in root function. Similarly, this same technique can be used to decompress exiting nerve roots when late myelography, tomography or oblique radiographs demonstrate foramenal encroachment by disk or bone. The anterior horn cells giving rise to roots exiting at a level of dislocation lie rostral to the dislocation; thus, although no change in cord function may be achieved, the root decompression may result in significant functional improvement for the quadriplegic patient.

MEDICAL AND NURSING CARE

Prolonged care of the patient with a severe spinal cord injury must be planned and well thought out from the time of the injury and the physician's first contact with the patient to his discharge from the hospital. The acute psychologic as well as medical problems must be dealt with expectantly to ensure early rehabilitation and return to productive life. Immediate considerations include care of the skin to prevent decubiti with treatment on alternating pressure mattresses, water beds or Stryker frames; assiduous care of the peroneal region; and maintenance of nutrition. Bladder care should be individualized for each patient and use be made of the fact that the bladder can be operated in an "automatic" manner because of its reflex innervation. Initially, the bladder will distend, and aseptic installation of catheter drainage should be performed immediately. Once the effects of spinal shock have gone, the bladder will revert to a reflex activity, provided that the injury exists above the S2–S3 nerve roots. Careful urologic evaluation with cystometrography, sphinctermetrography and cystoscopy should be carried out to determine if automatic bladder function can be successful in evacuating residual urine. In many cases, this is a satisfactory method of treatment. However, if significant residual urine is left in the bladder, infection will supervene and the need for diversionary urologic procedure may become apparent.

Care to prevent impaction should be taken from the onset, with enemas or suppositories every other day and range of motion exercises of the lower extremities performed every 2–3 hours by nursing personnel to decrease the incidence of phlebitis. We have not utilized prophylactic anticoagulation in the initial care of these patients, but believe that there may be a place for careful application of such treatment in those immobilized for prolonged periods.

Physical and occupational therapy programs should be mapped out for each patient and, if possible, attempts should be made to have them treated in units specializing in the care of paraplegic patients. It is important to begin planning for the rehabilitation of the cord-injured patient early in his acute hospitalization. Active therapy as early as spinal stability permits is essential to minimize the catabolic effects of denervation and to maintain the patient's psychologic and financial resources. The psychologic needs of the patient and his family must not be overlooked. The National Paraplegia Foundation is active in seeking to aid those with neurologic deficit as well as supporting research in the treatment of paraplegia.

BIBLIOGRAPHY

Adamkiewicz, A.: Die Blutgefässe des menschlichen Rückenmarkes. I. Die Gefässe der Rückenmarkssubstanz, S. B. Akad. Wiss. Wien, Kl. Abt. III, 84:469, 1882.

Albin, M. S., White, R. J., Acosta-Rica, G., et al.: Study of functional recovery produced by delayed localized cooling after spinal cord injury in primates, J. Neurosurg. 29:113, 1968.

Alexander, E., Jr., Forsyth, H. F., Davis, C. H., Jr., and Nashold, B. S., Jr.: Dislocation of the atlas on the axis. The value of early fusion of C1, C2, and C3. J. Neurosurg. 15:353, 1958.

Austen, G.: *The Spinal Cord.* Section I–Spinal Trauma (Springfield, Ill.: Charles C Thomas, Publisher, 1961).

Bolton, B.: The blood supply of the human spinal cord, J. Neurol. Psychiat., n.s. 2:137, 1939.

Bors, E., and Comarr, A. E.: *Neurological Urology* (Baltimore: University Park Press, 1971).

Cloward, R. B.: Treatment of acute fractures and fracture-dislocations of the cervical spine by vertebral body fusion, J. Neurosurg. 18:201, 1961.

Comarr, A. E., and Kaufman, A. A.: A survey of the neurological results of 858 spinal cord injuries, J. Neurosurg. 13:95, 1956.

Crosby, E. C., Humphrey, T., and Lauer, E. W.: *Correlative Anatomy of the Nervous System.* Chapter 2–Spinal Cord (New York: The Macmillan Company, 1962).

Dohrman, G. J., Wagner, F. C., and Bucy, P. C.: Fine structure of the microcirculation in traumatized spinal cord, Fed. Proc. 29:289, 1970.

Dohrman, G. J., Wagner, F. C., and Bucy, P. C.: Transitory traumatic paraplegia: Electron microscopy of early alterations in myelinated nerve fibers, J. Neurosurg. 36:407, 1972.

Ducker, T. B., and Hamit, H. F.: Experimental treatment of acute spinal cord injury, J. Neurosurg. 30:693, 1969.

Gelfin, S., and Tarlov, I. M.: Differential vulnerability of spinal cord structures to anoxia, J. Neurophysiol. 18:170, 1955.

Gillilan, L. A.: The arterial blood supply of the human spinal cord, J. Comp. Neurol. 110:75, 1958.

Guttmann, L.: Early management of the paraplegic. Symposium on spinal injuries, Royal College of Surgeons of Edinburgh, J. R. Coll. Surg. Edinb., 1963.

Hollin, S. A., Gross, S. W., and Levin, P.: Fracture of the cervical spine with rheumatoid arthritis, Am. Surg. 31:532, 1965.

Joyner, J., and Freeman, L. W.: Urea and spinal cord trauma, Neurology 13:69, 1963.

Kahn, E. A., Crosby, E. C., Schneider, R. C., and Taren, J. A.: *Correlative Neurosurgery.* Chapter 26–Trauma to the Spine and Spinal Canal (Springfield, Ill.: Charles C Thomas, Publisher, 1969).

Lemmen, L. J., and Laing, P. G.: Fracture of the cervical spine in patients with rheumatoid arthritis, J. Neurosurg. 16:542, 1959.

Matson, D. D.: *Neurosurgery of Infancy and Childhood.* Chapter 23–Spinal Cord Injury (Springfield, Ill.: Charles C Thomas, Publisher, 1969).

Munro, D.: The cord bladder. Its definition, treatment and prognosis when associated with spinal cord injuries, N. Engl. J. Med. 215:766, 1936.

Osterholm, J. C., and Mathews, G. J.: Altered norepinephrine metabolism following experimental spinal cord injury, J. Neurosurg. 36:386, 1972.

Queckenstedt, M. E.: Zur Diagnose der Rückenmarks Kompression, Deutsche Ztschr. Nervenh. 55:316, 1916.

Schneider, R. C.: The syndrome of acute anterior

cervical spinal cord injury, J. Neurosurg. 12:95, 1955.
Schneider, R. C.: Surgical indications and contraindications in spine and spinal cord trauma, Clin. Neurosurg. 8:157, 1962.
Schneider, R. C., Cherry, G. L., and Pantek, H. E.: The syndrome of acute central cervical spinal cord injury, J. Neurosurg. 11:546, 1954.
Schneider, R. C., and Kahn, E. A.: Chronic sequelae of spine and spinal cord trauma. I. The significance of the acute "tear-drop" fracture, J. Bone Joint Surg. 38-A:985, 1956.
Tarlov, I. M.: Spinal cord compression studies. III. Time limits for recovery after gradual compression in dogs, Arch. Neurol. & Psychiat. 71:588, 1954.
Tarlov, I. M.: Acute spinal cord compression paralysis, J. Neurosurg. 36:10, 1972.
Tarlov, I. M., and Klinger, H.: Spinal cord compression studies. II. Time limits for recovery after acute compression in dogs, Arch. Neurol. 71:271, 1954.
Tavares, J. M., and Wood, E. H.: *Diagnostic Neuroradiology* (Baltimore: The Williams & Wilkins Company, 1964).
Turnbull, I. M., Brieg, A., and Hassler, O.: Blood supply of cervical spinal cord in man: A microangiographic cadaver study, J. Neurosurg. 24:951, 1966.
Wagner, F. C., Dohrman, G. J., and Bucy, P. C.: Histopathology of transitory paraplegia in the monkey, J. Neurosurg. 35:272, 1971.

16 | Injuries to the Spine: Neurologic Considerations; Fractures and Dislocations

DONALD S. PIERCE and ROBERT G. OJEMANN

BONY INJURIES to the spine may occur in many forms. The bodies of the vertebrae may be crushed; fractures may involve the transverse or spinous processes, laminae or pedicles. Vertebrae may be dislocated as a whole or in part. Each of these injuries may involve but a single vertebra or several; they may occur in the cervical, the thoracic or the lumbar region. Forcible hyperflexion, hyperextension, side bending or rotation may result in 1 or more of these injuries.

CORD INJURY

Because the spinal cord is contained within the vertebral column, cord and nerve root damage from bone displacement due to injury is an ever present possibility, especially in the cervical spine. Probably 90% of persons who "break their backs" suffer not the slightest cord or nerve root injury.

The spinal injuries with which cord or nerve root damage may be associated are clearly defined. Usually they are those that decrease the anteroposterior diameter of the vertebral canal, but on rare occasions they are related to interference with major blood supply to the cord, such as compression of the vertebral artery[38] or artery of Adamkiewicz. These injuries include vertebral dislocations (Fig. 16-1), fracture-dislocations (Fig. 16-2) and bursting fractures of the vertebral body that result in backward displacement of fragments into the vertebral canal (Fig. 16-3). Uncommonly, forcible hyperextension injuries in the cervical region associated with extensive cervical spondylosis (Fig. 16-4) may be complicated by cord damage; and, also uncommonly, severe cervical and thoracic disk injuries with retropulsion of disk fragments may cause this serious complication.

On rare occasions complete vertebral dislocation may be followed by spontaneous reduction, apparently the result of the recoil of the hyperflexed spinal column. As the vertebra is dislocated, complete transection of the cord may occur, yet roentgenographically there may appear no other evidence of dislocation than a slight decrease in the intervertebral spacing at the level of the dislocation (Fig. 16-5). Less than complete reduction probably occurs spontaneously in some cases. Extensive cord injury in the presence of only slight displacement at the time of first x-ray examination is difficult to explain on any other basis unless there is associated pathology, such as cervical spondylosis.

In contrast the common wedge-compression fractures of the vertebral body without dislocation (Fig. 16-6), the com-

344 / Donald S. Pierce and Robert G. Ojemann

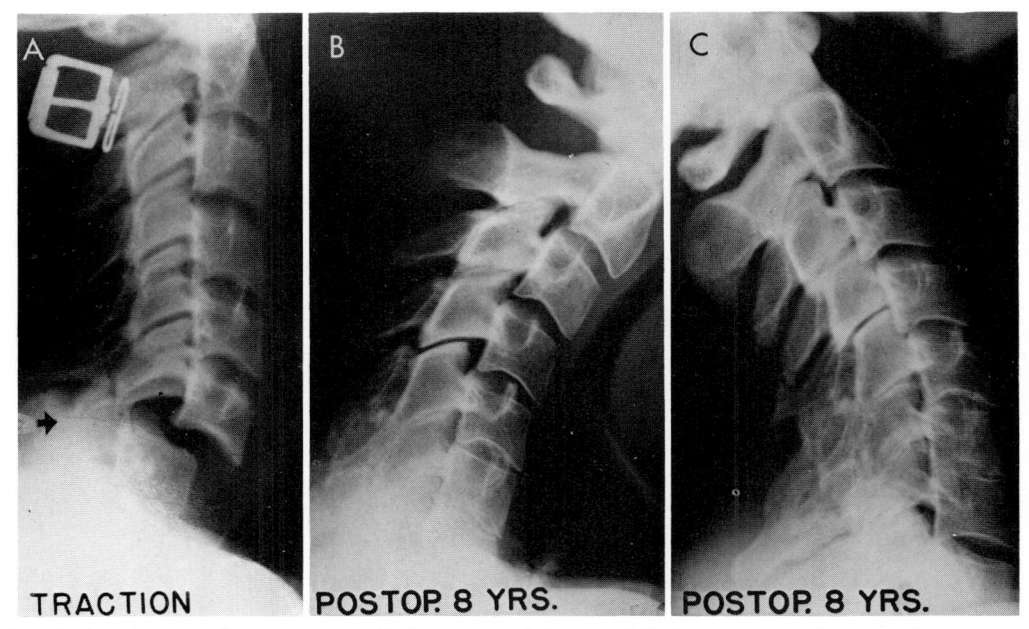

Fig. 16-1.—**A,** complete anterior dislocation of C6 on C7. Symptoms of partial loss of cord function were observed immediately after injury; improvement neurologically was noted shortly afterward. Reduction was easily completed at operation after several days of halter traction. **B,** result after 8 years. Roentgenogram made in maximal flexion. **C,** maximal extension. Fusion was solid. No neurologic symptoms and no complaints. Patient was carrying on full preinjury activities as a dairyman. (From Rogers, W. A.: Fractures and dislocations of the cervical spine: An end result study, J. Bone Joint Surg. 39-A:341, 1957.)

Fig. 16-2.—**A,** lateral and **B,** anteroposterior views of fracture-dislocation involving the T12 and L1. There was immediate complete (permanent) loss of cord function at the level of the injury.

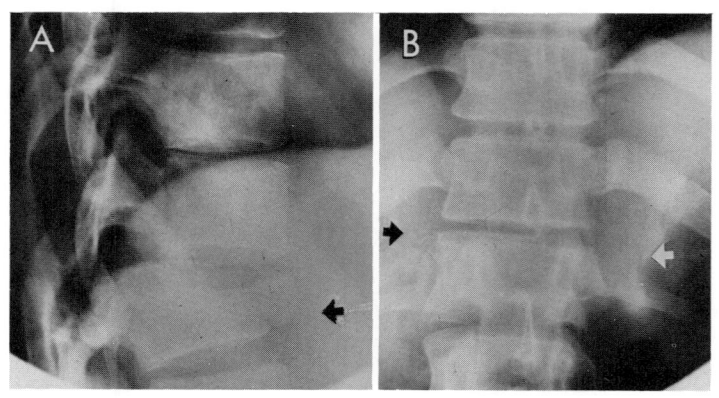

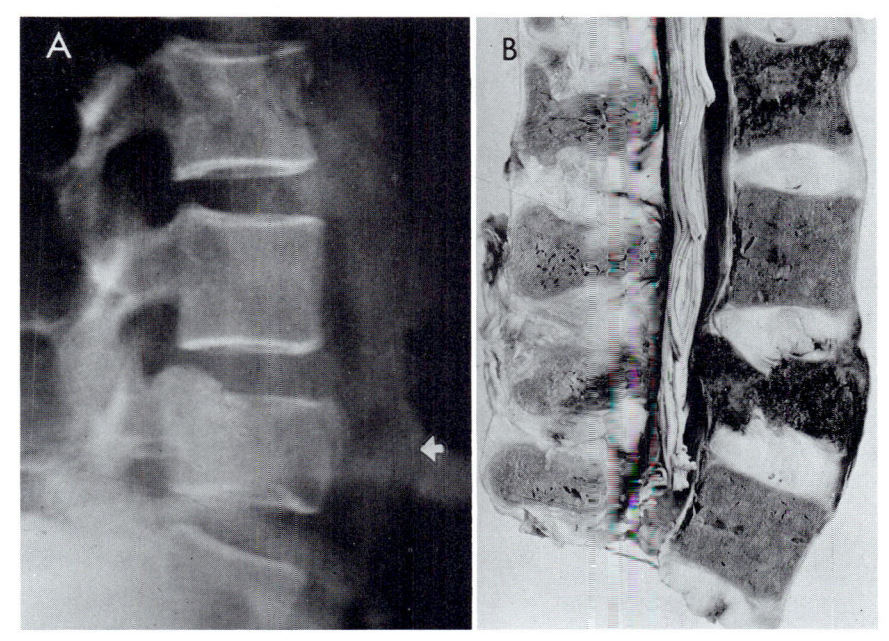

Chapter 16: INJURIES TO THE SPINE: NEUROLOGIC CONSIDERATIONS / 345

Fig. 16-3.—**A**, lateral roentgenogram showing a fracture of the body of L4. A careful check of the outline of the posterior wall of this vertebra reveals backward displacement of a large posterior fragment which might easily be overlooked. The patient had fallen 40 ft, sustaining multiple injuries, and died of shock shortly after admission to the hospital. **B**, sagittal section of spine shows marked decrease in anteroposterior diameter of vertebral canal and very little space remaining for nerve roots. A casual inspection of the x-ray film might result in the overlooking of a serious condition. (From Rogers, W. A.: Cord injury during reduction of thoracic and lumbar vertebral-body fracture and dislocation, J. Bone Joint Surg. 20:689, 1938.)

mon transverse process fractures and the isolated fractures of the spinous processes are almost never complicated by cord or nerve root trauma.

THE CERVICAL SPINE

Injuries Dangerous to the Cord

The spinal cord may be damaged in most of the more common injuries of the cervical spine. In a series of 85 patients treated for 87 injuries of the cervical spine at Massachusetts General Hospital, Rogers[33] reported complete interruption of cord function immediately following injury in approximately 1 in every 5 patients; immediate onset of partial loss of cord function in 1 in every 4 patients, and definite evidence of nerve root pressure immediately after injury in approximately 1 in every 5 patients. In only 28 of the 85 patients was there no sign of loss of cord or nerve root function. It is a sad commentary that 1 in every 10 patients had symptoms of cord compression or an

TABLE 16-1.—TIME OF ONSET OF NEUROLOGIC SYMPTOMS

	PATIENTS No.	%
Late onset of increase of cord symptoms (all were anterior dislocations	8	9
Immediate onset of symptoms of complete cord interruption	15	18
Immediate onset of symptoms of incomplete cord interruption	19	22
Symptoms of nerve root pressure only	15	18
No neurologic symptoms	28	33
Total	85	100

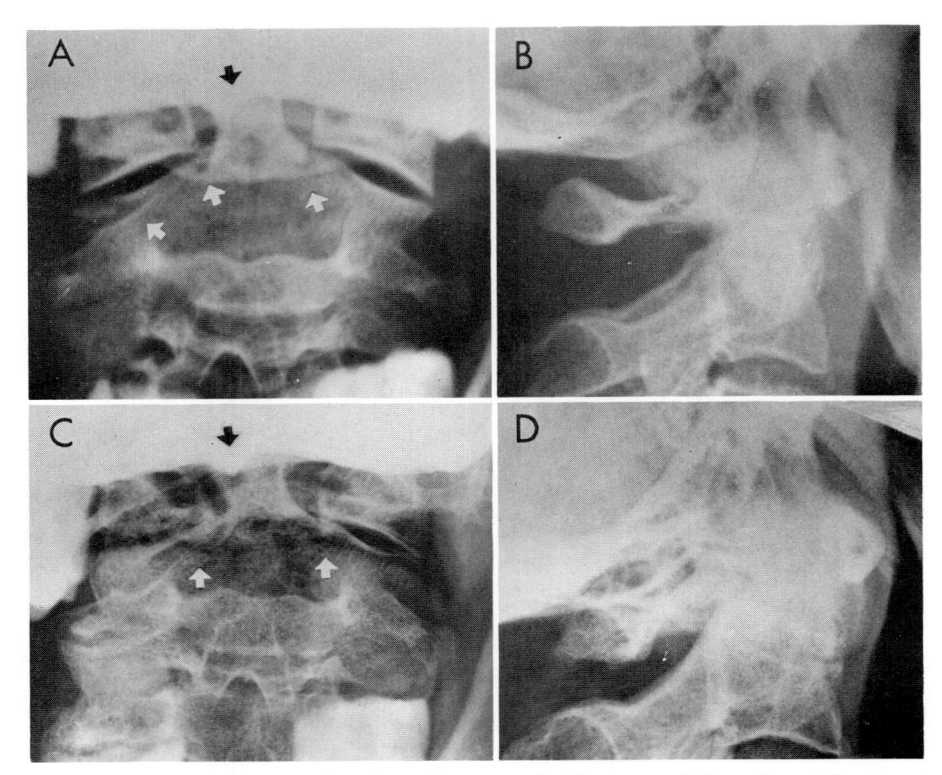

Fig. 16-4.—**A,** anteroposterior and **B,** lateral views of a fracture of the odontoid process. Moderate displacement, the process being inclined to the right, and a compression fracture of the right superior articular process of the axis. Union of the fracture occurred with traumatic changes in the right superior articular process of the second vertebra 3½ months after injury. **C** and **D,** roentgenograms made at follow-up examination 12 years after injury. (Figs. 16-4 and 16-5 from Rogers, W. A.: Fractures and dislocations of the cervical spine: An end result study, J. Bone Joint Surg. 39-A:341, 1957.)

increase of cord symptoms subsequent to the time of original injury—during emergency care, during the time when the diagnosis was being established, during definitive treatment or following reduction (Table 16-1). Little has changed to the present in most areas.

Bursting fractures of the vertebral body (longitudinal compression) commonly result in backward displacement of bone fragments (Fig. 16-7) and often there are immediate symptoms of cord compression. A. S. Taylor,[46] Schneider and Kahn[37] and Rogers[28] have reported the late onset of cord symptoms after failure to correct backward displacement of bone fragments. Relief of symptoms followed decompression. Elsberg,[16] Stookey,[43] Cramer and McGowan,[11] Bucy and associates[8] and Barnes[2] demonstrated that hyperflexion injuries of the cervical spine without vertebral fracture or dislocation may cause retropulsion of fragments of the intervertebral disk. It is also well known that disk displacements, disabling neurologically, may occur without specific injury. Anterior dislocation or unilateral rotatory dislocation may also result in cord damage (Figs. 16-1 and 16-8). In such dislocations, Barnes has shown that cord compression is not possible until the dislocation of 1 or both of

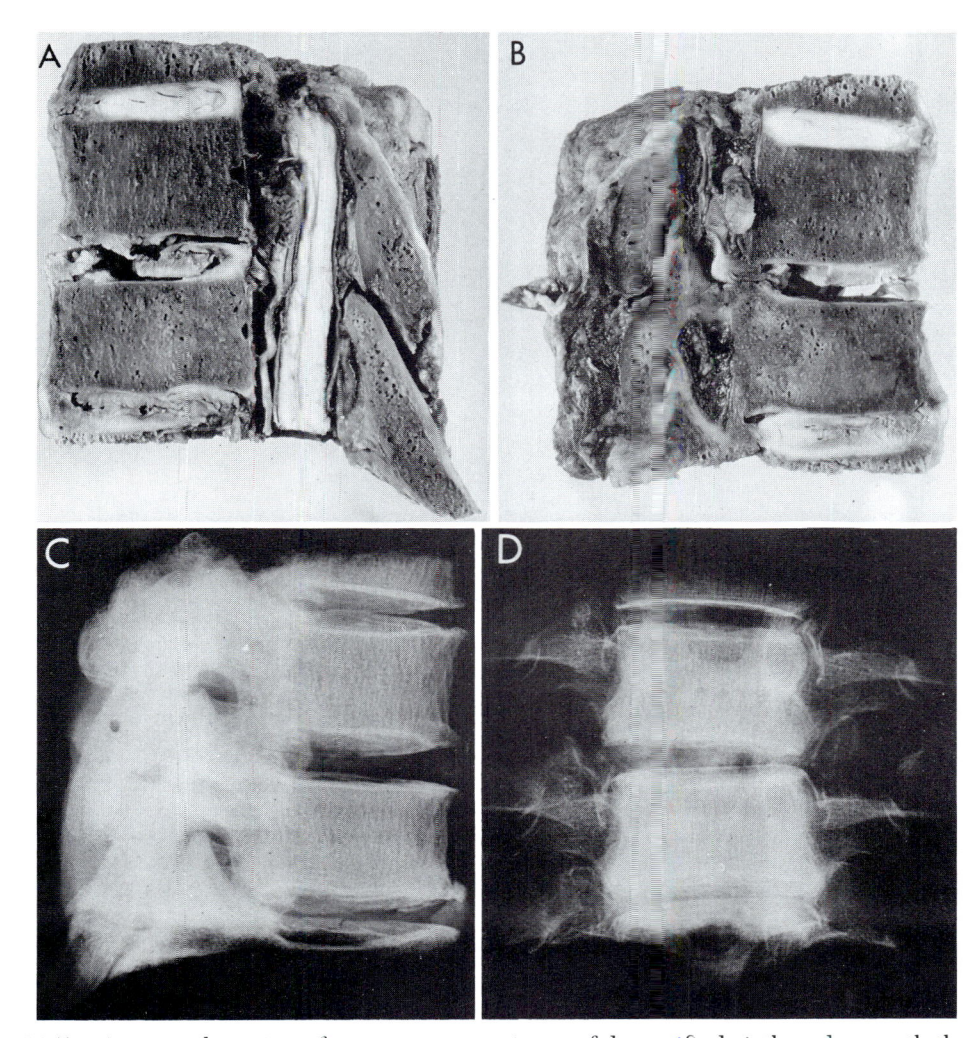

Chapter 16: INJURIES TO THE SPINE: NEUROLOGIC CONSIDERATIONS / 347

Fig. 16-5.—**A,** sagittal section of an autopsy specimen of decalcified sixth and seventh thoracic vertebrae (Warren Museum, Harvard Medical School, specimen no. 12736). The patient, aged 43, had fallen 4 stories from a roof to the sidewalk below. He had sustained a fractured skull, remained unconscious, and died the third day after injury. There is complete rupture of all binding ligaments and muscles. The sixth intervertebral disk is shattered. Fragments of the sixth disk and a hematoma are lodged between the dura and the posterior wall of the upper of these 2 vertebrae. Above, the disk fragments are seen lodged in the vertebral canal as high as the superior surface of the sixth vertebral body; below, disk fragments, including a fragment of the cartilaginous end-plate, are found as far distally as the sixth disk, to the remnants of which they are still attached by a band. The posterior longitudinal ligament has been torn across, opposite the middle of the sixth centrum. The mass of disk fragments presses on the crushed cord. **B,** paramedial sagittal section through one of the posterior articulations. **C** and **D,** roentgenograms of the specimen. No evidence of fracture in the vertebrae. Marked anterior dislocation of T6 on T7 must have occurred, reduction having taken place spontaneously through the recoil of the column when the force had been spent. (From Rogers, W. A.: Fractures and dislocations of the cervical spine: An end result study, J. Bone Joint Surg. 39-A: 341, 1957.)

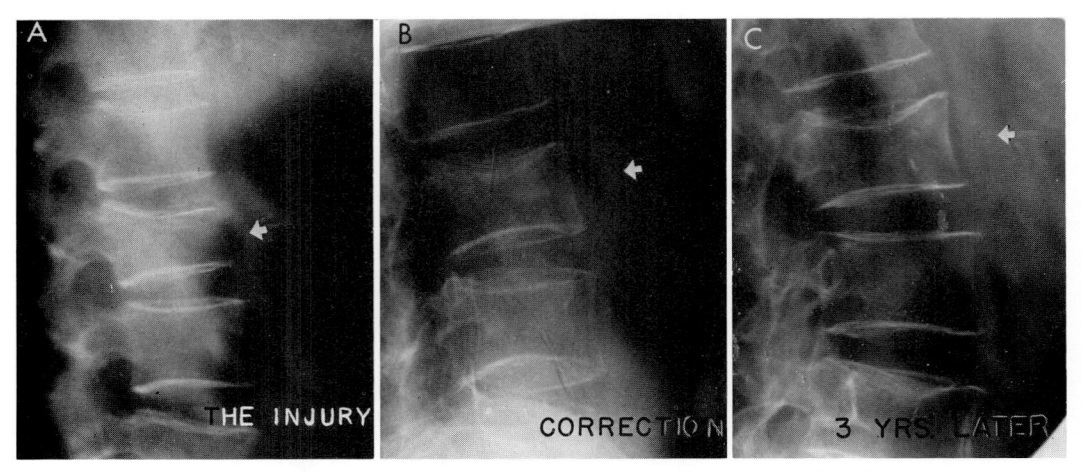

Fig. 16-6.—**A,** common wedge-compression fracture. No dislocation and no fracture of posterior wall of the centrum. Vertebral canal is normal. The apex of the wedge is usually directed forward. **B,** correction of the deformity. **C,** 3 years after injury the correction has been maintained.

Fig. 16-7.—**A,** bursting fracture of C5, the result of a dive into shallow water. Posterior fragments have been displaced backward into the vertebral canal. **B,** anteroposteriorly, the centrum appears split vertically in the sagittal plane. The lower part appears jammed into the concavity of the upper surface of the vertebral body below. In the upper part there is definite lateral displacement of fragments; the superolateral processes do not clasp the body above but have been pushed laterally. **C,** result 2 years later. Fusion was solid. There were complete and lasting freedom from cord symptoms at 11-year follow-up, no pain and full preinjury activities. (Figs. 16-7–16-9 from Rogers, W. A.: Fractures and dislocations of the cervical spine: An end result study, J. Bone Joint Surg. 39-A:341, 1957.)

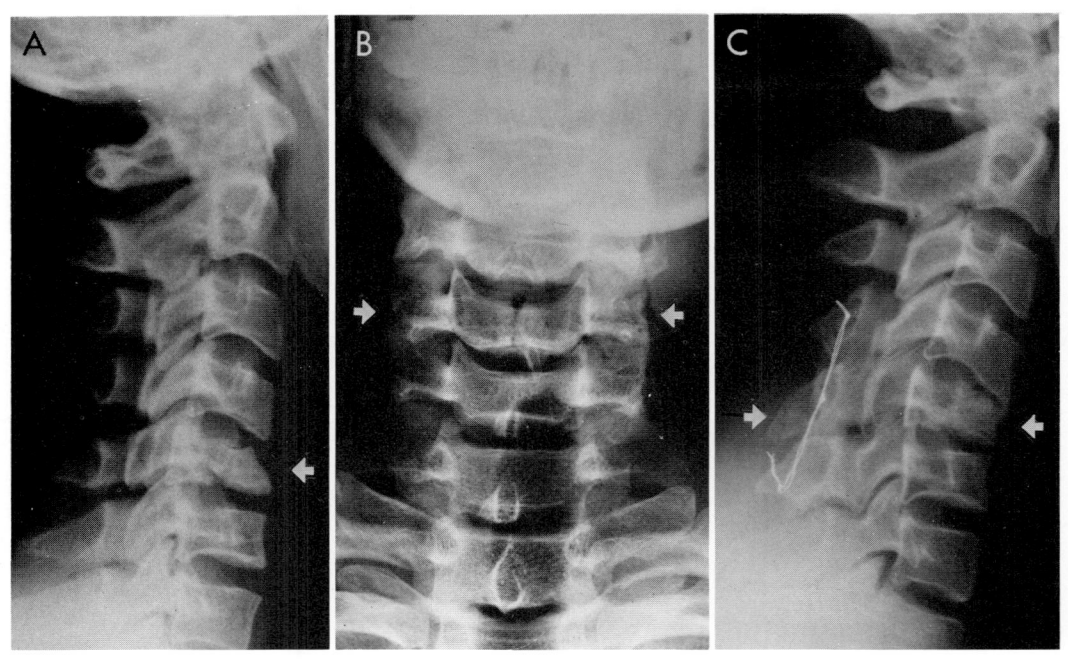

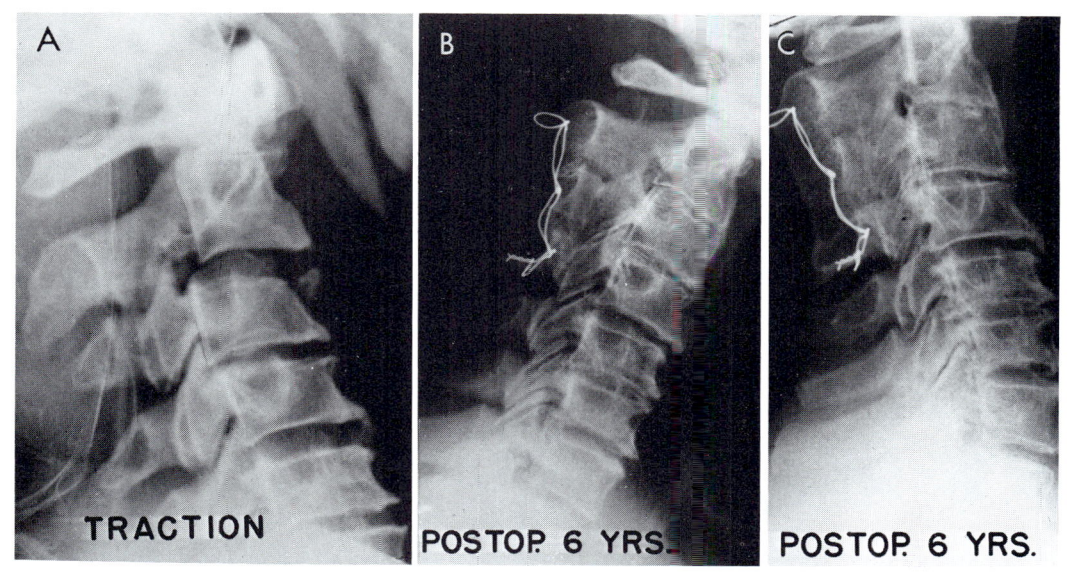

Chapter 16: INJURIES TO THE SPINE: NEUROLOGIC CONSIDERATIONS / 349

Fig. 16-8.—**A**, lateral view shows a unilateral rotatory dislocation of C2 on C3. Symptoms of partial interruption of cord function were noted immediately after injury but disappeared in a few days. Reduction was attempted by skull traction without success, but was achieved at open operation. **B**, result 6 years later. Maximal flexion. **C**, maximal extension. Fusion was solid. The patient resumed full preinjury activities as a truck driver in 10 weeks.

Fig. 16-9.—**A**, anterior dislocation of C4 on C5, 4 months after an automobile accident. Patient had received no treatment. No symptoms of loss of cord function. **B**, strong skull traction resulted in only slight improvement in position. **C**, result after 5 years. Fusion was solid. Full preinjury activities. No loss of cord function.

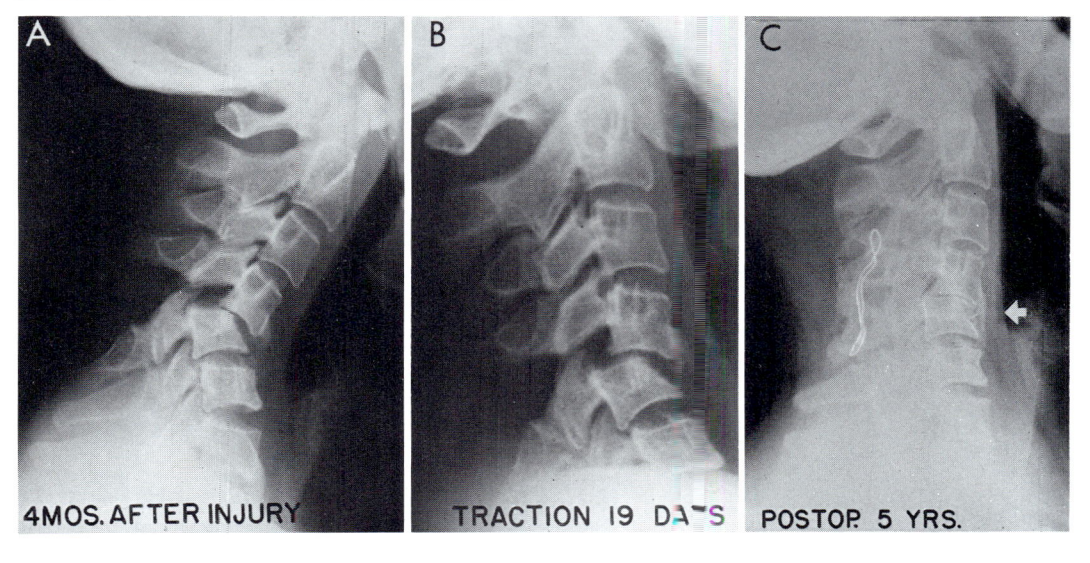

the inferior articular processes is complete and they lock. In the presence of complete anterior dislocation, there may be no cord damage whatever (Fig. 16-9). However, Barnes showed that, if the spine is extended while 1 or both of the inferior articular processes of the dislocated vertebra are anterior to the superior articular processes of the vertebra below, the lower border of the vertebral arch may move downward and forward into the vertebral canal and compress the cord from behind (Fig. 16-10). Posterior dislocation (Figs. 16-11 and 16-12) and hyperextension injuries may also result in cord damage. A. R. Taylor and Blackwood[45] demonstrated at autopsy that posterior dislocation of a cervical vertebra may cause transverse compression of the cord. The dislocation may undergo spontaneous reduction without any immediate roentgenographic evidence of injury. In Drake's series,[15] 11 of 45 patients had no x-ray evidence of bone damage. Taylor[44] also demonstrated on the cadaver that forward bulging of the ligamentum flavum through hyperextension of the cervical spine, especially when it occurs opposite a marginal osteophytic ridge on the front wall of the canal, may cause compression of the cord. There is ample autopsy and clinical evidence to support this finding (Fig. 16-13).

In order to explain cord damage in the absence of definite x-ray evidence of injury to the vertebral column, it was long

Fig. 16-10.—A, anterior fracture-dislocation of L1 on L2. The patient had been thrown from an automobile. There was little immediate evidence of root pressure. A few days later on transfer from a distant hospital there was an increase in motor and sensory paresis in both lower extremities. He could still move his lower limbs. Reduction was attempted by traction-extension without anesthesia. B shows extent of the replacement obtained. The flexion element of the dislocation had been corrected, but replacement posteriorly had been blocked by the superior articular processes of the vertebra below. At this point there was an abrupt and almost complete motor and sensory loss in the lower extremities. Open operative reduction was immediately carried out under local anesthesia. When the vertebral arches were exposed, the inferior articular processes of the dislocated vertebra lay anterior to the superior processes of the vertebra below. As a result of the extension, the arch of the dislocated vertebra had moved downward and slightly forward, decreasing the diameter of the canal and compressing the dura and cauda equina between its lower edge and the posterosuperior margin of the vertebra below. Finally, the posterior elements of the 2 vertebrae had locked, preventing further extension. The locked processes were disengaged by spinal flexion, were manipulated into normal alignment and then reduced by extension, decompressing the cauda equina. Subsequently there was full return of motor and sensory function.

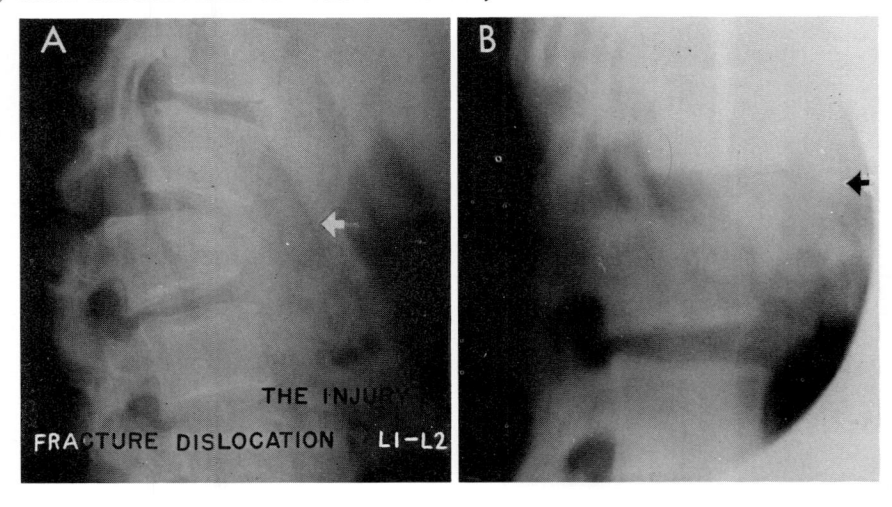

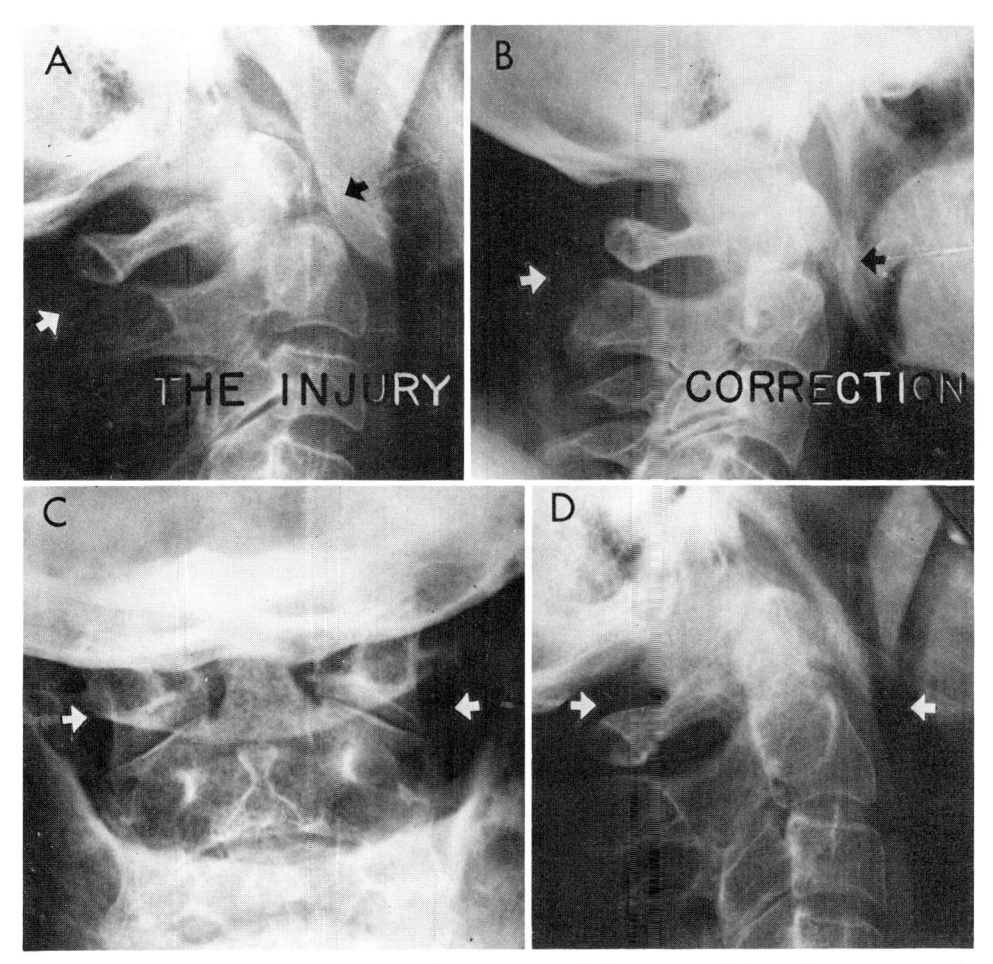

Chapter 16: INJURIES TO THE SPINE: NEUROLOGIC CONSIDERATIONS / 351

Fig. 16-11.—**A**, lateral roentgenogram of a posterior dislocation of the atlas on C2 with fracture of the odontoid process and the lateral articular processes of C2. Patient had fallen downstairs, landing on her face. Shortly after, on admission to the hospital, there was evidence of almost complete loss of cord function. **B**, reduction obtained by skull traction. **C** and **D**, same vertebrae 7 years later. Although greatly improved neurologically, the patient was unable to work; she was able to care for herself in an institution for the partially disabled. Range of cervical motion was normal. (Figs. 16-11–16-13 from Rogers, W. A.: Fractures and dislocations of the cervical spine: An end result study, J. Bone Joint Surg. 39-A:341, 1957.)

held that a dislocation had taken place, immediately followed by spontaneous reduction. The reduction was assumed to be due to recoil of the column resulting from muscle action; the dislocation was believed to cause the cord damage. No definite evidence in support of this explanation appears to have been reported, and the concept has been widely disclaimed as highly improbable. In 1939, however autopsy findings were reported in a thoracic spine which can be interpreted on no other basis than that of spontaneous reduction following dislocation (Fig. 16-5). It is also apparent from Figure 16-5 that, although the cord may have been compressed during the phase of dislocation, the obvious cause of

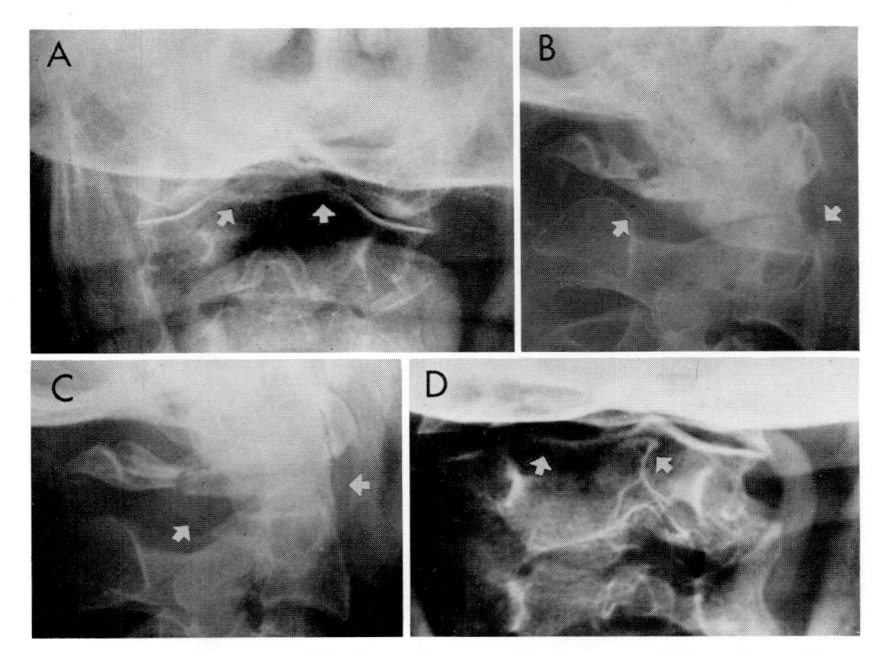

Fig. 16-12.—A, anteroposterior and B, lateral views of a fracture of the odontoid process. Posterior dislocation of the atlas on the axis; the odontoid process was displaced backward with the atlas. C, reduction was obtained by skull traction and was almost complete. D, although union of the fracture of the posterior arch had occurred within 3 months of injury, nonunion of the odontoid fracture was still present at follow-up examination 5 years later. Patient was symptom-free, normally active and had a normal range of cervical motion. The dislocation had not recurred. The examination was negative neurologically.

Fig. 16-13.—A, anterior dislocation of C5 on C6 in a man, 64, with marked hypertrophic changes (marginal lipping). B, While under halter traction for about 1 hour, he became paraplegic and a complete spinal fluid block developed. X-ray film shows reduction and hyperextension at the site of injury.

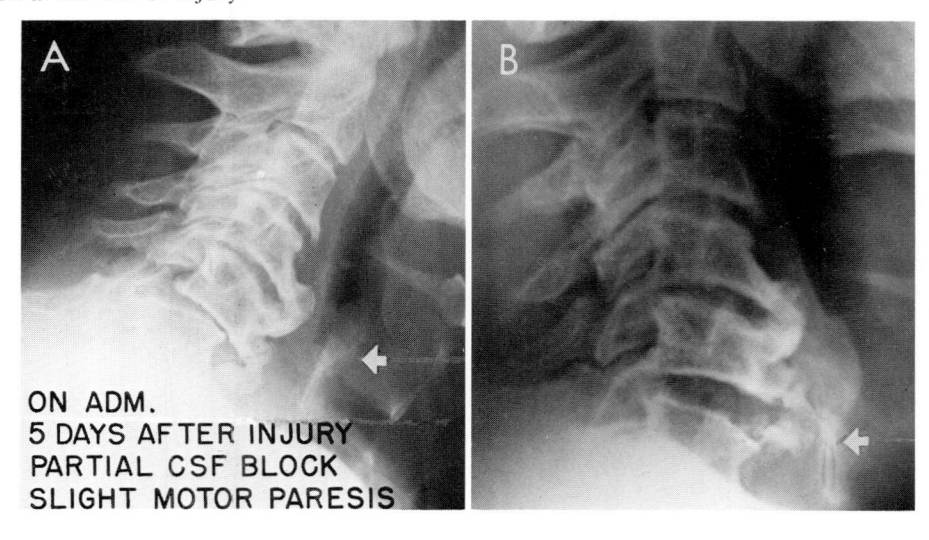

compression is the retropulsion of disk fragments into the vertebral canal. The roentgenograms show narrowing of the intervertebral space. It is well known, however, that backward displacement of disk tissue can occur without narrowing of the involved disk space.

Schneider, Cherry and Pantek[36] described the acute central cord syndrome with paralysis of the upper body and sparing of the lower extremities and pointed out its common etiology as the hyperextension injury of the spine, often without radiographic evidence of bony injury or dislocation. They elaborated a spectrum from central cord injury with recovery possible to permanent total transection secondary to ischemia from contusion and necrosis secondary to edema and microscopic hemorrhage.

Emergency Treatment

It is worth repeating that it is the responsibility of the person who is first called on to care for the patient with a cervical injury to institute emergency measures which will protect the spinal cord. Traction applied in the direction of the long axis of the spine in the neutral position will in many cases protect the cord, at least to some extent, if the cord has escaped injury at the time of, or subsequent to, fracture or dislocation of the cervical spine (Table 16-2); it will also prevent further cord and root injury if damage has already occurred. Traction is applied to the cervical spine, as first aid, by means of an adjustable traction neck brace (such a device should be available in an ambulance) or by any other available means such as a head halter, constructed on the spot from triangular bandages or clothing or straps. If a cervical brace is available, it affords the best means of immobilization. It should be noted, however, that cineradiographic studies by the author (DSP), testing many types of cervical braces and collars that did not involve skeletal fixation, showed that all allow considerable motion of the cervical spine, even when tightened to a maximal degree. As a temporary measure, an adjustable brace may be constructed so that it exerts a constant pressure against the chin and occiput in the cephalad direction and against the chest and shoulder girdle in a caudad direction, thus exerting mild traction on the cervical spine. The brace is worn at all times when the patient is being moved from place to place, as in transfer to and from the x-ray department or to and from surgery, and during the application of tongs or halo skeletal traction.

The traction force must be applied in the direction of the long axis of the neck in the neutral position. The importance of keeping the direction of traction in the neutral position cannot be overemphasized. The term "neutral," as applied to the cervical spine, may be defined as that position in which there is a slight amount of extension, i.e., one of slight lordosis. Since both flexion and extension from the neutral position have been demonstrated to cause cervical cord compression in injuries of the cervical spine, flexing and

TABLE 16-2.—RESULTS OF SKULL TRACTION IN REDUCTION OF FRACTURES AND DISLOCATIONS AND PROTECTION OF CERVICAL SPINAL CORD

Total number of patients	48
Total time of traction	326 weeks
Average time of traction	6.8 weeks
Cord injury during traction (patients)	0
Complete reduction (patients)	29 ⎫ 37 (77%)
Prior complete reduction maintained (patients)	8 ⎭
Satisfactory reduction maintained (patients)	6 (12.5%)
Failure of reduction (patients)	5 (10%)

extending forces are to be avoided, at least until the nature of the injury has been determined by x-ray.

It should be noted that for the brace to be effective, moderate pressure is necessary on the chin and occiput, making it possible to wear such a brace for only a few hours in the fully tight position. A soft pad on the chin piece of the brace will often make the wearing of the brace more bearable, and a foam rubber or plastic foam pad can add greatly to the wearer's comfort. The skin under the chin and the occiput and of the chest and shoulders should be checked frequently to prevent the development of pressure sores and should be gently massaged and kept powdered to prevent maceration. Pressure should be reduced for short periods, during which time the patient must be inactive and should be under careful surveillance by a trained attendant. When traction is resumed, the brace is shifted slightly to change the points of maximal pressure.

The traction brace should be worn from the earliest possible moment after injury until the patient is safely under care in the hospital and skeletal traction has been applied.

When there is sensory paralysis, hard objects, such as wallets and keys, must be removed from pockets as soon after injury as feasible, in order to prevent the development of pressure necrosis. In addition, great care should be taken to avoid pressure on areas such as the sacrum, iliac crest and heels during transport of the patient and while diagnostic procedures are being carried out. Full-thickness loss of skin around the sacrum and heels may occur in a period of 4–6 hours if pressure relationships on these bony prominences are not altered at least every 2 hours, even though a soft pad is placed beneath the prominent areas.

Initial Evaluation and Treatment

The diagnosis of cervical spinal cord injury and fracture and/or dislocation is made on the basis of x-ray and neurologic examinations. Anteroposterior and lateral roentgenograms of the entire cervical spine, as well as roentgenograms made through an open mouth to show the odontoid process, are essential. A surgeon must be present when the roentgenograms are being taken because of the danger of cord injury at the time the patient is moved. The surgeon himself should be the only one to position or handle the patient's head and neck during this period. The patient should not leave the x-ray department until satisfactory films have been made.

Before considering special radiographic studies such as laminagraphy and myelography, skeletal traction and immobilization is usually indicated. At the Massachusetts General Hospital during the past 2 years it has become increasingly common, when possible, to apply skeletal traction in the emergency ward, using a halo and 4 threaded pins or screws for traction at 4 points on the skull (Fig. 16-14). Subsequently the halo is locked into a traction frame supported on an aluminum brace. This consists of a well-padded, plaster girdle about the patient's pelvis, resting on Spence-gel (platinum silicone gel) pads over all bony prominences, with 4 uprights, 2 anterior and 2 posterior, connected to an adjustable aluminum hoop, also padded with felt and platinum silicone gel about the thorax. Two steel uprights from sockets on the anterior aspect of the thoracic hoop are attached to the halo from above by 3 vertical traction bars, through which traction can be applied to a single anterior point or 2 posterior points, thereby bringing about relative flexion or extension of the head and neck. The 3 vertical traction bars are also movable in an anteroposterior direction and laterally on the halo-supporting frame, making it possible to gain control of the neck and to position the cervical spine on a millimeter-by-millimeter basis better than by any other known means.

Experience has shown that it takes no longer to put on the halo and halo brace than to take the patient to the operating

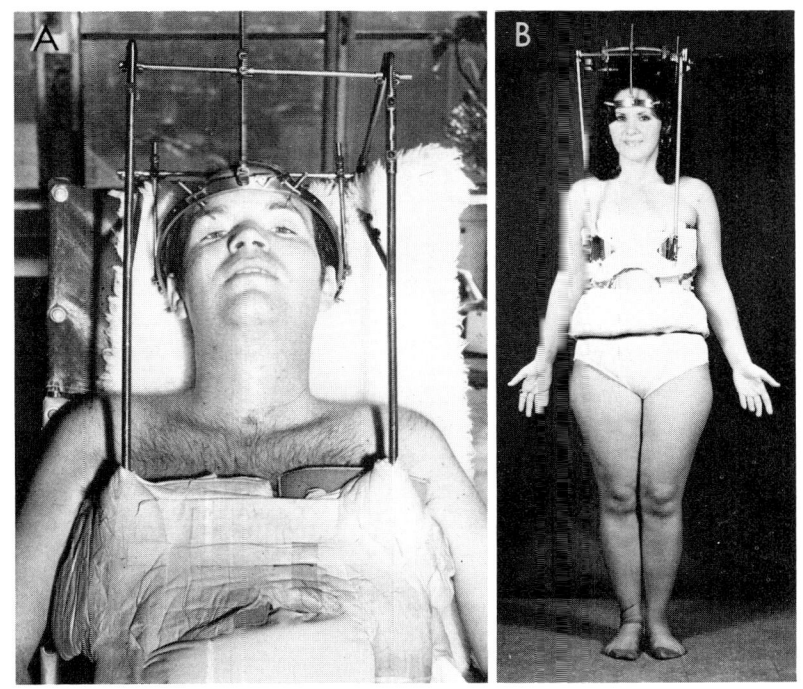

Fig. 16-14.—**A,** halo and frame. Note 4 pins entering skull supported by circular band (halo) and by 3 vertical screws, through which traction may be applied. Frame is attached to a cast. Traction screw carriage may be moved in the anteroposterior plane. **B,** ambulatory patient with vertical fracture of C2. No neurologic deficit. Patient was employed in hospital for 3 months while wearing halo and cast.

room and apply Crutchfield, Barton or Vinke tongs through surgical incisions, during which time there is only relative immobilization of the cervical spine. Once the halo and its supporting brace have been applied, the patient becomes a totally mobile unit and can be turned face down, on the side or in any other desired position to obtain a myelogram or laminagrams. Surgery from the anterior or posterior aspect can be done at will, as it is possible to remove a single upright of the halo frame for anterior surgery, and the neck is entirely exposed and held rigidly in traction for posterior exposure.

Definitive Treatment Methods

The first objective in the definitive treatment of a cervical injury is the protection of the spinal cord during reduction and stabilization. When the safety of the cord has been reasonably assured through properly applied and adequate skeletal traction, reduction of the fracture or dislocation becomes the surgeon's next responsibility. In attempting reduction, restoration of the anteroposterior diameter of the vertebral canal to as near the normal as possible is of primary importance. Restoration of the injured vertebra to a normal or stable relationship with the vertebrae immediately above or below is the next important step. Finally measures are undertaken to ensure lasting stability in the injured spine either through internal fixation and fusion or by adequate external fixation until bony healing is complete.

In many cases, fractures are through vertebral bodies without displacement and are found on adequate myelographic and laminagraphic studies to show no impingement on the spinal cord or nerve

	Electric arm	Electric hand splint	Elevated proximal arm—MAS	Wrist-driven flexor hinge—H.S.	Adapted feeding equipment	Electric razor	Electric toothbrush	Masticlean	Urinal (catheter) clamp	Pencil	Electric typewriter	Mouthstick	Hand controls	Special cuffs	Steering knob	Mirror	Button hook
C_4 level																	
Assisted with equipment in:																	
Hygiene activities	X					X		X									
Feeding	X				X												
Communication skills											X	X					
C_5 level																	
Assisted with equipment in:																	
Hygiene activities		X	X			X	X										
Feeding		X	X		X												
Upper extremity dressing		X															X
Communication skills (legal signature)		X	X							X	X						
C_6 level																	
Independent with equipment in:																	
Hygiene activities				X													
Feeding				X													
Dressing				X													X
Communication skills				X						X	X						
Bladder training and emptying bag									X								
Skin inspection				X												X	
Driving automobile				X									X	X			
Assisted with equipment in:																	
Homemaking activities				X													
C_7-C_8 level																	
Independent with equipment in:																	
Hygiene activities				X													
Feeding				X													
Dressing				X													X
Communication skills				X						X	X						
Bladder training and emptying bag									X								
Skin inspection				X												X	
Driving automobile													X	X			
Assisted with equipment in:																	
Homemaking activities				X													
Paraplegic level																	
Independent in:																	
Hygiene activities																	
Feeding																	
Dressing																	
Communication skills																	
Bladder training and emptying bag																	
Independent with equipment:																	
Skin inspection																X	
Driving automobile													X		X		
Homemaking activities																	

Fig. 16-15.—Functional goals and equipment needs of patients with spinal cord injury. (Courtesy of Rancho Los Amigos Hospital, Occupational Therapy Department, Downey, Calif.)

roots. These have good potential for healing with simple immobilization. The halo and halo brace can be used with the patient in a wheelchair, participating in an active program of rehabilitation from the first week postinjury, or ambulatory if there is no neurologic deficit. Recuperation at home in the halo device is possible. There is now rarely the need for a patient with a cervical spine injury to remain for more than a week in tong traction. If tong traction is used initially in treatment of cervical fracture, it should be converted as rapidly as possible to the halo brace device for rapid mobilization of the patient and progress of rehabilitation.

In situations in which simple bone healing over a period of time will not produce stability in the spine, other treatment methods are used. These include internal fixation by means of wire loops, binding together of the vertebral spinous processes, arches, and posterior or anterior fusion by grafting. When decompression is unnecessary, posterior fusion of the cervical spine is the treatment of choice in fracture or fracture-dislocation, when bone and/or ligament healing would not produce stability. In general, the method initiated by Rogers[32] in 1942 is used, with internal fixation by means of iliac crest grafts placed and wired against the spinous processes. When laminectomy makes it necessary to remove the spinous processes over a wide area, the method of Alexander et al.[1] using iliac bone grafts laid flat in the coronal plane on the facet joints and wired to the facet joints at each level is preferred.

In a series of 50 cases treated at our hospital in the past 4 years it was found that production of stability without decompression of the spinal cord itself, in the cervical area, can account for the improvement in the functional level of the patient in from 1 to 3 root levels. It should be emphasized strongly that whether it is assumed that a cord lesion is complete or incomplete at the time of initial examination does not mean that root recovery is not possible. In many situations in which the cord is actually severed, roots having origins above the level of cord injury have undergone contusion or stretch and appear to be nonfunctional at the initial examination. If stability of the spine can be re-established, even though cord function is beyond recovery these roots may recover. Since they represent a peripheral nerve injury rather than a central nervous system injury, the patient will have a significant level of functional recovery beyond that initially expected (Fig. 16-15). The addition of 1 or more root levels in such cases may spell the difference between a patient capable of functioning outside an institution and earning a living and a patient who is institutionalized. The importance of relief of compression of nerve roots at the site of a fracture-dislocation has also been stressed by Drake.[15]

Traction and Immobilization

The spinal cord is generally protected when the cervical spine is under traction. That this is true is attested by the fact that cord injury did not occur in a single instance in 48 patients in whom the neck was under traction for a total of 326 weeks (Table 16-2). The injuries in these patients represented almost every common type of fracture and dislocation of the cervical spine (Table 16-3). In 43 of the 48 patients (90%) complete reduction of the fracture or dislocation or a satisfactory position* of bone fragments was obtained as a result of the traction applied primarily to protect the cord. When reduction is followed by internal fixation and fusion continued skull traction is usually unnecessary.

In the past 4 years at Massachusetts General Hospital, patients who have

---

*One may arbitrarily accept as a satisfactory position one with less than a 3-mm decrease of the lumen of the vertebral canal, unless a congenital narrowing of the spinal canal is present. In the latter case, absolute measurement of canal diameter, using laminagraphy if necessary, is essential.

TABLE 16–3.—INJURY DISTRIBUTION

	NO. OF PATIENTS	NO. OF LESIONS	%
Wedge-compression fracture	6	9	10
Bursting fracture of atlas	2	2	2
Bursting fracture of vertebral body	10	12	13
Unilateral rotatory dislocation	8	9	10
Anterior dislocation	29	31	34
Anterior fracture-dislocation	8	9	10
Fracture of ankylosed spine	1	1	1
Posterior dislocation	2	2	2
Hyperextension injuries	2	2	2
Posterior fracture-dislocation (including odontoid process)	2	2	2
Anterior fracture-dislocation (including odontoid process)	2	2	2
Fracture of odontoid process	9	9	9
Unknown	3	3	3
	84*	93†	
	− 7	− 6	
Total	77	87	100

*Seven patients who had 2 different injuries were counted twice.
†Six lesions were counted twice; 2 anterior and 2 posterior fracture-dislocations of atlas on axis, and 2 hyperextension injuries.

undergone posterior fusion with wiring, in which the grafts are placed along spinous processes and wired in place, have been immobilized in a 4-poster brace, with a thoracic attachment for stability, or a heavy felt collar cut high over the lateral aspect of the mandibles to prevent rotation and reinforced with steel stays. When laminectomy has rendered the spine itself intrinsically unstable, or when anterior fusion with total body removal has been carried out, the halo device has been used preoperatively, during surgery and postoperatively for up to 3 months until healing is complete. In none of 30 patients in whom the halo device was used has there been an increase in neurologic deficit, nor has there been any case of osteomyelitis of the skull, even when 4-point fixation was maintained for a period up to 4 months. In over 50% of the 30 patients, simple application of the halo device, stabilizing the spine itself and making possible accurate reduction of the fracture and/or dislocation, brought about early neurologic improvement of a root type.

It should be noted that, although tong traction is still the rule in most centers for immobilization of cervical spine fractures, the tongs themselves fail to prevent motion in any direction. It is not uncommon to see a patient on a Stryker frame turn his head as much as 50 degrees to either side to see who is approaching the side of his frame at a time he is receiving oral alimentation. Even though no further cord damage may occur, this excessive motion, especially in rotation, may retard root recovery. Six patients received in the authors' unit, who had been treated for up to 3 months on Stryker frames with tong traction and had not improved, were placed in halos and showed marked improvement within a matter of 24 or 48 hours and progressive improvement in lowering of the effective spinal level by 2 or more root levels.

The halo device is the preferred treatment. However, if it is not available, cervical spine fractures should be treated with tong or wire traction, either on a Stryker frame or in traction in bed. With the Stryker frame the cord from the tongs

Chapter 16: INJURIES TO THE SPINE: NEUROLOGIC CONSIDERATIONS / 359

is passed through a hole in the end of the frame and runs over an attached pulley to weights suspended above the floor. To apply traction in bed, if the patient has a relatively stable fracture, the traction cord is passed through a pulley attached to a trolley that can move freely on a horizontal track fixed to the adjustable head element of the bed. This device makes it possible for the patient to be turned toward either side or on his back. He may also be raised to a semiupright position of about 45 degrees when the head of the bed is elevated. Reading and feeding are facilitated in this position. Recumbency is, however, required during the period

Fig. 16-16. — **A,** anteroposterior and **B,** lateral views showing anterior dislocation of the atlas on C2 with nonunion of a fracture of the odontoid process. The injury had occurred 7 months earlier, and diagnosis had not been made. Neurologically the examination was negative. **C,** reduction was by skull traction. The roentgenograms were made after 10 days of traction. **D,** result 3 years after operation. There was solid bone fusion; the patient was symptom-free and had been working for 2½ years. The fracture of the odontoid process did not unite. (From Rogers, W. A.: Fractures and dislocations of the cervical spine: An end result study, J. Bone Joint Surg. 39-A:341, 1957.)

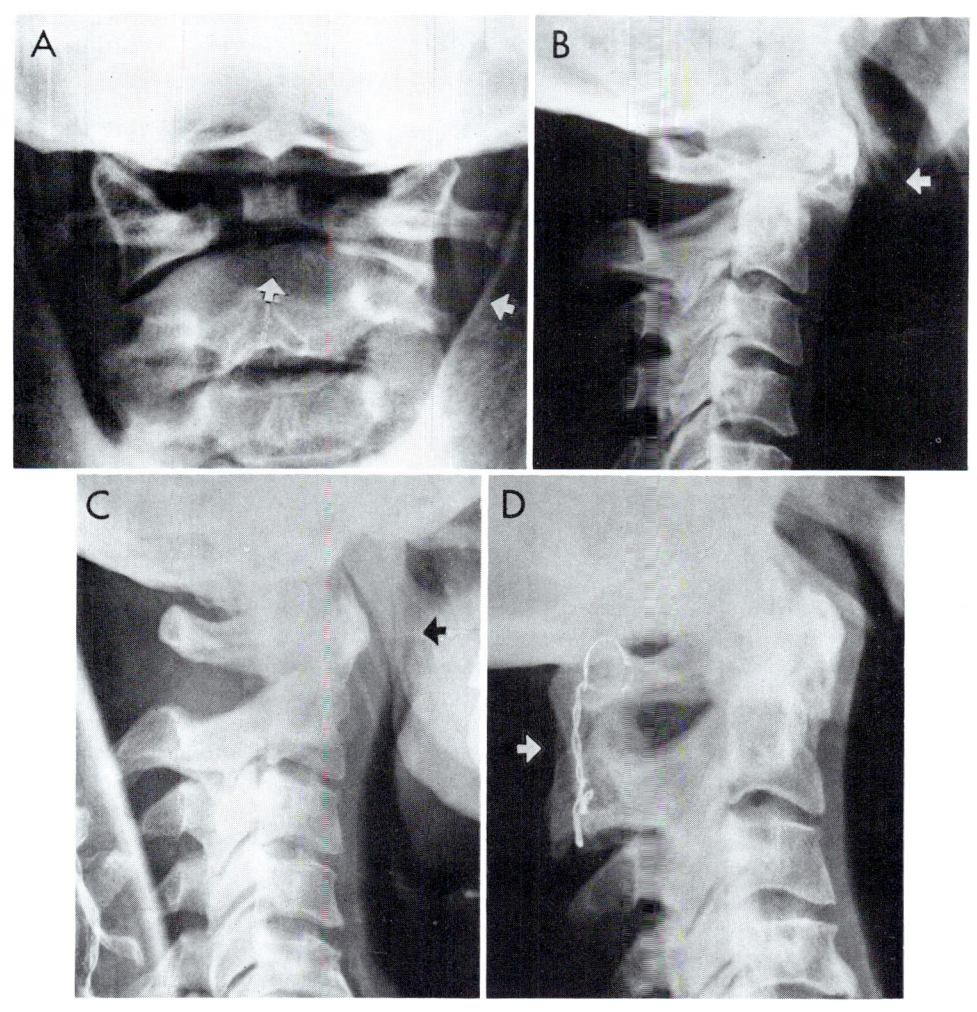

of bone healing. It should be noted that a patient in such a situation must be turned at least every 2 hours without fail, on a side-back-side routine, to prevent pressure sores.

In the 48 patients whose statistics are shown in Table 16-2, recumbency in bed or on a frame was required for 326 weeks. If a halo brace had been used in these 48 patients they would have required only an estimated 48 weeks of hospital time in a recumbent position.

The time during which a cervical spine fracture may remain unstable is notable; in 1 of the patients included in Table 16-2, partial anterior dislocation had been present for 7 months and was reduced shortly after the application of skull traction (Fig. 16-16). However, in another patient skull traction failed to reduce a partial anterior dislocation present for 4 months (Fig. 16-9). The spinal canal may be narrow on a congenital basis or may be narrowed either by old disk herniation posteriorly and/or by cervical spondylosis, making the cord much more susceptible to lesser degrees of displacement. A 3-mm decrease in the anteroposterior diameter of the cord may thus be excessive in some patients and necessitate surgery. Although reduction may appear to be adequate by the Rogers' criteria and neurologic deficit may not be present, or may disappear following reduction, there is a chance of a later cervical spondylosis with cord or root compression at the foramen at the level of injury. This is a distinct possibility and in 1 case reported by White[49] caused complete quadriplegia.

Surgical Treatment: Posterior Operation

The first principle of surgical treatment is to correct a significant decrease in the anteroposterior diameter of the bony spinal canal, if possible. This may require (1) reduction of the fracture or dislocation by traction (skull or halo brace) as noted previously, or, if necessary, open reduction, and (2) removal of bone or disk fragments which have narrowed the canal.

Morgan, Wharton and Austin's study[25] of spinal cord injured patients admitted to the Montebello State Rehabilitation Hospital in Baltimore demonstrates the grave risks associated with laminectomy in patients with incomplete spinal cord injuries. The authors feel there are few indications for this procedure. In their series of 70 patients with partial cord injury, 54% of 28 without operation improved and none deteriorated. However, in the 42 patients undergoing laminectomy, 33% improved and 52% were worse after surgery. The only indications the authors accept for laminectomy in such patients are: debridement of an open wound and open reduction of an irreducible fracture-dislocation. Of interest also is their finding that in laminectomy delayed over 48 hours after injury the percentage of patients improved was lower (24%) and the percentage of patients made worse was higher, compared to laminectomy performed in the first 48 hours (54% of these patients improved). No conclusion was reached regarding the effect of early operative stabilization on improving the likelihood of neurologic sparing or recovery; however, early stabilization was felt to be desirable because it allows early and progressive rehabilitation.

Removal of multiple spinous processes and laminae decreases the inherent stability of the spine, particularly in the cervical area. Unless a fusion is done, laying bone grafts on the lateral masses over the facet joints and wiring the grafts in place, healing and scar contraction will in almost all cases cause a swan-neck deformity of the cervical spine with a hyperextended segment at the area of laminectomy and compensatory curves above and below.

Recent studies with the halo brace in patients with incomplete lesions have shown that much of the paralysis believed to be due to insult to the cord may be due to continued cord and root edema, secondary to instability, and is relieved by complete immobilization. Laminectomy, unless it is done specifically for cooling of the spinal cord (see Chapter 15), or for the removal of compressing bone fragments, is generally contraindicated. Most particularly is this true when the laminectomy is done purely for the sake of "looking at the spinal cord." Especially to be condemned is the practice of performing a laminectomy alone with later fusion planned. There is great difficulty in approaching the spinal cord, uncovered by a previous laminectomy, with extensive scarring, without injury to the cord. Blood loss of 8–10 units is not uncommon in the course of such an exposure and a fusion over 4–6 vertebral segments. This situation can be avoided by doing the fusion at the time of laminectomy. It is rare that a patient who can tolerate anesthesia in the prone position for laminectomy cannot tolerate the additional 1–2 hours necessary for the fusion. Bone graft for the fusion may be taken while the neurosurgeon is exposing the spinal cord, therefore reducing to a minimum the extra time required for the spinal fusion.

In facet dislocation which cannot be reduced by skeletal traction (up to no more than 15 lb) or gentle manipulation, an operative approach under anesthesia with removal of bone as needed to allow reduction is the procedure of choice. Use of excessive traction is fraught with danger of further root or cord damage.

OPERATIVE TECHNIQUE. — When open reduction is performed with the patient prone, the head must be firmly supported either by a halo brace or an attached, well-padded head rest. The eyes must be carefully protected, and the head should be lifted slightly and the forehead massaged at regular intervals. The position of the eyes should be checked by the anesthetist every hour during the procedure to be certain there is no pressure on them.

General anesthesia is carried out, using an endotracheal or nasotracheal tube with cuff. In general, the nasotracheal approach is used to avoid hyperextension or any significant motion of the neck. When the patient is supported in a halo brace, the head is in a position such that laryngoscopic oral-tracheal intubation usually can be carried out. With skull traction, the nasotracheal route is almost mandatory.

Once the spinous processes and laminae are exposed, a marker is placed and the level is confirmed by a lateral x-ray film. The prominences of the spinous processes of the second, sixth and seventh cervical vertebrae are landmarks which may be used in identification, but exact identification is vital. There are cases on record in which the injured level has not been included in the spinal fusion. The neural arches of the involved vertebrae, including the articular processes, are exposed subperiosteally. Operation is aided greatly by the use of the Cobb spinal elevators. Reduction is then effected, usually by gentle manipulation, using instruments, and with force applied through the spinous processes. If necessary, the head may be moved by an assistant with the spine under direct vision. Partial excision of 1 or more articular processes may be necessary, particularly in long-standing dislocation, in order to accomplish the reduction without undue force.

Following reduction with a posterior approach, excellent internal fixation is provided by wiring the spinous processes of the injured vertebrae to those of the vertebrae next above and below. This is accomplished by drilling a hole through the base of the spinous process of each vertebra to be wired and included in the fusion. Care is taken not to fracture the spinous process. Anything smaller in diameter than 20 gauge is of little value in giving support to the spine while the fusion is healing.

If no more than 3 laminae and spinous processes have been removed at laminectomy, it is possible to lay 2 grafts, made up of the outer table of the ilium, on either side of the midline. The upper and lower ends of the grafts are wired to the bases of the spinous processes at the upper and lower limits of the laminectomy area, and cancellous bone is added laterally.

When a more extensive laminectomy involving 4 or 5 levels has been carried out, it may be necessary to abandon the idea of wiring to the spinous processes themselves. The grafts may be laid flat on the articular facets and wired directly to the facets. Before placing the graft and tightening the wires to hold the grafts in apposition to the lateral masses of the vertebrae, a Hall air drill with a small bur is used to roughen or partially decorticate the posterior aspect of the facet joints.

The wire ends should be bent down against the bone grafts, pointing laterally, and should not be allowed to protrude upward into the overlying musculature. In most cases, Gelfoam may be left in the defect over the cord. The wound should be copiously irrigated with normal saline or lactated Ringer's solution. A suction drain is then placed in the wound and the muscles closed in layers. Interrupted sutures are preferred.

Patients who have no neurologic deficit at the time of surgery or who have complete recovery after surgery may be allowed up, if the fusion is secure, in an adjustable cervical brace of the 3- or 4-poster type. The brace is carried down over the torso to a circumferential chest band, with supports going over the shoulders.

Cineradiography studies were carried out by the authors on use of the 4-poster brace, the felt collar with reinforcement, the adjustable 4-poster cervical brace with thoracic extension and the halo brace. It was found that relatively small motions of the head, particularly those involved with chewing, caused considerable motion between individual vertebral bodies in the cervical spine, even when the adjustable braces were tightened to the point of discomfort. Active motions of the head resulted in gross motion of the vertebral bodies at all levels down to C7–T1 in all braces studied except the halo brace, which prevented any observable motion in the cervical spine.

The adjustable 4-poster brace with thoracic extension was the next most stable device, followed by the adjustable 4-poster collar, which gave very little stability and essentially no control of rotation. The standard foam or felt collar provided virtually no immobilization.

A newer type of heavy felt collar, reinforced with steel struts, and cut high over the mandibles to help prevent rotation, has been shown to provide stability comparable to the 4-poster brace without thoracic extension.

When extensive cervical laminectomy is done and it is not possible to wire the grafts securely in place, the halo brace can be used for immobilization for periods from 6 weeks to 3 months. The halo is removed when signs of early bony union are apparent, and the 4-poster brace with thoracic attachment is used for 6 weeks, followed by the high-cut felt collar with steel reinforcement. When such immobilizing devices are used, it is usually possible for the patient to be up in a wheelchair, carrying on an active program of physical or occupational therapy. When there is no appreciable neurologic deficit, early ambulation and discharge from the hospital are possible. Ryerson and Christopher[34] have shown that unrestrained motion will result in erosion of bone by the wire or in breaking of the spinous processes and stability loss before the bony fusion has taken place.

In the past 4 years, 25 patients with fractures or fracture-dislocations of the cervical spine have been treated on our unit by anterior decompression and replacement of a vertebral body with a bone graft. The graft is taken either from the anterosuperior spine of the ilium or from the fibula. A comparable series at Rancho Los Amigos Hospital in Downey, California, numbers more than 60 such fusions. These have been carried out in some cases with the removal of as many as 3 vertebral bodies and their substitution with a fibular graft. Although the fibula is slightly smaller in diameter than the average vertebral body, in the midportion of the cervical spine, it provides an excellent vertical strut, which unites rapidly at both ends and is gradually incorporated throughout its length. For a total body replacement the fibular graft has shown itself preferable to a graft from the iliac crest.

Surgical Treatment: Anterior Operation

There is increasing recognition that delayed onset of neurologic symptoms or failure to regain function resulting from a damaged spinal cord following injury of the cervical spine is related to a decrease in the anteroposterior diameter of the neural canal. This decrease in diameter is in many cases caused by displacement of bone, disk, cartilaginous end-plates or ligamentous fragments against the anterior surface of the spinal cord. Often there is little or no disruption of the posterior longitudinal ligament, but dissection of this material anterior to it causes a bulge posteriorly against the spinal cord.

Often when there is anterior compression, decompression of the spinal cord and roots can only be done by removing the offending material from the spinal canal through an anterior approach. This method of treatment has been the subject of several reports, has been under development at Massachusetts General Hospital over the past 4 years and was presented as part of an American Academy of Orthopaedic Surgeons' Instructional Course Lecture in 1973. One of the most important adjuncts to the operative technique is immobilization in the halo for the operation and the postoperative period of healing. In this way the complication of angulation, noted where external support has been inadequate, can be avoided.

In the past 7 years, 25 operations have been performed at times varying from 3 days to 1 year following spinal injury. Patients who had mechanical compression of the cord and root showed improvement in motor function after decompression. In 2 patients, up to 3 previously nonfunctioning roots showed significant recovery.

OPERATIVE TECHNIQUE. — The technique of anterior decompression is to place the patient in a halo brace and to reduce the fracture or fracture-dislocation by traction and manipulation of the head and neck with the halo traction screws and movable supporting carriage. Thereafter, under endotracheal anesthesia, a transverse incision is made at the appropriate level from the midline to the border of the sternocleidomastoid muscle (Fig. 16-17) The edges are elevated, exposing the platysma, which is divided. The interval between the sternocleidomastoid muscle and carotid sheath laterally and the tracheoesophagus and overlying strap muscles is then opened and a virtually bloodless avenue of approach to the anterior cervical spine is available. The midline is exposed and the medial borders of the longus colli muscles are identified. There are often small veins in this region that require coagulation. The longus colli muscles are separated from their attachments to the anterior vertebral bodies, using a Cobb elevator. The exposure is facilitated by gentle retraction of the trachea and esophagus medially with a vaginal wall retractor and by keeping the carotid sheath lateral. Once the muscles are elevated from the vertebral bodies, the Cloward toothed retractor blades are introduced and are set carefully into the longus colli muscles on either side of the anterior cervical spine.

A no. 20 needle is then inserted into an exposed disk space and a lateral x-ray obtained for localization of the level of injury. When this has been carried out, the Hall air drill, curets and appropriate rongeurs are used to remove the damaged vertebral body as well as the disks above and below it. This may be carried

364 / Donald S. Pierce and Robert G. Ojemann

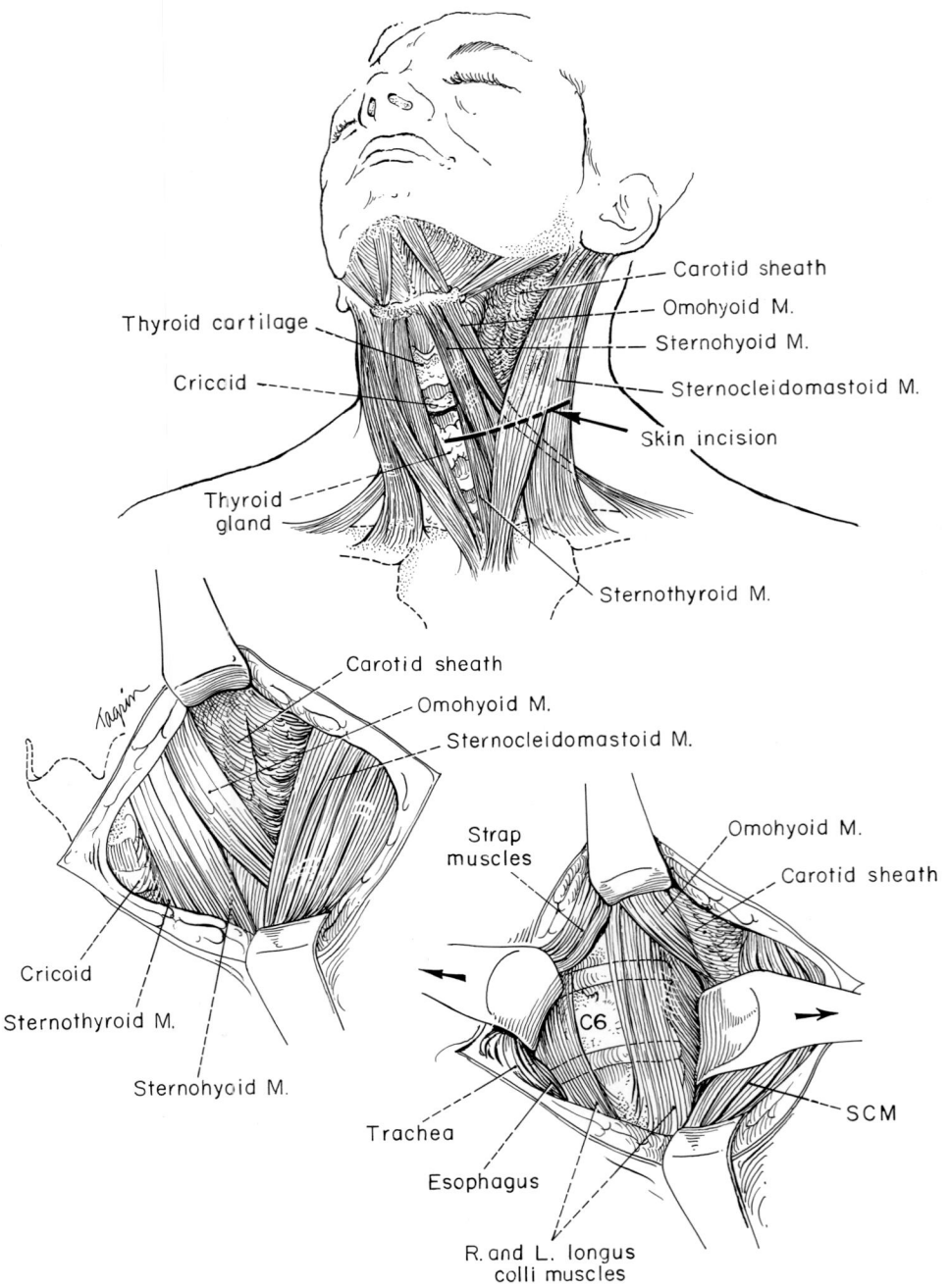

Fig. 16-17.—Anterior approach to the cervical spine.

Chapter 16: INJURIES TO THE SPINE: NEUROLOGIC CONSIDERATIONS / 365

out by the neurosurgical member of the team, who then explores the spinal canal and removes any herniated disk or end-plate material or bone fragments from the canal. The operation is greatly facilitated by the use of magnification and a headlight.

While the neurosurgeon is removing the vertebral body and exploring the foramina and disk spaces, the orthopedist removes a segment of fibula, which must be slightly longer than that needed to replace the vertebral body. The area at the junction of the upper and middle thirds of the fibula is chosen as most nearly equal in size to the cervical vertebral body. Care is taken in exposing the fibula not to injure the common peroneal nerve. In taking the fibular graft a lateral approach is used, going along the lateral intermuscular septum and dividing the musculature in the anterior and lateral compartments, down to the fibula, which is then exposed subperiosteally. Multiple drill holes are made at the top and bottom of the piece to be removed for the graft.

Following closure of the fibular wound, the height, depth and width of the area from which the vertebral bodies and disks have been removed are measured with a sterile paper ruler, introduced directly into the cavity.

The bone graft is then cut (Fig. 16-18) to give a pointed or toothed posterior aspect at the top and bottom ends. Corresponding holes are then drilled in the end-plates of the vertebrae above and below, just anterior to the posterior cortical bony rim using a Hall air drill with a 45-degree angle attachment. An assistant then applies traction to the skull through the vertical traction bars of the halo, distracting the space so that the graft can be slid into place with a minimal amount of instrumentation (Fig. 16-19). It may be easier to use the Cloward spreader for this purpose in certain situations, placing it as far lateral as possible on 1 side of the opening. Once the graft is in place, with the 2 slight projections in the proper corresponding holes above and below, the traction is decreased, either by removing

Fig. 16-18. — Cutting of bone graft.

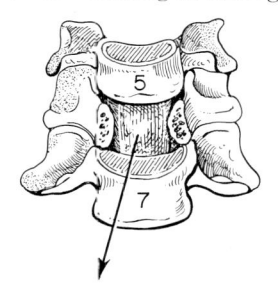

Body of vertebra removed anteriorly

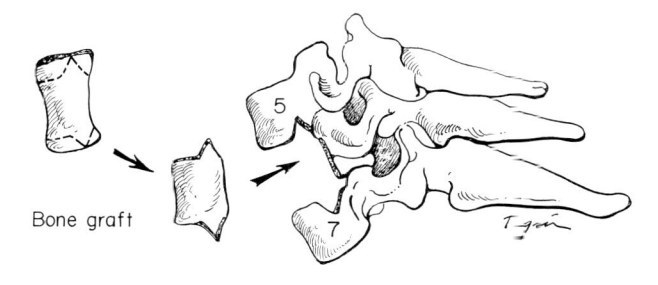

Bone graft

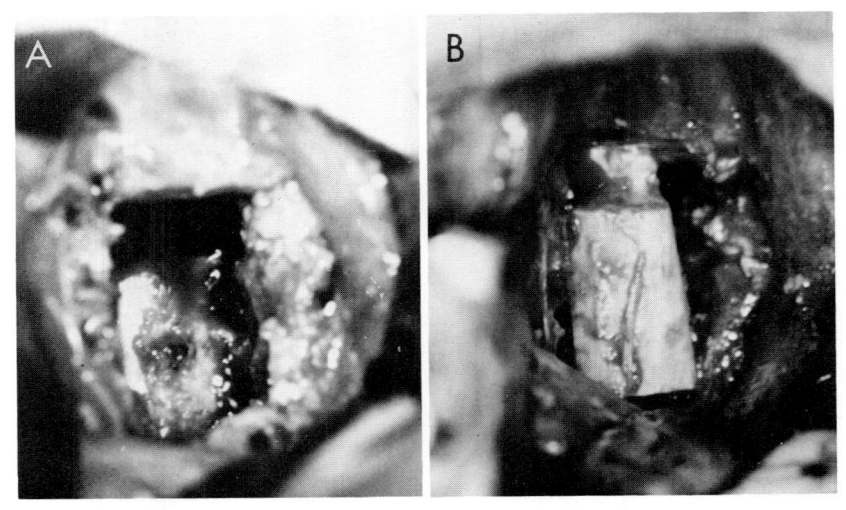

Fig. 16-19.—**A,** anterior decompression of cervical spine. Note remaining portion of lateral masses and undercut end-plate above. Note also perforation of posterior longitudinal ligament, through which disk material had herniated. Complete decompression of the spinal cord and roots was facilitated by removal of the destroyed vertebral body. **B,** fibular strut graft inserted in area of decompression.

the Cloward spreader slowly or by decreasing the traction on the vertical bars to a null-traction position of the halo. This puts the graft under compression and, at this point, generally provides excellent contact between the superior portion of the graft and inferior portion of the body and between the inferior portion of the graft and superior portion of the body below.

A lateral x-ray is then taken to be certain the graft is not impinging on the spinal cord in any area. A no. 4 Penfield instrument is passed behind the graft and on both sides to make certain there is no impingement posteriorly. A bloodless field is obtained by the use of Surgicel and Gelfoam, if needed, and by the judicious use of electrocautery with a low current setting or bipolar coagulation. The wound is irrigated with bacitracin solution, 500,000 units in 250 ml of normal saline or lactated Ringer's solution. This is sponged out and the wound is closed by closing the platysma with interrupted sutures of 00 chromic catgut, with the knots buried, and placing a single layer of 000 plain catgut in the subcutaneous tissue. The skin is closed with a running, subcuticular suture of 4-0 nylon, brought out through the ends of the wound. This is removed on the fourth postoperative day. The edges of the wound are painted with tincture of benzoin and Steri-Strips applied to prevent spreading.

The anterior approach to the cervical spine has been carried out in the past 4 years in 50 patients, including those with disk pathology. The described method of closure with subcuticular suture and burying of the surgical scar in a skin line has been eminently satisfactory; the scar at the end of 1 year could barely be seen.

More Common Types of Cervical Spine Injury

The common injury of the cervical spine is anterior dislocation of a vertebral body. Less common injuries are bursting fractures of a vertebral body, unilateral rotatory dislocations and uncomplicated wedge-compression fractures. Still less common are fractures of the odontoid process, fracture-dislocations of the atlas on the second cervical vertebra, bursting fractures of the atlas and posterior fracture-dislocations (Table 16-3).

Wedge-Compression Fracture

Wedge-compression fracture of a cervical vertebral body is caused by violent hyperflexion of the cervical spine, the mechanism being essentially the same as that in wedge-compression fracture of the lumbar spine. Uncomplicated by dislocation of the vertebra next above, this injury was found 9 times in 6 patients in a series of 87 injuries of the cervical spine. Four of the patients remained free of cord symptoms (Fig. 16-20).

Five of the fractures were reduced by traction. In these, reduction was almost complete. In 2 instances, restoration of shape of the deformed vertebra was satisfactory. Stabilization of the spine by fusion was effected in 2 of the 6 patients. All patients returned to work, 4 patients in an average of 5½ months after injury. One with multiple major injuries resumed work in 24 months; and 1 with cord injury in 14 months.

Patients with severe wedging of a single vertebral body, though there has been no proved dislocation of the vertebral body above, may require even after recovery a posterior fusion from 1 level above to 1 level below the injured vertebra. There is often extensive ligamentous damage as well as damage to the intervertebral disks above and below the fracture. Should a sudden blow to the back of the head be sustained or the patient subjected to a second flexion injury, severe neurologic damage may result and may be irreversible. The question of such a prophylactic fusion is an individual matter and must be decided by a surgeon of considerable experience with spinal injury.

Fig. 16-20.—**A**, wedge-compression fracture of the fifth cervical vertebral body shortly after injury. No cord damage. **B**, result at the end of 8 years. Flexion. **C**, extension. Bone fusion was solid; the patient had resumed work as a printer 6 weeks after injury. He had remained symptom-free since operation. (Figs. 16-20 and 16-21 from Rogers W. A.: Fractures and dislocations of the cervical spine: An end result study, J. Bone Joint Surg. 39-A:341, 1957.)

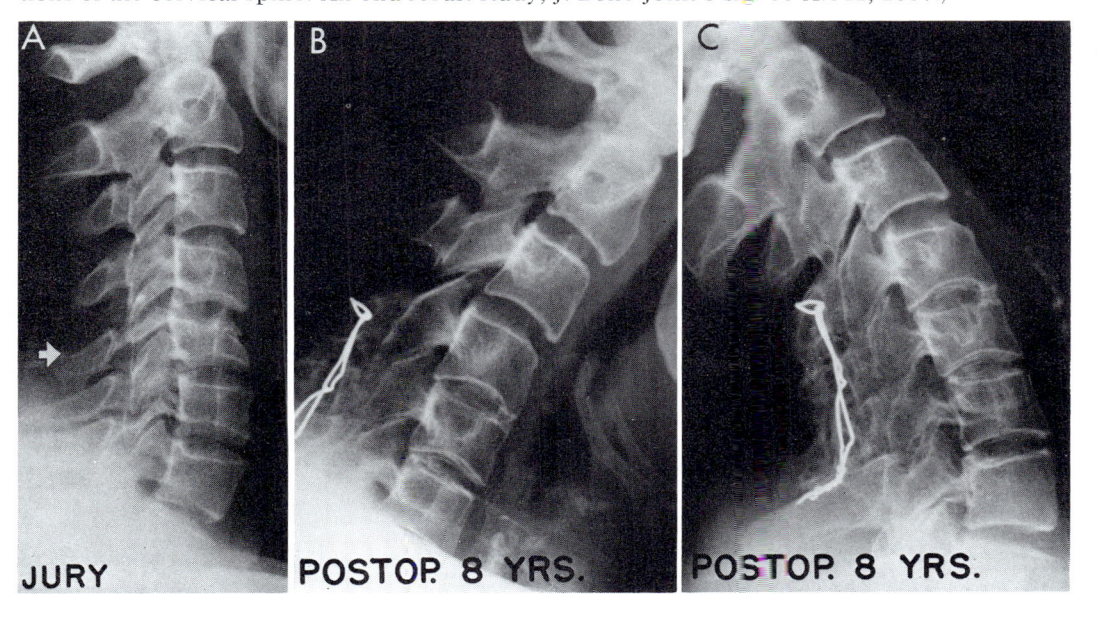

Bursting Fracture of First Cervical Vertebra (Jefferson's Fracture)

As with the bursting fracture of a vertebral body in the lumbar region, bursting fracture of the first cervical vertebra results from violent compression in the long axis of the spine. Usually the patient falls from a height in a manner such that he lands on the top of his head. The condyles of the occiput, which are directed distally and laterally, are forced against the superior articulations of the atlas. Acting as a wedge, the condyles burst the ring of bone which constitutes the atlas. The resulting fracture may be single or

Fig. 16-21.—**A**, anteroposterior and **B**, lateral views of a bursting fracture of the atlas. (The fracture occurred when the horse the patient was riding in a steeplechase refused a jump and the patient was thrown over the fence, landing on the top of his head and bursting the atlas. There were no cord symptoms.) Notable is fracture through the groove of the vertebral artery in the lateral view; also, the fracture through the right lateral mass, including the attachment of the anterior arch of the atlas to the right lateral mass of that bone, in the anteroposterior view. **C**, reduction obtained by skull traction. **D** and **E**, result 12 years after the accident. Patient was symptom-free.

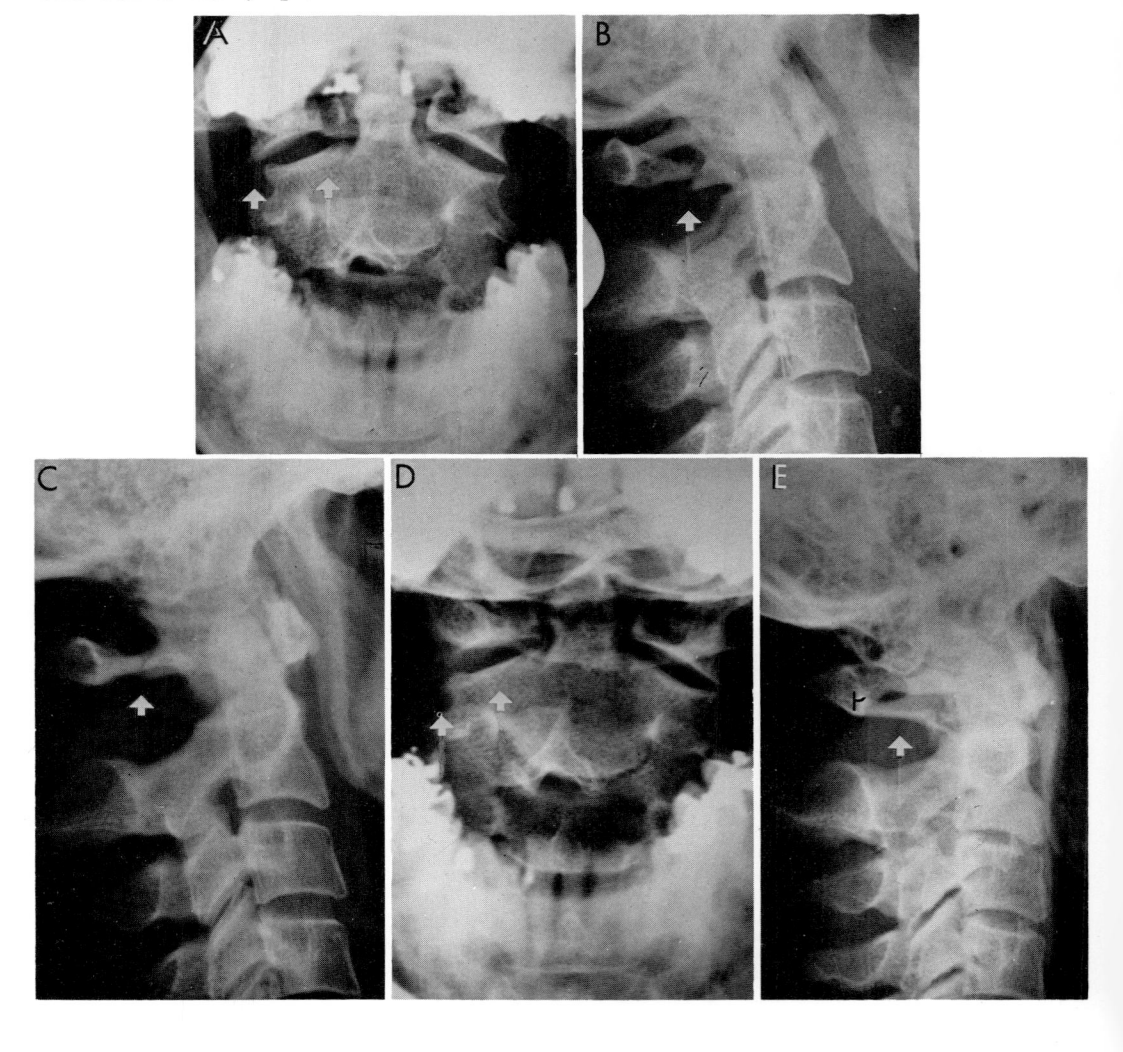

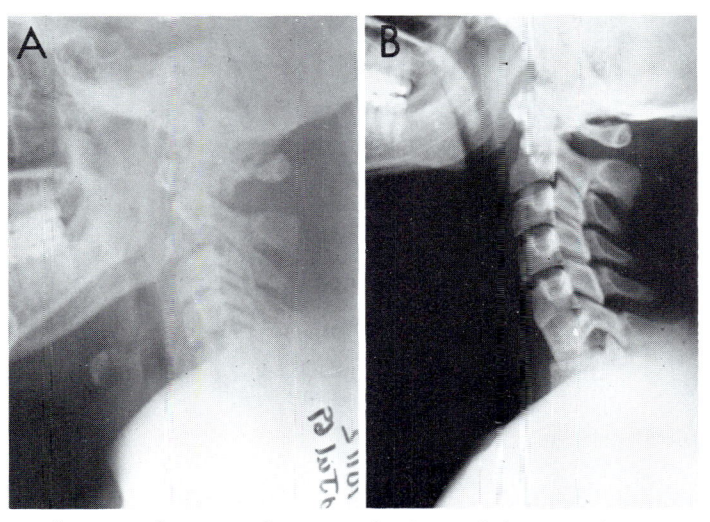

Fig. 16-22.—A, combination bursting fracture of atlas and fracture-dislocation of C5-C6. Patient immobilized in tongs and subsequently in a halo cast; anterior decompression and fibular graft. Patient remained in halo 3 months and recovered 2 full root levels. B, fusion is solid and fractures are healed.

multiple. Posteriorly the fractures occur through the grooves of the vertebral arteries (Fig. 16-21, A). Anteriorly they may occur on either side at the junctions of the anterior arch of the atlas with the lateral masses. The lateral masses of the atlas tend to become displaced laterally (Fig. 16-21, B). This fracture occurred twice in Rogers' series (Fig. 16-22).

It is rare for a patient who survives a Jefferson fracture to have significant cord injury. In 1 case a fracture-subluxation of C5 on C6, was accompanied by severe compression and vertical splitting of the body of C6 and quadriplegia below the C6 root level. The patient was immobilized in a halo brace, myelography and laminagraphy carried out and the body of C6 removed on the fourth postinjury day and replaced with a fibular graft. No treatment beyond the halo brace was given to the bursting fracture of the arch of C1, which healed in a period of 3 months in the brace, as the spinal fusion was also healing. Function of the C7 root returned on the right.

In Rogers' series reduction was accomplished by skull tong traction, and in each of 2 fractures union occurred.

The fracture is too uncommon to have statistical information as to how often pain occurs at the C1–C2 junction after healing. The authors' experience in 2 cases has been that it is severe enough that the patient should be warned at the beginning of treatment that a posterior fusion from occiput to C3 or from C1 to C3 may be necessary because of post-traumatic arthritic pain, secondary to changes in the relative position of the lateral masses.

Bursting Fracture of Vertebral Body

A bursting fracture of a vertebral body results from violent compression of the vertebra between the body of the vertebra above and the body of the vertebra below. Commonly the injury occurs on diving into shallow water. The force is applied directly in line with the long axis of the spine. As in lumbar bursting fractures, the nucleus pulposus of the disk above and that of the disk below are forced into the core of the body, causing it to burst. But unlike some bursting fractures of lumbar vertebrae, in fractures of the cervical vertebrae the cervical body breaks into several large fragments (Fig. 16-7, A). The centrum, as seen in the lateral roentgenogram, appears to have been split into 1 or more anterior fragments and 1 or more posterior fragments. The sharp anteroinferior lip of the centrum above appears to have been driven into the fractured vertebral body, splitting it in the coronal plane. The anterior fragments appear to have tipped backward and superiorly and to have become displaced forward inferiorly. The main posterior fragment is tipped forward and displaced backward inferiorly.

More important is the dangerous backward displacement of the main posterior fragments into the vertebral canal, which may cause cord compression by decreasing the anteroposterior diameter of the vertebral canal. Lateral displacements may cause nerve root compression.

As seen in the anteroposterior roentgenogram, the vertebral body appears to have been split vertically in the sagittal plane (Fig. 16-7, B). In the inferior portion of the vertebral body there may be little or no lateral displacement of the fragments. Presumably the upward lateral projections of the vertebra below prevent this. Superiorly, however, there may be slight but definite lateral displacement of fragments, for the lateral processes of the fractured vertebral body do not clasp the vertebral body above but are spread apart. Each lies lateral to the normal position.

In these fractures, in which such severe skeletal displacement takes place, neurologic symptoms are to be expected and occur frequently. Though often not so, the bursting fracture of a cervical vertebra can be an especially dangerous injury, as it is in other areas of the vertebral column. In Rogers' series there were 12 injuries (14%) in 10 patients, only 2 of whom escaped neurologic changes.

Although skull traction should be used when the halo brace is not available, the preferred treatment of a severe bursting fracture is the halo brace, in which careful manipulation of the fracture may be carried out through the vertical traction bars and the fracture reduced and stabilized in optimal position. Such stabilization alone has resulted in marked improvement in neurologic conditions from the point of view of root recovery in a significant number of patients, even before decompressive surgery was performed.

Removal of the compressing bone fragments and disk material through an anterior approach is recommended for these patients, with anterior fusion in the halo brace being accomplished using either iliac crest or fibular bone.

Unilateral Rotatory Dislocation

Unilateral rotatory dislocation is caused by forcible lateral flexion and rotation of the cervical spine away from the dislocation, as the result either of muscle action or of indirect violence (Fig. 16-8). The dislocation may occur spontaneously in the rheumatoid cervical spine or during sleep in children with upper respiratory tract infections. Such spontaneous dislocations appear to follow abnormal relaxation of the binding ligaments.

There were 9 unilateral rotatory dislocations in 8 patients in the Rogers series. In only 2 patients did symptoms of cord damage develop as a result of the injury. These symptoms, indicative of partial interruption of cord function, appeared in a patient who was struck on the head by a heavy plank and knocked down. They came on immediately after the injury and began to disappear in a few minutes. Motor power returned in 15 minutes. The second patient was thrown through the windshield of an automobile. He immediately became quadriplegic and remained so.

With this type of injury, traction failed to reduce the dislocation in each of the 5 patients on whom it was employed. In 1 patient, skull traction partially reduced the dislocation between the atlas and C2.

Six of the 8 patients in this group were operated on. Open manipulative reduction was successfully performed in 3 patients, and a fusion was carried out. The dislocated vertebra in each of the other 3 patients was fixed by a wire loop and successfully fused to the vertebra below. Fixation and fusion in the latter 3 patients were carried out without reduction because the superior articular process of the vertebra below had been fractured and could not, therefore, be relied on to prevent recurrence of dislocation and to immobilize the spine in the vicinity of the injury. There was no recurrence in the 3 patients in whom the dislocation was reduced. In 4 of the 6 patients operated on, fusion was obtained. Another, an elderly patient with marked marginal lipping died of cord damage during laryngoscopic tracheal intubation (intranasal intubation has been employed in all subsequent cervical spine operations). There was 1 apparent failure of fusion. Six of the 8 patients in this group resumed preinjury activities in an average of 5 months.

Anterior Dislocation

In the cervical spine, anterior dislocation without fracture of the body of the vertebra below occurs chiefly as a result of shearing forces which violently displace a vertebra forward on another; commonly the patient falls, landing on the back of the head. The ligaments which bind the vertebrae together posteriorly are insufficient to withstand such forces. At operation they are found to have been extensively ruptured. Unless muscles act to maintain stability, the dislocating vertebra, no longer held by the posterior ligaments, is displaced anteriorly, often carrying with it the disk above.

If the superior articular processes of the vertebra next below the dislocating vertebra do not fracture as a result of the

Fig. 16-23.—**A,** partial dislocation anteriorly of C5 on C3. The articular processes are still engaged, the dislocating forces having become spent before the displacement was complete. There had been partial loss of cord function immediately after the accident. Neurologically, recovery began soon after and was complete in a few days. Reduction was effected at open operation 4 months later. The vertebrae were fixed with wire, and bone grafts were applied. Fusion was solid in 8 weeks. **B,** appearance 1 year later. Flexion. **C,** extension. Patient had been regularly at work as a deep-sea fisherman for 8 months. (Figs. 16-23–16-28 from Rogers, W. A.: Fractures and dislocations of the cervical spine: An end result study, J. Bone Joint Surg. 39-A:341, 1957.)

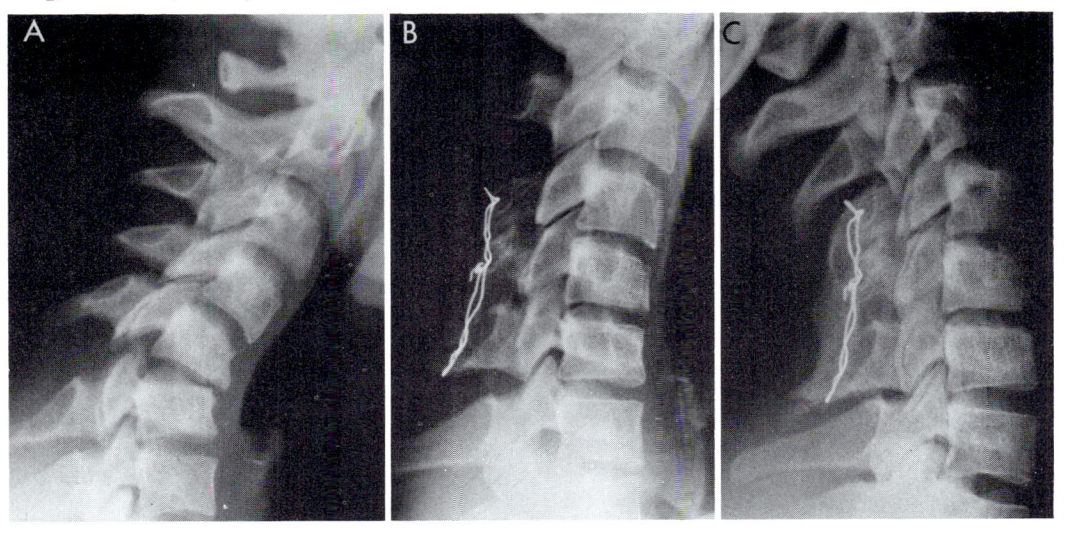

TABLE 16-4.—COMPLETE AND ALMOST COMPLETE INTERRUPTION OF CORD FUNCTION

	IMPROVEMENT TO NORMAL OR ALMOST NORMAL	MODERATE IMPROVEMENT	SLIGHT OR NO IMPROVEMENT	RETURN TO WORK	DEATH DURING OR AFTER TREATMENT	DEATH BEFORE DEFINITE RESULTS OF TREATMENT
Anatomic reduction and operative or spontaneous fusion (9 patients)	5 (55.5%)	..	4 (44.4%)	4	2 (Cord death, 1; pneumonia, 1)	..
Satisfactory reduction without operative or spontaneous fusion (11 patients)	1 (9%)	1 (9%)	9 (82%)	1	8 (Cord death, 5; urinary-tract infection, 2; pulmonary infarct, 1)	..
Unsatisfactory* reduction but operative or spontaneous fusion (1 patient)	1	..	..	..	..	..
Without result from treatment (4 patients)	..	..	..	..	..	4
Total (25 patients)	7 (28%)	1 (4%)	13 (52%)	5	10	4 (16%)

*More than 3-mm. decrease in diameter of vertebral canal.

violence, the posterior elements of the dislocating vertebra are tipped forward and upward by the inclination of the articular facets. The displacement may result in partial or complete dislocation, depending on the magnitude of the violence and the resistance of the column to it. When the inferior articular processes of the dislocated vertebra lie anterior to the superior articular processes of the next vertebra below, the dislocation is complete (Fig. 16-1, A). When they are still posterior, but displaced upward and forward, the dislocation is partial (Fig. 16-23).

In the thoracic spine, anterior dislocation may occur with complete rupture of the disk and of the binding ligaments, the cord is usually transected, and reduction may then take place spontaneously. It seems probable that similar spontaneous reduction may occur in the cervical spine (Fig. 16-5).

There were 31 anterior dislocations without fracture of the vertebral body in 29 patients in the Massachusetts General Hospital series. In 12 of the 29 patients, the symptoms of complete or partial interruption of cord function were present immediately after injury, and in 4 patients, cord interruption occurred subsequent to the injury but before definitive treatment could be established. Seven patients died as a result of complete interruption of cord function (Tables 16-4 and 16-5).

Reduction of the dislocation was effected or maintained by traction in 22 of the 29 patients on whom it was employed—16 by skull traction and 6 by halter traction. Open reduction was performed in 3 patients, in each of whom the reduction was complete. Following reduction, the dislocated vertebra was fixed to the vertebra below with wire, and bone grafts were applied in 15 patients. In another patient, an irreducible dislocation was fused with minor displacement. In each of these 16 patients, solid bone fusion was obtained; 13 of them returned to work, the average time to return being 5 months.

It is now felt that use of the halo and brace for immobilization is preferable, since it eliminates prolonged confinement to bed.

Recurrence of the dislocation followed reduction and prolonged external fixation in 2 patients in this series, in whom no internal fixation or fusion had been done. However, in both, spontaneous interbody fusion occurred in 8 and 9 months, respectively. More recently, when the halo brace has been used, the decision regarding operation has rested on whether or not there was disk and/or end-plate or bone fragments in the spinal cord anteriorly, causing cord compression. When this is felt to be the case, anterior removal of compressing material has been carried out, with an anterior interbody fusion as described previously. When there was no persistent anterior compression, a posterior fusion was usually carried out with wiring of the spinous processes and wiring of bone grafts onto the spinous processes. The cortices of the spinous processes and laminae are generally partially removed with a high-speed air drill.

Anterior Fracture-Dislocation

Anterior fracture-dislocation of cervical vertebral bodies is caused by forces similar to those which produce the anterior dislocation without fracture, with the notable exception that considerable longitudinal compression is present. As a result, a wedge-compression fracture is produced in the subjacent vertebra in

TABLE 16-5.—PARTIAL INTERRUPTION OF CORD FUNCTION

	No. of Patients
Satisfactory reduction and operative or spontaneous fusion	10
Improvement to normal or almost normal	8 (80%)
Marked improvement	1 (10%)
Moderate improvement	1 (10%)
Return to work	8 (av 6 mo)

addition to the forward displacement of the dislocated vertebra. If the injuring forces are then not spent, 1 or both pedicles of the dislocated vertebra may fracture, provided that the posterior articulations hold (Fig. 16-24). In the Massachusetts General Hospital series, there were 9 anterior fracture-dislocations in 8 patients. Pedicle fracture occurred in 2 of the patients.

Symptoms of interruption of cord function were present in 3 of 8 patients; 2 had complete interruption and 1 had partial interruption (Tables 16-4 and 16-5).

Reduction of the fracture-dislocation was effected by traction in 4 of the 8 patients. Open reduction was done in 1 patient. In the 2 patients in whom traction failed to effect a reduction, the injury had occurred 2 and 4 months prior to treatment.

Internal fixation and fusion were employed in 5 patients. In each, solid bone fusion was achieved, and in none was there recurrence. Four of the 5 patients in whom fusion was done resumed work in an average of 4 months. Spontaneous fusion occurred in 2 patients. These 2 patients returned to work in an average of 8 months.

As in anterior dislocations without fracture in the cervical area, the halo and halo brace have become the method of preference, when available, in fracture-dislocations of the cervical spine. The same criteria noted for dislocations of the cervical spine apply to fracture-dislocations. However, in these injuries, the anterior approach with removal of the vertebral body and disks above and below and interbody fusion has been more valuable than in simple dislocations. In compression fractures of the cervical spine without dislocation, posterior fu-

Fig. 16-24.—**A,** an anterior dislocation of C2 on C3, together with a wedge-compression fracture of the body of C3. The pedicles of C2 were fractured. No dislocation of the posterior articulations between these 2 vertebrae was present, and there was no evidence of interruption of cord conductivity. **B,** reduction was effected by traction. The first, second and third vertebrae were wired together, and bone grafts were applied posteriorly across the vertebral arches of the three segments. **C,** roentgenogram 6 months after the operation shows maintenance of reduction and bone fusion. There were no symptoms; patient had been at work for 3 months.

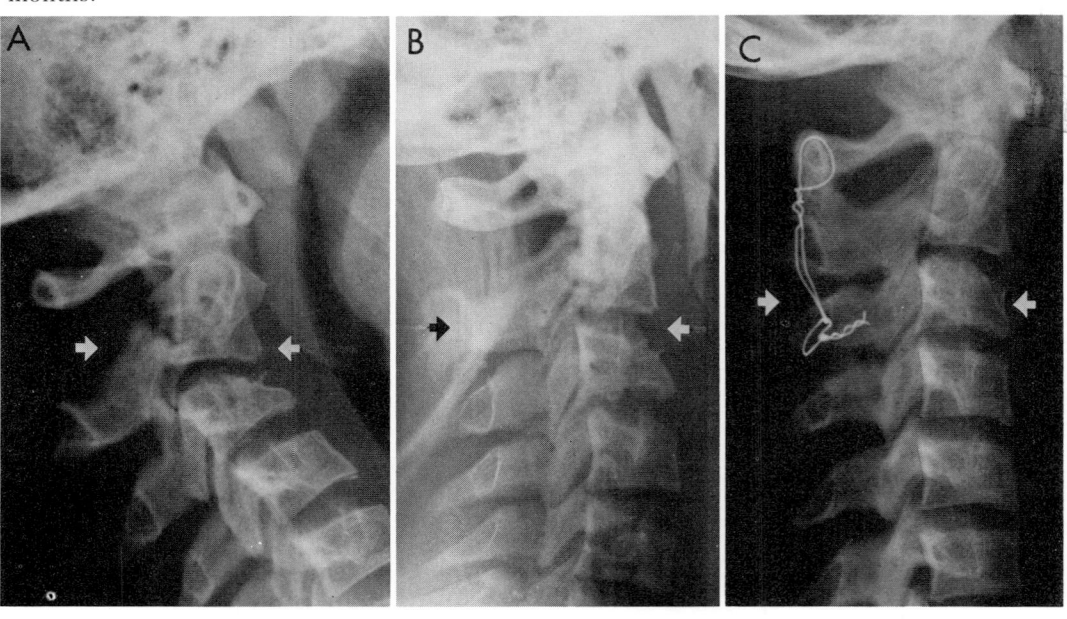

Fracture of Ankylosed Cervical Spine

When a patient with rheumatoid ankylosis of the cervical spine falls, striking his head against an unyielding object, fracture of the ossified longitudinal ligament of the cervical spine may occur between 2 vertebral bodies. Angulation at the fracture site may be forward or backward, depending on the direction of the fracturing forces.

One patient who sustained this injury (Fig. 16-25) had fallen face down, striking his forehead. There were no symptoms referable to the cord and no root symptoms. Correction of the pre-existing flexion deformity was easily effected by skull traction. Refusion occurred spontaneously in 8–10 weeks in a much improved position. The patient returned to work 10 months after the injury.

Similar cases have been reported by Rogers and by Lemmen and Laing,[23] who also found that the previously ankylosed spine usually fused spontaneously after fracture in 6–10 weeks.

Posterior Dislocation

Posterior dislocation is the result of a shearing force applied to the face, as in a fall forward, head first, displacing 1 vertebra backward on another. A. S. Taylor[46] demonstrated the clinical aspects of this injury in severe form and reported autopsy findings. The anterior longitudinal ligament is ruptured at the intervertebral disk immediately below the dislocating vertebra. This disk is completely torn transversely. In turn, the flaval and interspinal ligaments rupture and the vertebra is dislodged backward, drawing with it the intact posterior longitudinal ligament. Marked narrowing of the vertebral canal results, and the cord may be

Fig. 16-25.—**A,** an extension fracture of the ankylosed cervical spine through the level of the fourth intervertebral disk. Despite complete ankylosis of the spine in flexion, the patient had managed to earn a living as a truck driver. Shortly before admission he had fallen from his truck, striking his forehead on the tailboard. There were no neurologic symptoms. The extended position was maintained by skull traction, with some improvement in posture. **B,** refusion took place spontaneously in the improved position in 10 weeks, and the patient resumed work 10 months after injury.

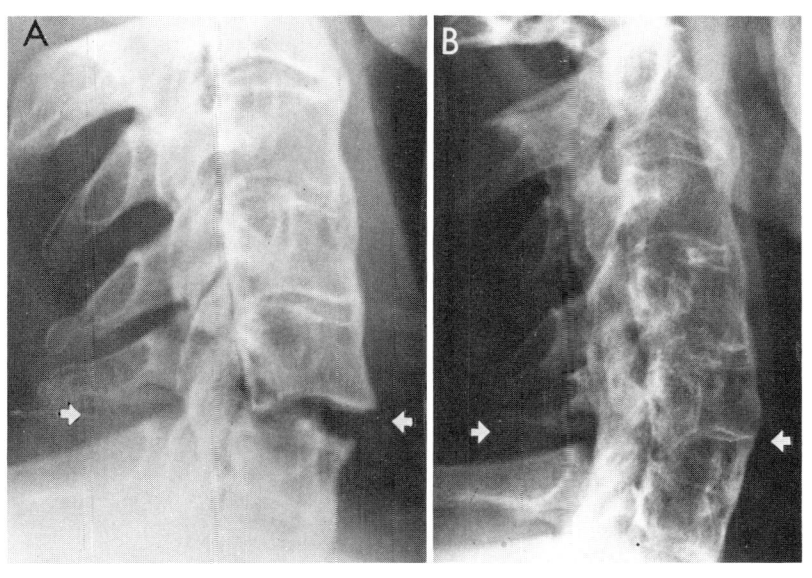

crushed. Spontaneous reduction of the dislocation had occurred in Taylor's patient; the roentgenograms were negative although there was a complete transverse lesion of the cord. In Rogers' series reported here there were 2 patients with posterior dislocations. The lateral view of the cervical spine in 1 patient is shown in Figure 16-26; slight posterior displacement of the third upon the fourth vertebra remains. Both patients had immediate symptoms of cord injury. In 1 of the 2 cases reported, spontaneous interbody fusion occurred and there was rapid improvement in neurologic status to normal; the other patient had no neurologic return and died of urinary tract infection after 7 months. Patients with such injuries who were managed earlier in skeletal traction on Stryker frames are now managed in the halo brace.

Fig. 16-26.—Lateral view of a healed posterior dislocation of C3 on C4 which had been almost completely reduced 6 years before. Interbody fusion occurred between C2 and C3, C4 and C5, and C5 and C6. Patient had recovered almost to normal following quadriplegia.

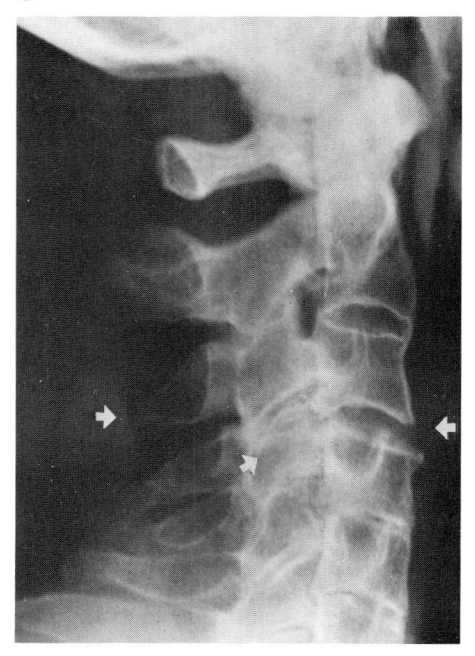

Hyperextension Injuries

Reference has been made earlier to the work of A. R. Taylor, in which the role of extension of the cervical spine in cord injury was demonstrated. As a result of hyperextension the flaval ligaments are compressed, causing them to bulge forward. This may result in cord compression, especially if there is narrowing of the canal due to marginal lipping anteriorly along the posterior borders of the vertebral body. Such lipping is present in many elderly people. There were 2 such cases in Rogers' series. Both patients became quadriplegic through hyperextension, and both died as a result. Both patients were aged and had advanced marginal lipping; in each, hyperextension occurred during treatment of the dislocation. Permission for autopsy was denied.

One of the patients, aged 64, was admitted with a complete anterior dislocation of C5 on C6. He had fallen downstairs 1 week before, striking the back of his neck. There were mild symptoms of nerve root pressure bilaterally in the distribution of the C6 and C7 nerves. There was advanced marginal lipping (Fig. 16-13). Halter traction was applied. Soon after, the patient was reported to have become very restless, tossing about in bed. When re-examined an hour after application of the halter traction, he was found to have become quadriplegic from the C5 level downward. There was a partial block of the cerebrospinal fluid. X-ray films showed reduction with hyperextension of C5 on C6.

The other patient, a woman, aged 62, was admitted with a unilateral rotatory dislocation of C5 on C6; she had fallen downstairs an hour before. There was advanced marginal lipping. Halter traction was applied without effecting a reduction, and 8 days later skull traction was applied for 6 days without success. She was then operated on, open reduction being easily effected with the neck under skull traction. During tracheal intubation with the aid of the laryngoscope for endotracheal anesthesia, the patient's neck was accidentally hyperextended. When she recovered from the anesthesia, she was found to be quadriplegic from the C5 level.

Because of the hazard of hyperextension injuries, laryngoscopic tracheal intubation is contraindicated in surgery of the cervical spine.

Skull traction is indicated in cervical injuries in elderly people, especially in the presence of hypertrophic arthritis with marginal lipping of the vertebral bodies posteriorly.

Halter traction beyond emergency care is contraindicated in all cervical spine injuries, except those in children. If at all effective, it causes discomfort because of undue pressure on bony prominences. Because of skin pressure it is removed from time to time, placing the patient in a situation in which there is neither traction nor any form of immobilization. The use of the halo brace or skeletal traction is by far preferable.

Posterior Fracture-Dislocation

Posterior fracture-dislocation is caused by forcible hyperextension. A backward-displacing force is combined with compression in the long axis of the spine to drive 1 vertebra backward and downward on another, next below, fracturing the latter and dislocating the former posteriorly. A fall downstairs, head foremost, the victim landing on the face, is the usual type of accident. Cord damage may occur (Fig. 16-11).

Fracture of Odontoid Process with and without Dislocation of Atlas

When fracture of the odontoid process occurs without dislocation of the atlas, the fracturing forces seem to be complex. Blockey and Purser[7] have studied the mechanism of fracture of the odontoid process in a series of 46 adults. They feel that any force which violently flexes, extends or rotates the head on the neck may avulse the odontoid process. In the Massachusetts General Hospital series the x-ray appearance of the injured second vertebra suggested the injuring mechanism in 3 of 5 patients with this injury to be forcible flexion and rotation. In each of the patients there appeared to be a crushing of the superior articular process of the second vertebra on 1 side, in addition to the typical odontoid fracture described by Blockey and Purser (Figs. 16-4, A, 16-27 and 16-28, A). In 2 of the 5 patients in this category, a fracture of the odontoid process had occurred without displacement or crushing of either superior articular process.

In only 1 of the 5 patients were there neurologic symptoms, either of cord or nerve root origin. This patient complained of unilateral occipital pain, which proved to be temporary.

Two cases have come to the authors' attention in which 20 and 30 years, respectively, following fractures of the odontoid process with nonunion severe cord symptoms developed. In 1 patient there was migration of the odontoid process into the foramen magnum, reducing the diameter of the cervical spinal canal to 11 mm and causing symptoms of quadriparesis and pain whenever the patient moved the head forward. In the other, syncopal attacks and weakness in both arms occurred on flexion of the neck. In both patients, posterior fusions from occiput to C3 gave relief of symptoms (Fig. 16-29).

Fracture of the odontoid process with anterior dislocation of the atlas apparently results from a violent shearing force directed anteriorly. The ligaments which bind the lateral articulations of the atlas to the second vertebra rupture and the atlas is displaced forward on the axis, carrying with it the odontoid process, which fractures across its base. Should the odontoid process not fracture, the inevitable result must be death from high cord transection.

Alexander et al.[1] found that the majori-

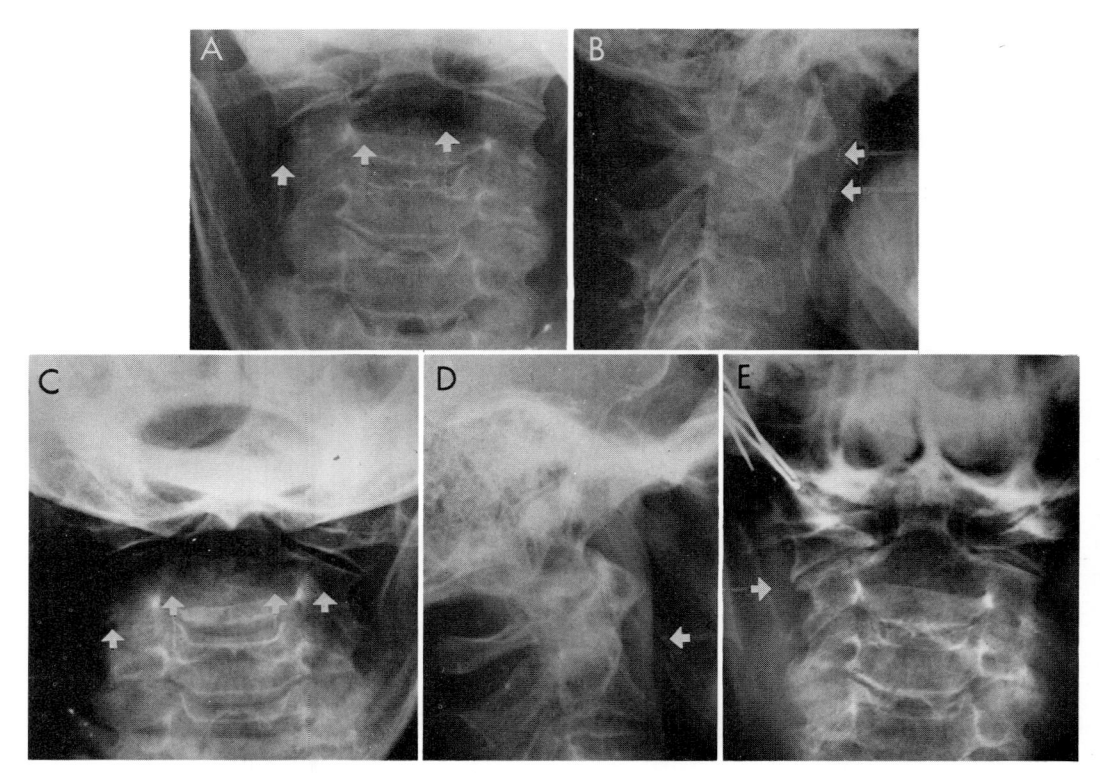

Fig. 16-27. — **A,** anteroposterior and **B,** lateral views of a fracture at the base of the odontoid process and a crush fracture of the right superior articular process of C2. **C** and **D,** only partial correction of the deformity was obtained by skull traction. **E,** result 3 years after injury. There is evidence of traumatic arthritis of the right lateral articulation between the axis and the atlas and depression of the right articular process of the axis. Patient was symptom-free.

ty of surviving patients with this injury have little or no immediate neurologic deficit. However, they summarized the numerous reports in the literature of late complications of nonunited fractures of the odontoid processes, finding recurrent neck stiffness, episodes of neurologic deficit secondary to cord compression and chronically progressive compression of the high cervical cord.

Once the diagnosis is established by x-ray examination, the dislocation is reduced by placing the patient in skeletal traction, preferably a halo apparatus. In cases of acute injury, early fusion is done as soon as the patient's general condition permits, with early ambulation in the halo brace. In chronic dislocation, reduction and fusion can also be accomplished in many cases, since the mechanism of injury is probably the excessive mobility of the upper cervical spine.

Alexander and co-workers prefer fusion of C1, C2 and C3. In 12 patients there was no detectable movement in postoperative flexion and extension films. Satisfactory immobilization has also followed fusion of C1 and C2, as reported by several surgeons, although in 2 cases reported by Alexander x-rays revealed slight residual mobility.

There were 9 fractures of the odontoid process in the Massachusetts General Hospital series. Five occurred without dislocation of the atlas upon the axis; 4 occurred with dislocation of the atlas, 2

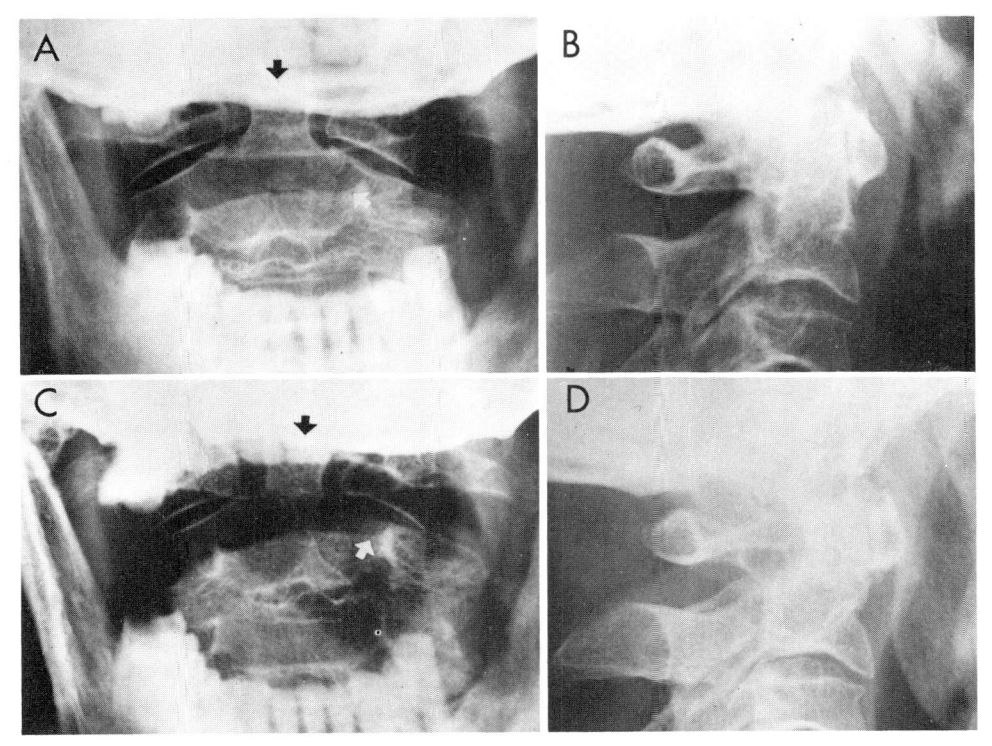

Fig. 16-28.—A, anteroposterior and B, lateral views of a fracture of the odontoid process. Moderate displacement, the process being inclined to the left; and a compression fracture of the left superior articular process of the axis. C and D, union of the fracture occurred with traumatic changes in the left superior articular process of the axis, 4 months after injury. X-ray films were made at follow-up examination at 9 years. (From Rogers, W. A.: Fractures and dislocations of the cervical spine: An end result study, J. Bone Joint Surg. 39-A:341, 1957.)

anteriorly and 2 posteriorly. When displacement of axis fragments was present or there was dislocation of the atlas, skull traction alone was successful in effecting reduction. Wire internal fixation and fusion seem indicated in the presence of old irreducible dislocation, old dislocation following reduction and atlantoaxial instability.

Nonunion of the odontoid process resulted in 4 of the 9 patients. Failure occurred despite there being no displacement of the odontoid process in 2 patients. One had been treated by halter traction and brace fixation; the other had been recumbent under skull traction for 10 weeks. Neither patient had any untoward symptoms as a result; both resumed work. These patients were under observation for 5 and 7 years following injury, 1 first reporting for treatment with established nonunion. The other 2 instances of nonunion were in patients who had received no treatment for their anterior fracture-dislocations. One had been injured 15 years before; the other, 7 months before. Both spines were fused; both united posteriorly, but in each the odontoid failed to unite even after the surgical fusion.

Essential Points

The following factors are important in the treatment of fractures and dislocations of the cervical spine:

380 / Donald S. Pierce and Robert G. Ojemann

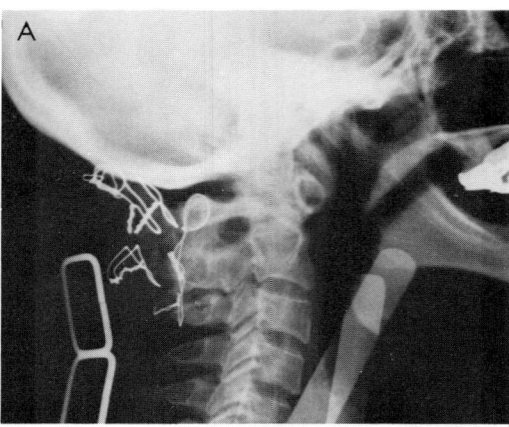

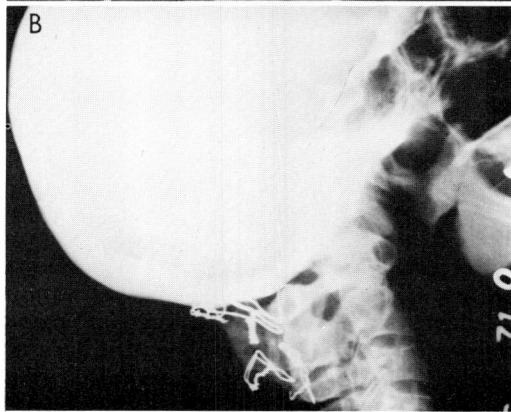

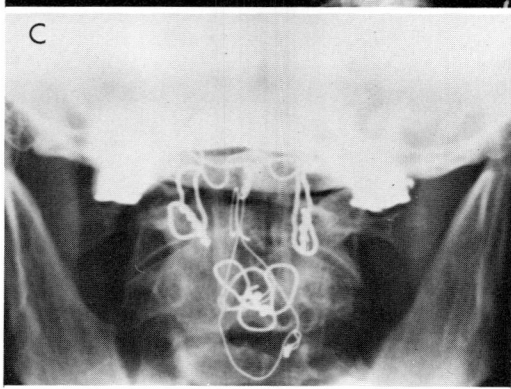

Fig. 16-29.—**A**, odontoid fracture, which occurred 20 years before in teacher, now 55. Note migration of odontoid through foramen magnum. Previous fusion of C2-C3 failed, producing symptoms of quadriparesis and pain in flexion. **B** and **C**, fusion extended to occiput with relief of symptoms.

1. For the dangerous period between the time of injury and definitive treatment, and while the patient is being moved about during definitive treatment, he should at all times be held recumbent, either on a stretcher, bed or frame. An adjustable-traction neck brace should be worn during these times, applied in the long axis of the spine in neutral position. Effective immobilization of the cervical spine in the emergency room prior to detailed study should be the goal of all teams treating spinal injury.

2. Skull traction is the best proved means of protecting the cord during definitive treatment of cervical spine injuries.

3. Skull traction will accomplish reduction and maintain it in a high proportion of injuries. However, rotary motion is still possible with the conventional skeletal traction using tongs or long wires. Frequently a posterior spinal fusion must be done for stabilization, since, even after several months of immobilization in skeletal traction, subluxation of the cervical spine may recur.

The preferred method of reduction and maintenance of reduction of a fracture of the cervical spine is with the halo and halo brace. Rigid immobilization of the cervical spine can be obtained immediately and the patient mobilized. Spinal fusion is then possible, if necessary.

4. Fracture of the cervical spine often results in compression of the cervical spine and root by fragments of disk, endplate and bone. When these compress the spinal cord roots from the front, they can be removed using an anterior approach while maintaining spinal stability in the halo and halo brace.

Reduction in the halo and halo brace has been followed by root recovery and is the procedure of choice. Anterior cervical fusion for fracture is indicated when compressing material lies anterior to the cord. Spontaneous bony healing without surgery may be allowed to take place with the spine securely fixed in the halo brace without surgical fusion.

5. Internal fixation and surgical fusion provide reliable stabilization of the injured vertebrae. These procedures appear to protect the cord against attrition in patients with a vertebral canal of less than normal diameter and to allow root recovery in instances in which continued motion would cause irritation, inflammation and swelling and prevent such recovery.

6. The treatment of cervical spine injuries is highly specialized; technical errors in treatment may be fatal. A trained and experienced team is essential.

THE THORACIC SPINE (UPPER 10 THORACIC VERTEBRAE)

In the upper 10 thoracic vertebrae, fractures and fracture-dislocations are less common. Stability characterizes this segment of the spine, with its narrow intervertebral disks, relatively flat vertebral end-plates and attached rib cage. As a result, the thoracic spine is comparatively rigid and compression-flexion forces are transmitted to the more mobile, less stable lumbar or cervical segments, where these injuries are far more apt to occur.

Wedge-Compression Fracture

When the spine is significantly osteoporotic, wedge-compression fractures are not uncommon in the thoracic vertebrae. They may occur singly or be multiple, and they may be found in association with the same type of fracture in the lumbar region. Biconcave vertebrae also may be found in both of these segments in the osteoporotic spine, owing to the vertical compression of the soft bone above and below by the nucleus pulposus. These fractures may be overlooked because they result from minor traumas, such as a mild lifting strain when the spine is in the forward-bent position, or even from rising suddenly from a chair or bed, or sitting down heavily. Rest in bed (for several days to several weeks) will usually suffice to relieve the pain, and gradual resumption of activity is then permitted. Reduction is unnecessary, and immobilization in extension in plaster-of-paris jackets is inadvisable. The support will only cause further bone atrophy.

Uncommonly, a thoracic vertebra (upper 10) of normal density becomes compressed into a wedge shape. Correction of such fractures and fixation in extension with the plaster-of-paris jacket, often important in the lumbar spine, are usually unnecessary when the fracture is in the thoracic spine. The reason for this lies in the innate stability of this segment of the vertebral column. Patients become symptom-free and resume preinjury activities after a shorter period of disability without reduction and jacket fixation. Rest in bed until the patient is free from pain, early active exercises to develop the spinal extensors, and a gradual resumption of activities will yield consistently good results.

ADOLESCENT EPIPHYSITIS. — The wedge-shaped deformities seen in the lateral roentgenograms of thoracic vertebrae resulting from active or healed adolescent epiphysitis (Scheuermann's disease) are not to be mistaken for wedge-compression fractures. They may be distinguished by the presence of characteristic hernial protrusions of disk tissue into the involved centra, by the absence of convexity of the anterior walls of these bodies and, in individuals over 35 years of age, by proliferative bone changes along the margins of the disks.

Fracture-Dislocation

Fracture-dislocation in the thoracic region is not common for the same reason that wedge-compression fracture is not common — the high degree of stability of the thoracic spine (Fig. 16-30). Great violence is necessary to produce this injury, and the spinal cord may be irreparably damaged when it occurs. Open reduction, on the front or laterally through a

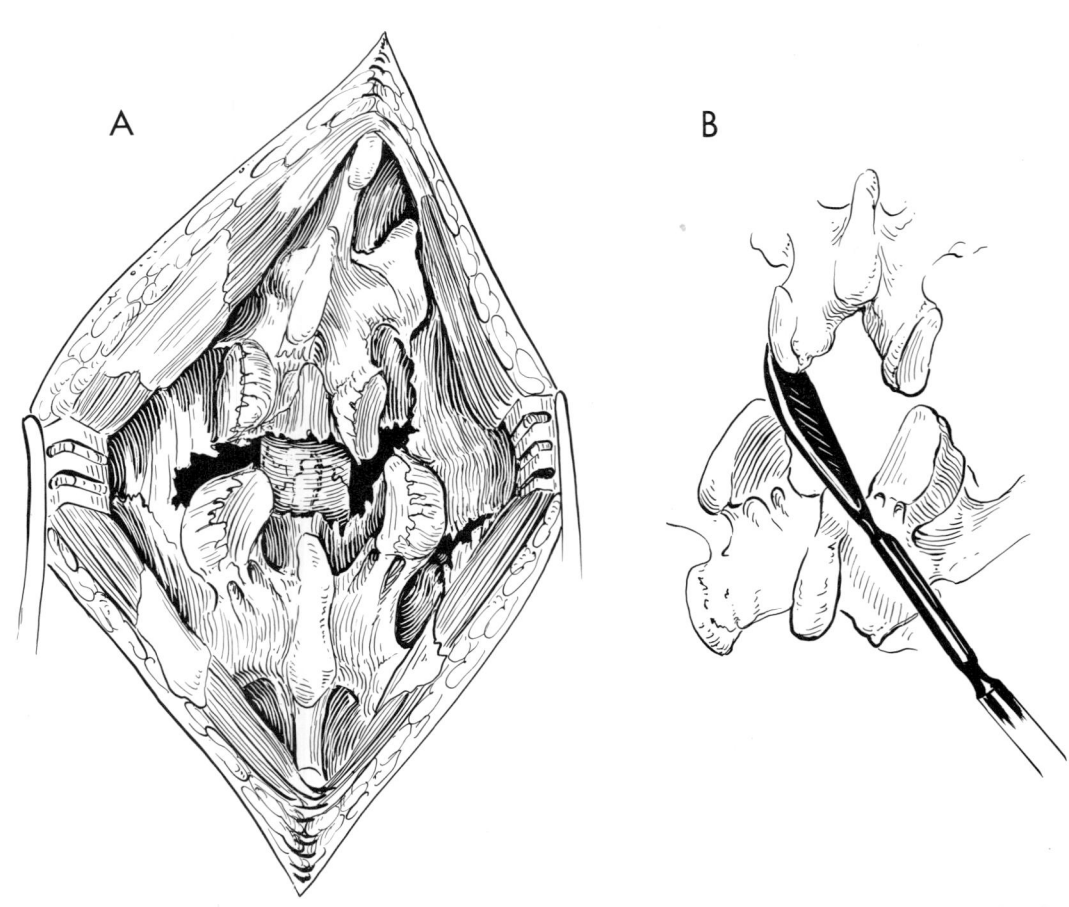

Fig. 16-30.—By flexing the spine the articular processes are disengaged. **A**, as seen by the surgeon. **B**, the inferior articular processes of the dislocated vertebra are pried into normal alignment. The spine may then be extended and the reduction completed by raising the ends of the table.

costotransversectomy approach, should be carried out in preference to a laminectomy, unless there is actual damage to posterior elements. In the series of Morgan, Wharton and Austin[25] a number of patients with thoracic spine fractures worsened after laminectomy. A laminectomy in this area, as in the cervical spine, tends to destabilize the spine itself. If the compression is from the front, caused by a bolus of herniated disk material, endplates and bone fragments, the laminectomy may not effectively decompress the cord. The further bony deformity that may result from the removal of ligaments and muscles posteriorly in the area of laminectomy may cause additional injury to the spinal cord and/or root or may in fact bring about injury where little or no injury was present. Removal of the offending bolus of compressing material can easily be accomplished anteriorly, and if the semicircular arcades, which give supply to the anterior spinal arteries from the thoracic area, particularly from T6 to T9, are not cut across, there need be no fear of devascularizing the spinal cord.

Partial or total reduction of the fracture may be accomplished at this time and anterior interbody fusion carried out with

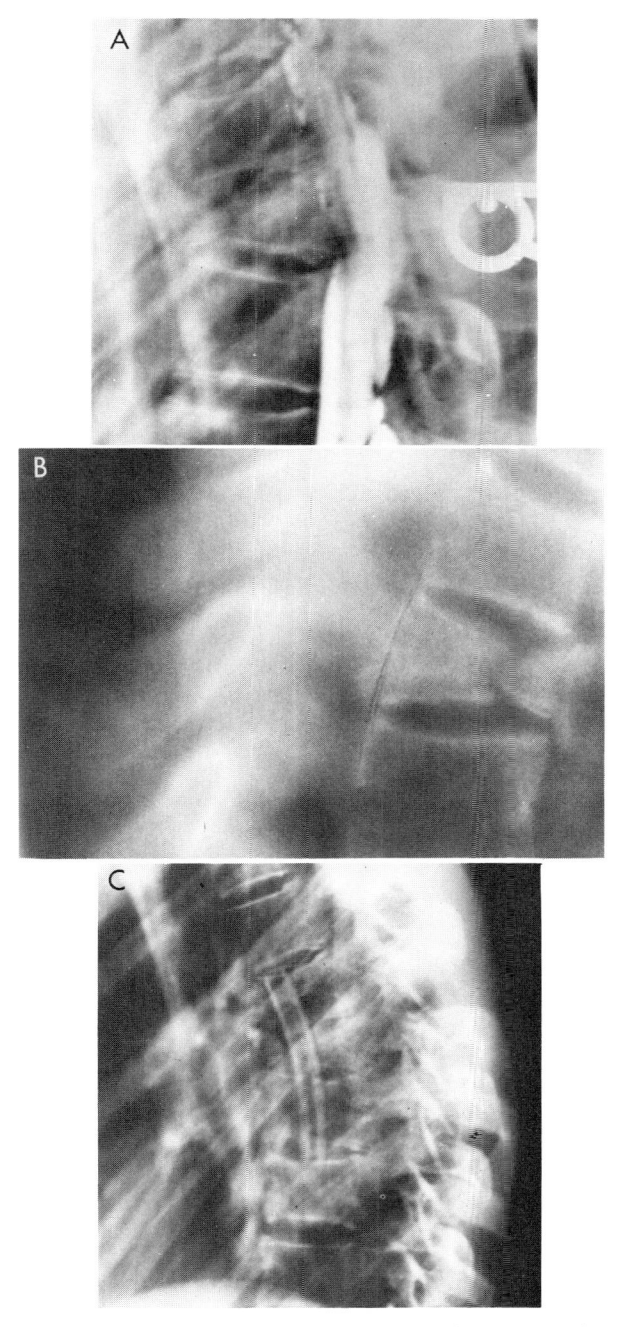

Chapter 16: INJURIES TO THE SPINE: NEUROLOGIC CONSIDERATIONS / 383

Fig. 16-31.—A, lateral view of T6. Apparent compression fracture with partial myelographic block and symptoms of cord bladder. B, laminagram reveals a bursting component with potential for instability. C, transthoracic decompression of cord and fusion with rib graft and cancellous bone 3 weeks after injury. Total neurologic recovery followed surgery.

a rib graft and/or iliac bone. (Fig. 16-31). In 1 patient, such a procedure was done 1 month after laminectomy and posterior fusion without neurologic return and yielded within 5 days complete return of function 8 levels below the injury. In a second patient, who had nearly total dislocation of the spine at the T10–T11 level, root recovery 4 levels below the level of injury followed anterior decompression and fusion 6 months after the initial injury when posterior laminectomy and fusion had yielded no return.

In another case involving total transection of the spine at T3–T4, a thoracotomy was carried out at the T4 level. Incision was made over the fourth rib and was carried up along the midline of the spine posteriorly. Initially, the fracture-dislocation was explored anteriorly, and a rib strut placed centrally across the fracture anteriorly. Subsequently, in the same operation, Meurig-Williams spinal plates were applied posteriorly across the area where the posterior elements were completely shattered, and iliac bone was laid across this area as well. The patient was in a wheelchair 2½ weeks later, pulling weights with his arms in physical therapy. A 5-month follow-up showed both fusions going on to solid union and no movement of the Meurig-Williams plates. As the cord was totally transected at the time of injury, there was no danger of further neurologic injury; the anterior grafting gave initial stability to an otherwise unstable spine, allowing early mobilization.

Patients who had such a procedure previously were kept supine, with the head of the bed elevated no more than 45 degrees, for a period of 6 weeks to 3 months or until there was x-ray evidence of fusion.

It has been the authors' practice in the past 2 years to do a single operation, as noted above for extreme instability, for the anterior and posterior stabilization of a thoracic fracture or to do either a posterior stabilization with Meurig-Williams spinal plates and posterior fusion or an anterior decompression and interbody fusion with rib graft inlaid across the area of injury, whichever procedure would yield the greater early stability. With these procedures, which give early spinal stability, the patient can be mobilized almost immediately. A Jewett or Norton-Brown brace with anterior horns across the chest is utilized during the early stages of mobilization in a wheelchair.

THE LUMBAR SPINE (INCLUDING T11 AND T12)

The 2 common fractures of the lumbar spine are the wedge-compression fracture of the vertebral body and the fracture of the transverse process. Less common is the bursting fracture of the vertebral body. The fracture-dislocation is uncommon. As separate entities, fractures of the articular and spinous processes, of the laminae and of the pedicles are almost rarities. The hyperextension vertebral body fracture is rare compared to the flexion type.

Wedge-Compression Fracture

Forcible hyperflexion of the lumbar region of the spine results in compression of the vertebral body into a wedge shape. The apex of the wedge is usually directed forward; less frequently it points laterally (Figs. 16-32 and 16-33).

It is usually the anterosuperior portion of the centrum which is compressed. Uncommonly, the anteroinferior portion is involved. Since most of the vertebral body is composed of cancellous bone, much of the compression takes place through meshing of the trabeculae. The superior articular end-plate of the compressed vertebra is usually fragmented, and there is often tearing of the fibers of the annulus fibrosus. Through the rents in the annulus the nucleus pulposus of the damaged disk is sometimes forced along the fracture fissures into the core of the centrum. These changes often result

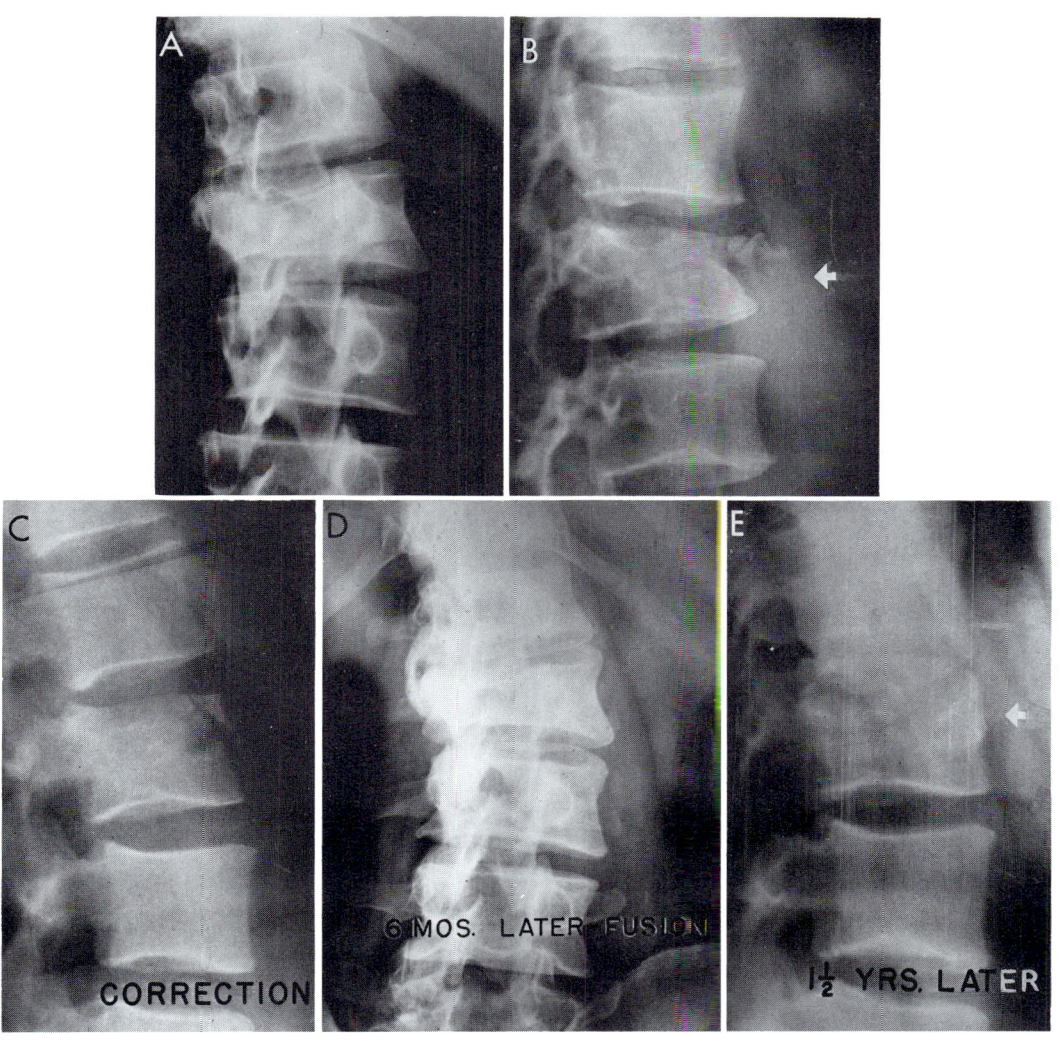

Fig. 16-32.—A, the common wedge-compression fracture with apex of the wedge pointing anterolaterally. B, with apex of wedge directed forward—the usual case. C, correction of the anterior crushing. D, lateral crushing persists; bone bridging complete 6 months later. E, lateral view 1½ years after injury. (From Rogers, W. A.: Treatment of fractures of vertebral bodies uncomplicated by lesions of the cord, Arch. Surg. 30:284, 1935.)

in replacement of the disk by scar tissue, with loss of the normal disk mechanics, and a decrease in the intervertebral spacing results. Such changes were noted in 26 of a series of 31 patients at the Massachusetts General Hospital (Figs. 16-6 and 16-33). The later changes are degenerative, with marginal lipping, subchondral bone sclerosis and spontaneous intervertebral fusion.

In the wedge-compression fractures there is no element of dislocation of the vertebra as a whole, the vertebral canal is not decreased in diameter and the posterior wall of the centrum remains intact. The interspinal and flaval ligaments at-

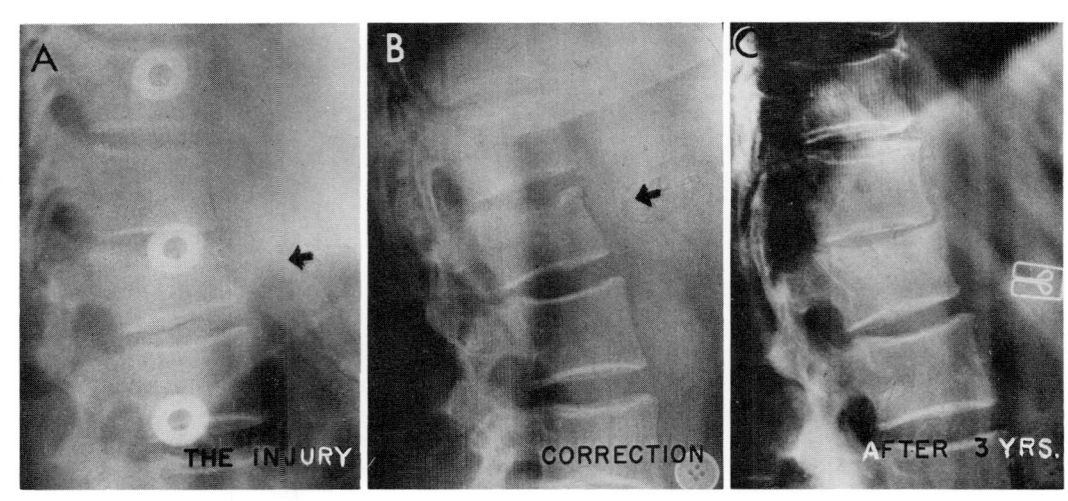

Fig. 16-33.—**A,** wedge-compression fracture of L1. Slight anterior dislocation, but posterior wall of the centrum is intact. **B,** hyperextension of the spine while under traction has restored the shape of the crushed vertebra almost to normal. **C,** the fractured vertebra 3 years later. No loss of bone correction. The intervertebral spacing is decreased.

tached to the posterior bone structures may be mildly sprained. If there is evidence of severe softpart injury posteriorly, one must at once suspect subluxation.

Compression fractures are common in osteoporosis.

Great violence is not necessary to produce this fracture. The usual history is of a fall, the patient landing on the feet, buttocks or shoulders; of an automobile accident; or of a heavy object falling on the shoulders. The spine is hyperflexed anteriorly or laterally.

In the thoracolumbar or lumbar region, pain and tenderness may be present, localized in the region of, and deep to, the spinous processes of the involved vertebra.

Painstaking examination with the aid of x-ray is indispensable. The usual lateral and anteroposterior exposures should be made. If there is any doubt, the x-rays should be directed obliquely through the posterior articulations on both sides. Vertebral subluxation must always be excluded. If 1 or more of the vertebral bodies are compressed into a wedge shape, the posterior wall of each of the involved centra should be carefully checked in the lateral roentgenogram for any evidence of fracture. If plain films leave any doubt, sagittal laminagrams must be resorted to. The presence or absence of fracture fissures or compression (as in bursting fractures) or subluxation must be determined beyond a doubt. (Figs. 16-2 and 16-3).

TREATMENT.—Mild wedge-compression fractures in which no element of dislocation and no fracture involving the posterior wall of the centrum has been demonstrated may be treated without reduction as a ligamentous injury. This method has been strongly advocated by Nicoll,[26] and it appears to have met with some success in Great Britain and on the Continent in more severe fractures of the vertebral bodies. The patient should be confined to bed for 2–3 weeks, but without other early immobilization. After a few days, as the pain subsides, active exercises may be begun which develop the erector spinae muscles. As the patient becomes ambulatory, a back brace must be worn for a period of 6 weeks to 3 months.

The results of treatment by this method

have been satisfactory, provided the degree of wedge deformity is slight (the amount of compression has been arbitrarily set at less than one-fourth the vertical diameter of the vertebral body at the anterior wall) and the patient does not resume an athletic or physically laborious life.

Since hyperflexion and compression forces produce the fracture and the deformity, restoration of the shape of the vertebra may be expected by reversing these forces. Actually, extension and traction may restore the wedge-compression centrum almost to its preinjury form (Fig. 16-32). During extension and traction the anterior longitudinal ligament gradually tightens. Through Sharpey's fibers, this ligament gains attachment not only to the cortex of the vertebral body anteriorly and laterally, but to cancellous elements deep within. Thus, as the ligament becomes taut, at the normal limit of extension, the compressed fragments of bone are decompressed and pulled back into almost normal position, the shape of the body being almost completely restored. Reductions carried out to the absolute limit of normal extension may restore the shape of the compressed vertebra to such an extent that gross angulation of the spine at the level of the fracture is avoided. Often, compressed vertebral bodies may be restored practically to normal. Extension of the spine to less than the absolute limit will fail to achieve a satisfactory reduction.

Fracture-Dislocation

When the lumbar segment of the spine is violently hyperflexed, the column is subjected to a bending force, directed forward or laterally, and to a compression force, exerted longitudinally. If an injury occurs in which the bending force almost wholly predominates, as in seat belt injuries, that portion of the column to which the force is being applied may be driven forward onto a fixed portion until the articular processes are sheared or slip off to become dislocated; posterior ligaments and muscles may sometimes rupture, laminae may fracture and dislocation of the vertebra and the portion of the column above may occur. Such injuries result from great violence. Usually the vertebral column is subjected to both forces, longitudinal compression combining with the horizontally directed force to drive a portion of the column forward and downward onto a fixed portion. If the hyperflexing forces are not spent in the production of sprain, where the portion of the column that is being driven forward contacts the fixed portion, fragmentation or simple wedge-compression of the uppermost fixed vertebral body will occur. If, then, the column is forced still further beyond the limit of hyperflexion, posterior ligaments, fascia and even the erector spinae muscles may rupture; articular processes may tear apart and become dislocated or fractured; laminae or spinous processes may fracture; and the vertebral body next above may dislocate forward or laterally on the fractured vertebral body. The cord or cauda equina may be compressed between the neural arch of the dislocated vertebra and the posterosuperior lip of the vertebra below, or may be compressed by disk tissue displaced as the result of the dislocation.

When the full extent of the fracture may not be appreciated in plain films, or when there is a question as to whether or not surgical intervention is necessary, laminagrams should routinely be employed.

One of the most common fractures of this area is the slice fracture-dislocation, usually seen at the thoracolumbar junction, in which a vertical compression force is combined with a rotatory one. The upper vertebra takes the disk below with it, as well as a "teardrop" fragment consisting of the upper anterior portion of the vertebra below. Often posterior elements are either fractured or dislocated in a rotary fashion, and in all cases ligamentous damage is severe. Such fracture-dislocations are notoriously unstable and do not heal unless accurately reduced by closed or open methods.

The neurologic injury is often severe. However, at this level a peripheral nerve, i.e., root, injury results in most cases, as it is the conus medullaris that occupies this area of the spinal canal. In incomplete neurologic injury, therefore, neurologic return is a possibility if orthopedic management provides a stable spinal column and proper alignment.

THE REDUCTION OF FRACTURE-DISLOCATION.—If 1 vertebral body is displaced forward on another and the dislocated inferior articular processes are out of alignment with their articulating fellows of the vertebra below, spinal extension without surgery will fail to reduce the dislocation. The articular processes of the 2 vertebrae may lock during attempted extension, blocking reduction; or they may cause compression of the cord or cauda equina. Manipulative extension, alone, to reduce this dislocation should never be attempted. With each increment of extension, the malaligned neural arch of the dislocated vertebra will either lock more tightly with the neural arch next below or will protrude further into the neural canal and ultimately compress the cord (Fig. 16-34) or cauda equina. Open operative reduction is indicated.

For open operative reduction the patient is placed on the surgical table in the prone position, with the dislocated vertebra directly above the break in the table (Fig. 16-35). Under general anesthesia with endotracheal tube, the spine is exposed in the area of injury and inspected. The neural arches of the dislocated vertebrae are exposed subperiosteally. The articular processes will be seen to have become dislocated, the inferior processes of the dislocated vertebrae being anterior to their articulating fellow below. One or both of each pair may be fractured; they may have become displaced to 1 side or the other. If there is a fracture of the body, the lower ones may actually have become widened (Fig. 16-36).

When the dissection of the 2 arches has

Fig. 16-34.—Drawings showing effect of extension on the anteroposterior diameter of the vertebral canal in fracture-dislocation when the pairs of articular processes do not engage normally. If the processes do not become locked to prevent further extension, 1 or both will rotate forward into the vertebral canal, as the spine is extended, until finally the cord is compressed. (From Rogers, W. A.: Cord injury during reduction of thoracic and lumbar vertebral-body fracture and dislocation, J. Bone Joint Surg. 20:689, 1938.)

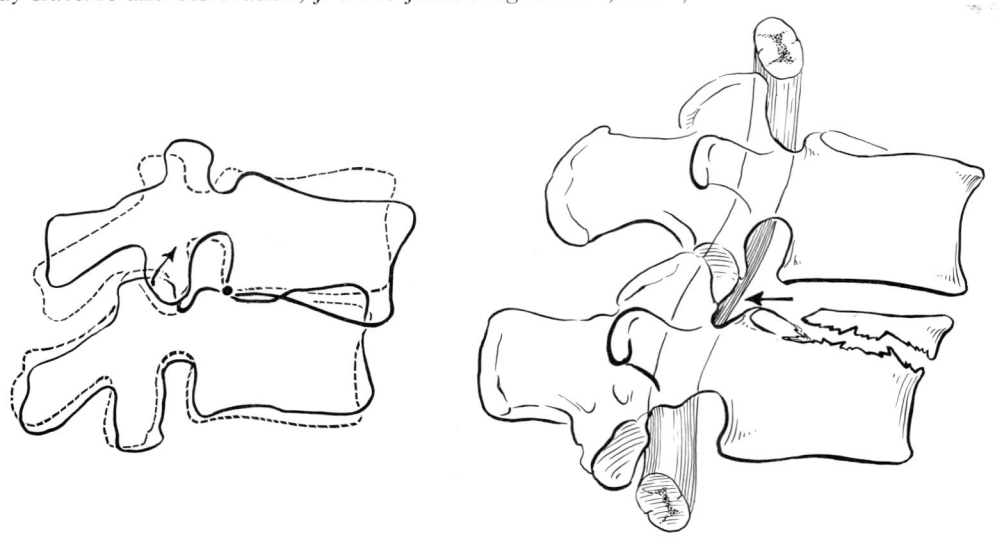

Chapter 16: INJURIES TO THE SPINE: NEUROLOGIC CONSIDERATIONS / 389

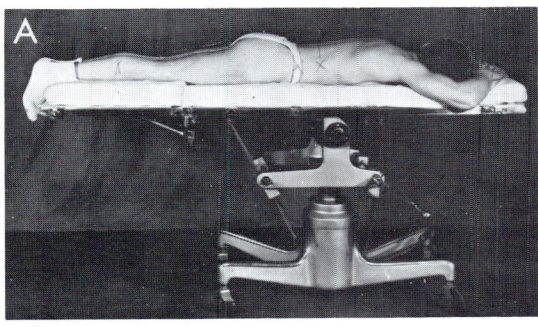

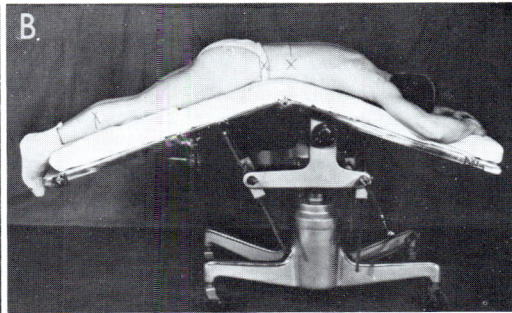

Fig. 16-35.—Position on the table for open reduction of fracture-dislocation (lumbar). **A,** level of the injury is directly above the axis, about which the ends of the table may be lowered. **B,** flexion may be obtained under complete control by lowering the ends of the table.

been completed, it becomes apparent that it is necessary to be able to see the disaligned articular processes before they can be maneuvered back into position. Reduction can hardly be accomplished without open operation. By

Fig. 16-36.—Drawing of a locked and overridden articular process as seen from behind.

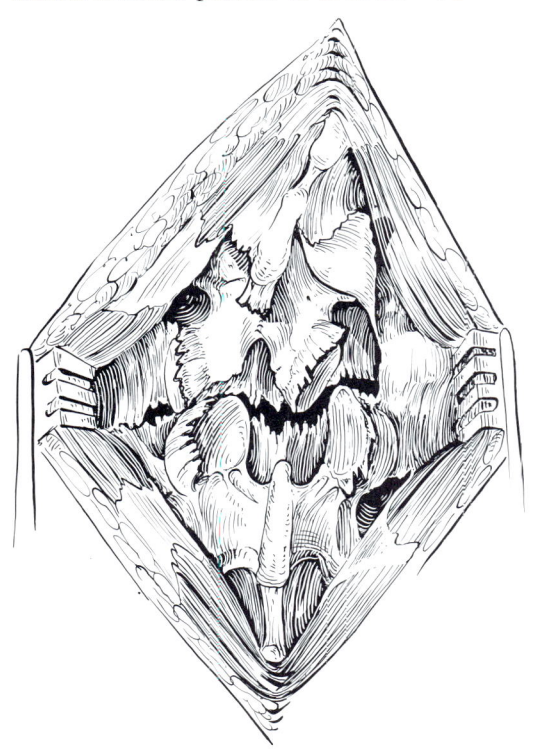

being able to see the dura mater, the surgeon can at all times be assured that the cord is not being injured during the manipulations necessary to reduction.

If there is overriding, the processes may be disengaged by powerful manual traction and countertraction applied under the surgical drapes by assistants. This method may fail of its object, however. In that event, enough bone should be trimmed from the articular processes to permit reduction by having the anesthetist hyperextend the operating table slowly under direct vision, with the ends under direct manual control. In some cases, locked processes may be freed by gently flexing the spine under direct vision (Fig. 16-30). Once freed and in normal alignment, these processes can be made to engage their articulating fellows. Once the articulating processes have been made to engage, the reduction is completed and held by hyperextension of the operating table. Meurig-Williams spinal plates are then applied across the area of the fracture-dislocation and are bolted through 2 normal vertebral spinous processes below the area of the dislocation (Fig. 16-37). The laminae and spinous processes are then denuded with a Hall drill or Cobb gouges and a posterior fusion with iliac graft performed. The plates should never be used as an immobilizing device alone. Cartilage should be stripped from the facet joints at this

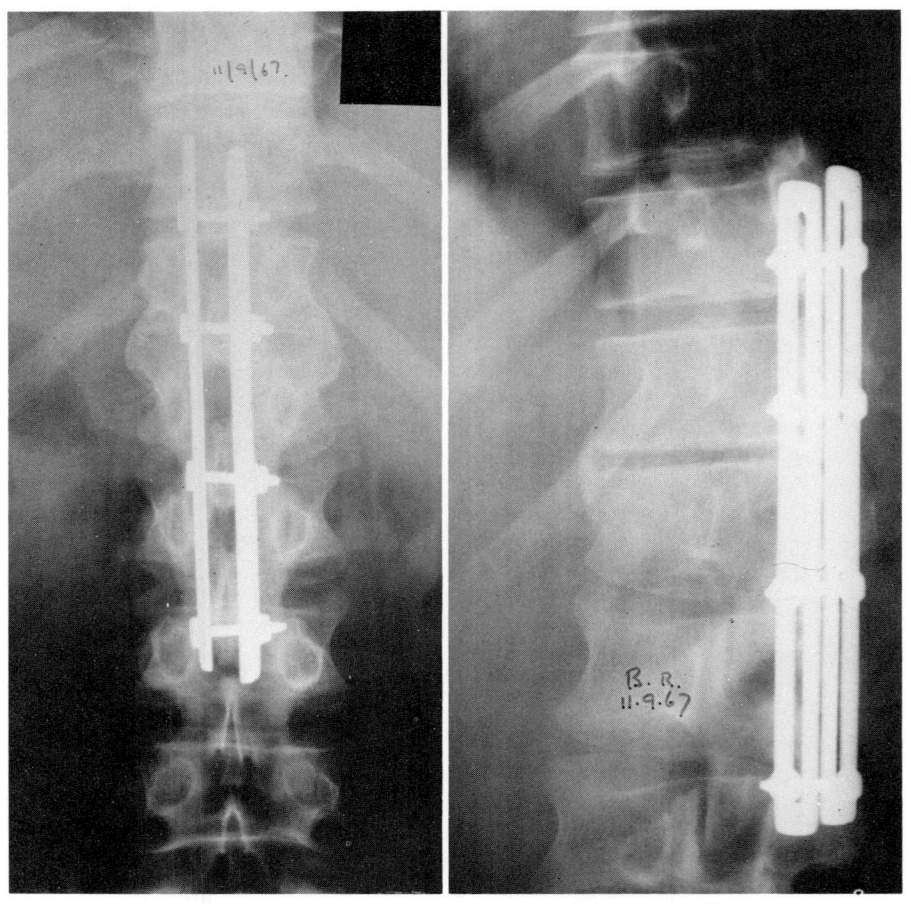

Fig. 16-37.—Fracture-dislocation of T12–L1 facets, totally dislocated, in man, 25. Operative reduction. Anesthesia lightened inadvertently, allowing patient to cough, and redislocation occurred under direct vision. Meurig-Williams spinal plates were applied to maintain reduction; iliac bone grafts were placed beside spinal plates. Patient was without pain and the spine was stable 6 months later.

time and all facet joints fused, with cancellous bone grafts placed between them.

Bursting Fracture of the Vertebral Body

A bursting fracture of the vertebral body in the lumbar spine is caused by longitudinal compression of the spine. The horizontal force component, predominant in wedge-compression fractures, is negligible or absent in this fracture. The nucleus pulposus of the intervertebral disk above and, in more violent injuries, the nucleus pulposus of the disk below are driven by the compressing force into the core of the vertebral body. One or both of the articular end-plates are fragmented and the vertebral body is compressed. If the compression force is not then spent, the walls of the centrum burst and bone fragments may be displaced outward in all directions (Fig. 16-38). If there is backward displacement of bone, the cord or nerve roots may be compressed. Fracture of the calcaneus is not uncommonly associated.

When there are no symptoms of cord or nerve root pressure and there is no very

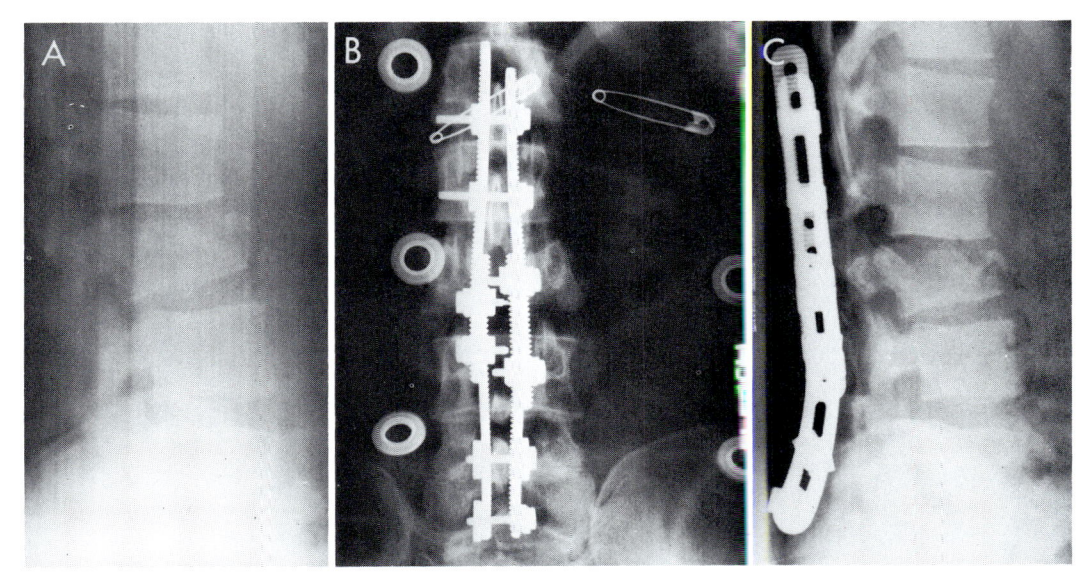

Fig. 16-38.—**A**, bursting fracture of lumbar vertebra in student, 18, who fell from a dormitory window, landing on the buttocks. Total paraplegia below the L4 level resulted. **B** and **C**, treatment included removal of bone fragments and disk material, stabilization with Meurig-Williams spinal plates and the addition of iliac bone grafts posteriorly.

definite decrease in the anteroposterior diameter of the neural canal, patients with this fracture may be treated by plaster-jacket fixation. Attempts at reduction have not been successful, although the advent of the Meurig-Williams plates makes stable fixation and operative fusion possible. The use of such plates is advocated when disruption of the vertebra is extreme.

Discarding of the jacket should be postponed until bone repair is adequate. This may require 4–6 months or longer.

When there is a definite decrease in the diameter of the vertebral canal but no symptoms of cord or nerve root pressure, spinal fusion is indicated to stabilize the spine and safeguard against late neurologic changes.

When symptoms of cord or root compression are present, decision must be made as to whether laminectomy or an anterior approach to the spine should be made. If a compressing material can be removed from the nerve root from a posterior approach, this is the procedure of choice. A foramenotomy and laminectomy are performed, after which Meurig-Williams spinal plates are applied and a posterior spinal fusion done. If there is central compression of the cauda equina and/or spinal root at the level of the lower thoracic or lumbar spine, operation through an anterior approach or posterolaterally through a costotransversectomy approach should be done. After the compressing material is removed, an anterior interbody fusion is carried out (Fig. 16-39).

The importance of early decompression of the traumatically compressed cauda equina is emphasized by the fact that some improvement in neurologic function may be found even when the compression is removed several months after injury.[22]

FRACTURES OF THE TRANSVERSE PROCESSES

In fractures of the transverse processes, the usual history is that of a fall, a blow on the back or a violent wrench of the trunk in an effort to maintain equilibrium, as

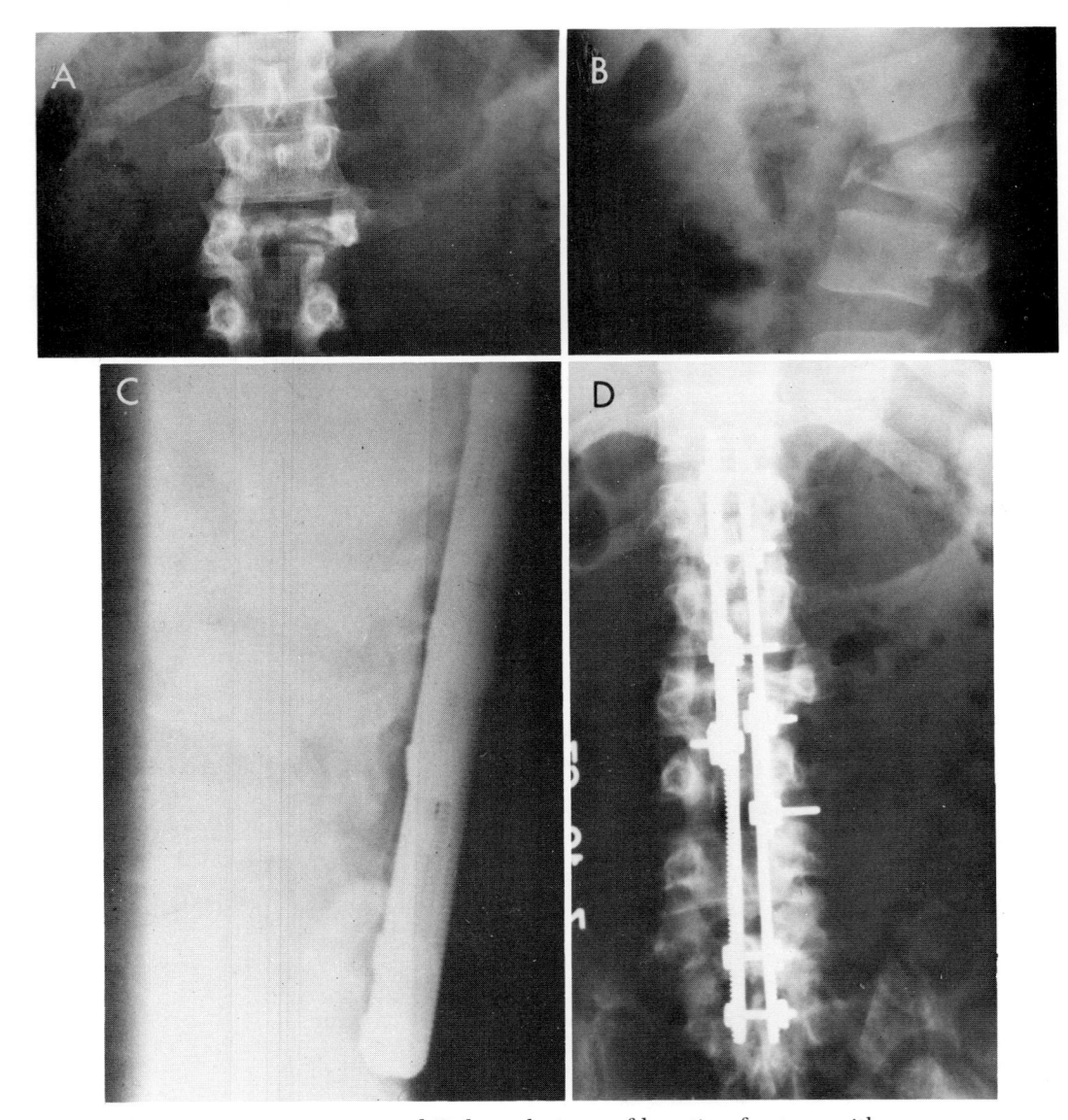

Fig. 16-39.—**A,** anteroposterior and **B,** lateral views of bursting fracture with severe compression of L2. **C** and **D,** nonunion stabilized with Meurig-Williams spinal plates. At time of injury small plates did not exist and 2 plates were bolted together on either side to obtain sufficient length to make it possible to place 2 bolts above and 2 bolts below vertebral spinous processes. Iliac bone grafts were added laterally throughout length of plating.

when a heavy weight borne on the shoulders becomes displaced. These fractures almost always occur in the lumbar spine; they are uncommon in the cervical region and rare in the thoracic spine.

Transverse process fractures are caused by violent muscular contraction of an involuntary protective nature. They may occur singly and without displacement. Commonly, however, they are

Chapter 16: INJURIES TO THE SPINE: NEUROLOGIC CONSIDERATIONS / 393

multiple (Fig. 16-40) when they are associated with especially violent muscular contraction. If the injury is severe, there may be considerable displacement of fragments, hemorrhage, hematoma and fascial and muscular tears. The soft part injury may be so extensive as to prolong convalescence and leave an excess amount of scar tissue. There is a tendency to exaggerate complaints. Often, however, the injury is not a serious one, some patients even preferring to continue their usual activities with little or no interruption.

The diagnosis is based on the history, localized tenderness and the aggravation of symptoms when torn structures are placed under tension. It is confirmed by x-ray films.

Fig. 16-40.—Anteroposterior roentgenogram of multiple transverse process fractures. Note the loss of outline of the psoas shadow on the left (due to a large hematoma). The psoas shadow on the right may be clearly seen. The left first, second, third, and fourth transverse processes are fractured.

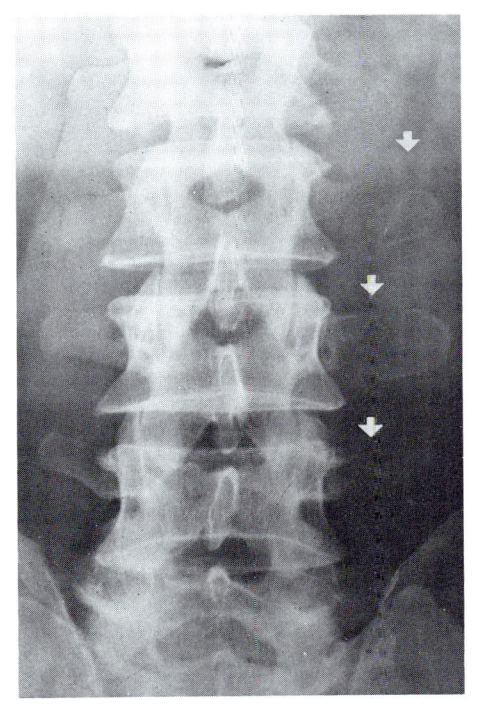

It is a fact that recovery takes place without regard to reduction of the fracture or to bone union. The surgeon should therefore direct his attention to the treatment of the soft part injury. At first, this will mean protection of torn periosteum, fascia, aponeurosis and muscles. How much support to provide will depend on the extent of the injury. Lumbar strapping with adhesive plaster or a well-fitting corset, with or without a few days of recumbency, will suffice in most of the milder injuries. A plaster-of-paris jacket may be necessary if there are much pain and muscle spasm. Jackets should not, however, be worn for more than 2 or 3 weeks, because refractory pain associated with excessive scar limitation may ensue.

As swelling subsides, gentle active exercises are instituted. Gradually the exercises are increased, so that, when soft part repair is complete in 6–8 weeks, a normal range of active motion may be present without pain.

When the injury is of moderate severity, 6–12 weeks may be required before repair is complete. When the fractures are multiple and accompanied by extensive rupture of fascia and muscle, there may be 4, or as much as 6, months of disability.

URINARY TRACT

Injury to the spinal cord in the cervical or upper thoracic area leads in most cases to a period of bladder flaccidity and subsequently to the development of a severely spastic bladder detrusor and sphincter. Injury to the cauda equina is a peripheral nerve injury and produces immediate and long-term flaccidity of the bladder detrusor and bladder sphincters.

The most successful care of the bladder following a spinal injury can be initiated by immediate, careful catheterization of the patient with a straight catheter, removing urine and studying the bladder, with radiopaque dye if there is a question of bladder injury at the time. Subsequently, the patient should be placed on a program of intermittent catheterization if adequate, trained personnel are available. Catheterization under sterile conditions should be done by a trained technician or a male nurse or physician every 2 hours. In most institutions, when such a pool of trained personnel is not available, a Foley catheter will have to be placed. As soon as it is practical and other injuries have been taken care of, attention is turned to bladder function. The bladder is filled with a radiopaque, water-soluble dye and the catheter is clamped under the direct supervision of a trained urologic technician or a physician. Under fluoroscopy it is noted whether there is competence or incompetence of the ureterovesical valve on either or both sides. Should reflux of urine up the ureter toward the kidney begin on either side, the catheter should be immediately unclamped and the bladder drained. If the patient can tolerate 350–400 ml or more of radiopaque material in the bladder without reflux and if a gentle Credé maneuver is carried out and there is still no reflux, it will be safe to remove the Foley catheter and begin a period of intermittent catheterization. This should be carried out with a straight catheter by well-trained personnel under aseptic conditions at the bedside every 2 hours after the patient has made an attempt to void. In the event the patient is unable to void spontaneously and even by moderate Credé maneuvers, a measurement of sphincter pressure should be carried out by a urologist. If the sphincter pressure is too great to allow voiding and overpowers the detrusor, the question of making radial cuts in the sphincter muscle itself to weaken it must be taken up by the urologist. In most cases, under 3–6 months postinjury, it would be wiser to reinsert a Foley catheter or to keep the patient on a program of intermittent catheterization. Studies carried out at Stoke-Mandeville in England and at Rancho Los Amigos and Long Beach Veterans hospitals in California have shown that a bladder can most readily be trained to function on a reflex basis by a Credé maneuver and/or stimulation of the abdomen with intermittent catheterization. When adequate personnel is not available, a Foley catheter may be used and a subsequent voiding trial, following cystometrography and determination that no reflux exists, carried out approximately 6 weeks to 3 months after the initial study.

In all instances, it is preferable to remove a catheter from the bladder as soon as possible. The presence of a foreign body definitely increases the probability of septic urine in the bladder, and its removal greatly decreases the chance of urinary tract infection.

The use of Urecoline, 5–10 mg subcutaneously (never intramuscularly), before the voiding trial may greatly facilitate the patient's ability to void initially and to become catheter-free.

Should the patient show reflux at the time of initial study, there should be no attempt to clamp the catheter or to allow the bladder to fill beyond the 200-ml level. It is far better in such a patient to irrigate the bladder with sterile saline or 0.25% acetic acid solution 3 times a day to a point of 200- or 250-ml expansion, and then to allow the bladder to drain slowly through the Foley catheter. Intravenous pyelography should be performed in every spinal injury patient with neurologic symptoms every 3 months for a period of 2 years and thereafter every 6 months for the rest of his life. Experience with the intermittent catheterization method in the authors' unit has shown that 85% of all patients with spinal injuries can be maintained catheter-free within 3–6 months of the time of injury or insult to the spinal cord from tumor by the intermittent catheterization method.

The use of the ileal loop in patients with spinal injury is generally to be condemned, as the quadriplegic patient is unable to change his own ileostomy bag and there have been a significant number of urinary tract infections even in patients with the ileal loop. Only in the face of increasing uropathy should the ileal loop be resorted to and then only when all other methods of draining the urinary tract satisfactorily have been exhausted.

In the patient with a lower motor neuron lesion, the intermittent catheterization program should also be carried out in the hope that some sort of reflex mechanism may possibly develop or that use of the Credé maneuver may actually empty the bladder entirely without difficulty. An external collecting device is worn and the patient is instructed to void as completely as possible by Credé's method every 2 hours. The tone of the bladder is assessed with a cystometrogram approximately every 6 weeks and completeness of voiding is tested with straight catheterization under aseptic conditions. The use of bladder pacemakers to stimulate either the sacral roots or the bladder detrusor itself is still in an experimental stage.

THE BOWELS

Immediately after the spinal injury has been taken care of and the bladder program established, the patient should be placed on a program of bowel regulation. Suppositories are used, beginning with glycerine suppositories and going, if necessary, to Dulcolax suppositories, or Vacuette suppositories.* The suppository program is continued in such a manner as to establish a bowel program for the patient, in which the bowels are moved by suppository insertion and later by digital manipulation with a gloved finger in the rectum, in the case of the patient who has the use of his hand, every second or third day.

The use of Colace or other stool softeners is sometimes necessary, and occasionally enemas and manual disimpactions may have to be resorted to but should be kept to a minimum.

In most patients it is possible to regulate the bowels completely with suppositories, so that the patient can be free of bowel accidents, go out in society, earn a living, and not worry about having difficulties.

A good bowel pattern, as in the case of a good bladder pattern, may be difficult initially to establish, but in most patients can be established within 6 weeks to 3 months.

PHYSICAL THERAPY

Every patient with a spinal injury in the cervical area that involves the nerve supply to the upper extremity should be seen by an occupational therapist within 6 hours of the time he enters the hospital. Resting splints should be made for the hands to prevent contracture of the web space between the thumb and first finger and to hold the thumb in a position of opposition to the first and second fingers. Functional training with dynamic splints to give a 3-jaw chuck pinch between the thumb and the index and long fingers should be carried out as early as practical by the occupational therapist if the patient has use of the wrist extensors.

If wrist extensors are missing but the patient has the ability to abduct and/or flex the shoulder, a mobile arm support should be used to support the forearm, and a power-driven splint, either with carbon dioxide or electric power, should be applied as soon as it becomes obvious that the patient is not going to recover the use of the wrist extensors. Patients supplied with such powered splints, and particularly those who can power their own splints with their wrist extensors, can be functional individuals in society again if they have the mental capacity to learn white-collar jobs. Even patients with quadriplegia as high as the C4–C5 level with only the fourth cervical root available can use wheelchairs with electric

---

*Vacuette suppositories are made of sodium bicarbonate and, when inserted slightly moistened, release a bolus of carbon dioxide, thereby expanding the rectal ampulla and bringing about evacuation of the lower bowel.

power and switches manipulated by the patient's tongue. The wheelchair can be driven forward, turned from side to side and moved in reverse. A surprising degree of accuracy can be obtained with such a device, to the point where the patient can drive the wheelchair through a doorway at 2–3 mph with 1–2-in. tolerance on either side.

In general, patients with thoracic and lumbar lesions should be encouraged to use all of the musculature available to them. However, if the lesion is above the level of T8, there should be no pressure on the part of the treating surgeon to have the patient ambulate. It is often reasonable, however, to construct long leg braces for such a patient simply as a method of preventing contractures. The braces should be worn at least at night or during some part of the day for a minimum of 12 hours. With a lesion at a level below T8, ambulation may be possible.

It has been the universal experience that patients with lesions above the level of T8 are not functional walkers, as the energy expended is so great that it is too tiring to walk except for a brief time, as during an exercise period. For this reason, hospitalization at high cost for gait training for this particular type of patient is not warranted, except in rare instances. If the patient is determined to walk, he should be provided with standing bars or a set of parallel bars at home, and arrangements made for a visiting nurse or private physical therapist to teach the patient to walk with braces and progress to crutches if he so desires and has the ability.

THE SPINAL INJURY TEAM

Modern treatment of the patient with a spinal injury requires a well-coordinated spinal injury care team. As soon as practical after emergency and definitive care of the acute spinal injury by the methods discussed in this chapter, the patient should be referred to a spinal injury treatment center. Here the manufacture of definitive hand splints and braces, overall occupational and physical therapy and bowel and bladder training can be carried out. Vocational counseling and planning for care outside the hospital are also a part of the services. Treatment is carried out by a team of persons accustomed to working together and with these patients and their families. It is not a job for the average hospital in which 1 or 2 cases a year are seen and where no such team exists. Proper treatment by a well-coordinated team can often result in a patient returning to society as an active, happy, employed and tax-paying citizen.

BIBLIOGRAPHY

1. Alexander, E., Jr., Forsyth, H. F., Davis, C. H., Jr., and Nashold, B. S.: Dislocation of the atlas on the axis: The value of early fusion of C1, C2 and C3, J. Neurosurg. 15:353, 1958.
2. Barnes, R.: Paraplegia in cervical spine injuries, J. Bone Joint Surg 30-B:239, 1948.
3. Barton, L. G.: The reduction of fracture-dislocation of the cervical vertebrae by skeletal traction, Surg. Gynecol. Obstet. 67:94, 1938.
4. Bedford, P. D., Bosanquet, F. D., and Russell, W. R.: Degeneration of the spinal cord associated with cervical spondylosis, Lancet 2:55, 1952.
5. Bergmann, E. W.: Fractures of the ankylosed spine, J. Bone Joint Surg. 31-A:669, 1949.
6. Burke, D. C.: Hyperextension injuries of the spine, J. Bone Joint Surg. 53-B:3:1971.
7. Blockey, N. J., and Purser, D. W.: Fractures of the odontoid process of the axis, J. Bone Joint Surg. 38-B:794, 1956.
8. Bucy, P. C., Heimburger, R. E., and Oberhill, H. R.: Compression of the cervical spinal cord by herniated intervertebral discs, J. Neurosurg. 5:471, 1948.
9. Cloward, R. B.: Treatment of acute fractures and fracture-dislocations of the cervical spine by vertebral-body fusion: A report of 11 cases, J. Neurosurg. 18:201, 1961.
10. Cone, W., and Turner, W. G.: The treatment of fracture-dislocations of the cervical vertebrae by skeletal traction and fusion, J. Bone Joint Surg. 19:584, 1937.
11. Cramer, F., and McGowan, F. J.: The role of the nucleus pulposus in the pathogenesis of so-called "recoil" injuries of the spinal cord, Surg. Gynecol. Obstet. 79:516, 1944.
12. Crutchfield, W. G.: Skeletal traction for dislocation of the cervical spine: Report of a case, South. Surgeon 2:156, 1933.
13. Davis, A. G.: Fractures of the spine, J. Bone Joint Surg. 11:133, 1929.
14. Davis, A. G.: Fractures of the spine, Am. J. Surg. 15:325, 1932.
15. Drake, C. G.: Cervical spinal-cord injury, J. Neurosurg. 19:487, 1962.
16. Elsberg, C. A.: *Tumors of the Spinal Cord and the Symptoms of Irritation and Compression*

of the Spinal Cord and Nerve Roots (New York: Paul B. Hoeber, Inc., 1925), p. 421.
17. Ewald, F. C.: Fracture of the odontoid process in a 17-month-old infant treated with a halo: A case report and discussion of the injury under the age of 3, J. Bone Joint Surg. 53-A:1636, 1971.
18. Hoen, T. I.: A method of skeletal traction for treatment of fracture-dislocation of cervical vertebrae, Arch. Neurol. Psychiat. 36:158, 1936.
19. Jefferson, G.: Fracture of the atlas vertebra: Report of 4 cases, and review of those previously recorded, Br. J. Surg 7:407, 1920.
20. Kahn, E. A.: The role of the dentate ligaments in spinal cord compression and the syndrome of lateral sclerosis, J. Neurosurg. 4:191, 1947.
21. Kahn, E. A., and Yglesias, L.: Progressive atlanto-axial dislocation, JAMA 105:348, 1935.
22. Landan, B., and Ransohoff, J.: Late surgery for incomplete traumatic lesions of the conus medullaris and cauda equina, J. Neurosurg. 28:257, 1968.
23. Lemmen, L. L., and Laing, P. G.: Fracture of the cervical spine in patients with rheumatoid arthritis, J. Neurosurg. 16:542, 1959.
24. McKenzie, K. G.: Fracture, dislocation and fracture-dislocation of the spine, Can. Med. Assoc. J. 32:263, 1935.
25. Morgan, T. H., Wharton, G. W., and Austin, G. N.: The results of laminectomy in patients with incomplete spinal cord injuries, Paraplegia 9:1:14, 1971.
26. Nicoll, E. A.: Redevelopment of muscle function (Surgeons' Conference of the Miners Welfare Commission), J. Bone Joint Surg. 30-B: 392, 1948.
27. Raynor, R. B.: Severe injuries of the cervical spine treated by early anterior interbody fusion and ambulation, J. Neurosurg. 28:311, 1968.
28. Rogers, W. A.: Cord injury during reduction of thoracic and lumbar vertebral-body fracture and dislocation, J. Bone Joint Surg. 20:689, 1938.
29. Rogers, W. A.: An extension frame for the reduction of fracture of the vertebral body, Surg. Gynecol. Obstet. 50:101, 1930.
30. Rogers, W. A.: Treatment of fractures of vertebral bodies uncomplicated by lesions of the cord, Arch. Surg. 30:284, 1935.
31. Rogers, W. A.: Fractures and Dislocations of the Vertebral Column, in Scudder, C. L.: *Treatment of Fractures* (11th ed.; Philadelphia: W. B. Saunders Company, 1939), p. 461.
32. Rogers, W. A.: Treatment of fracture-dislocation of the cervical spine, J. Bone Joint Surg. 24:245, 1942.
33. Rogers, W. A.: Fractures and dislocations of the cervical spine: An end result study, J. Bone Joint Surg. 39-A:341, 1957.
34. Ryerson, E. W., and Christopher, F.: Dislocation of cervical vertebrae: Operative reduction, JAMA 108:468 1937.
35. Schatzker, J., Rorabeck, C. H., and Waddell, J. P.: Fractures of the dens [odontoid process]: An analysis of 37 cases, J. Bone Joint Surg. 53-B: 392, 1971.
36. Schneider, R. C., Cherry, G., and Pantek, H.: The syndrome of acute central cervical spinal cord injury, with special reference to the mechanisms involved in hyperextension injuries of cervical spine, J. Neurosurg. 11:546, 1954.
37. Schneider, R. C., and Kahn, E. A.: Chronic neurological sequelae of acute trauma to the spine and spinal cord, J. Bone Joint Surg. 38-A: 985, 1956.
38. Schneider, R. C., and Schemm, G. W.: Vertebral artery insufficiency in acute and chronic spinal trauma, with special reference to the syndrome of acute central cervical spinal cord injury, J. Neurosurg. 18:348, 1961.
39. Smith, G. W., and Robinson, R. A.: The treatment of certain cervical-spine disorders by anterior removal of the intervertebral disc and interbody fusion, J. Bone Joint Surg. 40-A:607, 1958.
41. Stiasny, H.: Fraktur der Halswirbelsaule bei Spondylarthritis Ankylopoietica, Zentralbl. Chir. 60:998, 1933.
42. Stookey, B.: Compression of the spinal cord due to ventral extradural cervical chondromas: Diagnosis and surgical treatment, Arch. Neurol. Psychiat. 20:275, 1928.
43. Stookey, B.: Compression of the spinal cord and nerve roots by herniation of the nucleus pulposus in the cervical region, Arch. Surg. 40:417, 1940.
44. Taylor, A. R.: The mechanism of injury to the spinal cord in the neck without damage to the vertebral column, J. Bone Joint Surg. 33-B:543, 1951.
45. Taylor, A. R., and Blackwood, W.: Paraplegia in hyperextension cervical injuries with normal radiographic appearances, J. Bone Joint Surg. 30-B:245, 1948.
46. Taylor, A. S.: Fracture dislocation of the cervical spine Ann. Surg. 90:321, 1929.
47. Verbiest, H.: Anterior operative approach in cases of spinal-cord compression by old irreducible displacement or fresh fracture of cervical spine Contribution to operative repair of deformed vertebral bodies, J. Neurosurg. 19:389, 1962.
48. Watson-Jones R.: Treatment of fractures and fracture dislocations of the spine, Br. Med. J. 16:1:30, 1934
49. White, J. C.: Personal communication.

17 | Shoulder Girdle Injuries
CARTER R. ROWE

ANATOMY AND FUNCTION

Anatomy

THE SHOULDER is a suspended joint which functions from a movable base, the scapula, and from a yardarm, the clavicle. More specifically, the shoulder girdle consists of the following: 3 joints (the sternoclavicular, the acromioclavicular and the glenohumeral); 3 bones (the clavicle, the scapula and the humerus), and 20 muscles. The muscles are divided into 3 main groups, extending (1) from the thorax to the scapula and clavicle, (2) from the thorax to the humerus and (3) from the scapula to the humerus.

LIGAMENTS (Fig. 17-1).—Strong ligaments give support and stability to the sternoclavicular, acromioclavicular and glenohumeral joints. Of these, the most important stabilizers are the supra-articular ligament of the acromioclavicular joint and the coracoclavicular ligaments (the trapezoid and the conoid).

MUSCLES (Fig. 17-2).—The muscles of the shoulder comprise perhaps the most complex functional unit in the body. There are 2 primary layers: the musculotendinous short rotator-cuff group (the subscapularis, supraspinatus, infraspinatus and teres minor muscles) and the deltoid muscle. The primary function of the short rotator muscles is to depress the humeral head and hold it in the glenoid fossa, thus allowing the deltoid muscle to elevate the arm.

NERVES.—The shoulder has an adequate overlapping nerve supply. The trunks of the brachial plexus pass posterior to the middle third of the clavicle into the axilla and thence to the arm. Gardner[27] has demonstrated clearly the complete nerve supply to the capsule and rotator muscles of the shoulder, arising from C5 and C6 through the supraspinatus nerve and the axillary nerve.

BLOOD SUPPLY.—The shoulder is generously supplied with blood except for 1 important area, the tendinous portion of the supraspinatus muscle. This poorly nourished area shows attritional changes in advancing decades, owing to its repetitious motion under the overlying acromion.

Function

Codman[16] in his book illustrates uniquely the functional development of the shoulder. In quadrupeds the shoulder functions as a swinging pendulum. In the erect position of bipeds (as in man), however, the shoulder must function as a lever arm, thus adding definite strain to the shoulder mechanism. Codman also describes "scapulohumeral rhythm," the smooth reciprocal functioning of the shoulder girdle muscles.

Inman, Saunders and Abbott[32] in 1944 supplied further information regarding the mechanism of total shoulder motion. The important points concerning shoulder motion are the following.

400 / Carter R. Rowe

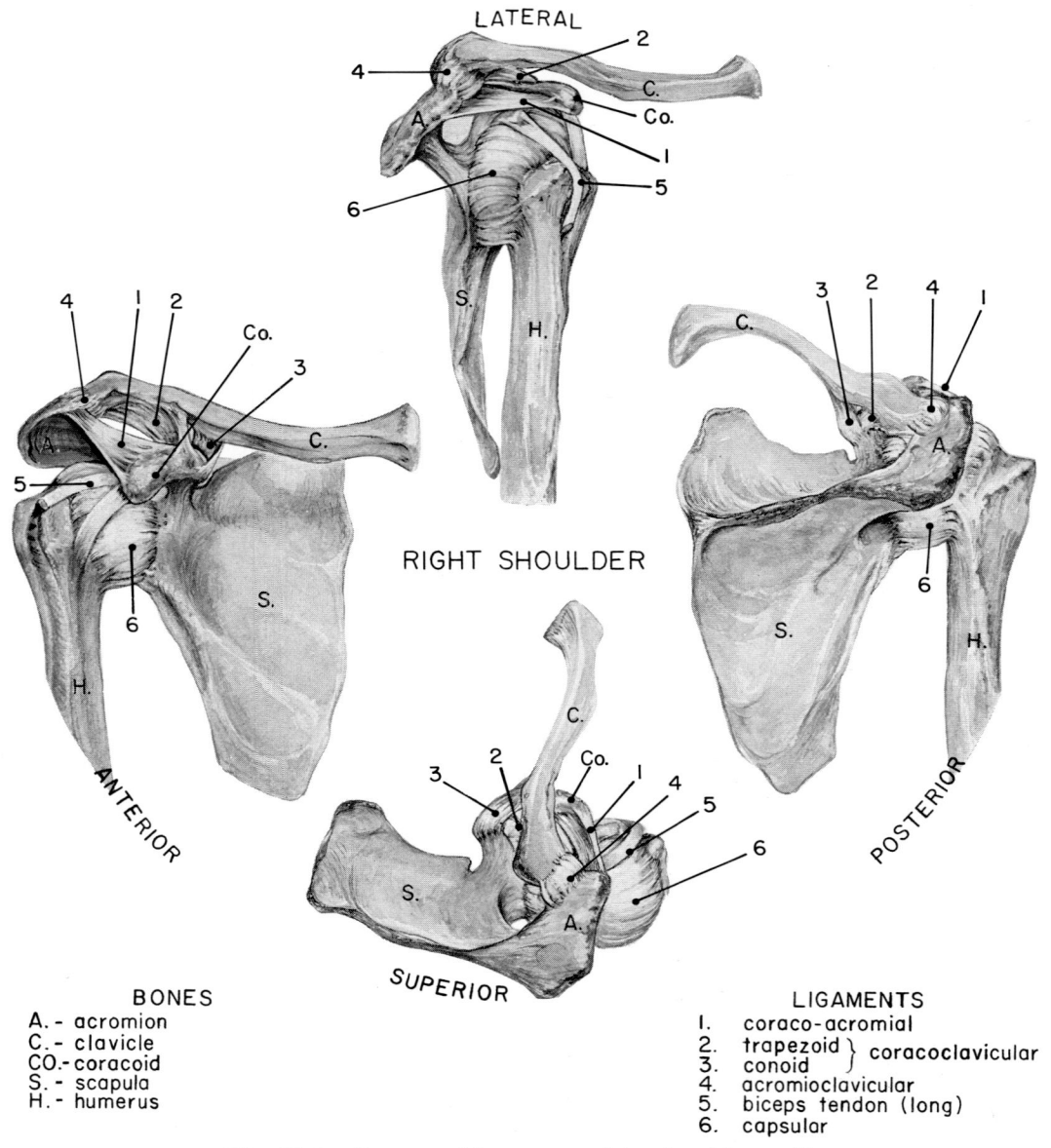

BONES
A. - acromion
C. - clavicle
CO. - coracoid
S. - scapula
H. - humerus

LIGAMENTS
1. coraco-acromial
2. trapezoid } coracoclavicular
3. conoid
4. acromioclavicular
5. biceps tendon (long)
6. capsular

Fig. 17-1.—Bones and ligaments of the shoulder girdle.

1. *In the first 45 degrees of abduction,* the scapula does not rotate, but "sets itself" (Fig. 17-3, A). The short rotators depress the head of the humerus, allowing the deltoid muscle to elevate the arm. Early motion is noted in the sternoclavicular joint. The clavicle is gradually elevated 25 degrees in the first 110 degrees of abduction.

2. *Between 45 and 90 degrees of abduction,* scapular rotation begins and continues, with a 1:2 ratio, to the humerus (Fig. 17-3, B).

3. *From 90 degrees to complete eleva-*

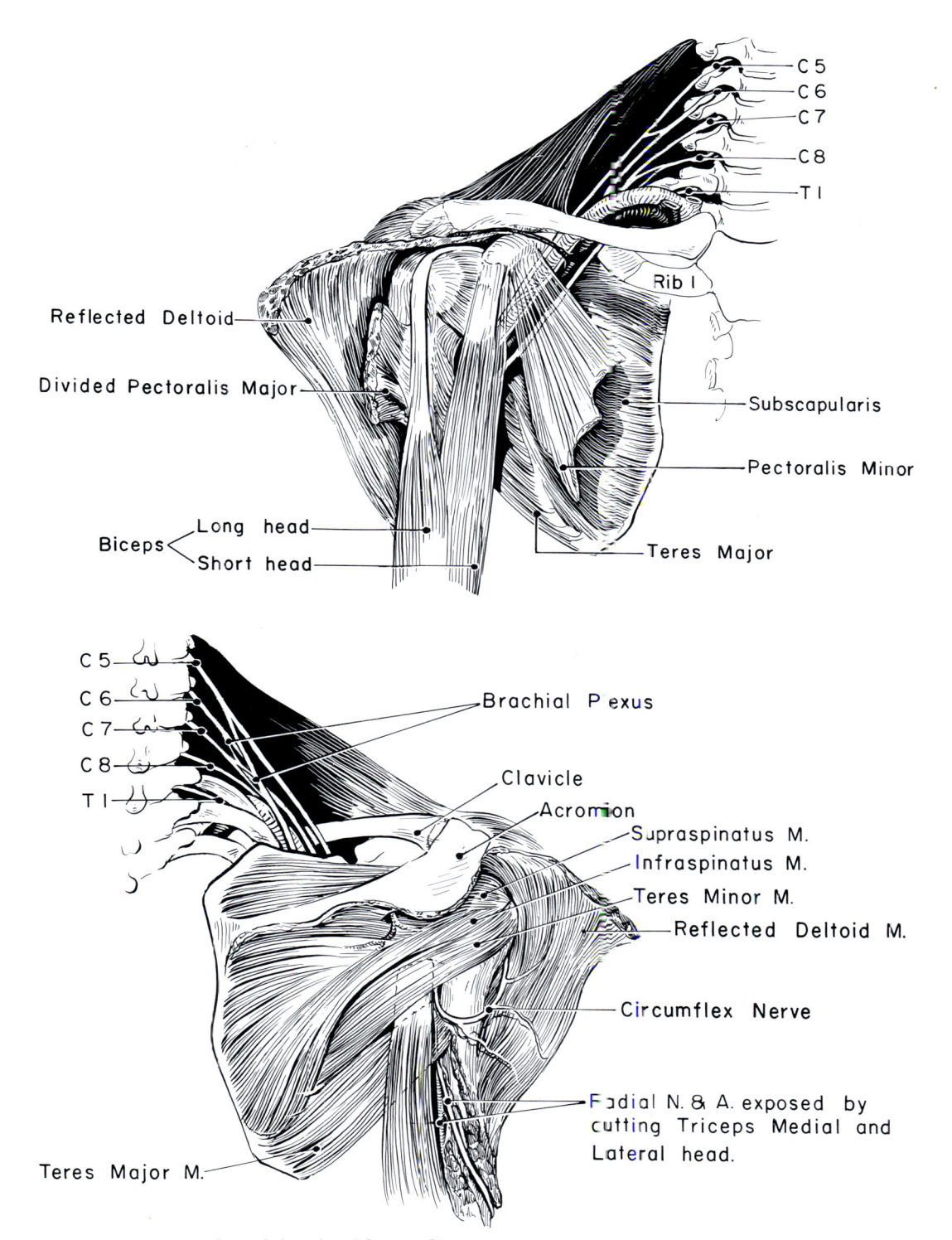

Fig. 17-2.—Muscles of the shoulder girdle. **Top,** anterior aspect. **Bottom,** posterior aspect.

401

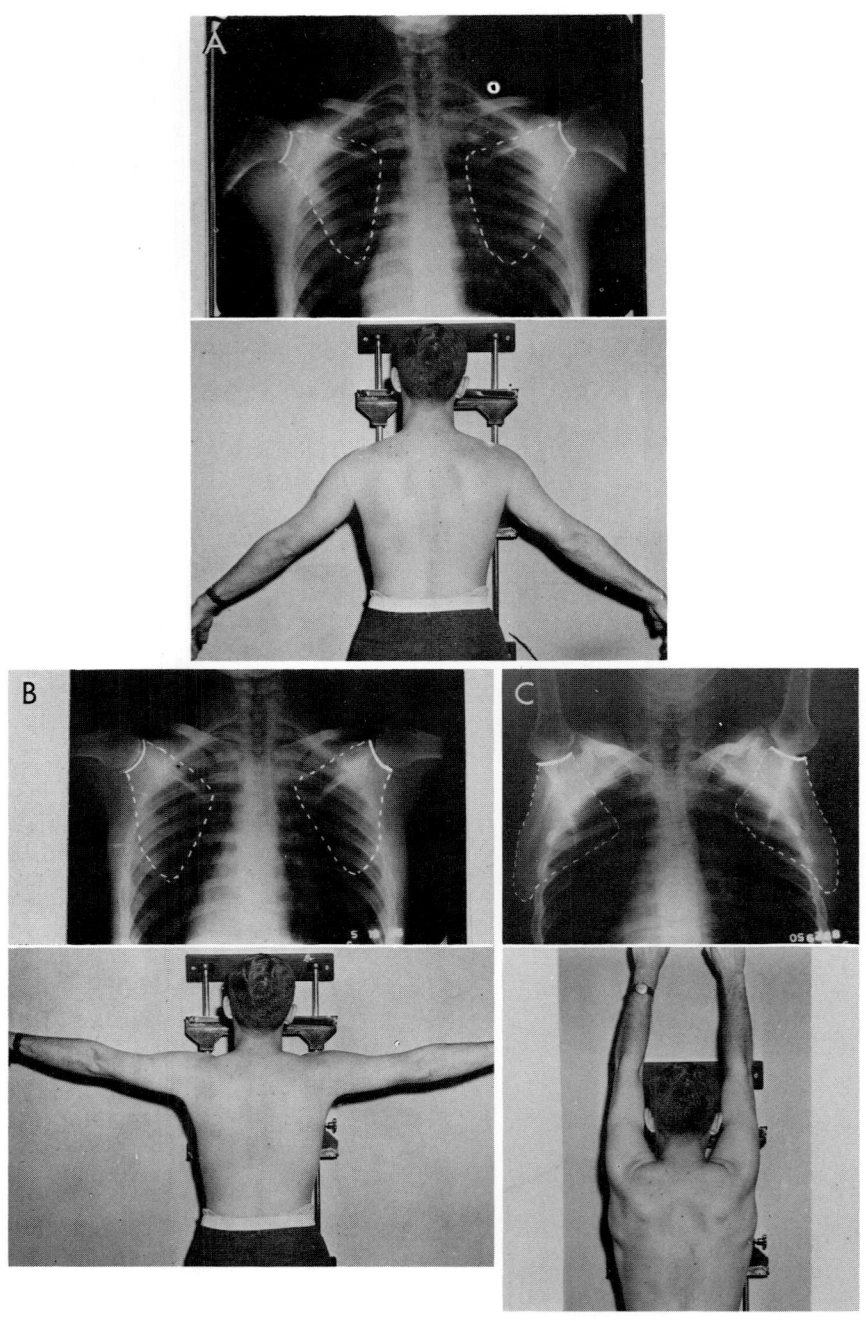

Fig. 17-3.—Total shoulder motion. **A,** zero to 45 degrees of elevation. **B,** 45 to 90 degrees of elevation; note that the scapula has moved very little. **C,** 90 degrees to complete elevation (complete rotation of scapula).

tion, the scapula rotates or pivots upward and forward on the chest wall, thus placing the glenoid fossa directly under the head of the humerus (Fig. 17-3, *C*). This quick and efficient adjustment to an optimal mechanical position is an important factor in shoulder stability.

The clavicle at 110 degrees elevation rotates 45 degrees. Unless this rotation takes place, shoulder elevation may be limited.

CLINICAL EXAMINATION

Inspection.—Much can be learned from careful inspection of the shoulder girdle, noting bony landmarks, alignment, atrophy and hypertrophy.

Palpation.—The examiner should gently palpate the entire shoulder—the joints, muscles, tendons and bones—for painful or unstable areas. The rotator-cuff tendon can be examined by placing the fingers just beyond the acromion and rotating the arm at 45 and 90 degrees of abduction. Sometimes a crunch, eminence or sulcus can be felt. The point of insertion of all muscles and tendons should also be palpated gently.

Motions.—1. The patient should be instructed to bend forward at the waist, to let the arms hang loosely, and then to swing them gently forward and backward. Next, he should stand erect, extend the arms in full elevation and then *slowly* lower the arms in wide abduction. The examiner should watch from behind the patient, noting the motions of the scapula, muscles and joints; then he should repeat the instructions, observing from the front. This is the "scapulohumeral rhythm," the most useful step in shoulder examination.

2. The examiner should next instruct the patient to stand erect, elbows at side; to flex the forearms to 90 degrees, and to execute external and internal rotation. The patient should abduct the arm to 90 degrees and repeat the foregoing procedure in this position. Then he should put the hands behind the back.

Neurologic examination.—With pin and cotton, the examiner should map out areas of anesthesia or hyperanesthesia. Loss of muscle power and atrophy should be noted, and the biceps and triceps reflexes should be tested.

Cervical spine, elbow, wrist and hand.—These should be examined in order to complete the shoulder examination. Figure 17-4 shows an analysis of 1,603 shoulder girdle injuries (fractures and dislocations) treated at Massachusetts General Hospital.

Fig. 17-4.—Analysis of 1,603 shoulder girdle injuries, showing the number and distribution of fractures and dislocations.

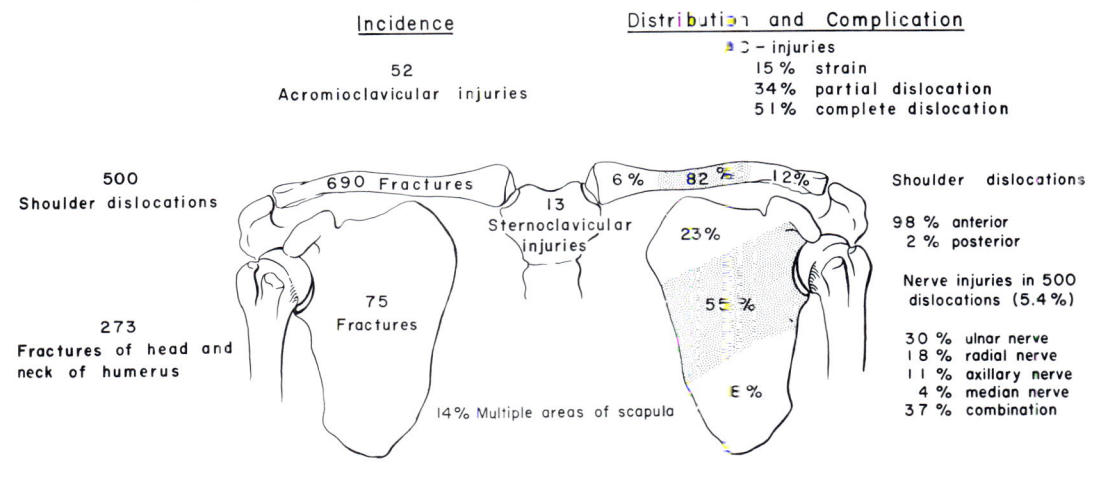

Incidence	Distribution and Complication
	A C – injuries
52	15 % strain
Acromioclavicular injuries	34 % partial dislocation
	51 % complete dislocation
500 Shoulder dislocations	6 % 82 % 12 % Shoulder dislocations
690 Fractures	98 % anterior
13 Sternoclavicular injuries	2 % posterior
	23 %
75 Fractures	Nerve injuries in 500 dislocations (5.4 %)
273 Fractures of head and neck of humerus	55 %
	30 % ulnar nerve
	18 % radial nerve
	11 % axillary nerve
	6 %
	4 % median nerve
14 % Multiple areas of scapula	37 % combination

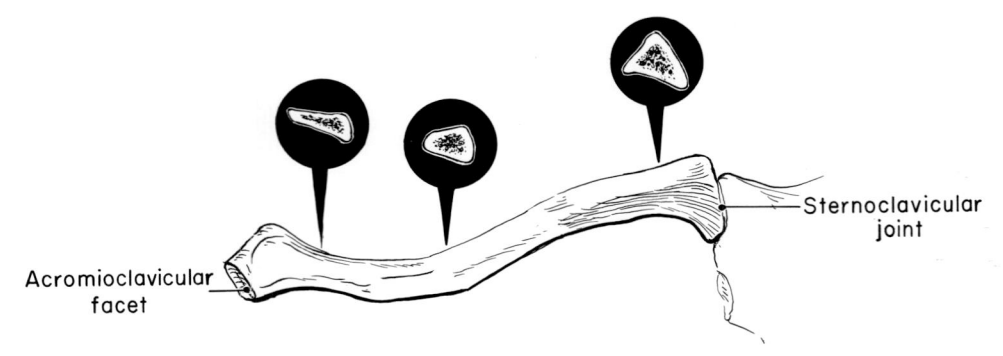

Fig. 17-5.—Cross section of the clavicle.

THE CLAVICLE: ANATOMIC CONSIDERATIONS

The clavicle is a curved, dense bone that serves to protect the brachial plexus and lends efficiency to the function of the glenohumeral joint. The bone is larger and more curved in the male than in the female. It presents a double curve; its lateral third is flattened horizontally, whereas the medial two-thirds is rounded or prismatic in shape. Its cross section varies, as shown in Figure 17-5.

The clavicle articulates to the sternum with a well-developed joint, the sternoclavicular joint, and to the acromion with a less perfect joint, the acromioclavicular joint. The stability of these joints is produced principally by their superior articular ligaments and the coracoclavicular ligaments (the conoid and trapezoid). Stability and mobility are desirable in both the sternoclavicular and acromioclavicular joints in order more effectively to elevate and rotate the clavicle.

ACROMIOCLAVICULAR INJURIES

INCIDENCE.—It has been found that the acromioclavicular joint is injured approximately 4 times as frequently as the sternoclavicular joint. Anatomically, the acromioclavicular joint is weaker and more vulnerable to injury than the sternoclavicular joint. Massachusetts General Hospital data indicate that most acromioclavicular injuries occur in the second decade of life but that otherwise there is a fairly even distribution from 20 to 60 years of age.

MECHANISM.—Injury to the acromioclavicular joint is usually produced by a forceful depression or blow to the tip of the shoulder.

TYPES OF INJURY.—An analysis of the acromioclavicular injuries treated at the Massachusetts General Hospital reveals the following types: strain, 15%; partial subluxation, 34%, and complete dislocation, 51%. In acromioclavicular strains, incomplete tears of the acromioclavicular articular ligaments occur. Partial acromioclavicular subluxation usually is accompanied by partial rupture of the capsule ligament and the coracoclavicular ligaments. In complete upward dislocation of the clavicle, there is complete rupture of both the acromioclavicular articular ligaments and the coracoclavicular ligaments.

Diagnosis

Diagnosis of an acromioclavicular injury usually is not difficult.

Inspection.—The patient should be stripped to the waist for examination of both shoulders. In complete dislocations, the injured shoulder will show a marked prominence of the outer end of the clavicle. Local ecchymosis may be present.

Palpation.—Local tenderness is elicited on palpation over the acromioclavicular joint. The prominence of the clavicle may be increased by a downward pull of the arm and decreased by an upward and backward positioning of the shoulder.

X-ray. — With the patient standing, anteroposterior films of both shoulders should be taken. Weights held in both hands may increase the displacement of the injured side.

Treatment

Treatment of acromioclavicular injuries depends on the severity of the injury, the age and the occupation of the patient. Strain and partial subluxations are more common in the younger age groups and respond well to strapping and rest (Fig. 17-6).

The usual direction of complete dislocation of the clavicle is superior, although the clavicle may dislocate inferiorly. In superior dislocation, closed reduction can best be accomplished by supporting the arm upward and applying anteroposterior pressure to the outer end of the clavicle, rather than direct superoinferior pressure. However, complete reduction is seldom maintained by external support as it loses much of its effectiveness in the reclining position.

Satisfactory results are reported whether the dislocation is reduced or remains unreduced. When the dislocation remains unreduced or is partially reduced, the deformity persists and symptoms of strain or discomfort may be experienced in performing heavy lifting or in working with the arm elevated in adduction or abduction. Yet, this does not constitute a major disturbance, and unless traumatic changes in the joint occur, the long-term prognosis is favorable.

OPERATIVE TREATMENT. — The purposes of open reduction should be to produce stability of the acromioclavicular joint, eliminate the deformity and preserve clavicular motion. The surgical exposure must be adequate, so that both the cora-

Fig. 17-6. — Mechanical principles of the sling used for acromioclavicular separation. (After Goldberg, D.: Acromioclavicular joint injuries — a modified form of treatment, Am. J. Surg. 71: 529, 1946.)

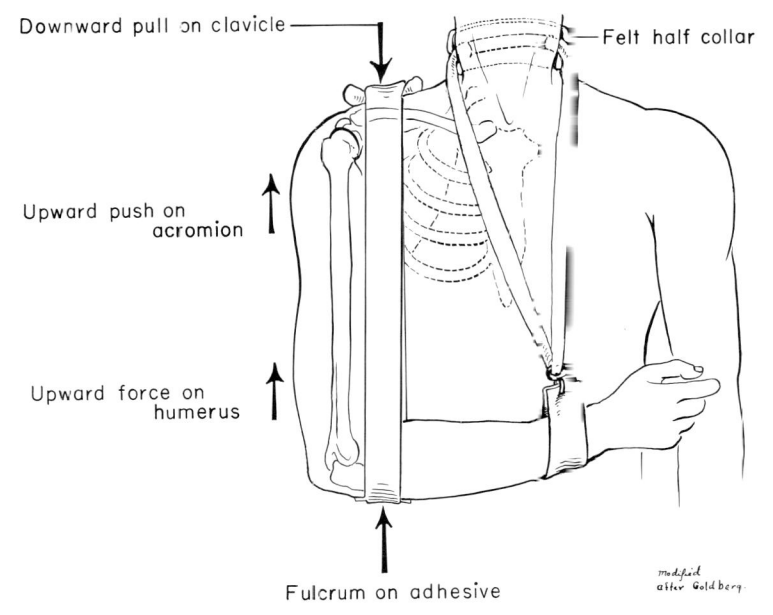

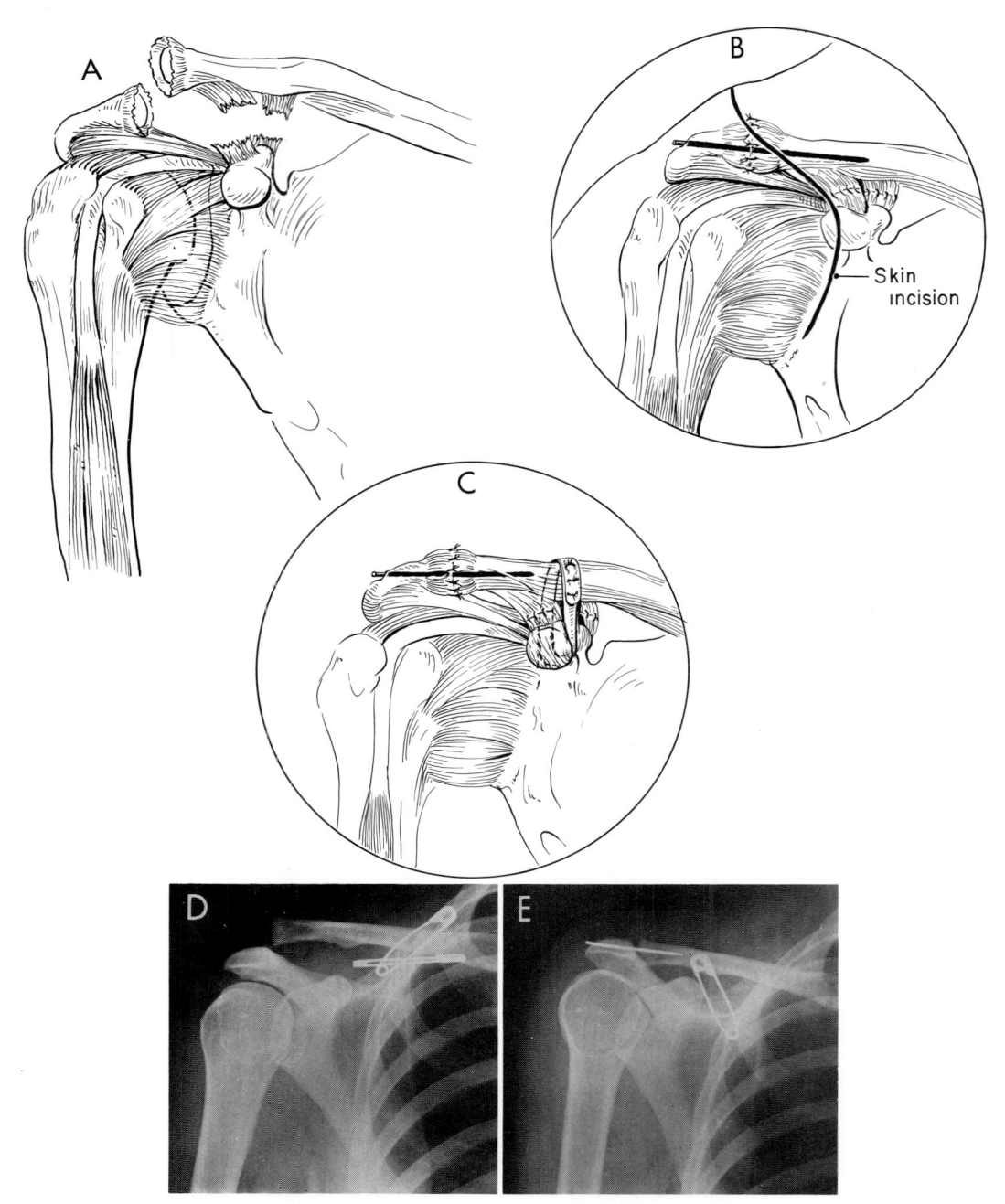

Fig. 17-7.—Open reduction for complete separation of the acromioclavicular joint. **A,** diagram of dislocation. **B,** 3/32-in. Kirschner pin fixation with direct repair of supra-articular acromioclavicular ligaments and coracoclavicular ligaments. **C,** repair with fascia lata. **D,** roentgenogram showing complete separation of acromioclavicular joint in a woman, aged 52, who had been thrown from a horse. **E,** direct repair of ligaments and temporary Kirschner pin stabilization. Follow-up rating 1 year later was excellent.

coclavicular and the acromioclavicular ligaments can be thoroughly inspected.

The technical steps for open reduction are as follows:

1. *Position of the patient:* Semisitting position with the affected shoulder elevated.

2. *Exposure:* Superoanterior shoulder exposure should be carried out to facilitate complete inspection of the acromioclavicular and coracoclavicular ligaments.

3. *Repair:* It is important to repair both the superior articular ligament and the coracoclavicular ligaments. Some means of internal fixation is usually necessary during the healing period. This may be accomplished very effectively with a 3/32-in. Kirschner pin, introduced under direct vision across the acromioclavicular joint from the acromion into the clavicle (Fig. 17-7). The pin should be left in situ for 4–8 weeks. The superior articular ligament of the acromioclavicular joint and the coracoclavicular ligaments are then repaired with cotton sutures. At Massachusetts General Hospital, repair of the coracoclavicular ligaments has often been reinforced with fascia lata, although this is used much less frequently in recent years. The fascia lata is obtained through a 1-in. incision on the lower thigh, using a fascial stripper. The strip of fascia is passed over and around the clavicle and down around the coracoid; it gives added stability but does not eliminate the rotation action of the clavicle. We have not found it necessary to pass the fascia through the clavicle or through the acromioclavicular joint.

Late follow-up studies have shown calcific deposits in the fascia between the clavicle and coracoid, which may somewhat limit complete elevation of the arm. Alldredge[3] does not transfix the acromioclavicular joint but uses heavy stainless steel wire around the clavicle and coracoid and omits fascia. He reports 90% good results. The wire is usually removed in 6–8 weeks under local anesthesia.

Neviaser[47] transfixes the acromioclavicular joint with a 1/16-in. Kirschner wire, detaches the coracoid attachment of the coracoacromial ligament, turns it upward and uses it as a ligamentous reinforcement to the superior acromioclavicular ligament.

In 1968, Simmons and Martin[62] reported the successful use of a special pin-screw transfixion of the acromioclavicular joint. The smooth inner end of the screw allows the clavicle to slide against the acromion as well as to rotate. They advise removing the screw under local anesthesia in 3 months.

In *chronic dislocations* of the acromioclavicular joint that are symptomatic or have caused symptomatic traumatic changes in the joint, *resection* of the distal inch of the clavicle has proved most successful in our hands. The technical

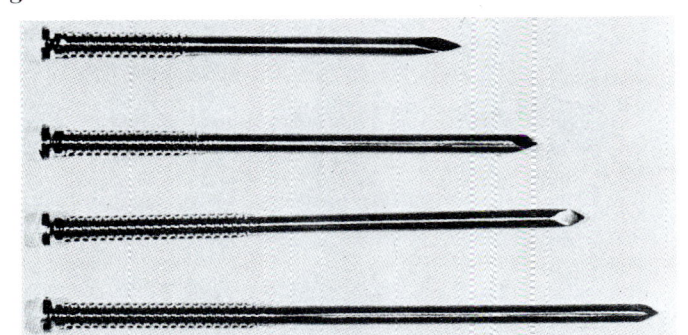

Fig. 17-8. — The Simmons-Martin acromioclavicular pin-screws.

steps are important (Fig. 17-9). The incision is made so that the superior acromioclavicular ligament, capsule and periosteum can be double-breasted over the beveled end of the distal end of the clavicle, thus eliminating the deformity. In the past few years, this technique has been used by the author in *acute complete dislocation* of the acromioclavicular joint with very satisfactory results. In the acute dislocation, special care should be given to repair of the disruption between the trapezius and deltoid muscles. This technique will permit early use of the arm, and no external support is needed. It also eliminates a second operation for removal of internal fixation material, such as wires, screws or pins, as well as the possible late complication of traumatic joint changes.

AFTER-TREATMENT.—The type of aftercare will depend on the method of treatment. For the patient who has had the distal end of the clavicle removed, only a sling is needed for a few days for soft tissue healing, after which the patient has a full range of painless shoulder motion.

When internal fixation material is used, sling support is needed for 10 days to 2 weeks. The patient is cautioned not to elevate his arm fully until the pins or

Fig. 17-9.—Resection of distal end of the clavicle.

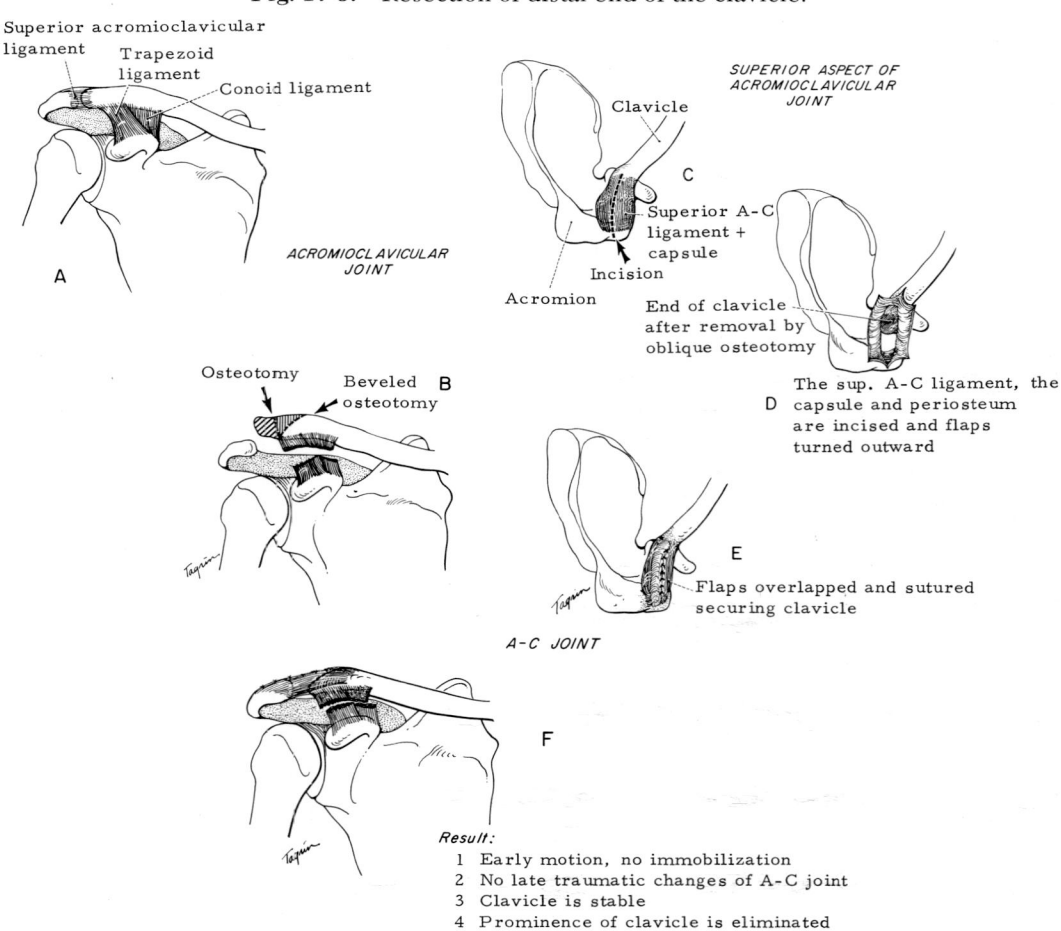

Result:
1 Early motion, no immobilization
2 No late traumatic changes of A-C joint
3 Clavicle is stable
4 Prominence of clavicle is eliminated

wires are removed. Light work may be undertaken in 6–8 weeks or after removal of internal fixation materials, and heavy work probably in 3 months.

Complications

Fractures were associated in 6% of acromioclavicular dislocations at Massachusetts General Hospital, and nerve injury was recorded in only 1 case. There were no serious vascular complications. End-result x-ray films usually indicated a mild degree of ossification of the fascial strips, when these were used for repair.

STERNOCLAVICULAR DISLOCATIONS

Dislocations of the clavicle at the sternoclavicular joint may be acute, chronic or recurrent, superior or posterior. The clavicle is usually dislocated upward, although in rare instances it may dislocate posteriorly. In the acute posterior dislocation, the clavicle has, in some instances, exerted pressure against the trachea. We have had 2 patients in our series in whom dypsnea was critical. Two patients in our series had bilateral recurrent upward dislocations of the clavicle. One patient was able to produce the dislocation voluntarily on either side.

Diagnosis

The diagnosis is made with little difficulty.

Inspection.—A prominence is present at the sternal end of the clavicle. Local ecchymosis and swelling may be present.

Palpation.—Local pain and instability of the inner end of the clavicle are present.

X-ray.—Anteroposterior and oblique views will usually demonstrate the dislocation of the sternoclavicular joint.

Treatment

CLOSED REDUCTION.—Closed reduction of the upward or superior dislocation can be easily accomplished by extension and outward traction of the shoulder and downward pressure on the inner third of the clavicle; however, maintenance of reduction may prove more difficult. We have had good success in securing reduction by the use of the wraparound shoulder support (see Fig. 17-22). Very unstable dislocations are best treated with the patient supine for a week or 10 days.

Reduction of the posterior dislocation may be more difficult than that of the usual superior dislocation. Local procaine infiltration may be necessary, and a towel clamp used to reduce the clavicle. If this fails, open reduction should be performed. Recurrent posterior dislocations are usually accompanied by a fracture of the sternal or clavicular articular surface, rendering the joint unstable.

OPEN REDUCTION.—One of the most reliable techniques of open reduction in our hands consists of repairing the suprasternoclavicular ligament and capsule and reinforcing this repair by using the intra-articular disk if it is still attached to the first rib (Fig. 17-10). This may be reinforced by lashing fascia lata over the inner end of the clavicle to the first rib. Although the sternoclavicular joint can be transfixed by threaded 3/32-in. Kirschner pins, this technique has the potential complication of pin migration.

Old, painful, partial or complete dislocations of the sternoclavicular joint may be the source of continuous discomfort and disability. Resection of the inner end of the clavicle has not, in our hands, been associated with the good clinical results usually obtained by resection of the outer end of the clavicle. A painful, thickened, indurated mass may remain after resection of the inner end, and this may prove to be as bothersome as the original problem.

Recurrent posterior dislocation of the clavicle that produces dangerous pressure against the trachea and has not been successfully stabilized by open reduction may respond safely and effectively to to-

REPAIR OF DISLOCATION OF STERNOCLAVICULAR JOINT

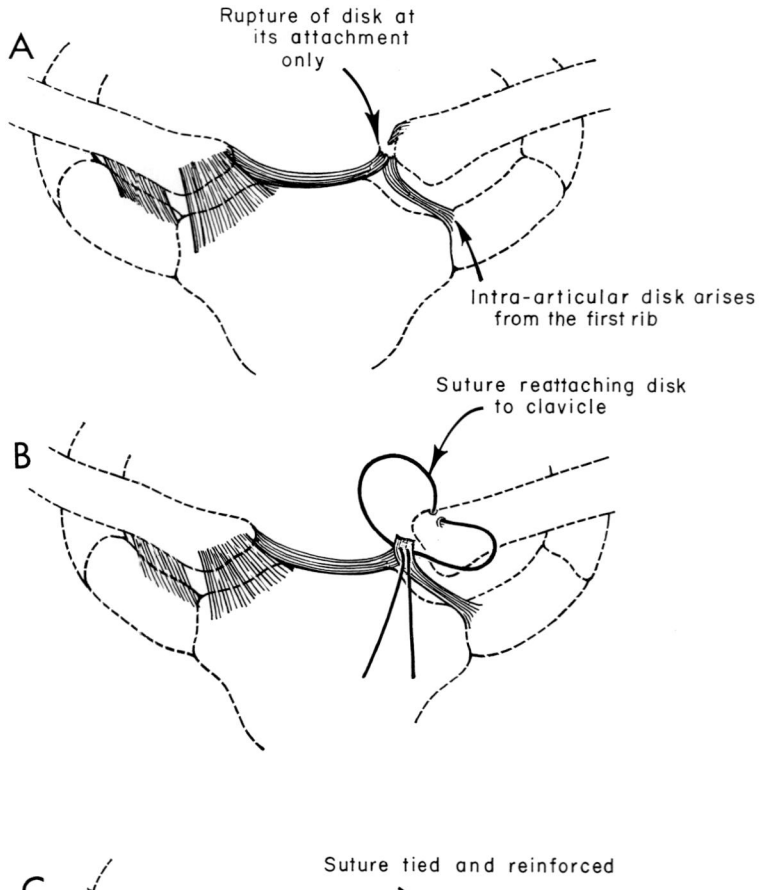

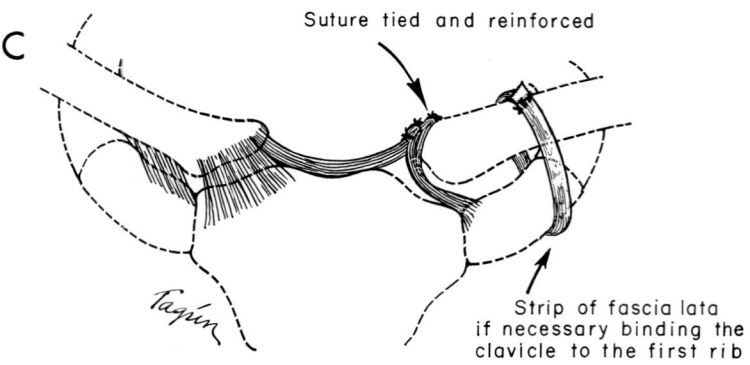

Fig. 17-10. — Repair of superior dislocation of the sternoclavicular joint.

tal resection of the clavicle. If total resection is planned, the surgeon should carefully observe the following technical points.
  1. The skin incision should be made just above and in line with the clavicle. The incision is carried down directly to the clavicle, dividing the periosteum and leaving all muscles attached to the periosteum.
  2. The clavicle is then completely removed from its periosteal bed.
  3. Several strips of Gelfoam are placed in the periosteal bed to eliminate hematoma formation.
  4. The periosteum is then carefully closed, using #40 cotton sutures, securing all muscle attachments to the periosteal bed.
  5. The shoulder is supported by means of a Velpeau dressing for 2–3 weeks, after which graduated exercises are begun.

FRACTURES OF THE CLAVICLE

MECHANISM OF INJURY.—Fractures of the clavicle usually follow a fall on the extended arm or a direct blow to the shoulder. They occur most frequently at the junction of the middle and outer thirds of the bone. The typical deformity is a downward and inward displacement of the shoulder and an elevation of the proximal end of the clavicle (Fig. 17-11).

Diagnosis

Inspection.—The patient with a fractured clavicle has a typical appearance. He leans forward slightly, supporting the injured arm at the elbow and holding it close to the body. Any change in this position may cause pain.

Palpation.—Local pain, swelling and crepitation are usually present over the fracture site.

Fig. 17-11.—Typical deformity of clavicle fracture, with upward pull on the medial fragment and downward displacement of the distal fragment. **A,** transverse fracture. **B,** comminuted fracture.

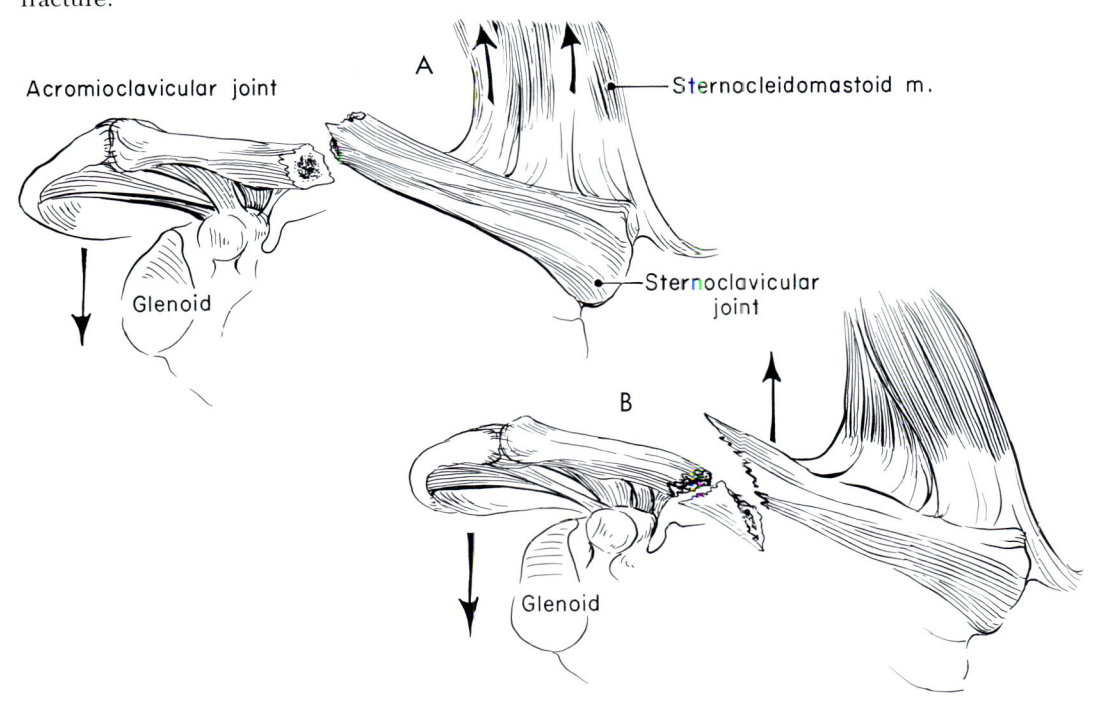

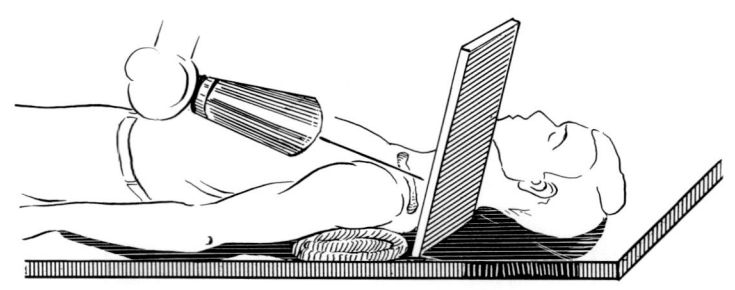

Fig. 17-12.—Oblique view of the clavicle is taken with the tube resting on the patient's chest and the film in the vertical position behind the shoulder.

X-ray.—At times the diagnosis of a fractured clavicle can be difficult. Anteroposterior films of the clavicle may fail to show a fracture line. However, lateral or oblique views will often demonstrate a fracture line that may not be clearly visualized in routine films (Fig. 17-12).

Treatment

Because the typical deformity is depression of the shoulder, reduction is achieved by replacing the shoulder upward and backward. Reduction may not be necessary in infants and in young children, but it is desirable in adolescents and adults. It is usually accomplished by placing the patient on a stool and drawing the shoulders back, or by having the patient lie supine on a fracture table with a small perineal rest, or bar, between the shoulder blades. As a rule, an anesthetic is not necessary. If needed, 5–10 ml of 1% procaine may be used locally.

Methods of immobilizaton.—The methods of immobilization vary with the age of the patient (Fig. 17-13).

Infants.—Usually a hank of knitting wool, used in a figure of eight around the shoulders, will be effective.

Children.—A figure-of-eight webbing, made from Webril and Ace bandages, will give comfort and support. However, frequent adjustments are necessary.

Adults.—In adults the problem is to maintain reduction. The simplest method is complete rest for 3 weeks, the patient flat in bed on a firm mattress, with a slight raise between the shoulder blades. Bed rest is usually impractical and some ambulatory device is required. Interscapular rings or adjustable shoulder braces with figure-of-eight webbing around the shoulders can be effective but require frequent adjustments. One must also watch for axillary irritation or pressure from the figure-of-eight apparatus.

A clavicular cross or a modified shoulder plaster spica can be used. The latter can be applied with the patient sitting or lying. Before the plaster sets, the patient should be upright, so that careful molding of the jacket posteriorly between the scapulae and anteriorly in the pectoral region will maintain the shoulder upward and backward. Clothing can be worn over the spica, and the patient may return to many of his usual activities. As a rule, no change in the plaster is necessary until the fracture has healed.

DURATION OF TREATMENT.—The expected period of healing for fractures of the clavicle may be estimated as follows:

Infants	10–12 days
Children	2–3 weeks
Young adults	4 weeks
Adults	6 weeks or longer

OPERATIVE TREATMENT.—In certain cases in which there is marked displacement and angulation of the fragments, open reduction and intramedullary pinning may be required. The operative technique described here is illustrated in Figures 17-14 and 17-15.

Chapter 17: SHOULDER GIRDLE INJURIES / 413

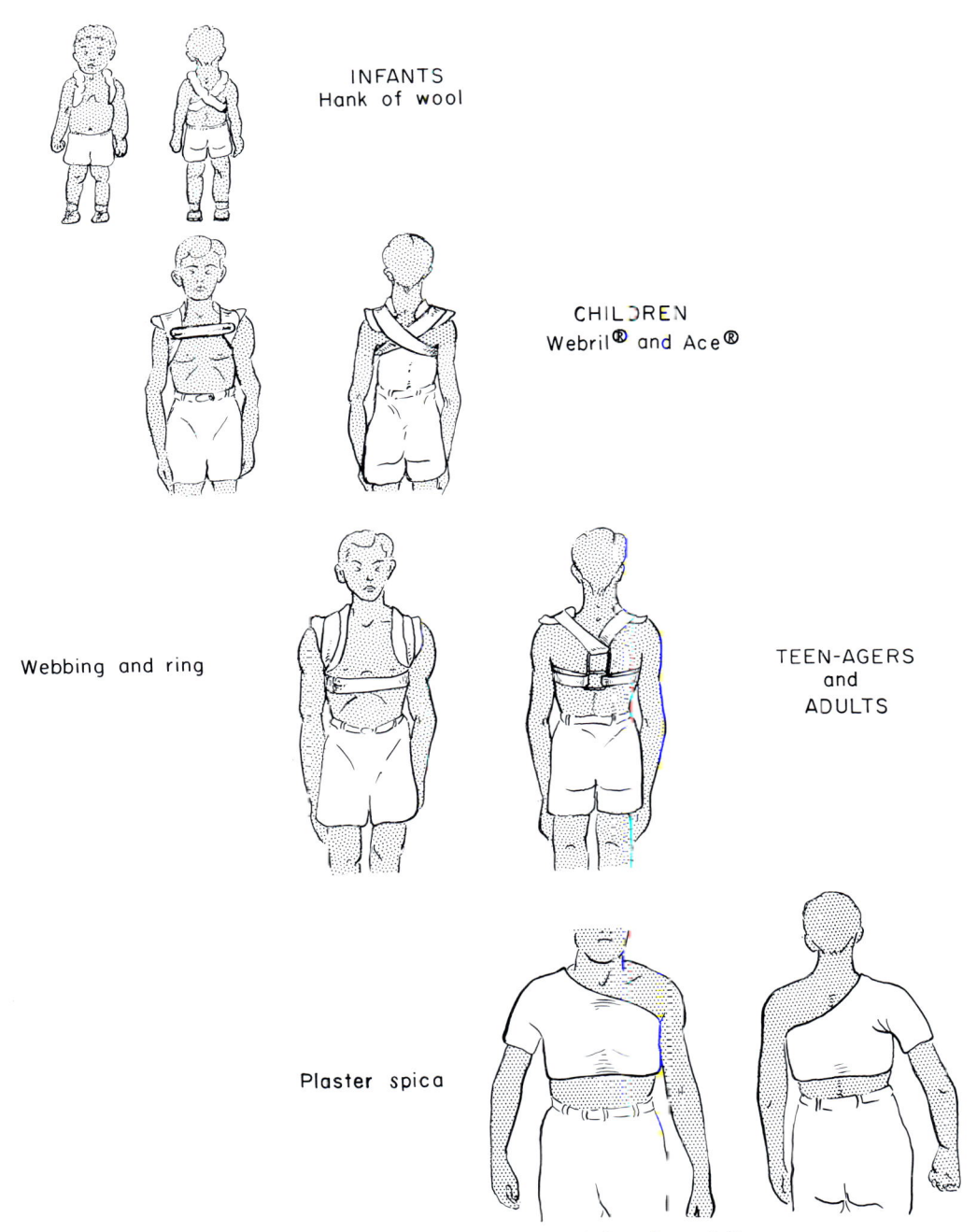

INFANTS
Hank of wool

CHILDREN
Webril® and Ace®

Webbing and ring

TEEN-AGERS
and
ADULTS

Plaster spica

Fig. 17-13. — Typical splints for fractures of clavicle at different ages.

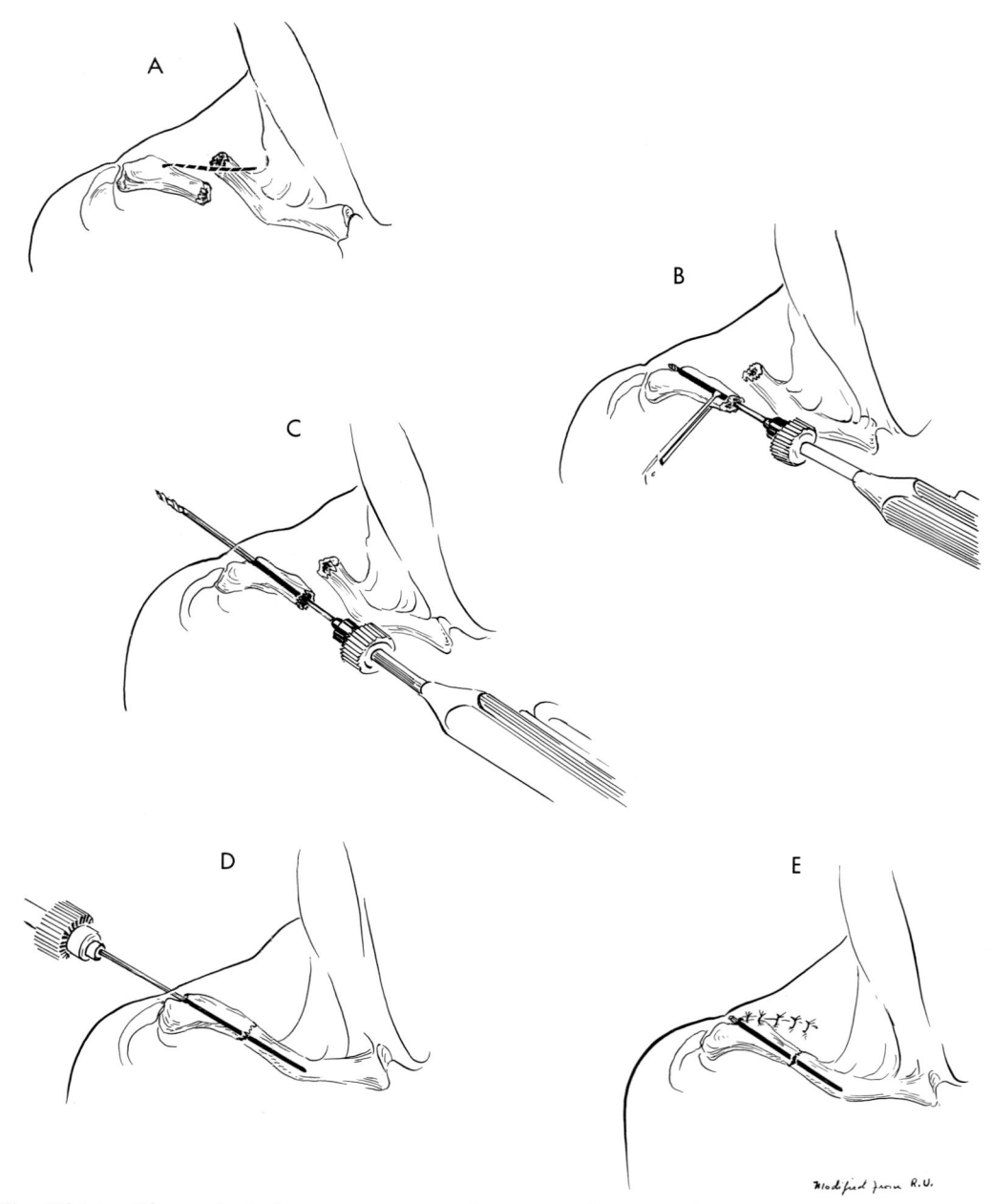

Fig. 17-14.—The technical steps in open reduction and intramedullary fixation of a fractured clavicle, using a 3/32-in. Kirschner pin (see text).

The patient is placed in a semisitting position, with elevation of the injured shoulder. Sandbags or folded blankets are placed under the shoulder blades. The tip of the shoulder should point toward the ceiling. The entire extremity is prepared and draped.

A 2- to 3-in. linear incision is made parallel to, and just above or below, the clavicle (Fig. 17-14, A). Extreme care must be taken in exposing the fragments to avoid injury to the subclavian vessels or brachial nerves.

A 3/32-in. Kirschner wire, or pin, is drilled from the fracture site through the medullary canal of the outer fragment until it pierces the skin behind the acromion (Fig. 17-14, B and C). The Kirschner pin is drilled outward until the base of the pin is at the fracture site.

With the Kirschner pin driven to the fracture site, the drill is removed from the pin. The fracture is then reduced under direct vision.

The drill is next attached to the projecting pin behind the acromion. The pin is then "backed" into the medullary cavity of the proximal fragment of the clavicle for a distance of 2–3 cm, until it strikes the cortex of the middle third of the clavicle (Fig. 17-14, D). *The blunt end of the pin must not penetrate the cortex.* The posteriorly projecting pin is finally cut off below the skin (Fig. 17-14, E).

Nonunion has not occurred in any case at Massachusetts General Hospital following this technique, although several instances of delayed union were experienced because the pin was removed too early. The pin should be left in for 8–10 weeks. If the pin works out, it will extrude posteriorly or *in the line of least resistance.* No instance of extension of the pin proximally into the chest space occurred in this series. Such extension cannot occur if the cortex of the proximal fragment is not penetrated and if the procedure is carried out by direct exposure of the fracture site. In cases of nonunion of the clavicle, iliac or rib grafts are placed subperiosteally around the fracture site. Figure 17-15 illustrates open reduction of a fractured clavicle with intramedullary pin fixation.

Some authors prefer a threaded pin, which will not migrate backward through the skin. However, the disadvantage of a threaded pin is the difficulty in removing it if bent or broken.

A word of warning to the uninitiated surgeon performing this procedure for the first time: the clavicle consists of dense, hard bone. Drilling or passing a pin through the clavicle is difficult and at

Fig. 17-15.—**A,** unsuccessful closed manipulation of a fractured clavicle in a male, aged 19, due to interposition of muscle at fracture site. **B,** open reduction with a 3/32-in. intramedullary Kirschner pin.

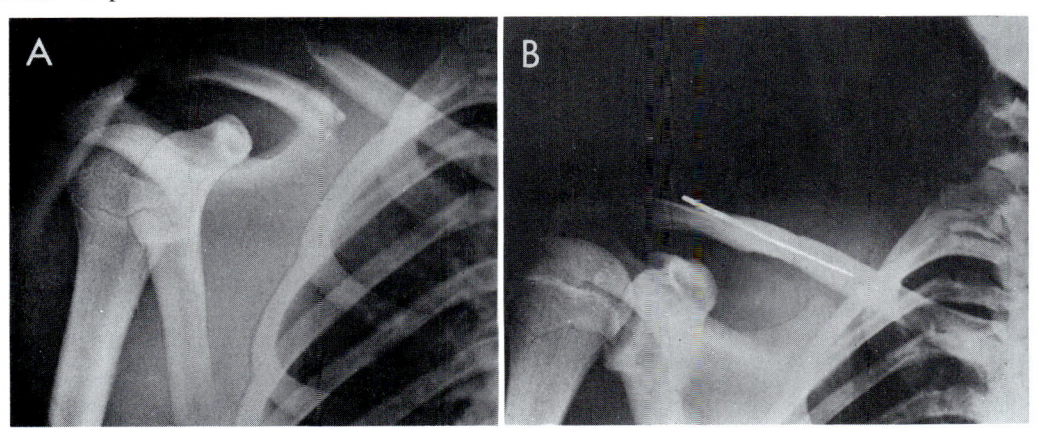

times very frustrating to the uninitiated surgeon.

FRACTURES OF THE SCAPULA

INCIDENCE. — In a series of 75 fractures of the scapula treated at Massachusetts General Hospital, the majority of patients were 40–60 years old; 32% were in their 50s. Most of the fractures involved the middle third of the scapula, including the glenoid, and the neck of the scapula.

COMPLICATIONS. — A fracture of the scapula may be considered a fracture with associated injuries, for some type of associated injury occurred in 71% of patients in this series. Of the associated injuries, 45% were fractures other than the scapular fracture. This is understandable, since the scapular fracture is usually the result of a forceful, direct blow to the torso. Pneumothorax and subcutaneous emphysema occurred in 3% of the patients and injuries to the brachial plexus in 4%. Dislocations complicating this fracture occurred in 12% of the patients; 7% had dislocated shoulders.

Diagnosis

Much may be gained from a careful inspection. Local contusion or subcutaneous hematoma formation may indicate scapular injury. A consistent sign is marked limitation of all shoulder motions because of pain. The patient usually supports the arm close to the body. In evaluating patients with scapular fractures, the examiner must be mindful of other injuries, particularly injuries to the ribs and lungs.

X-rays. — Anteroposterior and oblique tangential views will usually demonstrate scapular fractures.

Treatment

In general, fractures of the scapula heal readily and respond satisfactorily to conservative measures.

FRACTURES OF THE BODY. — Fractures of the flat surface of the scapula are treated with rest and support. As a rule, overlying subcutaneous hematomas will absorb. Support is given to the shoulder by means of a sling for 3 weeks, followed by active exercises.

FRACTURES OF THE SPINE OF SCAPULA AND OF THE ACROMION. — Displaced fractures of the acromion, in which there is interference with the motion of the humeral head, require manipulation or open reduction. Such treatment is rarely necessary if the acromial fragment is small. If it is large, the fragment may be removed. In general, depressed fractures of the spine of the scapula do well with little treatment.

FRACTURES OF THE GLENOID FOSSA AND NECK OF SCAPULA. — All degrees of glenoid fractures may occur, ranging from linear, undisplaced fractures of the fossa to severe bursting fractures with mesial displacement of the humeral head (Fig. 17-16). In x-ray views, these are distressing looking, but little can be gained by open reduction to improve the final, functional result. Initial traction in abduction may give comfort. This may be followed in 10–12 days with early, mild, pendulum exercises in the standing position,

Fig. 17-16. — Complicated scapular fracture with mesial displacement of the glenoid. This patient did very well on conservative treatment.

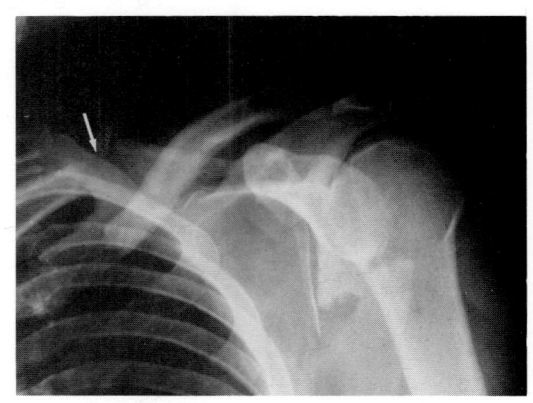

with support to the shoulder by means of a strapping dressing or a sling.

Open reduction may be necessary in rare instances. This should be carefully considered, since closed treatment usually brings good response, with early active function. The most direct approach to the glenoid fossa is through the posterior shoulder exposure.

DISLOCATIONS OF THE SHOULDER

INCIDENCE.—From a study of 500 dislocations of the shoulder at Massachusetts General Hospital in 1956[54] it was found that the *initial*, or primary, dislocation occurred as frequently after 45 years of age as it did before. However, the incidence of *recurrent* dislocation of the shoulder in the author's series[57] was found to be highest in youth, diminishing in each succeeding decade (Table 17-1). McLaughlin and MacLellan's follow-up study in 1967 confirmed this.[41]

TYPES OF DISLOCATION.—It is important to recognize that all dislocations are not the same. Causative factors and pathologic anatomy differ, as does the response to treatment. Therefore, it is essential to recognize that each type of dislocation has its specific treatment.

In general, shoulder dislocations are divided into (1) *traumatic* dislocations (85%) and (2) the *atraumatic* group (15%). The traumatic group usually has typical bankartian lesions, consisting of separation or avulsion of the capsule and labrum from the anterior glenoid rim and erosion, or at times fracture, of the glenoid rim. This group is predictable as to its response to treatment. Atraumatic dislocations, on the other hand, are produced by a minor injury or strain. These do not demonstrate the Bankart lesion injury to the humeral head, or evidences of soft tissue injury, and are notably unpredictable in their response to treatment, whether it be conservative or operative. A small subgroup of atraumatic dislocation is the *voluntary* dislocation, which is most unpredictable. These will be referred to in the discussion of treatment.

Posterior dislocations occurred in 3% of our series, and bilateral dislocations in 2.4%. Fifteen per cent of dislocations were associated with fractures of the

TABLE 17–1.—INCIDENCE OF RECURRENCE OF SHOULDER DISLOCATION IN RELATION TO AGE OF PATIENT

AGE OF PATIENT	NO. OF PRIMARY DISLOCATIONS	NO. OF RECURRENCES	% RECURRENCE
1–10	4	4	100
11–20	49	46	94
21–30	64	51	79
31–40	16	8	50
41–50	33	8	24
51–60	63	9	14
61–70	50	8	16
71–80	32	2	6
81–90	10	0	0
	321	136	42

Total no. shoulders (3 bilateral cases) 324

Under 20 years — 94% recurred
20–40 years — 74% recurred
Over 40 years — 14% recurred

greater tuberosity. The incidence of recurrence was lowest (5.6%) in this group.

The acute *transient dislocation* or recurrent subluxation, which is generally unrecognized, occurs in a small group of patients, usually good athletes, who experience a sudden agonizing pain when suddenly elevating an arm, or when throwing a ball.[9] This type, when recognized, responds successfully to surgical repair. The Bankart lesions are consistently present, indicating a traumatic subluxation or complete dislocation of the shoulder. These dislocations are characterized by spontaneous reduction, thus are never documented by x-ray findings as dislocations. This is often the source of much frustration to the patient, as well as to the physician.

Chronic or *unreduced dislocations* may occur anteriorly, posteriorly or inferiorly. These also present problems in recognition and management and will be discussed under treatment.

Anterior Dislocations

Diagnosis

The patient with an anterior dislocation assumes a typical appearance (Fig. 17-17). On inspection, prominence of the acromion is noted. The natural roundness of the shoulder is lost; there is a depression or hollow under the acromion, and the displaced arm is slightly longer than the normal (opposite) arm. The elbow cannot be brought to the side of the body. In thin subjects, the head of the humerus may be palpated anteriorly in the position in which it comes to rest.

X-rays.—Routine anteroposterior views as a rule show the position of an anterior dislocation, but axillary views (Fig. 17-18) will give more specific information.

Acute Anterior Dislocation

Before manipulating the shoulder, the surgeon should know the following:
1. The position of the humeral head.

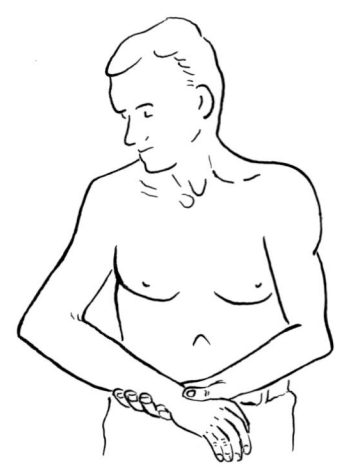

Fig. 17-17.—Typical appearance of patient with an anterior dislocation of the right shoulder.

2. The condition of the humeral head; i.e., the presence or absence of fracture.
3. Whether the dislocation is primary or recurrent.
4. The length of time the shoulder has been dislocated.
5. The presence or absence of nerve injury.

In several instances, patients with old, unreduced dislocations have been admitted to the emergency ward because of superimposed trauma to the shoulder. The resident was greatly embarrassed to find, after several completely unsuccessful attempts at reduction, that the shoulder had been dislocated for 10 years or more.

Reduction of Anterior Dislocations

Since the first edition of this book, we have changed the technique of reduction of shoulder dislocations. In the past, attempts at reduction were carried out with the arm at the side of the body (the hippocratic method with the heel in the axilla or the Kocher method), in which position the surgeon is pulling against strong scapulothoracic and thoracohumeral muscles that are in painful spasm. When the surgeon finds he is unable to overcome

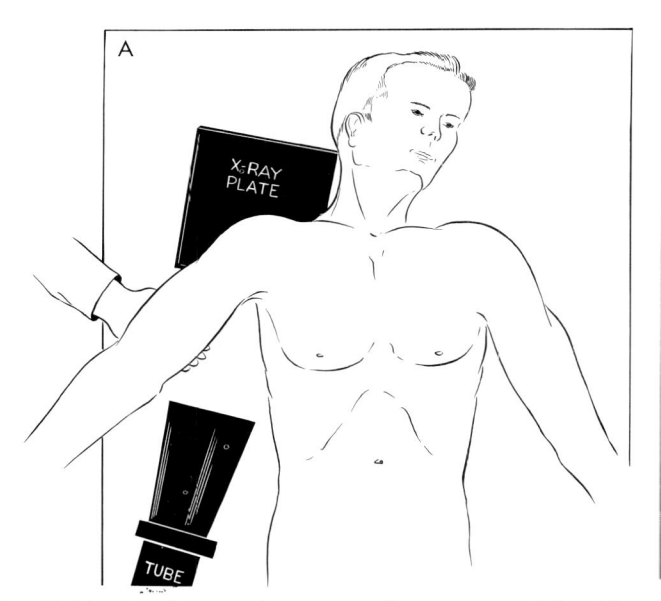

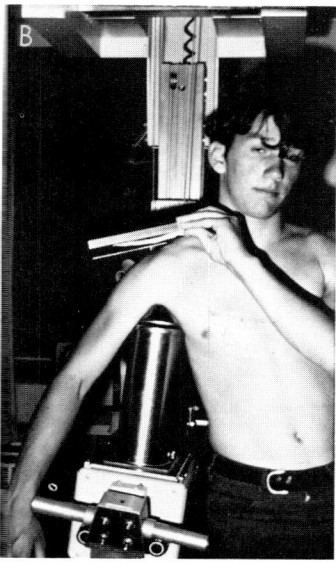

Fig. 17-18. — Technique for true axillary views of shoulder. **A,** supine: With the arm supported, the x-ray tube is placed in the axilla and the film placed over the top. **B,** standing: The patient leans lateralward, the injured arm is supported away from the body, and the x-ray tube is inverted and focused up through the axilla to the film, which is placed superior to the shoulder.

the pull of these muscles, he then resorts to an anesthetic. In the past 10 years, we have had consistent success using the principles pointed out in 1825 by Sir Astley Cooper[17] and in 1934 by E. A. Codman[16] that, when the arm is in complete elevation, the controlling muscles of the shoulder are neutralized or powerless and offer little resistance to the surgeon. Thus, in the overhead position, muscle spasm is eliminated and reduction of the dislocation is relatively easy and painless. Milch,[42] in 1963, also recommended the overhead method to reduce fracture-dislocations of the shoulder.

The residents in our emergency ward have been taught this method. Seldom is medication or an anesthetic needed, unless the shoulder has been unreduced for several days.

STEPS IN REDUCTION. — 1. The patient is placed supine on the treatment table.
2. The maneuver is explained to the patient. He is told to relax as his arm is slowly and gently elevated (Fig. 17-19, *A*) in forward flexion (not in abduction) to full elevation or the direct overhead position. If the patient complains of numbness or tingling in his hand or arm, further manipulation is not carried out. We have *not* had this occur to date.
3. With the arm in complete elevation, gentle upward and outward traction is produced in 25–30 degrees of abduction (Fig. 17-19, *B*). This displaces the head of the humerus lateralward from beneath the coracoid to the edge of the glenoid.
4. The surgeon's thumb is then placed under the humeral head, and the head is gently lifted into the glenoid (Fig. 17-19, *C*).

Another method that may be used and that observes essentially the same principles as the overhead method is the Stimson traction method (Fig. 17-20). After 10–15 minutes in this position the shoulder may be reduced by gentle downward and upward traction.

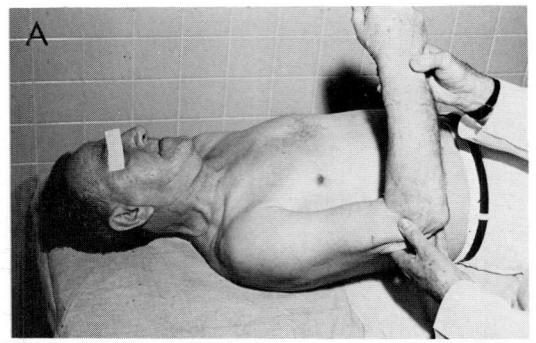

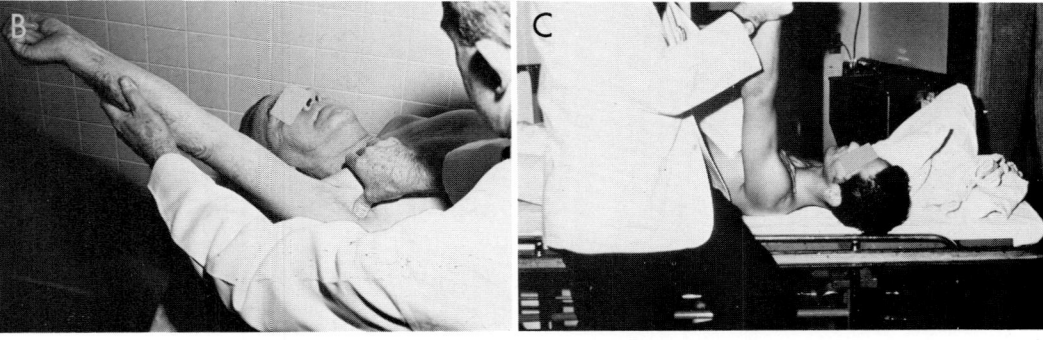

Fig. 17-19.—Reduction of anterior dislocation of the shoulder by the *elevation method.* **A,** arm is gently elevated to the overhead position. **B,** upward and outward pull is applied by the operator in full elevation. Pressure is then applied from below to the humeral head, reducing the shoulder. **C,** reduction of anterior dislocation, without pain medication, in a jockey who had dislocated his shoulder 1 hour prior to admission.

Fig. 17-20.—Stimson method of reduction of an anterior dislocated shoulder.

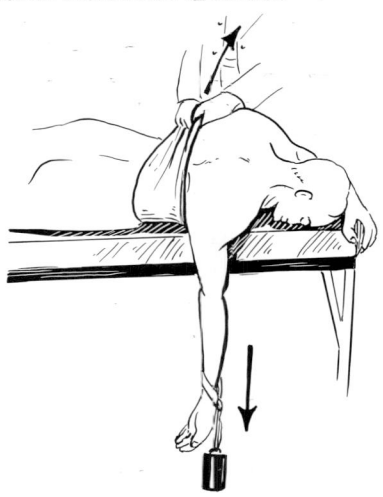

KOCHER METHOD.—Although this method is used infrequently in our hospital, the Kocher maneuver (Fig. 17-21) is described for those who may prefer it.

1. Gentle traction is applied in line of deformity with the elbow flexed to 90 degrees. Gradually the arm is externally rotated.

2. With the arm in external rotation and under steady traction, the extremity is adducted across the chest and then internally rotated. This will usually reduce the shoulder. A rapid, grinding maneuver should be avoided. *A word of warning:* Avoid force. The surgeon must be mindful of the possibility of fractures of the humerus occurring when this maneuver is used in elderly patients or in old dislocations.

Chapter 17: SHOULDER GIRDLE INJURIES / 421

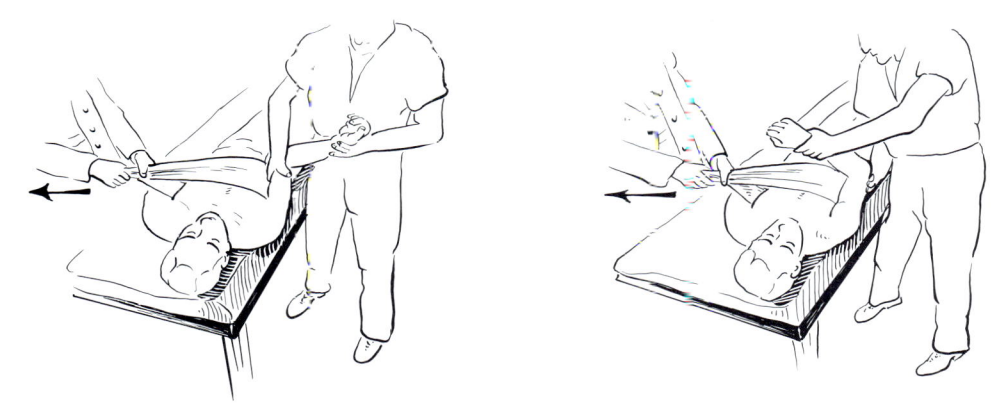

Fig. 17-21.—Kocher method of reduction of anterior dislocation of shoulder.

Fig. 17-22.—Simple methods of shoulder support. **A,** front and back views of the sling-and-swathe, or double sling, support. **B,** the wraparound sling.

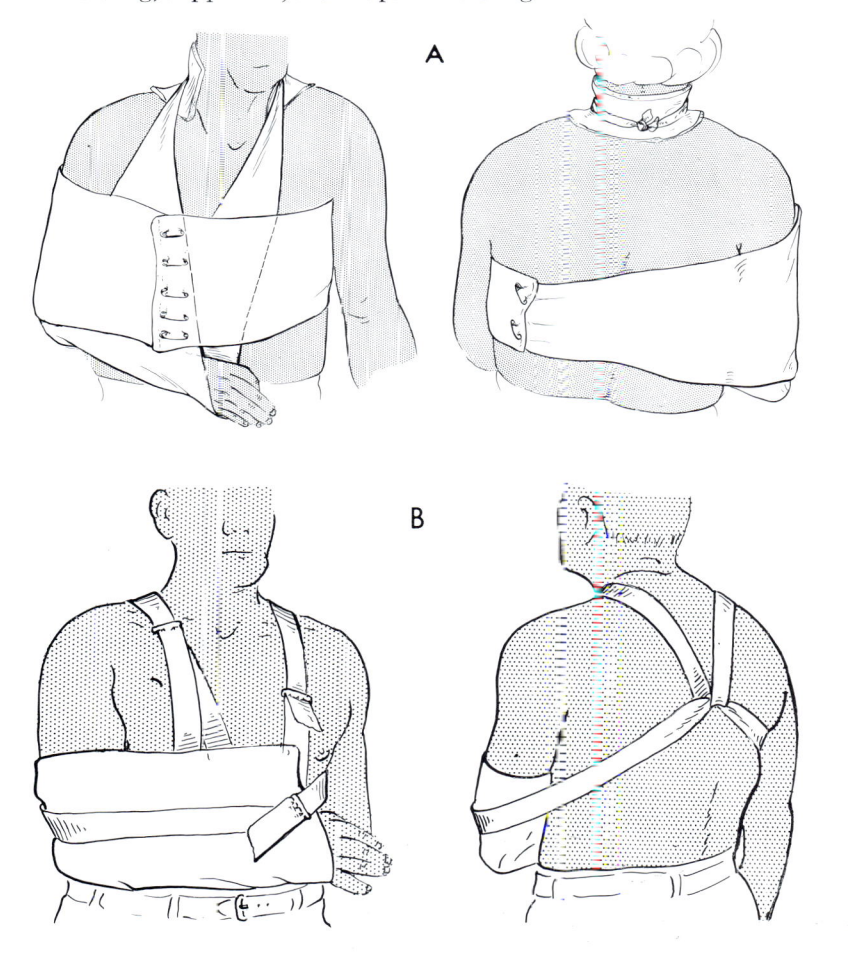

Reduction of Posterior Dislocations

The usual position of the upper extremity in a posterior dislocation is one of internal rotation and adduction. To reduce a posterior shoulder dislocation, the arm should be gently brought into a position of forward flexion and abduction. While traction is applied in this position, the surgeon places his thumb *behind* the humeral head and, with lateral pressure, replaces the head into the glenoid.

After-Care

After reduction, x-rays should be taken to show the position of the humeral head in relation to the glenoid and the presence or absence of fractures. The axilla should then be powdered and the shoulder supported in 1 of the following ways.

For an *anterior* dislocation, the shoulder should be supported in a position of adduction and internal rotation. We have used the wraparound sling (Fig. 17-22), which is made in the hospital sewing room, and have found it to be comfortable and efficient.

For the *posterior* dislocation, the arm should be simply supported posterior to the coronal plane of the body (Fig. 17-23). We have found the use of Elastoplast a simple and effective way to accomplish this.

LENGTH OF IMMOBILIZATION. — Follow-up statistics in the author's series indicate that the incidence of recurrent dislocations drops off rapidly at 50 years of age. Therefore, in persons over 50, the shoulder should be immobilized for a short time only. Active exercises should be begun early, in order to maintain maximum range of motion and function. The incidence of recurrence following the initial dislocation is high in the teenager and young adult. Our follow-up studies indicate that 3 weeks of immobilization in adduction and internal rotation lowered the incidence by 15%. However, periods of immobilization *longer* than 3 weeks, surprisingly, were associated with a higher incidence of recurrence.

EXERCISES. — During immobilization, active use of the hand, wrist and elbow should be begun immediately, with deltoid-setting exercises for the shoulder. To be effective, these exercises are best

Fig. 17-23. — A simple and effective method of supporting the arm after reduction of a posterior dislocation. Note: The arm should be maintained *posterior* to the coronal plane of the body.

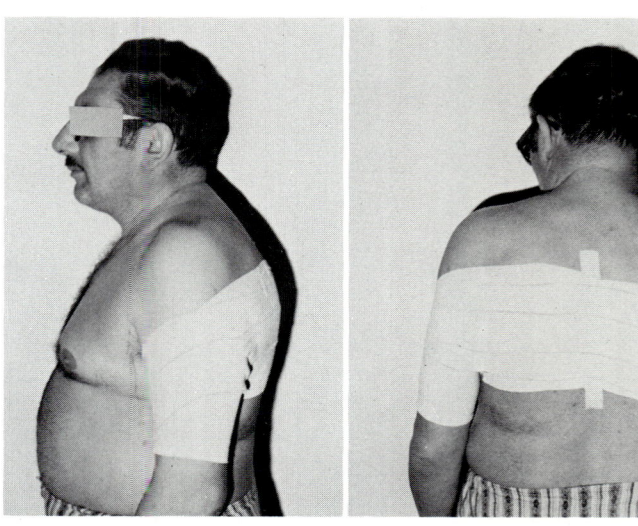

performed slowly and repeatedly during the day.

Following immobilization of the shoulder, a period of resistive exercises is most important in restoring muscle strength and stability to the shoulder. The exercise program should be planned to strengthen the muscles of abduction, external rotation and internal rotation. These can be carried out as illustrated in Figure 17-24.

Recurrent Anterior Dislocations

Pathologic Factors

It is generally conceded that no single pathologic finding accounts for recurrent shoulder dislocations. Rather, they result from traumatic factors, individual predisposition and the natural unstable structure of the shoulder.

The checking forces that prevent dislocation of the shoulder are a combination of muscle tone, the enveloping short rotators, the protective pivoting of the scapula and the checking elements along the anteroinferior glenoid rim, consisting of the labrum and the attached capsule. In elevation and external rotation of the shoulder, the capsule tenses; with adequate attachment, plus the glenoid labrum, it functions as a check to the forward riding of the humeral head. The subscapularis muscle is also a definite

Fig. 17-24.—Specific resistive exercises in abduction, in internal rotation and in external rotation will strengthen the supporting muscles of the glenohumeral joint.

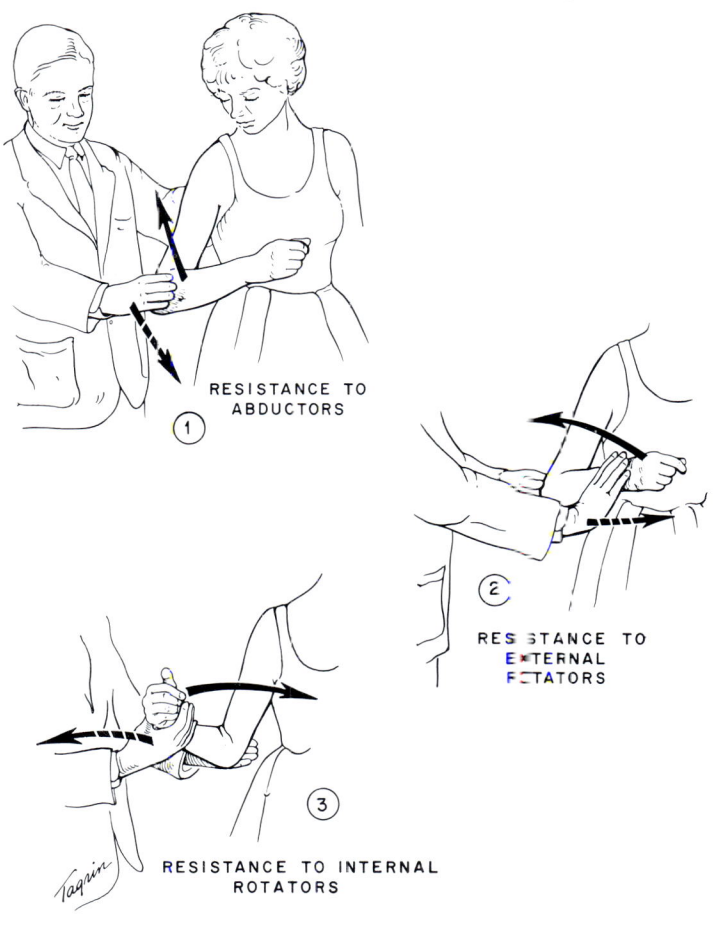

factor in checking the humeral head, particularly in the position of elevation and external rotation of the shoulder. However, in extreme elevation and external rotation, the subscapularis muscle moves upward and leaves the anteroinferior part of the humeral head unprotected. In the position of elevation, also, the neck of the humerus is in close contact with the acromion, a leverage point to force the head out of the joint.

Separation of capsule and labrum (the medial and inferior capsular folds) from the anterior glenoid rim (the Bankart lesion).—This lesion (Fig. 17-25) is present in a high percentage of recurrent traumatic dislocations. In the atraumatic recurrent dislocations, this lesion is usually not present.

Compression fracture of the superior lateral surface of the humeral head (Hill-Sacks lesion).—This lesion (Fig. 17-26) occurred in our series[53] in 38% of primary traumatic dislocations and in 57% of recurrent traumatic dislocations.

Constitutional factors.—A relatively small group of persons are predisposed, by constitutional factors, to have recurrent shoulder dislocations. Such dislocations occur with little or no trauma to the shoulder.

Surgical Procedures

Operative repair is indicated in dislocations that recur frequently and thus become a disability. The primary requirement for operative repair, regardless of the method employed, is an adequate surgical exposure; for without this, the pathologic anatomy associated with the dislocation cannot be identified and thereby corrected. The operation should have as its aim the restoration of a stable shoulder with a useful range of motion.

The method of shoulder repair used by the majority of the staff at the Massachusetts General Hospital is Bankart's operation or some modification. This operation has proved extremely satisfactory.

From our experience and from reports of operative procedures in follow-up

Fig. 17-25.—The Bankart lesion, illustrating separation of the capsule (and labrum) from the anterior glenoid rim and neck.

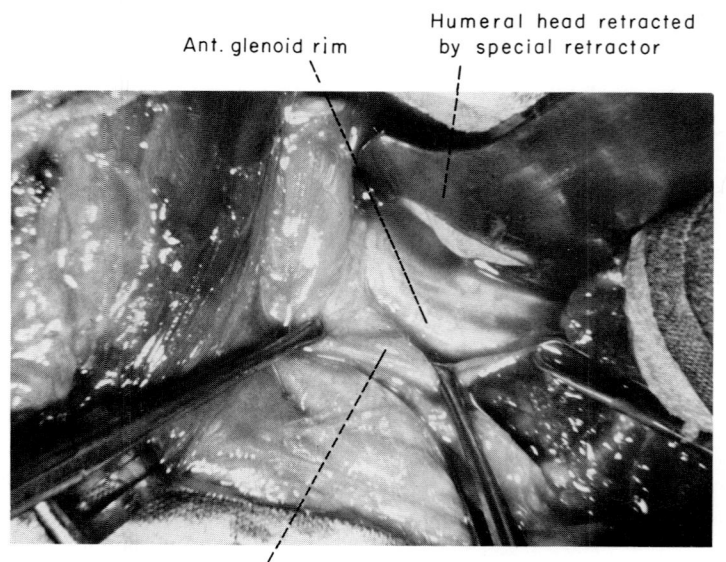

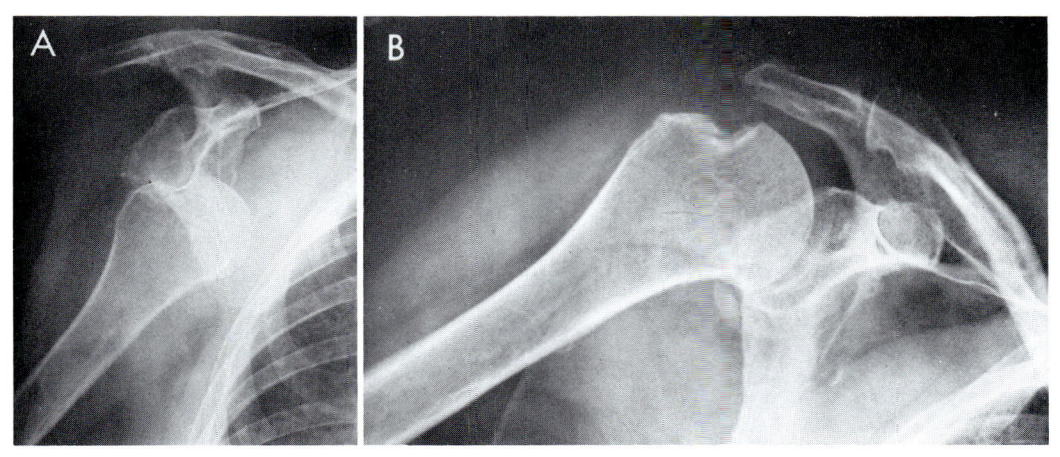

Fig. 17-26.—Anteroposterior views of right shoulder showing the typical "hatchet" defect in the humeral head. **A**, subglenoid dislocation before reduction. **B**, postreduction. (From Rowe, C. R.: Prognosis in dislocations of the shoulder, J. Bone Joint Surg. 38-A:957, 1956.)

studies in the literature, the following techniques are standing the test of time and have a relatively low rate of recurrence for traumatic anterior recurrent dislocation of the shoulder: the Bankart (1–5% recurrence); the Putti-Platt (5% recurrence); the Gallie-LeMesurier (4% recurrence); the Hybbinette-Eden (6.3% recurrence); and the Magnuson-Stack (2.45% recurrence). The Rowley-Bristow procedure has been popularized by Arthur Helfet[28] and, although results are encouraging, we do not have to date a series with a long-term follow-up.

The Nicola procedure has a high rate of recurrence in young active individuals (59% in our series). The Dickson operation has not had an adequate test. The Henderson sling operation and the Clairmont-Ehrlich procedure have been uniformly unsuccessful in the experience of the staff at our fracture clinic.

The foregoing techniques have their loyal supporters. The design of the Putti-Platt and the Magnuson-Stack procedures is to limit external rotation. The Rowley-Bristow operation relies on the sling effect of the short head of biceps and coracobrachialis muscles across the anteroinferior glenoid. We prefer the modification of the Bankart procedure, for this repair goes directly to the source of the shoulder's instability—the anterior rim of the glenoid.

THE BANKART PROCEDURE.—*Object.*— Direct reattachment of the capsule to the anterior rim of the glenoid; reinforcement of the attachment by double-breasting the mesial flap of capsule over the lateral flap, thus producing a strong buttress along the bony rim, allowing restoration of an excellent range of motion.

Position of the patient.—The patient is placed with a rolled blanket under his shoulder and the injured shoulder elevated. The entire extremity is surgically prepared and draped (Fig. 17-27), so as to be available for maneuvering by the surgeon. The anesthetist should be positioned on the opposite side of the operating table, thus giving more space to the surgeon and his assistant.

Skin incision.—We recommend that the incision begin at the anterior fold of the axilla and extend upward toward the coracoid (Figs. 17-28 and 17-29, A). In females the incision may be short and still adequate. In heavy muscular males it is necessary to extend the incision up to the coracoid or to the clavicle for adequate exposure. We do not use the true

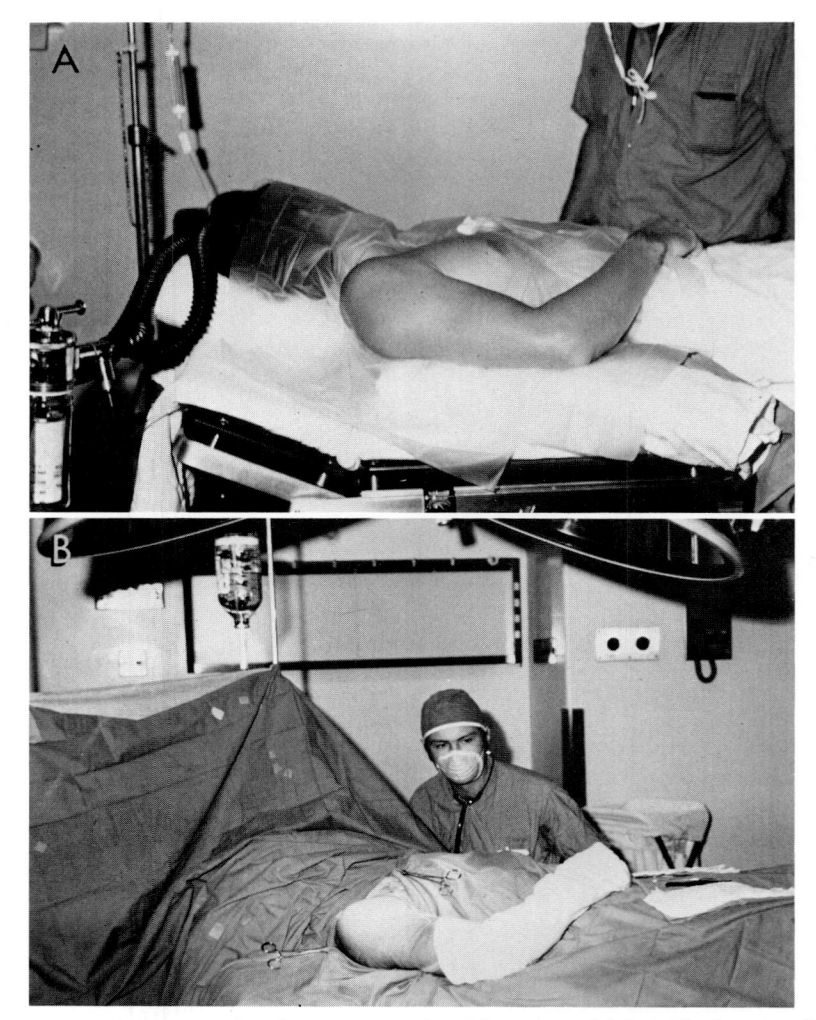

Fig. 17-27.—Surgical draping for the anterior shoulder. **A,** a folded blanket is placed under the shoulder and arm. Plastic drapes are applied before prepping. **B,** the anesthetist is positioned on the opposite side of the table, giving more room to the surgeon and his assistant at the head of the table.

"axillary approach," preferring to keep out of the armpit. We also advise that the incision not be extended down the arm lateral to the axillary fold, because the incision in this area invariably spreads.

Shoulder exposure.—The deltopectoral space is identified and developed. The cephalic vein should be picked up here; it may be retracted or, if troublesome, it can be ligated "high and low" and discarded. As a rule, it is not necessary to detach the deltoid from the clavicle. However, when necessary for exposure, the inner 2–3 in. can be separated from the clavicle by sharp dissection.

The coracoid process may, or may not, be osteotomized (Fig. 17-29, *B*). As a rule, osteotomy is preferred because it allows the attached muscles to retract mesially toward the chest wall. Prolonged traction

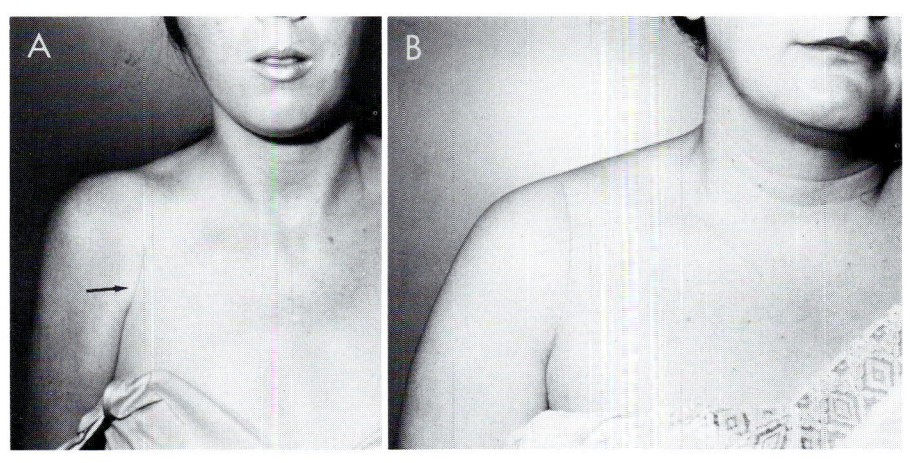

Fig. 17-28.—Anterior incisions. The incision for an anterior approach to the shoulder should begin in the anterior axillary fold, and extend upward toward the coracoid in line with the natural skin lines **A**, a short incision may be adequate in a thin patient. **B**, a longer incision may be required for heavier individuals.

on these muscles may injure the musculocutaneous nerve which supplies the biceps and the coracobrachialis muscles. Before osteotomizing the coracoid, a hole should be made through it with a small gouge.

The subscapularis muscle is outlined by externally rotating the arm. The lower border of the muscle is identified by the "marginal veins" (the anterior humeral circumflex veins). These are ligated separately with a suture ligature (Fig. 17-29, C). Removing the subscapularis from the capsule is a most important step and can be performed simply and easily. However, it has proved a difficult obstacle to many surgeons, causing them either to cut completely through the muscle and capsule and perform a Putti-Platt procedure or to split the subscapularis muscle in the line of its fibers, modifying the Bankart technique.

A helpful suggestion in removing the subscapularis muscle cleanly and completely from the capsule is first to do a complete external rotation of the arm, then to bevel the knife almost horizontally and, beginning at the tendinous attachment to the lesser tuberosity, to separate the musculotendinous attachment from the capsule (Fig. 17-29, D). This is the only difficult part, as the muscle belly of the subscapularis is not densely adherent beyond its tendon and can be easily separated by blunt dissection. The subscapularis muscle is then marked and allowed to retract toward the chest wall. There are a number of advantages of complete separation of the subscapularis muscle from the capsule. (1) The surgeon has complete exposure of the shoulder lesion. (2) The capsule is available to direct repair. (3) The entire subscapularis muscle is available for reattachment lower or more laterally, if necessary.

One now has the capsule completely exposed. When this has been accomplished, the surgeon is surprised to find that it is a much more developed tissue, thicker and stronger than he had expected. With the arm in external rotation, 2 Allis forceps are applied to the capsule approximately ¼ in. lateral to the glenoid rim (Fig. 17-29, E). The capsule is then opened in line with the rim and the joint is inspected (Fig. 17-29, F). In traumatic dislocations the capsule is usually separated from the anterior glenoid rim and the labrum is nonexistent. In those patients who have experienced many re-

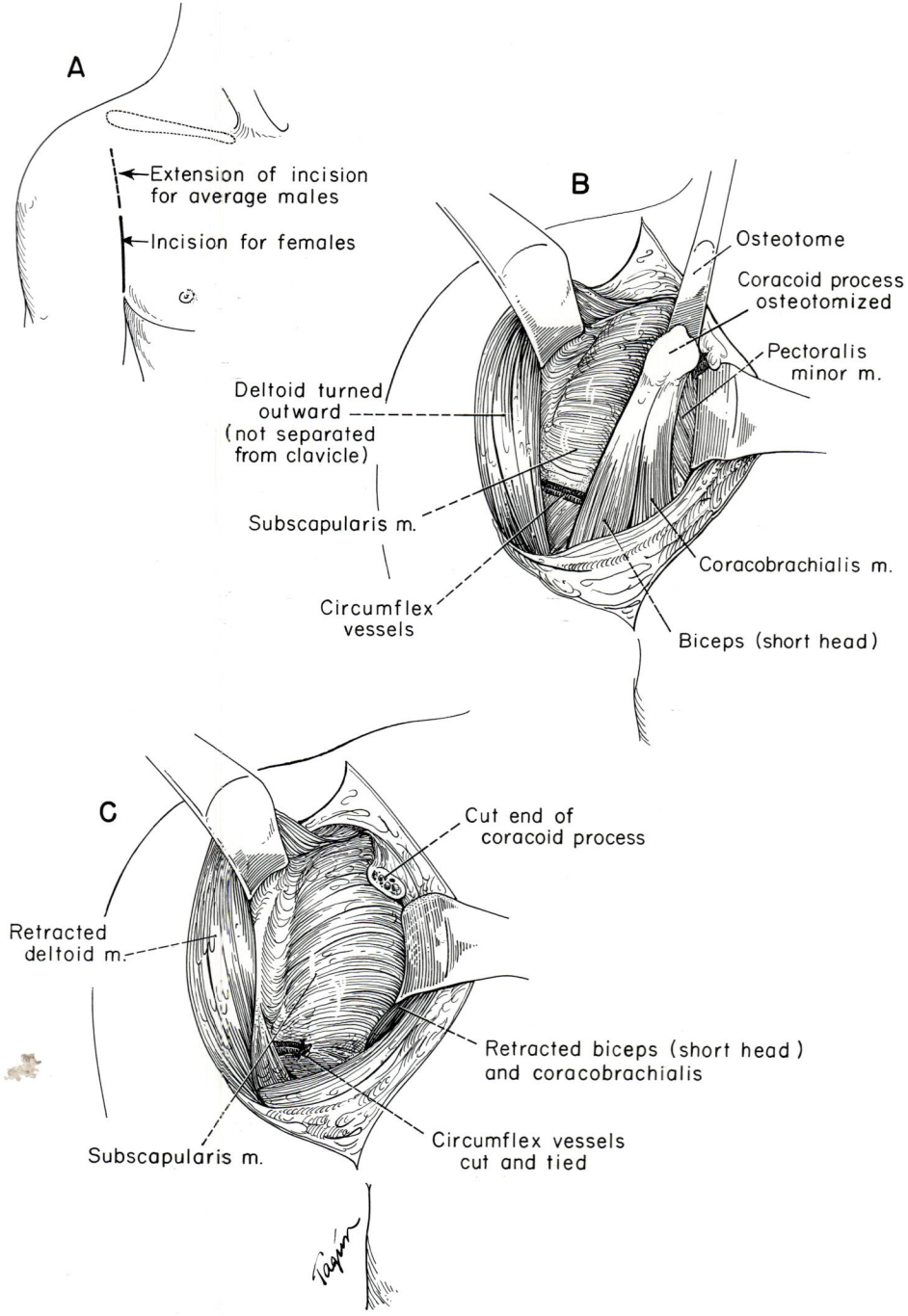

Fig. 17-29.—Operative steps in the modified Bankart procedure (as used by the author).

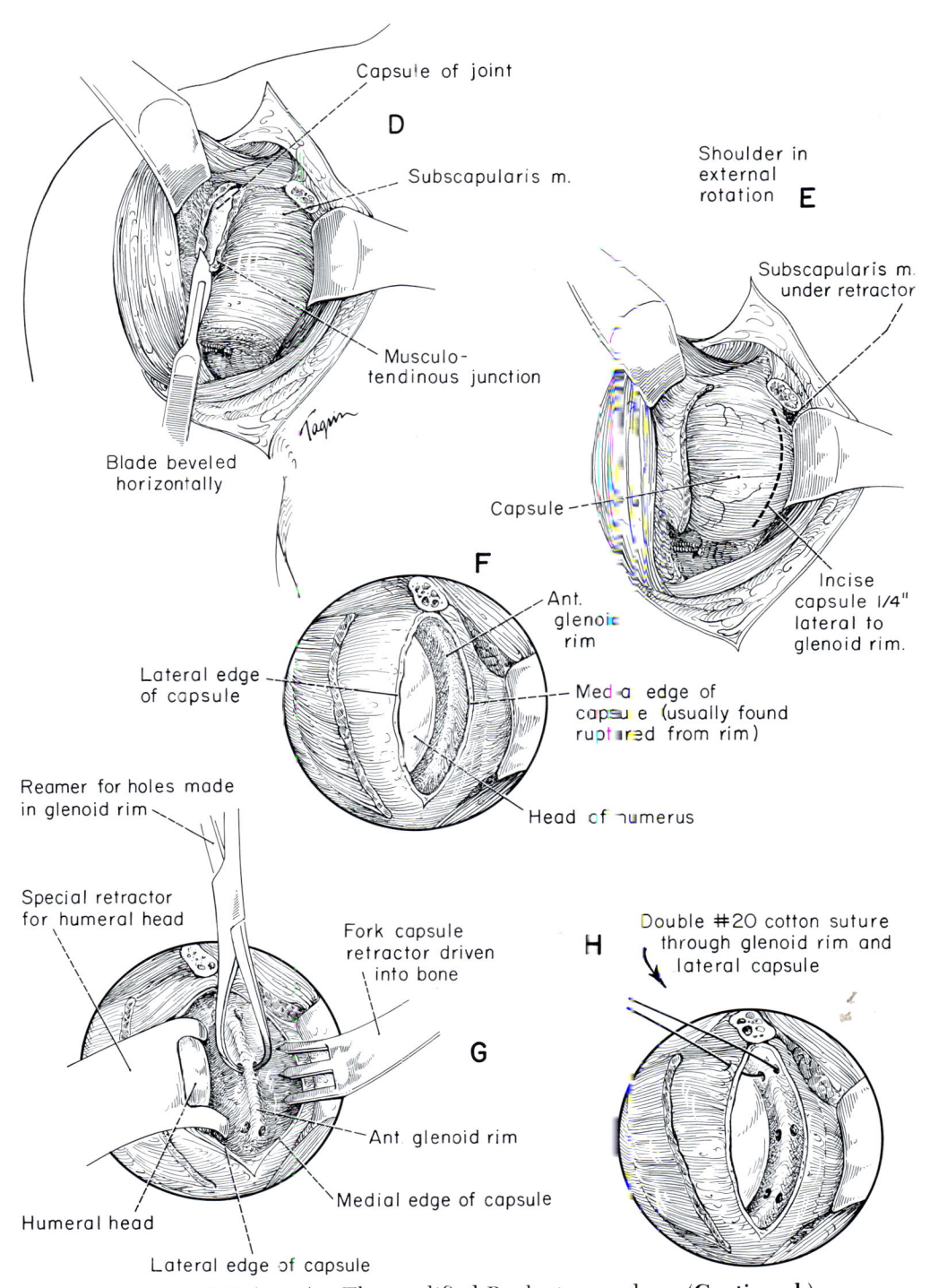

Fig. 17-29 (cont.).—The modified Bankart procedure. (Continued.)

I Direct suture of lateral flap of capsule to glenoid rim.

J Medial capsule is then double-breasted over lateral capsular repair

K Subscapularis m. resutured to its insertion (or reinforced downward or more laterally)

L Reattachment of coracoid process by 3 double cotton sutures

Subscapularis m.

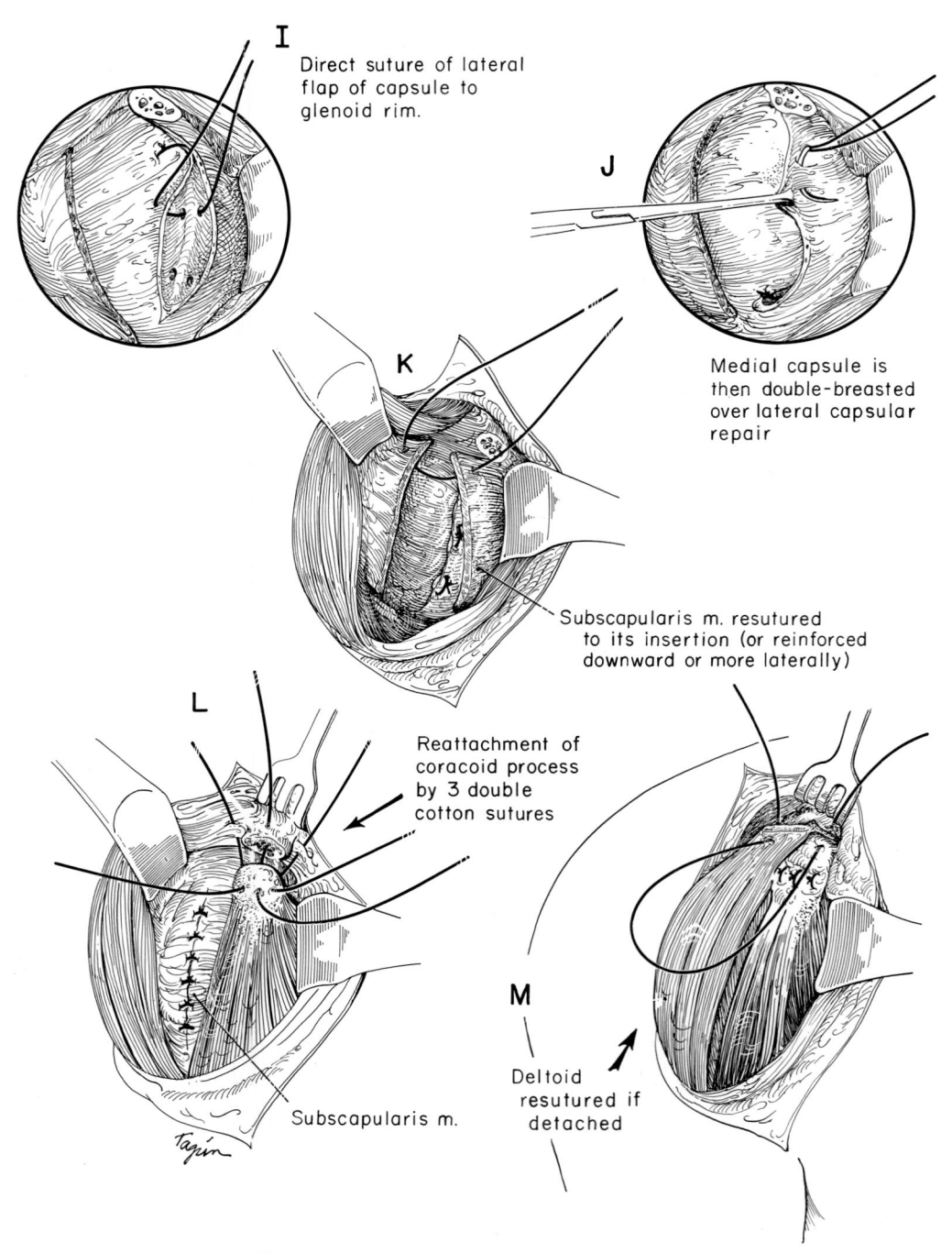

M Deltoid resutured if detached

Fig. 17-29 (cont.). — The modified Bankart procedure.

currences, the bony rim is eburnated, worn down and, in some instances, actually fractured off.

Of great assistance are the humeral head and fork capsule retractors (Figs. 17-29, G, and 17-30). The former is inserted with its prongs over the posterior glenoid rim, displacing the head laterally. The fork is inserted into the neck of the scapula to retract the mesial fold of the capsule. With these 2 instruments, there is no need for other retraction in the wound.

The bony rim is then freshened, and 3 holes are made in the rim, in the upper one-third, the middle and lower one-third of the glenoid or, on a right shoulder, at 1–3–5 o'clock. These holes can be easily made with a specially devised pincer sharpened on 3 sides. When the holes are completed, 2 strands of #20 cotton are inserted onto a small curved needle (a no. 5 Mayo trocar needle), which is "backed through" the 3 holes. The head retractor is then removed, the suture passed through the lateral flap of capsule (Fig. 17-29, H) firmly tied down to the bony rim (Fig. 17-29, I). The mesial capsule is then double-breasted over the repair for extra strength (Fig. 17-29, J). This will permit unrestricted external rotation of 25 or 30 degrees at the time of surgery, a great advantage in regaining complete external rotation postoperatively. Eyre-Brook,[23] instead of reattaching the capsule to the rim of the glenoid, designs 3 holes along the neck of the scapula just mesial to the rim and sutures the lateral capsule to the scapular neck.

The subscapularis muscle is then resutured to its original insertion or, when indicated, a bit more inferiorly or laterally (Fig. 17-29, K). The coracoid process is reattached by 3 double #20 cotton sutures, 1 through the bone and 2 at the lateral and mesial tendinous junctions (Fig. 17-29, L). The deltoid muscle is resutured to the periosteum of the clavicle (Fig. 17-29, M). The deltopectoral junction closes naturally and may be secured by a few interrupted 000 plain catgut sutures.

A wraparound sling (Fig. 17-22, B) is applied at surgery, which is comfortable and effective.

After-treatment.—Early motion of the

Fig. 17-30.—A, instruments used for the modified Bankart repair. *1*, the humeral head retractor; *2*, the fork to hold the capsule off the neck of the scapula; *3*, pincers used to make the glenoid rim holes; *4*, curved instruments to complete the holes. B, the glenoid pincers have 3 sharpened edges to facilitate making holes in the glenoid.

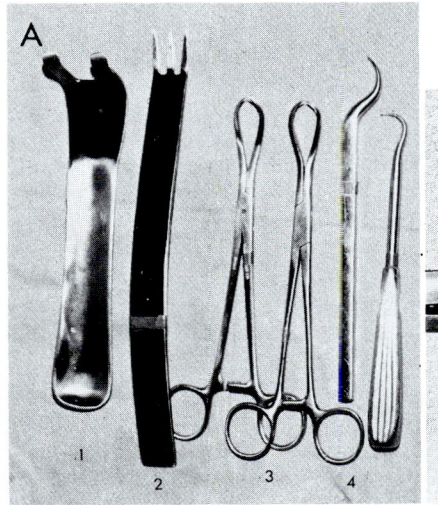

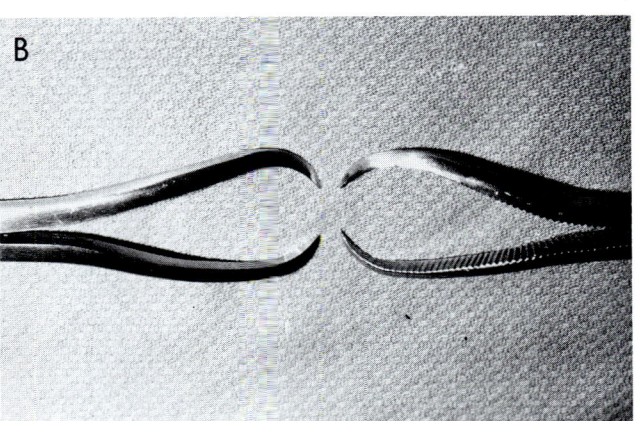

shoulder is begun by removing the sling during the second or third postoperative day. In fact, the patient may take a shower on the fourth or fifth day. The patient is usually discharged the fifth day and is instructed to wear the sling part time for 3 weeks. Pendulum exercises are begun and the arm is free during the day for increasing activities. The patient is encouraged to use the arm as tolerated, increasing its range of motion and function over the first 6 weeks. Useful motion is expected at 6 weeks and near full range of motion within 3–6 months. The patient is then allowed to participate in heavy work and athletics.

THE PUTTI-PLATT PROCEDURE (Fig. 17-31). — *Object.* — Overlapping and shortening ("double-breasting") the subscapularis tendon.

Approach. — The anterior portion of the shoulder is used.

Division of the subscapularis tendon. — The arm is then externally rotated and the upper and lower portions of the subscapularis muscle identified. The surgeon passes his finger or a blunt instrument under the subscapularis muscle and divides the tendon approximately 1 in. medial to its insertion into the lesser tuberosity. The incision is carried down directly through the muscle and capsule. The joint is opened and inspected.

Repair. — The lateral stump of the subscapularis tendon and capsule is attached to the anterior glenoid rim or the neck of the scapula. This is done with the arm in internal rotation. Here the technique varies somewhat. Some surgeons suture the tendon to the labrum (if intact), to the glenoid rim or to the periosteal tissues along the scapular neck. The mesial portion of the capsule and of the subscapularis muscle is then "double-breasted" over this repair and attached to the lesser tuberosity or bicipital groove. This operation has given very stable reduction, but external rotation is more limited than after the Bankart procedure.

After-treatment. — The arm is supported at the side of the chest for 3 or 4 weeks. This treatment is followed by a program of active exercises.

THE GALLIE-LEMESURIER PROCEDURE

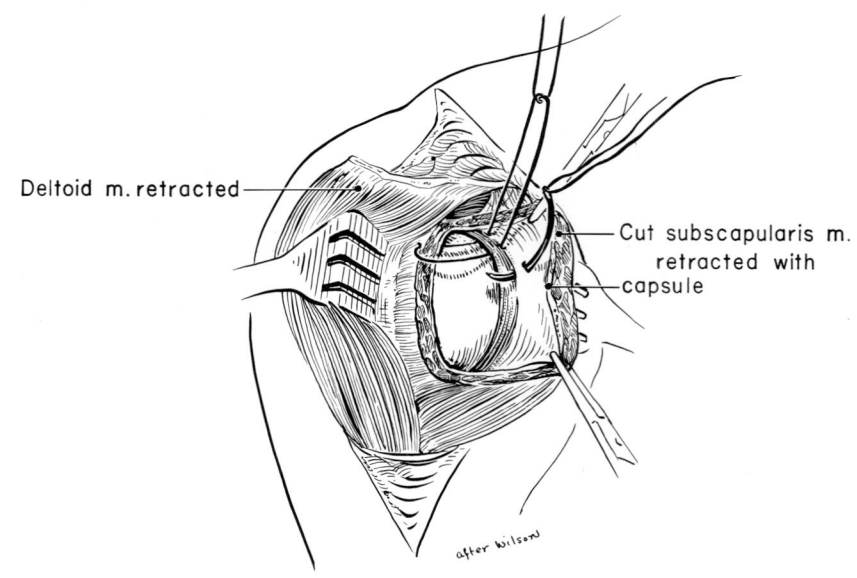

Fig. 17-31. — The Putti-Platt procedure. (From Osmond-Clarke, H.: Recurrent dislocations of the shoulder, J. Bone Joint Surg. 30-B:19, 1948.)

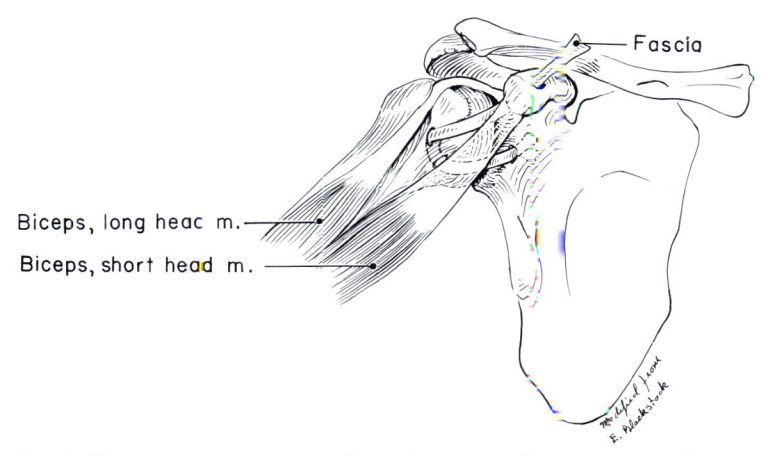

Fig. 17-32.—The Gallie-LeMesurier procedure. (From Gallie, W. E., and LeMesurier, A. B.: Dislocations of the shoulder, J. Bone Joint Surg. 30-B:9, 1948.)

(Fig. 17-32).—*Object.*—Reconstruction of a "new ligament" (fascia lata) for the anterior capsule and the glenohumeral ligament.

Approach.—The anterior approach to the shoulder is similar to the Bankart approach, except that the subscapularis tendon is left attached and is retracted upward from its lower border, exposing the underlying capsule.

Repair.—With the forefinger of the left hand on the anterior glenoid rim, a 3/16-in. drill is driven through the neck of the scapula from a point 1/2 in. from its lower border. The drill is tapped gently onward until it reaches the skin below the scapular spine. A 1-in. incision will expose the point of the drill. A strip of fascia 1/2 in. wide and 10 in. long is removed from the thigh. In 1 end a single knot is tied. The fascial strip is passed anteriorly through the drill hole, leaving the knot posteriorly. The fascia is next passed through the tunnel in the anterior humeral neck, then through the coracoid. The fascia is then split and sutured anteriorly to itself.

After-treatment.—The arm is supported across the chest. Abduction and external rotation are avoided for a month, after which active exercises are begun. Gallie states that at first there is marked limitation of external rotation and abduction but that after 3–4 weeks only slight limitation of external rotation persists.

THE HYBBINETTE-EDEN PROCEDURE (AFTER IVAR-PALMER AND ANDERSON) (Fig. 17-33) —*Object.*—"Fixing" a bone graft (iliac crest) in the periosteal pocket of the anterior glenoid rim.

Approach.—The anterior shoulder approach is used.

Repair.—With the joint open, the humerus is pulled down and outward, allowing inspection of the glenoid and anterior joint capsule. A subperiosteal pocket is made with a rasp or osteotome along the anterior glenoid rim. If the labrum is found attached, the pocket is made be-

Fig. 17-33.—The Hybbinette-Eden procedure.

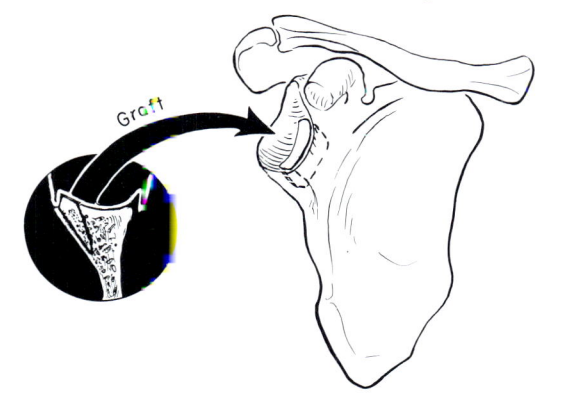

tween the labrum and the rim. A bone graft usually measuring 1 × ¼ in., but varying according to the size of the pocket, is taken from the iliac crest. The graft is pressed down into the subperiosteal pocket so that the projecting part is lodged on the rim, forming an anterior wall of bone. For stability, Eyre-Brook transfixes the graft with a metal screw.

After-treatment.—The arm is supported in a sling for 2 weeks, after which active motion of the arm is begun, but external rotation is avoided.

THE MAGNUSON-STACK PROCEDURE (Fig. 17-34).—*Object.*—"The formation of a cup of muscle or tendon around the lower or anterior part of the head of the humerus."

Approach.—The anterior approach to the shoulder is used as in the preceding exposures.

Exposure.—The subscapularis tendon is identified and its borders above and below are freed. The tendon, with a wedge of bone, is detached from its insertion at the bicipital groove. The tendon is retracted mesially, exposing the anterior capsule and humeral head and also the glenoid rim.

Repair.—The arm is then internally rotated and the tendon is pulled around to a position below the greater tuberosity to the upper portion of the shaft of the humerus and is attached here to a wedge-shaped gutter in the humerus. The tendon may be sutured to the capsule or to the external rotator cuff for reinforcement. This procedure extends the wraparound effect of the subscapularis muscle and tendon to a lower position, thus becoming more effective when the shoulder is in elevation and external rotation.

After-treatment.—The arm is supported across the chest by a Velpeau bandage for 2 weeks and then by a sling for 2 weeks. Active exercises are then begun, but external rotation and elevation of the shoulder are avoided for 8 weeks postoperatively. Permanent external rotation of 50% may be present, but function is good.

THE NICOLA PROCEDURE (Fig. 17-35).—*Object.*—Transplantation of the long head of the biceps tendon through the head of the humerus.

Fig. 17-34.—The Magnuson-Stack procedure.

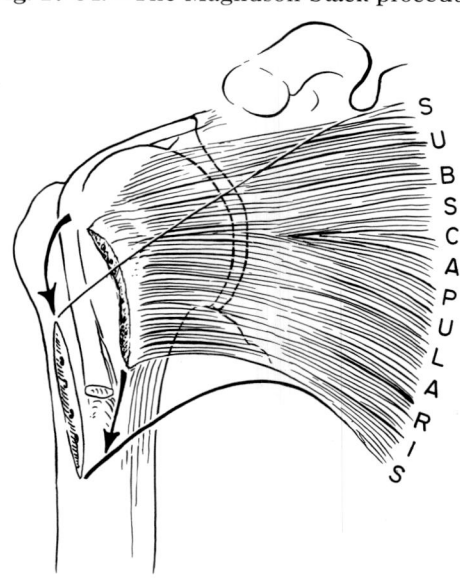

Fig. 17-35.—The Nicola procedure.

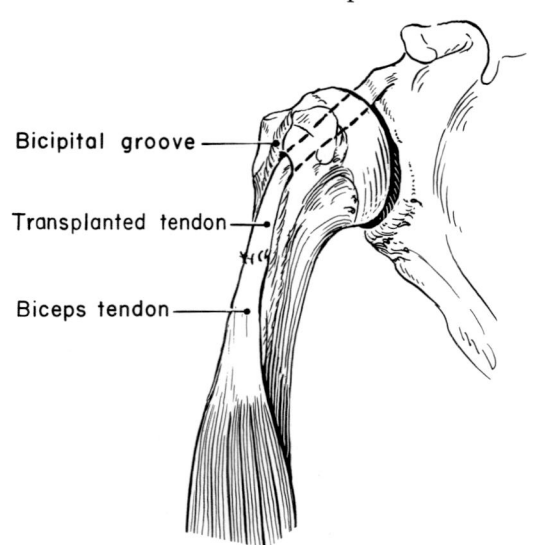

Approach.—Anterior approach to the shoulder.

Exposure.—The tendon to the long head of the biceps is exposed by division of the transverse humeral ligament or the "roof" of the bicipital groove. Stay sutures ¼ in. apart are placed through the tendon 1 in. below the cut margin of the transverse humeral ligament. The tendon is divided proximally to the sutures.

Repair.—Just below the transverse humeral ligament, a ¼-in. hole is drilled through the humeral head to the center or approximate center of the articular surface of the head. Some surgeons aim for a point halfway between the center of the head and the articular border. By means of a tendon passer, the proximal tendon is passed from the joint through the humeral head and is reattached to its fellow tendon at the base of the groove.

After-treatment.—The shoulder is supported for a period of 2–3 weeks with a double sling (Fig. 22, A) or Velpeau bandage, after which active exercises are begun.

THE ROWLEY BRISTOW PROCEDURE (HELFET MODIFICATION) (Fig. 17-36).—In this procedure the terminal ½ in. of the coracoid process, with its attached conjoined tendon of the short head of the biceps and the coracobrachialis, is osteotomized and transplanted through the tendinous portion of the subscapularis muscle to the neck of the scapula, just medial to the glenoid rim. Thus, when the arm is elevated and externally rotat-

Fig. 17-36.—The Rowley Bristow procedure (Helfet modification). **A**, exposure of coracoid process and conjoined tendon. **B**, coracoid process is divided and peeled downward with conjoined tendon. Slit is made through tendon of subscapularis, and scapular neck is rawed through this slit. **C**, coracoid process is passed through slit and lies in contact with rawed area of scapula. Subscapularis is closed around the transplanted bone and attached muscles. (From Helfet, A. J.: Coracoid transplantation for recurring dislocation of the shoulder, J. Bone Joint Surg. 40-B:198, 1958.)

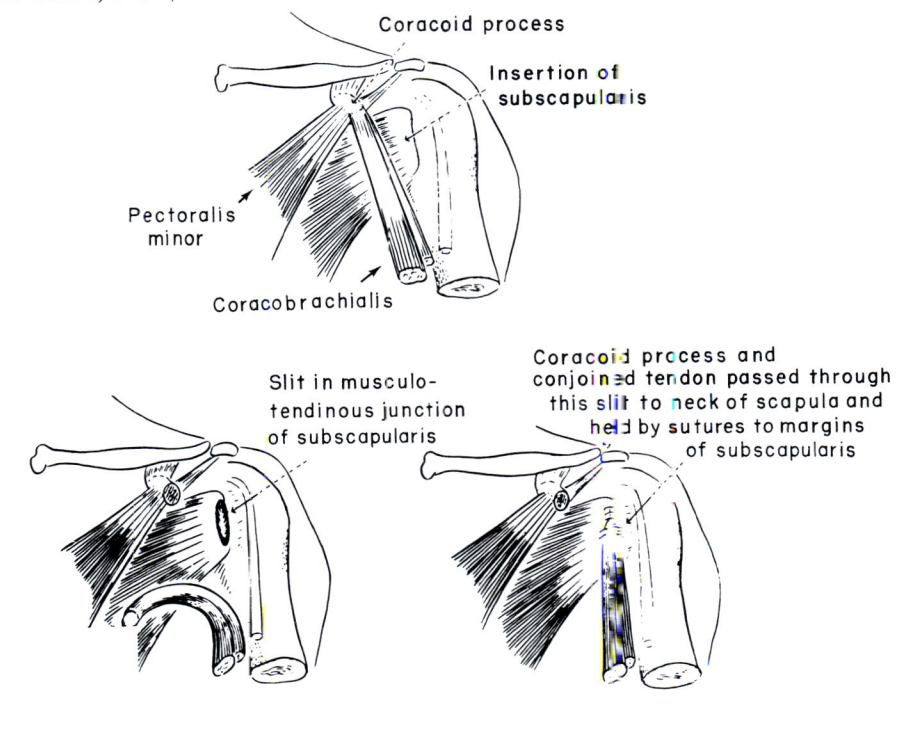

ed, the attached muscles form a buttressing sling across the weak area, the anteroinferior surface of the capsule.

The shoulder is protected for 6 weeks, after which the fixation of the coracoid process is firm and the patient is allowed to increase the motions and use of the arm as tolerated.

Transient Recurrent Anterior Subluxation

This syndrome is becoming more frequently recognized at present and is included under traumatic dislocations. The patient is usually a good athlete, who complains that when he suddenly elevates or externally rotates his arm, or when he throws a ball, he experiences a sudden "paralyzing" pain in his shoulder and arm, causing the arm temporarily to "go dead." The patient becomes frustrated and disappointed, as x-rays are read as "negative" and his physician has not been able to document a dislocation or reproduce the shoulder complaint on physical examination. Thus, lacking a diagnosis, usually no treatment is offered. The author and others[9] have explored the shoulders of a number of these patients and have found a typical Bankart lesion, indicating that the patient has experienced a transient subluxation, which reduces immediately and leaves few identifying traces. Fortunately, this painful syndrome responds well to procedures used for the usual traumatic, recurrent anterior dislocations. In the author's hands, the modified Bankart procedure is preferred.

Fig. 17-37.—**A**, unrecognized posterior dislocation of left shoulder of 3 months' duration. The patient was seen because "he had not responded to physical therapy." With arms at the side of the body and elbows flexed 90 degrees, he is unable to externally rotate the left arm. Note atrophy of left anterior deltoid muscle. **B**, view of shoulders from above illustrates absence of normal anterior contour of left shoulder and the abnormal prominence posteriorly. **C**, anteroposterior views may be deceiving; these were read as normal. **D**, true axillary views, however, clearly demonstrate the posterior dislocation of the *left* shoulder.

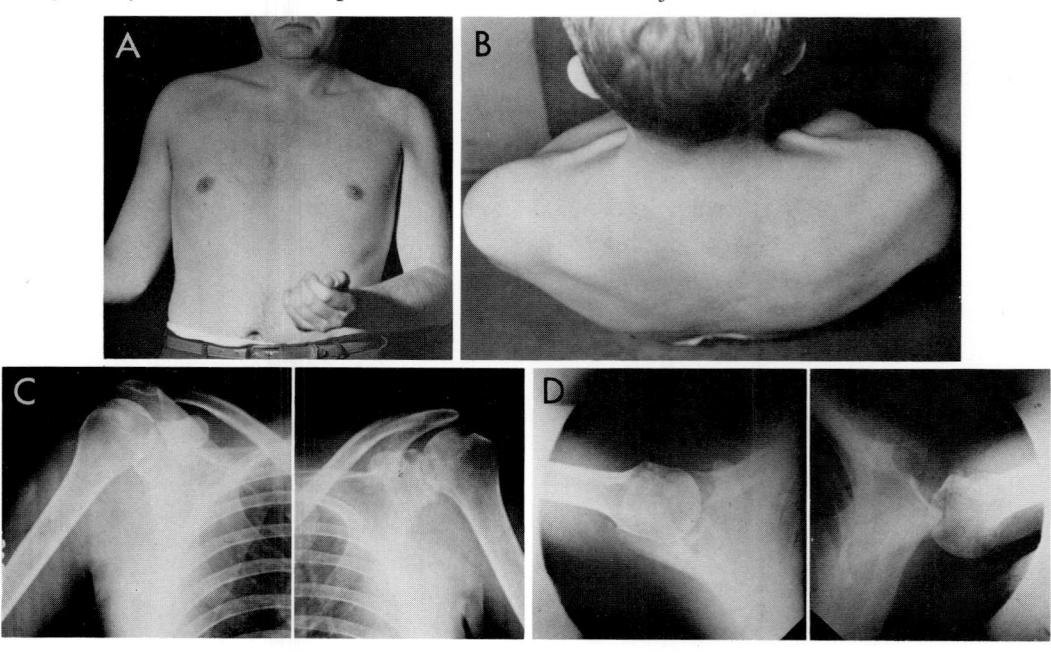

Posterior Dislocations

Traumatic posterior dislocations may be divided into 2 types, the primary and the recurrent.

DIAGNOSIS. — Posterior dislocations are often difficult to diagnose and sometimes go unrecognized for months or years. This has been the experience of the staff at Massachusetts General Hospital and has been emphasized by Wilson and McKeever[69] and by McLaughlin.[38] On casual inspection, the examiner may see little. However, there are several helpful signs: The patient's arm is in a position of complete internal rotation. The arm *cannot* be externally rotated (Fig. 17-37, A). A helpful diagnostic procedure is to have the patient sit in a chair and to observe his shoulders from above. The injured shoulder will show loss of the normal anterior roundness and possibly slight fullness posteriorly in the infraspinous fossa (Fig. 17-37, B). On palpation in thin subjects, the head of the humerus may be felt in the posterior position.

X-rays (Fig. 17-37, C and D). — In routine anteroposterior roentgenograms the shoulder may appear perfectly normal. Axillary views, however, will demonstrate the posterior dislocation. If necessary, transthoracic or oblique views may be taken, but as a rule good axillary views are sufficient (Fig. 17-18).

PRIMARY TRAUMATIC DISLOCATION. — This injury is commonly accompanied by history of a definite, severe blow to the shoulder. The head of the humerus is usually found wedged over the posterior glenoid rim.

When there has been delay in recognizing the dislocation, open reduction is necessary. The utility shoulder incision is used (Fig. 17-38). Adequate exposure is necessary because there may be some difficulty in replacing the head of the humerus in the glenoid fossa. Reduction usually can be maintained by overlapping the external rotators. When in doubt, a bone graft may be wedged posteriorly, as in the anterior Hybbinette-Eden procedure, or as below for recurrent posterior dislocation.

RECURRENT DISLOCATION. — This condition occurs with little initiating trauma and is frequently associated with some degree of muscle imbalance. Recurrent posterior dislocations are usually produced from a position of forward elevation and internal rotation of the arm with some adduction. In most instances, the patient is able to reduce the dislocation. Operative repair of this condition has been successfully carried out at Massachusetts General Hospital by using the Bankart technique along the posterior glenoid rim or performing osteotomy of the posterior glenoid neck and inserting a wedge graft (Fig. 17-39), taken from the curve of the posterior acromion.[61]

Old Unreduced Traumatic Dislocations

MANIPULATION. — Closed manipulation, if performed with care and gentleness, may be attempted for dislocations which have been unreduced up to a period of 6 weeks. With complete relaxation and prolonged traction and countertraction, and with complete understanding on the surgeon's part of the inherent dangers of this maneuver, reduction has been obtained in a number of old dislocations. Force must never be applied, and repeated manipulations should be discouraged, especially in elderly patients.

OPEN REDUCTION. — The decision for open reduction should be based on the amount of pain and functional disability the patient is experiencing. Actually, the unreduced shoulder functions as an arthrodesed shoulder. If it is not painful and if the patient is satisfied with the limited motion he has, as so many elderly patients may be then one should not recommend open reduction. If, however, the patient is in constant discomfort, is experiencing sensory or motor irritation

438 / Carter R. Rowe

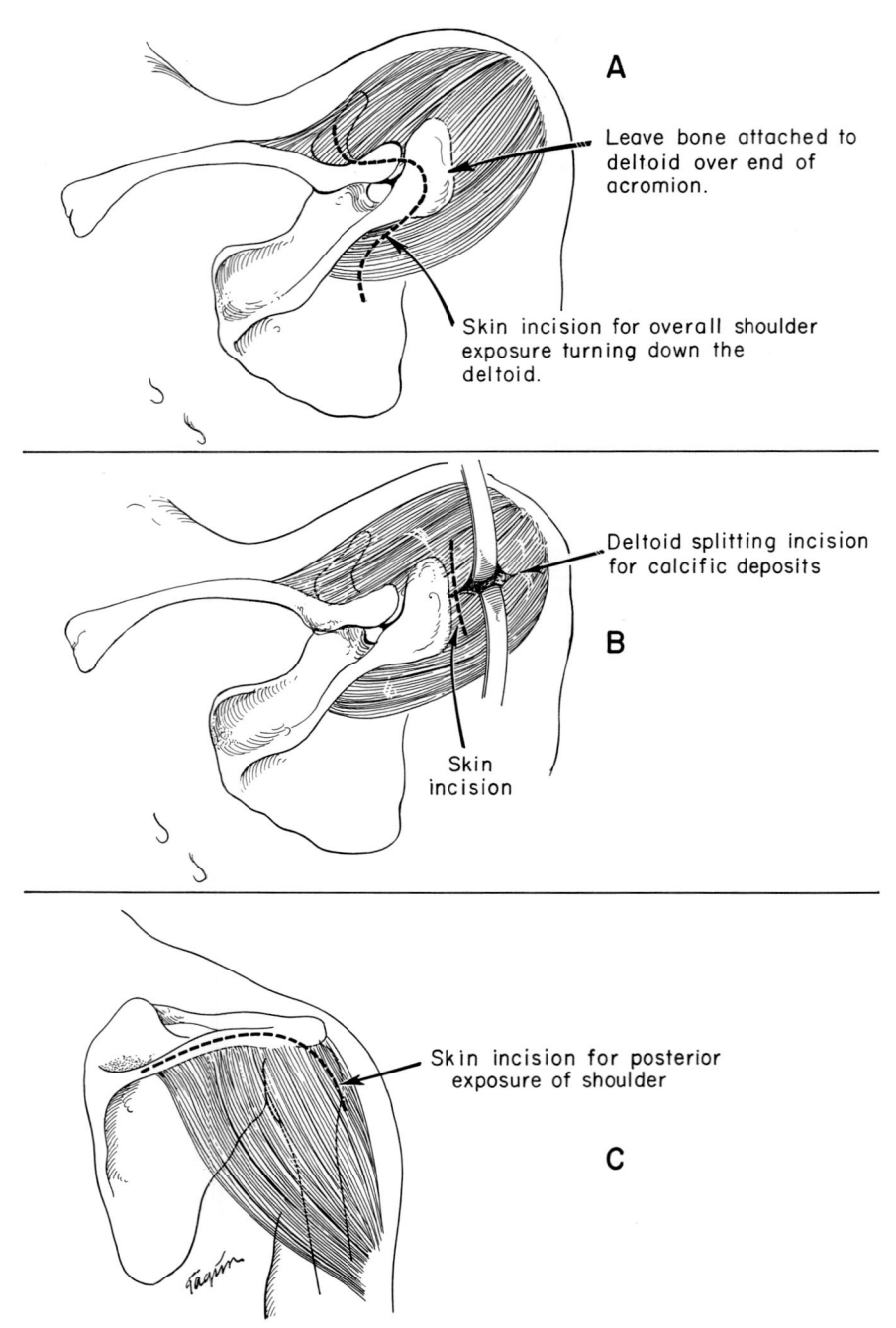

Fig. 17-38.—Superior and posterior shoulder exposures. **A**, utility incision for exposure of the entire glenohumeral joint. **B**, horizontal incision for removal of calcium from rotator cuff. **C**, posterior incision.

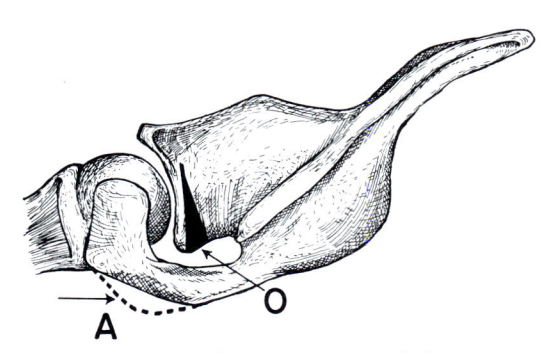

Fig. 17-39.—Wedge osteotomy of the scapular neck as described by Scott (shoulder viewed from above). *A* is part of acromion removed during exposure and used as graft. Wedge-shaped area *O* is site of the osteotomy; the location of the apex may be varied to suit the operator. (From Scott, D. J., Jr.: Treatment of recurrent posterior dislocations of the shoulder by glenoplasty, J. Bone Joint Surg. 49-A:471, 1967.)

of the brachial plexus and is a young or middle-aged individual, open reduction should be considered. When open reduction is planned:

1. Adequate skin preparation is mandatory, consisting of antiseptic soap washes twice daily for a week prior to surgery.

2. The utility incision, with the patient on his side, should be used (Fig. 17-38, A). The deltoid muscle should be turned down so that the anterior and posterior aspects of the shoulder can safely be exposed. *Caution*: When using this incision, the surgeon should be certain to leave a portion of the acromion attached to the central tendon of the deltoid muscle to insure a stable repair; otherwise, the deltoid muscle may pull off and retract down the arm.

3. The rotator cuff is divided at its tendinous insertion to open the joint and give an exposure adequate to clean out the glenoid fossa of organized clot and fibrous tissue.

4. The humeral head is then reduced and the rotator cuff tendons resutured to their insertions. *No* transarticular fixation is advised. In our experience, postoperative stability can be maintained by position of the arm in relation to type of dislocation; thus, if the chronic dislocation is *anterior*, the arm will be secure if held in adduction and internal rotation (Fig. 17-22). If the dislocation is *posterior*, it will be secure if the arm is maintained posterior to the coronal plane of the body. In this position it is impossible to dislocate posteriorly. This can be simply supported with Elastoplast strapping (Fig. 17-23).

5. Pendulum motions may be started gently in 10 days and activities increased gradually during the ensuing 3–4 weeks.

6. A good result should be anticipated if the surgical procedure is carefully done and transarticular fixation is avoided.

Recurrent Atraumatic Dislocations

The identification of the dislocation which occurs initially *without* trauma, or from a minor strain, is most important because the treatment and prognosis of this small group will differ markedly from that for the usual traumatic dislocation.

We emphasize again that in this group the Bankart lesion is absent and instability of the shoulder is related to generalized relaxation of shoulder musculature, capsule and ligaments rather than to a specific traumatic lesion.

Also in this group the surgeon may find that his favorite procedure for a traumatic (or usual) recurrent dislocation works less well on the atraumatic dislocation. He may experience the disappointment of having repaired the shoulder anteriorly, only to have the patient return later with a dislocation of his shoulder posteriorly. A small subgroup of atraumatic recurrent dislocations is the *voluntary*, or spontaneous, recurrent subluxation or dislocation of the shoulder (Fig. 17-40). This syndrome is at present under study by Drs. Donald Pierce, John Clark and the author at Massachusetts General Hospital. Our findings to date would prompt us to advise the surgeon:

1. To avoid, if possible, surgical pro-

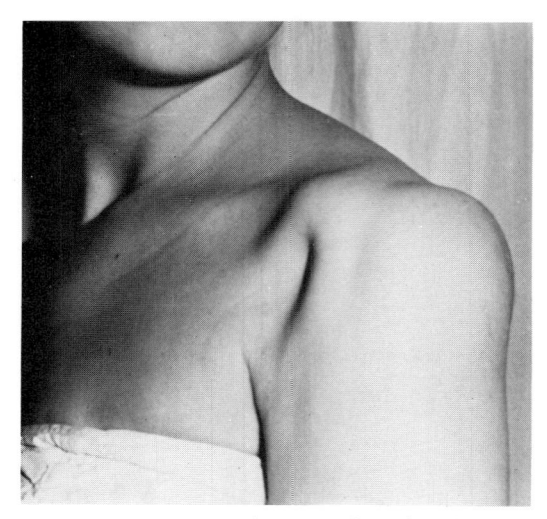

Fig. 17-40.—Typical example of voluntary recurrent posterior dislocation of the shoulder.

cedures in this group, as conservative treatment (resistive exercises and cooperation by the patient) may prove more successful.

2. If surgery is resorted to, the usual shoulder repairs may prove unsuccessful.

3. If your first surgical repair proved unsuccessful, do *not* repeat the surgery.

4. A number of these patients have psychologic or emotional problems that must be identified.

Complications of Traumatic Dislocations

INJURY TO THE ROTATOR CUFF.—It is reasonable to assume that some degree of injury to the rotator cuff may occur in many traumatic dislocations of the shoulder, particularly in elderly persons. McLaughlin and Asherman[40] have called attention to this possibility. The dislocation may enlarge cuff tears which have been present prior to the dislocation, or may create an entirely new tear.

NERVE INJURIES.—In a series of 500 dislocations treated at Massachusetts General Hospital in a period of 20 years, nerve injuries occurred in 27 instances. Of these nerve injuries, 23 (85%) were temporary, whereas 4 (15%) were permanent. Of the single nerve injuries, the ulnar nerve was injured in 30%, the radial nerve in 18%, the axillary in 11% and the median nerve in 4% of the total nerve injuries. The other 37% consisted of combinations of nerve injuries. It was of interest to note that all single nerve injuries were temporary, whereas combinations of nerve injuries included the permanent nerve injuries.

ADHESIVE CAPSULITIS.—This was an uncommon incident in the younger age groups but was usually noted after age 35–40. Varying degrees of this condition were present.

RECURRENT DISLOCATIONS.—A number of definite factors are related to the incidence of recurrent dislocations. Listed in order of importance, these are: (1) age of patient, (2) trauma in relation to initial dislocation, (3) defects in the superior lateral surface of the humeral head and (4) constitutional factors.

Age.—The most significant factor in relation to the incidence of recurrent shoulder dislocation was found to be the age of the patient at the time of the first dislocation. The findings of McLaughlin and Cavallaro,[39] reporting on 101 consecutive patients in 1950, and of Rowe,[57] reporting on 112 primary dislocations in 1963, are summarized in Table 17-2.

The significant fact is the high incidence of recurrence in the second and third decades of life and the sudden drop at age 40.

Trauma.—Perhaps the next most sig-

TABLE 17–2.—INCIDENCE OF RECURRENT SHOULDER DISLOCATIONS IN RELATION TO AGE

AGE OF PATIENT	INCIDENCE OF RECURRENCE McLAUGHLIN AND CAVALLARO	ROWE
Under 20	90%	93%
20–40	60%	63%
Over 40	10%	16%

nificant factor relative to the incidence or recurrence was the degree of injury at the time of initial dislocation. Studies at Massachusetts General Hospital suggest that the greater the initial injury causing the dislocation, the less likelihood of recurrence. It was interesting to note the low incidence of recurrence (4.5%) when the shoulder dislocation was associated with a fracture of the greater tuberosity.

Humeral head defects.—The presence of a defect in the superior lateral surface of the humeral head was associated with an increase in the incidence of recurrence.

Constitutional factors.—A relatively small group of persons is predisposed, by constitutional factors, to have recurrent shoulder dislocations. Such dislocations occur with little or no trauma to the shoulder.

FRACTURES OF HEAD AND NECK OF THE HUMERUS

Diagnosis

Clinically, there are no characteristic signs differentiating the various types of fractures of the head and neck of the humerus. In general, patients with these fractures present a painful, swollen, disabled shoulder. There is local pain on palpation and motion of the shoulder. The patient holds the arm close to his side.

In undisplaced fractures, there is no unusual change in the contour of the shoulder.

In displaced fractures, such as fracture-dislocation of the head or shaft of the humerus, there is flattening of the shoulder contour. The injured arm may be shorter than the opposite extremity. Although fracture-dislocation of the shoulder is a severe injury, it is surprising how frequently this condition is not recognized initially by the examining physician or surgeon. In a number of patients with this injury, the initial diagnosis was "severe sprain" or even "acute bursitis of the shoulder." Alteration of the contour of the shoulder may not be noted because of swelling and local tissue induration. The appearance of ecchymosis within 48 hours should suggest a fracture.

X-ray.—When the diagnosis is in doubt, x-rays should be taken, including an anteroposterior view and a *true* axillary view. The axillary view may be taken with the patient lying or standing over

Fig. 17-41.—Types of fracture-dislocation of the shoulder. **A** displacement of the humeral shaft. **B**, displacement of the humeral head. **C**, bursting fracture of head and tuberosities.

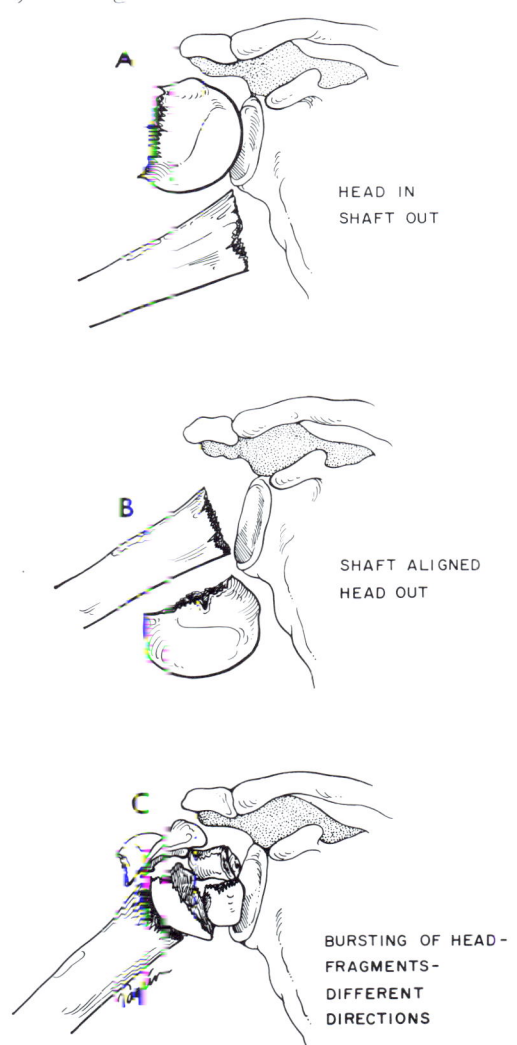

A — HEAD IN SHAFT OUT

B — SHAFT ALIGNED HEAD OUT

C — BURSTING OF HEAD — FRAGMENTS — DIFFERENT DIRECTIONS

the inverted x-ray tube (Fig. 17-18). These views will demonstrate the degree of comminution and anteroposterior displacement, as well as the anterior or posterior position of the displaced head or shaft of the humerus. Only with this knowledge can one reasonably manipulate the shoulder.

Treatment

Fracture-dislocations of the shoulder may be divided into the following types:
1. The impacted humeral neck fracture or minimally displaced tuberosity fracture
2. The displaced tuberosity fracture
3. Fracture-dislocation of the head and shaft of the humerus (Fig. 17-41)
    a) With the humeral shaft displaced from the humeral head
    b) With the humeral head displaced from the glenoid
    c) Complete shattering of all elements of the shaft and head.

Impacted Surgical Neck or Minimally Displaced Tuberosity Fractures

The impacted neck fracture is a stable fracture; therefore, it responds well to sling support and early pendulum exercises. The prognosis is good. Bigelow, in 1869, concisely summarized the treatment of impacted neck fractures: "Pad in the axilla, Elbow at the side, Arm in sling." Even though early activity may be possible in impacted and greater tuberosity fractures, maximum motion may not be obtained for 6–8 months.

Displaced Tuberosity Fractures

It is generally accepted that many displaced tuberosity fractures do well clinically, although some limitation in abduction or complete elevation may result. With a tuberosity fracture that is appreciably displaced in a young adult or an active middle-aged patient, the patient would have a better functioning shoulder if the tuberosity were replaced by open reduction. In an elderly inactive patient open reduction most likely would not be indicated.

Fracture-Dislocations Of the Shoulder

Treatment of the 3 types may be discussed together. In most of these fracture-dislocations an initial attempt at closed reduction should be made within the first 24 hours, if possible. If this is not successful, the author does not recommend open reduction at the time of injury, for the skin and soft tissue are not in optimal condition for major surgery. Time should be allowed for the muscles and soft tissues to recover from the trauma and for an adequate skin preparation to be accomplished by daily washing with an antiseptic soap. After 4–6 days of preparation the shoulder will be in far better condition for surgery than on the day of admission.

CLOSED MANIPULATION. — Every orthopedic surgeon has his own technique for closed manipulation of a fracture-dislocation, which works best for him. The author's routine is as follows:

1. Good anteroposterior and *axillary* roentgenographic views are mandatory; otherwise, we do not know the actual position of the head in relation to the shaft, i.e., which is anterior and which is posterior?

2. With this information in mind, the extremity is gently brought into the overhead position in full elevation, the position in which the muscles of the shoulder are most relaxed. In all manipulations of the shoulder it is most important that the surgeon keep in mind the nerve and vascular elements of the brachial plexus. Any defects should be noted early and corrective steps taken.

If the head of the humerus is in the glenoid fossa and the shaft displaced anteriorly or posteriorly (Fig. 17-41, *A*), the surgeon can gently align the displacement.

If the shaft is in normal relation to the glenoid, and the head dislocated anteriorly, posteriorly or inferiorly (Fig. 17-41, *B*), the surgeon places his thumb under the displaced head and lifts it back into the glenoid. It is most important to know exactly where the humeral head is. A good axillary x-ray view will demonstrate this. The surgeon is fortunate when the long head of the biceps tendon has not been ruptured from its groove (Fig. 17-42). In this instance, when the arm is extended upward, the intact biceps tendon aligns the head to the shaft.

Fig. 17-42.—When the biceps tendon has not been torn from its groove, it will aid in obtaining reduction.

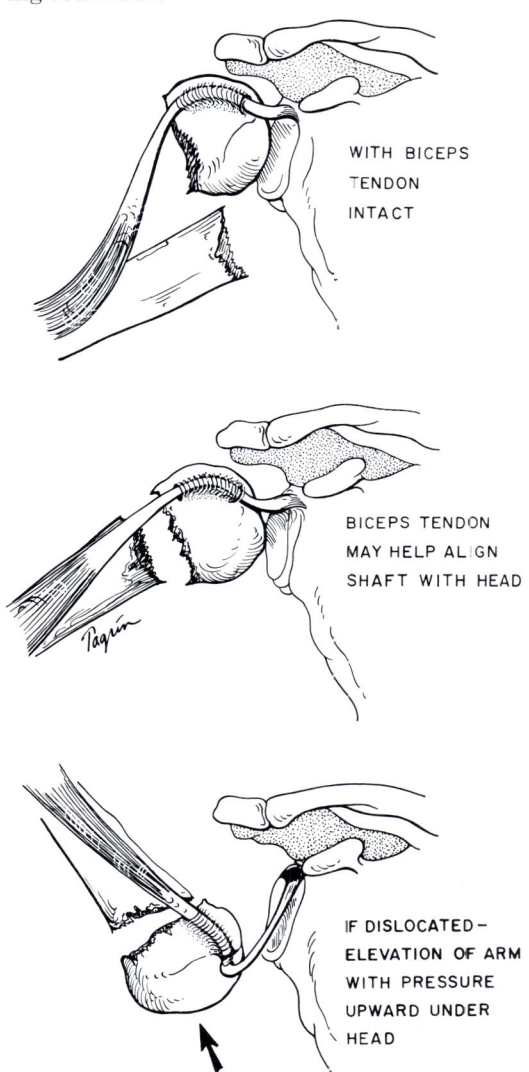

WITH BICEPS TENDON INTACT

BICEPS TENDON MAY HELP ALIGN SHAFT WITH HEAD

IF DISLOCATED— ELEVATION OF ARM WITH PRESSURE UPWARD UNDER HEAD

In the shattered fracture, i.e., a dislocation in which the head and tuberosities are in many pieces (Fig. 17-41, C), again a clear axillary view is necessary to indicate the direction of the displaced bone fragments. The surgeon in helped by tendinous and ligamentous attachments to the bone fragments. We have had greatest success in reassembling the displaced fragments by carrying out the maneuver described for dislocation of the head (Fig. 17-43).

In the elderly, poor-risk patient, the wisest decision may be to leave the shoulder as it is, apply a sling support and initiate motion and use of the hand as early as possible. In many of these, results are surprisingly good.

Position of arm after manipulation.—After manipulation, the arm is placed in the neutral position at the side of the body and is supported by the wraparound shoulder sling. This permits early gentle pendulum exercises. We advise against use of the airplane splint, as it leaves the arm in an abnormal position (Fig. 17-44). We also would not recommend the hanging cast, since it is apt to distract the unstable bone fragments.

Follow-up care.—The wraparound sling can be removed at any time for skin care of the axilla. This is easily accomplished by instructing the patient to lean forward, thus moving the body away from the arm, rather than the arm away from the body. Exercises and use of the arm are gradually increased over the ensuing 3–4 weeks, during which time the surgeon may decide when to discontinue the use of support.

OPEN REDUCTION.—As previously emphasized, open reduction of a fracture-dislocation of the shoulder is *seldom an emergency*. Time should be taken for adequate skin preparation and recovery of soft tissue. Emergency exploration may be necessary if there has been major blood vessel injury, such as a laceration of the axillary vein or artery indicated by an expanding hematoma, or an arterial embolism. Evidence of major nerve inju-

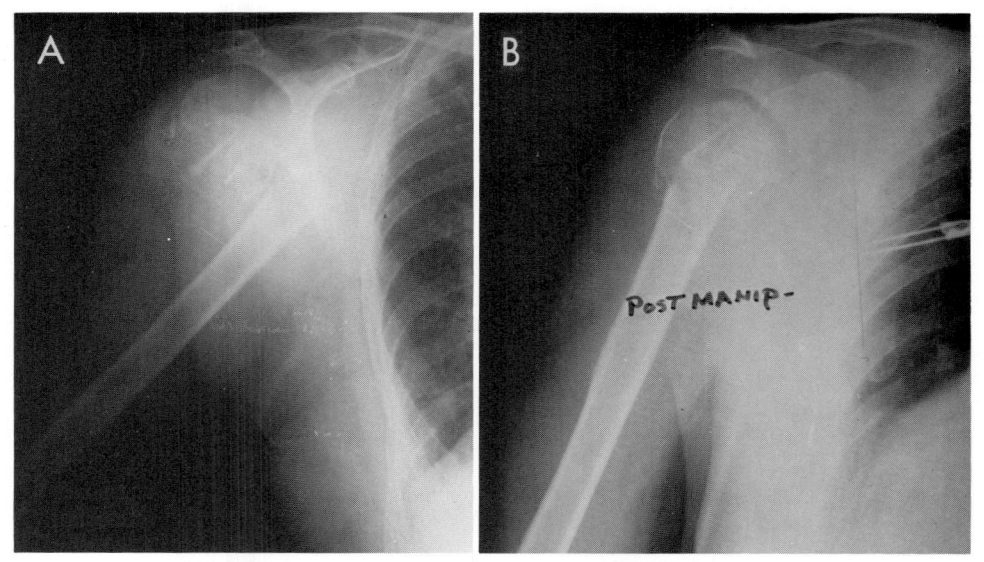

Fig. 17-43. — **A,** shattered fracture of the shoulder in a 79-year-old woman. **B,** after closed manipulation; a very satisfactory result was obtained.

ry will require a careful investigation and evaluation prior to exploration.

Two considerations should stay the hand of the surgeon in performing open reduction of the shoulder: (1) In the *growing child,* the common injury is epiphyseal separation. The more experience the surgeon has, the more he will appreciate the remarkable remodeling power of nature in the growing child.

Fig. 17-44. — **A,** angulation of a humeral neck fracture in an abduction (airplane) splint. **B,** satisfactory alignment is obtained when the arm is brought to the side of the body.

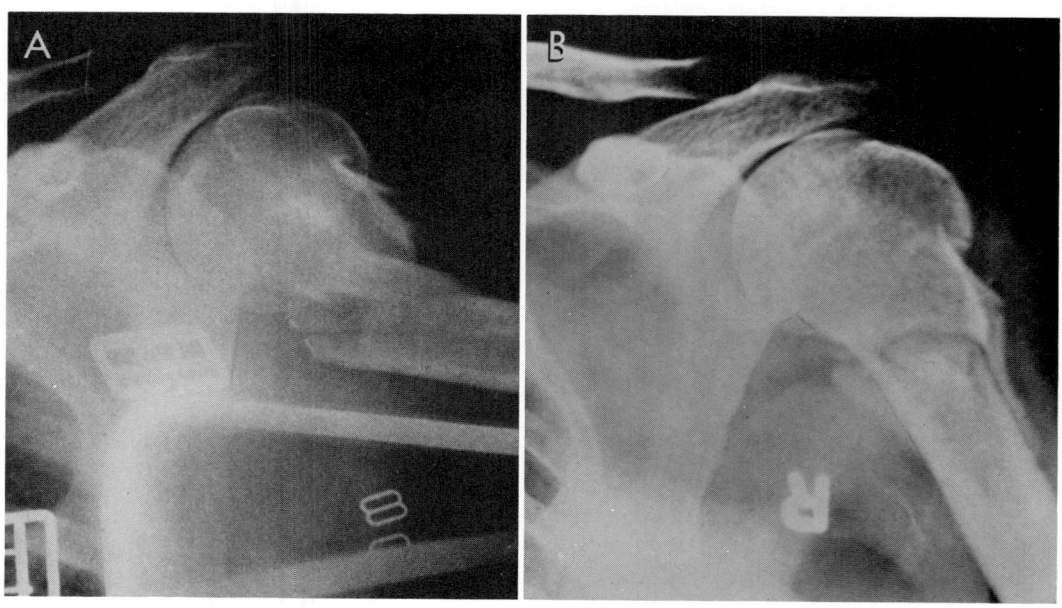

(2) In the *elderly patient,* likewise, experience will teach the surgeon that he would best treat the patient, not the x-ray film. Nature again comes to the patient's aid in non-weight-bearing joints.

Epiphyseal separation.—In the growing child (before age 10), it would be unreasonable to perform an open reduction so long as there is contact between the epiphyses and shaft, as nature will remodel rather markedly displaced fragments in the child. In the growing adolescent, 10–12 years and older, marked displacement may not be completely remodeled and open reduction may be indicated. When the head is completely separated from the shaft and manipulation has failed, open replacement is indicated.

Complete separation of humeral head and shaft not reduced by manipulation.—Exposure.—As a rule, the anterior shoulder exposure may be adequate for most fracture-dislocations. The incision may be extended down the shaft as far as necessary. There will be instances, however, when the utility incision will be necessary, in which the deltoid is turned down to give anterior, central and posterior exposure (Fig. 17-45).

INTERNAL FIXATION.—The following methods of internal fixation have been used.

1. A lag screw (Fig. 17-46) gives good stability and allows early motion.

2. The use of a Rush rod (Fig. 17-47) must be accepted with due consideration. In a number of patients in whom the Rush rod was inserted through the humeral head into the shaft, a backing up of the rod occurred. On the other hand, the rod can be a useful means of temporarily stabilizing the humeral head to the shaft. Care must be taken to place the rod off center from the dome and to bury it in the rotator cuff. The tendon is then repaired over the head of the rod. The rod should not protrude. The patient should also be cautioned to avoid reaching over 45 degrees upward until union has occurred, at which time the rod may be removed.

3. A small-blade plate or flange nail can be used in a similar manner.

4. The Nicola procedure may be effective.

5. Single or multiple screws have been used, perhaps best when adequate bony extensions of the head and shaft fragments permit secure screw fixation (Fig. 17-48).

6. In those instances in which the head fragment is merely a shell of cartilage, it should be discarded. In the past, the Laurence Jones technique of discarding

Fig. 17-45.—By turning down the deltoid, complete exposure of the glenohumeral joint is possible.

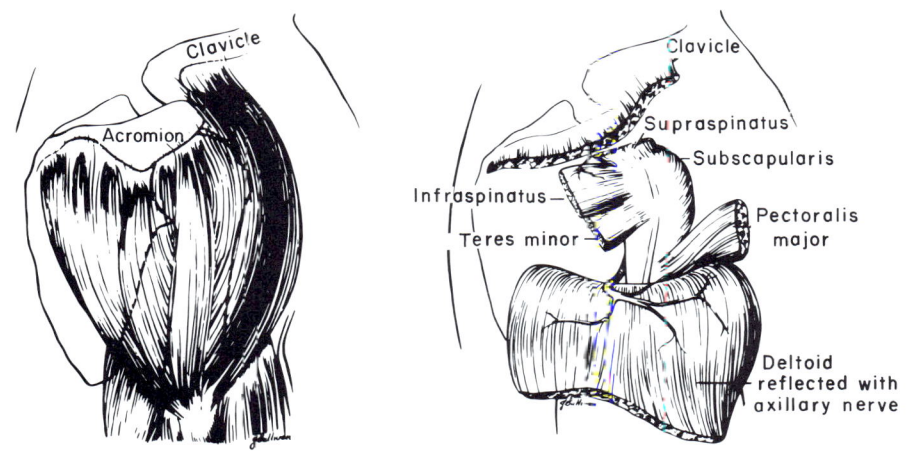

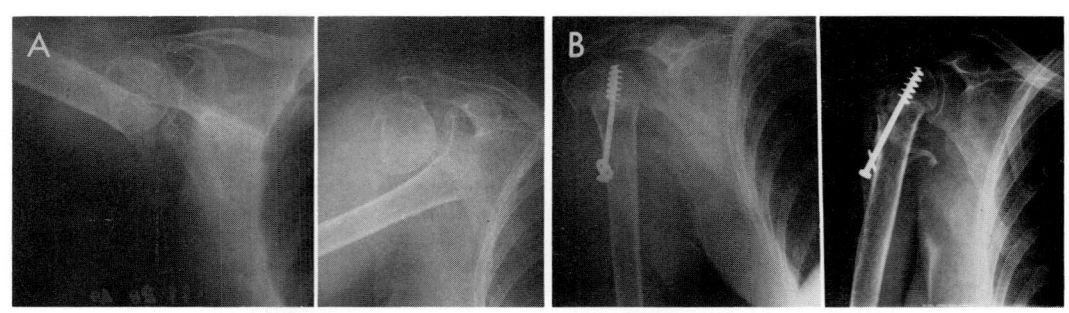

Fig. 17-46. — **A,** displaced humeral neck fracture. **B,** lag-screw fixation.

the head fragment and securing the tuberosities with rotator cuff attachments to the humeral shaft proved very effective (Fig. 17-49). In recent years, the use of a replacement prosthesis has become popular. The Neer prosthesis (Fig. 17-50) is preferred in our hospital. We recommend careful reading of Neer's technique, with special reference to the retroposition of the prosthesis, the preservation and reattachment of the tuberosities or rotator cuff and the degree of snugness of the prosthesis in the glenoid.

7. We strongly advise *against* primary arthrodesis as a form of treatment of the severely comminuted fracture-dislocation of the shoulder. A trial of other forms of treatment is mandatory before arthrodesis is decided on.

INJURIES TO THE ROTATOR CUFF

Tears of the rotator cuff may be caused by a specific injury, such as a fall or a sudden lifting strain. They may also result from attritional changes, without specific injury. An injury, on the other hand, may extend or increase a pre-existing rent in the cuff. DePalma as well as McLaughlin and Asherman have catalogued these findings.

Codman was one of the first surgeons

Fig. 17-47. — **A,** posterior fracture-dislocation of the humeral head. **B,** a Rush nail was used successfully.

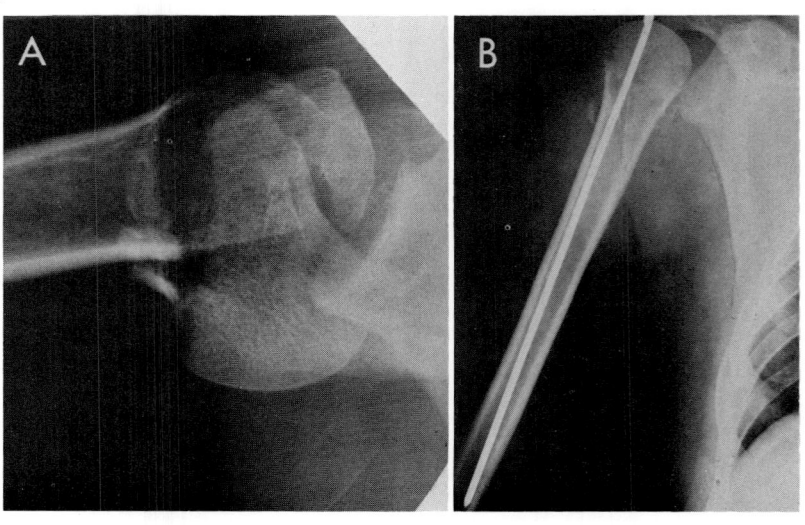

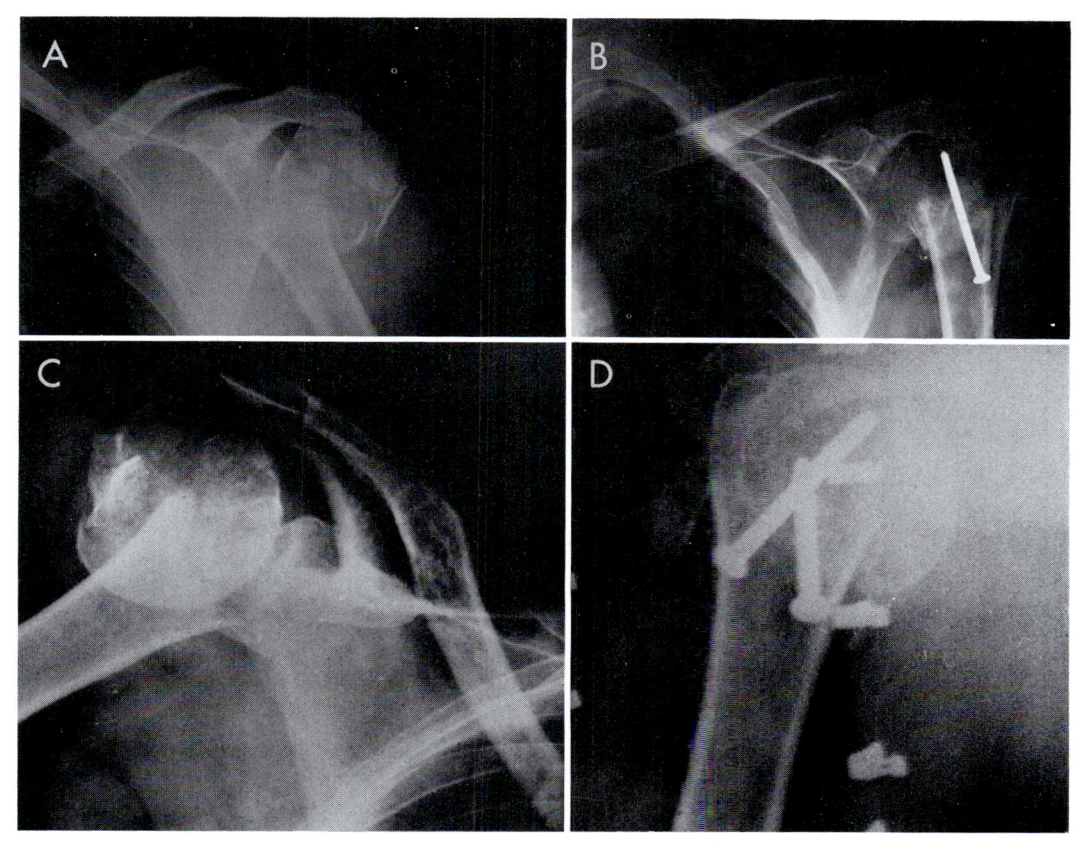

Fig. 17-48.—Fixation of displaced surgical neck fractures by means of 1 (**A** and **B**) or multiple (**C** and **D**) screws.

to investigate the rotator cuff injuries thoroughly.

Diagnosis

A careful study should be made of the following list, which covers the 18 significant factors in the diagnosis of a ruptured supraspinatus tendon or rotator cuff. This list is from Codman's book, *The Shoulder*.[16]

Conditions, symptoms and signs which indicate complete rupture of the supraspinatus tendon and which should be present within 24 hours after the accident:

1. Occupation—labor.
2. Age—over 40.
3. No symptoms in shoulder prior to accident.
4. Adequate injury—usually a fall.
5. Immediate sharp, brief pain.
6. Severe pain on following night.
7. Loss of power in elevation of the arm.
8. Negative x-ray findings.
9. Little, if any, restriction when stooping.
10. Faulty scapulohumeral rhythm.
11. A tender point,
12. A sulcus and
13. An eminence
14. At the insertion of the supraspinatus,
15. Which cause a jog,
16. A wince and
17. Soft crepitus as the tuberosity
18. Disappears under the acromion

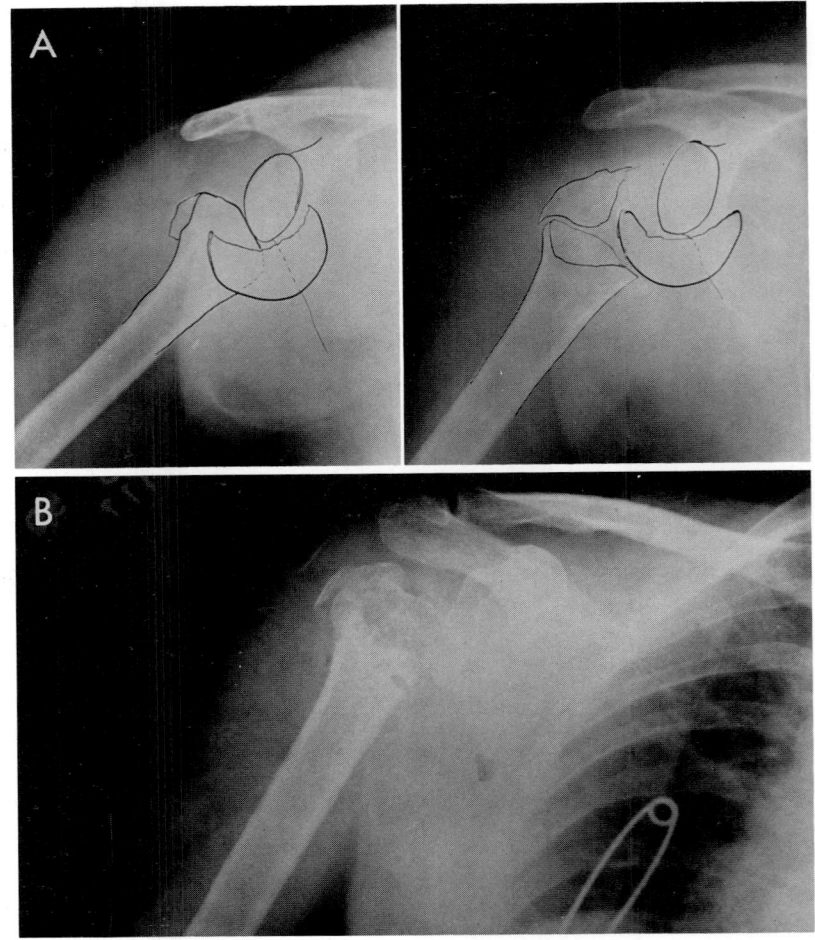

Fig. 17-49.—**A**, complete shattering of the humeral head treated by **B**, the Laurence Jones technique of resecting the shattered head and reattaching the rotator cuff (with tuberosities if attached) to the shaft of the humerus.

when the arm is elevated, and usually, also, as it reappears during the descent of the arm.

In addition to the history and physical findings, arthrograms may give added information regarding the presence or extent of rotator cuff tears.

Treatment

The over-all treatment of rotator cuff tears by the orthopedic service of Massachusetts General Hospital is conservative. Specific therapy depends on the extent of the tear and the age of the patient.

In our opinion, most patients with a partial or incomplete rotator cuff tear will do well on conservative treatment. This would consist of initial rest to the shoulder with a sling, followed by a program of graduated exercises. Inman, Saunders and Abbott have demonstrated that a partial tear or a tear involving, for instance, only the supraspinatus tendinous portion of the cuff tendon does not eliminate

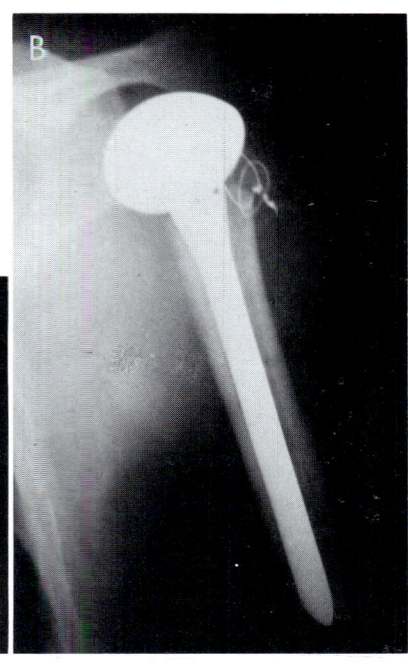

Fig. 17-50. — **A**, complete shattering of the humeral head treated by **B**, a Neer replacement prosthesis.

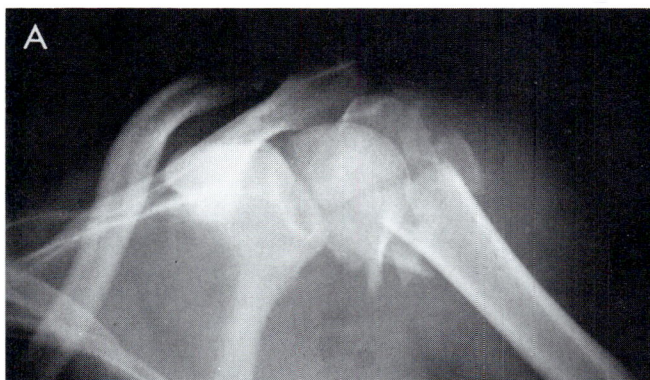

efficient abduction of the shoulder. They have shown that the teres minor, infraspinatus and subscapularis are the chief depressors of the humeral head, which allow the deltoid muscle to elevate the shoulder. DePalma also found varying degrees of rotator cuff tendon tears at autopsy in patients who had not complained of shoulder weakness or disability.

Symptoms from a partial rotator cuff tear may be due more to impingement of the thickened edges of the torn tendon under the acromion, than to the rupture or tear per se. We have had very good results in selected cases by performing an acromioplasty and smoothing down the rough furrows of the rotator tendon. This gives the shoulder mechanism more clearance on abduction and less impingement of tissues.

When, however, by clinical findings or arthrograms a complete avulsion of the rotator cuff attachment to the humeral head is demonstrated, which would include the supraspinatus, infraspinatus and varying portions of the teres minor or subscapularis tendon attachments, disability of the shoulder will result unless the tendons are effectively reattached to the humeral head or tuberosities. In these instances there is loss of "depressor" power to the humeral head or of a stabilizing effect to allow the deltoid muscle to function.

In youth and young adulthood, the blood supply to the rotator cuff is adequate, and satisfactory repair has been excellently demonstrated by Laurence Jones and by McLaughlin and Asherman. The tendon should, if possible, be reattached to viable bone, even if some portion of the humeral head has to be sacrificed to obtain a satisfactory bed.[6, 7] Postoperatively, the shoulder is supported in a plaster spica with the arm in 40 degrees of abduction and 40 degrees of forward flexion (position "salute"). It is safe to protect the repair in this position for 6–8 weeks before permitting shoulder motion.

When a complete rotator cuff avulsion

occurs in the patient aged 45 and older, we are faced with a somewhat different problem. In this age group the blood supply to the rotator cuff tendons is not as adequate as it is in youth. Our experience is that surgical repair of severe cuff avulsion in the older age group requires 2 assists: (1) fascia lata to reinforce the rotator cuff and (2) introduction of the tendinous repair into fresh bone. To accomplish these 2 requisites, the author has used, and recommends, the technique proposed by Bateman,[5, 6] in which the rotator cuff is approached through the acromioclavicular junction, removing a small portion of the inner side of the acromion (but leaving its deltoid attachment to the outer border) and the outer ½ in. of the clavicle. The deltoid is split for a distance of 3 in., which is safe, and gives excellent exposure of the entire rotator cuff.

A cleft is then cut in the dome of the humeral head, into which the stump of the rotator cuff is sewn by means of a strip of fascia lata. The coracoacromial ligament should be sectioned, when repairing the rotator cuff; otherwise, the repaired tendon impinges under the tight ligament on abduction or elevation of the arm. Instead of fascia lata, Neviaser uses a portion of the long head of the biceps tendon to fill the gap between the rotator stump and the humeral head attachment.

SURGICAL APPROACHES TO SHOULDER JOINT

In general, all surgical approaches to the shoulder should follow the cleavage lines and natural folds of the skin. If these lines are crossed horizontally, the incision will widen and become unsightly. Another general rule is to avoid splitting the deltoid muscle 4 in. below the tip of the acromion or clavicle, as the axillary nerve may be injured.

DELTOID-SPLITTING INCISION. — This is used for *limited exploration* for calcium in the rotator cuff (Fig. 17-38, *B*). The skin incision, 3 in. in length, should cross the outer tip of the acromion. The deltoid muscle is then split in the line of its fibers for not more than 2–3 in., thus avoiding injury to the circumflex nerve. Through this window the rotator cuff can be examined completely by rotating the head of the humerus.

ANTERIOR APPROACH. — This has been described in detail under the Bankart procedure (Fig. 17-29).

UTILITY INCISION. — This approach will permit exploration of the anterior, medial and posterior aspects of the shoulder by completely turning down the deltoid muscle (Fig. 17-38, *A*), thus preserving its nerve and vascular supply. We emphasize *again* that the tip of the acromion should be osteotomized, leaving the common middle tendon of the deltoid attached; otherwise the muscle repair is not secure and may pull off, gliding down the arm. The middle third of this approach may be used for acromionectomy or exposure of the acromioclavicular joint.

POSTERIOR APPROACH. — The approach described by Rowe and Yee[55] in 1942 has proved satisfactory for a limited posterior approach. The incision begins along the spine of the scapula and extends lateralward, curving down the posterior shoulder (Fig. 17-38, *C*). The deltoid muscle is released along the spine of the scapula and turned down, exposing the entire posterior aspect of the shoulder. By turning down the deltoid and *not* splitting it, the nerve supply is kept intact, and no atrophy of the muscle will result.

SHOULDER EXERCISES

Exercises for the shoulder may be divided into 3 general types: early pendulum, stretching and resistive (Fig. 17-51).

1. The earliest shoulder exercises may best be rhythmic pendulum exercises. These should be performed with minimal muscle action, but they must be carried out in a position of moderate forward flexion of the body, so as to eliminate

Chapter 17: SHOULDER GIRDLE INJURIES / 451

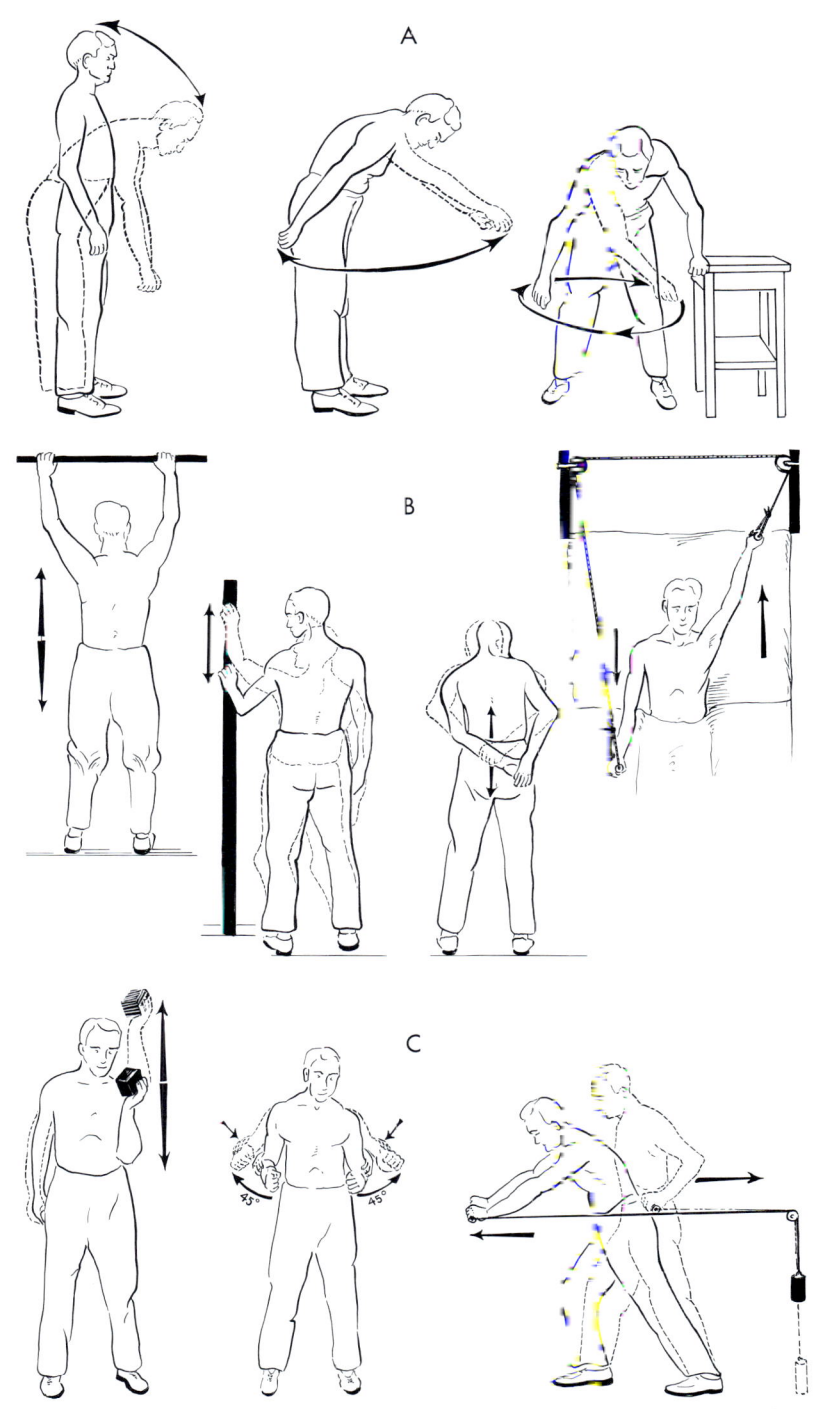

Fig. 17-51.—Exercises for the shoulder. **A,** early pendulum exercises. **B,** stretching exercises. **C,** resistive exercises.

impingement of the humeral head on the undersurface of the acromion.

2. The second group of shoulder exercises may be called the "stretching" exercises. These should be carried out gently and frequently, so as gradually to regain shoulder motion without producing reaction in the tissues stretched.

3. The third group is the strengthening or active "resistive" exercises. If instituted too early, these may produce pain and irritation of the shoulder mechanism. Maximal benefit is obtained from the resistive group if time is allowed to regain a useful degree of motion for active exercises.

Exercises that should be avoided are repetitious forceful shoulder motions carried out at shoulder level or at 90 degrees of abduction. In this position, the short rotator tendons and protective subacromial bursal tissues are impinged against the undersurface of the acromion. In like manner, push-ups are a poor exercise for the shoulder and are more apt to precipitate painful syndromes than to alleviate them.

BIBLIOGRAPHY

1. Abbott, L. C., Saunders, J. B. M., Hagey, H., and Jones, E. W.: Approaches to the shoulder joint, J. Bone Joint Surg. 31-A:235, 1949.
2. Adams, J. D.: Recurrent dislocations of the shoulder, J. Bone Joint Surg. 30-B:26, 1948.
3. Alldredge, R. H.: The surgical treatment of acromioclavicular dislocations, J. Bone Joint Surg. 47-A:1278, 1965.
4. Allen, A. W.: Living suture grafts in repair of fractures and dislocations, Arch. Surg. 16:1007, 1928.
5. Bankart, A. S. B.: Br. Med. J. 2:1132, 1923; Br. J. Surg. 26:23, 1948.
6. Bateman, J.: *The Shoulder and Environs* (St. Louis: C. V. Mosby Company, 1955).
7. Bateman, J.: Rotator cuff repair (personal communication).
8. Biebl, R.: Therapy and prognosis of fresh dislocations, Arch. Orthop. Unfallchir. 35:381, 1935.
9. Blazina, M. E., and Satzman, J. S.: Recurrent anterior subluxation of the shoulder in athletes —a distinct entity. Read at meeting of American Academy of Orthopaedic Surgeons, Chicago, Ill., January, 1969.
10. Bost, F. C., and Inman, V. T.: Pathological changes in recurrent dislocations of the shoulder, J. Bone Joint Surg. 3:595, 1942.
11. Bosworth, D. M.: Acromioclavicular dislocation—end result of screw suspension treatment, Ann. Surg. 127:98, 1948.
12. Brav, E. A.: An evaluation of the Putti-Platt procedure, J. Bone Joint Surg. 37-A:731, 1955.
13. Bunnell, S.: Fascial graft for dislocations of the acromioclavicular joint, Surg. Gynecol. Obstet. 46:563, 1928.
14. Bunnell, S.: *Surgery of the Hand* (Philadelphia: J. B. Lippincott Company, 1944).
15. Cave, E. F., and Rowe, C. R.: Capsular repair for recurrent dislocation of the shoulder: Pathological findings and operative technique, Surg. Clin. North Am. 27:1289, 1947.
16. Codman, E. A.: *The Shoulder* (Boston: Thomas Todd Company, 1934).
17. Cooper, Sir Astley: *A Treatise on Dislocations and Fractures of the Joints* (Philadelphia: Carey & Lea, 1825).
18. Cubbins, W. R., Callahan, J. J., and Scuderi, C. S.: Reduction of old or irreducible dislocations of the shoulder, Surg. Gynecol. Obstet. 58:120, 1934.
19. DePalma, A. F.: Recurrent dislocations of the shoulder, Ann. Surg. 132:1052, 1950.
20. DePalma, A. F.: *Surgery of the Shoulder* (Philadelphia: J. B. Lippincott Company, 1950).
21. Dickson, J. A., and O'Dell, H. W.: Recurrent dislocations of the shoulder: Phylogenetic study, Surg. Gynecol. Obstet. 95:357, 1952.
22. Eden, R.: Deutsche Z. Chir. 144:268, 1918.
23. Eyre-Brook, A. L.: Recurrent dislocations of the shoulder, J. Bone Joint Surg. 30-B:39, 1948.
24. Fairbanks, J. J.: Fracture-dislocation of the shoulder, J. Bone Joint Surg. 30-B:454, 1949.
25. Flower, W. H.: Tr. Pathol. Soc. London 12:179, 1861.
26. Gallie, W. E., and LeMesurier, A. B.: Dislocations of the shoulder, J. Bone Joint Surg. 30-B:9, 1948.
27. Gardner, E.: Innervation of the shoulder joint, Anat. Rec. 1:102, 1948.
28. Helfet, A. J.: Coracoid transplantation for recurring dislocation of the shoulder, J. Bone Joint Surg., 40-B:198, 1958.
29. Henderson, M. S.: Tenosuspension operation for recurrent dislocation of the shoulder, Surg. Clin. North Am. 23:927, 1943.
30. Hill, H. A., and Sachs, M. D.: Grooved defect of humeral head, Radiology 35:690, 1940.
31. Hybbinette, S.: Acta Chir. Scand. 71:511, 1932.
32. Inman, L. T., Saunders, J. B., and Abbott, L. C.: Observations on the function of the shoulder joint, J. Bone Joint Surg., 26:1, 1944.
33. Jones, L.: The shoulder joint: Reconstruction operations following extensive injury, Surg. Gynecol. Obstet. 75:433, 1942.
34. Lange, M.: *Orthopädisch-Chirurgische Operationslehre* (Munich: Verlag J. F. Bergmann, 1951), pp. 248–260.
35. Lowman, C. L.: Operative correction of old sternoclavicular dislocations, J. Bone Joint Surg. 10:740, 1928.
36. Magnuson, P. B.: Treatment of recurrent dislocations of the shoulder, Surg. Clin. North Am. 25:14, 1945.
37. Masland, H. C.: Positive lift for fractured clavicle, Am. J. Surg. 60:154, 1943.
38. McLaughlin, H. L.: Posterior dislocations of the shoulder, J. Bone Joint Surg. 34-A: 584, 1952.
39. McLaughlin H. L., and Cavallaro, W. U.: Primary anterior dislocation, Am. J. Surg. 80: 615, 1950.

40. McLaughlin, H. L., and Asherman, E. G.: Lesions of the musculotendinous cuff on the shoulder, J. Bone Joint Surg. 33-A:76, 1951.
41. McLaughlin, H. L., and MacLellan, D. I.: Recurrent anterior dislocation of the shoulder—a comparative study, J. Trauma 7:191, 1967.
42. Milch, H.: Pulsion-traction in reduction of dislocation in fracture-dislocation of the humerus, Bull. Hosp. Joint Dis. 24:147, 1963.
43. Moseley, H. F.: *Shoulder Lesions* (Edinburgh: E. & S. Livingstone, Ltd., 1969).
44. Neer, C. C., Brown, T. H., Jr., and McLaughlin, H. L.: Fracture of humerus with dislocation of head fragment, Am. J. Surg. 85:252, 1953.
45. Neer, C. S.: Articular replacement of humeral head, J. Bone Joint Surg. 37-A:215, 1955.
46. Neviaser, J. S.: Adhesive capsulitis of the shoulder, J. Bone Joint Surg. 27:211, 1945.
47. Neviaser, J. S.: Acromioclavicular dislocation—treated by transference of the coracoacromial ligament, Arch. Surg. 64:292, 1952; Bull. Hosp. Joint Dis. 12:46, 1951.
48. Nicola, T.: Acute anterior dislocation of the shoulder, J. Bone Joint Surg. 31-A:153, 1949.
49. Nicola, T.: Anterior dislocation of the shoulder, J. Bone Joint Surg. 24-A:615, 1942.
50. Osmond-Clarke, H.: Recurrent dislocations of the shoulder, J. Bone Joint Surg. 30-B:19, 1948.
51. Palmer, I., and Widen, A.: Bone block method for recurrent dislocation, J. Bone Joint Surg. 30-B:53, 1948.
52. Phemister, D. B.: Treatment of acromioclavicular dislocations with threaded wire fixation, J. Bone Joint Surg. 24:166, 1942.
53. Quigley, T. B.: Management of simple fractures of the clavicle in the adult, N. Engl. J. Med. 243:286, 1950.
54. Rowe, C. R.: Prognosis in dislocations of the shoulder, J. Bone Joint Surg. 38-A:957, 1956.
55. Rowe, C. R., and Yee, L. B. K.: A posterior approach to the shoulder joint, J. Bone Joint Surg. 26:580, 1944.
56. Rowe, C. R.: Fractures of scapula, Surg. Clin. North Am. 43:1565, 1963.
57. Rowe, C R.: Anterior dislocation of the shoulder—prognosis and treatment, Surg. Clin. North Am. 43:1609, 1963.
58. Rowe, C. R.: The surgical management of anterior recurrent dislocation, Surg. Clin. North Am. 43:1633, 1963.
59. Rowe, C. R.: The results of operative treatment of recurrent dislocation of shoulder, Surg. Clin. North Am. 43:1667, 1963.
60. Saha, A. K.: Recurrent anterior dislocation of shoulder—a new concept (Calcutta, India: Academic Publishers, 1969).
61. Scott, D. J., Jr.: Treatment of recurrent posterior dislocations of the shoulder by glenoplasty, J. Bone Joint Surg. 49-A:471, 1967.
62. Simmons, E. H., and Martin, R. F.: Acute dislocation of the acromioclavicular joint, Can. J. Surg. 11:473, 1968.
63. Speed, J. S.: Recurrent anterior dislocations of the shoulder: Operative cure by bone graft, Surg. Gynecol. Obstet. 44:468, 1927.
64. Tyler, G. T.: Acromioclavicular dislocation fixed by Vitallium screw through joint, Am. J. Surg. 57:245, 1952.
65. Urist, M. R.: Complete dislocations of the acromioclavicular joint, J. Bone Joint Surg. 28:813, 1946.
66. Watson-Jones, R.: Recurrent dislocations of the shoulder, J. Bone Joint Surg. 30-B:49, 1948.
67. White, M.: Late results of shoulder dislocations, Tr. Roy. Med.-Chir. Soc. Glasgow 22:243, 1929.
68. Wile, I. S. *Handedness, Right and Left* (Boston: Lathrop, Lee and Shepard, 1934).
69. Wilson, J. C., and McKeever, F. M.: Traumatic posterior dislocations of the shoulder, J. Bone Joint Surg. 31-A:160, 1949.
70. Wilson, J.: Plaster shoulder spica for fracture of clavicle (personal communication).

18 | Humeral Shaft Fractures
ROBERT J. BOYD

As a rule, closed humeral shaft fractures heal rapidly and are rarely problems if operative treatment can be avoided. Spiral oblique and comminuted fractures of the shaft usually become stable very rapidly with the simplest form of immobilization. Simple transverse fractures, particularly of the middle-distal third junction, are more apt to be troublesome, with delayed union and nonunion likely to occur unless carefully handled. This failure to heal may be related to problems in maintaining satisfactory reduction or to problems of local blood supply, since the main nutrient artery of the humeral shaft usually enters at the middle-distal third junction.

Nonunion presents an extremely difficult therapeutic problem, with the patient significantly disabled until the nonunion is successfully corrected.

Considerable amounts of shortening, angulation and rotational malalignment are surprisingly well tolerated in the middle third of the humeral shaft. Occasionally, proximal third fractures unite with excessive medial and anterior angulation, resulting in significant limitation of shoulder abduction and external rotation. Correctional osteotomy is then required.

ANATOMIC CONSIDERATIONS

The shaft of the humerus is cylindrical in its upper half and gradually broadens and flattens in its distal portion. Beneath the biceps muscle anteriorly lies the coracobrachialis and its insertion proximally, with the brachialis distally arising broadly from the lower third of the anterior humeral shaft (Fig. 18-1). Along the medial aspect of the humerus courses the main neurovascular bundle, with the brachial artery and vein and the median, musculocutaneous and ulnar nerves. These lie in the anterior compartment, which is divided from the posterior compartment by the medial and lateral intermuscular septa. The primary posterior landmark is the fusiform triceps, the medial and lateral heads of which have their origin in the posterior humeral shaft. Between these heads, next to bone, lies the radial nerve, which travels obliquely downward and lateralward as it passes from the posterior axilla to the anterolateral epicondylar region. The triangular deltoid muscle caps the shoulder joint; its anterior, lateral and posterior elements converge into a single tendon. This tendon inserts into the deltoid tuberosity, which is easily palpable on the lateral midshaft of the humerus. The deltoid muscle flexes, abducts or extends the upper arm. The broad, fan-shaped pectoralis major muscle, which forms the anterior axillary border, originates in the upper anterior chest wall and converges into a flat tendon which inserts into the lateral lip of the bicipital groove of the humerus (Fig. 18-1). This muscle acts conjointly with the other muscles in depressing the elevated arm to the side of the chest and as a strong adductor and internal rotator of the upper arm.

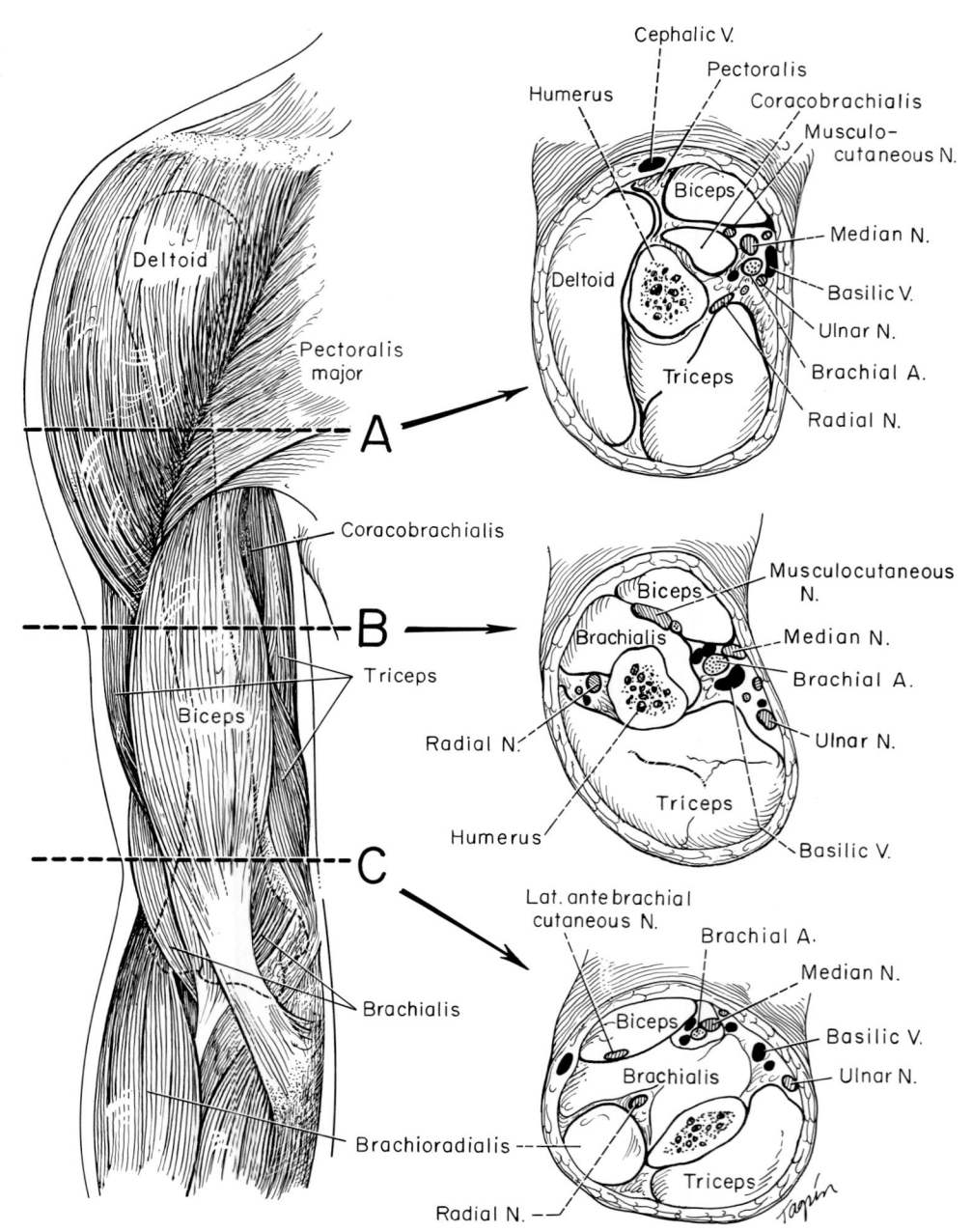

Fig. 18-1.—Details of surface and cross-sectional anatomy with important relationships.

Beneath the body of the deltoid muscle, the muscles of the rotator cuff surround the humeral head. (See Chapter 17.)

The essential elements in humeral shaft fracture analysis are the abduction action of the supraspinatus and deltoid muscles, the internal rotation function of the subscapularis, and the adduction action of the pectoralis major.

PHYSICAL EXAMINATION

The examiner must be alert, not only for the obvious evidence of a humeral shaft fracture, including swelling, pain and deformity, but also for possible secondary or associated trauma. Radial nerve injury, carpal and metacarpal fractures, forearm and elbow abnormalities, as well as shoulder girdle and vascular problems, have all been reported as complicating features. A methodical palpation and a testing of the joint functions of the entire upper extremity may reveal an area of tenderness that has been obscured by the more severe pain of the obvious injury. The injury may be of soft tissues only, but x-ray confirmation is mandatory when doubt exists. X-rays must provide adequate visualization of the entire humeral shaft. Neurologic evaluation of the extremity is essential. A comprehensive and thoughtful initial examination will often save the examiner future embarrassment and will serve as a baseline in later evaluations, particularly of progressive nerve or vascular injury.

ETIOLOGY AND TYPES OF FRACTURES

Fractures of the humeral shaft may be in the upper, middle or lower third and are transverse or spiral oblique. Segmental fractures occasionally occur. A direct force is apt to produce a transverse, short oblique, or comminuted fracture; an indirect force, a spiral oblique fracture with or without comminution. If the blow is severe, the possibility is greater that the resultant fracture will be comminuted or open. Indirect violence, such as a fall on the outstretched hand or on the elbow, may result in a spiral oblique shaft fracture, with secondary fractures of the radius, navicular, clavicle or other bones of the upper extremity. Forceful muscular action, such as that in gymnastics or throwing a baseball, may produce a spiral fracture.

Fractures of the humeral shaft most often occur in the middle third, and the degree of displacement is variable. The proximal one-half of the humerus is a common site for metastatic tumor and pathologic fractures.

TREATMENT

GENERAL CONSIDERATIONS.—If alignment of a humeral shaft fracture is good, then perfect end-to-end apposition is unnecessary and one-third to one-fourth contact at the fracture ends is sufficient. Strict immobilization is not necessary and almost all of these fractures unite with the minimum of external splinting. Rigid external immobilization is discontinued when evidence of clinical union is present and comfort allows; usually this is 3–6 weeks after injury. A sling alone offers a reasonable transition support, with exercises encouraged out of the sling when progress of union allows.

Conservative management of the humeral shaft fracture is employed whenever possible since open operations are among the most common causes of failure in bone healing.

Based on an analysis of the mechanism of injury, physical examination, x-ray findings and the muscle forces producing the deformity, a decision can be made as to management of the fracture. The age of the patient and the dominance of the involved extremity must also be considered. A moderate deformity of a left humeral fracture in an elderly right-handed woman may be more readily acceptable than the same fracture in the dominant arm of a young male laborer.

Ambulatory versus recumbent methods of treatment must be taken into consideration. Can the patient cooperate with the hanging cast type of treatment? Will the medical condition of the patient permit general anesthesia? Are there associated injuries? All factors must be weighed in determining specific treatment.

Hanging Cast

The hanging cast is one of the most successful and widely accepted methods for treatment of humeral shaft fractures and can be employed for almost all varieties, if properly used. It permits early active exercise, and the small amount of motion at the fracture site does not appear to interfere with callus formation, or the progress of healing. In principle, it consists of partial immobilization of the fracture by means of a light-weight long arm cast, applied so as to produce mild extrinsic traction aimed at relaxing the musculature and aiding in the reduction and alignment of the fracture elements. The plaster must be light and *must not distract the fracture ends*. It is applied with the elbow flexed 90 degrees and the forearm in neutral position, and it extends from the midpalm to, or slightly above, the fracture site (Fig. 18-2).

It must first be determined whether reduction of the fracture is necessary. If displacement of the fragments is minimal, the position may be accepted without specific manipulation, or in anticipation of slight reduction by traction from the cast. However, whenever there is marked deformity (shortening, rotation or angulation), reduction under anesthesia or intravenous analgesia is mandatory prior to application of a cast. The hanging cast may contribute substantially to the length of the upper arm and to the alignment of the fragments, but its purpose is primarily to maintain, rather than produce, reduction. If the cast weight is excessive, distraction occurs and delayed union may result. If the forearm support is incorrectly placed or the upper arm is in a position of abduction due to obesity, angulation deformity usually occurs. The sling support is attached at wrist level and lateral angulation can be corrected by moving the loop to the dorsum of the wrist (Fig. 18-3). Medial angulation can be corrected by placing the loop along the volar aspect of the wrist. Lengthening the sling will usually correct posterior angulation, and shortening the sling will correct anterior angulation.

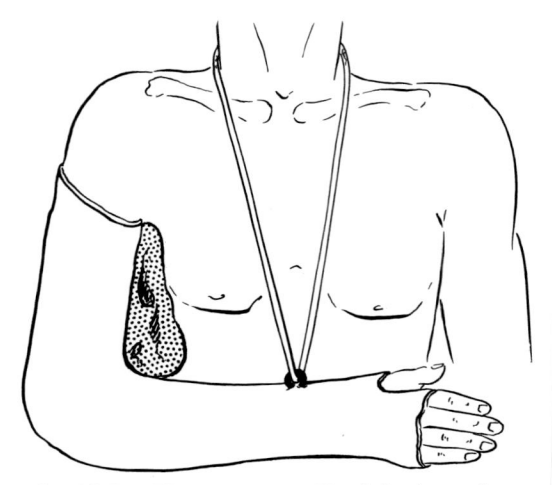

Fig. 18-2.—Hanging cast. Useful when alignment of the fracture can be maintained with partial immobilization and by following the principle of the "vertical sector." Note axillary wedge. (See also Fig. 18-3.)

The arm should be continuously dependent; if the patient must remain recumbent, light traction can be applied to the cast in the line of the long axis of the humerus. Fractures just below the deltoid insertion produce abduction of the proximal fragment, and alignment can be improved by attaching the sling to the dorsum of the wrist, as just noted. Angulation of fractures in the distal third of the shaft can be corrected, according to Stewart and Hundley,[13] by placing the forearm in pronation and attaching the sling to the ulnar border of the wrist. Frequent x-ray examinations are important in the early stage of treatment with the hanging cast.

The hanging cast method is ideal in comminuted fractures of the lower two-

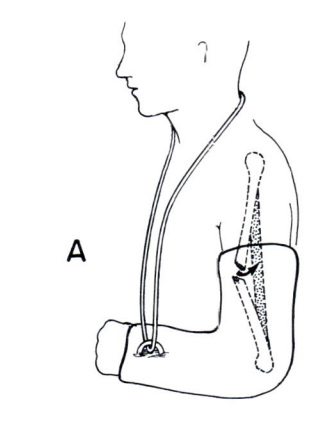

A
Loop attachment at dorsum of wrist to correct lateral angulation

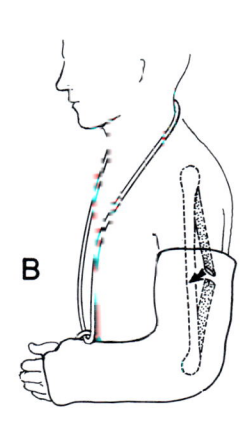

B
Loop attachment at volar aspect of wrist to correct medial angulation

HUMERUS IS INTERNALLY ROTATED 60°

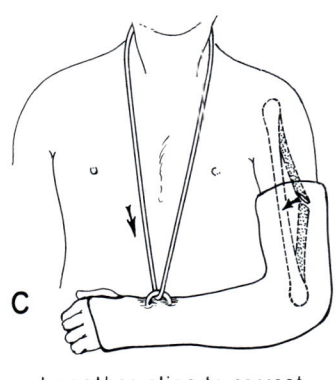

C
Lengthen sling to correct posterior angulation

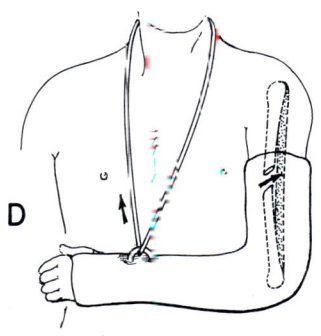

D
Shorten sling to correct anterior angulation

Fig. 18-3.—Correct placement of forearm support is imperative in maintaining alignment.

thirds of the humerus and in long spiral oblique fractures. The method appears best adapted to those fractures which have a broad fracture suface. It is less well adapted to the transverse shaft fracture, and considerable experience is needed for proper management of fractures of the proximal third of the shaft where angulation deformities are apt to occur.

Because a vertical vector is required at all times with the hanging cast, the patient must initially sleep in a semireclining position without support beneath the elbow, although a wedge may be inserted between the elbow and trunk if necessary (Fig. 18-2). Shoulder exercises should be started early, using gentle pendulum motions that swing the cast away from the body (Fig. 17-51).

The hanging cast method has been proved in practice, is widely applicable and is adaptable to essentially all humeral shaft fractures.

Coaptation Splint

Another acceptable method for treatment of humeral shaft fractures is the coaptation splint or plaster splint applied to the arm and a collar and cuff (Fig. 18-4). This method is preferred by many members of the Massachusetts General Hospital orthopedic staff. The splint is applied either after reduction has been achieved or primarily in instances of minimal displacement where the vertical weight of the arm is sufficient to maintain position. The coaptation splint is often used in humeral shaft fractures in children, in whom an intact periosteal tube

Fig. 18-4. — Coaptation splint.

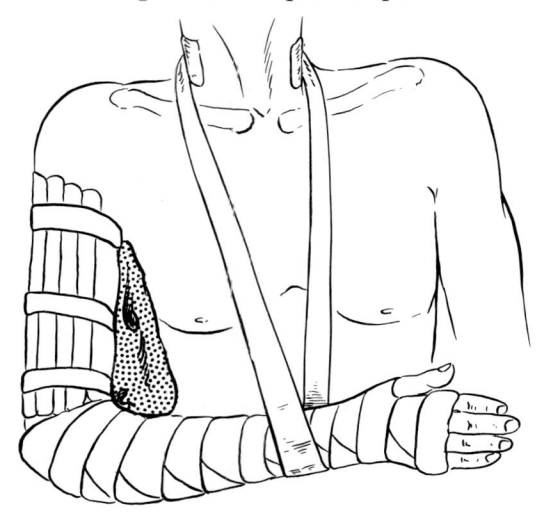

can act as a firm internal aligning element and moderate deformities are acceptable in view of the extensive remodeling possibilities. The method is well adapted for use during convalescence, as a transition method after the more radical splinting has been removed and before allowing the patient complete freedom.

Plaster Spica

In some instances the use of a spica is indicated, particularly in children who cannot cooperate in the use of a hanging cast. The plaster spica is cumbersome and often difficult to apply; consequently, it is a less adaptable form of treatment. When used, it is essential that the iliac crests be included in the spica and that care be exercised in molding to the body contours.

Use of the plaster spica is most strongly indicated in the early healing stage of the unstable fracture, e.g., after a period of traction. It is replaced by a simpler form of treatment as soon as the fracture elements show evidence of stability adequate to maintain reduction. The spica is also indicated occasionally when delayed union or nonunion appears imminent and more complete immobilization is desired. Its purpose can be defeated unless care is taken to assure form-fit.

Skeletal Traction

Only rarely is the use of traction indicated in the treatment of humeral shaft fractures. Skeletal traction is a difficult method of treatment, requiring close supervision by the doctor as well as cooperation by the patient. The necessary apparatus, whether for ambulatory or recumbent use, is complex and has the disadvantage of possibly producing distraction, leading to nonunion or even damage to neurovascular elements. Skeletal traction may be effectively used in an open fracture when observation and dressing changes are necessary, and if comminution and shortening have occurred. It is indicated most strongly

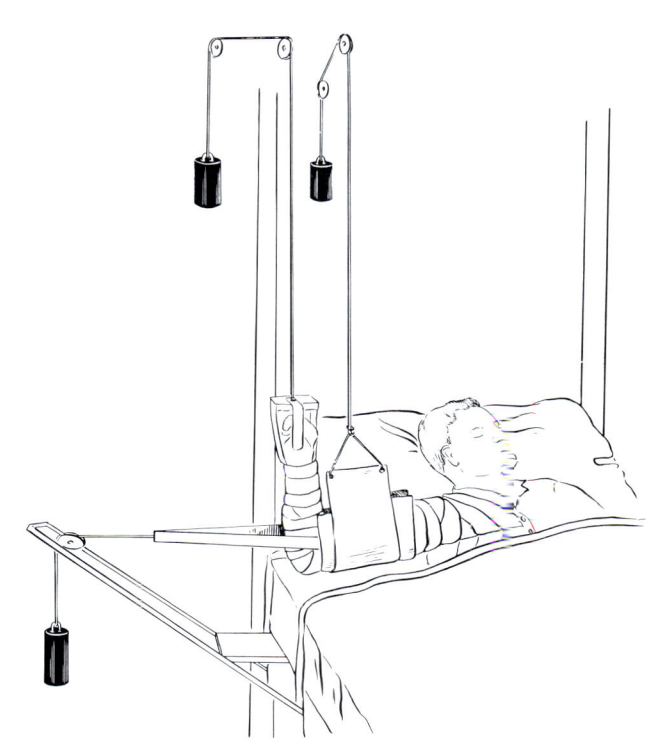

Fig. 18-5.—Axial traction in recumbency, skin-adhesive technique. Skeletal technique may also be used (see Fig. 19-14).

when recumbency is necessary because of other injuries.

Probably the simplest method of applying skeletal traction is through the olecranon, with suspension of the forearm and hand (Figs. 18-5 and 19-14). Countertraction by the patient's body is obtained by tilting the bed. Checking the circulation in the hand and frequently reminding the patient to exercise the fingers are essential adjuncts of this type of treatment.

Open Reduction

Before deciding to perform open reduction of a humeral shaft fracture, the surgeon must carefully consider all factors involved. Open reduction has the advantage of obtaining anatomic alignment with internal fixation; it may allow early exercising of the elbow and shoulder, and the period of discomfort is shortened. This form of reduction is indicated in situations in which interposition of soft parts prevents adequate reduction; in potential nonunion or delayed union; when actual nonunion exists, and when there are severe associated neurologic or circulatory problems. However, it is important to remember that where firm internal fixation has been obtained, both the doctor and the patient may have a false sense of security. It is essential that some form of external protection be maintained until there is x-ray evidence of progressing union. Delayed union is present when there is absence of clinical union 8–10 weeks following injury.

Exposure of the humeral shaft is most readily accomplished through the classic anterior approach. The proximal shaft is readily available through the deltopectoral approach, whereas the middle and

462 / Robert J. Boyd

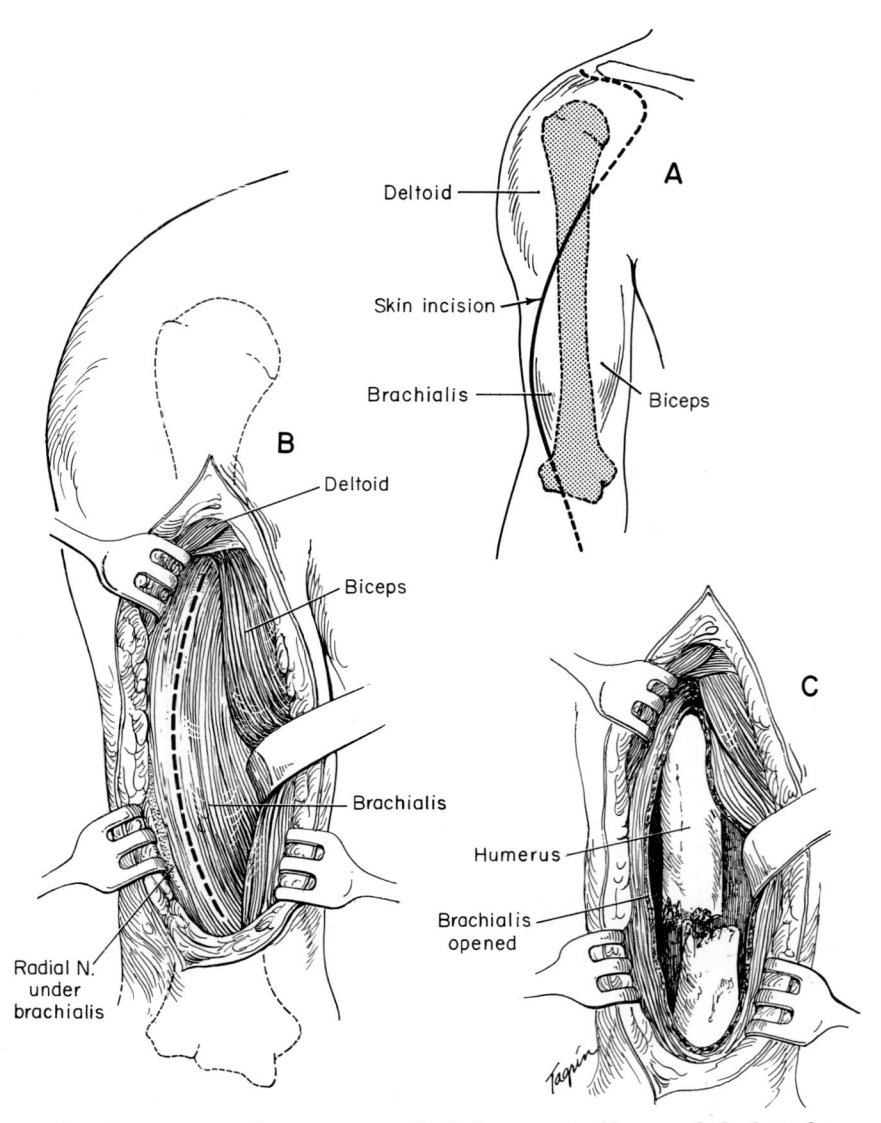

Fig. 18-6.—**A**, utility incision for exposure of whole or part of humeral shaft. **B**, biceps muscle displaced to identify brachialis muscle directly over shaft. **C**, exposure of shaft, with radial nerve protected in the brachialis muscle. (Adapted from Banks, S. W., and Laufman, H.: *An Atlas of Surgical Exposures of the Extremities* [Philadelphia: W. B. Saunders Company, 1953].)

distal shaft may be visualized by medial displacement of the biceps muscle and direct incision through the brachialis muscle (Fig. 18-6). This exposure avoids the radial nerve, but care must be taken so that the nerve is not traumatized by heavy retraction.

Numerous methods of internal fixation are available and each has its preferred application. Multiple screws adapt well to long spiral oblique fractures (Fig. 18-7), whereas plate and screws best fix the transverse fracture (Fig. 18-8). A combination of both methods may sta-

Chapter 18: HUMERAL SHAFT FRACTURES / 463

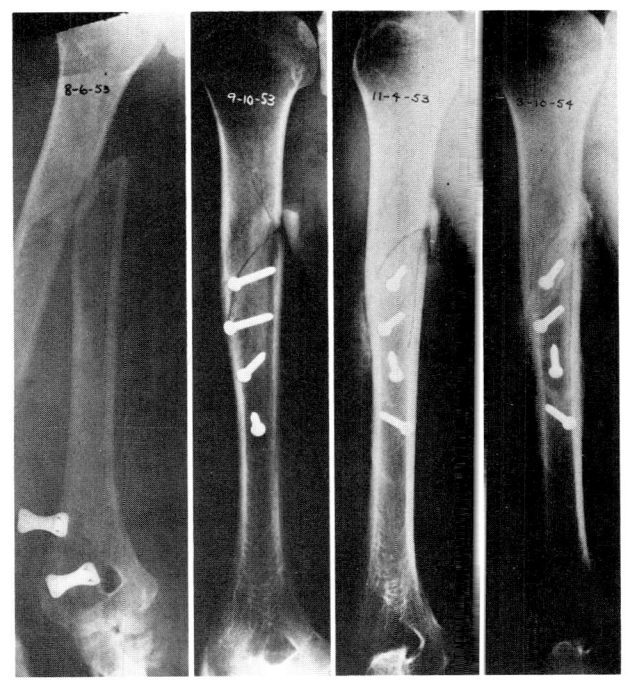

Fig. 18-7.—Open reduction elected on long spiral oblique fracture because of forced confinement to bed for secondary injuries. Postoperative support with sling and swathe. Good functional use in 3 months.

Fig. 18-8.—**A,** segmental fracture (proximal and middle thirds of shaft). Unable to maintain a closed reduction. **B,** open reduction with plate and screw fixation and without grafting. Note delayed union at midshaft fracture and early union in unexposed proximal shaft fracture.

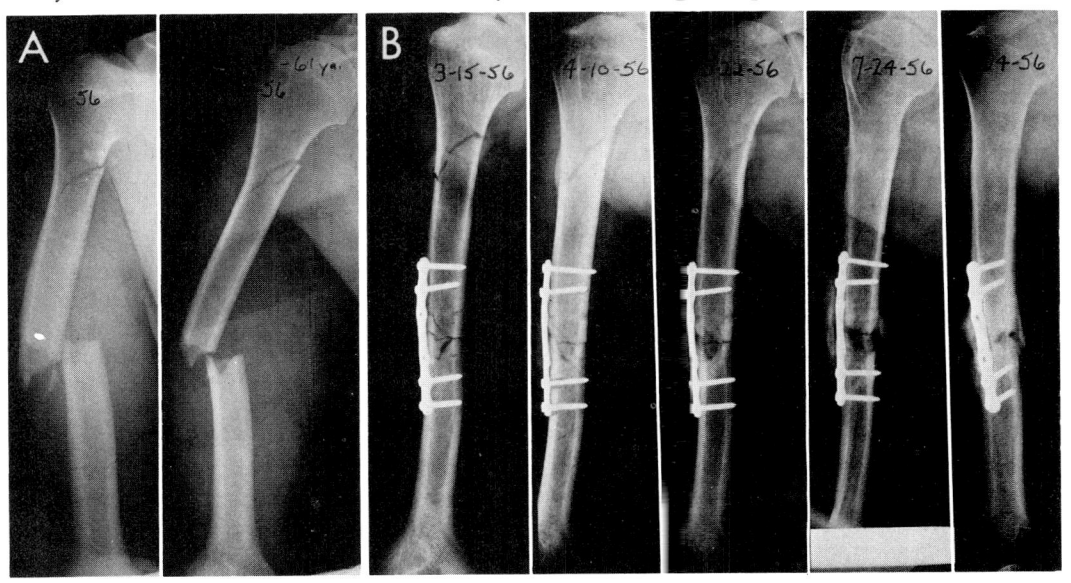

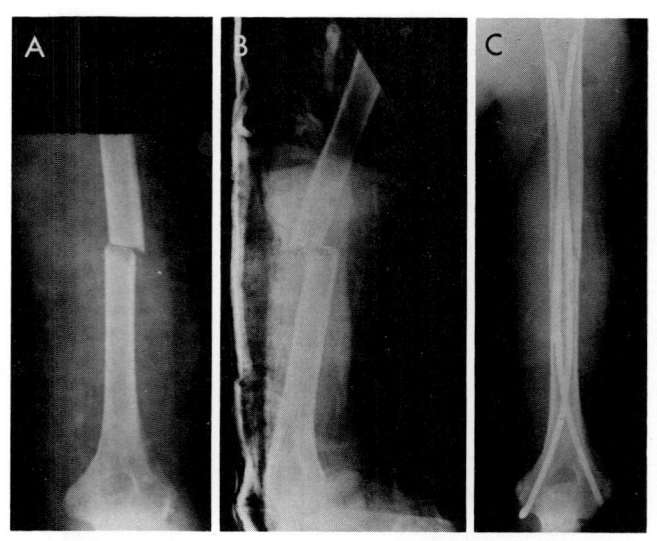

Fig. 18-9.—Shaft fracture in an uncooperative 65-year-old male; unreliable fixation. **A,** transverse fracture of middle third of humerus. **B,** poor maintenance of reduction with posterior plaster splint and cravat. **C,** 2-month postinsertion of Rush nails by "blind" technique. Full shoulder and elbow motion. Clinically healed.

bilize the comminuted fracture with a butterfly fragment. Intramedullary nails are useful in segmental and transverse fractures for maintaining length and alignment (Fig. 18-9). Frequently, however, they are difficult to introduce, may fail to stabilize rotation and may keep fracture ends apart. When used in conjunction with Parham bands, the medullary nail often effectively controls the markedly comminuted fracture, although usually additional external support is required. Bone grafting is commonly indicated in nonunion, and the fibula or tibia serves as an acceptable source for the graft (Fig. 18-10). Such a graft does well when firmly applied to a raw area of superficially denuded cortical bone and when cancellous onlay grafts are placed opposite the fracture site. In those instances in which osteoporotic cortical bone is unable to support screws, plates or nail fixation, it may be necessary to telescope the fragments of the fracture, holding them with circumferential wires or Parham bands (Fig. 18-11), and to accept shortening of the humerus. Variations and combinations of the foregoing techniques may be necessary in unusual instances. Compression plating is an excellent method of fixation with good initial stability, and the strength of the apparatus allows early mobilization. Fracture healing is difficult to assess with compression fixation, however, and the apparatus should not be removed for at least 12–18 months.

COMPLICATIONS

Complications in the healing of humeral shaft fractures are common and include some of the most difficult problems in the field of trauma. Nonunion of these fractures is a major tragedy and requires the maximal skill and judgment of the surgeon to overcome. Radial nerve and vascular injuries, which are common, require a high index of suspicion and careful examination to detect. The examination must be thorough enough to determine any concomitant upper extremity injuries and avoid later complications.

Chapter 18: HUMERAL SHAFT FRACTURES / 465

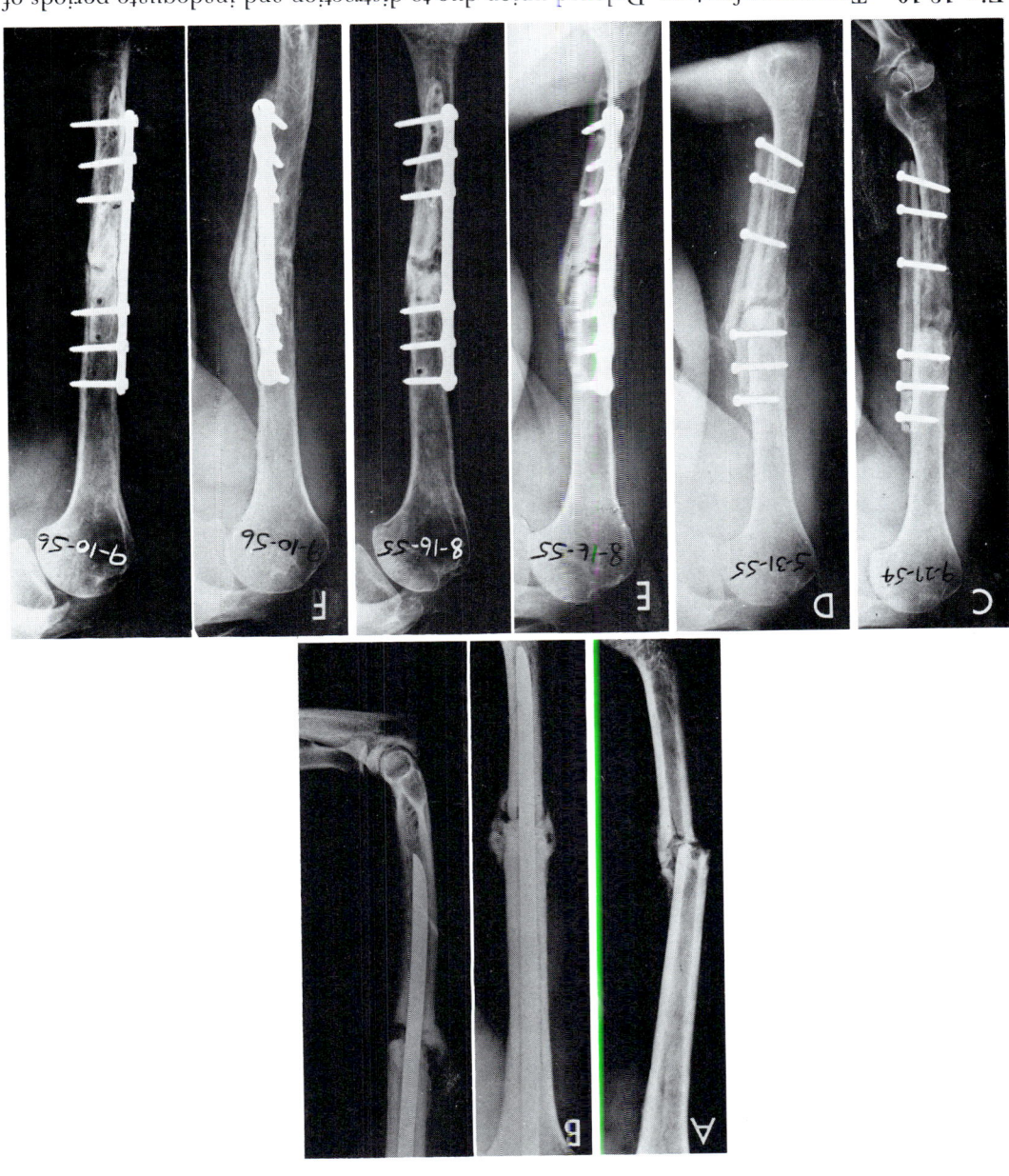

Fig. 18-10.—Transverse fracture. Delayed union due to distraction and inadequate periods of immobilization. Initial olecranon wire traction for 3 weeks, followed by 6 weeks with a hanging cast. A, 9 weeks postfracture. Distraction, delayed union. B, intramedullary nail fails to correct distraction. Subsequent treatments included: spica, iliac grafts, fibular grafts and screw fixation. C, 2 years postfracture with nonunion. Open reduction with screw fixation of full-thickness fibular graft plus iliac grafts. D, nonunion with fracture through fibular graft 8 months postoperatively. E, operation: removal of screws; fixation with Vitallium plate; osteoperiosteal tibial grafts. F, ultimate union after 4 years and 7 operations.

ered. Union may be achieved only by supplemental cancellous bone grafting, taking care to keep to a minimum any disturbance of the healing process that may already be present.

Radial nerve injury accompanying fracture of the mid- or lower third of the humeral shaft has an incidence of approximately 5 to 10%. Radial nerve paralysis results in sensory deficit in a small area on the radial side of the dorsum of the hand, but there are significant motor losses, with paralysis of extensor muscles of the wrist, fingers and thumb as well as of the brachioradialis and supinator muscles. The surgeon can be optimistic about the chances for spontaneous recovery in a high percentage of radial nerve paralyses in closed injuries. However, the following points are worthy of note.

Partial radial nerve paralysis associated with closed fracture has an excellent prognosis, although lack of evidence of spontaneous recovery at 2 months justifies nerve exploration. In complete radial paralysis, which developed at the time of fracture satisfactorily reduced by gentle manipulation, exploration should be considered if evidence of recovery has not been noted by 2 months. If a humeral shaft fracture, either closed or open, requires open reduction and internal fixation, at the time of operation the radial nerve should be explored for all partial or complete paralyses. Treatment of the nerve which is found to be crushed, but in continuity, may safely be delayed for 8 weeks. If, at the end of that time, recovery is not evident, exploration, excision of the neuroma and neurorrhaphy or neurolysis are indicated. If at exploration following acute injury the nerve is found to be divided, the nerve ends should be loosely approximated and definitive repair done several weeks later.

One should be suspicious of radial nerve injury in the overriding spiral oblique fractures of the distal third of the humeral shaft. If complete or progressive paralysis of the radial nerve develops aft-

suspected, early surgery must be considered. Revascularization and restoration of trabecular continuity may be hampered by interposition of soft parts. When this is suspected, early surgery must be considered. Union may be attributable to discontinuance of immobilization before adequate time for healing has been allowed. Nonunion may be attributable to discontinuance of immobilization before adequate time for healing has been allowed. Occasionally, nonunion may be attributable to discontinuance of immobilization before adequate time for healing has been allowed. Occasionally, nonunion may be attributable to discontinuance of immobilization before adequate time for healing has been allowed.

Delayed union of the humeral shaft fracture occurs most frequently in 2 circumstances: in the transverse fracture where open surgery has been performed and in distraction of fracture elements by the ardent use of a heavy hanging cast or by excessive traction through an olecranon wire (Fig. 18–10, A). Occasionally, nonunion may be attributable to discontinuance of immobilization before adequate time for healing has been allowed. Revascularization and restoration of trabecular continuity may be hampered by interposition of soft parts. When this is suspected, early surgery must be considered.

Ultimate limitation of motion of the shoulder and elbow can usually be avoided if early active exercises are begun under supervision as soon as discomfort lessens. Early active exercises are also of great importance for the wrist, hand and fingers. It is essential that the surgeon be aware of potential dangers and practice prevention.

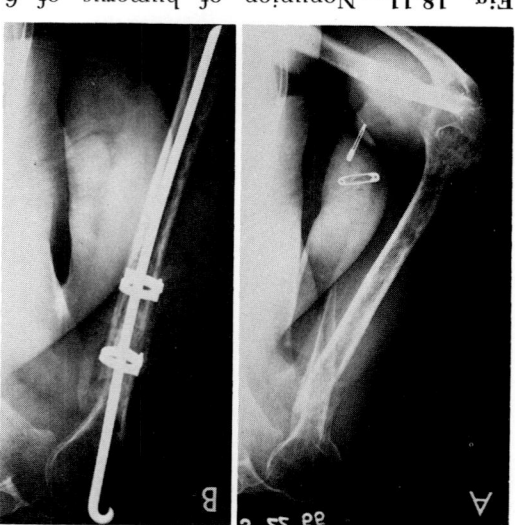

Fig. 18–11.—Nonunion of humerus of 6 months' duration in a housewife, 46, with multiple sclerosis. A, anteroposterior view 6 months after injury and treatment with external splinting. B, 4 months after open reduction, insertion of a Rush pin and Parham bands, and application of iliac bone slabs subperiosteally.

Chapter 18: HUMERAL SHAFT FRACTURES / 467

er manipulation of this type of fracture, immediate surgical exploration is indicated. It should be emphasized that great caution must be used in manipulating this type of fracture.

In neglected cases, when suture of the radial nerve is impractical or when recovery does not occur, function can be markedly improved by suitable tendon transfers to restore wrist, thumb and finger extension (see Chapter 47).

Vascular damage, such as laceration or severance of the brachial artery or vein, may occasionally have severe complications. Early recognition and treatment by ligation or anastomosis are necessary.

BIBLIOGRAPHY

1. Banks, S. W., and Laufman, H.: *An Atlas of Surgical Exposures of the Extremities* (Philadelphia. W. B. Saunders Company, 1953).
2. Billington, R. W.: Nerve injuries complicating fractures, J. South. M. A. 21:91, 1928.
3. Blum, L.: Double pulley traction in the treatment of humeral shaft fractures, Surg. Gynecol. Obstet. 65:812, 1937.
4. Caldwell, J. A.: Treatment of fractures of the shaft of the humerus by hanging cast, Surg. Gynecol. Obstet. 70:421, 1940.
5. Campbell, W. C.: Un-united fractures of the shaft of the humerus, Ann. Surg. 105:135, 1937.
6. Holstein, A., and Lewis, G. B.: Fractures of the humerus and radial-nerve paralysis, J. Bone Joint Surg. 45-A:1382, 1963.
7. Klenerman, L.: Fractures of the shaft of the humerus, J. Bone Joint Surg. 48-B:105, 1966.
8. Laferte, A. D., and Rosenbaum, M. C.: The "hanging cast" in the treatment of fractures of the humerus, Surg. Gynecol. Obstet. 65:230, 1937.
9. Laing, P. G.: The arterial supply of the adult humerus, J. Bone Joint Surg. 38-A:1105, 1956.
10. Rush, L. V., and Rush, H. L.: Intramedullary fixation of fractures of the humerus by the longitudinal pin, Surgery 27:268, 1950.
11. Scientific Research Committee, Penn. Orth. Soc: Fresh midshaft fractures of the humerus in adults, Pa. Med. J. 62:848, 1959.
12. Shaw, J. L., and Sakellarides, H.: Radial-nerve paralysis associated with fractures of the humerus: A review of forty-five cases, J. Bone Joint Surg. 49-A:899, 1967.
13. Stewart, M. J., and Hundley, J. M.: Fractures of the humerus: A comparative study in methods of treatment, J. Bone Joint Surg. 37-A:681, 1955.

19 | Fractures and Dislocations of the Elbow

WILLIAM R. MACAUSLAND, JR.

DISLOCATIONS

DISLOCATIONS OF THE ELBOW are very common, occurring next in frequency to dislocations of the shoulder. In type, the injuries are classified as posterior, anterior, medial, lateral or divergent dislocation, depending on the relationship of the ulna to the humerus. On occasion, the radial head alone is dislocated (Monteggia). By far the most common is the posterior or posterolateral type of dislocation. Anterior dislocations without an accompanying fracture are rare.

Any injury to the elbow, particularly dislocations, may be followed by troublesome complications that impair functional recovery. Therefore, exact diagnosis based on clinical examination and x-ray investigation is of utmost importance. Reduction should be carried out as soon as possible, even as an emergency measure, to prevent neurovascular complications. Important bone anatomy is noted in Fig. 19-1.

Posterior Dislocation

Backward dislocation (Fig. 19-2) may occur at any age, usually as the result of a fall on the outstretched hand. The line of force transmitted through the forearm causes the olecranon to lever the lower end of the humerus forward, passing over the coronoid process and tearing the anterior capsule of the joint. At the same time the radius and ulna may be shifted outward or inward. Accompanying damage to soft tissues varies with the degree of displacement. The brachialis anticus is often partially torn or even avulsed from the coronoid process when it is stretched over the distal humeral articular surface. The median and radial nerves may be damaged from stretching or contusion.

The diagnosis of posterior dislocation is usually made without difficulty from a careful examination. There are considerable hemorrhage and swelling. Flexion-extension of the elbow is restricted and extremely painful, while rotation is usually performed more easily. On palpation, the abnormal relationship of the olecranon to the epicondyles is revealed. The olecranon is easily palpated posteriorly, and the sulcus may be felt between the olecranon and the posterior lower humerus. Precise evaluation of damage to sensory and motor nerves at and distal to the elbow is vital, as is careful appraisal of circulation.

Posterior dislocation must be differentiated from a supracondylar fracture of the humerus, which presents similar deformity. Distinguishing features are the degree of mobility possible with a supracondylar fracture and the undisturbed relationship of the olecranon to the epicondyles.

X-rays are an absolute necessity to confirm the diagnosis. The deformed elbow should be visualized in at least 2,

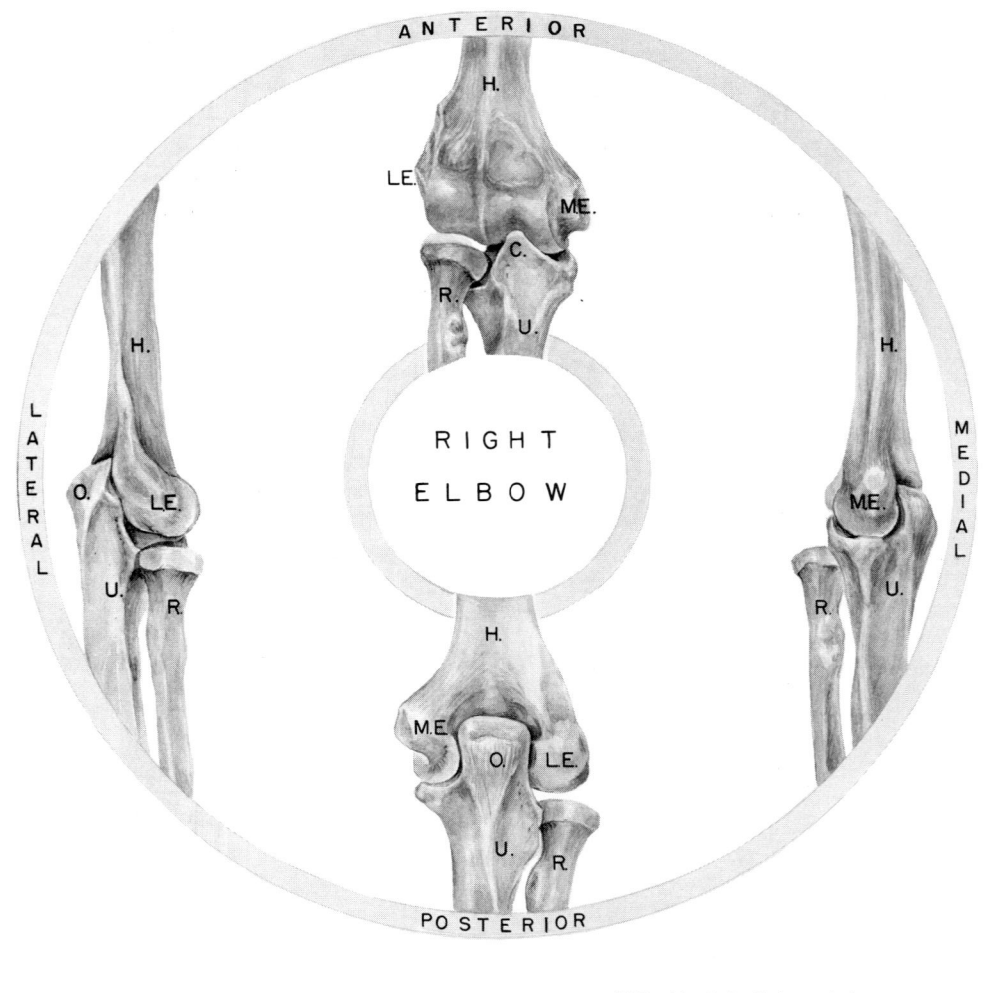

H - Humerus
R - Radius
U - Ulna

M.E. - Medial Epicondyle
L.E. - Lateral Epicondyle
O. - Olecranon
C. - Coronoid process

Fig. 19-1. — Anatomy of the elbow.

and preferably 4, views (anteroposterior, lateral, obliques).

Because of pain and deformity, it is usually extremely difficult to obtain standard x-rays in the anteroposterior and lateral positions. If the patient is under age 16, views of the corresponding elbow should be obtained for comparison of the epiphyseal plate, which will vary with different age groups, to aid in determining the exact type of dislocation.

Reduction of most dislocations calls for appropriate regional or general anesthesia. The dislocation is usually reduced without difficulty by manipulation and traction. Lateral displacement, if present, is corrected first. With one hand the surgeon applies traction distally on the

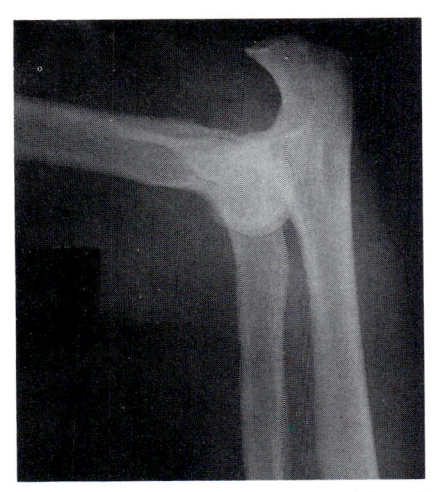

Chapter 19: FRACTURES AND DISLOCATIONS OF THE ELBOW / 471

Fig. 19-2.—Posterior dislocation of the elbow.

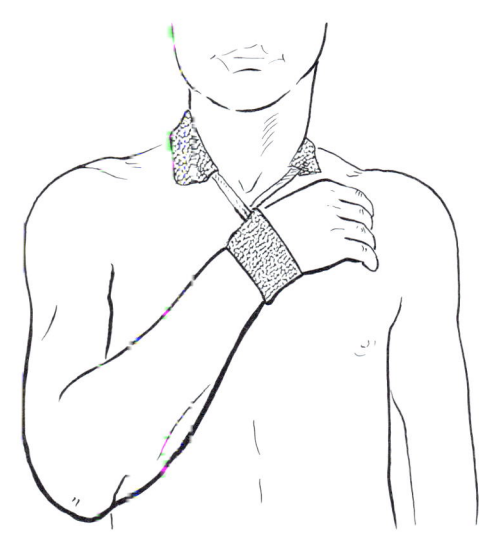

Fig. 19-3.—Immobilization by a collar and cuff sling following reduction of dislocated elbow.

lower forearm in the line of deformity, while with the other hand, he—or his assistant—establishes countertraction on the lower end of the humerus. The traction force can be supplemented by the surgeon's pressing on the tip of the olecranon with his thumb as his fingers surround the lower part of the humerus and thus apply countertraction. A definite impact is usually felt when reduction is accomplished. The range of motion in supination, pronation, flexion and extension should then be tested. The humeral condyles and tip of the olecranon should be palpated to make certain that the anatomic relationship is satisfactory. True anteroposterior and lateral x-ray views are taken to confirm the reduction and rule out the possibility of small chip fractures previously undetected.

Following reduction, the elbow is immobilized in a posterior plaster slab or a collar and cuff sling (Fig. 19-3) in a position of approximately 110 degrees of flexion and midpronation. Immobilization is maintained for approximately 7 days, during which period range of motion exercises for the shoulder, hand and fingers are practiced. On removal of the splint, the patient begins guarded active elbow exercises in flexion-extension and rotation to increase the range of motion. At no time should passive exercises of the elbow be allowed or heavy weights carried in order to increase the range of extension.

The status of the neurovascular structures should be carefully checked at the time of reduction and at intervals throughout after-care. Further damage to adjacent soft tissues, with resulting myositis ossificans, may be avoided by prompt reduction of the dislocation, using gentle traction, and careful supervision afterward. Yet in some cases, particularly in adults, despite the best possible care the patient is left with a permanent flexion contracture of from 10 to 20 degrees, the result of soft tissue contractures. No attempt should be made to overcome these contractures by passive exercises or stretching. In fact, in the first few months the contracture may increase if treated by such measures in the first weeks after reduction.

Old unreduced dislocations, diagnosed within a month of the injury, may at times be treated by closed reduction. After a month has elapsed, however, open reduction is probably indicated. This may be best performed through the Boyd incision, taking care to preserve the articular surface, or by transection of the olecranon to achieve more adequate exposure.

Anterior Dislocation

Anterior dislocation of the elbow without an associated fracture of the olecranon is extremely rare. The injury is due to hyperextension of the forearm or to a fall on the flexed elbow with the point of impact at the olecranon. The neurovascular structures in the antecubital median nerve are especially liable to damage in this injury.

The dislocation is easily reduced under anesthesia by applying strong traction on the forearm in the position in which it lies and providing countertraction by pressing backward on the upper

Fig. 19-4.—**A,** anteroposterior and **B,** lateral views of anterior dislocation of the elbow without fracture (5 weeks' duration). **C,** reduction. **D,** function 6 months after operation.

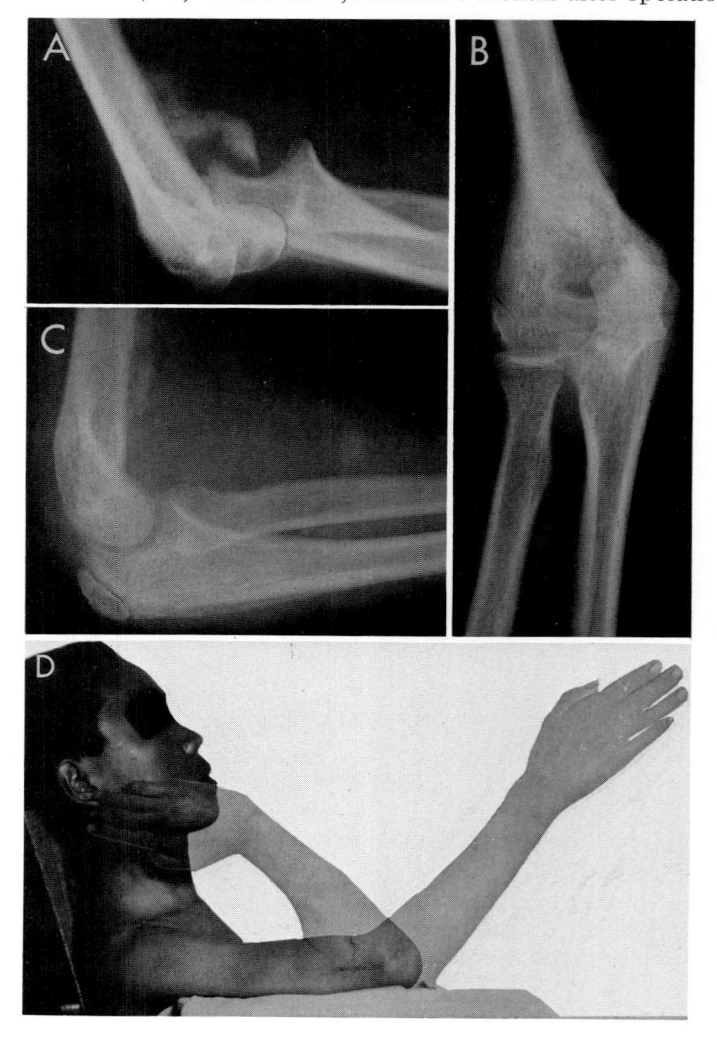

portion of the forearm. The humeral condyles serve as a point of counterpressure during reduction. The elbow, once reduced, is immobilized by a posterior plaster slab in the position of 90 degrees for approximately 10 days. Active motion is then begun. Preservation of the neurovascular integrity is of vital importance.

The development of myositis ossificans in the brachialis anticus muscle may limit the flexion-extension range of motion following anterior dislocation (Fig. 19-4). No attempt should be made to remove this bony block until at least 2 years after the injury. Earlier excision will result in prompt recurrence of the bony block.

Lateral Dislocation

A purely lateral dislocation of the elbow is rare (Fig. 19-5) and is usually associated with fracture of the lateral condyle. The diagnosis is established by careful palpation of the bony landmarks, the pronounced lateral instability of the joint and, in particular, x-rays.

Reduction is accomplished without difficulty, with appropriate anesthesia, by gentle lateral pressure on the displaced olecranon. The after-care follows that given for posterior dislocation of the elbow.

Dislocation of Head of Radius

Traumatic dislocation of the radial head is of common occurrence in children under age 4. It is often referred to as a "pulled elbow" or "nursemaid's elbow."

The mechanism of the entity is not fully understood, but it is presumed that the radial head is dislocated from under the orbicular ligament as the result of a longitudinal pull on the forearm when the elbow is in extension. The injury is seen as the result of suddenly lifting a child by the hand to prevent his falling or of jerking him back out of the path of an oncoming car. Occasionally, older siblings play "airplane" by grasping the child by both forearms and spinning him around in a horizontal plane, causing considerable traction on the elbows.

Diagnosis is established from the fixed position of the elbow in flexion of approximately 35 degrees and midpronation and, in particular, from the fretful crying

Fig. 19-5.—**A**, anteroposterior and **B**, lateral views of lateral dislocation of the elbow without fracture.

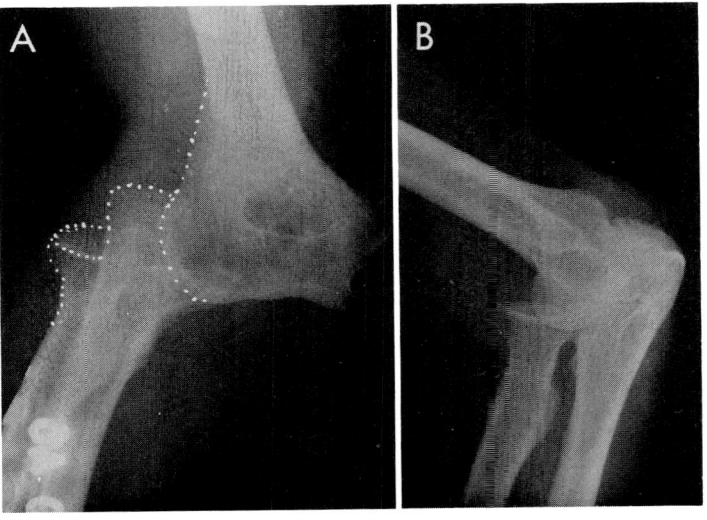

of the child. Palpation reveals little in the way of deformity. Results of x-ray examination are negative. An attempt at passive motion is met with resistance. In essence, the diagnosis is based on a high index of suspicion.

Reduction is accomplished by gently forcing the forearm into full extension and supination while pressure is applied simultaneously on the anterior radial head with the thumb. A gentle click may be experienced under the thumb as the radial head slips into normal position. Following this maneuver, the child will usually flex the elbow and permit passive examination of the elbow in flexion, extension and rotation. If indicated, the procedure may be repeated. After reduction, the elbow should be protected by a sling for 4 or 5 days to prevent recurrence and to let the soft tissue reaction subside.

Occasionally an old dislocation of the radial head is seen. The diagnosis is easily made from x-rays and by comparison of the involved elbow with the corresponding joint. Surprisingly, the elbow has an excellent range of motion; indeed, the only significant abnormal physical findings may be a permanent flexion contracture of 10–15 degrees and prominence of the radial head behind the capitellum.

No attempt should be made at open reduction in childhood. The untreated elbow has excellent functional capacity, and surgery might damage the proximal radial epiphysis, disturbing growth and resulting in Madelungs deformity at the wrist. When full growth has been established, and if cosmesis is of concern, excision of the head of the radius may be performed. Most patients, however, are quite satisfied with the functional ability of the elbow and do not desire surgery.

FRACTURE-DISLOCATIONS

Posterior Dislocation with Fracture of Coronoid Process

Posterior dislocation is often associated with a fracture of the coronoid process due to avulsion of the brachialis anticus insertion. The injury is treated as a simple dislocation, on reduction of which the coronoid fragment usually falls into satisfactory position. If the fragment is exceptionally large, threatening the stability of the joint, the elbow should be immobilized in flexion for 3 or 4 weeks. A varying degree of permanent flexion contracture must be anticipated to follow this injury. If the coronoid fragment is especially large and significantly displaced, open reduction of this fragment may be necessary.

Posterior Dislocation with Fracture of Radial Head

A marginal or comminuted fracture of the radial head and, occasionally, a complete separation of the radial head from the shaft of the bone may accompany a posterior dislocation of the elbow (Fig. 19-6). The first step in treatment is to reduce the dislocation; then treat the radial head injury. In marginal or comminuted fracture, which produces gross incongruity of the articular surface, it is generally felt that excision of the radial head should be performed. Immediate removal is advisable and, for practical purposes, while the patient is under the same anesthesia. When separation of the

Fig. 19-6. — Posterior dislocation of the elbow with fracture of the head of the radius.

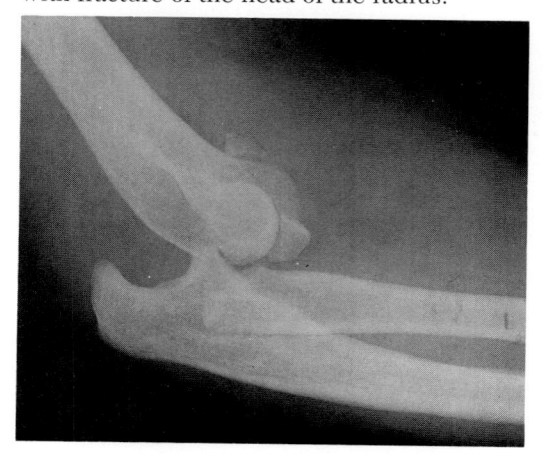

radial head from the shaft occurs, the type of treatment depends on whether the radial epiphysis has closed. In adults, the radial head may be removed. If the injury occurs before closure of the proximal radial epiphysis, the radial head should be restored to normal position. Postoperatively the elbow is immobilized for 10 days to 2 weeks in a posterior plaster splint, with the forearm flexed 90 degrees and in midrotation. Exercise of the forearm in rotation should be started immediately. *Never excise the radial head epiphysis.*

Posterior Dislocation with Fracture of External Condyle

The separated fragment (capitellum) is carried backward with forearm bones; the relationship between the radial head and the capitellum remains normal.

The dislocation is first reduced and subsequently the fracture of the external condyle is manipulated. The elbow, if necessary, is immobilized in a posterior plaster splint to permit union of the fractured condyle. Immobilization is maintained approximately 5 weeks if the patient is an adult; 3 weeks if the patient is a child.

Anterior Dislocation with Fracture of Olecranon

Fracture of the olecranon and anterior dislocation of the elbow usually occur in combination. Treatment consists first in reducing the dislocation. If the olecranon fragment fails to fall into satisfactory position, operative reduction may be indicated. Because neurovascular complications of the hand and forearm are likely after anterior dislocation, care must be taken to check for incipient Volkmann's contracture.

Lateral Dislocation with Avulsion of Internal Epicondyle

This common elbow injury, occurring between the ages of 8 and 16, is frequently overlooked. The avulsion of the medial epicondyle is the result of a valgus strain of the joint, at which time the elbow dislocates laterally. At the same time, the flexor pronator group of muscles arising from the medial epicondyle laterally avulses the epicondyle off the shaft of the humerus. The joint capsule on the medial side of the elbow may be torn simultaneously, so the medial epicondyle may be sucked into the joint space and trapped, as the dislocation spontaneously reduces (Fig. 19-7).

Avulsion of the medial epicondyle is usually obvious if looked for. Careful palpation reveals areas of maximal tenderness and swelling along the medial aspect of the elbow. There is occasionally an associated ulnar nerve injury. The x-ray evidence is clear if the dislocation is unreduced when the patient is first seen. The bony epicondyle is visualized between the articular surfaces of the olecranon and trochlea. On the other hand, the x-ray evidence may be deceiving if the dislocation has spontaneously reduced itself and the epicondyle is trapped in the joint (Fig. 19-7, *B*). Unless multiple oblique views of the normal elbow are taken for comparison, the epicondyle is not readily apparent.

When the elbow is still dislocated at the time of first examination, an effort should be made to extract the medial epicondyle from the joint space. With the patient under general anesthesia, the valgus deformity is slightly increased and, with the forearm supinated to the maximum, the wrist and fingers are extended. As tension is exerted on the flexor pronator muscle group attached to the epicondyle, it may slip out of the joint. Faradic stimulation of the flexor muscle belly is advocated by some. Reduction of the dislocation is then easily accomplished. The freed bone fragment is then manipulated as close as possible to its normal position. The elbow is maintained in the position of 90 degrees of flexion, with the forearm pronated to relax the muscle pull on the attached epicondyle.

476 / *William R. Macausland, Jr.*

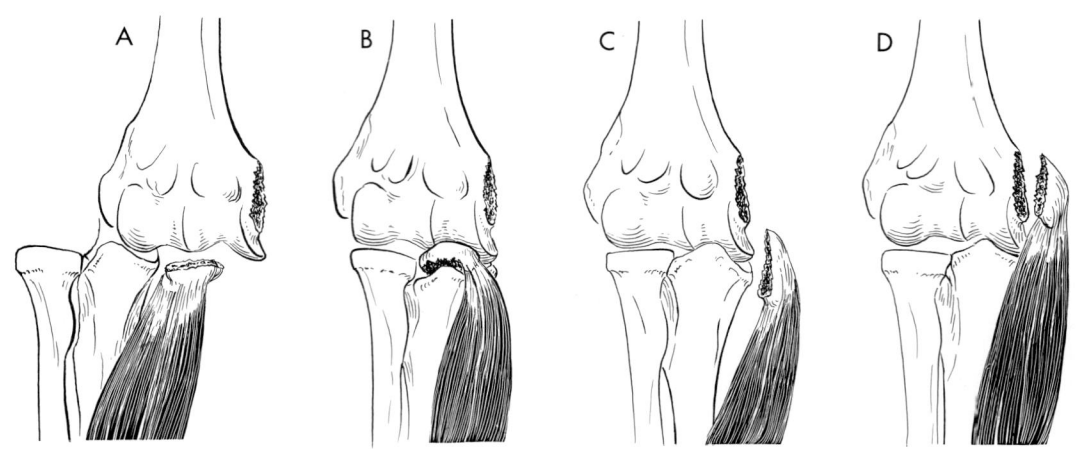

Fig. 19-7.—Degrees of displacement of internal epicondyle. **A,** displacement of internal epicondyle following lateral dislocation of the elbow. **B,** incarceration of internal epicondyle in the joint after reduction of lateral dislocation of the elbow. **C,** fracture of internal epicondyle with wide separation of the fragment. **D,** fracture of internal epicondyle with minimal separation of the fragment.

Fig. 19-8.—Operative view of internal epicondyle incarcerated in elbow.

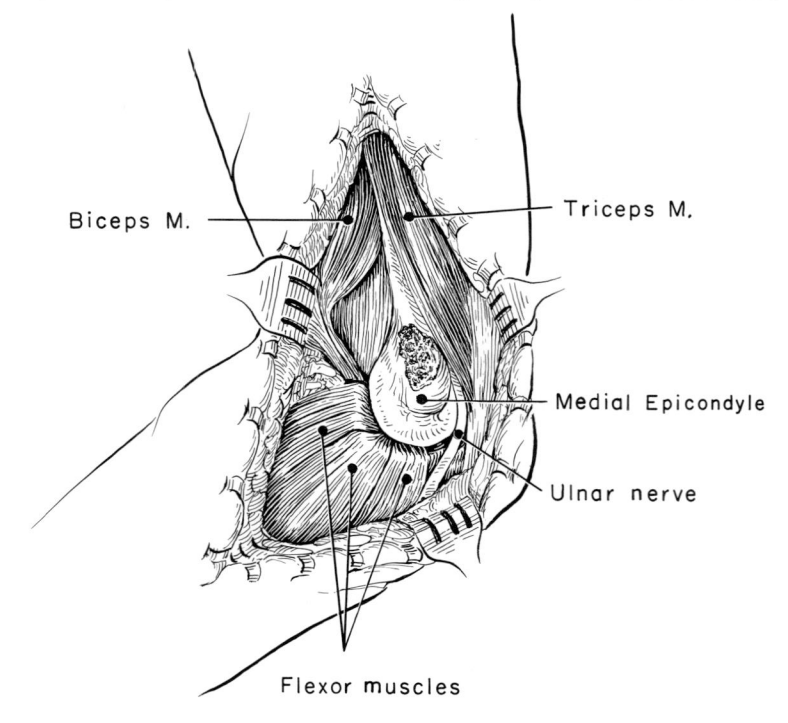

When removal of the medial epicondyle is not possible by manipulation, open reduction must be performed promptly. A medial approach to the elbow, with care taken to avoid trauma to the ulnar nerve, exposes the muscle that turns into the joint through the defect in the medial capsule (Fig. 19-8). Simple traction on the muscle withdraws the epicondyle and allows reduction of the dislocation. The epicondyle is then reattached at its point of origin by 2 Kirschner wires, which are left sufficiently long to present subcutaneously for ease of removal in 3 or 4 weeks. Postoperatively, the elbow is immobilized in about 90 degrees of flexion and neutral rotation. Gentle active range of motion exercises are begun in 2 weeks, care being taken to avoid excessive force.

Dislocation of Radial Head with Fracture of Ulna (Monteggia's Fracture)

The injury consists of a fracture of the proximal shaft of the ulna with dislocation of the radial head and rupture of the orbicular ligament (Fig. 19-9). It is an unusual injury, presenting problems in diagnosis and treatment and characterized by complications which may preclude obtaining good functional results.

This complex injury is often overlooked. Though there is no difficulty in diagnosing the fracture of the ulna from the gross deformity, which is apparent both clinically and on x-rays, the dislocation of the radial head may not be appreciated. Special care must be taken in interpreting the x-rays. It should be borne in mind that a fracture of the upper ulnar shaft seldom occurs without an associated dislocation of the radial head. In x-ray views a line drawn through the shaft of the radius and its articular surface normally bisects the capitellum. The angular deformity of the ulna always points to the direction of the dislocation of the radial head (Fig. 19-10). The subtle dislocation of the radius-capitellum articulation produces significant functional loss if untreated.

When the injury is seen within the first 2 weeks, it is usually possible to perform a closed reduction of the radial head. Under general anesthesia, the elbow is gently extended and fully supinated.

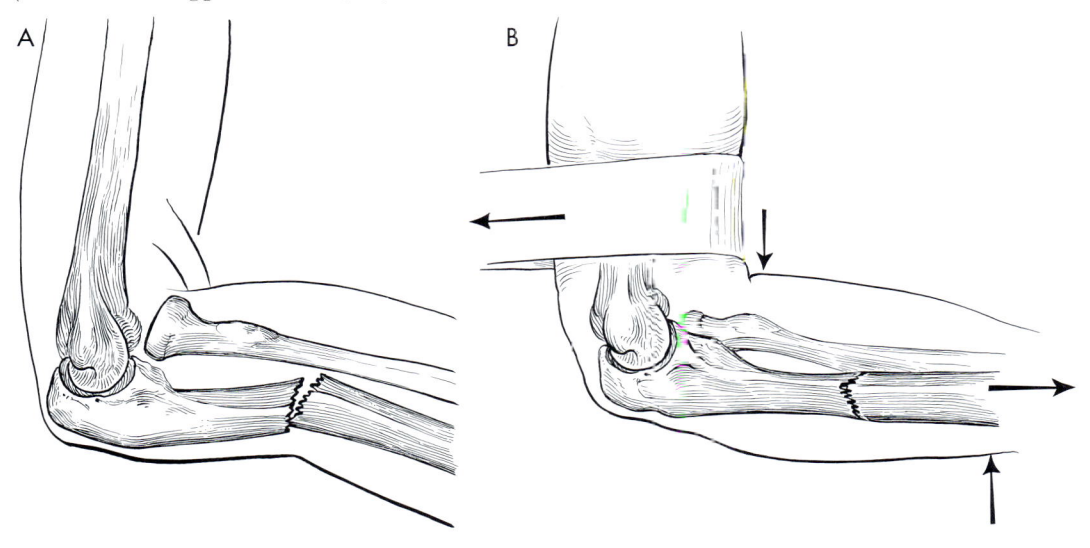

Fig. 19-9.—Fracture of the shaft of the ulna with anterior dislocation of the head of the radius (anterior Monteggia's fracture). A, before reduction. B, after reduction.

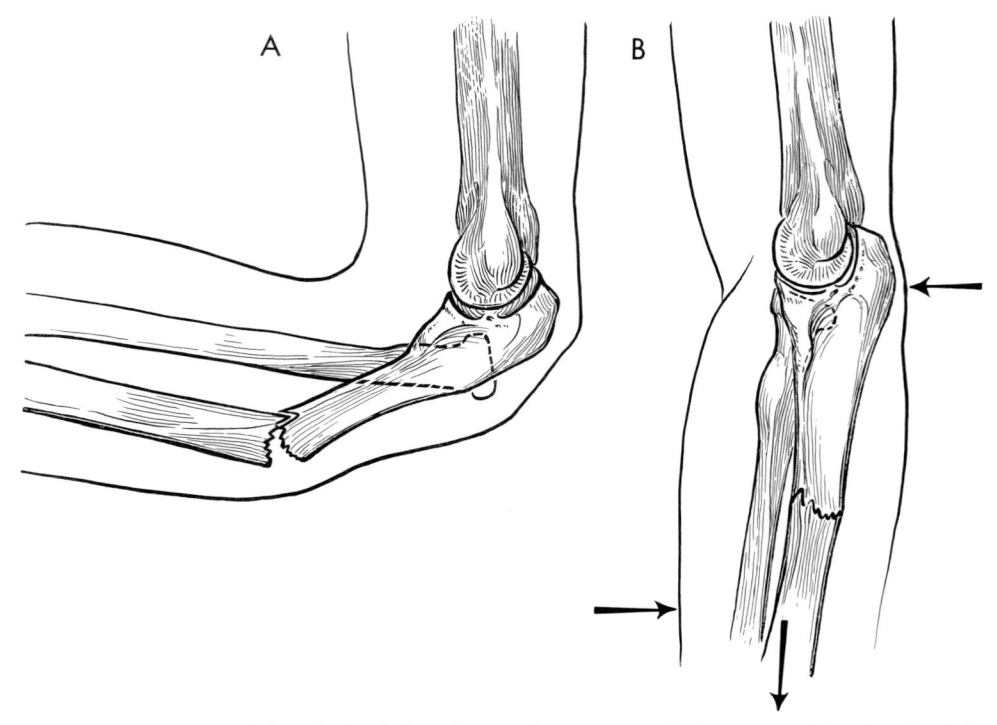

Fig. 19-10.—Fracture of the shaft of the ulna with posterior dislocation of the head of the radius (posterior Monteggia's fracture). **A,** before reduction. **B,** after reduction.

Gentle pressure on the radial head results in satisfactory reduction of radial capitellar dislocation. The ulnar shaft fracture may need internal fixation to assure restoration of ulnar length.

FRACTURES OF THE ELBOW

The fractures of the elbow may be classified as (1) fractures of the lower end of the humerus, e.g., supracondylar fractures of the humerus (extension-flexion and malunited types), transcondylar fractures of the humerus, fractures of the capitellum (chip, hemicapitellar and old ununited fractures and capitellar epiphyseal separation), fractures of the external condyle of the humerus in the adult, and intercondylar T and Y fractures of the humerus; (2) fractures of the upper ulna (fractures of the olecranon), and (3) fractures of the upper end of the radius (radial head fractures and separation of the upper radial epiphysis).

Supracondylar Fractures of Humerus

Probably the most common fracture of the elbow, especially in children, is the supracondylar fracture. It is of 2 types, depending on the position of the broken bone fragments. If the distal fragment lies behind the lower end of the humeral shaft, the fracture is termed the "extension" type (Fig. 19-11), whereas if it lies in front of the humerus, it is known as the "flexion" type. The extension type is the most frequently seen and is also the most favorable from the point of view of treatment. The flexion type, fortunately, is quite rare; it is much more difficult to treat, particularly if unrecognized as to type of supracondylar fracture.

The deformity produced by these frac-

Chapter 19: FRACTURES AND DISLOCATIONS OF THE ELBOW / 479

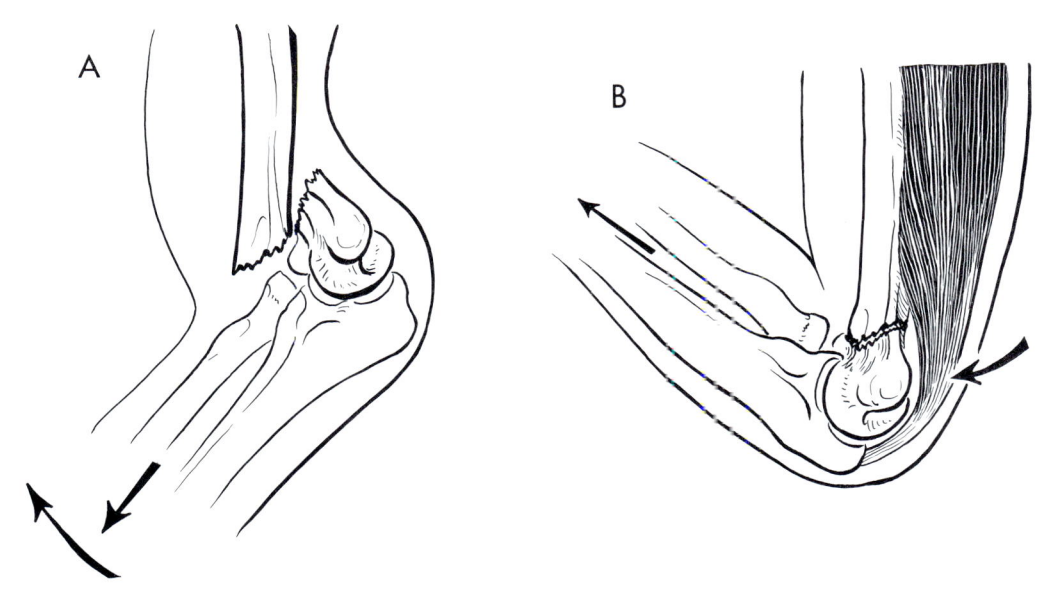

Fig. 19-11.—The usual extension type of supracondylar fracture of the humerus. **A,** before reduction. **B,** after reduction.

tures is quite similar to that of a posterior dislocation of the elbow and, when marked swelling is present, it may be difficult or impossible to differentiate clinically between the 2 conditions. In general, it can be said that supracondylar fractures show a greater amount of mobility than do posterior dislocations and that the anatomic relationship of the olecranon with the internal and external epicondyles is not disturbed in these fractures as it is in dislocations. On careful, gentle palpation, the 3 bony prominences in the normal elbow—the external condyle, the internal condyle and the tip of the olecranon—present as an equilateral triangle. This relationship is maintained with most supracondylar fractures despite the swelling and angular deformity at the fracture site. However, with posterior dislocations of the elbow, this equilateral triangular relationship is lost due to the displacement of the olecranon.

As a general rule, in dealing with the extension type of supracondylar fracture, the displacement of the distal fragment is corrected by immobilization of the fragments with the elbow flexed. In the opposite type of fracture, the so-called flexion injury, the distal fragment may have to be immobilized with the elbow in extension.

Usual (Extension) Type of Supracondylar Fracture

During the initial examination of the injured elbow a careful and exact examination of the neurologic and circulatory status of the extremity is of extreme importance. This particular injury is notorious for producing severe neurovascular complications in the form of Volkmann's ischemic contracture if treatment is not immediate and appropriate.

TREATMENT.—Under general or regional anesthesia, the patient's upper arm is held by an assistenat while the surgeon grasps the elbow with the left hand and the wrist with the right. The general alignment of the arm is corrected by gentle pressure and manipulation with the surgeon's left hand. Then strong traction is applied as the arm is gradually completely extended. The manipulation plus traction should draw the distal fragment down into proper relationship with the proximal fragment. Then, and not until then, the elbow is flexed to maintain the reduction by tightening the triceps musculature. In other words, flexion of the elbow should never be attempted until the manipulation and traction have been first performed, because if it is done before, it may produce extremely serious consequences by encroachment on the neurovascular supply in the antecubital fossa (Fig. 19-12).

It is well to remember that, in supracondylar fractures of the elbow, the movement of flexion does not reduce the fragment and may do irreparable damage. Flexion should only be used as a final maneuver to maintain the reduction.

As the surgeon flexes the elbow while maintaining traction, he must be careful to avoid any rotatory displacement of the distal fragment. To prevent such displacement, the arm should be held with the forearm in supination and the antecubital space facing upward as the movement of flexion is carried out. Once the desired degree of flexion is obtained, the surgeon should immediately check the patient's pulse to be sure that it is present and bounding. The degree of elbow flexion for immobilization purposes is determined by the pulse; should the position of acute flexion result in absence or weakening of the pulse, the forearm should be lowered and the degree of elbow flexion lessened until the pulse beat is strong. Sometimes the elbow is so swollen or the injury is so severe that flexion beyond a right angle cannot be obtained without obliterating the pulse. When such a situation arises, it is well to use another method of treatment, such as Dunlop's traction (Fig. 19-13) or overhead skeletal traction (Fig. 19-14). Either of these methods will maintain traction on the arm and keep the fracture reduced. At the same time the circulation

Fig. 19-13.—Dunlop's traction. (Tracing of a photograph.)

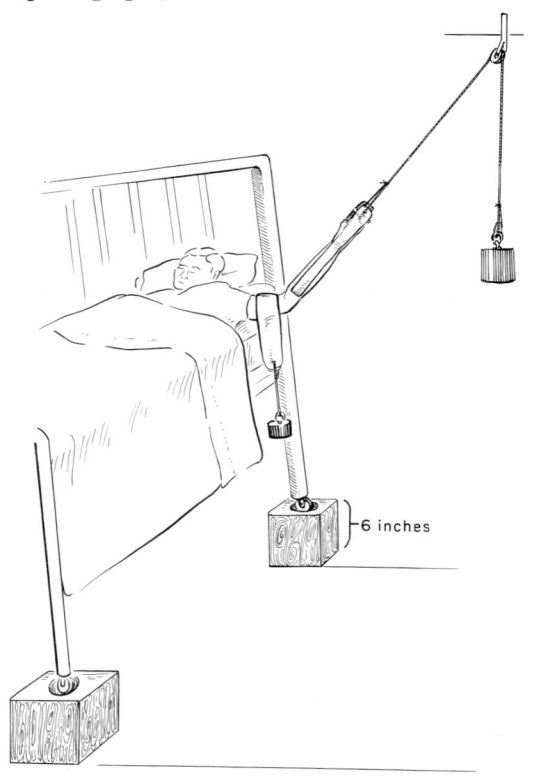

Fig. 19-12.—Diagram illustrating the danger to blood vessels of flexing the elbow in supracondylar fracture before applying traction. Traction must always be applied first.

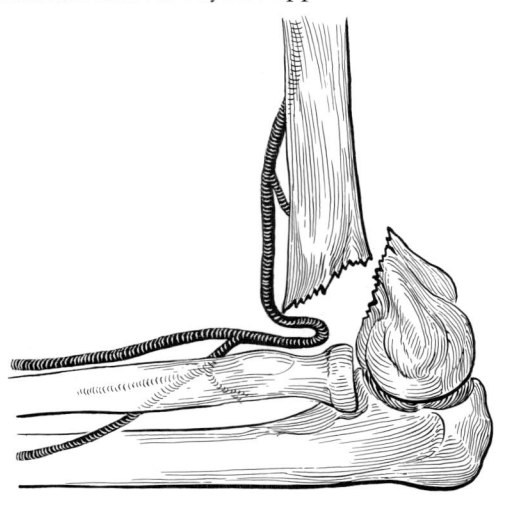

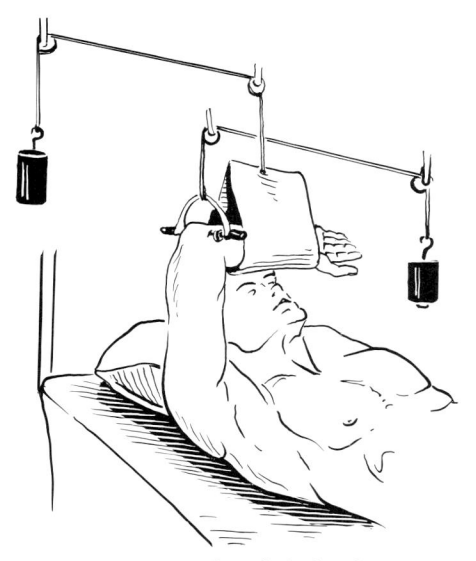

Chapter 19: FRACTURES AND DISLOCATIONS OF THE ELBOW / 481

Fig. 19-14. — Overhead skeletal traction.

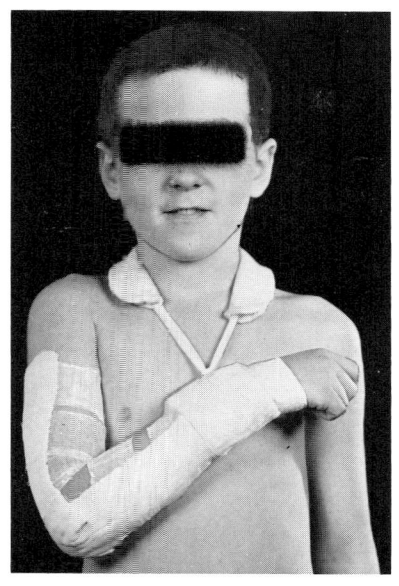

Fig. 19-15. — Immobilization of supracondylar fracture by a plaster-of-paris slab and a collar and cuff, following reduction.

will be aided by elevation of the extremity, thereby reducing the risk of Volkmann's contracture. It is a wise practice to use either Dunlop's traction or overhead skeletal traction whenever there is any doubt regarding the circulation.

In most instances, the patient's arm can be safely flexed into a comfortable position. It can be supported and the position maintained by a collar and cuff sling (Fig. 19-15), suspending the wrist from the neck. A strip or 2 of sheet wadding should be placed in the antecubital fold of the elbow as it is being flexed, in order to avoid maceration of the skin. In addition, a plaster-of-paris splint should be carefully molded to the posterior surface of the flexed arm from the posterior axilla to the metacarpophalangeal joints and secured by a lightly applied gauze bandage.

This posterior plaster-of-paris slab should be applied immediately after the flexion of the elbow with the forearm supinated and the antecubital space facing upward and after a strong radial pulse is verified at the wrist. The arm is held in this position until the plaster is well set before the arm is allowed to rotate against the chest wall and be suspended by the collar and cuff sling. If further fixation or reinforcement is desired, an encircling wide strip of adhesive plaster or figure-of-eight bandage can be used to bridge the space between the midforearm and upper arm.

AFTER-TREATMENT. — After the fracture has been reduced and the arm immobilized, x-ray films should be made to determine if the reduction is satisfactory. If it is not, a second attempt should be made, either immediately or after the swelling has subsided, depending on the degree of displacement and the severity of the injury. Sometimes several repeated attempts at reduction are necessary before success is obtained; as a rule, however, these fractures can almost always be reduced without resorting to skeletal traction or operation.

When the x-ray examination shows the reduction to be satisfactory, the elbow should be placed in the optimal position of 125 degrees of flexion if possible. If the amount of swelling does not permit this degree of flexion at first, as swelling subsides, flexion should be increased and new plaster splints applied until the optimal position is reached.

Finger and shoulder exercises should be started at once. Repeated x-ray examinations during the first 3 weeks are necessary to assure maintenance of the previously achieved reduction. After 3 weeks, the collar and cuff sling with the plaster splint can be discarded and only an ordinary arm sling retained for another week to 10 days. The arm is taken out of the sling at regular intervals for active exercises and mobilization. Under no circumstances should passive exercises, massage or stretching be employed, since these measures may encourage the development of myositis ossificans. The family must be carefully instructed in this matter.

The complications which are likely to occur in supracondylar fractures are Volkmann's ischemic contracture, injury to the nerves and blood vessels, vascular obstruction from tight bandaging or splinting and myositis ossificans. These complications are so dangerous and so tragic in their nature that every caution should be taken to avoid them. For this reason, it is often advisable to have patients with supracondylar fractures hospitalized and kept under observation for at least 24 hours.

The prognosis of supracondylar fractures in children is, as a rule, excellent. Careful, gentle manipulation and traction are usually successful in obtaining a satisfactory reduction, and the position of acute elbow flexion maintains it. If, because of marked swelling or vascular disturbance, the elbow cannot be safely flexed to a right angle, Dunlop's traction or overhead skeletal traction should be employed to secure the reduction and reduce the swelling. After 2 weeks, the arm may be safely brought to the side and treated as previously described. It is of utmost importance in after-care to avoid forcing the joint motion or using massage and passive stretching.

In adults, the prognosis of supracondylar fractures is not so favorable as in children. It may be anticipated that a permanent flexion contracture and limitation of full flexion may develop.

Flexion Type of Supracondylar Fracture

The flexion type of supracondylar fracture, in which the distal fragment is displaced upward and anterior to the lower end of the proximal fragment, is fortunately quite rare (Fig. 19-16). It is also less likely to be complicated by blood vessel and nerve damage than is the extension type of fracture.

TREATMENT. — This fracture is not nearly so easily reduced as is the usual extension type of supracondylar fracture. Reduction may be difficult to accomplish and maintain. Because of this, no one method of manipulation is considered ideal and several different procedures are suggested in the textbooks. Key and Conwell,[5] for instance, prefer the position of right-angle flexion for immobilization after the fracture is reduced by traction and manipulation. They do mention as a possible alternative acute flexion of the elbow if the fragments are stable in this position. Watson-Jones,[12] on the other hand, believed that it is clearly wrong to treat this fracture in the flexed position and strongly advised complete extension. He contended that traction followed by complete extension will reduce the fracture with no difficulty and that, in the extended position, it is easy to judge the carrying angle and to apply any lateral pressures that may be necessary to correct any tilting of the lower fragment. Following reduction, a posterior plaster-of-paris slab is applied to the extended arm for 3 weeks. Then, if reduction is perfect, full movements are easily recovered. It is apparent from the foregoing statements that there is a difference of opinion regarding treatment of this rare fracture. It would seem, however, that the position of complete extension offers the best chance for reduction; if, by

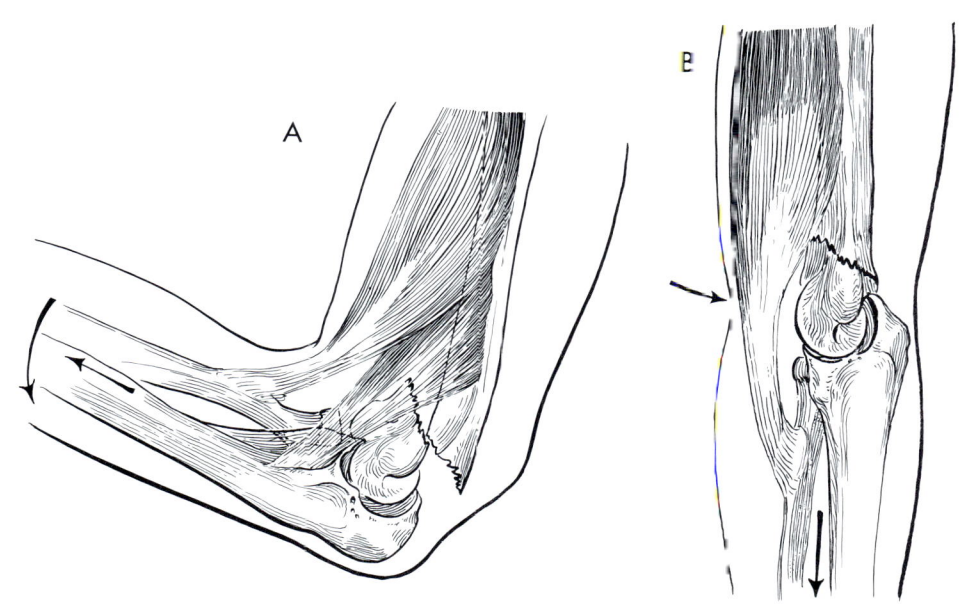

Fig. 19-16. — The rare flexion type of supracondylar fracture. **A**, before reduction. **B**, after reduction.

chance, this should fail, then a reduction with x-ray control will best determine what position is optimum for immobilization. The after-treatment is essentially the same as that for other supracondylar fractures.

Malunited Supracondylar Fracture

If the fracture is more than 3 weeks old and is displaced, there are 2 alternatives in treatment — immediate operative reduction or delayed osteotomy. The deformities most likely to occur are cubitus varus, cubitus valgus and a flexion block deformity. Cubitus varus and cubitus valgus are the result either of incomplete reduction or of epiphyseal growth arrest and, when the deformity is severe, should be corrected by osteotomy. It is well to defer the corrective osteotomy until normal joint motion is regained and until full growth is obtained, unless the degree of deformity is marked.

Corrective osteotomy, when undertaken, should be done with extreme care and precision. In order to obtain the desired results, a paper tracing of the x-ray film should be made and cut to exact measurements so that the surgeon, noting the proper correction necessary, will know the exact size of the wedge of bone to be removed from the humerus to produce a normal carrying angle. Following removal of the wedge of bone, the 2 bone fragments should be brought into apposition and held in their corrected alignment by some form of internal fixation, preferably a small bone plate. In this way the surgeon can be certain of the proper degree of correction, and motion of the elbow can be started at an earlier date. Should the deformity be one of flexion block, the treatment will depend largely on the age of the patient. In young children, this deformity is usually outgrown and operative measures are unnecessary. In adults, however, this is not the case, and operative resection of the projecting mass of the lower end of the humerus is necessary to bring about improved motion.

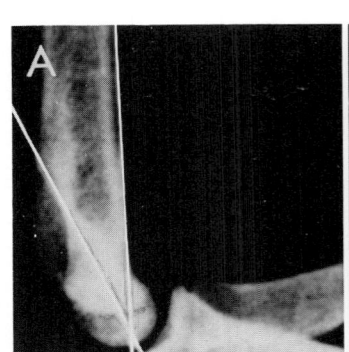

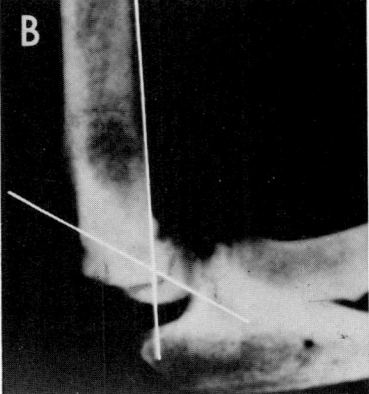

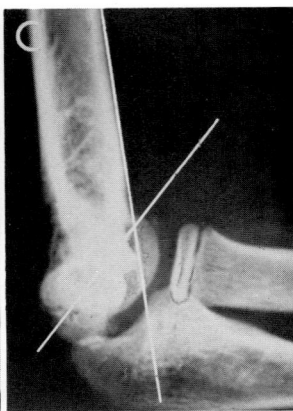

Fig. 19-17.—Greenstick type of intercondylar fracture. **A**, normal elbow. **B**, flexion type. **C**, extension type.

Transcondylar and Dicondylar Fractures

These fractures occur at the level of the epicondyle and extend through the olecranon fossa (Fig. 19-17). They may be of the greenstick type or may show separation, in which case the lower end of the humerus has the appearance of a fishtail. They are intra-articular fractures and therefore should be reduced as accurately as possible to avoid the danger of bony block. In other respects, they are similar to the supracondylar fractures and should be treated in the same way.

Fractures of Capitellum

There are 3 usual types of capitellar fractures: chip fractures, hemicapitellar fractures and capitellar epiphyseal separations with or without rotational displacement.

Chip fractures are frequently associated with a fracture of the radial head and they are usually the result of the radial head striking the capitellum at the moment of injury. They are characteristically moon shaped or elliptic and generally they lie detached as a loose fragment of bone. Since they are detached from the

Fig. 19-18.—Typical hemicapitellar fracture before, **A**, and after, **B**, closed reduction.

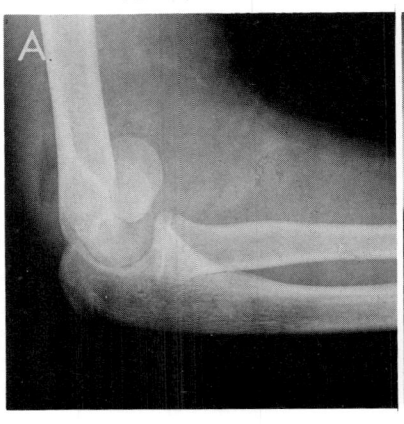

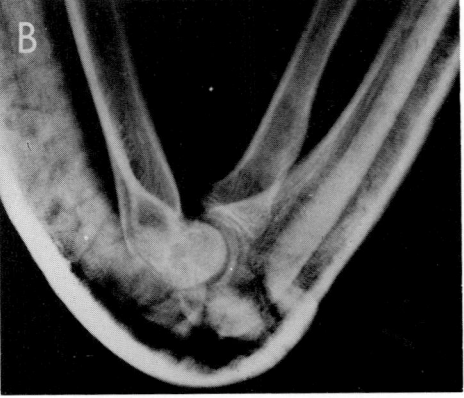

Chapter 19: FRACTURES AND DISLOCATIONS OF THE ELBOW / 485

capitellum and therefore deprived of blood supply, they should be removed through a small incision over the outer side of the joint.

Hemicapitellar fractures involve the anterior half of the capitellum and a considerable portion of the trochlea as well. As a rule, they are much larger than they appear in the x-ray film. The fracture fragment is displaced directly upward on the lower end of the humerus, hugging the shaft so that it may not be visible in the anteroposterior x-ray view and may be overlooked. The lateral view, however, reveals the displaced fragment clearly; it usually shows the fractured base in apposition with the anterior cortex of the humerus and the articular surface facing forward just as if the capitellum had been split in its sagittal plane and the anterior portion had slid upward out of its bed (Figs. 19-18–19-20). Sometimes the displaced fragment becomes rotated so that its articular surface faces the

Fig. 19-19 (left).—Capitellar epiphyseal separation with rotational displacement.
Fig. 19-20 (right).—A, 2 views showing fracture of capitellar epiphysis with rotational displacement in a child, aged 7. B, 2 views taken 4 years after closed reduction. Note the presence of aseptic necrosis. Despite this, function was the same as in the normal opposite elbow.

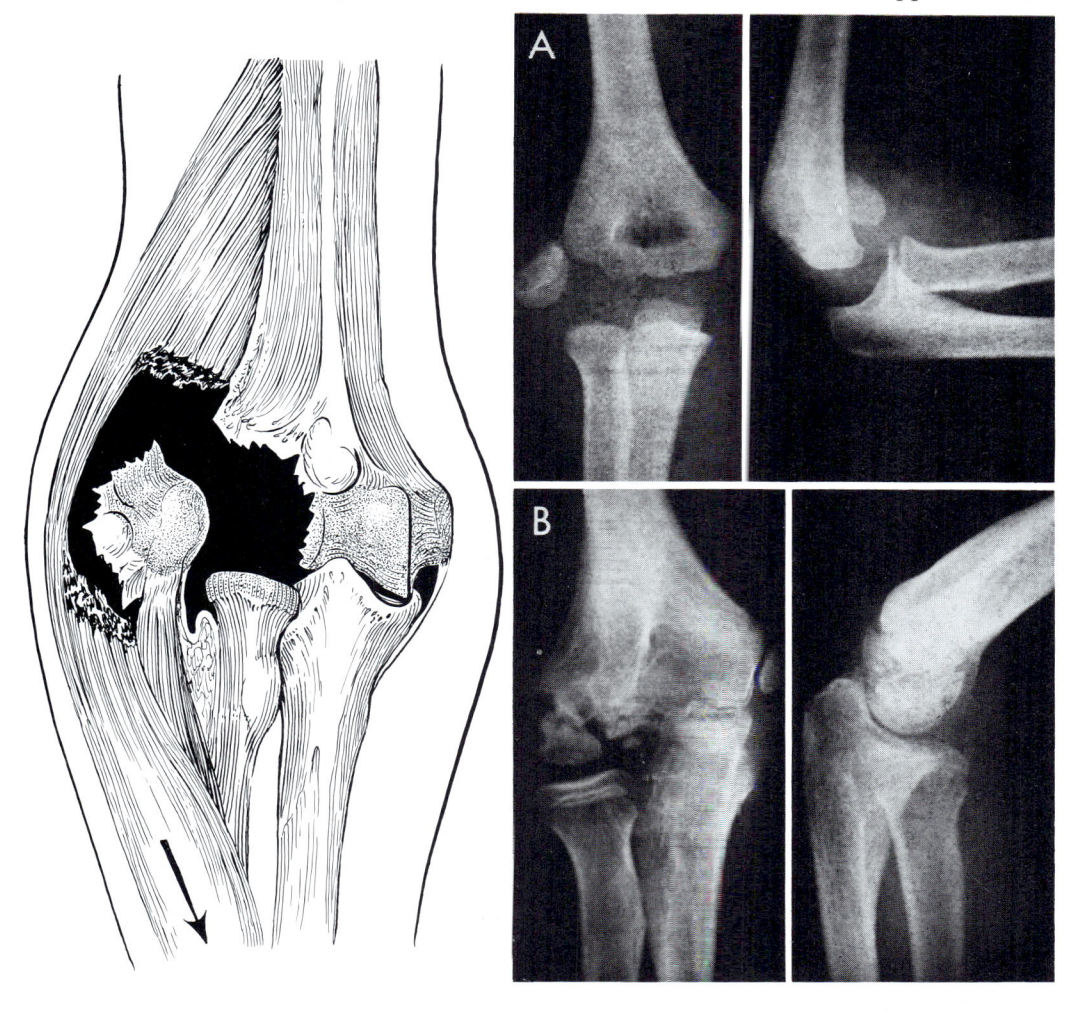

head of the humerus, but this is not the usual finding.

TREATMENT.—The aim of treatment in the hemicapitellar fractures is to slide the detached portion of the capitellum downward into the bed from which it arose and then to hold it there by acute flexion of the elbow. The forearm is extended and adducted at the elbow to widen the space from which the displaced fragment came; then, with steady traction exerted on the extended arm, local digital pressure is applied on the loose fragment, pressing it down into its proper anatomic position. Because of the marked swelling that may be present, reduction may require the aid of fluoroscopy. Otherwise, it is not always possible to apply digital pressure to the exact point desired to effect reduction. Following reduction, the elbow should be held in acute flexion; careful and exact evaluation of the neurovascular supply of the hand should be carried out as previously discussed. Immobilization should be continued for approximately 4 weeks.

Occasionally, the fracture fragment may become slightly rotated. This makes closed reduction more difficult, but it should be attempted before resorting to open reduction.

Should all attempts at manipulation fail, operative reduction is indicated, through an anterolateral approach. When the joint has been opened, the size and character of the broken fragment will determine whether it should be removed or replaced. If the fragment is quite small or is comminuted and has no soft part attachment, it should be removed. If, as is usually true, it consists of 1 piece of bone avulsed from a corresponding other half, it should be carefully and accurately placed and held in position by flexing the elbow. Elbow flexion ordinarily supplies a stable reduction for this type of fracture, although it may be necessary to stabilize the fracture further by the introduction of 1 or 2 fine Kirschner wires.

Some authors feel that capitellar fragment excision is the treatment of choice. This, however, is predicated on the observance of occasional avascular necrosis of the capitellar fragment that has been reduced. Excision, however, leads to the potentiality of valgus deformity, instability and loss of strength of the elbow, particularly if the fragment excised is a large portion of the capitellar surface.

Fractures of External Condyle of Humerus in Adults

This fracture is sometimes associated with a fracture of the capitellum and is of unusual importance because of its possible effect in producing a lateral dislocation of the radius and ulna which may not be recognized (Fig. 19-21). If the fracture is complete and includes the radial ridge of the trochlea, then a closed reduction may be impossible to maintain because of the lack of articular support of the ulna, which depends on this ridge for its stability. Without this support, the ulna slips laterally and is likely to remain in the dislocated position along with the radius unless it is replaced accurately and secured by open reduction.

The importance of this fracture depends on its location with reference to the trochlea. If the fracture line extends into the midportion of the joint and is medial to the radial ridge of the trochlea, the situation is serious; dislocation of the forearm bones on the lower end of the humerus is a probable complication. Should it occur, open reduction will probably be necessary. Reduction should include not only hairline replacement and internal fixation of the bone fragment, but repair of the internal lateral ligament which is usually found to be severed. If, on the other hand, the fracture line does not extend so far into the joint as to include the radial ridge of the trochlea, the broken fragment may be treated by either closed or open reduction without fear of dislocation.

After either closed or open reduction of this fracture, the elbow should be immobilized in flexion and a posterior plaster-of-paris molded splint applied for 2 or 3

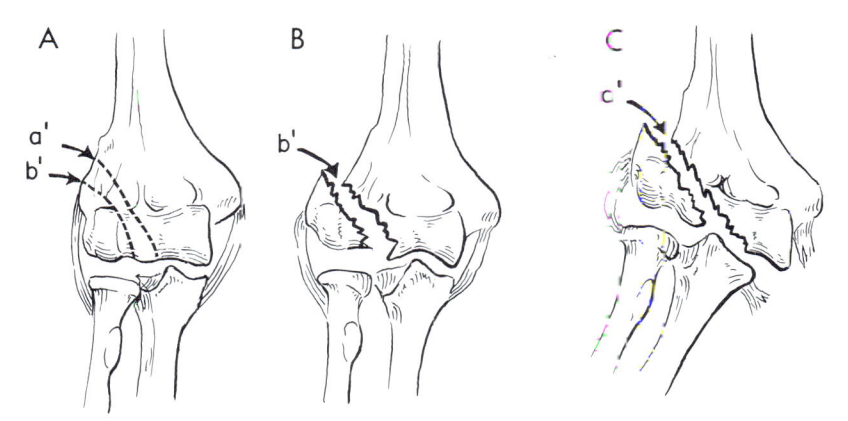

Fig. 19-21.—Two types of fracture of the external condyle of the humerus in adults. **A,** normal bone. **B,** stable type of fracture (represented by *b'*), which does not include the lateral lip of the trochlea and can be safely treated by closed reduction. **C,** unstable type of fracture (shown by *a'*), which includes one-half the trochlea and offers no possible fixed support for the ulna or radius. This type of fracture usually requires open reduction with internal fixation and possibly repair of the ruptured internal lateral ligament.

weeks. The splint should then be retained for night use; during the day a sling will be sufficient. Active exercises should be begun, keeping within the limits of pain.

Intercondylar T and Y fractures of Humerus

These fractures occur most frequently in adults (Fig. 19-22) and are caused by a blow or force striking on the undersurface of the upper ulna, driving the wedge-shaped olecranon between the humeral condyles and separating them. There may also be a transverse fracture of the lower humeral shaft as well as various degrees of comminution of the bone fragments and damage to the articular surface of the joint.

TREATMENT.—Treatment will depend on the character and severity of the fracture. If separation of the broken fragments is only slight and satisfactory alignment is present, a closed reduction

Fig. 19-22.—Anteroposterior and lateral views of a T or Y fracture of the humerus. Attempt at closed reduction was unsuccessful.

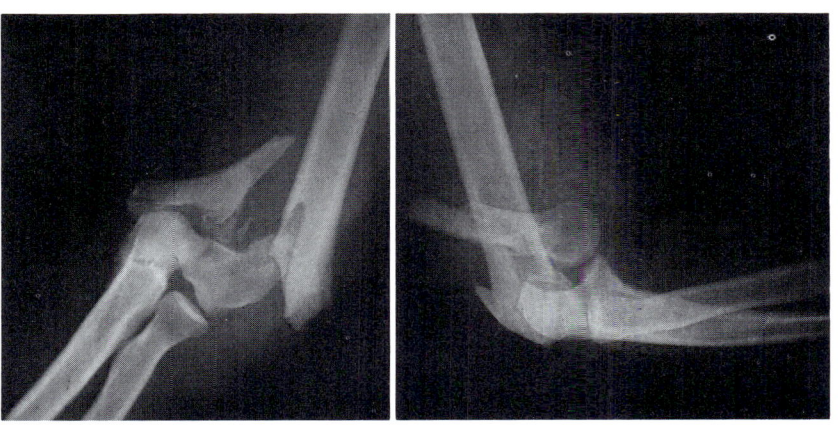

with plaster-of-paris fixation is all that is necessary, the elbow being held in a position of right-angle flexion.

If, however, there is wide separation of the fragments with overriding and disalignment, overhead skeletal traction with a Kirschner wire in the upper end of the ulna is indicated. This method of treatment will restore the proper length to the humerus and correct any malalignment. Further manipulation of the comminuted bone fragments, if thought necessary, can be carried out while traction is being continued. Also, it will permit a certain degree of early active motion.

If, however, the fracture consists of no more than 2, 3 or 4 separate large discrete fragments, which are separated by soft parts, which resist any attempt at closed reduction or which are so displaced as to disrupt the articular surface of the humerus, the treatment recommended is open reduction and internal fixation. (Fig. 19-23). In making this last recommendation,

Fig. 19-23.—**A**, fracture of humerus following open reduction and internal fixation. **B**, 2 views show function 1 year after open reduction of intercondylar T fracture of humerus.

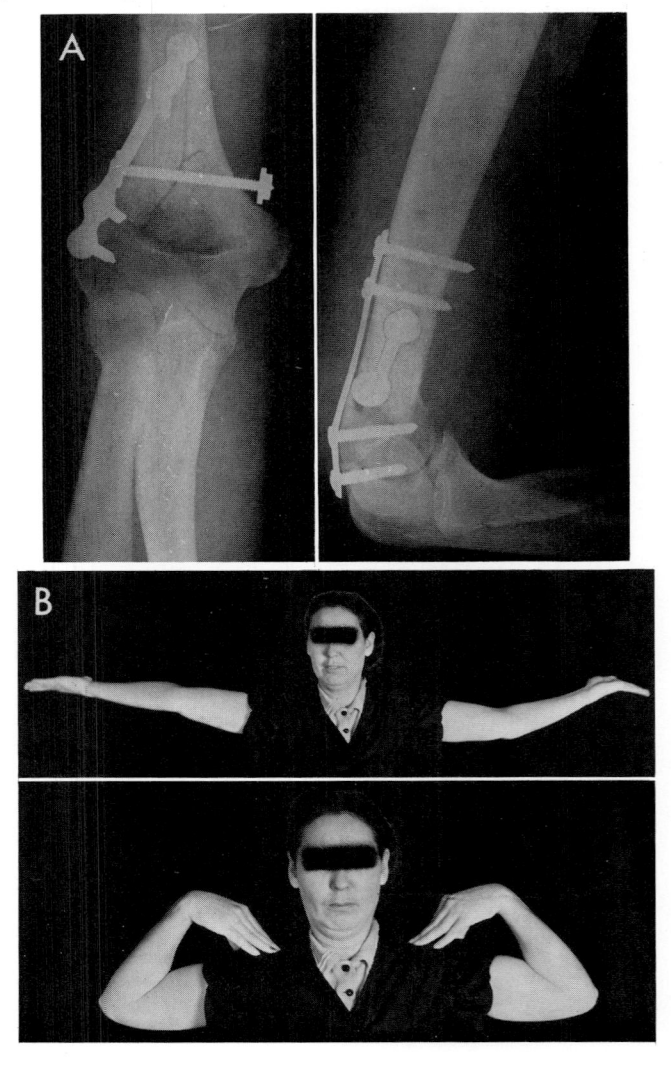

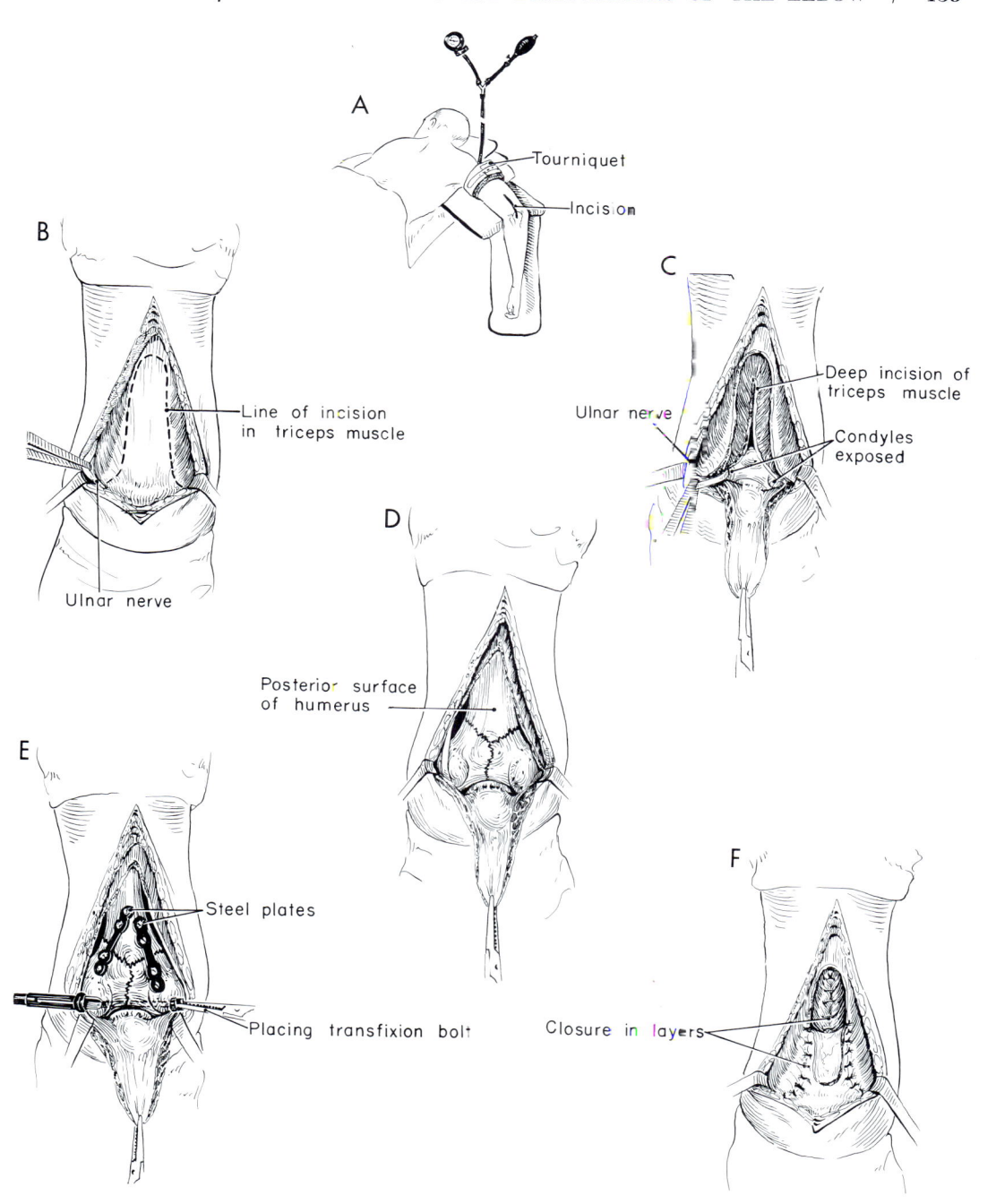

Chapter 19: FRACTURES AND DISLOCATIONS OF THE ELBOW / 489

Fig. 19-24.—Operative technique for reduction of supracondylar T and Y fractures of the humerus. **A,** proper position of the patient (face down) on the operating table for posterior exposure of the elbow. **B,** exposure of the triceps fascia and isolation of the ulnar nerve. **C,** dissection of fascial tongue and further exposure of the ulnar nerve. **D,** retraction of all soft parts and exposure of fracture area. **E,** internal fixation of the fracture with stainless steel plates and transfixion bolt. **F,** closure of fascial tongue before subcutaneous tissues are approximated.

it is assumed the surgeon has had a large and adequate experience in fracture surgery and that the necessary specialized armamentarium for internal fixation is at hand. Also, that the operation has been planned and studied before it is undertaken. The surgeon must analyze the x-rays and establish the feasibility and practicality of achieving rigid internal fixation at the end of the contemplated operative procedure As a rule, this is possible only when the 3 or 4 fragments are of considerable size and there is no comminution of the articular surfaces of the trochlea and capitellum. If one cannot be assured of achieving rigid internal fixation by an operative procedure, skeletal traction is the treatment of choice.

When an operative procedure is indicated, the widest exposure of the fracture area with least involvement of important soft part structures should be obtained. These requirements are most easily satisfied by a posterior surgical approach to the elbow (Fig. 19-24). If, at the time of operation, the bone fragments are accurately reduced and firmly fixed by plates, screws, bolts or wires, the elbow can be mobilized almost at once and convalescence will be greatly shortened.

A posterior plaster-of-paris splint or bivalved plaster casing should be used for immobilization immediately after operation. After a few days to a week, it should be removed during the day to allow active range of motion exercises and reapplied for night protection for a period of 3 weeks. After that time a sling may be used, if necessary, being removed for active exercises and finally discarded completely at 4 to 5 weeks.

Fracture of Olecranon

This injury is usually associated with distraction of the proximal fragments due to the pull on the triceps attachment. It is commonly seen in the adult, being relatively rare in the child. There is little separation at the fracture site, occasionally avulsion of the epiphysis occurs.

In the treatment of simple fractures in the adult, manipulative reduction is first attempted. If accurate apposition of the articular surface is not achieved, internal fixation is advisable. Various types of fixation have been used. A figure-of-eight suture of stainless steel wire has been advocated. A long screw may be used. Internal fixation has not always proved entirely satisfactory in treatment of the simple fracture. A study of patients treated at Massachusetts General Hospital revealed a significant number of complications caused by these operative techniques.

In simple fractures in which the proximal fragment is small, excision of the fragment and suture of the triceps to the proximal ulna is a most satisfactory method of treatment. Indeed, at Massachusetts General Hospital, excision has produced more acceptable results with many fewer complications than internal fixation with screw or wire.

In comminuted fractures proximal to the coronoid process, operative excision of the fragments (Fig. 19-25) is the treatment of choice. Nonmetallic sutures are passed through the distal triceps tendon and then through drill holes in the proximal ulna. A wire suture is likely eventually to fragment around a movable joint, necessitating operative removal of the fragments. When satisfactory repair of the triceps mechanism is accomplished, the integrity of the surgical repair is tested by flexing the elbow to 90 degrees before the incision is closed. Postoperatively, the elbow is immobilized for 3 weeks by a posterior plaster slab, with the joint at approximately 60 degrees of flexion. Active motion is then begun.

Grossly comminuted fractures of the olecranon involving the coronoid process, and complicated at times by an associated fracture of the radial head, require special handling. The stability of the elbow is often lost. Attention is first given to treating the fracture of the radial head. If grossly comminuted, this should be excised promptly. The comminuted ulnar

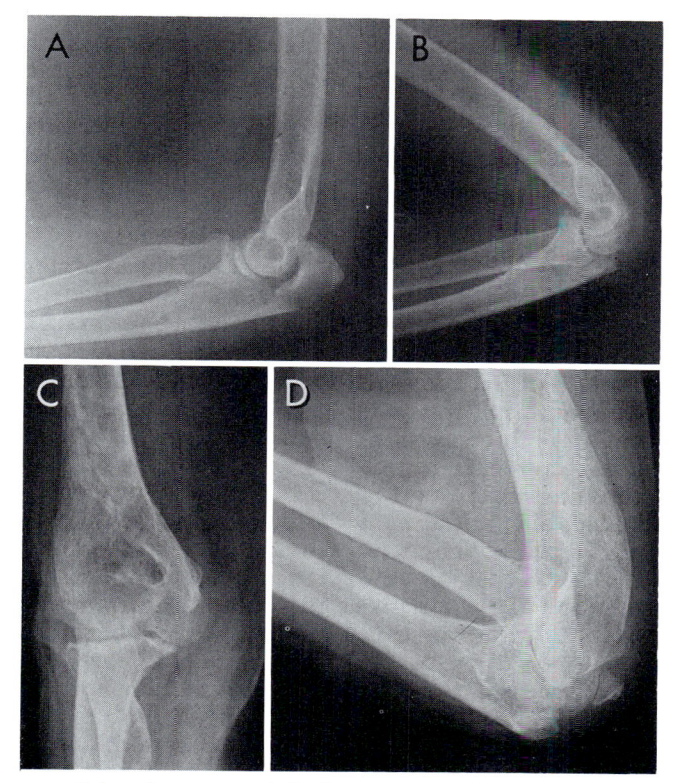

Chapter 19: FRACTURES AND DISLOCATIONS OF THE ELBOW / 491

Fig. 19-25.—Fracture of the olecranon. **A,** before operation. **B,** after excision of proximal fragment. **C,** extension and **D,** flexion 1 year after excision of proximal fragment; excellent function.

fragments are not excised. To decrease the danger of distraction of these fragments due to the pull of the triceps, the elbow is immobilized for 6–8 weeks by a posterior plaster splint, with the joint in approximately 60 degrees of flexion. The posterior splint should allow exercise in range of motion, both supination and pronation. Once the ulnar fracture is healed, active flexion-extension exercises are started. If, after several months, flexion-extension motion is limited significantly, delayed excision of the olecranon and suture of the triceps mechanism may be performed. The advantage of a delayed excision of the olecranon is that stability of the elbow in the first few weeks is preserved in the severely comminuted fracture.

In the child, treatment of olecranon fractures consists of immobilizing the elbow in approximately 30–50 degrees of flexion to relax the pull of the triceps. In the rare case with significant displacement of the fragments, immobilization in the fully extended position is indicated to reduce the fracture. Immobilization is continued for approximately 4 weeks, and then a program of gradual exercises should be started. There is little danger of a stiff elbow occurring in the fully extended position in the child, and recovery of a normal range of motion may be expected within a short period.

In the unusual fracture in a child in which the ulnar fragments are widely displaced, open reduction may be indicated. Care must be taken to avoid damage to the ulnar epiphysis. Usually suture of adjoining soft tissues provides sufficient fixation without resorting to internal devices that might traumatize the epiphysis. If internal fixation is considered necessary, the device should be promptly removed following union to avoid arrest of growth.

Fracture of Head of Radius in Adult

This fracture, which is of fairly common occurrence, is due to a fall on the outstretched hand or to a direct blow on the lateral side of the joint. Diagnosis is made without difficulty from precise clinical evaluation. There is a varying degree of hemarthrosis and distention of the joint. Palpation elicits point tenderness over the radial head, more pronounced on attempts at rotation of the forearm. Limitation of the flexion-extension depends on the degree of hemarthrosis. Multiple x-ray views should be taken; otherwise, transverse fissures of the radial neck may not be discerned. Minor fractures may be overlooked, and the injury incorrectly diagnosed as a sprain.

The treatment depends largely on the type of fracture, i.e., whether or not there is comminution of the articular surface. In general, if there is minimal disruption of the articular surface, conservative treatment gives most satisfactory results. When gross comminution disrupts the articular surface or when the bone fragment is depressed and tilted, total excision of the radial head should be performed (Fig. 19-26).

Conservative treatment includes, first, aspiration of the hemarthrosis at the elbow to relieve pain and allow better evaluation of the active range of motion. The bony landmarks of the elbow, tip of the olecranon, medial epicondyle and radial head may be palpated, regardless of the degree of swelling. They form an approximate equilateral triangle, the center of which designates the level of the joint. Aspiration at this point often produces as much as 20 ml of hemorrhagic joint fluid; the patient can immediately, then, demonstrate a much better range of motion. If motion seems satisfactory the joint is immobilized for approximately 2 weeks by a simple plaster slab that allows supination and pronation. Rotation should be started as soon as pain permits. Following removal of immobilization, active exercises, particularly in extension and

Fig. 19-26.—Comminuted fracture of head of radius before (**A**) and after (**B**) excision. Perfect function 1 year later.

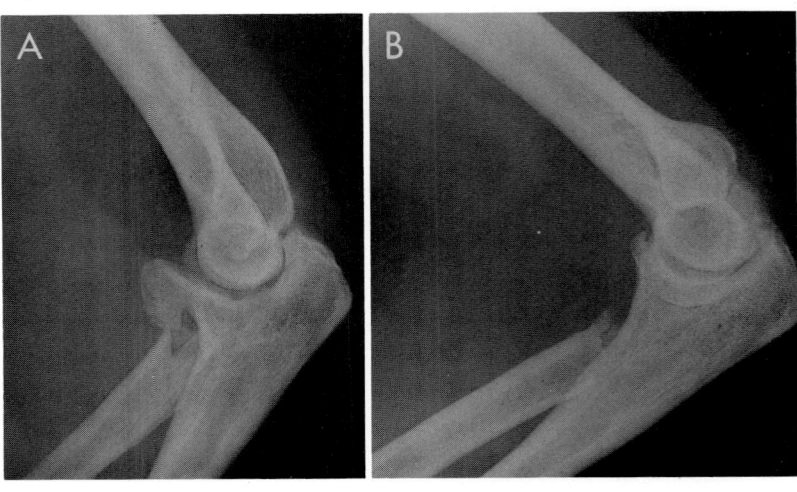

supination, should be carried out to regain full motion.

Excision of the radial head, when indicated, should be carried out promptly, if possible within 24 hours of injury. Delayed excisions of the radial head are followed by less than satisfactory functional results.

The operative approach is through a short oblique incision running from the lateral epicondyle to approximately 1/2 in. below the radial head. Care must be taken to avoid the radial nerve as it winds around the radial head in the belly of the supinator muscle. Once the radial head is removed, the fragments must be carefully matched to make certain that none are left behind. Small fragments may easily become loose bodies in the depth of the elbow. An x-ray check should be made at the time of operation. Postoperatively, the elbow is immobilized by a posterior plaster slab, which permits early active supination and pronation. It is usually possible to discontinue rigid immobilization after the tenth postoperative day. Exercise programs emphasize restoration of full extension and supination.

EPIPHYSEAL INJURIES

Epiphyseal Separation of Radial Head in Children

The injury is usually the result of a fall on the outstretched hand (Fig. 19-27). The displaced epiphyseal fragment often includes a fragment of the adjacent diaphysis.

Reduction may usually be obtained by closed manipulation. The elbow is gently extended, the forearm is brought into the varus position and direct pressure is applied with the surgeon's thumb over the displaced epiphysis. Following reduction, plaster immobilization with the elbow flexed in midposition is continued for approximately 3 weeks. Gentle active exercise is necessary for an extended period before a satisfactory range of motion is regained.

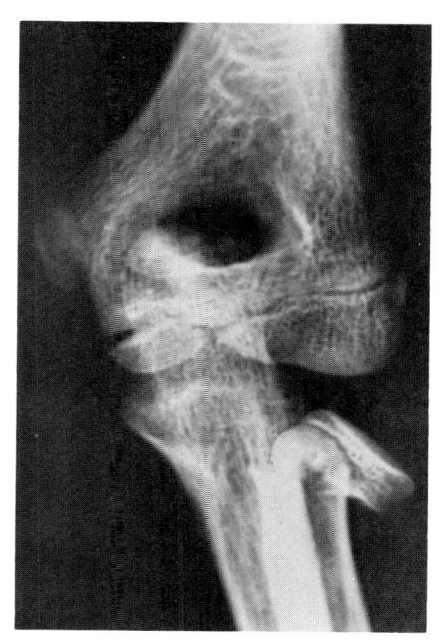

Fig. 19-27.—Slipped upper radial epiphysis with characteristic deformity.

If normal alignment of the fragment cannot be restored by closed manipulation, operative reduction with gentle manipulation of the fragment into position is indicated. Internal fixation is not necessary and should be avoided.

It is to be noted that under no circumstances should the proximal radial epiphysis be removed in treating the initial injury. Excision of the fragment results in a loss of radial growth and a subsequent deformity of the hand and forearm due to the continued growth of the ulna (Madelung's deformity).

In an epiphyseal displacement of more than 3 weeks' duration when first seen, no attempt should be made at reduction. The subsequent growth of the radial epiphysis may correct the relationship at the elbow to a surprisingly significant degree. If there is marked functional impairment, excision of the radial head

Avulsion of Medial Epicondyle Epiphysis

Avulsions of the internal epiphysis of the elbow are common in adolescents, occurring as the result of a valgus strain of the joint. The epiphysis may be merely separated without displacement or it may be displaced distally to a varying degree, even to the joint level. In severe injuries, it may be included in the joint (see lateral dislocation with avulsion of internal epicondyle, p. 475).

Conservative treatment is satisfactory in the majority of cases. When the displacement is slight, the joint is immobilized by a plaster cast, with the elbow in midposition. After 10 days, active exercises are begun. In pronounced displacement, and particularly when the fragment is at or in the joint, the epiphysis should be replaced by manipulative or operative reduction. Because of the disfigurement caused by the operative scar, the patient may prefer to accept distal displacement of the epiphysis. Functional impairment is usually negligible and only occasionally is there a slight limitation of extension. In old injuries the displaced fragment may be excised.

Displacement of External Condylar Epiphysis

The displaced fragment consists of the entire external condyle of the humerus, including the epiphysis of the capitellum and the metaphysis above and a portion of the trochlea (Fig. 19-19). The fragment may be displaced laterally with the fractured surfaces little disrupted, or it may be rotated from the pull of the common extensor muscles and rotated 90 degrees in 2 planes (Fig. 19-20).

Slight displacements require little in the way of treatment, and bony union takes place when the fragment is simply

Fig. 19-28 (left).—Cubitus valgus deformity of right elbow (2 years' duration) following nonunion of capitellar epiphyseal displacement.
Fig. 19-29 (right).—**A,** nonunion of old capitellar epiphyseal separation before operation. **B,** correction of deformity by iliac bone graft and screw fixation (7 years postoperative). Function excellent.

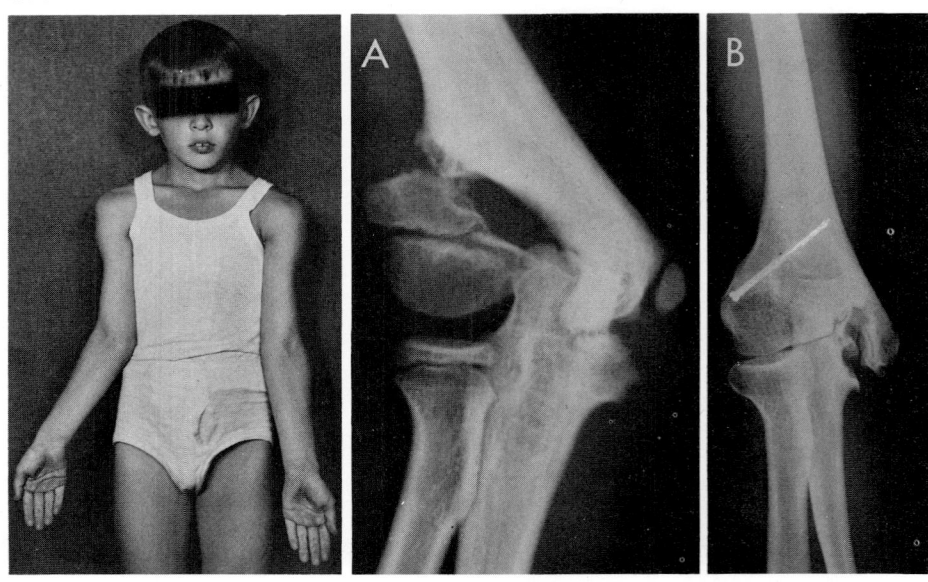

pressed into position. Rotated fragments must be restored to normal position; otherwise, valgus deformity and delayed ulnar nerve palsy may develop. If treated promptly, it may be possible to manipulate the fragment into position. If x-rays show that reduction is not accurate, open reduction should be performed without delay by internal fixation with screw or Kirschner wires. (Figs. 19-28 and 19-29.)

BIBLIOGRAPHY

1. Böhler, L.: *Textbook on the Treatment of Fractures* (4th ed.; Baltimore: William Wood & Company, 1935), p. 208.
2. Boyd, H. B.: Monteggia fracture: Operative technique, Surg. Gynecol. Obstet. 71:86, 1940.
3. Dunlop, J.: Transcondylar fractures of the humerus in childhood, J. Bone Joint Surg. 21:59, 1939.
4. Evans, E. M.: Pronation injuries of the forearm with special reference to the anterior Monteggia fracture, J. Bone Joint Surg. 31:578, 1949.
5. Key, J. A., and Conwell, H. E.: Flexion Type of Supracondylar Fracture, in *Fractures, Dislocations and Sprains* (5th ed.; St. Louis: C. V. Mosby Company, 1951), p. 572.
6. McKeever, F. M., and Buck, R. M.: Fracture of the olecranon process of the ulna, JAMA 135:1, 1947.
7. Rombold, C.: A new operative treatment for fractures of the olecranon, J. Bone Joint Surg. 16:947, 1934.
8. Smith, F. M.: Displacement of medial epicondyle of humerus into the elbow joint, Ann. Surg. 124:410, 1946.
9. Van Gorder, G. W.: Surgical approach in old posterior dislocation of the elbow, J. Bone Joint Surg. 14:127, 1932.
10. Van Gorder, G. W.: Surgical approach in supracondylar T fractures of the humerus, requiring open reduction, J. Bone Joint Surg. 22:278, 1940.
11. Watson-Jones, R.: Excision of Olecranon Fragment and Triceps Repair, in *Textbook in Fractures and Other Bone and Joint Injuries* (2d ed.; Baltimore: Williams & Wilkins Company, 1941), p. 346.
12. Watson-Jones, R.: Flexion Type of Supracondylar Fracture, in *Textbook on Fractures and Other Bone and Joint Injuries* (2d ed.; Baltimore: Williams & Wilkins Company, 1941), p. 353.

20 | Fractures of the Forearm
WILLIAM N. JONES and JOSEPH S. BARR, JR.

ANATOMY

IN FRACTURES OF THE RADIUS AND ULNA the preservation of forearm rotation requires exactness in treatment. Both bones are curved in 2 planes. In the position of full supination the radius has a faint lateral bow, the ulna has a slight medial bow, and both are somewhat concave volarward (Figs. 20-1 and 20-2). In his study of cadaver radii, Sage[11] found the average radial bow to be 9.3 degrees and the dorsal bow to be 6.4 degrees. When the posterior bow of the radius or of both bones is increased, supination is limited by impingement of the radius against the ulna. When anterior bow of the radius or of both bones exists, pronation is restricted.

Except for the pronator quadratus muscle, which causes appositional deformity, all the forearm muscles pull in a direction which produces shortening or bowing of the radius and ulna. Rotational deformity of both bones, or of the radius when the ulna is intact, may also exist; in fractures of the radius above the insertion of the pronator teres, the supinator will tend to pull the proximal radial fragment into supination while the pronator will pull the distal radius into pronation. This counterrotatory effect is somewhat suppressed by the interosseous membrane and by the extended insertion of the supinator muscle if the radial fracture is within the area of the supinator insertion (Fig. 20-3).

In a bone as curved as the radius is, malrotation alone cannot exist. In common, fresh forearm fractures with disrup-

Fig. 20-1.—Bony anatomy of the forearm. The radius and ulna curve away from each other. Fractures through the area where the fibers of the interosseous membrane are dense are more likely to cause loss of rotation than fractures at the extremities of the shafts.

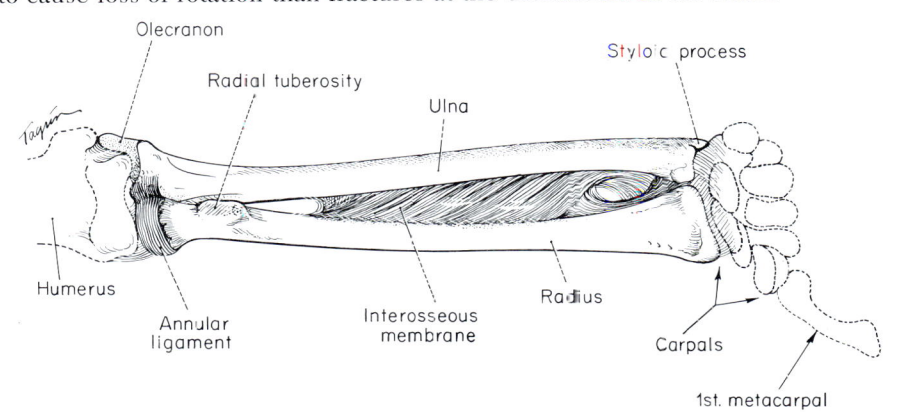

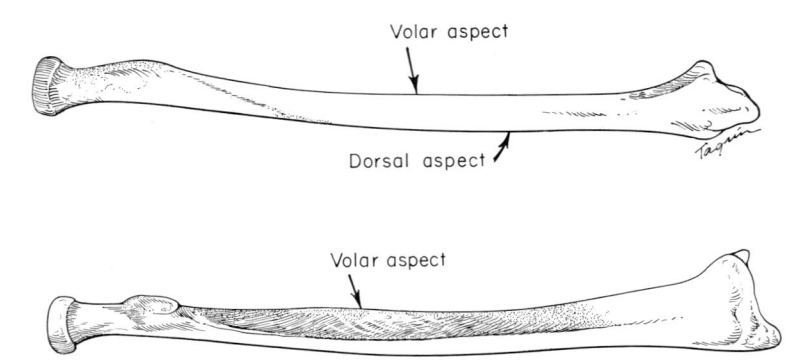

Fig. 20-2.—Curves of the radius. The radius is curved in 2 planes. The medullary canal is wide only in the distal third. In the midportion of the radius much of the breadth is the interosseous crest—thin, dense cortical bone.

Fig. 20-3.—Rotatory pull of forearm muscles. In a fracture of the radius above the insertion of the pronator teres and below the insertion of the supinator (**left**), rotational deformity is a consequence of biceps and supinator pull on the proximal fragment and pronator teres and pronator quadratus unopposed pull on the distal fragment (**right**).

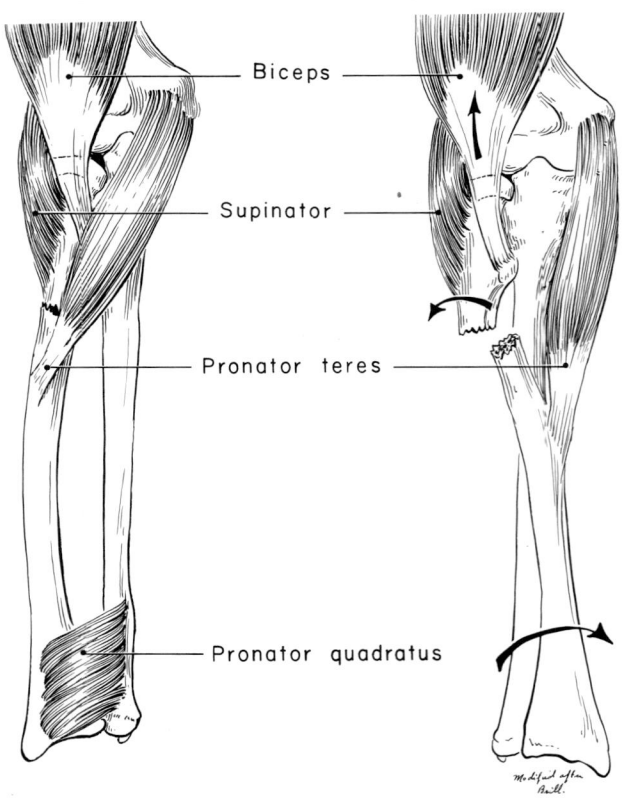

Chapter 20: FRACTURES OF THE FOREARM / 499

tion of bone at a single site or in a limited area but without distortion of the natural curving contours of the fragments, reduction of the fractures to normal linear alignment and normal bow will achieve proper rotatory alignment. If proper rotational alignment has not been achieved, there will be flattening or reversal of the normal curve, or in the distal radius discrepancy in the widths of the fragments may result. In old malunited or callus-surrounded ununited fractures, special care must be taken to insure that a normal rotatory relationship of the proximal to the distal radius is achieved. Evans[3] has described a special method of radiologic examination that is valuable in establishing this relationship: it identifies the rotational position of the proximal radius by reference to the bicipital tuberosity, which in full pronation faces directly radialward, in full supination ulnarward, and in neutral rotation about in midposition.

The interosseous membrane which joins the distal three-fourths of the radius to the distal two-thirds of the ulna can become tightened by scarring around the fractures in these areas. When infection or poor reduction has delayed healing of forearm fractures, the scarring will restrict the recovery of rotation even though a late open operation may achieve union in excellent position. Scarring or excessive callus on the ulnar side of the interosseous membrane will restrict motion more.[10]

Injuries to the distal radioulnar joint may be a cause of pain and disability in some forearm fractures as well as in wrist fractures (see Chapter 21).

INCIDENCE: AGE AND SEX DISTRIBUTION

Fractures of forearm bones have comprised about 5% of all fractures treated at Massachusetts General Hospital. Of these, only 15% occurred in adults, with more fractures in men than in women. In children the fractures were divided equally between the sexes.

MECHANISM OF INJURY

Most forearm fractures result from falls on an outstretched arm. When direct blows break forearm bones, the fracture is often comminuted, as in high-speed automobile and motorcycle accidents.

X-RAY EXAMINATION

Proper x-ray examination of a fractured forearm requires anteroposterior and lat-

Fig. 20-4.—Positioning of forearm for **A**, lateral, **B**, oblique and **C**, anteroposterior projections during radiography. The forearm maintains a constant relation with the arm and is not rotated during changes of position.

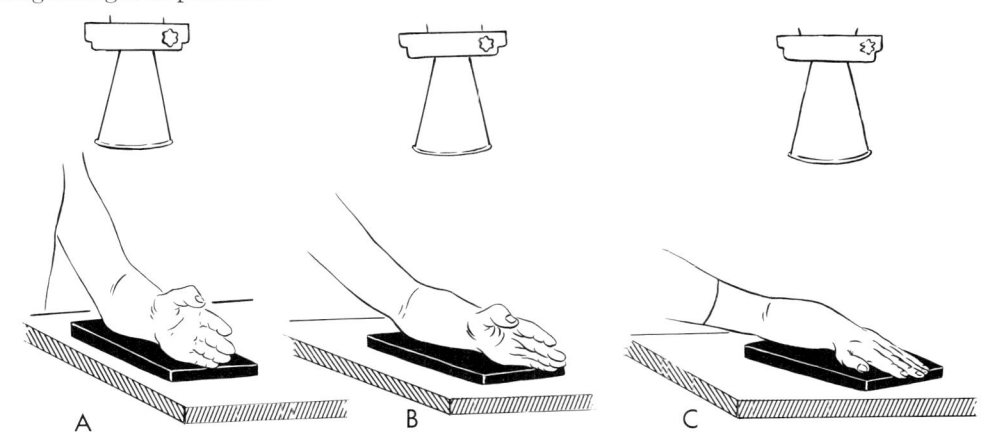

eral views, including the elbow and the wrist. Oblique views are often helpful, and views of the opposite forearm are valuable at times, particularly in children. Films taken before and after rotation of the forearm on the elbow through a 90-degree arc will give 2 projections of the radius but will yield duplicates of a single view of the ulna. Such an examination is not adequate. A true 90-degree change of position of the whole upper extremity is necessary (Fig. 20-4).

TREATMENT

Anesthesia

The complete muscle relaxation necessary for manipulation and reduction of most forearm fractures requires either general anesthesia or brachial plexus block.

Closed Reduction by Manipulation

In closed forearm fractures in children, except in most unusual circumstances, only closed reduction by manipulation, or traction as used by Blount,[2] should be considered proper treatment. The consequences of infection after open treatment can be truly catastrophic when incompletely developed bones are affected.

In adults, fractures in the distal thirds of both bones, isolated ulnar fractures and some radial fractures may be treated by closed manipulation often enough to make this method fairly regularly worthwhile. Oblique fractures of the distal radius with an intact ulna (Galeazzi's fracture) seldom can be treated closed, and repeated attempts to do so are not justified. Displaced fractures in the midportion of both bones rarely can be treated successfully by closed reduction. What may appear to be an acceptable position of fragments immediately after manipulation and cast application often deteriorates within a few days.

Manipulation is best done after sustained traction against countertraction. Traction can be obtained by the pull of assistants or by mechanical devices. With the patient supine, the hand can be suspended by various devices to secure the 3 middle fingers, such as clove hitches, wire finger traps or a pencil in the fingers kept flexed by adhesive tape; countertraction is applied by hanging a weight from a broad band placed across the arm above the flexed elbow (Fig. 20-5). Ordinarily a traction force of 10 lb exerted for 10 minutes fatigues muscles sufficiently to allow relaxation. Manipulation is done at the fracture site by the surgeon's fingers. After traction has been applied, angulating or increasing the deformity of the fracture may allow reduction of 1 bone, which may then be used as a fulcrum for reduction of the other.

The site of the fracture may have indi-

Fig. 20-5.—Traction for reduction of forearm fractures. The finger traps are attached to a fixed point, such as the ceiling or an IV pole, and the traction is varied by changing the amount of weight on the upper arm sling.

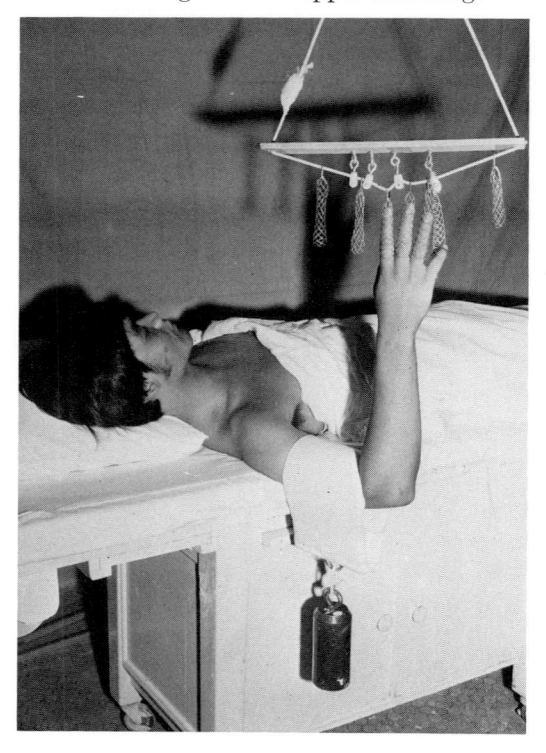

cated the expected position of rotation of the proximal radial fragment and the rotation of the hand and wrist been adapted to it, but portable x-ray studies are required to determine alignment as well as rotation of the fragments. In some fractures, such as a comminuted gunshot fracture of the mid- or upper radius, Evans' views will be required to assess suitability of positions of rotation, and for many fractures this is a useful study.

Plaster splints are applied to the hand and forearm over padding. Thick slabs will not mold closely to the forearm; if heavy splints are required, they should be applied in layers, molded carefully as each is laid on.

The strap and weight are removed from the arm. A light casing of plaster can be applied to the axilla, either incorporating the forearm splint entirely or extending only from the upper forearm portion.

Position is lost easily. In more than half of all forearm fractures, after what initially appeared to be stable reduction, some degree of redeformity occurred at various times after reduction, even as late as the fourth week.

Maintenance of reduction is more likely if adjustment of the plaster is done as swelling subsides and muscles atrophy. Snugging of splints by rewrapping bandages or guttering both sides of solid casts will accomplish this.

Patrick[10] points out that atrophy of the brachioradialis as well as the proximal forearm muscle mass is rapid and that a collar and cuff or a sling that supports the distal forearm tends to cause the casing to drop away from the elbow and lead to redeformity. The cast should be suspended from a ring attached just below the elbow (Fig. 20-6).

In adults, reduction is acceptable only if there is no overriding and if the natural contour of the bones is restored and maintained. Moderate displacement of 1 fragment on the other in the lateral or anteroposterior planes will not jeopardize functional recovery. Angulation of more than a few degrees may be expect-

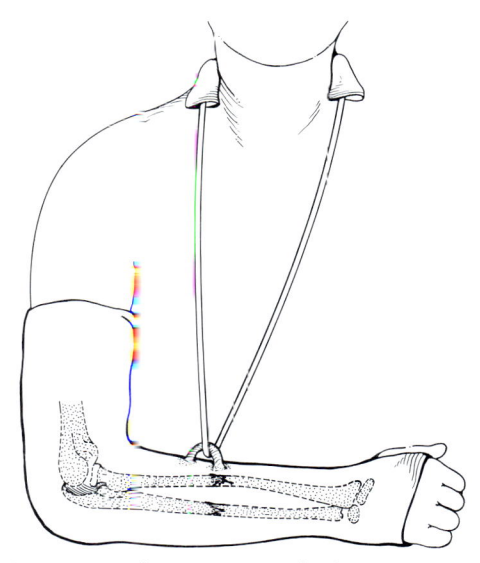

Fig. 20-6.—The cast extends from the metacarpal necks to the axilla. The cast is suspended from a ring placed just below the elbow.

ed to increase in the early postreduction period when it affects the upper and middle thirds of the bones, and such angulation will interfere with rotation. Recheck x-ray studies should be done; if important position loss has occurred in children, remanipulation is indicated; in adults, open fixation is usually indicated.

Immobilizing all fractures of both bones after closed reduction in a position of supination has been recommended,[7, 10] since supiration loss generally is greater than pronation loss. In fractures that by their nature would be expected to entail substantial or severe loss of rotation, a neutral position is preferable.

Although in our experience with only slightly displaced or distal forearm fractures, the period of healing with closed reduction has been less, the usual time required for healing in adults has been found to be 4½–5 months.

Open Reduction

Accurate reduction of forearm fractures in adults is mandatory to restore length, alignment and rotation. When both bones are fractured, operative treatment is necessary in most adult patients. In fractures that are oblique or comminuted, the decision for operative treatment can be made without first attempting closed manipulation.

Operation should be carried out within a few days of the injury, if possible. Occasionally, vascular or nerve injury may demand urgent operation in closed forearm fractures.

OPERATIVE TECHNIQUES.—General anesthesia or supraclavicular (brachial plexus) block is used. A tourniquet is used unless there is arterial injury or severe swelling. Separate incisions should be used for the radius and ulna. The ulna may be approached directly, as it is subcutaneous throughout its length.

The entire radius may be exposed by the anterior approach of Henry.[4] There are several posterolateral techniques for exposure of the proximal radius and, in all, care must be taken to protect the deep branch of the radial nerve lying in the fibers of the supinator muscle. Thompson's[12] approach is useful for the proximal and middle thirds of the radius.

Firm internal fixation is necessary for healing without loss of position. Fixation devices are available in a variety of plates and intramedullary rods. The use of tibial or iliac bone grafts fixed by screws is now generally reserved for complicated cases of nonunion or bone loss. With fractures of both bones, open reduction of one and

Fig. 20-7 (left).—Intramedullary fixation of the ulna led to union, but closed treatment of the radius led to marked angulation, resulting in complete loss of forearm rotation. Open reduction of the radius should have been carried out.

Fig. 20-8 (right).—Use of Sage pins. The curves of the radius are well maintained.

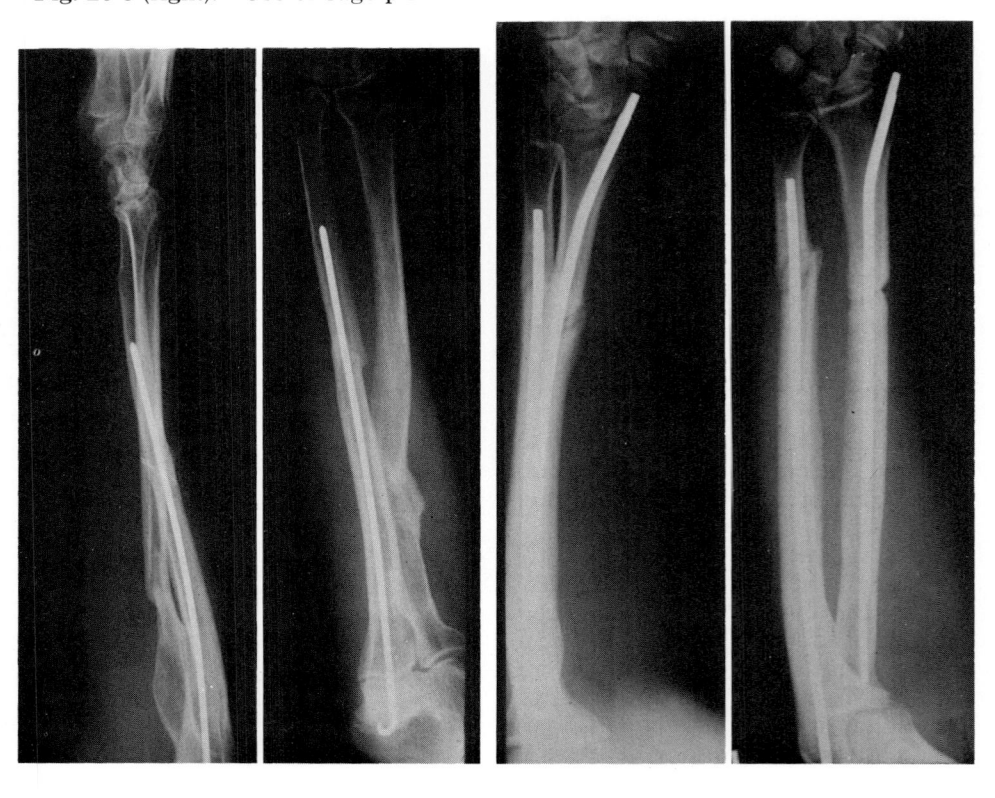

closed treatment of the other is not recommended (Fig. 20-7).

The controversy as to whether plates or rods are superior has not been resolved. Intramedullary rods require less soft tissue exposure for insertion, but they may become jammed in a small medullary canal. A rod in the medullary canal impairs endosteal healing, and if the canal is reamed, endosteal blood supply is severely damaged. Rods do not provide secure fixation in comminuted fractures. "Closed" or blind intramedullary nailing is possible with fluoroscopic control.

Of the types of rods available, the Sage[11] pin is triangular in cross section and is straight for the ulna and shaped to fit the contour of the radial medullary canal (Fig. 20-8). Insertion of the radial pin requires close attention to Sage's techniques. Rush rods do not provide good rotary stability and are not prebent to fit the radius (Fig. 20-9). Diamond-shaped and cloverleaf rods are also available.

In recent years, the concept of rigid fixation through the use of compression plates has gained much popularity. The Association for the Study of Internal Fixation (ASIF) group in Switzerland deserves credit for developing the method and instrumentation. The plates are strong and the screw holes in the cortical bone are threaded by a sharp tap, providing excellent purchase for the screws. A special compression device is used to impact the fracture ends tightly before screws are placed on both sides of the fracture. ASIF equipment also includes semitubular plates that fit well on the forearm bones but are not as strong as regular plates (Fig. 20-10). These plates have oval holes and, by placing the screws against the side of the holes away from the fracture site, the fracture is compressed as the screws are tightened. A somewhat smaller incision and less periosteal stripping are possible when the compression device is not needed. Four-hole plates of the compression type provide excellent fixation, but in comminuted fractures longer plates are pre-

Fig. 20-9.—**A,** closed fractures of radius and ulna. **B,** stabilization by Rush rods. Note the loss of radial bow.

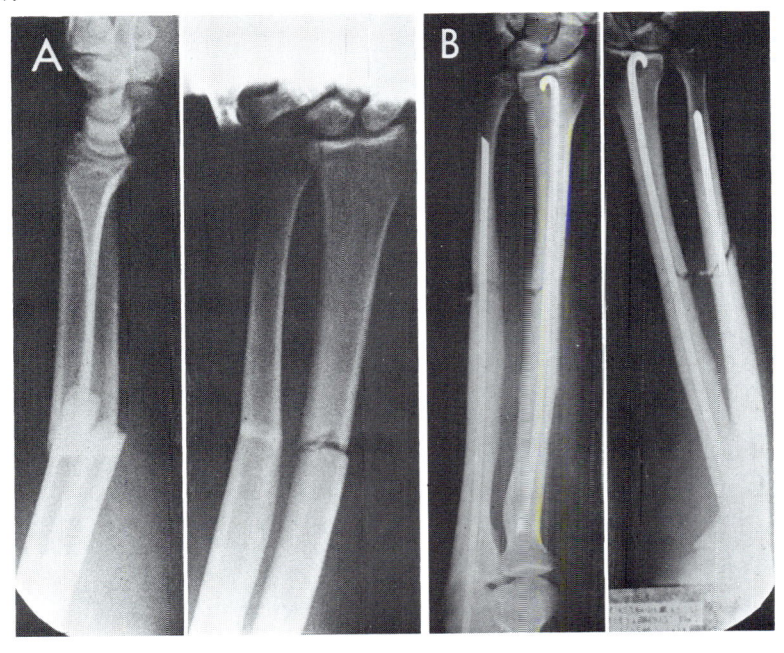

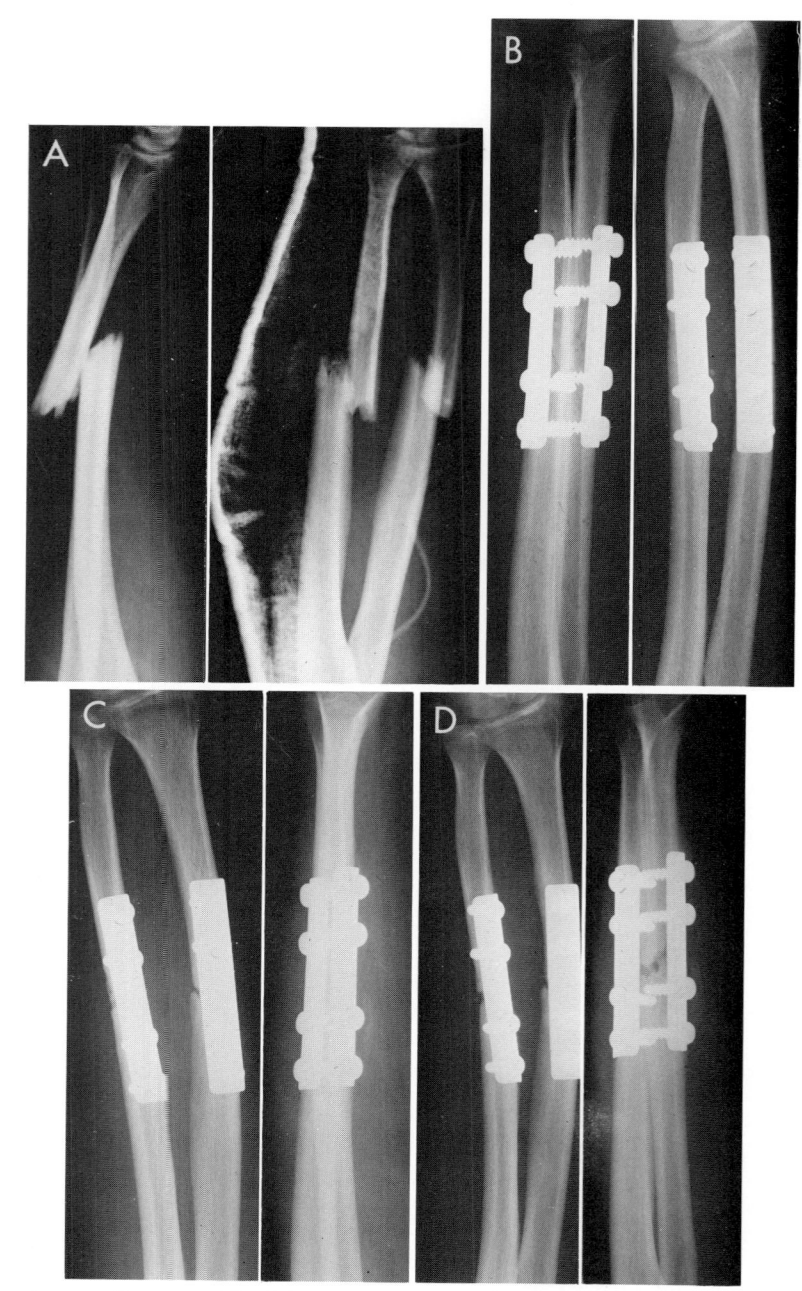

Fig. 20-10.—**A,** open fracture of both bones sustained by man, 21, in motorcycle accident. Initial debridement and wound closure were performed. At 10 days postinjury open reduction was carried out, using 4-hole semitubular plates. **B,** 6 weeks postfracture. Fracture lines are well compressed. Cast protection was discontinued at this time. **C,** at 3 months, there is evidence of resorption at fracture line. Lateral film is inadequate to show the fracture. **D,** at 4½ months, further resorption is evident. Immobilization should have been resumed. (**Continued.**)

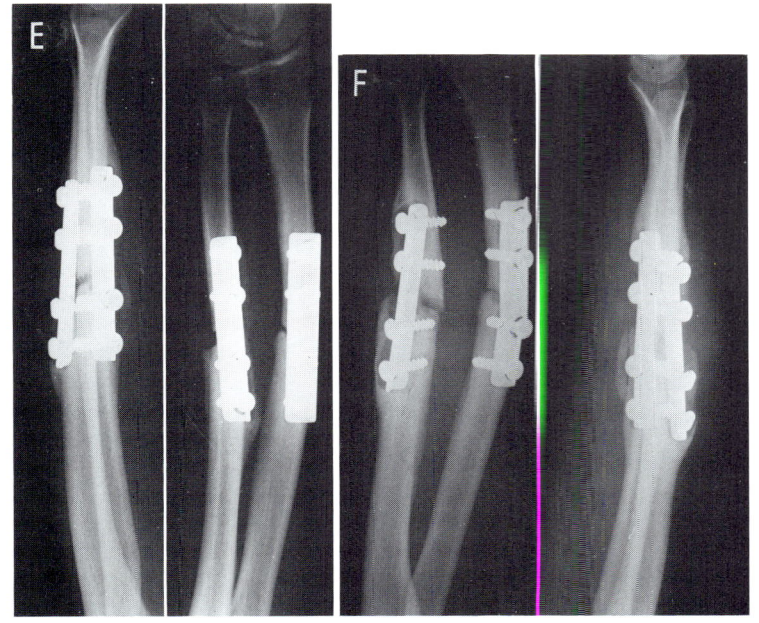

Fig. 20-10 (cont.).—E, at 6 months, periosteal callus and reaction indicate nonrigid fixation. Bone grafting should have been done at this time. F, 1 year; the patient fell and had gross motion at the fracture site. The radial plate is broken at the second screw hole. At a second operation, longer and stronger plates were used with iliac bone graft; union resulted. The short semitubular plates are inadequate for early function in a young, vigorous patient.

ferable. In general, longer (6-hole) plates are superior to the semitubular type and will allow earlier function with less risk of nonunion. When both forearm bones are plated, the plates should be applied to lie opposite, rather than facing, each other. Screw size should be chosen carefully, so that the screw tips do not protrude into muscle and interfere with rotation.

In comminuted fractures the compression technique cannot be used, but the plates still provide excellent fixation and rigidly hold the fracture ends until healing occurs. In cases of bone loss or severe comminution, it is wise to add autogenous iliac bone graft at the time of operative fixation of the fracture.

The operative insertion of plates requires more soft tissue dissection and periosteal stripping than are needed for intramedullary rods. However, in general, plates provide more rigid fixation, and Anderson[1] has advanced experimental evidence that plates do less harm to the blood supply of bone. Plating generally allows the patient to begin early motion of the forearm, particularly rotation. Early restoration of function is obviously important in forearm fractures.

Postoperatively, the arm is immobilized in splints or a cast according to the surgeon's judgment as to the rigidity of the internal fixation. Gentle guided motion, especially rotation, is begun when possible and the healing of the fractures is checked by radiographs at appropriate intervals. In tightly compressed fractures, there is little resorption of cortical bone and sparse callus in many instances. Healing is evaluated by the obliteration of the fracture line. Large amounts of callus or cortical resorption indicate loosening of the metallic device and require prolonged immobilization or secondary surgery with bone grafts and replacement of the rod or plate with more rigid fixation.

Fracture of Radius with Dislocation of Distal Ulna (Galeazzi's Fracture)

The Galeazzi fracture is an oblique fracture of the radius at the junction of the middle and distal thirds, combined with disruption of the distal radioulnar joint. Hughston[5] pointed out the poor results of closed treatment of this fracture. Open reduction with fixation of the radius is mandatory (Fig. 20-11).

OPEN FRACTURES OF FOREARM

These should be treated according to the principles described in Chapter 37. Thorough debridement and irrigation are done meticulously. Bone fragments are sacrificed only if they are severely contaminated and impossible to clean. Wound closure may be primary or delayed. At times, primary full- or split-thickness skin grafting is done.

Immediate fixation by plates or rods may be carried out if contamination of the wound is not severe. Otherwise, the bone ends may be reduced and the fracture held in traction or plaster until the wounds have healed and are clean. Once healing has occurred, metallic devices may be placed, often with supplementary bone grafts.

Kirschner wires placed above and below the fractures may be useful to maintain length and stability while awaiting soft tissue healing.

Nonunion of Forearm Bones

In the period since the first edition of this book, an appreciation of the lessons of the previous decades regarding poor results of closed treatment of forearm fractures in adults and the introduction of superior devices for internal fixation have considerably diminished the incidence of malunion and nonunion.[1, 11] These are encountered still, however, and the same methods now commonly used in primary treatment are equally useful in the treatment of unsatisfactory results.

Before the introduction of the ASIF compression equipment and of intramed-

Fig. 20-11.—**A,** 1 year after a Galeazzi fracture was treated inadequately with a wire loop. Note radial shortening and disruption of the distal radioulnar joint. **B,** restoration of radial length accomplished by onlay iliac graft. Forearm rotation limited to 25 degrees pronation and 15 degrees supination. This fracture should have been treated with a secure plate or rod fixation initially.

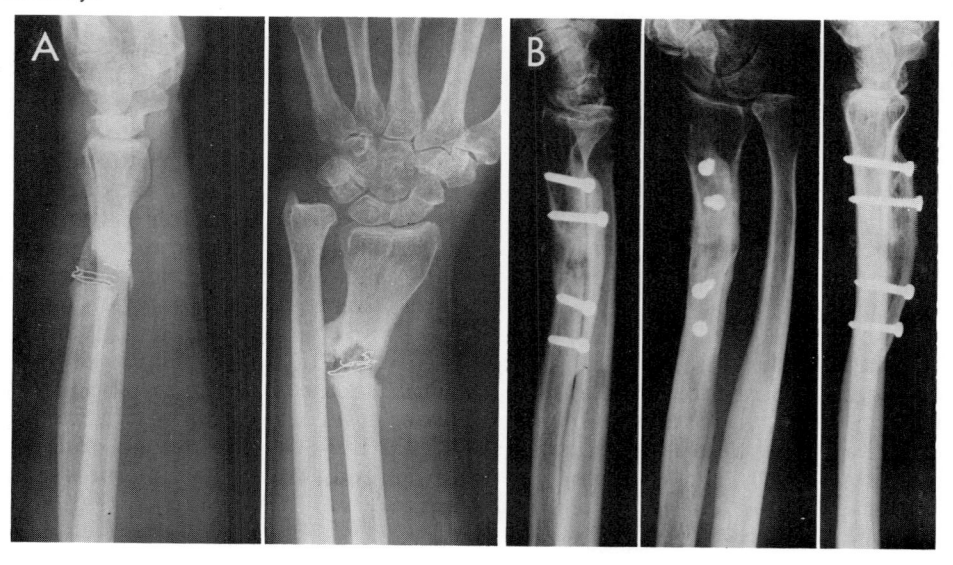

Chapter 20: FRACTURES OF THE FOREARM / 507

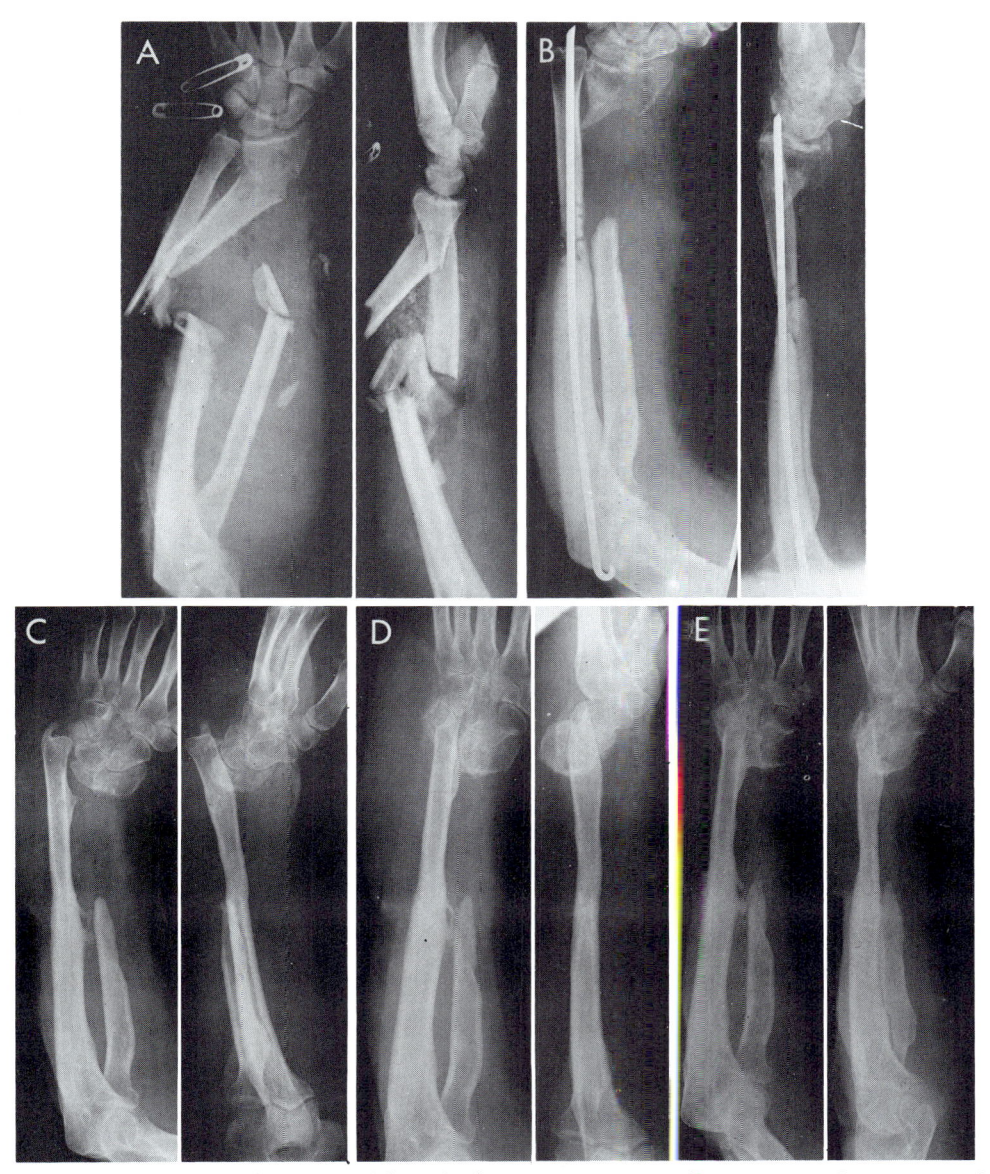

Fig. 20-12.—**A,** original fracture. Although there was massive damage to soft tissues and intense soiling of bone which required resection of large fragments, function and sensation of the hand were preserved well enough to justify its preservation. **B,** instability of bone fragments during use of the hand interfered with healing of wounds. Insertion of a Rush nail in the ulna at 8 weeks stabilized the forearm sufficiently to allow continuing hand exercises, union of the ulna and closing of skin. **C,** the ulna united. **D,** the soft tissue shadow of a full-thickness pedicle graft applied preparatory to radiocarpal grafting can be seen. Hand function is good. An attempt to reconstitute the defect of the radius by the use of a tube of fibula stabilized by a Rush nail did not succeed. This graft was removed, and the distal ulna has been inserted into the carpus with the expectation of fusion. **E,** end-result after failure of the fibular transplant to the radius. The graft was removed through a separate incision from the ulnar side of the wrist. The distal end of the ulna was imbedded in the central portion of the carpus and fusion obtained.

ullary rods—square, triangle or diamond shaped in cross-section contour—onlay or double onlay autogenous grafts fixed with screws alone yielded a high incidence of successful treatment of established nonunion or malunion. The newer types of metal devices, used with autogenous onlay grafts, now succeed as well.

The common causes of nonunion are insufficient time of effective immobilization, insecure internal fixation after open operation and especially a combination of these 2 circumstances. Poor position and soft tissue interposition may be influences in failure of union.

The usual time for healing of radial and ulnar fractures in adults is 15 or more weeks when satisfactory closed reduction can be accomplished. When compression plates provide rigid immobilization, or intramedullary devices suppress endosteal healing, roentgen evidence of union appears much more slowly. Even after 5 months, if there are not signs of pseudarthrosis at the fracture site and position has not deteriorated, it may be assumed that union eventually will become firm; healing usually can be accelerated by the addition of cancellous bone about the fracture.

Treatment of established nonunion is grafting at the fracture site with firm fixation of fragments. Motion at the fracture site and some deformity ordinarily exist. In forearm bones restoration of almost normal contour is required to anticipate good functional recovery. Weak devices usually will not succeed; in most ununited forearm bones the ASIF plates are preferable, even though in some instances, as when there has been bone loss or resorption creating a gap, compression is not used. In some instances, use of an intramedullary rod may have advantages over a plate, as soft tissue dissection may be less; the rod must secure fragments against rotation, or an additional device, such as wire or screws, must be used. External immobilization is necessary until union is firm.

In instances of major loss of bone substance (Fig. 20-12), soft tissue defects and scarring may exist. Before bone grafting is attempted, relaxed soft tissue with good vascular supply should surround the area for bone transplant. A pedicle graft or other plastic procedure may be a necessary step preliminary to bone grafting.

When an intact or stable ulna exists with reasonably good wrist and elbow joint surfaces, efforts should be made to bridge even large defects of the radius.

For large defects, tibia cortex and split fibula as onlay grafts, or whole fibula and full-thickness iliac crest inserted in the defect and skewered by an intramedullary rod, will be required.

Dual tibial onlay grafts have been used successfully for many years; however, removal of even a moderate-sized slab of tibial cortex does weaken the bone enough that fracture may occur, and protection against this may be required for many months. A semitubular iliac crest onlay graft may be used to bridge a gap of 1½ in. or a little more.[9]

Recovery of forearm function after such reconstruction is almost never complete. If it has not been possible to restore normal radial length, mechanical impingement and pain at the wrist joint may hamper rotation; improvement may be gained by limited resection of the distal ulna.

When attempts fail to re-establish a radius, the distal ulna may be fused to the carpus. Although the hand maintains a fixed position, varied only by shoulder and trunk motions, the arm can function satisfactorily in activities of daily living.

Malunion of Forearm Bones

In making a decision as to whether or not operative correction of malunion is indicated, one must consider especially what the functional loss to the patient's total activity is, and what can be expected to result from operation. When solid union in malposition has existed for more than a brief period, contractions of the interosseous membrane and adaptive changes at the elbow and wrist will probably sharply limit recovery of rotation. Motion indeed may be lost after operation, but functional or cosmetic improvement occurs by the derotation-osteotomy effect achieved.

If the deformity affects both radius and ulna, operation carries some risk of synostosis. Considerable deformity often involves apposition of bone, and completely separate incisions to reach the fractures cannot be made. Wide stripping of soft tissue necessary to free and fix fragments favors ossification of soft tissues, even though bone separation is achieved by internal fixation.

Cross Union of Forearm Bones

The treatment of cross union after trauma, fortunately relatively rare, is as difficult as is treatment of congenital synostosis, and the techniques used are similar. These include: resection of the bone bridge with interposition of fascia, tantalum foil or other substances; derotation of both bones; resection of a segment of ulna at the level of the bone bridge, with wrist fusion and distal ulnar resection; resection of the bone bridge and a segment of 1 bone, with suture of flexor to extensor muscles and late graft of the bone defect; and implants of metal mechanical devices.[6] Recovery of rotation in any case is likely to be disappointing.

Fig. 20-13.—Restoration of normal contour in a 14-year-old boy after reduction of midshaft radial and ulnar fractures in which the fragments were displaced but not angulated. **A**, original fracture. **B**, 6 weeks after stable reduction with moderate displacement. In the lateral projection, less than half the fragment ends of the radius are apposed. Linear alignment is good, with no bow. **C**, 1 year after fracture there is expected restoration of normal contour and normal function.

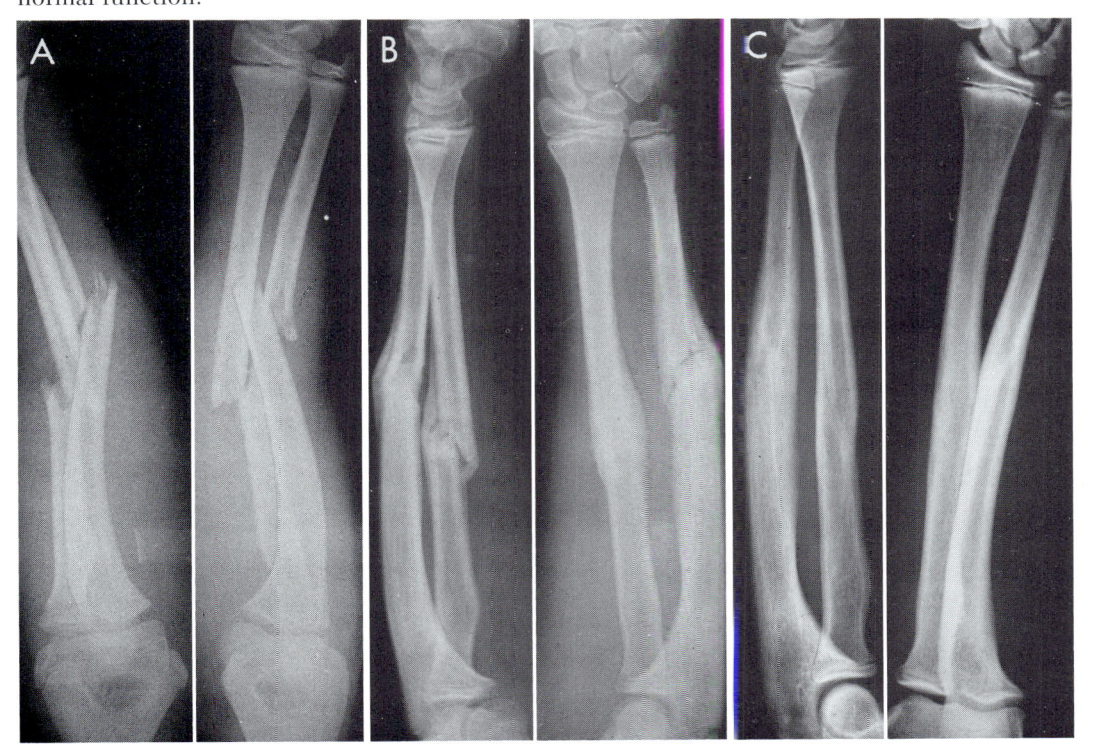

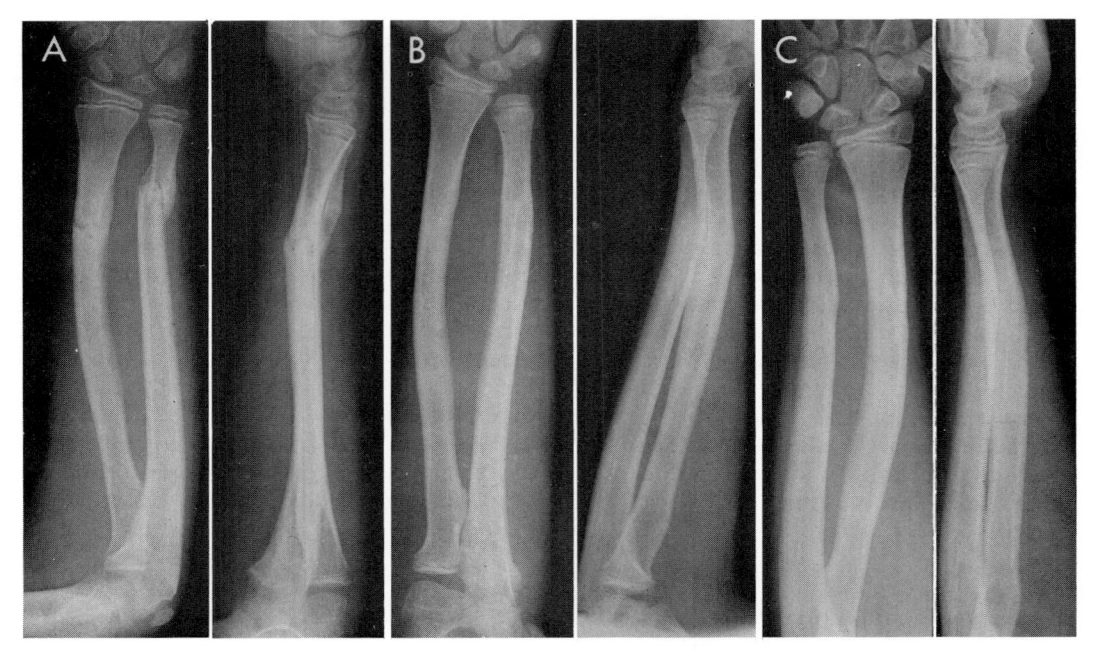

Fig. 20-14.—Persistent anterior bow of forearm bones in an 11-year-old boy after fracture at junction of middle and lower thirds of radius, and of ulna in distal third. **A**, 5 weeks after satisfactory reduction; angulation apparent, but considered likely to be corrected rapidly during growth. **B**, 1 year after fracture; anterior bow persists. **C**, 3 years after fracture; anterior bow limits pronation to 35 degrees.

Forearm Fractures in Children

In most forearm fractures in children under age 12–14, satisfactory reduction can be achieved by traction and manipulation. Residual deformity after reduction may, in some instances, diminish as growth proceeds. Ordinarily, slight overriding will not permanently limit functional recovery (Fig. 20-13). Depending on the level of the fracture, there is a considerable difference in the amount of recovery to be expected from angulation deformity. Bow deformity of 15 degrees or more in the middle and upper thirds of the radius and ulna is likely to persist with some permanent limitation of rotation (Fig. 20-14). In the lower third a bow of even 35 degrees may be reduced during growth to a normal contour with recovery of normal function. This difference is evident through most of childhood, i.e., a midshaft bow in a 6-year-old child may be a permanent deformity, whereas a more severe bow in the distal third affecting an adolescent with only a year or so of growth remaining may in that year be reduced to a normal bone contour. Rotatory deformities do not correct with growth.

GREENSTICK FRACTURE.—Because cortical bone is less brittle in the young, and the periosteum is considerably thicker, greenstick fractures of the forearm shafts are common. Ordinarily these are the result of a twisting injury when the patient falls on the outstretched hand. The distal forearm is fixed with the hand on the surface that the hand strikes, and the proximal forearm either supinates or pronates to a degree sufficient to cause fracture of the forearm bones. With a twisting of the extremity into supination, the forearm is deformed with an anterior bow at the fracture site (Fig. 20-15, A).

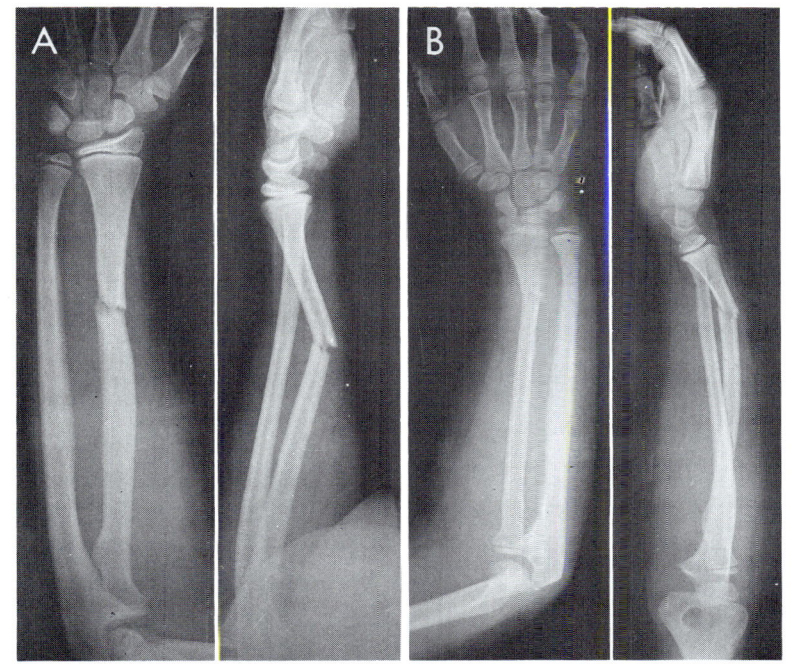

Fig. 20-15. — Supination and pronation fractures. **A,** fracture of the distal radius in 10-year-old child, caused by supination of the extremity on the hand. **B,** greenstick fracture of right arm of a 7-year-old girl in which the extremity was pronated on the hand. The fracture was reduced by supination of the hand.

The reverse deformity is caused by a pronating injury. Occasionally only the radius is fractured (Fig. 20-15, *B*).

In greenstick fractures, simple manipulation by rotation of the distal fragment on the proximal one will achieve reduction of the bow, as well as of the rotatory deformity. If the fracture can be reduced by rotation, it is not necessary to immobilize the forearm in extreme pronation or supination to hold stable reduction. The usual length of time required for plaster fixation is 4–8 weeks, depending on the age of the child.

It is usually necessary to break the periosteum on the concave side in order to obtain complete reduction and stability of a greenstick fracture. Otherwise, a recurrence of deformity is apt to occur.

As swelling about a fracture site subsides and muscles atrophy, the fixing plaster must be adjusted to be sure it fits the size and shape of the arm closely. The more perfect the fracture reduction, the less likelihood there is of displacement. But even with the rapid healing of children, if firm fixation is not maintained, loss in position of forearm fractures can occur as late as the third week after reduction. The position of fragments should be examined by x-ray frequently after reduction; if satisfactory position is lost, remanipulation should be done promptly. Either a circular cast or plaster splints bandaged to the arm may be used for fixation; in both forms, fixation should extend from the necks of the metacarpals to the axilla, usually with the elbow flexed to 90 degrees and the forearm in the position of rotation in which reduction is most stable.

If closed manipulation does not result in satisfactory position, or reduction cannot be maintained, a banjo splint with elastics taped to the fingers for traction, as described by Blount,[2] should be used and open reduction avoided. Such traction is well tolerated in children, and there is no loss of finger function in the relatively few weeks required for the fracture to become stable.

REFRACTURE OF FOREARM BONES. — Refracture of the radius and ulna in children is common, especially when reduction is incomplete. After remanipulation and reduction, plaster fixation must be prolonged for at least 8–10 weeks.

BIBLIOGRAPHY

1. Anderson, E. D.: Compression plate fixation and the effect of different types of internal fixation on fracture healing, J. Bone Joint Surg. 47-A:191, 1965.
2. Blount, W. P.: *Fractures in Children* (Baltimore: Williams & Wilkins Company, 1954).
3. Evans, E. M.: Rotational deformity in the treatment fractures of both bones of the forearm, J. Bone Joint Surg. 27:373, 1945.
4. Henry, A. K.: *Extensile Exposure* (Edinburgh: E. & S. Livingstone, Ltd., 1957).
5. Hughston, J. C.: Fractures of the distal radial shaft, J. Bone Joint Surg. 39-A:249, 1957.
6. Kelekian, H., and Doumanian, A.: Swivel for proximal radioulnar synostosis, J. Bone Joint Surg. 39-A:945, 1957.
7. Knight, R. A., and Purvis, G. D.: Fractures of both bones of the forearm in adults, J. Bone Joint Surg. 31-A:755, 1949.
8. Müller, M. E.: Allgöwer, M. and Willenegger, H.: *Technique of Internal Fixation of Fractures* (Springer-Verlag, New York, Inc., 1965).
9. Nicoll, E. A.: The treatment of gaps in long bones by cancellous insert grafts, J. Bone Joint Surg. 38-B:70, 1956.
10. Patrick, J.: A study of supination and pronation with especial reference to the treatment of forearm fractures, J. Bone Joint Surg. 28:737, 1946.
11. Sage, F. P.: Medullary fixation of fractures of the forearm, J. Bone Joint Surg. 41-A:1489, 1959.
12. Thompson, J. E.: Anatomical methods of approach in operations on the long bones of the extremities, Ann. Surg. 48:309, 1918.

21 | Fractures of the Distal End of the Radius

JOSEPH S. BARR, JR. and EDWIN T. WYMAN, JR.

FRACTURES of the distal end of the radius are common, accounting for 10–20% of all fractures. In 1814, an Irish surgeon, Abraham Colles,[4] wrote about distal radial fractures, and since that time the term "Colles' fracture" has been used commonly. Colles' original description referred to a fracture of the radius 4 cm above the wrist, but this is an uncommon fracture, and Colles' fracture has come to refer to a fracture of the distal radius within 3 cm of the wrist, with dorsal angulation or displacement of the distal fragment. Fracture of the ulnar styloid may or may not be present.

ANATOMY

The distal radius is widened and consists of cancellous bone with a thin covering of cortical bone. The radius articulates with the navicula and lunate to form the radiocarpal joint. The distal ulna does not articulate with the carpus but with the ulnar notch of the radius to form the distal radioulnar joint. These joints have thin capsules reinforced by ligaments (Fig. 21-1). The articular disk is a triangular structure from the ulnar styloid to the ulnar notch on the radius. It strengthens the distal radioulnar joint.

Pronation and supination occur at the distal radioulnar joint. The radiocarpal joint allows wrist flexion, extension and radial and ulnar deviation.

The radial and ulnar styloid processes are useful bony landmarks and from them collateral ligaments extend distally to increase the stability of the wrist. Flexor and extensor tendons, vessels and nerves are closely associated with the distal radius and ulna, but are not often injured in typical wrist fractures.

MECHANISM OF INJURY

These fractures usually are caused by a fall on the outstretched hand. Experimental efforts to reproduce wrist fractures have shown that if the wrist is less than 40 degrees dorsiflexed, a forearm fracture may result; with 40–90 degrees of dorsiflexion, clinical types of distal radial fractures occur, and more than 90 degrees of dorsiflexion can produce fractures of the carpal bones. Forearm rotation and radial or ulnar deviation of the wrist at the time of impact also may influence the resultant fracture.

The "silver-fork" deformity (Fig. 21-2) typically occurs The distal radius and hand are displaced dorsally, obliterating the normal straight-line relationship of the dorsum of the radius and hand. The usual dorsal prominence of the ulna disappears. The radial styloid is shortened in relation to the ulnar styloid and the hand may be deviated radially. Swelling occurs rapidly and ecchymosis appears, particularly on the volar aspect of the wrist.

Motion of the wrist is impaired but fin-

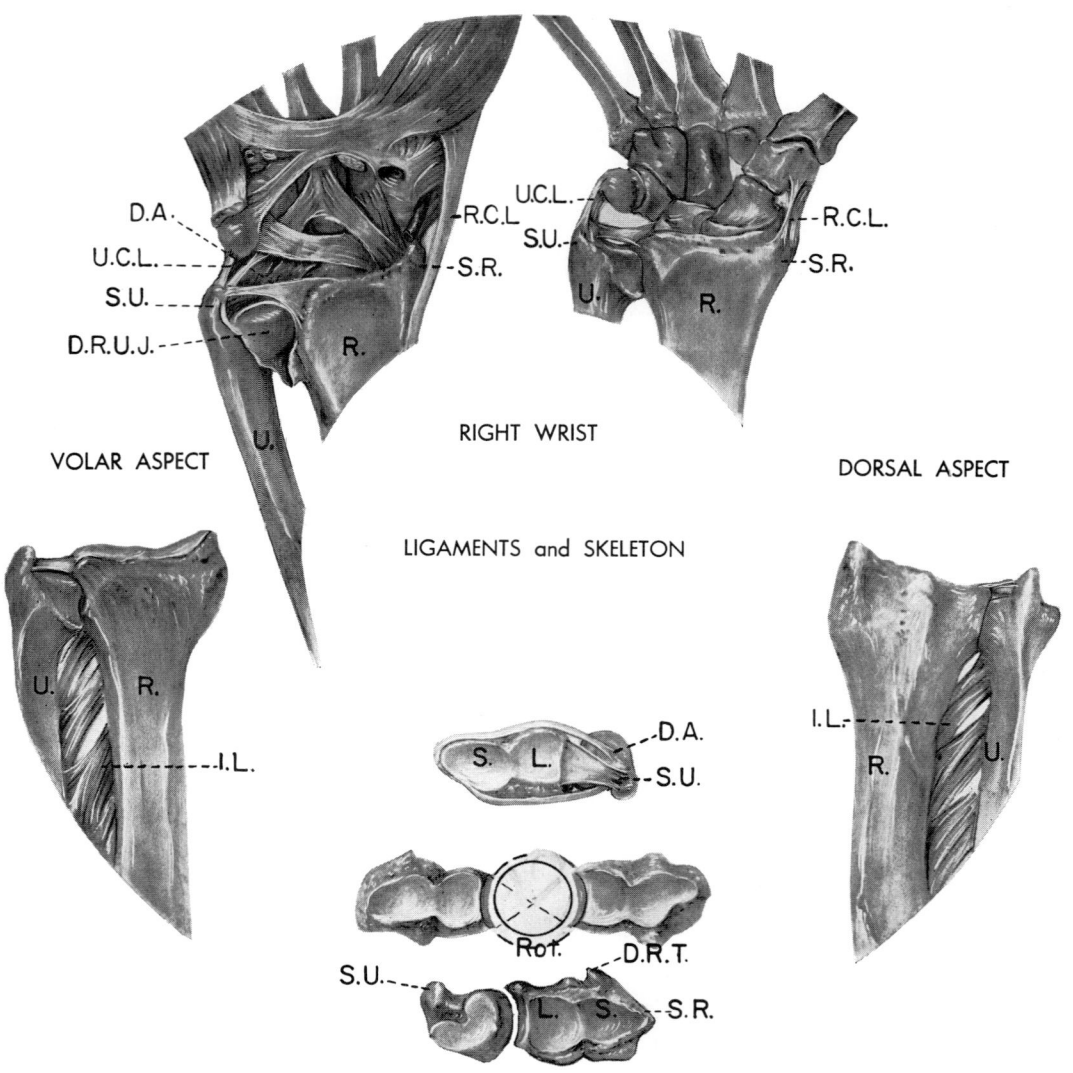

Ligaments—Volar Aspect

U.C.L. — Ulnar collateral ligament
R.C.L. — Radial collateral ligament
I.L. — Interosseous ligament
D.R.U.J. — Distal radioulnar joint
D.A. — Discus articularis

Distal Extension of Radius and Ulna

S. — Articulation of scaphoid
L. — Articulation of lunate
D.A. — Discus articularis
Rot. — Rotation of radius around ulna
S.U. — Styloid process of ulna
S.R. — Styloid process of radius
D.R.T. — Dorsal radial tubercle

Skeleton—Dorsal Aspect

U. — Ulna
R. — Radius
S.U. — Styloid process of ulna
S.R. — Styloid process of radius

Fig. 21-1.—Anatomy of the wrist.

Chapter 21: FRACTURES OF THE DISTAL END OF THE RADIUS / 515

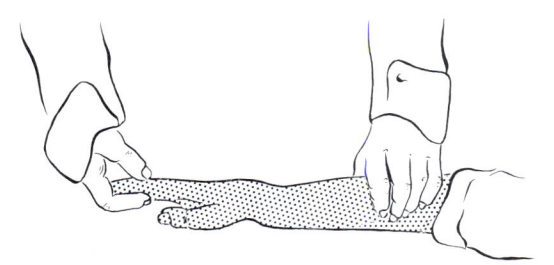

Fig. 21-2. — Diagram of silver-fork deformity.

ger motion usually is possible if the wrist is splinted or stabilized.

Careful sensory examination should be done, particularly in the median nerve distribution. Complaint of numbness occurs often, but rarely is there marked loss of sensation on neurologic testing. Capillary circulation of the nail beds should be evaluated also.

The undisplaced fracture may be difficult to diagnose but, on careful examination, tenderness over the fracture line dorsally can be elicited.

Fig. 21-3. — **A**, comminuted Colles' fracture with fracture of the carpal navicula. **B**, reduction in plaster. **C**, healed fracture of radius and healing fractured navicula with graft in site (graft done because of nonunion of the navicula).

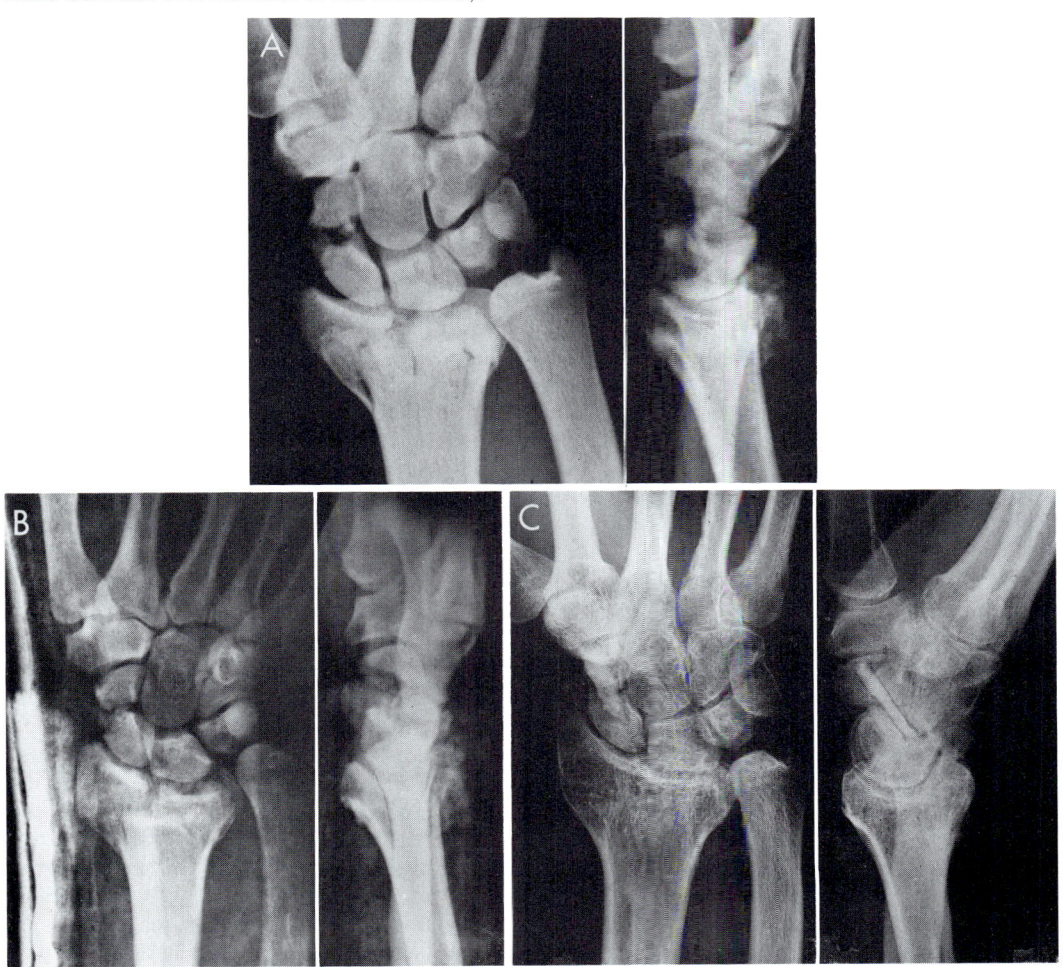

ASSOCIATED INJURIES

It is not uncommon to find other fractures or dislocations accompanying a Colles fracture in the same arm. Careful physical examination of the remainder of the extremity is mandatory. Fracture of the carpal navicula may occur with distal radial fractures, necessitating prolonged immobilization (Fig. 21-3). Transmission of force through the forearm may cause a variety of elbow injuries, including fracture of the distal humerus. Dislocation of the shoulder or fracture of the surgical neck of the humerus also occurs with distal radial fractures.

X-RAY EXAMINATION

Anteroposterior and lateral radiographs of the injured wrist should be examined carefully. If fracture or dislocation of carpal bones or epiphyseal injuries are suspected, films of the opposite (normal) wrist may be helpful. X-ray films of the elbow and shoulder should be obtained if physical examination suggests injury to these areas.

TREATMENT

Undisplaced fractures in adults and dorsal buckle fractures of the distal radius (torus fractures) in children may be simply immobilized in plaster splints or light circular casts for 2 or 3 weeks.

Displaced fractures must be reduced. Even in patients with multiple severe injuries, treatment of a wrist fracture should not be compromised, as, with good medical care, many of these patients will survive and the most disabling injuries are likely to be those to the musculoskeletal system.

Anesthesia is necessary for satisfactory reduction of the displaced fracture and several varieties of anesthesia are suitable. Infiltration of the fracture site with a local anesthetic agent is used widely. Scrupulous sterile precautions must be observed and the anesthetic agent must be introduced into the fracture hematoma and around the ulnar styloid if it is fractured. As with any method of local infiltration or block anesthesia, the surgeon must wait at least 15–20 minutes for diffusion and full effect of the anesthetic agent. This time can be spent profitably by applying traction and preparing splints. Intravenous regional anesthesia is reliable, but proper dosage and technique of tourniquet application must be fully understood by the operator. Axillary and supraclavicular (brachial) blocks may be used and provide excellent anesthesia if proper technique is followed. Supraclavicular block should not be used on an outpatient basis because of the possibility of pneumothorax. General anesthesia is best for securing muscle relaxation but is contraindicated in the patient who has eaten recently. As the majority of patients with these fractures are treated as outpatients, some form of local anesthesia is used most commonly.

Once adequate anesthesia is induced, reduction is carried out. Forceful traction, with an assistant providing countertraction at the elbow, is used to regain radial length and disimpact the fragments (Fig. 21-4). The hand and wrist then are manipulated into flexion and ulnar deviation. Dorsal pressure over the distal radius is helpful to mold the fragments. Adequacy of reduction is checked by palpating the radial styloid process to ensure that radial length has been regained. Dorsal prominence of the distal ulna should be restored. If, with the forearm held in a vertical position, the hand and wrist hang passively in a position of 60 degrees of flexion, it is a reliable indication that reduction has been achieved.

The fracture then is immobilized in plaster splints that are padded with a layer or two of sheet wadding and wrapped on carefully with gauze bandage to avoid wrinkling or buckling of the splints, especially on the volar aspect of the wrist (Fig. 21-5). The dorsal splint extends from the metacarpophalangeal joints on the dorsum of the hand to just below the

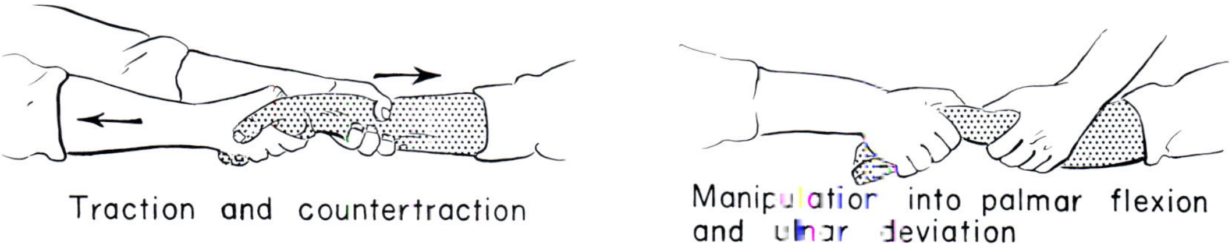

Chapter 21: FRACTURES OF THE DISTAL END OF THE RADIUS / 517

Traction and countertraction

Manipulation into palmar flexion and ulnar deviation

Fig. 21-4.—Manual method of reduction.

elbow and the volar splint from the distal palmar crease to below the elbow. The splints are molded carefully while the plaster hardens. The plaster must be trimmed back in the palm to allow full flexion of the metacarpophalangeal joints. Alternatively, a radial gutter splint or sugar-tong splint can be used. With unstable fractures, the elbow should be immobilized to prevent forearm rotation.

The hand and wrist are held in pronation, ulnar deviation and some palmar flexion. A position of extreme flexion and ulnar deviation may be responsible for median nerve compression in the carpal tunnel, as well as excessive stiffness of the fingers, and should be avoided.

Once reduction and immobilization have been completed, x-ray films are obtained. They should be examined carefully with several thoughts in mind:

1. Has radial length been restored?
2. Has the normal 10–15 degrees of volar angulation of the distal radius been achieved?
3. Is the distal ulna in a slightly dorsal position?
4. If the fracture involved articular surfaces, has congruity been restored to the radiocarpal and/or distal radioulnar joints?

Once a satisfactory reduction has been achieved, the patient is instructed to elevate the hand and wrist for a majority of the time during the next several days. This helps to prevent excess swelling of the hand and fingers. The patient must also carry out active finger exercises frequently and should remove the sling several times a day in order to put the shoulder through a full range of motion. The disabling sequelae of stiff fingers and frozen shoulders are largely preventable.

It is advisable to check the maintenance of the reduction with radiographs at 24–48 hours and again at 7–10 days postreduction. If a significant loss of position occurs during this time, the fracture can be remanipulated. The splints may be tightened as swelling subsides.

At 2½–3 weeks, x-ray films out of plaster are obtained and a short arm cast applied with the amount of wrist flexion decreased but ulnar deviation maintained. At 5–6 weeks, healing usually is sufficient to allow active exercises out of

Fig. 21-5.—Plaster splints applied after correction of the deformities to maintain position.

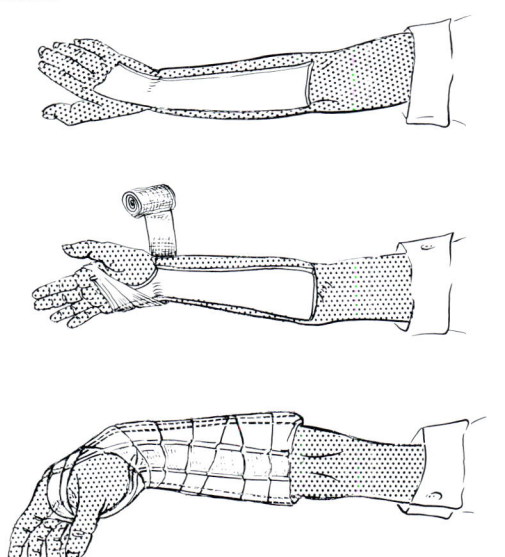

plaster. Active treatment must be continued until the patient has regained joint mobility and muscle power. Most patients will rehabilitate themselves with the physician's encouragement, but a few will require concentrated physical therapy to ensure recovery.

Traction

Traction may be used to achieve reduction of the Colles fracture (Fig. 21-6). Traction on the thumb for 10–15 minutes reduces the fracture and pulls the hand into ulnar deviation. The traction is maintained as the plaster splints are applied and the operator can flex the wrist slightly and mold the dorsal fragments.

Operative Treatment

It is uncommon for the Colles fracture to be open (compound), but if such is the case it usually may be treated by wound

Fig. 21-6.—Method of thumb traction for reduction of Colles' fracture. (From Cave, E. F.: Injuries to the wrist joint, Am. Acad. Orthop. Surgeons Lect. 10:1, J. W. Edwards, Inc., Ann Arbor, Mich., 1953.)

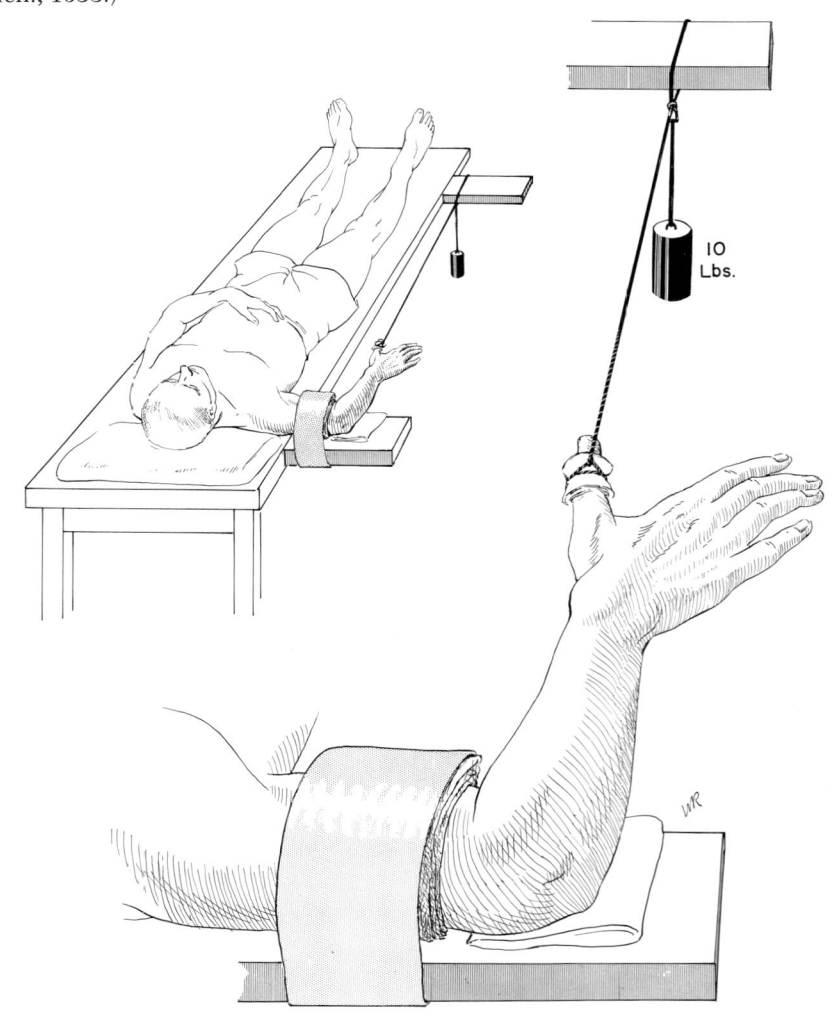

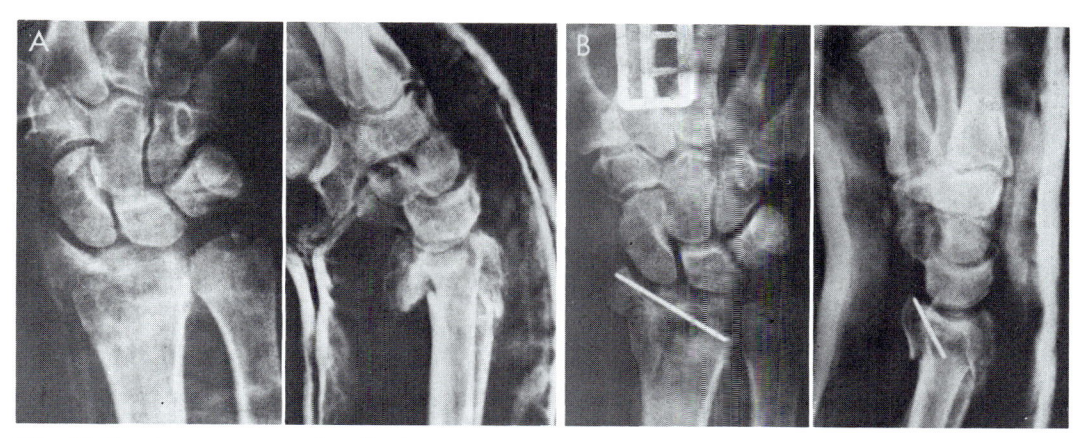

Chapter 21: FRACTURES OF THE DISTAL END OF THE RADIUS / 519

Fig. 21-7.—**A,** comminuted Colles' fracture after attempted closed reduction with unsatisfactory position. **B,** open reduction and internal fixation with a Kirschner wire and plaster splints.

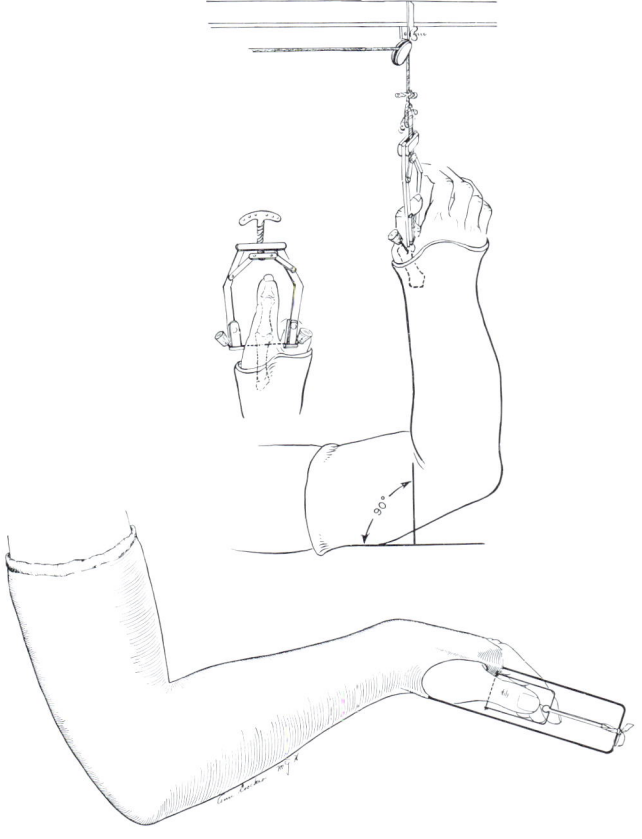

Fig. 21-8.—Diagrammatic sketch of skeletal thumb traction in treatment of Colles' fracture. **Top,** suspension in bed. (From Cave, E. F.: Injuries to the wrist joint, Am. Acad. Orthop. Surgeons Lect. 10:1, J. W. Edwards, Inc., Ann Arbor, Mich. 1953). **Bottom,** an extension attached to the cast, used in skeletal fixation.

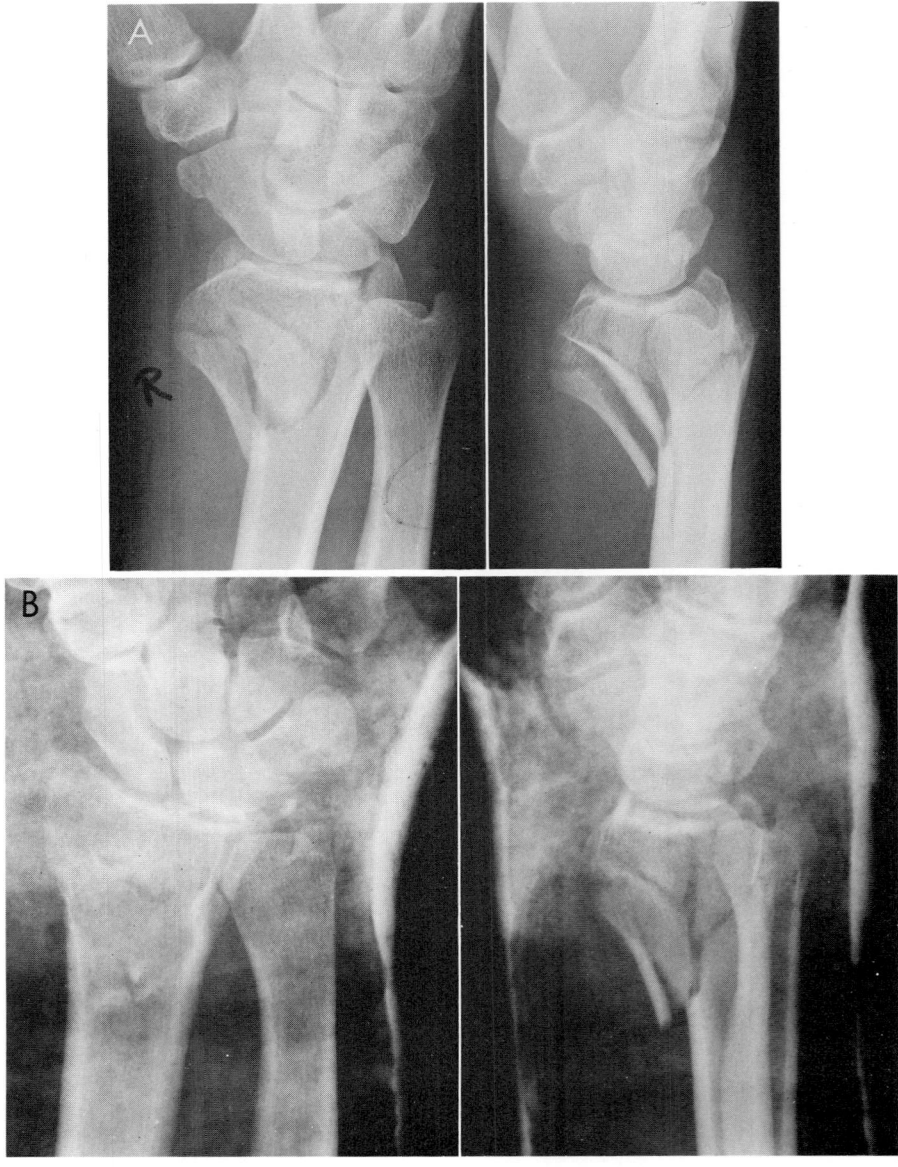

Fig. 21-9.—A 55-year-old shipping clerk suffered this wrist injury when his arm was pinned against a wall by a loaded cart. **A,** the original fracture. Volar and radial subluxation of the carpus. Note also the undisplaced fracture of the navicular tuberosity. **B,** attempted closed reduction. Volar subluxation unreduced and it was believed that further deformity would occur. **(Continued.)**

debridement and closure, followed by closed reduction. Occasionally, a Colles fracture has one or two fragments that may be fixed with Kirschner wire if closed reduction fails (Fig. 21-7). With severe comminution, closed reduction and plaster immobilization may lead to unacceptable deformity and radial shortening, especially in younger patients. In this situation, skeletal fixation may be

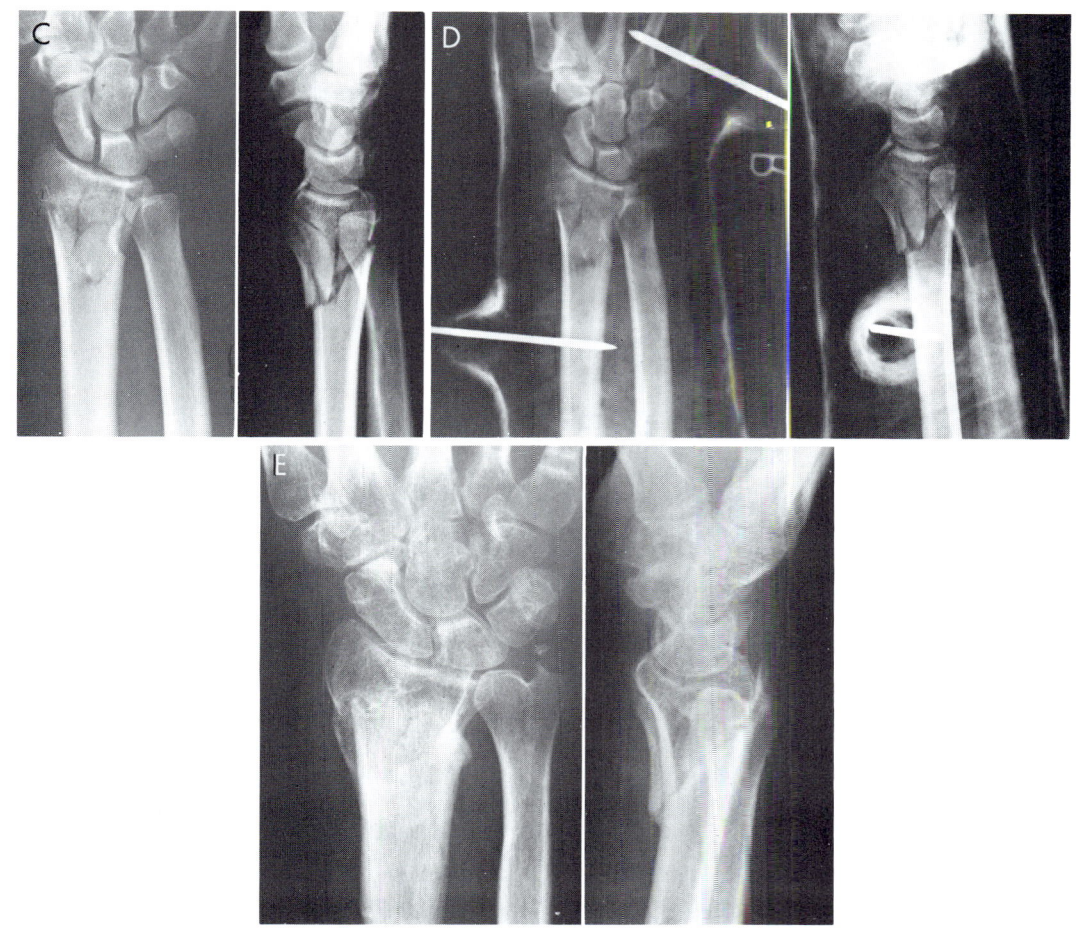

Fig. 21-9 (cont.).—C, reduction in traction, fingertraps and countertraction (10 lb) at elbow. Note slight distraction of the wrist and carpal joints. D, skeletal fixation in short arm cast. Maintained for 8 weeks. E, 4 months postfracture. At this time the patient had full painless motion and returned to work.

necessary to maintain the reduction. This may be done in a variety of ways (Figs. 21-8 and 21-9). Cole and Obletz[3] have described a technique that uses traction to reduce the fracture and skeletal fixation with one wire in the radius and another in the fourth and fifth metacarpals. These wires are incorporated in a short arm cast, which is kept on for a minimum of 6–8 weeks to allow for consolidation of the fracture. The patient can pronate and supinate some while wearing the cast and may use the fingers freely. This method has produced excellent results in unstable comminuted fractures (see Fig. 21-9).

PROGNOSIS

In his original article, Colles stated that although the deformity will remain, the limb eventually will regain free motion and be pain-free. This optimistic view is not borne out by large follow-up series (Frykman,[8] Lindstrom[9]), in which 20–25% of results were graded poor or fair. Approximately 50% of patients report subjective symptoms of weakness or pain in the hand and wrist. Objectively, 50–75% of patients have some loss of mobility of the wrist and approximately 15% will have laxity of the distal radioulnar joint.

There are a number of factors that favor a poor result:

1. Shortening of the radius causes prominence of the distal ulna and disturbance of the distal radioulnar joint. In contrast, loss of volar tilt of the distal radius of up to 20 degrees is not particularly associated with residual symptoms.

2. Intra-articular fractures of the radiocarpal joint are less favorable than extra-articular ones.

3. Fracture of the ulnar styloid that fails to unite indicates injury to the articular disk and often is associated with symptoms.

4. Injury to the distal radioulnar joint by intra-articular fracture or ligamentous disruption carries a particularly unfavorable prognosis. Pain on forearm rotation is the most prominent and disabling symptom.

5. Injury to nerves and tendons and residual swelling also adversely affect the prognosis and are discussed below.

COMPLICATIONS

The most common complication is some loss of position of the fracture following reduction. Fortunately, radial shortening of up to 4 mm and dorsal tilt of the distal radius of 20 degrees often are compatible with good wrist function.

Severe residual dorsal angulation may be corrected by a dorsal open-up wedge osteotomy of the distal radius, and some increase in radial length can be achieved also (Fig. 21-10).

Dislocations of the distal radioulnar joint may be responsible for pain on pronation and supination and for pain on compression of this joint. Excision of the distal ulna (Darrach[5] procedure) has been suggested for this problem, but in our experience it rarely is indicated. Functional recovery of the wrist following fracture usually is such by 1 year postinjury that excision of the distal ulna becomes unnecessary.

Residual stiffness of the fingers, especially in elderly patients who have some osteoarthritis, is preventable by diligent early exercise of the fingers. Once established, however, there may be some residual loss of finger motion despite vigorous physical therapy.

One of the most severe complications following Colles' fracture is post-traumatic reflex dystrophy, also called Sudeck's atrophy, or the shoulder-hand-finger syndrome. This condition occurs in approximately 2% of Colles' fractures and may also be seen after soft tissue injuries of the hand or arm. It is characterized by the onset of marked swelling and pain in the hand and fingers several weeks after injury. Skin creases and lines are obliterated and finger motion decreases markedly, especially in the metacarpophalangeal joints. The skin is warm and hyperemic. X-ray films demonstrate a spotty rarefaction in the carpals and metacarpals. The palmar fascia almost always is thickened and may progress to a typical Dupuytren's contracture. Sudeck's atrophy can result in almost total loss of function of the extremity. The etiology is not known but has been ascribed to a disturbance in the autonomic nervous system or failure of the muscles to pump venous blood and lymph out of the extremities. Vigorous and prompt treatment is necessary once the syndrome appears. Stellate ganglion blocks often are helpful. Active exercises must be encouraged and the use of a sling and dependent position of the arm discouraged.

Nerve injuries complicate approximately 3% of Colles' fractures. It is rare for the nerve to be injured at the time of fracture. Acute wrist flexion brings the sharp proximal edge of the transverse carpal ligament closer to the radius and also causes rotation and volar projection of the lunate. When edema and fracture hematoma are added, it is obvious why

Chapter 21: FRACTURES OF THE DISTAL END OF THE RADIUS / 523

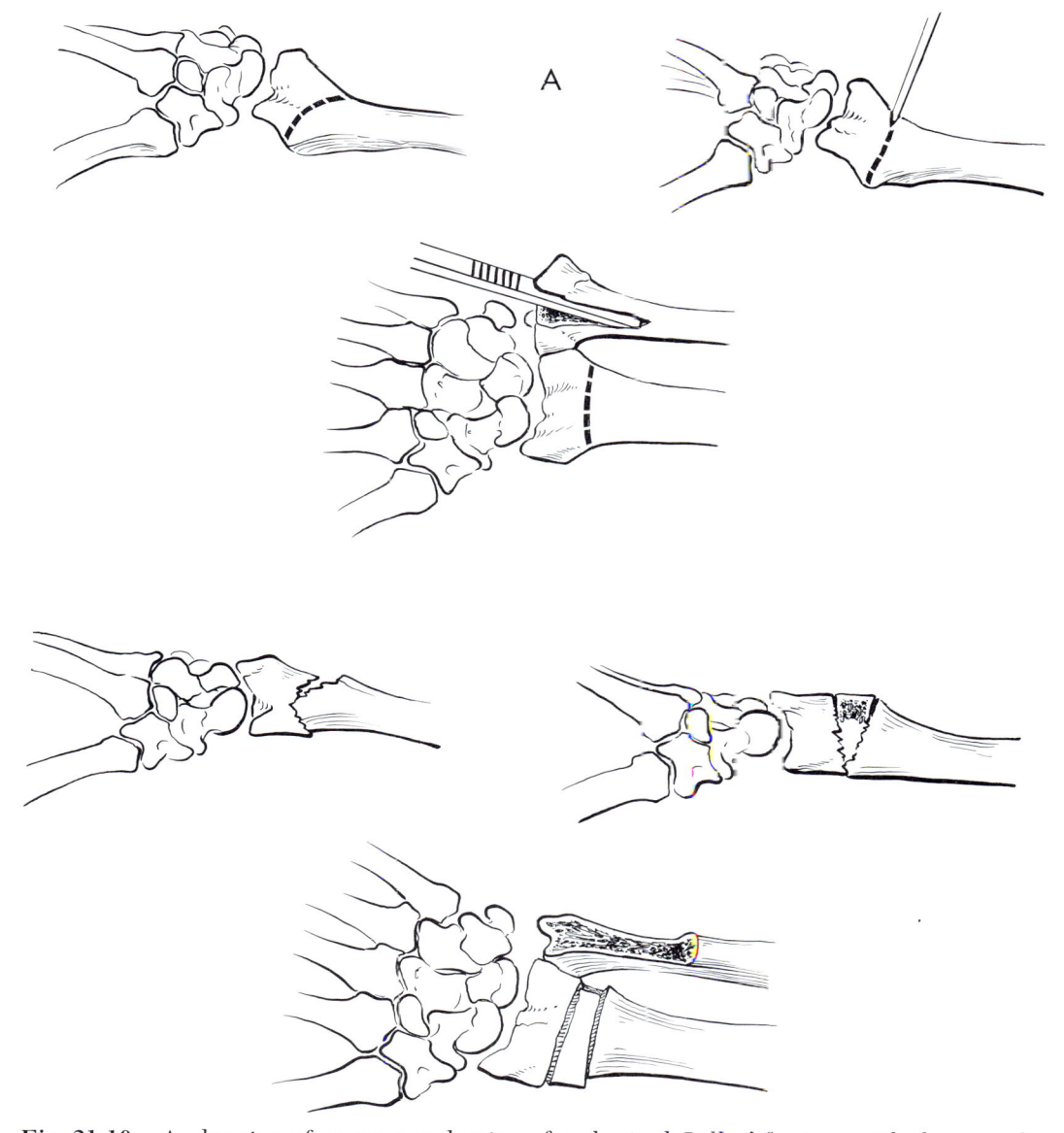

Fig. 21-10.—**A**, drawing of an open reduction of malunited Colles' fracture with the use of a portion of the distal ulna as a graft. (**Continued.**)

immobilization in acute wrist flexion may cause median nerve compression. The median nerve may also be irritated if there is residual dorsal displacement of the distal radius with volar projection of a bone fragment, or voluminous volar callus formation. Most cases of median nerve injury subside spontaneously, but, if sensory changes persist or if atrophy of the thenar musculature occurs, the transverse carpal ligament should be sectioned.

The ulnar nerve is involved less frequently than the median nerve in wrist

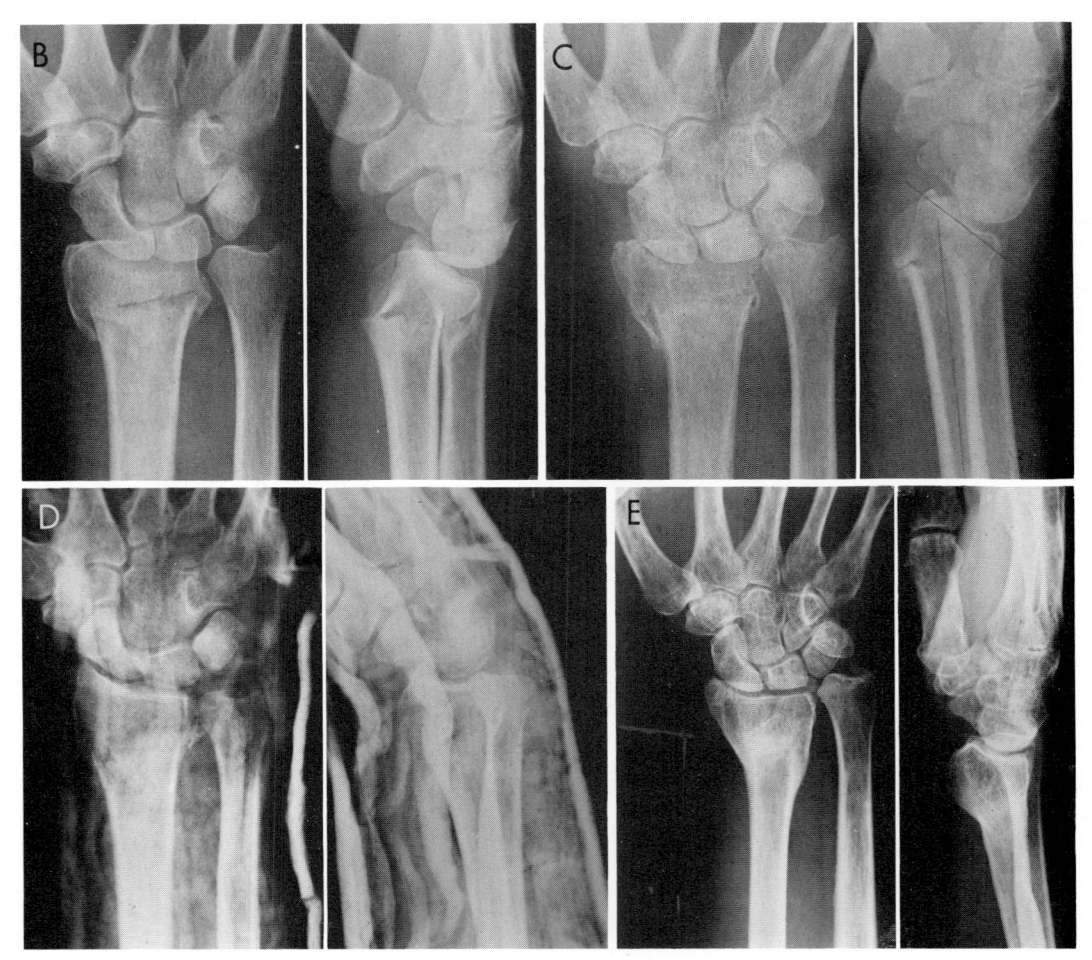

Fig. 21-10 (cont.).—B, roentgenogram of typical Colles' fracture. C, healed in malposition 6 months after injury with symptoms of median nerve irritation. D, x-ray view in plaster following open reduction and insertion of wedge graft. E, 4 years after open reduction. Dorsal displacement has been corrected. Median nerve symptoms have been relieved, but there still is some radial shortening.

fractures. Disruption of the distal radioulnar joint, even with dorsal displacement of the distal ulna, rarely causes ulnar nerve paresis, although if this does result, release of the tunnel of Guyon may be required.

Last, rupture of the extensor pollicis longus tendon occurs in somewhat less than 1% of cases. Occasionally the tendon is lacerated at the time of fracture by a sharp bone fragment. More commonly, however, the tendon ruptures several weeks after the fracture. This late rupture is due to edema in the fibro-osseous tunnel, which interrupts the tendon's blood supply and causes attrition and eventual rupture. The diagnosis may be missed, as the abductor pollicis brevis can extend the interphalangeal joint of the thumb. Repair may be end-to-end suture, tendon graft or transfer of the extensor indicis proprius.

SMITH'S AND BARTON'S FRACTURES

Smith's and Barton's fractures have been the subject of a good deal of confusion in regard to both nomenclature and treatment. In 1847, Robert William Smith[11] of Dublin described a fracture in which the distal radial fragment was displaced volarward after a fall on the back of the hand. Smith's fracture is the reverse of Colle's fracture. It occurs about one-twentieth as often. In fact, few patients can recall falling on the back of the hand, and Evans[7] has suggested that rotation plays an important part in the resultant fracture. If one falls backward onto the palm of the hand with the forearm supinated, body weight will further supinate the arm with the hand fixed to the ground. This combination of twisting and compressive forces theoretically will cause the fracture of the distal radius to angulate dorsally (distal fragments displaced volarward) and produce Smith's fracture.

Reduction of Smith's fracture is attained by traction, full supination of the hand and forearm and slight wrist flexion. Thomas[12] recommends immobilization in a long arm cast in full supination for 6 weeks.

In 1838, John Rhea Barton[2] of Philadelphia described two types of fracture-dislocation of the wrist. His principal discussion dealt with a posterior (dorsal) marginal fracture of the distal radius with dorsal displacement of the carpus. He also mentioned volar marginal fracture of the distal radius. Both of these have become known as Barton's fracture, creating confusion. It is best to refer to them in anatomic terms. Both are rare, the volar type being the more common. In recent years, it has been well demonstrated by a number of authors that the volar marginal fracture is stable if reduced and held in full supination and wrist flexion. The fragment can be pushed back into place and the wrist flexion relaxes the radiocarpal ligaments. As with Smith's fracture, immobilization in a long arm cast is necessary for 6 weeks. Ellis[6] has described the use of a small volar buttress plate to stabilize these fractures (volar marginal and Smith's) and allow for early mobilization.

The dorsal marginal fracture may be immobilized in supination and wrist extension.

BIBLIOGRAPHY

1. Anderson, R., and O'Neil, G.: Comminuted fractures of distal end of radius, Surg. Gynecol. Obstet. 78:434, 1944.
2. Barton, J. R.: Views and treatment of an important injury of the wrist. Med. Examiner and Rec. of Med. Sci. 1:365, 1838.
3. Cole, J. M., and Obletz, B. E.: Comminuted fractures of the distal end of the radius treated by skeletal transfixion in plaster cast, J. Bone Joint Surg. 48-A:931, 1966.
4. Colles, A.: On fractures of the carpal extremity of the radius, Edinb. M. J. 10:182, 1814.
5. Darrach, W.: Forward dislocation at the inferior radio-ulnar joint, with fracture of the lower third of the shaft of the radius, Surgery 56:801, 1912.
6. Ellis, J.: Smith's and Barton's fractures, J. Bone Joint Surg. 47-B:724, 1965.
7. Evans, E.: Fractures of the radius and ulna, J. Bone Joint Surg. 33-B:548, 1951.
8. Frykman, G.: Fracture of the distal radius including sequelae—shoulder-hand-finger syndrome, disturbance in the distal radio-ulnar joint and impairment of nerve function, Acta Orthop. Scand., Supp. 108, 1967.
9. Lidström, A.: Fractures of the distal end of the radius, Acta Orthop. Scand., Supp. 41, 1959.
10. Mills, T. J.: Smith's fracture and anterior marginal fracture of the radius, Br. Med. J. 2:603, 1957.
11. Smith, R. W.: A Treatise on Fractures in the Vicinity of Joints (Dublin: Hodges & Smith, 1847), pp. 162–163.
12. Thomas, F.: Reduction of Smith's fracture, J. Bone Joint Surg. 39-B:463, 1957.

22 | Injuries to the Carpal Bones

EDWIN F. CAVE and ROBERT J. BOYD

FRACTURES AND DISLOCATIONS of the carpal bones comprise approximately 2% of all fractures and dislocations treated at Massachusetts General Hospital. The injuries occur most commonly in the late teen-age and early adult group, whereas Colles' fractures are more frequent in the middle-aged and older group. Carpal injuries are common in males and extremely uncommon in females, owing, undoubtedly, to the trauma to which males are subjected. The usual cause is a fall or blow on the dorsiflexed hand. Of all the carpal injuries (see Table 22-1), the most common are, in order of frequency: fracture of the navicular bone, dislocation of the lunate bone and retrolunar dislocation of the capitate bone with rotation or fracture of the navicula (transcarpal dislocation) Other injuries occur much less frequently. Chip fractures of the dorsum of the lunate, capitate or other carpal bones are rather frequent, but usually they do not cause severe disability or require prolonged treatment. The symptom is pain in the wrist joint and the signs are swelling, limitation of motion and tenderness localized to the particular bone injured. The diagnosis is based on a history of the fall, local examination and —above all—properly taken x-ray films.

TABLE 22-1.—TYPES OF INJURIES IN A SERIES OF 218 CARPAL BONE INJURIES AT MASSACHUSETTS GENERAL HOSPITAL

Fractured navicula	
Recent without other carpal injuries	70
Old (4+ mos.) without other carpal injuries	47
With other carpal injuries	18
Dislocated lunate	13
With other carpal injuries	6
Dislocated ulnocarpal joint	1
Retrolunar dislocation of capitate bone	21
Fractured lunate bone	5
Subluxated midcarpal joint	1
Kienböck's disease of the lunate	9
Miscellaneous fractures, including chip fractures	24
Cyst of lunate bone	1
Cyst of navicular bone	1
Congenital fusion of triangular and lunate bones	1
TOTAL	218

DEVELOPMENT OF THE CARPUS

The carpal bones usually develop according to a definite plan, and anatomic variations are infrequent. The bones are cartilaginous at birth, and during the first year the ossification centers of only the capitate and hamate bones appear. The remaining centers are visible by x-ray between the second and eighth years, except for the center of the pisiform bone, which does not appear until the tenth year or later. Inflammatory processes may cause the ossification centers to appear earlier than normal. Poliomyelitis or prolonged congestion of the extremity from any cause may have the same effect. Delayed development of the carpus may occur in the chondrodystro-

528 / Edwin F. Cave and Robert J. Boyd

phies and as a familial characteristic. Normally, these bones develop from a single ossification center, but there are exceptions. The most common of the anatomic variations is the bipartite navicular bone. Variations may also occur in the capitate bone. Usually these anomalies are bilateral, and there may be no history of injury.

BLOOD SUPPLY OF THE CARPUS.—The blood supply of the carpus is derived from terminal twigs of the ulnar and radial arteries. These twigs, after being carried along supporting ligaments, enter the fibrous covering that represents the periosteum.

ANATOMY

A thorough knowledge of the anatomic arrangement of the carpal bones (Figs. 22-1 and 22-2) is essential to the surgeon who expects to treat carpal injuries. Indistinct fractures and subluxations frequently are overlooked, not through failure to take roentgenograms but through the surgeon's lack of knowledge of the anatomy of the parts in various positions of the

Fig. 22-1.—Skeletal anatomy, showing carpal bones and x-ray positions.

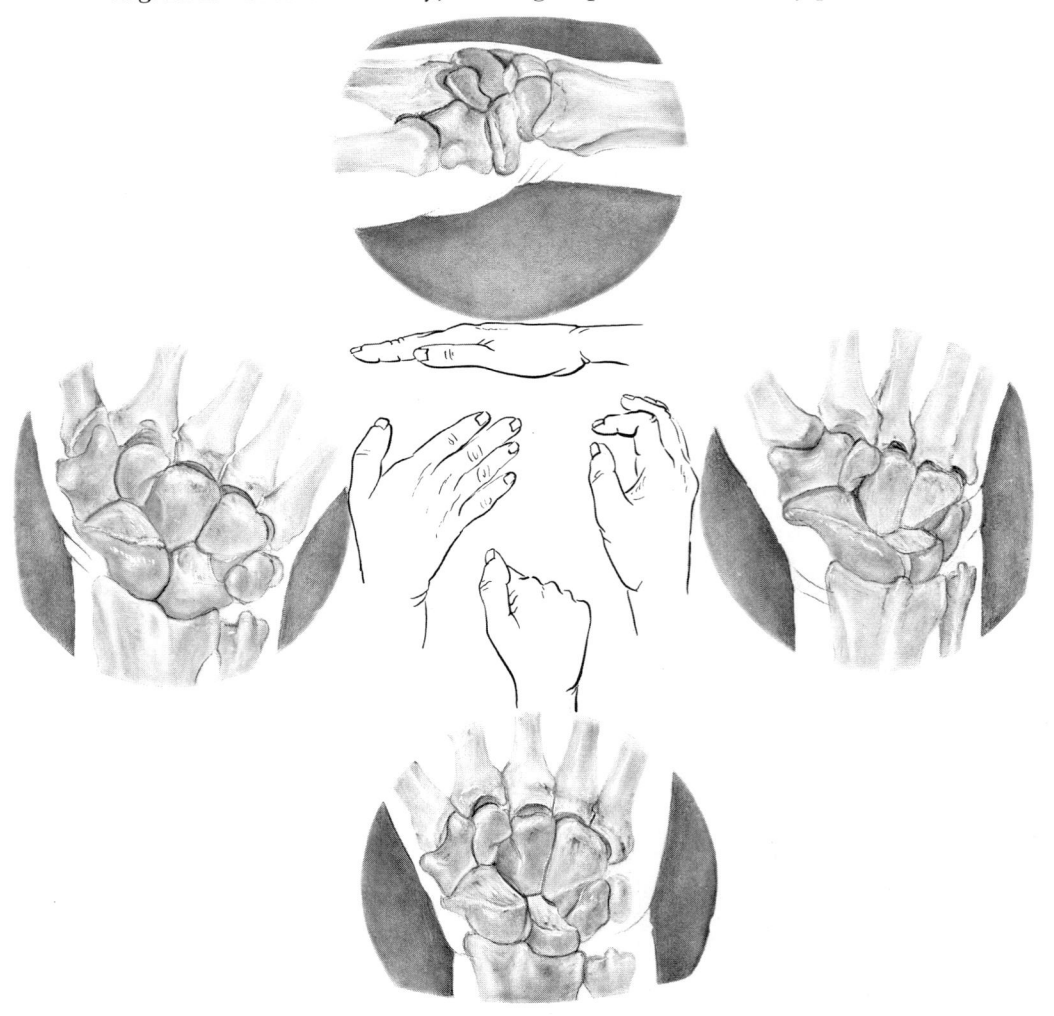

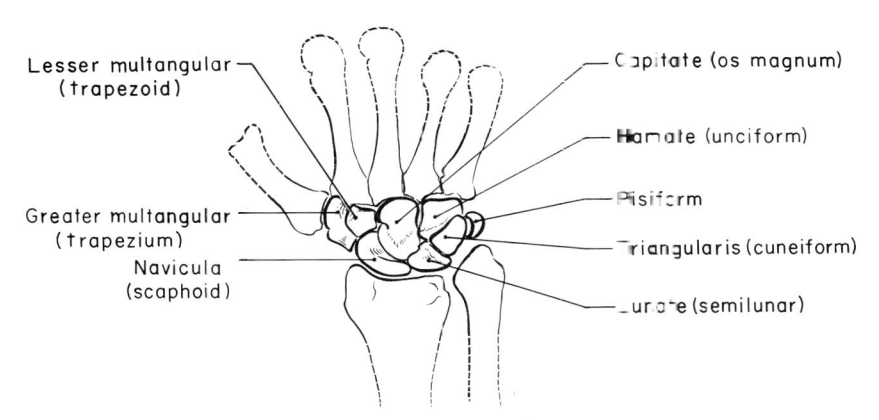

Fig. 22-2.—Anatomy of carpus

hand. The surface of the bones in the first row of the carpus, consisting of the navicular, lunate, triangular and pisiform bones, is largely cartilaginous. The remaining portions of the surface serve for ligamentous attachments. The second row, made up of the greater and lesser multangular bones and the capitate and the hamate bones, is less cartilaginous but is covered more extensively by the ligamentous attachments. This row is held together more firmly by the supporting ligaments than are the navicular and lunate bones, which are more exposed to trauma because of their location and their movable articulations with the radius. On the volar surface there are tendinous attachments only to the pisiform, hamate and greater multangular bones; on the dorsal surface there are no attachments. The navicular bone articulates, on its dorsal surface, with the radius, the greater and the lesser multangular bones and the lunate bone. On its volar surface, the navicula is in contact with the greater and the lesser multangular bones, the capitate bone, the lunate bone and the radius.

DIAGNOSIS BY X-RAY EXAMINATION

The hands may be placed in so many varied positions that in the roentgenogram the bones may appear to have an abnormal relationship. If the anteroposterior view of the navicular bone is made with the wrist in radial deviation, the bone may appear shortened or subluxated, whereas with the wrist in ulnar deviation, the true long axis of the bone is visible and any abnormality is seen more easily. It is important, therefore, not only to have the standardized methods of roentgen technique but also to have adequate knowledge of the relationships of the carpal bones in the various positions of the hands. For studying the carpal bones, both hands should be photographed on the same plate.

Routine anteroposterior and lateral views of the wrist joint are not sufficient to make a diagnosis of a fracture in the navicular bone. Because of the overlap of one bone on the other in the lateral view and the change in relationship of the carpal bone in the anteroposterior view, special positions are necessary. The following views are required (Fig. 22-3):

1. Posteroanterior view with hand in extreme ulnar deviation. (At times, this is not feasible because of pain.)
2. Oblique view with thumb and forefinger together and remaining fingers resting on the film.
3. Posteroanterior view with fist closed.
4. Direct lateral views.
5. Midsupination view with plane of the palm at an angle of 45 degrees to the film.

Views taken with the wrists in extreme

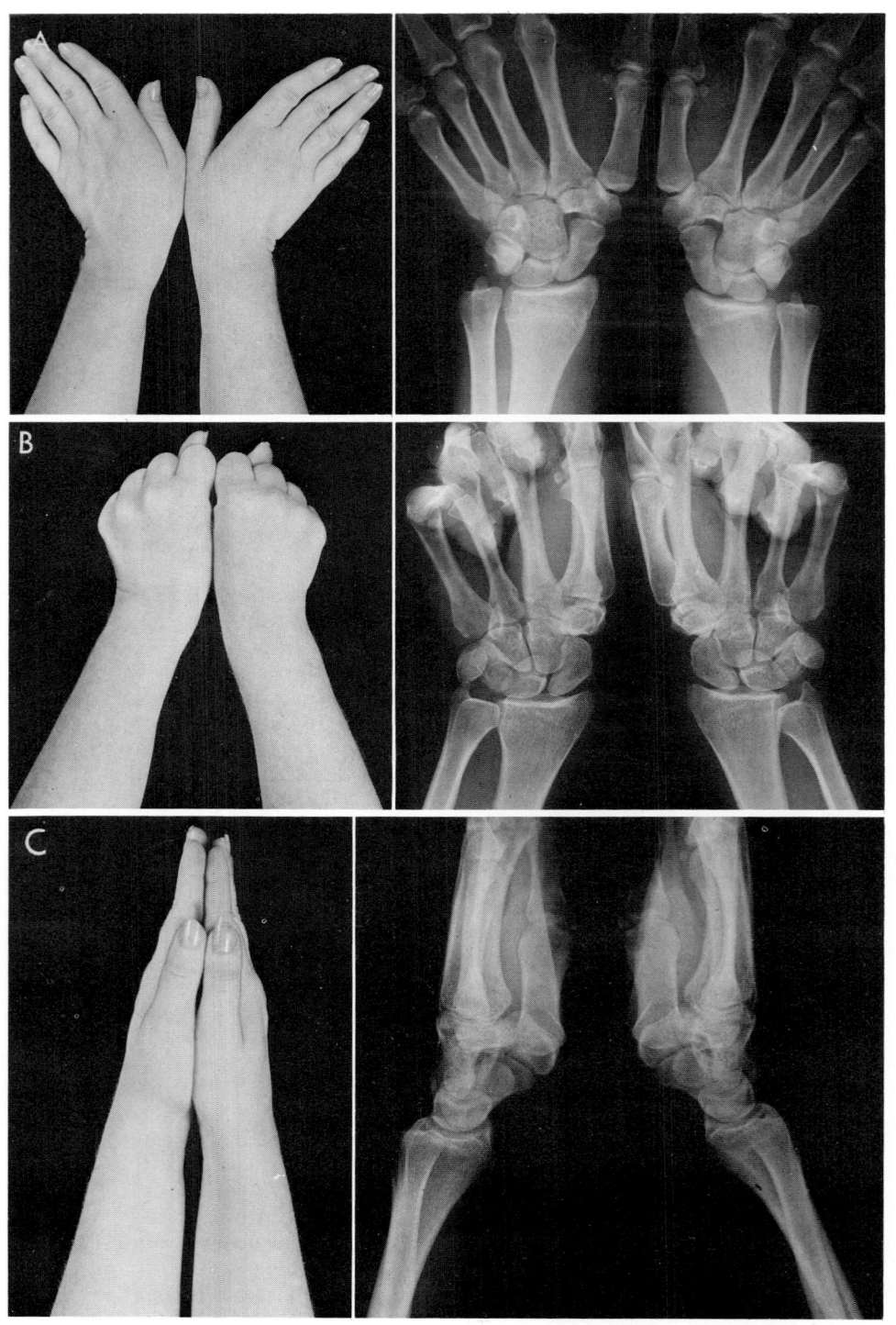

Fig. 22-3.—Positions of hands for x-ray of carpus, with accompanying x-ray views. **A,** ulnar deviation. **B,** clenched fist. **C,** lateral. (**Continued.**)

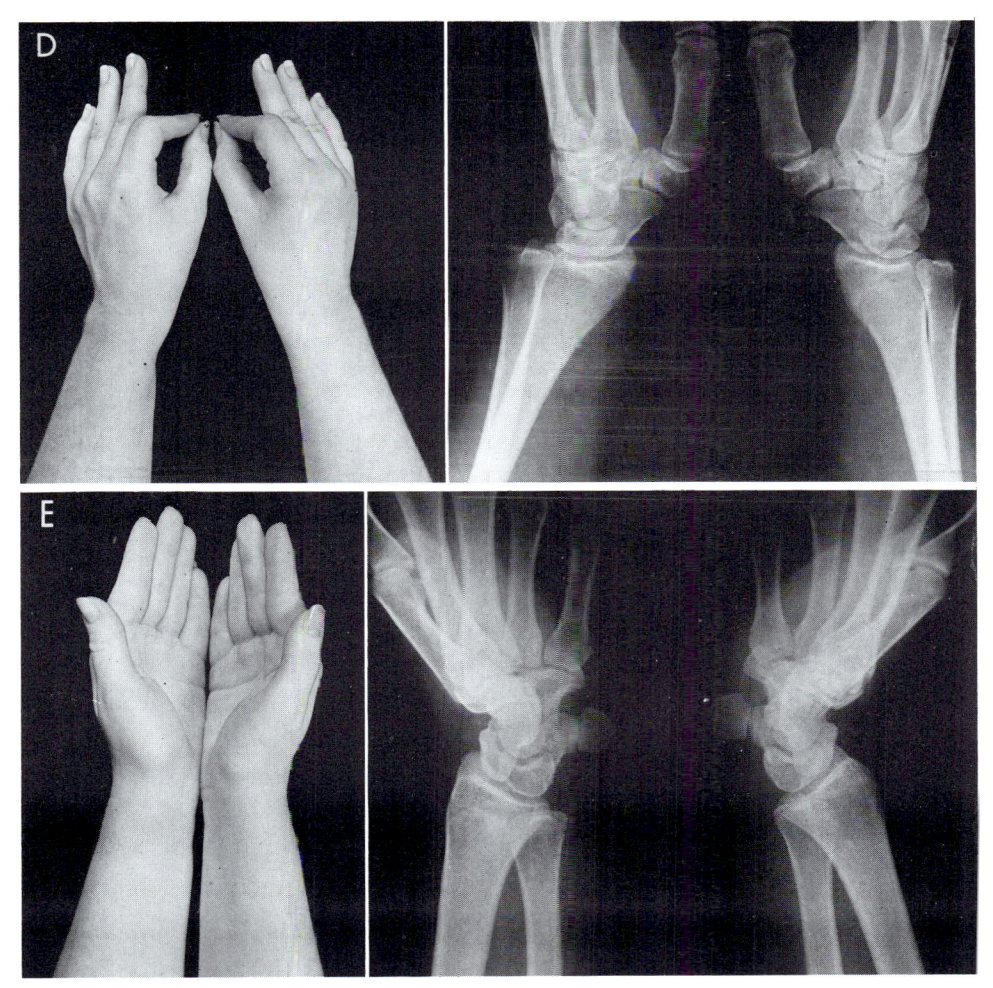

Fig. 22-3 (cont.).—D, oblique. E, midsupination.

supination may be of value occasionally, but very often the acute stage of the injury makes it impossible to place the wrist in this position.

TREATMENT

Fresh Navicular Fractures

Fracture of the navicula is by far the most common carpal injury (see Table 22-1).

When any bone is fractured, the blood supply to the fragments is temporarily interrupted, but this is particularly true of the carpal navicular bone (Fig. 22-4). If the fracture line runs directly through the bifurcation of the main artery, which enters the midportion of the navicular bone, nutrition to the proximal fragment is interrupted; the distal fragment is nourished, however, by the artery entering the tubercle. Such interference with the blood supply to the proximal fragment explains the failure of union in a large percentage of navicular fractures in the middle and proximal regions if prompt treatment is not initiated. If immediate

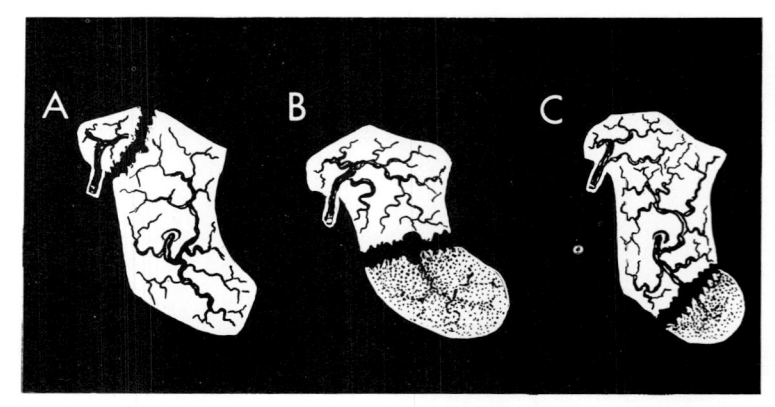

Fig. 22-4.—Diagram showing interruption of circulation in navicular fractures. **A,** fracture through the tubercle or distal portion of the bone is favorable for union because each fragment has a nutrient artery. **B** and **C,** fractures through central portion or proximal third are very slow to unite because the proximal portion of the bone usually has no nutrient vessel.

reduction and fixation are carried out, there usually is restoration of blood vessels across the fracture line. If treatment is delayed, a scar forms and the blood channels are sealed off. Even after several weeks have elapsed, it is possible to promote blood supply to the fracture if immobilization is carried out for a sufficient length of time.

The navicula usually fractures through the waist of the bone or at the junction of the proximal and middle thirds. As a rule, displacement is not great, and the only treatment indicated is plaster immobilization with the wrist in a neutral position. The plaster should include the proximal phalanx of the thumb and should run from the palmar crease to just below the elbow (Fig. 22-5). If the diagnosis of fracture is made early and immobilization is instituted at once, a high percentage of these fractures will unite within 10–16 weeks. The plaster should be renewed at 4-week intervals, and x-ray films should be made each month to determine whether union is present. This opinion must be based entirely on the roentgenogram (Fig. 22-6).

Fig. 22-5.—Plaster immobilization for navicular fracture, including thumb in position for grasping.

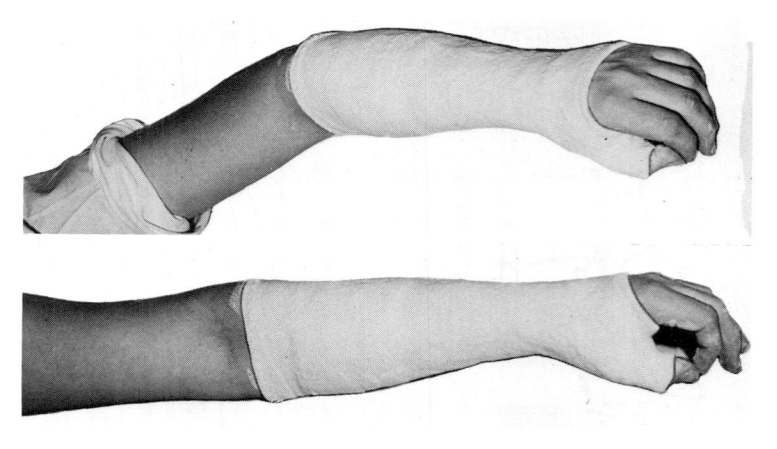

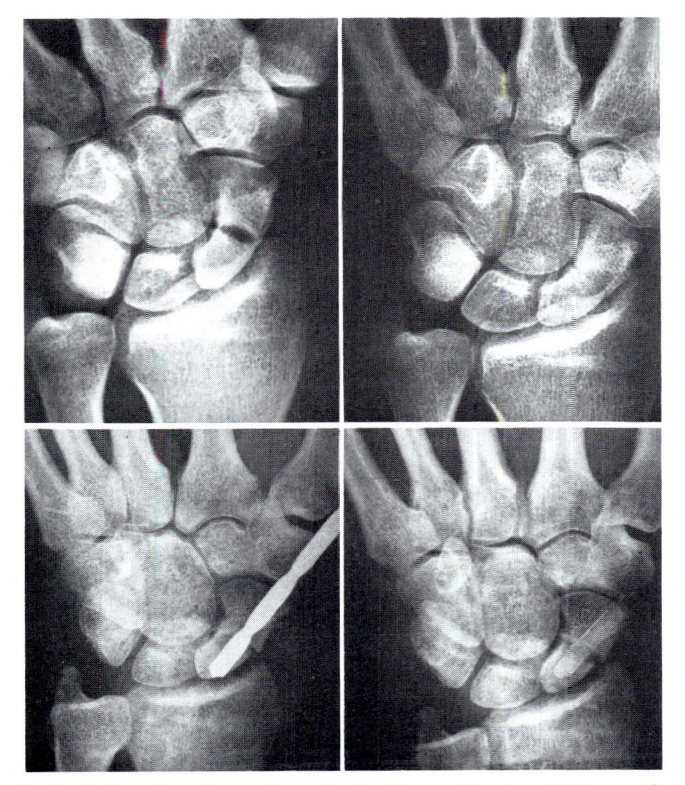

Fig. 22-6 (top).—**Left,** delayed union of navicular bone fractured 5 months previously. Note same density of two navicular fragments, indicating maintenance of circulation to both. **Right,** healed fracture 4 months after immobilization in plaster of Paris.

Fig. 22-7 (bottom).—Technique for inserting tibial graft for ununited navicula. **Left,** drill in position. **Right,** tibial graft inserted from distal fragment into proximal fragment.

Nonunion of the Navicular Bone

In cases of prolonged nonunion of the navicula, a reasonable form of treatment is a dowel graft directed from the distal to the proximal fragment (Fig. 22-7). Following this operation, the lesion is treated as a fresh fracture and immobilization is prolonged until union is complete. If there is an associated extensive traumatic change in the wrist joint, along with the fractured navicula, wrist fusion may be the acceptable form of treatment. In old cases, excision of the navicula and the lunate does not give a satisfactory result, and this operation is to be condemned. Böhler[6] stated:

I have never seen a case in which the usefulness of the hand has returned to normal after removal of the navicular bone. Kemper has collected 60 cases of removal of the navicula and lunate bones; in all of these, function of the hand was poor. In cases operated on early, the mobility of the wrist may remain good, but the strength of the hand is always weakened.

Barnard and Stubbins[4] advised removal of the radial styloid in cases of nonunion of the navicula (Fig. 22-8), particularly in those cases not suitable for grafting because of traumatic changes in the wrist joint. The Fracture Clinic at Massachusetts General Hospital has had no experience with this form of treatment but, on occasion, has excised the radial styloid

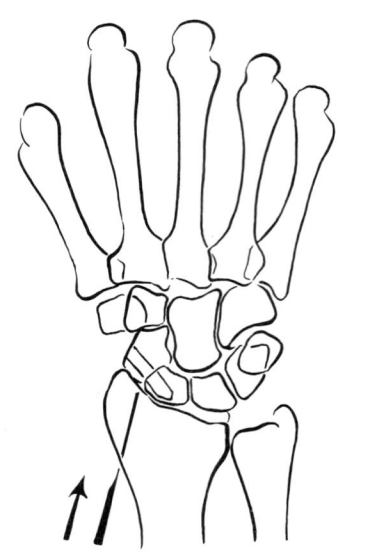

Fig. 22-8.—Barnard's operation: resection of radial styloid.

when exposure of the fracture site of the navicula was particularly difficult to accomplish.

Steele[33] advocated exposing the carpus on the dorsum and, with osteotomes or a specially devised reamer, cutting a circular piece, including portions of the navicula, capitate and lunate, and rotating the section through an arc of 90 degrees, thus serving to promote union between the three bones. He immobilized his patients for only 3 weeks. Of the 36 cases reported, bone union had occurred in the 32 that were followed up.

DRILLING.—Another method of treatment of the ununited navicular bone has been that of drilling; however, as the years have passed, drilling has been largely abandoned as a treatment in favor of some form of graft.

AUTOGENOUS BONE GRAFT.—The most satisfactory method of treating nonunion of the navicular bone is that of the autogenous tibial bone graft. The first advocate of this procedure was Adams,[2] who, in 1928, demonstrated a case in which bone union had been established by introducing a slot graft from the radius into the navicular bone. Murray[27] inserted the graft through a drill hole from the tubercle through the distal fragment into the proximal portion. Others have also advocated this method. In considering the reasons for frequent nonunion of the navicular bone, one must think in terms of blood supply and of the free motion through which the navicular bone normally travels, as compared with the other carpal bones. Therefore, the combination of drilling and introducing a bone peg offers the best chance of re-establishing blood supply and, at the same time, securing fixation of the fragments. In initial cases at Massachusetts General Hospital, the graft was placed in a slot on the dorsum of the navicular bone across the fracture line. The objections to the slot graft are that it is necessary to expose too much of the dorsum of the bone and to interfere with the blood supply to this region, that too much bone is sacrificed from the navicular bone and that the method of fixation with the slot graft is not as secure as that with the dowel graft.

Technique of bone graft of the navicula.—A pneumatic tourniquet is placed around the arm. After the usual preparation and draping of the forearm and hand, a sterile Esmarch bandage is applied to the extremity. The pneumatic tourniquet then is inflated to 275 or 300 mm Hg pressure and the Esmarch bandage is removed. A curving incision with convexity toward the volar surface is made over the radial aspect of the wrist (Fig. 22-9). The superficial branch of the radial nerve is identified lying on the sheath of the abductor pollicis longus and extensor pollicis brevis. The capsule of the wrist is opened to the dorsum of these tendons, and the nerve and tendons are retracted toward the palm. If there is difficulty in exposing the distal fragment of the navicula, the tendons can be retracted toward the dorsum. The distal fragment then is identified. A spatula is introduced between the navicula and the radius (Fig.

Chapter 22: INJURIES TO THE CARPAL BONES / 535

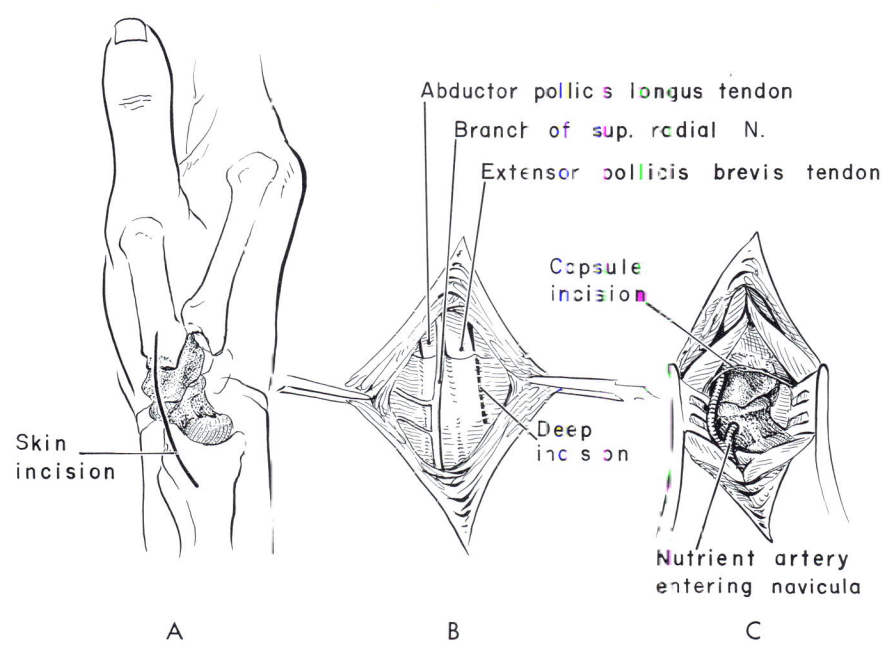

Fig. 22-9.—Radial approach to navicula. **A,** curved radial skin incision. **B,** exposure of tendons and sensory nerve. **C,** exposure of navicular bone.

22-10) and the fracture line is viewed. With the spatula in place, a small 1/8-inch drill hole is begun well toward the tubercle of the bone and is carried across the fracture line into the proximal fragment. With the hand in maximal ulnar deviation, the drill should be about parallel with the first metacarpal bone. Portable x-ray films then are taken in anteroposterior and lateral views. If the drill point is in the desired position, the hole is enlarged with larger drill points to accommodate the largest possible graft without disturbing the articular surfaces of the navicula. A full-thickness tibial graft, 3/8 inch wide and 3 inches long, is removed with the motor saw. It is shaped to proper size with a rasp. The advantage of a graft of this length is that it can be held more easily by a clamp or the surgeon's fingers as it is inserted into the drill hole. After the graft has been driven gently into the proximal fragment, portable films are taken again. The graft is cut with a rongeur at its entrance to the navicula. The

Fig. 22-10.—Spatula holding navicula.

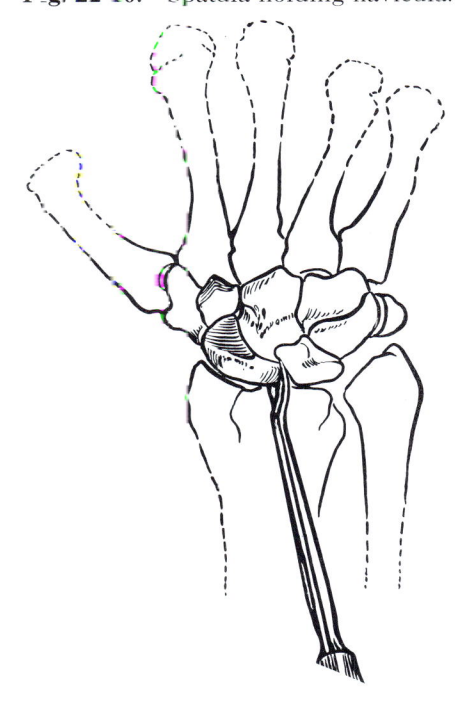

tourniquet is released and the wound is made dry and sutured. A dressing and plaster of Paris are applied with forearm, wrist and thumb immobilized in a neutral position. The fracture then is treated as a recent fracture would be and is protected in plaster until union is firm (Fig. 22-11).

Presently, good results have been obtained in several cases at Massachusetts General Hospital by internal fixation of the fractured carpal navicula, using the exposure outlined and inserting a small lag screw across the fracture fragments, as described by Müller, Allgöwer *et al.* in *The Manual for Internal Fixation.*

Fig. 22-11.—Nonunion of navicula 1 year after fracture. **Top,** oblique and anteroposterior views, showing fracture in "waist" of bone with increased density of proximal fragment. **Bottom,** 6 months after graft; healing of fracture and incorporation of tibial bone graft.

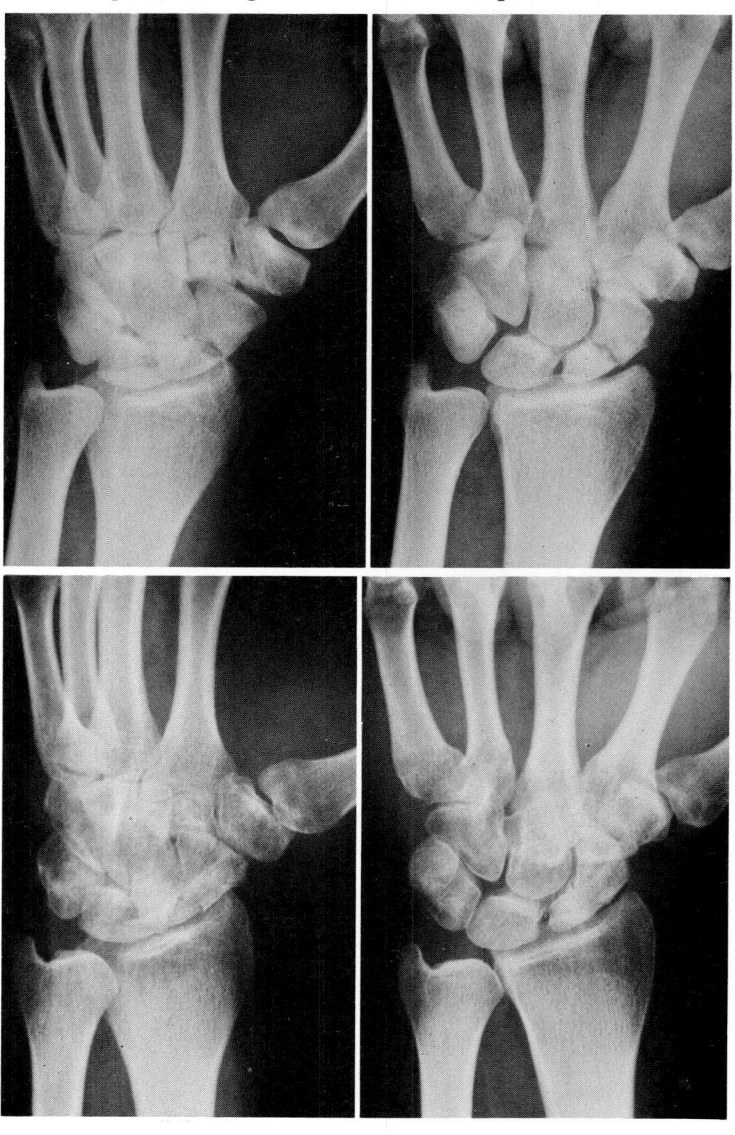

Chapter 22: INJURIES TO THE CARPAL BONES / **537**

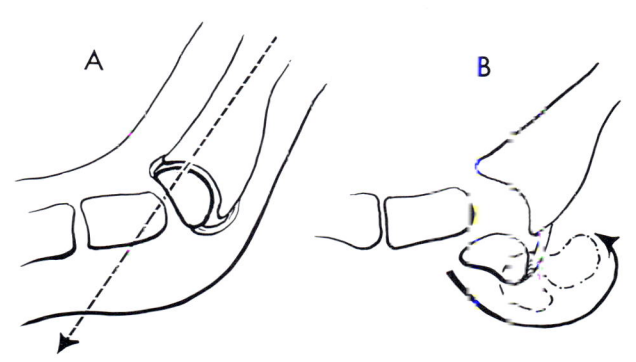

Fig. 22-12.—Dislocation of lunate—practically always to volar side and sometimes as much as 180 degrees. **A,** normal. **B,** dislocation.

Dislocation of the Lunate

Second in frequency of carpal bone injuries is dislocation of the lunate bone. This injury occurs most commonly in young adult males. The mechanism of production usually is sharp dorsiflexion of the wrist, secondary to a fall on the hand. The displacement practically always is toward the palm, and the degree of dislocation varies from a slight tilt to complete volar rotation of 180 degrees or more (Fig. 22-12). At Massachusetts General Hospital the lunate has not been seen displaced toward the dorsum except in those cases in which the injury was associated with other carpal fractures or dislocations.

The symptoms and signs are pain and swelling distal to that seen in Colles' fractures but quite similar to that manifested by fracture of the navicula, and so

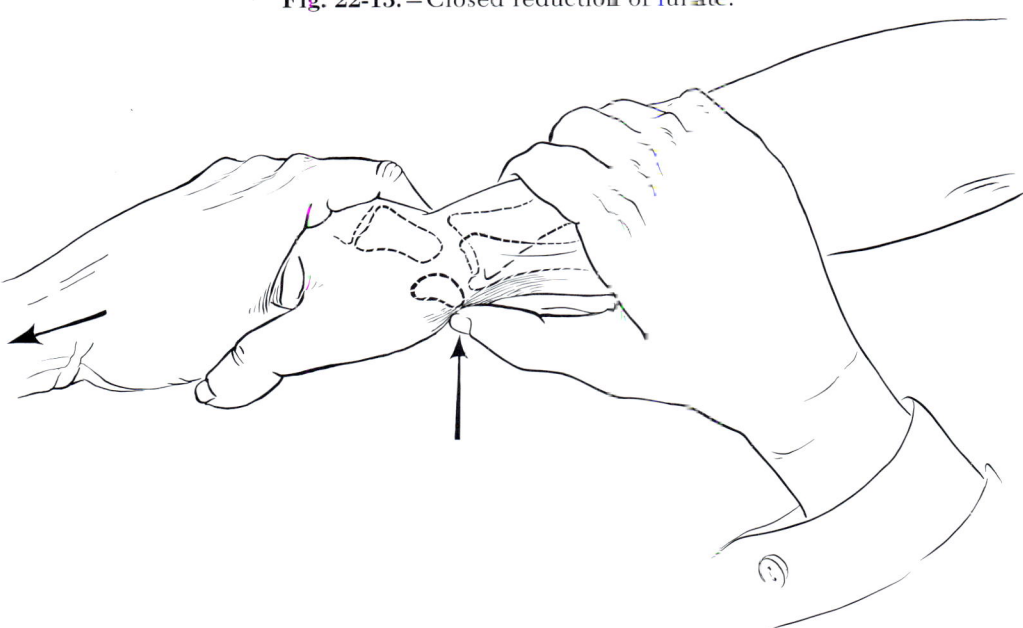

Fig. 22-13.—Closed reduction of lunate.

an accurate diagnosis cannot be made without roentgenograms.

The important x-ray view is a true lateral projection, but other routine exposures should be made to rule out associated fractures or subluxations of the carpus. Usually the dislocation is uncomplicated.

CLOSED REDUCTION.—Immediate reduction should be attempted. If manipulation is delayed longer than a few hours, the wrist will become swollen and tense, making any closed maneuver difficult. For anesthesia, the choice lies between brachial block and a general anesthetic in order to produce maximal relaxation.

Method of reduction.—With manual traction on the fingers and countertraction on the flexed elbow (Fig. 22-13), the carpus is distracted from the radius and ulna. As this is done, the wrist is brought into dorsiflexion and the operator's thumb is placed on the dislocated lunate, which is pushed back into place. As traction is maintained, the wrist is brought down into moderate palmar flexion. Before any splinting is applied, portable x-ray films are taken; if reduction has been accomplished, anterior and posterior plaster slabs are applied and held with a supporting bandage for 2 weeks.

TREATMENT OF OLD DISLOCATIONS.—If treatment has been delayed for longer than a few days, manipulation may be unsuccessful, in which case open replacement or possibly excision of the bone is indicated.

Fig. 22-14.—Dorsal approach to carpus. **A,** longitudinal skin approach between radial styloid and dorsal prominence on radius. **B,** exposure of dorsal tendons. **C,** incision into capsule. **D,** exposure of navicula and lunate.

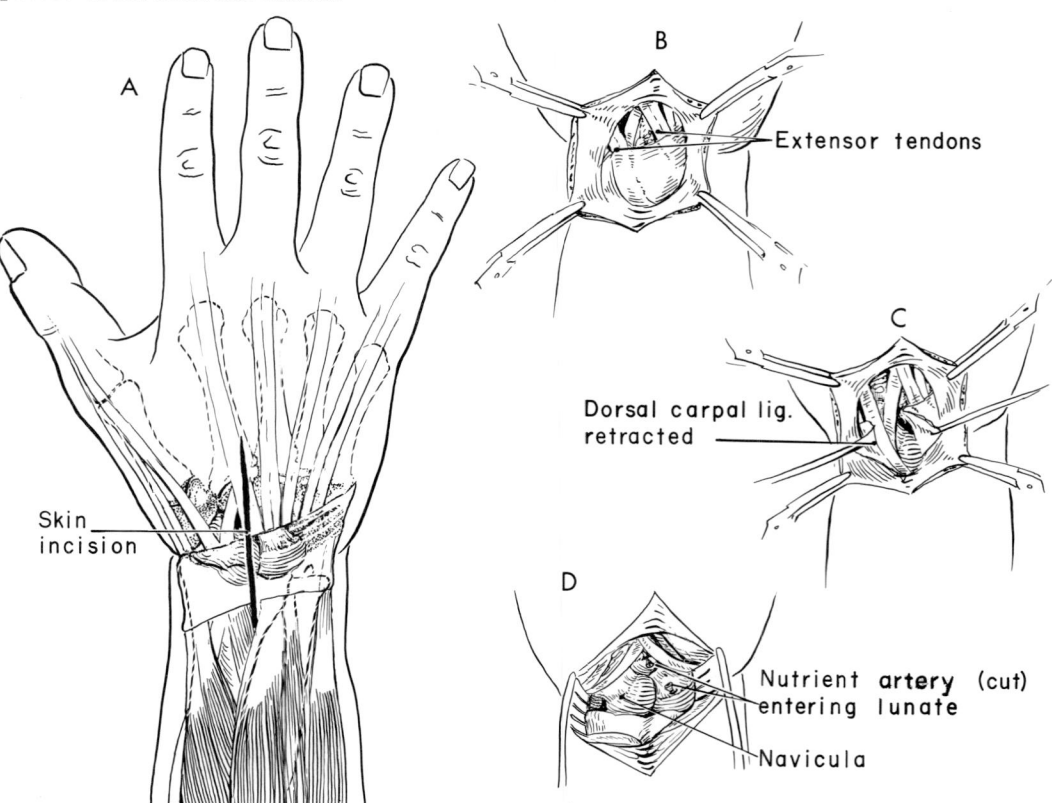

If reasonable attempts at manipulation have failed, the surgeon should proceed at once with an open operation. It is best to use a pneumatic tourniquet on the arm. If replacement of the bone is contemplated, a dorsal incision should be used in order to clear the space formerly occupied by the lunate (Fig. 22-14). The skilled surgeon may be able to accomplish this operation through a transverse incision, but if doubt exists as to the possible exposure, a longitudinal approach should be used. Occasionally, incisions on both the dorsal and volar surfaces are necessary.

If the surgeon believes that replacement of the bone is impossible because of scar tissue, he may elect to excise the bone. This is accomplished best by means of a transverse volar incision through a crease in the wrist. The structures encountered are the transverse carpal ligament, under which lie the palmaris longus tendon and the median nerve, and the flexor tendons. These are retracted, the joint capsule is opened and the displaced lunate is easily excised by dividing its remaining ligamentous attachments.

LATE EFFECTS OF LUNATE DISLOCATION. — If the lunate can be carefully replaced (Fig. 22-15), it practically always survives despite the severe ligament laceration and partial interruption of blood supply associated with the injury. Aseptic necrosis (Fig. 22-16) of the bone or traumatic arthritis, or both, are possible late complications to be anticipated. If either does occur, excision of the lunate, or possibly wrist fusion, may have to be done.

Kienböck's Disease of the Lunate[22]

The term "Kienböck's disease" indicates a condition in which the lunate undergoes a slow, progressive but incomplete degeneration with absorption of necrotic bone lamellae, followed by fibrous-tissue replacement (Fig. 22-17). The condition is not common. Fewer than 100 cases have been recorded in the literature. It is probable, however, that often the diagnosis is not made because the symptoms frequently are not severe and, unless roentgenograms are taken, the disease is not recognized.

ETIOLOGY. — Severe trauma is not necessary to produce necrosis of the lunate. In 3 of 9 cases at Massachusetts General Hospital there was a history of a direct blow resulting in immediate acute disability, and in 2 other cases in this series there was no known injury. In all 9 cases, however, partial necrosis of the lunate

Fig. 22-15. — Open reduction of lunate through dorsal incision, using Davis skid. **A**, lunate. **B**, capitate.

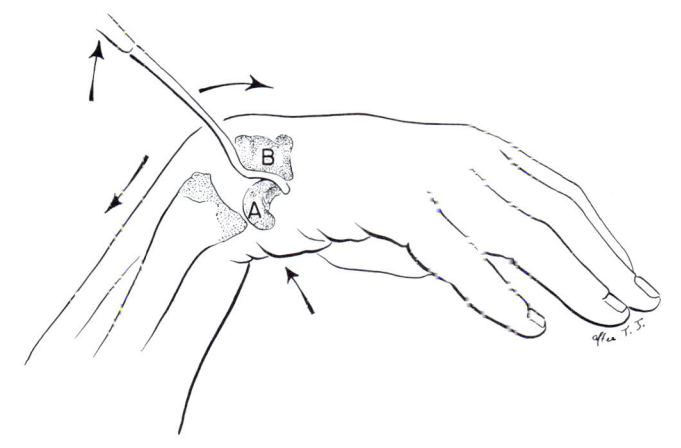

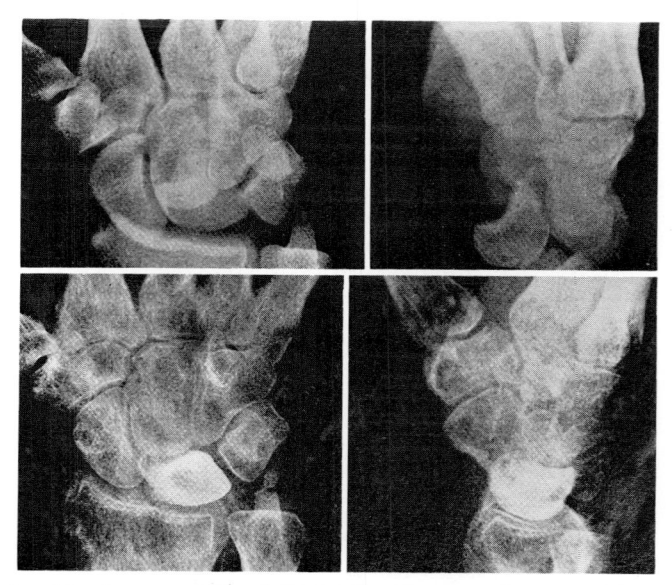

Fig. 22-16.—Kienböck's disease following dislocation of lunate. **Top,** anteroposterior and lateral views showing the dislocation, which was promptly reduced by manipulation. **Bottom,** same views 2 years later, showing aseptic necrosis of lunate. (Although this illustration is far from perfect, it is reproduced because of the unique character of the case.) (From Cave, E. F.: Kienböck's disease of the lunate, J. Bone Joint Surg. 21:858, 1939.)

Fig. 22-17.—Kienböck's disease of the lunate (lateral and anteroposterior views). Note compression of lunate bone.

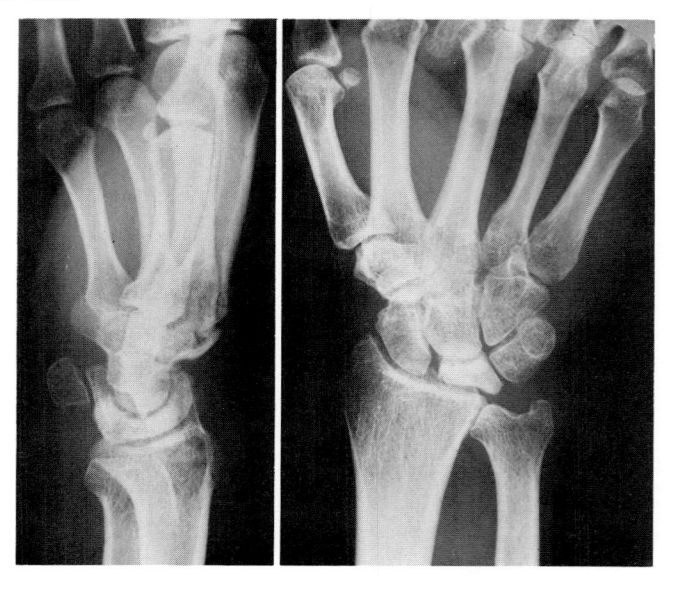

resulted. The nature of the trauma may be a crushing force applied to the bone, resulting in a fracture of the bony contour, or simply a contusion of the cartilaginous surfaces. Or there may be a subluxation of the bone, which reduces spontaneously but results in tearing of the dorsal ligament and subsequent interruption of the blood supply, followed by aseptic necrosis of the bone. In a series of 19 cases of dislocation of the lunate, there was only 1 case in which Kienböck's disease subsequently developed. McBride[24] reported 8 cases of old palmar dislocation of this bone, and Kienböck's disease did not develop in any. In 1 of his cases, the dislocation had been present for 3 years.

PATHOLOGY. — In 1 case at Massachusetts General Hospital, the report on the microscopic sections was as follows:

Much of the articular surface is essentially negative, although patchy degeneration is evident (Fig. 22-18). Immediately subjacent to the cartilage, however along one entire edge of the bone, penetrating its substance for about one half of its diameter, there is an extensive necrotic process. This varies considerably in its appearance. There are foci with complete necrosis consisting entirely of amorphous eosinophilic substance with relatively little exudative reaction. The undersurface of the articular cartilage shows discrete shaggy areas of chondrolysis. Elsewhere in the osseous substance there are spicules of nonvital bone and an occasional focus of apparently new bone formation. Save for the region of complete necrosis, the involved marrow substance exhibits dense fibrosis associated with a variable degree of lymphocytic and phagocytic infiltration. Several groups of foreign-body giant cells are observed.

ROENTGENOGRAPHIC APPEARANCE. — The changes usually are more marked at the proximal portion of the bone. In the anteroposterior view, early cyst formation and irregularity of the radial surface may be seen, with some localized areas poor in calcium and others showing a marked increase in calcium content. As the disease progresses, the bone becomes more dense, smaller and irregular in outline, taking on the appearance of a sequestrum. Usually it remains in this state — a dead bone. In certain patients, the destroyed portion of the bone be-

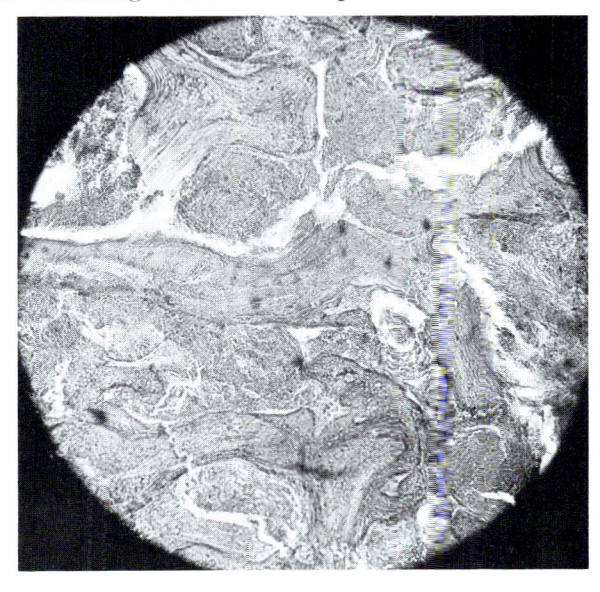

Fig. 22-18. — Pathologic section from a patient with Kienböck's disease.

comes fragmented. In the lateral roentgenogram, the density of the bone is increased and the proximodistal diameter of the bone is lessened whereas the anteroposterior diameter is increased.

SYMPTOMS AND SIGNS. — The onset of the disease is insidious. Frequently there is no history of injury that the patient can recall. Other patients remember that their symptoms began with a severe strain of the wrist while lifting a heavy object; still others give a history of a direct blow on the wrist or a fall on the hand with the wrist in dorsiflexion. Characteristically, the disease occurs in young males who do heavy work. There may be a slow but definite increase in pain, moderate stiffness and thickening of the wrist joint. All symptoms are made worse by use of the wrist and improve with its rest and support. Sudden forced motions may bring on severe pain.

On examination, the wrist is found to be moderately swollen and thickened in the anteroposterior diameter. Thickening is most marked over the dorsum of the wrist in the central portion. Local tenderness usually is acute and sharply localized to the center of the dorsum of the wrist. The amount of limitation of motion varies greatly in the individual case. In the acute stage, active motion in any direction may be painful, and passive motion may be carried out only to a moderate degree. Dorsiflexion and palmar flexion are the motions most likely to be restricted, and in the cases seen at Massachusetts General Hospital, ulnar deviation was more limited than motion to the radial side. Making a complete fist often is impossible.

DIAGNOSIS. — The diagnosis of Kienböck's disease depends primarily on the roentgenogram, for the history and examination only arouse suspicions of the lesion. The changes from the normal are confined to the lunate. The condition conceivably may be confused with tuberculosis. Tuberculosis, however, does not remain confined to a single bone of the carpus; with this disease there probably is more generalized atrophy of the bones of the hand and the wrist. Also, in tuberculosis there usually is more synovitis of the wrist joint and possibly evidence of tuberculosis elsewhere in the body.

TREATMENT. — If the diagnosis is made early, and before the degenerative changes in the bone have become advanced, conservative measures consisting of support from a plaster or leather wristlet may help to restore nutrition to the bone and to prevent advance of the process. When the bone is permanently deformed, however, and has the appearance of an irregular sequestrum, or when it has disintegrated, the only logical form of treatment is excision (Fig. 22-19). This operation should be done with great care in order to avoid trauma to surrounding structures. If the changes have remained confined to the lunate — that is, if traumatic arthritis of the wrist joint has not developed — we may expect good recovery of the wrist-joint function with little or no pain after the diseased lunate has been carefully removed.

Gillespie[17] describes 88% excellent or good results in excision of the lunate in Kienböck's disease. These results appear to be as good as those reported by Agerholm and Goodfellow[3] with prosthetic replacement of the lunate for avascular necrosis. There appears to be little advantage in prosthetic replacement compared with excision alone. The early results of dorsal flap arthroplasty after excision of the lunate as described by Nahigian et al.[28] appear promising in relieving pain sufficiently to allow light work activities.

Retrolunar Dislocation of the Capitate with Fracture or Subluxation of the Navicula

Dislocation of the capitate bone with fracture or subluxation of the navicula was third in frequency of occurrence in a series of 218 cases of carpal injuries treated at Massachusetts General Hospital.

Chapter 22: INJURIES TO THE CARPAL BONES / 543

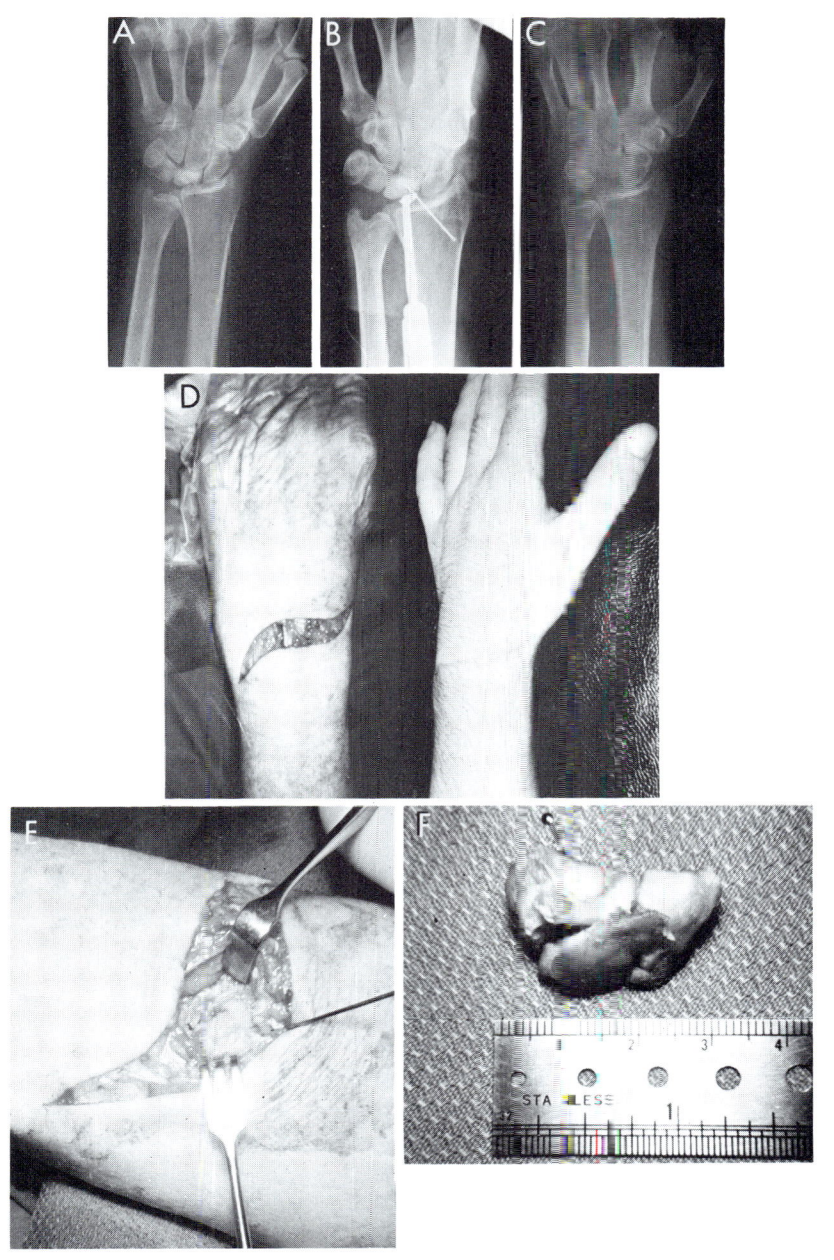

Fig. 22-19.—Kienböck's disease of the carpal lunate bone. Pain in the wrist following a fall on the outstretched hand 1 year prior to admission. No previous treatment. **A,** anteroposterior view, showing aseptic necrosis of the lunate bone. **B,** at the time of operation. Lunate is identified by portable x-ray film. The spatula is in place for removal of the lunate. **C,** appearance of wrist after complete removal of lunate bone. **D,** surgical approach through the dorsum of the wrist. Needle is in lunate. **E,** appearance of lunate at the time of operation. **F,** the excised lunate, showing partial disintegration. Patient obtained an essentially painless wrist but slight restriction of motion.

MECHANISM.—Retrolunar dislocation of the capitate, sometimes referred to as "transcarpal dislocation," is produced by a blow that suddenly forces the hand into dorsiflexion. The most common type of injury is a fall on the outstretched hand. The force may be transmitted through the third metacarpal or may be received directly by the distal portion of the capitate. The dislocation of the capitate always is accompanied by a fracture of the navicular bone or rotation luxation of this bone (Fig. 22-20). Usually, great force is required to bring about such an injury. When the injury occurs, the ligamentous structures between the lunate and the capitate are ruptured and the blood supply is interrupted. The lunate retains its

Fig. 22-20.—Severe carpal injury, secondary to fall on outstretched hand. Injuries sustained: retrolunar dislocation of the capitate, displaced fracture of the navicular bone and fracture of the radial styloid. Treated by attempt at manipulation and traction. This failed (**A**). Kirschner wire inserted for skeletal traction. Open reduction through dorsal incision (see Fig. 22-14). Result: reduction of displaced capitate to articular surface of lunate; replacement of the navicular fracture. Stability maintained by threaded Kirschner wire through the articular surface, proximal portion of the proximal fragment of the navicular bone, while traversing the fracture line. Also, maintaining reduction of the dislocation and the radial styloid fracture (**B**). Although the dislocation is replaced satisfactorily, there remains nonunion of the navicular bone. Primary grafting would have been the treatment of choice.

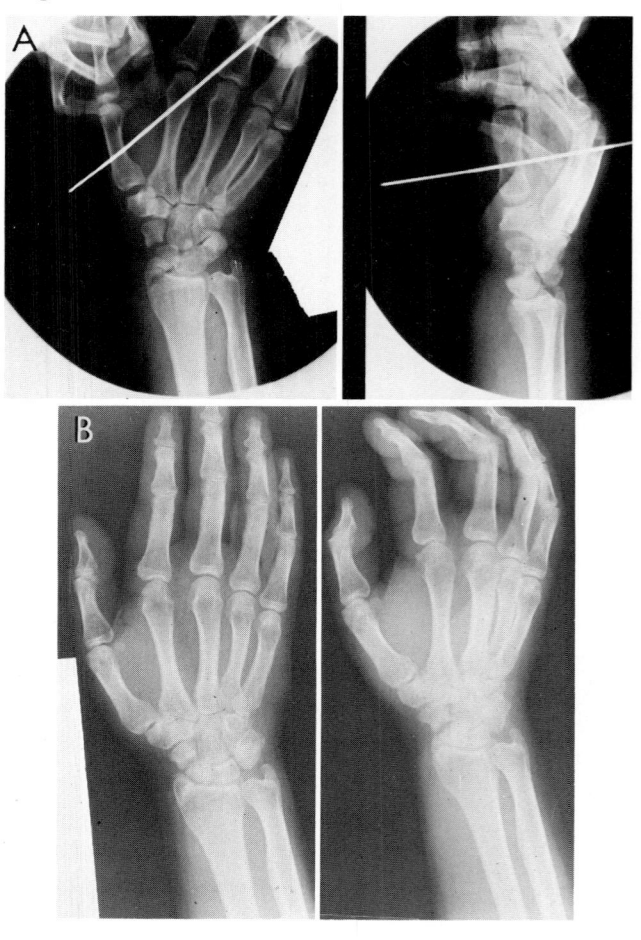

Chapter 22: INJURIES TO THE CARPAL BONES / 545

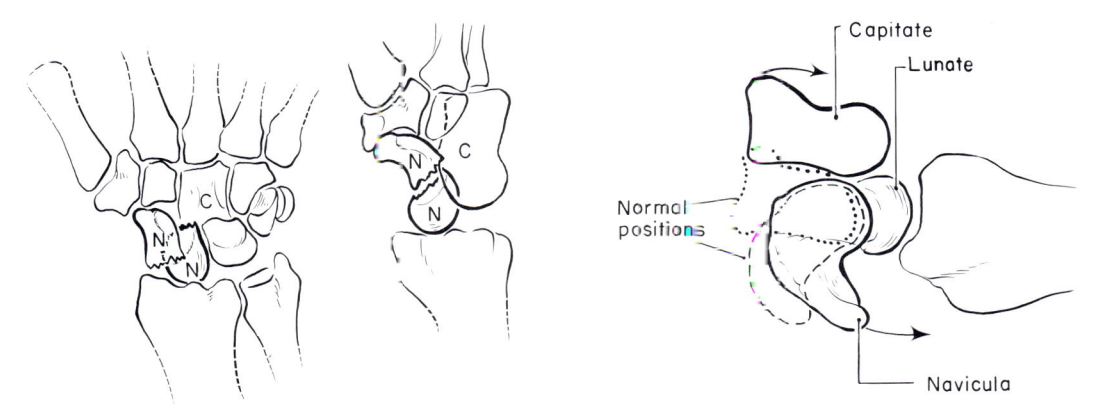

Fig. 22-21.—**Left,** retrolunar dislocation of capitate (*C*) with fracture of navicula (*N*). **Right,** retrolunar dislocation of capitate with rotation of navicula. Note that capitate is dorsal to lunate, which maintains its normal relationship to radius.

Fig. 22-22.—Retrolunar dislocation of capitate with fracture of navicula. Treated by closed reduction of capitate and by open reduction and graft fixation of navicula. **A,** anteroposterior views of the injured and uninjured wrist. **B,** lateral views of the injured and uninjured wrist (*L,* lunate; *C,* capitate). **C,** end-result 1 year later; bone union of navicula and excellent return of function.

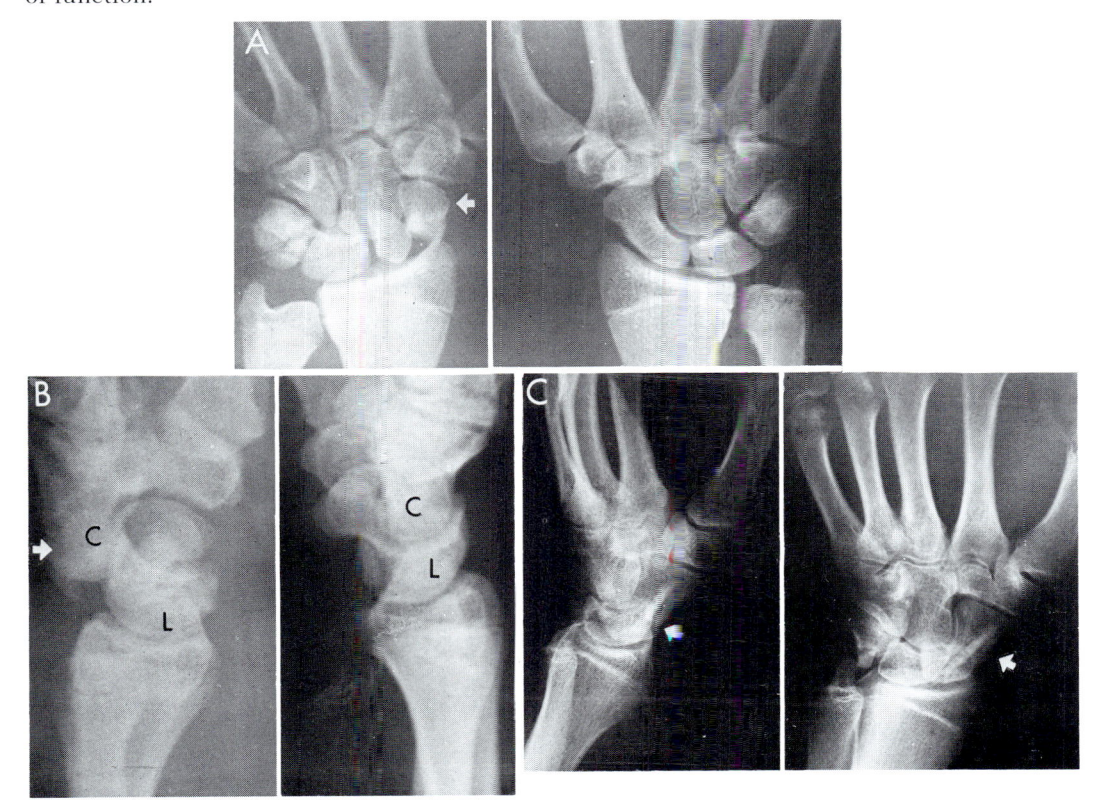

normal relationship to the radius, or it may be tilted slightly toward the palmar surface (Fig. 22-21). The capitate is displaced dorsally to the lunate bone. At the same time, because of the shortening of the distance between the radius and the second row of the carpus, the navicula must either fracture transversely or rotate through its long axis (Fig. 22-22). If the navicula has been fractured, the distal portion of the bone moves dorsally and upward with the displaced capitate whereas the proximal fragment continues to maintain its normal relationship to the radius. More frequently, the navicula may be subluxated rather than fractured; rarely is it completely dislocated.

DIAGNOSIS.—As with all other carpal injuries, the diagnosis is based entirely on the roentgenograms. Standard exposures should be made. Retrolunar dislocation of the capitate frequently is confused with dislocation of the lunate bone.

TREATMENT.—With this injury, immediate closed reduction is indicated by traction in hyperextension, then in extension and finally in flexion. The earlier the maneuver is attempted after injury the more likely it is to succeed. If it is delayed beyond a few days, open reduction may be necessary (Fig. 22-23), and if many days or weeks have passed, even an operation may fail to replace the bones to their normal positions. If closed reduction is successful, immobilization with an anterior splint for 10 days is sufficient unless there is an associated fracture of the navicula, in which case immobilization must be prolonged until union of the navicula is complete. If there has been only rotation luxation associated with the capitate dislocation, 10 days of immobilization is sufficient, as in the following case, treated at Massachusetts General Hospital.

A 37-year-old man was admitted to the emergency ward with a retrolunar dislocation of the capitate, rotation luxation of the navicula and fracture of the ulnar and radial styloids, following an automobile accident (Fig. 22-24). Reduction had been attempted under ether anesthesia but had failed. Five days later an incision was made over the dorsal aspect of the wrist. The capitate was found to be displaced backward on the lunate, and the navicula was rotated so that it occupied partially the normal position of the capitate. The capitate was reduced to its normal relationship with the lunate, and this brought the navicula into normal position. A plaster splint was discarded at the end of 2 weeks. One year later the patient was working at his old job. He had no pain; motions were three-quarters normal and still improving.

Treatment of retrolunar dislocation of the capitate with fracture of the navicula.—When, in addition to the dislocation of the capitate, there is a fracture of the navicula, the fracture may reduce spontaneously as the displaced capitate is restored to its normal position, but if accurate reposition of the navicular fragment is not obtained, open reduction should be done and the fragments of the navicula should be realigned and held with a dowel graft (see Fig. 22-21).

The graft operation must be performed within a few days; otherwise, it may be impossible to realign the navicular fragments satisfactorily, even though the dislocation of the capitate may have been reduced. If it is necessary to reduce the dislocation of the capitate by open operation as well as to graft the navicula, a bayonet type of incision is used. Postoperative fixation in plaster in this type of injury should be carried out until union of the navicula is complete.

Treatment of old retrolunar dislocation of the capitate with or without fracture of the navicular bone.—The old dislocation probably cannot be treated satisfactorily by attempting to restore normal position of the carpal bones. The surgeon must choose between (1) excision of the lunate and navicular bones and (2) wrist fusion. Excision of these two bones may result in improved motion and less pain in the wrist but will produce a weakened wrist, probably necessitating the use of

Chapter 22: INJURIES TO THE CARPAL BONES / 547

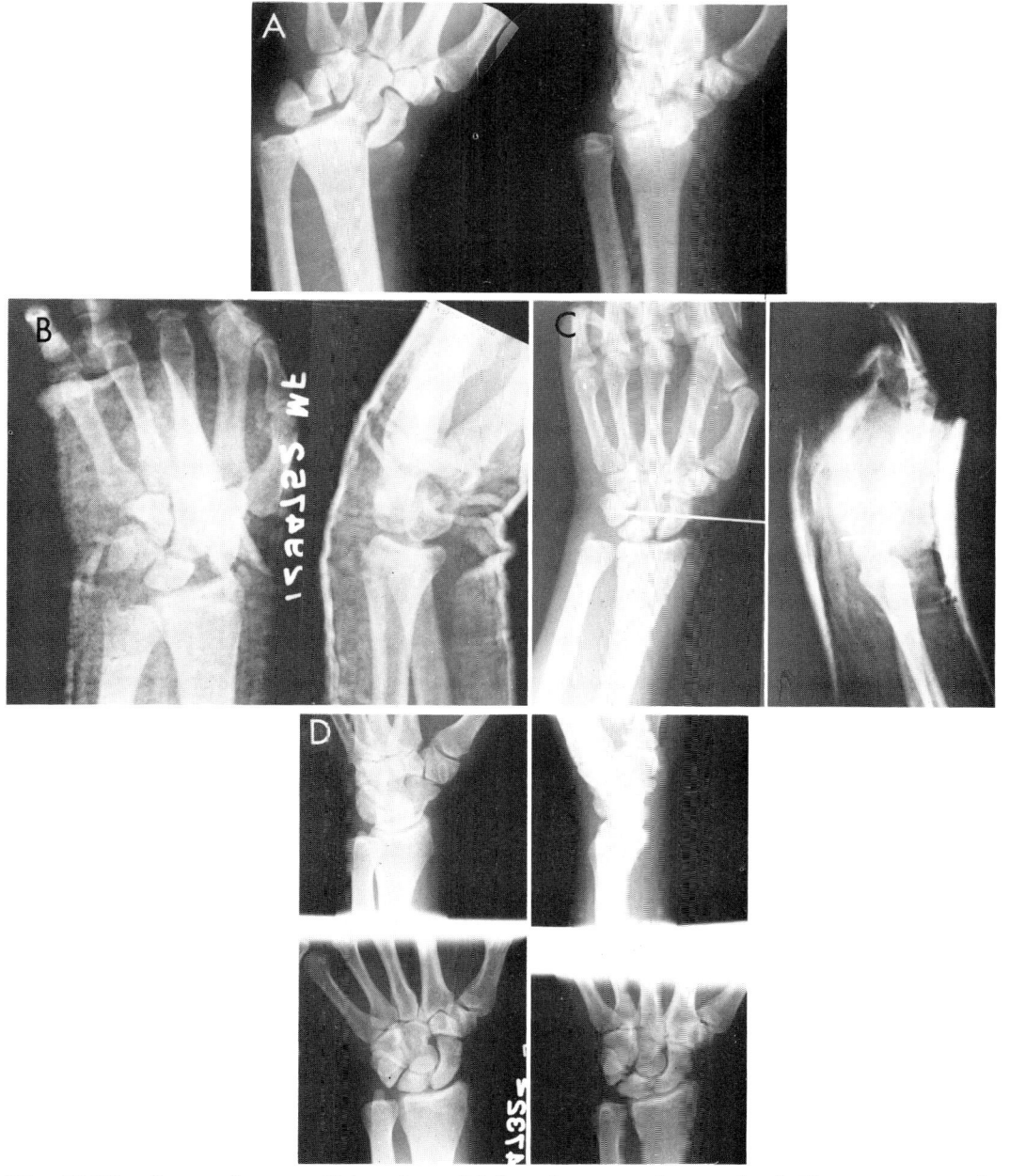

Fig. 22-23.—Severe fracture-dislocation of left wrist, secondary to football injury. Patient's wrist was crushed under a pile of players. Injuries sustained: radial dislocation of carpus and fracture of radial styloid (**A**). Treatment: attempt at closed reduction, revealing successful replacement of radial carpal articulation but persistent retrolunar dislocation of the capitate (**B**). Following open reduction with replacement of capitate to normal articulation with lunate. Stabilization by a Kirschner wire inserted through the navicular bone into capitate (**C**). End result 4 years after injury, revealing normal appearance of all carpal bones (**D**).

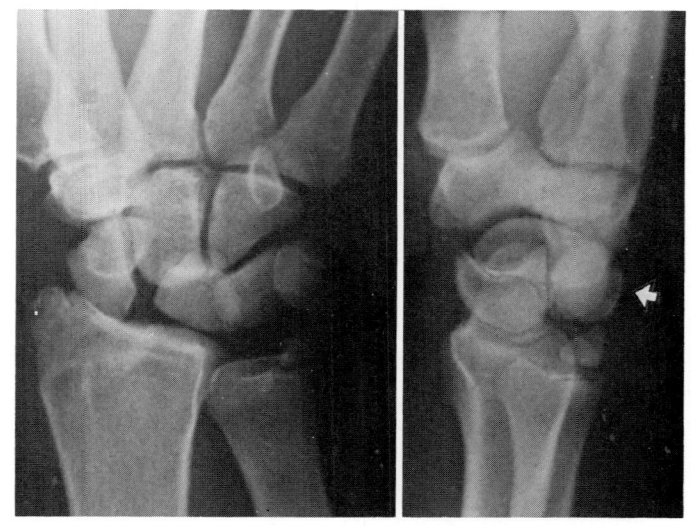

Fig. 22-24.—Anteroposterior and lateral views showing retrolunar dislocation of capitate *(arrow)*, rotation subluxation of navicula and fracture of radial and ulnar styloids.

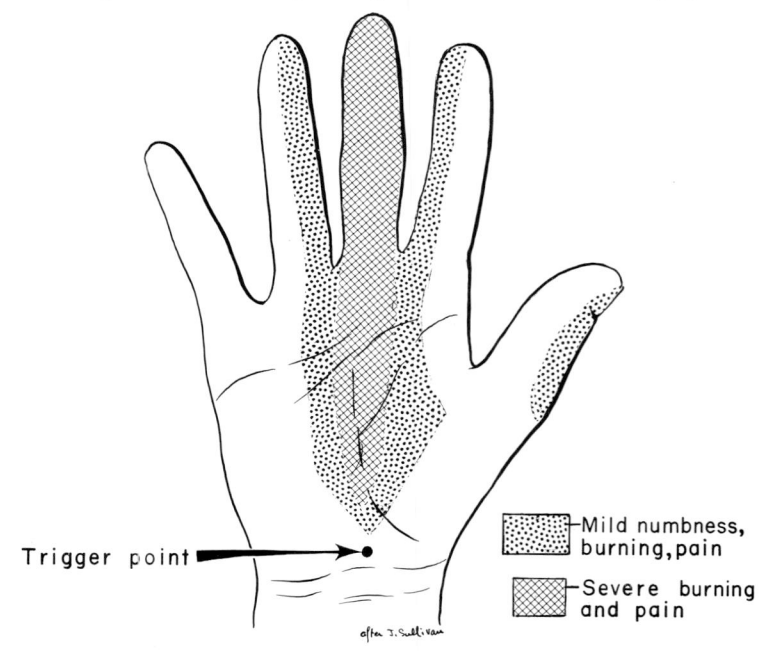

Fig. 22-25.—Sensory changes with median-nerve injury.

Chapter 22: INJURIES TO THE CARPAL BONES / 549

external support for heavy work. Wrist fusion is the alternative to the excision operation. Fusion will produce strength, and, although motion in dorsiflexion and palmar flexion will be eliminated, pronation and supination can be maintained, since fusion is carried out only between the radius and the carpus.

Traumatic Neuritis of the Median Nerve

A rare but very painful complication of wrist injuries is traumatic neuritis of the median nerve (Fig. 22-25). The injury occurs at the volar aspect of the wrist as the nerve is compressed between the transverse carpal ligament and the radius or carpus. Usually the difficulty is manifested only by a transitory numbness in the hand, and it may be short-lived after injury and manipulation of the wrist. This symptom requires no treatment because it usually disappears after days or weeks and does not recur.

In an occasional case, however, symptoms of pain and burning in the palm may be extremely severe and may require immediate attention. The onset may be gradual or immediate. In one patient, the pain came on overnight, even though the wrist injury was of long standing. An examination of the wrist and hand may reveal little except for moderate fullness of the hand owing to misuse. On palpation directly over the course of the nerve under the level of the carpal ligament, the pain and burning are aggravated. Percussion in this area produces "shock-

Fig. 22-26.—Approach to median nerve.

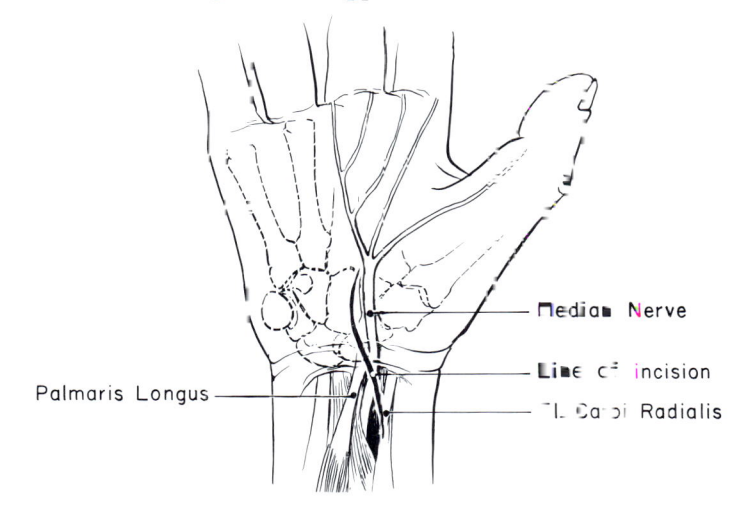

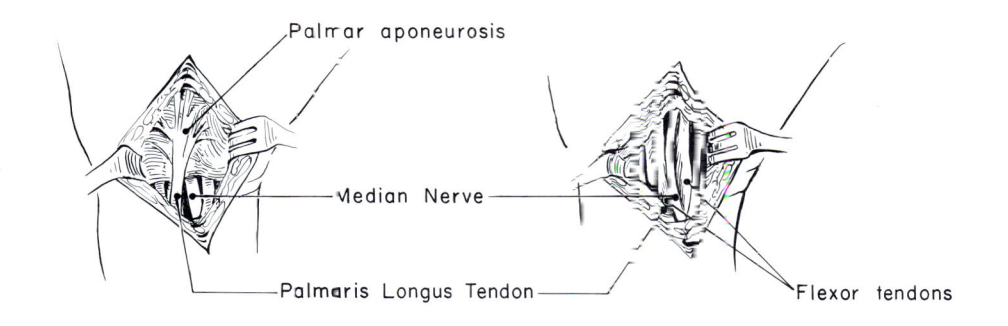

like" sensations into the palm (Tinel's sign). The x-ray film may show evidence of old injury, possibly with excess bone production on the volar aspect of the wrist.

If pain and burning are severe and persistent, division of the transverse carpal ligament gives complete and immediate relief (Fig. 22-26). If there has been motor weakness of the muscles supplied by the median nerve, recovery may be prolonged. Cannon and Love[10] of the Mayo Clinic reported their observations on 38 cases in 1946. They emphasized the necessity to distinguish the lesion from conditions involving the cervical portion of the spinal cord, such as protruding cervical disks, cervical ribs, neuritis of the brachial plexus and progressive muscle atrophy. The outstanding symptoms and signs in their cases were paresthesia, pain, atrophy, sensory impairment and muscle weakness in the hand. Operation was performed in 9 of the 38 cases with satisfactory results. In several cases, true enlargement of the median nerve was found proximal to the transverse carpal ligament. In a further personal communication, Cannon[9] has written:

Twenty-two cases of tardy median palsy were carefully studied as to etiology. Eleven of these were corrected by division of the transverse carpal ligament. Many factors, such as external trauma, bone deformity, arthritis and acromegaly, seemingly contributed to the pathogenesis of this entity. Observations on this group of cases, however, implicated nocturnal or early-morning swelling of the hands as the important factor in initiating median nerve compression. This swelling, along with numbness and paresthesia in the hands, comprised the symptom complex of "waking numbness," a condition apparently due to intermittent vascular compression at pectoral level. "Waking numbness" was characteristically present in these cases and appeared as the precursor of the median nerve constriction found within the carpal tunnel.

Combined Wrist Injuries

Severe trauma to the wrist may result in a combination of injuries, some of which are illustrated in Figures 22-27

Fig. 22-27.—Anteroposterior and lateral views showing a severe carpal and wrist joint injury due to a fall on the wrist from a height of 10 feet. Injuries are: (1) fracture of proximal portion of navicula; (2) fracture of radial styloid; (3) retrolunar dislocation of capitate; and (4) fracture of ulnar styloid.

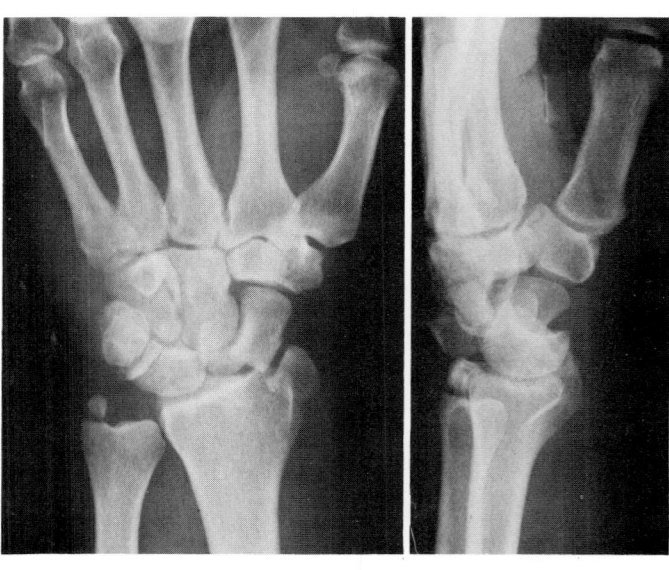

Chapter 22: INJURIES TO THE CARPAL BONES / 551

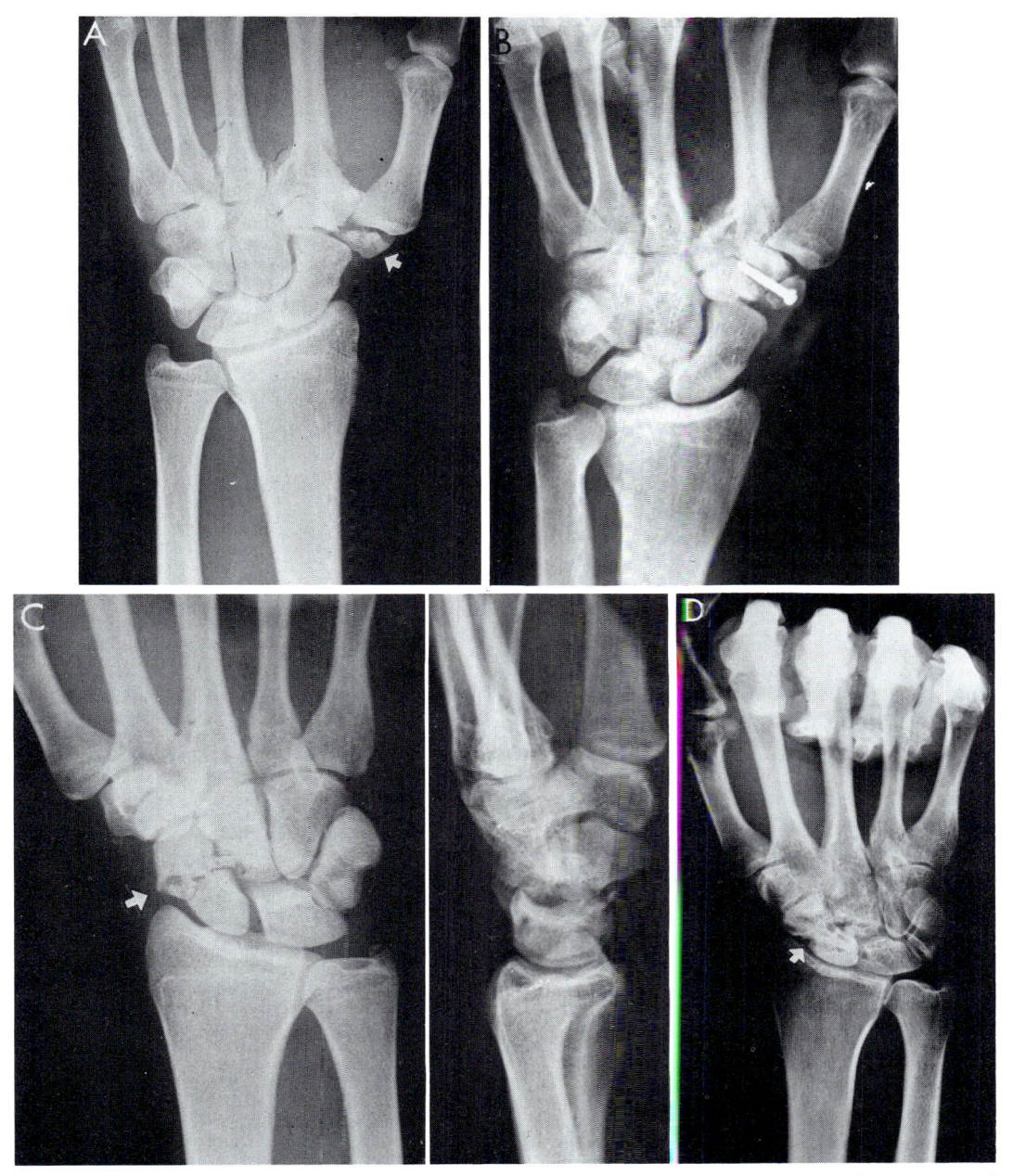

Fig. 22-28.—**A**, fracture of greater multangular bone (*arrow*) associated with dislocation of base of first metacarpal and fracture of base of second metacarpal. **B**, correction of multangular fracture and dislocated first metacarpal by open reduction and screw fixation of greater multangular. **C**, anteroposterior and lateral views of fracture of navicula of opposite wrist in same patient. **D**, after treatment by open reduction and tibial bone graft.

and 22-28. There may be associated fractures and dislocations of the carpus along with fractures of the radius or ulna or both. Such combined injuries require more than ordinary experience in the interpretation of the roentgenograms. It is well to emphasize again the absolute necessity to make films in the various projections described (see Fig. 22-3) and to include the opposite wrist for comparison. No one method can be recommended for handling such complicated injuries, but, in general, the following principles are applicable:

1. If there is an open wound, it should be debrided and sutured, if possible.

2. In general, closed manipulation should be tried.

3. If a closed maneuver is not successful and if the surgeon believes that there is a reasonable chance to gain a stable reduction by open operation, surgery is justified.

4. If open replacement and stability are not possible, excision of fragments or an entire carpal bone may be justified, but experience has shown that excision of the first carpal row does not give a strong, painless wrist.

5. In the very severe injuries, when replacement and stability are not possible and when trauma to cartilaginous surfaces is great, fusion between the radius and the carpus may give the best result—that is, a strong and painless wrist with dorsiflexion and palmar flexion eliminated but pronation and supination preserved.

With a combination of injuries involving the carpal bones and other injuries to the upper extremity, it is important to evaluate carefully, by physical and x-ray examination, the shoulder, the elbow and the wrist in order to rule out the possible associated fractures or dislocations.

BIBLIOGRAPHY

1. Adams, J. D.: Displacement of the semilunar carpal bone: An analysis of twelve cases, J. Bone Joint Surg. 7:665, 1925.
2. Adams, J. D., and Leonard, R. D.: Fracture of the carpal scaphoid: A new method of treatment with a report of one case, N. Engl. J. Med. 198:401, 1928.
3. Agerholm, J. C., and Goodfellow, J. W.: Avascular necrosis of the lunate bone treated by excision and prosthetic replacement, J. Bone Joint Surg. 45-B:110, 1963.
4. Barnard, L., and Stubbins, S. G.: Styloidectomy of the radius in the surgical treatment of nonunion of the carpal navicular: A preliminary report, J. Bone Joint Surg. 30-A:98, 1948.
5. Barr, J. S., Elliston, W. A., Musnick, H., DeLorme, T. L., Hanelin, J., and Thibodeau, A. A.: Fracture of the carpal navicular (scaphoid) bone: An end-result study in military personnel, J. Bone Joint Surg. 35-A:609, 1953.
6. Böhler, L.: Konservative oder operative Therapie der Fraktur der Os naviculare carpi?, Wien. Med. Wochenschr. 85:1085, 1935.
7. Böhler, L.: *The Treatment of Fractures* (trans. by E. W. Hey Groves) (4th English ed.; Baltimore: William Wood & Company, 1935).
8. Burnett, J. H.: Fracture of the (navicular) carpal scaphoid, Surg. Gynecol. Obstet. 60:529, 1935.
9. Cannon, B. W.: Personal communication.
10. Cannon, B. W., and Love, J. G.: Tardy median palsy; median neuritis; median phenar neuritis amenable to surgery, Surgery 20:210, 1946.
11. Cave, E. F.: The carpus, with reference to the fractured navicular bone, Arch. Surg. 40:54, 1940.
12. Cave, E. F.: Kienböck's disease of the lunate, J. Bone Joint Surg. 21:858, 1939.
13. Cave, E. F.: Retrolunar dislocation of the capitate with fracture or subluxation of the navicular bone, J. Bone Joint Surg. 23:830, 1941.
14. Davis, G. G.: Treatment of dislocated semilunar carpal bones, Surg. Gynecol. Obstet. 37:225, 1923.
15. Dwight, T.: *A Clinical Atlas: Variations of the Bones of the Hands and Feet* (Philadelphia: J. B. Lippincott Company, 1907).
16. Finsterer, H.: Zur Kasuistik und Therapie der Verrenkungen des Mondbeins, Beitr. klin. Chir. 62:496, 1909.
17. Gillespie, H. S.: Excision of lunate bone in Kienböck's disease, J. Bone Joint Surg. 43-B:245, 1961.
18. Goldsmith, R.: Kienböck's disease of the semilunar bone, Ann. Surg. 81:857, 1925.
19. Hess, A. F., and Abramson, H.: Familial retardation in ossification of the carpal centers, J. Pediatr. 3:158, 1933.
20. Hirsch, M.: Konservative oder operative Therapie der Fraktur der Os naviculare carpi?, Wien. Med. Wochenschr. 85:803, 1935.
21. Johnson, R. W., Jr.: A study of the healing processes in injuries to the carpal scaphoid, J. Bone Joint Surg. 9:482, 1927.
22. Kienböck, R.: Über traumatische Malazie des Mondbeins and ihre Folgezustände: Entartungsformen und Kompressionsfrakturen, Fortschr. Geb. Röntgenstrahlen 16:77, 1910.
23. MacAusland, W. R.: Perilunar dislocation of the carpal bones and dislocation of the lunate bone, Surg. Gynecol. Obstet. 79:256, 1944.
24. McBride, E. D.: Dislocation of the carpal semilunar bone: A report of eight cases, M. J. & Rec. 124:82, 1926.
25. McBride, E. D.: Dislocation of the semilunar

bone: Neuroplastic fixation of the hand, a deformity characteristic of the injury, Arch. Surg. 14:584, 1927.
26. Mouat, T. B., Wilkie, J., and Harding, H. E.: Isolated fracture of the carpal semilunar and Kienböck's disease, Br. J. Surg. 19:577, 1932.
27. Murray, G.: End results of bone-grafting for nonunion of the carpal navicular, J. Bone Joint Surg. 28:749, 1946.
28. Nahigian, S. H., Li, C. S., Richey, D. G., and Shaw, D. T.: The dorsal flap arthroplasty in the treatment of Kienböck's disease, J. Bone Joint Surg. 52-A:245, 1970.
29. Soto-Hall, R., and Haldeman, K. O.: Treatment of fractures of the carpal scaphoid, J. Bone Joint Surg. 16:822, 1934.
30. Speed, K.: Fractures of the carpal navicular bone, J. Bone Joint Surg. 7:682, 1925.
31. Speed, K.: Fractures of the carpus, J. Bone Joint Surg. 17:965, 1935.
32. Speed, K.: Small bone repair, Surg. Gynecol. Obstet. 64:9, 1937.
33. Steele, F. B.: Personal communication.
34. Todd, A. H.: Fractures of the carpal scaphoid, Br. J. Surg. 9:7, 1921.

23 | Soft Tissue Injuries of the Hand

JOHN P. REMENSNYDER

HAND INJURIES are major problems in the lives of patients, as they affect their functioning as useful human beings. Who should treat hand injuries depends less on a surgeon's particular specialty than it does on his interest and willingness to equip himself properly to meet the acute and long-term challenges posed by this form of trauma. Management of hand injuries demands changes in pace and timing: acutely, one must think in terms of rapid small time units in an urgent sense; reconstructively, one must shift to a longer time base commensurate with a slower pace of such biologic events as wound healing, scar softening and joint mobilization. One must be able to visualize from start to finish not only the end result but also the many alternative pathways of getting there.

The sine qua non of the care of the acutely injured hand is gaining useful early healing. This chapter will focus on the period from initial injury through the operative care to the time of complete wound healing, at which point the patient has returned to normal activity or progressed to subsequent elective reconstruction.

NATURE OF HAND INJURIES

Hand injuries may be divided into four major groups:

1. EDEMA ONLY.—Examples of this are contusions, superficial burns, closed fractures, etc. Edema produces important effects on deeper structures, which are not always evident in the acute phase but may show up later in the form of secondary joint stiffness.

2. INCISED WOUNDS.—This group includes superficial lacerations of the skin only and deeper lacerations of tendon and nerve. Lacerations are one of the major pitfalls in caring for hand injuries, since a superficial laceration may hide a deeper injury to major tendons and nerves. Essential to the proper management of this type of wound is accurate, anatomic diagnosis of the function of the deep structures of the hand.

3. TISSUE LOSS.—There are several varieties, such as slicing injuries, crushing injuries, full-thickness burns and degloving injuries. The major problem is to diagnose accurately the extent of tissue injury and microvascular insult and to decide whether more tissue will be lost following the acute injury. For example, in crushing injury, one frequently has secondary tissue necrosis due to edema and ischemia, which produces more tissue loss in the days following injury.

4. OPEN INJURIES.—These include the most severe forms of hand injuries: blast wounds, crushes, avulsions and gunshot

wounds. In this group one sees injuries to all the tissues of the hand, each of which brings its own special problems to the surgeon undertaking repair.

PRINCIPLES OF REPAIR

In the over-all management of hand injuries there are certain general and specific principles underlying a sound approach to all. The approach to any hand injury should embody the following *general principles:*

1. Cleaning and debriding the wound in order to produce a healthy, well-vascularized wound.
2. Stabilizing skeletal structures, frequently by internal K-wire fixation.
3. Connecting vital structures, such as tendon and nerves, when indicated.
4. Providing appropriate coverage, usually by the simplest method possible.
5. Minimizing edema formation at each step.
6. Planning for future reconstruction at the time of initial injury. The final result should be envisioned at the time of injury so as to carry out any appropriate maneuvers early to lay the ground work for later reconstruction.

In the execution of any repair of major hand injury, the above general principles should be observed. In striving for these goals, several categories of *specific principles* should be observed.

1. HISTORY AND PHYSICAL EXAMINATION. — An accurate history of the injury should be obtained, including mechanism of injury, time prior to being seen and any treatment already carried out. In addition, other important elements of the history should include the handedness, age, prior injuries to either hand, general medical history and concomitant illness, medications and allergies, especially to local anesthesia and antibiotics. A general physical examination should be performed. Recorded examination of the hand should include a careful description and, when possible, a sketch or photograph of the general appearance and gross function of the hand. It is not necessary to expose the wound extensively or probe the wound in the emergency ward, since one should be able to determine much of the functional loss without undue wound exposure. Examination of the motor, sensory and vascular status of the hand should be recorded in detail and the history and physical examination on appropriate forms. X-ray films are indicated in virtually all hand injuries except the simplest of soft tissue injuries. These help in delineating fractures, dislocations and the presence of foreign bodies, as well as recording bone age in children, which may serve as a basis for following functional growth. Insurance companies frequently request x-ray films to help determine the nature of the patient's injuries. Special examinations, such as arteriography and graded functional hand evaluations, may be included when appropriate.

2. ANESTHESIA. — Skillful application of anesthesia permits the appropriate amount of time to be employed in the initial operative treatment of the hand. When anesthesia is not adequate, the surgeon cannot bring to bear his best effort in the initial operative treatment. Since there are several types of anesthetics that might be employed in the treatment of hand injuries, each with its varying duration, one would prefer to employ a technique giving somewhat more time than necessary rather than be caught short.

A small distal injury can be handled satisfactorily using a local anesthetic. Xylocaine in 2% concentration containing *no epinephrine* is suitable for a short anesthetic without tourniquet, giving 20–30 minutes. Adequate amounts infiltrated widely initially obviate the necessity for repetitive and uncomfortable injections. Ethyl chloride plays no role as a local anesthetic in acute hand injuries.

There are several regional conductive-type anesthetics that are effective. In injuries limited to a single digit, digital block carried out with 2% Xylocaine containing no epinephrine is highly satisfactory. Utilizing a single needle puncture with a #25 needle over the metacarpal head volarly, the digital nerve to each side of the finger may be infiltrated satisfactorily using approximately 1 ml of anesthetic. A field block at the midportion of the proximal phalanx dorsally blocks the more diffuse fibers of the dorsal innervation of each finger. Injuries limited to the median nerve distribution may be treated satisfactorily by blocking the median nerve at the wrist. Two per cent Xylocaine may be instilled satisfactorily around the median nerve, utilizing the landmarks of the flexor carpi radialis longus tendon and the palmaris longus. Care should be taken not to inject local anesthetic into the nerve itself. However, paresthesias elicited at the time of needle puncture are useful. When the lesion is confined to the ulnar nerve distribution, this may be treated using an ulnar nerve block at the level of the elbow. Radial nerve distribution is more difficult to block because of the diffuseness of the fibers. In the radial portion of the hand, sensory branches discrete enough to be blocked satisfactorily exist where the nerve crosses the extensor pollicis longus tendon just distal to the wrist crease.

An axillary block is used frequently, since many hand injuries are not confined to a single nerve area. The technique consists of carefully prepping the axilla of the patient with the arm in an abducted, externally rotated position. Palpating the brachial artery high in the arm against the head of the humerus, approximately 30 ml of a mixture of Pontocaine and Xylocaine is infiltrated around the brachial artery pulsation. In this fashion, each of the major nerves of the forearm may be anesthetized satisfactorily. At the completion of a satisfactory nerve block, a ring of anesthetic may be instilled around the upper arm if a tourniquet is to be employed. With the availability of axillary block anesthetic there is virtually no indication for a supraclavicular brachial block because of a significant incidence of the complication of pneumothorax. Recently, blocks at the interscalene level have been shown to be effective, but the occasional appearance of a cervical extra-dural block makes it mandatory that it be administered by a skilled anesthetist.[23]

Regional intravenous anesthesia is another satisfactory anesthetic for hand injuries. A double-tourniquet technique is used to trap Xylocaine in the venous system of the forearm and hand. The arm is exsanguinated after placement of an intravenous needle. Thirty to 40 ml of 0.5% Xylocaine is injected and the upper of the two cuffs inflated. After the arm is anesthetized, the lower cuff is inflated and the upper cuff deflated, leaving the inflated cuff in an anesthetic area. The duration is limited only by tourniquet time. At the conclusion of the procedure, occasional central effects have been noted if the unfixed anesthetic gains the general circulation. Observing the safeguard of a minimal time of 20 minutes to allow virtually complete fixation of the Xylocaine, almost no complications have been noted in the use of this technique at Massachusetts General Hospital in 10 years.[9, 14]

General anesthesia is preferred in most instances of extensive and complicated hand injuries. Although optimal regional anesthesia can give satisfactory anesthesia for up to 2 or 3 hours, many complicated hand injuries including those requiring primary flaps for closure, need longer periods and may involve incisions on other parts of the body. Prior to the induction of general anesthesia, the patient should be determined to be in good general health, have normal laboratory values of routine blood and urinalyses, have blood volume replaced and show evidence of an empty stomach. Appropriate premedication is indicated, as in any general anesthetic.

3. EQUIPMENT. – The hand represents a limited volume of tissue with many intri-

cately detailed bits of anatomy, and when attempting the repair of an acute hand injury, continued bleeding and oozing obscures the field. For this reason, a pneumatic tourniquet is employed to give a clear, dry field during repair. An exception is where the viability of large areas of tissue is in doubt; here, it probably is wiser not to limit circulation with the use of a tourniquet. Digits should not be subjected to tourniquet ischemia by use of a rubber band twisted around the base of the finger, which runs the risk of thrombosis due to direct injury of small vessels. If it is essential to have ischemia of the finger during the operative procedure, a broad 1-inch Penrose drain may be secured against the base of the finger with a large clamp. A large clamp and drain cannot be inadvertently enclosed in a hand dressing.

The use of an upper-arm pneumatic tourniquet is a very satisfactory procedure when certain safeguards are observed. Employment of an Esmarch bandage tourniquet no longer is indicated because of the danger of subsequent neuropathies. The pneumatic tourniquet should be applied with appropriate underlying padding in the upper half of the upper arm. A strip of adhesive tape is placed beneath the padding prior to applying the tourniquet, and after the tourniquet is applied, is turned back on itself and taped onto the shoulder in the manner of a halter. In this way, the tourniquet is prevented from slipping down across the lower humerus on the radial nerve.[8] Reinforcing the tourniquet with adhesive tape prevents a bothersome, spontaneous release of the tourniquet during the procedure. Prior to inflation of the tourniquet, blood should be expressed in the entire forearm with an Esmarch bandage, which then is discarded. Tourniquet pressures for adults range from 250 to 280 mm Hg pressure. This form of ischemia may be employed safely for periods of 60–90 minutes, after which the tourniquet should be released for a 5–8-minute period. The tourniquet may be used to prolong the action of local anesthetics in the hand.

For the appropriate execution of the entire repair procedure, a large-size hand table should be available. Such a table should be of suitable size and stability, permitting 3 or 4 individuals around the operative area. This table should be easily available in the operating room. An additional feature of the table is a sliding top and pan holder beneath for the irrigation of the wound postoperatively. Appropriate instruments should be available and sterile at the time of exploration; otherwise, much time can be consumed in requesting, getting and sterilizing instruments during the procedure. Valuable time can be saved by prethinking the operative setup so that all the instruments necessary to handle the various kinds of tissue involved in extensive hand injury are in the kit at the beginning of the procedure.

4. PREOPERATIVE CARE OF THE WOUND. —Care of the wound begins at the time of entry to an emergency ward or hospital. In general, it is not necessary to unduly expose the wound in the emergency ward, where the dangers of contamination and infection are great. Diagnostic exploration of the wound itself should be saved for the operating room. If there is significant bleeding, blindly probing into the wound with the hemostat to gain control runs the risk of compounding the injury by crushing an adjacent nerve. Direct pressure applied evenly is as effective and is much safer. Before the patient is transferred to the operating room, as much excessive dirt as possible should be removed from the skin of his hand and forearm. Nails should be trimmed back and cleaned and hair removed from the surrounding areas.

Once in the operating room, closed injuries should be prepped as in the elective hand case, the guiding principles being thoroughness and the use of abundant time and effort in the scrub. Although the specific prep solutions may vary, a good combination is tincture of green soap and ether, followed by 70% alcohol. In the preparation of open injuries for operation, it is essential to keep the prep agents from direct contact with the wound. The practice of inundating an open wound with tincture of green soap or alcohol is to be condemned, since it creates excessive tissue injury of its own, leading to additional tissue death and postoperative edema. The studies by P. Branemark are very impressive in this regard.[3] His studies of the effects of various types of common prep solutions on the microvasculature should be consulted before even using the gentlest of agents in open wounds. Frequently, in open wounds of the hand, there is a good deal of foreign matter, such as grease, oil, printer's ink, road grime and the like. In general, the best form of removal is mechanical, i.e., a combination of irrigation, gentle gauze removal and subsequent sharp surgical excision. Occasionally, some specific solvents are useful that do not have injurious effects on the tissue, such as mineral oil used as a solvent for heavy road tars and other long-chain hydrocarbons.

The draping of the arm should be a wide one to allow adequate exposure of all possible areas. The drape should be smooth enough to permit the effective use of the Esmarch bandage in conjunction with the pneumatic tourniquet and allow the limb to move freely in any direction without risking contamination of the field.

5. INTRAOPERATIVE PRINCIPLES OF WOUND CARE.—Irrigation is one of the customary events preceding the mechanical debridement of the wound. It is used not only for mechanical cleansing effect but also for its dilutional effect on contaminated wounds. The usual solution to be employed is normal saline; however, balanced electrolyte solutions, such as Tisusol or Ringer's solution, have been suggested. The latter are safer in terms of tissue reaction but more expensive when used in volume. Distilled water should never be used because of its hypotonic, cytotoxic effect. Although irrigation of hand wounds, employed judiciously, is an essential for appropriate cleansing of the wound, enthusiastic use of large volumes of solutions is not necessary and may compound tissue injury. (Normal saline is a well-known liberator of histamine for mast cells.)

Gentleness is essential for the handling of all wounds. Sterling Bunnell[5] recognized this principle prior to World War I and wrote of it in 1918 in his first paper dealing with hand surgery. This technique involves the use of fine instruments, sharp dissection, skin hook or stitches used as retractors and wet sponges to prevent drying of tissue, especially when using a tourniquet. Atraumatic technique is more than just a matter of using fine instruments; it is also a state of the operator's mind.

Adequate exposure and exploration are essential goals of early operative care of the wound. Elective extension of incisions should follow natural lines in the hands, being designed to avoid postoperative skin contractures and to avoid the immediate underlying structures, such as the motor median nerve. In exploring an extensive hand injury, one of the first maneuvers should be the identification and protection of all uninjured structures adjacent to the field, particularly the nerves These should be identified early in the course of exploration and can be protected easily. In virtually any wound of a hand, a *normal-to-normal* technique of exploration should be employed. This means that one begins in normal tissue at one extreme of the wound and explores systematically through the wound, identifying all injured structures, on into the normal tissue of the opposite side of the wound. In this way, one will not miss significantly injured structures. This is a three-dimensional concept and should be carried out in more than one direction. For example, in a major avulsion injury of the palm, one should explore from side to side, superficial to deep and proximal to distal.

At the conclusion of the operative procedure, the wound should be closed by a monofilament material (nylon, wire), since it lacks a capillary action of a multistrand suture and pain on suture removal is reduced. Wound suture is not always indicated. For example, in major crushing avulsion injuries where flap viability is in doubt, a delayed closure is indicated. Drainage should be employed whenever there is a possibility of postoperative accumulation of serum or blood. A 24-hour drain is far safer to employ than to deal with effects of postoperative hematoma. Use of suction drainage is not necessary or desirable because it is not always technically satisfactory and may produce additional trauma due to unregulated negative pressure.

6. POSTOPERATIVE CARE.—Hands swell over the first 48–72 hours after injury or operation and much of the postoperative care seeks to minimize edema.

Dressings or plaster casts should be appropriate to the individual situation or injury. The hand in any dressing should be placed in a position of rest, which is basically a position of muscle balance: wrist somewhat extended, metacarpophalangeal joints flexed approximately 60 degrees, interphalangeal joints flexed and the thumb in abduction and some opposition. The position of the hand in the dressing must, of course, be modified to the type of injury; for example, in the repair of multiple flexor tendon injuries, less wrist extension should be used. A resilient hand dressing usually is employed. One of the most important characteristics of this dressing is that it permits the take-up of pressure increases as edema accumulates in the hand. Resilient materials, such as dry cotton, synthetic fiber or even steel wool pads, are useful as pressure buffers. Appropriate plaster splints may be incorporated within the hand dressing as indicated. A special form of postoperative hand dressing is the wet dressing. This is extremely useful in injuries in which there is extensive crushing and the wound is being left open for delayed closure. Use of a wet dressing, with normal saline as a wetting agent, is an effective method of ensuring drainage of an open wound by establishing a gradient of capillary action from the site of wound exudate into the dressing itself. The dressing is left intact for periods up to 48 hours before renewing. In any dressing it is important that the finger tips be visible so as to follow circulation of the hand.

During the postoperative period, the hand should be elevated at all times—an essential maneuver to minimize postoperative edema. Virtually any mechanism suffices that fulfills the following requirements: (1) elevates the hand above the right heart level; (2) produces no constriction anywhere in the hand, forearm or arm; (3) is comfortable for the patient. Figure 23-1 shows the type of hand bag used by Dr. Raymond Curtis, which is an excellent device to allow continued elevation of the hand while maintaining a degree of freedom for the patient. A stockinet sling that is applied smoothly from the axilla out to beyond the finger tips and suspended from a pole is a simple and readily available mechanism for elevation. After the first few days following major hand injury, the patient may be up and about with his arm in a sling for continued elevation.

Early mobilization of the patient's hand following a major hand injury is, in general, desirable; however, many times early mobility may lead to more pain and edema than the gain in joint function warrants. If early mobility is sought, moving the joints in question only a few times per day will suffice. This should minimize the amount of pain and edema. After the first few days, mobilization usually is a desirable feature and should be supervised carefully by the surgeon himself or by a physical therapist who is quite familiar with the problems involved and the surgeon's aims.

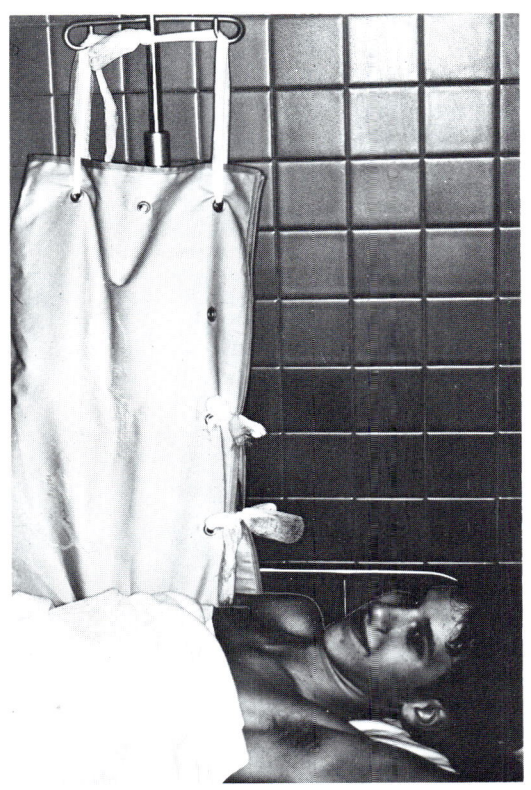

Fig. 23-1.—Hand bag designed for postoperative elevation. The top and one side are open and there are no restricting points on the arm while the hand rests easily in an elevated position.

Pain following an acute hand injury and operative repair always is significant and requires analgesics early in the postoperative course. Motion itself will be painful at this time, and if early motion is desirable, analgesics should be continued. With the hand at rest in an appropriate dressing or cast, the patient should be comfortable within a few days. Any increase in pain in the postoperative period should be looked on as a danger signal and investigated actively. Three important causes of early increases in postoperative pain are: (1) too tight a dressing, which may restrict circulation; (2) significant hematoma formation in the operative wound; (3) early sepsis. (Streptococcus may cause an established infection within 24 hours.) The most common of these three is the tight dressing on a hand that is continuing to swell. This is relieved easily by simply splitting the dressing through *all layers* to the skin and then rewrapping in a looser position.

7. ANTIBIOTICS.—The use of antibiotics in injuries of the hand in the acute phase can be considered prophylactic only, since no specific infection exists at the time. Reliance on antibiotics solely to prevent infection is a foolish and dangerous maneuver, since the primary defenses against postoperative sepsis in such situations are adequate wound cleansing, debriding, hemostasis and drainage. Prophylactic use of antibiotics is justified because even limited sepsis of the hand produces devastating damage. Antibiotics used prophylactically should be started prior to surgery and given intravenously, when possible, to get an early high level so that the wound will receive maximal amounts of the antibiotic. Penicillin in high doses intravenously is a reasonable choice, since this is a bactericidal drug that will be effective against most gram-positive nonhospital organisms, especially beta hemolytic streptococcus.

Tetanus prophylaxis in some form is essential in all open hand injuries, since many injuries are sustained in environments favoring tetanus contamination. History is most important in determining what form of immunization should be employed. Tetanus antitoxin or toxoid is essential when there is a clear indication that tetanus contamination may have occurred. The older horse serum-based forms of tetanus antitoxin, which run the danger of hypersensitivity, serum sickness and major anaphylactic reactions, no longer are used. The newer forms, based on human globulin, obviate these dangers. Effective duration of protection probably is up to at least 10 years following an average immunization.[13] If the patient has not been previously immunized against tetanus, the first dose of tetanus toxoid then should be followed up with the second and third doses at monthly intervals, followed by a booster of tetanus toxoid at 1 year. In patients with a history of prior immunization against tetanus, the toxoid booster is effective in maintaining immunity if used within 10 years of the last dose.

In the case of postoperative wound infections of the hand, indicated antibiotics should be used aggressively and in sufficient time periods to be effective. The choice of antibiotics should be based on the smear of the wound exudate and specific cultures with sensitivity determinations. The duration of the use of antibiotics should be maximal rather than minimal because of the low order of vascularity of some of the vital tissues of the hand. A partially treated infection will continue to wreak its devastating functional effects on the hand.

8. FOLLOW-UP CARE. — Late care of the patient with hand injuries is dictated by the usual considerations implicit in any surgical procedure, but there are a few special needs. It is useful to follow these patients at closer intervals in their early postoperative course to be sure that their progress is satisfactory. In as little as a week or 10 days, valuable function can be lost by incorrectly performed physical therapy.

Records and reports should be maintained. Careful recording of the physical examination of the hand on each postoperative visit is essential. One of the modern accompaniments of the postoperative care of a patient's hand injury, especially industrially induced, is a necessity for careful and continued reports to the responsible insurance carriers. A release for medical information still is required from the patient himself, and his release must be made a part of the record. Reports are essential to permit disability and lost-work payments to the patient. Reports eventually must deal with the patient's disability, both as to his hand function and disability to himself as a whole person. Such determinations are made only after careful description of residual loss of function and matching this against appropriate disability tables.[1, 18]

9. PSYCHOLOGIC PATTERNS. — Each person varies in his emotional make-up, but certain reactive patterns are seen commonly following major traumatic injuries. Because the hand is an area of high emotional significance, the patient with a major hand injury may show brisk emotional response that, to the inexperienced observer, seems to be out of proportion to the volume of tissue injury.

There is a normal emotional pattern discernible among patients with major hand injuries. Taking as a prototype the industrial worker with a family who has suffered an acute major hand injury, the normal reactive pattern breaks down into three parts. The initial reaction is characterized by *anger*. In this phase, rage, frustration, anxiety and even guilt are evident. This usually is a brisk and observable reaction modified by the individual's make-up, circumstances of the injury and other factors. His initial reaction may make the patient extremely difficult to manage, especially for the nursing and ancillary personnel. The patient may be demanding and unreasonable in his behavior, even irrational and childlike at times. Following the initial reaction, one usually finds some form of *denial*. Most patients at some time in the course of their care will employ denial in order to manage their feelings of anxiety concerning the injury and its consequences. Denial in this case means the involuntary suppression or nonrecognition of obvious physical impairments. This mechanism is important to the patient and usually is a temporary means of dealing with unacceptable reality. Because it is a temporary mechanism, it is not necessary for the surgeon to force the patient to "face up" to his situation. Surgeons and nurses may observe a certain optimistic, unreal approach on the patient's part during this phase. For instance, the patient who has suffered multiple phalangeal amputations may talk about expecting to return to his old job of delicate electronic circuitry work. At some time in the normal course of events, the patient will come to a gradual *acceptance* of his hand injury Eventually, most patients will come around to a greater or lesser degree of acceptance of their injury. As the patient becomes able to deal with his injury in a real sense and put denial behind him, the surgeon's job of rehabilitation becomes a good deal easier because the patient, now handling his injury at the conscious level of intellect, will be more likely to follow directions, work harder in his own behalf and formulate more realistic plans for the future.

All too often, the normal emotional pattern is disrupted pathologically. Knowledge of the general sequence of emotional reactions is essential in the effective and complete management of a patient with a major hand injury. This knowledge is essential also because departure from the normal pattern may signal serious abnormal reactions that will severely complicate the patient's recovery. There are at least three types of pathologic reactions. *The neurotic pattern:* For a variety of reasons, the patient may persist in one of the early phases of the normal reaction pattern. The immature patient may remain unduly angry, resentful or upset about his injury, and begin to blame those around him for his lack of progress. *Compensation neurosis* is a term that is used to mean that the patient is claiming unreasonable disability and manifesting a lack of expected progress as a result of expecting monetary compensation so long as he persists in such a state. Complaints may be bizarre, and exaggeration is a prominent feature. Frank *malingering* is a legal term that implies a deliberate attempt to feign illness or disability in order to receive compensation that is not legitimate. Manifestations vary widely. One clear example is the patient who, following relatively minor trauma to his dominant hand, which was swollen for a short time, began to tie a silk stocking tourniquet around his upper arm under the cover of his sleeve while at work in the morning. Within an hour or two, he would demonstrate impressive edema to his boss, claiming it was due to this injury, and take the rest of the day off.

Symptoms of pathologic patterns of behavior vary widely. Certain general symptoms signal departure from the normal behavior pattern: a sudden change in the patient's attitude toward his injury or his surgeon; missed or repeatedly tardy appointments; failure of the patient to act in his own behalf—for instance, not carrying out his own home physiotherapy; recurrence of symptoms without physical basis; and exaggeration of relatively minor physical problems.

The management of well-developed pathologic emotional reaction patterns to hand injury almost always is difficult, largely because the patient is in the frame of mind that he no longer wishes to get better; his motivation to get better has been converted into a wish to stay disabled. This difficulty is further complicated because of the number of people who begin to figure in the patient's problem: the surgeon, the insurance company representative, spouse, physical therapist and lawyers, at the least. The pathologic patient finds himself in a position to take advantage of an increasingly large web of relationships and communications. Psychiatrists may be of value in serious situations that have clear pathologic patterns, particularly in evaluating symptoms and recommending treatment. Actual psychiatric treatment rarely is necessary for the usual case and difficult to obtain when indicated. Most psychiatrists point out that it usually is impossible to substantially alter the life patterns of the immature patient who may be affected also with limited insight and intelligence. Settlement of the claim in the financial sense has been suggested as a specific remedy for the patient with either compensation neurosis or frank malinger-

cult to execute from a legal and insurance standpoint. Thus, solutions of the management of these difficult problems come from the rare psychiatrists who are specifically interested in patients with hand problems.[12]

SPECIFIC INJURIES*

Simple Injuries

EDEMA.—Edema is a common accompaniment of all forms of hand trauma. The exudate from damaged capillaries and venules accumulates in the hand, producing increased interstitial pressure within a confined space. This may produce circulatory embarrassment to the fine musculature, and in its full-blown state actually may cause ischemic damage to muscle, subcutaneous tissue and skin. The edematous hand assumes a "position of comfort," with the metacarpophalangeal joints in extension and the interphalangeal joints in flexion—clearly not a "position of function."

Edema presents several problems for the hand. The hand assumes an imbalanced state. Protein-rich edema fluid accumulates and leads to the laying down of excess scar tissue throughout the hand, especially around the joints themselves. Capsular fibrosis ensues, producing stiff joints and nonfunctional positions, especially in the proximal interphalangeal and metacarpophalangeal joints. Exaggerated edema and scar actually may cause neural compression and acute carpal tunnel symptoms. At the very least, edema compounds venous obstruction, which then may go on to produce additional tissue loss.

Essential to the treatment of edema is elevation, which has been discussed previously. Compression dressings, when used judiciously, are useful. Resilient material incorporated in the dressing is a pressure equalizer in the acute phase. Use of wet dressings to take up exudate in open injuries is indicated also. Steroids, enzymes and low molecular weight dextran do *not* have sufficient benefit to be utilized in this instance.

LACERATIONS.—Lacerations of the hand and fingers are common and have added significance when major deep structures have been injured also. Depending on the direction of laceration, secondary scar contracture can develop, especially when laceration crosses active flexion creases of the hand at a right angle. Treatment for simple lacerations is primary suture after appropriate cleansing. If the laceration lies in a poor position across flexion creases, the line of the incision should be redirected during the closure to avoid secondary scar contractures.

Tendon Injuries

Uniformly good results still elude us in tendon injuries, especially those of the flexor tendons, largely because of the failure on the part of the individual first seeing the wound to appreciate the magnitude of the problem and factors that must be controlled to ensure the patient a good functional recovery.

Diagnosis of a tendon injury is made by employing a knowledge of functional anatomy. By simple inspection, many times one can diagnose divided tendons. In fact, in the infant and young child, this usually is all one has to go on. At rest, the uninjured normal hand should show a smooth progression of increasing flexion of the fingers from the index to the little finger. A finger whose flexor tendons are divided will lie outside its normal flexion arcade (Fig. 23-2). Likewise, the location of the laceration gives a clue as to the tendons that possibly may be involved, as does the history of the type of injury, wounding agent and position of the hand at the time of injury. Each tendon in the suspect area should be tested individually, remembering that the partially divided tendon still may produce the

---

*Skeletal and ligamentous injuries are discussed in Chapter 24.

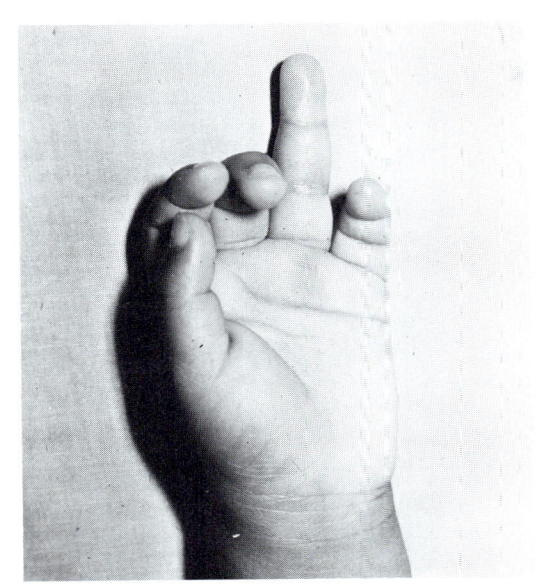

Fig. 23-2.—Divided flexor tendons. A 1½-year-old girl with an 8-week-old division of both flexor tendons of the ring finger. The digit lies well outside the normal resting flexion arcade of the fingers, suggesting the diagnosis by inspection alone.

expected function. Operative examination still remains the only final means of accurately diagnosing the partially divided tendon. The examination of the distal function in the hand with an open injury should be carried out without looking into the wound itself until one is ready for formal exploration under the aseptic conditions of the operating room.

FLEXOR TENDONS.—Timing is the immediate problem of flexor tendon repair. The question as to whether a given flexor tendon injury should be repaired primarily or some form of secondary reconstruction elected depends on many factors: the patient's age and general condition, time after injury, condition of the wound, experience of the operator and equipment available. Perhaps the most important factor is the anatomic location of the injury (Fig. 23-3). Each anatomic zone of the flexor surface of the hand has its own considerations as to timing and method of repair.

Area 1 is the terminal phalangeal area located from the midportion of the midphalanx distally in each finger. The flexor digitorum profundus is the only tendon liable to injury in this area, the flexor digitorum sublimis having been inserted proximally. Primary repair usually is possible by advancing the cut end of the profundus tendon and reanastomosing it to the area of insertion on the distal phalanx. This is done using a Bunnell criss-cross stitch, drawing the tendon into a gouged hole in the phalanx and securing a button on the fingernail (Fig. 23-4). In the normal adult finger, advancements of up to 1.5 cm may be done safely without producing flexor deformity in the involved digit.

Area 2 is the well-known "no man's land," described by Bunnell[5] in 1918. No more troublesome problems arise in the field of hand surgery than those stemming from the ill-advised repair of tendons in this region. This area is defined by the tough fibrous tunnel that conducts both flexor tendons from the palm into the fingers and usually begins at the level of the metacarpal neck in the palm and extends to the midportion of the middle phalanx, in the region of the insertion of the flexor digitorum sublimis on the lateral aspects of the middle phalanx. In the proximal portion of Area 2, injuries produce severance of both tendons, whereas more distally in this area the profundus tendon alone may be injured, the sublimis having decussated over the proximal phalanx prior to its insertion. In primary repairs, tendon ends heal not only together but also to the thickened tendon sheath and underlying periosteum and volar plates. Secondary tendon grafting has given the most consistently good results in flexor tendon injuries in this region.[2]

The primary treatment of tendon injuries of Area 2 should be operative cleansing of the wound, confirmation of the tendon pathology, repair of any divided digital nerves and skin closure. During the period of healing, the joint must be

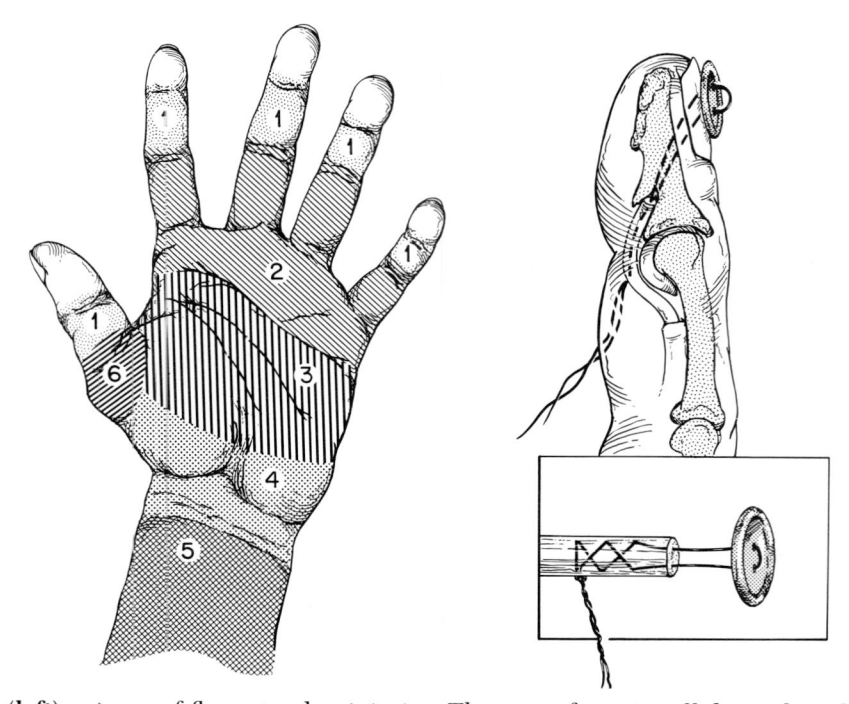

Fig. 23-3 (left).—Areas of flexor tendon injuries. The type of repair will depend on the area in which the flexor tendons are injured. For details see text.
Fig. 23-4 (right).—Method of anastomosing tendon to terminal phalanx. This method was developed by Bunnell and is applicable to both tendon grafting and advancing of severed tendons. Inset shows details of stitching method and pull-out wire.

kept mobile with passive guided motion. Six to 8 weeks later, the tendon mechanism should be explored under appropriate anesthesia and tourniquet control. The injured profundus tendon should be excised from the terminal phalanx proximal to the midpalmar region. The sublimis should be left and, indeed, if severed, the spontaneous tenodesis of this tendon may serve to avoid a later recurvatum deformity of the proximal interphalangeal joint. The proximal profundus tendon must be freed as far as necessary to ensure that no adhesions remain to impair its normal excursion. This excursion is measured when the tendon has been freed completely. The tendon sheath should be excised except for broad pulleys—one left over the region of the metacarpophalangeal joint and another left over the midportion of the middle phalanx. If the area is not scarred excessively, tendon grafting may be carried out directly using either the palmaris longus or the plantaris tendon to span the area of injury. A strong proximal anastomosis is created using the interweaving technique described by Pulvertaft,[20] and the distal anastomosis done as described for tendon advancement. Tension is adjusted by positioning the wrist and fingers in neutral and drawing the graft out from zero tension to a distance corresponding to that previously measured for the amplitude of the tendon in question. The tendon is marked in this position opposite the site desired for insertion. If done carefully and all proximal adhesions are released, the involved finger at the completion of the procedure should resume its proper position in the normal flexion arcade of the fingers.

If the tendon sheath, at exploration, is found to be unduly scarred and fibrotic, the excision should be completed as described, but instead of placing a tendon graft, a silicone rod should be placed. Either a 3- or 4-mm solid silicone rod is used and is tacked by a single, nonabsorbable suture to the distal phalanx and to the proximal tendon stump with the fingers and wrist in neutral. At the end of 2–3 months, a fine tunnel of flattened, fibrous tissue resembling tendon sheath has been laid down around the rod, thus re-creating a slippery tunnel (Fig. 23-5). The rod is removed and a tendon graft then placed as described above. Using the silicone rod technique many functional hands have been obtained under circumstances unfavorable to direct tendon grafting.[16]

Area 3 is the midpalmar or lumbrical portion of the flexor surface extending from the metacarpal neck proximally to the distal extent of the transverse carpal ligament. Injuries in this area respond well to primary treatment. In clean, early wounds, the tendons should be joined primarily, using either the Bunnell pull-out wire technique or a buried, nonabsorbable weaving stitch.[6] Excellent results occur in this area, presumably because of the lack of tissues, such as the tendon sheath of "no man's land," which may immobilize the repair.

Area 4 represents the region beneath the volar carpal ligament and Area 5 begins at the proximal edge of the volar carpal ligament and extends to the tendomuscular junction in the forearm. Careful primary repairs with buried nonabsorbable suture in both these areas yield gratifying functional results. The carpal ligament is not reconstituted in Area 4 injuries.

In the thumb, injuries of the flexor pollicis longus in Area 1 respond well to primary advancement as in the fingers. In the zone defined by the thenar musculature, results are excellent with primary repair, similar to the midpalmar injuries of digital tendons. Injuries to the flexor pollicis longus in Area 3 should be explored first proximal to the carpal ligament because the proximal cut end of the tendon retracts completely out of the hand and into the wrist, since there are

Fig. 23-5.—Silicone rod in place after removal of flexor tendons. There was extensive scarring from an old injury, making a successful direct tendon graft unlikely. When the rod was removed in 3 months, a slippery, well-developed tunnel had been formed to receive the tendon graft.

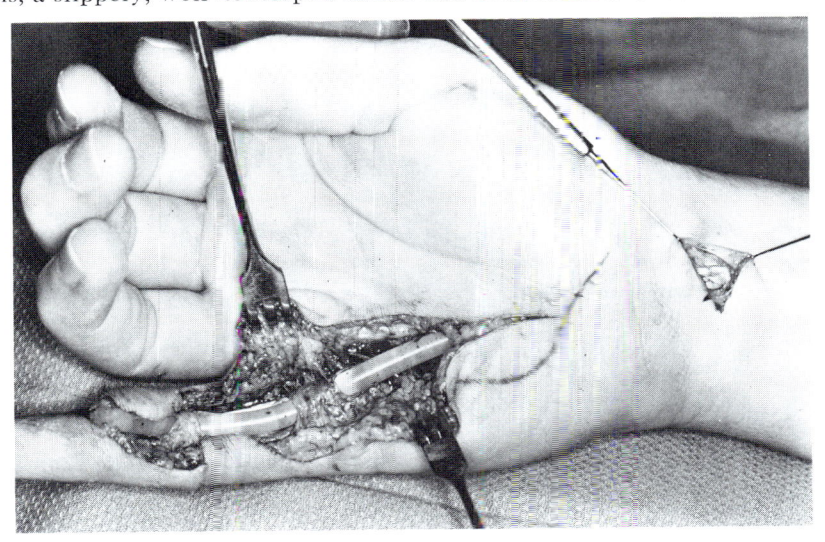

no restraining vincula at that level of the flexor pollicis longus.

Area 6 of the thumb, the sesamoid area, is a narrow, tight zone defined by the insertions of the thenar intrinsic muscles with their sesamoids through which the flexor pollicis longus courses. If the tendon is divided at this level, 1.0–1.5 cm of the distal stump should be resected and a primary repair carried out in the proximal part of Area 1. This obviates the possibility of the repair becoming immobilized by adherence to the structures of the sesamoid tunnel.

In combined tendon and nerve injuries of the wrist, one must face the difficult question as to whether simultaneous, primary repair should be carried out. The argument concerning primary and secondary nerve repair is presented elsewhere. In combined injuries, absolutely optimal conditions must be obtained for one to consider the possibility of attempting nerve repair in addition to the suture of multiple tendons. It usually is best to complete the tendon repairs in such injuries and to tag the nerve ends together with a single nonabsorbable suture to preserve length. Six to 8 weeks later, when the patient has in large part regained tendon motion, a secondary nerve repair should be carried out as an isolated repair procedure.

Flexor tendon repairs, in general, should be immobilized 3 weeks and then begun on protected active and passive motions, progressing to active resistance exercises over a 1–2-week period.

EXTENSOR TENDON INJURIES.—The extensor surface of the hand, as in the flexor, may be divided into areas with differing requirements for repair of lacerations. Unlike the flexor surface, however, virtually all extensor tendon lacerations are amenable to direct primary repair, except in the most unfavorable circumstances or when there has been actual tendon loss with avulsion or gouging. The extensor tendons and mechanisms are immediately accessible beneath the skin and are not constrained in narrow fibrous tunnels.

The complexity of the extensor mechanism to the fingers makes analysis of the treatment of injuries of this area more detailed and varied. The intrinsic-lateral band-retinacular system governs interphalangeal extension whereas the extrinsic long extensors are responsible for metacarpophalangeal extension. Injuries of the dorsal region of the fingers and hand must take into account these two systems.

Trauma to the terminal insertion of the extensor mechanisms into the dorsum of the distal phalanx is common. Both an open laceration and closed avulsion of the tendon over the distal interphalangeal joint will produce the typical baseball, or mallet, finger (Fig. 23-6). If the injury has been produced by an acute laceration, direct repair offers the best chance for a functional result. The wound should be explored and, if the tendon is available, a Bunnell type of zigzag wire suture can be used to advance the tendon to its insertion into holes drilled in the distal phalanx. Either type of repair should be supported by fixing the joint in extension by a single K-wire, to be removed in 6–8 weeks.

Closed injuries producing a mallet finger frequently respond to nonoperative treatment if carried out for a sufficient length of time. Small thimble casts, incorporating the proximal interphalangeal joint in some flexion to take tension off the terminal tendon, may be used and must be renewed for a period of 6 weeks. A simple technique of taping a mallet finger to maintain proximal interphalangeal joint flexion and distal interphalangeal joint extension is illustrated in Figure 23-7. Immobilization should continue for approximately 6 weeks. Likewise, the distal interphalangeal joint may be immobilized in full extension with a single buried K-wire to permit the separated tendon ends to heal during the same period.

If conservative therapy fails, the area

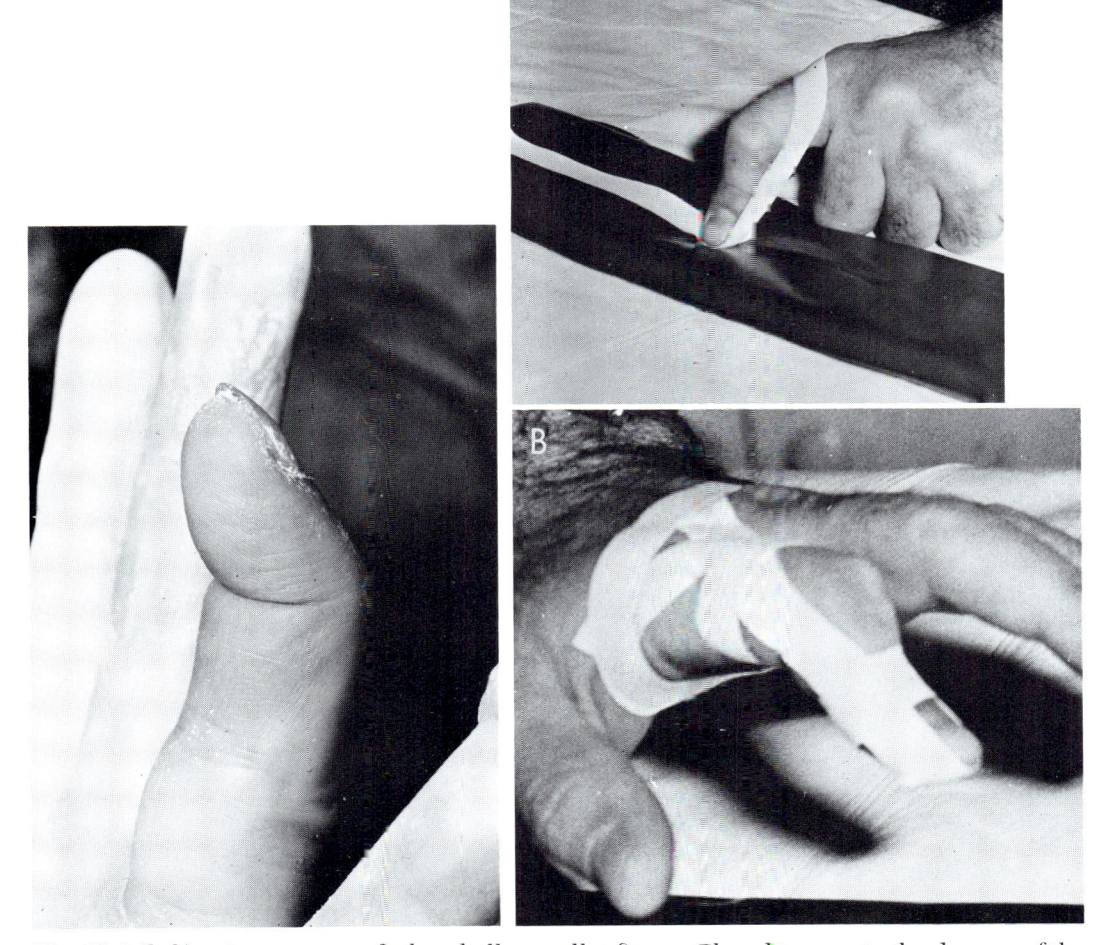

Fig. 23-6 (left).—Appearance of a baseball or mallet finger. Closed trauma to the dorsum of the distal interphalangeal joint had produced disruption of the terminal fibers of the extensor mechanism. The patient was unable to extend his finger tip.

Fig. 23-7 (right).—A simple technique for treatment of a mallet finger by taping.

must be explored and repair carried out much as in the acute laceration, but depending, in this instance, on suturing the well-developed scar. In instances of closed injury in which more than one-third of the joint surface of the distal phalanx is avulsed with the tendon, excellent results may be obtained by operatively replacing the fragment and fixing it with a small K-wire until the fracture is solidly healed.

Acute lacerations more proximally over the proximal interphalangeal joint produce the well-known "boutonniere" deformity (Fig. 23-8). With open injuries in the region of the joint, the central tendon of the extensor mechanism is divided, permitting the lateral bands to slip volarly from their normal position dorsal to the pivot point of this joint. In addition, the central tendon retracts proximally from the injury. Thus, the deformity is one of

570 / *John P. Remensnyder*

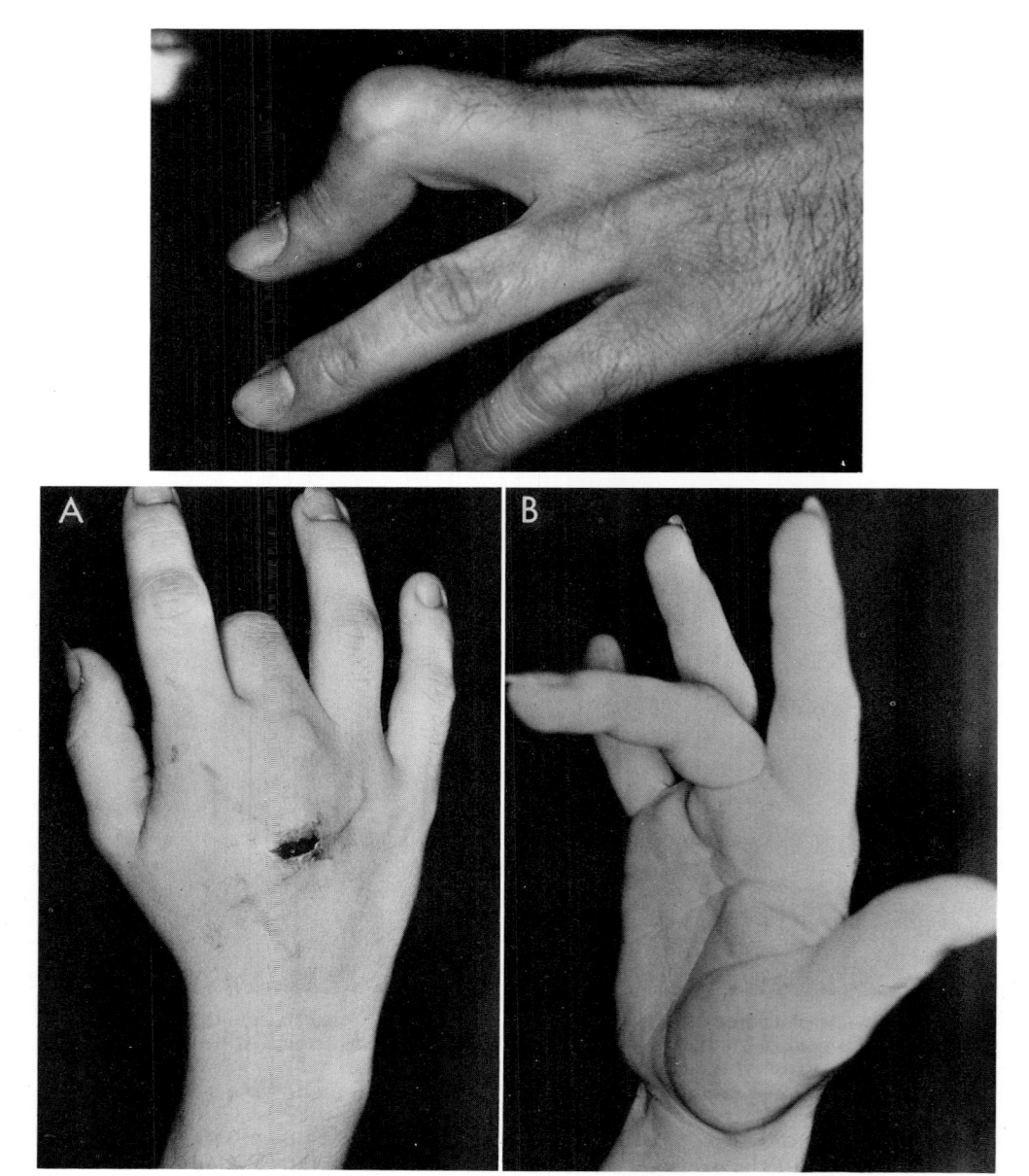

Fig. 23-8 (top).—Typical "boutonniere" deformity resulting from a closed injury 6 months before. The proximal interphalangeal joint is held in flexion by the displaced lateral bands and ruptured central tendon; the finger tip is unstable due to lack of effective extension.
Fig. 23-9 (bottom).—Acute laceration of the extensor communis tendon of middle finger (**A**) producing characteristic drop-finger deformity (**B**). Interphalangeal extension still is possible due to intact intrinsics. Occasionally, variations of the intertendinous connections between the extensor communi will permit weak metacarpophalangeal extension.

hyperflexion of the proximal interphalangeal joint and extension of the distal interphalangeal joint. Immediate repair is indicated, with operative repositioning of the lateral bands with fine nonabsorbable sutures. In addition, the central tendon must be advanced and reinserted into the base of the middle phalanx, either by suturing tendon to tendon or by advancing the tendon into drill holes placed into the bone. The joint should be immobilized for 5–6 weeks until solid healing has taken place. A subsequent period of vigorous mobilization may be necessary to achieve full active flexion after this type of injury.

Closed ruptures of the central tendon over the proximal interphalangeal joint unfortunately are not often seen early and usually present as an established deformity with functional loss due to inability to straighten the finger. This deformity at this stage is difficult to correct satisfactorily, due in part to the secondary changes involving the joint capsule and retinacular system. Essential prerequisites to any operative attempt to correct this deformity are full passive mobility and a normal appearance of the joint on x-ray. Dolphin[10] recommends a simple form of correction that can give very useful results: tenotomy of the distal extensor mechanism, which permits the tendons to slide proximally, releasing the volar tension on the lateral bands. Both of these advantages tend to restore the extensor pull to the proximal interphalangeal joint at the expense of creating a mallet finger. Although the repair is incomplete, a useful finger can result. A successful, complete repair depends on adequate release of the structures that maintain the deformity and restoration of the central tendon and dorsal portion of the lateral bands. The lateral bands must be freed up completely, and shortened, oblique, retinacular fibers sectioned. In addition, particularly in longstanding cases, volar capsulectomy, release of the volar plate and flexor tendolysis may be necessary to give complete release to the deforming forces on the proximal interphalangeal joint. The central tendinous mechanism can be restored either by the "turn of the key" method of advancement described by Verdan[22] or by interlacing a free tendon graft. Such repairs must be held for 5–6 weeks by a transarticular K-wire and then intensive mobilization begun. Some patients lack full flexion of the proximal interphalangeal joints after such procedures, and this must stand as a major limitation of such procedures.

Lacerations in the dorsal hood area of the metacarpophalangeal joint (Fig. 23-9) produce the characteristic drop finger deformity and should be dealt with by immediate direct repair. Lacerations through the hood necessarily enter the joint, which must be washed out carefully and freed of any foreign bodies prior to repair. The tendon may be repaired satisfactorily by direct fine wire, figure-of-eight sutures, including skin and tendon, or, occasionally, a Bunnell pull-out wire repair. The metacarpophalangeal joint should be held in extension for 5 weeks after restoration to permit full healing. Of particular concern in the dorsal metacarpophalangeal joint area are the tendon lacerations produced by human bites, as when a closed fist strikes the mouth and teeth of an adversary. Immediate repair, despite careful lavage, debridement and antibiotic protection, all too often results in a septic joint. A more prudent course is to cleanse, debride and only close the deep structures, leaving the skin open to close secondarily, using wet dressings. The divided tendon and resultant deformity then may be dealt with as a secondary problem when healing is complete.

Lacerations and wounds more proximally in the dorsum of the hand and forearm respond favorably to immediate direct repair. For divided long extensor tendons in the dorsum, Bunnell advocated a figure-of-eight suture, including the tendon and skin and support for 5–6 weeks.[6] Removal of the skin stitch removes the tendon stitch, thereby reducing the chance of tenodesis. Extensor tendon divisions in the forearm should be repaired with a buried interweaving stitch and splinted for a similar period. With lacerations near the dorsal retinacular ligament of the wrist, the repair should be prevented from adhering to the ligament by judicious resection of the retinacular ligament to permit free excursion of the repaired tendon.

Injuries with Soft Tissue Loss

Skin and soft tissue deficits in the hand are divided into two types: primary loss and delayed loss. In *primary losses*, the defect is obvious and usually is the result of a slicing or avulsing type of injury (Fig. 23-10). There is immediate need for appropriate coverage, which is determined by the structures exposed by the injury: if only the soft tissue or muscle is exposed, a free skin graft should be elected; if the loss uncovers joints, fracture lines or tendons, pedicled flap tissue is indicated. *Delayed loss of skin* and soft tissue occurs with crushing or blast injuries and occurs as the result of edema, venous congestion and arteriolar occlusion, producing a delayed ischemic necrosis. With such injuries, coverage frequently is best delayed for a few days until the diagnosis of the extent of tissue death becomes certain. During that time, the hand should be immobilized in a bulky wet-to-dry dressing to help remove exudate from the wound surface by capillary action. Appropriate antibiotics and tetanus prophylaxis are essential. The extent of tissue loss may be obvious as early as 48 hours or may not be evident for 6 or 7 days; in either case, definitive coverage is delayed until the extent of loss is known. Again, the type of coverage is dictated by the type of structures exposed. It is possible, of course, to recognize certain situations early in the course of injury that are sure to go on to secondary loss—the large, crushed, distally based flap is a

Fig. 23-10.—**A**, severe flaying injury in a 26-year-old man due to milling machine injury. All the hand skin had been degloved in the machine and the terminal joints amputated. Deep strictures and muscles intact. **B**, wound was treated by immediate debridement and delayed split-thickness skin graft coverage was accomplished 3 days later. At 12 days, the graft had taken well and the patient was exercising in the whirlpool.

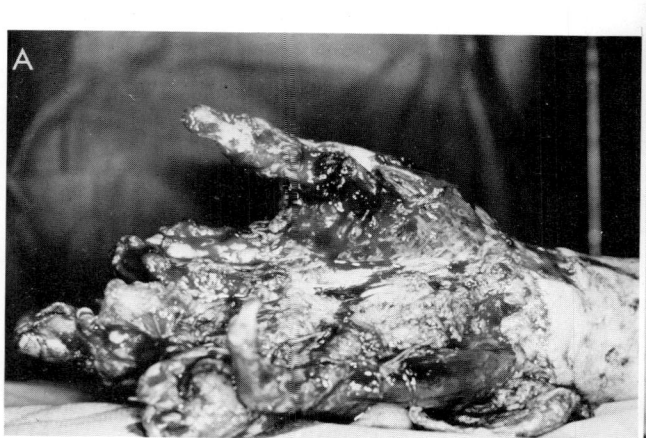

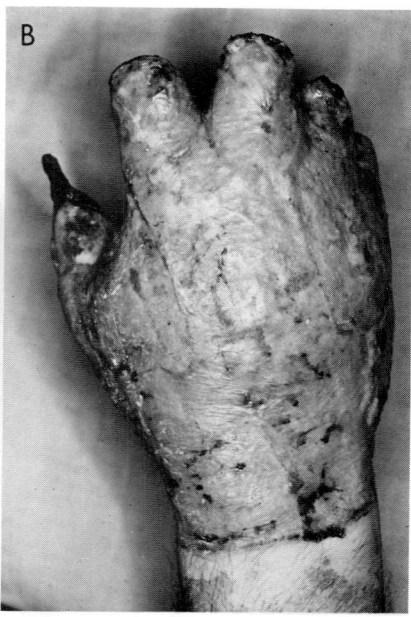

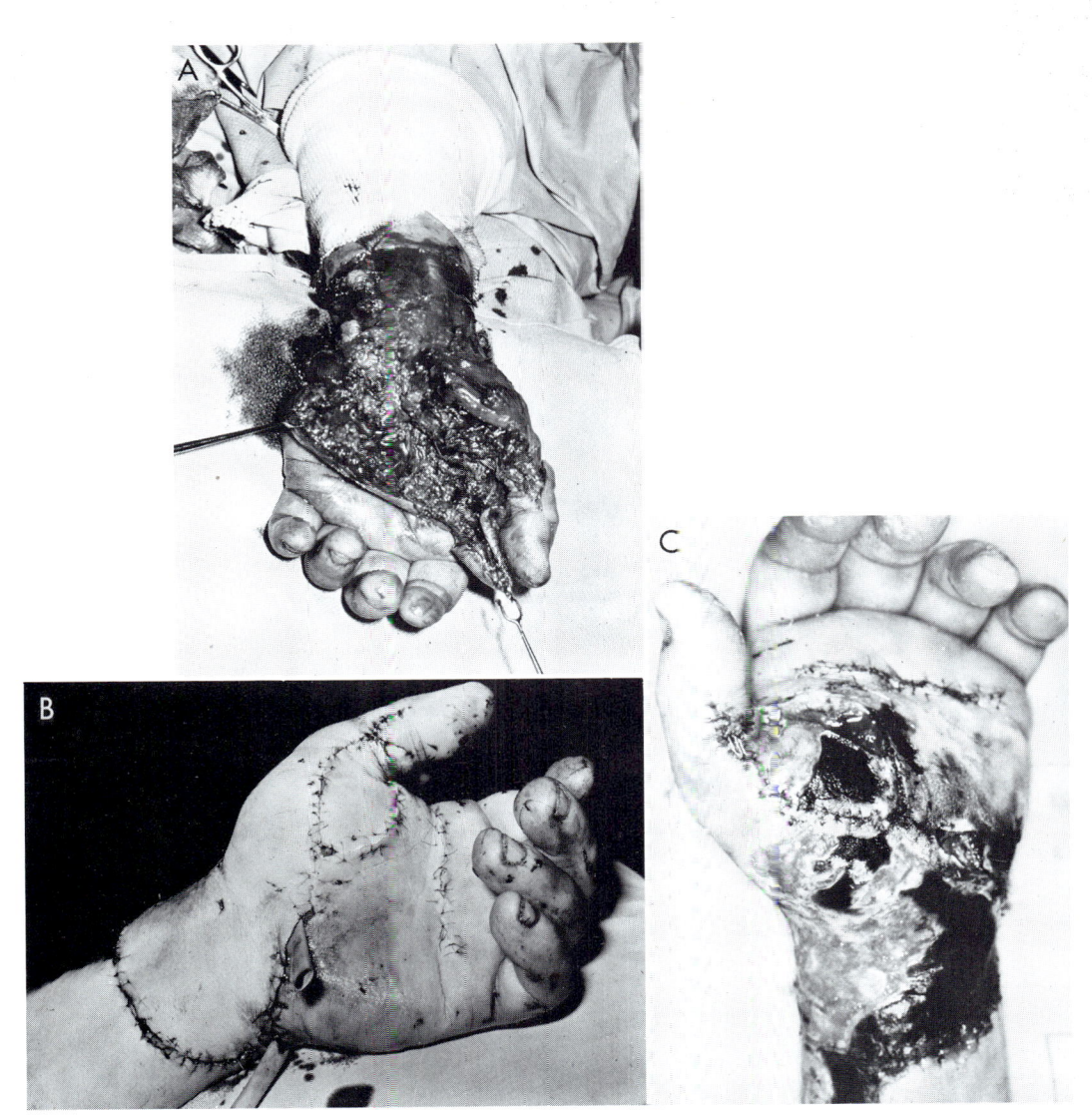

Fig. 23-11.—**A,** severe crushing, avulsing injury in the hand of a 48-year-old man, sustained in printing press. Distally based flaps should be regarded with great suspicion as to viability. **B,** same patient 3 days after primary debridement and suture with drainage. Central portion of avulsed flap already was dusky. **C,** loss of much of the avulsed skin by the sixteenth day. With distally based flaps, conservative debridement, wet dressings and no suture may preserve more tissue.

prime example (Fig. 23-11). By early removal of such jeopardized tissue, definitive coverage may be achieved sooner.

DIGITAL TISSUE LOSS.—Primary loss of the skin and pulp of the finger tip is a significant injury because it causes major impairment in the sense of touch of that finger. Likewise, as an area richly endowed with sensory nerves, injuries and subsequent healing may be quite painful, disabling the hand for periods up to 8 weeks, even with successful treatment.[4]

If the injury is confined to the distal

third or less, one may elect to simply dress the wound and permit wound healing to occur, with subsequent contracture drawing the innervated well-padded tissue distally to provide a good touch surface. If bone is exposed, this can be rongeured back to below the level of soft tissue. Such healing, because it may require 8–10 weeks, is ideal for children and nonworking people. Working people may insist on active treatment, even though the result may be the same.

A split-thickness skin graft applied immediately to the damaged finger tip must be regarded as the easiest and perhaps the best method of gaining early wound closure in the finger tip with tissue loss (Fig. 23-12). Sewn on and care-

Fig. 23-12 (top left).—Clean slicing injury of finger tip of a 36-year-old meat cutter. This may be closed in many ways, but split-thickness skin grafting in this type of injury gives early secure wound closure while not impeding the normal wound contraction mechanism, which will progressively draw volar pad dorsally.

Fig. 23-13 (top right, bottom).—**A,** sharp loss of radial aspect of dominant index finger exposing distal interphalangeal joint and flexor tendons sustained by a 32-year-old engineer. Flap coverage indicated to preserve joint and tendon function. **B,** flap from adjacent middle finger raised, based on lateral blood supply, and tailored to defect. Cross-finger flap must lie without tension. Skeletal fixation not necessary—simple soft dressing technique will hold the fingers in position for 2–3 weeks. **C,** final result 3 months later, showing flap well healed into place in index finger. Donor site was resurfaced with full-thickness skin graft taken from groin crease.

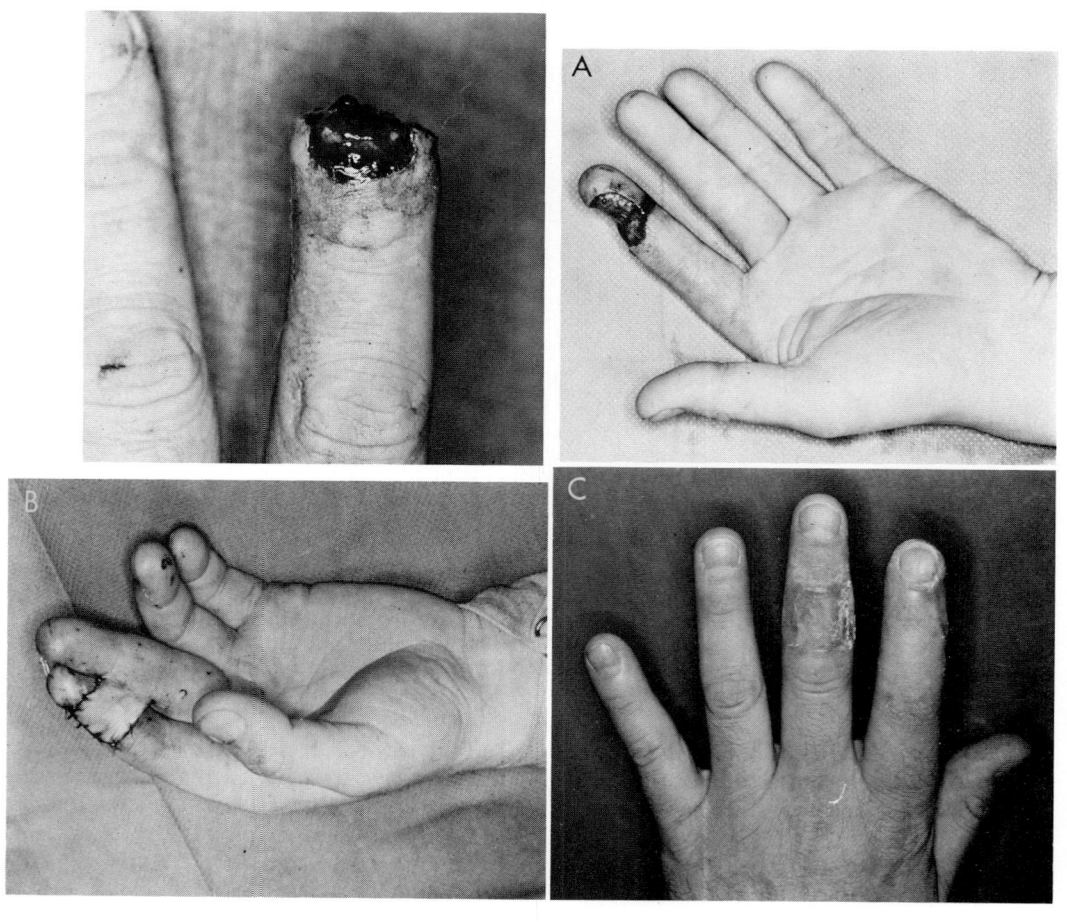

fully stented in a surgically clean wound, the graft should take well and ensure wound closure by the time of dressing on the seventh to the tenth day. An added advantage of using a split-thickness skin graft is that the mechanisms of wound contraction are not substantially impaired and, in the succeeding months, one will observe that the normally innervated skin and pulp will be drawn distally and the graft correspondingly will shrink and wrinkle. The graft should be taken from a hidden donor site, such as the upper inner arm or groin crease—*not* in an exposed area, such as the volar aspect of the forearm. In a black individual, a good color match may be obtained by taking the graft from between the two volar wrinkles in the ulnar aspect of the wrist. Full-thickness skin grafts have no significant advantages over the split grafts in acute injuries, and may retard later wound contraction and impair the quality of sensation.

Flap coverage is necessary when tendons or joints of important fingers are exposed by the injury. Free grafts will not take, in such a situation, and a cross-finger flap will give full-thickness coverage and padding to preserve joint and tendon function (Fig. 23-13). Although the area and volume of tissue transferred by a cross-finger flap is not large, the same principles that apply to the transfer of larger tissue masses must be observed: (1) a safe base-to-length ratio for tissue involved must be used—1:1 in the case of the finger; (2) the donor area must be able to afford the loss of the full-thickness tissue and function well with the coverage provided; and (3) the pedicle should remain in place only long enough to pick up a good blood supply before being divided—2–3 weeks in the case of a cross-finger flap. The flap is raised below the level of the subdermal plexus, which is the critical vascular network supplying the flap, and is stitched loosely into the defect to prevent undue tension. The dorsum of the adjacent finger is the usual site of election, although the dorsum of the proximal phalanx of the thumb also serves as an admirable donor site for injuries to the index finger. The use of cross-finger flaps necessitates some degree of disability to the donor finger, with some residual stiffness being noted in the donor digit in up to 20% of cases.[15] In deciding as to the use of the cross-finger flap, one must balance the gain to the injured digit against the loss and potential disability in the donor digit. Flaps raised from the thenar eminence for coverage of finger-tip injuries have limited usefulness for two reasons: (1) the donor site, if painful, limits thumb action and hence a major portion of hand function and (2) the motor median nerve lies very superficially and may be injured in raising such a flap.

Other flaps have specific indications in acute finger-tip injury. At times, a neurovascular island flap may be indicated in the treatment of acute injuries to the dominant thumb or index finger tip (Fig. 23-14). An island of tissue of appropriate size is raised from the side of a minor finger and the neurovascular bundle to this island dissected. This is passed subcutaneously to the injured area and the donor site is covered with a free graft. Such an island carries its own blood supply and sensation and will satisfactorily cover exposed bone and tendon. The patient still identifies sensation as part of the function of the repaired finger. The donor finger is, of course, hemianesthetic. The island transfer should be used only in special instances, as noted, and it is imperative that the patient's requirement for high-grade sensation be known and that he be aware of the loss to the donor finger before employing this method of repair.

Avulsions of skin and subcutaneous tissue from a finger, caused by catching a ring on a moving object and thereby stripping the distal tissue, present special types of problems for coverage (Fig. 23-15). Bones, joints and tendons usually are exposed in such an injury, and some form of flap coverage is indicated. Unfortu-

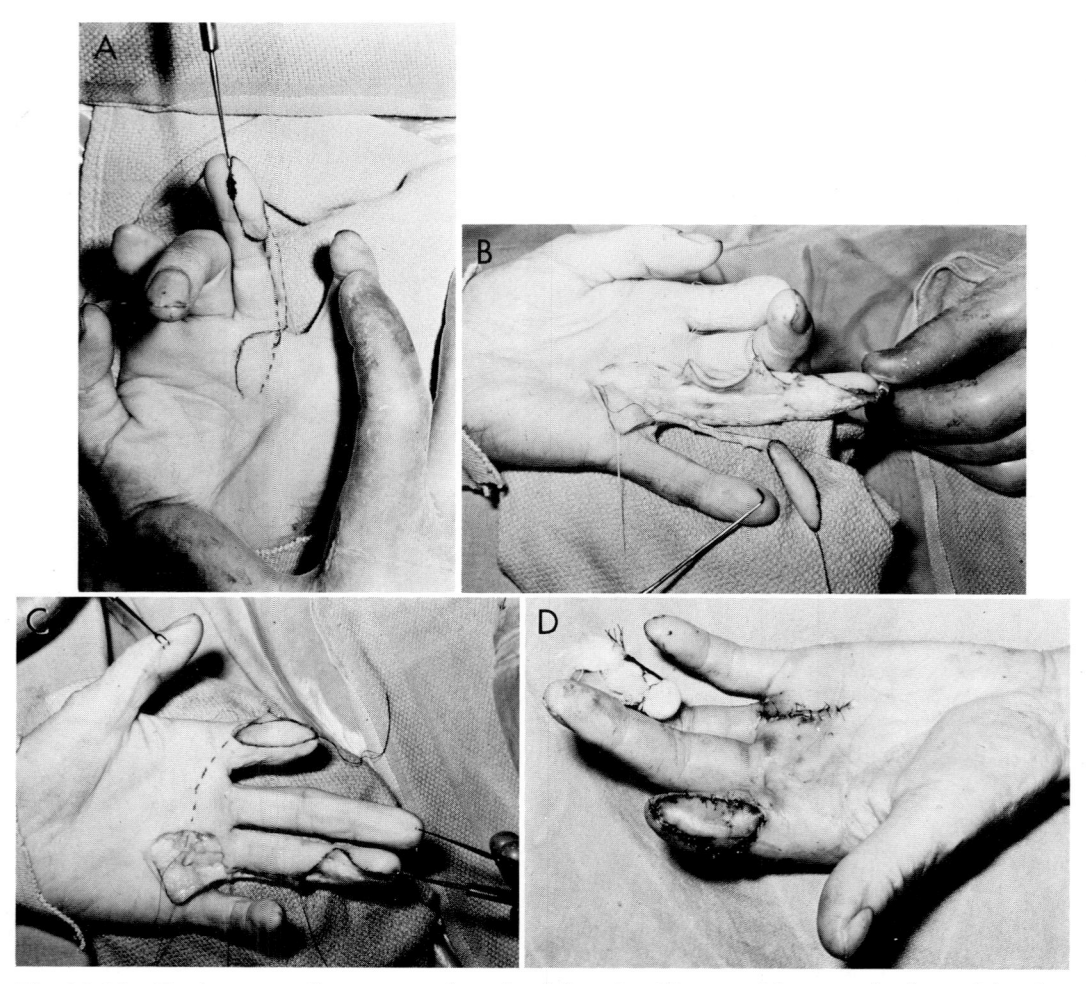

Fig. 23-14.—Techniques of neurovascular island flap. **A,** a 52-year-old painter had painful index finger amputation stump of dominant hand. Island of expendable skin from ulnar border of ring finger outlined. **B,** skin island has been removed and its supporting neurovascular supply dissected into the palm. In order to sufficiently mobilize the neurovascular stalk it is necessary to divide the palmar arch ulnar to the vessels in question. The common digital nerves may be gently split back well into the palm to gain mobility. **C,** the island of skin has been drawn under the palmar skin and brought out to fill the defect in the index stump resulting from removal of the thin, painful scar. **D,** neurovascular island sutured into place on index finger, showing good circulation. Digital-palmar incision of ring finger closed primarily. Defect in ring finger resurfaced with full-thickness skin graft with tie-over stent.

nately, although it is easy to apply a flap to such a finger, the results are unusable because of bulk and instability. A free split-thickness graft will not take acutely on the hard tissues exposed. A method to gain a well-covered, relatively slender, usable finger is to utilize the "crane principle.[11, 19] Initially, the finger is buried in the subcutaneous tissue of an appropriate location. After 2 weeks, the finger is removed, carrying with it a thin layer of fatty, vascularized tissue, and a split-thickness skin graft is immediately applied to this. When healed, this provides both

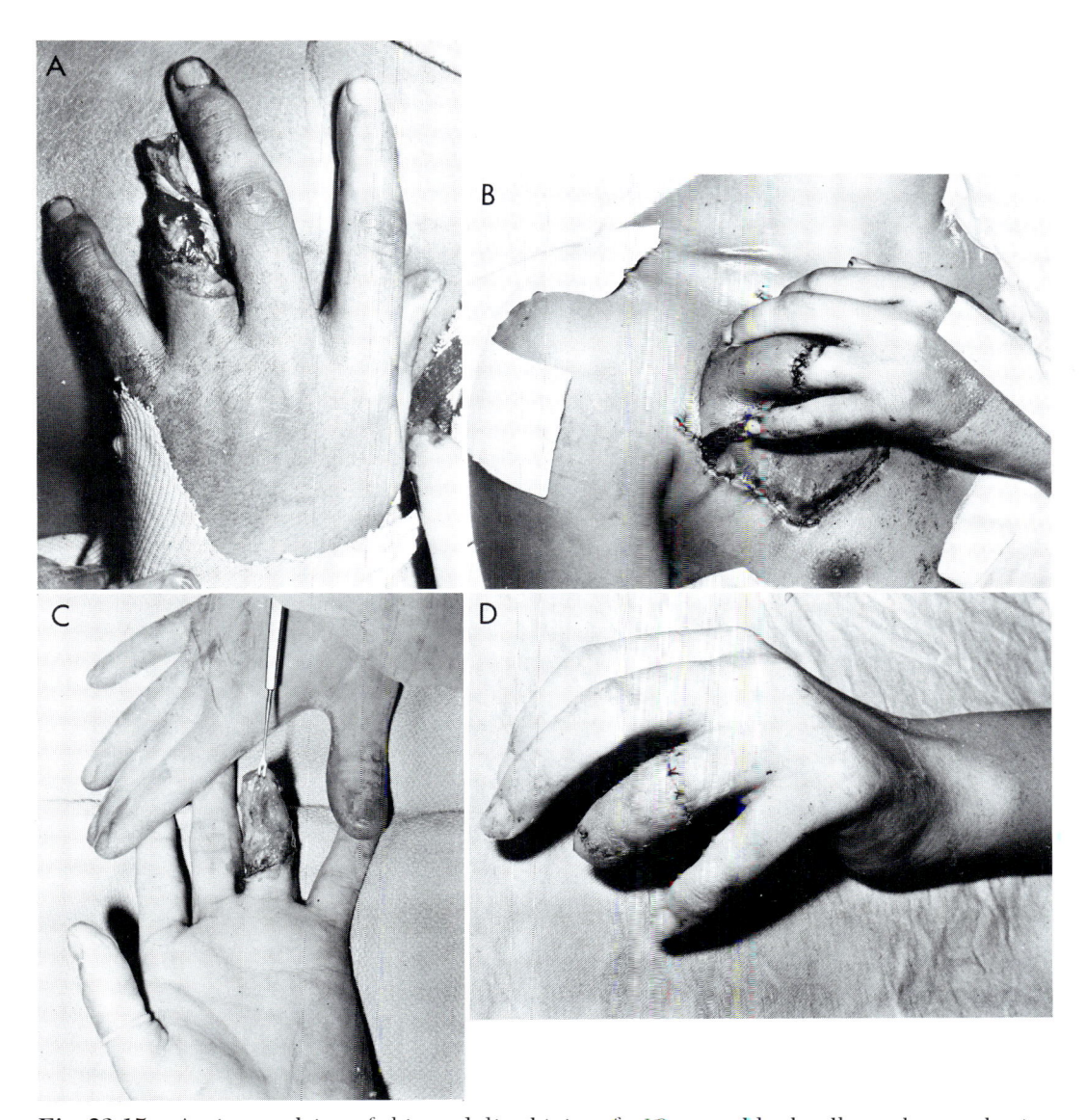

Fig. 23-15.—**A,** ring avulsion of skin and distal joint of a 15-year-old schoolboy who caught ring on top of a fence he was scaling. Sublimis tendon and proximal interphalangeal joint intact. The problem is to gain coverage without adding disabling bulk to finger. **B,** acute coverage gained by covering open portion with upper-chest pedicle flap. **C,** at 3 weeks, finger detached from flap, carrying only a thin layer of adherent fat and subcutaneous tissue rather than the whole bulky flap. This tissue will sustain a split-thickness skin graft. **D,** at the time of detachment (see **B**), a split-thickness skin graft was applied. Eight days later the graft had taken well and provided thin, appropriate coverage for the finger.

578 / John P. Remensnyder

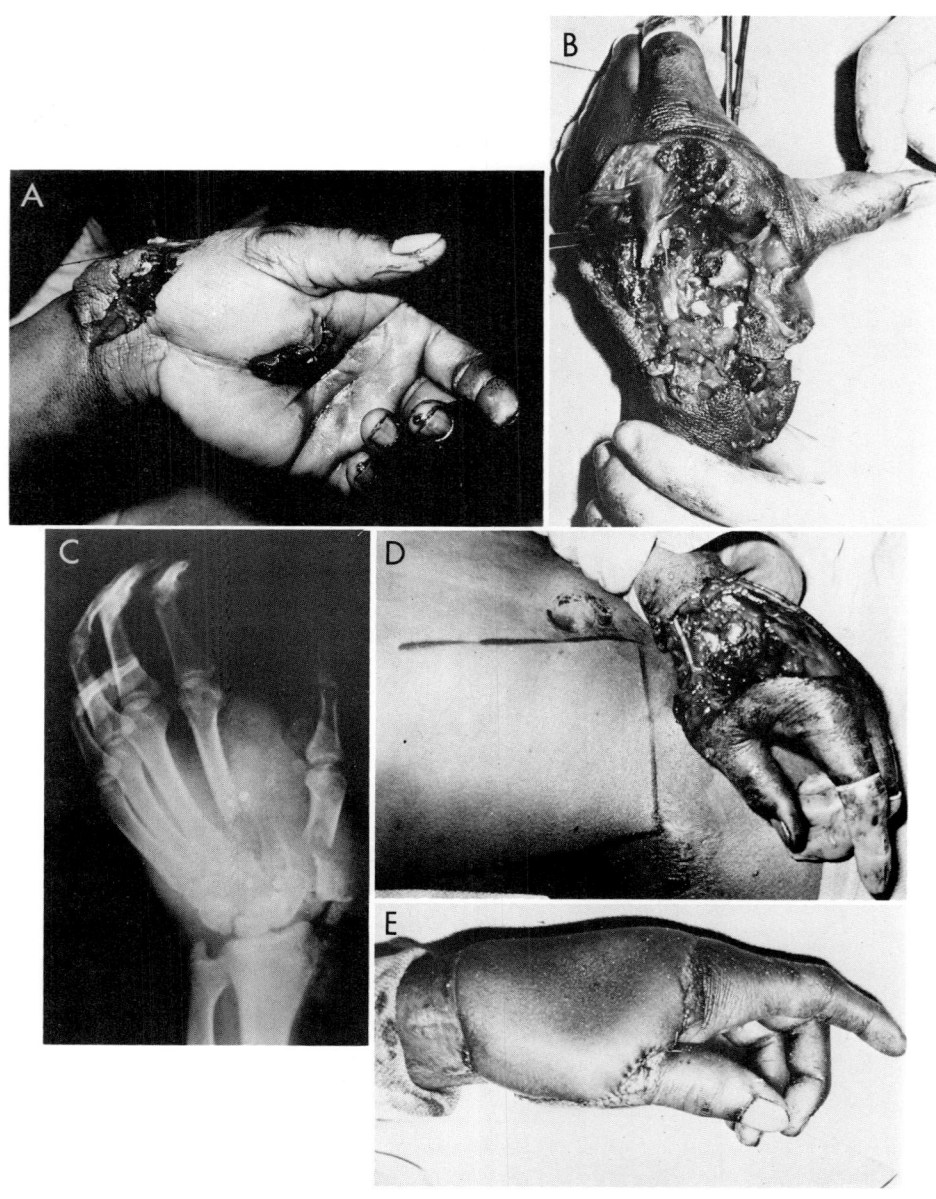

Fig. 23-16.—**A,** shotgun injury of hand of an 18-year-old boy, showing wound of entrance and laceration at edge of dorsal wound of exit. **B,** wound of exit showing blown-out dorsal radial portion of hand. All structures of this area of hand involved and immediate flap coverage indicated to cover fractures, joints and tendons and provide good tissue for later reconstruction. **C,** x-ray film showing fractures of thumb and index finger metacarpals and disorganized and missing carpal structures. **D,** after debridement of devitalized tissue and stabilization of bones with internal K-wires. Flap from right upper quadrant of abdomen with conservative base to lengthen ratio is outlined for immediate application. **E,** 3 weeks later, the flap has been divided and sewn into place while the hand was on the abdomen. Further reconstruction of thumb index complex may be done on an elective basis.

Chapter 23: SOFT TISSUE INJURIES OF THE HAND / 579

protection to the hard tissues and skin coverage. In such ring avulsions, if joints are open or there are significant tendon lacerations, serious consideration must be given to primary amputation in order to avoid a salvaged but still senseless finger.

Major Losses in the Hand and Forearm

Open injuries of the hand involving virtually all the tissues of the hand, exposing bone, joint and tendon, usually require the application of large pedicle flaps from a distant location. There are

Fig. 23-17.—**A,** large abdominal flap placed on forearm and hand of a 19-year-old boy who had sustained deep destructive burns of forearm and hand 13 months previously. Necessary nerve and tendon reconstructions could not be done through the thin adherent scar, which was excised and replaced by healthy flap tissue. **B,** flap and donor site. The flap had been raised in a single stage without delay. The defect in the abdominal wall had been resurfaced immediately with split-thickness skin grafts, which healed during flap application to arm.

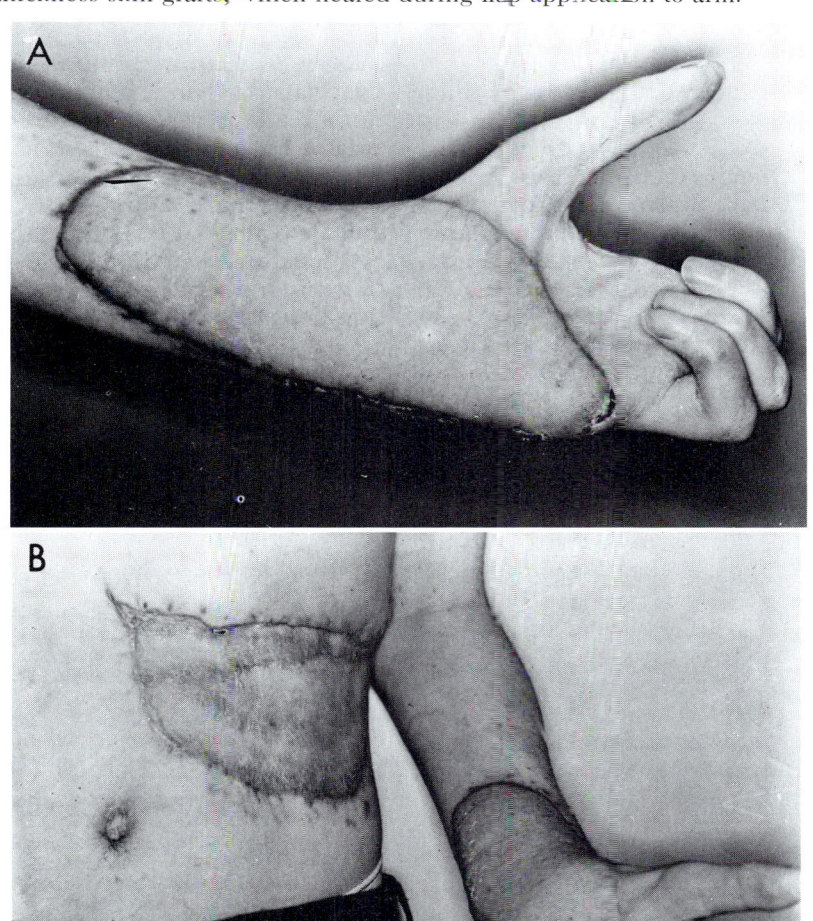

special instances in which split graft coverage is indicated to gain wound closure on either a provisional or a definitive basis. Whether using flaps or grafts, it is imperative to recognize the extent of tissue loss. In crushing or blast injuries, the true extent of tissue loss may not be known for several days and coverage must be delayed until debridement is complete. If coverage is elected before all nonviable tissue is removed, the entire wound will not be closed, placing the patient in jeopardy of continuing inflammation, open, raw areas and possible sepsis, all of which guarantee additional scar and crippling.

There are certain instances of open wounds in which gaining wound closure by a split-thickness skin graft is the wisest course.[7] Such examples are those of extensive crush, burn, blast or sepsis where the wound is either unstable enough or infected such that a potential donor site likewise would be at risk. In extensive, degloving injuries of the entire hand, split graft coverage is indicated, since flap coverage in such an injury results in a floppy, unusable situation. If bone or joints are exposed in such a situation, the "crane principle" could be employed. In general, if there is doubt concerning tissue viability, it is wiser to gain early wound closure by the use of split grafts and replace them later with definitive flaps.

In injuries with exposed bones and joints and with the diagnosis of tissue loss certain, immediate flap coverage is indicated (Fig. 23-16). The flap should be of undoubted viability and in such a position that the arm will rest comfortably for the ensuing 3 weeks, while permitting access to the wounds. The donor site should be closed—either primarily or by the use of free grafts. Healthy, well-vascularized flap tissue brought into an acute wound by this method not only provides secure, appropriate wound closure but provides tissue through which later reconstructive procedures may be done. Secondary revisions of the flap and thinning may be necessary at later operations. One problem in the use of flaps, especially from the abdomen, is that they tend to be unnecessarily thick and do not match the supple skin of the normal hand. Additionally, abdominal flaps gain weight as the individual does. To avoid this, one may elect to use the skin of a primarily defatted abdominal flap.[17] Flaps survive largely in the subdermal plexus, the fat being largely a metabolic load the flap must sustain. By thinning the flap initially and preserving the vital subdermal plexus, a thick abdominal flap may be transformed into tissue more appropriate to hand function. Lower abdominal flaps based inferiorly are appropriate for coverage of dorsal defects, whereas basing such a flap superiorly makes it more appropriate for palmar defects (Fig. 23-17). Large flaps from special locations occasionally are necessary to gain coverage prior to the reconstruction deficits left by acute injuries.

BIBLIOGRAPHY

1. Boyes, J. H.: *Bunnell's Surgery of the Hand* (4th ed.; Philadelphia: J. B. Lippincott Company, 1964), pp. 112–119.
2. Boyes, J. H., and Stark, H. H.: Flexor tendon grafts in the fingers and thumb, J. Bone Joint Surg. 53-A: 1332, 1971.
3. Branemark, P. I., and Ekholm, R.: Tissue injury caused by wound disinfectants, J. Bone Joint Surg. 49-A: 48, 1967.
4. Brody, G. S., Cloutier, A., and Woolhouse, F. M.: The finger tip injury—an assessment of management, Plast. Reconstr. Surg. 26:80, 1960.
5. Bunnell, S.: Repair of tendons in the fingers and description of two new instruments, Surg. Gynecol. Obstet. 26:103, 1918.
6. Bunnell, S.: Treatment of tendons in compound injuries of the hand, J. Bone Joint Surg. 23: 240, 1941.
7. Cannon, B.: Open grafting of raw surfaces of the hand, J. Bone Joint Surg. 40-A: 79, 1958.
8. Curtis, R. M.: Personal communication.
9. Davis, N.: Personal communication.
10. Dolphin, J. A.: Extensor tenotomy for chronic boutonniere deformity of the finger, J. Bone Joint Surg. 47-A: 161, 1965.
11. Edgerton, M. T., and Snyder, G. B.: Combined intracranial-extracranial approach and use of two-stage split flap technique for reconstruction with cranio-facial malignancies, Am. J. Surg. 110:595, 1965.

12. Edgerton, M. T., Snyder, G. B., and Webb, W. L.: Surgical treatment of congenital thumb deformities (including psychological impact of correction), J. Bone Joint Surg 47-A: 1453, 1965.
13. Furste, W., Scudder, P. A., and Hampton, O. P.: The evolution of prophylaxis against tetanus from the Civil War to the present, Bull. Am. Coll. Surgeons 52:277, 1967.
14. Harris, W. H., Slater, E. M., and Bell, H. M.: Regional anesthesia by the intravenous route, JAMA 194:1273, 1965.
15. Hoskins, H. D.: The versatile cross finger pedicle flap, J. Bone Joint Surg. 42-A: 261, 1960.
16. Hunter, J. M., and Salisbury, R. E.: Flexor tendon reconstruction in severely damaged hands, J. Bone Joint Surg. 53-A 829, 1971.
17. Kelleher, J. C., Sullivan, J. G., Baibak, G. J., and Dean, R. K.: Use of a tailored abdominal pedicle flap for surgical reconstruction of the hand, J. Bone Joint Surg. 52-A: 1552, 1970.
18. McBride, E. D.: *Disability Evaluation and Principles of Treatment of Compensable Injuries* (6th ed.: Philadelphia: J. B. Lippincott Company, 1963).
19. Millard, D. R., Jr.: The crane principle for the transport of subcutaneous tissue, Plast. Reconstr. Surg 43:451, 1969.
20. Pulvertaft, R. G.: Tendon grafts for flexor tendon injuries in the fingers and thumb, J. Bone Joint Surg. 38-B 175, 1956.
21. Shaw, F. S.: Pathological malingering: The painful disabled extremity, N. Engl. J. Med. 271:22, 1964.
22. Verdan, C. E.: Primary and Secondary Repair of Flexor and Extensor Tendon Injuries, in Flynn, J. E. (ed.): *Hand Surgery* (Baltimore: The Williams & Wilkins Company, 1966), Chap. 8, p. 238.
23. Winnie, A. P.: Interscalene brachial plexus block, Anesth. Analg. 44:455, 1970.

24 | Skeletal and Ligamentous Injuries of the Hand

EDWARD A. NALEBUFF and
LEWIS H. MILLENDER

THE SIGNIFICANCE of fractures, dislocations and ligamentous injuries encountered following trauma to the hand often is not fully realized. Every year, many patients are seen in hospital emergency rooms with hand injuries that if diagnosed correctly and treated properly would be minor problems. Unfortunately, many of these are poorly managed, causing prolonged morbidity and permanent disability. The busy house officer often does not have enough experience to examine the hand adequately. Very often after a "negative" x-ray report, the patient is discharged with a diagnosis of a simple sprain. The sprain may, in fact, be either a torn collateral ligament or a volar plate rupture. Misdiagnosis of this type would occur less frequently if the examining physician, using basic knowledge of the anatomy of the hand, carried out certain clinical examinations to determine whether the bone and supporting structures of the joint were intact. In addition, special x-ray views often are necessary to clarify the diagnosis. Only when the full extent of the injury is known can proper treatment be carried out. The aim of this chapter is to emphasize certain basic principles that we find helpful in the diagnosis and management of skeletal and ligamentous injuries of the hand.

LIGAMENTOUS INJURY*

JOINT ANATOMY.—Before discussing ligamentous injuries in detail, we will review briefly some aspects of digital joint anatomy that aid in the understanding of these injuries.

The distal and proximal interphalangeal joints are basically hinge joints that allow only flexion and extension. Lateral motion is limited by strong collateral and accessory collateral ligaments, a portion of which are tight in all positions of flexion and extension.[5] In contrast, the metacarpophalangeal joints of the second to the fifth fingers have a different anatomic arrangement that allows motion in two planes.[1,2] When the metacarpophalangeal joint is extended, lateral motion is possible due to the laxity of the collateral ligaments. However, with flexion of the metacarpophalangeal joint, the collateral ligaments become taut and little lateral motion is possible because of the anatomic configuration of the metacarpal head, as shown in Figure 24-1. This anatomic difference in the collateral ligaments of the metacarpophalangeal and interphalangeal joints explains why lateral forces frequently will injure the interphalan-

---

*Other soft tissue injuries of the hand are described in detail in Chapter 23.

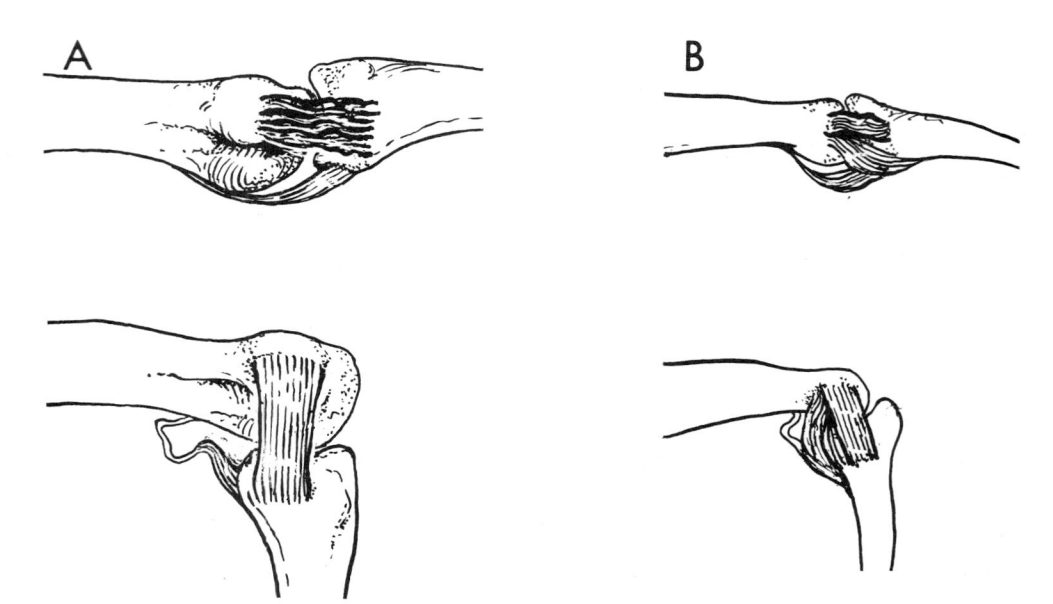

Fig. 24-1.—Comparison of the collateral ligament anatomy of the metacarpophalangeal and the proximal interphalangeal joints. **A,** as the result of the eccentric shape of the metacarpal head, the collateral ligaments are lax in extension but taut in flexion. This allows lateral mobility of the joints when the fingers are extended. **B,** ligaments of the proximal interphalangeal joints differ, in that a portion of the collateral ligament is taut in all positions. With the joint extended, the accessory collateral ligament is tight. When the joint is flexed, the main collateral ligament is tight and restricts lateral mobility.

geal joints. In contrast to the metacarpophalangeal joint of the finger, the metacarpophalangeal joint of the thumb has support characteristics similar to the interphalangeal joint with limited lateral mobility. Because the lateral motion at the metacarpophalangeal joint is minimal, lateral stress injuries frequently occur at this level.

The synovia-lined capsules of the fingers and thumbs are reinforced not only by radial and ulnar collateral ligaments but also by thickened volar plates. Whereas the collateral ligaments protect the joint against lateral stress, the volar plate protects the joint against dorsal stress. The volar plate is composed of a distal cartilaginous portion and a proximal membranous portion, which fold like an accordion during flexion.

Although the collateral ligaments and volar plates can resist ordinary stresses applied to the joint, they do have a limit. Unexpected blows from athletics or from other forceful activities may cause too much stress. The direction of the force applied to the joint determines which structure will tear. A careful history emphasizing the mechanism of injury often will clarify this point. Because there may be no associated bone injury, the x-ray appearance can be deceptively negative.

When a hand with a swollen, tender or painful joint is examined, the diagnosis first must be considered from an anatomic point of view. Are the collateral ligaments intact? Is there an injury to the volar plate? What about the extensor mechanism? Considered in this way, it is unlikely that the correct diagnosis will be overlooked.

We will now consider the common ligamentous injuries around the joints of the hand and elaborate on their diagnosis and management.

Chapter 24: SKELETAL AND LIGAMENTOUS INJURIES OF THE HAND / 585

COLLATERAL LIGAMENTS.—Collateral ligament injuries result from forceful lateral stresses applied to the extended digit. The radial aspect of the proximal interphalangeal joint is injured more frequently than is the ulnar side. The reverse is true at the metacarpophalangeal joint of the thumb, where the ulnar collateral ligament is injured most frequently.

A history describing the direction of stress applied to the joint is helpful, but a diagnosis still can be made without this information. On examination, the involved joint usually is swollen, with some limitation of motion. In addition, there usually is localized tenderness laterally at the site of injury. Routine x-ray examinations should be carried out even

Fig. 24-2.—Examples of recent and old collateral ligament injuries of the proximal interphalangeal joint. **A,** normal lateral stability on radial stress. **B,** note the bone fragment, which represents an avulsion of the ulnar collateral ligament with wide displacement. **C,** the same patient demonstrates gross instability when the torn ligament is stressed. **D,** chronically swollen proximal interphalangeal joint as a result of a collateral ligament injury that occurred 20 years previously. **E,** x-ray appearance, showing lateral subluxation of the proximal interphalangeal joint. Note the telltale bone fragment, which indicates a collateral ligament tear. **F,** a positive stress test, indicating that time alone does not restore ligament stability following a tear with displacement.

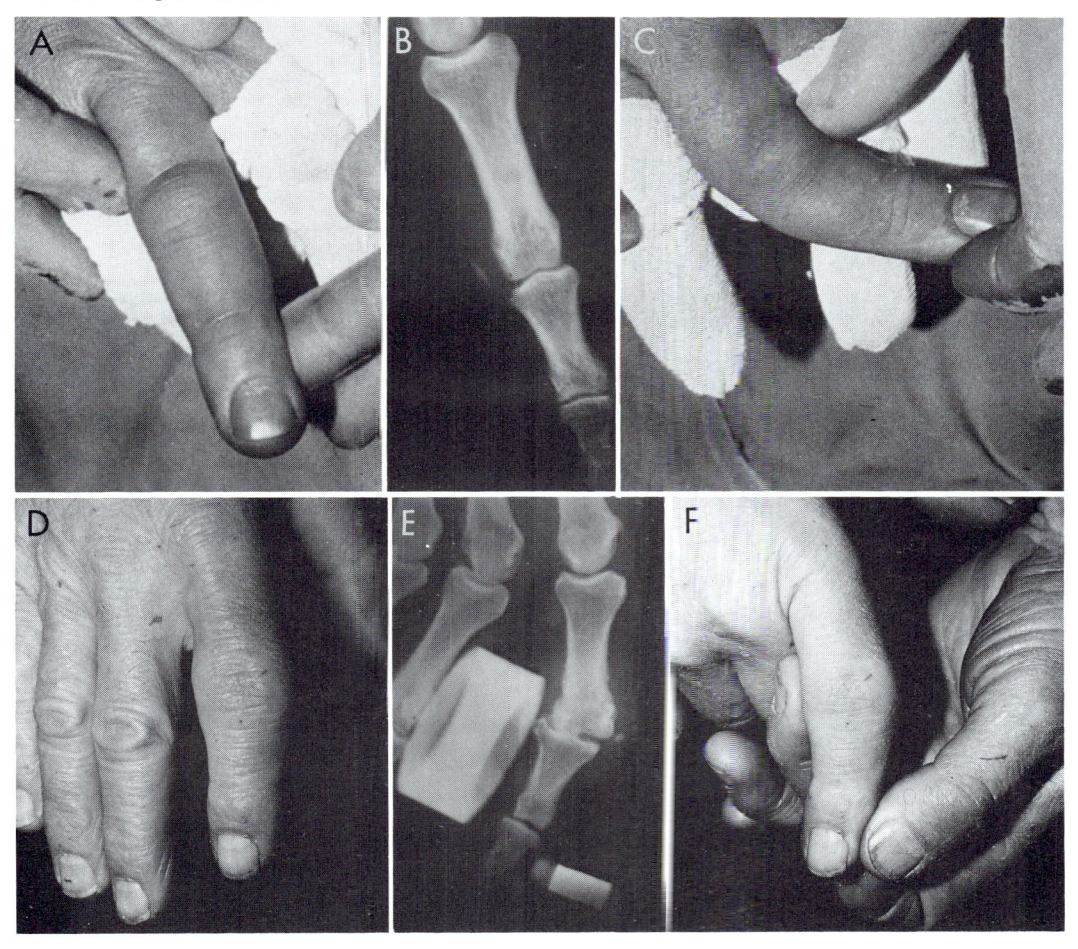

though they often are negative. In some cases, a small chip fracture may be noted, which represents an avulsion of the collateral ligament. The important point is to differentiate between an *incomplete* ligamentous injury, often referred to as a sprain, and a *complete* rupture of the ligament. This is done best by laterally stressing the joint to determine its stability. With a complete tear, the joint can be felt to open easily without anesthesia. If this maneuver is too painful to the patient, a metacarpal or a wrist block should be used, and the stress reapplied. Stress x-ray films can be very helpful in determining the diagnosis. If the joint feels stable to lateral stress or opens only minimally, the injury is, at most, a partial tear and conservative treatment is indicated. Most collateral ligament injuries are of this type. The involved finger with a partial tear should be splinted in moderate flexion to allow the soft tissues to heal. After 10 days, gradual motion of the joint may be started. Full function usually will return in 4–6 weeks.

On the other hand, if the joint is unstable and opens on stress, the patient has a complete tear and one should consider a surgical repair. The so-called conservative treatment of splinting these *complete* ligamentous injuries very often is followed by permanent joint laxity with chronic synovitis. Later on, these patients may develop degenerative arthritis with pain, instability and limitation of motion. Redler and Williams[13] and McCue and Horner[7] have emphasized the need for early surgical repair of these complete ligamentous tears. At surgery, the damage almost always is more extensive than anticipated. The proximal attachment of the collateral ligament is involved more commonly than is its distal insertion. The collateral ligament may be found interposed between the joint surfaces or widely separated from its normal attachment. This is particularly common in collateral ligament injuries of the metacarpophalangeal joint of the thumb, as was pointed out by Moberg,[8]

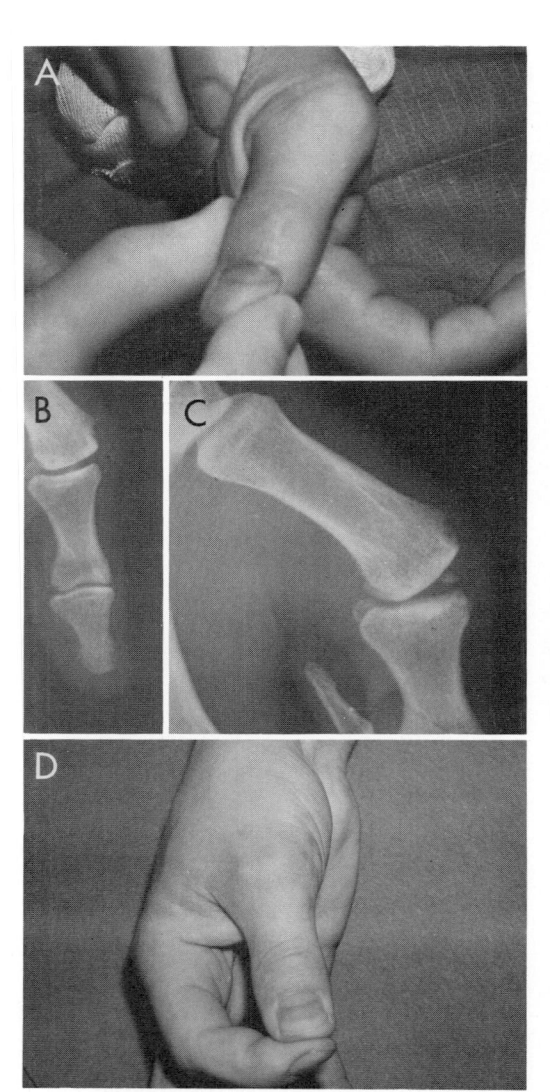

Fig. 24-3.—Radial collateral ligament rupture of the metacarpophalangeal joint of the thumb. **A,** injury to the radial collateral ligament, demonstrating lateral instability on stress. **B,** routine anteroposterior x-ray film, showing minimal abnormality. Note the irregularity of the metacarpal condyle, where the collateral ligament normally arises. **C,** stress x-ray film, showing gross lateral instability with a small bone fragment attached to the collateral ligament. **D,** following surgical repair of the collateral ligament, the patient regained good thumb stability.

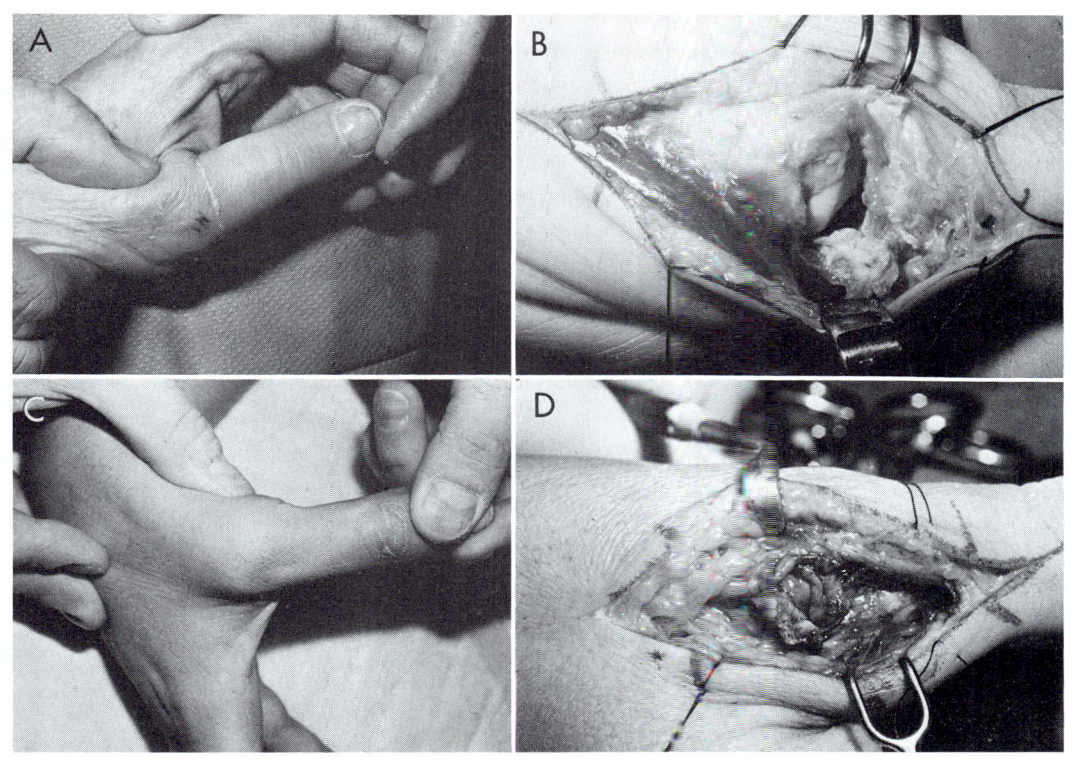

Fig. 24-4. — Pathologic findings in collateral ligament injuries of the thumb. **A**, tear of the radial collateral ligament. **B**, demonstrating a capsular tear at surgery with a portion of the ligament trapped within the joint. **C**, typical ulnar collateral ligament rupture with instability to lateral stress. **D**, note the abnormal position of the collateral ligament outside the adductor attachment.

Moberg and Stener[9] and Stener.[14] In these cases, the distal portion of the collateral ligament often is trapped proximally, with interposition of a portion of the extensor apparatus between the ligament and its normal point of attachment. Only surgery affords the opportunity to accurately assess this injury and to make the necessary anatomic corrections.

A midlateral incision is used for surgical repair of the collateral ligament of the proximal interphalangeal joint. The dissection is carried between the lateral band and the central slip, allowing the lateral band and the attached transverse retinacular ligament to be retracted volarly. This provides easy access to the lateral aspect of the joint and the collateral ligament. Tiny fragments of bone avulsed with the ligament should be removed and the ligament resutured in its normal position. A pull-out wire technique may be used, but ordinarily there is enough soft tissue remaining on the phalanx to carry out a direct suture. Postoperatively, the joint should be splinted in mild flexion for 2 or 3 weeks before gentle exercises are allowed. Vigorous activity should be avoided for at least 6 weeks. A midlateral incision is also used for collateral ligament injuries of the metacarpophalangeal joint of the thumb. The adductor pollicis or abductor pollicis brevis insertion is dissected from the extensor apparatus to provide exposure of the collateral ligament.

In our experience, the results of open repair of complete tears of the collateral

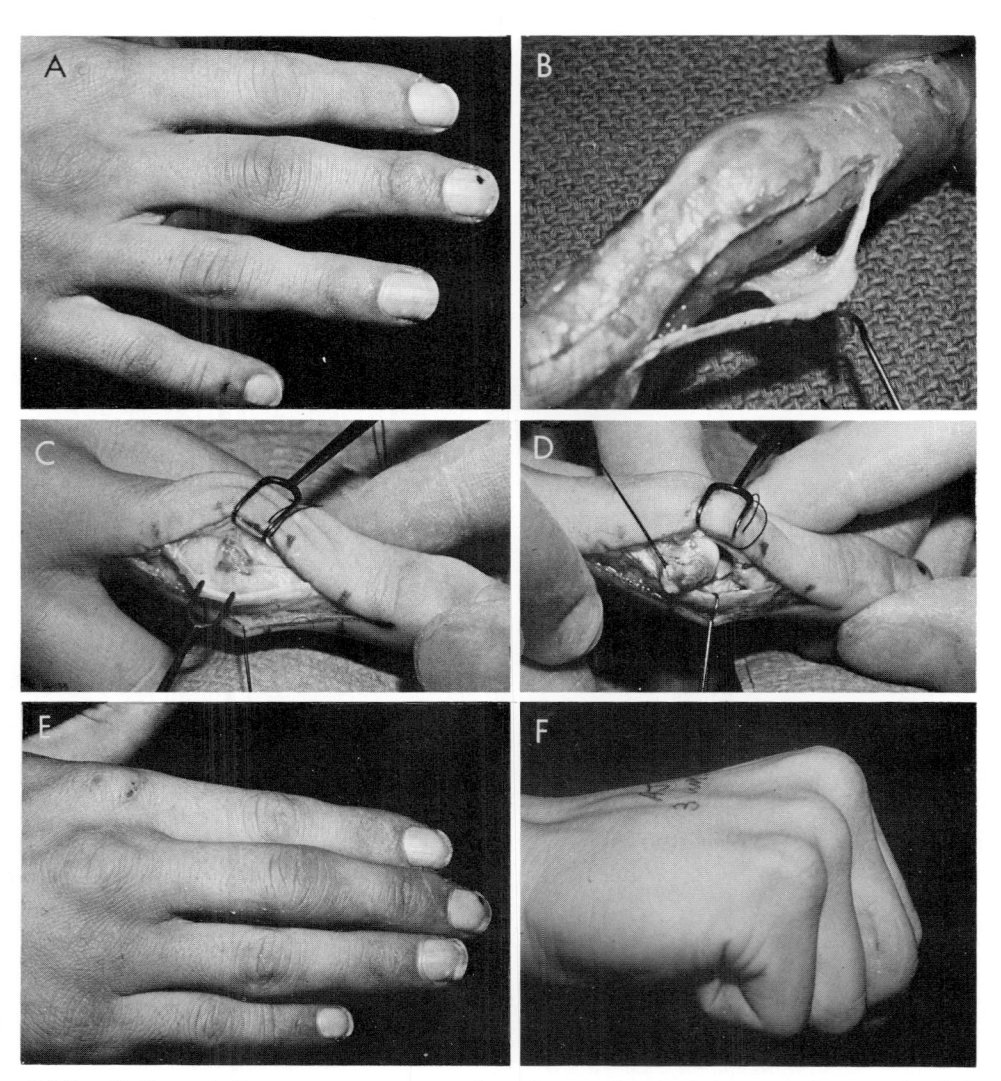

Fig. 24-5.—Collateral ligament rupture and early repair. **A,** injury to the proximal interphalangeal joint of the long finger. Note the swelling on the ulnar aspect of the joint. **B,** anatomic specimen, demonstrating the interval between the lateral band and the central slip mechanism. Note the retinacular ligament extending from the lateral band to the fibrous tendon sheath. **C,** the surgical approach to the collateral ligament usually is carried out between the lateral band and the central slip mechanism. There is evidence of hemorrhage in the soft tissues. **D,** typical appearance of a collateral ligament rupture at surgery. The ligament is avulsed distally and widely displaced. **E** and **F,** appearance of the hand 3 weeks following surgery. There was rapid disappearance of swelling and return of motion.

ligaments at both levels have been good. Ideally, surgery should be done as soon as possible after the injury. However, in the proximal interphalangeal joint, satisfactory results can be obtained, even in late cases. Patients undergoing early surgery for complete ligamentous tears usually regain normal motion as well as lateral stability. We have been impressed by the rapid disappearance of joint swelling following surgery.

Whereas we believe that late repairs of

collateral ligament tears in the proximal interphalangeal joint can be successful, arthrodesis is the procedure of choice for most old collateral ligament tears of the thumb. We have found that late soft tissue repairs have not held up as well against the lateral stresses applied to the thumb. Fusion provides a painless and stable metacarpophalangeal joint. This advantage outweighs the minimal disability from loss of motion at this level.

VOLAR PLATE INJURY.—A hyperextension force applied to a finger or thumb strains the supporting structures on the volar aspect of the joint. With a complete dislocation, one can assume that the volar plate is torn. However, tears of the volar plate can occur without joint dislocation. The diagnosis in these cases is more difficult. A small avulsion fracture noted on the volar aspect of the joint is helpful in localizing the site of injury. Given a history of hyperextension force applied to the proximal interphalangeal joint in a patient with a swollen, tender finger, a presumptive diagnosis of a volar plate tear should be made. Again, stress films would be helpful in demonstrating the extent of the injury. This is particularly true at the metacarpophalangeal joint of the thumb, where the position of the sesamoids affords additional information as to the exact site of the tear.[15] If these sesamoids retain their relationship to the metacarpal with the proximal phalanx in a hyperextended position, the tear is distal to the sesamoids. If, however, the sesamoids maintain their relationship to the hyperextended proximal phalanx, the

Fig. 24-6.—A volar plate injury of the metacarpophalangeal joint of the thumb treated by primary repair. **A**, illustrating gross instability of the metacarpophalangeal joint to hyperextension stress. **B**, x-ray film demonstrating distal migration of the sesamoid bones with the proximal phalanx. This indicates a volar plate tear proximal to the sesamoids. **C**, appearance of the tear at surgery, with the flexor pollicis longus retracted. **D** and **E**, postoperative result, showing good volar stability on pinch.

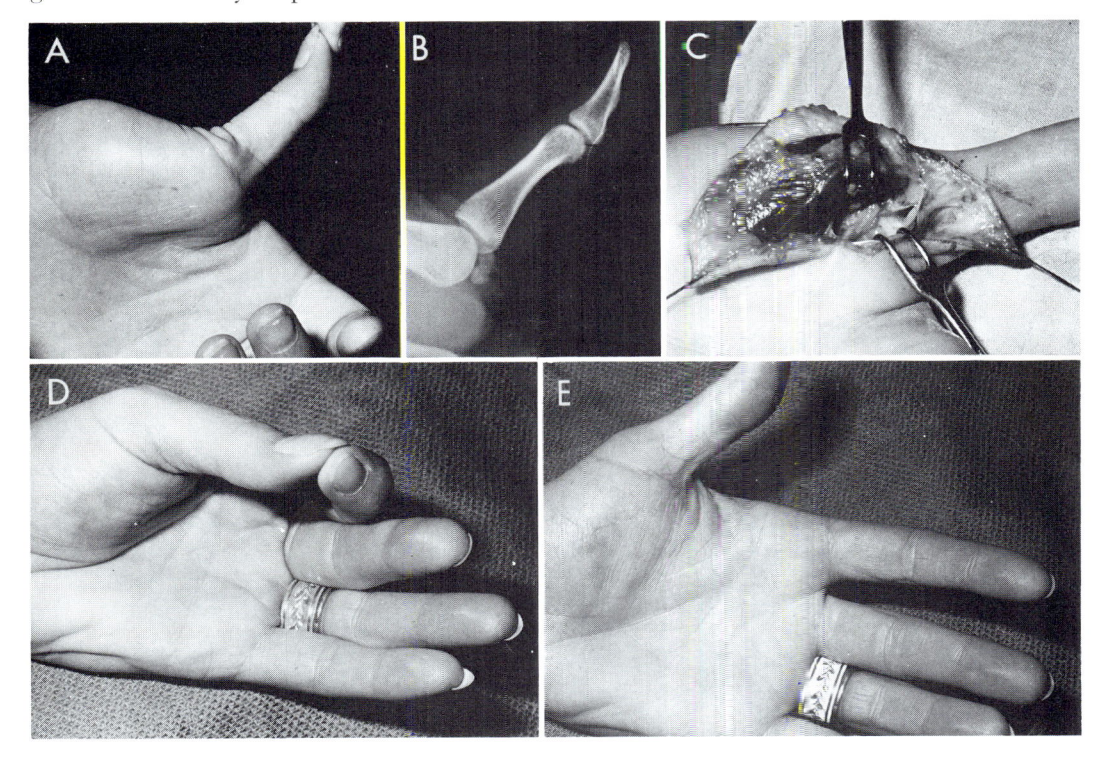

Fig. 24-7.—Swan neck deformity, secondary to an old volar plate injury of the proximal interphalangeal joint. **A**, note the hyperextension of the proximal interphalangeal joint with the finger at rest. **B**, demonstrating gross instability to hyperextension stress. **C**, a rent in the volar plate mechanism is repaired with a pull-out wire technique through a volar approach.

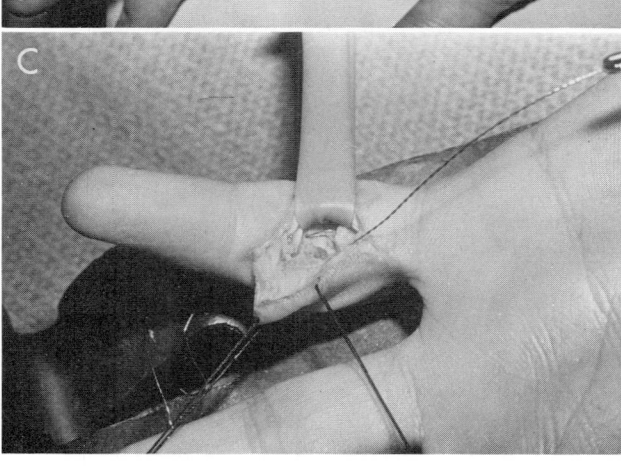

tear is proximal. In most volar plate injuries of the digits, joint stability is maintained. Splinting the finger in slight flexion will allow the volar plate to approximate and heal with little functional loss. Problems arise when the joint is incorrectly splinted in extension. This keeps the torn edges of the volar plate apart, and if healing occurs, it is with some laxity. However, splinting of the metacarpophalangeal joint of the thumb in a patient with a volar plate injury may not be adequate. Stener[14] has shown that the muscle pull on the volar plate tends to keep the edges apart despite splinting in flexion. Our experience with early repair of the volar plate of the metacarpophalangeal joint of the thumb has confirmed his findings.

Patients with incomplete healing of volar plate injuries gradually develop hyperextension of the involved joint and may be bothered later by repeated sprains as a result of minor trauma. Some patients gradually lose the ability to initiate flexion of the proximal interphalangeal joint. They are unable to flex the joint unless the proximal phalanx is stabilized or the distal joint is fully flexed. Flexion of the proximal interphalangeal joint then occurs but the normal smooth sequence of motion is lost. Treatment of an old symptomatic volar plate injury requires surgery. At the proximal interphalangeal joint level, an effort should be made to maintain motion while repairing or reinforcing the volar plate mechanism. At surgery, one finds that either the distal attachment is the site of injury or that there is a rent in the membranous portion of the volar plate. These tears can be closed with a fine suture material. In some cases, spontaneous healing with capsular laxity has occurred, making it necessary to excise a wedge of tissue to restore volar support. We often supplement the repair by using one slip of the superficial flexor tendon with its distal attachment intact to act as a checkrein against hyperextension. The tendon slip is passed obliquely across the joint surface and is either sutured to the margin of the fibrous tendon sheath or embedded into the proximal phalanx with a pull-out wire. Following this type of repair, performed through a volar zigzag incision, the finger should be splinted for 3 weeks. Our aim is to correct the hyperextension by creating a slight flexion contracture of the joint. In old injuries to the volar plate of the metacarpophalangeal joint of the thumb, we prefer to perform an arthrodesis of the joint to provide stability.

Dislocations

Dislocations of a joint represent the end stage in soft tissue injury. Unlike the collateral ligament and volar plate tears, the diagnosis is usually is evident. Dislocations are, for the most part, either dorsal or lateral, depending on the direction of thrust. One can assume that a dislocation represents a tearing of the volar plate with or without a collateral ligament injury.[2]

The most frequent digital dislocations occur at the proximal and distal interphalangeal joints, whereas in the thumb, dislocation of the metacarpophalangeal joint is more common. Dislocations at the metacarpophalangeal joints of the fingers also occur but are rather rare. One must also be aware of dislocations at the carpometacarpal joints. These often are overlooked, as the x-ray findings are less dramatic and pass unnoticed by the inexperienced examiner. There are certain features of dislocation at each level that deserve more attention.

INTERPHALANGEAL JOINT DISLOCATIONS.—Dislocations of the interphalangeal joints are the result of direct trauma, frequently occurring in contact sports. Clinically, the finger is distorted, with or without an open wound. X-ray films should be obtained to confirm the diagnosis and to rule out associated fractures before reduction is attempted. When seen early, before swelling and muscle spasm occur, these dislocations often can be reduced by gentle traction and manipulation. If, however, the patient experiences pain, a wrist or metacarpal block should be used. After reduction is obtained, it is wise to carry the joint through a complete range of motion to ensure completeness of reduction and to rule out interposed soft tissues. One should also gently check for stability of the collateral ligaments. Proximal interphalangeal joint dislocations that are stable should be immobilized in slight flexion for 2 weeks to allow healing of the volar plate. Then gentle range of motion exercises may be begun, but full extension should be avoided for an additional week. After 4–6 weeks, the patient may be allowed to resume his previous activities.

592 / Edward A. Nalebuff and Lewis H. Millender

Fig. 24-8.—Dislocations commonly encountered in the hand. **A**, dorsal dislocation of the distal interphalangeal joint. **B**, dorsal dislocation of the proximal interphalangeal joint. **C**, typical appearance of a dorsal dislocation of the metacarpophalangeal joint of the thumb. **D**, dorsal dislocation of the metacarpophalangeal joint of the index finger. This dislocation is not obvious clinically and can be overlooked. **E**, Bennett fracture-dislocation of the carpometacarpal joint of the thumb. **F**, reduction of the Bennett fracture is unstable and usually requires internal fixation. A Kirschner wire was used in this case. **G**, an example of a dorsal carpometacarpal dislocation. **H**, a volar carpometacarpal dislocation. These dislocations are not obvious on x-ray and often are not recognized.

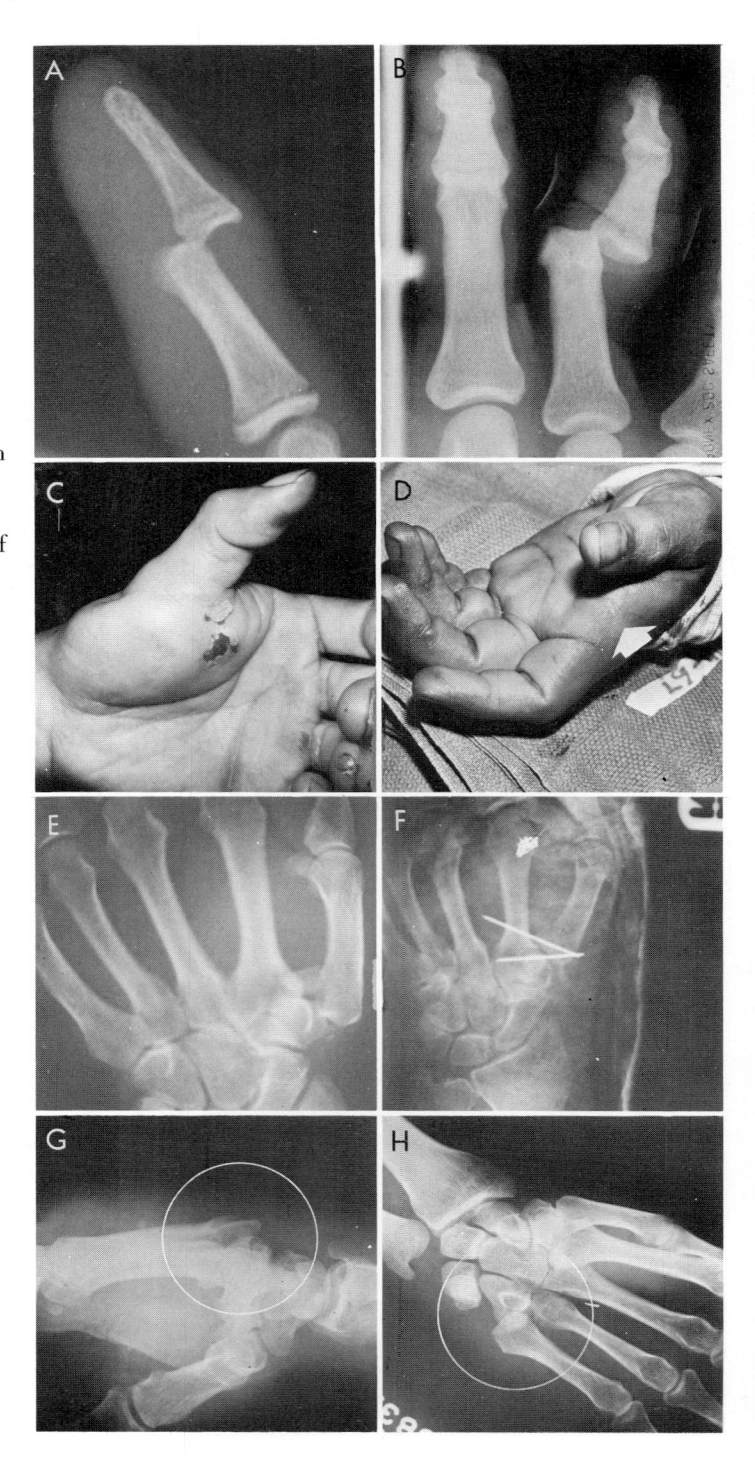

Dislocations of the distal interphalangeal joints frequently are unstable after reduction and tend to subluxate. In this situation, the reduction is maintained by a small Kirschner wire inserted across the joint for several weeks.

Most dislocations can be cared for in the emergency room, but there are conditions in which surgery is indicated. In open dislocations, it is preferable to carry out thorough cleansing and debridement in the operating room before reduction. In the occasional case in which closed reduction fails or in which reduction is incomplete, repeated manipulative attempts only further traumatize soft tissues. Therefore, open reduction should be carried out. Also, when there is an obvious complete tear of the collateral ligament, surgical repair is indicated.

METACARPOPHALANGEAL JOINT DISLOCATIONS. — Dorsal dislocations of the metacarpophalangeal joint of the thumb are relatively common. They result from a hyperextension force that tears the volar plate and allows the metacarpal to herniate through the capsule. Unlike digital dislocations, these often are impossible to reduce by closed methods. One gentle attempt at closed reduction is all that is justified. If this fails, open reduction through a volar approach should be carried out. We have been impressed at surgery with how the capsule acts as a buttonhole preventing reduction. Herniation of the metacarpal through two heads of the flexor pollicis brevis has been described. We have also found that the flexor pollicis longus can act as an obstruction to reduction until it is retracted to one side. After open reduction is carried out, the volar plate should be repaired because of its tendency to remain separated as described by Stener.[5] The joint should be immobilized for 3–4 weeks to allow adequate healing of the soft tissues before exercises are begun.

Metacarpophalangeal joint dislocations of the digits are much less common than the thumb counterpart. They are prone to resist closed reduction and almost always require open reduction. Kaplan[3] beautifully describes this particular dislocation in the index finger. He shows the volar plate interposed within the joint, with the long flexor and lumbricals surrounding the metacarpal head. The soft tissues form a Japanese finger trap, which tightens as reduction is attempted. Surgeons unfamiliar with this injury have attempted to reduce it from a dorsal approach and failed. One should expose the area through a volar incision, which reveals the distorted anatomy.[10] By opening the flexor tendon sheath, one can retract the flexor tendons laterally. The volar plate must be dislodged from within the joint before reduction is attempted. One or two sutures will repair the volar plate, after which immobilization of the joint in flexion permits soft tissue healing. The pathology is similar in other digits where a volar approach is advisable to achieve reduction.

CARPOMETACARPAL DISLOCATIONS. — Dislocations of the carpometacarpal joints occur in the thumb and in the digits. A force sufficient to dislocate the base of the thumb more frequently fractures the metacarpal shaft, producing the Bennett fracture-dislocation. In these cases there is an avulsion fracture of the radial articulating portion of the metacarpal, which remains attached to the radial collateral ligament. The shaft then dislocates proximally and dorsally. The thumb goes into adduction due to the overpull of the adductor pollicis.

These fractures are easily reduced with traction, but the position is quite difficult to hold. Sometimes it is possible to maintain the position with continuous skeletal traction or with a 3-point pressure cast applied to the thumb. However, we believe that a safer and more accurate method is to reduce the fracture by closed means and then to maintain position with a Kirschner wire passed percutaneously from the thumb metacarpal into the carpus. The thumb should be immobilized for 4 weeks before the wire is removed.

Dislocations of the carpometacarpal joint of the thumb without fracture do occur and, if treated early by closed reduction and immobilization in abduction, usually will heal with satisfactory stability. Chronic subluxations of the joint also occur and can be handled by reconstruction of a volar ligament. We have found that a portion of the abductor pollicis longus left attached to the metacarpal base can be passed through a drill hole in the greater multangular and then back on itself. Occasionally, arthrodesis of the joint is indicated in patients who have developed arthritic changes as a result of chronic subluxation of this joint.

Dislocations of the carpometacarpal joint of the digits are associated with crushing injuries and tend to be multiple. There is considerable soft tissue swelling, which obscures the diagnosis. Because neither the clinical nor the roentgenologic findings are obvious, the diagnosis frequently is overlooked. If this diagnosis is considered in *all* crushing injuries to the wrist, it will not be missed. Point tenderness over the carpometacarpal joint should lead to suspicion and if examined before swelling develops, the dislocated metacarpal can be palpated. Anteroposterior x-ray films show a loss of the normal joint space and a lateral or oblique film will show the dorsally displaced metacarpal. Comparison films of the uninvolved hand are helpful.

These dislocations are reduced easily when seen early but they are difficult to maintain. The joint surfaces are flat, and with torn capsules, the metacarpal tends to displace despite plaster immobilization. We tend to hold these with percutaneous wires until the soft tissues heal.

Old unreduced carpometacarpal dislocations cause pain, weakness and considerable disability. Displacement of the metacarpal base disrupts the longitudinal arch of the hand and may cause hyperextension at the metacarpophalangeal joint.

Old symptomatic unreduced dislocations of the second and third carpometacarpal joints should be treated by fusion.

Although carpometacarpal dislocations usually are dorsal and multiple, one should be aware of the fact that single dislocations can occur, and in the small finger they can be in a volar direction.[11] These isolated injuries are more difficult to diagnose. However, the prognosis following closed reduction is good. If the reduction is unstable, it should be supported with Kirschner wires.

FRACTURES

In the section describing ligamentous and soft tissue injuries it was stated that the proper diagnosis often is overlooked. However, once the correct diagnosis has been established, the treatment is not difficult. Conversely, in fractures of the hand, the diagnosis rarely is difficult but the treatment may be a challenge, even to the experienced surgeon. The difficulty one encounters in treating these fractures often is not anticipated. Many surgeons who would not attempt to treat a displaced femoral shaft fracture readily accept the responsibility for so-called minor hand fractures.

In the evaluation of any hand injury, a precise history and physical examination are mandatory. The history includes the method of injury and the magnitude of the force producing the trauma. The physical examination should be gentle. Evaluation of the soft tissue damage is of major importance. Although the diagnosis of displaced fractures is obvious, x-ray films still should be obtained before any attempt at reduction is carried out. X-ray examination is mandatory in any suspected fracture and represents an essential diagnostic tool. Both anteroposterior and oblique views should be taken. Lateral views of the *fingers* should be ordered instead of lateral views of the *hand* in order to prevent superimposition of the digits.

Although the bones within the hands are tiny, the difficulties that can occur are anything but small. Improper treatment of digital fractures can result in prolonged morbidity. Malunion and stiffness are the most frequent and serious complications. Malunion due to inadequate reduction may be either angular or rotary. Precise alignment is necessary in the treatment of digital fractures. This is treated best by flexing the fingers into the palm and noting that normally each digit points toward the tubercle of the navicula. The fingers function in sequence and a deviated or overlapping digit will seriously impair the entire function of the hand.

Stiffness, or limitation of motion, is another troublesome complication of digital fractures. Stiffness often results from prolonged immobilization, with adhesions of tendons within the fibrous tendon sheaths. As will be discussed, early motion and the avoidance of excessive immobilization of uninjured parts of the hand will reduce the frequency of this complication.

CLASSIFICATION. — In fracture textbooks, hand fractures commonly are classified according to their anatomic location. For example, all metacarpal fractures are grouped together whereas phalangeal fractures are subdivided into those of the proximal, middle and distal phalanx. This type of classification is not only complete but is helpful in explaining certain displacements that are the result of muscle pull on the fracture fragments. However, it is of less value in helping to determine the proper treatment. A simple classification that we have found useful is to divide hand fractures into the following groups: stable, unstable, intra-articular and open. Our method of treatment is influenced most often by these considerations.

Stable fractures. — Many hand fractures fall in the stable group. Included in this category are diverse fractures ranging from the linear cracks of the shaft of the phalanx to the comminuted fractures of the distal phalanx following a crushing injury. The mechanism of the injury may vary and the x-ray appearance and location may differ but the fractures have an inherent stability in common. This is best demonstrated by the lack of significant displacement of the fractured fragments as a result of the injury. Slightly displaced angulated fractures of the central metacarpals can also be included in this group, as they gain additional stability from the adjacent skeletal structure.

The basic consideration in the treatment of these stable fractures is a brief period of immobilization until the acute pain and swelling subside, followed by early active motion. These fractures ordinarily heal rapidly and usually are clinically united before the x-ray films show complete union. Complications in this group usually are the result of prolonged immobilization in a poor position. Ordinarily, we use molded plaster or aluminum splints, immobilizing as little of the hand as possible. The metacarpophalangeal joints are splinted in flexion with the collateral ligaments at their maximal length. The metacarpophalangeal flexion is also helpful in minimizing the risk of rotary malalignment. The latter problem is more common in the unstable fractures, but may also occur in stable metacarpal shaft fractures. With the digits held in flexion, it is easier to check for malalignment, which often goes unnoticed in extension. When adjacent fingers are splinted, it is necessary to insert cotton between the digits to prevent skin maceration. Repeat x-ray films during the first week are advisable to confirm the initial impression of fracture stability. After 10 days to 2 weeks of immobilization, the patient is allowed to remove the splint and start gentle exercises. Vigorous use of the hand should be avoided for a few additional weeks. By encouraging early motion in these fractures, one avoids joint stiffness.

In addition to the above stable fractures, crushing fractures of the distal

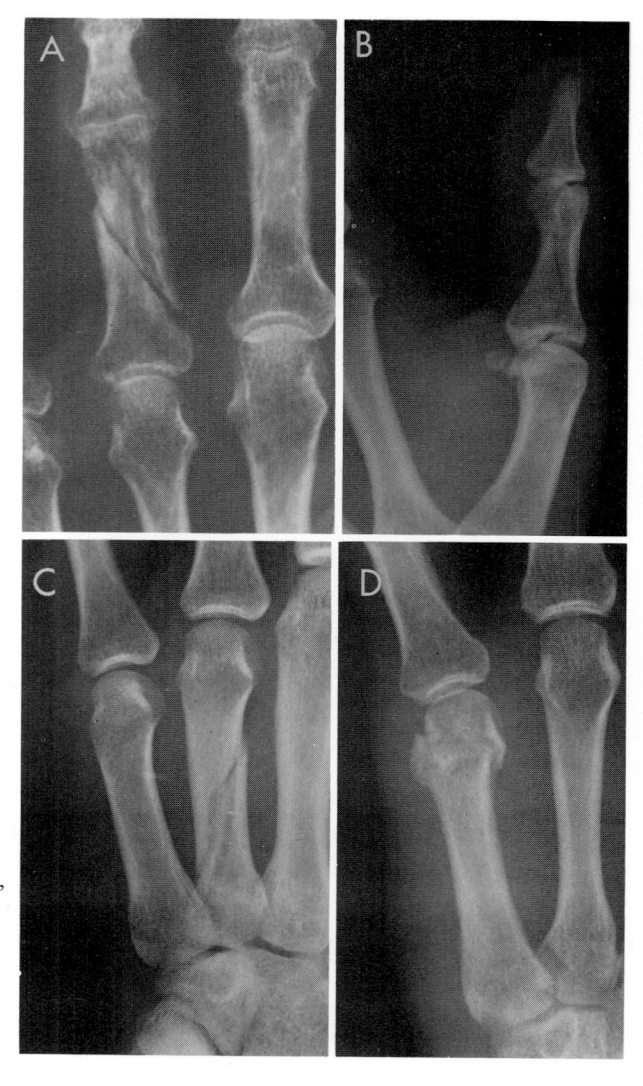

Fig. 24-9.—Stable fractures of the hand. **A** and **B**, typical examples of fractures of the proximal phalanges, which ordinarily do not displace significantly. **C** and **D**, additional examples of stable metacarpal fractures, which do not require prolonged immobilization.

phalanx are common injuries in which the soft tissue injury is more important than the fracture. These comminuted fractures require no reduction, and simple immobilization of the distal joint for a few weeks is adequate treatment. However, frequently they are associated with a painful, subungual hematoma, which should be relieved by drilling a small hole in the nail. Pain and increased sensitivity over the pulp may persist for a few months but usually will subside. Occasionally it is necessary to excise an ununited tender bony fragment.

Unstable fractures.—In contrast to stable fractures, in which early motion is indicated, unstable fractures need *immobilization* either to prevent displacement or to maintain the reduction achieved by the initial manipulation. Displaced fractures demonstrate their inherent instability by their initial displacement. In addition, certain fractures that appear well aligned initially in reality are unstable and may become displaced by muscle imbalance. This is especially true of short, oblique shaft fractures of the middle and proximal phalanges. These unstable fractures also show a greater degree of soft tissue injury than stable fractures and will, therefore, be associated with more swelling and more joint stiffness.

Displaced metacarpal and phalangeal fractures display a characteristic deformity due to the muscle imbalance. Unstable metacarpal shaft fractures show a dorsal angulation due to the tendency of the intrinsics to flex the distal fragment. Displaced fractures of the proximal phalanx angulate volarly due to the intrinsics flexing the proximal phalanx and the extensor central slip extending the distal fragment. In middle phalangeal fractures, the proximal fragment is pulled into flexion by the flexor digitorum superficialis.

These fractures demand accurate reduction and immobilization. Most of them can be reduced by closed methods and held in a position of function. A wrist block will give adequate anesthesia for manipulation. After traction and manipulation are carried out, the hand is placed in a position of function. Dorsiflexion of the wrist and moderate flexion of the metacarpophalangeal and proximal interphalangeal joints re-establish muscle balance and prevent redisplacement. Repeat x-ray examinations should be done during the first week to ensure maintenance of position.

If closed reduction cannot be obtained or if it is lost, open reduction with internal fixation is indicated. Kirschner wire fixation probably is the easiest and safest way to stabilize these fractures.[12, 16] Either longitudinal wires or transverse wires are preferred to cross-wires, which tend to prevent impaction. The fracture site can be exposed either laterally or dorsally by incising above or below the lateral bands. Careful sharp dissection and closure of the periosteal sheath will minimize adhesions of the extensor mechanism to the fracture callus.

Maintenance of position is not the only reason for open reduction and fixation. The stability achieved will also allow earlier motion, thereby reducing the risk of joint stiffness. Although open reduction has much to offer in the treatment of digital fractures, it should not be undertaken lightly. As is true in most surgical procedures, experience and proper tools are necessary for good results.

In our experience, traction seldom is indicated in the treatment of hand fractures. Pulling across the joint tends to lead to stiffness and seems to increase the tendency for tendon adhesion. Pulp traction seldom is indicated, as it can lead to considerable pulp atrophy, with diminished sensation in the finger tip. Therefore, we restrict our use of traction to the occasional case of severe comminution or contamination in which open reduction with internal fixation is not possible. By using *skeletal traction* in this situation, we are able to maintain length and alignment.

Intra-articular fractures.—These fractures represent some of the most difficult problems in fracture treatment. Regardless of the method of treatment, some limitation of motion or subsequent degenerative arthritis may develop. If the joint surface is allowed to heal in a displaced position, there will be not only impaired function but also painful instability. Because these fracture fragments are small, fixation in anatomic position often is difficult to achieve. However, our aim should be high in regard to restoring anatomic alignment, particularly with a large displaced fragment, which represents a significant portion of the joint surface.

These fractures result from either indirect forces or direct impacting injuries. The former often cause avulsion fractures in which the bony fragment is less important than the associated ligamentous injury. These can be fixed by reducing the fragment and transfixing it with a Kirschner wire or a pull-out suture. The more difficult fractures are those caused by direct blows to the phalanx. They are

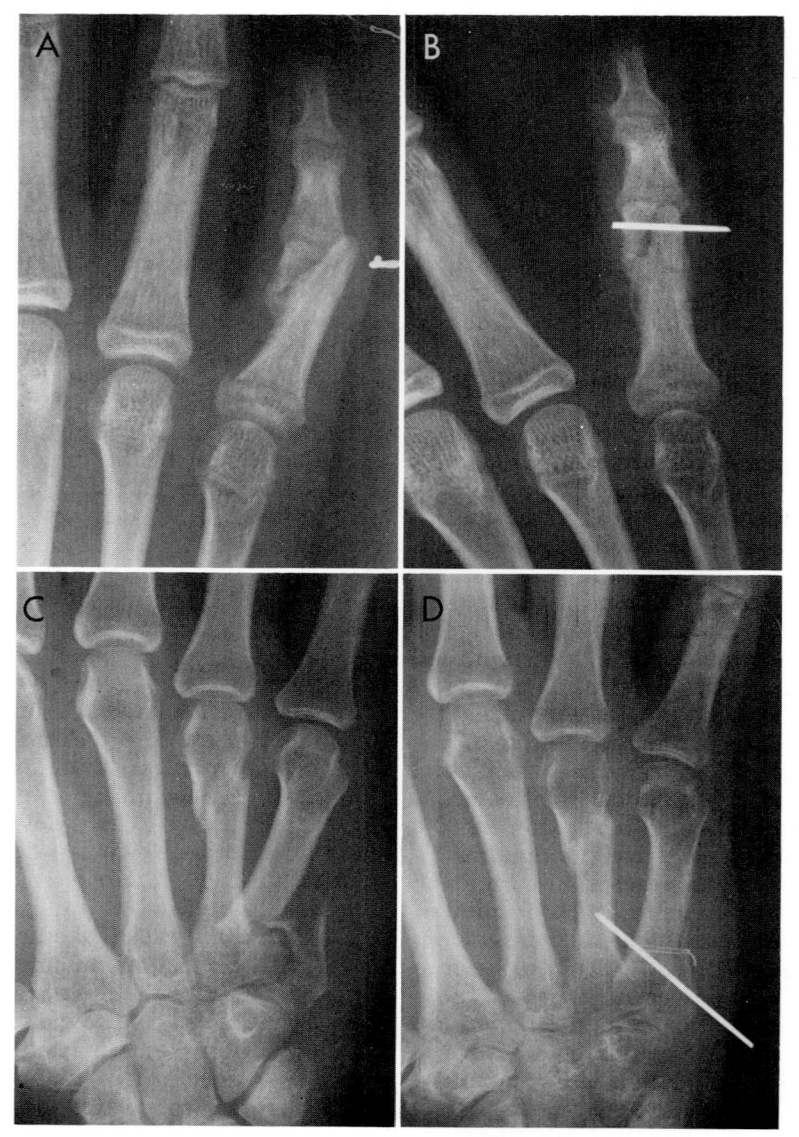

Fig. 24-10.—Examples of unstable fractures of the hand. **A** and **B**, unstable fractures of the proximal phalanx with proximal displacement of the fracture fragment. Reduction and internal fixation was necessary to maintain position. **C** and **D**, example of an unstable metacarpal fracture with medial displacement. Note the stable fracture of the adjacent metacarpal. The unstable fracture was reduced and held with internal fixation.

the large single condylar fractures, the more difficult "T" fractures and the badly comminuted fractures, which are so difficult to treat.

Large single or double condylar fragments can be replaced anatomically.

Usually we approach these dorsally, entering into the joint either between the lateral band and the central slip or below the lateral band. The collateral ligament is found to be attached to the fractured condyle, and efforts are made to preserve

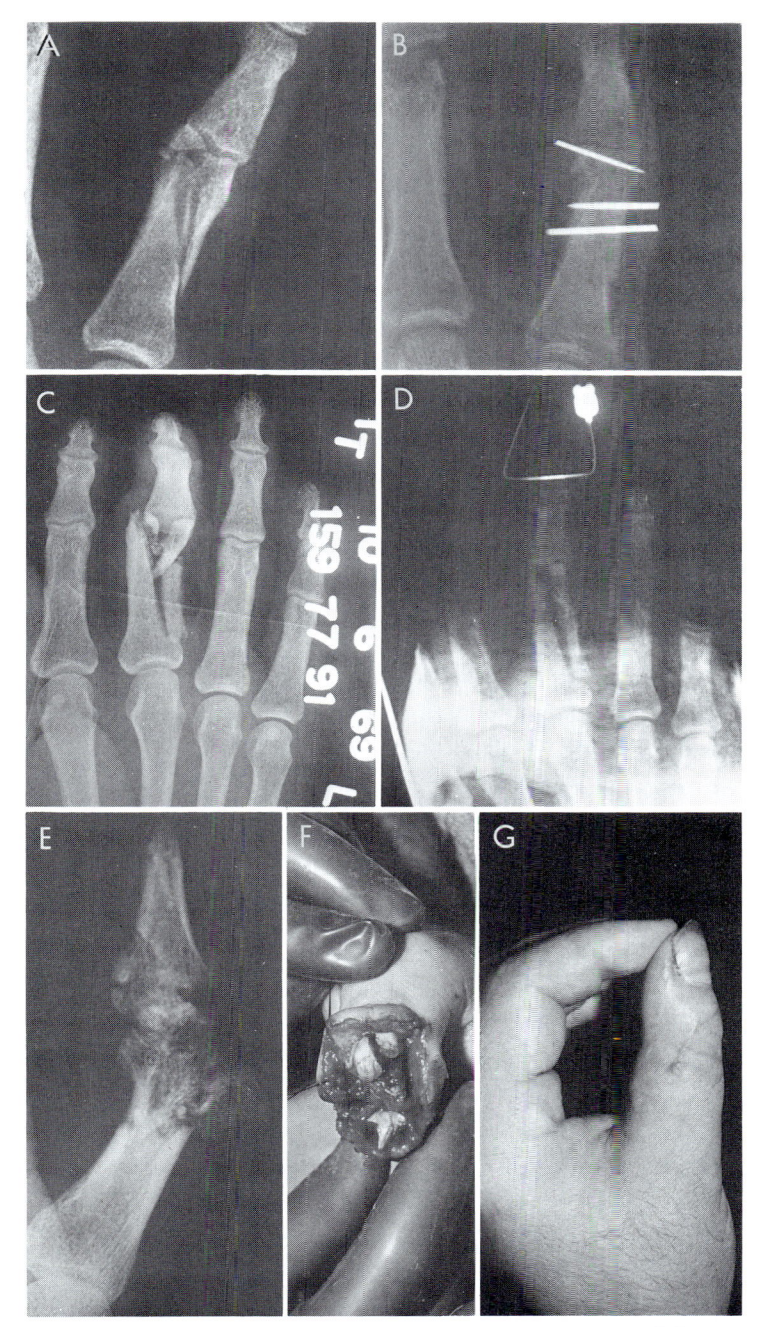

Fig. 24-11.—Examples of intra-articular fractures. A and B, comminuted fracture involving the proximal interphalangeal joint, treated by open reduction and internal fixation with Kirschner wires. C and D, grossly comminuted fracture of the proximal interphalangeal joint unsuitable for internal fixation, treated by skeletal traction to maintain alignment and length. E, severely comminuted fracture of distal interphalangeal joint of the thumb unsuitable for internal fixation. Appearance by x-ray. F, the articular cartilage was removed and primary fusion performed. G, showing a stable distal joint in good preservation.

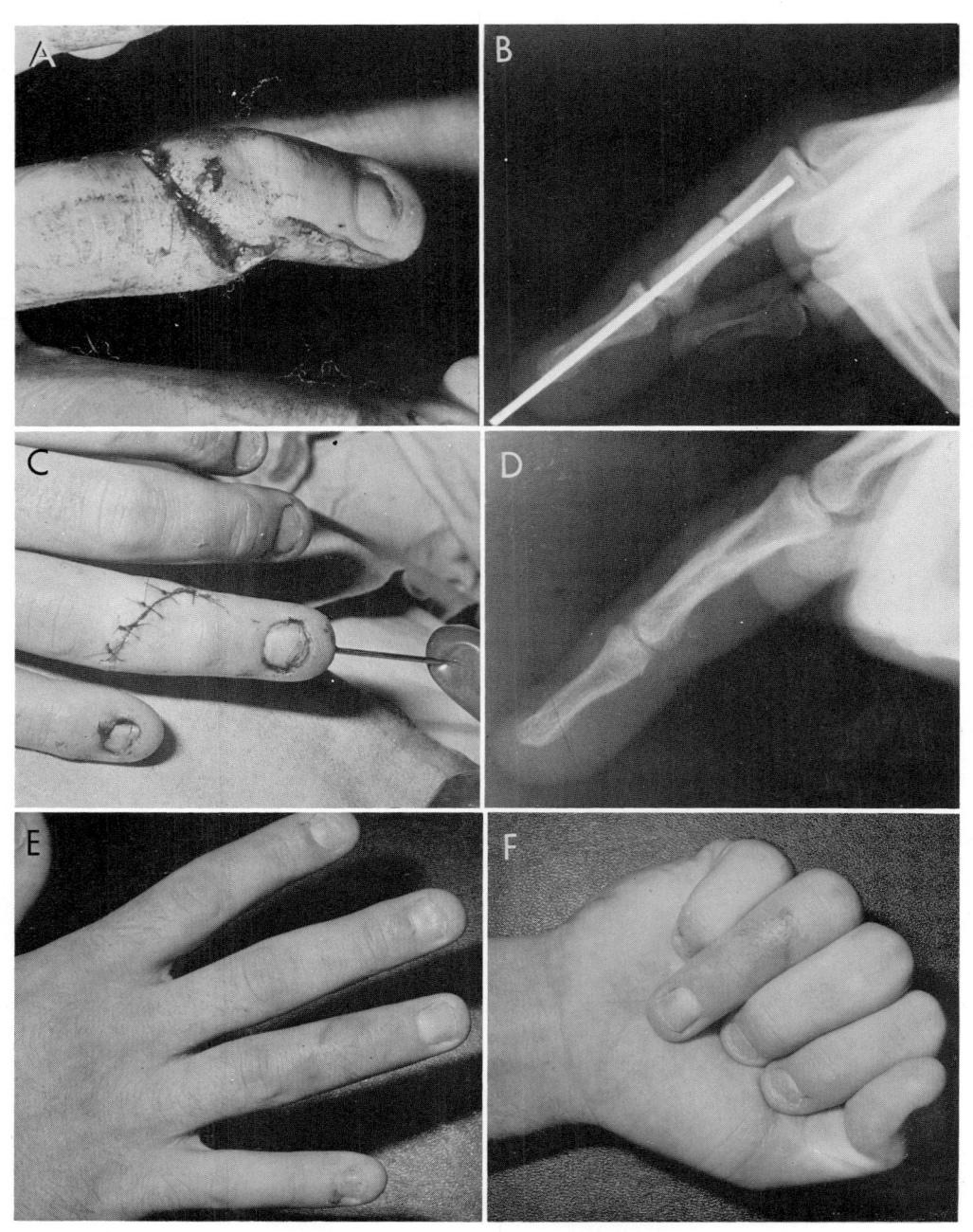

Fig. 24-12.—Typical open fracture, requiring wound cleansing, internal fixation and skin closure. **A,** open fracture of the middle phalanx with associated soft tissue injury, treated with retrograde insertion of a Kirschner wire. **B,** x-ray appearance, requiring surgery. **C,** appearance of the finger following primary stabilization of the fracture and soft tissue closure. **D,** x-ray appearance following fracture healing. **E** and **F,** excellent functional result was obtained.

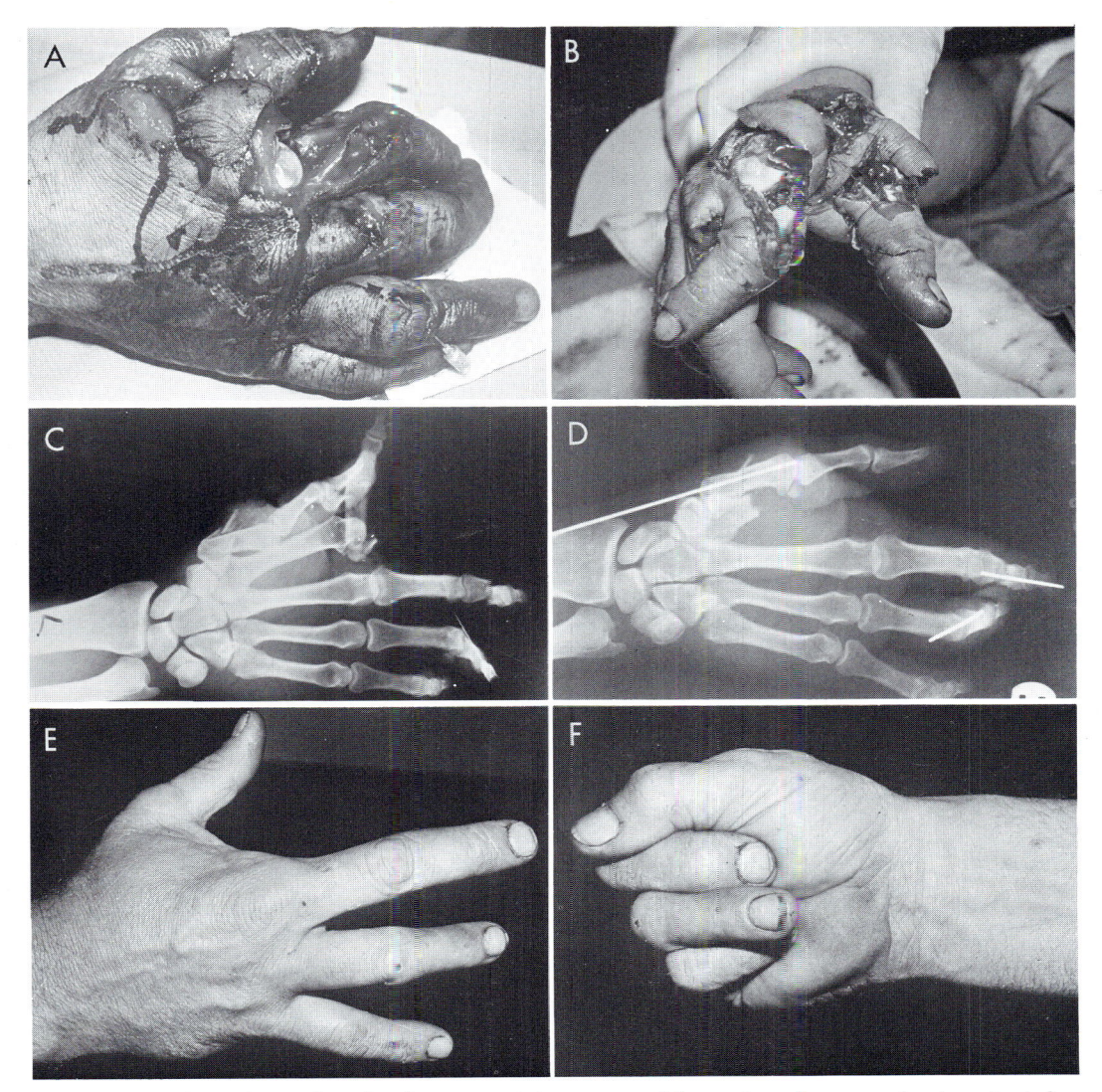

Chapter 24: SKELETAL AND LIGAMENTOUS INJURIES OF THE HAND / **601**

Fig. 24-13.—Complicated multiple tissue injury treated by using the same basic principles shown in Figure 24-12 for a single-digit injury. **A**, note the multiple fractures involving the thumb, index, long and ring fingers. **B**, appearance following initial cleansing of the wound. Note the skin defect in the thumb-index web space. **C**, x-ray appearance of the fracture. **D**, appearance following stabilization with Kirschner wires. Note the primary amputation of the index finger, with utilization of skin to close the thumb-index web space. **E** and **F**, early postoperative appearance, with recovery of excellent hand function, is shown.

this attachment. After the loose fragments and the hematoma are washed from the fracture site, the fragment can be anatomically replaced and fixed with a Kirschner wire. A decision regarding early motion is made only after determining the stability obtained at surgery. Although these fractures are difficult to treat, we have been impressed with the favorable results after open reduction and a carefully supervised postoperative exercise program.

Some intra-articular fractures result in severe comminution and destruction of the joint. In these, no attempt should be made to carry out open reduction. On occasion, an open crushing injury of this type is treated best by primary fusion. This certainly is true in the distal interphalangeal joint, where motion is not as important. At the proximal level, one can attempt to preserve motion by applying skeletal traction to prevent collapse while aiming for early motion. In a few cases of old fractures with painful joints in which motion is needed, we have inserted a silicone rubber joint prosthesis. This has become an added tool of treatment for this difficult injury.

Open fractures.—The problem of the open fracture with its associated soft tissue injury cannot be covered adequately in this chapter. However, there are certain basic principles that apply to all of these injuries despite their varying severity.[6] One cannot isolate the fracture treatment from the management of the overlying skin and adjacent tendons, nerves or vessels that have been damaged. The primary concern, of course, is to prevent infection. The wound should be cleansed with a bland soap solution and then irrigated with saline or Ringer's solution. Debridement of devitalized tissue completes the first stage of treatment. Attention then is directed to the skeletal injury. Stabilization is the key, and this is best and easiest achieved by the insertion of Kirschner wires. Retrograde insertion of the wires at the fracture site simplifies their use in shaft fractures. Kirschner wires are also helpful in stabilizing dislocations and articular fractures. The more complicated the injury the more the need for skeletal fixation. All of this should be accomplished prior to an attempt at tendon or nerve repair. When there are many fingers damaged, it becomes increasingly difficult to maintain the digits in proper alignment. Again, Kirschner wires across the flexed metacarpophalangeal joints or across the thumb-index web space will maintain a position of function. There is no better time to align and fix these fractures than at initial surgery. After the skeletal structures are positioned, attention may be directed to obtaining closure of the skin. This may require skin grafts or the application of a pedicle flap. Ideally, the wound should be closed initially. In badly contaminated wounds, however, it sometimes is advisable to clean, debride and stabilize and then carry out delayed closure after 3 or 4 days. This approach (delayed closure) is used extensively in war injuries and is also appropriate for many mangled hands seen in civilian practice.

In summation, hand injuries, like all trauma, deserve proper diagnosis and treatment in order to prevent subsequent deformity and disability.

Ligamentous and soft tissue injuries, dislocations and fractures require careful clinical examination and very often special x-ray views.

Whether the preferred method of treatment is traction, closed reduction or open reduction with internal fixation, one must try to avoid such complications as rotary malalignment, joint instability, joint stiffness and malunion.

Above all, one must consider the soft tissues, the bones, the tendons, the nerves, the vessels and the overlying skin on the hand as a single unit constantly interacting and intricately balanced.

BIBLIOGRAPHY

1. Bunnell, S.: *Surgery of the Hand* (5th ed.; Philadelphia: J. B. Lippincott Company, 1970).
2. Eaton, R. G.: *Joint Injuries of the Hand* (Springfield, Ill.: Charles C Thomas, Publisher, 1971).
3. Kaplan, E. B.: Dorsal dislocation of the metacarpophalangeal joint of the index finger, J. Bone Joint Surg. 39-A:1081, 1957.
4. Kaplan, E. B.: *Functional and Surgical Anatomy of the Hand* (2d ed.; Philadelphia: J. B. Lippincott Company, 1965).
5. Kuczuynski, K.: The proximal interphalangeal joint. Anatomy and causes of stiffness in the fingers, J. Bone Joint Surg. 50-B:656, 1968.
6. McCormack, R. M.: In Converse, J. M.(ed.), *Reconstructive Plastic Surgery. Acute Injuries of the Hand* (Philadelphia: W. B. Saunders Company, 1964), Vol. IV, p. 1574.
7. McCue, F. C., and Horner, R.: Athletic injuries of the proximal interphalangeal joint requiring

surgical treatment, J. Bone Joint Surg. 52-A:937, 1970.
8. Moberg, E.: Fractures and ligamentous injuries of the thumb and fingers, Surg. Clin. North Am. 40:297, 1960.
9. Moberg, E., and Stener, B.: Injuries of the ligaments of the thumb and fingers. Diagnosis, treatment and prognosis, Acta Chir. Scand. 106:166, 1953.
10. Murphy, A. F., and Stark, H. H.: Closed dislocations of the metacarpophalangeal joint of the index finger, J. Bone Joint Surg. 49-A:1579, 1967.
11. Nalebuff, E.: Isolated carpometacarpal dislocation of the fifth finger. Classification and a case report, J. Trauma 8:1119, 1968.
12. Pulvertaft, R. G. (Consultant Editor: *Operative Surgery. The Hand*, Rob, C., and Smith, R. (General Editors) (Philadelphia: J. B. Lippincott Company, 1970).
13. Redler, I., and Williams, J. T.: Rupture of a collateral ligament of the proximal interphalangeal joint of the finger. An analysis of 18 cases, J. Bone Joint Surg. 49-A:322, 1967.
14. Stener, B.: Displacement of the ruptured ulnar collateral ligament of the metacarpophalangeal joint of the thumb J. Bone Joint Surg. 44-B:869, 1962.
15. Stener, B.: Hyperextension injuries to the metacarpophalangeal joint of the thumb. Rupture of ligaments, fractures of sesamoid bones, rupture of flexor pollicis brevis, Acta Chir. Scand. 125:275, 1963.
16. Swanson, A. B.: Fractures involving the digits of the hand, Orthop. Clin. North Am. 1:261, 1970.

25 | Fractures of the Pelvis

WILLIAM N. JONES and WALTER S. KERR, JR.

BECAUSE THE FATAL OUTCOME of fractures of the pelvis almost always results from associated injuries, this chapter commences with a brief discussion of treatment of the severely injured patient who has a pelvic fracture. Details of treatment of the various associated injuries are described in other chapters and fractures of the acetabulum are considered separately.

PELVIC FRACTURES ASSOCIATED WITH OTHER INJURIES

Severe pelvic fractures often are associated with injuries to the head, chest, abdomen, genitourinary system and extremities. The care of such patients is a tremendous problem and should be a team effort of the orthopedic surgeon, general surgeon, urologist, radiologist, anesthesiologist, neurosurgeon and blood bank director. A number of things have to be done as rapidly as possible and some of them simultaneously. These include a history of the accident, physical examination, blood samples for cross matching, chemistries, complete blood count and blood gases, starting an intravenous with Ringer's solution or plasma until blood is available, central venous pressure line, abdominal tap for washings, x-ray films of the urethra, bladder and abdomen, infusion intravenous pyelogram and x-rays of other injured areas, notifying the blood bank,* the operating room, the anesthesia department and the angiography department of the problem at hand. An electrocardiogram should be done. A gravity suit† should be available. In order to accomplish these steps expeditiously and effectively, it is essential that one of the surgeons take over the direction of the care of the patient and coordinate the work of the other members of the team.

If possible, the patient should be put in a room large enough to hold 6–10 people. Often this many will be involved in caring for him. While the history and physical examination are being done, the blood lines should be put in, the Ringer's or plasma started and blood samples obtained. X-ray films should be obtained in the following order: (1) KUB, (2) urethrogram, (3) cystogram (if the urethra is intact), (4) then start the Renografin infusion urography. While this is running in, obtain the chest film and other indicated x-ray films. The 300 ml of Reno M-30 drip can be run in 5 minutes and film taken 5 minutes later. In most cases, unless the kidneys have been injured, a single film will give sufficient information concerning their number, location and state of function. The nephrogram will demonstrate parenchymal injury. All of these films should be finished in 30 minutes if done in the order outlined.

If there is evidence of an injured liver, kidney or spleen, celiac or renal angiography should be done. If severe continued blood loss from the pelvic fracture

---

*As many as 20 transfusions in 5 hours or less have been needed.

†The Kendall Co., Chicago, Illinois.

605

occurs, pelvic angiography (see Chapter 10) is indicated.

Massive uncontrolled hemorrhage is the most common cause of death in pelvic fractures.[7, 9, 10] Exploration of the retroperitoneum occasionally may be fruitful. Motsay et al.[5] reported finding lacerations of one external iliac vein and two common iliac veins in 3 patients explored. In 2 of these patients, hypogastric artery ligation did not control the bleeding and led to further exploration. Hemorrhage from an internal pudendal artery was controlled by spreading the symphysis pubis in one case. Byström et al.[1] have stopped bleeding from an obturator artery by ligation of the internal iliac artery in 1 patient. General efforts to control the hemorrhage usually have been unsuccessful. Hawkins et al.[2] found that suture ligation, hypogastric artery ligation, aortic cross clamping and packing are "not precise or specific." Ravitch[11] recommended an operative approach for direct control of bleeding only if the patient showed signs of continued bleeding after administration of more than 20 pints of blood. The source of fatal bleeding has been difficult to recognize at autopsy. Perry and McClellan[9] reported 15 patients with fatal pelvic fractures, of whom 8 died of hemorrhage, 1 of a severed iliac vein and 1 of a severed femoral artery. The site of fatal bleeding in the other 6 patients could not be identified.

Reynolds and Balsano[12] reported results of transfemoral venography in 25 cases of pelvic fracture. Localization of bleeding from venous plexus was not feasible. In 1 of these patients with dislocation of a sacroiliac joint, venography demonstrated an injured common iliac vein. Dislocation of the sacroiliac joint frequently is associated with major vascular injuries, especially venous, and is not uncommonly associated with nerve injuries.

The complexity of the care of such patients is illustrated by the following case report.

MGH CASE 174-91-89. — A 61-year-old white stevedore was admitted through the emergency ward having been struck by a 1,000-pound boiler top. There was a large hematoma of the left hip region. Blood pressure was 80/40 mm Hg and pulse 110 per minute. Examination of the chest, head and abdomen were otherwise negative. Peripheral nerve and arterial examinations were normal. Volume replacement was started. A urethrogram revealed complete separation of the membranous urethra. A catheter could not be passed into the bladder. An infusion intravenous pyelogram showed prompt bilateral function and marked upward displacement of the bladder. The pubic rami were severely fractured on both sides, with downward displacement of the fragment on the left side. Abdominal washing revealed no blood. Following infusion of 2,000 ml of whole blood and 4 units of plasma, he was taken to the operating room. The displaced bladder was identified and opened. A #20 Foley catheter with a 30-ml bag was introduced through the penis and put on 4 pounds of overhead tension. The pelvic hematoma was not disturbed. The peritoneum was opened. No visceral injury was identified. The patient had been in a gravity suit while waiting to go to the operating room. In the recovery room, he again was placed in a gravity suit inflated to 20 cm of water. Over the next 12 hours, blood requirements lessened. However, 22 hours after admission, fresh blood issued from around the Foley catheter at an alarming rate. Blood replacement reached 350–500 ml per hour. He received 17 units of whole blood by the time pelvic aortography was done. This demonstrated bleeding from a branch of the left obturator artery, and the artery stopped bleeding after the injection of 1 ml of the patient's clotted blood into the left internal iliac artery. The patient required only three transfusions over the next 24 hours and one further transfusion during his hospital stay.

The patient was maintained on 100% oxygen on a volume-controlled ventilator (Emerson). On the sixth hospital day, the patient was transferred from the recovery room to the respiratory intensive care unit, where he remained for 4 weeks. On the seventh postoperative day, his pulmonary problem improved to the extent that progressive weaning could be started; this was increased gradually over the next 4 weeks. On the fifteenth hospital day, the Foley catheter accidentally was pulled out. Septic shock developed, which responded to treatment. Because of an elevated bilirubin and a palpable mass in the right upper quadrant, on the same day a cholecystostomy was done for acute acalculous cholecystitis. The retropubic area was explored and no infection was discovered. Five weeks after admission, the patient was discharged from the respiratory unit to a surgical floor.

The patient was discharged on his sixty-fifth hospital day, walking quite well with crutches.

ANATOMY OF THE PELVIS

The combination of the two innominate bones and the sacrum forms the pelvic ring, which serves as a support for the trunk, either through the ischial tuberosities in sitting or through the acetabula in standing. The pelvic ring also supports and protects the pelvic viscera. The weight-bearing function is accomplished largely by the upper segments of the sacrum and the thick bars of iliac bone extending from the sacroiliac joints into the acetabula, forming a posterior arch, which joins the spine to the lower extremities. Both the bone masses and the ligaments of the sacroiliac joints are heavy and strong, and ordinarily they can be broken or torn only by violent forces.

The two obturator rings form an anterior arch that serves for visceral support and muscle attachments. Being thinner bone masses, the pubis and the ischium, along with the iliac wings, the lower sacrum and the coccyx, are likely to fracture by lesser forces.

Because of the encircling shape of the pelvis, wide separation or displacement at one point in the ring requires distortion of the ring at another point. Distortion may occur at any of the three pelvic joints — the symphysis pubis or the sacroiliac joints — by dislocation or tearing, or at a second site of pelvic fracture. Although the forces of injury determine, to a large extent, the deformity of a severely fractured pelvis, the trunk muscles inserting into the upper ilium pull a segment that is broken out of the pelvic ring up and through the posterior arch, tending to maintain proximal displacement. Strong contractions by the sartorius, the rectus femoris or the hamstring muscles may pull off their respective attachments in the anterior superior spine of the ilium, the inferior spine or the ischial tuberosity.

Although injuries to major nerves are not seen commonly, and when they are, usually are injuries of the sciatic nerve associated with acetabular fractures, bleeding more frequently is found to be a serious problem of treatment than was appreciated formerly.

This may be a result of more effective treatment now of other life-threatening injuries often associated with pelvic fractures — airway occlusion, chest and great vessel injuries, head and abdominal injuries and general resuscitative measures — so that patients survive long enough for bleeding associated directly with pelvic injuries to become the major hazard.

Although most commonly venous bleeding from a great number of points of vessel injury provides the requirement for massive blood replacement, arterial injury does occur in two particular and common patterns of pelvic fracture. Fracture through both sides of one or both obturator rings (when associated with violent injury) has a frequent enough incidence of obturator or pudendal artery injury to be recognized as a potentially serious injury — although, in comparison with many other injuries of the pelvis, it appears rather innocuous. A second type of injury also is associated with a fair incidence of arterial injury; that is, disruption of the external from the common iliac artery in fractures posteriorly close to the sacroiliac joint and displaced in the pattern of "opening like a book."

MECHANISM OF INJURY

Injuries involving those portions of the pelvis that have been fractured by less than violent forces—the obturator rings, the sacrum and the coccyx—result most commonly from falls and affect women more often. The severe fractures with displacement through the posterior arch formerly were incurred almost always in industrial accidents by men; in recent years, automobile accidents are a more common cause of these severe fractures, and men and women are injured with equal frequency.

Strong forces applied in the anteropos-

Fig. 25-1.—**A,** extreme widening of symphysis with tear of right sacroiliac joint and external rotation of right hemipelvis, the result of an automobile crash. Both the bladder and urethra were torn. Because of the massive damage to soft tissue structures, reduction of the dislocation could be achieved easily; but, owing to circumstances related to the other injuries, early mobilization was preferred to holding the joints reduced sufficiently long for healing. **B,** reduction of displacement by manual traction and compression of pelvis from side to side, followed by support from a pelvic sling for 6 weeks, when walking was permitted with crutches and with the support of a sacroiliac belt. At the end of 1 year, patient was doing heavy work without symptoms. **C,** end result 5 years later. Normal gait and no symptoms.

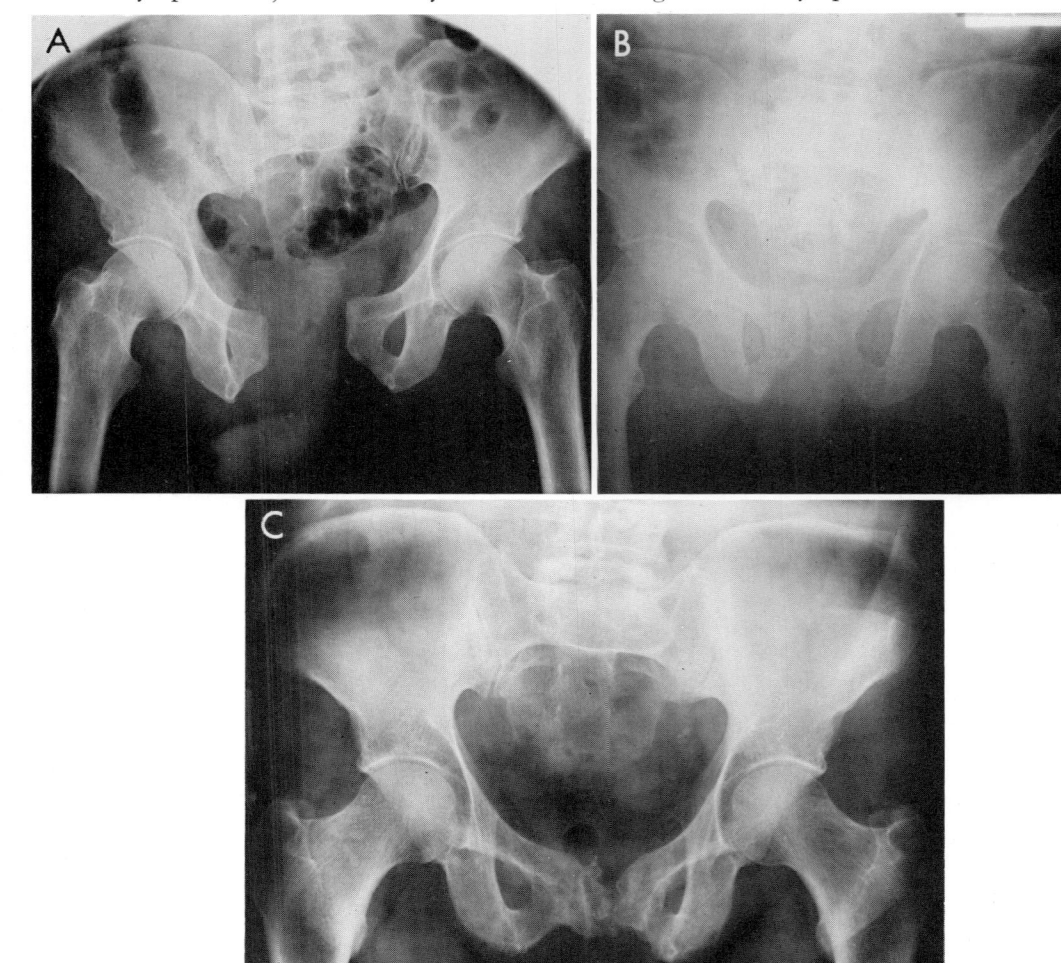

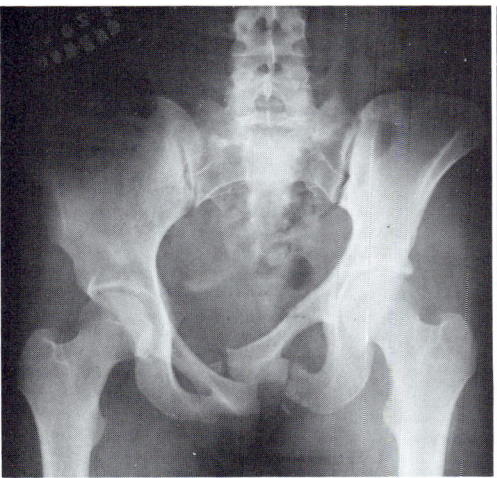

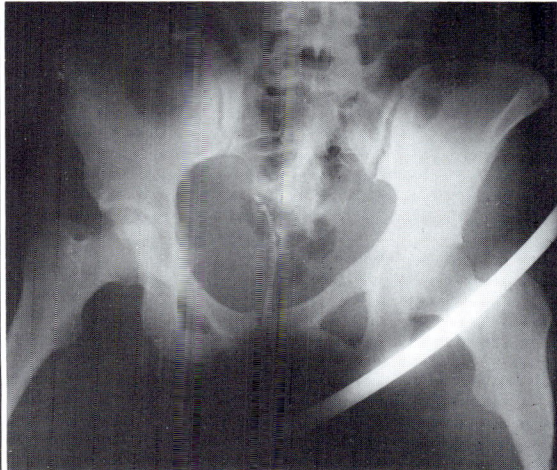

Fig. 25-2.—Left, inward collapse of pelvis by tear of left sacroiliac joint and inward dislocation of fractured left obturator ring, which occurred when patient was thrown from a horse, which fell onto her left side. This deformity is less common than an anterior opening of the pelvis. **Right**, after 48 hours with 25 pounds of traction applied through a Kirschner wire in distal left femur. Crutch walking was begun 1 month after injury. At 1 year, normal function and no symptoms.

terior plane ordinarily stretch out the circumference of the pelvic ring by opening it anteriorly; this is typical of crush injury, in which one or both of the innominate bones are rolled backward and out from a hinge-like base at or near the sacroiliac joints. Forces exerted from a lateral direction tend to diminish the ring circumference, with collapse of the anterior arch and a rolling inward and forward of the large iliac mass of the hemipelvis. Such a deformity occurs when a person is struck from the side or, when riding in a crashing vehicle, he is thrown heavily sideways against its wall. A combination of external rotation of one hemipelvis and internal rotation of the other may occur, producing rotation of the whole pelvis on the sacrum and spine.

With wide displacement of a hemipelvis inward or outward, i.e., by rotation in a coronal plane, some rotation ordinarily occurs in the sagittal plane as well, usually with tipping of the anterior obturator portion forward and of the top of the ilium backward.

A severely displaced vertical fracture of one large portion of the pelvic ring often occurs with rotation. Such an injury typically is caused by the heavy wheel of a car or truck running over the side of the pelvis after the person has been knocked down by the vehicle.

TREATMENT

Isolated Fractures of the Pelvis

Isolated fractures of the obturator rings, the lower sacrum, the coccyx and the iliac wings ordinarily are displaced only slightly and will heal readily without impairment of function. After rest in bed for several days to a few weeks, patients usually are comfortable enough to begin walking with crutches; early mobilization is desirable, especially in elderly persons. Discomfort in bed may be reduced by the use of a pelvic binder or belt. For patients with obturator ring fractures, a pillow placed between the thighs makes turning less painful. For those with such an injury as an iliac wing fracture, which might be expected to entail

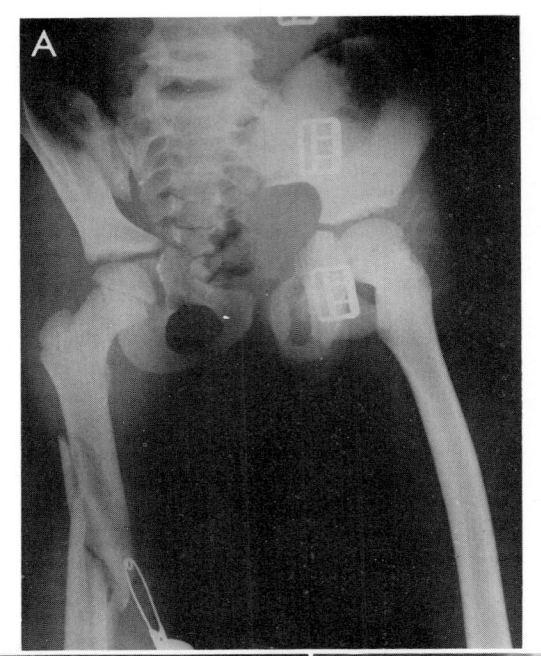

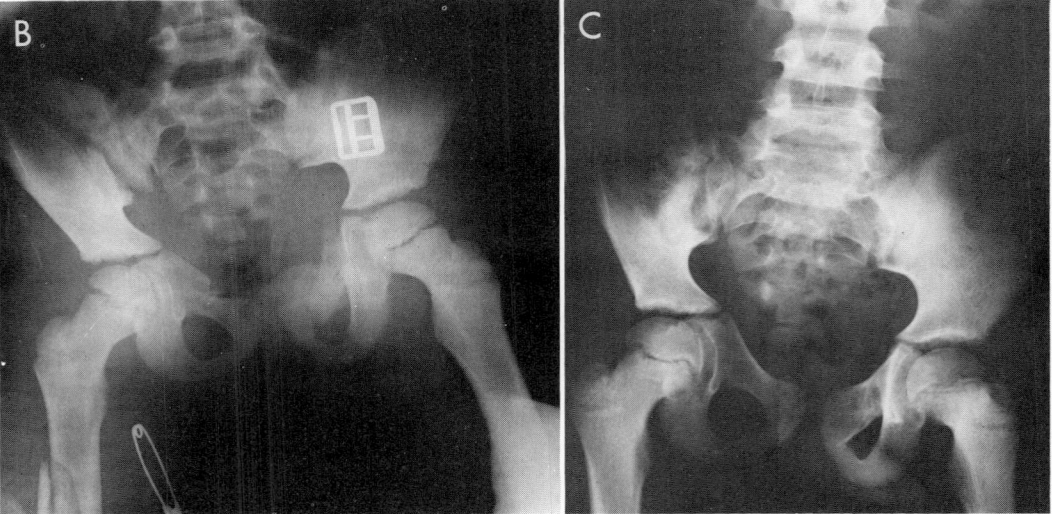

Fig. 25-3.—**A,** counterclockwise rotation of the pelvis on the spine in a 9-year-old boy as a result of fractures through the posterior right ilium and both obturator rings, with dislocation of both sacroiliac joints. The right ilium is rotated inward, the left outward, shifting the symphysis well to the left of the sacrum. The boy was struck from the right by an automobile. **B,** 48 hours after injury; deformity reduced by recumbency and traction on the fractured right leg. After 3 weeks, a plaster spica was applied and the child was discharged to care at home. **C,** at 1 year; pelvic contour mildly distorted but no defects of joint motions and no symptoms.

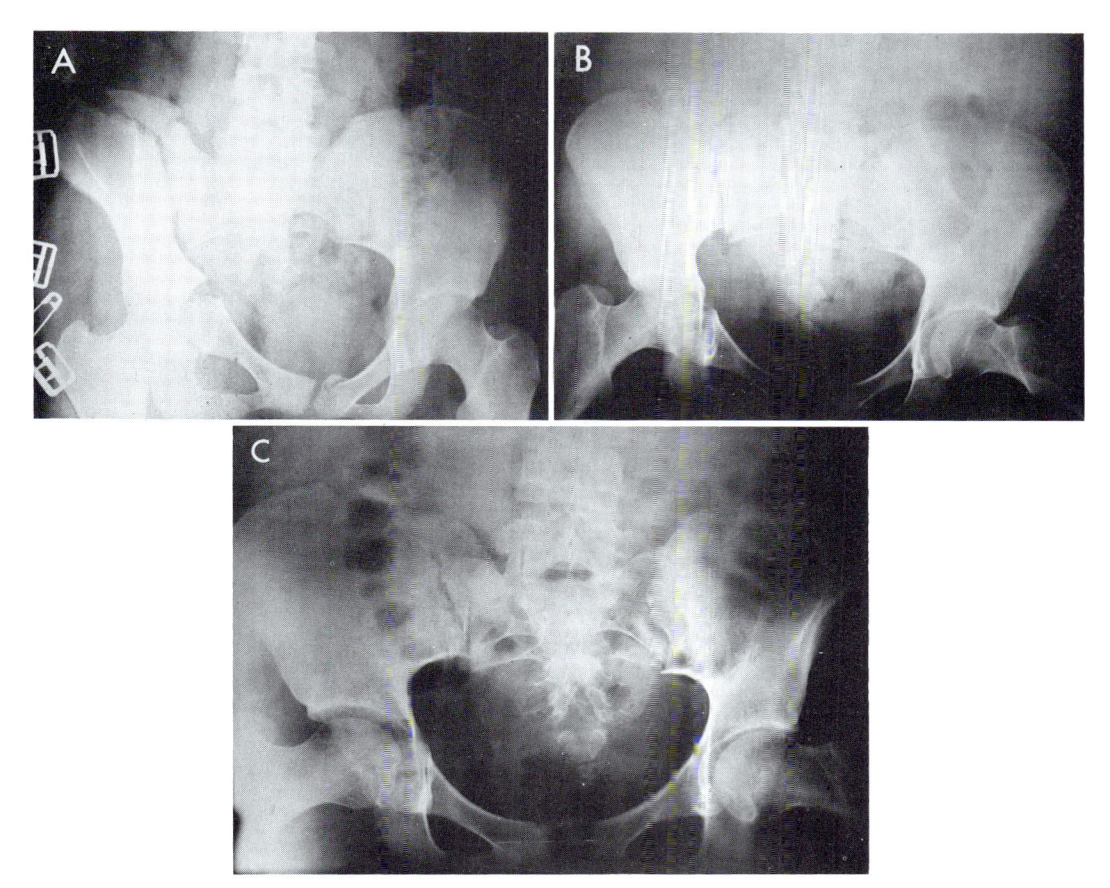

Fig. 25-4.—A, pelvic fracture in a 17-year-old girl who was thrown from a colliding automobile into a roadway, landing on her right side. The right iliac fragment is driven only slightly upward; the discrepancy between the inferior edges of the posterior right ilium and the sacrum is largely due to rotation of the iliac fragment in the sagittal plane. Both hemipelves are rotated counterclockwise on the spine—the left by tearing of the left sacroiliac joint and the right by fracture through the posterior ilium. The symphysis is rotated to the left. Fifteen pounds of traction was applied to the right leg through a threaded Kirschner wire, transfusion of 1 liter of blood was given and within 24 hours of the injury her general physiologic status became stable. There were no other serious injuries B, some reduction of deformity by manipulation (under anesthesia) 36 hours after injury. The manipulation included adduction of the legs over a bolster placed between the thighs in an effort to realign the acetabular fragments. The patient was returned to bed with 8 pounds of traction on the right leg. C, after 6 days in traction; considerable further change noted. Clockwise rotation to realign the symphysis and spine and improvement in the position of the iliac fragments occurred, with some overcorrection.

the development of ileus troublesome vomiting may be avoided by giving only parenteral fluids for a few days.

A cloth pelvic support of the sort customarily called a "sacroiliac belt" will make resumption of activity less uncomfortable and should be worn until symptoms subside. Lower-back exercises are prescribed during the period of convalescence.

Often fractures of the sacrum and of the coccyx are difficult to demonstrate by

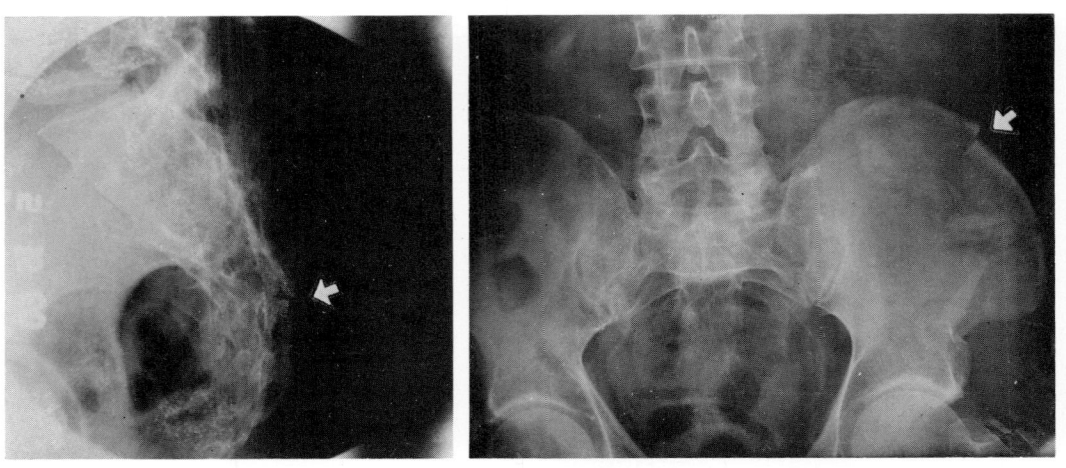

Fig. 25-5 (left).—Fracture of lower sacrum *(arrow)*, incurred when patient fell, striking the edge of a step. Previous standard x-ray examination of the pelvis had not disclosed the injury, and the patient's complaints had been untreated. Bed rest and sacroiliac corset sufficiently relieved the severe pain to allow the patient to begin walking after 1 week.
Fig. 25-6 (right).—Comminuted fractures *(arrow)* of the left iliac wing, which resulted when the patient was struck from the left by an automobile. The left kidney was contused. At rest in bed and wearing a pelvic binder, the patient soon was comfortable. At 2 weeks he began walking, wearing a sacroiliac belt.

Fig. 25-7.—A simple sacroiliac belt. Thin pads on the inner surface of the belt fit just lateral to posterior iliac crests. The top of the belt should rest just at the midpoint of the iliac crests, held there by garters (in women) or by perineal straps (in men, when necessary). For women, the top circumference of the belt is 4 inches less than the bottom; for men, only 2 inches less.

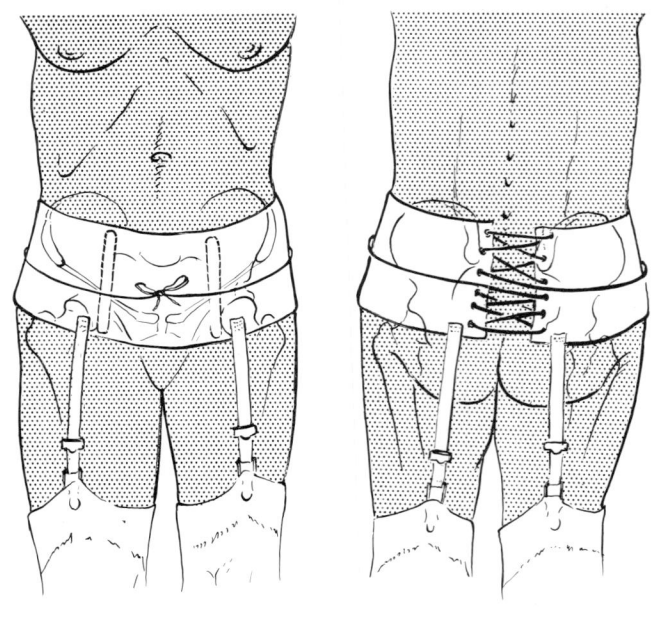

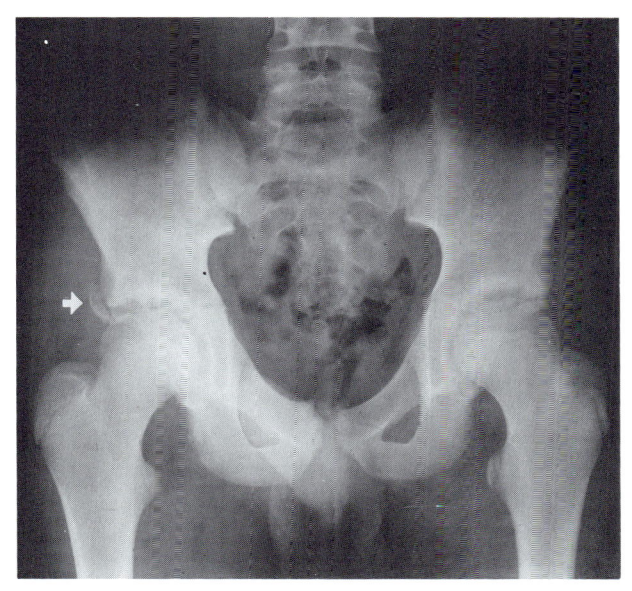

Fig. 25-8. — Avulsion of inferior iliac spine (*arrow*) in a 15-year-old boy who had suddenly felt severe pain in the right groin while running at high speed. The symptoms of the avulsion subsided rapidly with rest and heat. Function was normal 3 weeks after injury.

x-ray examination, and patients with these painful injuries sometimes fail to receive adequate protection in the early period after their injuries. Concern over the lack of an explanation for their pain may aggravate their discomfort.

In complete fractures of the coccyx, the distal fragment may be considerably displaced forward by the pull of the anal muscles. In rare instances, pain persists because of coccygeal deformity, which can be relieved by excision of the coccyx.

Avulsion Fractures

Avulsions of the anterosuperior or inferior iliac spines or of the ischial tuberosity may result from violent contraction of the muscles that originate from these protuberances. Such injuries usually occur in young athletes striving in competition. Ordinarily, the displacement of the avulsed fragment is slight and the fragment may be expected to reunite with the pelvis readily. With rest and protection of the injured area for 1 to several weeks, the symptoms subside completely. In the occasional wide displacement, particularly of the anterosuperior spine pulled off by the sartorius muscle, the natural healing process may be slow, with formation of large callus masses. In such an instance, surgical reattachment may be preferred.

Stress Fractures

Stress fractures of the obturator ring may occur when persons unaccustomed to strenuous exertion are subjected to unusual activity—for example, the long marches made in the early period of military service by formerly sedentary young men. Again, symptomatic treatment is sufficient.

Tear of the Symphysis Pubis during Childbirth

Occasionally during childbirth, the already relaxed ligaments of the symphysis pubis are torn by overstretching. Although there may be brief wide diastasis of the symphysis, the sacroiliac liga-

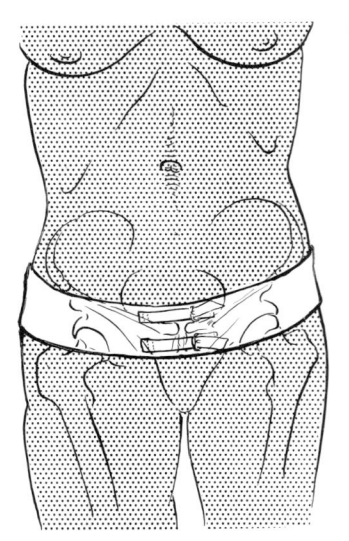

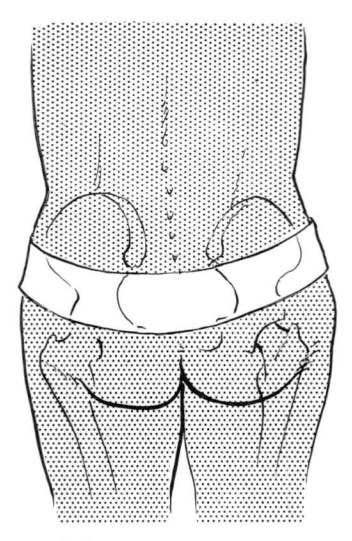

Fig. 25-9.—A pubic belt 3 or 4 inches wide. Fitting just over the trochanters and under the anterior iliac spines, this narrower belt is found to be more comfortable by some women with symphysis pain than is the wider sacroiliac belt.

ments stretch without tearing and spontaneous reapproximation of the symphysis is usual. Deformity of the sacroiliac joint will not be apparent by x-ray.

In the immediate postpartum period, a patient so injured often feels intense pain with any movement of the legs and so may lie immobile, as though paralyzed. A tight pelvic binder eases discomfort while the patient is recumbent, and ordinarily symptoms subside rapidly. Early mobilization will be easier when the pelvis is supported by a laced sacroiliac corset or a buckled pelvic belt. Low-back pain as a consequence of sacroiliac joint strain, as well as anterior pelvic pain, is usual, and the patients should be taught low-back exercises early. Recovery occurs after several weeks or a few months, and open wiring of the symphysis almost never is required for relief from pain.

Pelvic Injuries with Distortion of the Posterior Arch by Fracture or Sacroiliac Dislocation

Although functional impairment will not result from mild deformity of the pelvis, severe distortion of pelvic contour should not be allowed to persist. This is of especial importance in treating young women of childbearing age.

Four general patterns of deformity in severe injuries have been described earlier: (1) opening-out of the ring; (2) collapse inward of the ring; (3) in combination with either of the preceding, displacement of a hemipelvis in a vertical plane; and (4) rotation in a sagittal plane. These displacements may occur as a result of double or multiple fractures, of fractures with dislocation of a joint or of dislocations alone of a sacroiliac joint and the symphysis pubis.

Three particular considerations are important in the treatment of these severe injuries. Although a great variety of combinations of fractures and dislocations may be encountered, in almost every instance a large mass of innominate bone will be found intact, comprising at least a section of ilium extending from near the sacroiliac joint and running forward to and including the superior half of the acetabulum. With restitution of the normal relationship of this fragment of the sacrum, the other fragments of a hemipelvis usually assume an acceptable position. Even in the presence of acetabular fracture, sufficient hip capsule and muscle attachment to this major fragment remain to allow the use of the lower extremity for positioning the fragment; direct control by push or pull on the anterior portion of the iliac wing is possible. It should be remembered that this large fragment is displaced by bending or rotating it in or out anteriorly on a hinged base posteriorly, and not displaced as a whole in a lateral direction.

When extreme displacements exist, extensive ligament and fascial tearing has occurred. A completely ruptured and dislocated joint does not require great force for reduction, and usually fragments of a severely dislocated or fractured pelvis are not difficult to move. Slight subluxation of a sacroiliac joint is more difficult to reduce than is wide displacement.

Muscle attachments around the pelvis are very broad, with the points of insertion of the trunk muscles often fusing with the tips of the thigh muscles. Although the large trunk muscles attaching to the pelvis and the psoas muscle do tend to maintain proximal displacement of a hemipelvis or the major iliac fragment, displacement primarily because of muscle pull is not a regular problem in the treatment of these injuries.

Because violent forces are required to produce pelvic injuries with displacement through the posterior arch, additional serious injuries away from the pelvis are common. The displacement of pelvic fragments often results in injury to the soft tissue structure contained in and passing through the pelvis.

Unless it constitutes an impediment to treatment of critically urgent injuries during the period needed to assess damage and to bring the patient to physiologic stability, one or both legs, depending on the configuration of pelvic deformity, should be suspended and traction applied. An inverted half-ring Thomas splint with a Pearson attachment is a good suspension apparatus. With it, a threaded Kirschner wire through the lower femur with 15–20 pounds of traction is used, and the hips are moderately abducted and flexed and the legs maintained in neutral position.

Most of the severe deformities will be greatly improved or reduced completely by traction-suspension of the legs. The effect of traction-suspension on a collapsed ring with inward rotation of the ilium, an upward displacement in a vertical plane and on rotation in a sagittal plane, may be easily appreciated. This form of treatment is also effective in reducing the type of deformity that occurs when a proximal femur falls backward to a position behind the ilium at the time the pelvis is opened anteriorly by outward rotation of the ilium. By bringing the proximal femur forward from this position, suspension-traction acts, in a way, like a pelvic sling, which exerts its maximal force on the most prominent portions of the pelvic area, the greater trochanters.

Occasionally a pelvic sling assists in reducing or holding a widely opened pelvis. However, patients often find a sling uncomfortable, complaining of pressure over the trochanters; also, slings often make nursing care and treatment of genitourinary and other abdominal injuries awkward. A sling should not be used when an injured pelvis is collapsed inward or when the femoral head has been driven into or through the acetabulum.

Fractures involving the acetabulum associated with outward opening of the innominate mass sometimes are subjected to strenuous efforts of lateral traction applied to the proximal femur in an attempt to align the acetabular fragments to the displaced innominate and iliac fragment. Careful interpretation of x-ray evidence would indicate the proper treatment of inward-anterior rotation of the iliac-innominate fragment.

Although the effect of continuous traction-suspension is accomplished gradually, great improvement usually is apparent in 24–48 hours. In effect, the patient's movements act as limited manipulations during this period; but, as with other fractures treated by traction, major pelvic fragments may be positioned more delib-

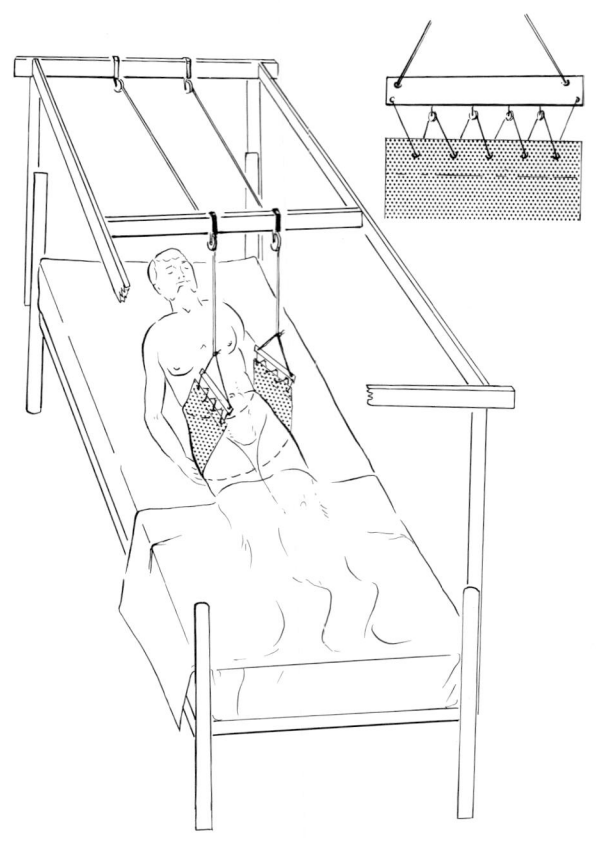

Fig. 25-10.—A pelvic sling. The force of lateral compression of the pelvis by the sling can be increased to some extent by suspending the sling's free ends in close approximation. The system of multiple pulleys allows the sling to fit the pelvic and hip contour closely.

erately manually. Because the fragments rarely are impacted and because with severe deformity there is severe relaxation of soft tissues, the fragments ordinarily are moved easily and anesthesia may not be required.

At times, early manipulation under anesthesia is desirable, and then it should be done as soon as the patient's general status allows it. This applies particularly to injuries in which displaced fragments jeopardize circulation to the lower extremity or prevent adequate treatment of visceral damage. It also applies to subluxation of the sacroiliac joints without severe ligament damage, since this sort of injury may require extreme traction force for reduction without anesthesia.

Because displacement of the ilium usually is posterior on the sacrum, manipulative reduction of this injury is done by placing the patient on his sound side with the thigh of the dislocated side rolled forward. Pressure applied directly over the ilium in an anterior direction will reduce the subluxation.

After manipulation, the patient is returned to traction-suspension, and often a position of incompletely reduced fractures is improved during the several days following. The reduced position is sustained, with gradual reduction of traction weight, for 4–6 weeks or longer when large fractures are involved. Injuries that are entirely joint dislocations may require a shorter period of 3–4 weeks if examination reveals sufficient stability to allow the patient to begin weight bearing with crutches. The pelvis then is supported by a sacroiliac belt and back exercises are begun.

In children, when the position of reduction has become sufficiently stable, a plaster spica may be used to shorten the period of hospitalization. In adults, traction ordinarily is continued until mobilization can be begun.

Although the method of reduction in lateral recumbency with the use of a plaster spica for immobilization is logical for patients who have fractures that are opened out anteriorly, its use often is precluded by the presence of other injuries, and traction-suspension is preferred.

Well-leg traction and turnbuckle casts of the legs, which aim to accomplish lateral distraction or coaptation of the hip joints as a force of reduction, do not take into account the hinge-like displacement of the major fragments. They also have the objection of possible damage to skin, nerves and blood vessels, damage that may accompany any strong force applied continuously.

Although, in general, open reduction with internal fixation of pelvic fracture fragments has not been used widely in the past, this circumstance has resulted from the usual acceptable results of closed treatment of the bone injuries and the prevalence of associated severe injuries of other structures and shock. There have been advocates of open treatment, however, and with advances in resuscitative treatment in general, in some cases open treatment may become the indicated procedure.

Results of Treatment

When grossly normal pelvic contour is restored, there is no appreciable impairment of function. Moderate bone deformity and moderate distortion of the symphysis pubis usually will not cause symptoms. Persistent sacroiliac subluxation, and sometimes the effects on the joint caused by the trauma of dislocation, even though reduced, may produce lasting backache, preventing the resumption of full activity. Sacroiliac arthrodesis may be required for the relief from pain. Fractures near or at the sacroiliac joint result in persistent pain less often.

BIBLIOGRAPHY

1. Byström, J., Dencker, H., Jäderling, J., et al.: Ligation of the internal iliac artery to arrest massive hemorrhage following pelvic fracture, Acta Chir Scand. 134:199, 1968.
2. Hawkins, L., Fomentantz, M., and Eiseman, B.: Laparotomy at the time of pelvic fracture, J. Trauma 10:619, 1970.
3. Holdsworth, F. W.: Dislocation and fracture: Dislocation of the pelvis, J. Bone Joint Surg. 30-B:461, 1948.
4. Margolis, M. N., Ling, E. J., Waltman, A. C., Kerr, W. S., Jr., and Baum, S.: Arteriography in the management of hemorrhage from pelvic fractures, N. Engl. J. Med. 287:317, 1972.
5. Motsay, G. J., Manlove, C., and Perry, J. F.: Major venous injury with pelvic fracture, J. Trauma 9:243, 1969.
6. Payner, H. F., and Hucherson, D. C.: Open reduction for fractures of the pelvic girdle, Arch. Surg. 55:339, 1947.
7. Peltier, L. F.: Complications associated with fracture of the pelvis, J. Bone Joint Surg. 47-A: 1060, 1965.
8. Pennal, G. F.: Personal communication.
9. Perry, J. F., Jr., and McClellan, R. J.: Autopsy findings in 127 patients following fatal traffic accidents, Surg. Gynecol. Obstet. 119:586, 1964.
10. Quinby, W. C., Jr.: Fractures of the pelvis and associated injuries in children, J. Pediatr. Surg. 1:353, 1966.
11. Ravitch, M. M.: Hypogastric artery ligation in acute pelvic trauma (Editorial), Surgery 56:601, 1964.
12. Reynolds, B. M., and Balsano, N. A.: Venography in pelvic fractures. A clinical evaluation, Ann. Surg. 173:104, 1971.
13. Selakovich, W., and Love, L.: Stress fractures of the pubic ramus, J. Bone Joint Surg. 36-A:573, 1954.
14. Spencer, F. C., and Robinson, R. A.: Division of the pelvis for massive hemorrhage from fractures of the pelvis, Arch. Surg. 78:535, 1959.
15. Watson-Jones, R.: Fractures and Joint Injuries (4th ed.; Edinburgh: E. & S. Livingstone, Ltd., 1955), Vol. 2, p. 634.

26 | Fractures of the Hip: Head, Neck and Trochanter

OTTO E. AUFRANC, J. DRENNAN LOWELL, HUGH P. CHANDLER and PAUL L. NORTON

THE MANAGEMENT of fractures of the proximal femur continues to be one of the most challenging areas in the field of trauma. This is as it should be, for despite our ever-increasing sophistication in the management of patients generally, improvement in anesthetic agents and techniques, and the singular contribution of successful methods of internal fixation, many patients with hip injuries do not survive the fracture, and disability due to unsatisfactory healing is common.

These are fractures primarily of the aged, in whom the incidence of serious associated disease is high and tolerance for prolonged immobilization and bed rest poor. With few exceptions, satisfactory outcomes will depend on successful surgery in patients who are members of a relatively high-risk group.

General principles of the care of a patient with a fractured hip require that the physician be prompt and aggressive each step of the way. Knowledge of the anatomy of the hips is essential. Protection by splinting of the injured member will do more than relieve the patient of pain. It will prevent further injury to soft tissue and perhaps prevent irreparable damage to the vascular supply of the femoral head. A rapid, thorough assessment of the general medical situation should be followed by the institution of therapeutic measures where needed. Surgery should not be delayed beyond the time necessary to accomplish these ends safely.

As the population ages, hip fractures will become more common and, as medical care improves, more of the patients will survive and more early and late complications will develop. It is crucial, therefore, that physicians, surgeons and researchers all retain an interest in this group of problems and work toward an ever-improving insight into their nature as well as better methods of treatment.

When surgery is required, a maximum of gentleness should be employed in the reduction of the fracture, and proper and secure fixation should be introduced in a minimum of time under adequate anesthesia. After operation, more than the usual attention to general details of cardiopulmonary, gastrointestinal and urologic functions will be needed, for these patients will not have the same potential for recovery as younger patients do.

Early mobilizing exercises, begun as soon as the patient awakes from the anesthesia, will be the first steps in a rehabilitation program. The program must be based on established knowledge of the healing processes associated with these fractures, as well as the properties of the fixation devices used. It will be directed progressively toward maximal functional recovery in the shortest possible time

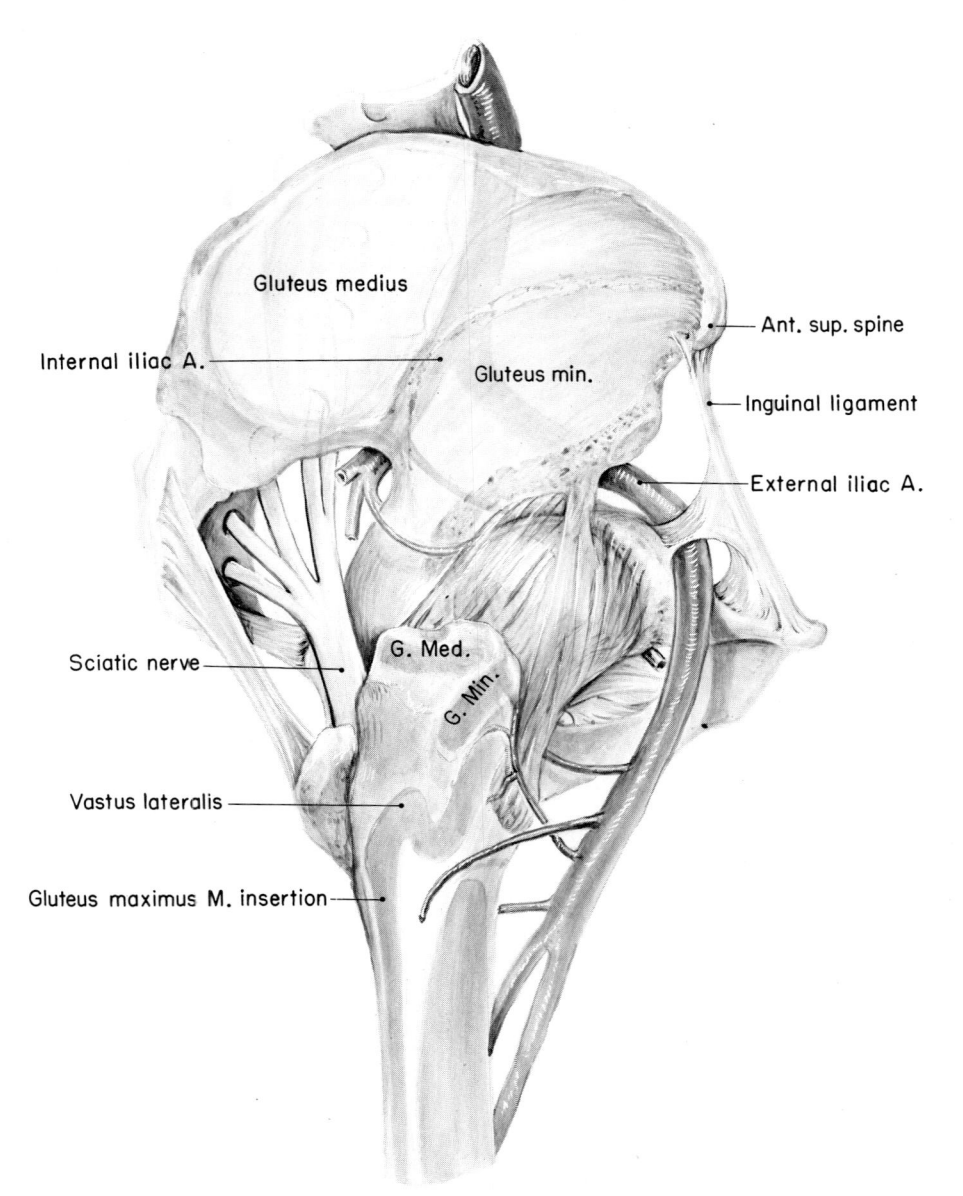

Fig. 26-1.—Anatomy of the hip.

consistent with the safety and well-being of the patient.

HISTORICAL CONSIDERATIONS

In a historical review of the literature, Peter Cordasco[18] found that Ambroise Paré[45] (1510–90) was the first person to recognize and make a written report on the recognition of a fracture of the hip. Freely translated, Paré's report reads:

I had observed the hurt thigh to be shorter than the whole, with the outward prominence of the ischium. I persuaded

Chapter 26: FRACTURES OF THE HIP: HEAD, NECK AND TROCHANTER

myself it was a dislocation of the hip. I then extended the thigh bone and forced, as I thought, the head into its cavity. The equalities of both legs which followed the point of this extension increased my persuasion that it was a dislocation. The next day I visited her and found her in great pain, her hurt leg shorter and her foot rested inwards. [This position may represent over-reduction, with the distal neck being dislocated behind the head fragment.] Then I loosened all her ligatures and perceived such a prominence as I did formerly. When I tried again to force the head of the bone as I did before, I heard a little crackling and also I considered there was no cavity or depression in the joint and by this sign I persuaded myself that the bone was broken at the hip and not dislocated. I therefore set the bone and joint and fragments together, laid splints thereon with compresses, made ligations with a rowler having two heads wrapped about the joint and the body crosswise, and I defended her foote with a case, that none of the clothes might press it. I fastened a rope to a post, and so let it come down into the midst of the bed and tied therein many knots, for the better taking hold and lifting up herself (Fig. 26-2)

From this description of a fractured hip and his care of the patient, Paré has given us the cradle to keep the bedclothes off the feet and the overhead rope for the patient to help himself about in bed. Since that time, the ideas of how to treat fractures of the neck of the femur have been about as varied as the number of surgeons who have written on the subject.

Hildanus (1537–1619) first applied the principle of extension and counter-extension through a system of multiple pulleys. This same principle had been applied by Hippocrates. Our present knowledge is improved by a clearer understanding of the details of anatomy of the hip and leg and the pathologic findings regarding fractures of the hip.

Pott[48] (1713–88) utilized the semi-flexed position of the hip and knee to neutralize the muscles of flexion and ex-

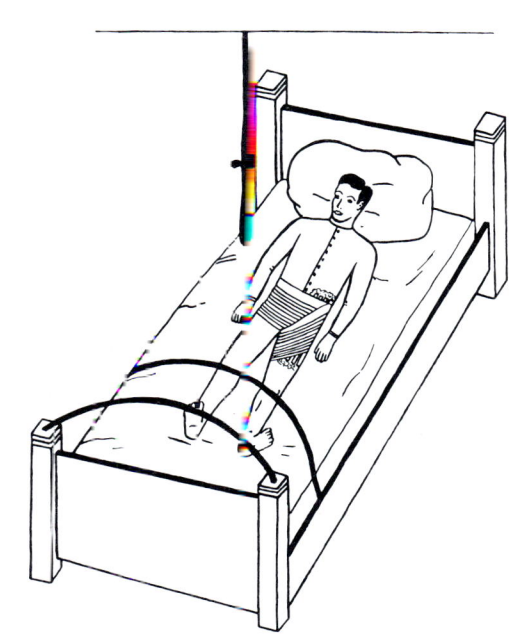

Fig. 26-2.—Illustrating Paré's description (the first recorded) of a fractured hip. Paré also gave us the cradle for keeping bedclothes off the feet and overhead ropes as aids for the patient. (From Colcasco, P.: Evolution of treatment of fracture of neck of femur, Arch. Surg. 37:371, 1938.)

tension to a point of balance. He also placed the patient on the affected side with the plane through the anterior iliac spine perpendicular to the horizon. The development of many complications led to the gradual abandonment of many variations in the methods of management. Cooper (1768–1841) used the double inclined plane, or pillow, under the knee. He was also the first to classify hip fractures into "intracapsular" and "extracapsular" types. And he brought out that the prognosis for union in the intracapsular type was very poor and in the extracapsular type very good.

In 1861, Buck described the application of traction to the thigh by pulling through the knee. Variations of this method are in use today—the wire traction through the tibia and Russell traction with the addition of the knee sling. All of the foregoing methods have left fragments of usefulness that are employed today.

The use of a metal nail to hold together the fragments of the femoral neck goes back to Langenbeck (1858). König (1875), Trendelenburg (1878), Lister (1880) and Lemon (1913) all used a nail for holding hip fractures. The nails used by these pioneers failed because they corroded in tissue and did not prevent rotation at the fracture site.

Whitman[73] in 1902 developed a method of reduction and a plaster hip spica that gave a definite improvement in the care of patients and a better prognosis for union of the fracture. Nine years later, Cotton[19] advocated artificial impaction of these fractures by a blow of a heavy mallet against the padded trochanter as an adjunct to cast treatment, but the attendant stiff knee and necessary prolonged immobilization left room for improvement.

Smith-Petersen[61] developed the unique idea of the flanged nail (Fig. 26-3) to hold the fracture in all planes. His first nail had 4 flanges, but it soon was obvious that 3 were enough. This nail, too, might have fallen into disrepute had not proper materials for use in its manufacture been developed. The first nails were of impure alloys, others a combination of steel for the flanges and brass for the cap on the protruding end. As might be expected, corrosion and soft tissue reactions frequently occurred. With the subsequent development of better materials

Fig. 26-3.—The Smith-Petersen nail. The blades of the nail are thin where they enter the head of the bone, and they are shaped like an osteotome so that they will compress bone as they advance. Note that the trabecular pattern in the femoral head is dense and the stress lines easily visible. Arrow A points to space occupied by 1 blade of the nail; this represents a lot of surface but only a small amount of space.

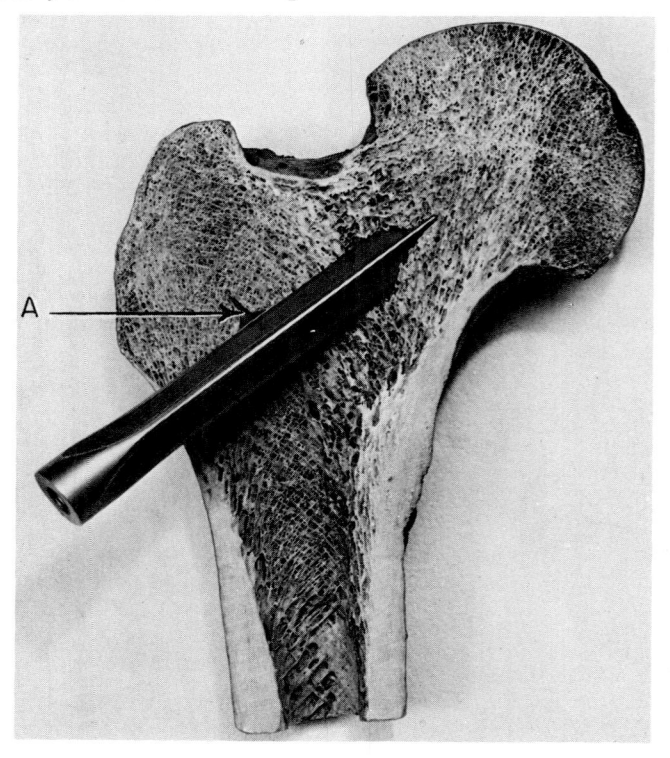

these problems decreased and the last objections to internal fixation of hip fractures disappeared. To the work of Venable and Stuck goes much credit for the impetus needed to bring this about.

The development of finer points in technique, together with proper use of x-ray control added to the more uniform adoption of internal fixation as the method of choice in management of fractures of the neck of the femur. The prognosis for life of a patient with a femoral neck fracture was reversed, the mortality rate of 50–90% being changed to 4–10% by these advances. With the advent of successful internal fixation, no longer did such an injury in the aged appear as a sign of impending death.

Wescott[70] in 1932 recommended closed reduction of the fracture, followed by nailing through a lateral incision. He also stressed the importance of anteroposterior and lateral x-rays as guides for more accurate nailing. Johansson,[33] also in 1932, devised the cannulated nail and guide wire to simplify nailing. There are, of course, numerous details of technique and new devices for fixation which have since been added and which greatly aid the surgeon, but the principal features of all methods consist of proper reduction, adequate fixation and careful postoperative management until union and function are restored.

Adequate fixation is the key that allows function during the period union is taking place.

MATERIALS AND DESIGN OF FIXATION DEVICES

Forty years after the development of the 3-flanged nail, we now have an ever-widening variety of devices for management of fractures of the hip. Each is satisfactory when used as indicated and each has its advocates. None is more simple and easy to introduce than the flanged nail, but many circumvent problems with which its use may be associated. At the same time, 3 different metals—stainless steel, cobalt-chromium alloys and titanium—have become the metals most commonly employed in their manufacture.

Much has been accomplished by interested orthopedists and the manufacturers of surgical appliances to improve the quality and reliability of the devices for internal fixation currently available. However, if failures with the use of any or all of them are to be avoided, the discrepancy between their inherent strength and that of normal bone must be appreciated.

One simple way of evaluating this is by the technique of static loading to failure, in which a test object is placed between 2 anvils and a measured load applied until the object breaks or bends beyond its elastic limit. This was done some years ago by Martz[40] or the proximal end of the human femur, on devices used for the internal fixation of fractures of this area and on specimens and devices in combination. Examples from the values he recorded follow.

The intact femur fails on the average with a load of 1,930 lb. A Moore blade plate and Jewett nail plate each fail at 108 lb. The Thornton nail plate fails at 175 lb and a Pugh nail plate at 203 lb. A fractured femoral neck with a Smith-Petersen nail fails at 350 lb. A Moore prosthesis fails at 1,870 lb and a fractured femoral neck with an Eicher prosthesis at 520 lb.

Static loading tests ultimate strength and not fatigue strength. The latter is determined by cyclic loading. Fatigue strength as a rule of thumb is only 50% of ultimate strength and is the more realistic value to take when the stresses that a recently fixed fracture may safely tolerate are under consideration. In addition, scratching of the surface of a device or bending it "to make it fit" may reduce its strength further, often to as little as 20% of ultimate strength.

Screws used to affix side plates to the femoral shaft will pull out when a force of 150 lb is applied in the direction of their long axis.

Although many of the above-named devices have since been redesigned and their strength improved, the principle still holds that they are not as strong as intact bone.

A few other figures must also be considered. In the stance phase of gait, the calculated force on the femoral head is 2.75 times body weight (Frankel) or 385 lb in the 150-lb adult. The forces applied across the hip joint by the abductors have been calculated to vary from 150 lb when the hip is used at neutral to 340 lb when used in 30 degrees of abduction (Merchant[42]). Should a patient be vigorous enough to jump, the force transmitted across the joint could reach 1,120 lb.[65]

Rydell[52] measured forces acting on a femoral head prosthesis by means of a strain-gauge supplied prosthesis in living persons. When standing on the prosthetic hip alone, the patient experienced a force on the prosthesis equal to 2.5 times body weight. As he stood on both legs equally, the force was one-third body weight. With walking, it varied from a maximum of 1.2 times body weight in stance phase, and while running it varied from 2.5 times body weight in swing phase to 4.3 times body weight in stance phase.

Consideration of these figures by the physician can be translated into words of caution for the patient, who may otherwise be deluded by the false sense of security accompanying the loss of pain after a fracture is internally fixed.

Potential tissue reaction to the metal used in the manufacture of the device selected also remains a consideration, though the problem is far less of an issue today than in years past. When a single implant is employed, tissue reaction with any of the 3 currently used materials will be insignificant. If there is more than 1 part to the implant, however, the problem is different, and stainless steel devices will be subject to electrolytic reaction in some measure if on insertion the parts in contact are subjected to scratching or deformation. Any metallic implant, if handled forcefully with a tool of dissimilar metal, will acquire in transfer some of its molecules by "cold welding," and this will give rise to formation of an electric cell and corrosion. Further discussion on the use and abuse of metal implants is included in Chapter 36.

EPIDEMIOLOGY

Alffram[1] reviewed some 1,600 hip fractures occurring over a 12-year period in Malmö, Sweden, a city of 209,000. This is an incidence of approximately 7 per 10,000 population per year. Cervical fractures were found to be twice as common as trochanteric fractures in women. In men, the numbers were equally divided. In women, the majority of cervical fractures were in the subcapital area, whereas in men they were divided equally between subcapital and midneck regions. One-fourth of the cervical fractures were stable. The mean age of the patients was 69 for men and 73 for women. Fractures were twice as common in women as in men. Moderate trauma was 9 times more common in women than severe trauma. In men, these were equally common. Age and skeletal fragility seemed to be the predominant factors in etiology and very likely lack of agility can be added.

Gyepes, Mellins and Katz[31] have commented on the low incidence of hip fractures in Negroes. Of 443 patients admitted to King's County Hospital Center with hip fractures, only 11 were black, yet Negroes account for approximately 50% of admissions of both male and female patients to this institution. No explanation for this finding was apparent.

St. Clair-Strange[65] stated that 1 in every 20 women who reach the age of 65 will sustain a fracture of the neck of the femur. He made 1 other interesting observation, and this concerned the rarity of intracapsular fractures in hips that are the site of osteoarthritis. He quotes Mason as seeing no instance in 100 patients.

INTRACAPSULAR FRACTURES

The division of fractures of the upper femur into 2 general categories, intracapsular and extracapsular (or trochanteric) is useful. The difference is more than that of location. It is one of age, incidence, mechanism of injury, treatment, mortality, morbidity, healing and the potential for vascular complication. The age range of patients in the intracapsular group is the middle to late 60s. For most of those with extracapsular or trochanteric fractures, it is the early to late 70s.

Although fractures in both groups are usually associated with a fall, the patients with intracapsular fractures often have an indirect mechanism of injury. The history suggests that the hip broke first from a twist and then the patient fell. In the patient with trochanteric fracture, the injury was generally the result of a direct blow to the trochanteric area. Precipitating causes of intracapsular fractures besides falls and muscular effort are tumors, radiation therapy, metabolic disease and electroshock therapy.

Although fractures in either the intracapsular or extracapsular area may be seen as a step in an inexorable process of dying, the mortality after intracapsular fracture is considerably less than that after extracapsular fracture. This is accountable on the basis of the younger age of the patients affected, the lower incidence of accompanying medical conditions, the lesser degree of injury sustained and the smaller magnitude of surgery required for repair. A lower incidence of postoperative complications is associated with these fractures for the same reasons.

Whereas most but not all intertrochanteric fractures heal with proper protection, and vascular complications involving the femoral head are almost unheard of, intracapsular fractures often fail to unite. Aseptic necrosis of the femoral head frequently occurs, both in the presence and in the absence of union.

Anatomic Deformity

The characteristic deformity of the leg in a patient with a fractured hip is one of adduction, external rotation and shortening. The amount of external rotation is usually of the magnitude of 30–40 degrees, since the intact capsule prevents the leg from achieving the extreme external rotation that is associated with trochanteric fractures that occur beyond its limits. The greater trochanter is prominent posteriorly and is higher than that on the normal side. Various degrees of this deformity are found. As a rule, the patient will be unable to lift the leg. The physical findings may consist of only minor changes, such as a small amount (¼–½ in.) of shortening, a few degrees of rotation deformity compared to the opposite hip, and only mild prominence and upward displacement of the greater trochanter. Any or all of these findings should lead the surgeon to suspect a fractured neck of the femur that either has impaled the capsule or is impacted in a poor position. Trying for crepitus is not indicated. The surgeon should rely on proper and adequate x-ray studies to confirm the diagnosis.

Variation from the classic deformity of a fractured hip may occur. In a patient who has fallen directly on the greater trochanter, the findings may reveal a slight increase in the length of the leg, a slight knock-knee deformity and a local hematoma over the greater trochanter. The trochanter may be lower and less prominent and the external rotation deformity may be absent. With these findings, it is almost certain that there is a fracture of the neck of the femur with impaction of the fragments in a valgus position. Loss of internal rotation may indicate impaction in external rotation. Loss of external rotation may indicate impaction in internal rotation. In most impacted fractures, the patient can move the leg about relatively freely, and he may have walked on it with minimal pain. The only complaint may be soreness or stiffness following a fall.

An unusual deformity associated with femoral neck fractures may be internal rotation of the extremity. This position may be due to displacement of the femoral neck behind the head of the femur, or it may indicate a base of the neck fracture in which the center of rotation is at the anterior capsule.

Emergency Treatment

As soon as a fracture is suspected, the affected limb should be splinted with a pillow bound between the limbs to protect the soft tissues and to minimize the possibility of further trauma to the vessels of the posterior retinaculum lying against the femoral neck. The use of a Thomas or Hodgen splint with traction through the foot and ankle is an equally good method in competent hands. Splinting will reduce the possibility of further hemorrhage within the joint, with accompanying increase in the intra-articular pressure, a condition that may contribute to the development of aseptic necrosis.[64] Splinting relieves the discomfort and much of the apprehension of the patient and makes transport considerably easier. Evaluation of the patient's general physical status should follow. Radiographs of the chest and hips and of other areas indicated by history and physical findings should be obtained with the pillow splint in place and the 2 legs bound together.

It is not difficult to take films of the affected hip in 2 planes by turning the patient toward the injured side for a lateral view. The quality of the films should be such that the surgeon can easily study the trabecular pattern in the head and neck of the femur. With such details visible on the films, he can more accurately plan the manipulative reduction or changes necessary to secure more favorable positions. If necessary, the binding and pillow may temporarily be removed during the x-ray examination, but this should be done by the surgeon or his assistant and not by the technician.

Radiographic Appearance

Much has been written about the radiographic appearance of intracapsular fractures and its relation to subsequent union, nonunion or aseptic necrosis. As a consequence of these observations, different forms of management have been suggested.

Pauwels[46] subdivided intracapsular fractures into 3 groups: those in which the obliquity of the fracture was 35 degrees or less from the horizontal (type I), those between 35 and 60 degrees (type II) and those between 60 and 90 degrees (type III). He found that fractures with the more horizontally placed fracture line united almost uniformly without internal stabilization. With both types II and III fractures, internal stabilization was mandatory, and as the obliquity of the fracture line became more nearly vertical, the rate of union diminished (Fig. 26-4).

Linton[38] and more recently Watson-Jones[69] interpret the radiographs somewhat differently and believe that the various types of fracture of the femoral neck represent different stages of 1 and the same displacing movement. Linton states that displacement first produces an abduction fracture, which ultimately terminates in an adduction or displaced fracture after passing through intermediary stages, and that simultaneously the head fragment angulates increasingly into retroversion as the fracture line opens anteriorly (Fig. 26-5).

Garden[28] divided intracapsular fractures into 4 groups, stressing the anatomic relationship of the proximal to the distal fragment rather than the apparent location or obliquity of the fracture line. The first group included those with a radiographically incomplete fracture line

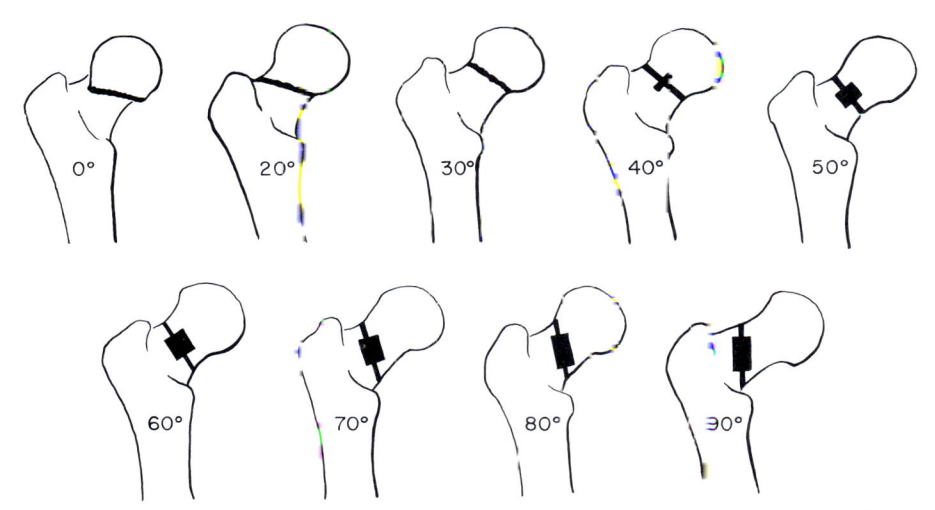

Fig. 26-4. — The range of fracture lines of the femoral neck — from almost horizontal to vertical. Fractures that are nearly horizontal seem more likely to unite than do those that are vertical. The vertical fractures also require more accurate reduction, extreme care in placing the nail and prolonged protection from weight bearing during convalescence. However, if these principles are followed, the percentage of bone union of vertical fractures will compare favorably with that of horizontal fractures.

but minimal or no displacement. The second group had a complete fracture line but again minimal or no displacement. The third group had displacement but an intact posterior retinaculum remained and tethered the proximal fragment so as to rotate it into varus with relationship to the acetabulum. The fourth group also showed displacement, but the retinaculum had torn, allowing the proximal fragment to swing back to normal relationship with the acetabulum. These initial observations were then equated to the subsequent fate of the fracture, with particular reference to the appearance of avascular necrosis,[26] and it was found that the frequency of this change was 13.3% with type II, 39.4% with III and 67.8% with type IV. This is useful information in deciding which fracture would be best treated with reduction and nailing or which with immediate prosthesis, particularly when the patient is old or infirm.

In our clinic, we have found interpretation of the obliquity of the fracture difficult, even after reduction. Seldom is the fracture line in 1 plane; more often it is helical, and frequently there is the added variable of posterior neck comminution, still another major determinant in the likelihood of union, as emphasized by Scheck.[56] A fracture line that on an initial radiograph appears to take 1 direction will after reduction appear to take another. The initial radiographs seldom are standard from 1 patient to the next due to different positions taken by the injured limb, a situation not practical to control. Therefore, except where the direction of the fracture line is clearly seen on the postreduction radiograph, our thinking parallels that of Linton,[38] Watson-Jones[69] and Garden.[28]

Anatomic Considerations

If a dried specimen of proximal femur is rotated through an arc of 180 degrees with the axis of rotation along the diaphysis and radiographs are taken at intervals along the arc, and then if the specimen is next rotated through a 180-degree

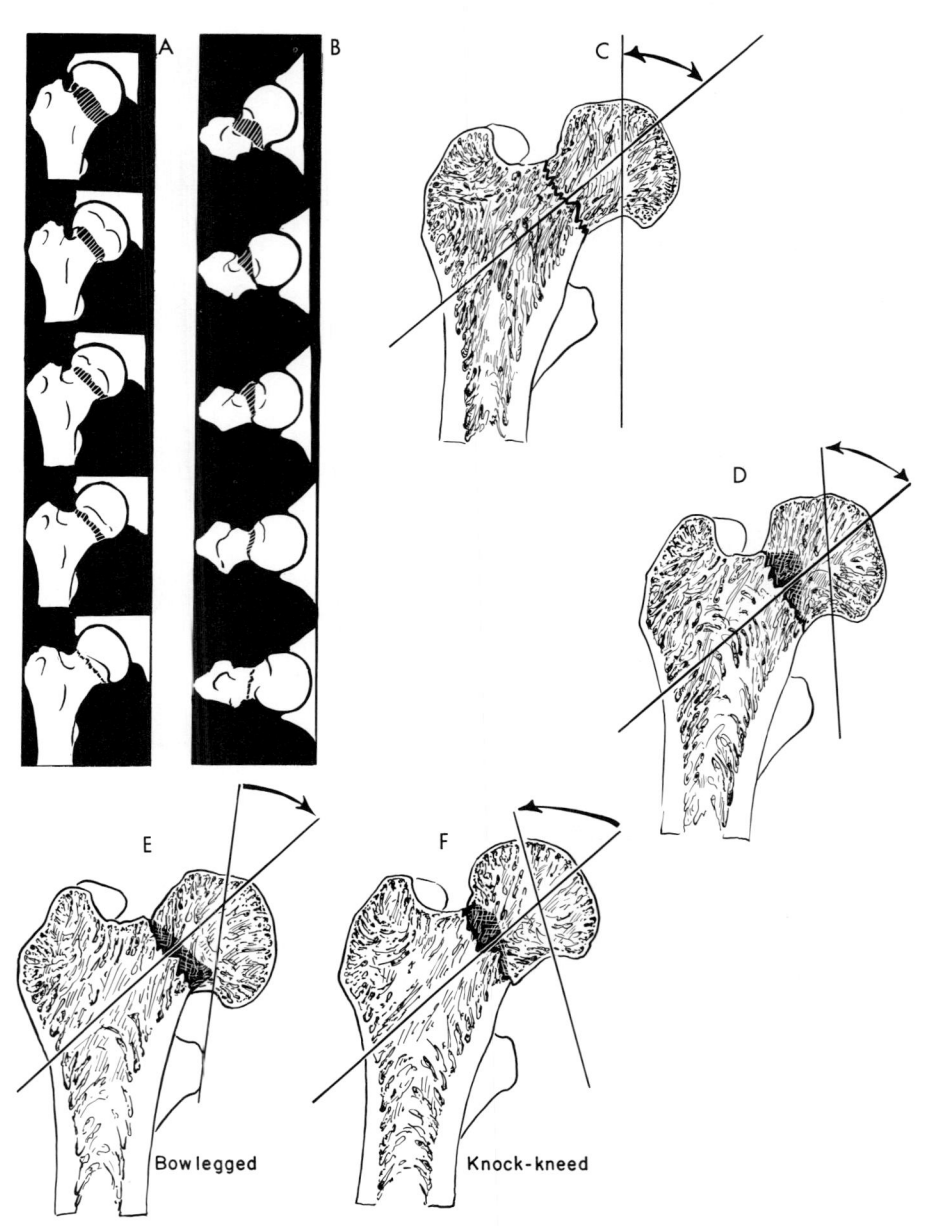

Fig. 26-5.—Mechanism of displacement of fractured neck of femur. **A,** progressive displacement of a fractured hip from below upward. **B,** the lateral displacements. It is noted here that favorably impacted fractures will represent a stage in any fracture. Widely displaced fractures probably go through a favorably impacted stage. The fracture in **C** progresses to a favorable valgus position, shown in **D.** Greater force will increase the valgus position, as in **F,** which is unfavorable and not stable. In this position of impaction the weight-bearing lines force the leg into a knock-knee. A displacement into a varus position (**E**) produces a bowleg position.

[Ed. note.—Some members of the Fracture Clinic of Massachusetts General Hospital do not believe that an increased valgus position is necessarily a hazard, since experience does not indicate that aseptic necrosis is caused by an increased valgus position. The varus position, is, of course, highly undesirable because the shearing force is increased. Note Fig. 26-19.]

Chapter 26: FRACTURES OF THE HIP: HEAD, NECK AND TROCHANTER / 629

arc with the axis of rotation along the midline of the neck and a similar series of radiographs taken, it will be noted that in all views a concave line formed by the cortical surface of the neck meets a convex line formed by the cortical surface of the head (Fig. 26-6). Together, these lines form an S or reversed S (Lowell) (Fig. 26-7). The curve is present above and below in all positions of the specimen. In the presence of a displaced fracture, to the extent that the distal arm of the S or its mirror image is flattened or changed to a C, the fracture lacks anatomic position or reduction and is unstable. When displacement is sufficient to disengage the fragments, continuity of the curve is lost. Consideration of these aspects of normal and abnormal anatomy in the relation between the head and the neck of the femur can be most helpful in the interpretation of radiographs in which a fracture is evident or suspected, both at the time of initial injury and throughout the course of its management.

Approximately three-fourths of femoral neck fractures will show a varus deformity, proximal displacement of the greater trochanter, rotation of the femoral head, a relatively right-angle relation between proximal and distal fragments, and 2 fragments separated. Approximately one-fourth will be in anatomic position or only moderately displaced in the direction of valgus and retroversion (rarely anteversion). Smallest of all will be a group of a few femoral neck fractures that will also show minimal displacement but into varus with minimal or no retroversion. The latter 2 groups make up the "impacted fractures."

Impacted Fracture of Femoral Neck

As noted in the preceding section, about one-fourth of all fractures of the femoral neck are impacted and these may be divided into 2 groups; the first is favorable for union, the other unfavorable. Of the favorable group 85–90% will pro-

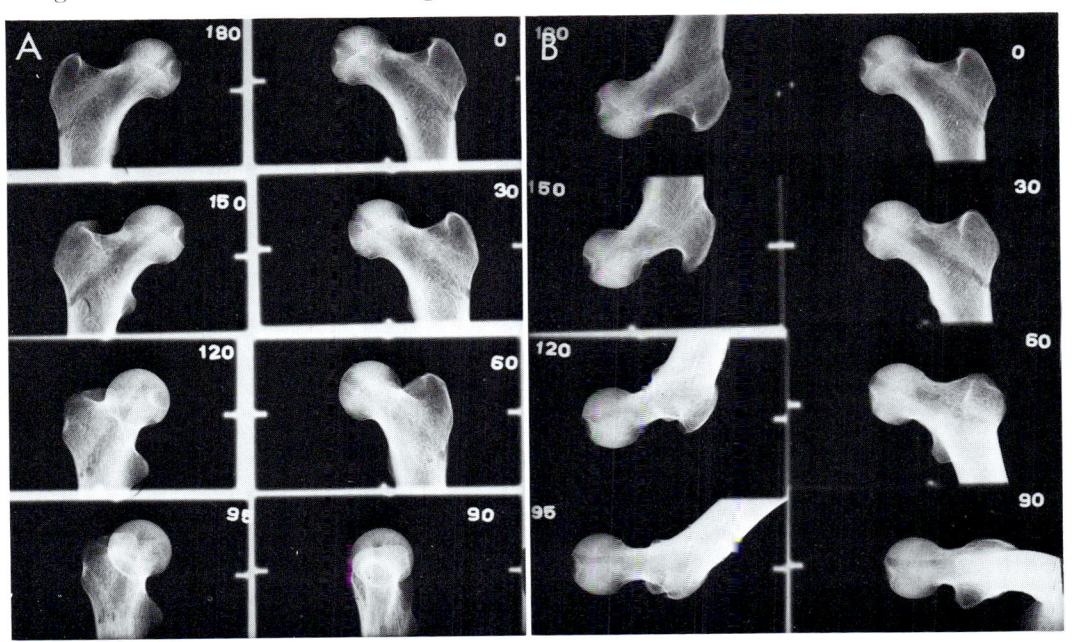

Fig. 26-6.—Anatomic relationships of the head and neck of the femur. Radiographs taken at 30-degree intervals in a normal adult dried femur rotated through an arc of 180 degrees: **A,** along the axis of the shaft and **B,** along the axis of the neck.

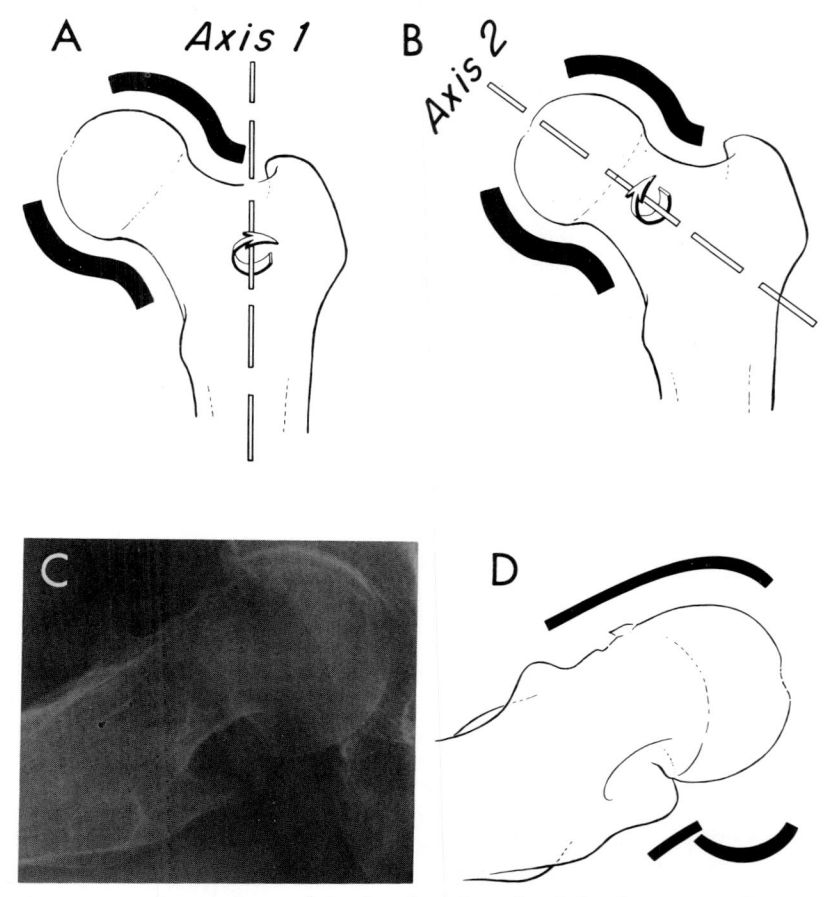

Fig. 26-7.—Anatomic relationships of the head and neck of the femur. In all positions of the specimen, a concave line formed by the cortex of the neck meets a convex line formed by the cortex of the head. **A** and **B**, together these lines form an S or reversed S curve. **C** and **D**, displacement after fracture progressively alters the contours.

gress satisfactorily to union without complication and without internal fixation (Figs. 26-8 and 26-9). As noted by Linton, these injuries generally represent the first stage in the displacement of any intracapsular fracture, and if certain features are present on the initial x-ray films and on physical examination, a given patient may be considered a suitable candidate for treatment within this group.

CONSERVATIVE MANAGEMENT.—Fragments should be in anatomic position or slight valgus on the anteroposterior radiograph. The S or reverse S curve formed by the junction of the cortical outline of the head and the inferior cortex of the neck should be present and not deformed beyond the degree in which its distal arm is flattened. The direction of the trabecular pattern within the head may also be rotated but should not be rotated beyond a vertical position. The fovea should be within the acetabular notch. On the lateral radiograph, modest retroversion or anteversion, as is occasionally seen, is not a contraindication to nonoperative treatment. However, posterior angulation of the head fragment should not exceed

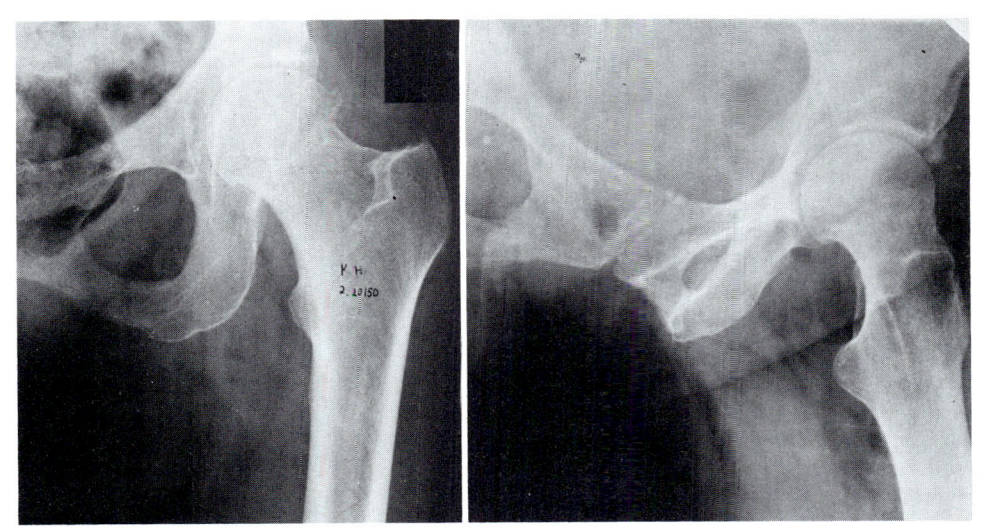

Chapter 26: FRACTURES OF THE HIP: HEAD, NECK AND TROCHANTER / 631

Fig. 26-8. — Impacted fracture of femoral neck in position favorable for union and function. Such a fracture should not be tampered with. During 18 years of follow-up, the hip has functioned practically normally.

20 to 30 degrees, and the S curve along the anterior neck line should not be converted to a C curve (Fig. 26-10). A wedge-shaped area of density should be present superiorly or posteriorly or both. Continuity of the fracture surfaces in all views is desirable although slight separation anteriorly or inferiorly will not make the fracture unsuitable for nonoperative treatment.

Crawford[21] reported a series of 50 cases in which he managed these patients with early mobilization on crutches, writing the word FRAGILE on the affected limb in large letters. He spent considerable time teaching the patient proper methods of sitting, standing, walking, and so forth. All degrees of obliquity of the fracture line were present in this series. At Massachusetts General Hospital, it is the practice of the fracture service to treat these patients on bed rest in traction for 10–14 days. If, at the end of this period, sensitivity has not left the hip joint and active motion without pain has not been regained, the fractures are fixed in situ with a 3-flanged nail or multiple pins. If the fracture is doing well, no operation is performed and a total period of 3–6 weeks of bed rest is completed. Crutch protection until union is complete, usually 4–6 months, follows.

In a series of 49 patients with impacted fractures reviewed at Massachusetts General Hospital, 36 received conservative treatment and 13 operative. Of those treated conservatively, all survivors had satisfactory union of the fracture if it was impacted in neutral or slight valgus position on the anteroposterior film and neutral or slight retroversion on the lateral film and if adequate protection was afforded during healing. Of the 8 patients who experienced separation of the fragments, 6 had a varus position of the fracture on the anteroposterior film, in retrospective review, 1 had an unrecognized fracture, and 1 patient, aged 80, was ambulatory at 7 days with inadequate protection. No varus fractures united satisfactorily (Fig. 26-11). All fractures with the medial weight-bearing trabeculae of the head angled beyond the vertical, whether treated conservatively or operatively, ultimately had avascular change (Fig. 26-12).

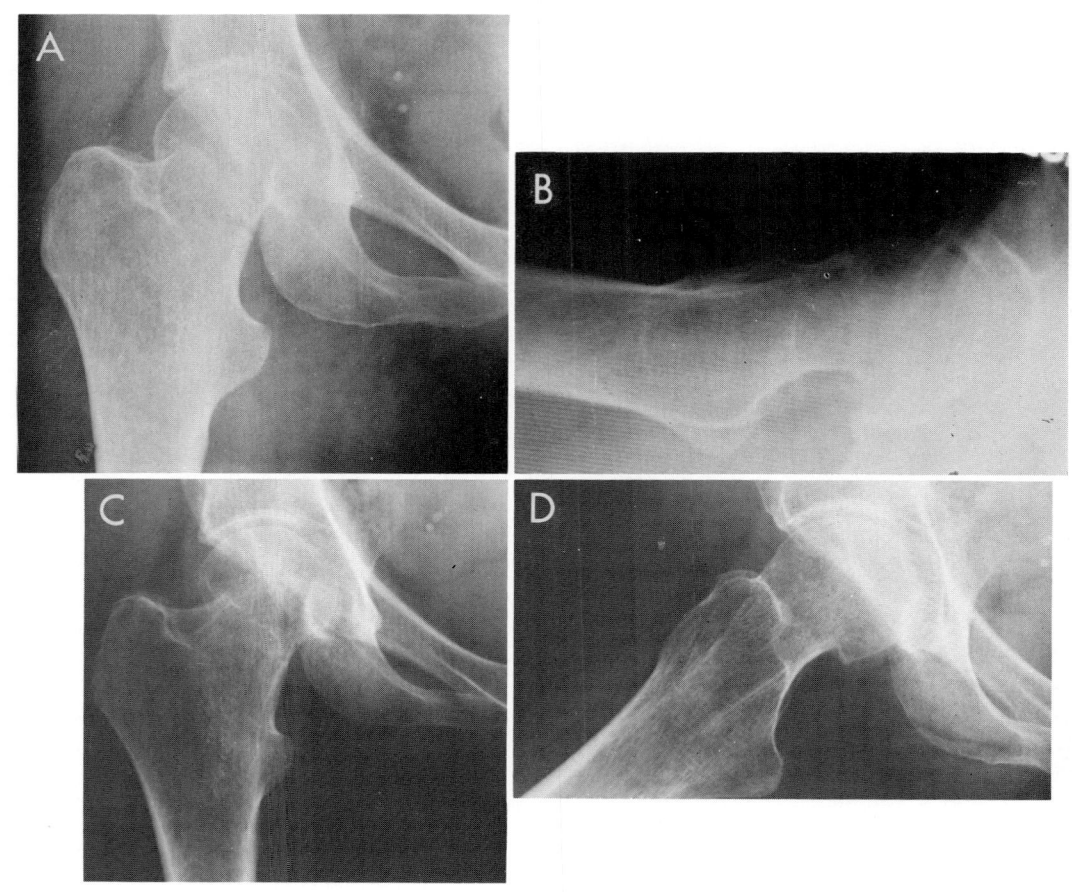

Fig. 26-9. — Favorable impacted fracture in woman, 54, who fell on her right hip. **A,** anteroposterior film shows slight valgus displacement with a wedge-shaped area of increased density superiorly, a minimal gap inferiorly, the fovea within the acetabular notch and the median weight-bearing trabeculae of the head displaced approximately 10 degrees. **B,** lateral film shows slight retroversion and a transverse line of increased density at the site of fracture. Impacted fracture favorable for treatment by nonoperative means. **C** and **D,** 1 year later, the fracture is solidly united.

Displaced Fracture of Femoral Neck

IS A DISPLACED FRACTURE AN EMERGENCY? — The question of whether or not a fractured hip is a surgical emergency is frequently raised. We believe that it is and for several reasons. At the moment preceding injury, the patient is usually in his best state of health; the pain and obligatory immobility that are present in the interval between fracture and fixation serve only to increase the severity of any associated medical conditions and slide him along a continuing path of deterioration. There are few common problems such as cardiorespiratory disease, diabetes and anemia that are seen in association with fractures that cannot be brought under satisfactory control to permit operation within 12–24 hours. In addition, data compiled by Brown and Abrami[8] strongly suggest that delay of treatment beyond 24 hours will adversely affect the expected rate of union. In their

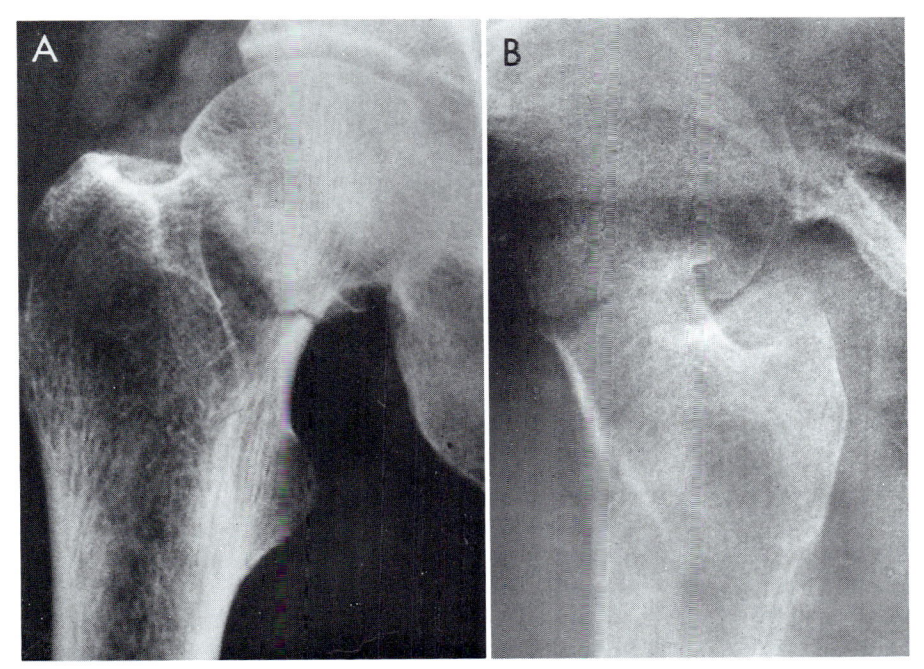

Chapter 26: FRACTURES OF THE HIP: HEAD, NECK AND TROCHANTER / 633

Fig. 26-10.—**A,** anteroposterior view showing area of increased density at fracture site, the upper portion of femoral neck. There were excellent range of motion and little pain. **B,** lateral view showing only 1 cortex intact. The impaction was not safe; accordingly, with a minimum of manipulation, the fracture was reduced and nailed.

series of markedly displaced intracapsular fractures in women over age 65, there were 80% union and 20% nonunion if operation was performed within 24 hours after injury. There was a 50% union, with 30% nonunion and 20% doubtful union, in patients with similar fractures and in a similar age group when operation was delayed beyond 24 hours.

To wait for days, "until the patient is in better general condition," is a delusion.

ANESTHESIA.—Less shock is produced in an elderly patient if anesthesia is started when he is in a traction splint in bed. During any transfer of the patient, the surgeon or a responsible member of his team should manage the fractured leg in order to prevent undue trauma or further displacement.

During the induction of anesthesia, the leg should be held and steady traction maintained in the line of deformity. As the patient relaxes under the anesthesia, a slow correction of the deformity can be obtained by simple maintenance of traction and correction of the position of deformity. Allowing a fractured leg to lie free on the table during the anesthesia permits additional damage and further deformity. This small detail may make a major difference in the reduction and the eventual outcome.

The anesthesia to be used for reduction and fixation of the hip fracture must be the combined choice of the surgeon and anesthetist. With the expanded variety of techniques and agents currently available, a combination of drugs is generally the rule. Spinal anesthesia has its place, but when difficulties are encountered, a supplementary general anesthesia is often needed.

In preoperative medication, opiates

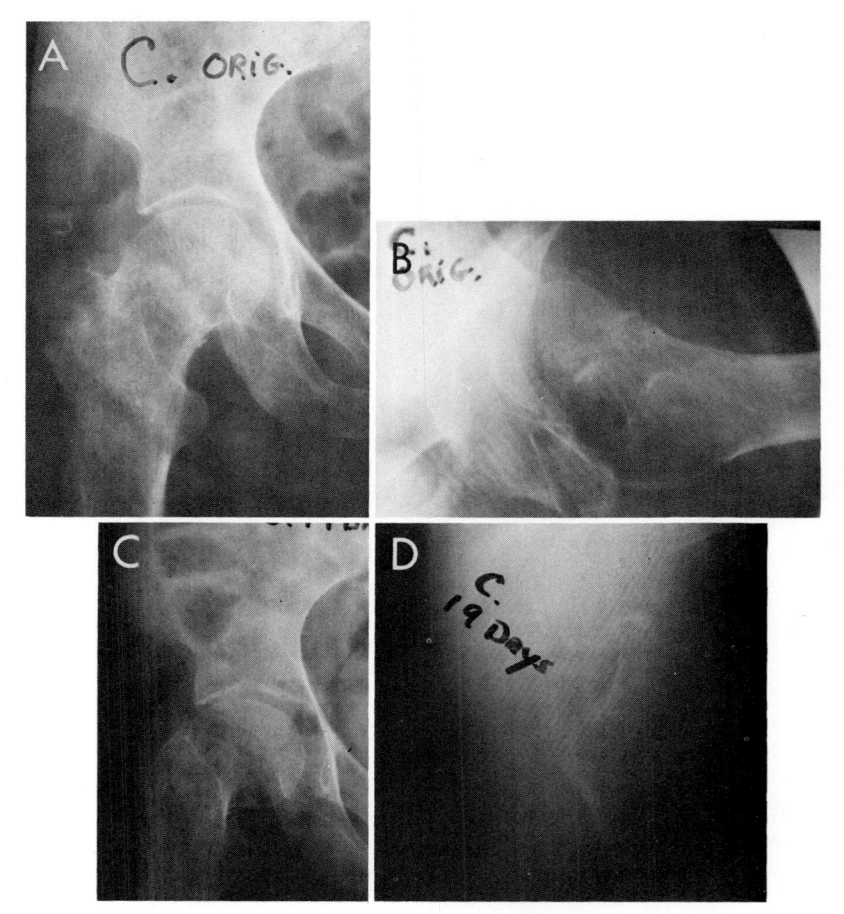

Fig. 26-11.—Unfavorable impacted fracture in 64-year-old man who fell on his right hip, sustaining a fracture of the midneck. **A,** anteroposterior radiograph shows a wedge-shaped area of increased density inferiorly; the cortex of the neck superiorly is nearly a tangent to the cortex of the head. Both features indicate a varus angulation. **B,** lateral radiograph shows retroversion of approximately 30 degrees. The fracture is unsafe and should be nailed even though the patient has been able to walk on the leg for 3 days. The patient was treated with crutches. **C** and **D,** radiographs 3 weeks later show further varus and retroversion. The hip has become painful and will no longer support even partial weight bearing.

that "snow the patient under" should be avoided.

Principles of Reducing a Fractured Neck of the Femur

The problem of reducing a fractured femoral neck is the same as that for any other fracture—to return the 2 fracture fragments to the anatomic relation. After reduction, the problem is one of holding these fragments until adequate healing has taken place.

Methods of accomplishing reduction and fixation are numerous, but certain common principles regarding reduction can be applied by all surgeons. Although it is true that, in the management of a particular case, clinical experience can become more valuable than theory, an understanding of theory can give added excellence to that experience.

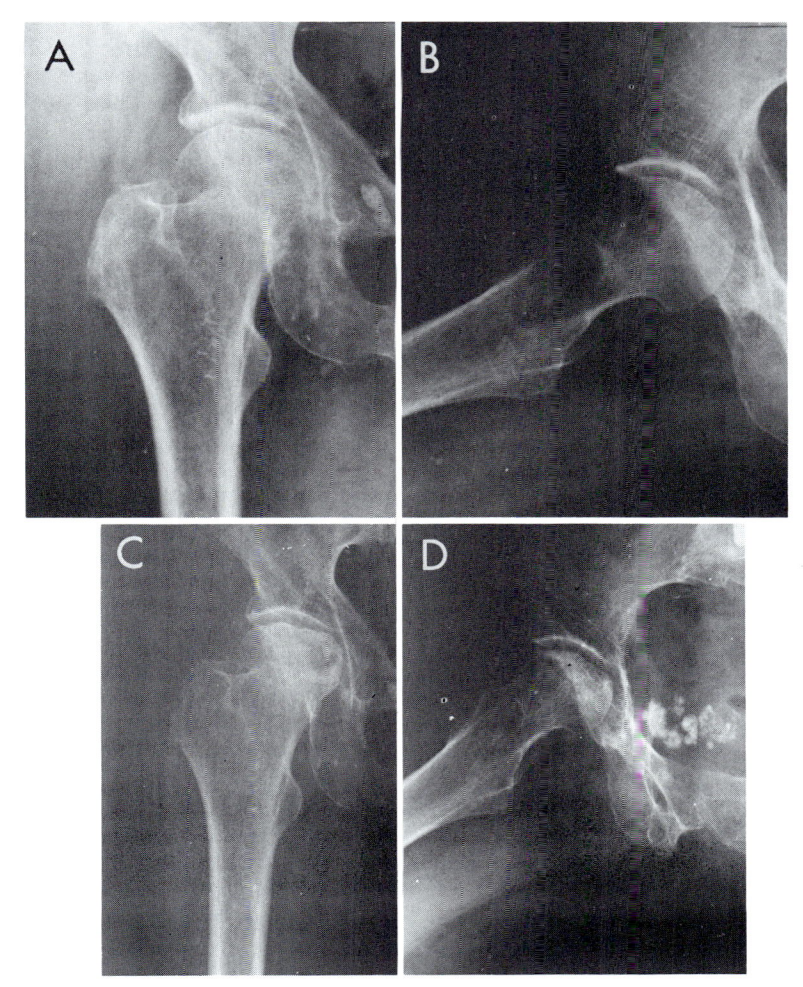

Chapter 26: FRACTURES OF THE HIP: HEAD, NECK AND TROCHANTER / 635

Fig. 26-12.—Unfavorable impacted fracture. Woman, 65, fell on her right hip but was able to walk with minimal pain. **A,** original radiographs show marked valgus displacement in anteroposterior view. The fovea is against the roof of the acetabulum. The median weight-bearing trabeculae of the head are angulated beyond the vertical position. Both features suggest a possibility of future trouble from avascular necrosis. **B,** lateral view shows good position. **C** and **D,** although the fracture healed, there was collapse of the superior segment of the head 2 years after injury. The hazards of breaking up a stable impaction outweigh the hazards of possible avascular necrosis. Treatment of this fracture was correct and this potential complication must be accepted. The patient had been warned of the possibility at the time of injury and a replacement prosthesis was inserted prior to the development of acetabular damage.

A thorough knowledge of the bony and muscular anatomy about the hip is a prerequisite to the reduction of a fractured neck of the femur. A certain amount of luck may occasionally result in a perfect reduction, but that luck will be more constant if the operator understands what the bony anatomy is like. There are more pitfalls in the reduction of a fractured neck of the femur than for any other bone.

Two factors make the manipulation difficult (1) The distal fragment is the larger one. (2) The proximal fragment is the smaller, and its hemispherical end lies in a slick socket and anatomically at an angle with weight-bearing lines. It is also easily capable of rotating through 180 degrees at the slightest touch because of its lack of muscular attachments after it has been fractured. The easy way to reduce a fracture would generally be to put the smaller portion onto the larger; but, in the fractured neck of the femur, the larger piece must be handled and placed on the smaller one, which is held only by negative pressure and the ligamentum teres. The friction coefficient of cartilage against cartilage is less than that of a skate runner against ice. This is a very movable target indeed!

Small spicules of bone at the fracture site will often rotate the head during the development of the deformity that is common with the fracture. Likewise, these same spicules will rotate the head in any manipulative attempts that are not thoughtfully carried out (Fig. 26-13). This rotation may or may not favor good reduction. The spicules may also interfere with reduction. A comminuted neck fracture with transverse fragments may be impossible to reduce properly by closed manipulation; open reduction then becomes necessary.

The most obvious maneuver is to restore length to the extremity in the line of deformity of the proximal head fragment. After traction has been applied in the line of deformity and length has been restored, and if the trochanter does not come forward with internal rotation, the external rotation should be resumed and the trochanter directly lifted forward before internal rotation is again attempted. This detail will often bring the distal fragment forward to meet the proximal head fragment without spinning the latter around. Thus, the opposing fracture surfaces will be opposite one another and can be firmly fixed on one another by internal rotation, abduction and extension. In this internally rotated, abducted and extended position, the muscle component forces are all in the line of the axis of the neck of the femur. The fracture can be made more secure or impacted by acute flexion of the knee beyond a right angle. This puts the rectus femoris muscle on considerable stretch and pushes the femoral shaft upward and toward the acetabulum, the component forces being along the axis of the neck of the femur. The internal rotation, abduction and extension position keeps the iliopsoas muscle under tension and thus aids in maintaining reduction.

After the manipulative reduction has been carried out, the position of the greater trochanter and its relationship to the anterior spine should be evaluated and compared with the opposite side, so that it can be fairly accurately assessed whether or not reduction has been satisfactory. The heel test of Leadbetter, to see whether or not reduction has been accomplished, is an inaccurate evaluation. Sometimes, by reducing the fracture with the Leadbetter maneuver, the neck of the femur can be displaced in such a manner that internal rotation will maintain itself without an adequate lateral reduction.

X-rays should be taken in both anterior and lateral projections, with an assistant sitting "frozen" to the injured leg in a comfortable chair, or with the patient's foot fixed to a low stool, knee flexed 90 degrees, hip extended and abducted and rotated slightly inward. The anterior view is taken with the cassette directly under the hip and with use of a tunnel cassette holder. The lateral view is taken with the x-ray tubes at a right angle to Poupart's ligament, with the cassette held above the crest of the ilium, between the crest and the ribs and perpendicular to the face of the x-ray tube. Adequate evaluation of the reduction can be made with these 2 views. External surface skin markings can be of great help in introducing the guide wire. Three uniform markers are placed along Poupart's ligament, with the central marker usually over the femoral artery and thus over the center of the

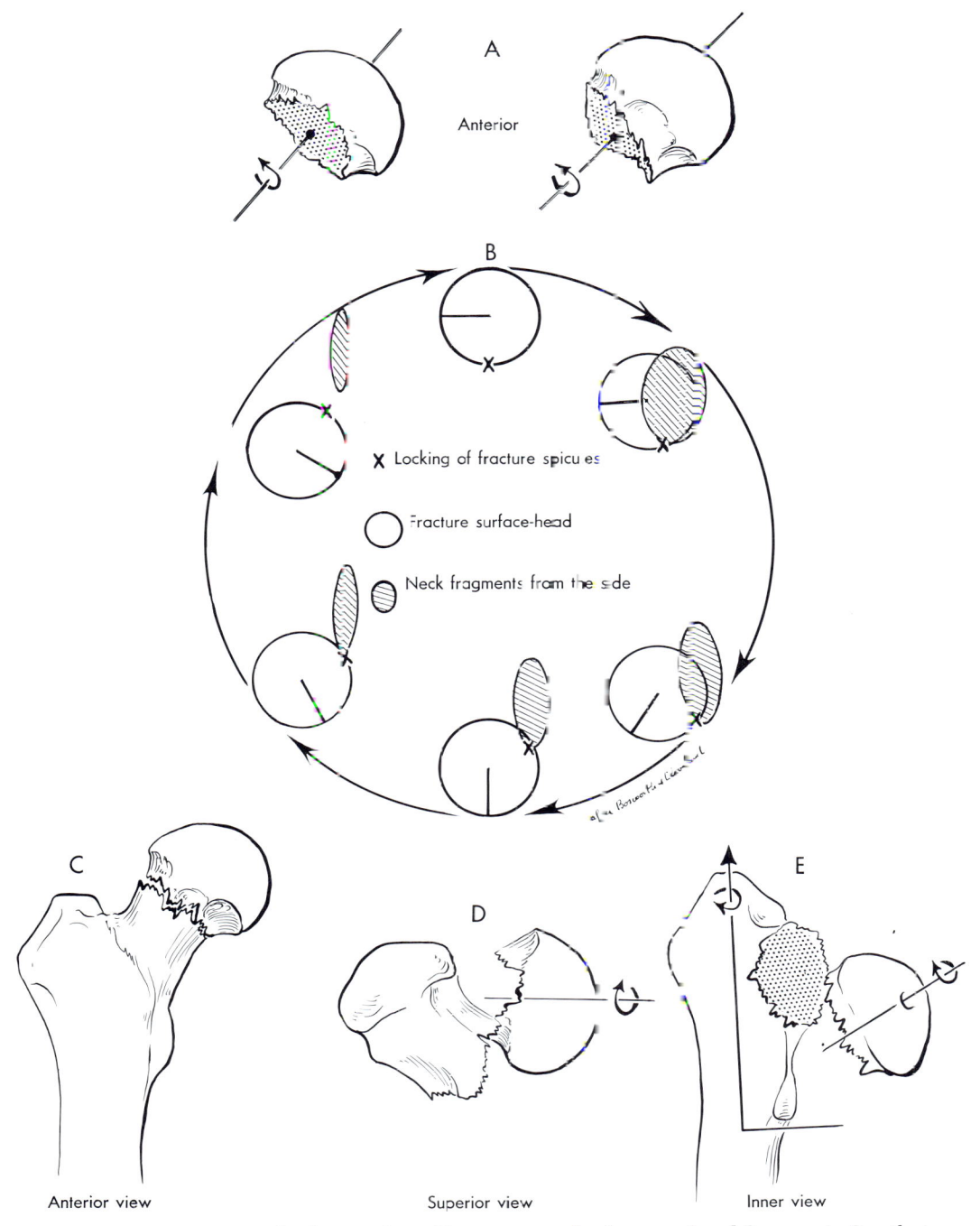

Chapter 26: FRACTURES OF THE HIP: HEAD NECK AND TROCHANTER / 637

Fig. 26-13. — Manner in which spicules of bone rotate the femoral head fragment. Gentle traction should restore length before the fractured surfaces are apposed by internal rotation. (From Cleveland, M. A., and Bosworth, D. M.: Fractures of the neck of the femur: A critical analysis of 50 consecutive cases, Surg. Gynecol. Obstet. 66:646, 1938.)

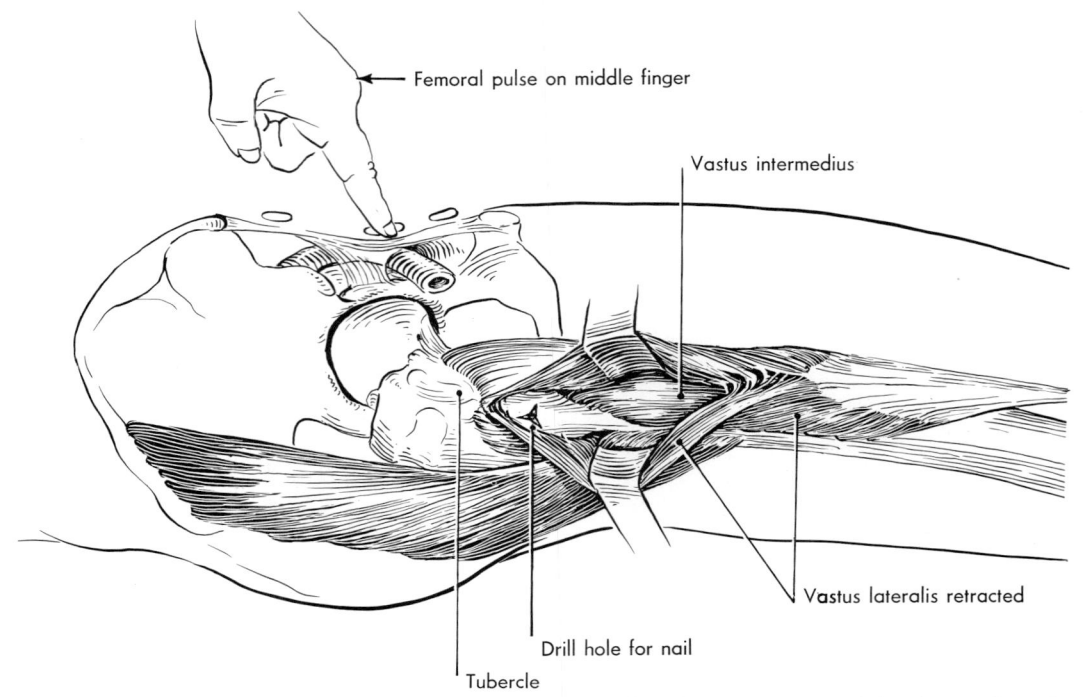

Fig. 26-14.—Helpful anatomic guides in reducing and nailing fractures of the femoral neck. In palpating the anatomy around the hip, the head of the femur may be marked on the skin by locating the femoral pulse at Poupart's (inguinal) ligament.

head, although too much abduction, adduction or rotation may change this position slightly. (Figs. 26-14 and 26-15). These markers, placed approximately 1 in. apart and ultimately visible on all the intraoperative anteroposterior radiographs, will serve as a useful reference for placing the guide wire accurately in the center of the femoral neck and head.

If the head fragment is revealed to be in too great a varus position, a valgus position can be obtained, without a full manipulation, by simply increasing abduction, using the hand as a fulcrum against the trochanter and applying counterpressure on the opposite pelvis. This maneuver, however, should be done only after extending and slightly adducting the thigh, maintaining traction throughout the entire procedure.

If too much of a valgus position has been obtained in the reduction, the leg can be extended again, counterpressure applied to the inner aspect of the upper thigh, and the leg slowly adducted against this fulcrum with the addition of traction and a gentle rocking of internal and external rotation. This maneuver will convert too great a valgus position to a more normal angle.

Anterior angulation of the neck at the fracture site can be changed by maintaining traction and bringing the leg (with the knee extended) into a neutral position, then using gentle flexion against the fulcrum (the heel of someone's hand) over the anterior neck and increasing the internal rotation. If this fails, the manipulation should be continued with the maintenance of traction, and the thigh adducted in right-angle flexion, directing the knee toward the opposite axilla.

If any of these maneuvers do not result in an improvement of the alignment of

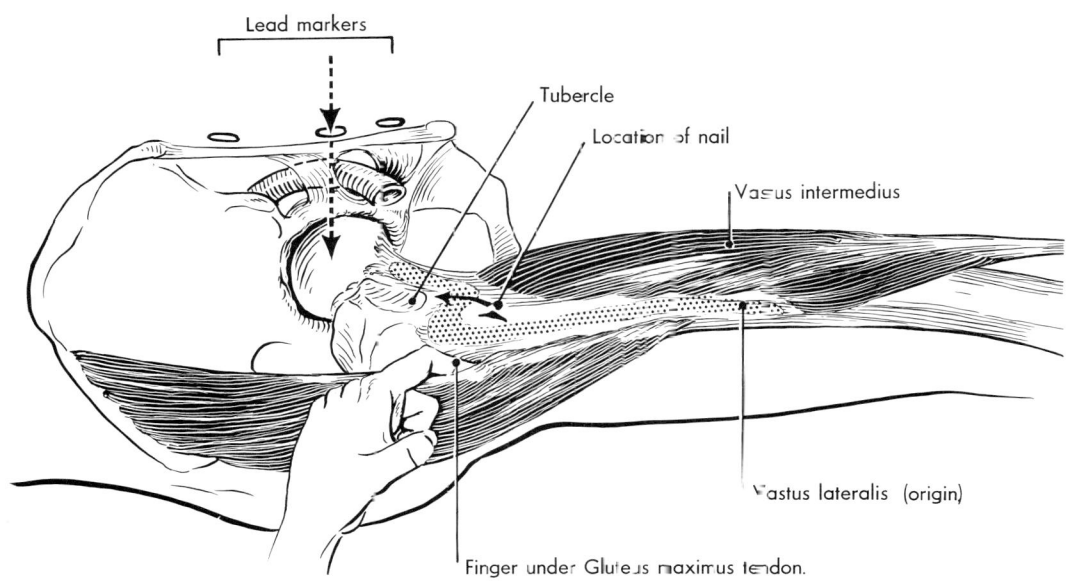

Chapter 26: FRACTURES OF THE HIP: HEAD, NECK AND TROCHANTER / 639

Fig. 26-15.—Lead markers placed along the inguinal ligament serve as guides in the x-rays for the angle of the nail. The usual site of entry of the nail is as indicated. Anatomically this area is opposite the insertion of the gluteus maximus tendon and usually about 1¼ in. below the tubercle.

the reduction, a gentle release of the maintained position should be accomplished and a remanipulation in more flexion and with longer traction should be carried out—with the restoration of length as the primary factor, the bringing of the trochanter forward as the secondary factor, and internal rotation, abduction and extension as the final factor.

Acute flexion of the knee in the final position serves to lock the fragments firmly in their reduced position. Multiple manipulations should be avoided. If 2 or 3 gentle tries fail to reduce the fracture properly, then open reduction is indicated. The main key to all these manipulations lies in the words of Ambroise Paré, "... to adjust that which is in default."

The maintenance of adjustment now relies on internal fixation and to accomplish this we have a wide selection of satisfactory devices. The specific choice among these must be based on the knowledge and experience of the surgeon. Some of the more common devices are multiple wires or small nails with or without lag bolts; spikes; nail-plate and screw-plate combinations designed to allow telescoping of the nail or screw into the modified upper end of the plate and thus to accommodate absorption and collapse along the fracture line. In recent years, the multiple pin fixation technique of Deyerle and the collapsible nails described by Clawson have produced gratifying results and impressive statistics. At Massachusetts General Hospital and at Peter Bent Brigham Hospital, the Smith-Petersen 3-flanged nail, 1 of the telescoping nails or the telescoping screw have all been found effective and simple to use in most patients. In selected cases, pins of the Austin Moore or Knowles type where no reduction is required are used in their stead.

Placement of Nail When Nail Alone Is Selected

After the reduction has been determined satisfactory by means of adequate x-ray films, the nailing can be carried out through a lateral incision. The placement of this lateral incision is aided by knowledge of the anatomy of the tip of the trochanter and the lateral shaft of the femur. A straight lateral incision down through the iliotibial band just below the tip of the trochanter and through the vastus externus muscle exposes the lateral shaft.

The point of entrance of the nail is usually 1¼ in. below the vastus externus tubercle and directly laterally. This point can be checked by its being opposite the superior margin of the tendon of the gluteus maximus as the tendon inserts into the linea aspera. These 2 points generally check within ¼ in. of one another.

The angle at which the nail is to be driven into the shaft can now be determined by use of a jig fixed to the lateral aspect of the shaft or by referring to the shadow on the x-ray film cast by 3 lead skin markers placed along Poupart's ligament prior to the skin prep. These markers can be covered by the drapes and then palpated through them or can be made visible by covering them with 1 or more layers of sterile transparent adhesive plastic.

The angle which the guide wire for the nail makes with the shaft generally falls within 43–47 degrees, with the average being about 45 degrees (Fig. 26-16). If,

Fig. 26-16.—The usual angle of the nail with the femoral shaft—between 43 and 47 degrees.

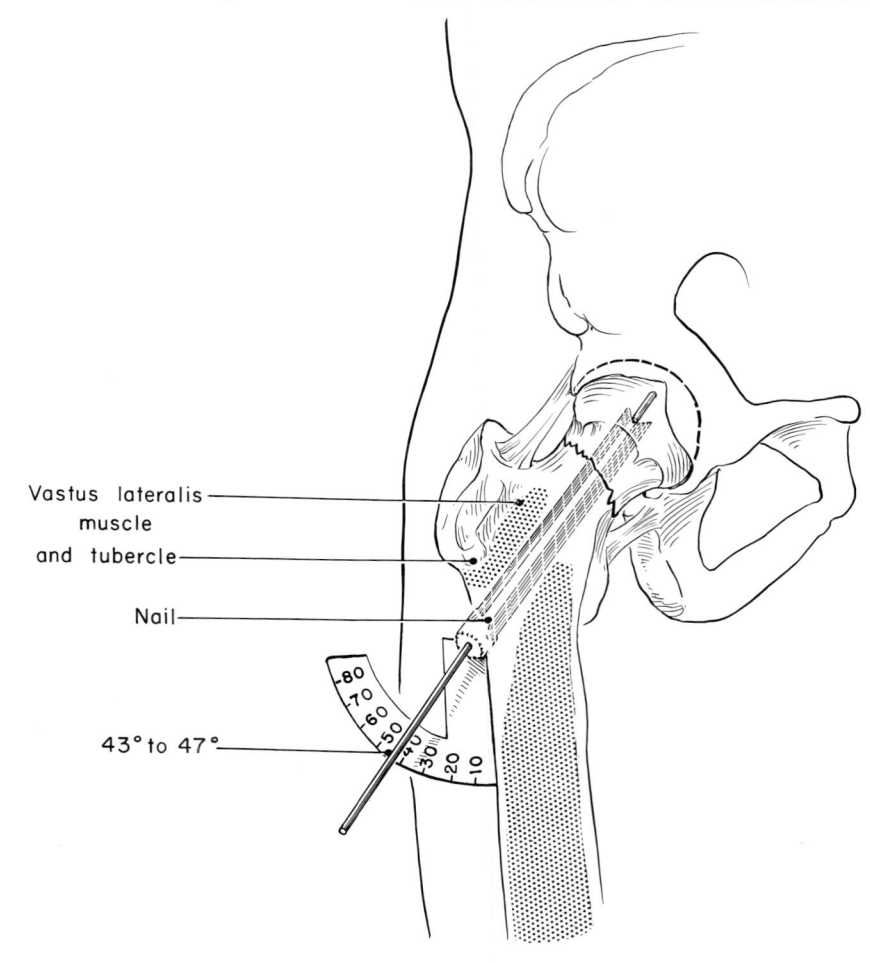

Chapter 26: FRACTURES OF THE HIP: HEAD, NECK AND TROCHANTER / 641

after checking these points with the skin markers and laying an external wire between the skin marker and the point of the anticipated entrance of the nail, this angle does not approach 45 degrees, a check on the x-ray should be made for a better point of entrance. Once this angle has been established, a ¼-in. drill hole should be made through the outer cortex of the shaft. Small wedge-shaped openings into the cortex in line with the 3 flanges of the nail are then made (Figs. 26-17 and 26-18). The single blade of the 3-flanged nail is best directed upward.

Following the placement of these 3 small openings and the drill hole, a 3/32 in. Kirschner wire can be drilled in by hand or driven in by the gentle tap of the mallet, aiming the wire at the optimal point in relation to the head that the markers have indicated. In driving this wire with a mallet (the most satisfactory method), a change in pitch is encountered as the wire crosses the fracture site and an increasing pitch gradually develops into a solid tone as the wire enters the head. With a well-placed wire, 3–3½ in. can be driven in before this point is

Fig. 26-17.—Technique for nailing hip to avoid splitting of femoral shaft. Wedges should be cut in the cortex for the nail blades.

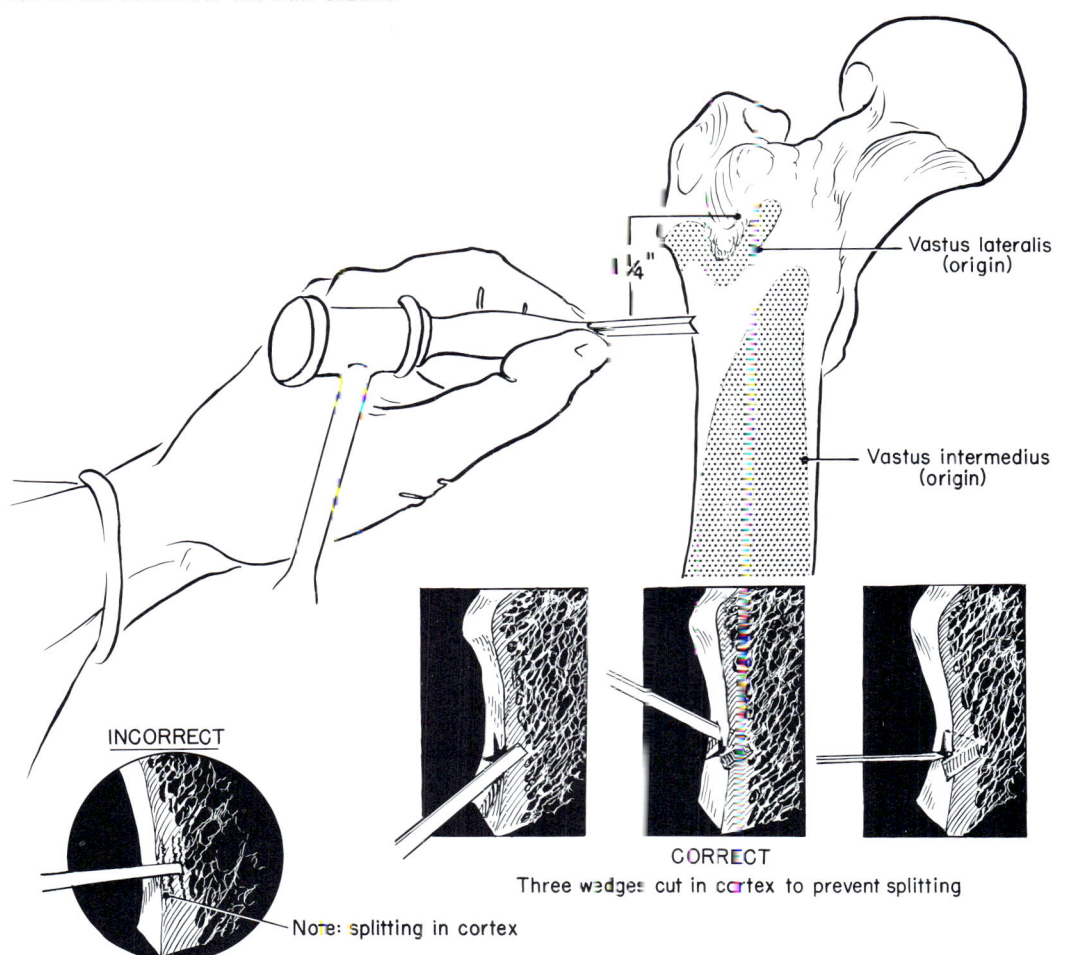

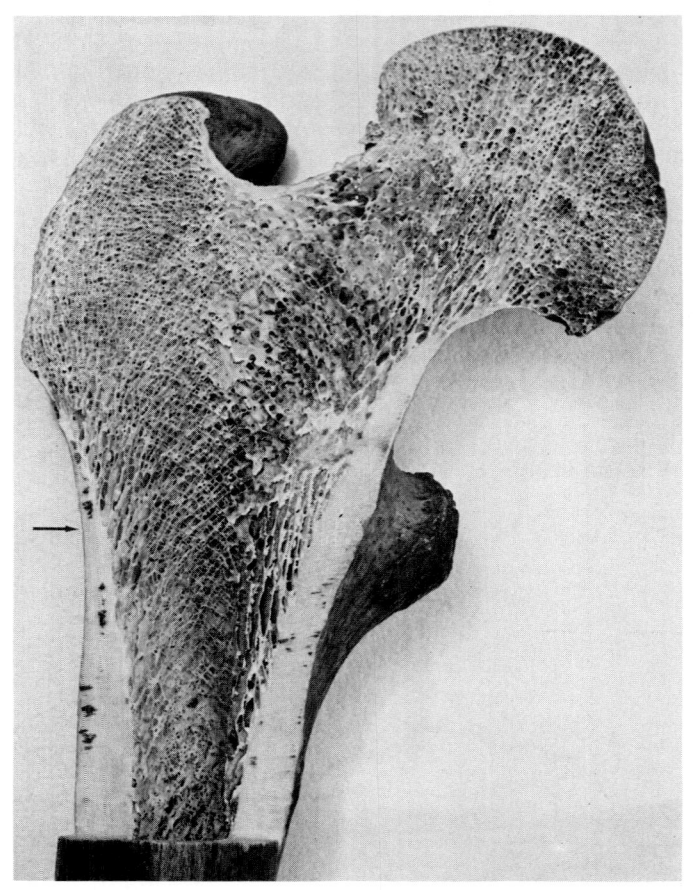

Fig. 26-18.—Internal architecture of neck of femur. Trabecular bone lends itself to compression by a 3-flanged nail, and this compression results in increasing holding power over the surfaces of the blades of the nail. Notice the heavy lateral cortex at the site where the nail is to be inserted *(arrow)*. To keep from splitting this cortex, small wedges of bone should be removed at this site before insertion of the nail.

reached. When viewed laterally the wire is generally parallel to the floor. Slight internal rotation at the conclusion of the reduction maneuver will have made the neck of the femur with a normal anteversion also parallel to the floor. Once the wire has been driven in, it should be checked by both anteroposterior and lateral x-rays to be certain of its position. It should lie directly in the center of the head in both views or slightly posteriorly and inferiorly.

POSITION OF THE NAIL.—An ideal reduction would be one that is perfect anatomically. Equally acceptable reductions are those in slight valgus position but in which the trabecular pattern does not cross the vascular channels of the neck. A very minimal varus deformity is acceptable, provided the angle of the neck with the shaft is not less than 135 degrees. More varus than this will consistently lead to trouble (Fig. 26-19).

An ideal tract for the nail would then be one in which the nail goes through the inferior neck and into the head slightly below its center of gravity and slightly in the posteroinferior quadrant. With such a position, any muscle pull or any very

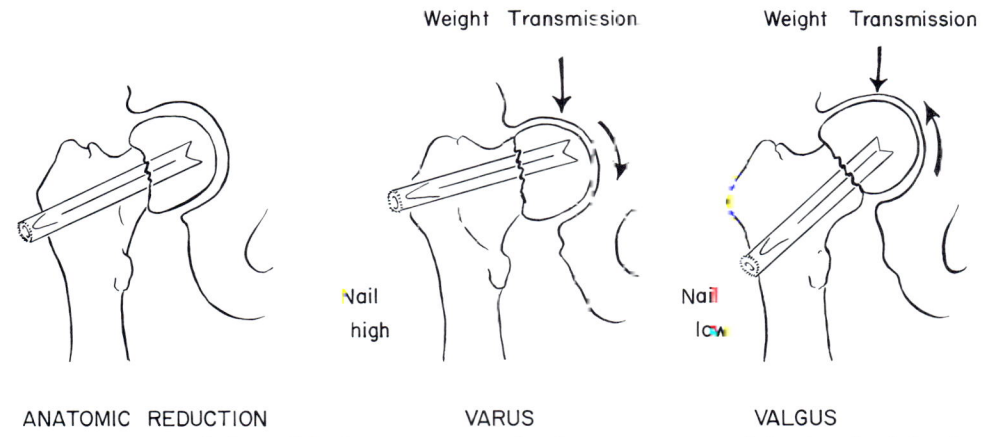

Chapter 26: FRACTURES OF THE HIP: HEAD, NECK AND TROCHANTER / 643

Fig. 26-19.—Acceptability of both anatomic and valgus positions of the head of the femur. The varus position, however, is not acceptable; nonunion will usually result unless the hip is protected through a prolonged period of non-weight-bearing. Even after union, traumatic arthritis in the joint is almost certain to develop.

slight weight bearing would impact the fragments. In any nail position which is less than a 45-degree angle, or one which traverses the superior position of the neck and enters the inferior portion of the head, the muscular and weight-bearing forces will tend to loosen the nail and have unfavorable shearing forces.

The proper length of the nail can be easily determined by use of 2 Kirschner wires of the same length, 1 of which is driven across the fracture as a guide and the other placed on the lateral surface of the femur and projecting outward. The difference in length of the 2 wires indicates the proper length of the nail (Fig. 26-20), provided the wire that has traversed the fracture line into the head is in the proper position and does not penetrate the cortex of the head.

As the nail is being driven over the guide wire into the head, a frequent check should be made, by loosening the extension apparatus, to be sure that the guide wire is not being driven into the pelvis. Any change in pitch or in the ease with which the nail progresses is indirect evidence that something is wrong. The surgeon should stop and check all factors. As the nail crosses the fracture line, there is a change in pitch and the percussion note of the mallet becomes higher as the nail penetrates farther and farther into the head. At any step in the procedure when there is doubt as to how the nail is entering the bone, a check x-ray will prove valuable. Once the nail has been driven into the flare at its base, a film should be made to determine whether or not disimpaction has occurred; if so, impaction should be carried out, (Fig. 26-21). This can be done by regular impactors or by any apparatus that permits striking the cortex of the femur and, thereby, pushing the shaft toward the head fragment. Impaction occurs when the nail protrudes a little after this procedure. When this occurs, the surgeon should not strike the nail again; such a procedure would undo the impaction. Impaction should be carried out when x-ray evidence indicates, in either view, that there has been separation of the fracture line by the process of nailing. It is not necessary to impact if separation has not occurred. A gentle clinical test of the security of the nailing and for reassurance regarding the efficiency of the procedure should be carried out while the patient is still under anesthesia (Fig. 26-22).

Many surgeons prefer the use of a fracture table for all hip nailings. One word of caution, however, is warranted in its

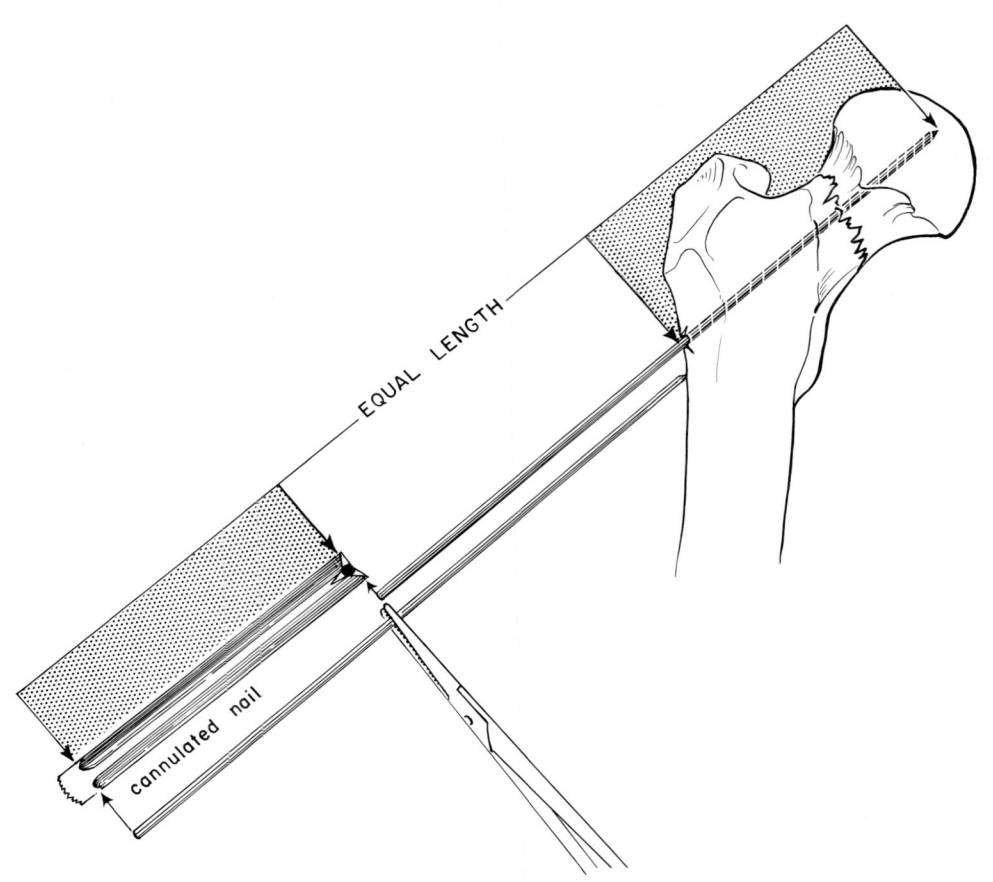

644 / O. E. Aufranc, J. D. Lowell, H. P. Chandler and P. L. Norton

Fig. 26-20.—Simple method for determining nail length. The simplest method is probably the best.

Fig. 26-21.—Importance of impacting a fracture of the femoral neck. **A** and **B,** as the nail is driven across the fracture line into the head, the fractured ends separate unless held together by some means. Even then, there is a tendency for them to separate. Impaction is usually indicated, as in **C.**

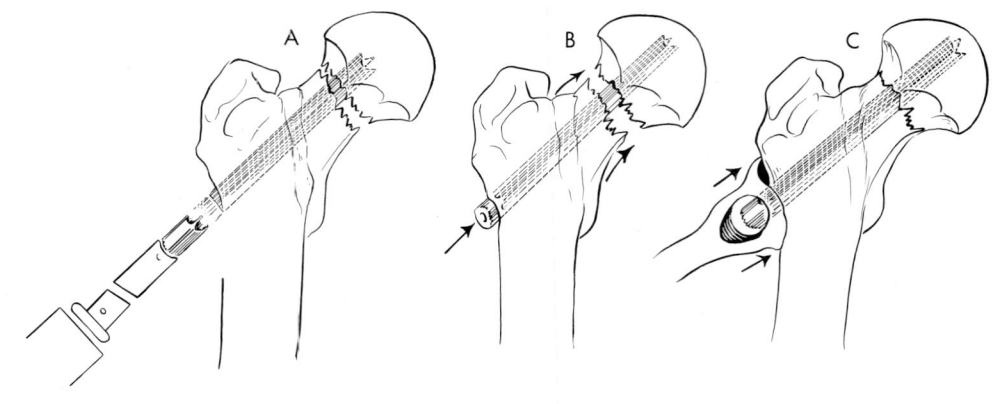

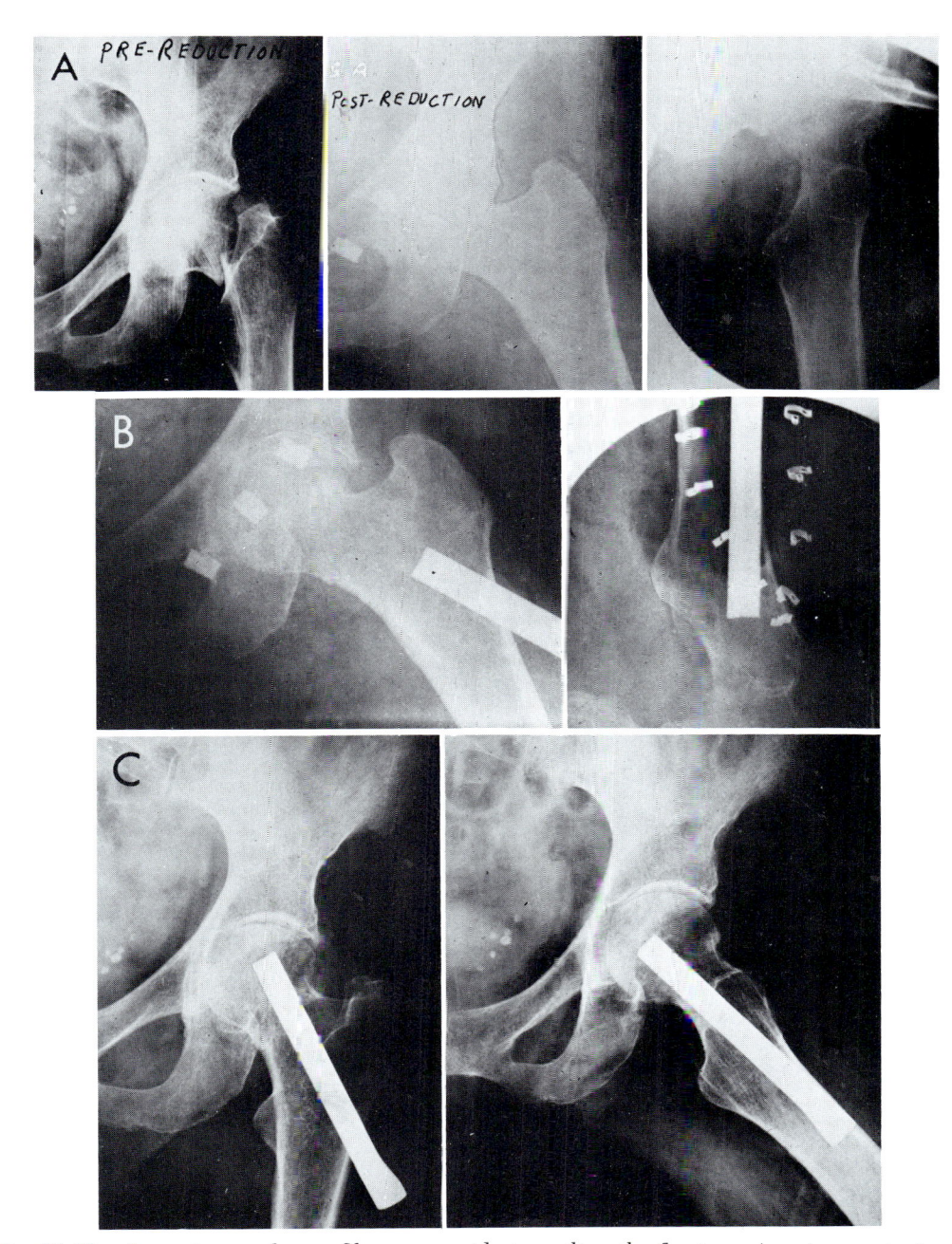

Chapter 26: FRACTURES OF THE HIP: HEAD, NECK AND TROCHANTER / **645**

Fig. 26-22.—Importance of x-ray films as a guide in nailing the fracture. **A,** anteroposterior and lateral x-ray films for reduction of a displaced fracture. Adequate films are a necessity to be sure of the reduction. **B,** films required for checking placement of nail (or other form of internal fixation). **C,** checking by x-ray, also a necessity before weight bearing is allowed.

use in management of the intracapsular fracture. If the table is used to maintain traction on the affected leg after reduction, the surgeon must appreciate that the fracture may well be distracted. As the nail is driven in, it has the potential to spin the head if it enters anywhere but in the very center. Use of the conventional table with the leg held by an assistant or fixed on a low stand or stool in the position of abduction, extension and slight internal rotation at the hip and right-angled flexion at the knee will put tension on the rectus femoris muscle, locking the fracture securely in its reduced position. The spinning of the head will then be avoided.

Fractures Difficult or Practically Impossible to Reduce by Closed Method

Whenever it is possible, the surgeon should carry out closed reduction and internal fixation of a fracture of the neck of the femur. There are instances, however, in which it is impossible to reduce the fragments into an acceptable position. When this occurs, an open reduction and nailing should be done. Such a procedure is long and at times difficult, and in an elderly, debilitated patient who has sustained a subcapital type of fracture in a very soft bone, the use of a replacement prosthesis should be considered.

No prosthesis can ever assume the good function of a well-healed fractured neck of the femur. In almost all fractures of the femoral neck, at least 1 attempt should be made at reduction and nailing. If, however, the condition of the patient warrants only minimal manipulation and the fracture is of the subcapital type, a femoral head replacement prosthesis seems to be the treatment of choice as the initial procedure.

The elderly, feeble patients, those with Parkinson's disease, spastic hemiplegia, pathologic fracture or an urgent need to become ambulatory because of blindness and those with a frankly unreducible fracture of the subcapital type are candidates for a primary prosthesis. Femoral neck fractures in which there is severe comminution or interposed transverse fragments are included in this classification. The lateral, the posterolateral or the anterolateral exposure of the hip is adequate for prosthetic replacement of the femoral head and is relatively atraumatic. Some consideration in choice of approach should be made in light of neurologic disease and any accompanying muscular imbalance that may be present. The posterior approach, for example, should rarely if ever be used in the patient with Parkinson's disease, since the flexion and adduction posture of the hip so frequently assumed by these patients postoperatively, often in spite of traction, leads to a high incidence of dislocation of the prosthesis from the acetabulum.

The desirability of using polymethyl methacrylate to obtain immediate secure fixation of the prosthesis in the proximal femur, thus allowing earlier unrestricted weight bearing, deserves comment. In the younger patient with more than 10–15 years' life expectancy, this is probably ill advised, because the tendency of any prosthesis to migrate centrally seems to be enhanced with the supplementary use of "cement" fixation. In the elderly and infirm, it appears to be a useful adjunct, but in employing it the surgeon must consider the increased risk to the patient and the possible consequences should infection ensue.

Surgical After-Care

The groundwork for the development of pressure sores is laid while the patient waits — on the floor after the injury, on the litter, on the x-ray table and lying in bed too deeply medicated following surgery. Frequent changes of position are necessary to avoid this disaster. Such care is as crucial to the patient as is the proper management of fluid and electrolyte needs and cardiac and pulmonary status.

Elderly patients with fractures need more attention in nursing care than do patients with other types of surgery.

Careful watching and attention to detail will be rewarding.

After operation, the patient will be more comfortable in Russell traction or balanced suspension with traction than he will be lying free in the bed, and it will be easier for him to move about, to receive proper skin care and to use the bedpan. As soon as he is able to cooperate, deep-breathing exercises and coughing should be started to expand the lungs and protect the patient from atelectasis or pneumonia. He should be doing arm, trunk and leg exercises, and he should begin moving the foot, knee and hip on the affected side as quickly as diminishing sensitivity of the muscles about the fracture site will permit. An overhead frame supporting a trapeze or hand grips was recognized as early as the time of Paré as an important adjunct in the care of the bedridden patient.

If the patient's condition warrants and the fixation of the fracture is secure, he may begin transfers to a chair within a day or 2 of operation. If, on the other hand, he is not medically fragile and is cooperative with an exercise program, he may be kept in bed 4 or 5 days or more to allow initial healing of soft tissues and return of muscle control. The patient is transferred first to a chair, then within a day or 2 to a walker and subsequently to crutches. In using both the walker and crutches, he is taught to put partial weight on the affected limb, usually 20–30 lb, or for the purpose of instruction, "the weight of the leg." He is maintained at this level of weight bearing until the fracture is healed. Before discharge from the hospital, he should be taught how to protect the leg not just in walking but in the act of getting in and out of bed, in and out of a chair, on and off a toilet, in and out of the tub and up and down a flight of stairs, both with and without the use of a banister. Follow-up radiographs are taken before discharge from the hospital, at 3 months, at 6 months from the date of injury and again at 1 and 2 years.

Fractures of the femoral neck heal differently from fractures elsewhere, healing primarily by callus arising from the marrow supporting structure. Banks[4] notes that Schmorl, in 1924, was the first to record that the periosteum of the neck of the femur contained no cambium layer and therefore was unable to form external callus. This lack of external callus is 1 reason it is often difficult to determine whether the intracapsular fracture is progressing satisfactorily to union and why it is often necessary to use arbitrary lengths of time before the fracture is considered healed sufficiently to permit unrestricted weight bearing or the withdrawal of a protruding nail that is painful. Generally speaking, no matter how satisfactory the status of the fracture appears on the x-ray film, it is wise to insist on crutch protection for at least 6 months from the time of fixation.

Prognosis

The prognosis of a fracture of the neck of a femur is influenced partly by mechanical factors and partly by physiologic factors; by the unknown amount of trauma to the circulation and by the unknown reparative ability of the individual patient. The manipulative efforts of the surgeon probably also affect the prognosis more than is generally appreciated.

Statistical information concerning the rate of union of these fractures varies widely among authors and often is not comparable because of the different parameters used in its determination. Boyd and Salvatore[7] noted 8–12% nonunion in displaced fractures in which internal fixation was employed. Charnley[13] reported union in 85% of displaced fractures in which a spring-loaded compression device was employed. Fielding and Zickel,[25] using a Pugh telescoping nail, report only 1 case of nonunion in a series of 38 patients. More recently, Deyerle[22] reported a 100% rate of union in a series of 112 personal cases using the device of his own design. Metz reported a 95.3% rate of union in 43 fractures also treated with the Deyerle device, and Meyers[43] and associates reported 97% rate of union using internal fixation with Hagie pins and supplementary insertion of a muscle pedicle graft on the posterior aspect of the femoral neck, a technique introduced by the Judets in 1962.

Complications

Reports concerning the frequency of avascular necrosis vary widely, but avascular necrosis is reported by all authors and certainly is common to our own experience. It will vary from a low of 7% when clinical radiographs alone are used to determine its presence to a high of 87.5% when information obtained by microscopic examination of specimens removed at operation 2 or more weeks after injury is included.[57]

Fortunately, the development of avascular necrosis does not mean that supplementary surgery is mandatory. Collapse of the weight-bearing portion of the femoral head may or may not follow in proportion to the degree of apparent involvement; even if present, symptoms may be minimal. In the series reported by Boyd and Salvatore, supplementary surgery was required in approximately half the cases in which this complication occurred. Minor degrees of avascular necrosis undoubtedly occur much more frequently than radiographs or the clinical course of the patient would indicate.

Other complications associated with intracapsular fracture of the femur may be directly related to the nailing procedure itself, such as loss of fixation by a nail that is too short, penetration of the joint space by one that is too long, or

Fig. 26-23.—**A,** anteroposterior and lateral views showing nailing of fractured hip of 93-year-old patient. Because of the patient's age, this nailing was accepted. **B,** 5 years later. Poor positions of fragments should not be accepted—regardless of age.

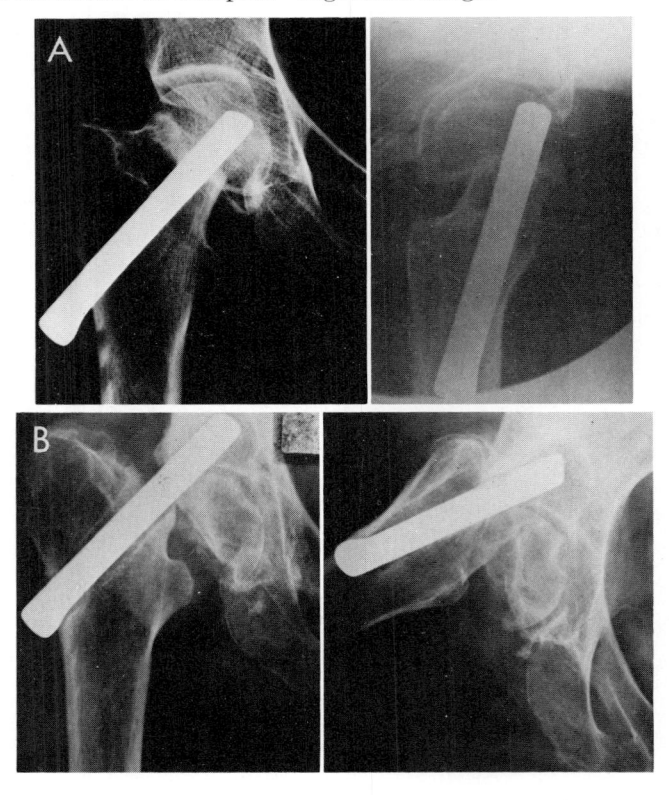

Chapter 26: FRACTURES OF THE HIP: HEAD, NECK AND TROCHANTER / 649

nonunion because the nail was directed either anteriorly or posteriorly and did not secure the fragments firmly (Fig. 26-23). In one case recently seen, a spring-loaded compression device had kept the fracture surfaces apart and held the proximal fragment in a position of malrotation of 90 degrees (Fig. 26-24). In another, multiple fixation wires had broken, some of the fragments had migrated and union had failed to occur (Fig. 26-25).

Deaths secondary to cerebrovascular accident, pulmonary embolism, myocardial infarction, pneumonia, hypertensive cardiovascular disease and less frequent causes are noted in each series reported. The over-all mortality rate ranges from a low of 7% among the gen-

Fig. 26-24 (top and bottom left).—Complication of internal fixation. **A** and **B,** fracture is impacted on original radiographs. Although valgus is extreme, a favorable outcome may well have followed treatment by conservative means. **C,** the device employed rotated the head fragment 180 degrees, causing the median weight-bearing trabeculae of the head to lie horizontally. The threaded portion of the device crossed the fracture line and held the surfaces apart. Nonunion and avascular necrosis followed.

Fig. 26-25 (bottom right).—Migration of wires. Three wires were used to secure a fractured femoral neck. All broke, and the proximal fragments of the wires migrated into the pelvis. This hazard must always be kept in mind when wires are used.

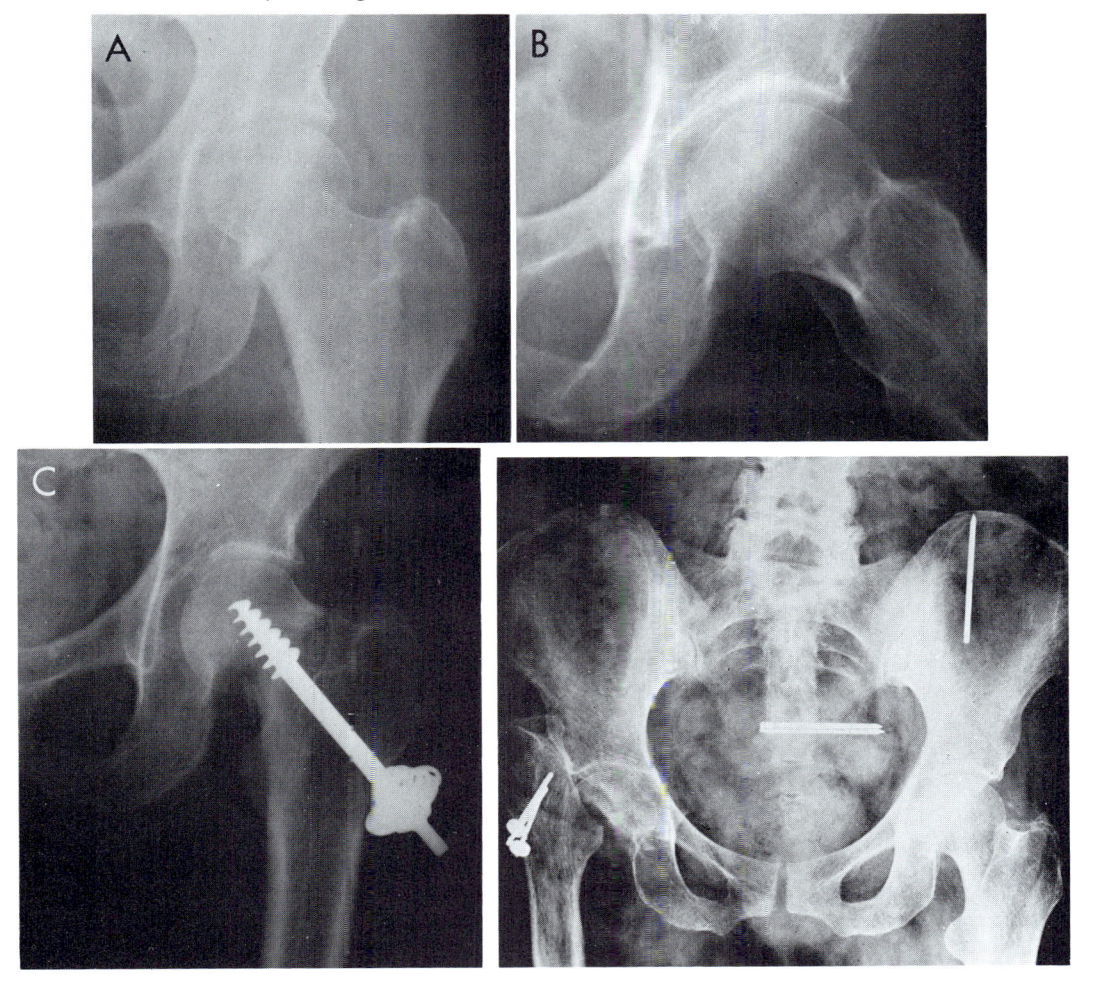

eral population in-hospital deaths to a high of 53% within the first 6 months after fracture in psychotic patients. These figures vary considerably, according to whether the author is reporting an in-hospital death rate, a death rate within 3 or 6 months after fracture or death before walking.

Infection, if deep, is a disaster. Its early signs are often subtle, consisting only of pain on motion or use, without accompanying fever or constitutional symptoms. An elevated sedimentation rate may be the only positive laboratory finding. Two or 3 months may elapse before radiographs show progressive loss of the cartilage space and demineralization of subchondral bone in the acetabular roof (Fig. 26-26). When the joint is involved, treatment requires exploration and removal of the femoral head if it is devoid of circulation and acting as a sequestrum. Thorough debridement and drainage, with appropriate antibiotic therapy, should follow. The proximal shaft should be allowed to lie against the side of the ilium after the method of Girdlestone, or an arthroplasty should be performed, with placement of the base of the neck into the acetabulum and transplantation of the trochanter distally along the shaft, with or without the interposition of a Vitallium mold. Fortunately, infection is rare.

AVASCULAR NECROSIS OF FEMORAL HEAD: ORIGIN, RECOGNITION AND PREVENTION. — Considerable interest is currently being shown in the problem of aseptic necrosis of the femoral head after intracapsular fracture. The research has been directed in 2 main areas. One is to learn as much as possible about the causes of the condition, so as to work out methods of prevention. The second is to determine whether destruction of the blood supply to the femoral head is already present at the time of operation, so that a replacement prosthesis procedure can be undertaken immediately rather than subject the patient to second surgery at a later date. Studies of the vascular

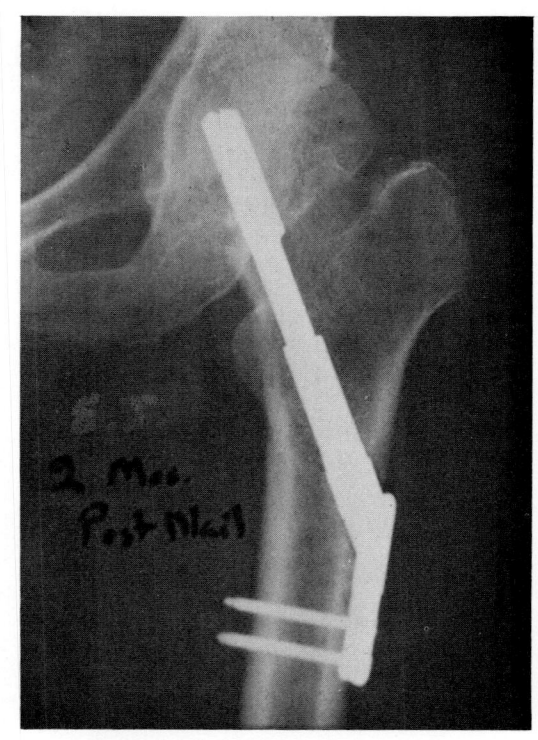

Fig. 26-26. — Septic arthritis after hip nailing. Loss of the cartilage space and demineralization of the subchondral bone of the acetabulum 2 months postsurgery are indicative of intra-articular infection. Patient's temperature and blood count were normal. Sedimentation rate was elevated and the hip was painful. A shaft cup arthroplasty eliminated the infection and gave the patient a painfree, stable, movable hip with good muscle control. The leg, however, is now 1½ in. short.

supplies to the femoral head have been carried out by Trueta and Harrison,[68] by Judet et al.,[34] by Banks[4] and by Smith.[59] Most investigators believe that the vessels of the ligamentum teres have a significant role in the ultimate viability of the femoral head in only a few cases and are grossly inadequate to replace other vascular structures that may be destroyed. Smith, however, from direct observations in the operating room found that 8 of 24 capital fragments, devoid of circulation except for that supplied by the artery of the ligamentum teres, bled actively, and that this bleeding could be shut off by either rotatory or valgus malpositions of the fragment. Related anatomic studies on fresh cadaver specimens revealed that it is impossible, in the intact hip, for the ligamentum teres to become sufficiently twisted, stretched or compressed to interrupt its supply of blood to the femoral head. According to Banks' investigation, the most important vessels to the femoral head are those contained in the inferior retinaculum. Other investigators considered those of the superior retinaculum to be most important. The blood supply coming through anastomotic channels within the neck itself is destroyed with displacement of the fracture.

Increased intra-articular pressure within the hip joint as a causative factor in aseptic necrosis has been investigated by Soto-Hall, Johnson and Johnson.[64] They pointed out the vulnerability of the retinacular vessels lying exposed along the posterior aspect of the neck and showed that, with the hip in a position of abduction, extension and internal rotation, intra-articular pressures of as much as 200 mm Hg could be produced. Woodhouse[75] has been able to produce aseptic necrosis of the dog femoral head by intracapsular injection of saline solution and maintenance of pressure of 50 mm Hg for 12 hours. Rokkanen[50] induced aseptic necrosis in the femoral head of the rabbit by constriction of the femoral neck and retinacular vessels by tight steel wire ligations. Soto-Hall and his coworkers frequently found increased intra-articular pressure within the hip in association with intracapsular fractures when the joint was aspirated at operation, and suggested that aspiration be carried out as a preventive measure or that an opening into the joint be created anteriorly at the time of surgery.

Investigations currently undertaken to determine the viability of the femoral head at the time of operation include measurement of the oxygen tension within the femoral head, thermal dilution studies, measurement of pressure within the femoral head itself, measurement of the rate of deposition or removal of various radioactive elements and angiography. Although many of these approaches show great promise, all are still in the experimental stage.

Dickerson and Duthie,[23] and Frankel and Derian[27] have reported on animal experiments using single vessels or muscle pedicles to bring circulation to devitalized bone. In man, the muscle pedicle graft technique recently reported by both Judet and Meyers et al.[43] uses the quadratus femoris muscle and the underlying segment of posterior cortex of the greater trochanter as both a source of blood supply and supplementary stabilization in fractures of the femoral neck and thus far shows great promise.

COMPLICATIONS WITH FIXATION DEVICE. —A device that has been driven in too far, particularly if it reaches the weight-bearing surface of the head of the femur, should be withdrawn and replaced by a shorter one. When a nail or pin tends to extrude, there usually has been absorption and settling down at the fracture site. The use of epaulets or transfixion screws or the countersinking of the head of a nail inside the cortex of the femur to prevent this extrusion is contraindicated because a certain amount of absorption may normally take place at the fracture surfaces; also, a small amount of extrusion of the nail is not detrimental because it allows the fractured ends closer apposition and a better chance to heal. A loss of position or a cutting out of a nail through the head may occur in an atrophic head or neck.

The development of avascular necrosis usually shows on x-rays as a relative increase in density of the weight-bearing portion of the head in comparison to both the neck region and the adjacent acetabulum. Ultimately, there will be loss of sphericity of the femoral head as the avascular portion collapses into the viable portion along the boundary line separating living from nonliving bone. There may also be accompanying absorption of the neck along the fracture line and around the distal portion of the nail, suggesting associated nonunion and motion of the fragments one against the other. Other than a relative increase in density of the avascular femoral head due to its failure to participate in surrounding osteoporosis, the earliest x-ray change is the so-called crescent sign, consisting of a thin radiolucent line of subchondral resorption usually noted at 1 margin of the avascular head because of resorption of bone by invading granulation tissue.

Removal of the nail is not necessary, however, unless there is protrusion of the nail into the acetabulum or extrusion, or the base of the nail becomes a source of irritation in the trochanteric area. All too often nails have been removed for the complaint of pain, when the pain arose not from the nail but from early avascular necrosis. Such added procedures not only provide no relief but on occasion have allowed a healing but not adequately healed fracture to fall apart.

TREATMENT OF COMPLICATIONS.—An area of aseptic necrosis which develops in a femoral head after the healing of a fracture may become an orthopedic reconstruction problem, but each case of aseptic necrosis must be treated on an individual basis. Reconstructive hip procedures, such as the femoral head prosthesis, total hip replacement, Vitallium mold arthroplasty, modification of the Whitman and Albee reconstruction operations using the mold, or modifications of the Colonna procedure using the shaft or the trochanteric area, are all indicated in appropriate situations. Routine procedures are not feasible, and the type of operation selected must suit the problem at hand.

The treatment of sepsis in and around a nailed hip, or of sepsis that has gone into the joint itself, is a complicated problem, requiring the efforts of a competent surgeon over a long period. Frequently, many operations are necessary before the sepsis can be brought under control. The surgeon must be aware of the possible complications of fractures of the femoral neck and be prepared to handle them as they arise. They may occur in the most carefully handled cases.

Summary

The management of fractures of the femoral neck may be summarized as follows:

1. Primary splinting of the patient with a fractured neck of the femur can be easily accomplished by placing pillows between the knees and ankles and bandaging the 2 thighs and legs together. This bandage may be left on while the patient is transported from the site of injury to the operating table, without loosening or changing the bandage while taking the necessary x-ray films. Such splinting reduces the amount of additional trauma that the patient might receive as a result of attempts to hold such a fracture in a Hodgen splint or other type of apparatus.

2. A responsible member of the team caring for the patient should supervise the taking of the necessary films without freeing the primary bandages.

3. The surgeon, or a competent associate, should maintain gentle traction on the fractured extremity during the time of induction of anesthesia, so that additional trauma from the effects of muscle effort during the induction stage are minimized.

4. In the manipulative reduction of the fractured neck of the femur, gentleness and steadiness are prime factors. There should be traction in the line of deformity, associated with an attempt to bring the distal fragment around to fit the small proximal fragment. The only remaining soft tissue attachments the head has are the ligamentum teres and possibly the posterior retinaculum. The leg is then held by a competent assistant or fixed to a low platform or stool, either preferable to tying it to a traction table or suspending it in a fracture apparatus.

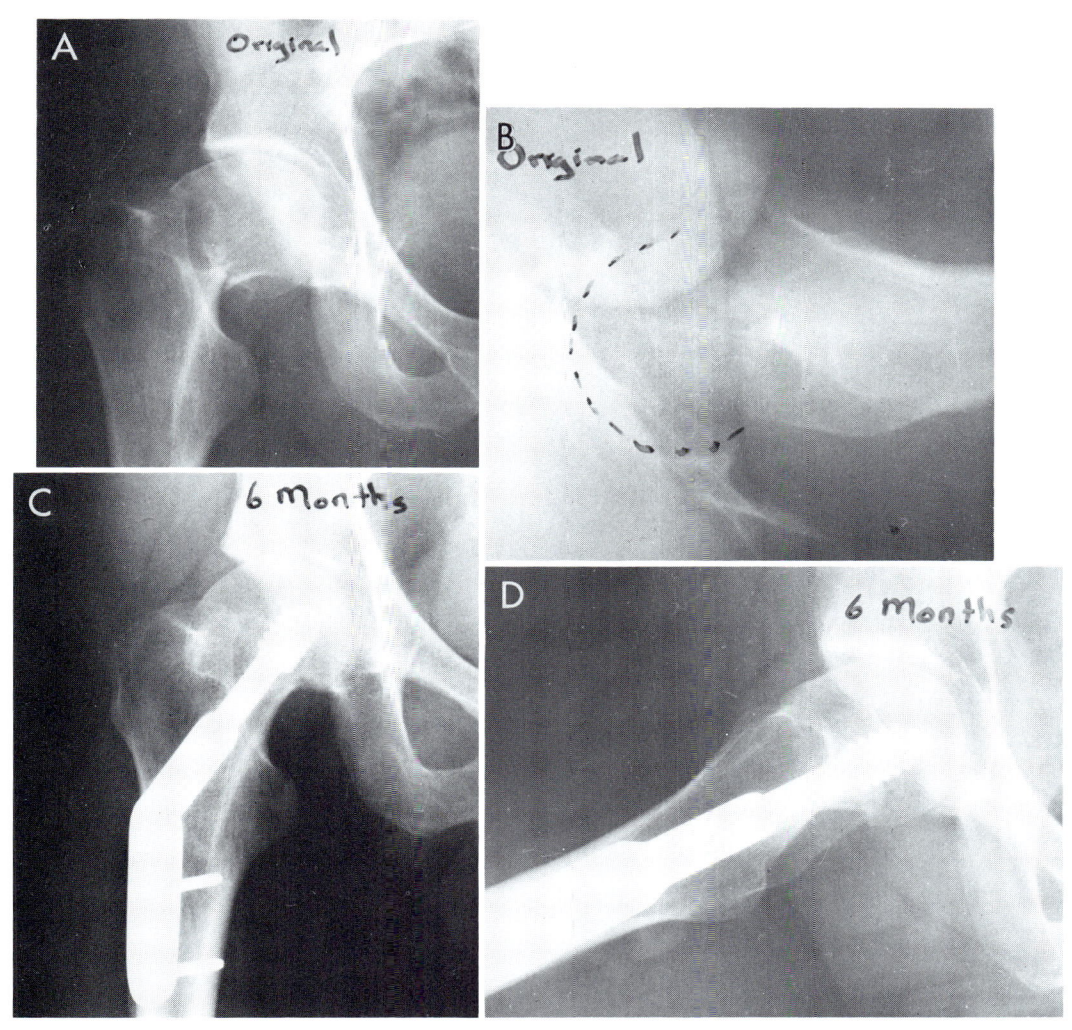

Chapter 26: FRACTURES OF THE HIP: HEAD, NECK AND TROCHANTER / 653

Fig. 26-27.—A 35-year-old man with right-sided cerebral palsy fell, sustaining an intracapsular fracture of the ipsilateral hip. **A** and **B**, original radiographs reveal varus and retroversion of femoral head. **C** and **D**, fixation was obtained with a sliding screw and sideplate. The patient, unable to use crutches effectively, was bearing full weight 8 weeks after injury. Solid union was evident at 6 months. The patient had returned to work at 1 month. This device is technically more difficult to use than a single 3-flanged nail and requires more soft tissue surgery. But it appears to be more tolerant of a patient's inability to follow a prescribed postoperative regimen than is the nail.

5. Adequate x-ray films of sufficient detail to allow proper interpretation of the reduction are necessary in both anteroposterior and lateral planes. Internal fixation with a 3-flanged nail, pins or a telescoping device seems to be the most satisfactory of the treatment methods available at present. The use of multiple wires, lag screws, bolts or ordinary wood screws may be preferred by some surgeons. Although large nails and other types of apparatus hold the fragments adequately, no apparatus displaces as little bone or has significantly more holding

power than the flanged nail. On the other hand, a singular advantage of the telescoping screw is that it lacks the capacity to act as an osteotome, a disadvantage of the nail which does not lose this ability simply because the mallet that drove it in has been set aside and the incision closed (Fig. 26-27).

6. A fracture of the femoral neck that heals with bony union and without avascular necrosis will give a better result than any reconstructive operation or prosthesis. For this reason, in the vast majority of fractured hips treatment should be reduction and internal fixation.

7. A femoral head replacement, with or without supplementary "cement" fixation, may be indicated in the subcapital type of fractures in elderly persons with osteoporosis, in fractures which have comminution in the neck and in certain other selected situations. Such a procedure should be treated as a reconstruction of the hip and so managed afterward.

EXTRACAPSULAR (TROCHANTERIC) FRACTURES

Extracapsular or trochanteric fractures include those occurring between the base of the neck along the trochanteric line and distally to an area just below the trochanteric line. Some are inherently stable and others tend to be quite unstable even with internal fixation.

These are fractures of the aged and infirm. In a series of 500 such fractures at Massachusetts General Hospital, the average age of the patients was 75; in another series, by Alffram, the average was 73. The fractures are twice as common in women as in men, and most are comminuted. They represent a greater trauma to the patient than an intracapsular fracture and thus carry higher mortality and morbidity rates, regardless of the method of treatment selected.

The usual mechanism of production is a fall directly on the hip. Findings on initial physical examination will closely parallel those associated with intracapsular fracture, except that there may be more shortening with a bruise over the greater trochanter. Since the joint capsule is proximal to the line of the fracture and does not tether the distal fragments, the leg will often lie in as much as 80 or 90 degrees of external rotation.

In years past, most of these fractures were treated in traction, a minimum of 3–4 months being required before adequate union occurred to allow mobilization. Though there is still a place for this approach in selected instances, improvement in the surgical management of the aged has been such that all but a few of these fractures are now treated with internal fixation. The rapid relief of pain, prevention of deformity, ability to mobilize the patient and economic savings are further powerful arguments in favor of this approach.

Emergency Treatment and Transportation

The details of emergency treatment and transportation are the same as those already outlined for intracapsular fracture. After adequate x-rays have been taken, the patient is transferred to his bed and Russell traction applied (Fig. 26-28). The important points to be noted in connection with Russell traction are:

1. The leg must be supported on a pillow with the knees flexed.
2. The pulleys must be free running, with traction applied.
3. The padded sling must be under the knee, away from the head of the fibula, and must be equipped with a spreader so that it will not act as a tourniquet.
4. The traction line should pass through 4 pulleys, giving the mechanical advantage of 2 pulleys minus the friction of the leg on the pillow and pulleys.
5. Sufficient weight should be used to prevent shortening. This should be about 15 lb of pull. If this amount of pull is used, then the traction straps should be extended above the knee in order to se-

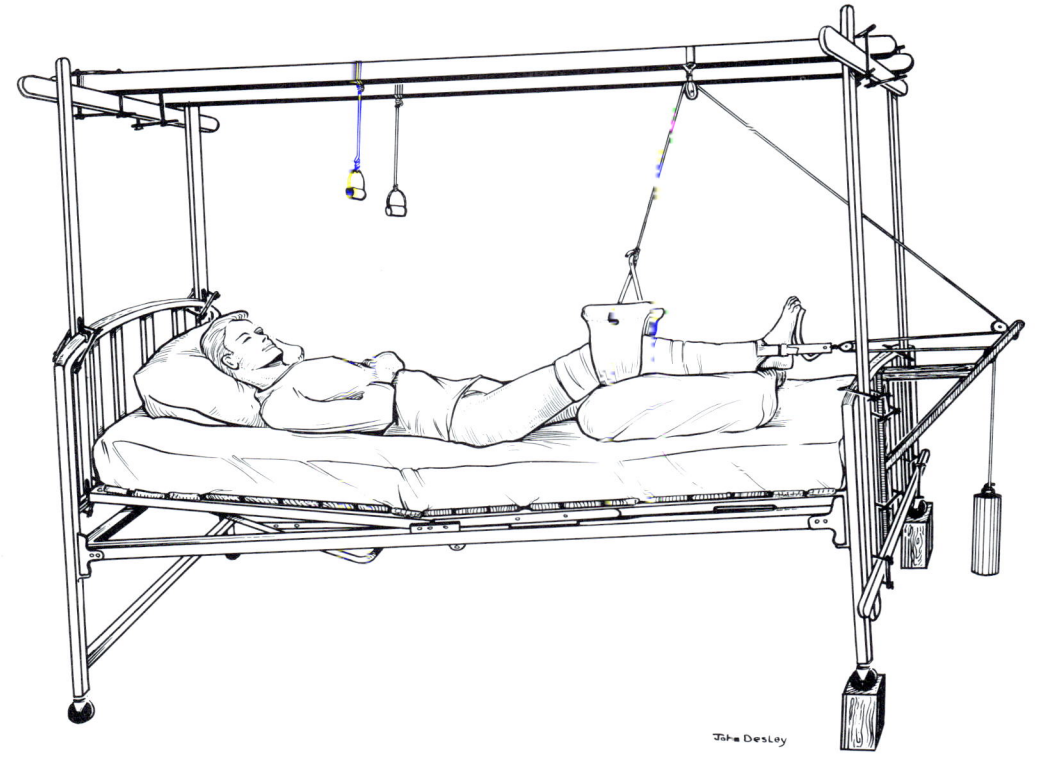

Chapter 26: FRACTURES OF THE HIP: HEAD, NECK AND TROCHANTER / 655

Fig. 26-28. — Russell traction.

cure a greater area of contact with the skin.

6. If traction is to be used for an extended period, a threaded Kirschner wire through the tibial tubercle should be used instead of moleskin.

Errors in the use of this type of traction include:

1. Failure to use a spreader. Such failure allows compression of the leg with obstruction of the circulation.

2. Failure to use a padded sling.

3. Allowing the sling to pull against the neck of the fibula with the leg in external rotation. In a thin subject, this may produce peroneal palsy.

4. Over 10 lb of pull with short traction tapes may cause skin damage. To avoid such damage, as large an area of skin as possible should be used for traction.

5. Incorrect position of the pillow. The pillow must be placed under the full length of the calf, not "balled up" under the knee.

6. Incorrect placement of the footpiece. The footpiece must not rest against the bedframe.

7. Failure to elevate the foot of the bed for countertraction. Low shock blocks should be used to elevate the foot of the bed.

After traction is applied, the physical status of the patient should be evaluated promptly and any deficiencies corrected, including the correction of possible dehydration. The cardiac and pulmonary condition of the patient also requires attention. Rapid digitalization or rapid control of unrecognized or uncontrolled diabetes is often needed. Preparation of the operative area is not done until after anesthesia has taken effect.

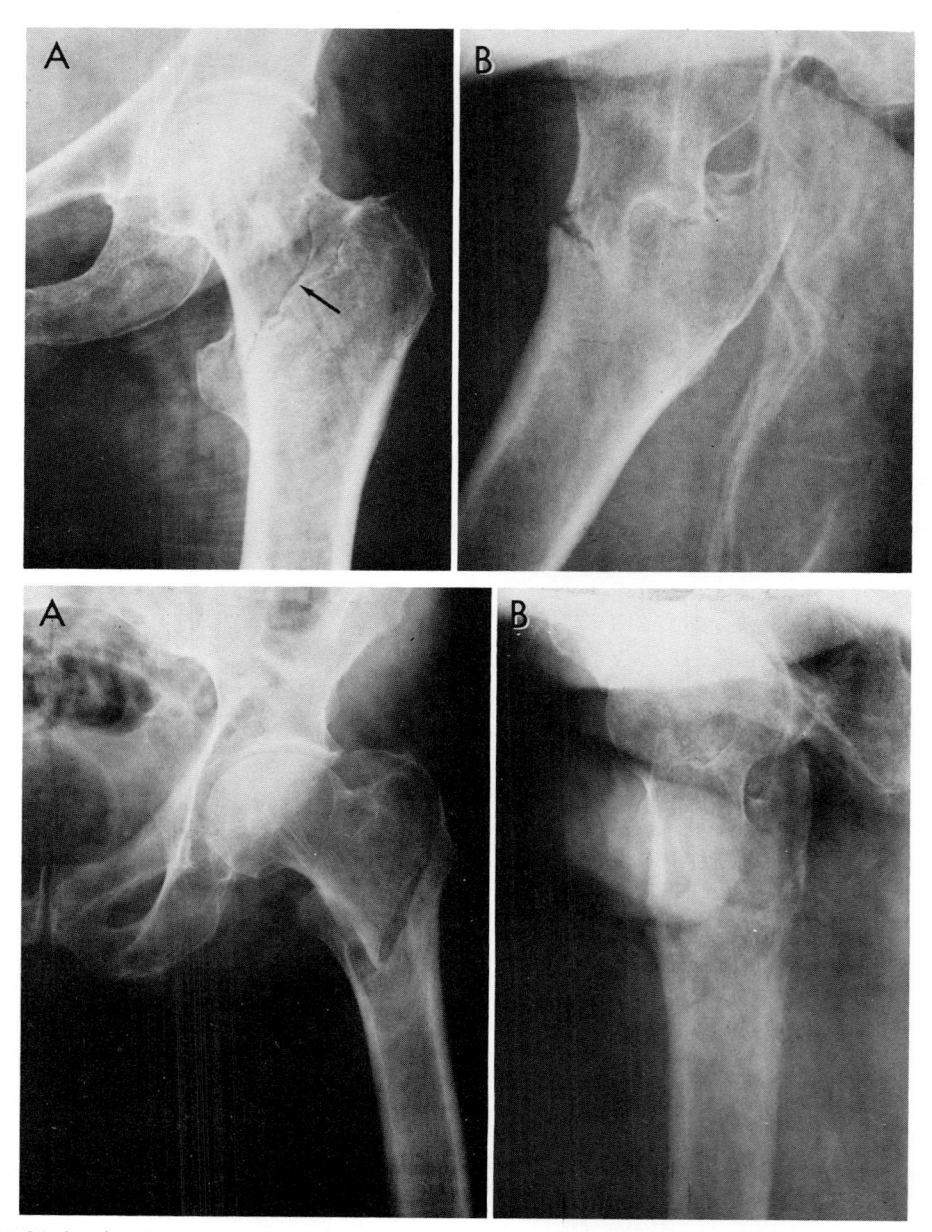

Fig. 26-29 (top).—Linear intertrochanteric fracture without displacement. **A,** anteroposterior view (arrow points to fractures). **B,** lateral view. A "stable" fracture.

Fig. 26-30 (bottom).—Pertrochanteric fracture with varus deformity and slight widening at fracture line, indicating external rotation of lower fragment. The lesser trochanter is intact. **A,** anteroposterior view showing fracture line passing into the trochanteric block. **B,** lateral view; not clear enough to tell whether greater trochanter is split vertically. Important to look for this! This fracture is "stable" and should be reduced anatomically.

Types of Extracapsular Fractures

The extracapsular fractures may be subdivided into the following types: (1) intertrochanteric, (2) pertrochanteric, (3) subtrochanteric (Figs. 26-29 to 26-33). In intertrochanteric fractures, the fracture line passes upward and outward along the intertrochanteric line; generally the trochanters are not involved. Variations in these fractures are determined by the deforming force that continues to act after fracture, producing external rotation and varus deformity at the fracture site. These fractures may vary from an undisplaced crack to a 90-degree varus deformity with marked external rotation. They are easy to repair, but they are not common.

Pertrochanteric fractures show a fracture line passing upward and outward into the greater trochanter. Both trochanters may be involved and comminution is frequent. About 70% of the extracapsular fractures in the Massachusetts General Hospital series were of the comminuted pertrochanteric type.

The subtrochanteric fractures are of multiple types and are found over a considerable age spread. In our patients with subtrochanteric fractures, the ages ranged from 9 to 92 years.

Trochanteric fractures may be further subdivided into those which are potentially stable after reduction and nailing and those which are potentially unstable. The hallmark of the latter group, consisting of about one-fourth of all trochanteric fractures, is that there are usually 4 parts to the fracture—a head-neck fragment, a lesser trochanteric fragment of varying size, a greater trochanteric fragment and a shaft fragment consisting of the remainder of the femur. Failure to recognize this group of fractures may lead to an attempt at anatomic reduction of the head-neck fragment, the greater trochanteric fragment and the shaft fragment, only to have the reduction and ensuing fixation followed by subsequent development of a "return to varus,"[35] cutting out of the fixation device or bending or breaking of the device[34, 39] (Fig. 26-34).

Treatment of Extracapsular Fractures

It is well known that a high percentage of trochanteric fractures heal without operation. If the surgeon and the patient elect conservative treatment, some form of Russell traction is the best means of regaining length and correcting deformity. Traction must be continued for 12–14 weeks in many cases; and even at the end of that time, varus deformity may recur.

The skin may not tolerate the prolonged use of the adhesive tape needed for effective traction. In such a case, a threaded Kirschner wire through the tibial tubercle is advisable. Use of a threaded wire eliminates sliding of the wire in the osteoporotic bone so frequently found in aged patients.

Operative Treatment

FIXATION DEVICES.—Numerous devices for holding the fracture fragments are available, including the adjustable nail-plate combinations of McLaughlin and Hubbard, sliding nails, telescoping screws, and angled nail-plate and blade-plate combinations. In the latter combinations, such as those of Moore, Neufeld and Jewett, the intramedullary portion of the nail and side plate are made from a single casting. Just as in intracapsular fractures, the selection of the device to be used must rest with the surgeon and be based on his knowledge and experience. At Massachusetts General Hospital and also at Peter Bent Brigham Hospital, the Jewett and McLaughlin nails or a telescoping device are currently those most frequently chosen.

OPERATIVE TECHNIQUE.—For the stable trochanteric fractures, the operative technique is the same for all. It consists of the use of a nail plate or screw plate, the length of the plate depending on the length of the fracture line. Occasionally,

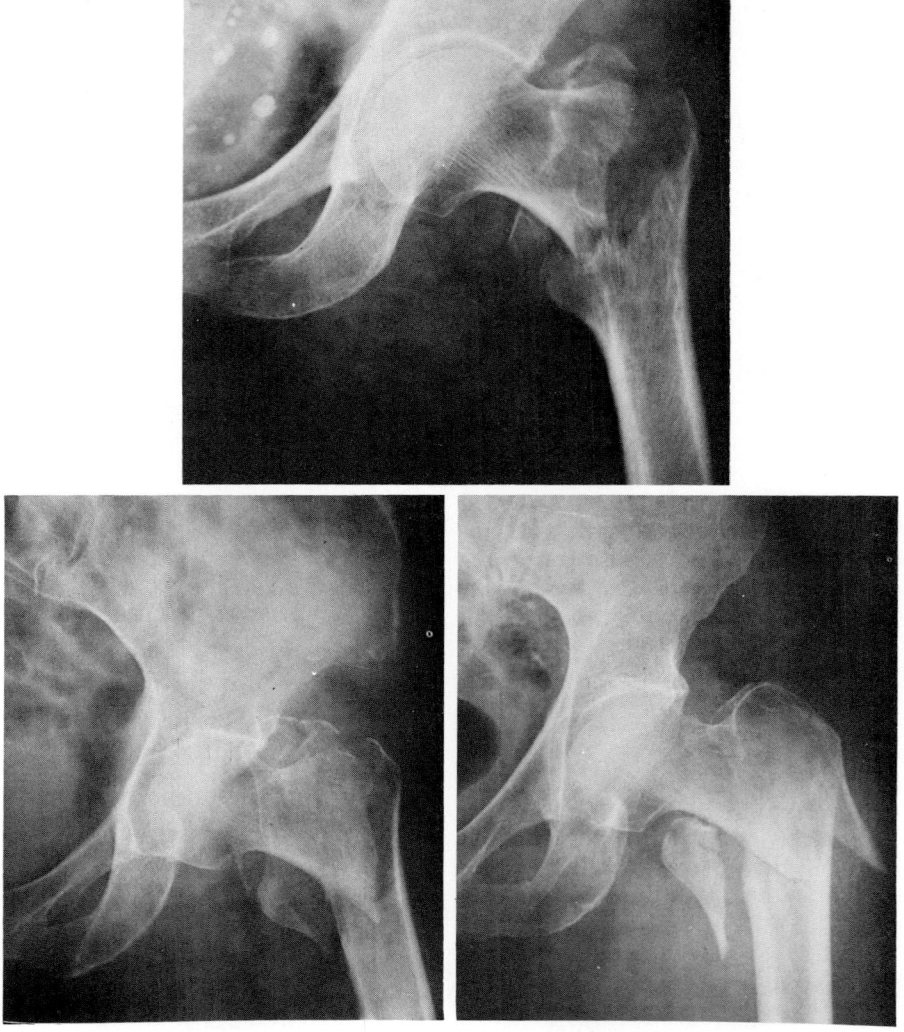

Fig. 26-31 (top).—Comminuted pertrochanteric fracture with (1) fracture through the greater trochanter with a loose posterior fragment, (2) fracture into lesser trochanter and (3) intact lesser trochanter. A stable fracture for which anatomic reduction should be sought.

Fig. 26-32 (bottom left).—Comminuted pertrochanteric fracture with varus deformity, external rotation, vertical splitting of greater trochanter and avulsion of the lesser trochanter. This is an unstable fracture; even with fixation and if anatomic reduction is selected, the fixation device should allow telescoping. Displacement fixation will achieve good bony contact and stability at operation.

Fig. 26-33 (bottom right).—Severely comminuted fracture, both pertrochanteric and subtrochanteric. Note the short, spear-pointed distal subtrochanteric fragment. Also the vertical splitting of the greater trochanter and the avulsion of the entire lesser trochanter. This fracture is "unstable" and requires fixation by displacement technique or with a telescoping nail or screw.

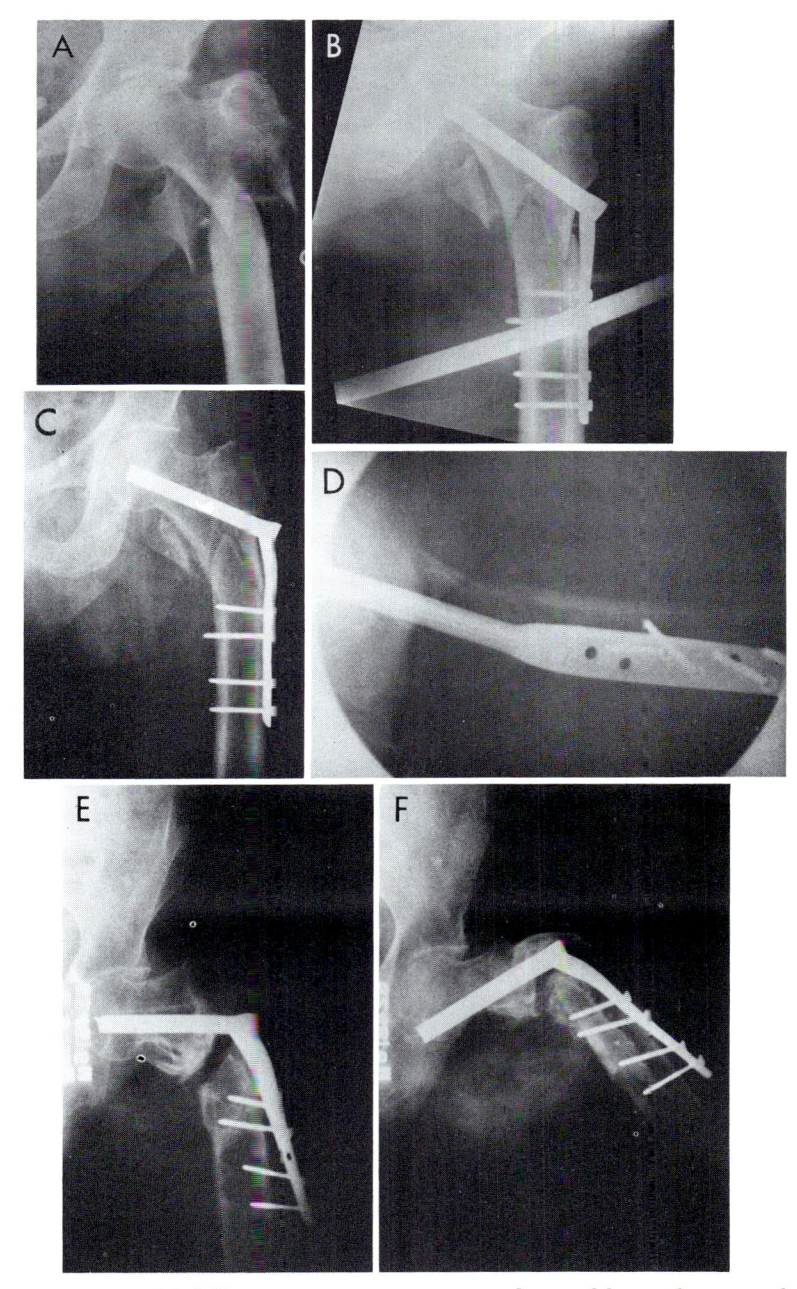

Fig. 26-34.—**A,** woman, 77, fell, sustaining a comminuted unstable trochanteric fracture of the left hip. **B,** an almost anatomic relationship of all but the lesser trochanteric fragment was achieved at time of internal fixation. **C** and **D,** 1 year later the fracture has assumed a varus alignment and the fixation device has started to bend. **E** and **F,** 3 years after operation, there is a nonunion; the screws have loosened and the side plate has pulled away from the femoral shaft. The fixation device could not compensate for the instability secondary to the displaced lesser trochanter.

reinforcement with a Parham band may be indicated. On occasion a Küntscher nail or Zickel nail is used for subtrochanteric fractures (Fig. 26-35).

The patient is placed on a regular operating table with a cassette tunnel under the hips. It is important to have the affected hip well over to the side of the table, since occasionally it may be necessary to nail the fracture with the leg in some degree of external rotation. This is an almost impossible task if the leg is toward the center of the table. A fracture table may be used.

The incision is made laterally from the tip of the trochanter distally for a distance of 8–10 in. The dissection is carried down to the fascia lata, which is split about 1 in. anterior to the linea aspera. The vastus lateralis muscle is split by blunt and sharp dissection also about 1 in. anterior to the linea aspera. Anterior reflection of the vastus lateralis is facilitated by curving the incision forward into the tendinous attachment of the muscle to the greater trochanter. Subperiosteal reflection is then done, and the muscle held forward by a Bennett retractor. The fascial attachment along the linea aspera is split by a knife sufficiently to allow the tongue of a Bennett retractor to be inserted through it and behind the upper shaft. It is helpful to locate this split at the level of anticipated entrance of the nail.

Adequate reflection of the upper reaches of the vastus lateralis and intermedius muscles will usually expose the fracture site anteriorly. Palpation of the fracture will disclose the situation to be remedied. Generally the fracture to be dealt with is one in which the distal fragment is externally rotated and the trochanter shows some degree of comminution. Not infrequently, the posterior portion of the greater trochanter may be split vertically and rotated externally and posteriorly as a free fragment. Reduction is obtained by traction on the leg in a slightly flexed position plus gentle internal rotation.

A word of caution about the use of rotation. In an unimpacted extracapsular fracture, the shaft of the femur rotates about

Fig. 26-35.—Transverse subtrochanteric fracture in Paget's disease. **A,** anteroposterior view showing varus deformity of proximal fragment. **B,** lateral view showing anterior angulation of proximal fragment at fracture site. **C,** fixation of fracture by a Küntscher nail with solid union. Note varus position of the head.

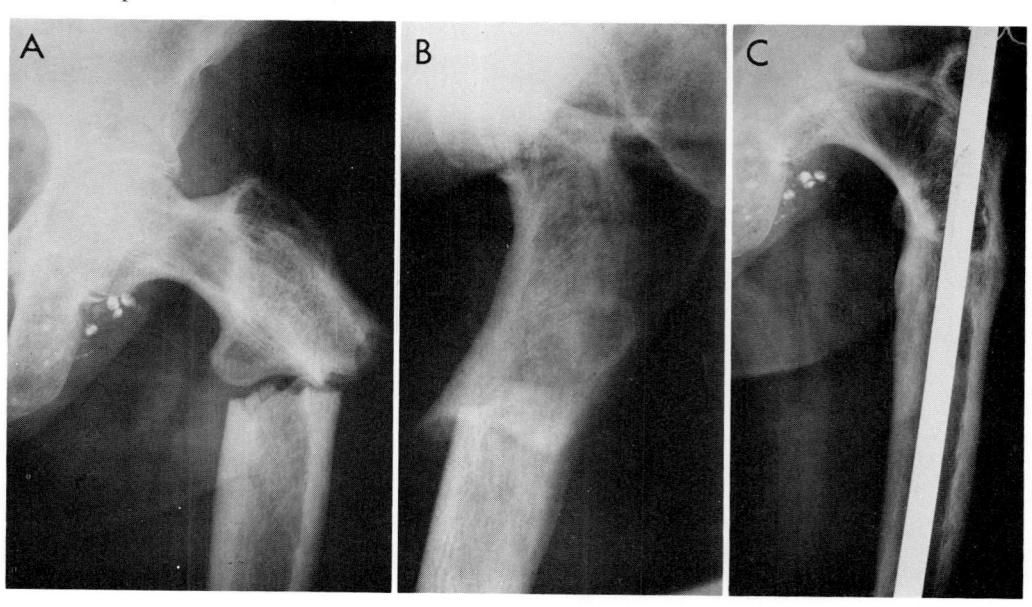

Chapter 26: FRACTURES OF THE HIP: HEAD, NECK AND TROCHANTER / 661

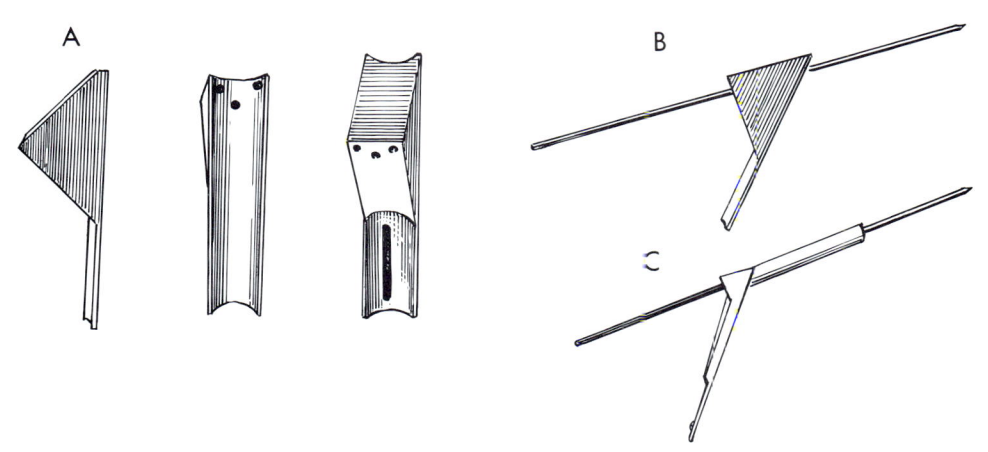

Fig. 26-36.—Jig for Jewett nail. **A**, three views of jig. Three holes are drilled in the jig to form an angle of 130 degrees, corresponding to the angle between the nail and plate elements of the Jewett nail. **B**, guide wire inserted through hole in jig. **C**, jig removed and Jewett nail placed over guide wire.

its own axis, whereas in the impacted extracapsular fracture and in the femoral neck fracture the shaft rotates on an arc with the center in the neck or head. The greater trochanter can be felt describing such an arc. The exception to this situation is the occasional intertrochanteric fracture in which the soft tissues overlying the fracture posteriorly remain intact and act as a hinge guiding the reduction and preventing overreduction. As in femoral neck fractures, internal rotation of the shaft will close the fracture line. Since in the comminuted extracapsular fractures the shaft revolves around its own long axis on rotation, the surgeon must be alert to the possibility of closing the fracture line in front and at the same time opening it too much posteriorly. This overreduction is prevented by placing the fingers of 1 hand behind the greater trochanter while rotation is performed. The optimal position of rotation is determined; then, to secure reduction, an assistant applies traction with slight flexion or abduction, or both.

If obtaining good reduction has required that the hip be markedly externally rotated, nailing may appear difficult or impossible. This situation can be met by placing 1 hand behind the greater trochanter and lifting the trochanteric block forward. By this maneuver, the guide wire can be passed into the neck in a

Fig. 26-37.—Anteroposterior and lateral views of head and neck of femur show jig in place with guide wire. Jig is placed on lateral aspect of femur with center hole at the point of election, usually 1¼ in. below the vastus externus line. Pilot hole is made in bone at this point. Jig is placed over the hole and a guide wire passed into the head. A Jewett nail can then be driven over the wire and its plate will fit flush against the femoral shaft. The lateral view shows holes posterior and anterior to the center to allow for change of wire in lateral plane.

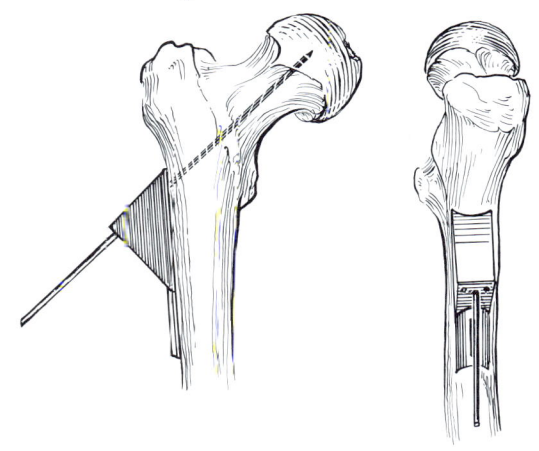

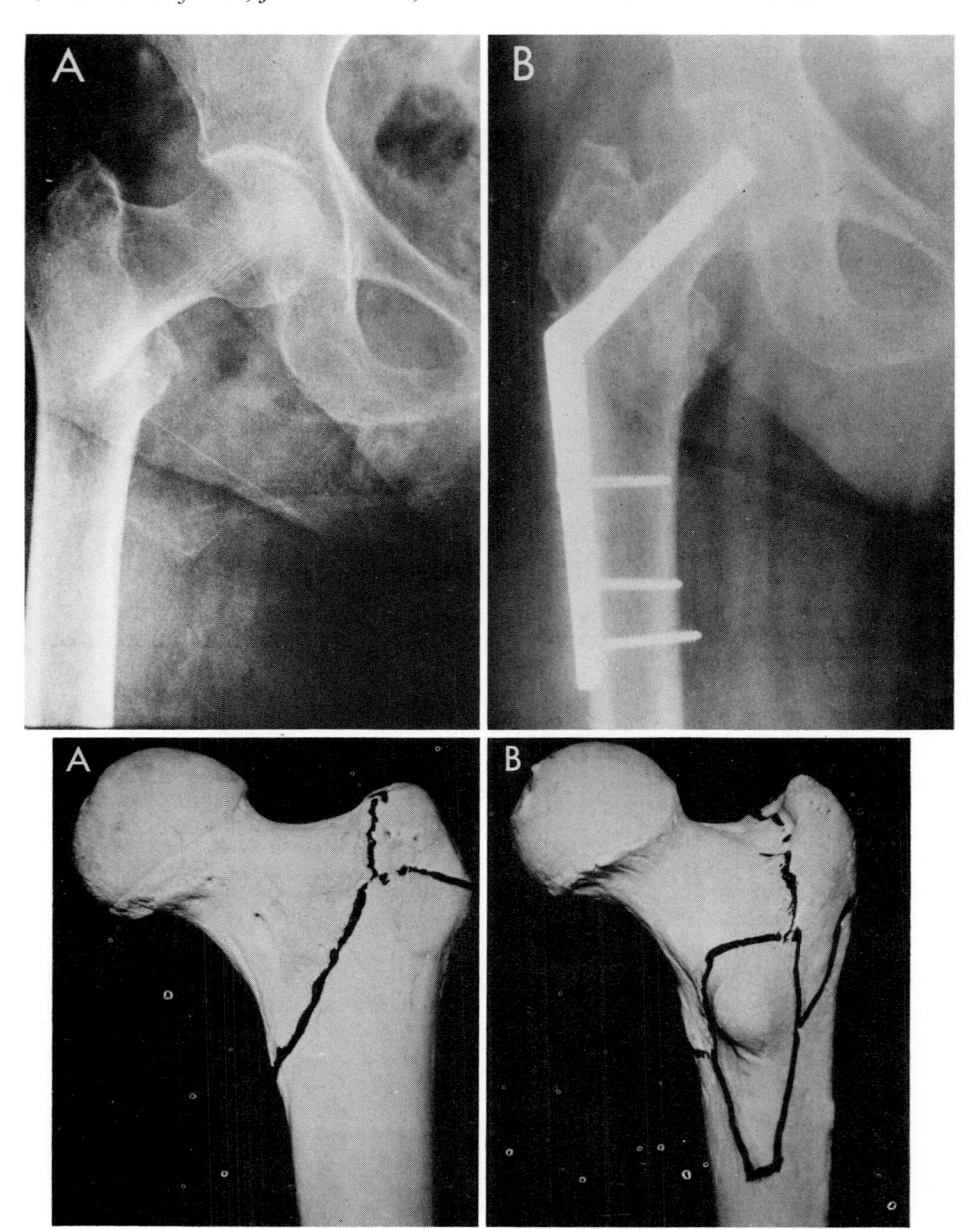

Fig. 26-38 (top).—Stable trochanteric fracture. **A,** initial radiograph in woman, 64; comminution of lesser trochanter is minimal in extent and degree. **B,** internal fixation after anatomic reduction almost uniformly leads to a satisfactory result. Protection until there is radiographic evidence of solid union is necessary unless specifically designed nails of extra strength are employed.

Fig. 26-39 (bottom).—Anatomy of a representative, 4-part, comminuted trochanteric fracture. The tracing was made on a dry specimen from original radiographs. **A,** from anterior view, the fracture lines do not reveal the major potential source of instability after nailing. **B,** viewed from behind, the strategic location of the lesser trochanter becomes more apparent and, if it becomes displaced due to injury, the loss of its function as a posteromedial buttress can be appreciated.

Chapter 26: FRACTURES OF THE HIP: HEAD, NECK AND TROCHANTER / 663

more horizontal plane. A pilot hole is drilled into the cortex of the shaft about 1¼–1½ in. below the vastus externus line. With the fracture reduced and held secure, if a Jewett nail plate is to be used, then a jig is placed against the femoral shaft and a ³⁄₃₂ in. guide wire is passed through 1 of the holes in the jig up into the femoral neck (Figs. 26-36 and 26-37). The wire may be drilled or tapped in by hand. If the wire is well centered, it may be pushed in by hand for 3–3½ in. without meeting appreciable resistance.

The holes in the jig are fixed at such an angle that the wire passed through 1 of the holes will form an angle with the shaft equal to that of the Jewett nail plate (130 degrees). The position and depth of the wire should be checked by anteroposterior and lateral x-rays. If the position of the wire is satisfactory, a second wire of the same length is placed against the first, with the tip of the second wire touching the edge of the pilot hole. The length of the second wire projecting laterally beyond the end of the first wire represents the length of wire in bone and is an accurate measure of the length of the nail to be used.

The length of the nail should be so calculated that the nail will project at least a full ¼ in. beyond the head-neck junction into the head itself. To allow it to terminate in the neck, in the area known as Ward's triangle, is to court disaster, for the trabeculae are sparse and offer poor support and poor grip and the nail will easily cut out of the bone superiorly. Adequate intrusion of the nail into the head for this distance will allow for secure fixation and will prevent the complication of overpenetration.

The nail plate is next driven home so that the plate section lies flush against the femoral shaft, to which it is then secured by screws. The plate section may vary in length from 3 to 6 in., depending on the extent of the fracture into the subtrochanteric region. When driving in a Jewett nail plate, the surgeon should watch for the tendency of the blade to rotate anteriorly.

Technique varies in the preparation of the cortex for nailing. Some surgeons pre-

Fig. 26-40.—Management of the unstable trochanteric fracture. **A**, most unstable trochanteric fractures consist of 4 parts: *1*, head-neck fragment; *2*, lesser trochanteric fragment of varying size posteromedially; *3*, greater trochanteric fragment posteriorly, and *4*, shaft fragment. **B**, osteotomy of the lateral fragment of the greater trochanter has been carried out and a nail with a fixed-angle side plate has been driven into the neck under direct vision. The nail should enter in the central axis of the neck and penetrate at least ¼ in. into the head of the femur. **C**, when the inferior neck spike has been inserted into the open upper end of the femoral shaft and the side plate brought against the lateral aspect of the shaft, a normal neck-shaft angle results. The fragment of the greater trochanter *(4)* released during the approach is sutured by means of its attached soft tissues back in position.

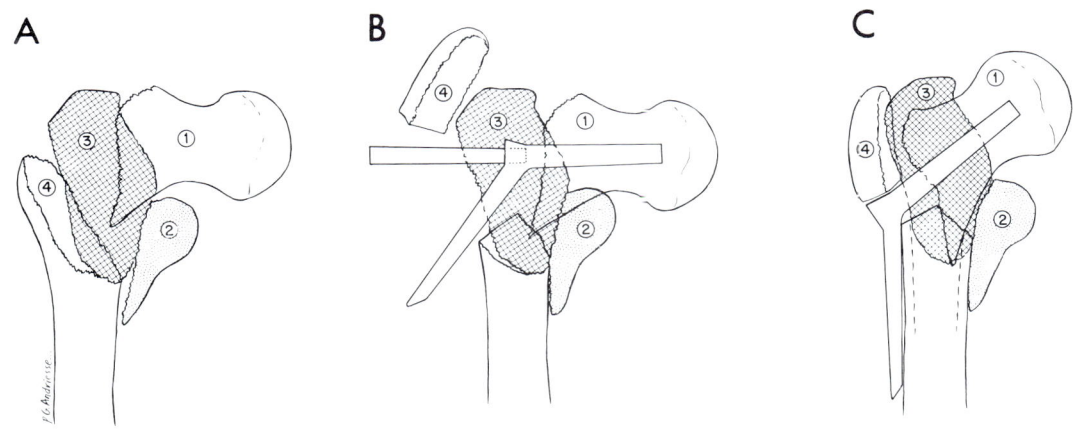

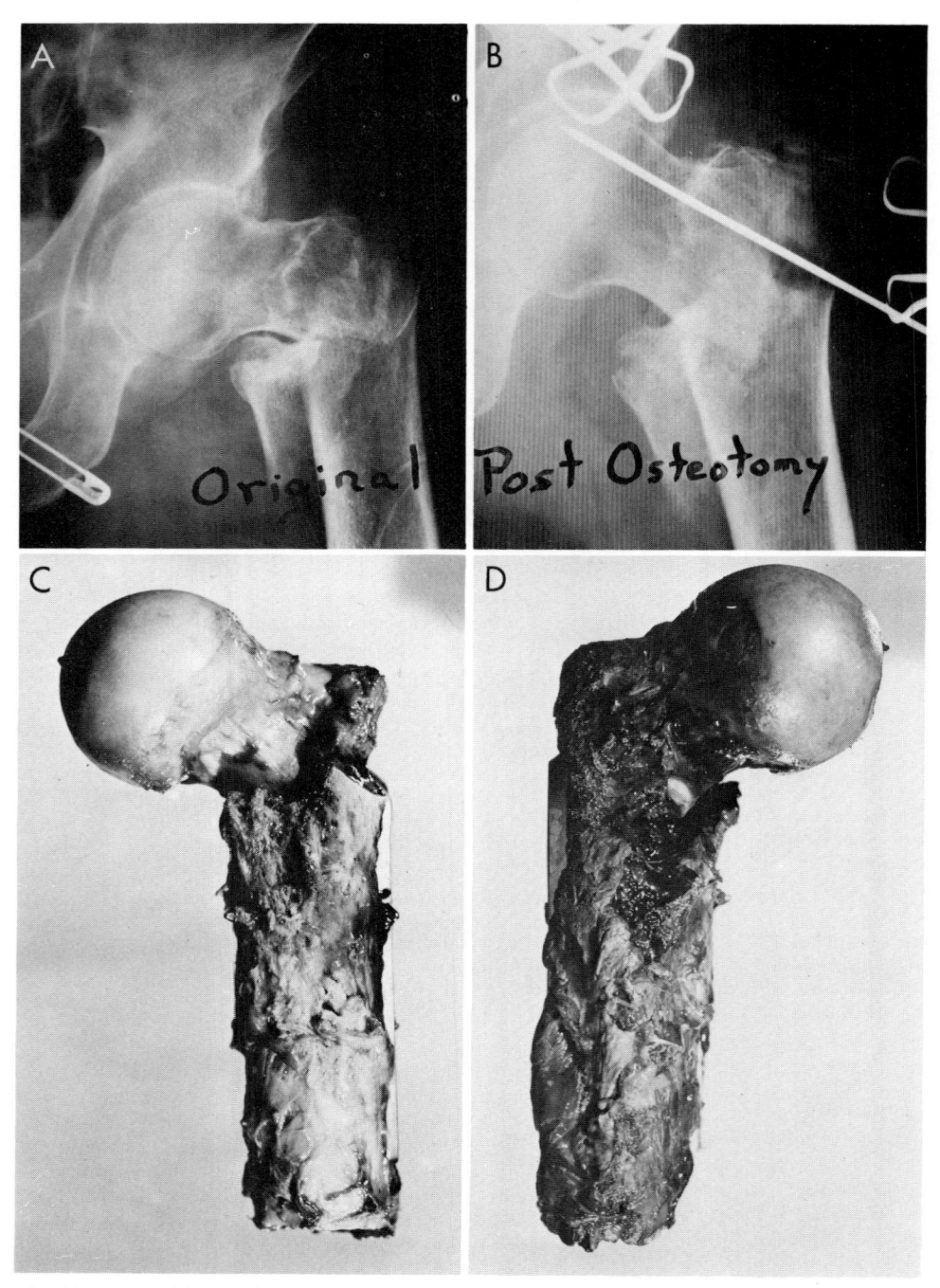

Fig. 26-41.—Unstable trochanteric fracture in a 73-year-old man with severe heart disease. **A,** original radiograph shows marked angulation and rotation of major fragments and a large subtrochanteric element. **B,** operative reduction after osteotomy of the anterolateral portion of greater trochanter. Patient died 1 week after operation. **C,** frontal view of specimen shows good contact between the head-neck fragment and upper shaft. **D,** posteromedial view shows the large defect left when the lesser trochanter is absent.

Chapter 26: FRACTURES OF THE HIP: HEAD, NECK AND TROCHANTER / 665

fer to ream out a hole, whereas others cut slots for the blades of the nail.

Fixation of the apparatus to the shaft is mandatory in all except the simplest undisplaced extracapsular fractures, in which a nail alone may occasionally be used with success.

Extensive stripping of the muscles should be avoided. It is preferable to accept a less perfect reduction than to deprive multiple fragments of their blood supply.

The avulsed lesser trochanter should be fixed if it can be reached without extensive dissection. The displaced lesser trochanter heals with abundant callus.

Check-up films are taken before closing the wound (Fig. 26-38).

When the lesser trochanteric fragment is large (Fig. 26-39) or when there is a medial cortical defect in the neck secondary to metastatic disease and a stable relationship between the fracture fragments cannot be achieved, management of the fracture is effectively accomplished by the technique of displacement fixation.[24, 39] With this method, the inferior neck spike, almost uniformly present on the proximal fragment, is levered into the open upper end of the shaft fragment after it is secured by a 3-flanged nail 2–3 in. in length (Fig. 26-40). Care must be taken, however, as the major fragments are approximated, to avoid rotational deformity.

Although ½ in. or more of shortening results from this technique, stability and good bone contact are immediately obtained (Fig. 26-41). The Jewett nail, the McLaughlin nail and the sliding nail or screw are all equally suitable as fixation devices, but an adequate selection of short sizes must be available (Figs. 26-42 to 26-44).

Sarmiento and Williams[54] have approached these problem cases effectively but in a different fashion. Their technique consists in creating a valgus relationship between the major fragments by use of a laterally based wedge osteotomy followed by fixation using a 135-degree I-beam nail plate.

Fig. 26-42.—Severely comminuted trochanteric fracture with large lesser trochanteric fragment in a 68-year-old woman. **A,** original radiograph reveals 4 separate fragments severely displaced. **B,** 4 months after displacement fixation, there is abundant callus and sound union.

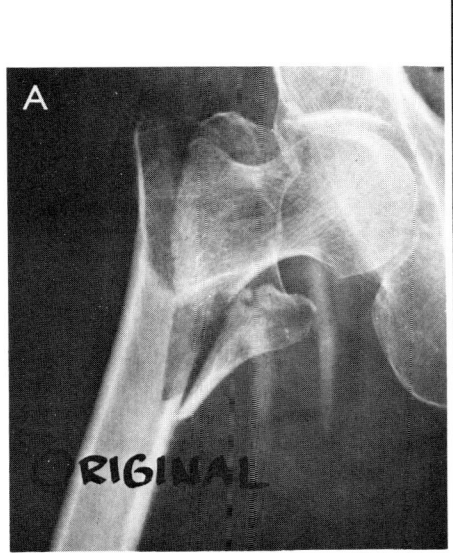

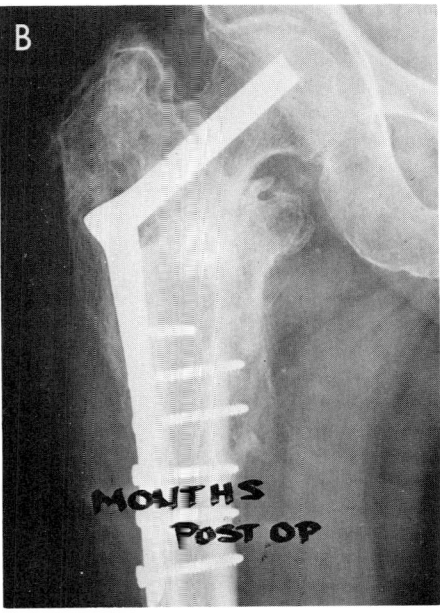

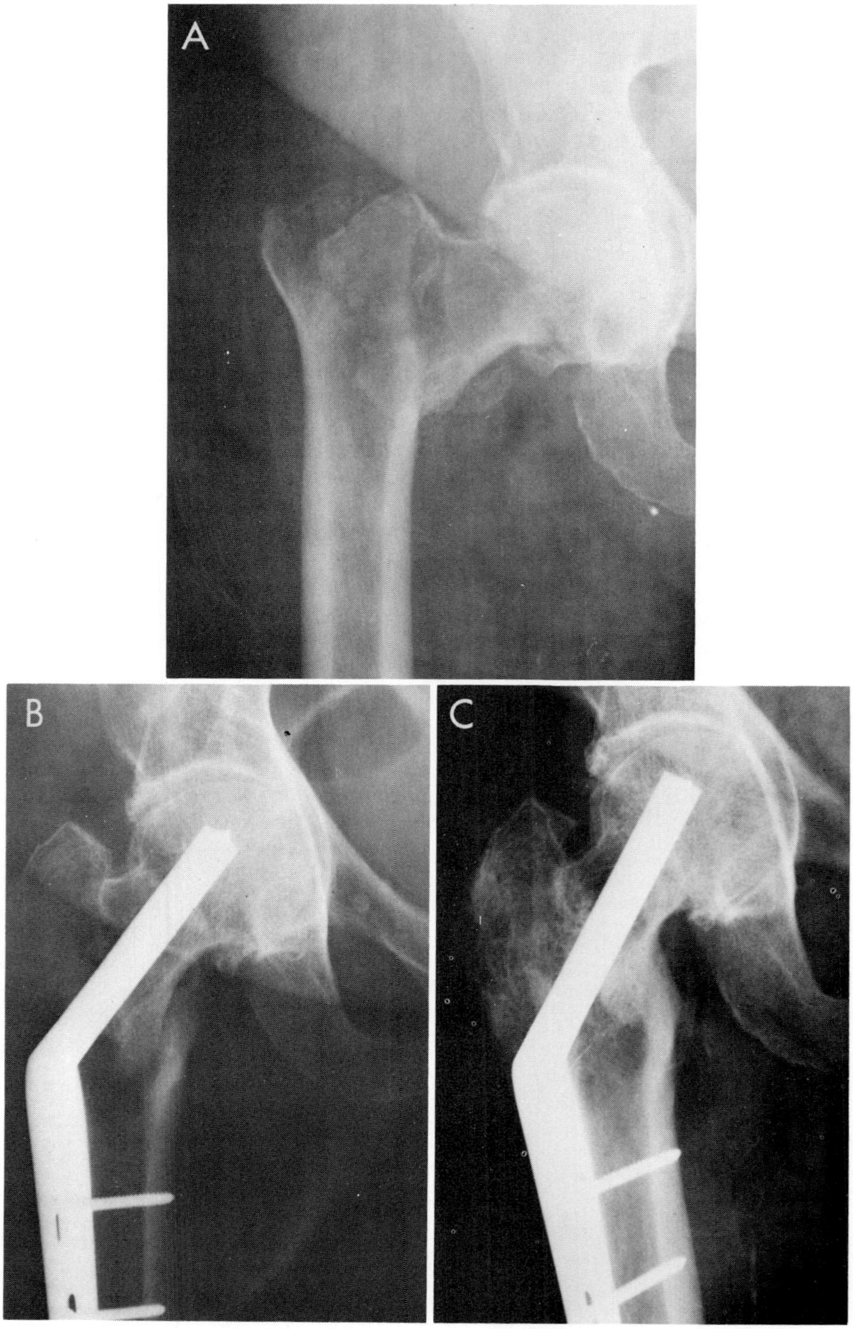

Fig. 26-43.—Comminuted, unstable trochanteric fracture in woman, 73. **A,** original fracture showing 4 major fragments. **B,** 1 month postoperatively, inferior neck spike is well seen within the upper end of the femoral shaft. **C,** at 6 months, there is solid union.

Chapter 26: FRACTURES OF THE HIP: HEAD, NECK AND TROCHANTER / 667

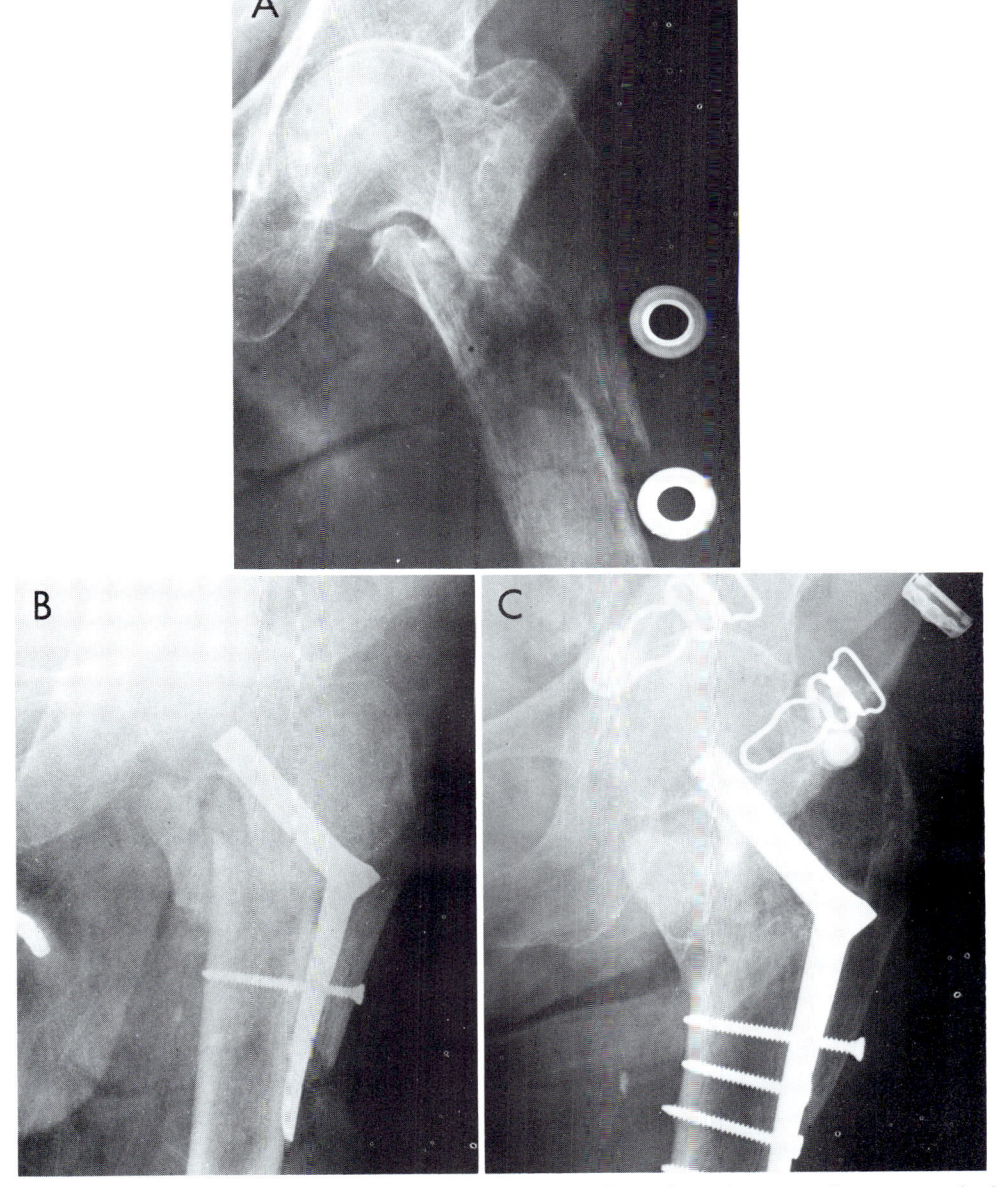

Fig. 26-44.—Unstable combination of a trochanteric and a subtrochanteric fracture with the obliquity of the fracture line the reverse of the usual. **A**, original radiograph in woman, 66. **B**, displacement fixation after osteotomy of the lateral spike. **C**, 18 months later, union and advanced remolding.

AFTER-TREATMENT.—The leg is bandaged, from toes to waist, with a pressure pad on the gluteal bursa region. One or more blood transfusions should be given, if indicated. Then the patient is returned to bed and placed in Russell traction with 2 lb of weight (4 lb of pull).

Postoperative Management

After operation the patient should be protected in Russell traction or in balanced suspension. It may be important for the general well-being of aged and infirm patients to transfer them to a chair the first or second day after operation. For the patient who is able to cooperate with a program of deep-breathing exercises and coughing as well as do exercises for the knee and hip on the affected side and for the upper extremities, trunk and normal leg, bed rest in traction for 2 – 3 weeks will allow soft tissue healing and return of muscle function. The patient will then be a better candidate for protected weight bearing in a walker or on crutches. Crutches are employed for 4 – 6 months or longer if healing is not adequate on x-ray study.

Holt,[32] by contrast, in his initial report on 100 cases of trochanteric fracture treated with his extra heavy nail, advocated the use of a walker at the end of 1 week and graduation to full weight bearing as soon as tolerated. In 80 survivors, all fractures united although in 7 cases 1 or more complications led to a poor result. There were no instances of bending or breaking of the nail. At the most, the nail advanced a few millimeters occasionally. Our experience with this approach has been similar with the stable trochanteric fractures, but we have seen progressive varus of the fragments and penetration of the device in the unstable group. Mulholland and Gunn[44] advocate a similar progression to tolerated weight bearing with the compression screw. They report settling of fractures but no failures to unite. Our experience with these sliding screws is still too limited to report, but to date results have been excellent, and there has been a reduced incidence of penetration or cutting out of the device (Fig. 26-45).

Complications

COMPLICATIONS DUE TO STRUCTURAL FAILURES.—Before use of the Jewett nail plate, most structural failures were due to the separation of nail-plate combinations. The bolts loosened; occasionally a bolt broke; and on rare occasions a plate fractured at the gooseneck, where it had been reshaped repeatedly to fit onto the nail.

Loosening of the bolts was due to several factors: (1) tightening the bolts with a screwdriver instead of a wrench; (2) variations in the depth of the well in the nail heads; (3) too short bolts.

Structural failures with the Jewett nail have been rare but on occasion nails have broken, plates have broken and screws have pulled out, particularly when the bony contribution to stability after nailing was poor (Fig. 26-46).

COMPLICATIONS DUE TO ERRORS IN TECHNIQUE.—The following observed errors in technique have been responsible for complicating the healing of some of these fractures.

1. Improper preparation of the nail bed in the cortex. Such an error may cause fracture of the femoral shaft at the point of nailing because the milled portion of the butt of the nail acts as a wedge to split the bone.

2. Overpenetration of the nail. The end of the nail should reach only $1/4 - 1/2$ in. beyond the head-neck junction.

3. Breaking of screws. The breaking of a screw may result from fixing the plate to the shaft under tension, a situation commonly produced by driving in the nail and then abducting the femoral shaft to fit against the plate. Unless the fracture is free, the screws will be under tension and may break.

4. Cutting out of the nail. This can

Chapter 26: FRACTURES OF THE HIP: HEAD, NECK AND TROCHANTER / 669

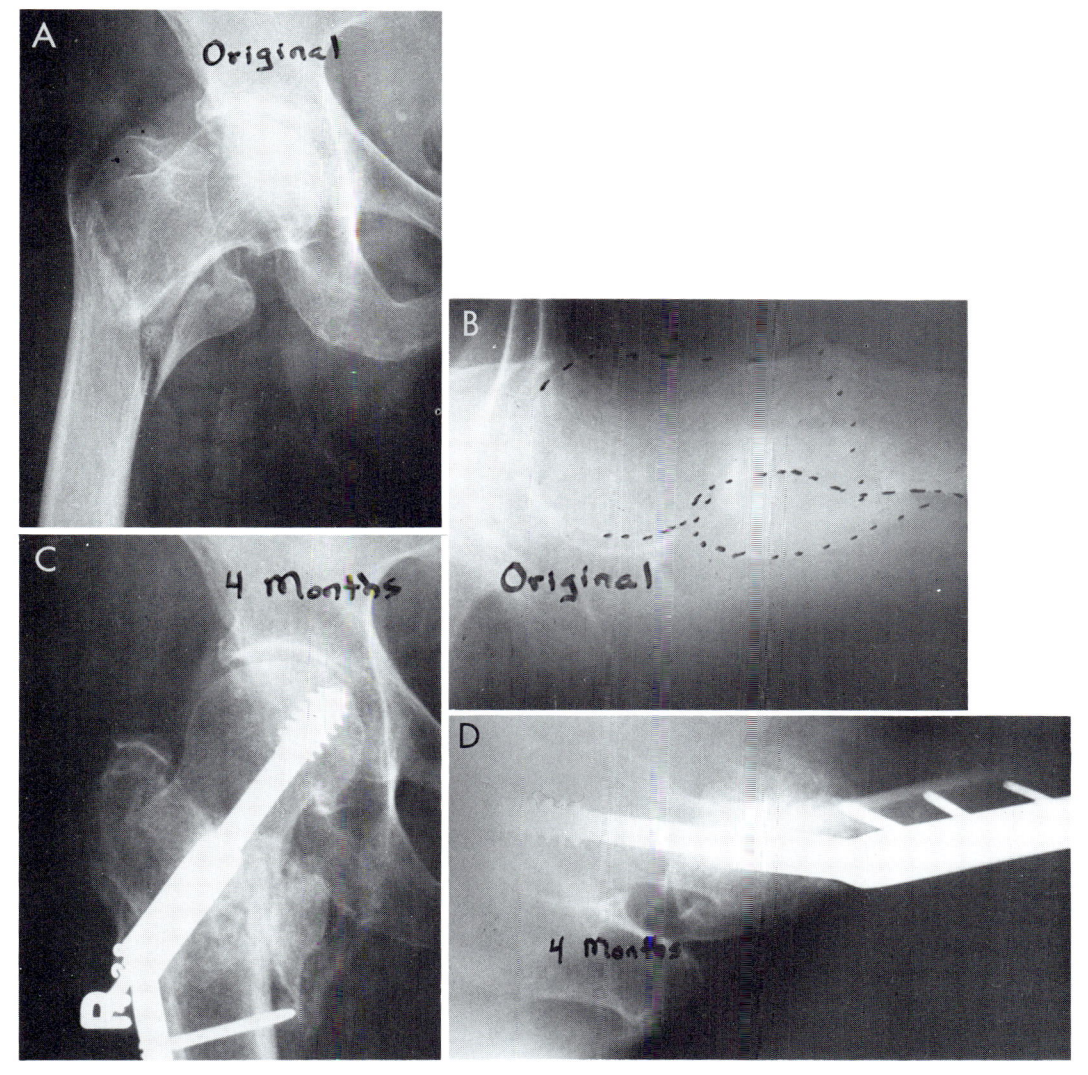

Fig. 26-45.—**A** and **B**, 4-part comminuted unstable trochanteric fracture in woman, 73. Note the large lesser trochanteric fragment that is displaced. **C** and **D**, 4 months after anatomic reduction of head-neck fragment and shaft fragment and internal fixation with a sliding screw. There has been approximately ½ in. of settling. There is advanced callus formation. To date, this technique appears to offer a viable alternative in the treatment armamentarium to the displacement method.

happen in osteoporotic bone with early weight bearing and should be considered as a possibility if the nail is off center superiorly in the lateral view, penetrates too short a distance into the femoral head, or lacks reaching it entirely (Fig. 26-47).
5. Broken drill points.
6. Inadequate fixation.
7. Loosening of bolts.

NONUNION OF TROCHANTERIC FRACTURES.—Although only 1–2% of trochanteric fractures fail to unite, those that fail may present a challenging thera-

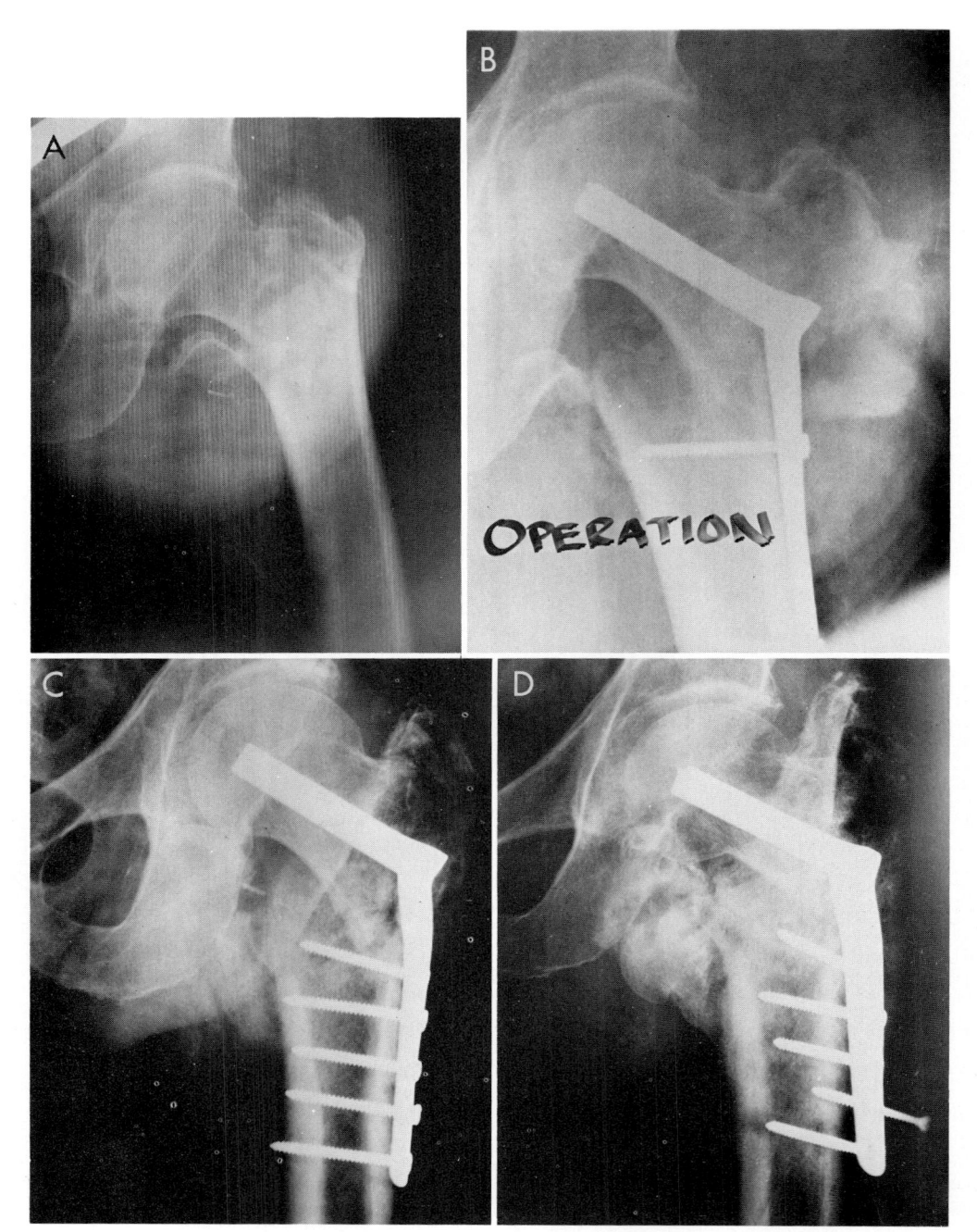

Fig. 26-46.—Unstable trochanteric fracture. **A,** original radiograph in 67-year-old woman with comminuted trochanteric fracture. **B,** in operating room, film shows good alignment of fracture and placement of nail, but the proximal fragment lies laterally more than half the width of the open end of the shaft. There appears to be little contact medially. **C,** 6 weeks later there is bending of the nail and varus angulation of the fracture. **D,** 6 months later the side plate has pulled away from the shaft and there is further varus angulation. The fracture healed. The achievement of good medial support is essential to the success of the procedure.

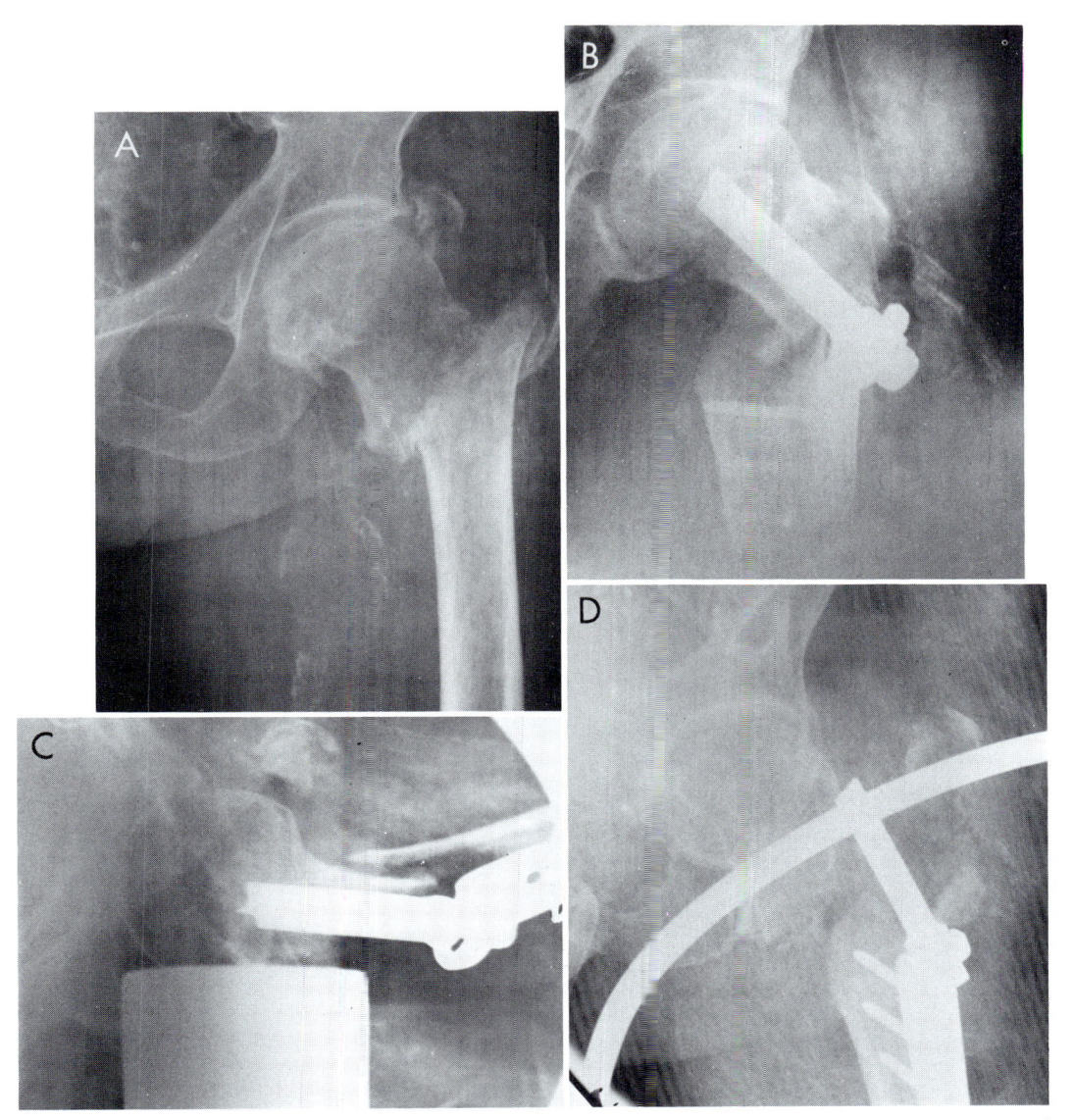

Fig. 26-47.—Failed displacement fixation. **A,** unstable trochanteric fracture in man, 73. **B** and **C,** radiographs at conclusion of operation suggest poor bony contact between the head-neck fragment and shaft fragment in both the anteroposterior and lateral projections. The nail barely penetrates the femoral head. **D,** 2 days later the nail has cut out and fracture fragments are again separated. Successful displacement fixation depends on achievement of good bony contact medially, good fixation laterally and adequate penetration of the nail into the femoral head. There is too little trabecular bone within the neck for satisfactory purchase by a nail.

peutic problem (Figs. 26-48 and 26-49). Recent experience with 8 such fractures revealed that by the time the patient came to reoperation, the nail was loose in the neck, the device frequently had broken, pulled out of the shaft or penetrated the head.

The Holt nail, a ½-in.-diameter Vitallium bar with attached side plate, has consistently been the answer to

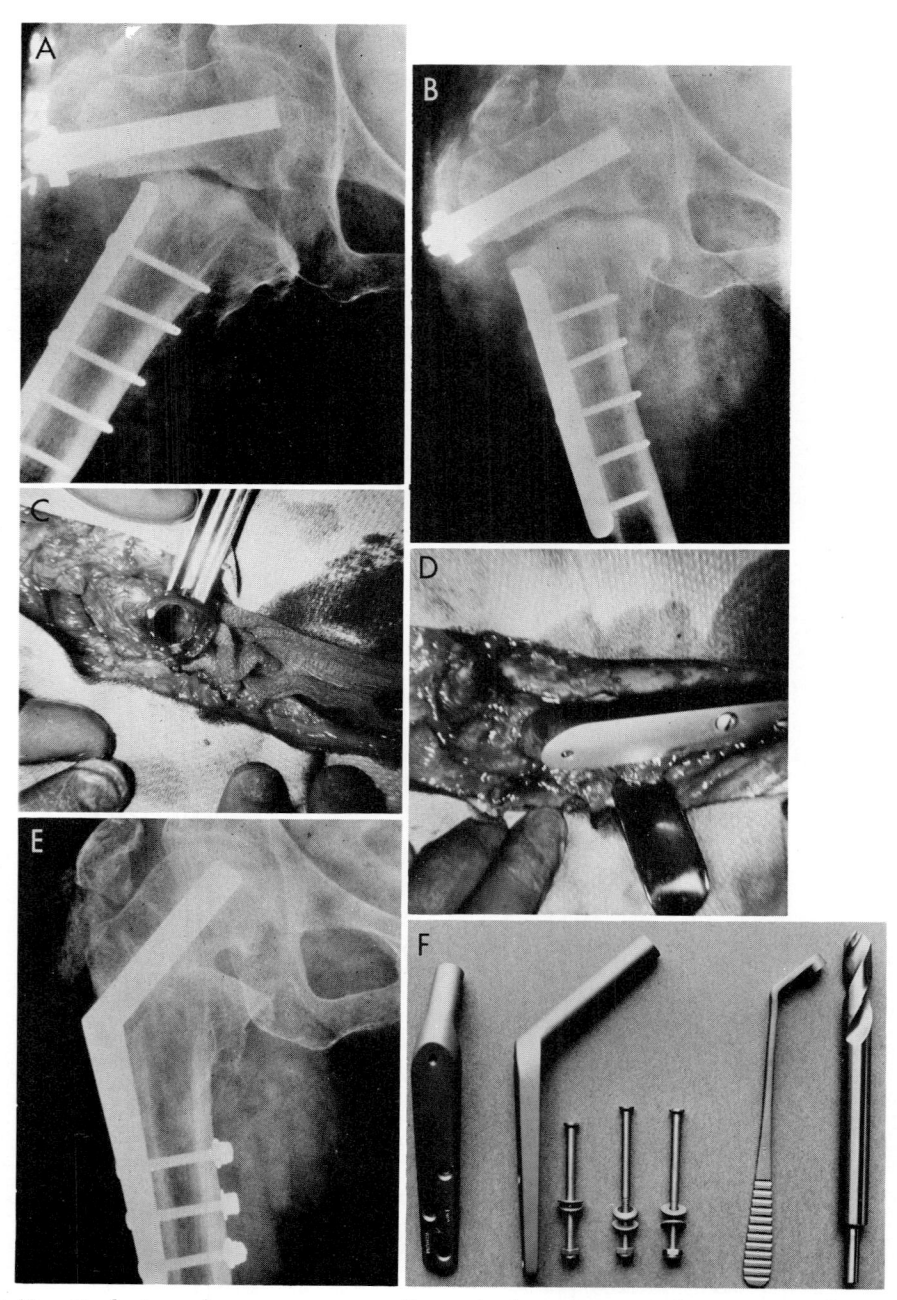

Fig. 26-48.—Technique for management of ununited trochanteric fracture. **A** and **B**, ununited trochanteric fracture in 79-year-old woman 3 years after injury. **C**, at time of reoperation the flanged nail was found to be loose in the neck and the tract in which it lay was nearly cylindrical. **D**, Holt nail, after a single pass of the ½-in. diameter drill point, fitted snugly. Freshening of the undersurface of the neck and upper shaft was followed by displacement medially of the shaft, autogenous iliac grafting and fixation of the side plate to the femoral shaft with Barr bolts. **E**, 6 months later fracture was solidly united. **F**, Equipment necessary for Holt nailing. Nails cut from 1¾ in. to 3 in. long in ¼-in. increments should be available.

Chapter 26: FRACTURES OF THE HIP: HEAD, NECK AND TROCHANTER / 673

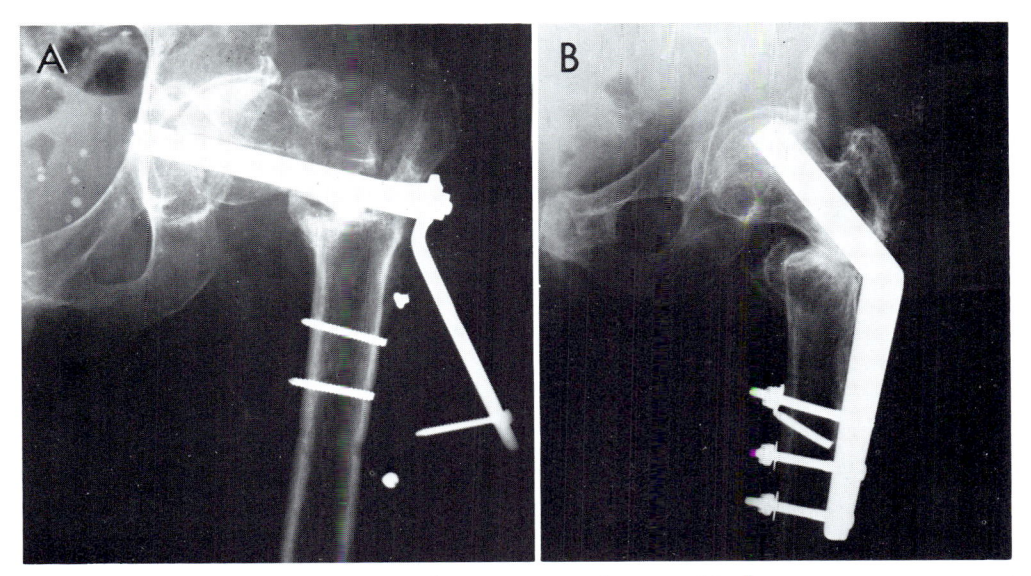

Fig. 26-49. — Nonunion of trochanteric fracture. **A,** in this unstable fracture, varus, penetration of the head by the nail and nonunion developed. **B,** union was obtained by open reduction, tailoring of the fracture surfaces, autogenous iliac bone grafting and insertion of a Holt nail along the old nail track. A shorter nail would have been preferable, although the one selected produced no symptoms.

securing the proximal fragment and allowing a new and stable relationship to be established between the major proximal and distal fragments. Some tailoring of the apposing bony surfaces is often required, and supplementary grafts of autogenous iliac bone should be added.

Union of all fractures treated by this technique was obtained.

In an elderly patient who cannot be expected to manage crutches successfully during convalescence, total hip replacement offers another alternative and has proved satisfactory.

CLINICAL COMPLICATIONS IN FRACTURES OF THE HIP

The common clinical complications are thrombophlebitis and embolism, vascular accidents, diabetes, cardiac failure and occasionally sepsis.

Smith, Dexter and Dammin[60] in autopsy studies at Peter Bent Brigham Hospital found pulmonary embolism to be the single most common cause of death. Almost all authors writing on the subject of fractures about the hip list embolism as a cause of death and embolism or thrombophlebitis as a complication. Thomas, in a recent review of the treatment of pulmonary embolic disease, states that venous ligation alone, whether at the level of the superficial femoral vein or the vena cava, does not prevent formation of further thrombi or emboli. He suggests that at least 2 pathogenic events are concerned in the formation of these thrombi — primarily local stasis and systemic altered coagulability of the blood. Thus, successful management of this condition and prevention of complications necessitate control of both factors. Numerous animal experiments and controlled studies in human beings are cited to show that both heparin and phenindione can be used effectively to this end. In a controlled study, Sevitt and Gallagher[58] demonstrated that prophylactic anticoagulant therapy could virtually abolish thromboembolic complications in elderly patients with fracture of the neck of the femur. Solonen,[63] using phenylindanedione between the second and fifth postoperative days, reduced the incidence of thromboembolic disease in patients with fractures of the lower extremity from 16% in the control to zero in the treated group. Pulmonary embolism occurred in 8% of the control and in 1% of the treated group. Salzman, Harris and DeSanctis[53] divided 187 patients into control and treated groups; there were 8 cases of emboli with 4 deaths in the control group, with no pulmonary embolism in the treated group.

Complications with anticoagulant therapy may occur. With the use of warfarin (Coumadin) derivatives, the prothrombin time should be maintained between 20 and 30% or 1½–2 times the control, and followed daily. The hematocrit should be checked twice a week and the urine and stools examined frequently for gross or occult blood, the anticoagulants being discontinued if adverse effects are evident. For patients in whom the drug is contraindicated, venous ligation at the appropriate level is the treatment of choice when evidence of thrombophlebitis or embolic disease appears. In the series of Salzman and associates, anticoagulant therapy has been discontinued at the time the patients become ambulatory. The drug is withdrawn without tapering of the dose. No rebound effect has been noted.

The routine followed at Massachusetts General and Peter Bent Brigham hospitals is an intramuscular injection of 10–15 mg warfarin on night following surgery, no warfarin the following day and then oral warfarin in a dosage scheduled directed at maintaining the prothrombin time between 20 and 30% of normal or 1½ times the control level. Preoperative prothrombin times are always obtained. No patient receives the medication who has a known blood dyscrasia or increased susceptibility to bleeding. When the dosage level is properly controlled, complications have been at a minimum.

Low molecular weight dextran and low dose heparin and aspirin are also used with satisfactory results, but the data on aspirin are still sparse and dextran, like warfarin, is not without hazards. Heparin has been both effective and free from problems to date. The choice of agent belongs to the surgeon, but there seems little justification for omitting use of some form of prophylaxis for every patient in whom there exists no specific contraindication to its use.

Vascular accidents, though common in the aged, have not increased in frequency in our experience with the routine use of anticoagulation.

Diabetes should be looked for and brought under control before surgery. In 1 recent year, 3 cases of major sepsis occurred in patients with severe diabetes.

Cardiac failure is listed as a frequent complication—often a final complication, in both operated and nonoperated cases. In the aged patient with whom we are so frequently concerned it may be unavoidable.

Each case of extracapsular fracture is a problem in itself, and statistics are valuable only in that they indicate trends. Over the years there has been a gradual decrease in mortality. At present, the mortality rate averages about 8% during the period of hospitalization and about 15% by 3 months after fracture.

The management of sepsis around a nailed hip can be 1 of the most difficult problems in orthopedic surgery and may require months of hospitalization and multiple operative procedures. If the infection is deep enough to involve bone or the hip joint itself, nothing short of complete removal of the fixation, of all devitalized bone and of scar can be totally effective. A Girdlestone procedure, Colonna-type reconstruction with or without a Vitallium mold followed by a prolonged period in a spica cast and a sustained antibiotic program has, in our hands, given the greatest measure of success.

Far more satisfactory is prevention, and here nothing exceeds in importance the gentle and careful handling of soft tissues locally and the restoration and maintenance of the patient in as good general health as possible.

Much attention has been given in recent years to the issue of prophylactic antibiotics. It is the practice of most members of this clinic to use them in all major surgery in and around the hip joint. To be effective, the antibiotic must be started prior to or during the surgery, given intravenously and be bactericidal rather than bacteriostatic. Reports in the literature as to the usefulness of this prophylaxis have at times been confusing and pessimistic, but at least part of this arises from the practice of some surgeons to use bacteriostatic agents given orally and starting as much as 24 hours after operation. This constitutes treatment and, in many instances, inadequate treatment.

Burke[11] has shown experimentally in the laboratory that systemic antibiotics, if they are to be used for the prevention of infection, must be given either shortly before, during or within 1 hour after contamination of a wound to have any significant effect. Antibiotics given after that time may modify, control or cure an existing infection, but they do not prevent it. Similar studies by Glotzer et al.[30] using topical antibiotics confirm the importance of timing and the need to employ bactericidal agents.

More recently a prospective study by Boyd et al.[7a] in patients with hip fractures treated at Massachusetts General Hospital and a retrospective study by Scales[55] at Royal National Orthopaedic and Queen Elizabeth II hospitals have shown a significant reduction in the incidence of infection in patients treated with prophylactic antibiotics compared to those who were not. More studies of this nature, however, continue to be needed.

PATHOLOGIC FRACTURES

Pathologic fractures of the hip occur secondary to metabolic disease, metastatic cancer, primary tumors within bone and pelvic irradiation. In a patient in the third or fourth decade of life, the presence of an intracapsular fracture of itself should raise the question of pathologic origin.

Local treatment of the postradiation fracture without displacement consists of bed rest, traction or crutches or occasionally, to quote Bickel et al.,[5] of "skillful neglect." Displaced fractures in this group will need reduction and internal fixation.

For fractures secondary to metastatic disease, the treatment must in each instance be individualized and a variety of forms may be required in any series of such patients. All therapy will be directed toward producing maximal comfort for the patient during his remaining life span and at the same time enabling him to be transported as necessary for appropriate treatment of the tumor.

Methods may include simple wire traction, nail and plate fixation, Knowles pins, prosthetic replacement of the head-neck and, more recently, internal fixation supplemented by polymethyl methacrylate insertion to fill large bone defects and obtain stability (Fig. 26-50). On occasion, total hip replacement will be appropriate when bone loss on 1 side or the other of the joint has been excessive. It is well to bear in mind that considerable bleeding may be encountered in open operations on pathologic fractures arising from metastatic disease, particularly those of renal origin.

HIP FRACTURES IN CHILDREN

Fractures of the hip in children are unique because the forces required, relative to the size of the patient, are much greater than those causing the average adult fracture. The incidence of fracture

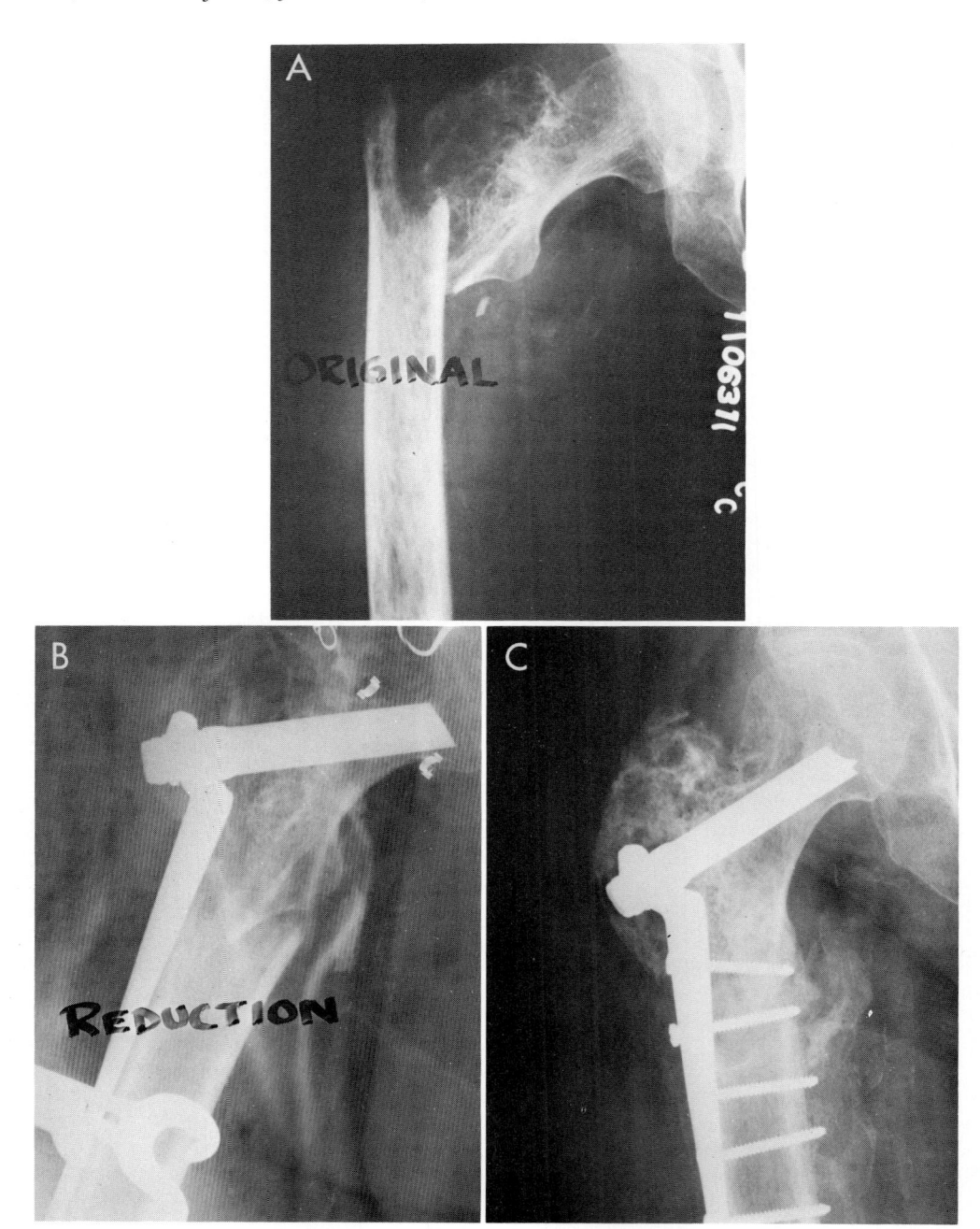

Fig. 26-50.—Pathologic fracture of the subtrochanteric areas secondary to a metastatic carcinoma of the breast in woman, 47. **A**, original radiograph shows extensive bone destruction. **B**, operating room radiograph shows the proximal fragment inside the distal and good alignment restored. **C**, 6 months later, after supplementary radiotherapy, the fracture is well healed.

is low, but there is a high morbidity, including aseptic necrosis, angular deformity, growth arrest, and delayed union and nonunion.

These fractures can be divided into 4 groups which include: type I, epiphyseal injuries; type II, neck fractures; type III, cervicotrochanteric or base of the neck fractures; type IV, intertrochanteric fractures.

Fractures through or including the femoral capital epiphysis are rare but may occur at any age from birth to epiphyseal closure. Epiphyseal separations at birth are sometimes confused both clinically and radiographically with congenitally dislocated hips, as the femoral capital epiphysis is not ossified. The excessive callus that forms within 7–10 days of injury confirms the diagnosis. Results are usually good with minimal treatment in infants and younger children. In older children, aseptic necrosis with permanent deformity is more common, particularly if there is significant displacement. With minimal displacement, fixation in situ with Knowles or other type of nondistracting pins is the treatment of choice. With significant displacement, closed reduction, either by gentle manipulation under anesthesia or by skeletal traction, followed by internal fixation with multiple pins is the treatment of choice.

Since these injuries often involve a great deal of force, there may be associated dislocation of the femoral capital epiphysis. Open reduction with multiple pin fixation will be required, although the prognosis for viability of the head is poor.

From 70 to 75% of all hip fractures in children are either type II (transcervical) or type III (base of neck). Varus deformity is common in patients with displaced fractures who are treated by spica immobilization alone. Avascular necrosis is more common in children than in adults. Manipulative reduction must be gentle. It is performed under general anesthesia or gradually by skeletal traction followed by pin fixation. The eventual result when the child reaches adulthood is greatly influenced by the gentleness of the reduction, the adequacy of the reduction and the adequacy of fixation. If a good reduction cannot be obtained by closed methods, there should be no hesitation to perform open reduction.

Intertrochanteric fractures are rare and usually constitute only 5–10% of fractures about the hip in children. Here the incidence of avascular necrosis is exceedingly low. Varus deformity may occur but almost always corrects with growth and remodeling. Intertrochanteric fractures in children are best treated either by skeletal traction until the fracture is stable or by internal fixation using a blade-plate device which does not cross the femoral capital epiphysis. We do not recommend a 3-flanged nail device in types I–III fractures as these may distract or damage the femoral capital epiphysis.

SUMMARY

Optimal management of fractures of the neck of the femur consists in prompt recognition of the condition, immediate splinting to prevent further injury and a careful and complete estimation of the patient's health, with institution of appropriate measures to control associated medical conditions, followed by definitive treatment of the fracture as soon as compatible with the safety and condition of the patient. Delay of operative treatment in hip fracture patients is acceptable only if one can reasonably anticipate improvement of the patient's medical condition, lessening of operative risk, or an increased likelihood of a satisfactory result.

Displaced fractures in the intracapsular area should be reduced and nailed, or a prosthetic replacement should be employed. In the trochanteric area, open reduction and internal fixation should be carried out unless conservative management and traction is elected as the treatment of choice. A thorough understanding of the use and limitations of the devices used for internal fixation must be part of the surgeon's armamentarium. Careful protection of the injured extremity after operation until adequate healing occurs is no less important than the operation itself. If antibiotics are to be used, the surgeon should appreciate whether these are to be given as prophylaxis or as treatment and guide his program accordingly. Anticoagulants appear to have a place in the prevention of thromboembolic disease in the bed-ridden patient but must be used with caution. Attention to detail along each step of the way will lead to increasing success in the management of these fractures. Although existing knowledge has by no means solved the problem of the fractured hip, a high level of success should be obtainable.

BIBLIOGRAPHY

1. Alffram, P. A.: Epidemiologic study of cervical and trochanteric fracture of femur in urban population: Analysis of 1,664 cases with special reference to etiologic factors, Acta Orthop. Scand. Supp. 65:1, 1964.
2. Anderson, R.: A new method for treating fractures, utilizing the well leg for countertraction, Surg. Gynecol. Obstet. 54:207, 1932.
3. Aufranc, O. E., Norton, P. L., and Rowe, C. R.: Fractures and Dislocations of the Hip, in Cave, E. F. (ed.), *Fractures and Other Injuries* (Chicago: Year Book Publishers, 1958).
4. Banks, S. W.: Aseptic necrosis of the femoral head following traumatic dislocation of the hip, J. Bone Joint Surg. 23:753, 1941.
5. Bickel, W. H., Childs, D. S., and Porretta, C. M.: Post irradiation fractures of femoral neck: Emphasis on results of treatment, J.A.M.A. 175:204, 1961.
6. Boyd, H. B., and Anderson, L. D.: Management of unstable trochanteric fractures, Surg. Gynecol. Obstet. 112:633, 1961.
7. Boyd, H. B., and Salvatore, J. E.: Acute fracture of femoral neck: Internal fixation or prosthesis? J. Bone Joint Surg. 46-A:1066, 1964.
7a. Boyd, R. J., Burke, J. F., and Colton, S. M.: A double-blind clinical trial of prophylactic antibiotics in hip fractures, J. Bone Joint Surg. 55-A: 1251, 1973.
8. Brown, T. T., and Abrami, G.: Transcervical femoral fracture: Review of 195 patients treated by sliding nail-plate fixation, J. Bone Joint Surg. 46:648, 1964.
9. Buck, G.: An improved method of treating fracture of the thigh, illustrated by cases, Trans. NY Acad. Med. 2:233, 1861.
10. Burke, J. F.: Effective period of preventive antibiotic action in experimental incisions and dermal lesions, Surgery 50:161, 1961.
11. Burke, J. F.: Pre-operative antibiotics, Surg. Clin. North Am. 43:665, 1963.
12. Catto, M. E.: Histologic study of avascular necrosis of the femoral head after transcervical fracture, J. Bone Joint Surg. 47-B:749, 1965.
13. Charnley, J.: Treatment of fracture of the neck of the femur by compression, Acta Orthop. Scand. 30:29, 1960.
14. Clawson, D. K.: Trochanteric fractures treated by the sliding screw-plate fixation method, J. Trauma 4:737, 1964.
15. Cleveland, M. A.: A critical survey of 10 years' experience with fractures of the neck of the femur, Surg. Gynecol. Obstet. 74:529, 1942.
16. Cleveland, M. A., and Bosworth, D. M.: Fractures of the neck of the femur: A critical analysis of 50 consecutive cases, Surg. Gynecol. Obstet. 66:646, 1938.
17. Colombot, C. P.: *Documents sur la Methode Osteotropique* (Paris, 1840).
18. Cordasco, P.: Evolution of treatment of fractures of neck of femur, Arch. Surg. 37:871, 1938.
19. Cotton, F. J.: Artificial impaction in hip fractures, Am. J. Orthop. Surg. 8:680, 1911.
20. Cotton, F. J.: *Dislocations and Joint Fractures* (Philadelphia: W. B. Saunders Company, 1924).
21. Crawford, H. B.: Conservative treatment of impacted fractures of femoral neck: Report of 50 cases, J. Bone Joint Surg. 42-A:471, 1960.
22. Deyerle, D. M.: Absolute fixation with contact compression in hip fractures (new fixation device), Clin. Orthop. 13:279, 1959.
23. Dickerson, R. C., and Duthie, R. B.: Diversion of arterial blood flow to bone: Preliminary report, J. Bone Joint Surg. 45-A:256, 1963.
24. Dimon, J. H., III, and Hughston, J. C.: Unstable intertrochanteric fracture of the hip, J. Bone Joint Surg. 49-A:440, 1966.
25. Fielding, J. W., and Zickel, R. E.: Pugh nail fixation of displaced intracapsular fracture of the femoral neck, Surg. Gynecol. Obstet. 118:1080, 1964.
26. Frangakis, E. K.: Intracapsular fracture of the neck of the femur, J. Bone Joint Surg. 48-B:1:17, 1966.
27. Frankel, C. J., and Derian, P. S.: Introduction of subcapital femoral circulation by means of autogenous muscle pedicle, Surg. Gynecol. Obstet. 115:473, 1962.
28. Garden, R. S.: Stability and union in subcapital fractures of the femur, J. Bone Joint Surg. 46-B:630, 1964.
29. Girdlestone, G. R.: Acute pyogenic arthritis of the hip giving free access and effective drainage, Lancet 1:419, 1943.
30. Glotzer, D. J., Goodman, W. S., and Lippman, H. G.: Topical antibiotic prophylaxis in contaminated wounds: Experimental evaluation, Arch. Surg. 100:589, 1970.
31. Gyepes, M., Mellins, H. Z., and Katz, I.: Low incidence of fracture of hip in Negro, J.A.M.A. 181:1073, 1962.
32. Holt, E. P., Jr.: Hip fractures in trochanteric region: Treatment with strong nail and early weight bearing; report of 100 cases, J. Bone Joint Surg. 45-A:687, 1963.
33. Johansson, S.: An operative treatment of medial fractures of the neck of the femur, Acta Orthop. Scand. 3:362, 1932.

34. Judet, J., Judet, R., LaGrange, J., and Dunoyer, J.: Study of arterial vascularization of femoral neck in adult, J. Bone Joint Surg. 37-A:663, 1955.
35. King, M. J.: Recent intracapsular fracture of the neck of the femur: A critical consideration of their treatment and a description of a new technique, Med. J. Aust. 1:5, 1934.
36. Laing, P. G.: The significance of metallic transfer in the corrosion of orthopedic screws, J. Bone Joint Surg. 40-A:853, 1958.
37. Leadbetter, G. W.: A treatment for fracture of the neck of the femur, J. Bone Joint Surg. 15: 931, 1933.
38. Linton, P.: Types of displacement in fractures of the femoral neck and observations on impaction of fractures, J. Bone Joint Surg. 31-B: 184, 1949.
39. Lowell, J. D.: Fracture of the hip, N. Engl. J. Med. 274:1418; 1480, 1966.
40. Martz, C. D.: Stress tolerance of bone and metal, J. Bone Joint Surg. 38-A:827, 1956.
41. Massie, W. K.: Functional fixation of femoral neck fractures: Telescoping nail technique, Clin. Orthop. 12:230, 1958.
42. Merchant, A. C.: Hip abductor muscle force: Experimental study of influence of hip position with particular reference to rotation, J. Bone Joint Surg. 27-A:462, 1965.
43. Meyers, M. H., Harvey, J. P. Jr., and Moore, T. H.: Treatment of displaced subcapital and transcervical fracture of the neck by muscle pedicle bone graft and internal fixation: A preliminary report on 150 cases, J. Bone Joint Surg. 55-A:257, 1973.
44. Mulholland, R. C., and Gunn, D. R.: Sliding screw plate fixation of intertrochanteric femoral fractures, J. Trauma 12:581, 1972.
45. Paré, A.: *Works* (translated by T. Johnson) (London: T. Cotes and R. Young, 1634).
46. Pauwels, F.: Der Schenkelhalsbruch ein mechanisches Problem, Z. Orthop. Chir., vol. 63, 1935.
47. Phemister, D. B.: Fractures of the neck of the femur, dislocations of the hip and obscure vascular disturbances producing aseptic necrosis of the head of the femur, Surg. Gynecol. Obstet. 59:415, 1934.
48. Pott, P.: *The Chirurgical Works of Percival Pott* (from the English ed. by J. Earle) (Philadelphia: J. Webster, 1819).
49. Pugh, W. L.: Self-adjusting nail-plate for fractures about the hip joint, J. Bone Joint Surg. 37-A:1085, 1955.
50. Rokkanen, P.: Role of surgical interventions of hip joint in aetiology and aseptic necrosis of femoral head, Acta Orthop. Scand., Supp. 58, 1962.
51. Russell, R. H.: Fracture of the femur: A clinical study, Br. J. Surg. 11:491, 1924.
52. Rydell, N. W.: Forces acting on the femoral head prosthesis: A study on strain gauge supplied prosthesis in living person, Acta Orthop. Scand., Supp. 88, 1966.
53. Salzman, E. W., Harris, W. H., and DeSanctis, R. W.: Anticoagulation for prevention of thromboembolism following fracture of the hip, N. Engl. J. Med. 275:122, 1966.
54. Sarmiento, A., and Williams, E. M.: Unstable trochanteric fracture: Treatment with valgus osteotomy and I-beam nail plate; preliminary report of 100 cases, J. Bone Joint Surg. 52-A: 1309, 1970.
55. Scales, J. T., Towers, A. C., and Roantree, B. M.: The influence of antibiotic therapy on wound inflammation and sepsis associated with orthopaedic implants: A long-term clinical survey, Acta Orthop. Scand. 43:85, 1972.
56. Scheck, M.: Intracapsular fracture of the femoral neck: Comminution of posterior neck cortex as cause of unstable fixation, J. Bone Joint Surg. 41-A:1187, 1959.
57. Sevitt, S.: Avascular necrosis and revascularization of the femoral head after intracapsular fractures, J. Bone Joint Surg. 46-B:270, 1964.
58. Sevitt, S., and Gallagher, N. G.: Prevention of venous thrombosis and pulmonary embolism in injured patients: Trial of anticoagulant prophylaxis with phenindione in middle-aged and elderly patients with fractured necks of the femur, Lancet 2:981, 1959.
59. Smith, F. B.: Effects of rotary and valgus malpositions on blood supply to femoral head: Observations at arthroplasty, J. Bone Joint Surg. 41-A:800, 1959.
60. Smith, G. T., Dexter, L., and Dammin, G. T.: Postmortem quantitative studies in pulmonary thromboembolism, in Sasahara, A. A., and Stein, M., (eds.), *Pulmonary Embolic Disease* (New York: Grune & Stratton, 1965).
61. Smith-Petersen, M. N.: Treatment of fractures of the neck of the femur by internal fixation, Surg. Gynecol Obstet. 64:287, 1937.
62. Smith-Petersen, M. N., Cave, E. F., and VanGorder, G. W.: Intracapsular fractures of the neck of the femur: Treatment by internal fixation, Arch. Surg. 23:715, 1931.
63. Solonen, K. A.: Prophylactic anticoagulant therapy in treatment of lower limb fractures, Acta Orthop. Scand. 33:329, 1963.
64. Soto-Hall, R. Johnson, L. H., and Johnson, R. A.: Variations in intra-articular pressure of hip joint in injury and disease: Probable factor in avascular necrosis, J. Bone Joint Surg. 46-A: 509, 1964.
65. Strange-St. Clair, F. G.: *The Hip* (London: W Heinemann Medical Books, Ltd., 1965).
66. Taylor, G. M., Neufeld, A. J., and Nickel, V. L.: Complications and failures in the operative treatment of intertrochanteric fractures of the femur, J. Bone Joint Surg. 37-A:306, 1955.
67. Thomas, D. P.: Treatment of pulmonary embolic disease: A critical review of some aspects of current therapy, N. Engl. J. Med. 273: 885, 1965.
68. Trueta, J., and Harrison, M. H. M.: Normal vascular anatomy of femoral head in adult man, J. Bone Joint Surg., 35-B:442, 1953.
69. Watson-Jones, R.: *Fracture and Joint Injuries* (4th ed.; Baltimore: Williams & Wilkins Company, 1955), Vol. 2.
70. Wescott, H. H.: A method for the internal fixation of transcervical fractures of the femur, J. Bone Joint Surg. 16:372, 1934; South Med. Surg. 96:458, 1934.
71. Wescott, H. H.: Preliminary report of a method of internal fixation of transcervical fracture of the neck of the femur in the aged, Va. Med. Mon 59:197, 1932.
72. White, J. W.: Instrument facilitating the use of

the flanged nail in treatment of fractures of the hip, J. Bone Joint Surg. 17:1065, 1935.
73. Whitman, R.: A new treatment for fractures of the neck of the femur, Med. Rec. 65:441, 1904.
74. Wilkie, D. P. D.: A new treatment for fractures of the neck of the femur, Surg. Gynecol. Obstet. 44:529, 1927.
75. Woodhouse, C. F.: Instrument for measurement of oxygen tension in bone: Preliminary report, J. Bone Joint Surg. 43-A:819, 1961.

27 | Dislocations of the Hip and Fractures of the Acetabulum

CARTER R. ROWE

DISLOCATIONS OF THE HIP

HENRY JACOB BIGELOW in 1869 was the pioneer in America to focus attention on the management of dislocations of the hip. Bigelow demonstrated that complete flexion of the hip, thus relaxation of the anterior iliofemoral ligament (Y ligament of Bigelow), was necessary in order to reduce most posterior dislocations of the hip.

Information is available on 107 dislocations of the hip and acetabular fractures which have been treated at Massachu-

Fig. 27-1.—Mechanism of anterior dislocation of hip.

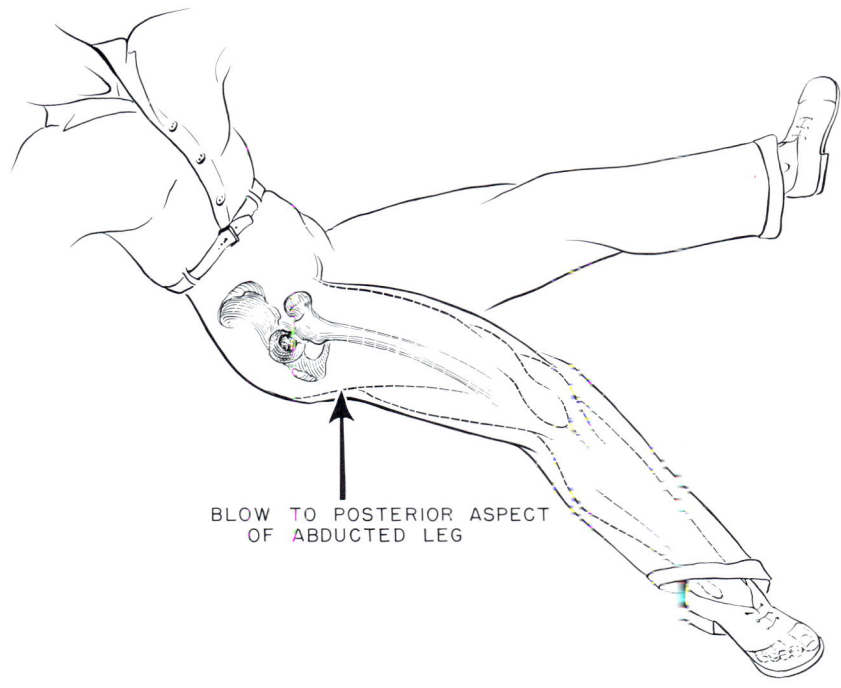

BLOW TO POSTERIOR ASPECT OF ABDUCTED LEG

setts General Hospital (Tables 27-1 to 27-3) during the past 20 years. Follow-up studies have been completed on 75 (70%).

Anterior Dislocations

MECHANISM OF INJURY.—The most frequent cause of anterior dislocation of the hip is a blow to the posterior aspect of the abducted and externally rotated thigh (Fig. 27-1). The blow is usually caused by a fall from a height.

DIAGNOSIS.—The typical deformity of the patient with an anterior dislocation of the hip is shown in Figure 27-2. The degree of deformity depends on the position of the femoral head. The femoral head may be palpated anteriorly.

X-ray examination.—An anteroposterior film of the pelvis is usually sufficient to establish the diagnosis of an anterior dislocation (Fig. 27-3).

TREATMENT.—Anterior dislocations are easier to diagnose and easier to reduce than are posterior dislocations. All anterior dislocations in the series were successfully reduced by closed manipulation.

Technique of closed reduction.—Figure 27-4 illustrates the closed reduction of an anterior dislocation of the hip. The procedure follows:

1. With the patient anesthetized and

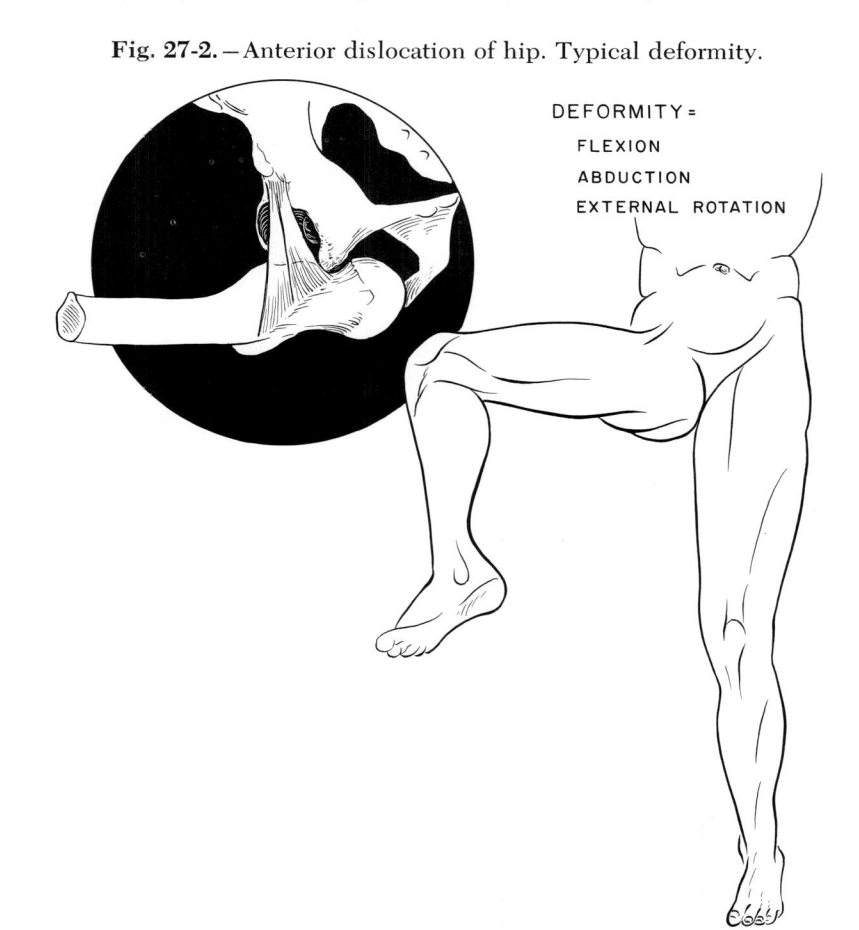

Fig. 27-2.—Anterior dislocation of hip. Typical deformity.

DEFORMITY =
FLEXION
ABDUCTION
EXTERNAL ROTATION

Chapter 27: DISLOCATIONS OF HIP AND FRACTURES OF ACETABULUM / 683

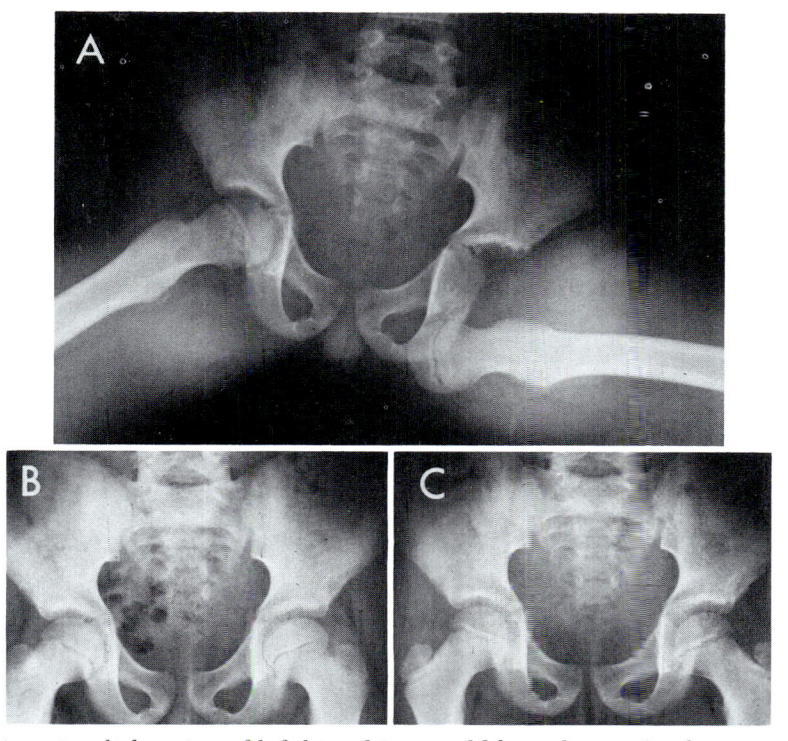

Fig. 27-3.—Anterior dislocation of left hip of 9-year-old boy, the result of a coasting accident. **A**, immediately after accident. **B**, follow-up at 1 year. **C**, follow-up at 2 years; excellent result.

lying supine on the floor, traction is applied to the hip in the position of deformity, i.e., in flexion and abduction.

2. When the femoral head "feels" free and is judged to be replaced on the inferior rim of the acetabulum, traction is applied in a more vertical position, and the hip gradually extended. The Y ligament will lever the head into the acetabulum.

3. Internal rotation usually completes the reduction.

Postreduction films are taken to determine the position of the femoral head and the presence or absence of loose bodies in the joint, since these have had a direct bearing on prognosis.

Posterior Dislocations (without Fracture of the Acetabulum)

MECHANISM OF INJURY.—A posterior dislocation of the hip is usually produced by a direct blow to the flexed and adducted knee (Fig. 27-5). This injury is more traumatic than is an anterior dislocation. In addition to rupture of the posterior joint capsule, the short external rotators of the hip (the piriformis gemelli and the obturator internus muscles) are usually perforated and the posterior acetabular wall damaged. Of the 24 posterior dislocations in the study reported, 21% required an open reduction.

DIAGNOSIS.—A patient with a posterior dislocation of the hip presents a typical deformity (Fig. 27-6). The extremity is usually shortened adducted and internally rotated. The extremes of this deformity depend somewhat on the high, middle and low positions of the femoral head. The head of the femur may be palpated posteriorly in thin persons. The lesser trochanter cannot be seen by anter-

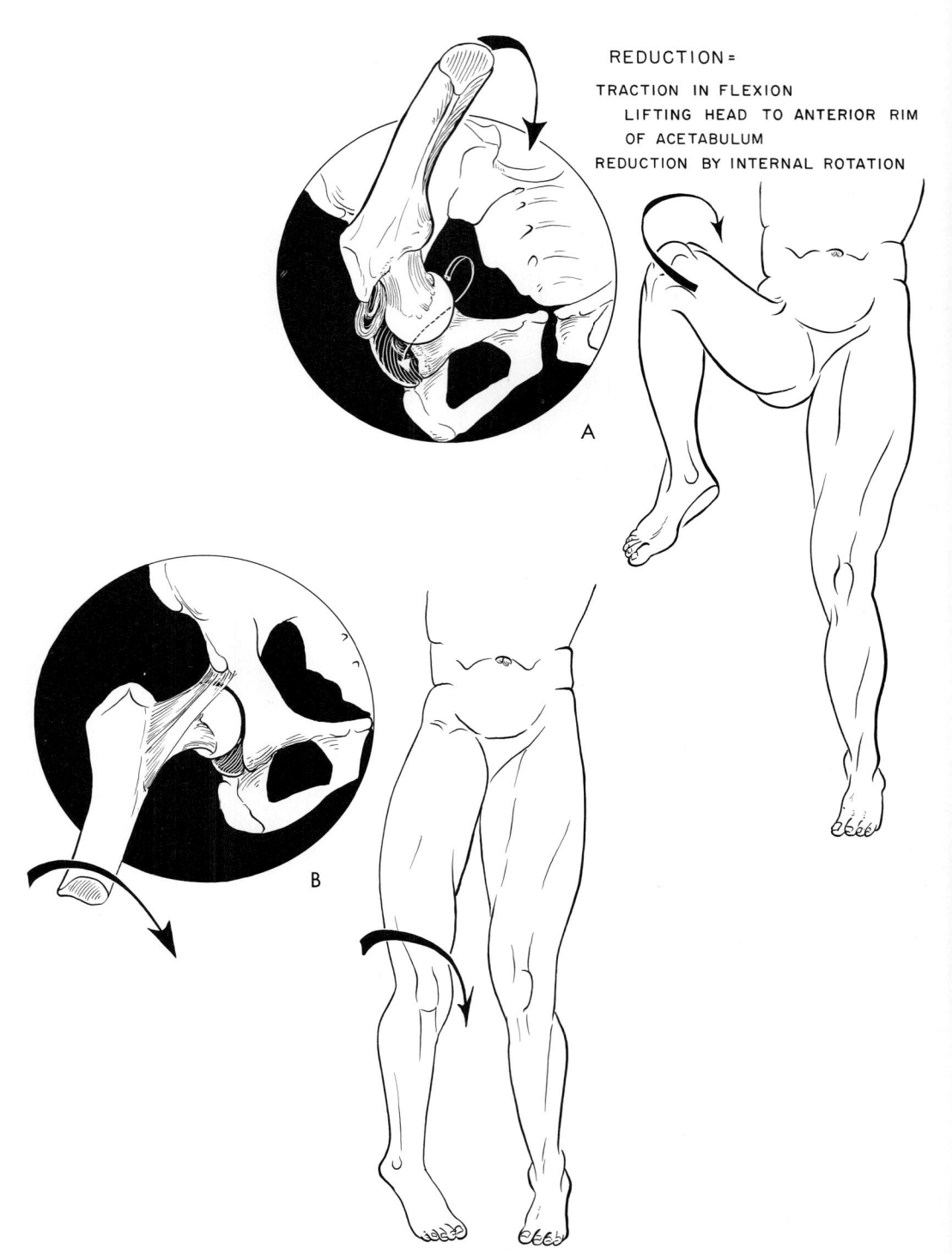

REDUCTION =
TRACTION IN FLEXION
  LIFTING HEAD TO ANTERIOR RIM
  OF ACETABULUM
REDUCTION BY INTERNAL ROTATION

Fig. 27-4.—Anterior dislocation of hip. **A**, closed manipulation. **B**, reduction completed by extension of leg.

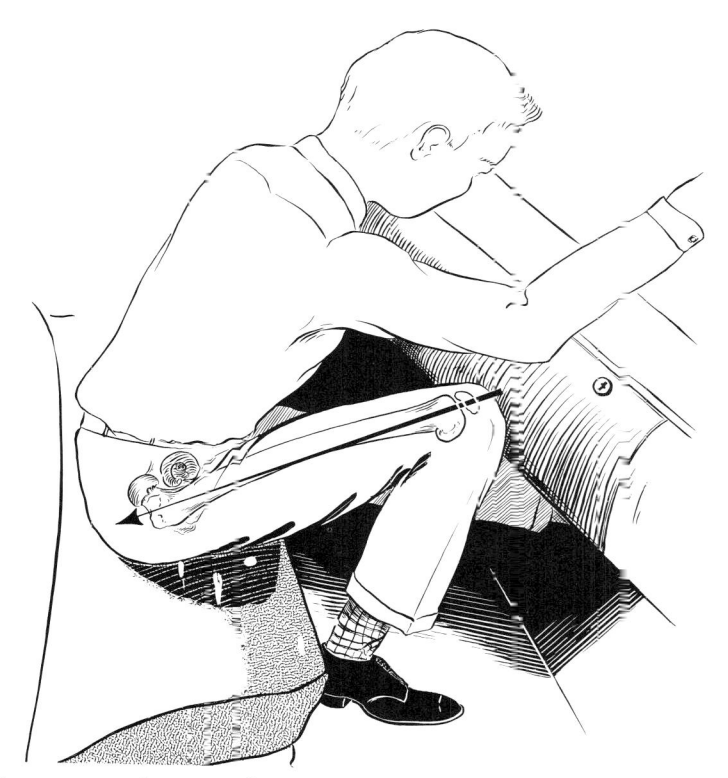

Fig. 27-5.—Common mechanism of posterior dislocation of hip—a direct blow to the knee.

oposterior x-ray examination on the dislocated side.

Bigelow observed that this position of deformity was due to the intact iliofemoral ligament, and noted that, when the ligament was ruptured, the characteristic deformity of the extremity was not present.

A posterior dislocation may be confused at times with a fracture of the femoral neck or of the femoral shaft. Sir Astley Cooper called attention to this in 1825. The deformity of the dislocated hip is "fixed," i.e., the position of the extremity cannot be corrected. If correction is attempted, the patient experiences acute pain and possibly sciatic nerve irritation. On the other hand, the deformity of a femoral neck fracture can be gently manipulated into a corrected position. This may be true also for fractures of the femoral shaft.

Signs of sciatic nerve injury should be noted. In addition, the knee should be examined for possible patellar or tibial table fractures.

X-ray examination.—An anteroposterior view of the hip is adequate for diagnosis (Fig. 27-7). In some instances, a true

TABLE 27-1.—ANALYSIS OF 107 DISLOCATIONS OF THE HIP AND FRACTURES OF THE ACETABULUM

Dislocation of the hip without acetabular fracture	27
Anterior dislocation 3	
Posterior dislocation 24	
Posterior dislocation of the hip with acetabular fracture	23
Central dislocation (intrapelvic protrusion)	25
Acetabular fracture, comminuted, without dislocation of the femoral head	17
Acetabular fracture, linear, undisplaced	15
Total	107

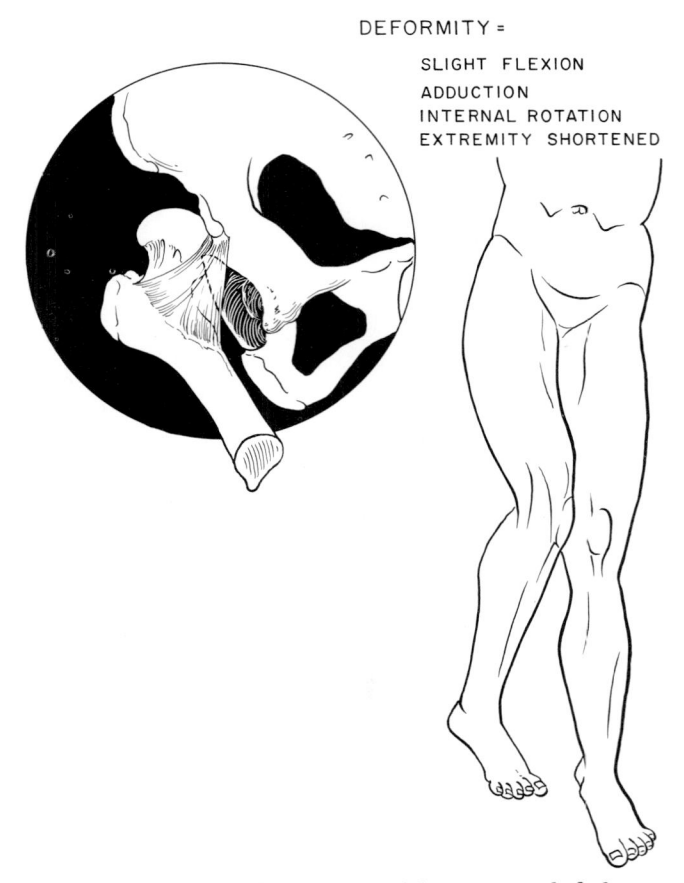

Fig. 27-6.—Posterior dislocation of hip. Typical deformity.

Fig. 27-7.—**A,** view of posterior dislocation of right hip (dashboard injury) showing posterior and high position of femoral head. **B,** follow-up 7 years later; no joint changes. Complete range of motion and no pain.

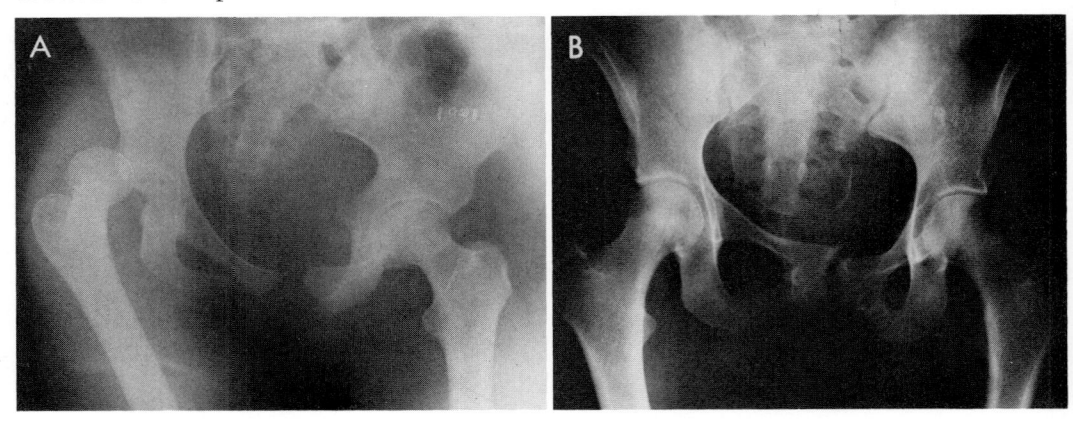

TABLE 27-2.—ANALYSIS OF 75 HIP DISLOCATIONS

Type		
Anterior dislocation	3	(4%)
Posterior dislocation	47	(63%)
(23 [49%] with fracture of the posterior acetabular rim)		
Central dislocation	25	(33%)
Position of femoral head in posterior and anterior dislocations		
Head in high position		(63%)
Head in midposition		(25%)
Head in inferior position		(12%)
Side of body		
Right		36
Left		35
Bilateral central dislocations		2
Sex		
Males	54	(72%)
Females	21	(28%)

Age	DISLOCATION		
	Anterior	Posterior	Central
Average	25 yr.	28 yr.	47 yr.
Youngest	12 yr.	9 yr.	11 yr.
Oldest	35 yr.	61 yr.	82 yr.

lateral view of the hip should be made. When a fracture of the posterior acetabular rim is present or if it is suspected, special oblique acetabular views should be secured (Fig. 27-8).

TREATMENT BY CLOSED MANIPULATION.—There are 3 essentials in the reduction of a posterior dislocation: anesthesia must be adequate; x-ray study must be thorough; and reduction must be carried out with the hip in 90 degrees, or more, of flexion.

Three methods of reduction are usually referred to for posterior dislocations: the Bigelow, the Allis and the Stimson methods. All three methods are based on reduction of the hip in flexion and with traction.

Bigelow's method (Fig. 27-9).—There is little difference between the Bigelow and the Allis methods. If one reads Bigelow's book carefully, one will find Allis' method described on several occasions. The procedure is as follows:

The patient is placed face up on the floor. Countertraction is applied to the anterosuperior spine by an assistant. If the operator does not have an assistant, he may remove his shoe and place his foot over the anterosuperior spine to give countertraction. The extremity is grasped with the knee flexed, and traction is applied in the direction of deformity—i.e., internal rotation and adduction—bringing the extremity gradually into 90 degrees of flexion. At this point, the thigh is gently "rocked" forward and backward in order to free the head from the rotator muscles and posterior capsule. In some instances it is helpful to flex the hip beyond 90 degrees, pointing the knee toward the opposite shoulder. When it is felt that the head has been freed posteriorly and elevated to the posterior rim of the acetabulum, 1 of 2 maneuvers may be used: (1) further internal rotation, and pull, to reduce the head into the acetabulum, or (2) gentle external rotation and extension of the thigh, which will tense the Y ligament and thus lever the head forward into the acetabulum.

All manipulations should be carried out gently. A rough manipulation with

TABLE 27-3.—ANALYSIS OF 80 ACETABULAR FRACTURES

Incidence		
Acetabular fractures associated with dislocation of the hip	48	(60%)
Posterior rim fractures with dislocation	23	
Central fractures with intrapelvic protrusion	25	
Acetabular fractures, comminuted without dislocation of femoral head	17	(21%)
Acetabular fractures, linear, undisplaced	15	(19%)
Total	80	
Sex		
Males outnumbered females 2 to 1.		
Side of body		
Right		59%
Left		41%
(Bilateral in 3 instances)		
Age		
Average for group		45 yr.
Oldest		82 yr.
Youngest		5 yr.

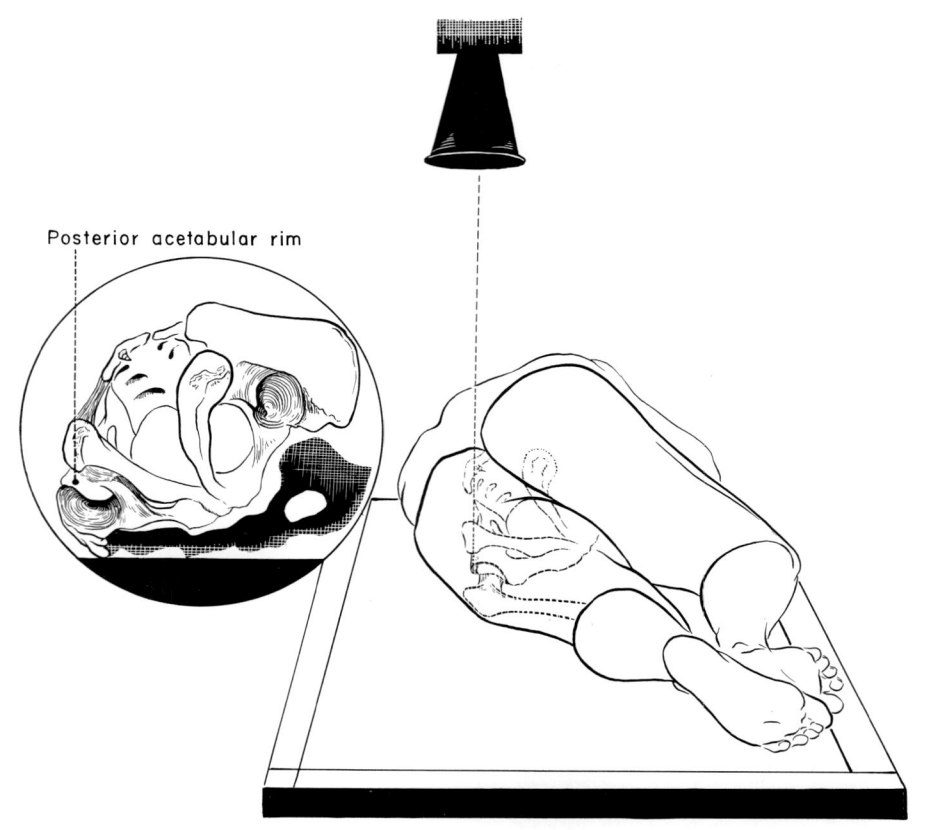

Fig. 27-8.—Technique for x-raying posterior acetabular rim. With the patient face down, the uninjured hip is elevated 45–60 degrees.

sudden and very forceful reduction of the femoral head may cause irreparable damage to the cartilage of the head. After reduction, a test for stability of the hip should be carried out. Postreduction x-ray films should be taken with great care to determine whether there is any visible bone injury to the femoral head or acetabulum or whether there are free bone fragments in the joint. This information is very important relative to prognosis.

Stimson's (prone) method (Fig. 27-10).—This method of reduction has perhaps been used too infrequently. It is a safe method.

The patient is placed face down on a table with the injured hip flexed, at 90 degrees or more, over the end of the table. Firm downward pressure is applied to the flexed leg—i.e., the thigh at 90 degrees and the knee at 90 degrees. A gentle rocking motion may be helpful in this maneuver, as in the Bigelow procedure. With thin patients, the operator may apply gentle pressure directly to the femoral head. By gradually increasing the downward traction on the leg, and with slight increase in internal rotation, flexion and adduction, the operator can position the head onto the posterior rim of the acetabulum, and reduction will be completed.

DISLOCATION OF HIP AND FRACTURE OF IPSILATERAL FEMORAL SHAFT.—In the management of a dislocated hip, it is well to keep in mind the possibility of a concomitant fracture of the femoral shaft.

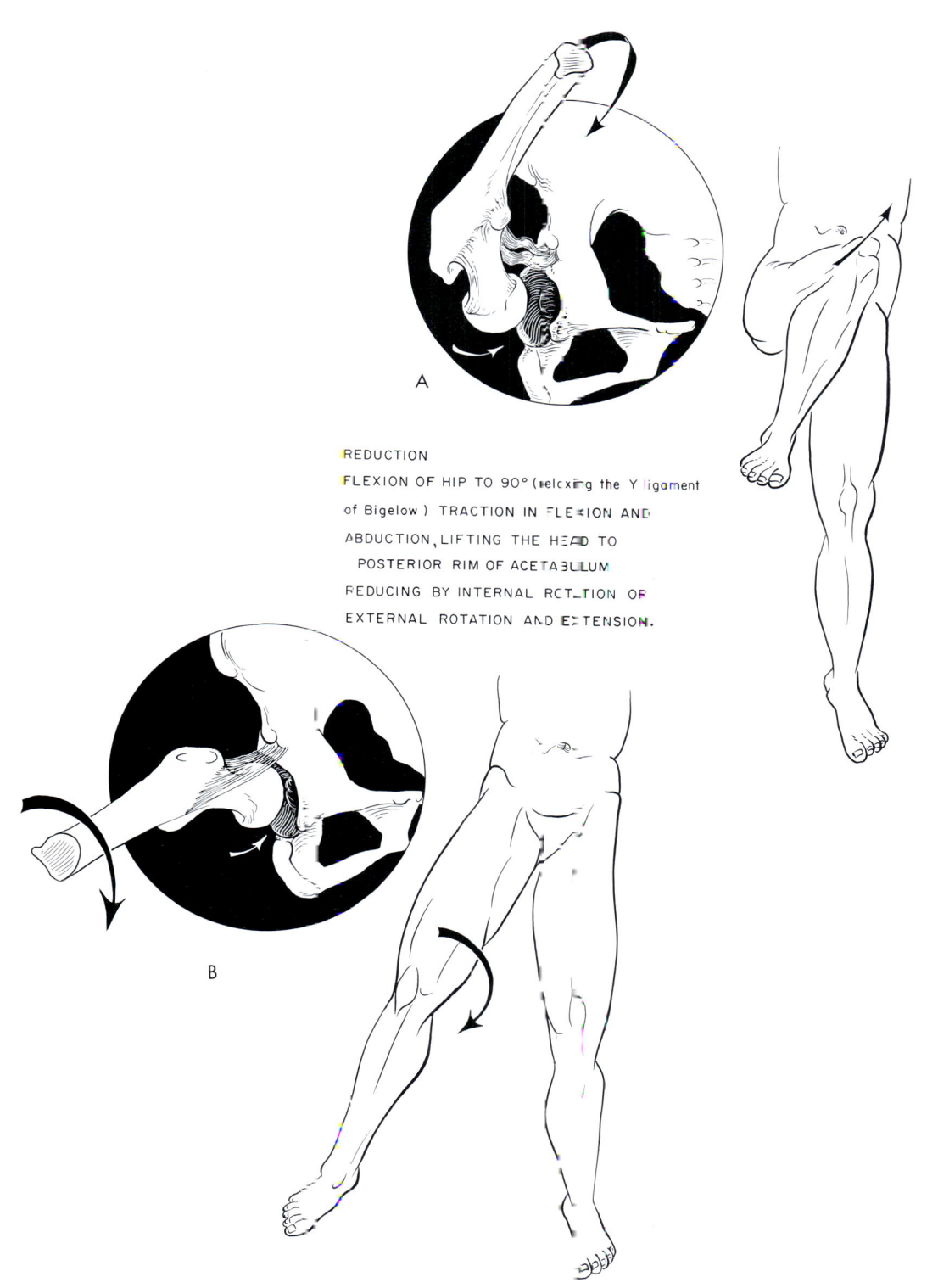

REDUCTION
FLEXION OF HIP TO 90° (relaxing the Y ligament of Bigelow) TRACTION IN FLEXION AND ABDUCTION, LIFTING THE HEAD TO POSTERIOR RIM OF ACETABULUM REDUCING BY INTERNAL ROTATION OF EXTERNAL ROTATION AND EXTENSION.

Fig. 27-9.—Posterior dislocation of hip. **A,** reduction **B,** reduction completed by extension of leg.

690 / Carter R. Rowe

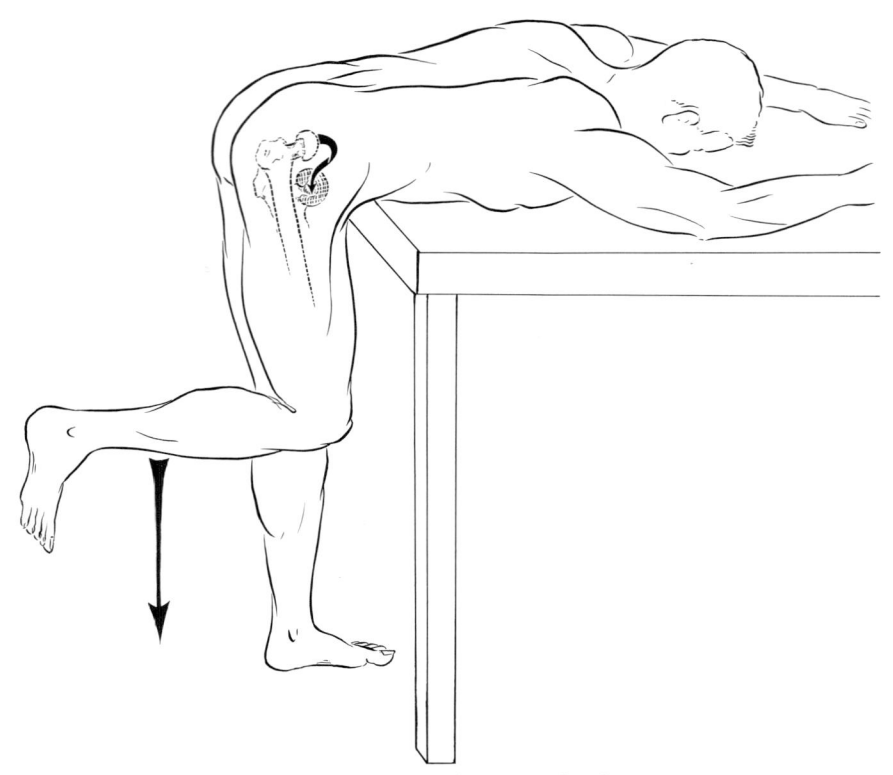

Fig. 27-10. — Prone technique of reduction.

This combination occurred in 4% of 107 hip dislocations and acetabular fractures at Massachusetts General Hospital. It is interesting to note that Bigelow also discussed this condition in 1869 and clearly stated that, when this combination occurs, "splinting" of the femur and a careful manipulation with manual pressure on the femoral head should successfully reduce the hip. His advice was sound, and the method should be tried. We would, however, suggest the following techniques to reduce the femoral head when the dislocation is complicated by a fractured femur.

1. Insert a Ray trochanteric screw (Fig. 27-11) into the lateral aspect of the trochanter and manipulate the head by flexion and by adduction of the trochanter and manual assistance upward to replace the femoral head into the acetabulum; or transfix the trochanter with a Steinmann pin to control the hip.

2. Prior to reduction of the hip, the femoral shaft may be stabilized with a Küntscher intramedullary rod; the hip may then be manipulated.

3. If the above methods prove unsuccessful, open reduction of the hip should be carried out.

TREATMENT BY OPEN REDUCTION. — The indications for open reduction are: (1) repeated unsuccessful attempts at closed reduction; (2) late or old dislocations; (3) recurrent dislocation of the hip; (4) in certain fractures of the acetabulum complicating a dislocation and producing instability of the hip.

The purpose of open reduction should be to return the head of the femur to the acetabulum with as little trauma as possi-

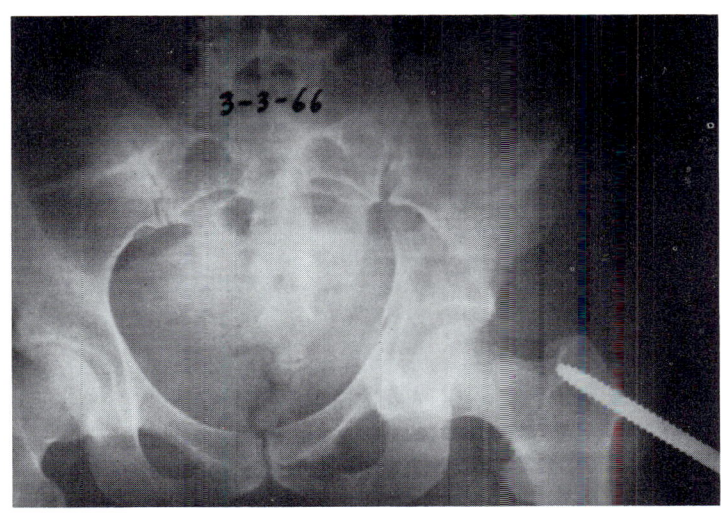

Fig. 27-11.—Use of the Ray trochanteric screw offers an effective method of stabilizing the femoral head under the superior dome of the acetabulum.

ble. Open reduction may be performed from the anterior, lateral or direct posterior approach to the hip (see p. 704). The approach will depend on the preference of the surgeon. Each approach has its indications and advantages.

AFTER-CARE.—Follow-up studies indicate that the method and schedule of after-care bear little relation to the final functional result of the uncomplicated dislocated hip. It seems important, however, to outline a schedule which is physiologic and reasonable. With this in mind, we emphasize the following.

1. The dislocated hip may be considered stable once reduction is accomplished, assuming that there is no fracture of the acetabulum.
2. Injury to the posterior capsule and short rotator muscles should heal within 3 weeks. During this time, painful motion and pressure on the posterior hip structures should be avoided.
3. Early active and passive joint motions, carefully performed, probably result in improvement of cartilage nutrition.

The following schedule is suggested.
1. Bed rest for a period of 3 weeks.
2. During this time, early active and passive motion of the hips and muscle-setting exercises should be undertaken. These may be started a few days after reduction and increased as tolerated by the patient.
3. Partial weight bearing on crutches for a period of 3 months. A longer period of partial weight bearing may be indicated, depending on the patient's progress.
4. The performance of light work by the patient is permitted 4–6 months after injury and full activities 10–12 months after injury.
5. Follow-up of the case. The patient should be followed carefully and examined periodically, with x-ray and physical examinations, for several years after injury.

PROGNOSIS.—Our follow-up studies indicated that the prognosis of a dislocated hip would be *unfavorable* if:

1. The dislocation were complicated by a fracture of the femoral head.
2. If loose bodies were present in the joint following reduction.
3. If fractures of the acetabular rim produce an unstable reduction.
4. If repeated unsuccessful manipula-

tions were carried out before the final closed or open reduction.

Recurrent Dislocations of the Hip

We have had 2 instances of recurrent, traumatic dislocations of the hip after initial reduction. One was a recurrent posterior dislocation, the other an anterior dislocation. Both responded successfully to surgical repair of the labrum and capsule to the rim of the acetabulum.

FRACTURES OF THE ACETABULUM

With increasing speed on the highways, the fractured acetabulum is rapidly becoming a major skeletal injury. In 1961, the experience at Massachusetts General Hospital was reviewed by Rowe and Lowell. From this new study and from our interest in the subject since the initial study, we have established certain helpful *guidelines* in the management of the fractured acetabulum. We may well preface a discussion of this injury by 2 summary statements: (1) Specific treatment will depend on the particular section of the acetabulum which has been injured. (2) The success or failure of treatment may depend on therapeutic steps taken *during* the first 48 hours following injury.

TYPES OF FRACTURES.—The primary divisions of the acetabulum are formed by the original epiphyseal divisions (Fig. 27-12):
 1. Inner wall (the pubic division)
 2. Superior dome (the iliac division)
 3. Posterior wall (the ischial division)

Most acetabular fractures will conform to these primary divisions. Furthermore, specific treatment in each division differs, one from the other.

In general, there are 4 typical fractures of the acetabulum:

Fig. 27-12.—The primary divisions of the acetabulum are formed by the original epiphyseal divisions.

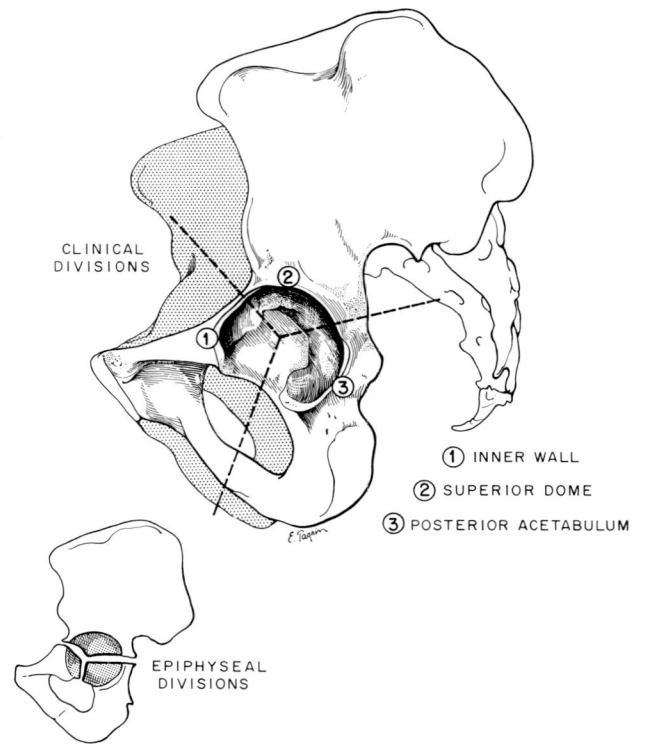

I. Fractures of the *inner wall* with and without intrapelvic protrusion.
II. Fractures of the *posterior wall* with and without posterior dislocation of the hip.
III. Fractures of the *superior dome* with and without displacement.
IV. *Bursting fractures,* including disruption of *all* divisions of the acetabulum.

EMERGENCY TREATMENT.—During the first 48 hours following injury (the "golden period"), prompt decisions must be made and rapidly implemented. During this time, the bone fragments are movable and will respond to manipulation. After 48–72 hours, the blood clots become organized, the bone fragments become less movable and closed reduction becomes progressively more difficult.

INVESTIGATION.—The extent of injury must be quickly determined, the vital signs constantly checked, adequate x-ray study obtained, and early steps instituted to prevent shock. Occult pelvic hemorrhage must be identified. In our series of 93 consecutive patients with acetabular fractures, 51% had 1 or more injuries involving the extremities, head, chest or abdomen. Seventeen per cent had sciatic nerve injuries and 6% genitourinary injury. Intravenous pyelograms and cystograms are made when indicated. The abdomen must be carefully observed and a general neurologic check made to rule out intracranial, spinal or peripheral nerve injury.

STABILIZATION.—The next step is to make the patient comfortable. The early use of skeletal, or adhesive, traction will prove most effective in comforting the patient, stabilizing the pelvic fragments and lessening hemorrhage and shock.

DECISION.—With adequate x-ray study, a plan of action is made. If manipulation is necessary, e.g., for a posterior fracture-dislocation or a displaced intrapelvic dislocation, manipulative reduction should be carried out as soon as the patient's condition will permit.

Fractures of the Inner Wall

Two anatomic features of the pelvis give this type of fracture a favorable prognosis. (1) The *inner* (or central) *wall* of the acetabulum is relatively thin, consequently little damage is inflicted on the femoral head (Fig 27-13). (2) When the inner wall is fractured, the important weight-bearing superior dome remains unharmed. Thus, once the femoral head is reduced back under the superior dome, with conservative treatment the outlook for a good hip is excellent (Fig. 27-14).

Fortunately, the fractured fragments of the inner wall, when healing, will conform to the contour of the femoral head (Fig. 27-15). An anatomic reduction and open reduction of the fragments are seldom, if ever, indicated.

TREATMENT.—Once the femoral head is replaced under the weight-bearing dome, it usually remains in place if the leg is *not* abducted or flexed beyond 35 degrees. The leg should be positioned in line with the body. Traction is best provided by means of a Kirschner wire

Fig. 27-13.—The thin wall of the acetabulum is shown. Fracture through this section produces very little injury to the femoral head.

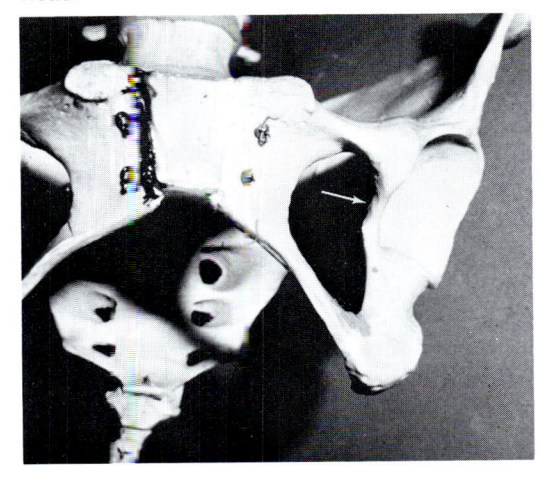

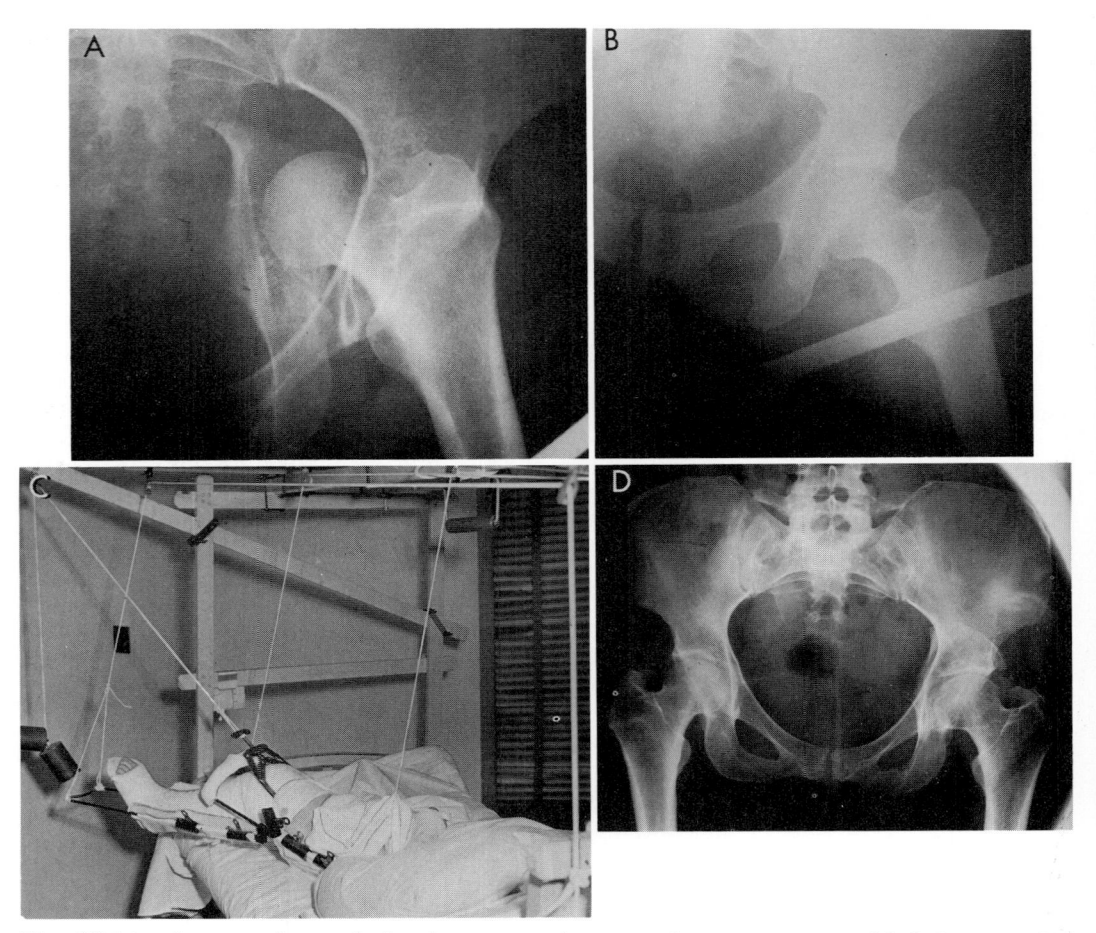

Fig. 27-14.—**A**, central acetabular fracture with intrapelvic protrusion of left hip; patient injured in automobile accident. **B**, immediate manipulation reduction of hip. **C**, postoperative traction and suspension. **D**, follow-up 2 years later; excellent function.

through the tibial tubercle. Early motion should be encouraged. In case the head drifts back into the pelvis, the lateral pull of a Ray trochanteric screw will stabilize the head under the superior dome (Fig. 27-11). This fracture is usually stable after 4–6 weeks, at which time traction may be removed and the patient allowed free motion of the hip in bed. Crutch walking with partial weight bearing follows for a period of 3 months or more.

We emphasize again that open reduction is seldom indicated in the inner wall fracture, even though the x-rays may be most inviting to the surgery-minded orthopedist. Of 29 consecutive inner wall fractures in our series reported in 1961, results in 90% were rated good to excellent with conservative closed treatment. Only 1 patient came to open reduction, and the surgeon in this case, on exposing the inner wall, closed the incision without internal fixation. Furthermore, our experience since 1961 strongly supports closed treatment for inner wall fractures. In a few of these, manipulation is necessary to replace the femoral head, but whether or not the *fragments* of the inner wall were reduced did not affect the prognosis.

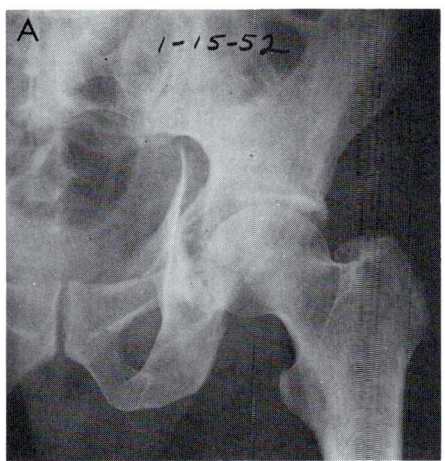

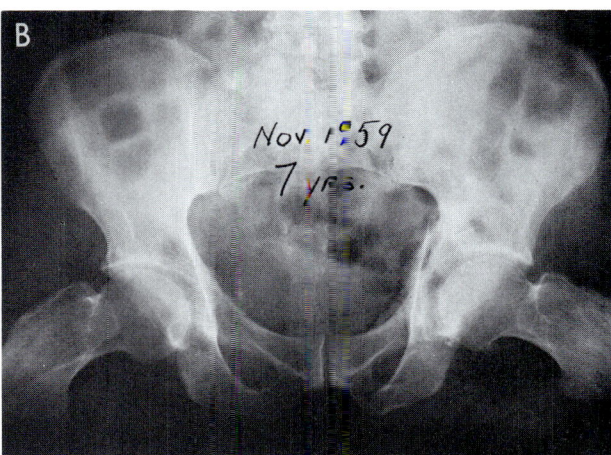

Fig. 27-15.—Molding of the acetabulum to the femoral head in an inner wall fracture, although the fractured fragments were not reduced initially. The patient, a 62-year-old man, had fallen on the left greater trochanter. A, unreduced inner wall fracture. B, follow-up roentgenograms 7 years after injury illustrate the even molding of the acetabulum to the femoral head. The hip is painless; there is no limitation of motion.

Fractures of the Posterior Acetabulum

The posterior wall of the acetabulum, in contrast to the inner wall, is thick and very strong. Its primary function is stability of the hip. Serious complications of fracture are injury to the femoral head and injury to the sciatic nerve. Follow-up studies, in general, indicate that the more promptly a posterior fracture-dislocation is reduced, the more favorable will be its prognosis.

The mechanism and the physical signs of injury are similar to those of complicated posterior hip dislocation. However, a posterior dislocation of the hip that has been reduced, with checkup x-rays interpreted as "satisfactory," may have an unrecognized fracture of the posterior acetabulum. The surgeon should be mindful of this possibility when a patient whose hip dislocation is reduced has signs of sciatic nerve irritation. Oblique posterior x-rays (Fig. 27-8) should clearly demonstrate whether or not a posterior wall fracture is present (Fig. 27-16).

TREATMENT.—Reduction is less difficult in a posterior fracture-dislocation than in an uncomplicated posterior hip dislocation because there is less obstruction to the femoral head. After reduction of the hip, the surgeon should gently test for posterior stability. If there is instability, special views of the posterior acetabulum should be taken at this time to identify the size and location of the displaced posterior acetabular fragment.

If the hip is stable and the posterior fragment small, the hip should be supported in traction and suspension, care being taken *not* to let the leg go into flexion beyond 25–30 degrees; otherwise the hip may redislocate. A few days following reduction the patient should be taken to the x-ray department for multiple views of the hip in order to identify possible bone fragments in the joint and to be certain that the femoral head escaped without fracture.

If oblique views at the time of reduction demonstrate a large displaced posterior fragment and the hip is unstable, open reduction should be planned. This should be performed a few days later when the patient's condition has improved and soft tissues have had a chance to recover. During the interim, a careful

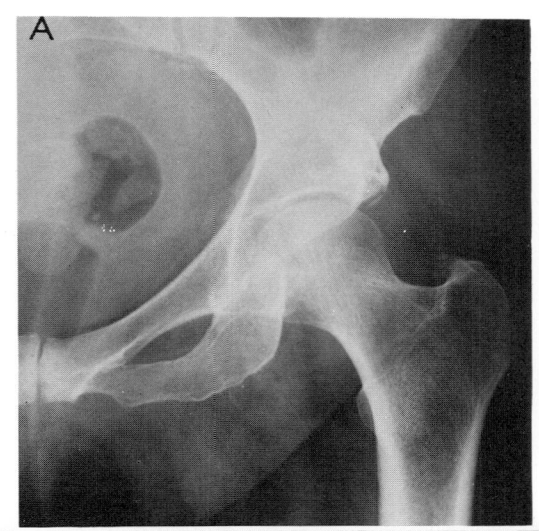

Fig. 27-16. — Deceptive appearance of an anteroposterior view of pelvis in a posterior rim fracture. **A,** "negative" anteroposterior roentgenogram of left hip following reduction of a posterior dislocation. Persistent pain in left hip and sciatic nerve pain when patient attempted to sit up led to further x-rays. **B,** 45-degree oblique view taken with patient positioned as in Figure 27-8. At operation the sciatic nerve was found to be displaced and stretched over the displaced bone fragment. **C,** internal fixation with 2 screws. At follow-up 5 years later, excellent function.

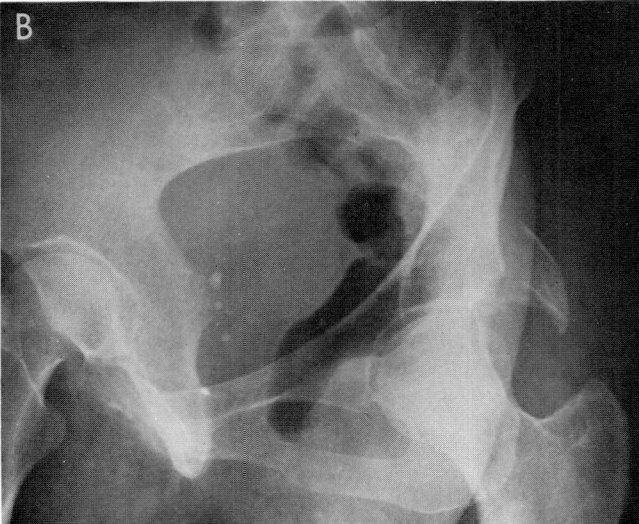

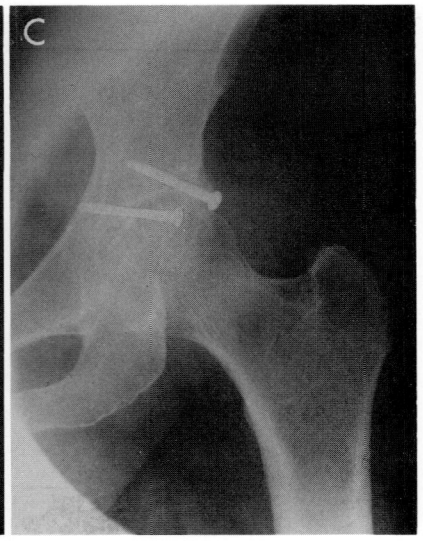

daily skin preparation should be carried out. A posterior fracture-dislocation which needed open reduction is shown in Figure 27-17. The posterior fragment was large and the hip unstable. Several days following injury, open reduction was carried out.

The technique of open reduction is detailed on page 690. A word of caution may be inserted here. The surgeon should exercise extreme care to avoid damage to the sciatic nerve, which should be identified and retracted from the field of surgery. Partial dislocation of the hip is carried out in order to irrigate the joint and remove any bone fragments which may remain. Failure to do this may lead to a poor result. Two screws will give excellent fixation. Avoid the use of threaded pins, since they may migrate.

AFTER-TREATMENT. — With firm fixation of the posterior fragment, the patient may be allowed up with crutches and light

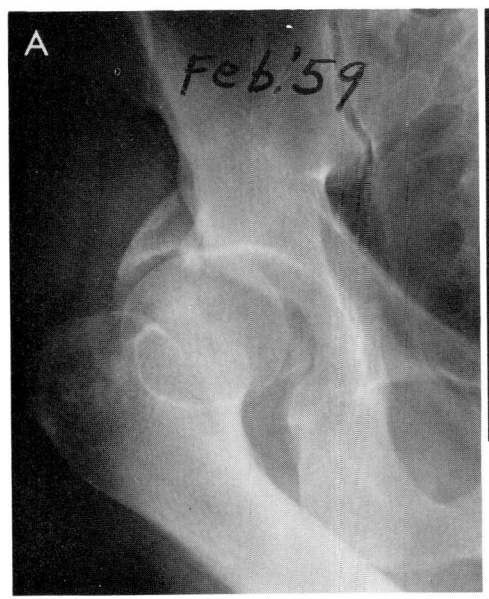

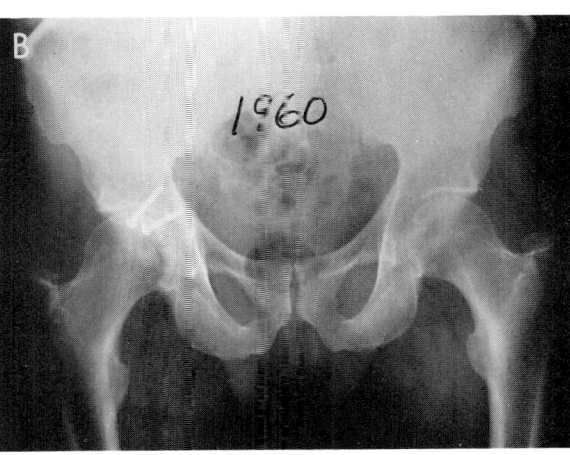

Chapter 27: DISLOCATIONS OF HIP AND FRACTURES OF ACETABULUM / 697

Fig. 27-17.—Posterior fracture dislocation in a 55-year-old man. A, posterior fragment was large, producing marked instability of the hip. B, open reduction was performed, using 2 screws for fixation. Result continues to be excellent.

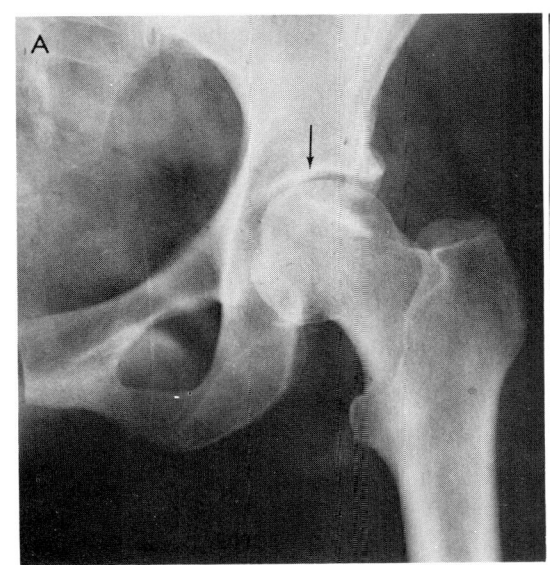

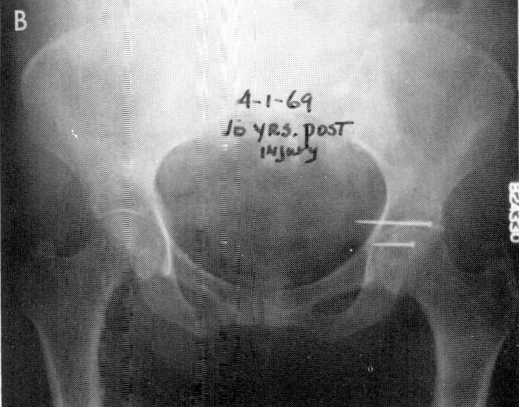

Fig. 27-18.—Superior dome fracture that appeared quite innocent on anteroposterior views. A stereoscopic view demonstrated a large section of the superior dome displaced. Open reduction secured accurate reduction of the dome. B, 16 years after surgery patient had a full range of motion and a painless hip.

weight bearing in 2–3 weeks. Crutches should be used for 3 months, after which they may be discarded if the patient has no pain or limp. However, use of crutches should be continued if there is pain, for the complication of avascular changes of the femoral head must be anticipated. Crutch protection from weight bearing should be continued until this possibility is eliminated.

Fractures of the Superior Dome

These fractures are produced by the upward thrust of the femoral head. In our follow-up study of 26 consecutive patients, results in 58% were evaluated as good to excellent and 42% as fair or poor. In those patients in whom fractures were adequately reduced, reconstructing a smooth articular surface for the superior dome had good results. Those patients in whom weight-bearing surfaces remained inaccurately reduced had poor results. In isolated superior dome fractures, manipulation is relatively ineffective. When the articular surface is unacceptable, an open reduction should be performed, using an anterior approach or a combination of an anterior and intrapelvic approach. Figure 27-18 illustrates a superior dome fracture in which stereoscopic views showed more disruption of the superior dome than did the anteroposterior film. An open reduction, using an anterior approach with multiple screw fixation, resulted in a good articular surface; 16 years after surgery hip function was rated as excellent.

A vertical cleft in the superior dome is illustrated in Figure 27-19. Manipulation proved ineffective and open reduction was carried out with an excellent functional result. In Figure 27-20 is shown the predictable result when the superior dome is *not* reduced by open or closed methods. Within 1 year the hip had deteriorated, necessitating a cup arthroplasty.

Bursting Fractures of the Acetabulum

In our series, bursting fractures proved to be the most serious type, with only 58% of them having results graded good to excellent at follow-up. The same principle was found to be true as in the superior dome fracture, namely that those patients in whom a smooth articular superior dome could be reconstructed did well, whereas those patients in whom the dome could not be reduced did poorly.

In this group, however, the "golden period" of the first 48 hours following injury was extremely important. We have been impressed with the success of early manipulation (within 48 hours) and the decreasing success of manipulation from

Fig. 27-19.—A vertical cleft of the superior dome in an 18-year-old male. **A,** closed manipulation was unsuccessful. **B,** open reduction was performed; using a bolt and screw fixation to secure reduction. Functional result 8 years later was good.

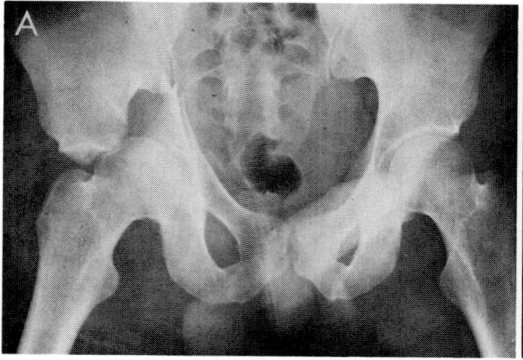

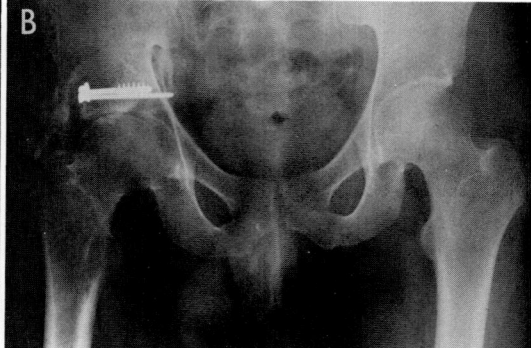

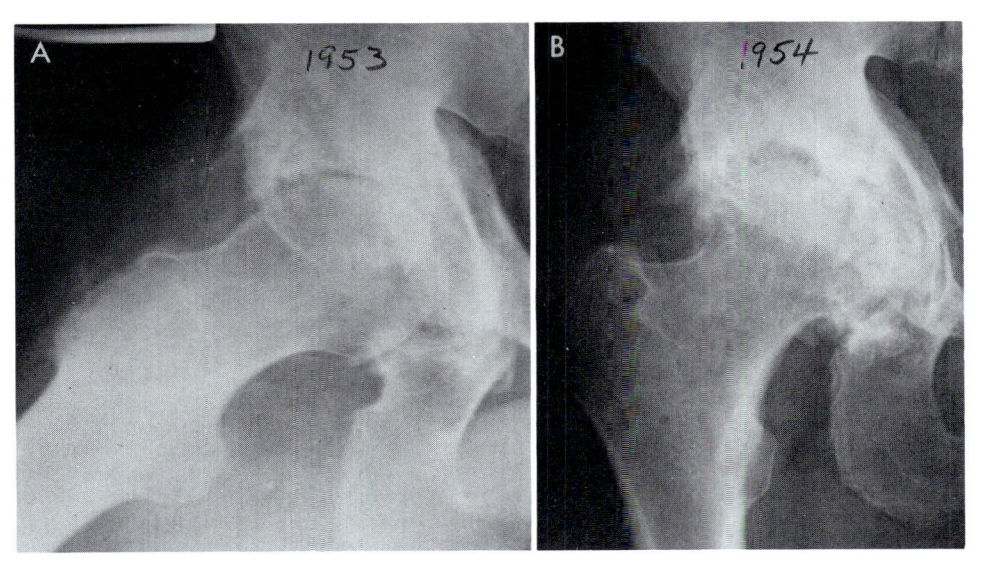

Chapter 27: DISLOCATIONS OF HIP AND FRACTURES OF ACETABULUM / **699**

Fig. 27-20. — Example of failure to reduce a superior dome fracture. **A**, fracture in which neither an open nor a closed reduction was attempted. **B**, 1 year later the hip had severely deteriorated, necessitating a cup arthroplasty.

48 hours on. If manipulation can be carried out before the large blood clots become congealed and organized, the surgeon has a good chance of obtaining a satisfactory reduction. In fact, in some instances, the early application of adequate (20–25 lb) skeletal traction will aid in the reduction of displaced fragments. We are apt to look at x-rays and *forget* that capsule, ligaments and muscles are attached to all displaced fragments (Fig. 27-21). Early traction and correct manipulation will reassemble these fragments via their soft tissue attachments. However, this must be done before the blood clot organizes; otherwise, traction and manipulation are relatively ineffective.

INITIAL TREATMENT. — The extremity should be placed in balanced traction,

Fig. 27-21. — The capsule and ligaments of the hip joint form strong attachments to the acetabulum; this may aid in reducing displaced acetabular fragments, provided *early* manipulation is carried out.

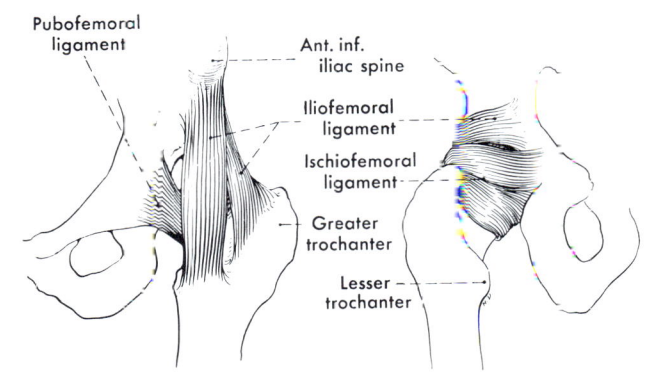

preferably skeletal traction (25 lb or more), with the leg in line with the body, avoiding flexion beyond 35 degrees. As soon as the patient has been thoroughly evaluated and the general condition stabilized, the hip should be manipulated. This sequence is well illustrated in a 26-year-old woman who was admitted to the emergency ward on a Saturday evening after an automobile accident. Examination revealed a patient in shock with sciatic nerve sensory and motor deficits to the left leg. X-rays revealed a shattered left acetabulum, including the pubic and ischial rami, with marked upward displacement of the left ilium (Fig. 27-22). Her general condition stabilized overnight, and at 9 A.M. the following day manipulation was carried out under light general anesthesia. Reduction was most satisfactory. She was maintained in skeletal traction for 10 weeks, during which time daily gentle motions of the hip were carried out. The sciatic nerve deficits

Fig. 27-22. — Severe bursting fracture of the left acetabulum in a woman 26. All elements of the socket were involved, with shattering and upward displacement of the left ilium. **A,** film of the pelvis on admission to emergency ward. **B,** postmanipulation (the following morning). The technique of manipulation is described in Figure 27-23, *A.* **C,** the appearance of the hip 4 months after injury. **D,** result 6 months after injury. At 3 years she has full range of motion and only minimal discomfort.

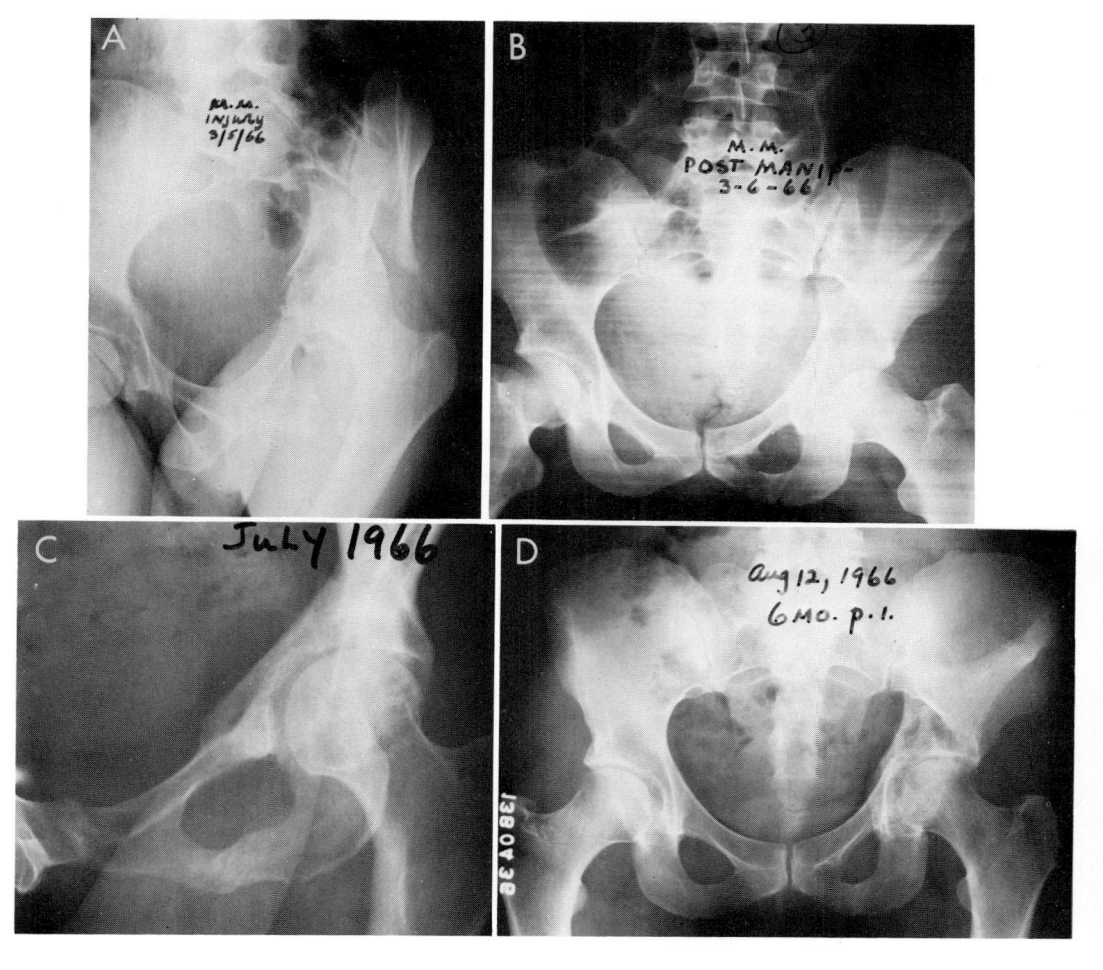

cleared up completely in 1 week. She has had excellent function for the past 3 years.

MANIPULATIVE TECHNIQUES.—The following techniques have been used to extract the femoral head from the pelvis and to reduce the displaced acetabular fragments. In all 4 techniques, the combination of skeletal traction in line of the extremity, plus lateral traction to the thigh in abduction, is used.

Rowe's method (Fig. 27-23, A).—With this technique, the surgeon applies skeletal traction to the leg. He then abducts the extremity laterally. Forceful lateral traction is then applied by a high thigh sheet and the leg is then internally rotated and adducted against the sheet to midline, thus delivering the femoral head from the pelvis. Internal rotation is applied during this manipulation in order to contract the strong obturator internus muscle, which wraps around the interior of the ilium. This technique was used in reducing the fracture-dislocation in Figure 27-22.

Kilfoyle's method (Fig. 27-23, B).— While traction in line of the extremity is being maintained by an assistant, lateral traction to the hip is applied by a sheet tied around the surgeon's waist.

Ray's screw method (Fig. 27-23, C).— Direct pull may be applied to the greater trochanter by means of a Ray trochanteric screw.

Bolster method (Fig. 27-23, D).—The abducting, or lateral, traction may be produced by *adducting* the thighs against a firm bolster placed between the legs.

FOLLOW-UP CARE.—"Early motion and late weight bearing" should be the aim in the management of a bursting acetabular fracture. Early passive motion carried out initially by the surgeon will aid in contouring the fractured fragments to the femoral head. It will also stimulate circulation to the femoral head. Later, the patient will be able actively to carry out motion of the hip. We emphasize again the necessity of keeping the injured leg in line with the body when carrying out motion of the hip. Skeletal traction should be continued for at least 8–10 weeks in severe bursting fractures, in order that the bony fragments may heal and a protective fibrocartilage layer cover the socket. After removal of skeletal traction, the patient should be allowed free active motion in bed, with the aid of slings, until satisfactory active muscle control of the extremity has been regained.

The patient's hip should be protected with crutches, with only light touchdown pressure on the injured extremity, for at least a year. Crutches should not be discarded until the patient demonstrates ability to walk without a limp and without pain. It is most important that x-rays are taken at intervals during the first year and at yearly intervals for 5 years. If pain and a limp occur during this time, the patient should return to the use of crutches and report for a checkup with the surgeon.

Prognosis in Dislocations of the Hip

The future function of a reduced dislocated hip depends primarily on the degree of injury sustained by the femoral head and acetabulum. This of course cannot always be accurately determined at the time of injury. To determine prognosis, hip dislocations may be classified into 2 groups: the uncomplicated and the complicated.

The *uncomplicated* cases are those in which the hip was reduced promptly and without undue trauma. The *complicated* are those in which 1 or all of the following conditions were present:

1. Reduction was delayed, or several unsuccessful attempts to reduce the hip preceded the final closed or open reduction.

2. There was x-ray evidence of fracture of the femoral head (Fig. 27-24).

3. Loose bone fragments in the joint were not removed.

4. Unreduced posterior or superior acetabular fractures complicated the dislocation.

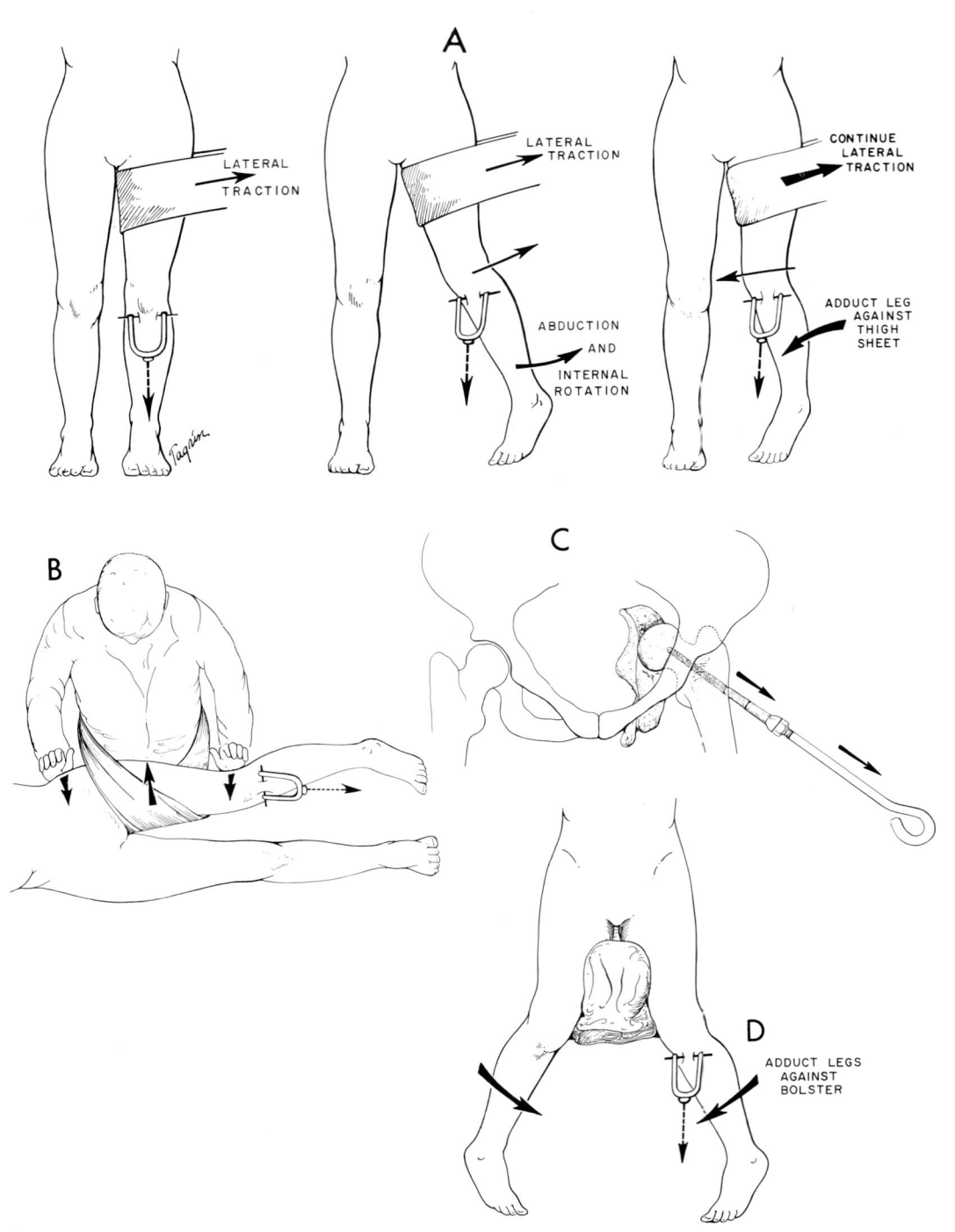

Fig. 27-23.—Manipulation techniques. **A**, the Rowe method; **B**, the Kilfoyle method; **C**, the Ray screw method; **D**, the bolster method.

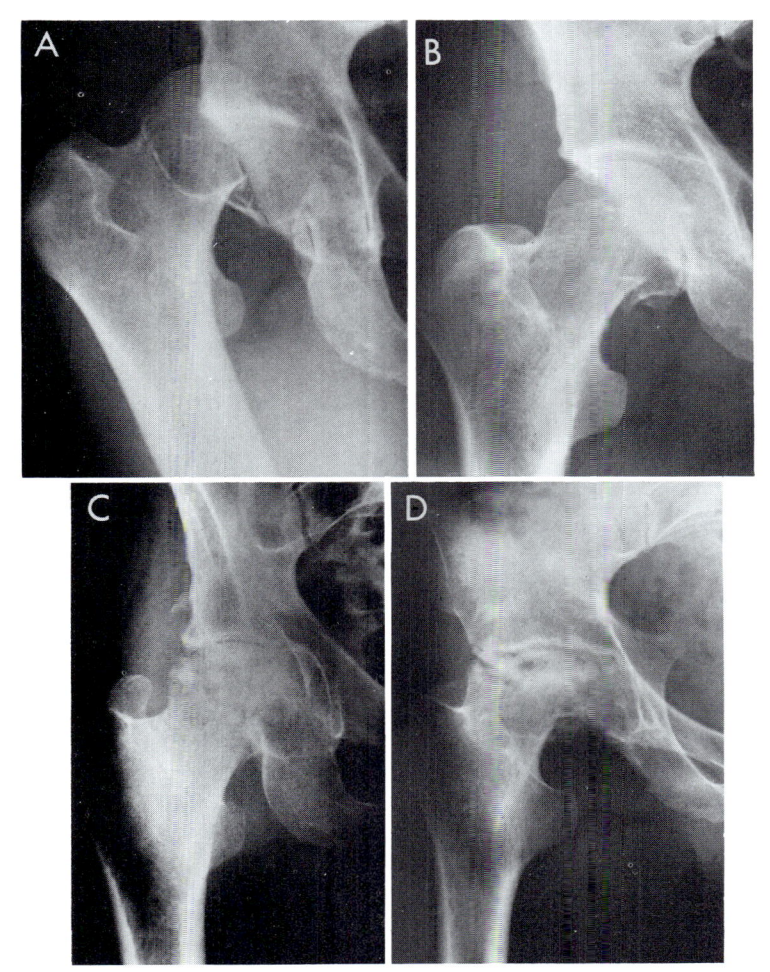

Fig. 27-24. — Importance in prognosis of injury to femoral head at time of dislocation of hip. **A**, posterior dislocation of hip. **B**, reduction of hip showing fracture of femoral head. **C** and **D**, views showing progressive aseptic necrosis of femoral head, for which an arthroplasty was later performed.

As shown in Table 27-4, the prognosis in the uncomplicated dislocations is excellent; whereas in the complicated dislocations the outlook is poor.

Prognosis in Fractures of the Acetabulum

The prognosis in acetabular fractures depends on the location of the fracture. Fractures of the superior or posterior quadrants generally carry a guarded prognosis. Those of the central area without dislocation of the femoral head usually do well.

In comminuted acetabular fractures in which a smooth superior articular surface was obtained either by manipulation or open reduction, 91% of the cases resulted in excellent or good hips. Of the hips with unreduced superior quadrants, 83% gave fair to poor hips.

TABLE 27-4.—FOLLOW-UP STUDY OF 37 HIP DISLOCATIONS

Uncomplicated dislocations (22 cases)		
Excellent	14	91%
Good	6	
Fair	0	9%
Poor	2	
Complicated dislocations (15 cases)		
Excellent	0	14%
Good	2	
Fair	3	86%
Poor	10	
Over-all prognosis (37 patients)		
Excellent	14	59%
Good	8	
Fair	3	41%
Poor	12	

Complications of Hip Dislocations and Acetabular Fractures

INTRA-ARTICULAR CHANGES.—The most common complications found in the series of 107 cases at Massachusetts General Hospital were intra-articular changes, which occurred in 47% of the cases. These changes were (1) traumatic arthritis, (2) aseptic necrosis of the femoral head, (3) fractures of the femoral head or (4) loose bodies. In some instances, both traumatic arthritis and aseptic necrosis of the femoral head occurred. The majority of aseptic necrosis complications developed in the hip dislocations. A significant finding was that clinical signs of aseptic necrosis and traumatic arthritis usually developed within a year of injury. An injured hip should be followed closely for several years. If, however, at the end of a year the patient is symptom-free and x-ray films are satisfactory, the patient stands a favorable chance of having a good hip.

SCIATIC NERVE INJURY.—Injuries to the sciatic nerve were next in frequency, occurring in 12% of the injured hips. All such injuries occurred in posterior dislocations. In fact, in 27% of the posterior dislocations there were symptoms or signs of sciatic nerve injury. Of these, 61% were temporary injuries and 29% were permanent partial injuries to the nerve.

VASCULAR INJURIES.—Vascular complications, primarily in the form of thrombophlebitis, were present in only 6.5% of the hip injuries. Pulmonary infarct occurred in 3 patients, with 1 death. The majority (43%) of the thrombophlebitic complications were in the simple, undisplaced acetabular fractures. No major vascular injury occurred at the time of dislocation of the hip or fracture of the acetabulum. Death due to vascular complications occurred in 0.9% of patients with hip injuries.

ASSOCIATED FRACTURES, OTHER THAN THE HIP.—Fractures of the femoral shaft were associated with dislocation of the hip in 5 instances (4.6%) and patellar fractures in 6 instances (5.6%).

SURGICAL APPROACHES TO THE HIP

Technique of Anterior Approach

A small sandbag or rolled towel is placed under the margin of the sacrum so that the injured hip is raised. In this position the surgeon can easily palpate the anterosuperior spine and the interval between the sartorius muscle and the tensor fascia lata (Fig. 27-25). The incision is started on the crest of the ilium at about the tubercle of the tensor fascia femoris and is carried down across the anterosuperior spine and distally and laterally along the anterior margin of the tensor out to the iliotibial band. The lower end of the incision ends just below a line horizontal to the symphysis pubis. Sharp and blunt dissection is carried out in the interval between the sartorius and the tensor. The tip of the tensor is then removed subperiosteally from the lateral margin of the crest of the ilium and brought down to and along the interval between the anterior and inferior spines of the iliac bone. The originating points

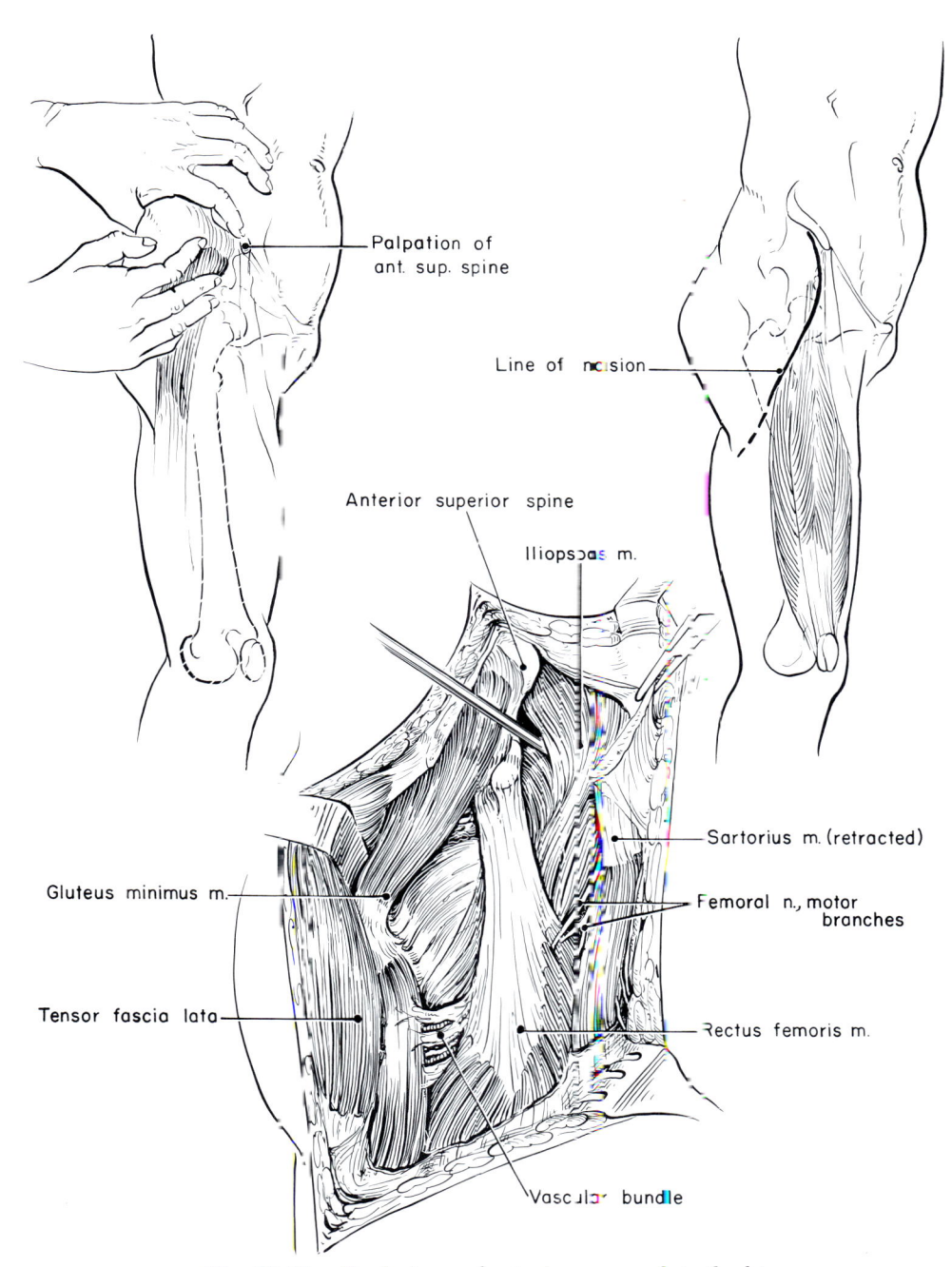

Chapter 27: DISLOCATIONS OF HIP AND FRACTURES OF ACETABULUM / 705

Fig. 27-25.—Technique of anterior approach to the hip.

of the sartorius and Poupart's ligament are reflected subperiosteally from the medial margin of the pelvis down to the anteroinferior spine of the iliac bone. This allows retraction of the sartorius muscle and Poupart's ligament medially, and of the tensor laterally, to expose the underlying straight and reflected heads of the rectus femoris muscle (Fig. 27-25). The anterior circumflex iliac vessels between the vastus externus and the tensor are then identified and ligated in the fascial sheath on the lateral margin of the vastus externus. The fascial compartment in this area is then split down to the vastus externus. The dissection is carried up along the anterior margin of the gluteus minimus tendon to the superior neck of the hip and toward the acetabulum. This allows exposure of the anterior capsule in its superior and lateral portions (Fig. 27-26). The medial side of the incision then is enlarged in the interval between the iliacus and capsular origin of the iliopsoas. The anterior acetabulum is then exposed to the inferior neck, and the dissection is carried bluntly and deeply to the lesser trochanter. With these 2 margins exposed medially and laterally, sharp dissection may be made into the capsule and synovia and through the straight and reflected heads of the rectus from the anteroinferior spine across the superior neck out to the greater trochanter. The tip of the rectus and the anterior capsule now can be turned down distally in 1 piece. This exposes the anterior acetabulum and the anterior margin of the

Fig. 27-26.—The anatomy, in the anterior approach, allows complete exposure of the hip.

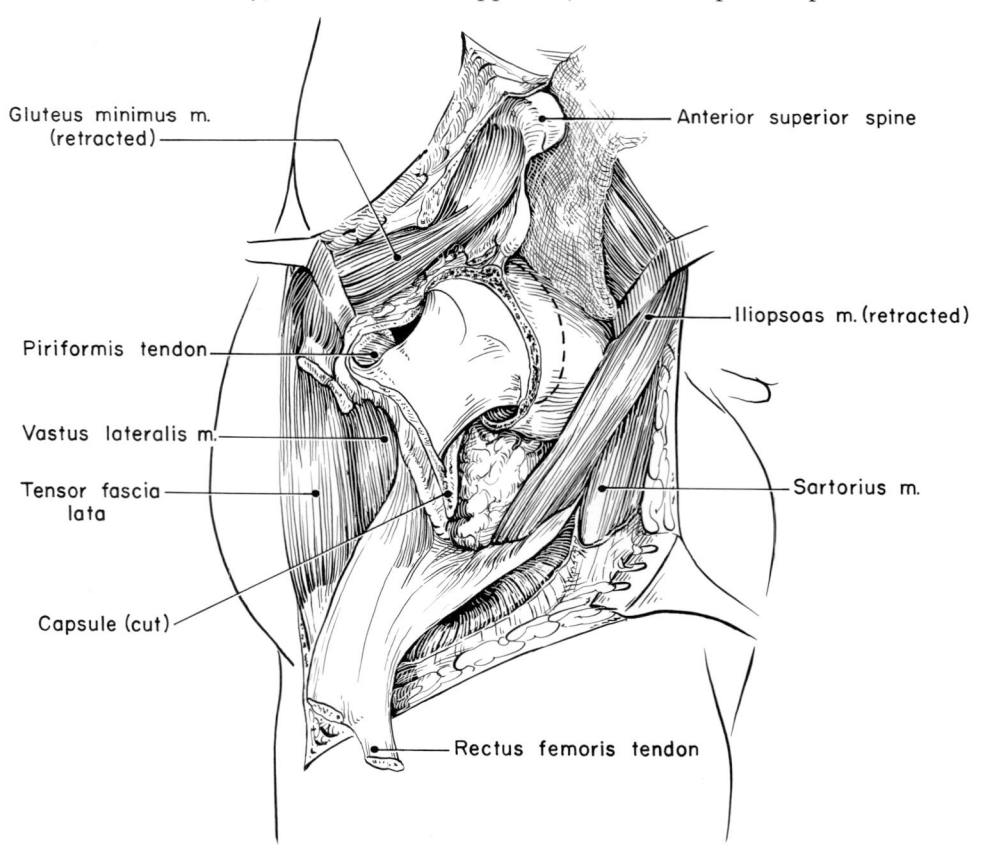

Chapter 27: DISLOCATIONS OF HIP AND FRACTURES OF ACETABULUM / 707

head and neck out to the greater trochanter. A tenotomy of the gluteus minimus tendon will facilitate greater exposure of the superior margin of the neck and allow more room superiorly. The head and neck can then be easily dislocated for any type of acetabular or neck surgery.

If more exposure of the posterior neck is necessary, such as in replacement prosthesis, complete capsulotomy is possible inferiorly and posteriorly. The base of the neck can be protruded into the wound by extending the thigh over the margin of the table laterally. In this position, the application of pressure to the sole of the foot directly in line toward the anterosuperior spine with the knee extended will dislocate the hip anteriorly. Then, by releasing the structures posteriorly, it is a relatively simple, mechanical job to replace a femoral head or do a femoral head prosthesis in this position.

Modifications of this technique which use only the interval between the tensor and the rectus for nailing are adequate in most instances. Such modifications constitute only the lateral portion of the incision without release of the structures from the crest of the ilium. By release of these muscles, however, it is possible to

Fig. 27-27.—The position of the patient and the incisions for lateral and posterior approaches to the hip.

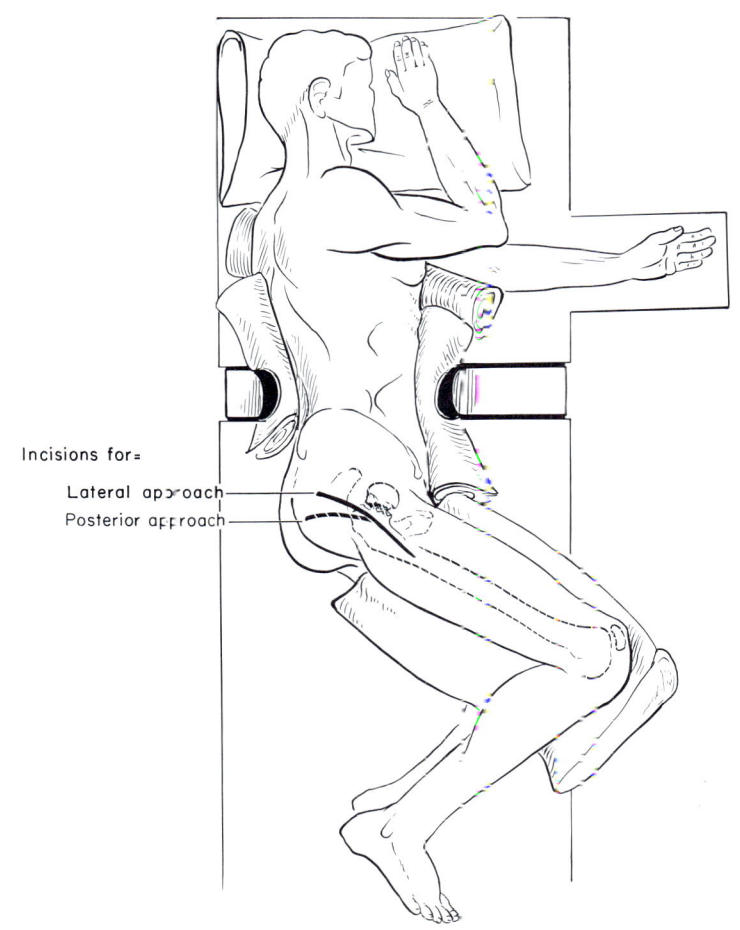

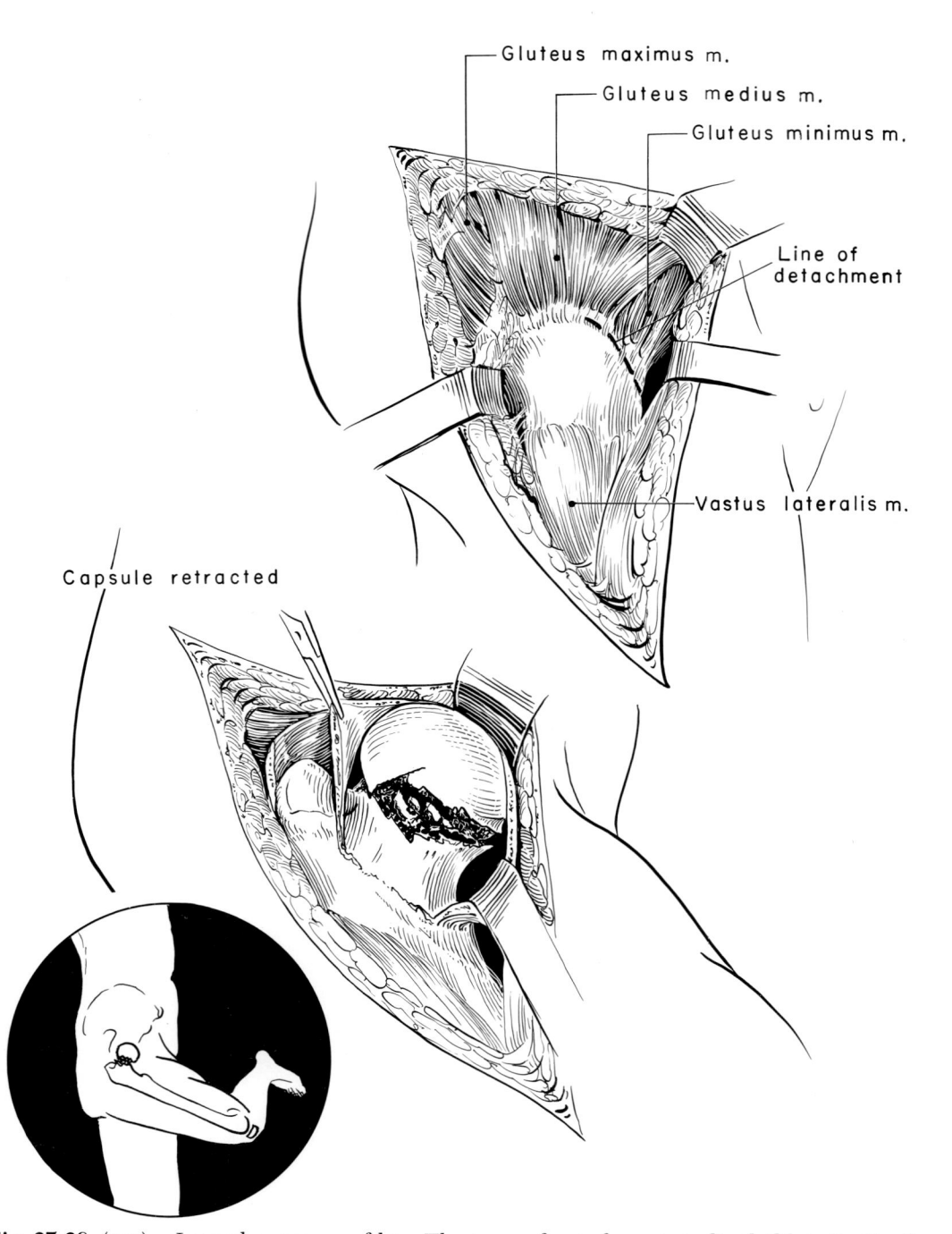

Fig. 27-28. (top).—Lateral exposure of hip. The tensor fascia femoris is divided longitudinally and retracted, exposing the attachments to the greater trochanter. The dotted line indicates the limited detachment of the gluteus minimus and medius muscles that is necessary to expose the capsule.

Fig. 27-29. (bottom).—Technique for presenting the intertrochanteric line. The hip is externally rotated and flexed, and the capsule is opened to expose the femoral neck and head. More extensive exposure can be obtained by completely separating the gluteus medius muscle from the greater trochanter.

Chapter 27: DISLOCATIONS OF HIP AND FRACTURES OF ACETABULUM / 709

get closer to the anterior acetabulum without undue retraction.

The surgeon should modify the incision into a joint according to the particular needs of the individual case. Such adaptation requires a detailed study of the anatomy and an understanding of what really needs to be exposed before beginning the procedure. More details of these surgical exposures may be obtained from any standard textbook on orthopedic surgery, and specific details from *Campbell's Operative Orthopaedics*.

Technique of Lateral Approach

The patient is turned on his side, with the injured hip upward, and is maintained in this position by rolled blankets placed anteriorly and posteriorly and fixed with kidney rests (Fig. 27-27). The incision begins above and posterior to the greater trochanter and extends distally over the trochanter and down along the shaft for 4–6 in. The tensor fascia femoris is divided longitudinally, exposing the greater trochanter (Fig. 27-28).

The attachment of the anterior capsule along the intertrochanteric line is exposed by reflecting posteriorly the gluteus minimus attachment and a portion of the gluteus medius attachment.

In fresh fractures of the femoral neck, it is not necessary to detach the entire gluteus medius; rather, the extremity is externally rotated and the capsule is opened by a ⊥-shaped incision and extended to the acetabular rim (Fig. 27-29). Through this exposure the head of the femur can be removed and a replacement

Fig. 27-30.—Posterior approach to the hip for exposing the external rotators of the hip and the sciatic nerve. The gluteus maximus muscle is separated in line of its fibers. The posterior hip and acetabular rim can be exposed by detaching the external rotators.

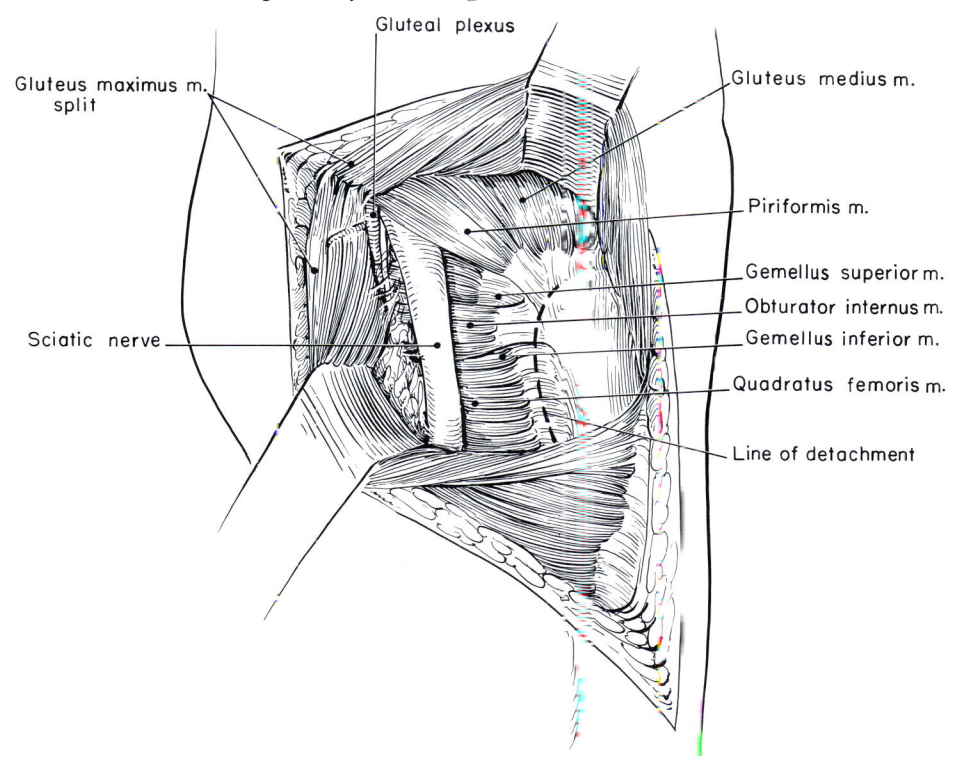

prosthesis inserted. For more extensive surgical procedures on the hip, it will be necessary to detach completely the gluteus medius from the greater trochanter, thus exposing the anterior, lateral and posterior aspects of the hip.

Technique of Posterior Approach

This approach is used primarily for exposure of the posterior acetabulum and the sciatic nerve. The patient is positioned as for the lateral approach, with the injured hip upward. The incision begins at a point midway between the posterior superior spine and the trochanter. It is angled forward and then distally over the greater trochanter and down the shaft for 4–6 in.

The tensor fascia femoris is divided longitudinally and retracted anteriorly. The belly of the gluteus maximus muscle is exposed. The gluteus maximus is divided in line of its fibers, exposing the external rotators of the hip. Care should be exercised to identify the sciatic nerve as it leaves the pelvis between the piriformis and gemellus superior.(Fig. 27-30). To expose the posterior capsule, the external rotators (gemullus superior, obturator internus, gemullus inferior, and obturator externus) are divided from their insertions to the greater trochanter. The capsule is then opened in a T-shaped manner and the joint examined.

BIBLIOGRAPHY

1. Armstrong, J. R.: Traumatic dislocation of the hip joint, J. Bone Joint Surg. 30-B:430, 1948.
2. Baker, W. J.: The management of the urinary tract in fractures of the bony pelvis, Am. Acad. Orthop. Surg. Instructional Course Lectures, XI, p. 245, 1954.
3. Bigelow, H. J.: *Mechanism of Dislocation and Fracture of the Hip with Reduction of the Dislocation by the Flexion Method* (Philadelphia: Henry C. Lea, 1869).
4. Cooper, Sir Astley: *A Treatise on Dislocations and on Fractures of the Joints* (Philadelphia: Carey & Lea, 1825).
5. Eichenholtz, S. N., and Stark, R. M.: Central acetabular fractures, J. Bone Joint Surg. 46-A:695, 1964.
6. Epstein, H. C.: Posterior fracture-dislocation of the hip, J. Bone Joint Surg. 43-A:1079, 1961.
7. Froman, C., and Stein, A.: Complicated crushing injuries of the pelvis, J. Bone Joint Surg. 49-B:24, 1967.
8. Hand, J. R.: Surgery of the Penis and Urethra, in Campbell, M. F. (ed.), *Urology* (2d ed.; Philadelphia: W. B. Saunders Company, 1963.)
9. Hawkins, L., Pomerantz, M., and Eiseman, B.: Laparotomy at the time of pelvic fractures. Read before Am. Assoc. Surg. Trauma, Oct. 2, 1969.
10. Holdsworth, F. W.: Dislocation and fracture-dislocation of the pelvis, J. Bone Joint Surg. 30-B:461, 1948.
11. Instructional Course, Am. Acad. Orthop. Surg., Chicago, January, 1968.
12. Judet, R., Judet, J., and Letournel, E.: Fractures of the acetabulum: Classification and surgical approaches, J. Bone Joint Surg. 46-A:1615, 1964.
13. Knight, R. A., and Smith, H.: Central fractures of the acetabulum, J. Bone Joint Surg. 40-A:1, 1958.
14. Miller, W. E.: Massive hemorrhage in fractures of the pelvis, South. Med. J. 56:933, 1963.
15. Moorehouse, D., and MacKinnon, K. J.: Urological injuries associated with pelvic fractures, J. Trauma 9:479, 1969.
16. Okelberry, A. M.: Fractures of floor of acetabulum, J. Bone Joint Surg. 38-A:441, 1956.
17. Pearson, J. R., and Hargadon, E. J.: Fractures of the pelvis involving the floor of the acetabulum, J. Bone Joint Surg. 44-B:550, 1962.
18. Peltier, L. F.: Complications associated with fractures of the pelvis, J. Bone Joint Surg. 47-A:1060, 1965.
19. Quinby, W. C.: Fractures of the pelvis and associated injuries in children, J. Pediatr. Surg. 1:353, 1966.
20. Rowe, C. R., and Lowell, J. D.: Prognosis of fractures of the acetabulum, J. Bone Joint Surg. 43-A:30, 1961.
21. Stewart, M., Jr., and Milford, L. W.: Fracture-dislocation of the hip, J. Bone Joint Surg. 36-A:315, 1954.
22. Stimson, L. A.: *A Practical Treatise on Fractures and Dislocations* (Philadelphia: Lea & Febiger, 1917).
23. Urist, M. R.: Injuries to the hip joint, traumatic dislocation incurred chiefly in jeep accidents in World War II, Am. J. Surg. 74:586, 1947.
24. Urist, M. R.: Fractures and dislocations of the hip: The nature of the traumatic lesion, treatment and 2 year end-results, Ann. Surg. 127:1150, 1948.
25. Urist, M. R.: Fractures and dislocations of the hip: Traumatic lesion, treatment, late complications, and end results, J. Bone Joint Surg. 30-A:699, 1948.
26. Winston, M. E.: Fractures of the floor of the acetabulum and traumatic central dislocation of the hip, Surg. Gynecol. Obstet. 113:479, 1961.

28 | Reconstructive Surgery of the Hip Following Trauma

WILLIAM H. HARRIS

MOST PATIENTS WITH FRACTURED ACETABULA or fracture-dislocations of the hip never require late reconstructive surgery. Even among those who do, there is usually a long period of useful function before reconstruction is needed. This frequently is true despite a very abnormal appearance of the hip on x-ray examination. For example, in a recent study of 39 patients with traumatic arthritis of the hip treated with cup arthroplasty, the average interval between injury and the reconstruction was 7.7 years.[3] This is the average duration in the group that did come to surgery. Obviously the patients with less severe symptoms have completely avoided surgery thus far.

In the chapters on fractures and fracture-dislocations of the hip, the key principle in the proper *early* management has been stressed, namely, the restoration of a stable, congruous weight-bearing dome. The prognosis will depend, of course, on the type and severity of the fracture or fracture-dislocation, on the success of the initial restoration of the joint and on whether or not avascular necrosis develops.

EARLY RECONSTRUCTIONS

Arthroplasty of the hip, in contrast to correction of the fracture damage and restoration of normal anatomy, is rarely indicated immediately after dislocation or fracture-dislocation. In essence, the only indication for arthroplasty is the irreparable disruption of the weight-bearing mechanism. This can take the following 3 forms: irreparable posterior acetabular instability (Fig. 28-1); demolition of the weight-bearing dome of the acetabulum, and severe fracture of the femoral head or neck. All of these are quite rare. Usually, despite severe injury, the posterior lip and the weight-bearing dome can be successfully reconstructed by appropriate surgery following the initial injury (Chapter 27).

If it is not possible to restore posterior stability or the weight-bearing dome, 2 options arise—total hip replacement and cup arthroplasty. Rarely will the conditions exist that will warrant a fusion. The selection of total hip replacement or cup arthroplasty will depend on both general and local factors. Total hip replacement is preferable because it provides better results in much less time. However, at present, since the known duration of successful use of total hip replacement is limited, this form of therapy should be confined to patients with a limited life span, for example, patients over 50 years of age. For younger patients, cup arthroplasty should be used. Cup arthroplasty

711

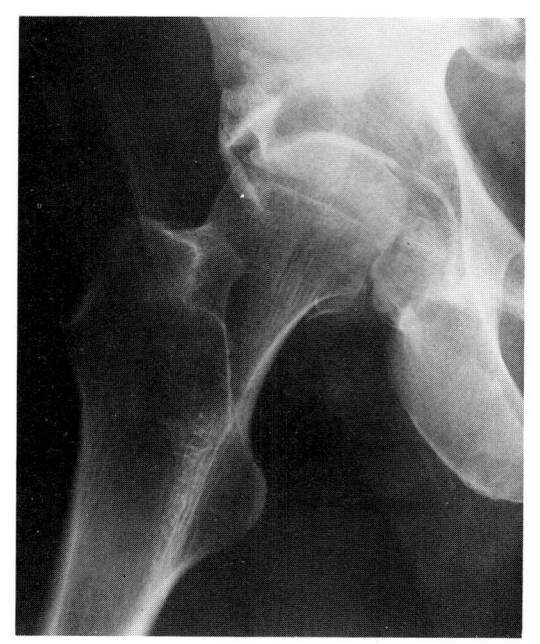

Fig. 28-1.—Anteroposterior film of hip in man, 53, who sustained a severe fracture-dislocation, gross disruption of the posterior lip of the acetabulum and fracture of the femoral head. Despite 2 closed reductions, the femoral head redislocated posteriorly because of the gross instability of the posterior lip.

has proved quite effective in the management of the small number of cases requiring early surgery because of recurrent instability (Fig. 28-2). It has also been used occasionally to restore a dome when the acetabulum has been massively disrupted (Fig. 28-3).

Several problems accompany reconstructive surgery in these patients. First, the acetabulum is so badly damaged that its reconstruction, whether by total hip replacement or cup arthroplasty, may be quite difficult and require considerable innovation. For posterior instability, the optimal approach is to move the dome of the socket medially, taking maximal advantage of the remaining intact acetabular stock. This medial transplantation of the socket is essential for a cup arthroplasty, since cartilaginous metaplasia must develop from the intact cancellous surfaces. It is also essential in total hip replacement, because placement of the socket component in a precarious position without lateral or posterior support carries with it a high risk of the socket breaking loose.

Similarly, with severe disruption of the dome, seating the cup or seating the acetabular component of the total hip replacement can be demanding. The methylmethacrylate can help hold fragments in position, but to do so effectively it must be well anchored into the stable acetabular stock at several other points.

LATE RECONSTRUCTION

For those patients requiring late reconstruction for traumatic arthritis, a clear distinction must be made between *cartilage damage* and *avascular necrosis* as the underlying pathology. This distinction is critical to the type of surgery required and the timing of the surgery.

Following the initial management of the injuries, reconstructive surgery falls into 5 broad categories:

1. The management of changes secondary to avascular necrosis.
2. The management of severe damage to the articular cartilage, with or without avascular necrosis of the femoral head.
3. The management of recurrent instability.
4. The management of postoperative sepsis.
5. The management of myositis ossificans.

Avascular Necrosis

In the management of the secondary changes of avascular necrosis, the key decisions are based on the condition of the articular cartilage of the acetabulum. Collapse of the avascular head will lead to destruction of the acetabular cartilage, if untreated. As the dead bone and repair tissue in the femoral head collapse, the articular surface of the femoral head buckles and becomes irregular. This irregu-

Chapter 28: RECONSTRUCTIVE SURGERY OF THE HIP FOLLOWING TRAUMA / 713

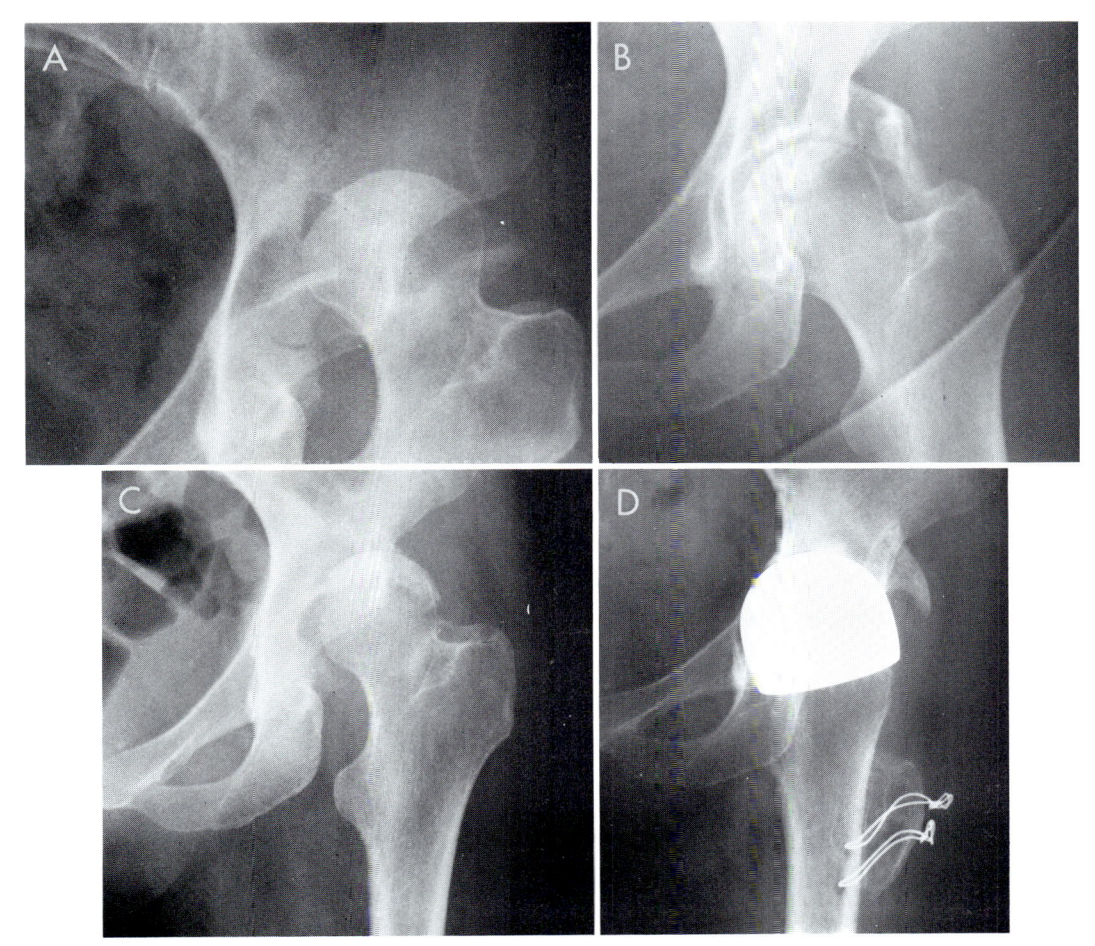

Fig. 28-2. — **A**, anteroposterior film of left hip of woman, aged 41, who sustained a severe fracture-dislocation in an automobile accident. In addition to disruption of the posterolateral acetabular wall, there is disruption of the superior weight-bearing dome. **B**, open reduction was carried out but no internal fixation was used. The patient was treated in traction for 16 weeks. **C**, 10 days after traction was discontinued the femoral head had dislocated again. **D**, the patient was transferred to Massachusetts General Hospital and a cup arthroplasty carried out. A new acetabulum was fashioned which provided stability by moving the acetabulum medially. The medial wall of the bony acetabulum was purposely removed to facilitate this medial translocation of the acetabulum. The greater trochanter was transplanted distally.

lar surface, in turn, will erode the acetabular cartilage. Because of this potentially destructive sequence, close follow-up of every dislocation and fracture-dislocation is required. The earliest signs of secondary change of avascular necrosis must be carefully sought. They are (1) a thin radiolucent line just beneath the subchondral cartilage in the femoral head,[1] (2) slight narrowing of the joint space, (3) loss of sphericity of the femoral head and (4) density changes. Tomography and occasionally pertrochanteric biopsy and arthrography are of value in establishing the diagnosis early. Close follow-up is required for at least 3 years, despite statements to the effect that most avascular necrosis will show up within 1 year.

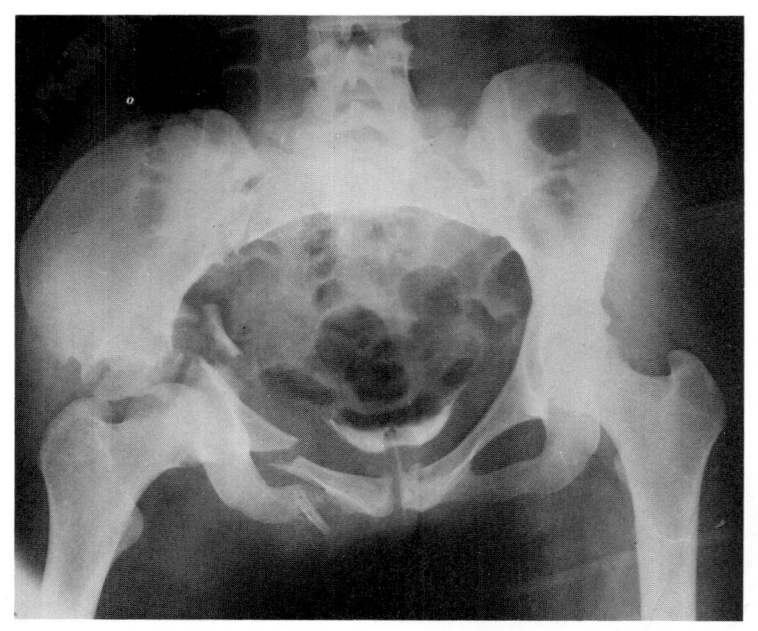

Fig. 28-3.—Anteroposterior view of hips and pelvis of 28-year-old woman who sustained a massive disruption of the right innominate bone. Under such rare circumstances as these, occasionally primary cup arthroplasty or, in older age groups, total hip replacement will be indicated.

Segmental collapse may first appear as late as 5 years after the dislocation (Fig. 28-4).

If the patient has a limited life span by virtue of age or other disease, asymptomatic avascular necrosis should be observed and operation not resorted to. It is well known that many patients with roentgenographically demonstrable avascular necrosis will remain completely or nearly completely asymptomatic until late in the course of the disease, sometimes long after the socket begins to fail. Thus, surgical intervention becomes a matter of judgment. In patients with a limited life span, expectant treatment is indicated, with total hip replacement to be undertaken subsequently if increasing pain or decreasing function demands a reconstruction.

The situation in patients too young for total hip replacement is far more intricate. In this group, progressive damage to the acetabular cartilage by the irregular necrotic femoral head should be prevented by early femoral head replacement. Cup arthroplasty is not indicated for 2 reasons: because the articular cartilage is intact and because marked shortening would result from removal of the avascular femoral head. Osteotomy is inappropriate treatment for avascular necrosis.

Following insertion of the prosthesis, the patient should remain on crutches until the prosthesis has solidified in the femur, as evidenced by the development of sclerosis, usually a minimum of 6 months.

Occasionally such surgery will even be indicated in patients who are asymptomatic or nearly so. In the young patient it is clearly indicated even in the absence of symptoms, once avascular necrosis is definitely established, in order to avoid progressive destruction of the intact acetabular cartilage. The aim is to preserve

Chapter 28: RECONSTRUCTIVE SURGERY OF THE HIP FOLLOWING TRAUMA / 715

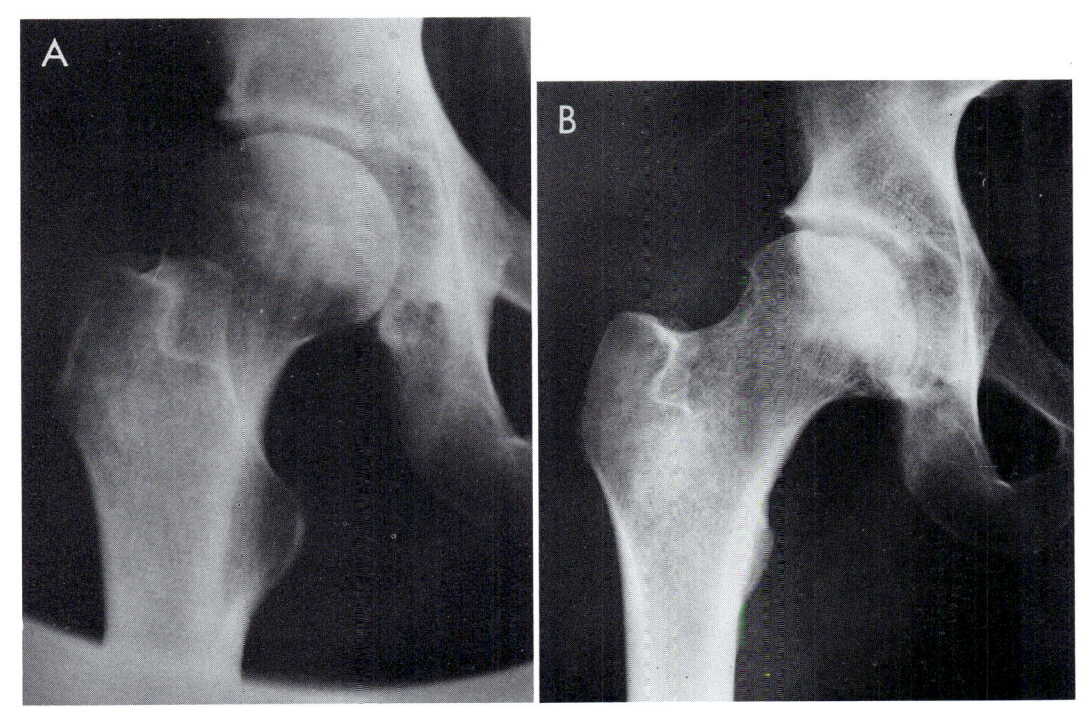

Fig. 28-4.—**A,** anteroposterior film of the right hip of 27-year-old man 2 years after closed reduction of dislocated hip. **B,** 7 years later there is clear-cut evidence of avascular necrosis with segmental collapse. (From Harris, W. H.: Traumatic arthritis of the hip after dislocation and acetabular fractures: Treatment by mold arthroplasty, J. Bone Joint Surg. 51-A:737, 1969.)

the intact cartilage by excising the avascular femoral head before it can destroy the socket. Prosthetic replacement has the advantages of preserving leg length, providing excellent function and preserving the normal acetabulum without the uncertainty of using a total replacement in the younger age group.

At surgery it is important to appreciate that the first change in the acetabular articular cartilage in avascular necrosis of the femoral head usually occurs at the lateral margin of the acetabulum. This is the most difficult area of the acetabulum to visualize, even with wide exposure. Careful inspection of this specific area is necessary before making a final decision that the acetabular cartilage is adequate to accept the prosthesis.

If in a young patient the x-ray films reveal that the acetabular contour or the acetabular cartilage is unsatisfactory, the urgency to perform prophylactic surgery to protect the socket from further destruction no longer exists. Under these circumstances, reconstructive surgery would be delayed until it is required on the basis of pain or limited function alone. Then the decision must be made whether to accept the shortening that would result from a cup arthroplasty or to do a total replacement. As the longevity of successful total hip replacement increases, this decision is swinging more and more toward total replacement. This is particularly true with the development of the easily replaceable acetabular component which makes wear of the prosthesis much less of a threat. In the face of avascular necrosis of the femoral head, fusion is difficult to obtain and in most instances is contraindicated.[6]

Cartilage Destruction

Destruction of the joint cartilage is the most common cause of symptoms following fracture of the acetabulum or fracture-dislocation. Most often it is due to inaccurate replacement of the fracture fragments, but there are other causes, such as the abrasive effect of small bits of bone and cartilaginous débris retained within the joint, the wearing that is secondary to segmental collapse of the femoral head or an irregular contour after femoral head fracture, and the effect of direct trauma to the cartilage at the time of injury. Although occasionally limited motion or deformity will bring the patient to surgery, usually pain or decreased functional capacity, such as limp or limited walking, is the chief complaint.[3]

The 3 types of surgery that warrant consideration are total hip replacement, cup arthroplasty and fusion. Osteotomy is rarely indicated. Patients over age 50 should have total hip replacement (Fig. 28-5), unless sepsis has been present. Until further data on the durability of the total hip replacement covers are available, it seems unwise to extend the indications for this type of surgery beyond this limit, unless special circumstances are present.

In the patients who are too young for total hip replacement, cup arthroplasty and fusion should be considered. Based on a long-term follow-up of 39 patients having cup arthroplasties for this condi-

Fig. 28-5.—**A,** anteroposterior film of right hip of 53-year-old man with a fracture-dislocation of the hip due to an automobile accident. He had severe pain and marked limitation of motion and required crutches. Because he had severe cardiac disease, total hip replacement was preferable to cup arthroplasty. **B,** appearance following Charnley-Müller type total hip replacement.

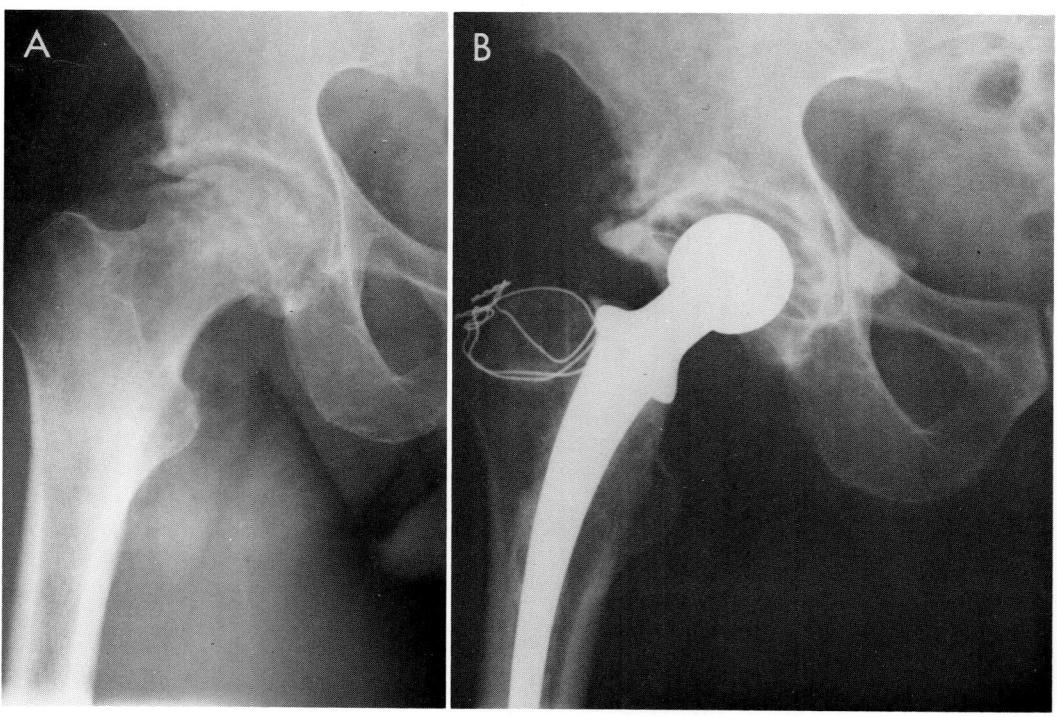

tion,[3] arthroplasty is preferable in most patients unless there is a specific indication for fusion, such as spasticity or the inability to carry out the rehabilitation program.

Sepsis

The incidence of sepsis following open reduction of fracture or fracture-dislocation of the acetabulum is higher than it is in many other major hip operations. This is understandable because of the massive tissue damage that may be present, the proximity of some incisions to fecal contamination and the other debilitating injuries that may have occurred simultaneously. When sepsis complicates open reduction, late reconstructive surgery will usually be required.

Total hip reconstruction is clearly contraindicated. Cup arthroplasty has been used quite successfully to solve both the joint problem and the septic problem and is preferable to hip fusion in most cases.[3]

A massive debridement is needed and 6 weeks of high-intensity antibiotic therapy should follow, during which the tissues are put at rest in a spica cast. Under selected circumstances, the use of a metal implant in the form of a cup arthroplasty in the face of infection can be carried out successfully in violation of the usual principle in the management of infection. Fusion is also appropriate in some of these patients, but a sound fusion may be difficult to obtain when sepsis is active, and it does not, per se, eliminate the possibility of recrudescence of infection.

Myositis Ossificans

Small or moderate deposits of ectopic, periarticular bone formation are common sequelae of dislocations, fractures of the acetabulum and fracture-dislocations. Open reduction increases the incidence and may increase the massiveness of the deposit. Hip function is rarely significantly compromised by this new bone formation. In the few instances in which it is, management may be difficult. If the joint itself is intact, excision of the myositis may be of considerable value. The procedure, however, is usually long and tedious, with rather large amounts of blood loss. The excision is often incomplete and recurrence is common. Excision should be delayed until 1 year after initial appearance of the ectopic bone.

If joint reconstruction is required in addition to removal of the ectopic bone deposit, the criteria detailed previously should be followed. In patients over 50, total hip replacement is the optimal treatment. In those under 50, cup arthroplasty should be carried out. Occasionally, a fusion will be indicated; if fusion has already been created by the ectopic bone formation but the position of the femur is unsatisfactory, a corrective osteotomy to improve the position may be the preferred solution.

Following cup arthroplasty for traumatic arthritis: the incidence of myositis ossificans prior to cup arthroplasty was 4 of 39 cases;[3] nine of 25 patients who were free of myositis prior to cup arthroplasty did have it after operation, but in only 1 was it of any clinical significance. In that 1 patient, revision of the arthroplasty led to excellent restoration of a satisfactory range of motion.

The incidence of myositis following total hip replacement is less than that after cup arthroplasty,[2] and usually it is of less clinical significance.

BIBLIOGRAPHY

1. d'Aubigne, M. R., Postel, M., Massabraud, A., Massas, P., and Cueguen, J.: Idiopathic necrosis of the femoral head in adults, J. Bone Joint Surg. 47-B:612, 1965.
2. Hamblen, D., and Harris, W. H.: Unpublished data.
3. Harris, W. H.: Traumatic arthritis of the hip after dislocation and acetabular fractures: Treatment by mold arthroplasty, J. Bone Joint Surg. 51-A: 737, 1969.
4. Harris, W. H.: A new total hip implant, Clin. Orthop. 81:105, 1971.
5. Harris, W. H.: Surgical management of arthritis of the hip, Semin. Arthritis Rheum. 1:35, 1971.
6. Watson-Jones, R., and Robinson, W. C.: Arthrodesis of the osteoarthritic hip, J. Bone Joint Surg. 38-B:353 1956.

29 | Fractures of the Femoral Shaft

DINESH PATEL and THORNTON BROWN

Fractures of the shaft of the femur are relatively common, serious injuries that may cause prolonged morbidity and severe permanent disability. Usually they are the result of automobile accidents, falls from a height, crushing, or other major violence, but they may also result from no more than a violent muscle contraction or from excess and unaccustomed activity, such as that sometimes observed in the fatigue fractures of military recruits. The femur is also a common site of pathologic fracture secondary to neoplastic involvement or bone disease.

Since fractures of the femoral shaft are usually the result of accidents involving high-energy dissipation, there are frequently other, associated injuries that may be overlooked if attention is focused on the obvious femoral fracture. Associated injuries therefore must be systematically identified, and priorities must be established for treatment of life-threatening visceral or other injuries while the fractured femur is treated in traction. At the same time, other skeletal injuries such as a dislocation or fracture-dislocation of the ipsilateral hip should not escape notice since their presence may be masked by the more obvious shaft fracture.

All types of fracture occur in the femoral diaphysis: transverse, oblique, spiral and comminuted. The degree of comminution varies considerably. There may be a third, "butterfly" fragment or merely a crack in 1 of the major fragments not visible on x-ray (Fig. 29-1). Such a crack may make intramedullary fixation unstable if additional fixation is not used or if the medullary canal is not reamed so that a large snug-fitting rod can be inserted.

A severely comminuted or shattered fracture (Fig. 29-2) usually signifies an injury associated with high-energy absorption and hence extensive damage to all the tissues of the thigh. This damage may impair wound healing and lessen resistance to infection after open reduction and internal fixation.

ANATOMIC CONSIDERATIONS

The anatomic characteristics of the femur and thigh account for some of the unique features of this fracture.

The femur is the largest bone in the body and its shaft is composed of dense cortical bone, which gives it sufficient strength to withstand the huge stresses caused by muscle forces, gravity and inertia during locomotor activities. Given these circumstances, it is not surprising that fractures of the femoral shaft are usually the result of major violence, that failure of internal fixation was frequent prior to the development of modern rigid devices, such as the medullary rod and compression plates, and that refracture is a not infrequent complication after closed treatment. It is also not surprising,

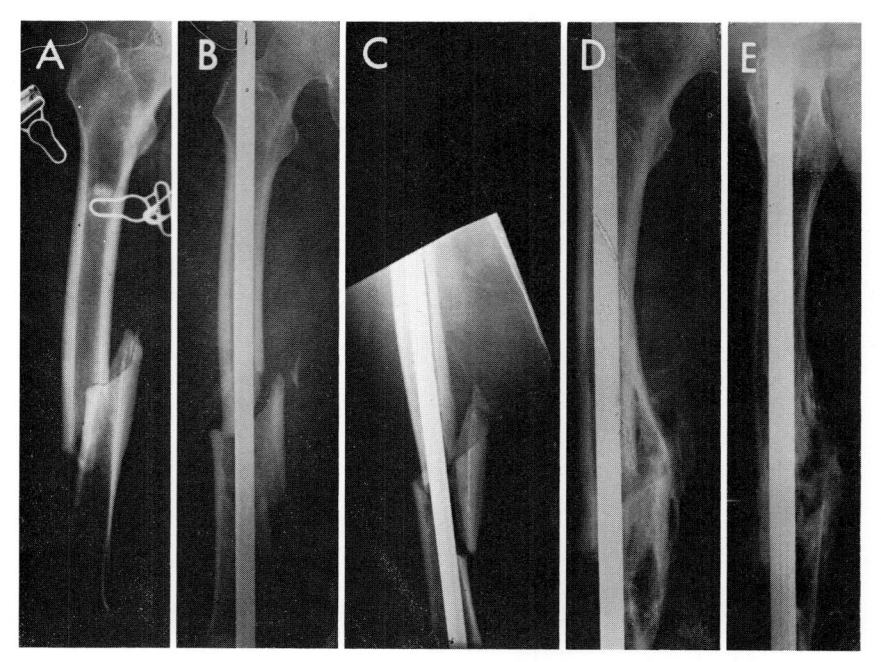

Fig. 29-1.—Oblique fracture of midshaft of femur. **A**, no "butterfly" fragment is visible on the initial roentgenogram. **B** and **C**, loss of position after open reduction and medullary fixation due to displacement of a "butterfly" fragment. Reaming of the canal and a larger nail would probably have prevented this complication. Additional fixation with Parham bands could also have been used. **D** and **E**, 1 year after fracture, healing is progressing slowly.

given these circumstances, that remodeling of the dense cortical bone at the fracture gap may require 2 years or more to restore full normal strength to the shaft.

The massive fascial and muscle envelope that surrounds the femoral shaft tends to obscure the extensive soft tissue injuries that are associated with the fracture. The 4 perforating branches of the profunda femoris artery which course around the posterior and lateral aspects of the femoral shaft are particularly vulnerable. Massive hemorrhage into the soft parts of the thigh, accompanied by a falling hematocrit, is not unusual. Even the femoral artery itself may be ruptured in association with fracture of the shaft (Fig. 29-3).

An adequate blood supply to the femoral shaft is, of course, essential for normal fracture healing. The initial injury and any subsequent surgical procedures may destroy this circulation. It is important to preserve it insofar as possible and, when planning treatment, to keep in mind the effects of various forms of treatment on the circulation already damaged by the injury or previous procedures.

The nutrient artery or arteries to the femoral shaft arise from 1 or more branches of the perforating vessels and enter the bone along the linea aspera. During open reduction, detachment of the soft tissues from the linea should therefore be kept to the minimum. When a medullary nail is used for fixation and the canal is reamed, the medullary circulation inevitably is destroyed. The inner two-thirds of the cortex is supplied by the medullary circulation.[43, 63] One would therefore anticipate profound changes in the circulation of the cortex not only as the result of the destruction of the medullary vessels but also as a consequence of occlusion of the intracortical and subperiosteal vessels by fat and bone marrow emboli forced into

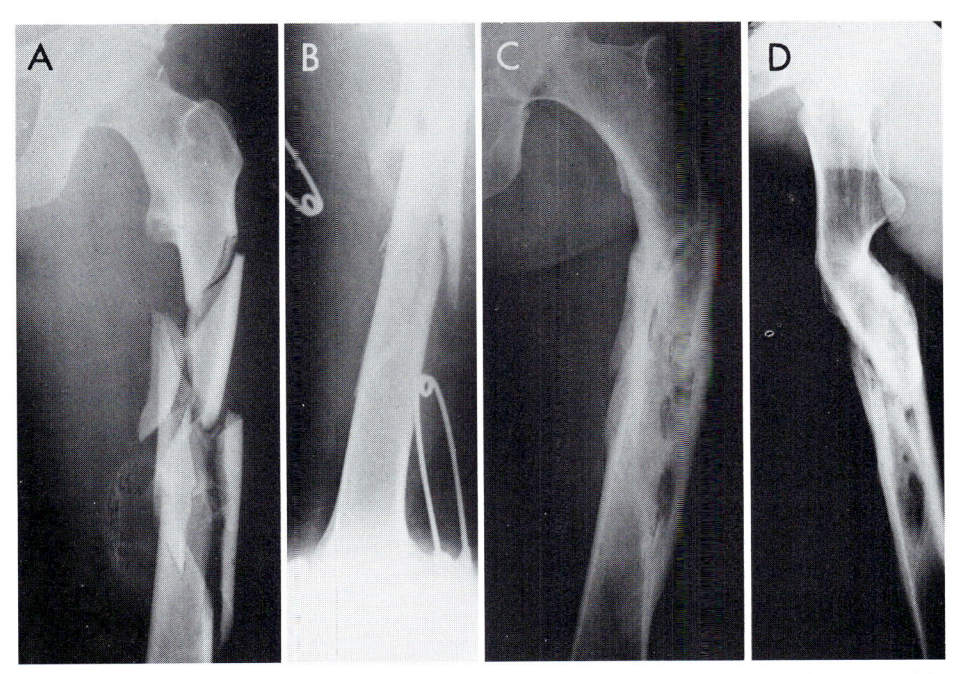

Fig. 29-2.—**A**, anteroposterior and **B**, lateral views of severely comminuted fracture of femoral shaft treated successfully by traction and a spica. **C** and **D**, 1 year after fracture; restitution of the cortex and medullary canal is progressing; normal function. Coxa vara and 1-in. shortening, although undesirable, are a small price to pay in view of the severity of the injuries.

these vessels in the process of reaming. Large cystic cavities and sequestration of part of the inner layer of the cortex, observed in animals after medullary nailing, have been attributed to the reaming process. This damage to inner cortex could be reduced by simultaneously reducing the intramedullary pressure by suction.[22] Furthermore, the simple placement of a medullary pin in the long bone of a rabbit without reaming has been shown to produce subperiosteal new bone formation along the length of the diaphysis.[62] These circulatory disturbances undoubtedly contribute to the delay in fracture healing seen when medullary fixation is used. However, this delay is offset by the fact that the patient can be ambulatory with the fracture still unhealed in the presence of stable medullary fixation.

The muscles and fascial layers enveloping the femur serve as "tension braces" which, during normal activity, reduce the bending stresses on the femoral shaft. This soft tissue support may be of some importance during convalescence from a fracture of the femoral shaft. Muscles atrophied as the result of prolonged immobilization do not support the shaft when activity is resumed. Treatment that permits the early resumption of activity either by internal fixation or by external support by means of a cast brace therefore tends to preserve this supportive function as well as the mobility of the knee. If prolonged immobilization has been necessary, restoration of normal muscle strength and mobility as rapidly as possible is an important phase of treatment. Of particular importance, from the functional viewpoint, is the extensor mechanism. For the knee to regain a full range of motion, the mobility of the quadriceps must not be limited by fibrosis, contracture or adhesions. Unfortunately, the massive hemorrhage into this muscle and the periosteal stripping associated

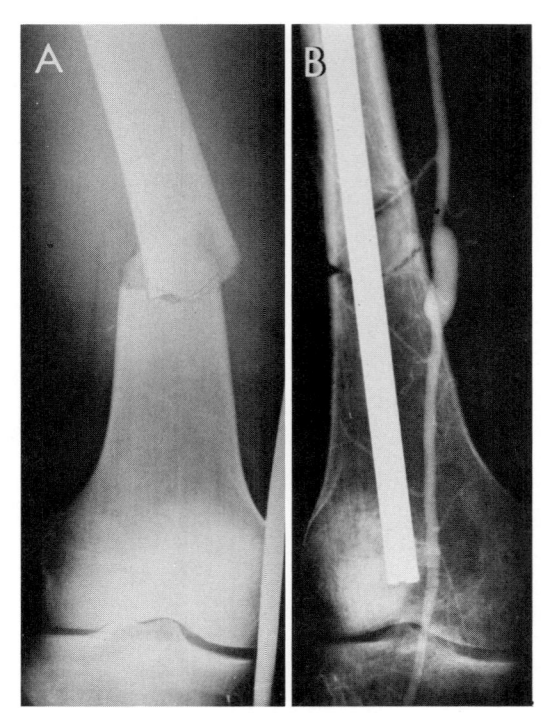

Fig. 29-3.—Vascular injury with fracture of the femur. **A**, femoral fracture which occurred when thigh was crushed between a piece of machinery and a wall. Patient complained of numbness in leg and foot, but dorsalis pedis and posterior tibial pulsations were present. Initial treatment was open reduction and internal fixation with Küntscher nail. On the following day increasing evidence of circulatory embarrassment required exploration of femoral artery; a 2½-in. thrombosed segment was excised and replaced by a graft from the corresponding femoral vein. **B**, arteriogram 3 months after operation. End result 17 months after injury revealed good pulsations, slight loss of knee and foot motions, and bone union of fracture.

with the fracture make it difficult to restore an elastic, freely mobile extensor mechanism when prolonged immobilization has been required.

Further sequels to prolonged immobilization are adhesions involving the knee joint itself and periarticular structures, with resultant fixation of the patella and loss of knee motion. If union is delayed, especially in the presence of sepsis, satisfactory knee motion may never be regained.

The massive muscles of the hip and thigh also play another role, since they tend to cause angulation and displacement of the fracture fragments. The proximal fragment, when the fracture is in the proximal third of the shaft, tends to flex, abduct and externally rotate due to the action of the gluteus medius and minimus, the iliopsoas and the short rotators. The distal fragment tends to displace medially due to the effect of the adductor and gracilis muscles and to move proximally under the influence of the long muscles arising from the ilium and ischial tuberosity—the hamstrings, rectus femoris, tensor fascia lata and sartorius. When fractures in the proximal part of the shaft are treated in traction, the distal fragment usually must be placed in a position of flexion, abduction and external rotation to achieve correct alignment of the 2 fragments.

SIGNS AND SYMPTOMS

When the femoral shaft is fractured, deformity—usually anterior and lateral angulation—is obvious. There is also abnormal rotation of the extremity. The patient complains of severe pain and is of course unable to move the extremity. Crepitus may be felt as the patient is moved or has painful muscle spasms in the thigh.

Massive swelling of the thigh may develop with surprising rapidity if there is arterial bleeding. The arterial pulses at the ankle should be checked, since rupture of the femoral artery is always a possibility (Fig. 29-3). Traumatic shock must also be anticipated and appropriate preventive measures instituted.

TREATMENT

First Aid

Further injury to soft parts and shock can, in large measure, be prevented by

Chapter 29: FRACTURES OF THE FEMORAL SHAFT / 723

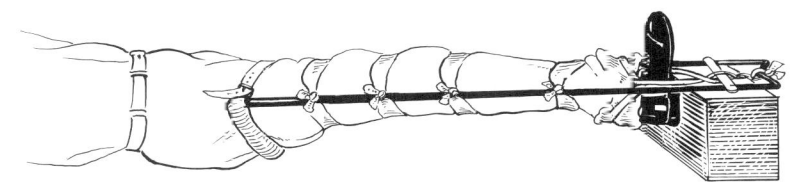

Fig. 29-4.—Keller-Blake splint for first aid immobilization of fractured femur. The ankle is carefully padded, and the leg is supported in the splint by encircling strips of cloth. The shoes and clothing are not removed, in order to avoid unnecessary, painful movement of the damaged extremity. Traction is maintained by means of a strip of cloth secured around the ankle, tied over the end of the splint and twisted taut by means of a stick. The distal end of the splint is supported to give some elevation.

proper first aid measures. The importance of this phase of treatment cannot be overemphasized.

The essential steps are, of course, gentle handling and efficient immobilization of the fracture so that the patient can be transported with the minimum of pain. The Keller-Blake or Thomas splints, if available, are certainly the best means of immobilization (Fig. 29-4). However, they are not essential. With ingenuity, a satisfactory splint can be improvised from poles or long boards suitably padded and fastened by means of bandages or strips of cloth. One board is placed medial, the other on the lateral aspect of the leg and trunk, extending from the axilla to the foot (Fig. 29-5). If nothing else is available, the other leg will serve as a useful splint (Fig. 29-6). By securing the injured extremity to the other leg with encircling bandages or strips of cloth, preferably with some form of padding (e.g., a folded blanket or clothing) between the legs, quite effective immobilization can be achieved. Bandaging the feet together will control rotation.

No attempt should be made to remove the patient's shoes or clothing, since this will result in unnecessary, painful manipulation. If feasible, some form of pressure dressing should be applied to the leg after immobilization because this may minimize blood loss into the soft tissues of the thigh. In an open fracture, after splinting is accomplished, enough clothing should be cut or torn away to permit the application of a sterile, or at least a clean, dressing, followed by a pressure bandage to minimize blood loss. Elevation of the lower extremities will also combat hemorrhage and shock.

Fig. 29-5.—Improvised splint, using boards or sticks, for fracture of the femoral shaft. The lateral splint extends distally from just below the axilla and is secured to the trunk; the medial one extends distally from the groin. All splints are padded to avoid pressure over bony prominences.

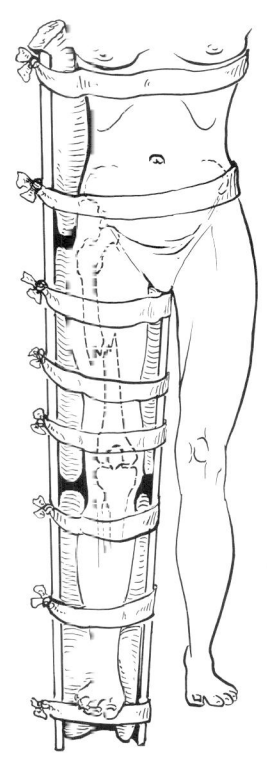

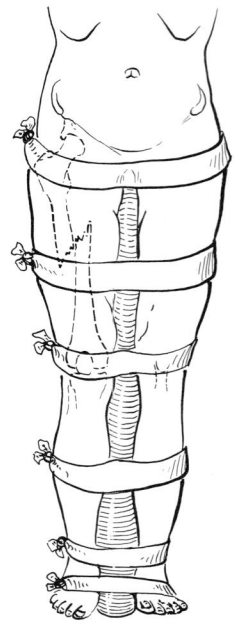

Fig. 29-6.—Improvised immobilization for fracture of femoral shaft when no splints are available. Legs, with padding between, are secured together. Feet are also bound together in order to control rotation.

Morphine or other appropriate analgesic should be administered and the patient should be kept warm. If there is an open fracture, 0.5 ml of adsorbed tetanus toxoid should be given intramuscularly. If the patient has been actively immunized more than 10 years previously and, in addition, there are soft tissue injury and contamination, 250 units of tetanus immune globulin (human) should be given as well.[1] An antibiotic or combination of antibiotics effective against both gram-positive and gram-negative organisms may also be given, especially if the wound has been neglected or treatment has been delayed. (See Chapter 35.)

Definitive Treatment

The method of treatment depends on such factors as (1) the age of the patient, (2) the condition of the skin and soft parts, (3) the degree of comminution, (4) the facilities available and (5) the training and preference of the surgeon.

In the child, delayed union or nonunion is rare, and loss of joint mobility seldom results even from prolonged immobilization. Furthermore, in the growing child, operative procedures carry some risk of damage to growth plates and, as emphasized by Blount[7] and more recently by Griffin and co-workers,[23] anatomic reduction in children between age 2 and 10 is contraindicated because of the overgrowth that occurs in the injured extremity after a femoral fracture in this age group. Healing with 1–2 cm of shortening is therefore desirable (Fig. 29-7), and treatment by traction followed by immobilization in a spica cast is preferred.

In elderly patients, on the other hand, prolonged recumbency, persistent pain and immobilization of joints may be disastrous. If rigid internal fixation of the fracture is feasible, permitting joint movement soon after injury and freedom of movement without pain, the risk of thromboembolic disease, pneumonia, pressure sores and similar problems is markedly decreased. Intramedullary fixation is therefore indicated in this age group whenever there are no contraindications.

In the healthy young adult the decision is less easy. For vigorous adults, either operative or closed methods may be used. Skeletal traction alone or supplemented by the use of a cast brace avoids the risk of postoperative sepsis and disastrous osteomyelitis. On the other hand, recent studies comparing the results of closed treatment by skeletal traction and a spica cast with those of medullary nailing indicate that better results at considerably less cost were achieved after intramedullary nailing.[13, 60] The best results after nailing are obtained with noncomminuted fractures located 5 cm or more below the lesser trochanter and 15 cm or more above the femoral condyles. Stable fixation of such fractures can be achieved consistently. The risk of sepsis is less, and there is less damage to the

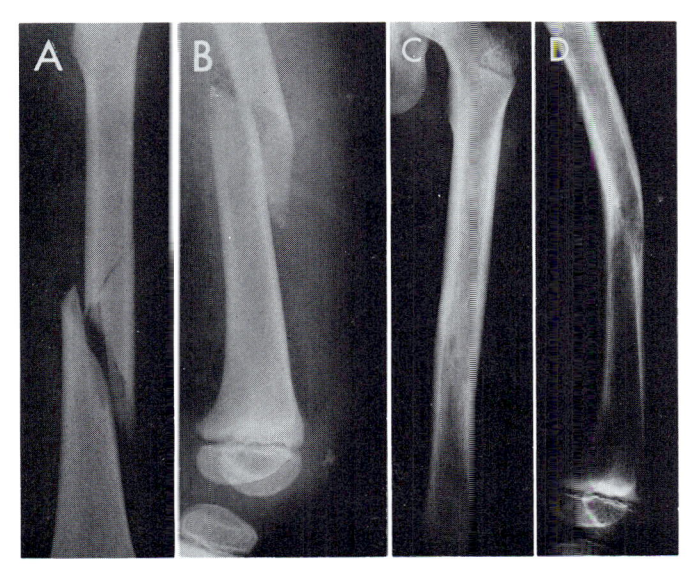

Fig. 29-7.—**A,** anteroposterior and **B,** lateral views of spiral fracture of midshaft of femur with a "butterfly" fragment, the result of a football injury sustained by a boy, aged 6. Treatment consisted of 3½ weeks in Russell traction plus 5 weeks in a plaster spica. **C** and **D,** teleroentgenogram 1 year after injury; solid union with slight anterior angulation and ⅛-in. overgrowth; function of extremity normal.

periosteal circulation with closed nailing. However, this procedure can only be used when the necessary special equipment and image amplification are available to gain and maintain exact positioning of the fragments prior to nailing.[8, 15, 31, 42]

Despite the shorter morbidity, decreased cost and shorter hospitalization associated with intramedullary fixation, the devastating effects of a postoperative infection and chronic osteomyelitis after intramedullary nailing argue strongly against its use as routine treatment in the healthy young adult. Delayed union, nonunion, malunion and refracture are indeed complications of closed treatment,[13] but they can be treated successfully in a high percentage of patients, whereas chronic infection with a resistant organism may condemn the patient to lifelong disability and intermittent drainage.

Fixation of fractures of the femoral shaft by 1 or 2 plates and screws or bolts has been used since the early days of internal fixation. Enthusiasm for this type of fixation has waxed and waned with each modification, starting with the Lane plate and progressing to the slotted plate of Eggers and more recently to the compression plates popularized by the AO group. It is now well established that fixation sufficiently strong to eliminate the need for immobilization cannot be achieved with a single plate. If dual plates are used, maximal strength is provided by parallel placement on the medial and lateral aspects of the shaft; this was pointed out by Bechtol[5] and practiced by Wenger[66] and Marshall[35] and others. However, the technical problems of such placement are great, so that anterior and lateral plates (at 90 degrees to each other) have been used by most proponents of double plating.[21, 34, 46] Even though such 90-degree plate fixation appears to provide adequate strength, there are significant disadvantages inherent in this method. These include: (1) the extensive exposure required to apply the plates, with the consequent impairment of the periosteal circulation and increased risk of postoperative infection; (2) the stress concentration at the ends of the plates that may result in secondary fracture at these levels unless the plates are removed, and (3) the fact that if both plates are removed together the risk of refracture is high. Accordingly, the plates must be removed separately with enough time between the removal of the first and the removal of the second to permit remodeling of the bone in the segment of shaft previously supported by the 2 plates. By such sequential removal, the strength necessary to withstand normal stresses in the absence of 2 plates is regained but the patient has had to undergo 3 operations. If postoperative sepsis occurs after plating, treatment may be difficult indeed. With an infection after medullary nailing the nail is unlikely to break, and it is feasible to wait until union slowly occurs and then treat the infection in a definitive fashion by removal of the rod, debridement, sequestrectomy and appropriate antibiotic therapy[33] (Fig. 29-8). With dual compression plates the same procedure may be followed, but the fixation is less reliable and removal of the plates is far more complicated. If the plate or plates do break or the screws pull out before healing occurs, the situation is quite desperate. In this event, the metal must be removed and an attempt made to clear up the infection with the patient immobilized for many months in a spica; another attempt must then be made to gain union by internal fixation combined with bone grafting when the infection is quiescent. Another method is to remove the plates and insert a medullary rod despite the sepsis, in the hope of getting union first and eliminating the infection at a later date. Both of these alternatives are desperate measures at best. A third alternative, whose effectiveness is not yet established, is the use of a cast brace after removal of the implant.

In general, then, plate fixation is not recommended. However, there are circumstances in which the use of plates may be the best solution. These circumstances include the following:

1. A spiral fracture in the proximal or distal third of the shaft in which adequate reduction is not achieved by closed methods and an intramedullary rod will not provide adequate fixation. Under these circumstances, use of an AO condylar blade plate and an anterior plate will provide very stable fixation.

2. An ununited fracture previously treated by closed or open methods. Although there are theoretical objections to the use of plates after an intramedullary rod has failed (because both the medullary and periosteal circulation are then damaged), experience has shown that compression plating under these circumstances is often successful.

3. Fractures in relation to the stem of an endoprosthesis in the hip or in the region of the femoral component of a total hip replacement. Fractures at these sites can often be adequately fixed with compression plates and screws.

4. Inadequate fixation after insertion of an intramedullary nail. Although with proper selection of cases, adequate reaming and use of a nail of proper size this situation should not occur, the addition of a compression plate with screws penetrating only 1 cortex as suggested by Burwell[11] may be a solution to this problem. Similarly, a nail supplemented by a plate may provide adequate fixation for fractures too far proximal or distal for fixation by the plate alone.

5. Comminuted fractures. With few exceptions, comminuted fractures are best treated in traction followed by immobilization in a spica cast or perhaps by mobilization in a cast brace if increasing experience demonstrates the practicality of this method. However, if satisfactory alignment of the femoral head-neck complex and condyles cannot be achieved in traction, or for some other reason there is a compelling need to resort to internal fixation, dual AO plating may be indicated. Iliac bone grafts should be used in addition and the fracture site should be

Chapter 29: FRACTURES OF THE FEMORAL SHAFT / 727

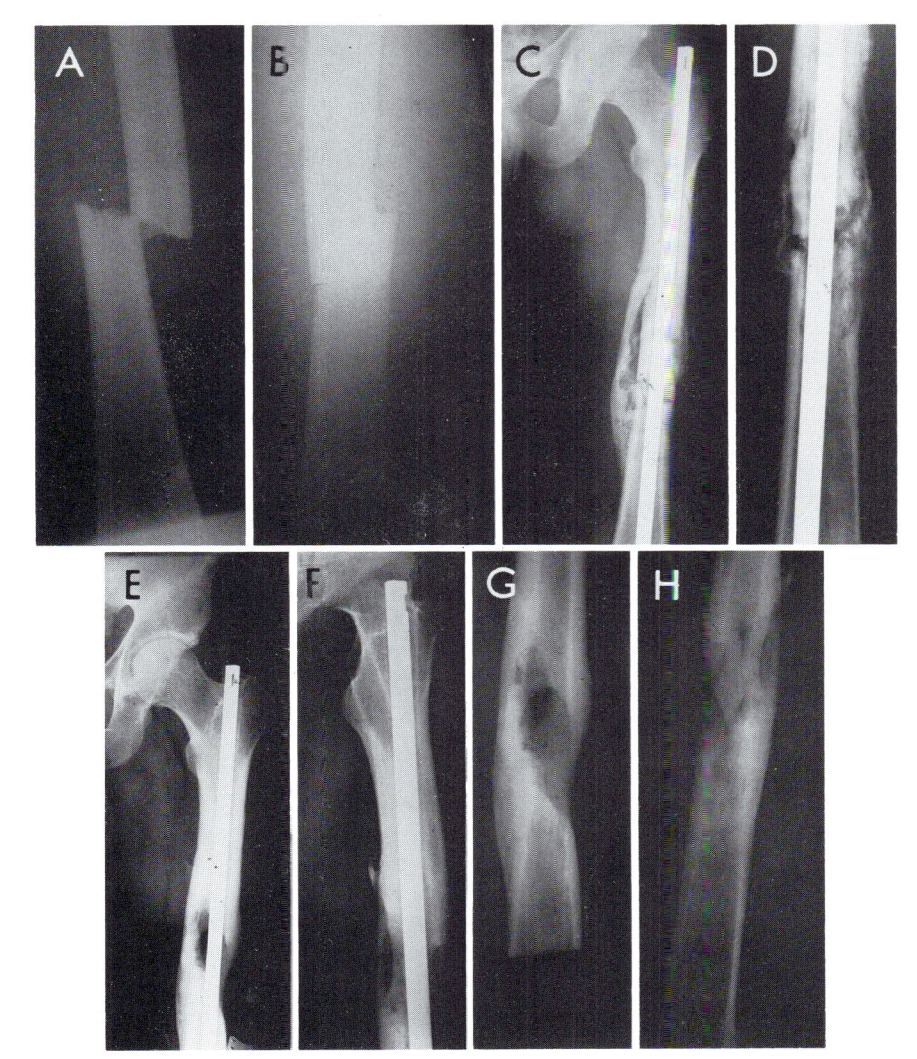

Fig. 29-8.—**A**, anteroposterior and **B**, lateral views of open fracture of femur received, with other injuries, in fall down elevator shaft. Initial treatment concerned the "other" injuries; the thigh wound was simply debrided and closed and the fracture immobilized by skeletal traction through the tibial tubercle. The thigh was well healed 11 days after injury, and open reduction and fixation with a Küntscher nail were performed. Wound sepsis resulted, and the wound was drained 10 days postoperatively. Walking on crutches, the patient was discharged 3½ months after injury. The wound was still draining, but the knee could be flexed 85 degrees. Sequestrectomies were performed 8 and 12 months after injury (**C** and **D**, fracture before first sequestrectomy; **E** and **F**, after last sequestrectomy). Two years after injury the nail was removed (**G** and **H** show fracture at this time); the sinus and scar tissue were excised and the wound closed. Several months later, at follow-up, the wound was found to be closed and the patient had knee motion from full extension to 45-degree flexion; he was able to be on crutches much of the time. This case illustrates the value of leaving the nail in place until bone union has taken place.

protected for many months, since union will be slow and the risk of refracture is high. When plates are used under these circumstances, they must be long enough so that at least 2 and preferably 3 or 4 screws are in intact bone both above and below the comminuted region.

Use of the cast brace or minispica cast brace in the regular treatment of acute fractures of the femoral shaft seems to be on the increase.[14, 30, 36, 37, 50, 53] It is clear that, in centers equipped to use the method, satisfactory results can be obtained with substantial reduction in duration of hospitalization and more rapid restoration of knee function. The method may also play an important role as a supplement to internal fixation when the stability provided by an intramedullary rod or plates is in question.

Manipulative reduction of acute fractures and immobilization in a plaster spica has seldom been considered feasible in our experience, even in young children, because of the difficulty in maintaining satisfactory alignment. However, as demonstrated by Irani, Nicholson and Chung,[27] in children 2–10 years of age immediate immobilization in a spica cast may give very satisfactory results. These authors accepted 2.5 cm of overriding, 15 degrees of lateral and 25 degrees of anterior angulation but no posterior or medial angulation. The cast was applied with the child sedated and alignment was corrected by wedging the cast; hospitalization was thus eliminated or reduced to a few days in their series. Because of the extent of remodeling of the femur associated with growth, considerable deformity can be accepted in this age group since it will be corrected as growth progresses.

Traction

Skin Traction

Although there are many satisfactory ways of applying traction to the skin, several principles should be emphasized.

The patient's skin and subcutaneous tissues must be healthy and able to tolerate traction. Atrophy due to advanced age, impaired sensation, dermatitis or skin damage due to injury are contraindications to this form of treatment. If careful questioning reveals that the patient has had a contact dermatitis from adhesive tape, compound benzoin tincture or resin skin adherent in the past, then skin traction should be avoided.

Finally, if skin traction is used, the extremity should be examined frequently. Should the areas where the straps are applied become tender to palpation, skin irritation should be suspected and the traction straps removed promptly. Similarly, complaints of persistent itching or burning are danger signals which require inspection of the traction straps. Early removal of the skin traction under these circumstances may avoid extensive damage to the skin.

The traction straps must be as large as possible in order to keep the tension per unit area of skin at a minimum. A good method is to use adhesive straps 2–2½ in. wide that extend along each side of the leg from a point 2–3 in. above the malleoli well up on the thigh. Oblique or transverse encircling adhesive straps are not advised. If the edges of the straps are too taut, ¼-in. and ½-in. oblique cuts, made with scissors at 1–2-in. intervals along each edge, will give a smooth fit (Fig. 29-9, C). An encircling elastic bandage will hold the tape in place (Fig. 29-9, D).

In general, not more than 10 lb of pull should be applied by skin traction. Excessive weight and uneven tension are common causes of skin breakdown.

Excess pressure on the malleoli may cause skin necrosis. Several turns of sheet wadding, 2 in. in width, placed just proximal to these bony prominences, will avoid this.

If the traction straps show evidence of slipping, all encircling bandages should be removed and the region of the ankle and dorsum of the foot inspected. Constriction and skin necrosis will thus be avoided. Usually the traction straps need not be disturbed, and all that is needed is to reapply the bandage in a more proximal position. However, new skin adherent and traction straps may be necessary.

External pressure or excessive tension on the skin and subcutaneous tissues in the region of the fibular head and common peroneal nerve may produce peroneal palsy. The palsy is characterized first by paresthesias and then by loss of sensation on the dorsum of the foot and weakness or paralysis of the dorsiflexors of the foot and toes. The common causes of palsy in a patient in traction are: tight bandages or traction straps; a narrow and inadequately padded sling when Russell traction is used; pressure on the region of the common peroneal nerve caused by an

Fig. 29-9.—Types of traction straps. Temporary straps can be made from strips of foam rubber ¼-in. thick. **A**, the edges are beveled and the strips are backed with moleskin (**B**), to which webbing straps are stapled. **C**, such straps can be made to fit the contours of the leg by multiple cuts. **D**, elastic bandages, applied from the toes to the top of the traction straps, can be used to maintain the contact of the traction straps with the skin.

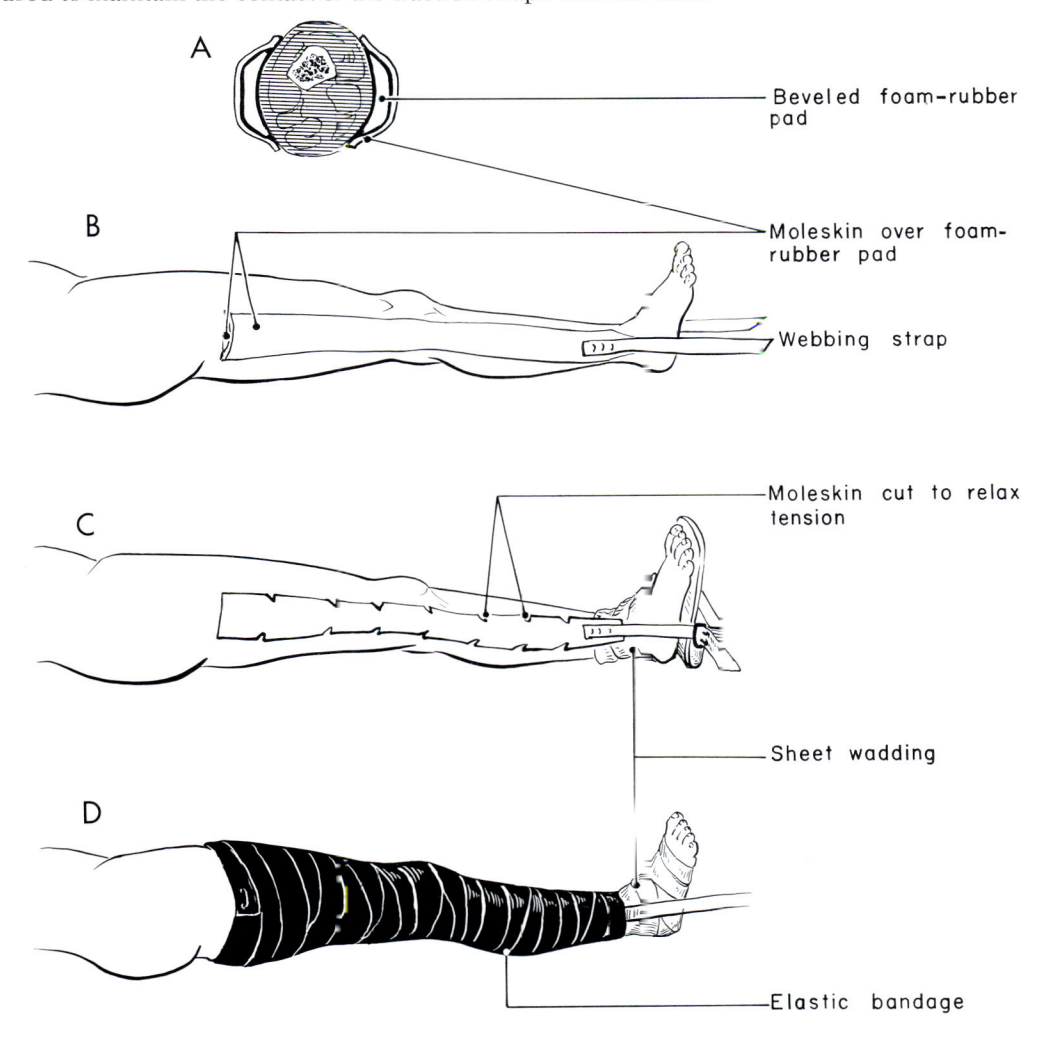

inadequately padded support for the leg or even by actual contact of the leg with the side bar of the suspension splint. If the limb is in external rotation, it is essential to palpate the region of the fibular head frequently to establish beyond doubt that there is no pressure on this region. The significance of paresthesias in the foot and the slightest weakness of dorsiflexion of the foot and toes must be appreciated by all those attending the patient.

An alternative method of applying skin traction but one not suitable for prolonged use is that accomplished with straps fashioned from strips of ¼-in. foam rubber backed with moleskin and held snugly in contact with the skin by an encircling elastic bandage (Fig. 29-9). These straps tend to slip gradually and usually must be reapplied every 24–48 hours.

Skeletal Traction

If traction for a prolonged period is anticipated, especially if heavy weights will be needed, skeletal traction is required. For this, a threaded Kirschner wire is preferred. Though the threaded

Fig. 29-10. — Sites for insertion of Kirschner wire for skeletal traction. In the tibial tubercle (**top**) the pin should be inserted 1 finger's breadth posterior to the prominence of the tubercle. By starting on the lateral side, accidental injury to the peroneal nerve can be avoided by careful placement of the wire; a wire inserted in the opposite direction may deviate during its course through the bone and damage the nerve. In the supracondylar region of the femur (**left**) the pin or wire is inserted as far posteriorly and as far distally as possible in order not to transfix the quadriceps mechanism and to avoid the synovial expansions of the knee. Great care is needed to avoid entering the knee joint with the wire. It is inserted just proximal to the most proximal palpable prominence of the lateral femoral condyle and is carefully directed at a right angle to the femoral shaft and in the frontal plane with the leg in neutral position. The wire will then emerge through the medial femoral condyle. In growing children, the point of insertion should be slightly more proximal to avoid injury to the epiphyseal plate. In the os calcis (**right**) the wire is started on the lateral side at a point approximately ¾ in. behind and ¾ in. below the tip of the lateral malleolus or at the midpoint of a line drawn between the tip of the lateral malleolus and the tip of the heel. (Adapted from Scuderi, C. S.: *Atlas of Orthopedic Traction Procedures* [St. Louis: C. V. Mosby Company, 1954].)

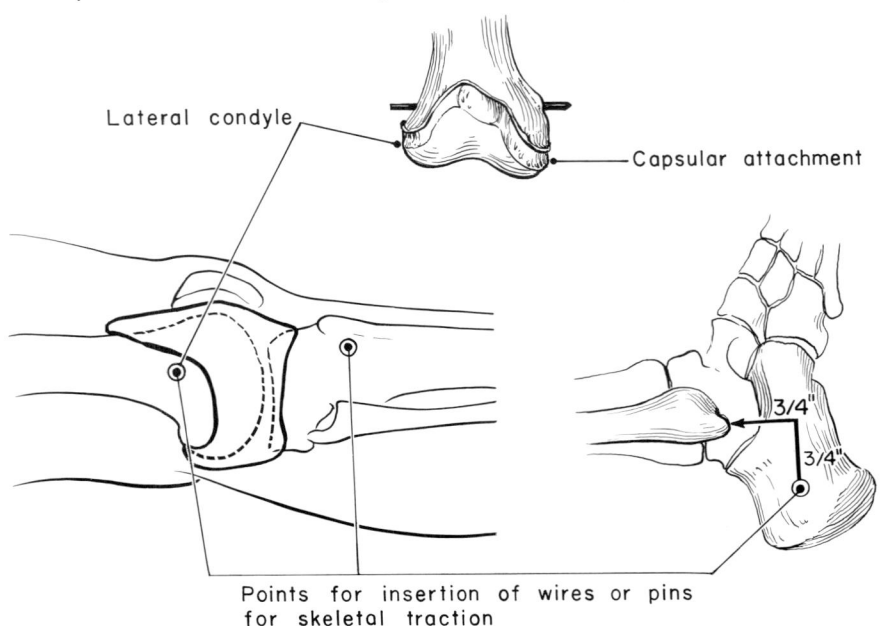

Points for insertion of wires or pins for skeletal traction

wire is somewhat more difficult to insert and remove, a smooth wire tends to loosen and slide medially or laterally, contaminating the pin tract. Soft tissue sepsis or even osteomyelitis and the formation of a ring sequestrum may result. If the bone is very porotic, a larger threaded Steinmann pin is less likely to cut through the bone.

Ordinarily, 3 points in the lower extremity are used for skeletal traction: the tibial tubercle, the supracondylar region of the femur and the os calcis (Fig. 29-10).

The tibial tubercle is the safest and most satisfactory site. Here the bone is dense; there are few soft tissues to be traversed, and sepsis or cutting out of the wire, should it occur, does not cause serious complications. The only disadvantage to the use of this site is that, if heavy traction is necessary for a considerable period, particularly with knee in flexion, stretching of the ligaments of the knee may occur, with resultant instability. The supracondylar region is used if heavy traction is indicated, or if extreme flexion of the knee is necessary, for example, with the so-called 90-90-90 traction. The chief objections to this location for skeletal traction are: the risk of damage to the epiphyseal plate in children; the danger of sepsis along the pin tract with scarring down of the quadriceps, and the possible contamination of the knee, should the wire cut through the cancellous bone after prolonged traction and enter the joint.

When the fracture is in the distal part of the femoral shaft, the associated hematoma may dissect distally to the supracondylar region where it will communicate with the tract of a supracondylar wire. Although Stewart et al.[58] reported no serious complication from this circumstance when using double pin traction for supracondylar fractures, severe infections have occurred in our experience, and supracondylar traction is not recommended for distal fractures. The use of the os calcis as a site for skeletal traction in the treatment of femoral fractures is seldom indicated. The wire is likely to cut through this cancellous bone, and pin tract infections at this site are particularly serious, leading to resistant chronic osteomyelitis of the os calcis or septic arthritis of the subastragalar joint. However in some situations the os calcis may be the only site available.

The wire should be inserted under the rigid aseptic conditions of the operating room. Although local anesthesia may be used, a general anesthetic will permit a manipulative reduction of the fracture at the time the traction is set up.

During insertion of a Kirschner wire the soft tissues may show a tendency to become wound around the wire as it is being drilled in. This may impede or even block the passage of the wire through the bone. This difficulty can be avoided by inserting a large-bore hypodermic needle down to the bone and threading the wire through the needle. The needle can be removed before the spreader is applied. An alternate measure, if a threaded wire is not being used, is to oscillate, rather than rotate, the wire

Fig. 29-11.—Bryant traction. The child is placed on a Bradford frame, and the traction is adjusted so that the buttocks are raised from the frame. By putting both legs in traction, rotatory movements of the pelvis are prevented. However, some surgeons prefer to put only the involved leg in traction, maintaining that more traction can be achieved in this way. Warning: Circulatory complications may occur with this treatment. (See text.)

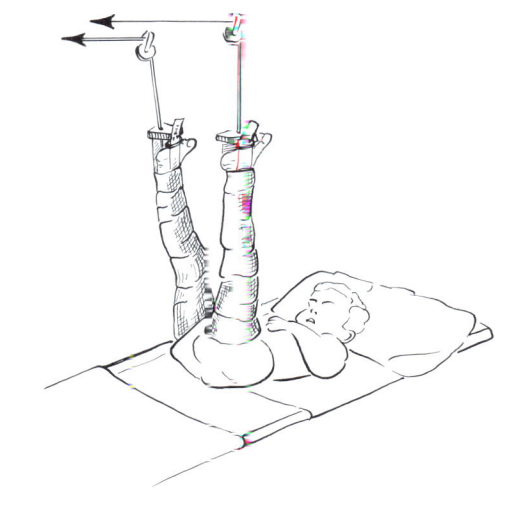

as it is driven through the bone and soft tissues.

The skin and subcutaneous tissues at the points of entrance and exit of the wire should not be under tension once the wire is in place, because persistent tension leads to necrosis and sepsis. To avoid this difficulty, a stab wound should be made with a scalpel at the point of insertion and also over the point of the wire as it tents the skin on the opposite side.

In order to place the wire accurately in the supracondylar region, it is well to use a guide if one is available.

Four types of traction commonly used are Bryant, Russell, suspension, and 90-90-90 traction.

BRYANT TRACTION.—For children under age 3 or weighing less than 30 lb, Bryant traction (Fig. 29-11) is convenient and effective. However, it should be emphasized that is is not without danger. Ischemic contracture has been observed in both the normal and the fractured limb of children treated by this method. When applying the traction straps and encircling bandages, great care must be taken that they are not too tight. Once the child is in traction the circulation and sensation of both feet must be checked at frequent intervals and the bandages loosened at the slightest suggestion of circulatory or sensory disturbance. One should not hesitate to use some other form of treatment if there is

Fig. 29-12.—Russell traction. The resultant of the vertical and horizontal forces is in line with the long axis of the femur. The leg rests on 2 pillows arranged to give support to the whole extremity, particularly the thigh. The sling beneath the knee is wide and well padded. The overhead pulley is placed slightly distal to the knee. The lower end of the bed is raised at least 6 in. to provide countertraction.

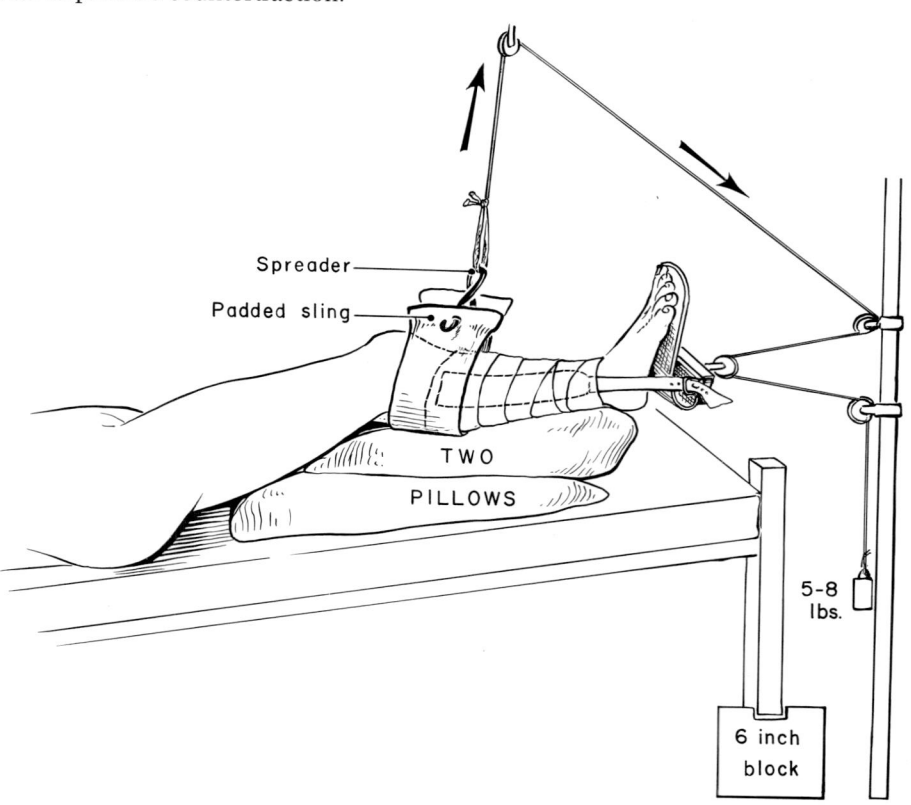

any doubt about the status of either limb.

RUSSELL TRACTION.—This type of traction (Fig. 29-12) is simple to apply and adjust and is free from serious complications except for peroneal palsy that may occur when an improper sling is used. The method is suitable for fractures in older children and some adults but is seldom utilized. When it is used, special measures to prevent posterior bowing at the fracture site are apt to be necessary since there is no external support under the thigh. A satisfactory method of providing support if it is needed is to use a second sling beneath the thigh, centered at the level of the fracture with upward traction perpendicular to the long axis of the femur. This sling is adjusted to provide enough support to restore the normal anterior bow of the femur. Needless to say, meticulous care to avoid pressure in the region of the common peroneal nerve is essential.

Russell traction may also be applied by means of a Kirschner wire through the tibial tubercle (Fig. 29-13). The vertical component of the traction is applied to the bow, while the horizontal component is secured to the projecting ends of the wire by means of webbing straps buckled to the foot piece. This arrangement avoids the need for a second wire in the os calcis as is sometimes used. The rotational alignment of the distal fragment can be adjusted somewhat by changing the direction of the upward component medially or laterally. The extremity may be suspended either by a Hodgen splint and Pearson attachment or by pillows and slings, as suggested by Rowe (Fig. 29-14).

SUSPENSION TRACTION.—For adults, sus-

Fig. 29-13.—Split Russell traction with a Kirschner wire through the tibial tubercle. Although a comparable pull could be achieved by a single rope and weight pulling in line with the femur, this more complicated method has some advantages. Rotation can be accurately adjusted and maintained simply by shifting the vertical component to 1 side or the other. The direction of pull can be shifted by increasing or decreasing the vertical or horizontal components as indicated. Note that the straps which transmit the horizontal pull to the wire in the tibial tubercle are attached distally to a spreader sufficiently wide to permit the Pearson attachment to move between the straps. Knee motion may thus be instituted early. A threaded Kirschner wire should be used to prevent the wire from sliding in the bone. (See Fig. 29-15 for details.)

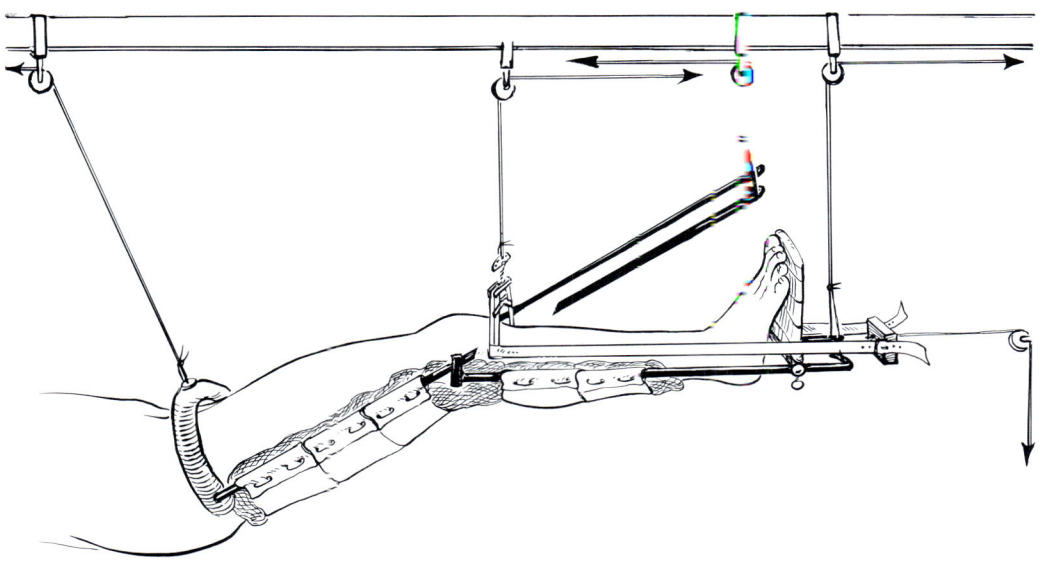

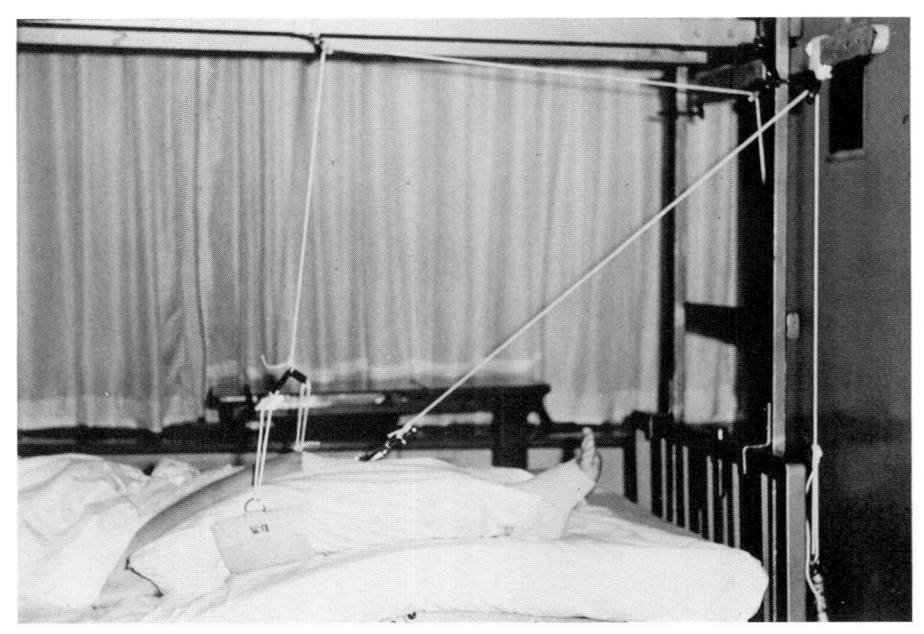

Fig. 29-14. — Pillow and sling suspension (method by Rowe). For elderly patients especially, this method provides comfort and maintains satisfactory alignment.

pension traction is usually preferred. The limb is supported by means of a Thomas half-ring splint or Hodgen splint fitted with a Pearson attachment (Fig. 29-15). With appropriate adjustment of the components of the splint and use of a pad behind the thigh, the tendency of the femur to angulate posteriorly at the fracture site due to the force of gravity can be corrected and the normal anterior bowing of the femur can be maintained. Properly counterbalanced, using well-lubricated ball-bearing pulleys, the suspended limbs should move up and down with the patient during nursing procedures, and from 30 to 40 degrees of active and passive motion of the knee should be possible.

Careful attention must be paid to rotary alignment, especially in patients with more proximally located fractures in whom the proximal fragment may tend to flex and externally rotate. Such external rotation can be estimated with some accuracy by palpating the position of the greater trochanter and placing the other leg in a position such that its greater trochanter is similarly located. The suspension can then be adjusted to hold the fractured limb in this position. If the extremity is placed in external rotation, as previously noted, extreme care is essential to avoid any pressure in the region of the fibular head. Peroneal palsy is an all too common complication of traction suspension.

Recently the 2-sling-2-pillow suspension advocated by Rowe (see Fig. 29-14) has become increasingly popular at Massachusetts General Hospital, especially for elderly patients. It is comfortable, easy to adjust and free from complications.

Traction should be applied by a Kirschner wire through the tibial tubercle in the great majority of cases. Skeletal traction through the supracondylar area is seldom necessary, in our experience.

90-90-90 TRACTION. — This method

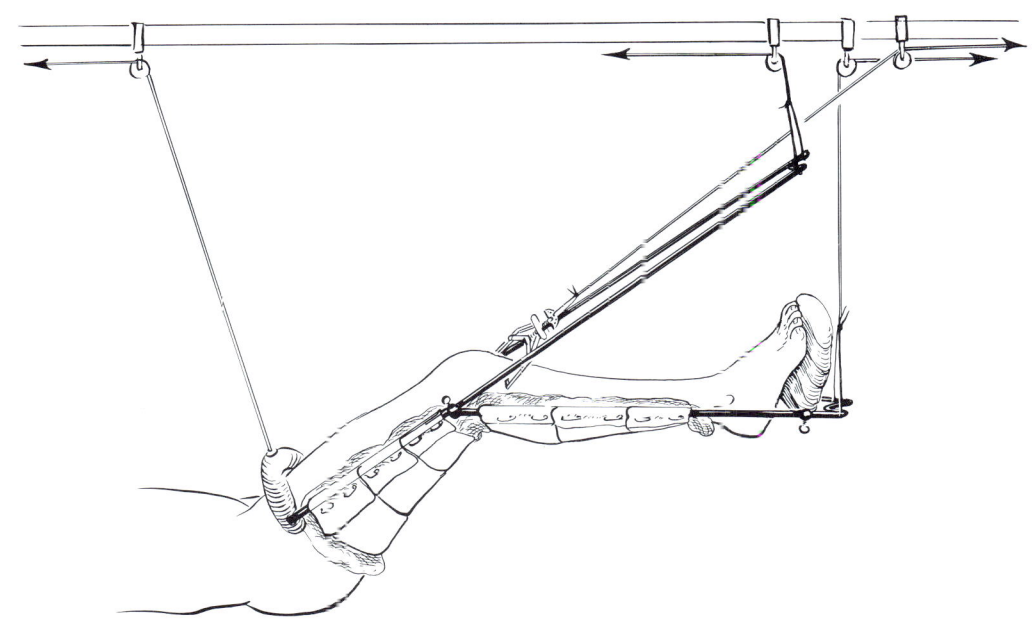

Fig. 29-15.—Suspension traction. The leg is supported on a felt pad, which is covered with stockinette and laid on top of webbing slings. The slings are secured to the Hodgen splint and Pearson attachment by means of large safety pins. The Hodgen splint is supported at both ends by sufficient weight just to balance the weight of the extremity. The Pearson attachment is supported by a rope at its distal end, to which sufficient weight is attached just to balance the weight of the leg. Traction is applied, usually through the tibial tubercle, as illustrated. With this arrangement for suspension, rarely is the pin or wire placed through the supracondylar region. Adjustments are made according to what the roentgenograms of the femur show. Anteroposterior angulation is corrected by (1) tightening or loosening the sling beneath the thigh, (2) sliding an additional pad beneath the thigh at the appropriate level if there is persistent posterior angulation or displacement of 1 of the fragments and (3) flexing or extending the knee, thereby relaxing or tightening the gastrocnemius muscle. The last maneuver is of particular value in distally placed fractures. Medial or lateral angulation is corrected by changing the direction of pull in such a manner as to align the distal with the proximal fragment. Shifting the position of the medial or lateral proximal ends of the Pearson attachment— either proximally or distally on the Hodgen splint, as indicated—may also correct angulation. The amount of rotation may be estimated by placing the opposite extremity so that the greater trochanters on the 2 sides are in comparable positions. The suspension is then adjusted so as to hold the fractured extremity in a position comparable to that of the normal one. This is usually in slight external rotation. In general, if the supporting ropes for the Hodgen splint pull in a slightly cephalad direction, there will be less tendency for the splint to slide off the leg.

(Fig. 29-16) is useful for proximal fractures when the proximal fragment is markedly flexed and externally rotated. With 90-90-90 traction it is relatively easy to align the distal with the proximal fragment. This method is also useful in children who are too old or too heavy to be placed in Bryant traction. Finally, in the presence of an open, infected fracture, for example, that in a gunshot wound, the 90-90-90 position may facilitate dependent drainage and wound dressings.

A Kirschner wire is inserted in the supracondylar region (see Fig. 29-10) and the leg is suspended in the horizontal position by means of a plaster boot and slings, so as to hold the knee, hip and ankle in 90-degree flexion. With this method the hamstrings are relaxed, and accurate control of the distal fragment is

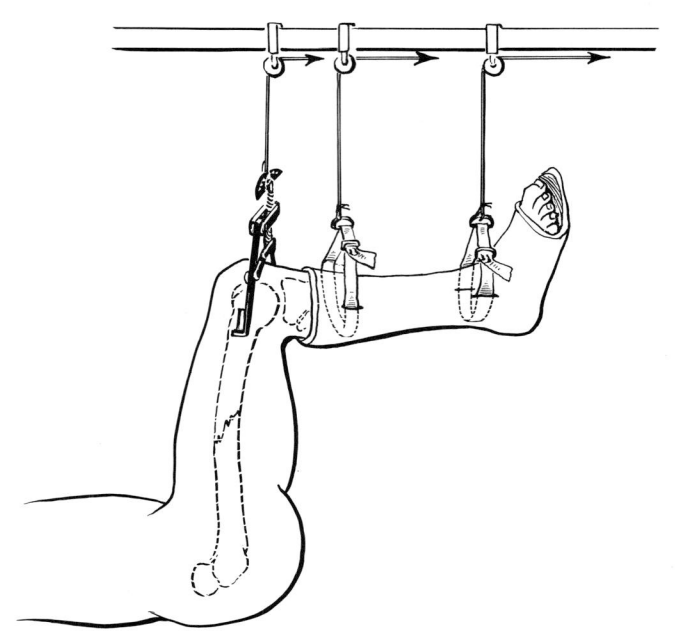

Fig. 29-16.—90-90-90 traction. Traction is applied to the femur in a vertical direction by means of a Kirschner wire inserted in the supracondylar region. The lower leg is merely suspended, the weights being adjusted to counterbalance the weight of the leg plus that of the plaster boot. With the pull of gravity in the axis of the femoral shaft, angulation can be controlled without the use of splints. Nursing care is relatively simple, and access to the thigh is made easy should daily dressings be required. The webbing straps supporting the cast are incorporated in the plaster.

assured by the traction wire and the suspended lower leg.

The disadvantages of this technique include the need for a supracondylar wire, with its attendant dangers, and the flexed position of the knee, which may be undesirable if prolonged traction is necessary.

Application of Traction and Closed Reduction

At the time traction is applied and the suspension apparatus is adjusted initially, it is highly desirable to reduce the fracture and to adjust the apparatus to maintain the desired position as shown by portable roentgenograms. This procedure is best carried out under general anesthesia so the manipulation and adjustments can be accomplished with the patient relaxed and free from pain.

Duration of Immobilization

In children, callus is formed rapidly and the fracture becomes stabilized in 3–5 weeks. At this time, good callus will be visible on x-ray film. It is then possible to apply a plaster spica without fear of losing position and to discharge the patient home. The duration of immobilization in this cast will vary, but ordinarily immobilization must be maintained for 8–12 weeks from the time of fracture or until an x-ray film shows that mature callus is present. A 1½ plaster spica, encasing the involved leg down to the toes and the normal leg to just above the knee, is applied at first. With fractures involving the distal femur the normal leg may occasionally be left free, but in general it is advisable to immobilize the pelvis, so far as possible, by having the cast include the normal hip and thigh. During the last 2 or

3 weeks of immobilization in plaster, the portion of the cast encasing the normal leg may be removed, thus converting it to a single spica.

For adults, traction must be maintained considerably longer, usually for 12–16 weeks. During this time, great care must be exercised to avoid distraction, particularly in transverse midshaft fractures. Once alignment has been obtained, the weight should be reduced gradually. However, the reduction in weight must be guided by periodic x-rays in order to avoid loss of position.

As soon as the position has become stabilized, especially if the bone ends are locked, quadriceps and hamstring exercises should be started.

Refracture, especially in adults, is a serious complication that may result in permanent loss of knee motion. Traction should not be discontinued until x-rays of good quality show adequate healing. Factors that delay healing and the restoration of strength at the fracture site, such as severe comminution with separation of the fragments, loss of bone substance and infection, should be given due consideration when the decision to discontinue traction is made. If any of these factors prevail, traction may have to be maintained for 16 weeks or longer.

The duration of traction and of hospitalization may be reduced by placing the patient in a 1½ spica once there is clinical union and the fracture gap is bridged by early callus. However, adults often tolerate recumbency in a plaster spica poorly and arrangements for care in a spica after discharge may be difficult. Hopefully the cast brace will provide a solution to this problem, since with this device it is possible for patients to be ambulatory after much shorter periods in traction.

A walking spica is another alternative, especially with distal fractures. If the patient is vigorous enough to manage the cast and not so obese that a snug, single spica cannot be applied, ambulation with crutches is quite feasible. A cast boot is worn on the fractured side and a raised shoe on the normal side. Unlike the cast brace, a spica does not permit knee motion. On the other hand, it does not require the specialized technique needed to apply an effective cast brace.

Another alternative, now seldom practical because of the high cost of hospitalization, is to decrease the amount of traction gradually until the leg is simply suspended. During this time the patient is encouraged to move the knee and gain muscle control. Once muscle control is satisfactory and union appears sufficiently solid, the limb may be removed from the suspension apparatus, first during the day only and then completely. Crutch walking with minimal weight bearing on the affected leg is started when there are 40–60 degrees of active knee motion and the patient has good muscular control as evidenced by his ability to do straight raising. Full weight bearing should not be allowed until mature healing is evident, usually about 6 months after fracture. Almost normal bone strength is probably not restored until roughly 2 years after fracture.

An ischial weight-bearing brace is sometimes prescribed as supportive apparatus during convalescence after fracture of the femoral shaft. This device is not very effective. Indeed, refractures have occurred while walking in such braces and even while putting them on or taking them off. Their use is not recommended.

The patient must be carefully instructed as to how to minimize the risk of refracture, and his activities must be closely supervised until he is able to walk with crutches skillfully and protect his injured limb.

A stiff knee, the result of prolonged immobilization or other cause, tends to increase the leverage on the fracture site, particularly if the patient slips or falls in such a manner as to cause knee flexion. When there is limited knee motion, protection must be prolonged and every effort made to improve knee motion by appropriate physical therapy. Too vigorous efforts to increase motion by passive stretching or progressive resistance exercises may cause refracture. Active exercises for both the flexor and the extensor muscles of the knee are the first and most important steps in rehabilitation of the knee after a fracture of the femoral shaft. The other measures must await restoration of sufficient strength at the fracture site.

A hip flexion contracture may also predispose to refracture. In the presence of this deformity, protection of the extremity should also be prolonged.

Much of what has been said about the duration of traction and the procedure for ambulation after traction is discontinued may have to be modified as experience with the cast brace technique increases.

Cast Brace

The treatment of fractures of the long bones of the lower extremities by early weight bearing is not new. The value of weight bearing and function in the treatment of fractures was recognized by Smith in 1855,[55] when he described his "artificial limb," a modified long leg brace with pelvic band. Recently the method has been revived, first for fractures of the tibia[17,50] and more recently for fractures of the femoral shaft.[14,36,37,50]

The cast-brace method is based on the concept that walking on a limb with an incompletely healed long-bone fracture is a positive factor, in that it encourages more rapid and secure fracture healing and maintains more normal muscle and joint function. Such weight bearing in the case of femoral fractures is believed to be possible because the total-contact thigh component converts the thigh into a semirigid fluid-filled tube in which the fluid is maintained under pressure as the thigh is compressed within the rigid conical external support. The resulting cylinder of compressed fluid (soft tissue) surrounding the fractured femur then tends to maintain length and alignment of the femur. However, as demonstrated by Connolly and associates,[14] using cineroentgenography and direct measuring techniques, there may be a startling amount of movement of the fragments as the patient walks in a cast brace. The thigh component with its quadrilateral brim contoured to fit the root of the limb probably tends to control rotation. During the swing phase of gait or when the braced limb is non-weight-bearing, this component is kept from displacing distally by the support provided by the hinged uprights at the knee, connecting the thigh component to the plaster boot.

The thigh component does not provide ischial weight bearing but rather encases the thigh to form the semirigid supporting cone. The snug-fitting cast with its quadrilateral brim controls rotation quite well. Indeed the measurements of Connolly and co-workers demonstrated that there was considerably less rotation of the fragments in a cast brace than in skeletal traction.

Indications.—The method is applicable to fractures in the middle and in the distal one-half of the femoral shaft (Figs. 29-17 and 29-18). It has been used satisfactorily for transverse, oblique, comminuted and segmental fractures in this region. It is also of value in the treatment of early delayed union and infected nonunions with some inherent stability.

Cast bracing is usually not suitable for fractures above the midshaft level since they tend to angulate. It is also not applicable to elderly patients who cannot walk in the brace. Similarly, obesity makes the brace ineffective. In the presence of significant skin abnormality or breakdown on the thigh, use of the brace may cause problems in wound healing (Burkhalter[14]). Finally, as might be expected, in the absence of sensory and motor function a cast brace will not be tolerated.

Technique.—Although the application of a cast brace is not difficult, it must be done correctly and for appropriate indications if excessive shortening and mal-

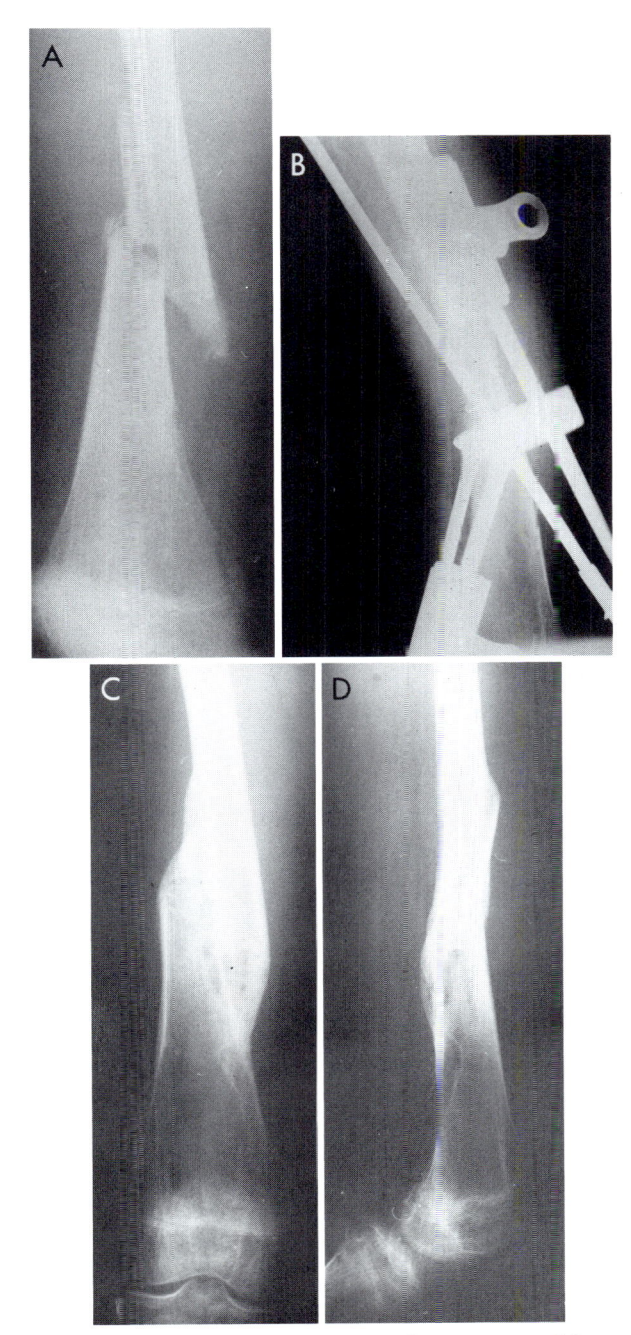

Fig. 29-17.—A, anteroposterior and B, lateral views of comminuted fracture of the mid-distal shaft of the right femur, sustained in a fall from a horse. Treatment initially was by skin traction and balanced suspension for 10 days, then by cast brace for 16 weeks. C, anteroposterior and D, lateral views on recent examination. Result: ½-in. shortening, 90-degree knee flexion, no angular deformity.

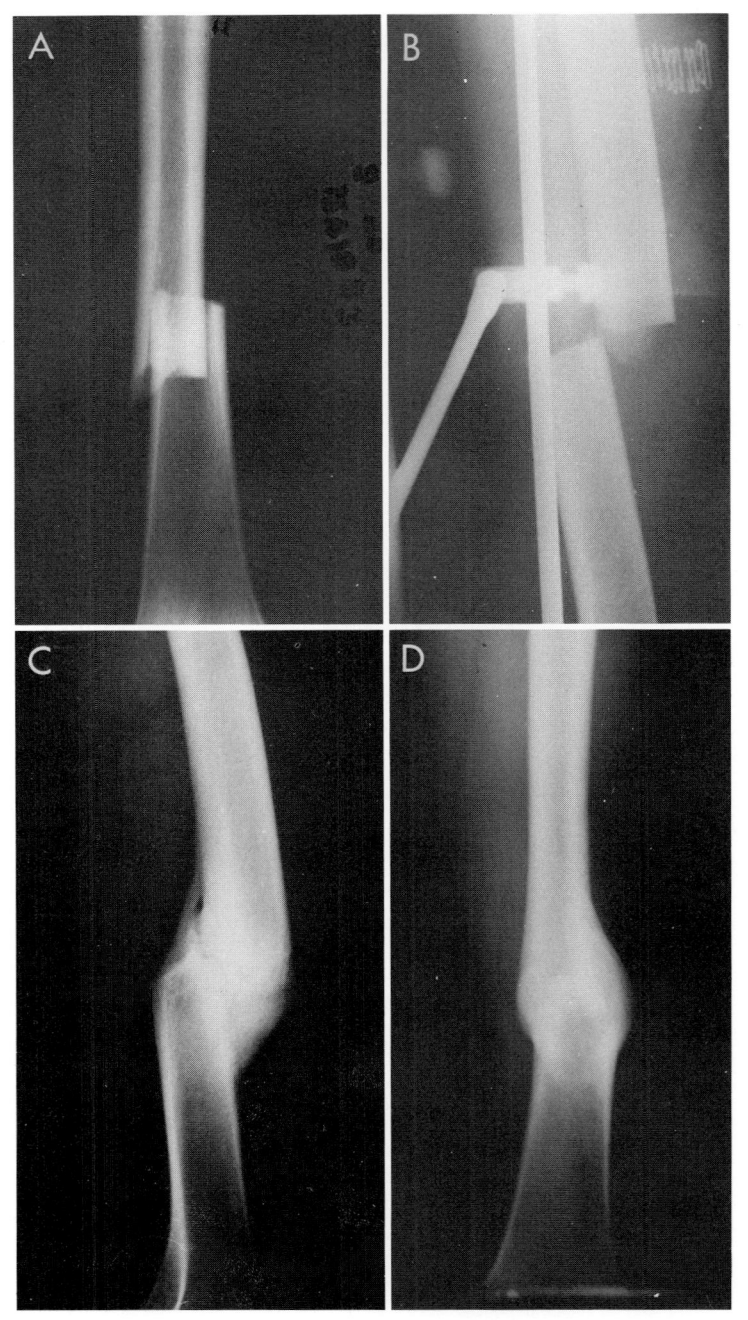

Fig. 29-18. — **A** and **B**, isolated closed transverse fracture of right femur at junction of mid and distal thirds of shaft, resulting from an automobile accident. Initial treatment was traction using a Kirschner wire through the proximal tibia and balanced suspension for 7½ weeks. Cast brace was used for 16 weeks. **C** and **D**, x-rays 4 months later show no shortening and 10 degrees of varus deformity, clinically not discernible.

union are to be avoided. Anyone planning to use the technique should first observe the application of the device by someone experienced in the method, or attend a continuing education course devoted to cast bracing. Only the briefest outline of the technique will be given here.

Initially the patient is treated with skeletal traction with a Kirschner wire through the tibial tubercle. Accurate alignment should be obtained and maintained until the fracture is clinically stable, i.e., until the fracture site is nontender and "rubbery" and no shortening occurs when traction is removed. This degree of stability is seldom achieved less than 8 weeks after fracture. The cast brace can then be applied, preferably with the patient under sedation or, rarely, with the patient under general anesthesia if the brace is applied within approximately 3 weeks.

While an assistant holds the traction bow to support the fracture, a total-contact cast is applied to the thigh over a Spandex sock or a single layer of Webril. A plastic-laminated quadrilateral socket jig incorporated in the cast is helpful, but is not essential if the cast is properly molded to form an ischial seat and fits snugly in Scarpa's triangle and over the greater trochanter. Elastic plaster-of-paris bandages are used for the first 2 layers, followed by rolls of conventional plaster. The plaster cylinder must be applied snugly and molded meticulously to provide a completely smooth inner surface and total contact. The thigh component should extend as far distally as possible and still permit knee flexion to 90 degrees when the cast brace is completed. If the thigh component is too short, angulation of the fracture may occur, especially when the fracture is distally placed.

Once the plaster in the thigh component has set, the plaster boot extending from toes to knee is applied. The Kirschner wire may be removed or may be incorporated in the plaster boot if there is any doubt as to the stability of the fracture and the need for further traction. After the plaster boot has set, the hinged knee joints are applied, using an alignment jig (Fig. 29-19). The axis of the hinges must be adjusted at the level of the adductor tubercle in both the sagittal and frontal planes. The hinges are secured temporarily to the 2 plaster components, using hose clamps, and knee motion is tested. With proper placement of the hinges, motion of the knee is smooth and pain free, the relationship of the plaster cast components to the thigh and lower leg do not change appreciably during knee flexion and extension, and the desired alignment with respect to valgus and varus angulation of the knee is maintained.

When placement of the hinges is correct, the hinges are secured with plaster bandages to the thigh and boot components. Cautious trimming of the cast sufficient to permit 90 degrees of hip and knee flexion is the final step.

After completion of the cast brace (Fig. 29-20), x-rays are obtained to check the position and alignment of the fragments as well as the position of the brace joints relative to knee joint and adductor tubercle. If the position of the fragments is not satisfactory, the thigh portion of the cast may be wedged by a single-cut, open wedge technique to achieve proper position. Using this technique, Mooney has had no skin problems.[38]

Swelling of the knee and exposed soft tissue between the 2 components of the brace will occur if elastic support is not provided. An Ace bandage or, preferably, an elastic knee cage applied to this area is sufficient support.

On the day following application of the cast, gait training with crutches and progressively increasing weight bearing are started. A canvas cast boot is used in preference to a conventional rubber heel. The patient should be instructed to extend the knee completely in the early stance phase to avoid walking with a bent-knee gait. He should start doing

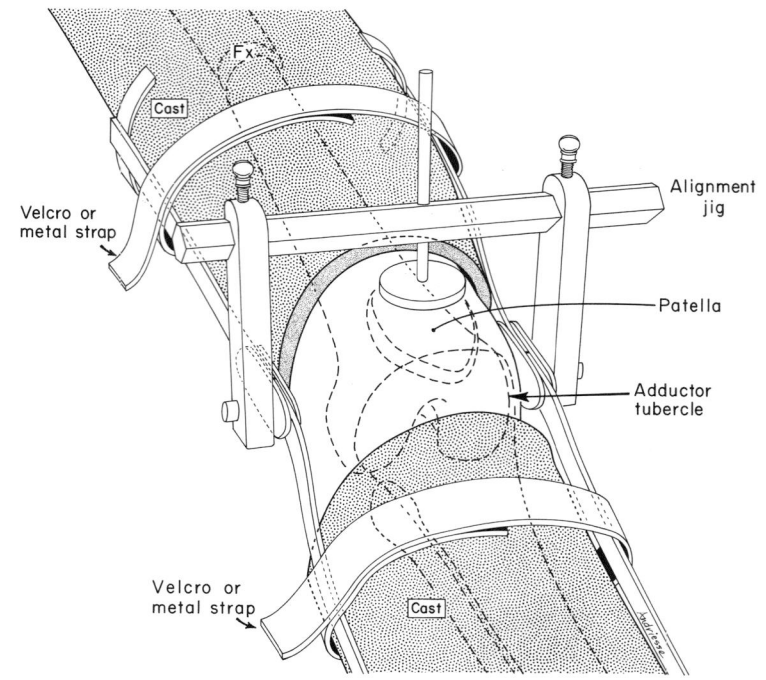

Fig. 29-19.—Application of polycentric hinged knee joints, using alignment jig and Velcro straps to hold hinges temporarily in position.

quadriceps setting and range of motion exercises as soon as possible.

The patient progresses to full weight bearing as tolerated and thereafter uses crutches only for balance. The patient normally has no pain after the first few days. If pain persists or recurs, the cast may be loose and a new snug cast should be applied. Similarly, if the cast becomes loose, it should be replaced. Such a change is rarely necessary. In the experience of Mooney and co-workers,[37] about 5% of over 300 cast braces had to be changed.

The cast brace is usually worn for 10–12 weeks until the patient can walk with full weight bearing without distress and has active use of the knee at the functional level. Serial x-rays are needed to monitor alignment. X-ray evidence of fracture healing, on the other hand, is relatively unimportant and indeed is ignored by Mooney and associates, who had no refractures or nonunion in 150 patients treated by preliminary traction and a cast brace. They also found no instance of measurable additional shortening while the cast brace was worn.

Although there is often limitation of knee motion at the time of removal of the cast brace, recovery of motion after removal is rapid. Thus, of the patients treated by Mooney and his associates, only 9% had knee flexion of less than 45 degrees 6 weeks after removal of the cast brace.

Treatment by traction and a cast brace has obvious advantages: none of the risks attendant on open reduction and internal fixation, continuing muscle and joint function, shortened hospitalization and convalescence compared to traction followed by immobilization in a spica cast, and a lowered incidence of nonunion and refracture. However, use of this device is only practical when personnel with experience in the use of total-contact plaster casts and the alignment of the joints of

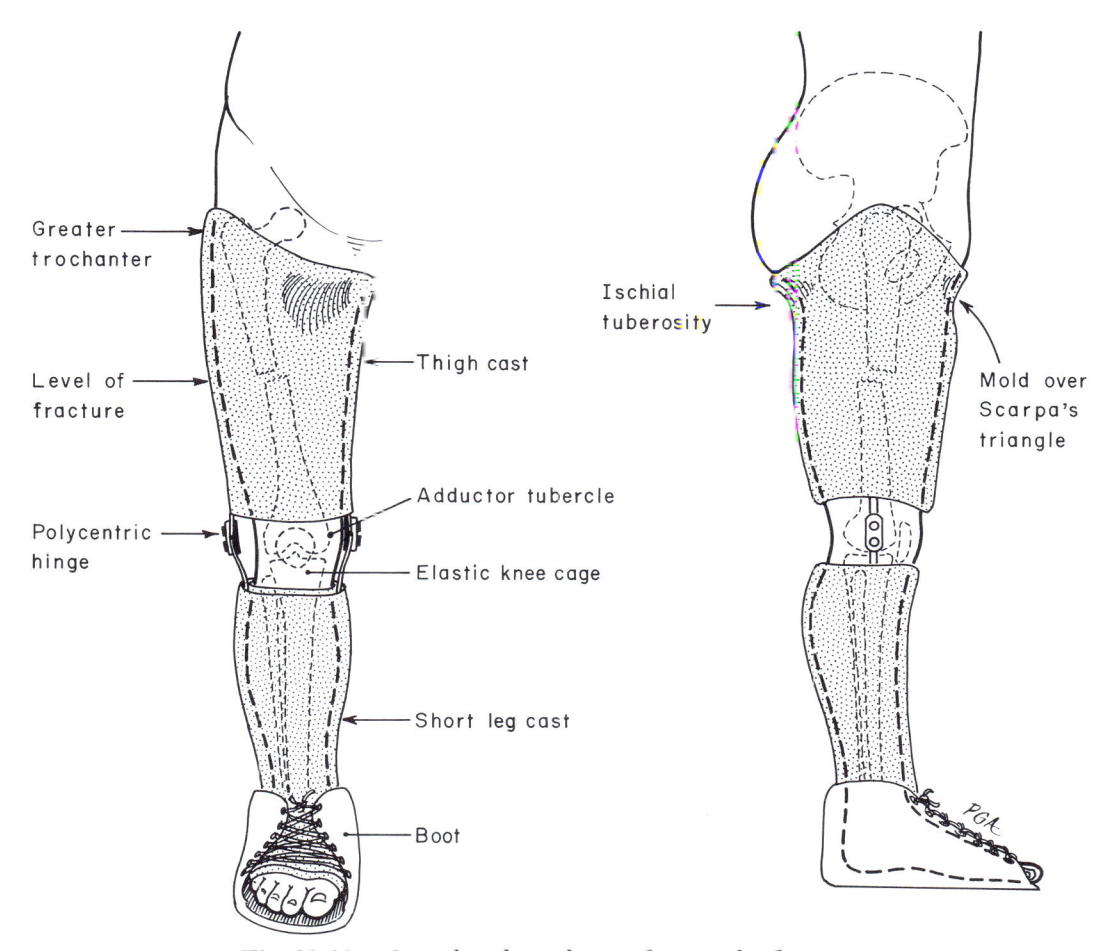

Fig. 29-20.—Completed cast brace; front and side views.

leg braces are available to apply the device. Application is a demanding and time-consuming procedure. Improperly applied, the cast brace can cause serious shortening and malunion.

Open Reduction

The technique for open reduction of a fracture of the femoral shaft using a medullary nail or compression plates is described in Chapter 35. Only some general comments will be made here.

Blind nailing as described by Küntscher,[31] Rokkanen,[45] Rascher and Nahigian[42] and Clawson et al.[15] has certain advantages, but it is only feasible when image-amplification x-ray equipment and other special apparatus are available. For most surgeons, limited exposure of the fracture site through a posterolateral approach is the most practical method. It has the advantage that the medullary canal can be reamed and the size of the nail tested under direct vision. Furthermore, if the bone ends are visualized, cracks or incomplete fractures which may not be visible on the x-rays may be found. If these are not secured by additional fixation or by sufficient reaming to produce extensive contact between rod and cortex above and below the fracture, displacement of the "butterfly" fragment with shortening and loss of fixation may result (Fig. 29-1).

Use of Rush pins or a Vesely rod may be advantageous for the fixation of more distally placed fractures.[47, 48, 64]

The self-broaching rods, such as the Hansen-Street and Schneider nails, eliminate the need for reaming.[51] However, nails of the proper length must be in stock, since they cannot be cut to the desired length as can the Küntscher nail. It is important to use a nail of the correct length, especially for the more distal fractures, if maximal stability is to be achieved. The lower end of the nail should engage the cancellous bone in the subchondral region at the distal end of the femur, while its proximal end should extend no more than 1 cm above the greater trochanter. A nail so placed achieves maximal fixation in the distal fragment and does not cause an antalgic limp because of a painful bursa formed about the projecting proximal end.

It is now generally agreed that the nail should be no smaller than 12 mm in diameter to minimize the risk of breakage and that, if the fixation is to be stable, the surface of the nail should be in contact with the inner surface of the cortex for a distance of at least 2.5 cm above and 2.5 cm below the fracture ends. In most femurs, reaming will be required, especially in the narrowest part of the canal just proximal to the midpoint of the shaft, in order to achieve this stable situation. On the other hand, in an osteoporotic femur it may be difficult to produce a tight fit even when a rod 18 mm in diameter is available. When the Küntscher apparatus is used, it is possible to nest 2 rods (half of each nail lying in the slot of the other) and thereby to obtain a tight fit in a medullary canal too large for the largest nail available.

With the fracture site exposed, the medullary canal can be reamed with ease both proximally and distally. The fracture is then reduced and held with clamps while the medullary nail is inserted. For the straight nail to traverse the anteriorly bowed medullary canal, the femur should be bowed posteriorly at the site of a fracture in the middle one-third as the nail is driven down the shaft. This maneuver will minimize the tendency of the nail to penetrate the thin anterior cortex in the supracondylar region. With a distally located fracture in a femur with considerable anterior bowing, the nail may jam in the canal during insertion or it may penetrate the anterior cortex of the proximal fragment. Under these circumstances, osteotomy at the apex of the curve may be necessary so that the shaft can be straightened to accommodate the rod (Fig. 29-21).

As the nail is driven along the medullary canal, it should move readily with each blow of the mallet. If the nail begins to bind, the cause of the binding must be determined and eliminated before the nail is driven further and becomes impacted, making removal or further insertion difficult or impossible. Most frequently, such a situation is due to the nail's being too large. Less commonly, it results from the nail's penetrating the cortex.

On rare occasions, as the Küntscher nail is driven over the guide rod, it may become constricted and grip the guide rod so firmly that further insertion or removal is difficult. This condition can be avoided by checking the guide rod periodically as the nail is inserted. If the nail binds or if the guide rod starts to move with the Küntscher nail, the guide rod should be removed before the nail is driven farther. In any event, the guide rod is removed when the nail is well past the fracture site.

Since the maximal bending stress on the femur during weight bearing tends to cause lateral angulation, an intramedullary nail should be placed so that it presents its maximal strength to stresses applied in this frontal plane. With the Hansen-Street nail, the long diameter should lie in this plane; with the Küntscher nail, the eye should be posterior and lateral and the slot anterior and mesial.

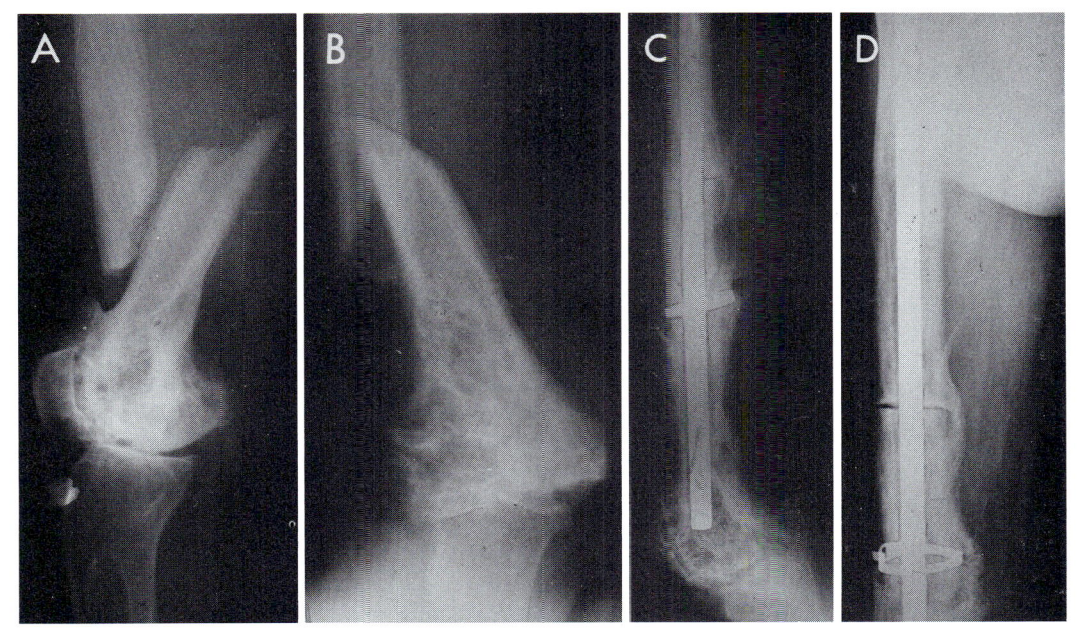

Fig. 29-21.—A, and B, posteroanterior views of pathologic fracture of femoral shaft in Paget's disease. Open reduction and fixation by means of a Küntscher nail and a Parham band were done after proximal osteotomy, which was performed to correct bowing of the shaft and to permit insertion of the nail. C and D, 3 months postoperative; healing progressing satisfactorily although the Parham band has pulled loose. At follow-up 1 year after the operation, there was bone union and good knee and hip function.

In some cases, bone grafts should be placed around the fracture site before the wound is closed. Shavings of cancellous bone obtained from the ilium at the time of operation are preferable for this purpose. An alternative can be shavings from the nearby femoral cortex, although these are less effective. Such grafts can probably be omitted in young adults, in whom union is almost certain to occur.

Postoperative Management

Traction should be avoided and efforts made to encourage impaction of the fragments. Simple suspension or support on pillows may be used during the immediate postoperative period. Muscle setting of the quadriceps, hamstrings and gluteal muscles should be started by the second or third day.

In the early days of medullary nailing, when reaming of the canal was not done and rods less than 12 mm in diameter were often used, rotary instability was occasionally observed. Some form of external immobilization, such as suspension with the knee flexed or a plaster cast with a rotation crossbar, was used to prevent rotation. With modern technique, such rotary instability is seldom a problem. If recognized during the procedure, it should be correctable by using a larger rod or a supplemental compression plate. If rotatory instability is first recognized postoperatively, a cast brace may well be the best solution.

Guarded weight bearing with crutches is ordinarily commenced as soon as the wound is healed. Non-weight-bearing with the leg dangling is contraindicated, since this may cause distraction with resultant delayed or even nonunion. Partial weight bearing is instituted from the start and continued until mature callus is visible on x-rays, or for 4–6 months as a rule.

For full weight bearing, it is safer to allow bone healing to progress to an advanced degree. In the absence of solid bone union, fracture or bending of the nail may occur, owing either to excessive stress, such as that from a fall or a misstep, or to fatigue of the nail.

Removal of the nail after the fracture has healed is not mandatory unless the nail is causing symptoms such as pain in the hip region or an antalgic limp. However, removal is advisable in most patients. Removal should be deferred until at least 1 year after nailing or until the cortex in the region of the fracture has been sufficiently remodeled to resemble that of the normal shaft. With the rod in situ the strength of the bone remains less than normal and refracture after removal of the nail is a real danger. If symptoms referable to the proximal end of the nail necessitate removal before adequate remodeling has occurred, the nail should be removed and a shorter and slightly larger one reinserted without exposing the fracture site.

Open Fractures of the Femoral Shaft

As in all open fractures, the first and most important step in the definitive treatment is an adequate debridement of the wound with removal of all foreign material and all contused and contaminated tissue. All the recesses of the wound should be thoroughly irrigated with sterile saline solution. The surgeon must then decide whether immediate internal fixation is indicated or whether the wound should be closed and traction instituted. In severely comminuted, or shattered, fractures, traction is unquestionably the method of choice. In transverse or short oblique fractures without gross contamination, in which debridement has been adequate and carried out within 6-8 hours of injury, fixation with an intramedullary nail may be indicated. If such ideal circumstances do not exist, it is safer to close the wound loosely or safer still to leave it open and do a delayed primary closure, treating the fracture in traction. When the wound is healed, the soft tissues have recovered from the effects of trauma and the danger of sepsis is much reduced, internal fixation or perhaps treatment in a cast brace may be indicated. If internal fixation is performed as a secondary procedure, autogenous iliac grafts should be inserted to expedite union. If the fracture is complicated by a vascular injury requiring repair or if for some reason traction is contraindicated, internal fixation may be done primarily when conditions are less than ideal. On occasion it may be desirable to fix the fracture simply to splint soft tissues that are in precarious condition and to promote their healing. This situation occurs rarely in the thigh.

Primary closure of the wound at the time of debridement is justified only when the debridement has been completely satisfactory, all dead space has been eliminated and the wound can be closed without tension. If the surgeon has the slightest doubt, the wound should be left open down to muscle and a delayed primary closure performed.

In addition to local treatment of the open wound and the fracture, the patient must receive antibiotics and prophylaxis against tetanus as previously described. (See Chapter 37.)

Pathologic Fractures

The treatment of pathologic fractures is discussed in Chapter 7. It need only be noted here that intramedullary fixation may be used for pathologic fracture of the femoral shaft consequent to metastatic disease, fibrous dysplasia, osteogenesis imperfecta, Paget's disease and the like. If there is extensive deformity of the femur 1 or more osteotomies may be required to straighten the shaft sufficiently to permit insertion of the intramedullary rod.

A significant advance in the treatment of fractures associated with metastatic disease would appear to be the use of methylmethacrylate to supplement the fixation provided by an intramedullary rod or other metallic device.[25] The acrylic can be used to fill defects and can be molded around the metallic implants to provide sufficient stability to enable the patients to be ambulatory and free from pain during the remaining months or weeks of their lives.

COMPLICATIONS

EMBOLIC DISEASE.—Once the acute effects of injury are past, perhaps the earliest major complication encountered in patients with fractures of the femoral shaft (as in all patients with major injuries) is fat embolism. The diagnosis and treatment of this condition are described in Chapter 54, but this complication is mentioned here to remind the reader that it must always be kept in mind while any patient with a fracture of the femoral shaft is being followed. If diagnosis is made promptly and treatment with respiratory support and intravenous administration of steroids is instituted early, the patient will almost invariably do well.

Another major, life-threatening complication is thromboembolic disease. Patients with fracture of the femoral shaft are likely candidates for this catastrophic complication. Prevention, diagnosis and treatment have been discussed by several authors[49] and discussed as well in Chapter 26.

SEPSIS.—Perhaps the most dreaded complication after an open fracture or after open reduction of a closed femoral fracture is sepsis[19, 20, 67] (Fig. 29-22). The treatment of infection after medullary nailing is discussed in Chapter 35. The same principles apply to infections complicating compression-plate fixation. In general, the goal of therapy is to bring the acute infection under control by the usual methods of dependent drainage and appropriate antibiotic therapy. Suction drainage may be useful as an adjunct in clearing up infections.[16] When the acute infection has been brought under control, the patient usually is left with a chronic infection and draining sinus. Under these circumstances, if there is stable internal fixation, union will gradually occur over the course of a year or more despite continuous or intermittent drainage. It is therefore desirable to defer definitive treatment of the infection until solid union has occurred. To do this may require repeated incision and drainage and perhaps sequestrectomy to keep the infection under control. Once solid union has occurred, a major effort should be made to eliminate the sepsis by removal of all metal, wound debridement and appropriate antibiotic therapy based on sensitivity studies.

In the presence of sepsis without internal fixation, e.g., in war wounds, similar attempts to control infection and gain union by external fixation are indicated. Traction, a spica or even a cast brace may be used for immobilization. Rarely, internal fixation of the fragments by a medullary rod, despite frank sepsis, should be considered. By making the patient more mobile and immobilizing the infected tissues, this salvage procedure may result in union as described by Brav[9] and by Carr and Turnipseed.[12]

If bone union occurs in the presence of a draining sinus but the bridge of bone is not sufficient to prevent refracture, it may be possible to approach the fracture site through clean tissue—usually anteriorly or medially—without entering the infected area. Autogenous onlay grafts can then be applied to the normal cortical bone exposed subperiosteally. This procedure may stimulate the formation of a stronger bridge of bone and permit earlier definitive treatment of the sepsis (removal of metal and sequestra) with less risk of refracture.

DELAYED UNION OR NONUNION.—For delayed union or nonunion in the absence of sepsis the usual aim of treatment is to provide rigid internal fixation and a stimulus to osteogenesis. If the faulty

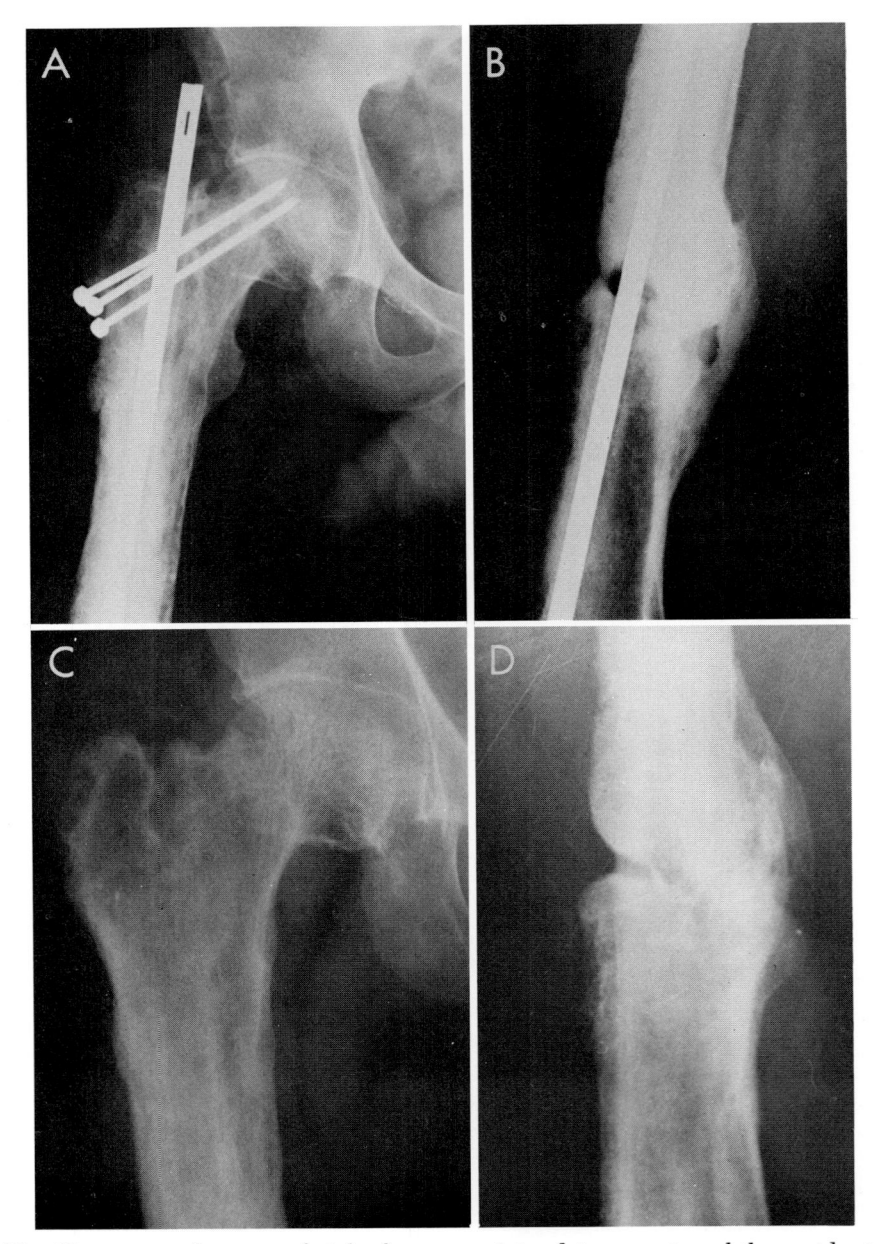

Fig. 29-22.—Transverse fracture of right femur, sustained in an automobile accident, treated elsewhere by open reduction and Küntscher rod. Postoperative drainage for 2–3 weeks treated by repeated surgical procedures and intermittent chemotherapy. Rod left in situ; persistent drainage and osteomyelitis. Two years later admitted with an undisplaced subcapital fracture of the right hip, treated by insertion of 3 Knowles pins (**A** and **B**). Uneventful healing of operative wound but drainage continued from midthigh sinus. Fracture was healed 22 months later, but patient was readmitted with *Staphylococcus aureus* septicemia, treated successfully with antibiotics intravenously. One month later the Küntscher rod and Knowles pins were removed (**C** and **D**); postoperative course uneventful.

union is a sequel to treatment in traction, a trial of a cast brace or a walking spica may be worthwhile. Usually medullary fixation supplemented by onlay autogenous cancellous bone grafts from the ilium is the preferred treatment. When the fracture site is exposed, especially if there is considerable callus in the presence of nonunion, elevation of a cuff of osteoperiosteal tissue (the osteoperiosteal graft of Judet and Patel[28] may be a sufficient stimulus to osteogenesis of itself or may be a worthwhile supplement to the onlay grafts which can be placed beneath the cuff.

If faulty union has developed after a previous open reduction, the old metallic implant must, of course, be removed and a new device inserted. A medullary rod or occasionally compression plates may be used, depending on the circumstances. The new internal fixation is supplemented by bone grafts, which are placed in a vascular bed produced by the debridement of scar tissue so far as it is possible. For discussion of the treatment of nonunion in the presence of a bent or broken medullary nail, see Chapter 31.

IMPAIRED KNEE FUNCTION.—If, for any reason, the knee has been immobilized for a prolonged period after fracture, especially if union has been delayed or sepsis has occurred, limitation of flexion and extension will result due to joint adhesions and to scarring and adhesions of the quadriceps mechanism. This is more likely to occur in distal fractures. When adequate intramedullary fixation has been achieved and active motion has begun early, this complication is rare.

In general, function plus prolonged physical therapy, including progressive resistance exercises when appropriate, will gradually restore a satisfactory, if not a complete, range of motion. If these measures fail, some form of quadricepsplasty should be considered if the knee is intact. The technique described by Thompson[61] for excision of the scarred portion of the quadriceps, usually the vastus intermedius, and release of the capsule and of the quadriceps expansions on both sides of the patella is probably the most satisfactory.

BIBLIOGRAPHY

1. American College of Surgeons Committee on Trauma: A guide to prophylaxis against tetanus in wound management, 1972 revision, Bull. Am. Coll. Surg. 57:32, 1972.
2. Anderson, L. D.: Conservative treatment, J. Bone Joint Surg. 49-A:1371, 1967.
3. Anderson, L. D.: Patient with multiple fractures, Minn. Med. 51:1091, 1968.
4. Barry, H. C.: Fractures of the femur in Paget's disease of bone in Australia, J. Bone Joint Surg. 49-A:1359, 1967.
5. Bechtol, C. O.: Engineering principles applied to orthopaedic surgeons, Am. Acad. Orthop. Surg. Instructional Course Lectures, IX, 1952.
6. Blichert-Toft, M., and Hammer, A.: Treatment of fractures of the femoral shaft, Acta Orthop. Scand. 41:341, 1970.
7. Blount, W. P.: *Fractures in Children* (Baltimore: Williams & Wilkins Company, 1954.)
8. Böhler, J. L.: Closed intramedullary nailing of femur, Clin. Orthop. 60:51, 1968.
9. Brav, E.: Modified intramedullary nailing in recent fractures of femoral shaft, J. Bone Joint Surg. 35-A:141, 1953.
10. Breck, L. W., and Bascom, W. C.: The dual plate, no cast, internal fixation of shaft fracture, South. Med. J. 37:582, 1944.
11. Burwell, H. N.: Internal fixation in the treatment of fractures of the femoral shaft, Injury 2:235, 1971.
12. Carr, C. R., and Turnipseed, D.: Experiences with intramedullary fixation of compound fractures in war wounds, J. Bone Joint Surg. 35-A:153, 1953.
13. Carr, C. R., and Wingo, C.: Fractures of the femoral diaphyses: A retrospective comparative study of treatment by intramedullary nailing and by traction-spica cast. J. Bone Joint Surg. 54-A:1344, 1972.
14. Cast bracing of fractures, National Academy of Sciences Workshop, 1971.
15. Clawson, D. K., Smith, R., and Hansen, S.: Closed intramedullary nailing of the femur, J. Bone Joint Surg. 53-A:681, 1971.
16. Compere, E. L., and Metzger, W. I.: The treatment of pyogenic bone and joint infections by closed irrigation (circulation) with a nontoxic detergent and one or more antibiotics, J. Bone Joint Surg. 49-A:614, 1967.
17. Dehne, E.: The natural history of the fractured tibia, Surg. Clin. North Am. 41:1495, 1961.
18. Delbet, P.: *Méthode de traitement des fractures: Annales de la clinique chirurgicale du Professeur Delbet*, No. 5 (Paris: Librairie Felix Alcan, 1916).
19. Dencker, H.: Shaft fractures in the femur: A comparative study of the results of various methods of treatment in 1003 cases, Acta Chir. Scand. 130:173, 1965.
20. Dencker, H.: Frequency of infection in treatment of femoral shaft fractures, Acta Chir.

Scand. 130:440, 1965.
21. Gant, G. C., Shaftan, G. W., and Herbsman, H.: Experience with the ASIF compression plate in the management of femoral shaft fractures, Trauma 10:458, 1970.
22. Goran, D., Lilliestrom, et al.: Intracortical circulation after intramedullary reaming with reduction of pressure in the medullary cavity: A microangiographic study on rabbit tibia, Acta Orthop. Scand., Supp. 134, 1970.
23. Griffin, P. P., Anderson, M. E., and Green, W. T.: Fracture of the shaft of the femur in children: Treatment and result, Orthop. Clin. North Am. 3:213, 224, 1972.
24. Grundy, M.: Fracture in Paget's disease of bone, J. Bone Joint Surg. 52-B:252, 1970.
25. Harrington, K. D., et al.: The use of methylmethacrylate as an adjunct in the internal fixation of malignant neoplastic fractures, J. Bone Joint Surg. 54-A:1665, 1972.
26. Humberger, F. W., and Eyring, E. J.: Proximal tibial 90-90 traction in treatment of children with femoral shaft fractures, J. Bone Joint Surg. 51-A:499, 1969.
27. Irani, R., Nicholson, J. T., and Chung, S. M. K.: Treatment of femoral fractures in children by immediate spica immobilization, J. Bone Joint Surg. 54-A:1567, 1972.
28. Judet, R., and Patel, A.: Muscle pedicle bone grafting of long bones by osteoperiosteal decortication, Clin. Orthop. 87:74, 1972.
29. Kaplan, I. W., and Craighead, C. C.: Two plate fixation of fractures of the femoral shaft with Eggers' plate, Am. J. Surg. 89:862, 1955.
30. Kaufer, H.: Nonoperative ambulatory treatment for fracture of the shaft of the femur, Clin. Orthop. 87:192, 1972.
31. Küntscher, G.: *Practice of Intramedullary Nailing* (Springfield, Ill.: Charles C Thomas, Publisher, 1967).
32. Lindquist, C. A.: Double plates in rectangular planes for internal fixation of fractures of the femur, Ann. West. Med. Surg. 2:93, 1948.
33. MacAusland, W. R., Jr.: Treatment of sepsis after intramedullary nailing of fractures of the femur, Clin. Orthop. 60:87, 1968.
34. Mann, R., and Sarmiento, A.: Two plate fixation for nonunion of fractured femur, Clin. Orthop. 38:93, 1965.
35. Marshall, D. V.: Three side plate fixation for fractures of the femoral and tibial shaft, J. Bone Joint Surg. 40-A:323, 1958.
36. Moll, J. H.: The cast-brace walking treatment of open and closed femoral fractures, South. Med. J. 66:345, 1973.
37. Mooney, V., Nickel, V. L., and Harvey, J. P., Jr.: Cast brace treatment for fractures of the distal part of the femur: A prospective controlled study of 150 patients, J. Bone Joint Surg. 52-A:1563, 1970.
38. Mooney, V.: Personal communication, 1973.
39. Parrish, F.: Surgical treatment for secondary neoplastic fractures: A retrospective study of 96 patients, J. Bone Joint Surg. 52-B:665, 1970.
40. Perez, C. A., et al.: Management of pathological fracture, Cancer 29:684, 1972.
41. Porter, M. F.: Delayed arterial occlusion, J. Bone Joint Surg. 50-B:138, 1968.
42. Rascher, J. J., and Nahigian, S. H.: Closed nailing of femoral shaft fractures, J. Bone Joint Surg. 54-A:534, 1972.
43. Rhinelander, F. W.: The normal microcirculation of the diaphyseal cortex and its response to fracture, J. Bone Joint Surg. 50-A:748, 1968.
44. Rich, N. M.: Internal vs. external fixation fracture with concomitant vascular injury in Vietnam, J. Trauma 11:463, 1971.
45. Rokkanen, P., Statis, P., and Vankka, E.: Closed or open intramedullary nailing of femoral shaft fractures: A comparison with conservatively treated cases, J. Bone Joint Surg. 51-B:313, 1969.
46. Ruoff, A. C., et al.: Dual plating in selected femoral fractures, J. Trauma 12:233, 1972.
47. Rush, L. V.: Dynamic intramedullary fracture fixation of the femur: Reflections on use of the round rod after 30 years, Clin. Orthop. 60:21, 1968.
48. Rush, L. V.: K rod early vs. late, Aust. N. Z. J. Surg. 40:44, 1970.
49. Salzman E. W., and Harris, W. H.: Anticoagulation for prevention of thromboembolism following fractures of the hip, N. Engl. J. Med. 275:122, 1966.
50. Sarmiento, A.: Functional bracing of tibial and femoral shaft fractures, Clin. Orthop. 82:2, 1972.
51. Schneider, H. W.: Use of the 4-flanged self-cutting intramedullary nail for fixation of femoral fractures, Clin. Orthop. 60:29, 1968.
52. Sevastona, A. A.: Comparative study treatment by traction and open fixation, R. I. Med. J. 54:144, 1971.
53. Scudese, V. A.: Femoral shaft fracture: Percutaneous multiple-pin fixation; thigh cylinder plaster cast and early weight bearing, Clin. Orthop. 77:164, 1971.
54. Slatis, P., Ryöppy, S., and Huittinen, V. M.: AOI osteosynthesis of fractures of the distal third of the femur, Acta Orthop. Scand. 43:162, 1971.
55. Smith, H. H.: On the treatment of ununited fractures by means of artificial limbs, Am. J. Med. Sci. 29:102, 1855.
56. Smith, J. E. M.: The result of early and delayed internal fixation of fractures of the shaft of the femur, J. Bone Joint Surg. 46-B:31, 1964.
57. Spinner, M.: Double spica treatment, Clin. Orthop. 53:109, 1967.
58. Stewart, M. J., Sisk, T. D., et al.: Fractures of the distal third of the femur, J. Bone Joint Surg. 48-A:784, 1966.
59. Street, D. M.: Medullary nailing of the femur: Comparative study of skeletal tractions, plating and medullary nailing, JAMA 143:709, 1950.
60. Stryker, W. S., and Russell, M. E.: Comparison of the results of operative and non-operative treatment of diaphyseal fractures of the femur at the Naval Hospital, San Diego, over a 5-year period, J. Bone Joint Surg. 52-A:815, 1970.
61. Thompson, F. R.: Quadriceps plasty to improve knee function, J. Bone Joint Surg. 26:366, 1944.
62. Trueta, J., and Cavadras, A.: Vascular changes caused by Küntscher type of nailing, J. Bone Joint Surg. 37-B:492, 1955.
63. Trueta, J., and Cavadras, A.: A study of blood supply of the long bone, Surg. Gynecol. Obstet. 118:485, 1964.

64. Vesely, D. G.: Technic for use of the single and the double split diamond nail for fractures of the femur, Clin. Orthop. 60:95, 1968.
65. Wade, P. A.: ASIF compression has a problem. Editorial, J. Trauma 10:513, 1970.
66. Wenger, H. L.: Shaft fracture immobilization without plaster, Am. J. Surg. 66:382, 1944.
67. Wickstrom, J. K., and Corban, M. S.: Complications following intramedullary fixation of 324 fractured femurs, Clin. Orthop. 60:103, 1968.

30 | Injuries Involving the Knee

WILLIAM R. MacAUSLAND, JR.

THE KNEE IS a weight-bearing joint which is subjected to a great variety of static and dynamic loads. Normal knee function is possible only if there is good muscle control, intact supporting ligaments and well-aligned articular surfaces.

Acute trauma to this exposed joint is common, particularly in the young adult who skis or plays contact sports, such as football. Automobile accidents produce tibial "bumper" fractures in the pedestrian and patellar or supracondylar fractures in the passengers.

GENERAL CONSIDERATIONS

Whether the primary injury is relatively minor and well localized or is more severe, the clinical pattern following injury is characteristically that of pain, joint effusion and hamstring muscle spasm, which produces a limping gait with the knee held rigidly in semiflexion. There is a widespread misconception that, if there is no fracture, "it is all right to walk on it." Although in mild soft tissue injuries recovery tends to occur spontaneously, in the moderate and severe injuries healing is extremely slow, and there may be permanent functional disability unless treatment is adequate. This implies correct diagnosis and the application of the necessary specific and general therapeutic measures. The specific measures will be discussed under the appropriate diagnostic headings. The general measures applicable to all types of knee injuries will be discussed here. The essence of skilled treatment lies in the use of rest and exercise at the proper time and in the correct amount.

Rest

The injured knee should be put at rest and protected from further trauma and from unphysiologic use until the injured tissues have healed and until good muscle control and joint function have been restored. The amount and type of rest that is necessary depend on the severity of the injury. In the acute severe injuries, such as occur in fractures or ligamentous ruptures, complete bed rest for a few days is indicated, with the knee elevated at or above heart level.

The method of protective immobilization will also depend on the severity of the injury. The Thomas or Hodgen splint, traction, plaster casing or a posterior splint are commonly used for severe injuries. Total immobilization should be discontinued as soon as it is safe to do so. Its prolonged use produces muscle atrophy, osteoporosis, fibrosis of the periarticular structures and thinning of the articular cartilage.

In mild and moderate injuries, crutches will protect the knee and still allow the patient to be quite active. It is not sufficient to prescribe the use of crutches. The physician must explain why they are necessary and see that the patient is instructed and drilled in their proper use.

In the acute phase of severe injuries in which the knee is immobilized in plaster, no weight is borne on the injured extremity and the foot does not touch the floor. In mild to moderate injuries and in the later phase of severe injuries, the patient places the foot on the floor as the knee goes through its normal motions, letting the crutches take the bulk of the body weight. In this way, smooth reciprocal flexion-extension muscle action is encouraged. This increases venous and lymphatic return and stimulates restoration of normal muscular physiology. As the injured tissues heal, the amount of weight borne on the crutches is gradually decreased until eventually the patient walks smoothly with full weight on the extremity. The occurrence of pain, muscle spasm or synovial effusion indicates that there is too much strain on the knee and that more weight needs to be carried on the crutches and less on the foot.

An elastic bandage applied over felt or sponge rubber is an efficient local support for most soft tissue injuries of the knee (Fig. 30-1). The patient is taught the proper application of this support using light, even pressure and to remove it for exercises several times daily.

Application of moist heat to the knee for 10 or 15 minutes several times daily will help remove the excessive synovial fluid and dissipate the soft tissue edema.

Exercise

The amounts of rest and exercise used in knee injuries bear a reciprocal relationship. In the acute phase, rest is maximal and exercise is minimal. As recovery occurs, rest is decreased and exercise increased.

Atrophy of the quadriceps extensor musculature is the inevitable sequela of an acute knee injury and leads to chronic weakness of the knee musculature unless vigorously combated by appropriate exercises. The exercises are continued until normal strength has been restored.

Quadriceps setting exercises should be instituted immediately, although in the presence of severe synovitis and effusion there may be difficulty in performing the exercises. They should be done even when the leg is encased in plaster.

TECHNIQUE OF EXERCISES. — Both knees are placed in the extended position. Preliminary application of heat is often helpful but not essential. The patient is taught to contract voluntarily and simultaneously the quadriceps muscle of both thighs to a maximal amount. Contraction is sustained for a count of 3 seconds, and the muscles are then relaxed for the same period of time. Emphasis is placed on slow, forceful, complete contraction with an equal period of relaxation. Beginning with 5 repetitions, the exercise is increased rapidly until the patient does 10 every hour during the day without diffi-

Fig. 30-1. — Application of an elastic bandage over sponge rubber. The suprapatellar pouch is obliterated, but no direct pressure is placed on the skin overlying the patella (*outlined in ink*). Note the pad in the popliteal space.

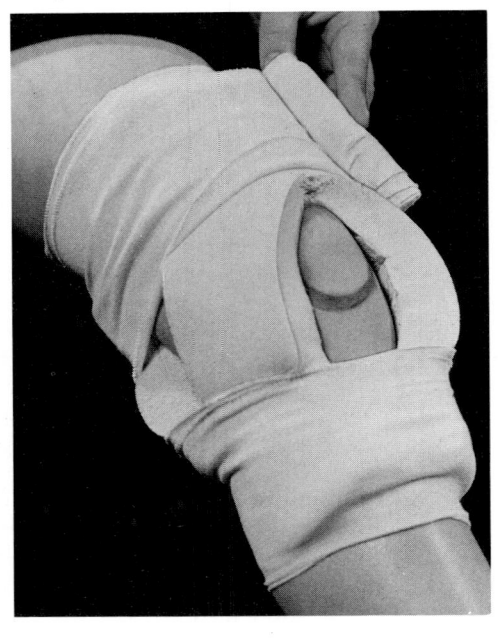

culty. This is followed by lifting the leg with the knee extended.

This type of quadriceps setting places no strain on injured tissues. When the synovitis has subsided, the exercise program is progressively increased until muscle strength has returned to normal, as shown by the measurement of the circumference of the 2 thighs.

The graduation of exercises is carried out as follows:

1. *Early phase.*—Quadriceps setting without resistance 5–10 times hourly.

2. *Convalescent phase.*—Quadriceps setting, lifting the leg off the bed with the knee extended 5–10 times hourly.

3. *Late phase.*—Quadriceps drill (progressive resistant exercise) 10 times once a day. The maximal amount of weight attached to the foot or ankle which can be lifted with the knee fully extended is determined. One-half this amount is used for this exercise. The weight is lifted with the knee fully extended. The exercise is done slowly, with the time of rest equal to the contraction time. The maximal weight which can be lifted is redetermined at weekly intervals and the amount of weight (one-half maximal) to be used for the exercise program is adjusted accordingly.

Knee motion.—As noted previously, complete immobilization of the knee should be discontinued at the earliest possible moment and carefully graded active motion should be instituted. Motion should be kept within the limits of pain and muscle spasm and should not be forced in the first few weeks of recovery. Underwater exercises and whirlpool baths are helpful.

In the later phase of recovery, lack of knee flexion may be gradually overcome by gentle assistive stretching over the edge of a table and by squatting exercises partially supported.

Occasionally, judicious gentle stretching under anesthesia is necessary to help restore joint motion. The aim of treatment is restoration of normal muscle strength, ligamentous stability and knee motion. The severity of the injury may in some instances make it impossible to regain a normal knee, but adequate treatment based on the proper use of rest, protection and exercise can almost always restore satisfactory function.

SOFT TISSUE INJURIES OF THE KNEE

CONTUSIONS.—Minor contusions occur frequently along the anterior aspect of the knee over the patella, the infrapatellar fat pad and the tibial tubercle, since these exposed sites are often injured by a direct blow. Severe injuries may result in hemorrhage into the synovial membrane, infrapatellar fat pad or the prepatellar bursa. The greatest potential danger from a minor blow on the knee is that the articular cartilage or the patella or femoral condyles may be damaged to such a degree that late degenerative changes, i.e., chondromalacia or osteochondritis, may occur.

TRAUMATIC HEMARTHROSIS.—Hemarthrosis of the knee usually denotes a severe injury. It is most commonly associated with fractures entering the joint, less frequently with tears of the cruciate or collateral ligament. After such injuries, swelling usually appears within the first 2 hours. The pain is severe and the local temperature is increased. Motion is limited and attended with pain. The bony landmarks are obliterated, and on palpation there is a sense of doughy firmness, particularly in the suprapatellar area.

TRAUMATIC SYNOVITIS.—Synovitis accompanies almost all injuries to the knee. It produces distention of the capsule with effacement of the anatomic landmarks. In simple cases of "water on the knee," little pain is experienced and the symptoms are those of mild discomfort from tension and restricted motion due to the effusion of the joint itself. The appearance of the swelling is often delayed for some hours after the injury. On palpation of the distended quadriceps pouch, less firmness is noted than is present with a hemarthrosis.

TREATMENT.—The treatment of contusions, hemarthrosis and traumatic synovitis of the knee must be modified to meet the needs of the given injury, but certain general principles are applicable to all types of knee injuries. Rest of the joint is of utmost importance. Avoidance of the strain of weight bearing by the use of crutches will prevent further damage to a weakened knee. The knee itself should be supported with an elastic bandage or a Jones dressing fitted over a felt or sponge rubber pad cut to fit around the patella. With more severe lesions, particularly if there is a tendency to flexion deformity, immobilization by means of a plaster cylinder and/or bed rest may be indicated. The application of ice bags for the first 24 hours following injury will lessen pain and reduce the degree of joint distention. When danger of further bleeding has passed, moist heat will produce a local hyperemia and aid in the phagocytosis of extravasated blood. The use of excessive heat is injurious and should be avoided. Applications for 10–15 minutes twice daily are sufficient.

Analgesics and sedation appropriate to the age of the patient and the severity of the injury should be given if necessary.

Aspiration of the knee may be indicated in severe effusions or traumatic hemarthroses and should be done with full sterile precautions. The use of an 18-gauge needle on a 50-ml syringe is usually adequate, the needle being inserted most easily between the patella and the femoral condyle with the knee extended, approaching either laterally or medially. Often, over 100 ml of blood may be removed, with great reduction in pain as a result.

INJURIES OF THE LIGAMENTS OF THE KNEE

Internal Collateral Ligament

A valgus strain of the knee, associated with twisting of the femur inward or of the tibia outward with the knee slightly flexed, is the usual cause of injury to the internal collateral ligament. The lesion varies from a minimal strain to a complete rupture of both the superficial and deep portions of the ligament. The ligament may tear at any level or may be avulsed from either its tibial or femoral insertion (Fig. 30-2). In femoral detachments, a piece of bone may be torn away with the ligament. If the producing force continues after the internal collateral ligament has ruptured, the anterior cruciate may likewise rupture and the medial meniscus may be injured. Rupture in varying degree of the medial and posteromedial aspects of the joint capsule frequently occurs with the more violent injury.

CLINICAL DIAGNOSIS.—It is important to determine the true nature and the severity of the injury in order to prescribe prop-

Fig. 30-2.—Tear of medial collateral ligament, avulsion of anterior spine and displacement of medial meniscus. This x-ray view, taken with knee forced into valgus position under anesthesia, demonstrates the wide gap at the medial joint line. Note also the avulsion of the bony tibial insertion of the anterior cruciate.

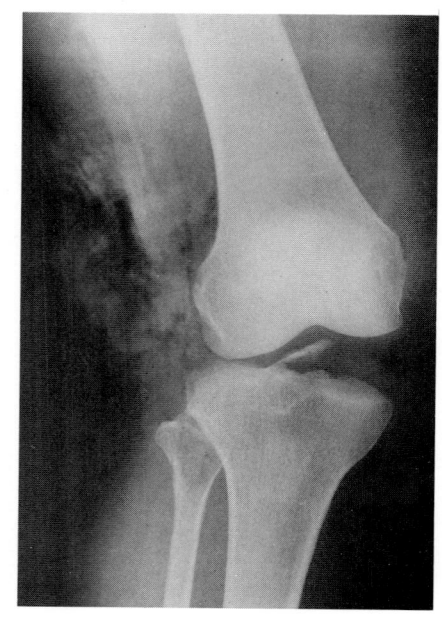

er treatment. With incomplete rupture or sprain of the internal collateral ligament, pain is experienced on the inner side of the knee over the ligament. Point tenderness is localized at the site of the lesion. The knee is held slightly flexed and no instability can be demonstrated on attempting to stress the knee into valgus position, although pain is increased by this maneuver. If the synovial lining is injured, effusion ensues. Hemarthrosis calls for diligent search to rule out the possibility of an unrecognized fracture, particularly an osteochondral fracture with a resulting loose body.

Should the ligament be completely ruptured both superficially and deep, there may be ecchymosis along the course of the ligament. Joint effusion may be present and the knee may lie in complete extension. A gentle valgus stretch of the knee may demonstrate a sulcus at the level of the joint; if the patient is seen in the first 2 or 3 hours following injury, this test may often be performed without anesthesia.

An estimation of the severity of the injury from the history together with the examination of the knee clinically, will usually satisfy a physician as to whether there is a partial or a complete tear of the ligament. However, if the surgeon is undecided as to the degree of injury, it is often advisable to test under appropriate anesthesia the integrity of the collateral ligaments, the cruciate ligaments and the menisci. Should the knee remain in a locked position of semiflexion following aspiration and appropriate anesthesia, a displaced meniscus or possibly a loose body must be suspected. To examine the knee for integrity of the medial collateral ligament, it is necessary to have the knee supported by the examining surgeon in approximately 10 degrees of flexion. At this position, valgus stress of the tibia will reveal the integrity of this ligament. If the knee, on the other hand, is tested in full extension, valgus deformity of the knee is prevented by the posterior capsule of the knee; thus, in full extension, the internal collateral ligaments are not adequately tested. One must flex the knee at least 10 degrees to relax the posterior capsule to get an adequate appraisal of the integrity of the internal collateral ligaments.

Roentgenograms in anterior, posterior, lateral and oblique views must be taken to rule out the possibility of avulsion fractures or of compression fractures of the tibial plateau.

CONSERVATIVE TREATMENT.—In partial tears of the internal collateral ligament, treatment is directed to protecting the ligament from further strain and, in particular, to relief of pain. It is usually advisable, when appropriate, to apply ice for the first 12–24 hours; following this, moist heat is beneficial in reducing local swelling and ecchymosis. The knee is immobilized in 5 degrees of flexion with either a Jones bandage, posterior molded splint or plaster cylinder, depending on the degree of discomfort. Crutches are used for protection until the gait is normal. Quadriceps exercises are practiced from the outset of treatment.

OPERATIVE TREATMENT.—Certain surgeons advocate immediate operative repair of internal collateral ligaments in all complete tears, whether isolated or associated with other injuries, since experience has shown that the ruptured ligament, when treated by plaster immobilization, may heal with a certain degree of laxity. Operative repair aimed at the restoration of a strong ligament is carried out as soon as possible after the injury and before reparative changes have occurred in the damaged soft tissues. Operative repair should be undertaken only if abnormal mobility can be demonstrated by examination—under anesthesia if necessary. At this time, the knee should be tested for rotatory instability (Fig. 30-3) to determine the advisability of advancing the pes anserinus anteriorly and distally (Slocum's procedure).

Technique.—A longitudinal bayonet incision is used to permit full visualization of the medial collateral ligament, the

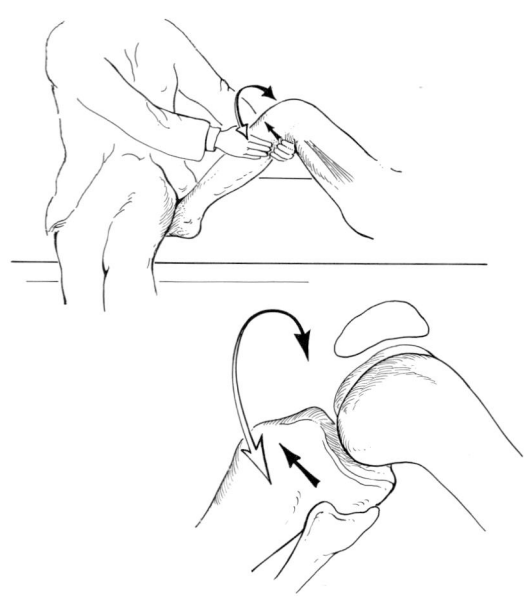

Fig. 30-3.—Test for rotatory instability of the knee. (After Slocum, D. B., and Larson, R. L.: Rotatory instability of the knee: Its pathogenesis and a clinical test to demonstrate its presence, J. Bone Joint Surg. 50-A:217, 1968.)

posteromedial capsule and the pes anserinus. The fascia is incised. The site of the lesion is inspected and particular attention is paid to the amount of damage to the medial and posteromedial capsule. Examination of the medial semilunar cartilage and anterior cruciate is usually possible through this incision at the site of capsular tear. Should the capsule be intact, an elective incision is made through the anterior portion of the capsule. If the medial semilunar cartilage is damaged, it should be removed before suture of the medial collateral ligament. If there is avulsion of the anterior cruciate ligament from its bony insertion, this, too, should be repaired.

If both deep and superficial layers of the internal collateral ligament are torn, each layer should be sutured separately. If the posteromedial capsule is torn, it should likewise be sutured with specific effort made to tighten the posterior capsule by overlapping the capsular suture line. When the internal ligament is avulsed from its tibial or femoral insertion, it may be resutured to its bony attachment through drill holes. When the medial ligament is then repaired, advancement of the pes anserinus is performed if clinically indicated to prevent rotatory instability.

External Collateral Ligament

The external collateral ligament is injured much less frequently than is the internal collateral. The injury usually occurs at the fibular attachment of the ligament and often it pulls with it a fragment of bone. There may be associated damage to other nearby structures, i.e., the capsule, popliteus tendon or iliotibial band and the cruciate ligaments. In rarer instances, the peroneal nerve may be stretched, with a resulting palsy. A tear of the lateral collateral ligament is suggested by history of varus strain followed by the clinical manifestations of localized pain, swelling and tenderness. As in the case of the medial collateral ligaments, should the severity of the injury by history and physical examination suggest a complete avulsion of the ligament, examination under anesthesia should be undertaken, comparing the injured knee to the normal joint. Definite widening of the lateral joint space may be demonstrated in roentgenograms. Surgical repair of complete ruptures is effective by methods similar to those used for repair of the internal collateral ligament. If there is evidence of peroneal nerve involvement, the nerve should be exposed at the time of surgical repair of the ligament. Usually the nerve is stretched rather than divided, but the prognosis for functional recovery is poor in either case. In late cases, neurolysis may result in some improvement in function.

Anterior Cruciate Ligament

AVULSION FRACTURE OF TIBIAL SPINE — ISOLATED LESIONS.—Isolated lesions of the anterior cruciate ligament may result from a direct blow on the posterior aspect of the tibia, displacing the tibia forward on the femur, or, conversely, from a blow to the anterior femur. A ligament may be stretched or ruptured at its upper attachment in the central portion or at its tibial insertion; in the latter case, there may be detachment of a fragment of bone from the tibial spine. Severe torsional strains produce combined lesions involving semilunar cartilage, anterior cruciate and medial collateral ligaments.

Examination reveals a joint effusion

Fig. 30-4.—**A**, sketch demonstrating the cruciate ligaments. **B**, posterior "drawer" sign for rupture of the posterior cruciate ligament. **C**, anterior "drawer" sign demonstrating anterior cruciate rupture.

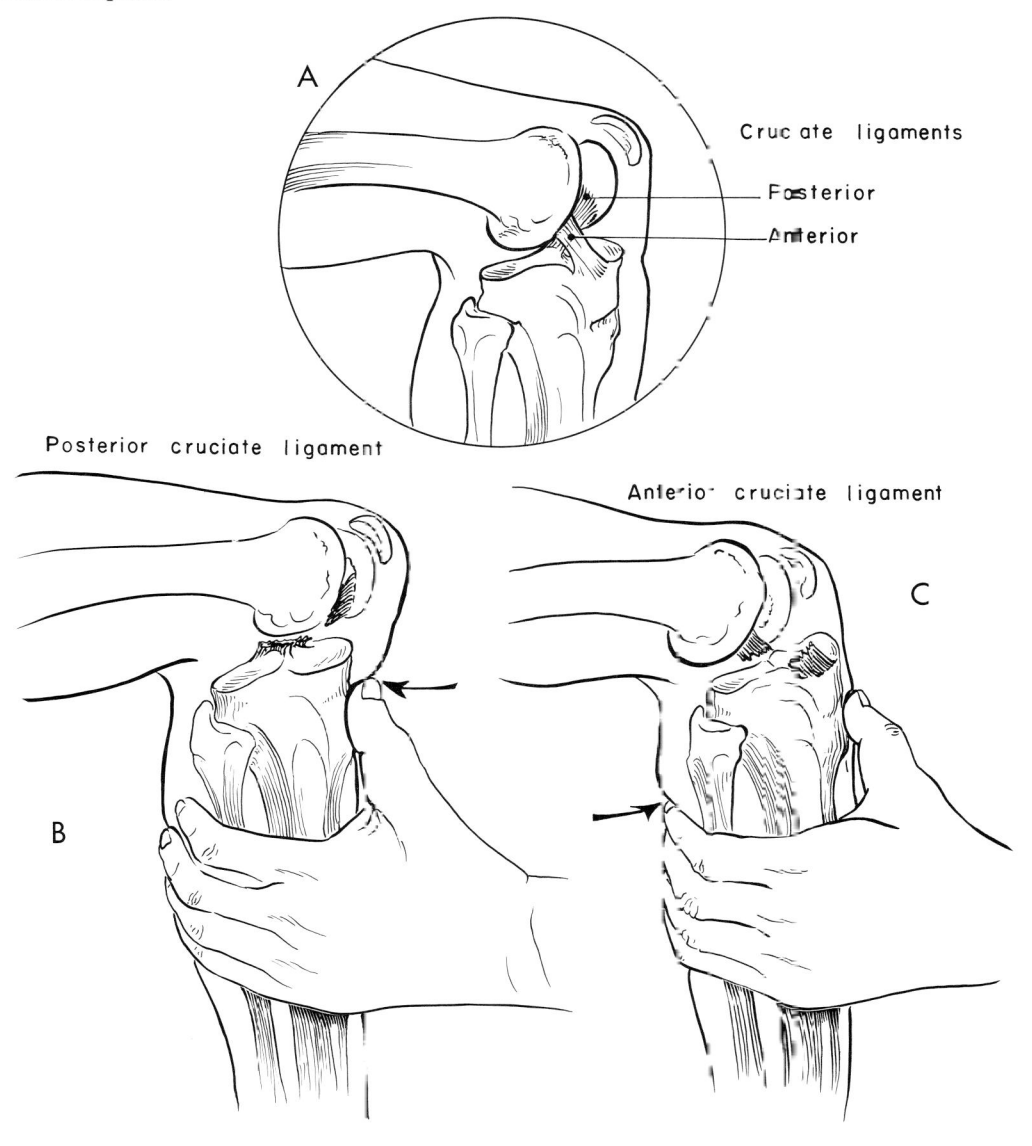

and restricted motion. Satisfactory clinical examination may be impossible until the joint has been aspirated and until muscle spasm has been eliminated by general anesthetic. The characteristic sign of stretching or rupture of an anterior cruciate ligament is an abnormal forward mobility of the tibia on the femur, compared with that on the uninjured side, when the knees are examined in the position of 90 degrees of flexion—the "drawer" sign (Fig. 30-4). Roentgenograms may demonstrate a fragment of bone detached from the tibial spine (Fig. 30-5). This finding is much more reliable in establishing the diagnosis than is the "drawer" sign, which some surgeons have found an invalid test.

Conservative treatment.—The treatment of avulsion of the tibial spine depends on the degree of displacement of the fragment. When the displacement is slight, operative intervention is not necessary. In such a case, the joint is immobilized in a plaster cylinder with the knee in the position of extension for a period of 6–8 weeks. Aspiration of the joint before application of the plaster cylinder helps to reduce the acute pain.

Operative treatment.—In avulsion fractures of the tibial attachment of the anterior cruciate ligament with displacement, the knee cannot be fully extended. An operative reduction and fixation of the fragment site is necessary.

The knee is approached with an anteromedial curved incision. The fascia and capsule are incised and the patella is displaced laterally to allow full inspection of the injury. If the semilunar cartilage attachments are damaged, 1 or both of the semilunar cartilages may need to be removed. The fracture of the tibial spine is then replaced and secured as shown in Figure 30-6. A plaster cylinder is applied and the knee is kept in extension for 3 weeks. Quadriceps exercises are practiced throughout the course of treatment. Consolidation of the fragment must be complete before unprotected weight bearing and full activity are resumed. Usually a period of 6–8 weeks is required.

Fig. 30-5.—**A**, lateral and **B**, anteroposterior views of avulsion fracture of the anterior tibial spine, showing fragment of the anterior spine lying within the joint. The anterior cruciate ligament is attached to this fragment.

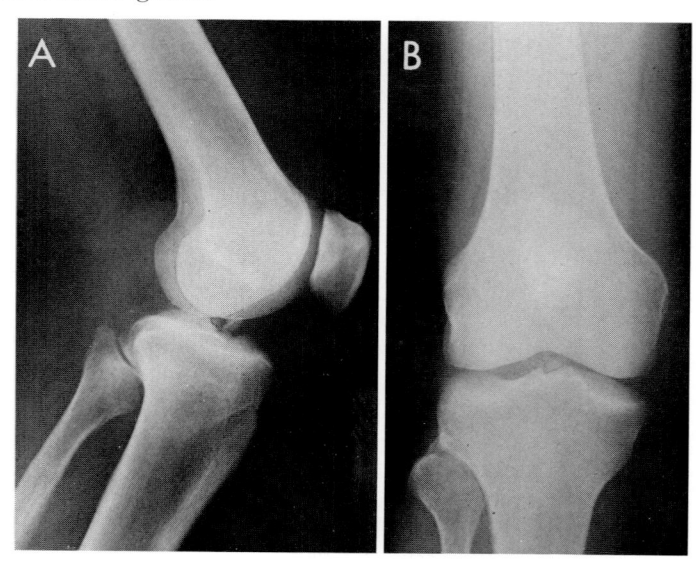

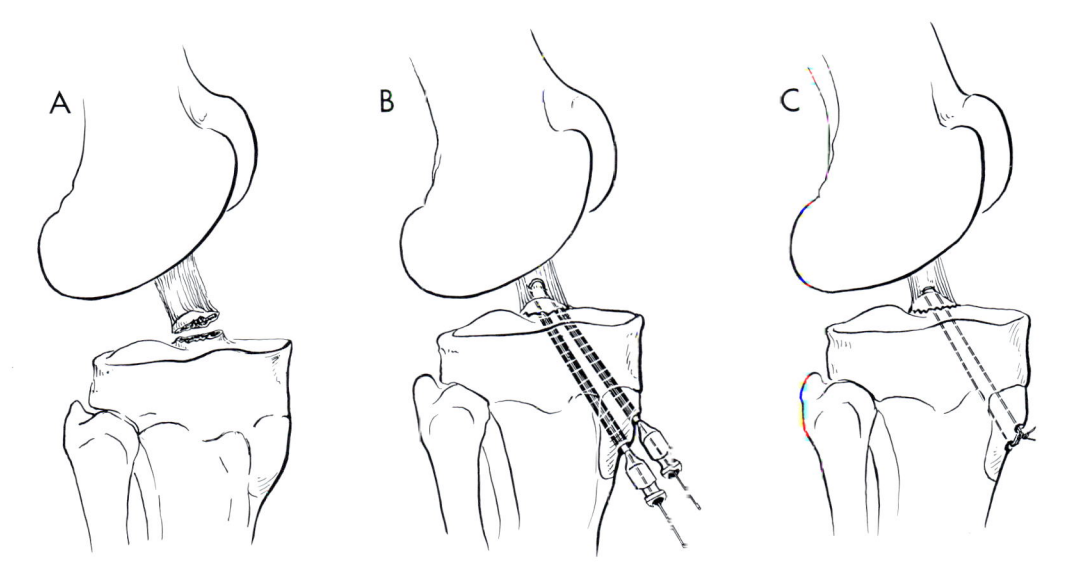

Fig. 30-6.—Repair of avulsed anterior tibial spine. **A,** lateral view. Pulling off of anterosuperior spine by anterior cruciate ligament. **B,** suture of spine by inserting a no. 28 stainless steel wire through no. 15 intravenous needles, placed in drill holes and through the avulsed fragment. **C,** needles are removed, wire is tightened, apposing displaced tibial spine, and 2 ends of wire are twisted snugly together.

Posterior Cruciate Ligament

AVULSION FRACTURE OF ATTACHMENTS OF LIGAMENT.—A direct blow on the semiflexed knee forcing the tibia backward is the usual cause of this type of injury. The lesion is sometimes observed following an automobile accident in which the person is thrown forward, striking the knee against the dashboard. Avulsion of the ligament may take place at its tibial insertion, lifting a fragment of bone from the tibial surface, or a rupture may occur at the attachment of the ligament on the medial femoral condyle. The history of an injury of the type described followed by instability and hemarthrosis of the joint suggests damage to the posterior cruciate ligament. A positive diagnostic sign is abnormal backward mobility of the tibia on the femur with the knee in 90 degrees of flexion—the posterior "drawer" sign (Fig. 30-4). On physical examination, the knee will be noted to assume the position of recurvatum when the heel is held elevated and the knee left unsupported. Aspiration of the joint and appropriate anesthesia will further demonstrate the gross instability of the tibia on the femur in an anteroposterior direction.

Treatment.—An avulsion fracture of the tibial attachment of the posterior cruciate ligament with no displacement may be treated by aspirating the joint and then applying a plaster cylinder with the knee slightly flexed. Immobilization is continued for at least 6 weeks. Surgical repair of the posterior cruciate ligament has its proponents, but by and large it is generally accepted that surgery is not satisfactory and is rarely indicated. Following removal of the plaster, quadriceps exercises and range of motion drills should be practiced regularly. Full recovery may be anticipated in 10–12 weeks but there may be some permanent residual instability of the knee due to relaxation of the posterior cruciate ligament.

INJURIES OF THE SEMILUNAR CARTILAGE

Traumatic lesions of the menisci have a well-recognized etiology in the form of rotatory strain of the knee. Such strains are often sustained in running or dodging movements, in contact athletics such as football or in the kicking movement of soccer, in certain occupations requiring a crouching position and a twisting of the body, such as telephone-line repairing and mining. Hence, injuries of the menisci are most common among males and in persons aged 18–40, the period of greatest physical activity.

Statistically it has been shown that injuries of the medial meniscus are far more prevalent than lesions of the lateral meniscus. The greater frequency may be explained by the variation in the anatomic relations of the menisci. The medial semilunar cartilage is firmly attached to the tibial collateral ligament and is also bound to the articular capsule along its peripheral border, whereas the external meniscus is not closely adherent to the capsule or the fibular collateral ligament. The internal meniscus glides backward and forward on the tibia and may be pinched between the opposing articular surfaces of the tibia and femur during a rotatory strain.

Medial Meniscus

The mechanism of injury is usually an inward twisting of the femur on the tibia combined with a weight-bearing strain when the foot is in a fixed position and the knee is forcibly extended from the flexed position. The medial meniscus may be torn longitudinally, transversely or obliquely in varying patterns. A split may occur in the posterior, central or anterior segment or along the periphery of the cartilage. If the capsule attachment of the meniscus is unusually relaxed or there is a marginal tear in its periphery, the meniscus as a whole or its major part may be displaced toward the center of the joint (the "bucket-handle" tear). At the time of injury, there is considerable pain, invariably accompanied by the feeling that the knee has given way. Following the trauma, the joint becomes swollen and tender and motion is restricted. In many instances, it is impossible to straighten the knee, the so-called locking of the joint.

Often a person fails to consult a physician after the initial attack unless the joint remains locked. Return attacks are experienced, however, although the symptoms tend to be less severe and subside more rapidly, even locking of the joint being only transitory. Conversely, subsequent attacks may occur on slight twisting movements of the knee. A person experiencing these recurrences has a constant fear that the joint may give way at any time.

The diagnosis of the meniscal disorder is made without difficulty in most cases although it is not always possible to determine the extent, the exact location or the type of the lesion. If a history of a twisting strain is obtained and the joint is locked, there is little doubt that the cartilage is torn and a segment displaced. A patient with a locked knee is unable to extend the joint fully, and any attempts to straighten the extremity cause pain and are met with a rubbery resistance. In view of the fact that a similar limitation of extension of the joint is encountered in traumatic synovial effusion subsequent to other lesions, it may be necessary to aspirate the joint to determine the presence of true locking. Differentiation is particularly important when a patient is unable to give a reliable description of the initiating injury.

In cases without locking, the most dependable diagnostic feature is the history. This will detail: the primary injury of a twisting strain accompanied by pain and swelling; tenderness and limitation of motion; the recurrence of similar attacks, and ever present fear that the knee may give way at any time.

Clinical evaluation of the knee with a suspected meniscus injury requires not only a careful analysis of the mechanism of injury involved but also a detailed local physical examination, consisting of inspection, palpation and testing for motions and stability as well as observation of stance and gait. Palpation of the joint line may reveal thickening anteriorly to the lateral ligament, usually more evident as the knee is brought from flexion through the extended position. Palpable thickening over the posterior portion of the internal semilunar cartilage indicates a probable tear of that portion of the meniscus.

If the lesion is of long standing and has gone untreated, disability is increased by repeated damage to the joint The capsule and collateral ligaments may be weakened from the intermittent effusion. There may be chronic or recurrent joint effusion. The quadriceps muscle may be atrophied, causing the patient to limp. The articular cartilage of the joint may be fibrillated and bony exostoses may develop as a late sequela. Roentgenograms should be taken to rule out other lesions, such as calcified cartilaginous loose bodies.

In recent years, 2 further techniques have been made available to aid in the establishment of the correct diagnosis of internal derangement of the knee. Arthrography, using a double contrast media instilled into the joint, has with experience proved reliable in determining the location of the meniscus tear and, incidentally, in ruling in or out the presence of further intra-articular pathology, such as loose bodies, popliteal cysts, etc.

Arthroscopy of the knee, utilizing a special optical instrument inserted through a small stab wound, permits accurate visualization of approximately 80% of the joint. It has been a particularly useful tool in evaluation of the pathology prior to any considered surgical exploration. As yet, the instrument is expensive and only a few individuals have mastered the technique of this particular examination. Certainly it holds promise for the future.

The newer techniques of arthroscopy and arthrography when combined with appropriate physical examination should permit an almost perfect evaluation of the pathology of the knee preoperatively. This should assist in planning more specific approaches or even possibly in avoiding surgical treatment entirely.

CONSERVATIVE TREATMENT.—Aspiration of the joint is indicated in the presence of a severe joint effusion. If the joint is not locked, the extremity may be immobilized in a posterior plaster splint in a position just short of maximal extension. Quadriceps setting exercises are initiated immediately and the patient carefully instructed to continue with them at stated intervals throughout the waking hours. Walking with crutches with partial weight bearing is permitted in approximately 10 days. Immobilization for 3 weeks is adequate on the average. On removal of the plaster cylinder more intensive exercise of the quadriceps muscles is begun. Throughout the entire course of treatment, the importance of improving the tone of the thigh musculature should be impressed on the patient. When normal muscle strength and a full range of motion have been regained, the patient is allowed full athletic activity.

OPERATIVE TREATMENT.—Surgical excision of a damaged meniscus is indicated when there is a history of recurrent episodes of locking or giving way of the knee joint, with accompanying pain, swelling and tenderness. If the cartilage is not removed, damage to the joint structures may result from repeated displacement of the meniscus and lead to degenerative changes of the articular surface. Operative excision of the cartilage is also indicated in an initial derangement, with locking of the joint, which proves to be irreducible by manipulative measures.

Prior to operation, attention should be focused on improving the strength of the quadriceps muscles. The patient should be instructed in quadriceps contraction and resistance exercises, and these should be practiced faithfully for several days before the operation.

Technique.—The surgical approach may be made with or without a tourniquet, and the type of incision should be one that will allow adequate inspection and complete removal of the meniscus, including its posterior attachment. The Fisher and the Robert Jones approaches permit free access to only the anterior compartment, and with these incisions it is not possible to remove adequately the posterior portion of the meniscus. The Cave incision permits removal of the entire meniscus without damage to the articular surface or the collateral ligaments. None of the foregoing incisions, however, is adequate for complete inspection of the opposite side of the knee. When complete exploration is required, the use of 2 incisions is recommended, 1 medial and the other lateral. Two such incisions give better access to the joint with less trauma than the single, extensive median parapatellar incision.

Postoperative care.—The knee is mobilized by means of a compression or Jones dressing or a posterior plaster splint. The quadriceps contraction exercises are practiced as soon as the patient is comfortable. In about a week or 10 days the patient may begin to walk with the aid of crutches, bearing partial weight. On removal of the compression bandage, usually within 2–3 weeks, active knee motion is begun. When quadriceps strength is considered to be sufficient to support the extremity and allow the patient to walk without a limp, crutches may be discarded.

Lateral Meniscus

Lesions of the lateral meniscus occur far less frequently than injuries of the internal semilunar cartilage, owing principally to the anatomic variation in mobility of the 2 structures and to the rarer occurrence of the reverse rotatory strain which damages the external meniscus. A lesion of the lateral meniscus is usually the result of an internal rotatory strain of the tibia on the femur. Not infrequently, the tear occurs in the posterior segment of the cartilage. As a rule, the symptoms are mild. Pain, usually localized at the outer end of the joint, is slight and effusion is minimal. Locking of the joint is not common, but there may be a history of recurrent attacks of giving way of the joint. Tenderness may be elicited along the lateral joint line. Lesions located in the posterior or anterior segments of the cartilage may often be identified by a click that is elicited when, in the case of posterior horn damage, the knee is fully flexed and then slowly extended.

TREATMENT.—The same principles apply in the management of injuries of the external meniscus as in the treatment of internal meniscal damage.

COMBINED LESIONS OF MEDIAL MENISCUS AND INTERNAL COLLATERAL AND ANTERIOR CRUCIATE LIGAMENTS

It has been pointed out earlier in this chapter that rupture of the anterior cruciate ligament and injury of the medial meniscus may be associated with a tear of the medial collateral ligament. In some cases, the meniscus is displaced into the intercondylar notch, locking the joint. This triad of lesions should be suspected in all severe injuries and is particularly common as a result of the "clipping" football injury (Fig. 30-2). Symptoms and signs pointing to a lesion involving each of these structures, as described, will be found if the knee is carefully and completely examined. Aspiration of the knee and examining under anesthesia will often be helpful. If the knee is examined in 0 degrees of extension, stability during a valgus strain may give a false sense of security referable to the medial collateral ligament. In full extension, the valgus stability of the knee is maintained primarily by the posterior capsule of the joint. In order to test appropriately the integrity of the medial collateral ligament, it is necessary to place the knee in 10 degrees of flexion and then produce a valgus stress to the joint. Significant false motion in this maneuver becomes diagnostic of a tear of the medial collateral ligament.

TREATMENT.—Acute severe injuries involving the internal collateral ligament, the anterior cruciate and the internal meniscus usually call for operative intervention. The collateral and cruciate ligaments are repaired, and if the internal meniscus is torn or displaced, it should be removed.

Conservative treatment of the combined lesions is the method of choice if the knee is not locked and if, on examination under anesthesia, there is *minimal* lateral and anteroposterior instability. The conservative treatment outlined for medial collateral ligament tears is then followed.

If surgical intervention is undertaken, repair of the anterior cruciate may be more or less successful, depending on the location of the tear. Particular attention should be paid to the posterior medial capsule of the knee to ensure that it is firmly reinforced. The medial collateral ligament should be repaired, both deep and superficial layers, at the site of separation. In most instances a pes anserinus transfer (Slocum's procedure) should be performed at the initial surgery.

LESIONS OF THE KNEE EXTENSOR APPARATUS

Disruption of the quadriceps extensor apparatus may occur at various levels (Fig. 30-7). For example, there may be avulsion of the proximal attachment of the rectus femoris at the anterior inferior iliac spine, rupture of the muscle components at any point in the thigh, rupture or avulsion of the quadriceps tendon at the upper margin of the patella with or without a small fragment of the patella itself, transverse fracture of the patella, and rupture of the patellar tendon with avulsion of its bony insertion. Each is a characteristic injury of a certain age group, and surgery is a necessity in many of these injuries.

Fig. 30-7.—Common injuries of extensor mechanism of the knee. **A**, tear of quadriceps muscle. **B**, avulsion of quadriceps tendon. **C**, fracture of patella (tear of quadriceps expansion not shown in sketch). **D**, laceration of patellar tendon. **E**, avulsion of tibial tubercle.

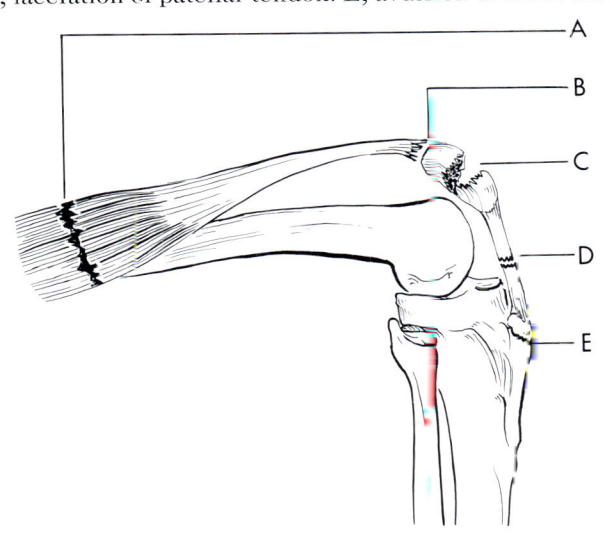

Muscle Ruptures

Young adults participating in contact athletics often sustain this type of injury as a result of a direct blow to the quadriceps muscle at the level of the midshaft of the femur. Occasionally, in an older age group, violent contractions of a single muscle group will result in a small tear. The vastus intermedius and rectus femoris muscles are the usual site of trauma, the degree varying from simple contusions to deep lacerations.

The clinical diagnosis of a fresh lesion is based on the history of an injury in the form of a blow or violent contraction of the quadriceps muscle, with subsequent pain, local hemorrhage and swelling. Tenderness may be elicited over the involved area. Ecchymosis is visible 2–3 days after the injury. When the symptoms are mild, there is seldom an opportunity to diagnose a recent rupture because the average person with the well-known charley horse rarely seeks medical advice unless complications develop.

TREATMENT.—Treatment consists of the simple measures of bed rest or use of crutches, depending on the severity of the injury, and the application of a compression bandage and cold compresses. With the subsidence of pain, exercises are instituted to restore joint function and muscle strength.

The instillation of procaine and hyaluronidase into and around the area of maximal swelling and the application of a firm pressure dressing to hasten the dispersion of the hematoma may be of some value.

The possibility of late development of myositis ossificans traumatica in ruptures of the quadriceps muscle, and particularly subsequent to lesions of the vastus intermedius group, must be kept in mind. In the event that such a complication does develop, treatment is conservative, consisting of immobilization and rest of the involved area until the metaplasia ceases. Surgical removal of the new bone formation should not be undertaken in the early stages of ossification. Such surgery is rarely, if ever, necessary. Resection prior to maturation will only lead to a new and more extensive bone formation. Physiotherapeutic measures, such as massage, passive motion and diathermy, are strictly contraindicated during this acute stage. The extremity should be carefully protected from further injury.

The differential diagnosis between myositis ossificans and osteogenic sarcoma may be difficult. A careful history and physical examination and a roentgenologic study will usually establish the correct diagnosis.

Rupture of the Quadriceps Tendon

This injury usually occurs in older persons whose muscles and tendons are losing their strength and elasticity and who may be overweight. Sudden contraction of the quadriceps muscle against the opposing resistance of the knee fixed in flexion is the usual mechanism of injury. The patient gives a history of having stumbled when going downstairs and of making a violent effort to keep his balance. The rupture may be accompanied by intense pain as the knee gives way.

The tendon may be torn completely across, often taking with it small fragments of bone from the superior pole of the patella, or the tear may occur through the tendon or at the musculotendinous junction. Diagnosis depends on the history and the clinical findings of local tenderness, displacement of the patella distally, the presence of a possible sulcus and loss of active extension of the knee. It should be borne in mind that extension of the knee may be possible if the tear is incomplete. With the tendon torn, the sulcus becomes more distinct on contraction of the quadriceps. Also, the contour of the thigh changes because of the abnormal function of the quadriceps muscles during contraction. Ecchymosis of varying extent is usually observed in injuries of this type.

TREATMENT.—Operative intervention is indicated to repair complete tears. The earlier the operation is performed, the easier the repair and the better the prognosis. When the lesion is treated promptly, healing is complete in 5–6 weeks. However, the strength of the quadriceps, and therefore the stability of the knee, will be impaired for many weeks. There are many methods of repair, e.g., the Campbell and McLaughlin methods. The surgical technique and suture material vary according to individual preferences. A thin strip of fascia lata woven across the defect is a very satisfactory method of repair.

Avulsion of Ligamentum Patellae

Avulsion from the lower pole of the patella in contradistinction to rupture of the quadriceps of the upper pole of the patella appears in youth. The mechanism of injury, however, is the same; namely, forcible contraction of the quadriceps with the knee flexed and the leg in a fixed position. As a rule, not only are the tendon fibers avulsed from the patella, but the lateral expansions of the quadriceps are also torn. Diagnosis in acute cases is made without difficulty. Intense pain, inability to extend the leg, local tenderness, swelling and ecchymosis are indicative features. Displacement of the patella proximally on contraction of the quadriceps mechanism is obvious. A defect is probably between the patella and the detached tendon.

TREATMENT.—Early operative repair of the tendon defect is indicated. Surgical methods of choice are the approximation of the tendon directly to the patella by wire or silk and the pull-out method described by McLaughlin.[25a] Tears in the lateral expansion of the quadriceps mechanisms must also be carefully repaired.

Avulsion from the Tibial Tubercle

Occasionally the quadriceps extension mechanism is avulsed from its bony insertion into the tibial tubercle, or the tubercle itself is fractured. In either instance, clinical examination will reveal swelling, local tenderness and displacement of the patella proximally, with a probable defect at the insertion of the patellar tendon into the tibial tubercle. A roentgenogram may demonstrate a detached fragment of bone.

TREATMENT.—Early operative repair is indicated. When a large fragment of the tibial tubercle is detached from the tendon, it is usually possible to replace the fragment in normal position and stabilize it by means of a screw. In cases of isolated avulsion, when only a small fragment of the tibial tubercle is avulsed through the ligament, a new anchorage for the tendon may be created as described by Palmer.[34] As with all previously described extensor tendon injuries, thoroughly active joint motion is encouraged on subsidence of the acute symptoms. For this reason, the surgical repair must be secure. It is well to test the integrity of the fixation at the time of surgery by flexing the knee to 90 degrees under anesthesia, during which time direct visual examination of the suture line may be undertaken.

TRAUMATIC DISLOCATION OF THE PATELLA

Traumatic dislocation of the patella in a normal knee is not a common injury (Fig. 30-8). Luxation is practically always to the lateral side and usually is the result of a blow to the medial surface of the patella or of sudden adduction and flexion of the knee. If trauma occurs when the quadriceps muscle is relaxed, dislocation may be complete. Damage to the quadriceps expansion (vastus medialis insertion), capsule and synovial membrane on the inner side of the knee accompanies such a lateral dislocation. Reduction is often spontaneous on extension of the knee, or a bystander may thrust the patella back into normal position. Occasional-

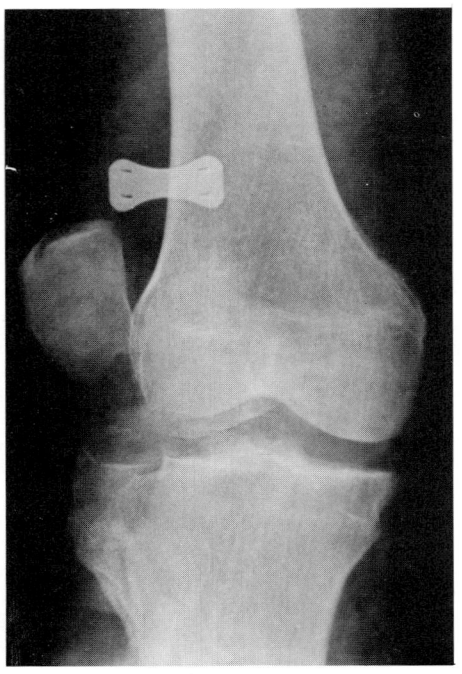

Fig. 30-8.—Traumatic dislocation of patella associated with lateral plateau fracture.

ly, general anesthesia may be necessary before reduction can be carried out.

The surgeon consequently seldom sees the patella in its dislocated state. Diagnosis therefore must be based on the history and the clinical findings of swelling, synovitis and tenderness of the medial aspect of the patella. Since these manifestations are equivocal, the differentiation of patellar dislocation from an injury of the internal meniscus can sometimes be quite difficult.

TREATMENT.—A dislocation of the patella, except in an unusual case, may be reduced by manipulation without general anesthesia. It is only necessary to extend the knee and restore the patella to the anatomic position by general pressure. Surgical intervention is indicated only rarely when the medial parapatellar structures and capsule have been severely lacerated and must therefore be repaired.

If the patella has already been reduced when the surgeon first sees the patient, the extremity is immobilized in a walking cylinder for 3 weeks. Restoration of the extensor muscle power is obtained by quadriceps exercises. Recurrent dislocation of the patella is not as a rule a direct result of trauma and is not discussed in this chapter.

Occasionally associated with traumatic dislocation of the patella are osteochondral fractures that arise from the medial facet of the patella or the femoral condyle during the act of dislocation. Diligent search for these should be made on roentgenograms taken in multiple projections. If such a fragment is noted, arthrotomy of the knee and removal of the loose body are indicated, with tight repair of the medial capsular structures.

FRACTURES OF THE PATELLA

Fractures of the patella may be divided into 2 major groups, the transverse fracture and the comminuted fracture, distinguished by the mechanism of the fracture, the associated pathologic process and the method of treatment.

The transverse fracture (Fig. 30-9) in most instances is produced by a sudden and violent contraction of the quadriceps muscle. The patella is snapped cleanly across in 2 fragments almost equal in size. Less often, the fracture line is near the upper or lower pole of the patella. A transverse fracture is likely to occur when a person tries to prevent himself from slipping or falling as his heel is caught. Less frequently, a direct blow may be the cause. Such a fracture has occurred in an attempt to mobilize a stiff knee when manipulation under general anesthesia was too forceful.

Tears of the quadriceps expansion to the medial and lateral side of the fracture site are usually associated with the displaced transverse fragment. At times, the

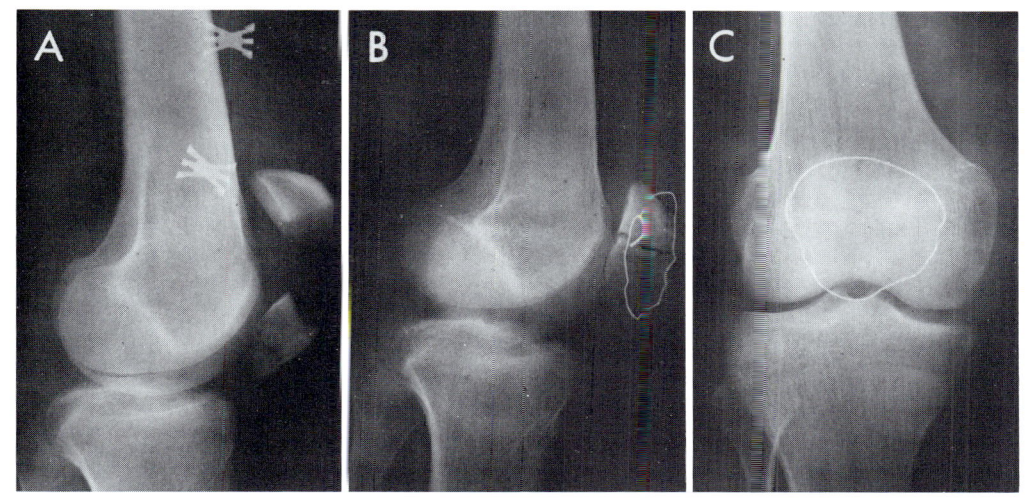

Fig. 30-9.—A, transverse fracture of patella. B and C, treatment with encircling wire. Note the separation of the fragments, denoting capsular tears. Fascia lata may be used in place of wire.

tears may extend from 2 to 3 in. radially from the fracture and usually they include both the joint capsule and its synovial lining (Fig. 30-10). Because the fracture communicates with the joint there are effusion and exudation of blood into the joint cavity. Roentgenograms fail to show the severe associated soft tissue damage associated with a transverse patellar fracture.

Retraction of the quadriceps muscle pulls the proximal fragment up. The degree to which the fragment separates depends on the extent of the tear, the quadriceps expansion and the joint capsule. It is not unusual for the fracture surface of the distal fragment to be tilted anteriorly and to be covered by fibers of the prepatellar fascia.

The second category of patellar fractures is the comminuted type (Fig. 30-11) which is produced by a direct blow, crushing the patella against the femoral condyle. The bone is broken into 3 or more fragments or is completely shattered. The displacement may be slight. In contrast to transverse fractures, the quadriceps expansion and joint capsules are seldom extensively lacerated. However, the articular surface of the patella and its opposing femoral surfaces are usually damaged and this affects the long-term prognosis.

The diagnosis of a recent fracture of the patella can usually be made without difficulty from the study of the mechanism of injury and the clinical manifestations of pain, local tenderness, limited motion and the inability to bear weight. The quadriceps mechanism has a direct connection to the patellar tendon through the lateral and medial quadriceps expansion. If these are not significantly torn, the patient may be able to hold the extremity extended against gravity or even to extend the knee in the flexed position. Roentgenograms must always be taken. Transverse fractures with separation of the fragments usually have a palpable sulcus between the fragments. Active extension of the leg is impossible and the attempt is painful.

A fracture of the patella must not be confused with congenital bipartite or tripartite patella (Fig. 30-12). Careful study of the roentgenograms will reveal the sharply delineated fracture line of a traumatic lesion, in contrast with a smooth,

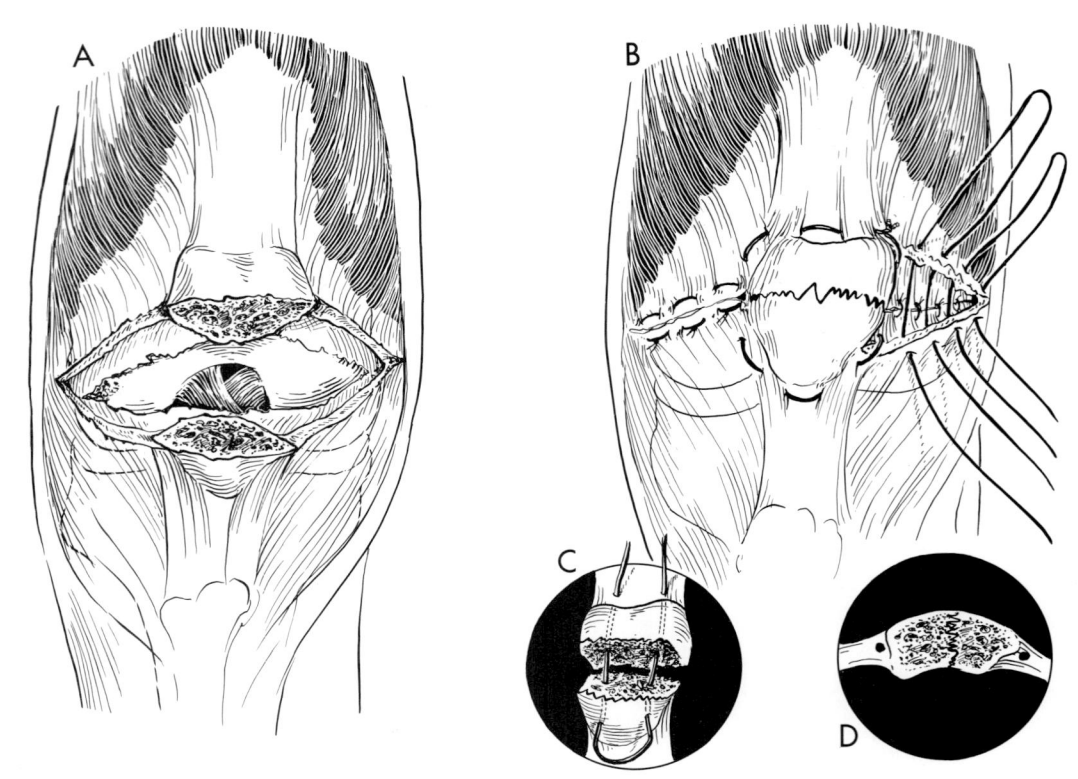

Fig. 30-10.—**A,** fracture of patella with separation. There are associated tears of the quadriceps expansion and underlying synovia. **B,** synovia closed with interrupted sutures. Heavier mattress sutures are placed in expansion and tied, following accurate approximation of the patellar surface under direct vision. The patella may be fixed with encircling fascia lata or stainless steel wire. **C,** alternate method of patellar fixation. **D,** central placement of the encircling wire to prevent angulation of the fragments.

often angulated, line of cleavage and zones of increased density found in the developmental variations. Differentiation must likewise be made from Larsen-Johansson disease, in which secondary ossification is present, usually at the inferior border of the patella. The correct diagnosis should be readily established from the history and clinical examination, together with the x-ray examination. Anatomic variations of the patella are frequently bilateral and therefore films should include both knees.

Care must be taken not to overlook a fracture of the patella when attention is directed to more obvious injuries. For example, a patellar fracture may be associated with a posterior dislocation of the hip in a dashboard type of injury.

Fractures of the patella call for prompt definitive treatment to ensure rapid functional restoration of the knee. Operative intervention, if necessary, should be carried out as soon as possible. Usually the local conditions are more favorable in the first few hours after injury. If operation is delayed, joint effusion, ecchymosis, tissue swelling and local necrosis or bleb formation of the skin make operation difficult and add the hazard of postoperative infection.

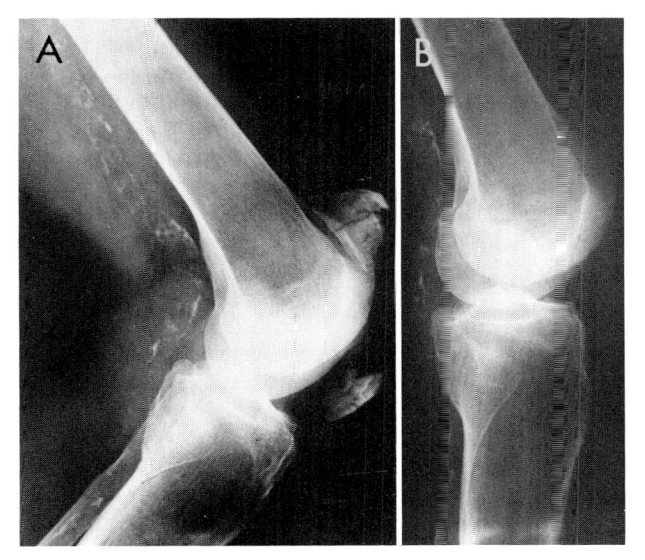

Fig. 30-11.—**A,** lateral view of comminuted fracture of patella. Note the multiple fracture lines. In this case the wide separation of fragments indicates tears of the quadriceps expansion. **B,** treatment consisted of patellectomy and repair of quadriceps expansion.

Transverse Fractures of Midpatellar Region

CONSERVATIVE TREATMENT.—When roentgenograms reveal little or no separation of the fragments, indicating that the quadriceps mechanism is intact, conservative treatment may be elected. Attention is first directed to aspiration of the blood from the knee. If necessary, aspirations may be repeated every 24 hours for the first 2 or 3 days. This will aid considerably in the general comfort of the patient by relieving the distention of the joint. The extremity is protected by a posterior plaster splint extending from ankle to groin with the knee in extension. When the pain subsides, the patient's function-

Fig. 30-12.—Bilateral tripartite patella. Tangential views of both patellas. Note the smoothness and round corners of the cleavage planes. This is an anatomic variation and is not to be mistaken for a fracture.

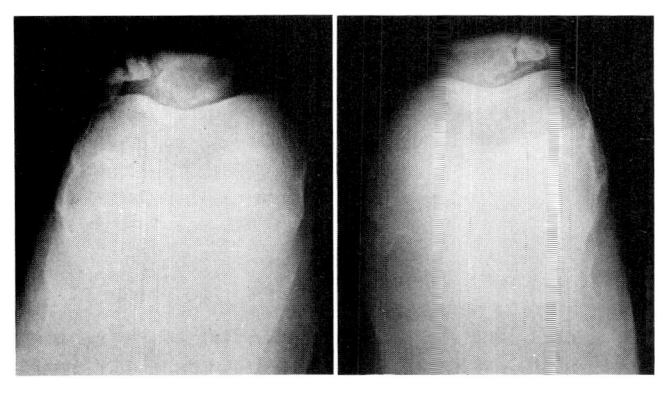

al recovery will be helped by early quadriceps exercises, gentle assisted motion, ambulation with crutches and partial weight bearing. Within 6 weeks the fragments are usually consolidated so that graduated active exercises against resistance may be commenced, with the objective of restoring full quadriceps strength and knee motion. Full weight bearing is permissible when range of motion of the knee and the strength of the quadriceps mechanism permit a smooth gait.

OPERATIVE TREATMENT.—When the fracture line divides the patella into nearly equal fragments which are separated, operative reduction is indicated if the condition of the patient warrants. The success of the procedure depends on 2 factors: (1) accurate realignment of the articular surface of the fragment, and (2) precise repair of the quadriceps expansion apparatus. The fragments must be fixed in a perfect anatomic position, for otherwise chondromalacia and osteoarthritis will develop. Attention has already been called to the tears in the strong quadriceps expansion on either side of the patella that are always associated with transverse fractures with separation of fragments. Unless these structures that are vital to the strength and function of the knee are perfectly repaired, active motion in the joint will be considerably impaired, particularly in the last 15 degrees of extension.

Technique.—A shallow U-shaped incision just below the lower pole of the patella will expose not only the entire patella but also the quadriceps expansion on either side. The fractured surfaces are separated and the knee inspected. Blood clots, bone chips and tags of fibrous tissues and cartilage are removed from the joint, which is then thoroughly irrigated with a sterile saline solution. A fine continuous catgut suture is used to approximate the synovial edges. The capsular edges are repaired with interrupted silk or catgut sutures placed so that the suture material itself does not end at the joint. The sutures are placed but are not tied until the bone fragments have been fixed. The fragments are accurately reduced and held by means of a clamp or large towel clip. Internal fixation is always used to maintain the bone fragments and their articular surface in exact position. The most popular suture material is stainless steel wire. Several different methods of placing the suture material have been advocated. Any method, to be satisfactory, must permit tightening of the suture without danger of producing angulation or rotation of the bone fragments (Fig. 30-10, *D*). At completion of the repair and before the operative incision is closed, the knee should be flexed to at least 90 degrees to test the integrity of the suture line.

Postoperative care.—The method of postoperative immobilization will depend on the decisions and judgments as to the security of the fixation of the fragments. When there is no question as to stability, the extremity may be placed on a Hodgen splint with a Pearson attachment, thus permitting quadriceps exercises and active flexion and extension of the knee within limits of pain. If there is doubt concerning the security of the fixation, a plaster cylinder is applied with the knee in extension.

After the operative reaction has subsided, quadriceps exercises are begun promptly. The cylinder is removed within 3 or 4 weeks and graduated exercises are begun to restore the quadriceps strength and range of motion of the joint. In the average patient, it will be at least 4–6 months before a satisfactory range of motion and full quadriceps power are regained. In some severe injuries, normal muscle power and a normal range of motion are never fully regained.

Polar Fractures

TREATMENT.—Fractures of the upper or lower pole of the patella with displacement or communition of the small frag-

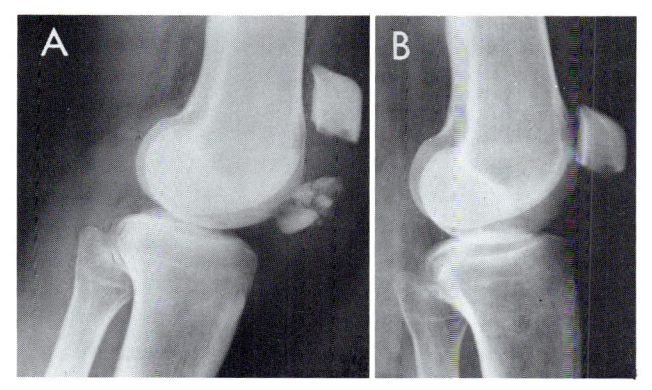

Fig. 30-13.—A, polar fracture of patella with comminution. B, view after excision of distal pole and suture of patellar tendon into proximal fragment. In this case, an acceptable alternative procedure might have been total patellectomy.

ments are treated by excision of the polar fragment or fragments and reattachment of the quadriceps or patellar tendons to the remaining larger portion of the bone (Fig. 30-13).

Comminuted Fractures of the Patella

Total patellectomy is the treatment of choice for comminuted fractures in which the patella is shattered into many pieces of varying sizes (Fig. 30-11). Anatomic reduction of the fragments is impossible and a smooth articular surface cannot be expected.

TECHNIQUE OF PATELLECTOMY.—In the fresh comminuted fractures of the patella, the joint may be approached through a vertical parapatellar or slightly curved transverse incision. The skin and subcutaneous tissues are retracted, exposing the patella and the quadriceps expansion. The fragments are removed by sharp dissection, care being taken to retain all viable soft tissue. The joint cavity and quadriceps pouch should be thoroughly explored and all fragments of cartilage and bone removed. The synovium is approximated with fine, plain catgut. After placing the interrupted sutures in the tears of the lateral expansion, the quadriceps and patellar tendons are sutured to each other with heavy, nonabsorbable suture material, while the 2 ends of the quadriceps and patellar tendons are held in close approximation by a clamp or tension sutures. On completion of the repair, a gentle testing of range of motion to 90 degrees is vital to ensure the integrity of the suture line.

Postoperative care.—Immobilization is established by means of a plaster cast or a posterior splint. When the surgeon is confident of the integrity of the suture line, a Hodgen splint with Pearson attachment may be used to permit earlier active motion. Quadriceps contraction exercises are commenced as soon as the surgical reaction has subsided. The rest of the treatment is essentially the same as that outlined for fractures of the patella.

Unusual Fractures of the Patella

Two other types of patellar fractures are occasionally encountered: (1) fracture of the periphery of bone, i.e., marginal fracture and (2) osteochondral fracture.

MARGINAL FRACTURE.—A fragment may be sheared off the rim of the patella as a direct result of trauma (Fig. 30-14). There is little displacement and the quadriceps extensor apparatus is not damaged. Linear fractures of the periphery of the patella are easily diagnosed by a proper x-ray examination. A long-standing lesion must

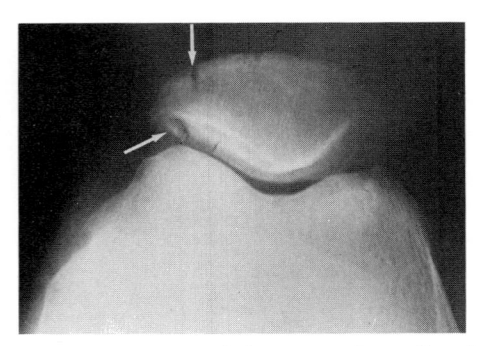

Fig. 30-14.—Marginal fracture of patella, the result of direct trauma, revealed only by the skyline (tangential) view.

be differentiated from a congenital bipartite patella, which usually is a bilateral condition. The bipartite and tripartite patella's opposing surfaces are usually smooth and dense (Fig. 30-12).

Treatment.—Marginal fractures may be treated by conservative measures, provided it is possible to ensure the restoration of a smooth articular surface. In other cases, operative removal or reduction and fixation of the fragment by suture or screw is indicated. The exposure need not be extensive and only a small incision over the small fragments is necessary.

OSTEOCHONDRAL FRACTURE.—Essentially, this lesion involves the articular cartilaginous surfaces of the patella. It is caused by contusion of the femoral condyle by the patella. Indirect violence, such as a twist, or a direct blow on 1 side of the patella may force the kneecap to move obliquely across a condyle, traumatizing its articular cartilage. A portion of the cartilage may be torn loose. Sometimes the cartilage may be bruised severely. In these cases, areas of degeneration resembling those seen in osteochondritis dissecans eventually may develop.

Osteochondral fracture usually occurs in childhood and adolescence. The symptoms are not unlike those of a sprain or contusion of the knee. There is a history of injury followed by pain, swelling and impaired function. The symptoms may subside rather rapidly, but the loose piece of cartilage within the joint space acts as a loose body, blocking motion and often causing the joint to lock. The diagnosis is made from a study of the history, from clinical examination and from axial roentgenograms, in which any incongruity in the articular surfaces of the patella may be demonstrated. Occasionally, diagnosis is established only after arthrotomy.

Treatment.—The patella is exposed through a median parapatellar incision. The articular surfaces are inspected, the loose pieces of cartilage are removed, and the irregularities of the cartilaginous surfaces are smoothed.

TRAUMATIC SEPARATION OF DISTAL FEMORAL EPIPHYSIS

Separation of the distal femoral epiphysis is usually a result of a torsion injury or a forceful hyperextension of the knee. The injury is seldom encountered today, but it was fairly common in the days of the horse and wagon, when youngsters slipping off the back of the cart caught the leg in 1 of the spokes of the revolving wheel. Occasionally it is seen today on the athletic field.

The typical displacement of the epiphysis is anterior, and the fragment is tilted backward by the pull of the medial head of the gastrocnemius muscle. The distal end of the femoral shaft presses dangerously close to the vital structure of the popliteal space, endangering popliteal vessels and nerves. In rare cases, the epiphysis is displaced backward (Fig. 30-15), and there may also be unusual instances of lateral displacement, in which a fragment of the metaphysis accompanies the epiphysis.

TREATMENT.—The injury calls for immediate reduction because of the potential

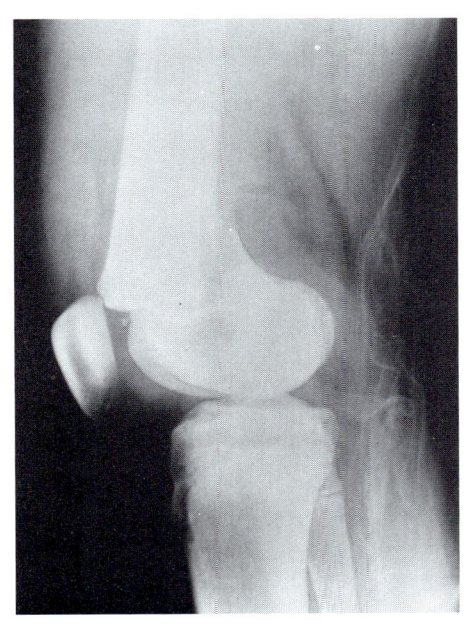

Fig. 30-15.—Posterior displacement of distal femoral epiphysis, carrying a portion of the metaphysis.

danger to the structures of the popliteal space. Reduction is carried out even if vascular impairment already exists. Thrombosis of a major popliteal vessel or findings indicative of an actual tear demand immediate operative exploration of the popliteal space (Fig. 30-16) and appropriate treatment of the vascular damage.

Typical anterior displacement of the distal epiphysis can usually be reduced by manipulation. General anesthesia provides effective muscle relaxation. If the knee is markedly distended, it is aspirated. A Kirschner wire is inserted through the proximal tibia, and strong traction is applied with the knee flexed at 30–50 degrees. The fragments are gently pressed back into position as the knee is further flexed to 90 degrees or more. The lateral and anteroposterior displacement is corrected and the reduction checked by roentgenograms.

Immobilization is established by means of an anterior plaster splint or casing with the knee flexed to approximately 90 degrees. The fragments are usually stable in this position because of the pressure of the quadriceps apparatus. This fixation is analogous to the triceps helping to maintain reduction of supracondylar fractures of the humerus when the elbow is flexed. Following reduction, circulation of the foot should be closely and repeatedly observed.

The plaster shell is removed after 3 or 4 weeks and a Hodgen splint with Pearson attachment is applied to permit gradual attainment of the extended position. Protected weight bearing on crutches is begun 6–8 weeks after reduction and full weight bearing is allowed after 10–12 weeks.

Occasionally, reduction will be unstable unless internal fixation is used. Satisfactory transfixion of the fragments during the early stage of healing may be obtained by use of cross-threaded wires, which apparently cause no damage to the epiphyseal plate. The wires are removed in 4 weeks. Operative replacement is required in the unusual case in which soft tissue is interposed between the fragments or a spicule of bone is caught in the muscle.

Disturbances of growth are common following traumatic separation of the distal femoral epiphysis. In at least 25% of the children with this injury angular deformity or inequality of leg length develops. For this reason, a guarded prognosis should be given and the importance of regular follow-up examination and x-ray studies should be impressed on the parents. Only by systematic follow-up during the entire period of growth is it possible to detect premature closure of the epiphyseal line at an early stage. If a valgus or varus deformity is developing, a stapling operation may be performed on the growing segment of the epiphysis. In order to obviate the development of unequal leg lengths when the epiphysis closes prematurely, the staplings of Blount

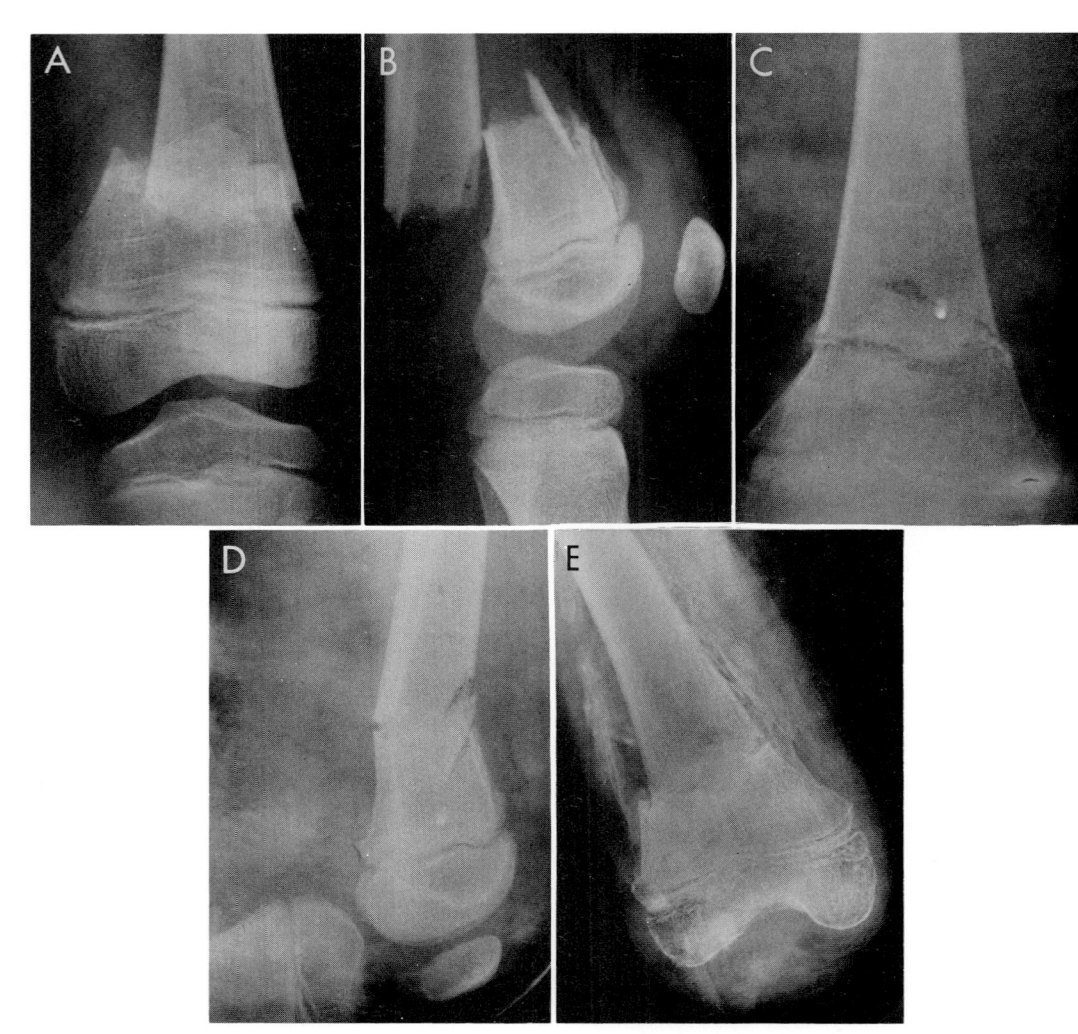

Fig. 30-16.—**A,** anteroposterior and **B,** lateral views of fracture of lower end of femur with displacement of proximal fragment into popliteal space. **C** and **D,** after closed reduction and application of plaster spica, holding knee at 70 degrees of flexion. **E,** healing fracture after disarticulation of knee, necessitated by thrombosis of popliteal artery.

or epiphysiodesis of Phemister may be performed on the normal extremity.

FRACTURES OF THE LOWER END OF THE FEMUR (SUPRACONDYLAR)

Fractures in this region present a distinct problem in management. Not only is it difficult to overcome the displacement produced by muscle pull, but vascular structures are endangered and may be damaged by displaced fragments (Fig. 30-17). The concomitant injury of the quadriceps extensor apparatus often produces marked scarring, and permanent limitation of knee motion is common after this fracture.

The short distal fragment of the femur is usually tilted posteriorly to almost 70

Chapter 30: INJURIES INVOLVING THE KNEE / 777

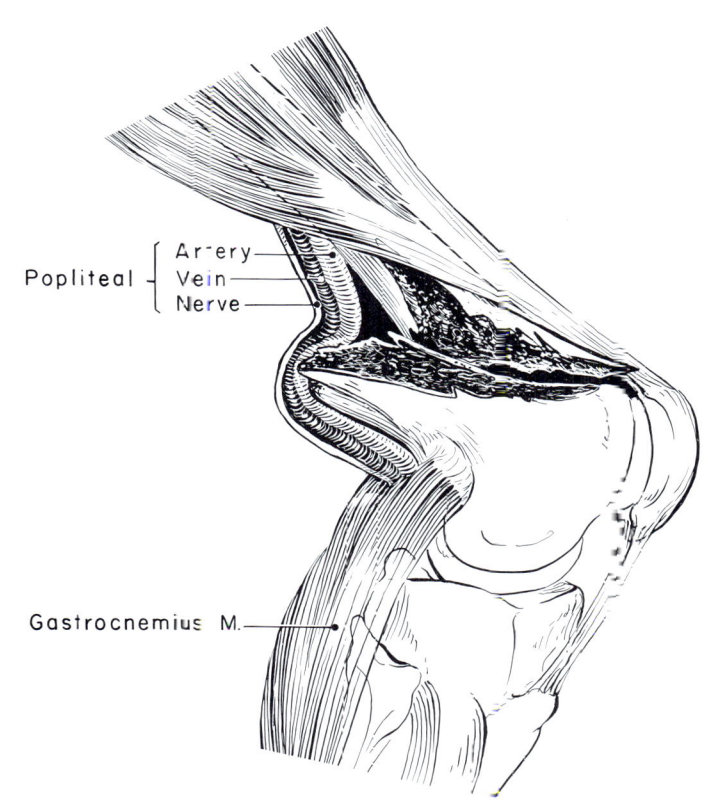

Fig. 30-17.—Supracondylar fracture of the femur. Note the proximity of the popliteal neurovascular bundle to the sharp edge of the distal fragment. The gastrocnemius muscle has flexed the free distal fragment. The proximal shaft often pierces the quadriceps tendon.

degrees by the strong pull of the gastrocnemius muscle. This places the serrated proximal end of the femur in direct contact or in close proximity to the popliteal artery. The vascular structures are sometimes severely contused or ruptured at the time of trauma, and there is always a danger of further injury to the popliteal artery by injudicious emergency therapy or forceful attempts at manipulative reduction.

The proximal fragment often penetrates or severely damages the quadriceps musculature, especially the vastus medialis. Severe hemarthrosis may be produced, with resulting synovial thickening. The quadriceps may become firmly bound to the lower end of the femur and seriously limit the motion of the knee.

Immediate evaluation of the circulatory function of the extremities is of prime importance. The absence of pulsation below the site of injury is indicative of severe contusion, laceration or pressure on the popliteal artery. If pulsations are absent, restoration of the fragments to anatomic position is of utmost urgency. Occasionally, mere pressure of the bone on the popliteal artery will occlude the pulsation. However, if on reduction the pulsation does not return, laceration of the popliteal vessels is probably present. In this case, arteriography followed by immediate surgical exposure with suture or appropriate graft replacement of the

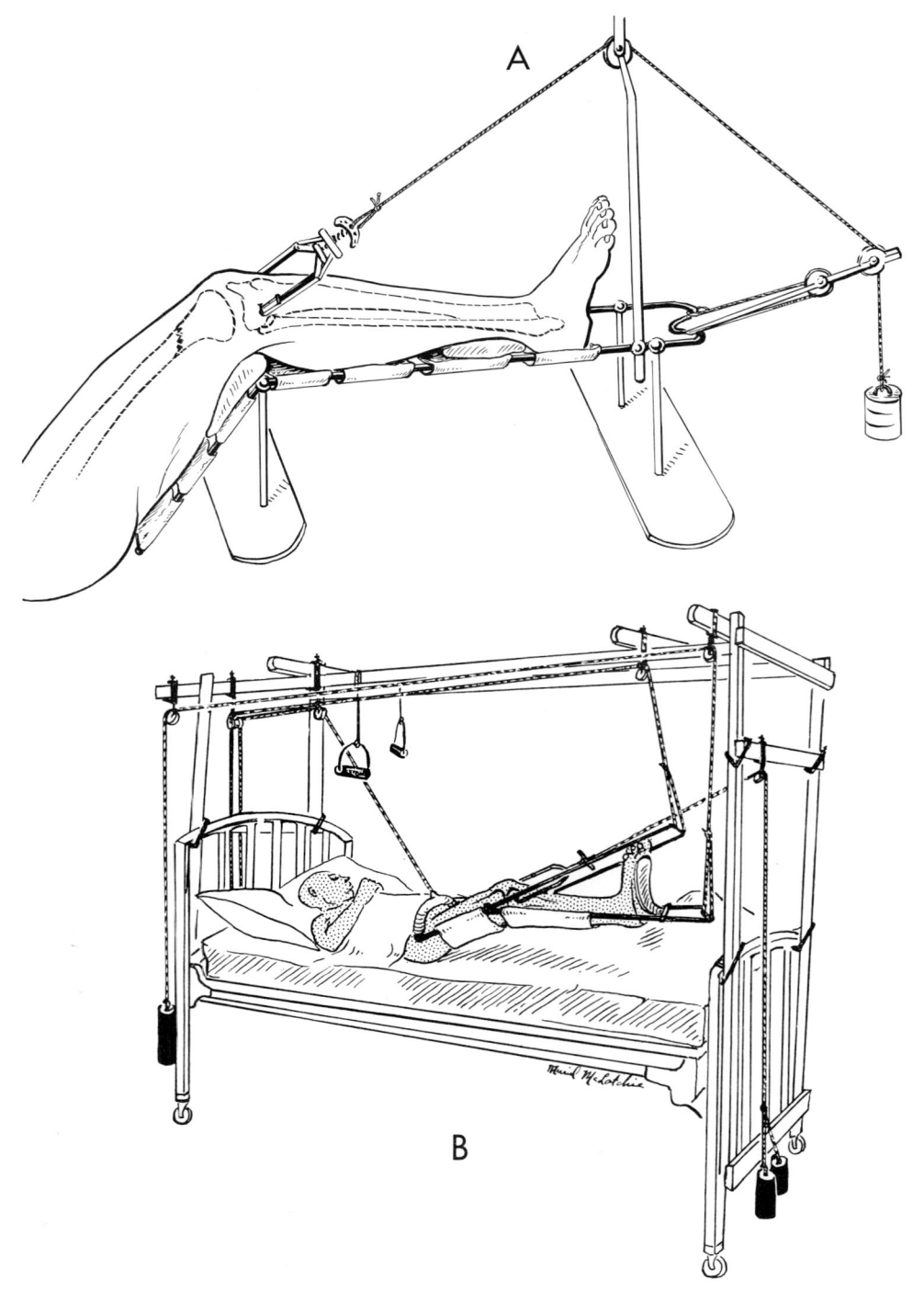

Fig. 30-18.—**A,** Böhler-Braun frame for immobilizing supracondylar fractures of femur. Note position of sandbag proximal to fracture line. **B,** Hodgen splint with Pearson attachment.

traumatized segment is the only procedure that holds any hope for salvage of the extremity, and even this operative measure has a guarded prognosis.

Supracondylar fractures are usually best managed by closed methods, but open reduction is occasionally indicated when satisfactory closed reduction has not been achieved. Malposition of the joint fragments may produce permanent impairment of knee function.

CONSERVATIVE TREATMENT.—Reduction of a supracondylar fracture can usually be achieved by manipulation. The reduced fragments can then be maintained in position by skeletal traction. The Böhler-Braun frame, in which the angle is proximal to the fracture site and not at the knee, is 1 of the most efficient forms of apparatus for postreduction support.

Technique.—The reduction is accomplished as follows: A general anesthetic is administered and the joint, if distended, is aspirated. A Kirschner wire may be inserted at the tibial tubercle and a spreader attached. Continuous traction is maintained throughout the manipulation. At first the pull is exerted in the line of deformity, and an assistant provides general continuous countertraction in the midportion of the thigh while the hip is flexed at approximately 25 degrees. Sufficient traction is established to restore the length of the femur. The surgeon gently manipulates the distal fragment into position with the proximal fragment, at the same time correcting any varus, valgus or rotational deformity of the lower extremity. Extreme caution must be exercised throughout the procedure because of the danger of traumatizing the popliteal artery. Once reduction has been achieved, traction is decreased to allow fracture site impaction. The position of the fragment is then maintained by placing the extremity in the corrected position on the Böhler-Braun frame (Fig. 30-18, *A*) or Hodgen splint with a fixed Pearson attachment (Fig. 30-18, *B*). A firmly rolled flannel bandage is placed just proximal to the fracture site and the limb is so adjusted on the splint that the angle of the frame lies at the level of the fracture. The position is checked by roentgenogram and maintained by traction of 10–12 lb in the average adult (Figs. 30-19 and 30-20).

Postreduction care.—Roentgenograms should be taken every 3–4 days during the first 2 weeks and at regular intervals thereafter until there is no longer danger of displacement of the fragments. The soft tissue of the posterior thighs as well

Fig. 30-19.—**A**, anteroposterior and **B**, lateral views of supracondylar T fracture of femur. Treatment consisted of closed reduction and traction. **C** and **D**, 1 year later; slight valgus position persists but excellent function is present.

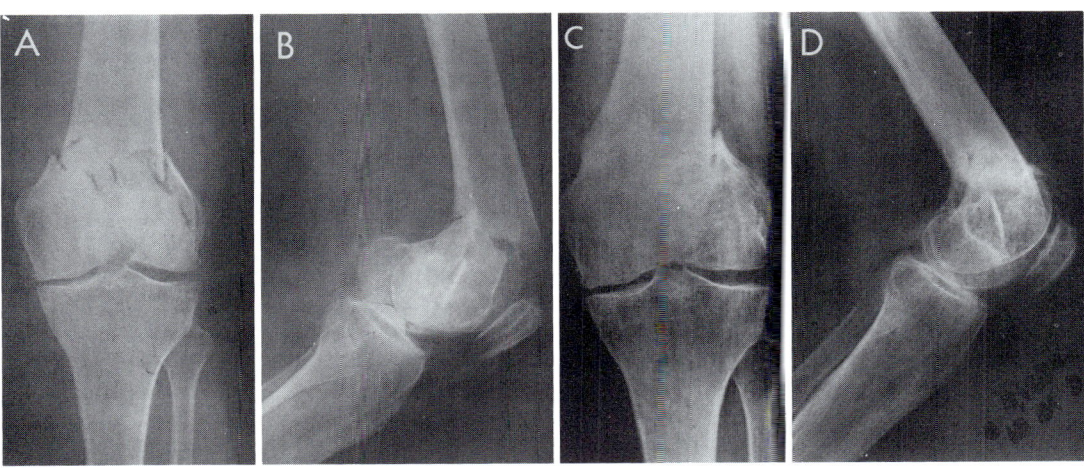

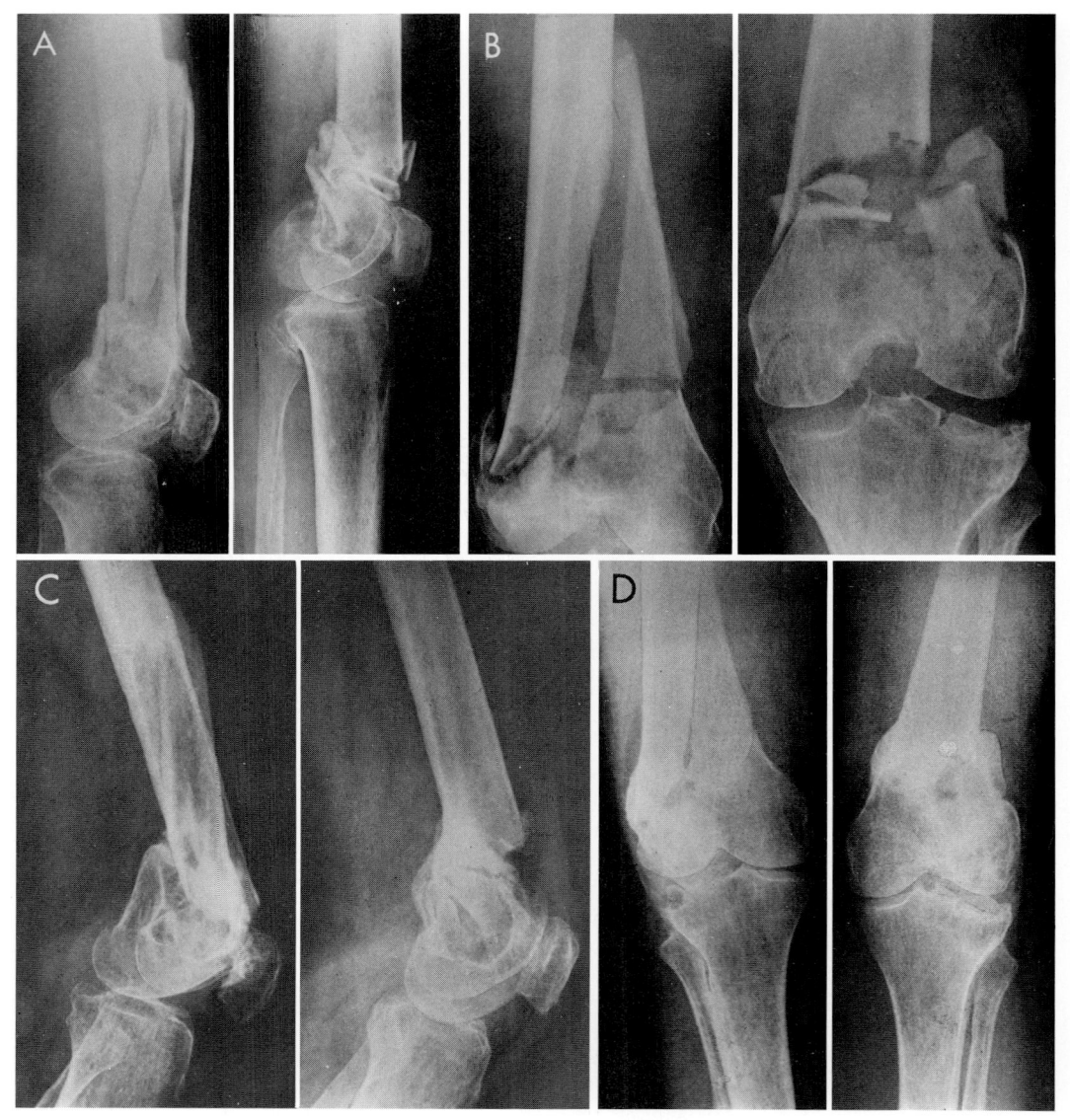

Fig. 30-20. — **A**, lateral and **B**, anteroposterior views of both femora, showing extensively comminuted fractures sustained in automobile accident; closed reduction and traction. **C** and **D**, 1 year later. Motions were: left, 5 degrees fixed flexion, further flexion 75 degrees; right, complete extension, flexion 85 degrees.

as the circulatory and neurologic status of the extremities should be frequently checked to make certain complications are not developing. The apparatus is inspected twice daily and is readjusted if necessary. After the acute symptoms subside, quadriceps setting without joint motion should be permitted. The maintenance of the reduction during the first 3 or 4 weeks is often facilitated by increasing the anterior bow at the fracture site. At the end of the third week, when the fragments are beginning to consolidate, the anterior bow may be restored to normal by careful reduction of the degree of knee flexion.

In the usual supracondylar fracture, healing has progressed sufficiently by the sixth week to permit decreasing the amount of knee flexion and beginning the quadriceps exercises with a little joint motion. Accordingly, the Kirschner wire is removed and the extremity is placed in suspension. Extension of the knee is

Fig. 30-21.—**A**, lateral view of supracondylar fracture. Treated by early open reduction and internal fixation with plate and screw. **B**, postoperative views showing fixation material. **C**, showing failure of internal fixation, which did not hold because of porosity of bone. The situation was complicated by severe pernicious anemia and poor nutritional state. Closed reduction and skeletal traction would have been more satisfactory.

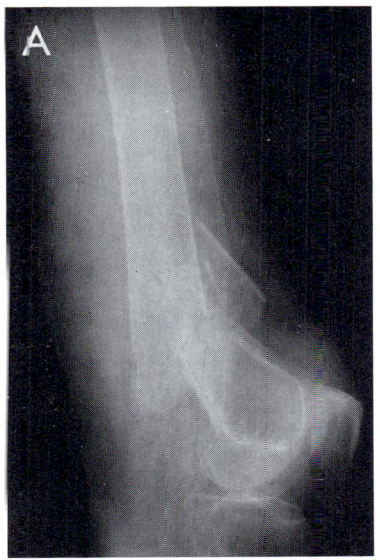

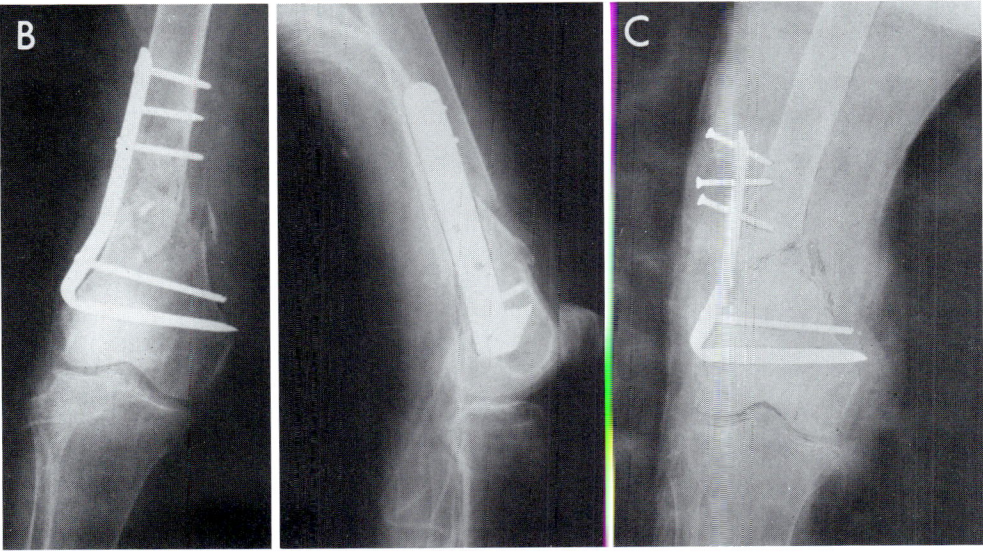

gradually achieved and active exercises of the quadriceps are performed under supervision. When good range of motion and extension is possible and the roentgenograms show the fragment to be firmly united, which is usually at the end of 8–10 weeks after injury, partial weight bearing is permitted with crutches. Active exercises are continued during this stage of convalescence. At the end of 12 weeks consolidation of the fragments is, as a rule, complete and quadriceps power has recovered enough to control motion at the knee. At that time, increased weight bearing may be permitted and the crutches gradually eliminated.

OPERATIVE TREATMENT.—Open reduction of supracondylar fractures is seldom advisable except in a few carefully selected patients in whom it is desirable to reduce the period of incapacity to a minimum or in whom closed reduction is unsatisfactory. The general condition of the patient must be satisfactory (Fig. 30-21), and the fracture must show little comminution if open reduction and internal fixation of the fragment are to be undertaken.

Technique.—The fracture may be exposed and reduced through a posterior lateral incision, in which the vastus lateralis is retracted anteriorly. In some instances, both medial and lateral incisions are used. Several types of fixation are available (Figs. 30-22–30-25). Two Rush nails are suitable in some cases (Fig. 30-23). One nail is passed through the cortex of the medial condyle, the tip prebent to match the flare of the femoral condyle. In a similar fashion, a second nail is passed through the lateral condyle. Once the nails are at the fracture site, they are straightened and then passed into the proximal shaft. The nails are tapped alternately so they progress proximally at about the same rate. When the Rush nails are within 2 in. of final insertion, the hooked ends are bent to a small curve by bending irons prior to final seating. This permits matching the flare of the femoral condyle. This technique usually gives rigid fixation and permits early range of motion exercises and ambulation. Occasionally, the use of a slotted plate is preferred. Again, care must be taken to bend the plate to fit the contour of the distal fragment. If there is a T fracture, i.e.,

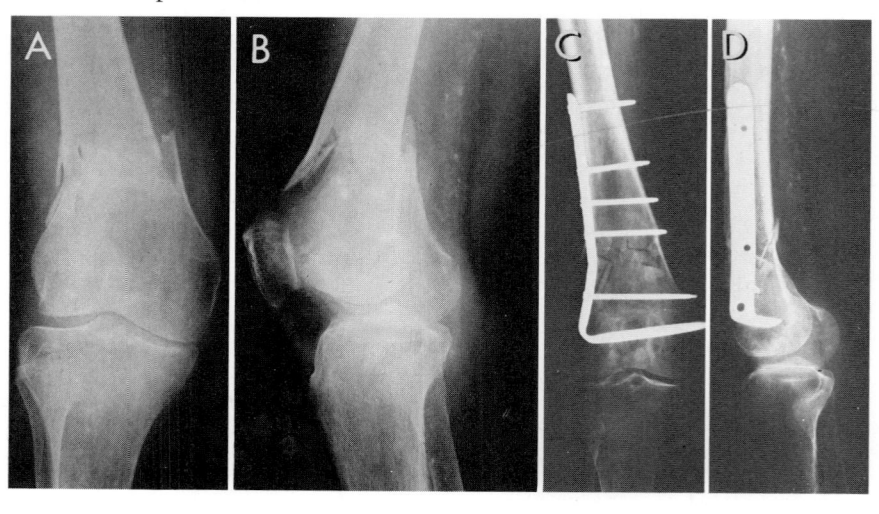

Fig. 30-22.—**A**, anteroposterior and **B**, lateral views of supracondylar fracture. **C** and **D**, angulated blade and screw fixation, the blade bent to match the normal flare of the lateral condyle. Early knee motion is permitted.

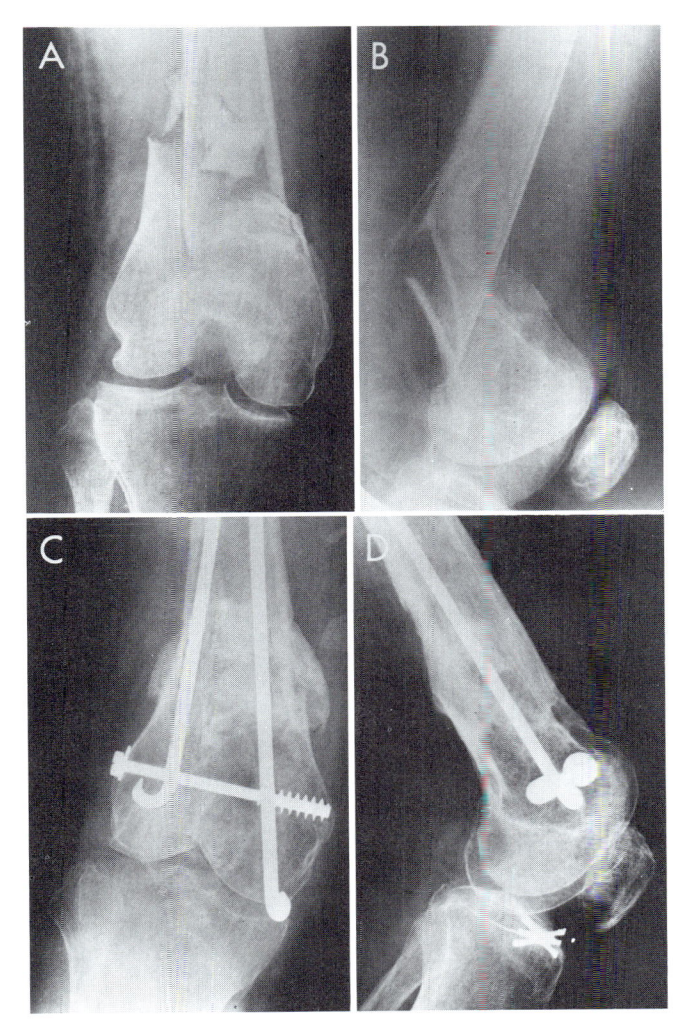

Fig. 30-23.—**A**, anteroposterior and **B**, lateral views of comminuted supracondylar T fracture of femur. **C** and **D**, after open reduction and fixation with 2 Rush nails. The lag screw converts a T fracture to a supracondylar fracture by fixing the condyles.

one in which the condyles are split and a vertical line extends into the joint articular surface, the condyles must be replaced anatomically by a bolt or screw before inserting the Rush rails or Elliot plate (Fig. 30-22).

Postoperative treatment.—The choice of postoperative management depends to a great extent on the surgeon's opinion of the stability of reduction. A Hodgen splint with Pearson attachment is a satisfactory means of immobilization and has the advantage of permitting general exercises of the quadriceps to be performed early. After operative reduction, just as after conservative handling, the circulatory and neurologic status of the extremity and soft tissue of the posterior thigh should be under close observation. Crutch walking with increased weight

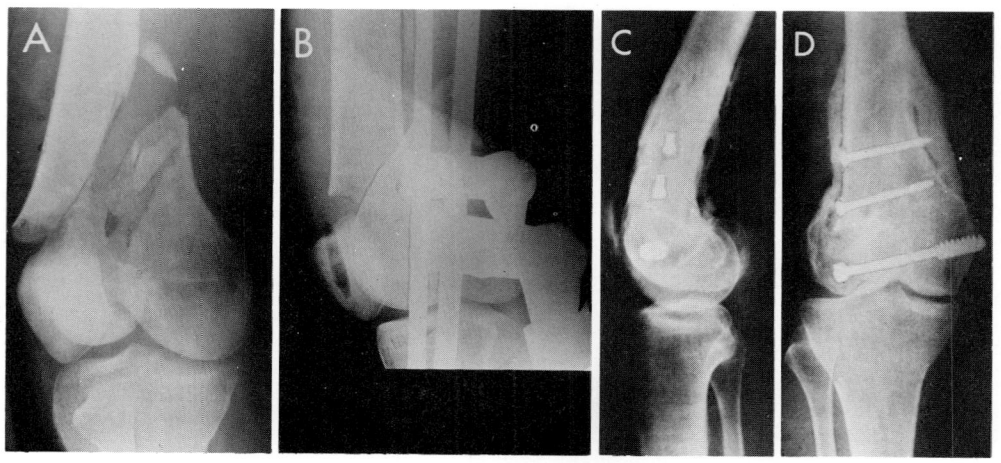

Fig. 30-24.—T fracture treated with a lag screw and 2 stainless steel screws. **A**, anteroposterior and **B**, lateral views show markedly displaced fractures. **C**, lateral and **D**, anteroposterior views after open reduction and screw fixation; the lag screw stabilizes the condyles.

bearing may be permitted when the joint motion, muscle strength and union of the fracture have progressed to the point that such physiologic activity will be beneficial.

DISLOCATION OF THE KNEE

Traumatic dislocation of the knee is a rare lesion that is produced by great force, either directly or indirectly applied. The tibia, with respect to the femur, may be dislocated backward, forward or to either side and may be rotated as well (Fig. 30-26). The dislocation may be complete or incomplete. Concomitant damage of the surrounding structures is usually extensive. In complete dislocation, both the cruciate and collateral ligaments are ruptured, the capsule is torn, and accompanying fractures of the tibial spine or condyles or of the femoral condyles are not uncommon. Neurologic and vascular complications are often present. The lateral popliteal nerve may be stretched and the popliteal vessels damaged. Diagnosis of dislocation of the knee presents little difficulty. The nerve complication is evident from both motor and sensory disturbance, and the circulatory disruption from the absence of pulsation and the extreme swelling that rapidly results. The foot is cold, senseless and may have a mottled, cyanotic appearance. Except in a posterior dislocation in which the pressure on the popliteal artery precludes any delay in treatment, an x-ray film is made to confirm the diagnosis and verify the existence of fractures. On the whole, the prognosis is grave.

Fig. 30-25.—**A**, fracture of lateral femoral condyle. **B**, treated by internal fixation. Early motion without weight bearing is thereby possible.

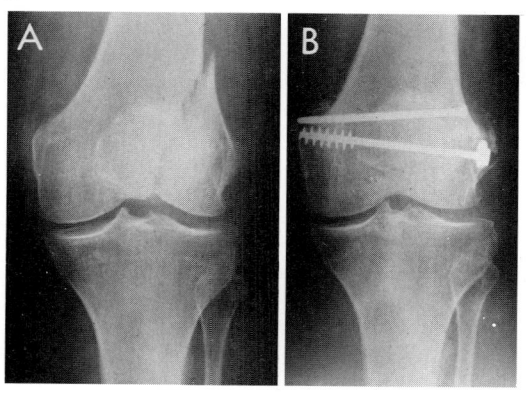

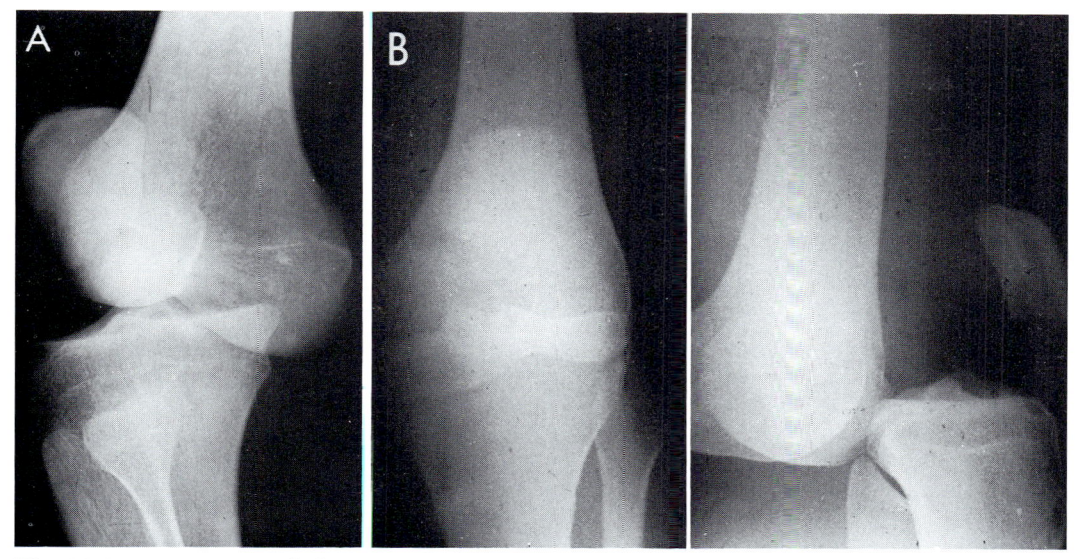

Fig. 30-26.—**A**, rotatory dislocation of knee. Closed reduction restored peripheral circulation. **B**, anteroposterior and lateral views of posterior dislocation of the knee, sustained when patient hit a tree while skiing at a high rate of speed. Vascular damage of the popliteal space was so severe that despite prompt reduction of the dislocation, gangrene of the foot and leg developed and supracondylar amputation was necessary.

TREATMENT.—A posterior dislocation must be reduced immediately, even without administering an anesthetic agent, if necessary, to relieve the pressure on the popliteal artery. The other types of dislocations should be reduced as soon as possible after the injury. As a rule, reduction may be obtained by applying traction and countertraction and pressing the tibia into the normal position in relation to the femur. General anesthesia is used if time permits. If there is difficulty in reducing a medial and lateral dislocation by manipulation, it is usually due to interposition of soft tissue between the articulating surfaces. In this case, operative intervention is required. Failure to achieve reduction of a lateral dislocation may also be due to displacement of the medial hamstrings into the intercondylar notch. In the latter condition, closed reduction may succeed as the knee is flexed to a right angle and traction and manipulation then applied.

AFTER-TREATMENT.—The joint is aspirated and then immobilized in a bivalved plaster cylinder with the knee flexed slightly and the leg elevated. A careful watch of the circulatory status is imperative. Immobilization may be discontinued in 6–8 weeks from the time of injury. Intensive quadriceps exercises should be performed throughout the period of treatment, and crutches are used until full quadriceps power has returned. If there are associated ruptures of the popliteal artery, immediate repair of the vascular injury is necessary. Saphenous vein or artery grafting may save the extremity.

Operative reduction and repair of the completely dislocated knee are advocated by some authors. If undertaken, the medial and lateral capsule and its associated collateral ligament must be thoroughly exposed and the appropriate soft tissue repair performed. The value of an attempted repair of the posterior cruciate in such an injury is to be questioned.

FRACTURES OF THE PROXIMAL FIBULA

Isolated fractures of the upper end of the fibula occur only occasionally and result from direct violence to the lateral aspect of the knee. The fracture may be transverse or oblique, and usually there is little or no displacement. Avulsion of the styloid process of the fibula with its attachment to the lateral collateral ligament is sometimes encountered. The lesion, which is produced by severe varus strain of the knee or by muscular pull at the insertion of the biceps, is occasionally associated with peroneal palsy.

Diagnosis of fracture of the fibula due to a direct blow is easily made from the history of injury, from the symptoms of localized pain, tenderness and spasm and from the x-ray examination. It is important to look for injury to the peroneal nerve manifested by paralysis of the anterior tibial, extensor and peroneal muscles of the foot and sensory loss on the dorsum of the foot.

TREATMENT.—Since there is seldom little displacement, reduction is rarely necessary. Unless pain is severe, treatment consists of permitting the patient to be ambulatory with partial weight bearing on crutches. The fracture is usually healed within a few weeks. If there is separation of fragments from the pull of the attached biceps femoris muscle, occasionally plaster immobilization is indicated.

DISLOCATION OF THE PROXIMAL FIBULA

Occasionally, following direct trauma or a twisting injury, the proximal fibula may dislocate either posteriorly or anteriorly on the tibia. The patient presents with acute pain and an inability to move the knee, resembling the locked knee of a "bucket-handle" tear of the medial meniscus. Roentgenograms are difficult to interpret, and only the clinical examination can really confirm the diagnosis. The fibular head may be more prominent or more posterior when compared with the opposite side.

TREATMENT.—General anesthesia is usually necessary for reduction. A firm, gentle pressure on the proximal fibula toward the normal position will result in a probable reduction of the fibula. Then treatment of acute symptoms can be aided by the use of a Jones dressing and crutches for a week to 10 days.

FRACTURES OF THE PROXIMAL TIBIA

The flaring end of the tibia is frequently subject to fracture because of its anatomic structure and its exposed position. The 2 plateaus overhanging the tibial shaft are largely cancellous and their lateral margins are not well supported by cortical bone. The slight concave articular surface of the tibia receives the convex femoral condyles, which may act as a punch to depress the opposing tibial plateau. This is a common mechanism of injury which occurs when a person falls from a height, landing on his feet.

The "bumper" fracture, in which the margin of the lateral tibial plateau is separated and its central portion is depressed, may occur when a person falls, twists his knee forcibly or is struck by an automobile on the lateral side of the knee.

Although certain surgeons have noted that the medial collateral ligament may be damaged in fractures of the lateral tibial plateau, at Massachusetts General Hospital it has been found at operation that the medial collateral ligament is usually intact. The anterior cruciate ligament is often involved, and fracture of the neck of the fibula may likewise be an associated injury. In severe cases, the lateral meniscus may be torn and displaced between the fragments or into the joint space.

The medial aspect of the knee is protected from direct blows by the opposite knee. Therefore, fractures of the medial tibial plateau that are caused by an adduction strain of the knee are far less common than those of the lateral tibial plateau. As an injury to the lateral plateau, the fragments may be displaced to a varying degree, and there may be comminution and disruption of the articular surfaces.

Comminuted fractures of both tibial plateaus usually result from a violent force acting directly down the line of the tibia, such as occurs when a person falls from a height, landing directly on his feet. The tibial plateaus may be split apart vertically or fractured in a form of a reversed T or Y with considerable separation and downward displacement of the condylar fragments and upper displacement of the shaft of the tibia into the intercondylar notch of the femur.

In tibial plateau fractures the first aim of treatment is restoration of a smooth joint surface by replacing the fragments in as near anatomic position as possible. The second objective is to protect the extremity until union has occurred and, at the same time, to take steps to ensure recovery of joint motion. This is a difficult problem in which the urgency of restoring joint motion by early exercise must be weighed against the possible further displacement of the tibial fragments if immobilization is prematurely discontinued.

Medial or Lateral Plateau Fracture with a Displaced Noncomminuted Fragment

In these fractures, a single large fragment of the tibial plateau is separated from the main portion of the plateau to a varying degree, but the fragment may be only slightly depressed. As a rule, weight-bearing surfaces are relatively undamaged, as the line of the fracture enters the joint in the region of the tibial spine. Invariably, the fracture line extends through the cortex distally.

CONSERVATIVE TREATMENT. — In most cases, the fracture may be successfully treated by manipulative reduction, followed by application of a plaster cylinder and a regulated system of exercises to preserve muscle tone.

Technique (lateral plateau). — General anesthesia is administered and traction is applied with the knee fully extended. The extremity is forced into the bowleg or varus position to open the joint and thus permit repositioning of the tibial fragment. As the genu valgum is corrected, the lateral collateral ligament and capsule become tense, drawing the fragment into position. If the fragment remains laterally displaced, further correction can be achieved by manual compression. Post-reduction films should be obtained and studied before the cast is applied. If the reduction is unsatisfactory, open reduction and fixation may be advisable.

Postreduction care. — A plaster cylinder extending from toes to groin is applied. As soon as the acute reaction has subsided, the patient should practice quadriceps exercises regularly. At the end of 6 weeks, the fracture is generally sufficiently healed to permit removal of the plaster cylinder and the start of active exercises to restore joint motion. A posterior plaster shell should be used at night to prevent recurrent varus or valgus deformity. Walking with crutches is begun but no weight bearing should be on the extremity. It is usually 10–12 weeks before even partial weight bearing is allowed. By this time the fracture is partially consolidated and the quadriceps extensor mechanism should have developed sufficiently to give good control of the joint. As a rule, full weight bearing is permitted at the end of 16 weeks if x-rays show sufficient healing.

Fractures of the medial condyle are treated in a comparable manner.

Comminuted Fractures of the Tibial Plateau

These fractures are difficult to treat. In addition to fracture of the cortical margin of the tibial condyle, many small fragments are driven into the cancellous head of the tibia. It is impossible to restore the central fragments to their normal positions by nonoperative methods. Lack of anatomic restoration of the articular surface of the tibia predisposes the joint to degenerative arthritis and to angular deformity with abnormal mobility.

CONSERVATIVE TREATMENT. — When the marginal fragment is sizable and displacement is not severe, closed treatment is the method of choice. Methods of reduction and postreduction management are similar to those outlined for the non-comminuted fracture of the tibial plateau. The compression force must be sufficiently strong to mold the loose fragments into reasonable weight-bearing alignment.

In older and obese patients, when careful examination of the roentgenograms fails to reveal any appreciable benefit from operative reduction, the patient may be immobilized in a Hodgen splint and Pearson attachment with approximately 4–5 lb of skin traction. On subsidence of the acute pain, active range of motion exercise is initiated in this apparatus and continued until such time as the patient has at least 90 degrees of flexion and musculature control of the extremity. Then a plaster cylinder may be applied and ambulation permitted in a non-weight-bearing regime until at least 16 weeks have passed since the time of injury.

OPERATIVE TREATMENT. — Fractures that cannot be satisfactorily reduced by closed reduction, as well as certain unstable fractures, should be treated by open reduction. In most instances, the earlier an operation is performed the better, because the condition of the skin of the knee usually deteriorates in 2 or 3 days following trauma, with resultant extensive ecchymosis and blister formation. If surgery can be carried out before these complications occur, the operation is less difficult and the danger of postoperative infection is reduced.

Technique.—At Massachusetts General Hospital, general anesthesia is preferred. A pneumatic tourniquet on the upper thigh may prove helpful by producing a bloodless field. The incision line for a lateral plateau fracture starts lateral to the patella at its upper pole and is carried distally just lateral to the patellar tendon to the joint level, from which point the distal portion of the incision swings laterally over the neck of the fibula. The skin and subcutaneous tissues are reflected laterally. The knee is then entered and carefully inspected. Blood clots and debris are removed by irrigation. The lateral meniscus is inspected and, if damaged, is excised. The articular surface of the tibial plateau is inspected. If the central depression is severe, the fracture line in the tibial shaft is exposed by making a right-angled periosteal incision, with the vertical limb of the incision just lateral to the tibial crest and the horizontal limb carried through the proximal origin of the extensor muscles. These muscles are then gently stripped laterally until the fracture line comes into view. The large lateral fragment with its muscular attachment intact is then retracted laterally, opening the fracture line. The central fragments are generally elevated into place, making certain by inspection of the joint that the articular cartilage is properly realigned. Additional bone may be packed beneath the articular fragments to support their position. This bone is usually obtained from the iliac crest or from the femoral condyle of the same knee. Fixation of the fracture is secured by a bolt inserted through a drill hole of appropriate size on the lateral side (Figs. 30-27 and 30-28). Through a second small incision on the medial aspect of the joint, the bolt is tightened over a lock nut and washer. Care must be taken not to tighten the bolt excessively. The protruding portion of the bolt is cut off with a heavy bolt cutter. Roentgenograms should be taken on the operating table to check the position of the fragment.

An alternate method of fixation is the

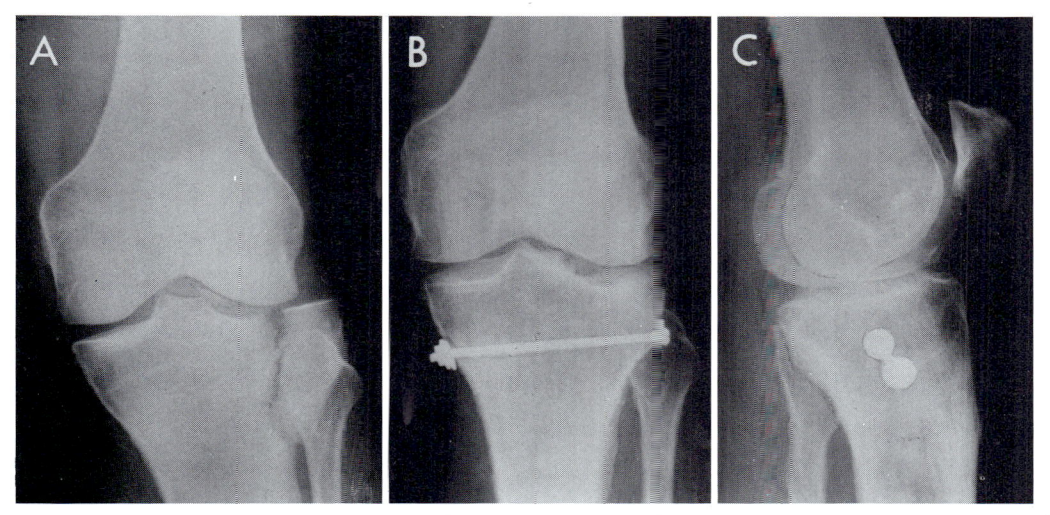

Fig. 30-27.—**A,** anteroposterior view of fracture of lateral tibial plateau. **B,** anteroposterior and **C,** lateral views postoperatively. Treated with open reduction and fixation with bolt, nut and washer.

use of heavy steel wire passed through large spinal needles and tied over buttons.

Postoperative care.—If the fragments appear to be stable, the limb is supported on a Hodgen splint with a Pearson attachment. This permits systematic carrying out of quadriceps exercises and general motion. On the other hand, if the fragments tend to be unstable, plaster immobilization should be continued for 8–10 weeks.

Quadriceps exercises are instituted immediately after operative reaction has subsided. Protected weight bearing with crutches may be started at 12 weeks, but full weight bearing should not be permitted for at least 16 weeks.

Medial Plateau Fracture

OPERATIVE TREATMENT.—In general, the same method of operative treatment is carried out as described for the lateral plateau fragment.

Dicondylar Fractures

CONSERVATIVE TREATMENT.—Treatment consists of applying traction to lengthen the leg to normal, replacing the

Fig. 30-28.—Diagrammatic sketch of a lateral plateau fracture of tibia treated with bolt, nut and washer.

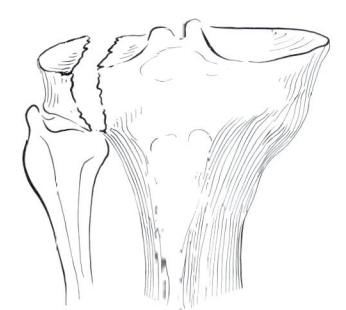

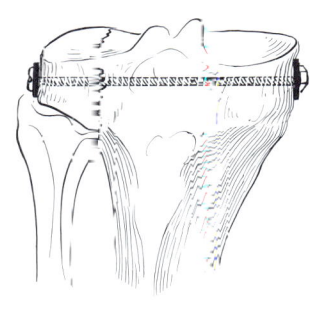

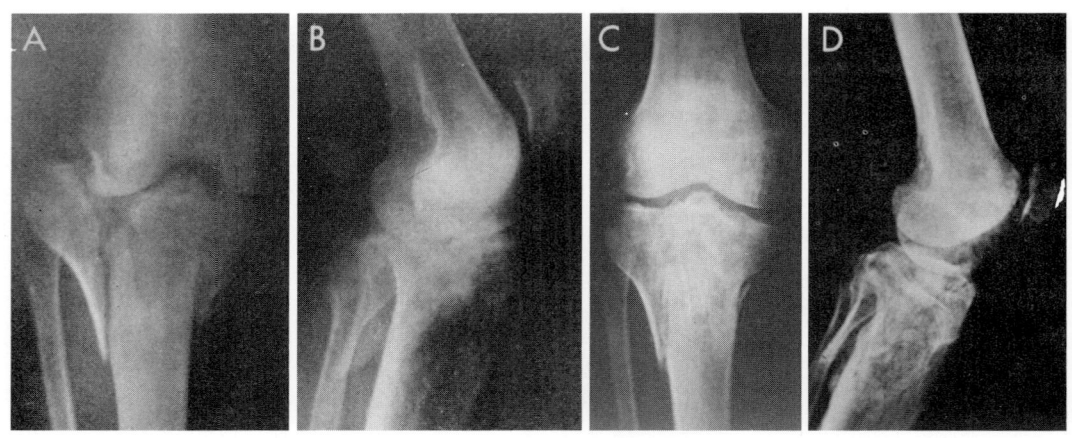

Fig. 30-29. — **A**, anteroposterior and **B**, lateral views of comminuted fracture of both tibial plateaus. **C** and **D**, 1 year after treatment with manipulation and traction.

plateaus by manipulation and compression and immobilizing the extremity with traction maintained until the fragments are consolidated (Fig. 30-29). Attention must also be directed to preserving the quadriceps function and restoring joint function as soon as possible. Under general anesthesia, traction is applied through a Kirschner wire inserted through the lower end of the tibia or the os calcis. Any separation of fragments is corrected by manual compression following the application of traction. With the traction somewhat reduced, the extremity is then placed in a Hodgen splint with a Pearson attachment or on a Böhler-Braun frame. When the fragments have consolidated, mobilization exercises are started.

OPERATIVE TREATMENT. — Operative reduction is occasionally indicated when closed reduction fails to achieve satisfactory anatomic restoration of the joint line and when the surgeon feels that appropriate rigid fixation is feasible and possible to restore anatomic alignment of the articular surface of the tibia. The incision is made on either side of the patella, the capsule is opened and the blood clots removed. The menisci are excised, if damaged, traction is applied, and the depressed fragments are elevated into position, manual compression being used if necessary. A transfixion bolt or bolts or lag screws are then passed parallel to the articular surface, traversing the entire width of the condylar region. Light traction is maintained with the extremity on a Hodgen splint with Pearson attachment, or a cast is applied, depending on the stability achieved.

Postoperative care is similar to that described for treatment of the single plateau fracture.

BIBLIOGRAPHY

1. Abbott, L. C., Saunders, J. B. D. M., Bost, F. C., and Anderson, C. E.: Injuries to ligaments of the knee joint, J. Bone Joint Surg. 26:503, 1944.
2. Barr, J. S.: New technique, Br. Med. J. 2:365, 1938.
3. Bennett, G. E.: Fascia for re-enforcement of relaxed joints, Arch. Surg. 13:655, 1926.
4. Boyd, H. B., and Hawkins, B. L.: Patellectomy: Simplified technique, Surg. Gynecol. Obstet. 86:357, 1948.
5. Bradford, C. H., Kilfoyle, R. M., Kelleher, J. J., and Magill, H. K.: Fractures of lateral tibial condyles, J. Bone Joint Surg. 32-A: 39, 1950.
6. Brantigan, O. C., and Voshell, A. F.: Mechanics of ligaments and menisci of knee joint, J. Bone Joint Surg. 26:793, 1944.
7. Brooke, R.: The treatment of fractured patellae by excision: A study of morphology and function, Br. J. Surg. 24:733, 1936–37.
8. Cave, E. F.: Combined anterior-posterior approach to the knee joint, J. Bone Joint Surg. 17:427, 1935.

9. Cave, E. F.: Fractures of tibial condyles involving the knee joint, Surg. Gynecol. Obstet. 86:289, 1948.
10. Cave, E. F., and Rowe, C. R.: The patella: Its importance in derangement of the knee, J. Bone Joint Surg. 32-A:542, 1950.
11. Cave, E. F., Rowe, C. R., and Yee, L. B. K.: Chondromalacia of the patella, Surg. Gynecol. Obstet. 81:446, 1945.
12. Cave, E. F., Rowe, C. R., and Yee, L. B. K.: Selection of cases for arthrotomy of the knee in an overseas general hospital: Two year follow-up study, J. Bone Joint Surg. 27:603, 1945.
13. Coonse, K., and Adams, J. D.: New operative approach to the knee joint, Surg. Gynecol. Obstet. 27:344, 1943.
14. DeLorme, T. L.: Restoration of muscle power by heavy resistance exercises, J. Bone Joint Surg. 27:645, 1945.
15. Fairbank, T. J.: Knee joint changes after meniscectomy, J. Bone Joint Surg. 30-B:664, 1948.
16. Fisher, A. G. T.: *Internal Derangements of the Knee Joint: Their Pathology and Treatment by Modern Methods* (2d ed.; London: H. K. Lewis & Co., Ltd., 1933).
17. Groves, E. W. H.: The crucial ligaments of the knee joint: Their function, rupture, and the operative treatment of the same, Br. J. Surg. 7:505, 1919–20.
18. Hohl, M.: Tibial condylar fractures, J. Bone Joint Surg. 49-A:1455, 1967.
19. Hughston, J. C., and Eilers, A. F.: The role of the posterior oblique ligament in repairs of acute medial (collateral) ligament tears of the knee, J. Bone Joint Surg. 55-A:923, 1973.
20. Kennedy, J. C.: Complete dislocation of the knee (discussion), J. Bone Joint Surg. 51-B:196, 1969.
21. Kennedy, J. C.: The anatomy and function of the anterior cruciate ligament: As determined by clinical and morphological studies, J. Bone Joint Surg. 56-A:223, 1974.
22. Lewin, P.: *The Knee and Related Structures* (Philadelphia: Lea & Febiger, 1952).
23. Lipscomb, P. R., and Henderson, M. S.: Internal derangements of the knee, JAMA 135:827, 1947.
24. Lucht, U., and Pilgaard, S.: Fractures of the tibial condyles, Acta Orthop. Scand. 42:366, 1971.
25. MacAusland, W. R.: Study of derangement of the semilunar cartilages based on 850 cases, Surg. Gynecol. Obstet. 77:141, 1943.
25a. McLaughlin, H. L.: Repair of major tendon ruptures by buried removable suture, Am. J. Surg. 74:758, 1947.
26. Mansoor, I. A.: Concealed epiphyseolysis of the distal end of the femur and both ends of the tibia, Clin. Orthop. 62:226, 1969.
27. Myers, M. H., and Harvey, J. P.: Traumatic dislocation of the knee joint: A study of eighteen cases, J. Bone Joint Surg. 53-A:16, 1971.
28. Neer, C. S., II, Grantham, S. A., and Shelton, M. L.: Supracondylar fracture of the adult femur, J. Bone Joint Surg. 49-A:591, 1967.
29. Nicholas, J. A.: The five-one reconstruction for anteromedial instability of the knee: Indications, technique and the end results in fifty-two patients, J. Bone Joint Surg. 55-A:899, 1973.
30. O'Donoghue, D. H.: Reconstruction for medial instability of the knee: Technique and results in sixty cases, J. Bone Joint Surg. 55-A:941, 1973.
31. Palmer I.: On injuries to ligaments of the knee joint: Its pathogenesis and a clinical test to demonstrate its presence, Acta Chir. Scand. Vol. 81, Supp. 53, 1938.
32. Rasmussen, P. S.: Tibial condylar fractures: Impairment of the knee joint stability as an indication for surgical treatment, J. Bone Joint Surg. 55-A:1331, 1973.
33. Roberts, J. M.: Fractures of the condyles of the tibia, J. Bone Joint Surg. 50-A:1505, 1968.
34. Shields, L., Mital, M., and Cave, E. F.: Complete dislocation of the knee: Experience at the Massachusetts General Hospital, J. Trauma 9 3:192, 1969.
35. Slocum, D. B., and Larson, R. L.: Rotatory instability of the knee, J. Bone Joint Surg. 50-A:211, 1968.
36. Slocum, D. B., and Larson, R. L.: Pes anserinus transplantation, J. Bone Joint Surg. 50-A:226, 1968.
37. Smillie I. S.: *Injuries of the Knee Joint* (2d ed.: Baltimore: Williams & Wilkins Company, 1951).
38. Soto-Hall, R.: Traumatic degeneration of the articular cartilage of the patella, J. Bone Joint Surg. 27:426, 1945.
39. Voshell, A. F., and Brantigan, O. C.: Bursitis in the region of the tibial collateral ligament, J. Bone Joint Surg. 26:793, 1944.

31 | Fractures of the Tibia and Fibula

EDWIN T. WYMAN, JR.
and JOSEPH S. BARR, JR.

FRACTURES OF THE TIBIAL SHAFT have evoked a great deal of therapeutic interest over the years. Undoubtedly this is because of the disability caused by fracture of this weight-bearing bone, the high incidence of open fractures and the long healing time. Let it be said at the outset that under most conditions closed treatment will afford quicker and surer union of tibial fractures than any operative fixation.

MECHANISM AND TYPE

Since the tibial shaft lies through its length on one surface immediately beneath the skin and is composed of heavy cortical bone, relatively minor displacement of fracture fragments may produce opening of the fracture from within and relatively superficial lacerations opening from without.

Transverse, segmental or comminuted fractures result from force in direct lines and oblique or spiral fractures by torsional forces (Fig. 31-1). It is important to note the displacement of fragments initially, as this will give important information as to the force absorbed at the time of fracture and therefore the amount of periosteal stripping, muscle tearing and other soft tissue damage. These are important factors in both stability of the fracture after reduction and length of healing time. In general, it may be said that unstable tibial fractures will tend to displace into their position prior to reduction, especially in regard to shortening, but not beyond that point. Fractures of the distal third of the tibia may be especially long in healing, since blood supply to the distal tibia comes from above and often is damaged by the fracture.

In fractures that have absorbed large amounts of force, swelling with ischemia similar to that in the forearm (Volkmann) may occur in any fascial compartment in the leg. Most commonly it occurs in the anterior compartment and must be recognized and treated by early fasciotomy if progressive.

INITIAL EVALUATION AND X-RAY EXAMINATION

Because of the proximity of bone to skin in the tibia, nowhere is the principle of early splinting to avoid further soft tissue damage more important. After evaluation of the neurocirculatory status distal to the fracture, the leg should be grossly aligned by gentle but firm traction and placed in a splint. Pillow splints, padded cardboard gutters with box ends to hold the foot and air splints are the most effective for this.

The condition of the skin is important,

STABLE FRACTURES

Transverse   Proximal tibia   Distal tibia

UNSTABLE FRACTURES

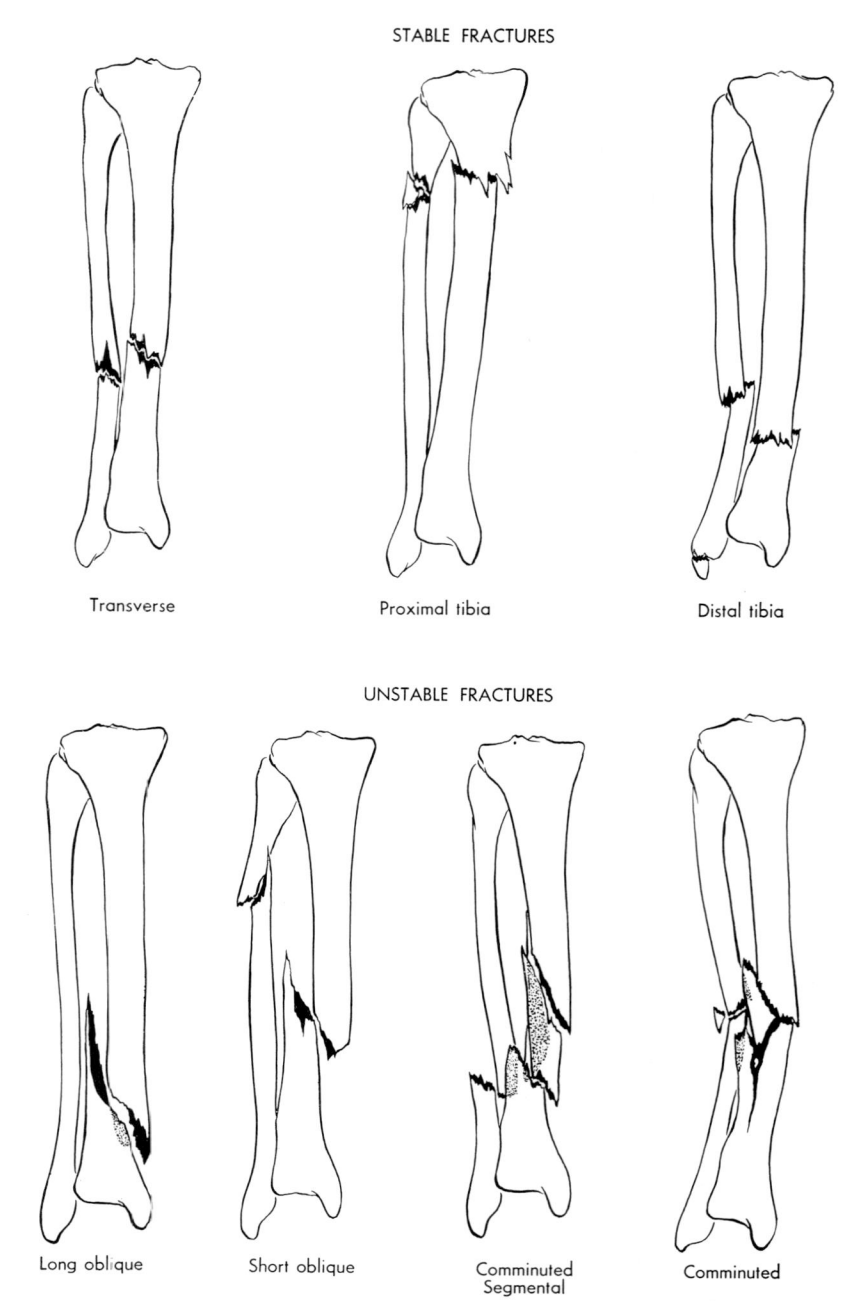

Long oblique   Short oblique   Comminuted Segmental   Comminuted

Fig. 31-1.—Some examples of relatively stable and relatively unstable fractures of tibia and fibula.

Chapter 31: FRACTURES OF THE TIBIA AND FIBULA

especially over the pretibial area. Badly contused or abraded areas may affect later treatment and should be noted. If an open wound is present, it is important to evaluate whether it was made from inside or outside. In all tibial fractures, the skin should be cleansed thoroughly before cast application in order to prevent contamination of fracture blisters or skin breaks from later swelling.

X-ray examination may be required in several planes. It must be kept in mind that any single x-ray film shows the fracture in one plane only. Since we are dealing here with a tubular bone that can displace in any direction, including rotational change, radiographic evaluation may be needed in more than the usual anteroposterior and lateral planes. Although 45-degree oblique views usually will be the only others needed to evaluate the fracture, occasionally other oblique views or evaluation under image intensifying fluoroscopy may be needed to show the fracture line most clearly.

One should note on x-ray the type of fracture, its displacement, any presence of foreign material (in open fractures), soft tissue swelling and its malalignment, including rotation. Careful inspection is needed to detect any small undisplaced cracks in the cortical bone indicating comminution, which, if not recognized, may become only too clear at the time of operation and prevent adequate fixation by any method. In general, transverse fractures tend to be stable, and spiral, oblique, comminuted and segmental fractures unstable. In addition, the farther displaced the fracture is initially the more unstable the reduction (Fig. 31-2). Displaced transverse fractures indicate greater injury force and more soft tissue damage.

Fig. 31-2.—A comminuted closed fracture on initial x-ray. Further displacement of fragments would indicate a longer healing time. Note undisplaced fracture lines extending nearly to ankle. This fracture is unstable. Treatment should be by closed methods because of the comminution.

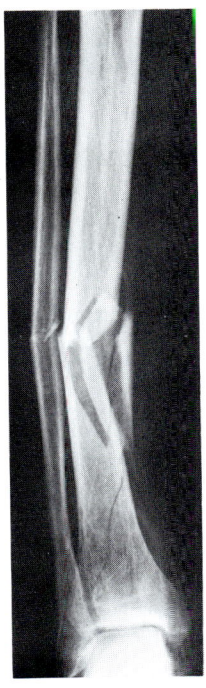

HEALING TIMES

Fractures through the cortical diaphysis of the tibia have a rather long healing time, being longest when the break is within the thick cortex of the distal third, because of relatively poor circulation, as noted before. Because of the great stresses on the tibia in weight bearing, functional healing time is as long as physiologic healing time and is in the range of 3–8 months. One cannot say that there is delayed union in this area under 6 months or nonunion in under 12 months. In the metaphyseal areas, where cancellous bone abounds and cortical bone is thinner, healing time decreases to 6–8 weeks. However, in the proximal tibia, the pull of the patellar tendon may separate the fracture enough to lengthen the time of union significantly. Healing time always is lengthened by opening a fracture, whether by injury or by operation.

CHILDREN.—The above healing times apply to adults in general, regardless of their age. Children heal faster, depending on size, and their powers of remodel-

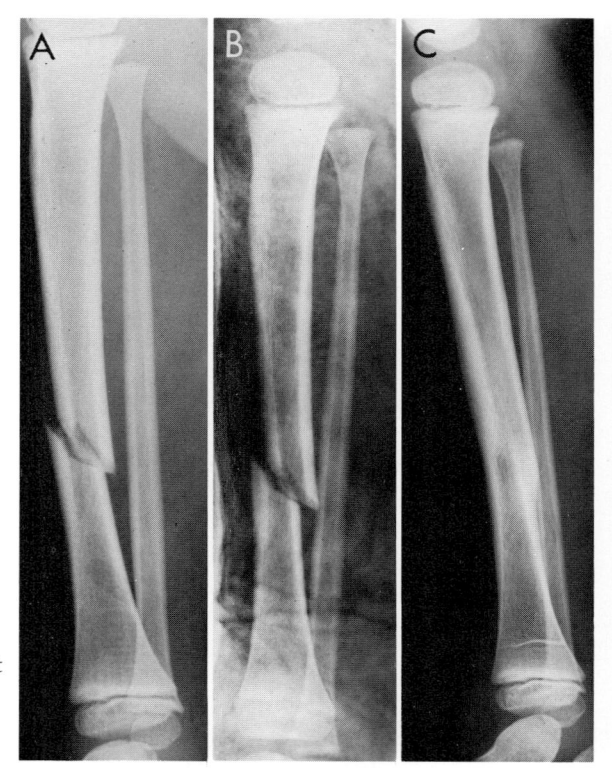

Fig. 31-3.—A 5-year-old boy with a tibial fracture (A) only partially reduced (B). Note remodeling apparent (C) in x-ray film 1 year after fracture.

ing work to great advantage in treatment of fractures of the tibia. Moderate amounts of angulation and displacement may be accepted and will remodel; however, rotational deformity is much slower to do this (Fig. 31-3). Shortening often will be overcome in the year following fracture by overgrowth of the tibia due to its temporarily increased blood supply. The thick periosteal covering acts as a shield for the tibia itself, and widely displaced and open fractures are unusual in children. Open reduction is not only unnecessary but undesirable. Healing time of diaphyseal fractures of the tibia approximates 2 months in children under age 10 and 3 months in those over 10.

TREATMENT

General Considerations

Questions that should come to mind in considering the course of treatment in tibial fractures are: Is the fracture open or closed? What is the alignment and expected stability? Can a satisfactory and stable reduction be obtained by closed methods? If open fixation is contemplated, what are the expected advantages to this method and are they worth the risks? It is difficult to answer these questions in generalities, since the *individual* with the fracture must be considered—his other medical conditions, his psyche, his occupation, his social situation and his individual reliability.

Closed Reductions

The pendulum swings in the treatment of this fracture, as in the treatment of most medical conditions. At present, the swing is toward the closed method, at least in the United States. This current swing began with Dehne's work in 1955, which showed conclusively that if tibial shaft fractures were aligned but allowed to remain in a stable (i.e., shortened) position, immobilized in long leg casts and allowed weight bearing early, the prior nonunion rate of 15% dropped to nearly zero. Sarmiento's work using a lightly padded short leg cast with plaster molds around the knee, resembling the weight-bearing surfaces of a below-knee prosthesis, confirmed Dehne's work (Fig. 31-4). More recent studies in the use of cast-brace techniques still must be considered experimental but probably will yield similar results when used properly. The early weight-bearing methods give quick and sure union of tibial fractures, with the disadvantage of shortening of about the same amount as was present after the initial fracture. If this is under three-fourths of an inch, the advantages outweigh the disadvantages.

If reduction is accomplished within 30–60 minutes after injury—which is unusual except in special situations, such as at a ski area—it frequently can be performed under light sedation only. Otherwise, general, spinal or effective regional anesthesia is needed. The fractured leg should be compared to the normal, in order to evaluate the patient's normal tibial varus bow, or lack of it, and tibial torsion (rotation). The principle of reduction then is traction to gain length and distract the fracture fragments and then a reversal of the mechanism of injury. This

Fig. 31-4.—Total contact cast. **A**, note position of hands to obtain proper triangulation and molds of the upper cast. **B**, cast should be lightly padded and trimmed along the line on cast.

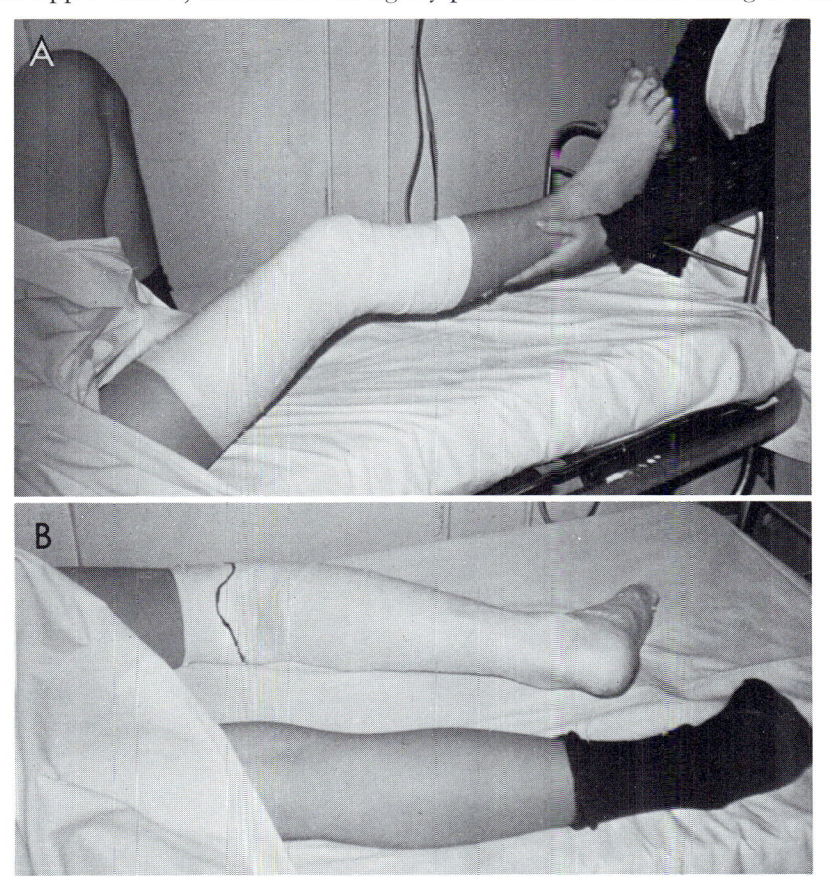

usually means lateral, medial or posterior force if the fracture is transverse and rotational (usually internal rotation of the distal fragment) if it is oblique. This can be accomplished by hand traction on the foot with the knee flexed over the side of a table. If more traction force is needed, skeletal traction with a wire through the distal tibia or os calcis may be used. The leg is manipulated to make it look like the normal leg. At this point, traction is released and stability tested gently. Then a lightly padded cast is applied below the knee with smooth hand molds in the plaster to maintain reduction. The leg then is raised to table height and the cast extended to above the knee with the knee in a few degrees of flexion, enough to prevent rotation of the cast in relation to the proximal fragments but also to allow later weight bearing. Closed reduction can also be carried out with the leg raised parallel to the table if enough help is available to hold the foot in position and apply traction (Fig. 31-5). With the knee flexed 30 degrees, countertraction is applied. With this method, however, the forces of gravity are working against the reduction rather than for it. All tibial fractures cause swelling to some degree, and

Fig. 31-5.—**Top,** by utilizing simple gravity, or with added weight through a temporary traction wire removed after the cast has hardened and been extended to above the knee, this position eases reduction. If further immobilization is needed, the wire may be left in place and similar wires placed above the fracture through the tibia and incorporated in the cast. **Bottom,** reduction can be accomplished in this position if enough help is available. Rotational alignment is checked at the time the cast is extended above the knee and held by flexing the knee slightly.

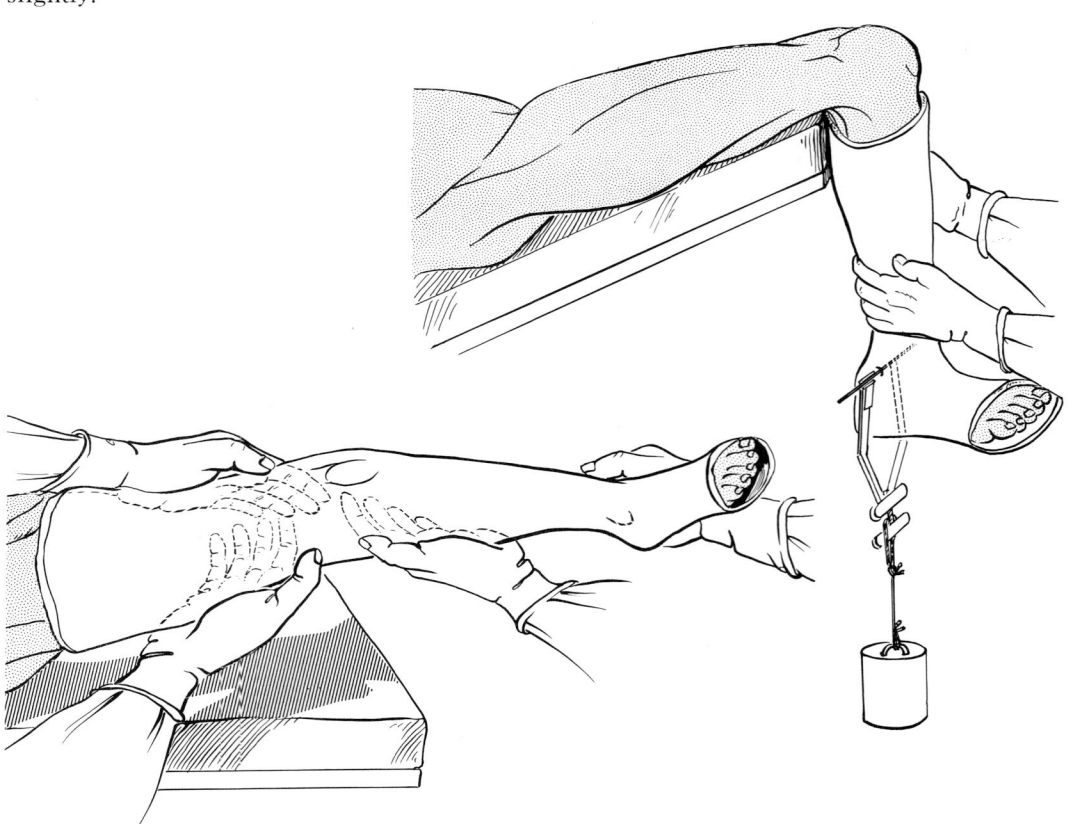

rest and elevation of the extremity with observance of motor, sensory and circulatory functions of the foot are essential for 48 hours. Hospital admission usually is necessary; if not available, the cast should be split below the knee and the plaster spread slightly. Postreduction films, including proper oblique views, are taken and evaluated.

ALIGNMENT.—One cannot judge alignment properly unless both the knee and ankle articular surfaces can be seen on the same film. Although perfect alignment is to be sought in the frontal and coronal planes, 15 degrees of malalignment on either the anteroposterior or lateral view can be accepted, with angulation of the distal fragment into varus on the anteroposterior and dorsiflexion on the lateral view being the least desirable. Rotational reduction is more difficult to evaluate by x-ray and is done best clinically by comparison with the normal side or the foot-knee relationship on the fractured limb (Fig. 31-6).

Fig. 31-6.—Fracture of both bones of leg, as seen immediately after injury. Note the external rotation deformity, which must be corrected at the time of fracture reduction.

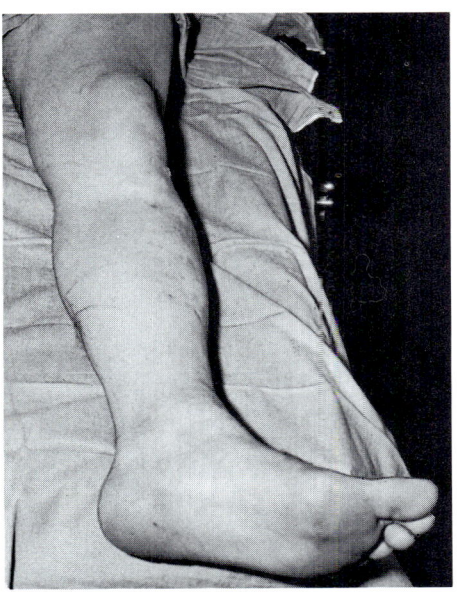

CONTACT.—The feeling of crepitus on reduction is important to obtain, since soft tissue interposition between fracture fragments can occur uncommonly. X-ray evidence of good contact can be misleading, and it is evaluated best by multiple oblique views, remembering that the worst view is the most accurate assessment of the actual fracture position.

DISPLACEMENT.—Except in unusual circumstances, if contact and alignment of the fracture are satisfactory, rather major amounts of partial displacement may be accepted (Fig. 31-7). Displacement is important only in its relationship to stability except for anterior displacement, in which the prominence of one fragment under the pretibial cutaneous surface may cause excess cast pressure or cosmetic deformity.

LENGTH.—In transverse fractures, length is not a problem if some end-on contact is established. Oblique and spiral fractures are a more difficult problem. In these fractures, length often can be restored initially by gentle traction, but the fracture will always shorten to its original position, even in plaster, over the following few days unless additional treatment is carried out to maintain length. One should carefully contemplate whether the added treatment to maintain length is really to the patient's advantage, since in order to gain, for example, ½ inch of length, it may be necessary to somewhat distract the fracture (unless rotational alignment is absolute) and increase the chance of delayed union or nonunion. In addition, maintaining full length will obviate the early weight-bearing treatment, which has been shown conclusively to be the quickest and surest pathway to fracture union (Fig. 31-8). If maintenance of full bone length is deemed to be necessary, the most useful techniques include the use of traction through Kirschner wires or open reduction and anatomic fixation. The latter will be discussed later. The former involves using a

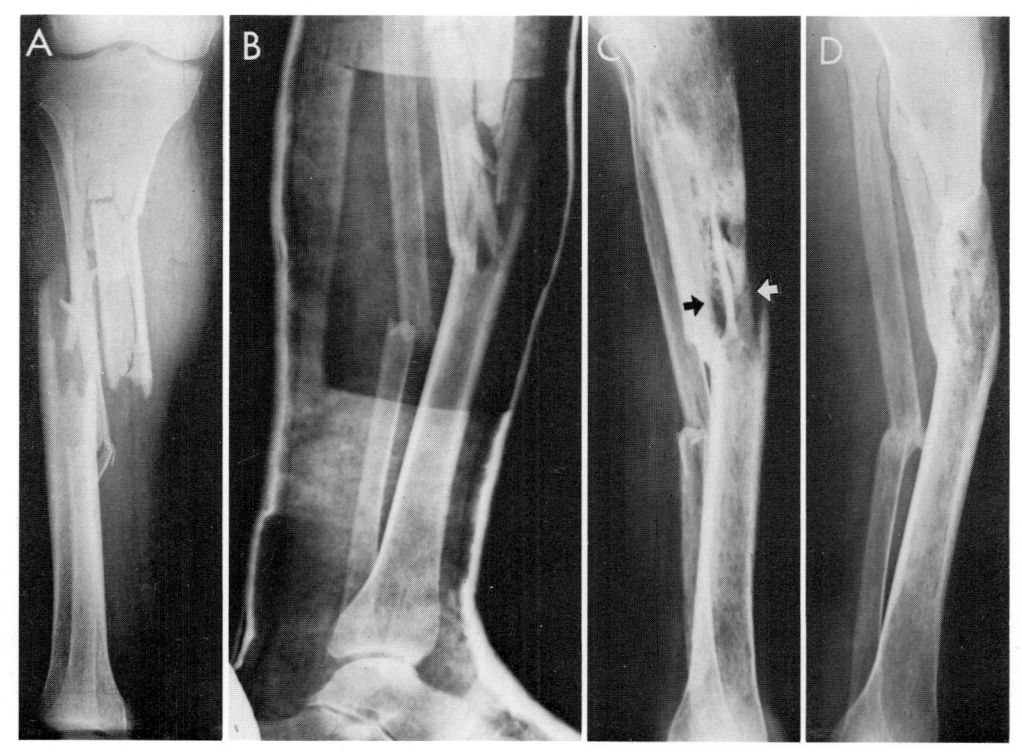

Fig. 31-7.—**A,** severely comminuted closed fracture of tibia and fibula before reduction. Note the marked comminution and displacement of small bone fragments. There is a 90-degree external rotation deformity; the proximal tibia is seen as an anteroposterior projection, the ankle as a lateral projection. **B,** after closed reduction. The general alignment is satisfactory, but there still is marked displacement of the smaller intermediate bone fragments. Delay in union is to be expected regardless of the type of treatment. **C,** 6 months after injury; union not yet complete. The two avascular cortical fragments noted in the fracture line *(arrows)* have contributed to the delay in bone healing. **D,** 26 months after injury; union finally complete.

Kirschner wire through the distal tibia for traction and two transverse wires through the proximal tibia, with incorporation of the wires in plaster to maintain length. These usually are left in place for 1–2 months and then are removed and the fracture treated by non-weight-bearing plaster immobilization until union occurs.

UNSTABLE FRACTURES.—Many fractures, especially if segmental or comminuted, display an extraordinary degree of instability. This usually will be obvious on initial reduction maneuvers (Fig. 31-9). Often, wrapping the first roll of plaster around the shaft of the tibia and allowing this to harden will afford enough stability to permit the remainder of the cast to be applied without loss of reduction. Occasional application of the upper portion of the cast first including the knee is helpful. Another method of cast application in unstable fractures is to align the leg in the supine position, using the normal side as a guide. An anterior splint is laid over the cast padding, gently molded and allowed to harden. The leg then can be elevated and the cast completed, reduction being maintained by the splint already applied. A third method used to combat gross instability is the use of trac-

Chapter 31: FRACTURES OF THE TIBIA AND FIBULA / 801

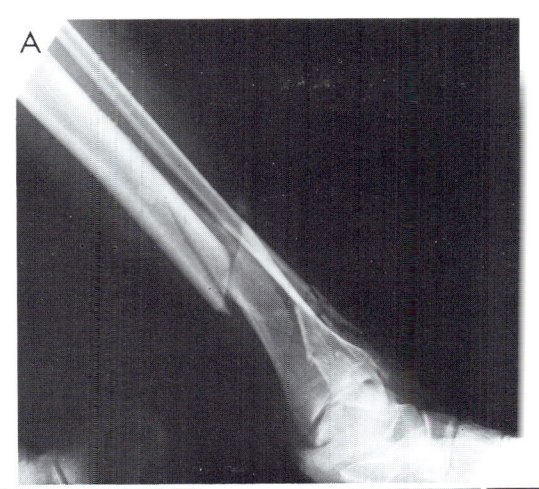

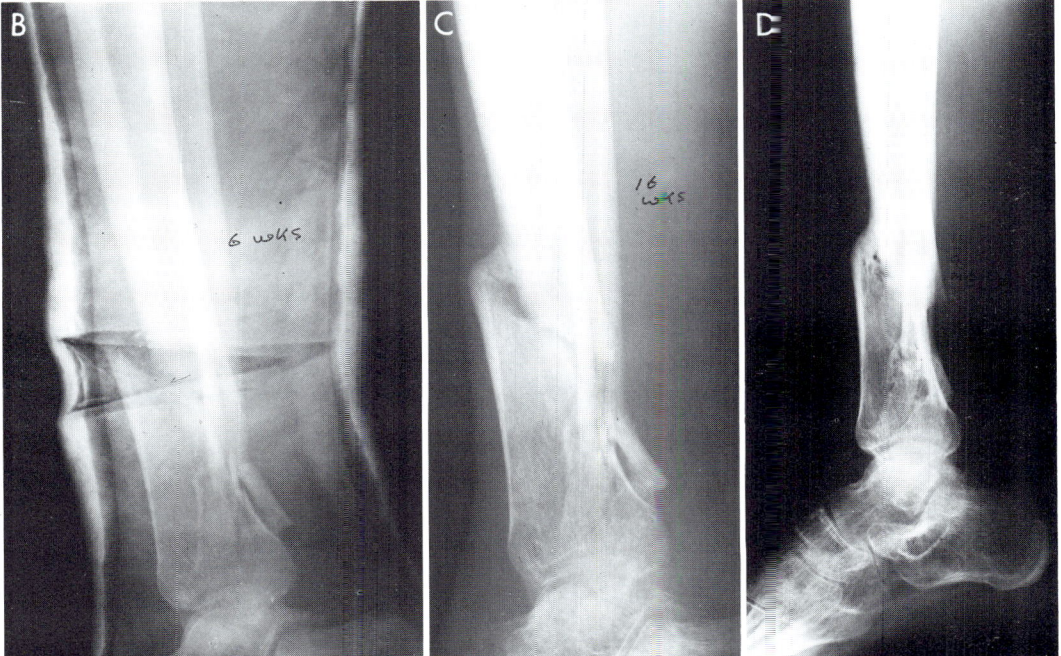

Fig. 31-8.—**A,** initial x-ray film of a comminuted fracture treated by **B)** closed reduction (with cast wedging to partially correct alignment) and early weight bearing. Patient released from plaster in 16 weeks (**C**) and obtained complete union (**D**).

tion through a wire in the os calcis with the leg on a Böhler-Braun frame for a period of about 2 weeks and then application of a cast after the fracture has become "sticky."

Open Fractures

In general, open fractures of the tibial shaft need to be carefully debrided and cleansed. Very small wounds of com-

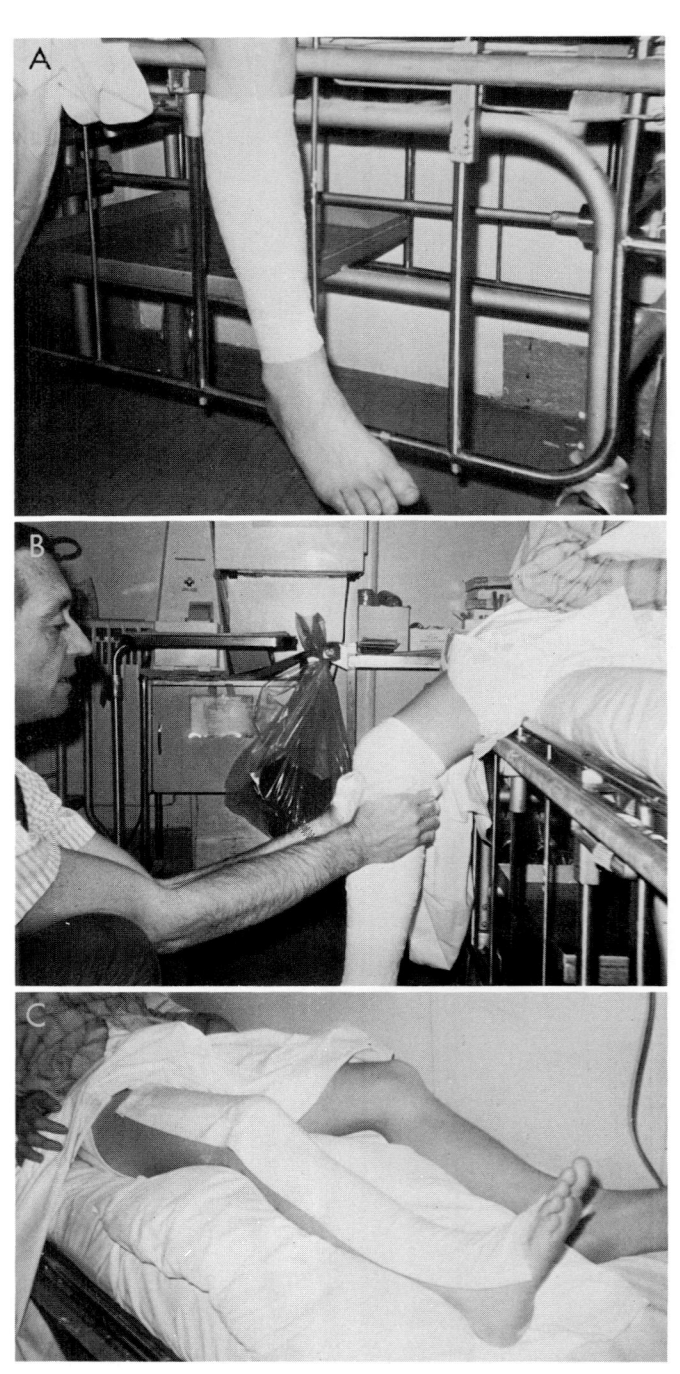

Fig. 31-9.—Reduction may be helped in unstable fractures by using an initial roll of plaster at the level of the fracture (**A**), placing the upper portion of the cast on first (**B**) or using an anterior splint placed on the leg in an aligned but unsuspended position (**C**). The leg and splint then are lifted as one and the cast completed.

pounding from within may be managed with skin cleansing, a dressing and antibiotic and tetanus immunization coverage, but this method should be the exception, not the rule. After debridement of an open fracture, the decision of whether to close the wound or not always comes up. Since the fracture usually lies directly beneath the skin, coverage of the bone is tempting and desirable. However, swelling and skin damage by trauma often make simple closure impossible or possible only under great tension. Whether the wound is to be closed or not is a matter for individual judgment. Certainly closure under extreme skin tension is doomed to failure. At times, the fracture itself can be allowed to assume a posterior bowed position, thus relaxing the pretibial skin for closure under less tension. Two weeks later, after skin healing, the fracture may be realigned. A "relaxing incision" may be useful to obtain skin coverage of the pretibial area, but it should be remembered that this is really a double-ended pedicle flap and is not a simple maneuver to be approached lightly. In general, under ideal circumstances, where the patient does not have to be immediately transported elsewhere, the wound is clean and well debrided, the fracture stable and closure without tension is possible, initial loose skin closure is indicated. When this is not possible, the safest and in the long run shortest course is the method proved effective in the military; that is, packing the wound open, applying a cast, elevation and antibiotics and, in 48–72 hours, carrying out a delayed primary wound closure. Where bone stability is not possible and there is likelihood of further skin, arterial or other significant soft tissue compromise by moving fracture fragments, fixation of open fractures may be considered, as long as the purpose of the fixation can be accomplished reasonably. Small metallic fixation devices (screws, wires, etc.) probably do not in themselves significantly increase the risk of sepsis in open fractures. In open fractures, antibiotic coverage should start by the intravenous route prior to debridement and continue for at least 48 hours. A culture of the wound should be taken before initiating therapy. The point of discontinuance of antibiotics varies, but in a wound in which no sepsis is evident usually is 5–14 days.

OPEN REDUCTIONS.—The open reduction and fixation of tibial shaft fractures may be considered generally if closed methods do not succeed in accomplishing the goals of reduction and fracture position outlined above in terms of displacement, alignment, contact, length and stability. Although operative reduction always is tempting in the tibia, where firm fracture fixation often is relatively simple and the operative approach uncomplicated, it should be remembered that open reduction always delays union, increases risk of infection and does not completely obviate the need for external fracture support, i.e., a cast.

The literature contains many methods of reduction and fixation that are meant to be used simply to provide an essential amount of contact or reduction of a tibial shaft fracture and must be used in conjunction with a cast for the full healing time. These methods occasionally are useful to maintain length in an oblique fracture or contact of a separated large butterfly fragment. They often are carried out with a small skin incision and minimal deep exposure, and for this reason often have been called "semiclosed" methods. This term is misleading, since any opening of the fracture site to achieve reduction must be considered an open reduction, with all the implications that brings forth. Fixation with two screws, circumferential wires and Kirschner wires are examples of this. In general, unless the problem of shortening is great, closed alignment and early weight-bearing therapy is preferable to partial fracture fixation.

Occasionally in unstable fractures of both bones of the leg, the fibular fracture, especially if transverse, can be opened and fixed. This often will increase the general stability of the tibial fracture without resorting to opening this major fracture. Fixation can be accomplished with an intramedullary rod or a plate and screws.

If true open reduction of the fracture is elected, the surgical approach is simple through the anterolateral route. The exposure should be kept toward the lateral side so as to be able to place any plate device along the lateral surface of the tibia, avoiding the subcutaneous surface, which may give closure problems or be uncomfortable later. Types of fixation devices may be generally classified into plate methods applied to the subperiosteal surface of the tibia or intramedullary methods. The former require more subperiosteal stripping for exposure and create more external mass, which may affect closure but can provide very firm fixation.

The latter methods cause considerable endosteal stripping, expose the entire medullary cavity to the operative area, are technically more difficult and may further comminute the fracture if one is not careful. However, occasionally a fracture can be fixed without actually opening the fracture site except through the medullary cavity and the proximal skin incision used to introduce the rod. In addition, the intramedullary method requires minimal local exposure if the fracture is opened and provides firm fixation except in comminuted fractures. The AO compression plate system probably is the best of the plate systems (Fig. 31-10), or its Vitallium equivalent, which negates the disadvantage of need for removal of the apparatus. The intramedullary fixation systems most applicable are the Lottes nail (introduced just medial to the tibial tubercle) and the Küntscher rod (introduced through the extra-articular

Fig. 31-10.—**A,** bilateral fractures fixed with compression-type plates (one should have another screw below the fracture site) and **(B)** a fracture fixed with a Lottes nail (Parham bands needed to increase fixation of a butterfly fragment).

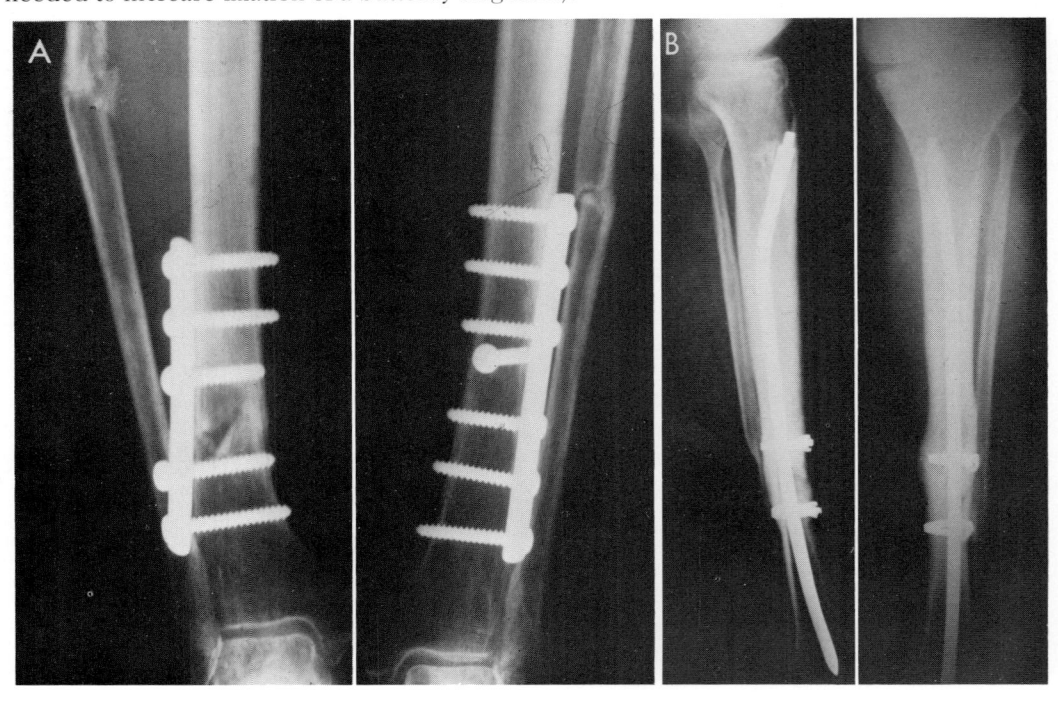

anterior lateral tibial plateau). All methods require considerable skill and practice and should not be attempted by the inexperienced.

Although the literature occasionally advises that a certain fixation method provides such firm support that cast support is unnecessary, this temptation should be resisted and cast support used after all open reductions, at least for a few weeks until the beginnings of union occur. It should be remembered that no metallic device can permanently take the place of firm bony union of the fracture, and that the holes made in the bone by the fixation device weaken the bone.

Also, the inelasticity of the fixation device places greater stresses on the bone adjacent to it.

Delayed Union and Nonunion

As mentioned before, the healing times of these fractures tend to be long. A tibial shaft fracture in an adult cannot be said to have delayed union for 6 months or nonunion for a year (and, even then, many fractures will progress to union after a year with further immobilization). The causes of delayed union in these fractures are the same as in other areas, i.e., malreduction with lack of bony contact

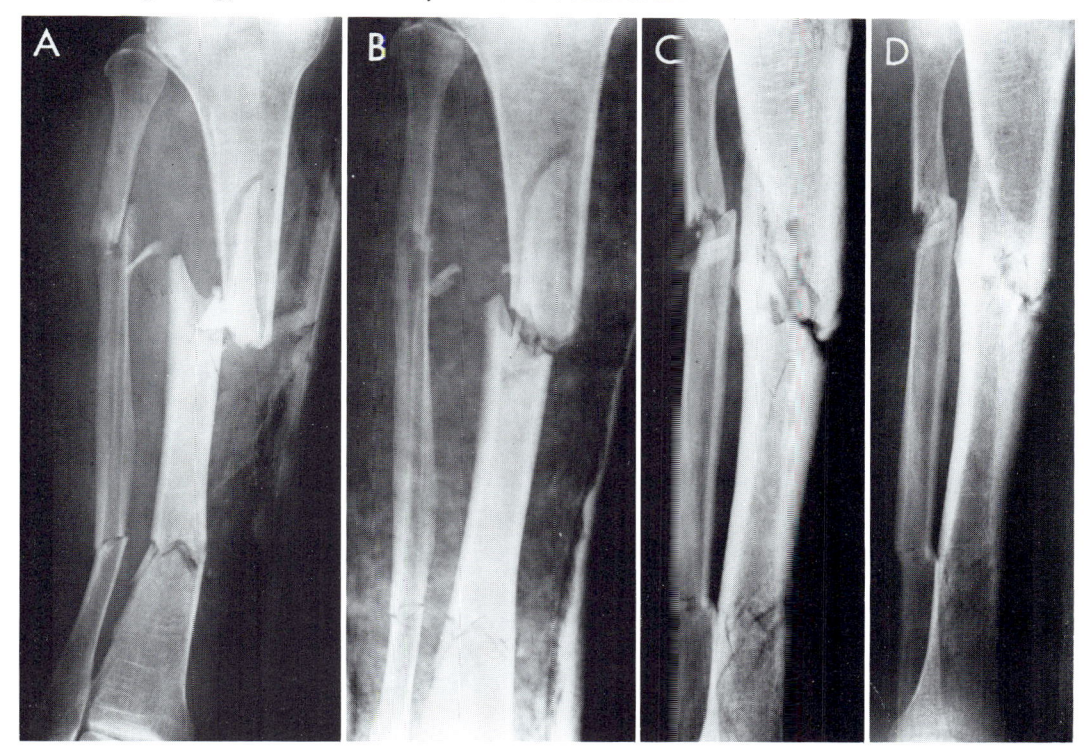

Fig. 31-11.—A, comminuted segmental open fracture of tibia and fibula immediately after injury. Note that the distal fracture shows minimal displacement and is relatively stable. The proximal fracture is comminuted, displaced and unstable B, 19 days after closed reduction and skeletal traction to maintain length and alignment. Distraction has occurred at the proximal fracture line, and delay in union may be predicted. C, 3 months after injury. The distal fracture is healing satisfactorily, but there is delay in healing of the proximal fracture. Note the cortical fragments not yet revascularized. The clinical and x-ray evidence of delay in union prompted the use of autogenous iliac onlay grafts. D, 10 months after injury, 7 months after bone grafting; union satisfactory. Excellent end result

of fragments, infection, open fractures and open reductions. Dr. Edwin Cave's admonition that the greatest cause of delayed union in tibial shaft fractures is testing the fracture to see if it is united must be remembered. Thus, cast changes and manipulative testing of the leg should be kept at a minimum during the healing period. Evaluation of callus production in healing fractures can be troublesome, since well-fixed fractures (especially with the AO compression system) can show very little external callus production while progressing to early firm union. On the other hand, exuberant external callus can be seen in delayed union.

The treatment of delayed union after 6 months is either further immobilization or bone grafting, usually without internal fixation (Fig. 31-11). The fracture site is not disturbed but Phemister-type grafts are placed along the back of the tibia bridging the fracture through a posterolateral approach (Fig. 5-37, p. 154). Onlay-type grafting is used much less frequently. Occasionally, fibular osteotomy to prevent further distraction of the fracture is useful. Further immobilization of the fracture is continued, with a high degree

Fig. 31-12.—**A,** open comminuted fracture of both tibia and fibula immediately after injury. **B,** after debridement and plating. Note the defect in the fracture line, indicating loss of a bone fragment. Unprotected weight bearing was started 7 months after injury, and at 1 year the result was rated excellent. **C,** 21 months after injury. The plate has broken, nonunion is present and there is massive excess callus. At a second operation, the plate and the excess callus were removed, the bone ends were freshened, autogenous iliac onlay grafts (Phemister) were applied and the fracture was immobilized by a Lottes nail. **D,** 5 months later. Clinically and by x-ray examination, healing appeared to be progressing satisfactorily. Patient was on full activity.

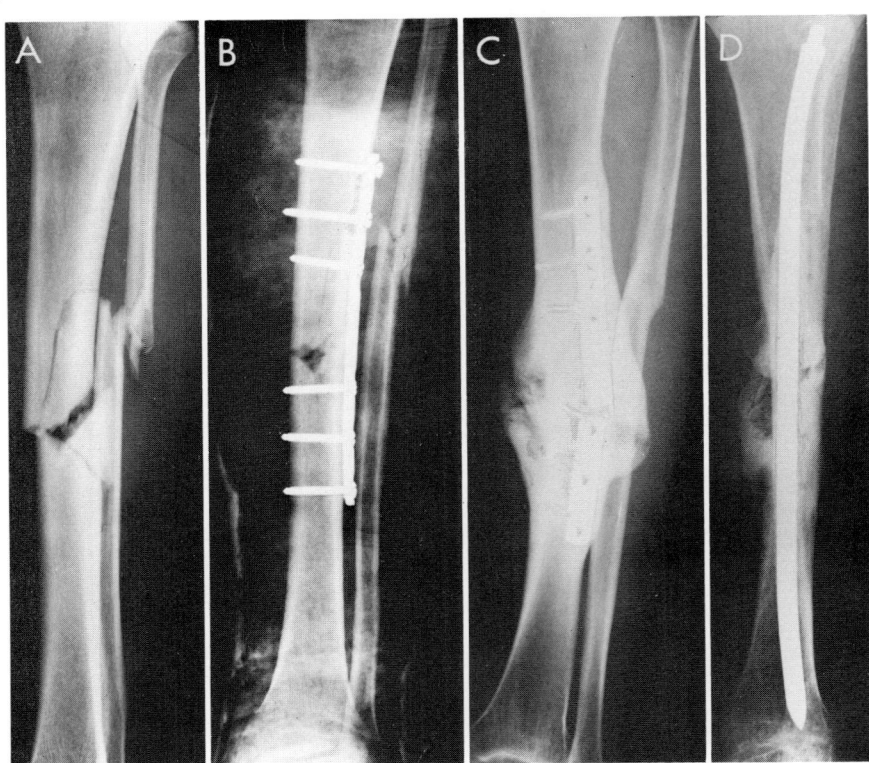

of union obtained (Fig. 31-12). Of course, grafting at this stage could be expected to yield excellent results, since many of these fractures would go on to union with further treatment without grafting.

Established nonunion of a fracture, with false motion, pain, redness and poor callus over 1 year postinjury, can be treated as described before, but more usually an internal fixation device is used. In order to insert this well, the nonunion area usually, but not always, is debrided to bleeding bone. The apparatus used is of the type described under open reductions. Grafting material usually is autogenous and of the Phemister type. Again, further immobilization until union occurs is mandatory.

In ununited fractures that have had several operative attempts to achieve

Fig. 31-13.—Appearance of a leg 3 years after injury prior to amputation. A severe crushing injury caused comminuted fractures, which were delayed in healing. Severe soft tissue injury and prolonged cast immobilization caused ankle stiffness, cavovarus deformity, clawtoes and impaired sensation. Function of this extremity was not as satisfactory as a prosthesis despite final fracture healing.

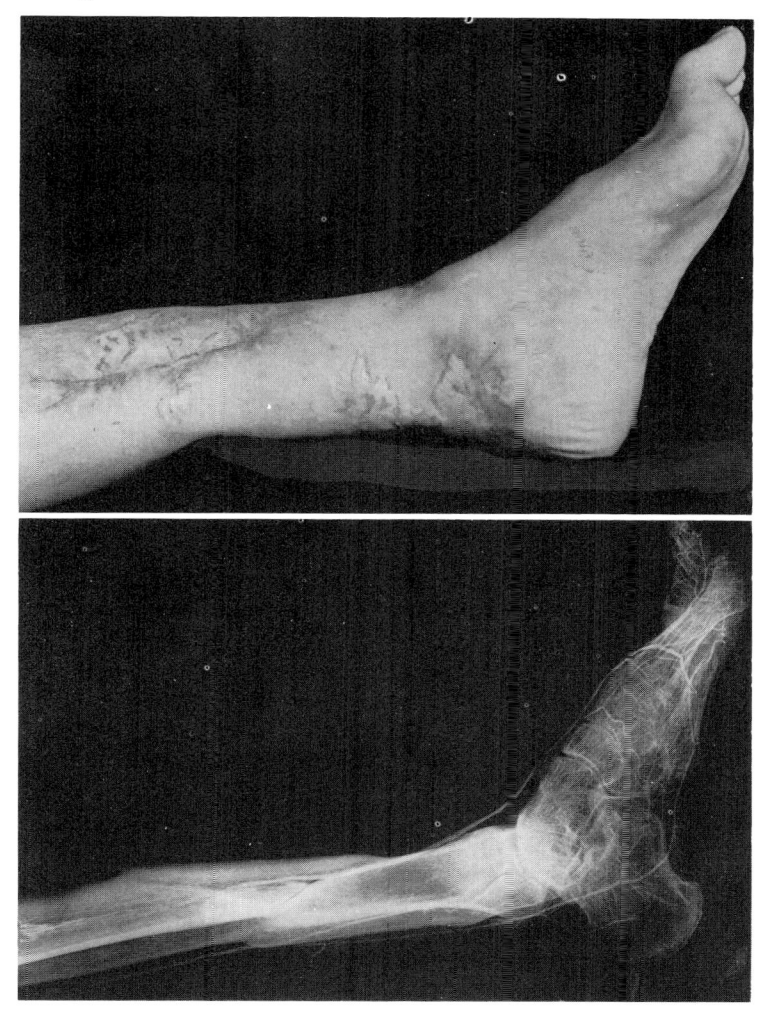

union, the method of McMaster sometimes is useful. This attempts to gain, with bone grafts, cross-union between the tibia and fibula above and below the fracture site. This method of treatment is especially useful in actively septic ununited fractures.

Occasionally, all attempts at gaining union seem to fail, at which time the total time of treatment of the fracture is measured in years. Since this time has been spent in long leg casts, knee and ankle stiffness is a great problem. Below-knee amputation then must be considered (Fig. 31-13). With the newer prosthetic developments, the disability caused by this amputation level has decreased considerably, so that it is less than that of a shortened leg with a stiff and perhaps painful foot and ankle, poor skin over the pretibial area and a stiff knee. The decision to amputate below the knee in difficult cases probably is made too late, often because of the great therapeutic investment in time and effort on the part of both patient and physician. Although no ironclad pronouncements can be made in this regard, it behooves the physician to keep in mind that the below-knee amputation level is extremely functional. One should advocate this procedure when it appears that function of the extremity will be less than that of a below-knee prosthesis, even if final union *is* attained, and not simply if union cannot be achieved.

If infection ensues, either after an open fracture or an opened fracture, the rate of nonunion will soar and chronic infection is common, even after union is obtained. High levels of the appropriate antibiotic, debridement and adequate drainage (with or without a suction-irrigation device) and prolonged immobilization are required. Fixation devices already in place at the time infection begins should be *left in place* until union occurs, since they afford immobilization of the fracture.

BIBLIOGRAPHY

Anderson, L. D., and Hutchins, W. C.: Fractures of the tibia and fibula treated with casts and transfixing pins, South. Med. J. 59:1026, 1966.

Boylston, B. F., and Milam, R.: Segmental fractures of the tibia. An analysis of thirty cases, South. Med. J. 50:1969, 1957.

Dehne, E., Metz, C. W., Deffer, P. A., *et al.*: Nonoperative treatment of the fractured tibia by immediate weight bearing, J. Trauma 1:514, 1961.

Edwards, P.: Fractures of the shaft of the tibia—492 consecutive cases in adults, importance of soft tissue injury, Acta Chir. Scand. Supp. 76, 1965.

Evans, E. B., and Eggers, G. W. N.: Internal fixation of the fibula in fractures of both bones of the leg, JAMA 169:321, 1959.

Hoaglund, F. T., and Statci, J.: Factors influencing the rate of healing in tibial shaft fractures, Surg. Gynecol. Obstet. 124:71, 1967.

Lottes, J. O., Hill, L. J., and Key, J. A.: Closed reduction, plate fixation, and medullary nailing of fractures of both bones of the leg, J. Bone Joint Surg. 34-A:861, 1952.

Moore, S. T., Storts, R. A., and Spencer, J. O.: Fractures of the tibial shaft in adults. A ten year survey of such fractures, South. Med. J. 55:1178, 1962.

Müller, M. E., Allgöwer, M., and Willenegger, H.: *Technique of Internal Fixation of Fractures* (New York: Springer-Verlag, 1965).

Nicoll, E. A.: Fractures of the tibial shaft. A survey of 705 cases, J. Bone Joint Surg. 48-A:257, 1966.

Olerand, S., and Karlstiow, G.: Secondary intramedullary nailing of tibial fractures, J. Bone Joint Surg. 54-A:1419, 1972.

Sarmiento, A.: A functional below the knee cast for tibial fractures, J. Bone Joint Surg. 49-A:855, 1967.

Weissman, L., Harold, H. Z., and Engelber, M.: Fractures of the middle two-thirds of the tibial shaft; results of treatment without internal fixation in one hundred and forty consecutive cases, J. Bone Joint Surg. 48-A:257, 1966.

32 | Ankle Injuries

EDWARD J. RISEBOROUGH
and OTTO E. AUFRANC

EARLY WRITINGS on fractures and dislocations of the ankle stressed the seriousness of these injuries. The authors reported only a rare cure, often permanent disability and not infrequently amputation or death as a consequence. Dupuytren (1777–1835) noted that even under favorable conditions fractures of the ankle almost always resulted in deformity and lameness, yet he reported cures in 202 of 207 of his own cases, with only 2 patients having deformity. Five of his patients died.

Dupuytren was the first to record experiments on the mechanism of the production of ankle fractures. His theories were totally accepted until a pupil of his, Maisonneuve, found an oblique fracture of the fibula in a cadaver. Maisonneuve discovered that external rotation was the force that opened the fracture. His work on the mechanism of ankle fractures was published about 1842. With his clear thinking and logic, he presented illustrations of the mechanical forces involved in external rotation injuries (Fig. 32-1).

Three others contributed to the early writings on ankle injuries. Hönigschmied (1882) produced by experimental means almost all the types of fractures of the ankle with the exception of fractures due to compression and Ashhurst and Bromer reported an extensive study on the classification and mechanics of fractures of the ankle (1922).

CAUSES AND MECHANISM OF ANKLE FRACTURES

A single misstep on a small pebble, an irregular path or a slippery surface often is all that is necessary to produce a severe ankle injury or fracture-dislocation. Falling, twisting or turning motions in which the foot becomes a fixed point and the body above becomes the long arm of a lever, with the talus as a movable, rounded and wedge-shaped fulcrum within the tibiofibular mortise, produce a variety of ankle fractures and dislocations. The direction of the body in motion above the relatively fixed point of the foot influences the type of fracture-dislocation. At the time of injury, the type of fracture will vary with the position of the foot and the direction in which the lower leg and body are moving.

A knowledge of the mechanism of the injury is useful in reducing the fracture. The use of a reversal of the forces that produced the injury often will result in an easy reduction of the fracture, and properly applied counterforces will maintain the position of the reduction without strain (Fig. 32-2).

EMERGENCY TREATMENT

Initial treatment should be guided by the principle of early splinting without doing additional harm. A pillow with side splints probably is the best apparatus for

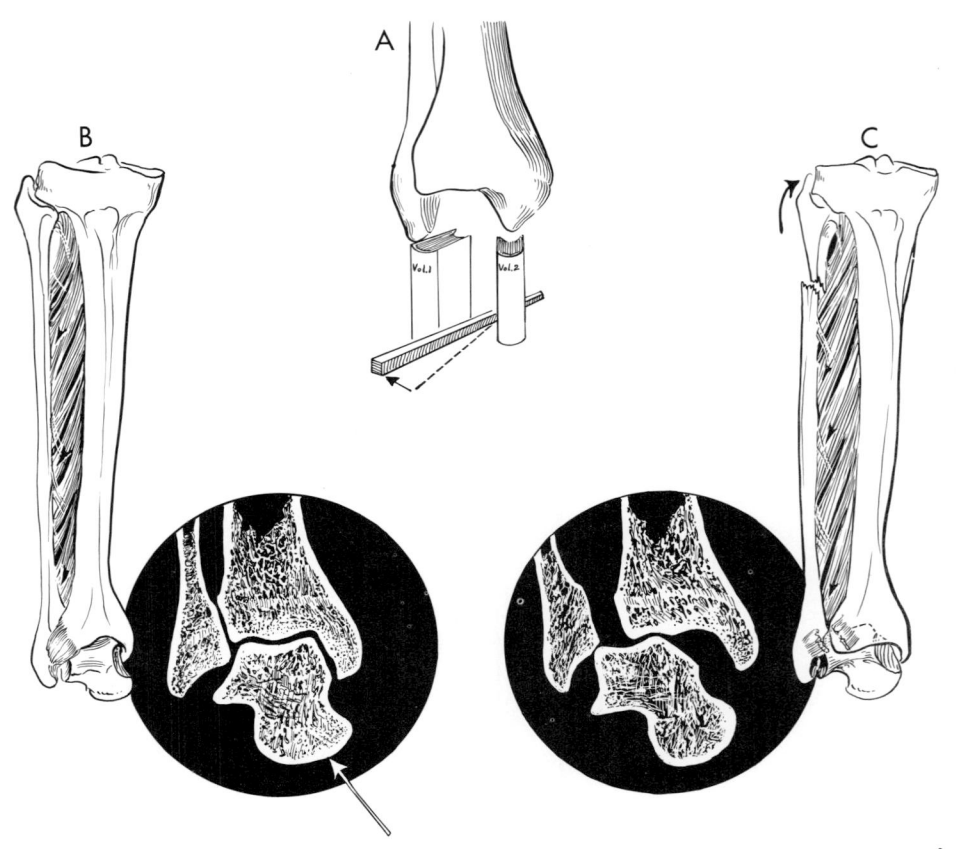

Fig. 32-1.—Leverage forces in external rotation violence. **A,** illustrating Maisonneuve's simple idea of external rotation violence: the malleoli are separated by the force derived from the rotation of the talus. **B,** showing direction of fibers of the interosseous membrane (tibiofibular) from tibia to fibula downward. The mortise of the tibia and fibula is grooved to fit the contour of the talus. **C,** indicating how an upward force with rotation may produce a high fibular fracture and widen the interosseous membrane and dislocate the talus into a lateral groove.

emergency treatment of ankle injuries. This splint can be applied by the inexperienced almost as well as by the experienced person. The pillow should be puffed to conform to the deformity, then firm wooden supports applied laterally and a third support applied posteriorly under the leg and heel. Side splints without padding are contraindicated, as their use very likely could produce malleolar necrosis of the skin. The use of metal side supports is not recommended, as they interfere with x-ray films being taken in the splint. Pressure over blanched or ischemic skin areas that are "tented" by the deformity should be avoided. It is desirable, if there is considerable deformity and the skin appears compromised, to apply traction on the foot and ankle in the line of the deformity and then align the foot beneath the tibia before applying the pillow splint.

Manipulation of the foot should not be performed when there is an open wound. A sterile bandage should be applied over the wound and the ankle splinted without reduction of its deformity.

Application of a pneumatic splint in emergency cases is a useful means of immobilizing the injured lower or upper

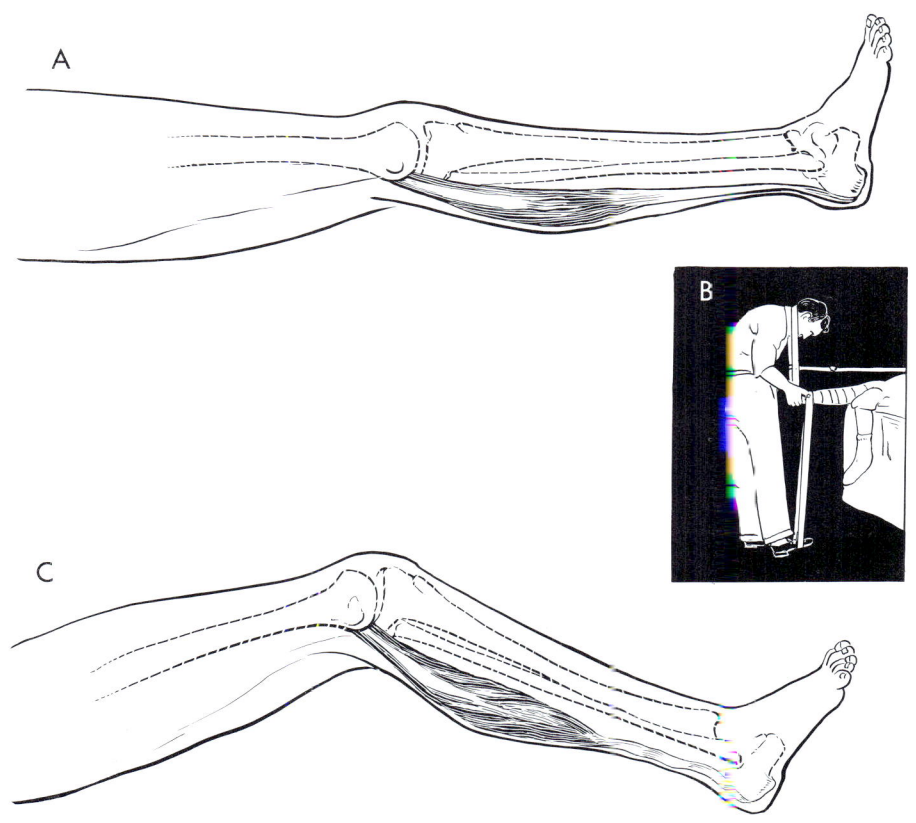

Fig. 32-2.—Manipulation for easy reduction. **A** and **B**, incorrect position, with gastrocnemius muscle taut and knee straight. With the leg in this position the muscles are not relaxed and the need for force is obvious. **C**, correct position. All muscles are relaxed by bending the knee and putting the foot in equinus.

extremity, including the distal femur, lower leg and ankle, humerus, forearm, etc. However, areas of ischemia may result from excessive localized pressure, and the pneumatic splint is viewed with disfavor by some surgeons because of its tendency to force the foot into an abnormal position of excessive dorsiflexion in lower-leg and ankle fractures.

X-RAY EXAMINATION

Anteroposterior, lateral and mortise views (anteroposterior view with the foot rotated internally 30 degrees) of the foot and ankle usually are sufficient x-rays for planning the management of the injury. The anteroposterior view will show the relationship of the tibia and fibula to each other. The mortise view shows the relationship of the talus to the mortise formed by the tibia and fibula and a view of the lateral side of the ankle will show the profile of the tibia with the fibula slightly behind. Other angle views should be taken when interpretation of the usual views is difficult. X-ray films of the uninjured ankle should be taken for comparative studies in unusual injuries and especially in children, in whom growth disturbances may follow epiphyseal injuries.

As first pointed out by Maisonneuve, external rotation violence may produce a

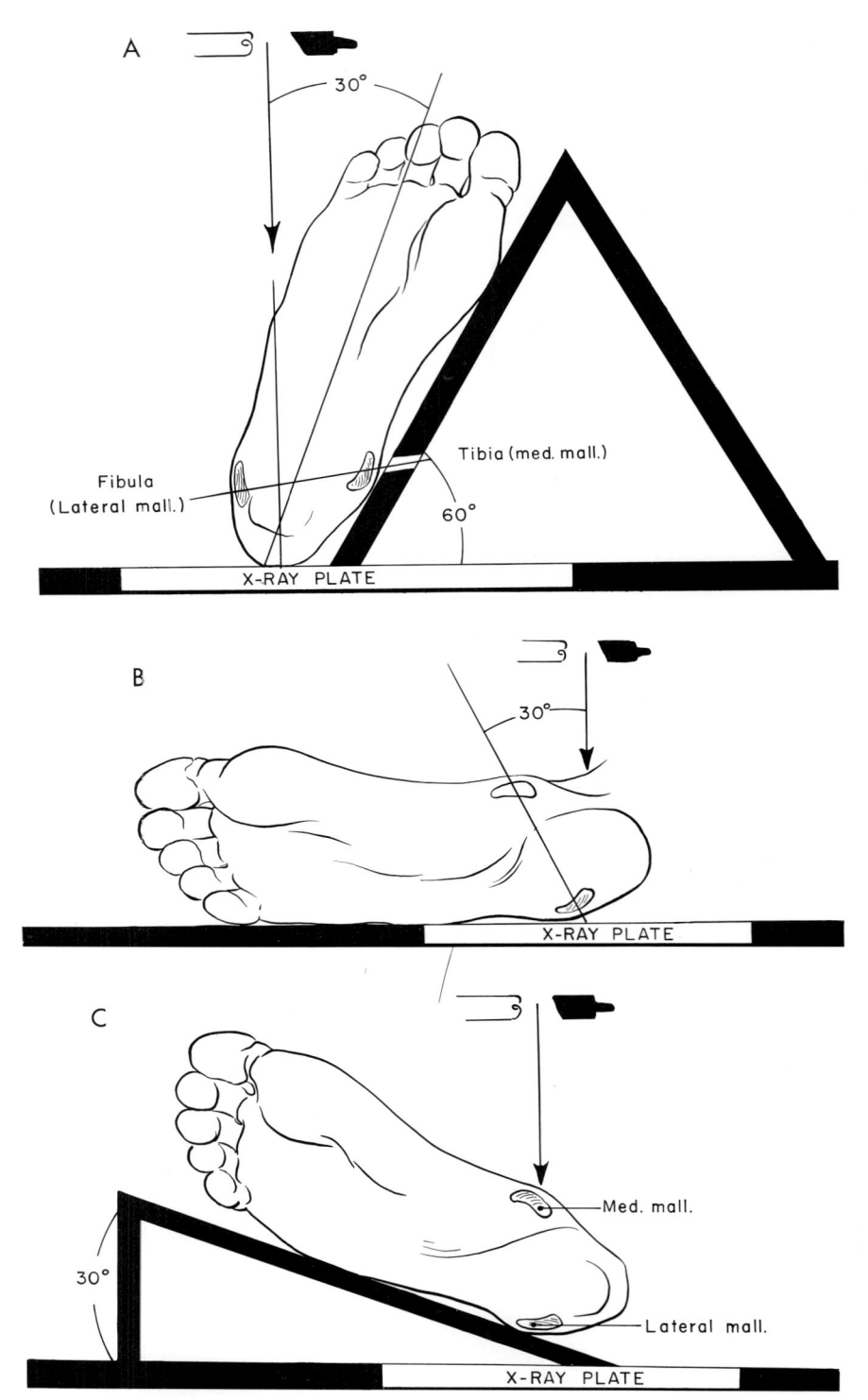

Fig. 32-3.—Positions of foot and ankle for taking an x-ray film. **A,** foot in internal rotation for true mortise view. **B,** lateral side of foot on plate for oblique view with fibula projected behind. **C,** toes elevated 30 degrees for a superimposed malleolus view.

high fracture of the fibula. Therefore, x-ray films should include the entire fibular shaft.

Further x-ray films of the fractures and dislocations are taken after reduction and repeated after plaster is applied. Later, the position of the bone fragments should be checked by x-ray examination as often as necessary. The stability of the reduced fracture and the amount of swelling are leads as to how often such viewing may be indicated. A change of plaster may be necessary as the swelling subsides to prevent displacement of fragments.

ANATOMIC POINTS OF CLINICAL SIGNIFICANCE AROUND THE ANKLE

The Talus

The key to the management and understanding of ankle fractures is the talus. Because of its wedge shape, the talus itself rarely is broken, but with excessive rotary movements the talus tends to break or dislocate the tibia and fibula. Because of its stability, the talus is used as the mold for reshaping a fracture of the ankle joint.

The superior articular surface of the talus is convex. The anterior surface is wider than the posterior—like a horizontal wedge with the base forward. The superior surface of the talus is also wider below than above, forming another wedge in the vertical plane, with the base inferiorly. These features constitute structurally a section of a quadrilateral pyramid with the top rounded and horizontally and transversely grooved from front to back. The groove is roughly in the center and runs over the entire articular convexity. The tibial surface thus is convex from front to back and concave from side to side. All of the articular edges are rounded. The anatomic plan permits the ankle mortise rotatory, rocking and tilting motion.

The fibular facet of the talus is longer and almost vertical and it is tilted more posteriorly than the shallow and more oblique tibial facet and in a more posterior plane than its medial counterpart. Thus, the ankle movements over the talus are not in a direct anteroposterior direction but along a plane inclined slightly externally.

In the anteroposterior x-ray view of the talus, the shallow groove, with slightly elevated and rounded ridges at each side, lies almost in the center of the weight-bearing ankle surface of the tibia, the concavity of the talus fitting a similar convexity of the weight-bearing surface of the tibia.

In the lateral x-ray view, the ankle weight-bearing surface is convex above, the surface appearing as a part of an arc of a circle. Flexion and extension motion of the ankle joint thus have an axis of movement transversely through the body of the talus at about the level of the tip of the fibular malleolus.

Ankle Articulation at the Distal End of the Tibia

At its distal end, the tibia enlarges from being roughly triangular in the midshaft to a quadrilateral shape at its distal end. This enlarged structure fits over the body of the talus. The lower end of the fibula fits in a shallow concavity on the lateral side of the tibia and projects distally as the lateral malleolus.

The inferior articular surface of the tibia is concave from front to back and roughly quadrilateral, broader in front than behind, and is slightly convex from front to back. This ridge seats itself in the concavity on the dorsal articular surface of the talus. Medially, the internal malleolus projects downward and has a shallow articulation with the talus.

Ankle Articulation at the Distal End of the Fibula

The lower end of the fibula forms the external malleolus and this malleolus is about twice as long as it is broad and projects beyond the tip of the medial malleolus. The articular facet of the fibular mal-

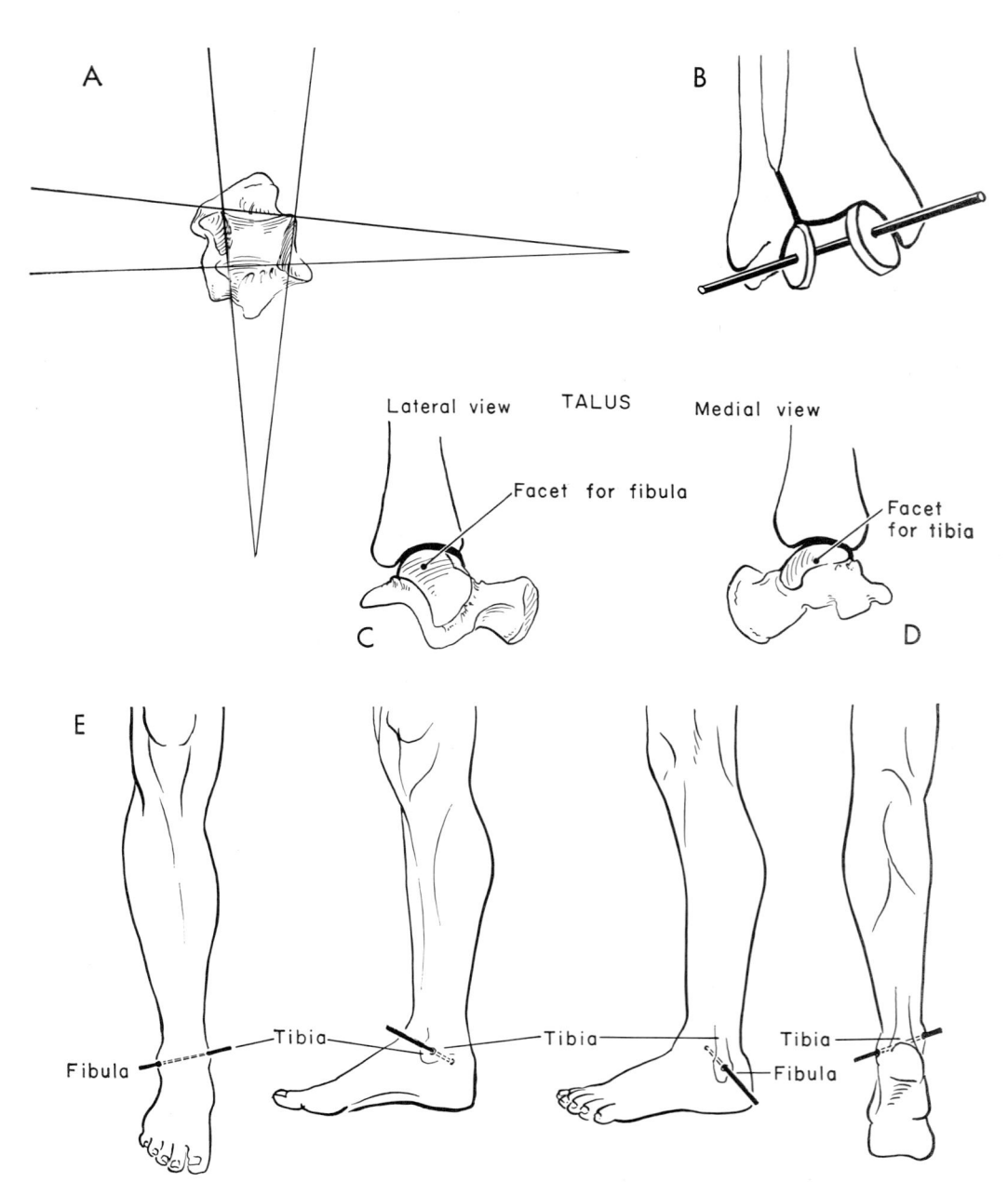

Fig. 32-4.—Important mechanical features of the talus. **A,** showing the talus as a part of a wedge, with a base in front in the anteroposterior plane and a base medially in the lateral plane. Note also that the direction of dislocation and fracture more often is toward the sharp edges of the wedges. **B,** left foot as viewed from behind, indicating, by the wheel of the fibular facet, how functional motions are toward the short arc of motion. **C,** facet of the fibula. In the vertical plane, the facet is elongated and narrow from front to back, allowing a rotation around this arc. The foot thus goes into valgus position in plantar flexion. **D,** indicating deficiency of tibia in front. The base of the talar wedge is forward and prevents anterior dislocation except in unusual violence. **E,** showing relationship of malleoli. These should be restored in reduction.

814

leolus is convex from above downward, but in horizontal cross section it is slightly concave. This structural feature adds to the strength and stability of the fibula in rotatory motion. The center of the fibular malleolus is slightly behind the transverse axis of motion. The bimalleolar axis and the axis of movement meet at an angle of about 30 degrees.

IMPORTANT LIGAMENTS OF THE ANKLE

The ankle joint is enclosed by an articular capsule. This capsule is thin and weak anteriorly and posteriorly. Laterally, it is strengthened by the anterior and posterior talofibular ligaments to form the fibular collateral ligament. Medially, it is strengthened by the triangular deltoid ligament (Fig. 32-5).

The fibula is attached to the tibia by strong anterior and posterior tibiofibular ligaments. The fibers, in general, run from the tibia above, outward and downward toward the fibular malleolus below. The interosseous membrane between the tibia and fibula has fibers running in the same direction. This arrangement allows the fibula to move out and slide upward a little on weight bearing, especially during dorsiflexion of the ankle.

The ligaments that should be considered in the functioning of the ankle are:
1. Mortise ligaments
   a) Anterior and posterior, tibiofibular
   b) Interosseous membrane, tibiofibular
2. Medial ligament, tibial collateral or deltoid ligament
   a) Anterior talotibial
   b) Posterior talotibial
   c) Calcaneotibial
3. Lateral ligament—fibular collateral
   a) Anterior talofibular
   b) Posterior talofibular
   c) Calcaneofibular
4. Cruciate ligament

A superficial ligament that encircles the ankle and holds the tendons in their sheaths is known as the cruciate crural band.

MUSCLES AND TENDONS AROUND THE ANKLE

The muscles and tendons around the ankle play an important part in fracture reduction. Tension on one muscle group and relaxation of the opposing one often are necessary to reduce and maintain the reduction of a fracture. In general, the tendons anterior to the ankle joint have little effect as deforming forces on ankle fractures. Those passing behind the joint are much more important in controlling the fracture fragments.

The *heel cord (Achilles tendon)* is taut when the knee is straight and the foot is at a right angle. A redislocation of the ankle or loss of reduction of a fracture may occur even in plaster unless the force through the heel cord is relaxed by bending the knee and letting the foot drop into equinus.

The *peroneal tendons* pass behind the fibular malleolus, under its tip and then forward to the foot; the fibula acts as a grooved pulley around which these tendons slide. In passive plantar flexion of the ankle the tendons are relaxed, and in dorsiflexion they are taut. If the distal fibula is fractured, the pressure exerted on the tip of the bone with the foot in dorsiflexion will displace or tilt the fragments backward at the fracture site. A slight equinus and varus position lessens this tension and diminishes the chance of redisplacement of the fragment.

The *posterior tibial tendon* passes behind the joint and in a groove on the medial malleolus. A slight equinus position will relax the tension on the posterior tibial tendon. In a fracture of the medial malleolus, this tendon, when taut, will push forward on the fracture, causing separation of the fragments anteriorly as the intact deltoid ligament holds the distal fragment down and acts as a fulcrum. Direct molding of the malleolus into

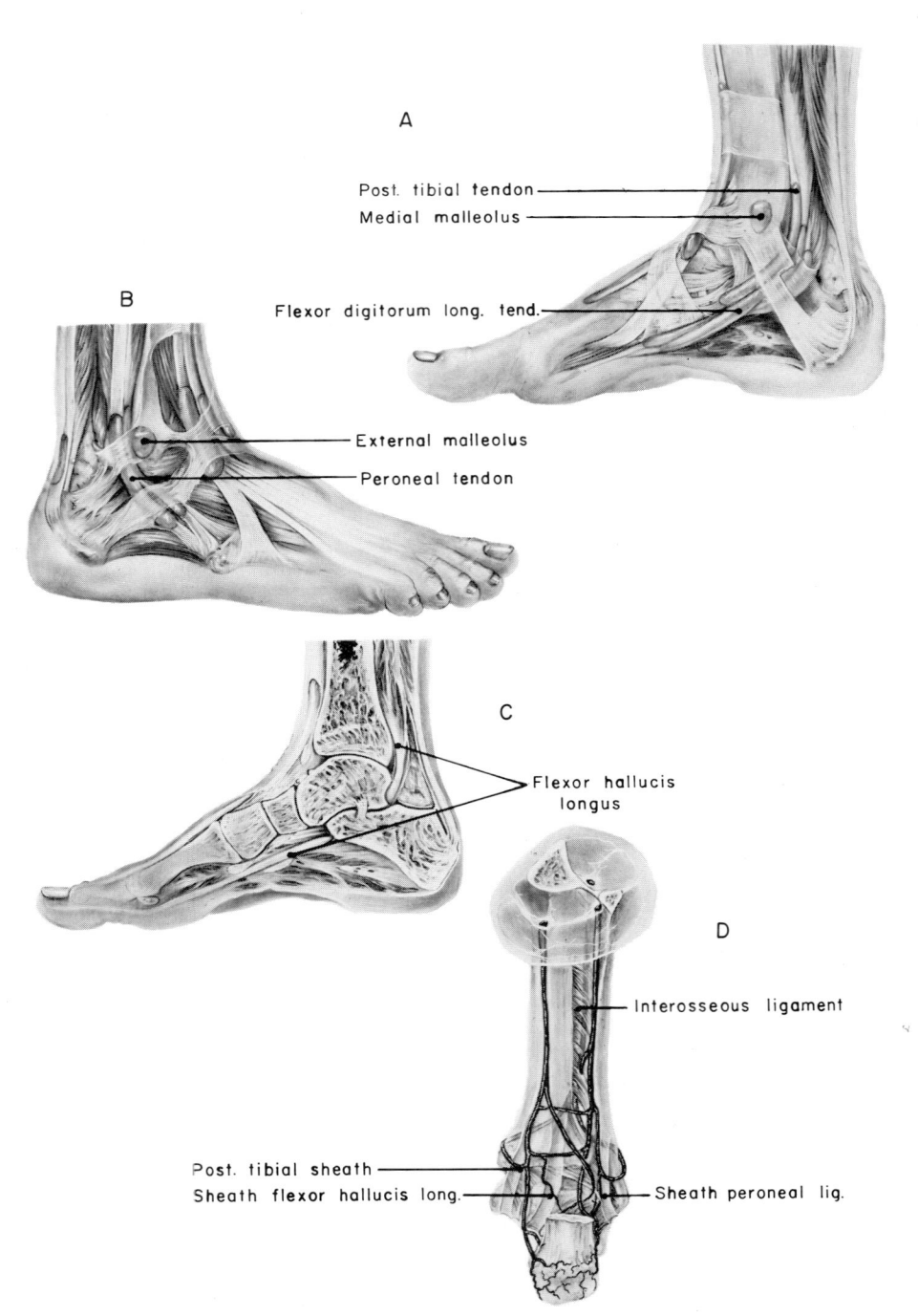

Fig. 32-5.—Surgically important anatomic features of the ankle. **A** and **B**, arrangement of tendons, which produces pulley forces on the malleoli. **C** and **D**, position of the flexor hallucis longus tendon in cross section and (below) its groove from behind. The strength and weakness of the ligaments and the abundance of the blood supply and anastomoses around the ankle should be understood by the surgeon.

Chapter 32: ANKLE INJURIES / 817

alignment thus often is possible in slight equinus and varus position. Interposition of periosteum, capsule or other soft parts may occur with this fracture and prevent unsatisfactory reduction.

The *flexor hallucis longus tendon* passes in a groove directly behind the tibia at the ankle level and obliquely from the lateral to the medial side. In the passive equinus position, the tendon is relaxed, but dorsiflexion of the great toe as the ankle is brought into dorsiflexion will pull the tendon downward and forward on the posterior margin of the tibia. The proper use of forces through this tendon occasionally will help to reduce a posterior tibial lip fragment and maintain its position.

MOTIONS OF THE ANKLE

In walking, as the foot hits the ground it becomes a fulcrum and the ankle joint acts as the hinge. The body above and the ankle have a tendency to continue forward because of the momentum. The weight of the body placed on the ankle thus would be transferred forward onto the dorsum of the foot were it not for the wedge-shaped talus with its base in front blocking further movement forward. As the tibiofibular mortise slides over the

Fig. 32-6.—The fallacy of rigid fixation of the lower end of the tibia to the lower end of the fibula. **A,** lateral and anteroposterior views of ankle showing injury with displacement. The films do not indicate a need for excessive internal fixation material. **B,** oblique and anteroposterior views reveal "rigid fixation" of tibia to the fibula. **C,** anteroposterior view showing bolt that broke with weight-bearing function. The surgeon should plan to remove all transfixation bolts that hold a ruptured tibiofibular ligament. **D,** anteroposterior view showing atrophy of bone around the broken bolt, attesting to the validity of not making the tibiofibular ligament solid.

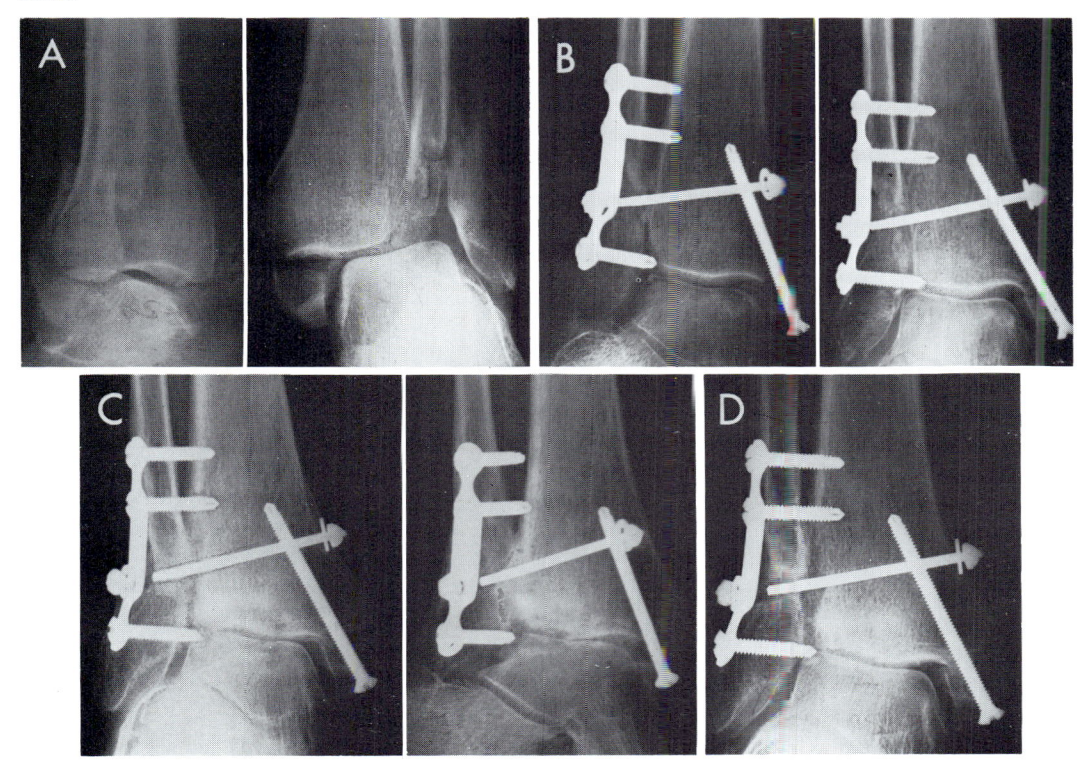

A ANTERIOR ANKLE LIGAMENTS

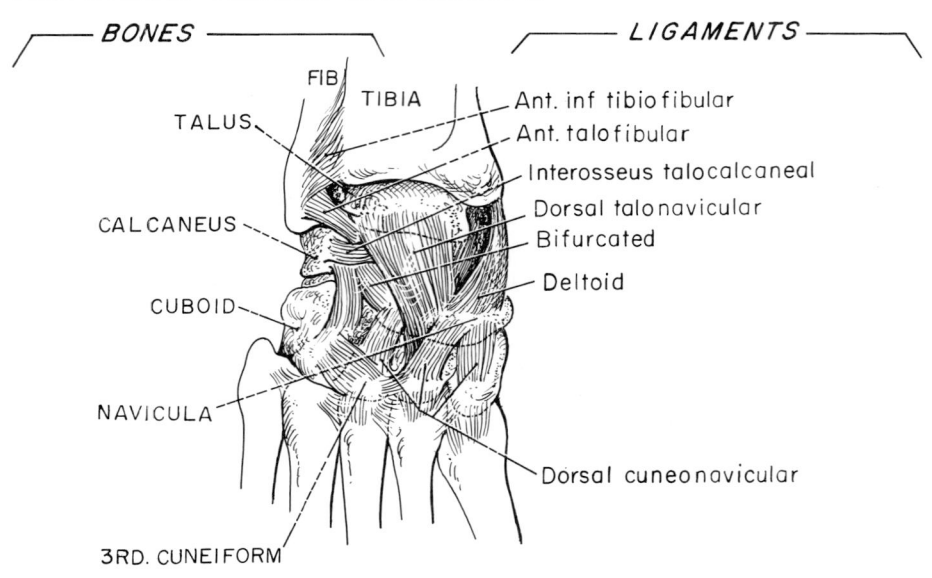

BONES: FIB, TIBIA, TALUS, CALCANEUS, CUBOID, NAVICULA, 3RD. CUNEIFORM

LIGAMENTS: Ant. inf tibiofibular, Ant. talofibular, Interosseus talocalcaneal, Dorsal talonavicular, Bifurcated, Deltoid, Dorsal cuneonavicular

B LATERAL ANKLE LIGAMENTS

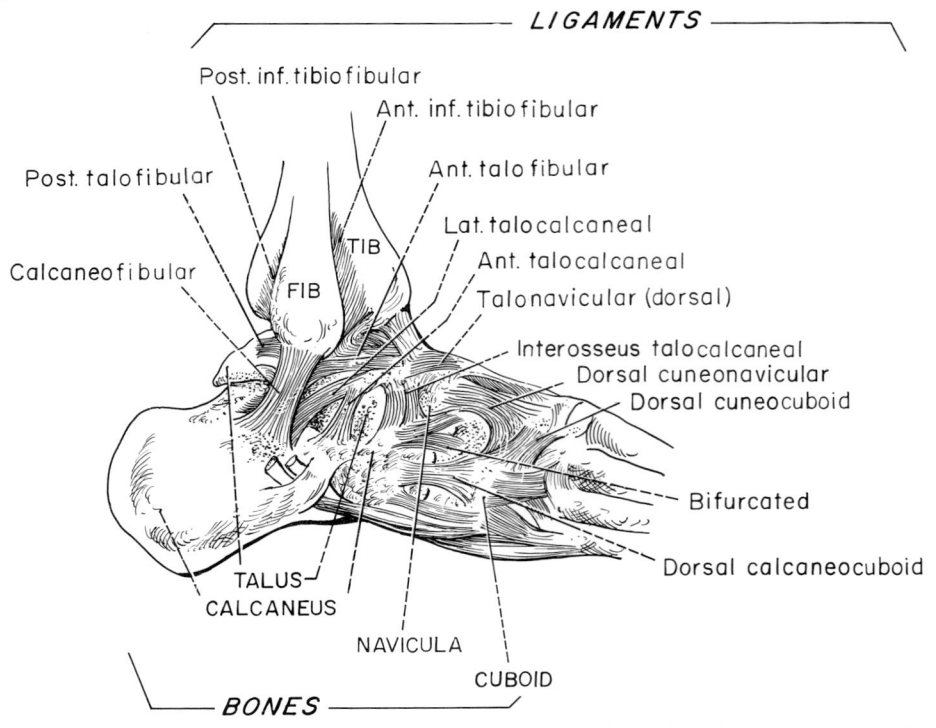

LIGAMENTS: Post. inf. tibiofibular, Ant. inf. tibiofibular, Post. talofibular, Ant. talofibular, Lat. talocalcaneal, Ant. talocalcaneal, Calcaneofibular, Talonavicular (dorsal), Interosseus talocalcaneal, Dorsal cuneonavicular, Dorsal cuneocuboid, Bifurcated, Dorsal calcaneocuboid

BONES: TIB, FIB, TALUS, CALCANEUS, NAVICULA, CUBOID

Fig. 32-7.—Anatomy of important ligaments around the ankle and midfoot. (**Continued.**)

C MEDIAL ANKLE LIGAMENTS

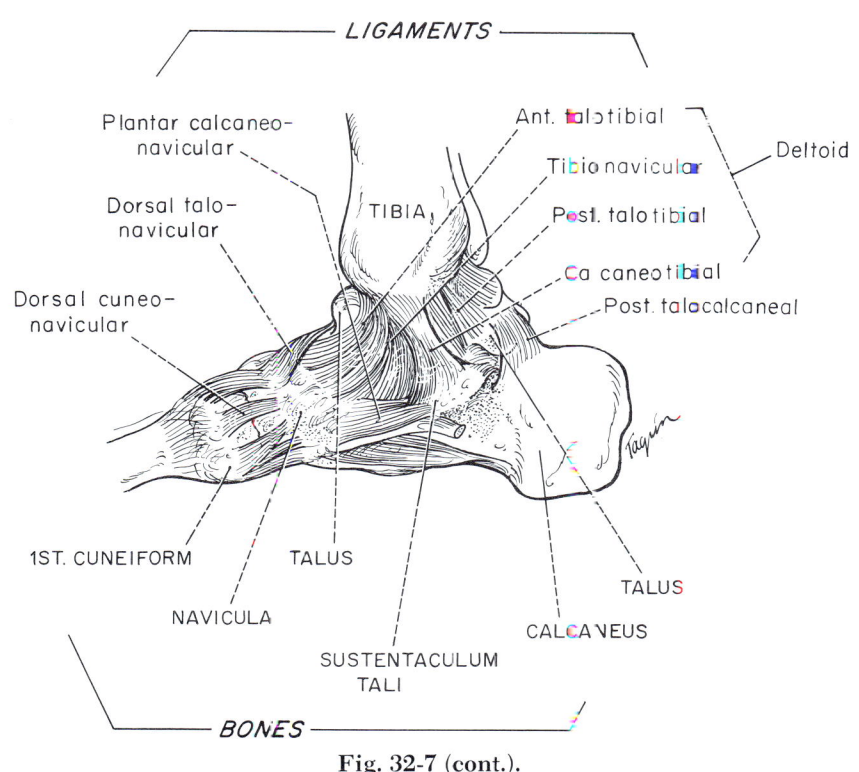

LIGAMENTS

- Plantar calcaneo-navicular
- Dorsal talo-navicular
- Dorsal cuneo-navicular
- Ant. talotibial
- Tibionavicular
- Post. talotibial
- Calcaneotibial
- Post. talocalcaneal
- Deltoid

TIBIA

BONES
- 1ST. CUNEIFORM
- TALUS
- NAVICULA
- SUSTENTACULUM TALI
- TALUS
- CALCANEUS

Fig. 32-7 (cont.).

talus from its narrow to its wide surface in front, the fibula rotates the articular surface slightly posteriorly. It also moves upward to adjust to the wedge-shaped talus, thus keeping articular surfaces opposed during flexion and extension. The direction of the fibers of both the tibiofibular and interosseous membrane (from tibia obliquely down to fibula) allows widening of the mortise and interosseous space on the ascent of the fibula.

There also is a slight external rotation of the fibular shaft as the foot goes into plantar flexion, bringing the posterior margin of the medial fibular talar facet against the narrower margin of the talus. This external rotation and downward motion of the fibular facet is aided by the flexor muscles attached high on the fibular shaft. The action of the peroneal tendons on the posterior margin and tip of the fibular malleolus also aid in narrowing the mortise.

Since ligaments are not elastic, the resilience of the ankle must be accounted for in the muscles themselves. The major portion of the soleus and posterior tibial muscle and all of the flexor hallucis longus muscle arise from the shaft of the fibula. Muscle tension on this group, as in plantar flexion, would push the fibula lower and against the sides of the talus at its narrow margin and, with the upward movement and posterior rotation, the fibula accommodates the wider margin of the talus. It is obvious that a rigid fixation of the fibula to the tibia is not possible with normal ankle function and therefore should not be attempted. The bolts, wires and screws that have broken after attempts at tibiofibular rigid fixation attest to the fallacy of this treatment. These agents may be used for temporary internal fixation during the healing time of ligaments and then should be removed. If not removed, they will break or loosen as function of the ankle is restored.

In any one position during walking, the tibia covers only about 50–60 degrees of the available 90–100-degree arc of the articular surface of the talus. The difference equals the true ankle motion from dorsi to plantar flexion of about 40–50 degrees.

LIGAMENTOUS INJURIES

Of all the ligamentous injuries of the body, those of the ankle are the most common.

Figure 32-7 details the anatomy of the important ligaments around the ankle and midfoot.

The ligaments of the ankle joint are of great importance and a knowledge of their anatomy is essential in dealing with

Fig. 32-8.—Patient twisted ankle when she stepped into a hole. **A,** comparative anteroposterior views of both ankles show widening of mortise on left. Fracture of fibula was found in midshaft area. Widening indicates tear of medial ligament. **B** and **C** show fracture subluxation reduced within an hour of accident and cast applied. **D** shows x-rays taken 1 week later in clinic. Reduction has been lost and talus displaced laterally. **E** and **F,** medial side of ankle joint was explored. Medial malleolus was found buttonholed through capsule. This was reduced and medial ligament repair and cast applied. Cast was removed after 6 weeks. **(Continued.)**

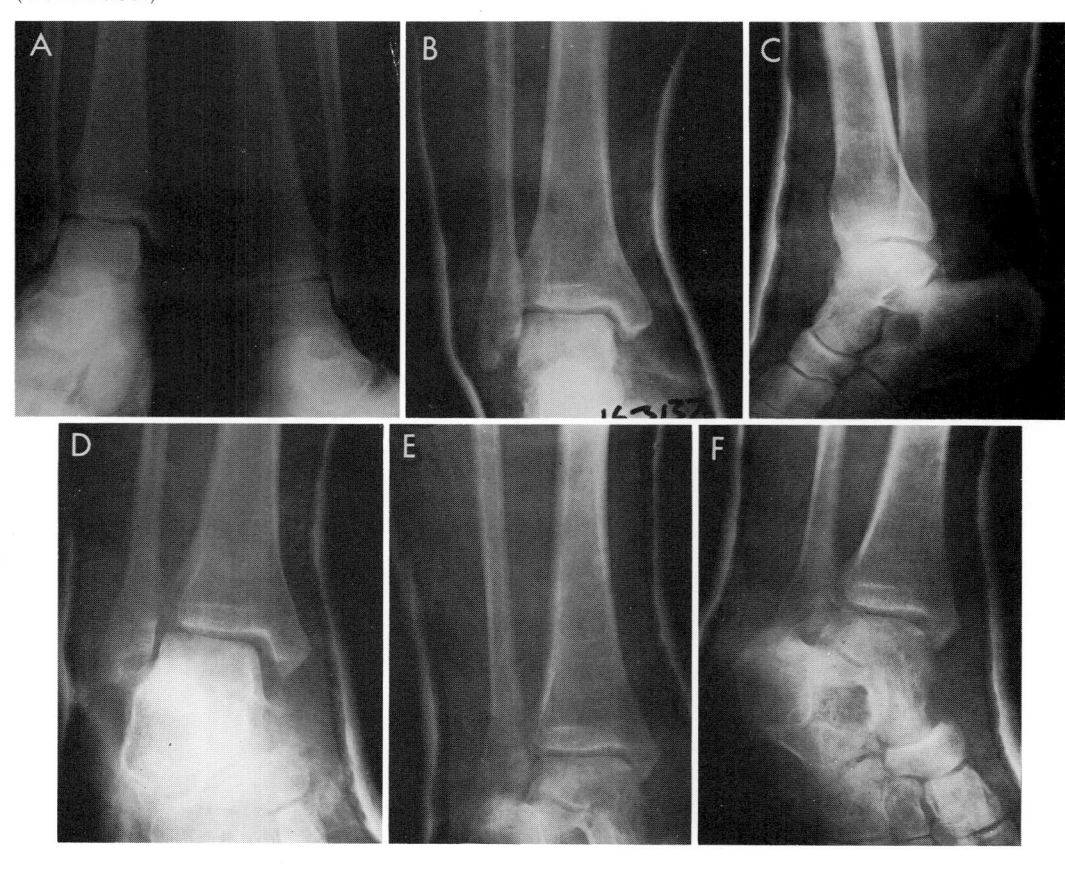

Chapter 32: ANKLE INJURIES / 851

by replacing and internally fixing the bone fragment. This may allow much earlier motion. Total disruption of major ligaments, including the calcaneofibular, deltoid, talofibular and tibiofibular ligaments, can be as disabling as fractures. If both medial and lateral ligaments rupture, dislocation usually occurs, with severe displacement possible. If ligaments on one side of the joint are disrupted, displacement usually is not severe, but operative repair and/or cast immobilization are essential.

The diagnosis of a sprain of the ligament is made by the history of the injury and by the fairly rapid swelling and stiffness of the joint that follows the injury plus the increased pain on walking. A local examination will reveal the point of maximal tenderness and swelling, with aggravation of pain at this point when the ligament is stretched or placed under strain. A combination of ligaments may be injured. Active and passive motion should be carried out, with gentle attempts at strain positions of inversion, eversion and rotation to check for a complete ligamentous tear.

A sprain may be treated symptomatically, the treatment being directed toward a reduction of the swelling by the use of elevation and gentle compression, with or without local application of ice.

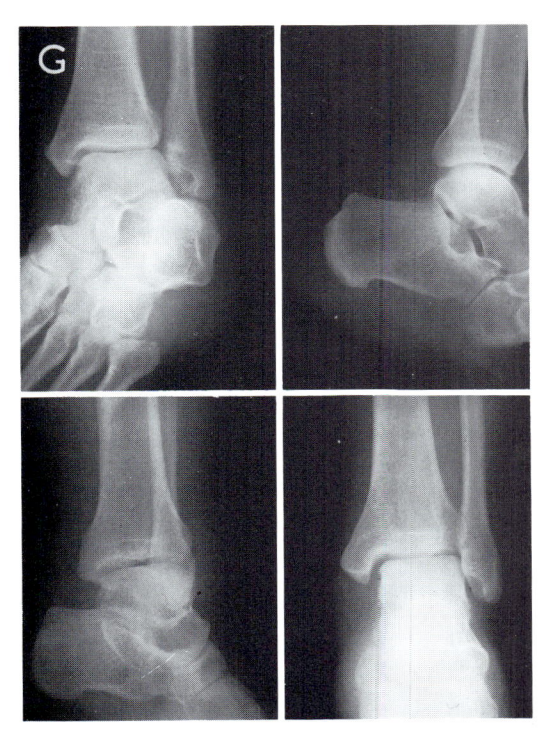

Fig. 32-8 (cont.).—**G**, shows ankle 1 year later. Normal range of painless motion.

ankle fractures. With other injury, often the ligaments remain intact and avulse the malleoli. In such cases, immediate stability of the fracture can be obtained

Fig. 32-9.—**A**, shows the transverse fibers of the medial capsule of the ankle joint. Inability to reduce a dislocated ankle joint following a tear of the medial ligament may be due to interposition of soft tissues between the talus and the medial wall of the ankle mortise or due to "buttonholing" of the medial malleolus through the transverse fibers of the capsule (**B**).

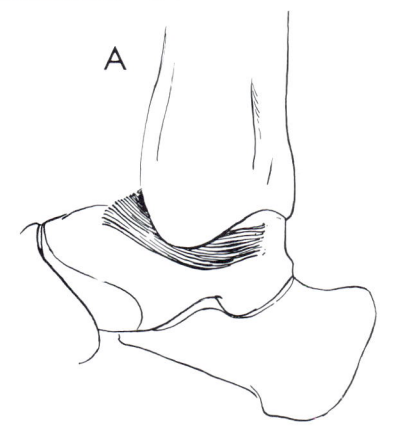

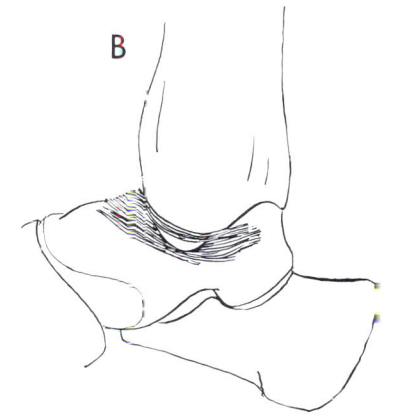

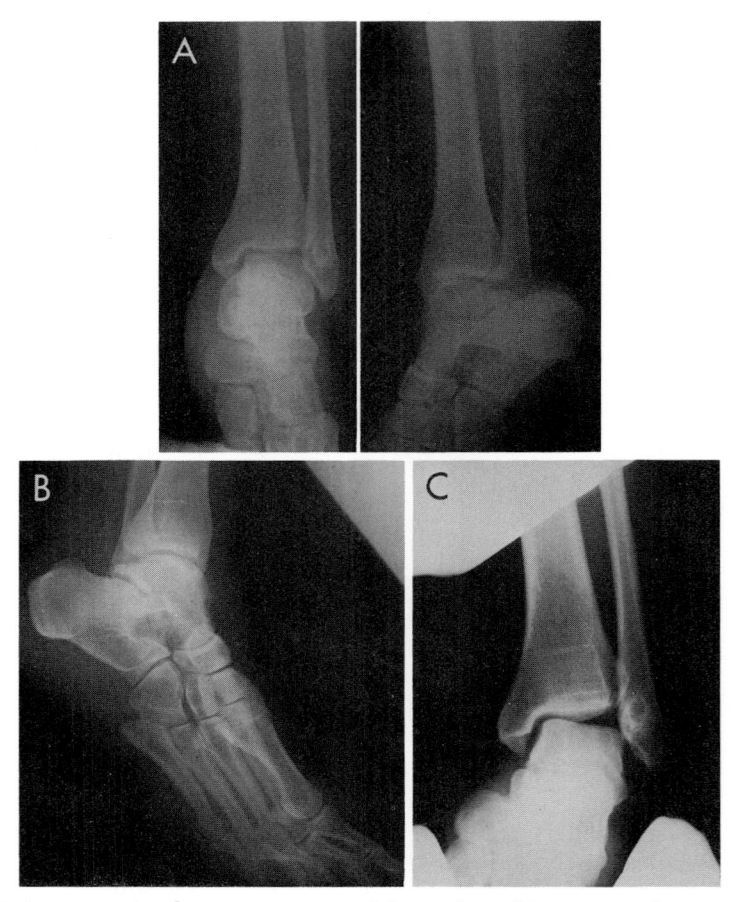

Fig. 32-10. — Patient sustained a severe twist of the right ankle coming downstairs. The ankle was swollen and very tender over lateral ligament. Initial x-ray films appear normal (**A** and **B**). After the ankle had been infiltrated with local anesthetic, stress x-ray films of the ankle were taken. These show instability of talus in mortise due to rupture of lateral ligament (**C**).

The return of ankle function can be accomplished by full or partial weight bearing with crutches and adhesive strapping. Ten days' to 2 weeks' time usually is sufficient for recovery without instability of the ankle joint. Active exercises should be started as early as possible.

A complete tear of either collateral ligament usually needs surgical repair. These can be difficult to diagnose. In those instances in which the diagnosis is not certain due to severe pain, it may be necessary to infiltrate the injured tissue with local anesthetic before a complete examination can be made. In a few cases, it may need a general anesthetic before the examination can be completed.

X-ray comparison of both ankles forced into inversion or eversion may be necessary to show instability of the talus within the mortise on the injured side.

Snug supportive plaster treatment for from 3 to 5 weeks is necessary for ligamentous healing. Experimental studies on healing show firm union of a ligament in 4 or 5 weeks but a persistence of cellular infiltration for 2–3 weeks more.

Restoration of function includes the

Chapter 32: ANKLE INJURIES / 823

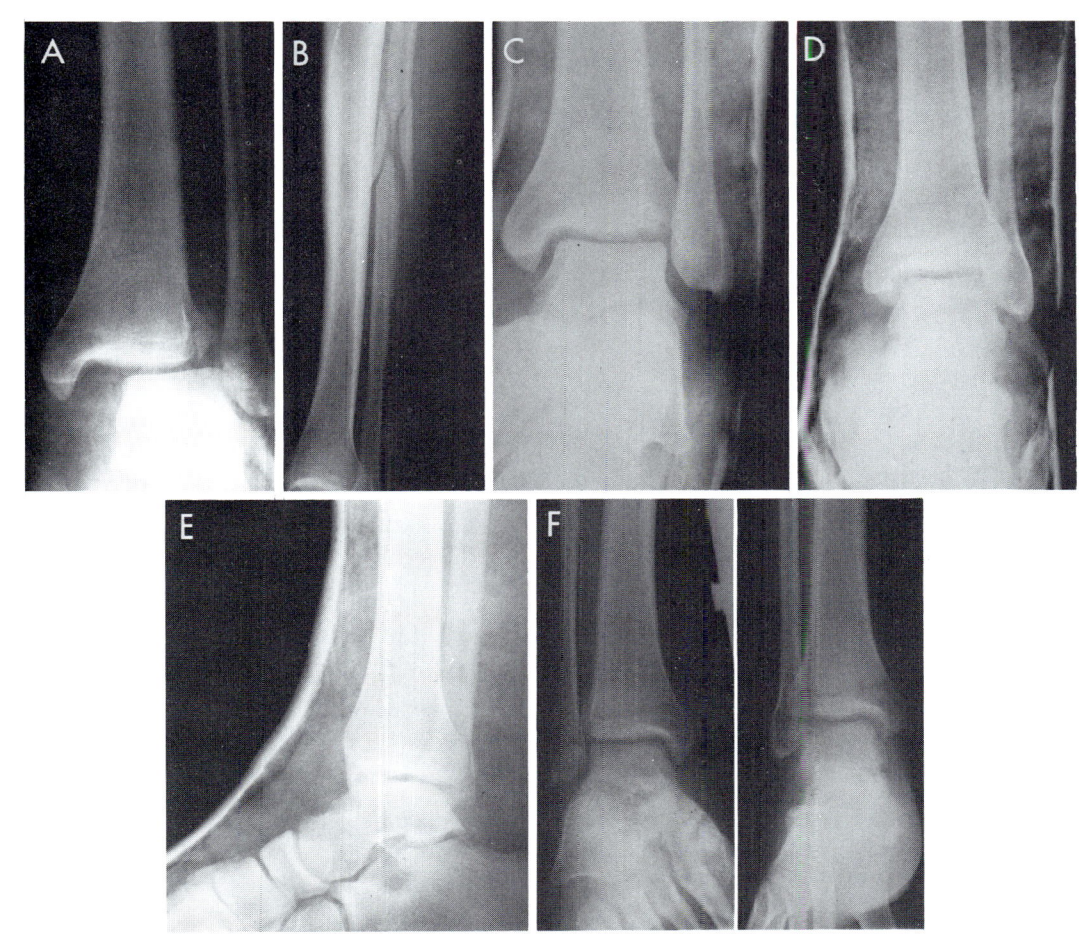

Fig. 32-11.—A, fracture dislocation of ankle with wide separation of the talofibular joint and rupture of medial ligament of ankle. B, x-ray film of the fibula showing fracture of midshaft. C–E show reduction of dislocation following repair of medial ligament of ankle and immobilization in cast. F, the cast was removed 6 weeks after repair of medial collateral ligament. X-ray film shows the result 6 months after accident. Note that the talofibular joint has been reconstituted without internal fixation.

regaining of muscle strength and the return of joint motion.

On occasions with marked instability of the ankle, open repair of the ligament may be necessary.

BONE INJURIES

Types of Bone Injuries

The diagnosis of bone injuries of the ankle is made by the history and physical examination. X-ray studies frequently will show the direction of the deforming force as well as give information concerning the best method of reduction.

I. *Malleolar fractures*
   A. Isolated
      1. Fibula (lateral)
         a) Malleolus alone
         b) With tibial collateral ligament injury
         c) With tibiofibular ligament injury

2. Tibia (medial)
     a) Malleolus alone
     b) With fibular collateral ligament injury
     c) With tibiofibular ligament injury
  B. 1. Medial malleolar with high fibular fracture
     2. Bimalleolar without dislocation
     3. Bimalleolar with dislocation
II. *Tibial weight-bearing surface fractures*
  A. Isolated
     1. Anterior marginal
     2. Posterior marginal
  B. Combined marginal fractures with malleolus fractures
     1. Anterior
     2. Posterior (trimalleolar fracture)
     3. Lateral margin of tibia
III. *Avulsion fractures*
  A. Tips of malleoli
  B. Tibiofibular ligament avulsion (usually with bony fragments attached)

Open Wounds Associated with Ankle Fractures

The injuries listed above may, of course, be complicated by open wounds and then will require the special care that is attendant to all open injuries with bone involvement. The surgical aim is to close viable skin over the reduced fractures without devitalizing tension to the skin.

The paucity of skin and soft tissue around an ankle, compared with the amount of bone, is most apparent in treatment of open ankle fractures and is obvious on a study of a cross section through the malleoli (see Fig. 32-7). Owing to these anatomic features, the skin should be preserved at the expense of other tissues, particularly bone, and even at the sacrifice of fracture position. A good reduction may be lost and joint function put in jeopardy by the loss of skin or by leaving open wounds around the joint into which infection can be introduced. Secondary operations to correct fracture position and restore joint function are more successful through healed skin; thus, accurate reduction of the fracture may assume a secondary role in open fractures.

Closed Manipulations

All ankle fractures deserve a well-thought-out attempt at closed reduction. It is helpful, although not always possible, to reconstruct the mechanism of injury and apply a reversal of forces in the reduction manipulation.

Only accurate reduction is compatible with good ankle function, and therefore it is essential that the ankle mortise is aligned and the upper surface of the talus must fit into the contour of the distal tibial articulation in all planes. Slight variations will not allow the talus to ride smoothly within the mortise and lead to loss of motion and cause pain.

The weight-bearing surfaces must be aligned to allow the heel to meet the floor squarely, and postreduction x-ray films therefore must be viewed to avoid valgus or varus deformities.

The best time to reduce any fracture is immediately after it occurs. If a severe fracture-dislocation of the ankle is seen within a few minutes after the injury, it is possible to reduce and maintain reduction, even without the use of anesthesia.

No ankle fracture is too swollen to be reduced and it is poor management to wait until the swelling goes down before a reduction is attempted. Persistent swelling may well jeopardize the skin in the area of the malleoli, and the development of fracture blisters, a not uncommon occurrence around the ankle, particularly following delayed reduction, may postpone surgery if an attempt at closed reduction fails. Swelling will go down after the fracture is reduced, and usually not very rapidly before. If there is extensive swelling, even with fracture blisters before there is an opportunity to treat the fracture, it is possible to use a compression dressing to reduce the swelling while the patient is being anesthetized. Often, in a very markedly swollen ankle, the use of an Esmarch bandage is instituted for 10–15 minutes to diminish swelling and the malleoli then can be felt easily and the plaster molded to the ankle contour as it is applied.

General Principles of Manipulation

To reduce the fracture deformity it is necessary to relax the muscles producing the deformity and/or resisting its correction. This can be done by applying traction in the line of the deformity. In the ankle, these muscles usually are the plantar flexors; therefore, the reduction should be attempted with the knee flexed to relax the gastrocnemius muscle and the foot should be in equinus to relax the plantar flexors. While the traction is maintained, a slight increase in the deformity should be produced before the distal fragments are manipulated to meet the proximal fracture surface (Fig. 32-12).

After restoration of length by traction, correction of the deformity is accomplished easily. Leverage forces against intact bone, pulley forces of tendons and traction forces through intact ligaments should be utilized to correct the deformity and to maintain the reduction. The pulley forces of the peroneal and posterior tibial tendons can be used to bring the malleoli forward. Too much force through these tendons by dorsiflexion of the foot may overcorrect and tilt the fibular fragments (Fig. 32-13).

After reduction, these forces should be released sufficiently to maintain position of the reduced fracture. Because of its posterior position in crossing the distal tibia at the ankle joint, the tendon of the flexor hallucis longus can be put under tension so that in some cases it will push forward on a posterior or marginal fracture, correcting its displacement and holding it in place.

For molding of fragments to form the mortise, direct pressure over bony prominences may be used during the manipulation.

During application of plaster, the foot should be held as nearly as possible in an angle of function, making allowances for the forces needed to hold the reduction. Plaster application should conform to the shape of the foot and ankle and should be molded smoothly around the Achilles tendon, the heel and the malleoli.

Immobilization of the Fractured Ankle

One of the chief problems in the management of ankle fractures is the maintenance of reduction. The position of the fragments may be lost as the swelling subsides. Therefore, the application of a well-molded plaster is as important as an accurate reduction

The position of reduction of the fracture should be held until the plaster has been rolled well above the ankle. The plaster should be molded to conform to the outline of the Achilles tendon and the two malleoli. Only enough padding should be used to protect the bony prominences.

If the lateral malleolus is fractured there should be gentle pressure through the plaster on the lateral side of the malleolus, and the foot should be in slight varus position to maintain the length of the fibula.

If the medial malleolus is fractured, the medial surface of the medial malleolus should have gentle pressure exerted to mold it to the talus and produce an accurate reduction of the mortise.

Postreduction Care of Fractures of the Ankle

Following manipulation or open reduction, the extremity should be protected from dependency for several days to prevent additional swelling within the plaster cast. It is advisable to keep the leg elevated until some wrinkling of the skin on the leg or foot is apparent. Increasing dependency then is allowed, depending

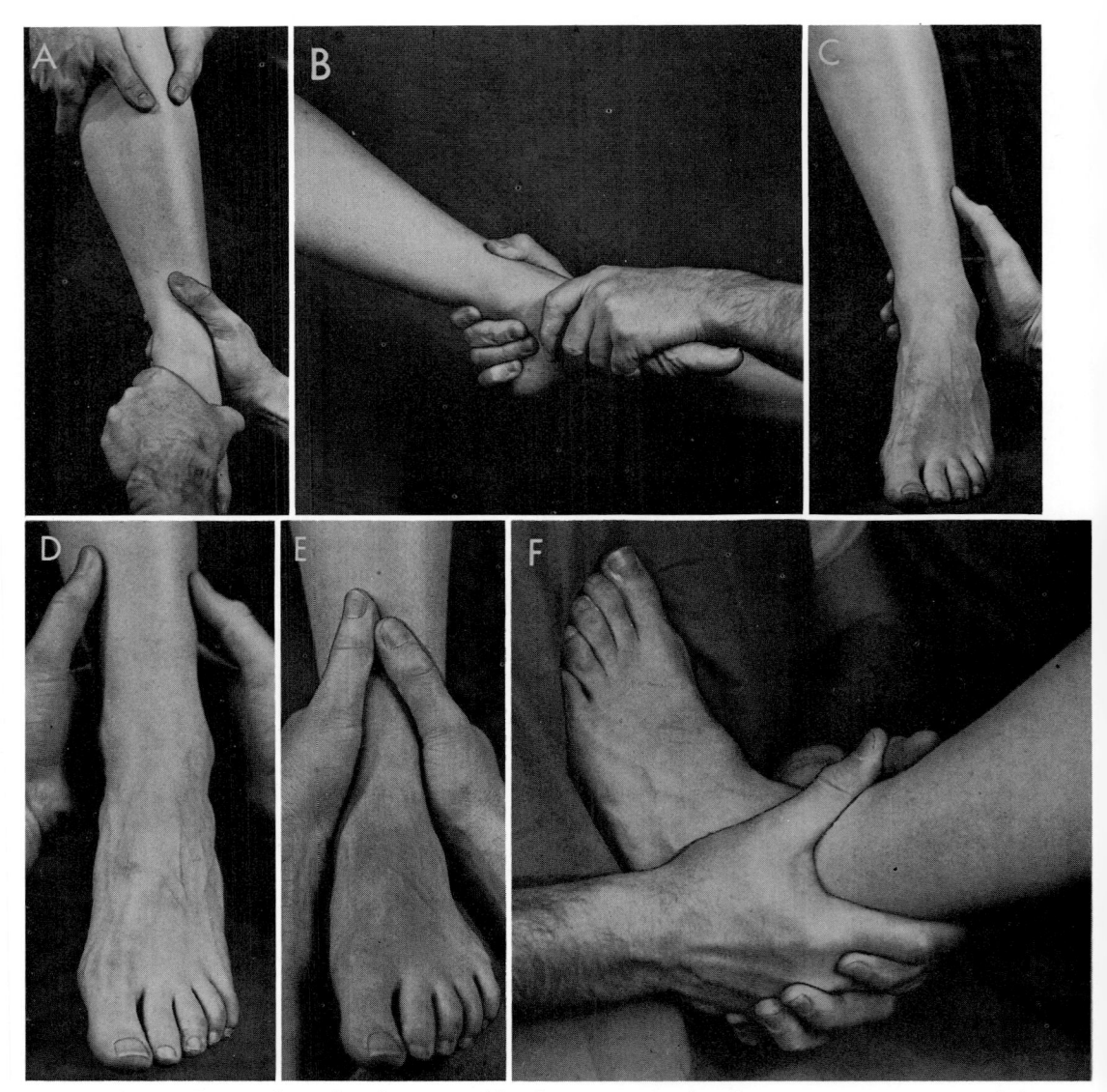

Fig. 32-12.—Principles of reducing ankle fractures. **A,** the first position, as viewed from above. The knee is supported in flexion for countertraction, either by an assistant or by flexion of the knee over a knee sling or support, or edge of table. The surgeon's hands are applied to the foot and ankle. The hand on the outer side of the foot grasps the foot and ankle over the fibula, the fingers hooking behind the heel and extending around to the medial malleolus. The hand on the inner side of the foot grasps the foot, palm of hand on dorsum of foot. (This traction position of the hands places the left hand on the top of the left foot.) In a more medial view (**B**), the fingers of the hand on the outer side hook behind the heel and end below the medial malleolus. The index finger remains behind the malleolus. **C,** showing the ease with which the relative positions of the malleoli can be outlined, and how naturally the contour of the palm of the hand can be adapted for molding the malleolus. **D,** position of hands for molding the malleoli. The concavity of each palm fits over each malleolus, and so a wide distribution of pressure can be placed evenly over these bony prominences. (This same positioning of the hands is used in molding the plaster casing.) **E,** closing the palms over the malleoli, the palm on the medial side of the foot is higher and more anterior than the one on the lateral side. The difference in height of the malleoli is approximately the length of a thumbnail, as shown in the illustration. **F,** the final positioning of the reduction: the finger locked above the →

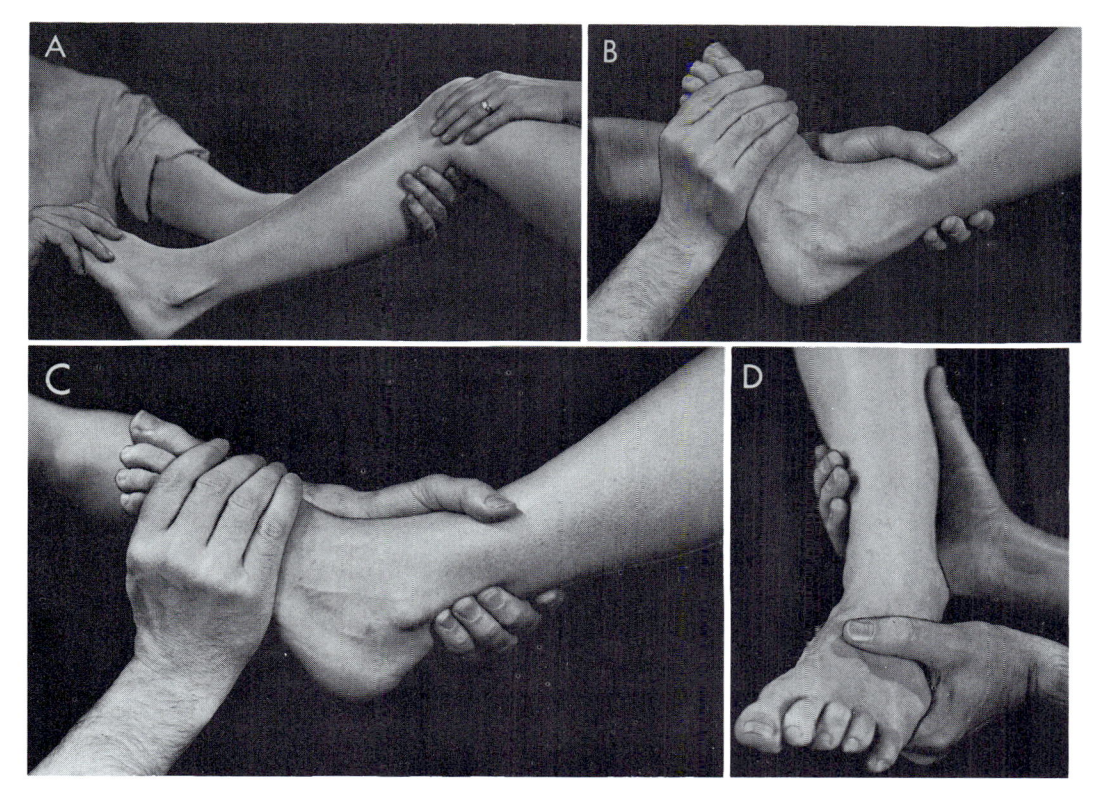

Fig. 32-13.—Tendon pulley forces on malleoli. A reduced fracture is most easily held by pressure toward the opposing ankle surfaces. **A,** the taut peroneal tendon with the foot at a right angle. A slight equinus position relieves this tension. The tendon pulley force of the peroneals can be seen when the foot is forced into dorsiflexion (**B**); this force will tilt a fibular fracture posteriorly. By lowering the foot into a few degrees of equinus and using pressure posteriorly over the fibula (**C**), a posterior angulation can be reduced. Rotatory positions can be controlled easily with the hands in this position. The most important position to obtain in fibulomalleolar fractures is a restoration of length and then a correction of the external rotation. These features can be controlled (**D**) by pulling on the tibia with the right hand and pushing with the left, and by pushing the calcaneus into varus position, internally rotating the foot and depressing the first metatarsal.

on the amount of swelling of the toes. The patient should be warned of the danger signs of vascular obstruction and should be instructed to check the color, sensation and function of the toes frequently during the first 24 hours. After reduction and immobilization, the extremity should not be very painful. If there is persistence of pain, blanching, cyanosis or loss of sensation in the toes and the symptoms are not relieved by properly positioning the leg in bed, a

---

←

heel and behind the Achilles tendon. The sole of the foot is supported on the surgeon's sternum. In this position, the ankle can be gently rocked in dorsal and plantar flexion while lateral pressure is maintained over the malleoli. Rotatory positions normally will be assumed by the seating of the talus into its normal grooves with the lower articular end of the tibia. An understanding of good x-ray films will help guide the surgeon during the application of gentle pressure toward the more intact articular surface.

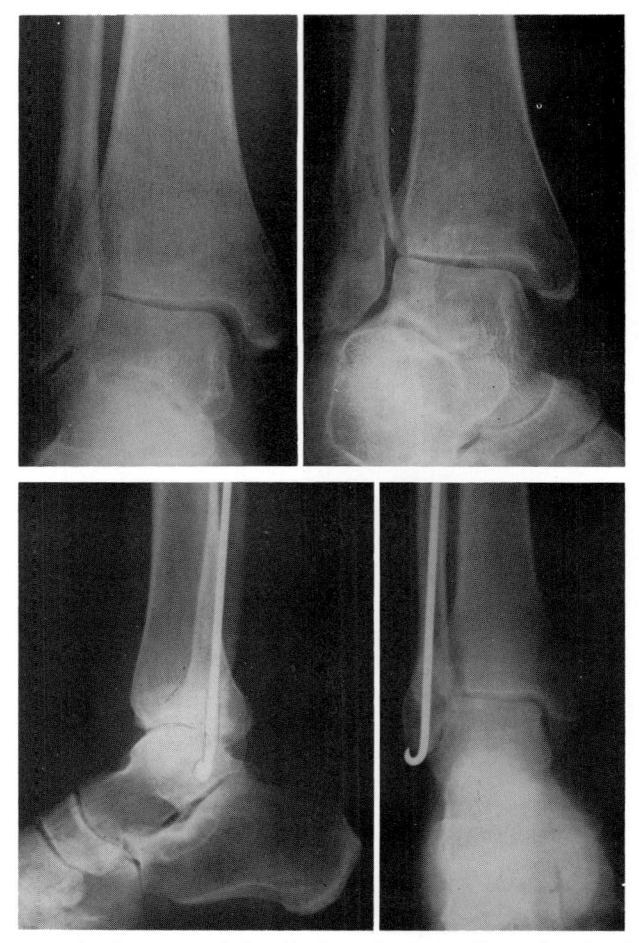

Fig. 32-14 (top).—A simple fracture of the fibula, which is allowed to heal in a slightly shortened position as this one has, will continue to give symptoms. Note the tilted talus and asymmetry of the tibiotalus articulation. At follow-up, the ankle was continuing to swell and gave painful symptoms after a minimal amount of function.

Fig. 32-15 (bottom).—A long intramedullary nail was used for fixation of this closed fracture of the fibula. The ankle was dislocated at the time of injury and was very unstable to closed reduction. It lost position in the cast. At the end of 1 year, the patient had symptoms of pain most of the time, with swelling on increased function. Complete fibular length was not restored, evidenced, in these views, by an upward tilt toward the fibula of the talar articular surface. The first aim of fibular fracture is restoration of length; the second, a reduction of the rotatory element.

thorough re-evaluation is indicated. The symptoms should not be treated with medication for pain. The causes of these disturbances are:

1. Inadequate reduction.
2. Too tight a plaster.
3. Improper elevation and a poorly fitting plaster.

Swelling within the cast is not uncommon and the surgeon should not hesitate to split and spread the plaster and the underlying padding to relieve constriction. With persistence of signs or symptoms after bivalving the cast, x-ray films should be taken to determine whether reduction has been maintained. It is not

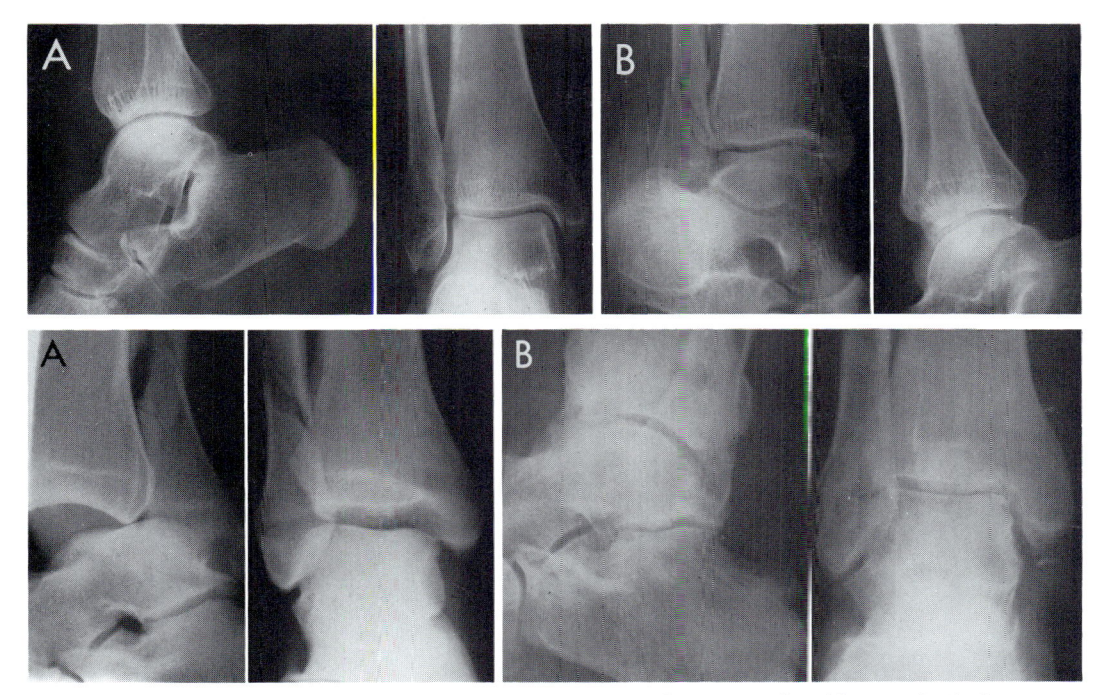

Fig. 32-16 (top).—A, lateral and anteroposterior views of an injured ankle in which the examiner had made a clinical diagnosis of a fractured fibula. B, oblique view, clearly showing the suspected fracture of the fibula. (This view is obtained by having the lateral side of the foot rest on the plate.) A walking plaster boot was applied.

Fig. 32-17 (bottom).—A, a fracture-dislocation, the result of a twisting injury produced by a fall on ice. Early weight bearing without support was allowed. Such a disruption of a joint requires 4–6 weeks of plaster and supported weight bearing until the patient can walk normally without pain or swelling. Disruption of mortise in A shows evidence of at least a partial tear of the medial ligament. B, 1 year later, the calcification below the medial malleolus is evidence of at least a partial tear of the deltoid ligament. The patient still had symptoms and swelling after a few hours of work.

uncommon for ankle fractures to require a second manipulation, and nothing is to be gained by delay.

Open reduction should be considered at an early stage in the treatment if closed reduction fails.

Fracture of the anterior lip of the tibia with an intact posterior articular surface should be held in slight equinus while the molding is accomplished. The ankle then is rocked through a safe arc of motion, with pressure directed posteriorly so that a redislocation anteriorly will not displace the fragments. The final position of forces is directed, without strain, toward the intact tibia in all tibial weight-bearing fractures. Early motion in comminuted articular surface fractures is essential.

Indications for Operative Treatment of Ankle Injuries

Open reductions are indicated whenever attempts at closed reduction have failed to produce realignment of the bone fragments into acceptable positions of function (Figs 32-14 to 32-17). The most common reasons for open reduction are:

1. Failure to obtain good position of the medial malleolus against the tibia.
2. Widening of the mortise in bimalleolar fractures.
3. Shortening of the fibula in a simple fibular fracture.

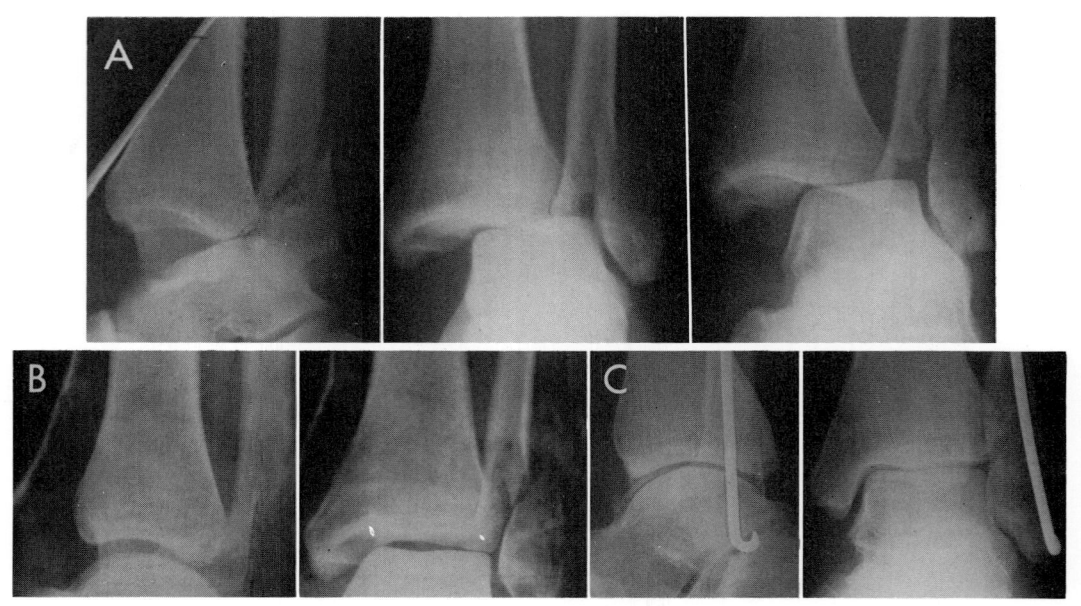

Fig. 32-18.—A, a severe rotatory fracture with dislocation. With this amount of lateral displacement, the deltoid ligament probably would be ruptured. An attempt at closed reduction (B) failed to reduce the ankle mortise to normal, and the proximal fibula remained behind. Operative treatment revealed the torn deltoid ligament, which was repaired. A medullary nail in the fibula (C) was sufficient for stabilization. Excellent function of the ankle joint resulted.

4. A displaced posterior lip, equal to one-fourth or more of the tibial articular surface, which cannot be reduced by manipulation.

5. The presence of intra-articular fragments or ligaments that do not allow the talus to assume a good weight-bearing position under the tibia (Figs. 32-18 and 32-19).

6. The fractured ankles should not be immobilized in a grossly abnormal position to maintain the reduction. If this cannot be achieved with the ankle in a good functional position, open reduction should be considered.

Medial Malleolus Fractures

Fractures of the medial malleolus can be divided into two groups (Figs. 32-20).

1. The fracture is distal to the angle of the mortise and there remains a lip of bone attached to the tibia. This leaves a shoulder for manipulation and these fractures usually can be treated by simple manipulation. The foot is brought into slight equinus and the heel held in varus position with pressure toward the fibula. The palm of the hand is used to mold the malleolus toward its fractured end. A final position of slight equinus will prevent the posterior tibial tendon from pushing the medial malleolus forward. An occasional nonunion usually produces minor symptoms, as the infracted base of the medial malleolus acts as a lip to the mortise and therefore maintains stability of the joint.

2. The fracture through the medial malleolus is at the level of the mortise or angled proximally from the mortise, leaving no lip for stability of the ankle joint (Fig. 32-21).

Closed reduction as described above should be attempted. If it is not possible to reduce or hold the reduced medial malleolus in accurate alignment for weight bearing or the ankle mortise re-

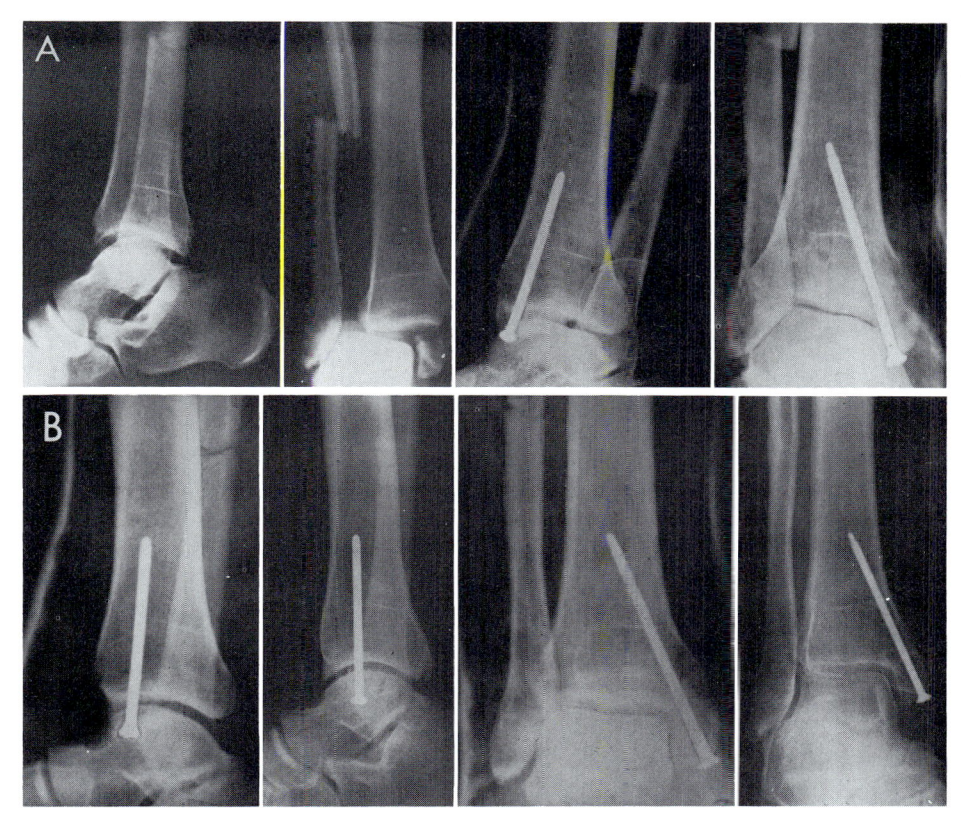

Fig. 32-19. — **A,** a fracture-dislocation sustained when the patient was struck by an automobile. Open reduction of the ankle joint alone was not sufficient to restore normal alignment in the ankle, and pain persisted. The fibular fracture remained displaced and was overriding. Open reduction of the overriding transverse fractured fibula (**B**) restored the normal length of the fibula and resulted in a normal restoration of ankle joint alignment. Pain was relieved.

mains widened, open reduction is advisable. The interposition of periosteum, joint capsule or tendons is a common finding at surgery and removal usually will allow an accurate reduction of the fracture. Once the fracture is reduced, the fragments can easily be held in place by a single screw or two crossed Kirschner wires, depending on the amount of comminution.

Bimalleolar or Potts Fractures

Closed reduction should be tried, but if the reduction fails to satisfy the criteria discussed above, open reduction should be performed (Fig. 32-22).

The medial fragment usually is stabilized and the lateral malleolus then can be reduced easily by closed manipulation against a firm medial border of the mortise. Occasionally it is necessary to fix the fibular fragment in addition. Those fractures that are associated with widening of the tibiofibular joint due to diastasis of the tibiofibular ligament usually can be handled closed when the medial and/or lateral malleoli are fixed. Occasionally, diastasis may remain after careful molding. This will require screw fixation across from the fibula to the tibia. The screw should be removed after 6 weeks or before weight bearing is allowed.

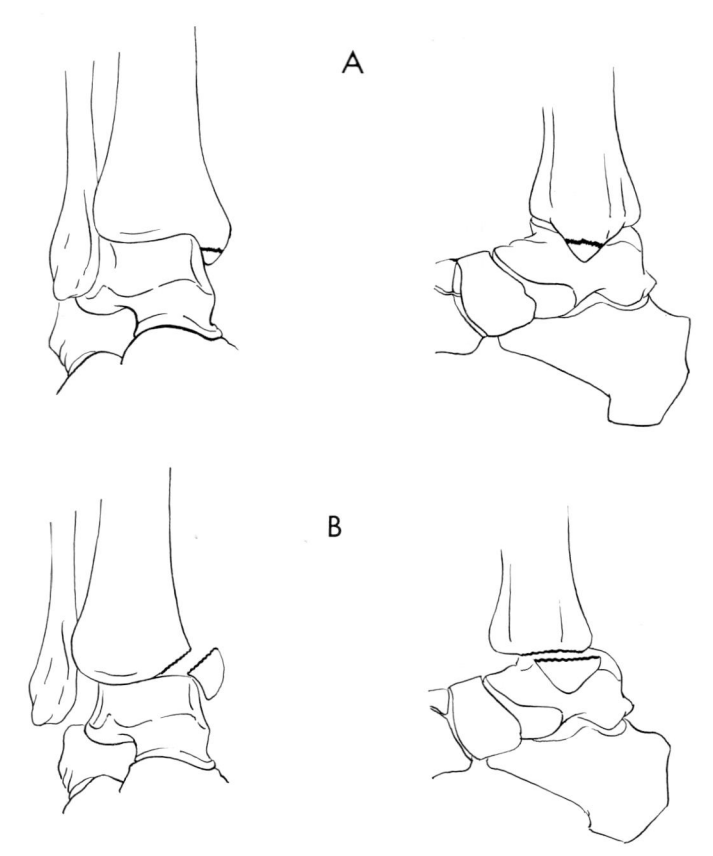

Fig. 32-20.—Fractures of the medial malleolus. **A,** those fractures of the medial malleolus that are distal to the mortise and leave a shoulder, maintaining the stability of the ankle joint, may be treated by closed methods. Nonunion, if it occurs, usually is pain-free. **B,** where the fracture is at the level of the mortise and there is no shoulder for stability of the ankle joint, open reduction is the treatment of choice. The fracture often can be reduced initially by manipulation, but this reduction frequently is lost within the first 2 or 3 days as the swelling subsides.

Trimalleolar or Cotton Fractures

Trimalleolar fractures require open reduction more than any other fracture around the ankle joint. The addition of a fracture of the posterior lip of the tibia leads to a very unstable joint. Open reduction and internal fixation of the medial malleolus usually is indicated. If the posterior fragment involves more than one-fourth of the articular surface, it should be reduced accurately. If this cannot be done by closed manipulation, open reduction and internal fixation is necessary. This frequently is the case, as posterior displacement is likely to recur.

Fractures of the Anterior Margin of the Tibia

The same principles of treatment applied to fractures of the posterior malleolus can be used with this fracture. It usually is not as severe as the posterior malleolus fracture and often can be treated by closed manipulation.

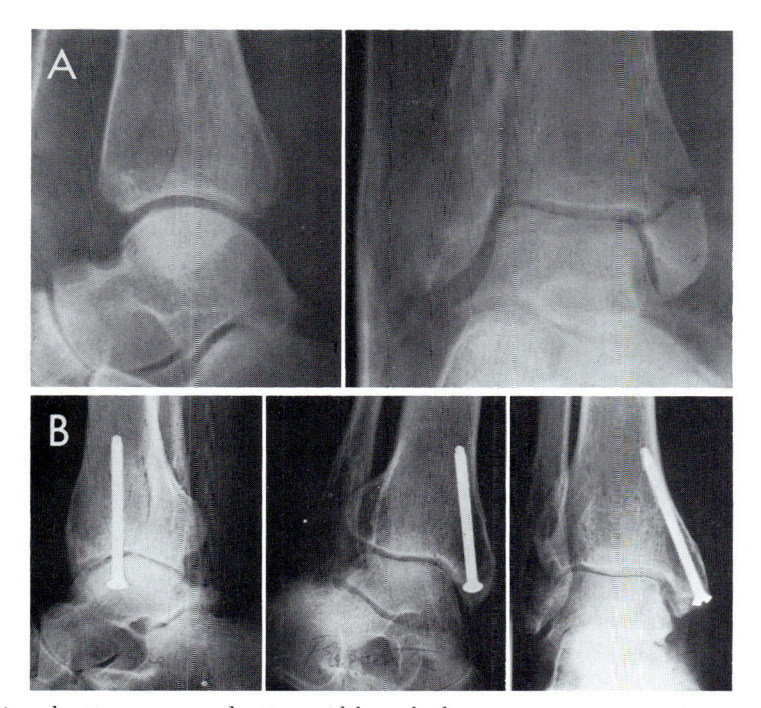

Fig. 32-21.—An elective open reduction. Although there was some question as to the advisability of carrying out an open reduction on this fractured ankle (A, lateral and anteroposterior views), the medial malleolus was stabilized (B, lateral, oblique and anteroposterior views). This provided a firm side to the ankle mortise. The fibular length thus was restored and maintained without fear of displacement of the talus medially. Although excellent function may have been obtained without medial malleolar fixation, function was ensured by the fixation.

Explosion Fracture of the Ankle Joint

These fractures usually are produced by a heavy landing on the heel causing a fracture of the distal and articular surface of the tibia and occasionally producing a fracture through the talus. Severe comminution usually is present and open reduction should be avoided. Manipulation is the treatment of choice, and an attempt is made to mold the many small fragments into as close a facsimile of the normal mortise as possible. Reconstruction and, in some cases, fusion of the ankle joint may be required, but it is best to wait until fracture healing has occurred. Occasionally, the fragments may be large enough to bring together by open reduction and fixed internally with screws or Kirschner wires.

Dislocations and Fracture Dislocations of the Ankle

Due to the stretching forces applied to the skin, dislocations of the ankle should be reduced as early as possible. If the dislocation is associated with fracture of the malleoli, it should be treated according to the methods described above.

Occasionally it may be impossible to reduce the dislocation by closed methods. This usually indicates that soft tissue is interposed within the mortise. Fractures of the medial malleolus and tears of the deltoid ligament and the posterior tibial tendons, sometimes accompanied by the posterior tibial nerves and vessels, may become trapped. This prevents reduction by closed manipulation.

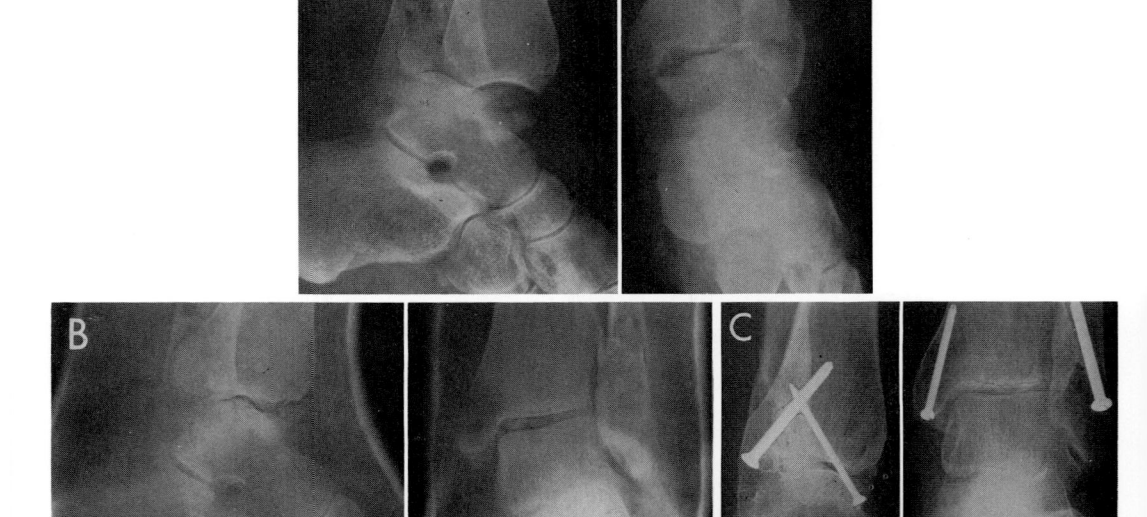

Fig. 32-22.—An unstable fracture requiring more than minimal fixation. **A,** bimalleolar fracture-dislocation sustained in a fall off a bicycle. The fragments are markedly comminuted, and the chances of bone fragments remaining in the joint after reduction are good. **B,** postreduction views revealing the fragments in the joint. (These roentgenograms should have been taken before the cast was applied.) Loose bone fragments in the joint over weight-bearing surfaces must be removed surgically. **C,** internal fixation with two screws in the malleoli. At follow-up, 1 year later, there were a few symptoms, but the patient was doing as much housework as formerly.

Open Fractures

As mentioned previously, there is practically no loose skin around the ankle, but skin closure without tension of the open ankle fracture is vitally important, even at the sacrifice of bone. Additional releasing incisions and skin grafts may be required to obtain initial skin closure. Screws, wire, nails or small plates of Vitallium or stainless steel may be used for internal fixation. The stabilizing of one malleolus often is sufficient to hold the entire ankle. Metal should be used sparingly. To hold a separated tibiofibular ligament, a bolt or screw may be used as a temporary fixture and removed in about 6 weeks. If left in, such a fixture may either break or become loose and impair ankle function.

Surgical approaches to the ankle should be as direct as possible, and the incisions generally should not cross the bony prominences of the malleoli but rather come below them. Incisions should be slightly curved at each end. With such an incision there will be less tension on retraction, and extension will be easier if the exposure needs enlarging. The skin should not be devitalized by strenuous retraction.

Length of Immobilization

Ankle injuries should be immobilized long enough to allow healing of sufficient strength to support the entire body. The form of immobilization will, of course, vary with the type of injury or fracture, from a simple bandage or adhesive strap-

Chapter 32: ANKLE INJURIES / 835

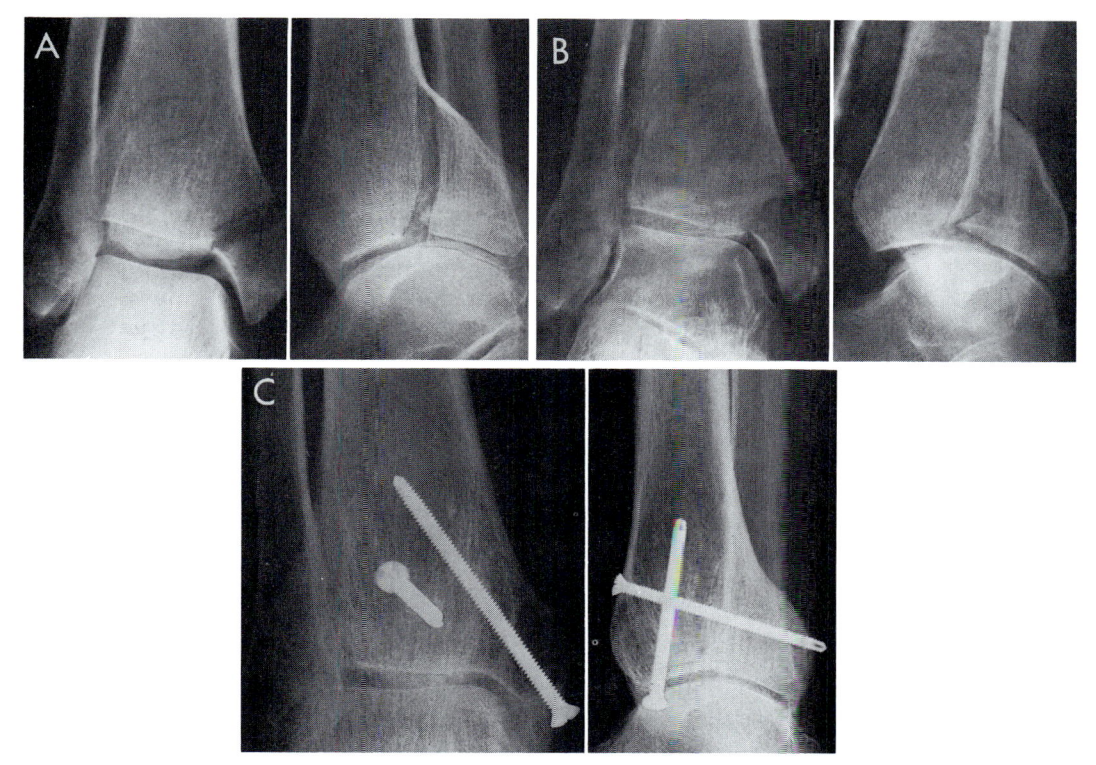

Fig. 32-23.—A definite indication for open reduction and internal fixation. The surgeon may be tempted to leave this trimalleolar fracture (**A,** anteroposterior and lateral views) as it is. However, since the posterior tibial lip fracture involves about one-half of the weight-bearing surface, an effort should be made to get as anatomic a result as is possible. **B,** the position attained by an attempt at closed reduction. It was decided to use the fractured medial malleolus in the surgical approach to the posterior lip fragment. Through an anterior medial malleolar incision, the malleolus was turned down at its fracture site and the tibial lip fragment line easily visualized. This fragment then was anatomically replaced. By the use of lag screws (**C**), the posterior lip fragment was held in place by turning the screw through a large hole in front to one of proper holding size behind. This maneuver snugged the fragments into anatomic position. The medial malleolus then was fixed with one screw. A normally functioning ankle was obtained.

ping to non-weight bearing for 12 weeks or more. Each ankle injury is an individual problem. Some ankle fractures, especially the explosion type, may need brace support for many months.

Management after Removal of Plaster Casing

The removal of a plaster cast from an injured ankle is followed by swelling, and the insecurity from the sudden loss of support is aggravated by muscle weakness. A patient who has been walking about in a weight-bearing plaster will, after removal of the casing, often have pain on walking and may need support in the form of adhesive strapping, elastic bandages or an arch support. Extensively injured ankles may require the support of a brace after the plaster is removed. The brace should be made with double uprights with an ankle hinge and it should be fastened to the heel of the shoe or into a sole plate.

In fractures of the ankle involving only

one malleolus and without displacement, and not involving a weight-bearing surface, early weight bearing in a plaster walking boot is advisable.

Simple malleolar fractures may be allowed to bear weight early (in about 3–4 weeks). If the weight-bearing surfaces are intact, early weight bearing is an aid to function.

A heel can be placed on the initial cast and weight bearing can be started as soon as it can be tolerated. Other types of fractures, particularly those involving the weight-bearing area, are protected until there is evidence of bone union. No matter how favorable the fracture appears, bone union must occur before complete weight bearing without support is allowed. In fractures of the medial malleolus, union takes place very slowly. Some type of support is necessary for 6–8 weeks.

Bimalleolar and trimalleolar fractures with satisfactorily closed reductions should be protected for as long as 6 weeks in plaster and after that by adhesive strapping. The duration of protection is dependent on the amount of soft tissue injury incurred at the time of the fracture. A trimalleolar fracture that has been widely displaced certainly must have support for as long as 4–6 months after the injury appears to have healed. A similar fracture that has not been displaced, and thus may be assumed to have had little soft tissue damage, should be immobilized only until bone union has occurred.

Fractures involving weight-bearing surfaces should be protected with some type of support for a period of 6–8 months, as indicated by the reaction of the joint to function.

After final removal of the plaster, the leg is protected by the use of either crutches or a cane until normal muscle strength has been recovered. The patient is given exercises designed to increase ankle motion and muscle strength and to improve circulation in the extremity. These exercises are active plantar flexion and dorsiflexion, eversion and inversion, heel cord stretching and toe pressing. Gait training is started early to prevent the development of habit limp. A Thomas heel with a slight inside wedge or an arch support may make the difference between a comfortable and an uncomfortable ankle. This simple program of rehabilitation should be continued until muscle strength is adequate for the patient to carry himself up on his toes and back on his heels unsupported by the other foot. Occasionally, the use of a stationary bicycle, foot rocker and an inclined plane may be necessary.

BIBLIOGRAPHY

Ashhurst, A. P. C., and Bromer, R. S.: Classification and mechanism of fracture of the leg bones involving the ankle, Arch. Surg. 5:51, 1922.

Böhler, L.: *The Treatment of Fractures* (4th ed.; Baltimore: Wm. Ward and Company, 1935).

Bonnin, J.: *Injuries to the Ankle* (New York: Grune & Stratton, Inc., 1950).

Bosworth, D. M.: Fracture dislocation of the ankle with fixed displacement of the fibula behind the tibia, J. Bone Joint Surg. 29:130, 1947.

Burgess, E.: Fracture of the ankle, J. Bone Joint Surg. 26:721, 1944.

Campbell, W. C.: In Crenshaw, A. H. (ed.), *Operative Orthopedics* (4th ed.; St. Louis: The C. V. Mosby Company, 1963), Vol. I, p. 404.

Close, J. R., and Inman, V. T.: The action of the ankle joint, TR #22, The Biomechanics Laboratory, U. of Calif., 1952. (Issued by Prosthetic Devices Research Project as Series II, issue 22.)

Coonrad, R. W., and Bugg, E., Jr.: Trapping of the posterior tibial tendon and interposition of soft tissue in severe fractures about the ankle joint, J. Bone Joint Surg. 36-A:744, 1954.

Denham, R. A.: Internal fixation for unstable ankles, J. Bone Joint Surg. 46-B:206, 1964.

Henry, A.: *Extensile Exposure Applied to Limb Surgery* (Edinburgh: E. & S. Livingstone, Ltd., 1948).

Isman, R. E., and Inman, V. T.: Anthropometric studies of the human foot and ankle, TR #58, The Biomechanics Laboratory, U. of Calif., 1968.

Magnuson, R.: On the late results in non-operated cases of malleolar fractures: A clinical-roentgenological-statistical study, Acta. Chir. Scand. (supp. 84) 1:129, 1944.

Parish, T. F.: Fracture-dislocation of the ankle. An unusual cause of failure of reduction: A case report, J. Bone Joint Surg. 41-A:749, 1959.

Patrick, J.: A direct approach to trimalleolar fracture, J. Bone Joint Surg. 47-B:236, 1965.

Ruth, C. J.: Surgical treatment of injuries of the fibular collateral ligaments of the ankle, J. Bone Joint Surg. 43-A:229, 1961.

Staples, O. S.: Injuries to the medial ligaments of the ankle. Result study, J. Bone Joint Surg. 42-A:1287, 1960.

Watson-Jones, R.: *Fractures and Joint Injuries* (4th ed.; Baltimore: The Williams & Wilkins Company), Vol. 1, 1952; Vol. 2, 1955.

33 | Injuries of the Foot
ROBERT J. JOPLIN

THE FOOT is a complicated assembly of 28 bones and multiple ligaments. Although roentgenograms taken after an injury may indicate the deformities of a fractured bone and the amount of displacement of the fragments, reduction is facilitated by a knowledge of the ligamentous attachments and the directional force of the muscles. (Fig. 33-1).

There are three major arches in a normal human foot: (1) the inner longitudinal arch, (2) the outer longitudinal arch and (3) the anterior metatarsal arch.

Three functions are performed by the human foot; (1) weight bearing, (2) locomotion and (3) shock absorption. For efficient performance of these functions following a fracture, restoration of the bones to as nearly normal configuration as possible is essential.

SOFT TISSUE INJURIES

Foot injuries vary in degree from a simple sprain or mild contusion to open, comminuted fractures and dislocation. A crushing or squeezing injury, such as may occur when an automobile wheel runs over a foot on soft ground, may not break the skin; yet it can produce a severe injury to soft parts. This has been called a "wringer foot" injury because the damage produced is similar to that caused when a person's fingers are caught in a wringer and the hand is pulled through the two rollers. A "wringer foot" is also of great concern because of the foot's dependent position, which can result in increased swelling.

The immediate use of a compression bandage may prevent the woody edema and scar formation that frequently limit early mobility and function. Inclusion of a foam rubber sponge over the contused or crushed area will hasten the return to normal size.

After 24 hours of gentle compression over the entire foot (including the tips of the toes, which otherwise may swell and become extremely painful), the bandages and sponges may be removed. With the extremity elevated, gentle massage from the toes toward the ankle may be started; heat must be omitted for the first 48-hour period. After 48 hours, a little heat may be applied before or during massage. The compression bandage then should be reapplied. Bed rest or the use of a wheelchair with the extremity elevated may be permitted as soon as the toes and forepart of the foot can be moved actively.

Elevation must be regulated, especially in the adult, because circulation can be diminished to the point of ischemia, which may lead to gangrene. Children can tolerate more elevation than can adults, who probably should have the extremity kept at or near heart level.

Berger exercises can be started early and continued as long as dependent edema is present. However, partial weight bearing with crutches may be permitted only when the dependent position can be tolerated. In early convalescence, putting the foot down causes rapid swelling and, almost instantaneously, throbbing pain. Later in the period of convalescence, these changes become

837

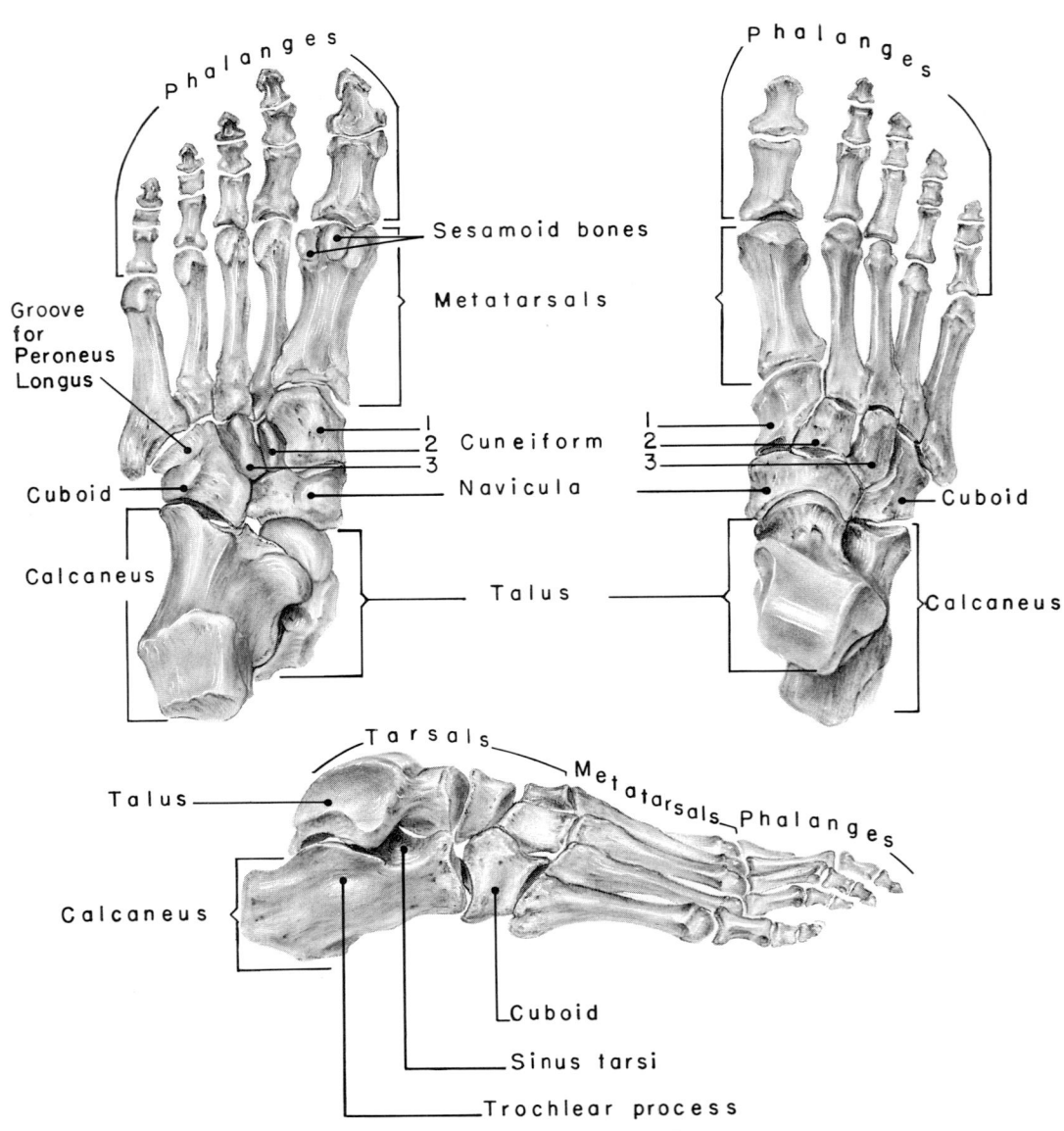

Fig. 33-1.—Anatomy of the foot.

less marked, and comfortable walking with crutches is possible.

Once ambulation has begun, the patient should be cautioned to avoid standing, or sitting with the foot resting on the floor, for prolonged periods. When he sits on a chair, his foot should be returned to the elevated position. Exercises can be carried out satisfactorily with the shoe on.

After a few weeks, a standstill in convalescence may be observed, and the patient may feel that normal recovery will never come. This is the time to encourage walking to the point of pain or even beyond to a mild degree, the "pain barometer" being used as the ultimate

Chapter 33: INJURIES OF THE FOOT / 839

guide. It is advisable to force activity to the point of slight pain each day. If pain from activity has persisted throughout the night and into the following day, exercise has been overstressed; if not, activity should be continued. Restoration of mobility of the joints of the foot and strengthening of muscular support usually are associated with diminishing pain.

FRACTURES OF THE OS CALCIS

A review of 111 cases of fractures of the tarsal bones showed 67 fractures of the os calcis (calcaneus). Most of the os calcis fractures occurred in persons between their third and sixth decades, with the peak incidence at 45 years. It seems that these fractures occur more frequently in adult males who have reached an age at which their agility is lessened and their resistance to bone injury is decreased; also, at this age, men are particularly exposed to industrial risk and accidents.

Of the 67 os calcis fractures, 6 were bilateral and 1 was an open fracture—all in males. In 5 cases (in males) there were complicating fractures of the spine, an incidence of 7% in the series.

Types of Os Calcis Fractures

Os calcis fractures may be insignificant or very complex. They are of two general types: those that do not enter the joint, such as the chip or "beak" and the avulsion types, and those that involve the subtalar joint, the "crush" or comminuted type.

Fractures of the posterior portion of the os calcis or tuberosity usually are the simplest to treat. The fracture line may pass longitudinally through the bone from the back forward, producing the so-called split, tongue, duckbill or avulsion fractures. The avulsion, or linear, fracture, where the Achilles tendon remains attached to the avulsed proximal fragment, may be treated simply by closed reduction and plaster fixation with the foot in plantar flexion and the knee

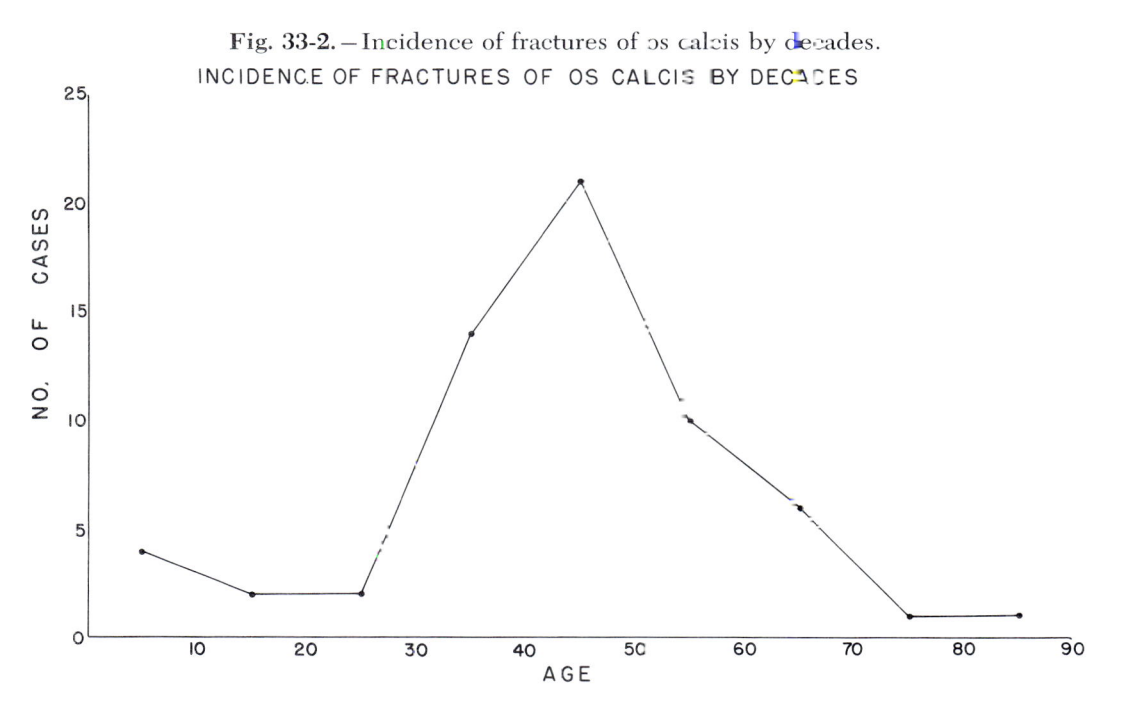

Fig. 33-2.—Incidence of fractures of os calcis by decades.

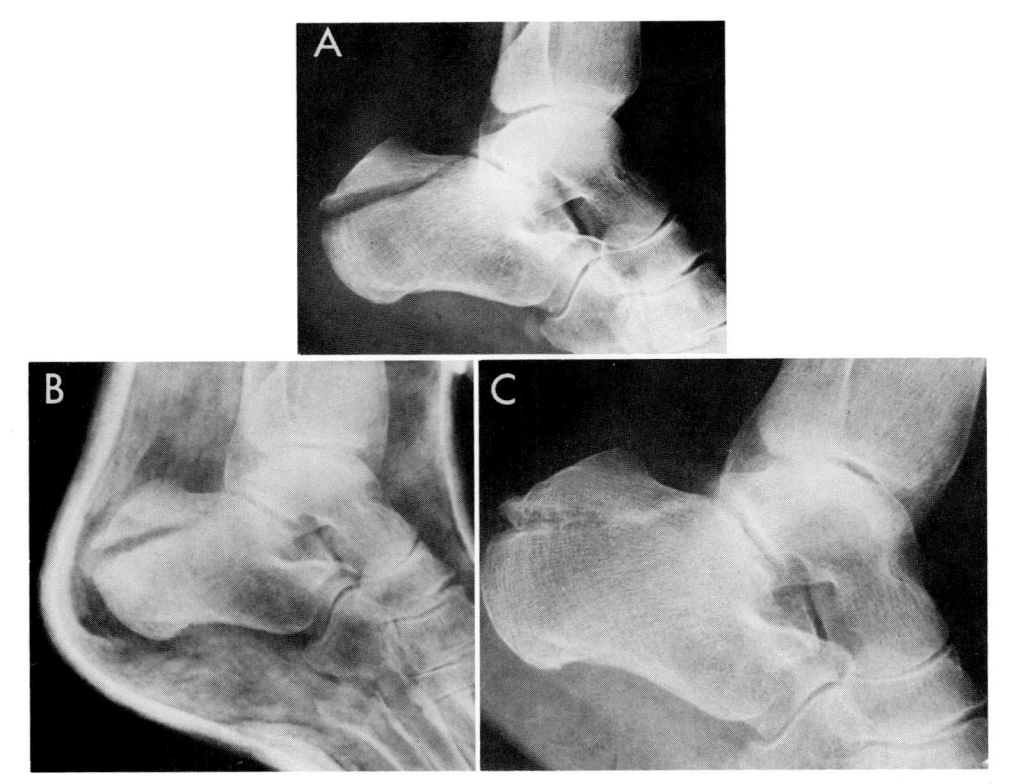

Fig. 33-3.—**A,** os calcis fracture ("duckbill" type), sustained when patient fell 4 feet, striking her left foot on the floor. **B,** immobilization in plaster-of-Paris boot. **C,** 5 months after injury; gap in os calcis almost completely filled in.

flexed* or it may be treated by open reduction and internal fixation, as with a screw.

A small linear fracture may occur in this region proximal to the attachment of the Achilles tendon. This also may be called a "duckbill" or "tongue" fracture, the difference being only that the Achilles tendon is attached to the avulsed fragment in the avulsion type and not in the other type. Union of this type of fracture is facilitated by simple plaster fixation for about 4–6 weeks with the foot in plantar flexion. If reduction then is not satisfactory, open reduction and internal fixation must be used.

*The normal adult gastrocnemius muscle may elongate as much as 10.5 cm, from the knee-flexion foot in equinus position to the knee-extended foot in dorsiflexion position.

Fracture of the anterior process of the os calcis, although rare, frequently is overlooked, Gellman believes, because of the difficulty of diagnosis and the failure to show the fracture clearly by roentgenograms. Since the mechanism of fracture probably is forceful adduction of the forepart of the foot or forceful extension (as when a person catches the forepart of his foot in a hole and falls backward), treatment may require a plaster-of-Paris boot, as described by Bradford and Larsen,[6] with the foot in slight valgus and dorsiflexion to appose the fragments and reduce the tension on the bifurcate ligament.

Of the 67 cases of os calcis fractures reviewed there were 3 fractures of the anterior process. In 2 cases, the small fractured portion was excised because of delayed union and malposition. In these

Chapter 33: INJURIES OF THE FOOT / 841

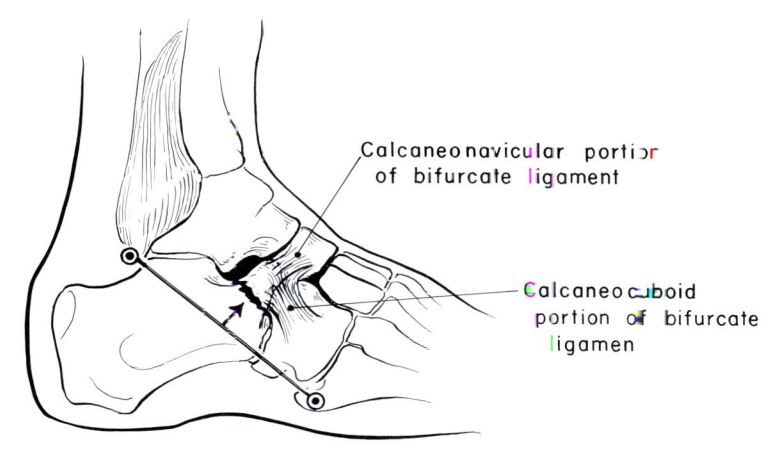

Fig. 33-4.—Schematic drawing demonstrating how the bifurcate ligament avulses the anterior process of the calcaneus when the foot is sharply inverted. If a line drawn from the tip of the external malleolus to the tip of the base of the fifth metatarsal bone (usually a distance of 3 inches) is bisected by a perpendicular line projected toward the top of the tarsus, the point of maximal tenderness will be found. (From Gellman, M.: Fractures of the anterior process of calcaneum, J. Bone Joint Surg. 33-A:382, 1951.)

2 patients, pain persisted for about 6 months, probably as a result of associated injuries to the subastragalar joint. Therefore, it is believed that operative removal is not the method of choice; plaster fixation certainly should be tried first and excision reserved as a last resort.

From both the clinical and the economic aspects, the os calcis is the most important bone in the foot. Not only is it

Fig. 33-5.—Technique for diagnosing fracture of anterior process of os calcis. If the examiner places his thumb on the tip of the external malleolus and the middle finger on the tip of the base of the fifth metatarsal bone, the slightly crooked index finger held equidistant between these two bones will fall directly on an exquisitely tender point. (From Gellman, M.: Fractures of the anterior process of calcaneum, J. Bone Joint Surg. 33-A:382, 1951.)

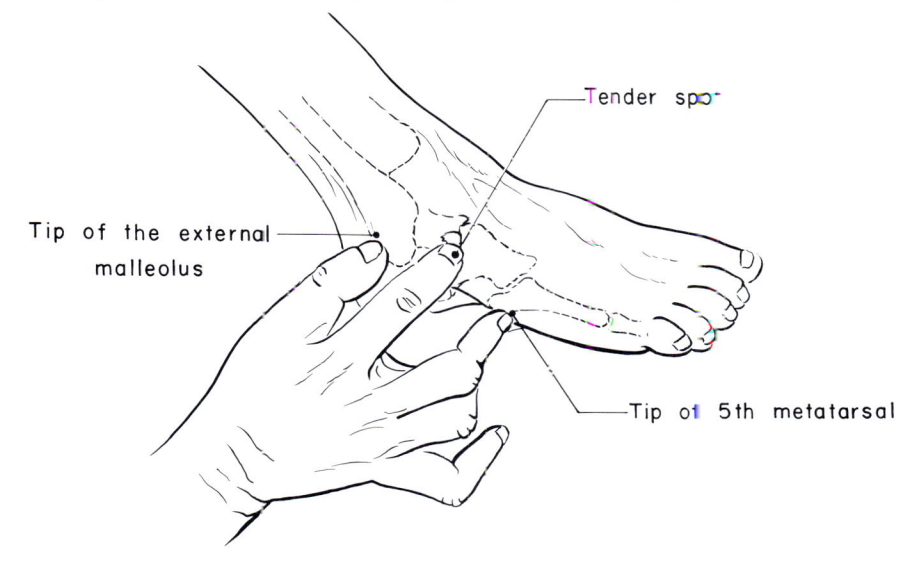

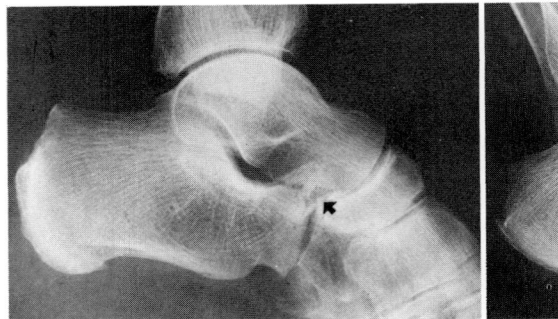

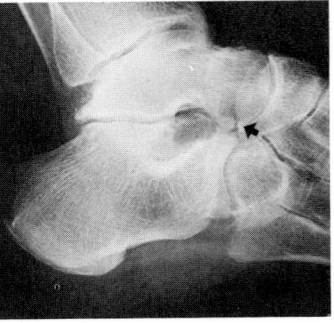

Fig. 33-6.—**Left,** fractured os calcis (anterior process) of left foot (*arrow*), sustained when patient fell off a chair while hanging curtains. Treatment consisted of the excision of anterior process of the os calcis, followed by plaster casing. **Right,** 2¼ years postoperatively. A small bone fragment has re-formed (*arrow*).

the largest bone in the foot but it is the one fractured most frequently and the one that causes the longest period of disability. Geckeler[16] reported in 1950 that an orthopedic consultant to an insurance company found, from a review of 100 cases, that the average time lost from work after a comminuted os calcis fracture amounted to 18 months, plus $1,561 paid in compensation. Furthermore, he stated that there was a decided permanent disability in almost every instance.

Serious efforts to restore the comminuted fractured os calcis to its normal anatomic configuration were started relatively recently. Cotton[12] of Boston pioneered the way in 1908 by introducing the technique of disimpaction and molding the fragments with a mallet. A rapid series of reports on the technique followed in surgical journals. Enthusiasm increased with continued improvement in technique both for anatomic restoration and for early rehabilitation.

Similar techniques were used in clinics both in the United States and abroad. Böhler[4] used a clamp for compressing the lateral bulging deformity. Harris[19] devised an adjustable circular apparatus that could produce skeletal traction in the

Fig. 33-7.—**Left,** Böhler clamp applied to foot. **Right,** same apparatus used on skeleton of foot, demonstrating correct position of pressure knobs.

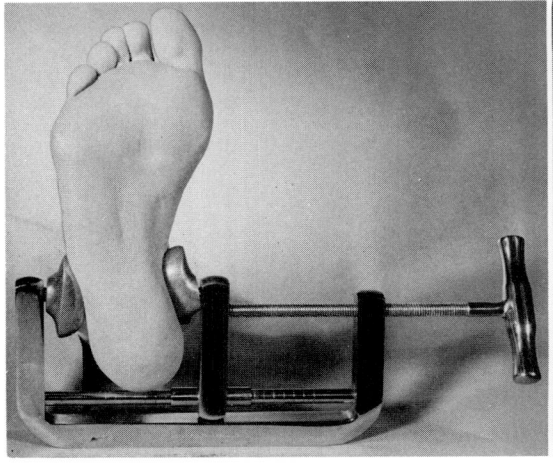

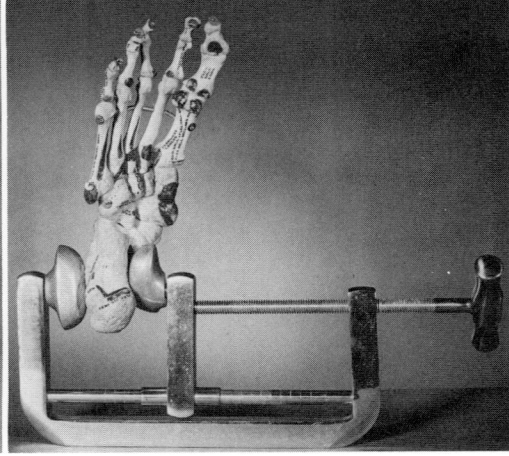

Chapter 33: INJURIES OF THE FOOT / 843

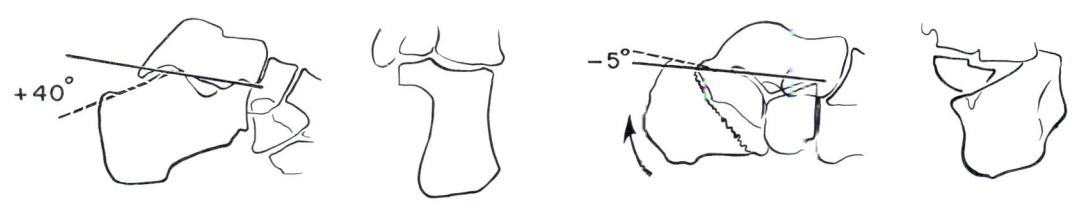

Fig. 33-8.—Left, normal foot, showing the tuber joint angle. Right, comminuted fracture with displacement of outer part of posterior joint, demonstrating reversal of tuber joint angle. (From Watson-Jones, R.: *Fractures and Joint Injuries* [3d ed.; Baltimore: The Williams & Wilkins Company, 1943].)

fragments in three different directions. But, unfortunately, accurate anatomic repositioning of the fragments was not the whole answer. Triradiate traction restored the alignment beautifully but not the blood supply. The resulting avascular necrosis required different treatment. Harris[20] then advocated subtalar arthrodesis after the technique of Gallie.[15] Conn[8] introduced a less-cumbersome reduction apparatus for the "squash" type of fractures and advocated 5 weeks' traction followed by a triple arthrodesis—still more surgery. Thus, the pendulum had swung too far. Not only did the use of such cumbersome apparatus and subsequent oper-

Fig. 33-9.—**A**, lateral and heel views of fractured os calcis (*arrows*). Treatment required little manual molding and the application of a plaster casing for 4 months. **B**, 2 years later; excellent result ($E_4F_4A_4$).

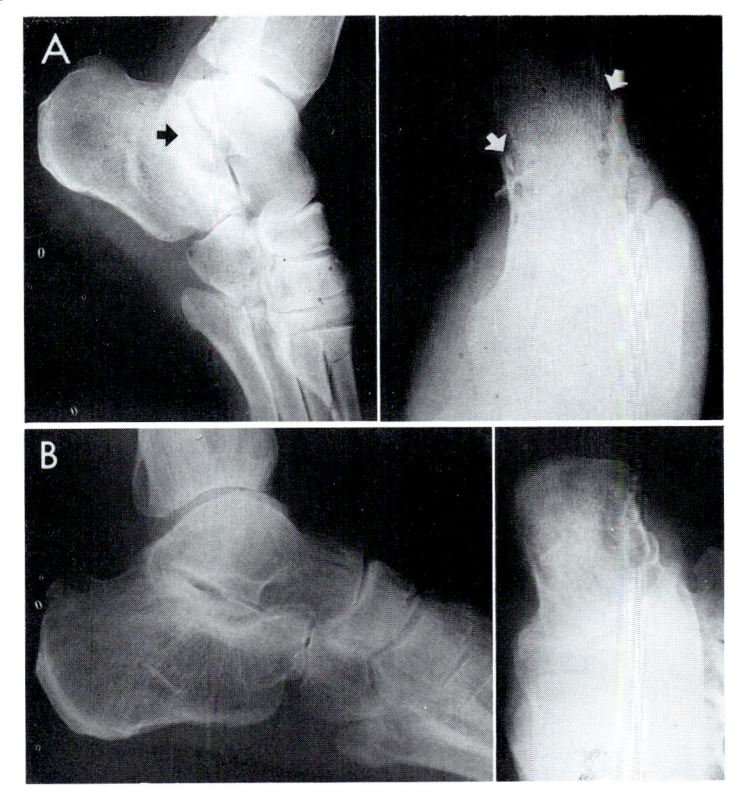

ations keep the patient in the hospital for too long a period but prolonged immobility often resulted in permanent stiffness. The result frequently was a deformed, immobile foot. In the search for a simpler method, Ivar Palmer suggested early open reduction with bone graft.

Mechanism of Fracture

When a person falls from a height and lands directly on his heels, or when an explosion beneath the deck of a ship suddenly produces an impact from below, the result is the same: two opposing forces, one transmitted through the tibia and the other from beneath the os calcis, cause the talus to be driven into the os calcis. The lateral wall of the os calcis is broken off; the medial wall with the sustentaculum tali may or may not be broken away and driven downward. The middle portion of the bone with its lateral fragment may be displaced laterally and appear as a hard mass below the lateral malleolus.

Furthermore, the tuberosity may be divided longitudinally, producing broadening. The normal tuber joint angle (salient angle) of about 40 degrees may be lessened or even reversed (Fig. 33-8).

Conservative Treatment

Most of the cases of os calcis crush fractures that have been reviewed were treated by the so-called conservative

Fig. 33-10.—**A**, lateral and posterior views of fractured right os calcis. Treatment by Palmer technique with bone graft, followed by 8 weeks in a plaster casing. Patient was back at work in 8 additional weeks. **B**, 1½ years postoperatively; excellent result ($E_4F_4A_4$).

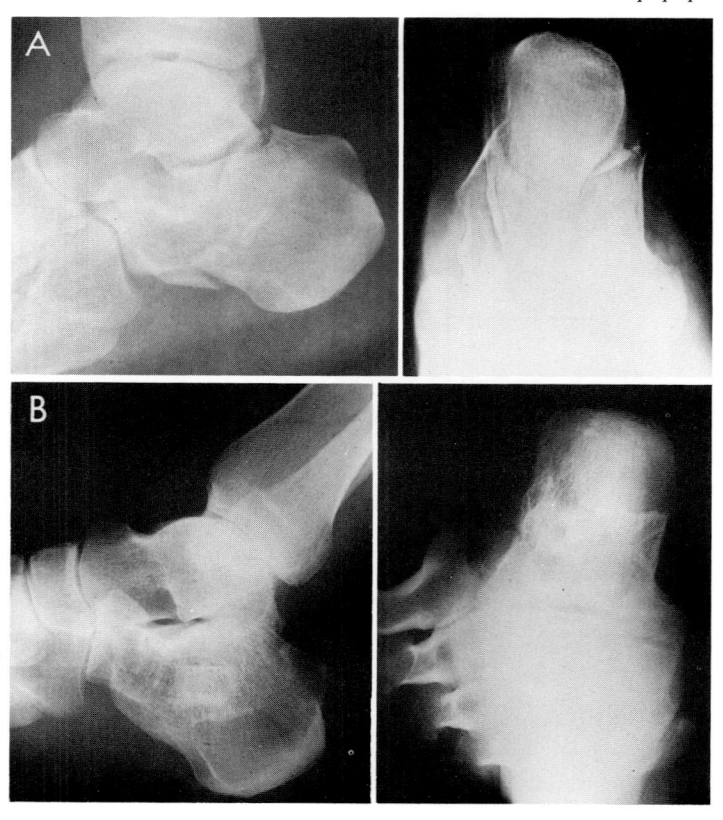

Chapter 33: INJURIES OF THE FOOT / 845

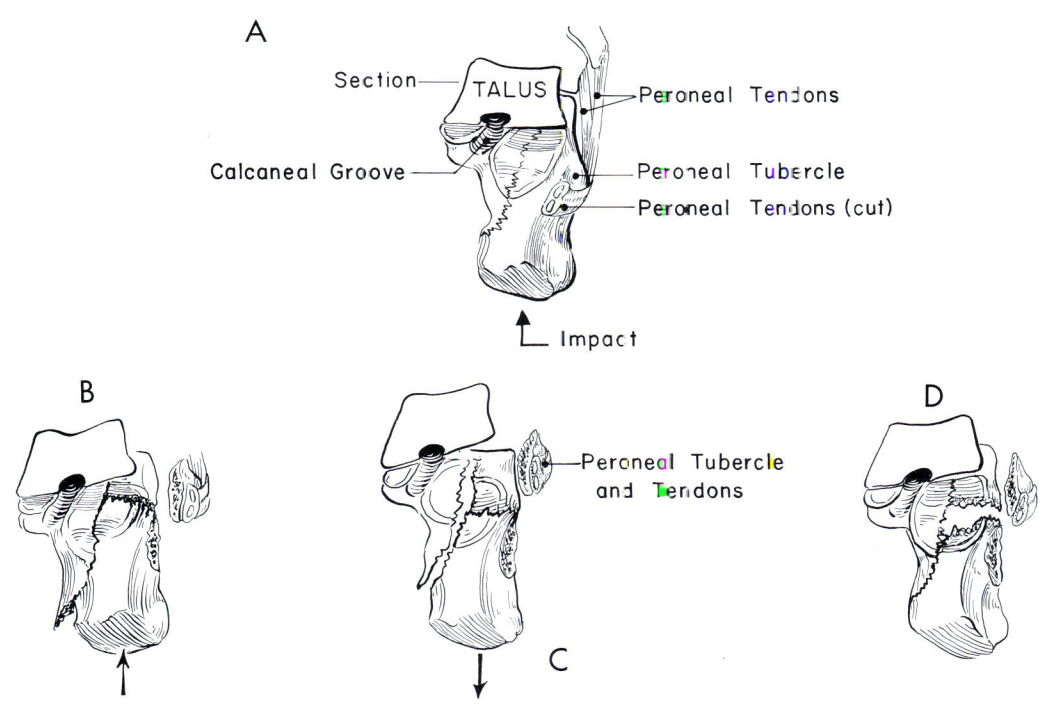

Fig. 33-11.—Deformities of fractured os calcis reduced and maintained by bone graft (after Palmer). **A**, position before displacement of fragments. **B**, immediate result after impact. **C**, position after traction. **D**, reposition after open reduction, demonstrating open space for insertion of bone graft.

method of manual molding of the os calcis and the application of a plaster-of-Paris boot or long-leg casing with the knee slightly flexed. For this treatment, the patient's knee is flexed over the end of the operating table. With the operator seated in front of the patient, the os calcis can be compressed through the "heels" of the operator's hands. With his fingers clasped, the operator catches the heel in this "manual vise" and applies pressure with traction until the impaction is broken up and the deformity corrected. A helpful trick is to apply liquid adhesive to the patient's heel and the operator's palms before the procedure is carried out; much more traction then can be applied. Next, felt rolls are placed carefully beneath each malleolus and plaster casing is applied. The casing is changed in a week or two if it becomes loose, and a snugly fitting plaster is kept on until heal-

Fig. 33-12.—Deformities of fractured os calcis reduced and maintained by bone graft (after Palmer). **A**, the step in the joint (right calcaneus). **B**, after reduction of lateral fragment. **C**, bone graft inserted.

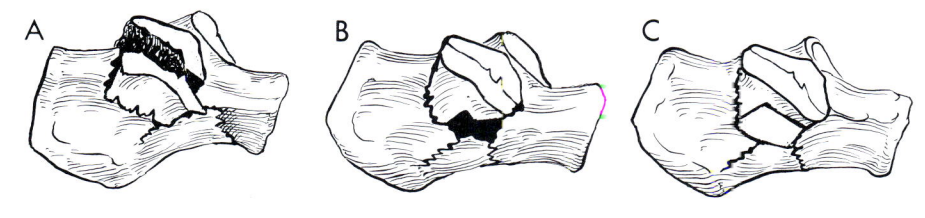

FRACTURE CLINIC

MASSACHUSETTS GENERAL HOSPITAL

END-RESULT RATINGS

All cases shall be rated at the end of 1 year from the time of injury, except for patients who have been treated primarily elsewhere and who come for reconstruction surgery —arthroplasty, arthrodesis, ostectomy, etc.

Amputations shall not be rated in the routine A, F, E manner.

The end results of certain cases cannot be established at the end of 1 year (e.g., epiphysial injuries); these cases must be followed for a longer period of time and rated at such time as the Fracture Clinic sees fit.

The *Percentage Rating* shall be as follows:

Rating 0,	from	0%	to	12½%
" 1,	"	12½%	"	37½%
" 2,	"	37½%	"	62½%
" 3,	"	62½%	"	87½%
" 4,	"	87½%	"	100%

The letters A, F, and E are used to signify: anatomical, functional, and economic result.

Anatomic Rating:

There are four factors which make up the total of an *anatomical* result:
 1. Length   3. Apposition
 2. Alignment   4. Angulation

The anatomical rating shall be based primarily on the roentgenogram—except for length.

Functional Rating:

There are four factors which make up the total of a *functional* result:
 1. Total functional result—subjective (asking the patient)
 2. "   "   "   —objective (by observation), muscle strength, and staying power
 3. Joint movement above the fracture, as compared to the other side
 4. "   "   below "   "   "   "   "   "   "   "

Functional rating shall apply to function of the part as a whole, with due evaluation of function of adjacent joints.

Economic Rating:

There are four factors which make up the total of an *economic* rating:
 1. Same work as before, lighter, or heavier work
 2. "   pay as before, more, or less
 3. "   hours of work, "   "   "
 4. "   volume of work, "   "   "

The economic rating shall be measured not only by the wage-earning capacity but also by the impairment of the person's general activities. In the case of a housewife, or of an elderly person, neither of whom was earning money before injury, any limitation of the person's activity subsequent to the fracture must be estimated in the economic rating.

Fig. 33-13.—A simple comprehensive fracture result rating scheme.

ing has occurred. After 4–6 weeks, a walking heel is applied for partial weight bearing.

Operative Treatment

The "squash" type of comminuted os calcis fracture, with its broadening, shortening and compression of the os calcis, is considered the worst type from the standpoints of both reduction and rehabilitation. The treatment of these fractures by the method of Ivar Palmer[25] reportedly gives good results. His technique can restore the tuber joint angle as well as correct the other deformities. The best results can be expected when the articular facets are not fractured or destroyed. If the facets are badly damaged, the prognosis is poor and the possibility of a subtalar arthrodesis or triple arthrodesis should be considered.

Postoperative treatment for the Palmer procedure consists of a long plaster-of-Paris casing for 4–6 weeks, depending on the weight of the patient. For example, a 200-pound man may be kept in plaster 6 weeks, a lighter person only 4 weeks. At the end of this period, the plaster is cut below the knee and the patient begins partial weight bearing with crutches and with a rubber heel attached to the bottom of the boot. At the end of 4 weeks, the casing is removed and a roentgenogram is made. If consolidation is apparent, the patient is permitted to start wearing his shoe with a molded steel arch support.

Of 14 cases treated by this method, 10 have been followed and rated. The end-result ratings (according to the method of rating shown in Fig. 33-13) were:

$E_4F_4A_4$ 4* $E_3F_3A_3$ 2
$E_4F_4A_3$ 1 $E_0F_3A_3$ 1
$E_4F_3A_3$ 2

A comparison of the functional progress of os calcis fractures according to type of treatment is shown in Table 33-1.

For the most seriously injured patients, where the os calcis is crushed beyond repair, Pridie[26] of England excises the entire fragmented os calcis and places the leg in plaster-of-Paris. Walking is permitted in 2 months, and the patients are permitted to return to work, wearing a high heel. Pridie has reported that one of his patients, after excision of the entire os calcis, walks without a perceptible limp.

There are two schools of thought concerning the treatment of os calcis fractures that apply to the postoperative management of those fractures treated by open reduction as well as those treated nonoperatively.

Long cast immobilization invites the chronic pain syndrome, which results

*One patient was over 60 years of age.

TABLE 33-1.—COMPARISON OF FUNCTIONAL PROGRESS OF OS CALCIS FRACTURES ACCORDING TO TYPE OF TREATMENT*

	TIME IN HOSPITAL (Days)	PARTIAL WEIGHT BEARING WITH CRUTCHES (Weeks)	FULL WEIGHT BEARING (Weeks)	WALKING WITHOUT CASING (Weeks)	BACK TO WORK (Weeks)
Noncomminuted fractures (10 years)	6.4 (25)	—	—	4.8 (7)	13.6 (6)
Comminuted fractures treated conservatively (10 years)	27.0 (41)	5 (6)	8 (5)	12.4 (9)	28.8 (16)
Comminuted fractures treated by Palmer method (5 years)	25.0 (14)	2.3 (6)	5.4 (7)	10.0 (8)	28.0 (5)

*Figures in parentheses indicate the number of cases.

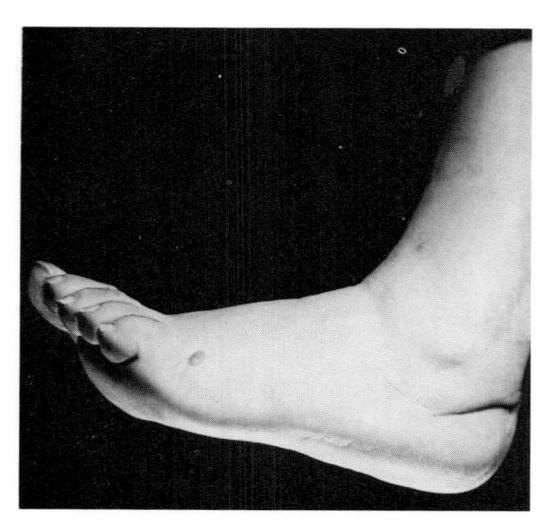

Fig. 33-14.—Foot after excision of os calcis. (Courtesy of Mr. K. H. Pridie.)

from an os calcis fracture treated by prolonged rigid fixation of the foot and ankle.

In recent years, another method of treating os calcis fractures has been used with increasing frequency by the members of the Massachusetts General Hospital Orthopedic Staff. Emphasis is placed on soft tissue components of the injury. The patient is admitted to the hospital. A closed manipulation is carried out to narrow the heel and to restore heel length. A soft dressing then is applied and the foot elevated. Motion of the foot and ankle is begun immediately, emphasizing inversion and eversion.

Usually within 1–2 weeks the swelling has markedly diminished and motions are quite free, as well as relatively painless. A soft sponge rubber arch support is made with a one-quarter-inch latex cupped heel and graduated weight bearing begun, with the use of crutches. Some of our staff members prefer the application of a patellar tendon-bearing short leg brace at this stage whereas others favor a short leg walking plaster, with a well-molded arch, until the patient can tolerate almost full weight bearing, which usually is within a few weeks.

FRACTURES AND DISLOCATIONS OF THE TALUS

Among the fractures of the bones of the foot, fracture of the talus ranks next to that of the os calcis in importance. (The findings from a review of 28 injuries to the talus are given in Table 33-2.)

There are many problems peculiar to the talus. The bone is intra-articular; three-fifths of its surface is covered with cartilage, which takes part in the formation of three joints (with the tibia, the os calcis and the navicula). Therefore, almost any fracture of the talus will involve a joint surface. This is all the more serious because the talus is a weight-bearing

TABLE 33-2.—Comparison of Functional Progress of Fractures of Talus According to Type of Treatment*

	Time in Hospital (Days)	Time in Casing (Weeks)	Partial Weight Bearing (Weeks)	Full Weight Bearing (Weeks)	Back to Work (Weeks)
Chip fractures	6.0[11]† or 1.2[10]†	3.0[1]‡	3.8[4]	3.2[4]	7.0[2]
Comminuted fractures	20[8]	24[4]	23[4]	31[2]	35[2]
Fractures with dislocation	53[4]	25[2]	11[2]	34[2]	43[3]
Dislocation without fracture§	12[5]	10[3]	8[2]	13[2]	20[2]

*Figures in parentheses indicate the number of cases.
†The first figure, 6.0[11], includes the case of a 73-year-old woman who was in the hospital 52 days; the second figure, 1.2[10], gives the average of the remaining cases.
‡Most chip fractures were treated by strapping.
§In 3 cases there were fractures of bones other than the talus—i.e., malleolus, fibula, etc.

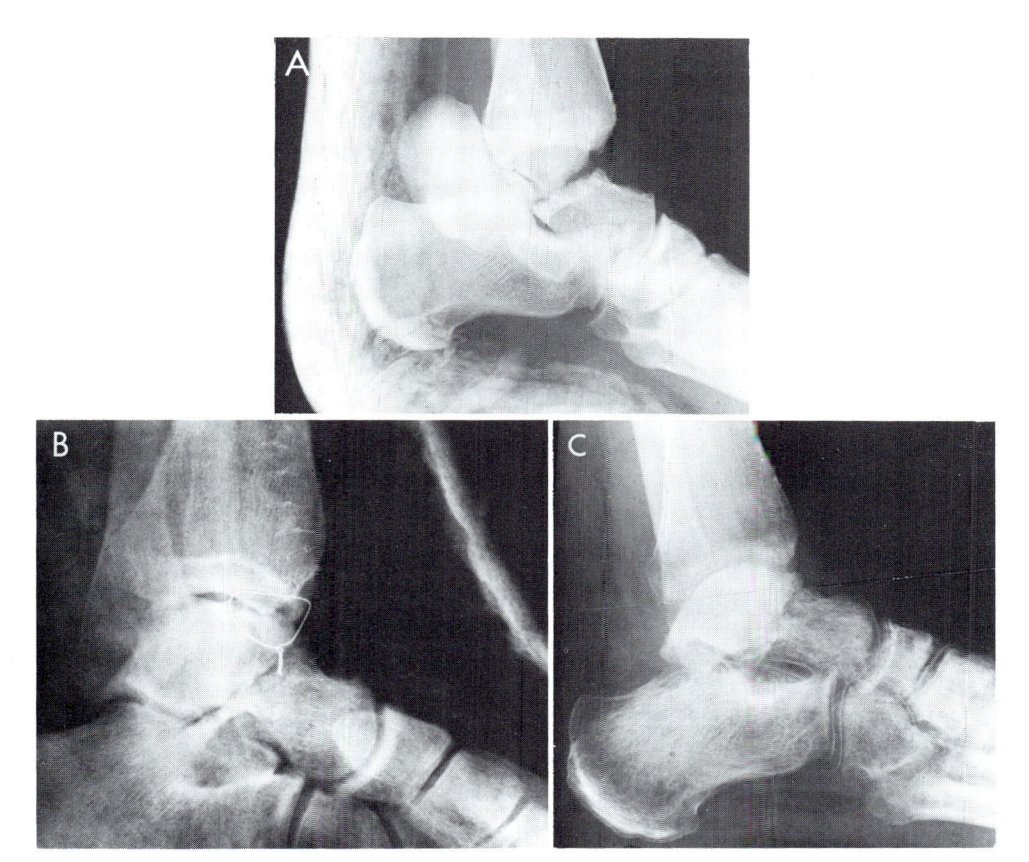

Fig. 33-15. — **A**, fractured left talus with dislocation sustained in an automobile accident. **B**, after treatment by open reduction and a wire loop in the medial malleolus. **C**, 4 months postoperatively, indicating nonunion with avascular necrosis. Rating 2 years postoperatively: failure ($E_0F_0A_0$).

bone; in fact, more weight per unit of area is borne by the superior surface of the talus than by any other bone in the body. Eventual traumatic arthritis is a constant danger.

Most of the nutrition of the talus is received through the neck of the bone (from a branch of the dorsalis pedis artery through the talonavicular ligament). By injecting 7 amputated limbs, McKeever[23] was able to demonstrate no other source of blood supply to the talus than that through the neck. The body of the talus, therefore, is subject to the hazards of avascular necrosis following fractures and fracture dislocations. Avascular necrosis usually follows backward dislocation of the body of the talus.

Although Gibson and Inkster[18] of Winnipeg, Canada, have attributed some of the talar blood supply to small arteries entering through the deltoid ligaments, they have also believed that a complete posterior dislocation of the body of the talus through a buttonhole between the flexor digitorum longus and the flexor hallucis longus will completely sever the body of the talus from its vascular connections.

The dangers of avascular necrosis in fractures of the talus with — and, indeed, occasionally without — dislocation cannot

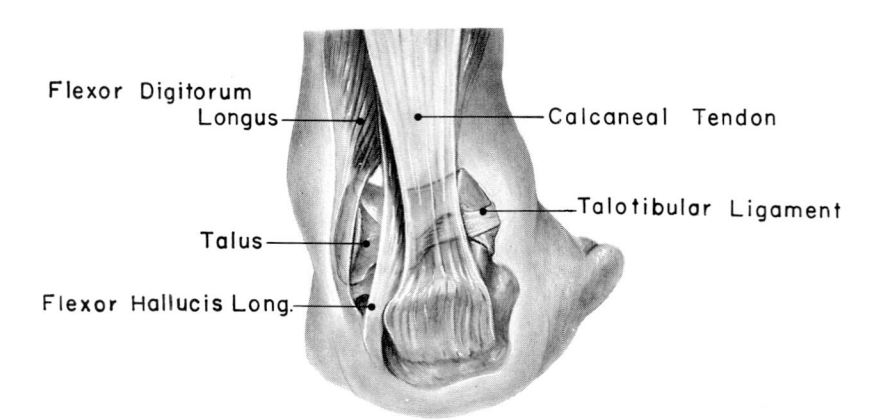

Fig. 33-16.—Diagram showing buttonhole formed by flexor digitorum longus and flexor hallucis longus through which talus may be squeezed in posterior dislocation, with shutting off of its blood supply. (From Gibson, A., and Inkster, R. C.: Fractures of the talus, Can. Med. Assoc. J. 31:357, 1934.)

be overemphasized; consequently, certain principles must be kept in mind constantly during treatment.

Impacted fractures of the head may respond satisfactorily to conservative measures. Incomplete fractures of the neck or fractures of the distal portion of the neck without displacement may be treated conservatively with plaster fixation. Fractures of the neck with displacement that do not respond to manipulation should be treated by open reduction and internal fixation (preferably a screw). Fractures of the neck with dislocation require treatment designed to avoid avascular necrosis.

The surgical approach for fusion of the tibiotalar joint is through an anterolateral incision. The soft tissues around the head and neck of the talus must be preserved as carefully as possible. Reduction, which is not difficult, is maintained by internal fixation. A plaster casing is applied from the toes to the knee for 8 weeks before weight bearing is permitted. A walking boot then may be applied for a month, followed by the wearing of a suitable shoe and arch support for 3 months longer. Comminuted fracture of the body of the talus with displacement requires either removal of all of the fragments or a calcaneotibial fusion. A simple excision of the talus is not as effective as fusion. However, sometimes it is advantageous to excise the talus and then later perform an arthrodesis of the tibia to the os calcis if painful function demands it.

FRACTURES OF THE TARSAL NAVICULAR

There are three different types of navicular fractures: fracture of the tuberosity, fracture of the dorsal lip and transverse fracture of the tarsal navicular.

Fracture of the tuberosity usually is an avulsion fracture caused by the pull of the posterior tibial tendon. This tendon has such a broad distribution that it is impossible for the fragments of bone to become widely separated. Treatment for this type of fracture consists of wearing a plaster-of-Paris boot for 8–10 weeks. Recovery of function usually is good.

In fracture of the dorsal lip, ordinarily only a piece of bone is flaked off. Immobilization in plaster or by adhesive strapping for 3 weeks usually gives excellent results.

The transverse fracture of the tarsal navicular is a different matter. In this

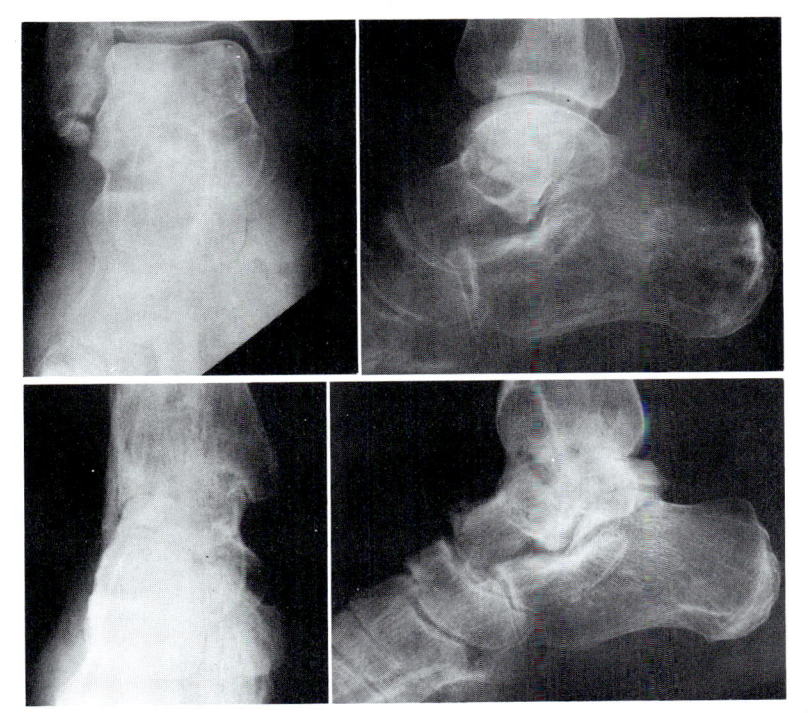

Fig. 33-17.—Top, anteroposterior and lateral views of right foot showing avascular necrosis 5 months after fracture through neck and body of the talus. Bottom, 3 years after injury, showing fusion following tibiotalar arthrodesis.

fracture there usually is a large dorsal and a small plantar fragment. If displaced, the dorsal fragment may be replaced by pressure of the thumb and held by a plaster casing, but displacement is likely to recur. No matter what the treatment, the fragmented bone may undergo absorption, with resulting arthritis and prolonged disability until dense fibrous union appears. Therefore, immediate arthrodesis of both the talonavicular and navicular-cuneiform joints with a tibial graft laid in a trough and immobilized in plaster for 10 weeks is considered the best and safest treatment. Other methods, however, such as wiring fragments together, have been successful. If the dorsal fragment is not displaced, transverse fractures may be treated successfully by plaster fixation for 4 weeks and later an arch support.

METATARSAL FRACTURES

Metatarsal fractures, such as stress, fatigue or march fractures, first described by Breithaupt in 1855, may not be seen in early x-ray films; however, several weeks later, repeat films will show the fractures clearly. In treating severe metatarsal strain fractures, bed rest may be necessary for a while. The usual regimen is plaster casing for 3 weeks, followed by the use of a carefully molded steel arch support.

A fracture of the neck of the metatarsal demands careful replacement, or a painful plantar callus may develop. All displaced metatarsal fractures should be corrected; in particular, the dorsal bow of the metatarsal should be restored.

The proximal end of the fifth metatarsal may be injured by turning the foot in-

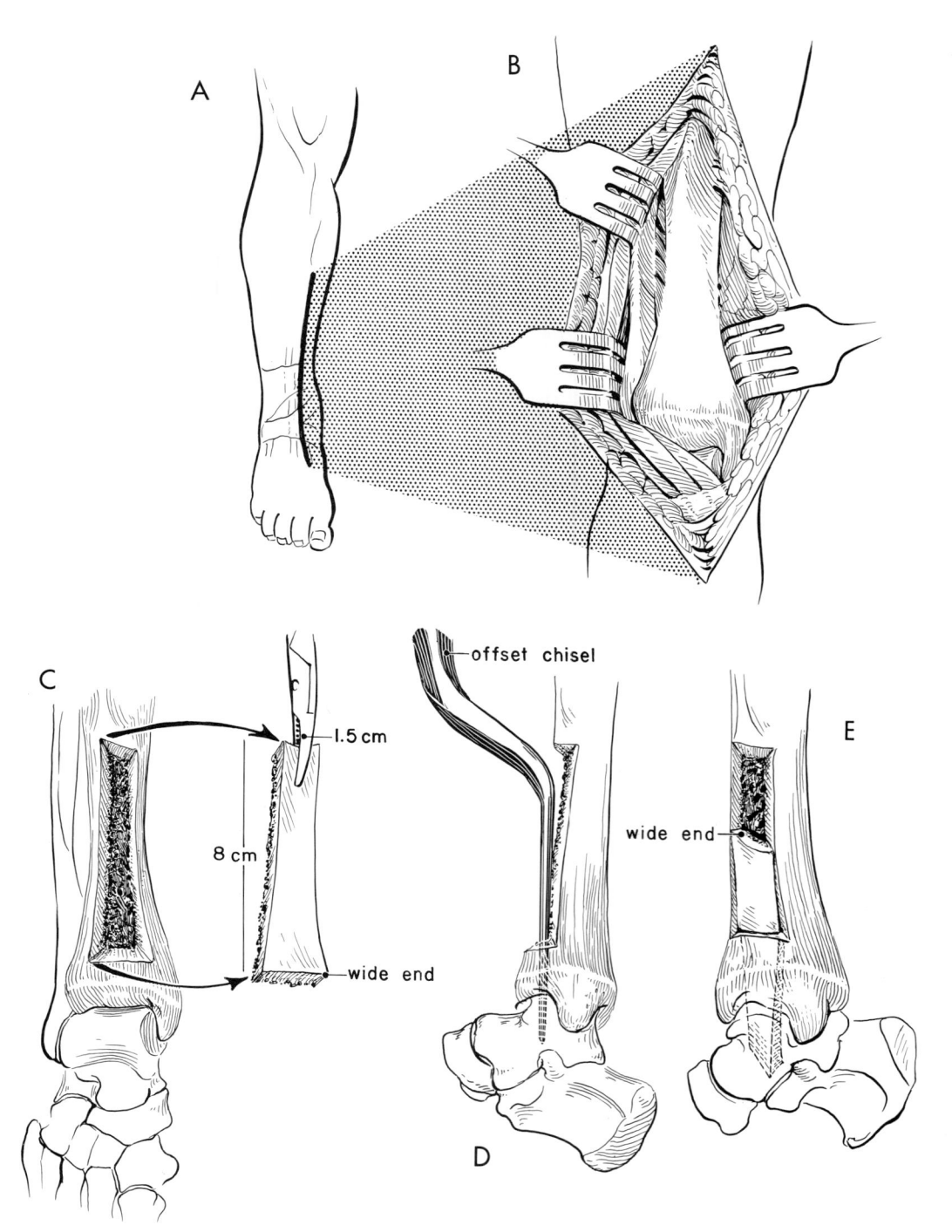

Fig. 33-18.—Operation for fusion of ankle joint. **A,** incision in skin. **B,** incision through the anterior tibial sheath and the periosteum to bone. **C,** articular surfaces destroyed; graft removed. **D,** bayonet-type osteotome forms tunnel for graft. **E,** graft driven through tunnel with bone set. (Adapted from Hatt, R. N.: The central bone graft in joint arthrodesis, J. Bone Joint Surg. 22:393, 1940.)

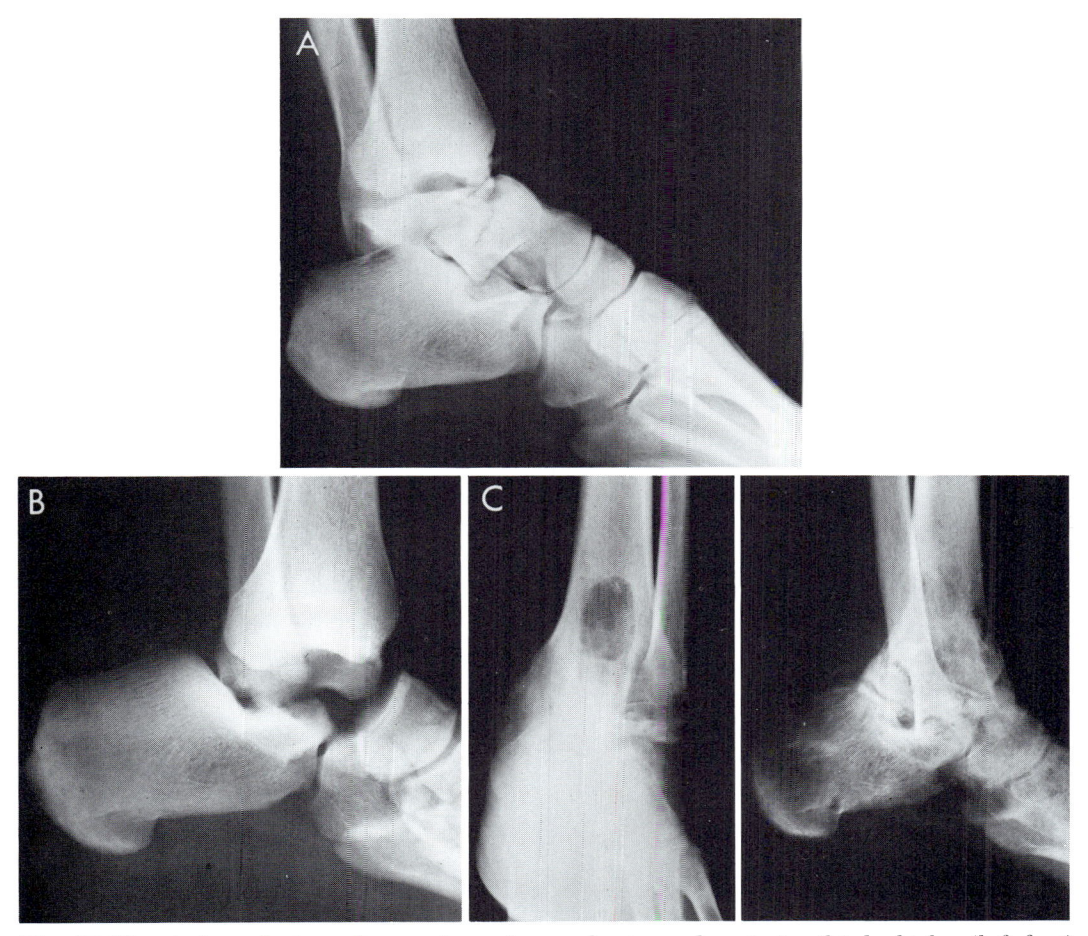

Fig. 33-19.—**A**, lateral view of comminuted open fracture of posterior third of talus (left foot) with complete detachment of this portion of bone from the remainder. **B**, after excision of talus. Arthrodesis was performed 1½ years later. **C**, anteroposterior and lateral views 6 months after arthrodesis.

ward and placing pressure on the proximal enlarged portion of the bone. The force from impact with the pavement or other firm surface, together with the increased pull of the peroneus brevis tendon, may produce a fracture. Usually, only slight separation of the fragments occurs. Treatment by simple adhesive strapping and arch support may be adequate in undisplaced fractures; however, if there is marked deformity, eversion of the foot, replacement of the displaced fragment by firm digital pressure and immobilization by a plaster boot may be indicated.

A review of 40 cases of metatarsal fractures revealed that of the 34 in which end results were available, results were excellent in 26 cases (75%).

METATARSAL FRACTURES WITH TARSOMETATARSAL DISLOCATIONS

If displacement is not severe, a satisfactory foot usually results from the reduction (open or closed) and molding of

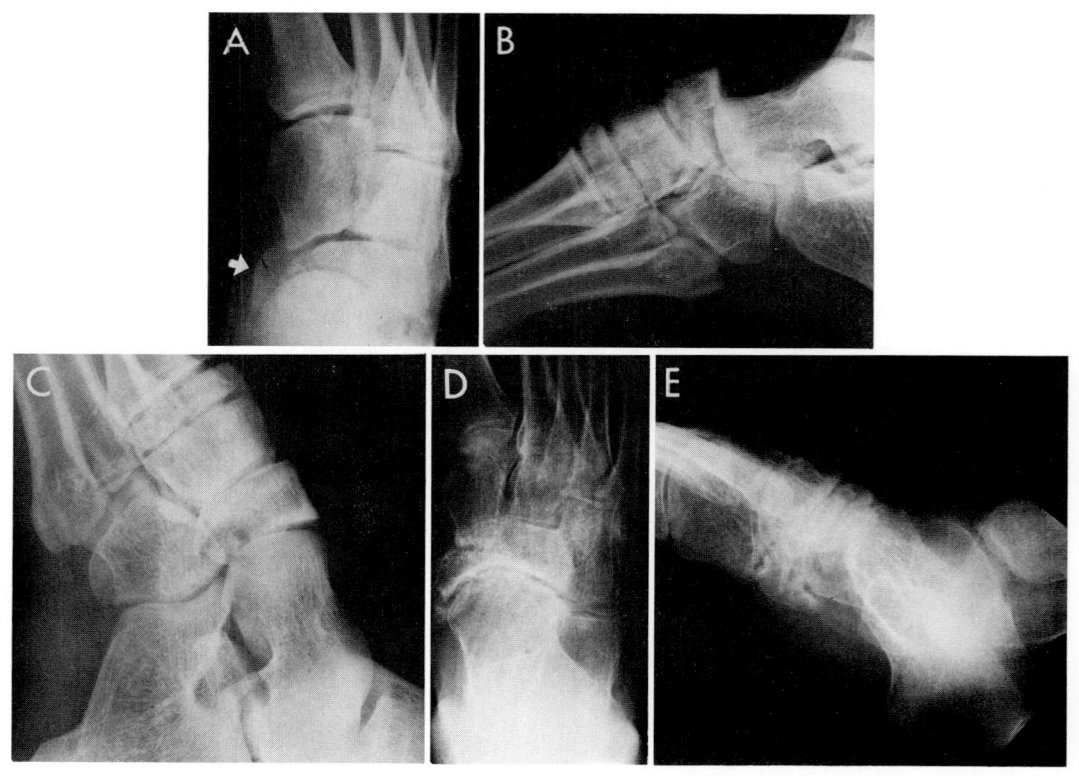

Fig. 33-20.—A and B, anteroposterior and lateral views of compression fracture of tarsal navicular bone (*arrow*). C, lateral view after closed reduction. D and E, anteroposterior and lateral views 2 years after injury, showing avascular necrosis of navicular bone and traumatic arthritis.

the displaced parts as accurately as possible, even though exact anatomic restitution may be impossible. This procedure is followed by immobilization in a plaster-of-Paris boot for 6–8 weeks, with partial weight bearing on crutches permitted after the fourth week. At the outset, it is imperative that the patient keep the foot elevated and do active exercises in order to avoid undue swelling. Improvement may continue over a period of 2–3 years if the patient wears a suitable shoe with arch support and elastic anklet and continues active exercises.

Falling objects frequently cause fractures of the metatarsals. The conscientious use of steel-toe-protector shoes, which many industries require of their workers, has lessened the incidence of these fractures considerably. A typical example of such an injury follows.

A steelworker was standing on the ground when a strip of steel fell from a height of 5–6 stories. It missed his head by only a fraction of an inch and struck his second and third toes near the junction with the foot, causing open fracture-dislocation of the second and third toes, severing all blood and nerve supply and leaving the toes attached by a small piece of skin with insufficient blood supply. Although the patient was seen approximately 1 hour after the injury, the second and third toes were cold and avascular, and no blanching could be demonstrated on any portion of either toe. Immediate amputation and closure of the skin were done, after debridement of the metatarsal

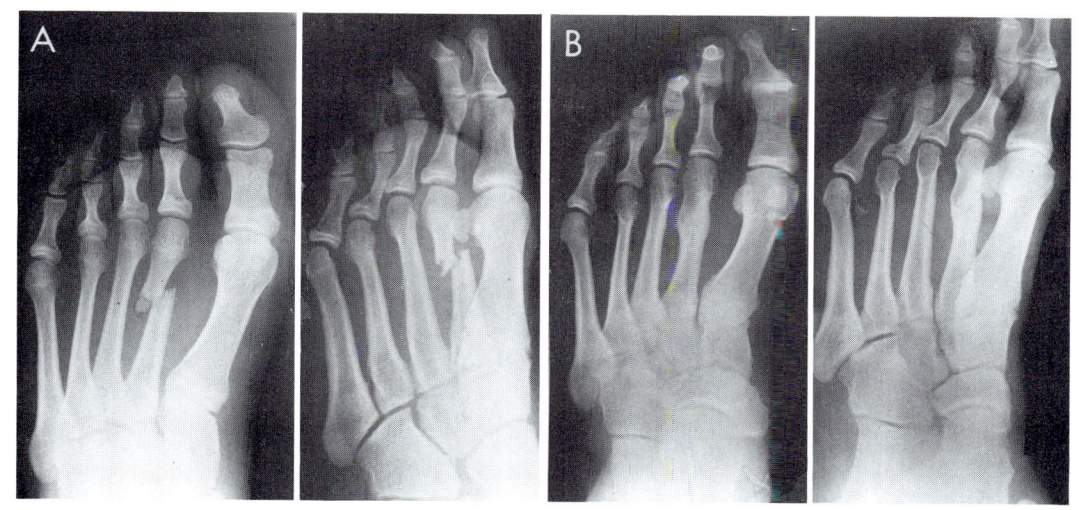

Fig. 33-21.—**A,** anteroposterior and oblique views of complete transverse comminuted fracture of left second metatarsal. Treatment by closed reduction (apposition not complete) and plaster casing. **B,** 1 year after injury; excellent result ($E_4F_4A_4$).

heads. Nevertheless, continued formation of painful neuromas on the dorsum of the foot eventually demanded further plastic surgery, consisting of the excision of most of the second metatarsal and a mass of scar tissue composed of tendons, nerves and blood vessels. Following this procedure, the patient remained asymptomatic and he returned to work approximately 8½ months after injury.

Fig. 33-22.—**Left,** oblique view of fractured proximal end of the left fifth metatarsal sustained when patient twisted her foot while walking. Treatment by strapping for 1 month. **Right,** 1 year later; excellent result ($E_4F_4A_4$).

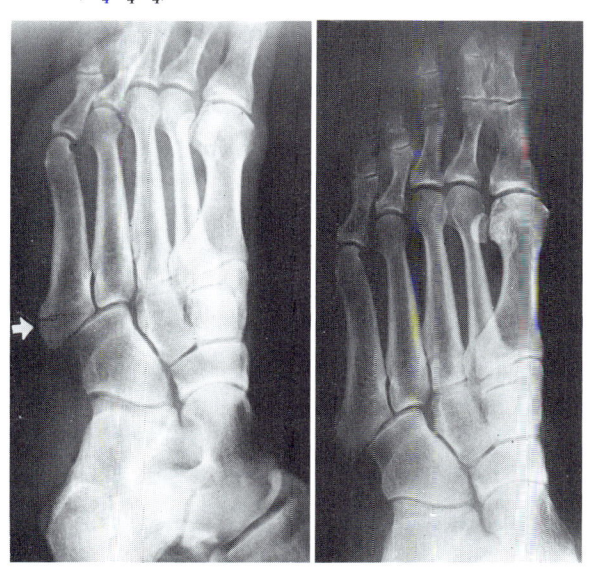

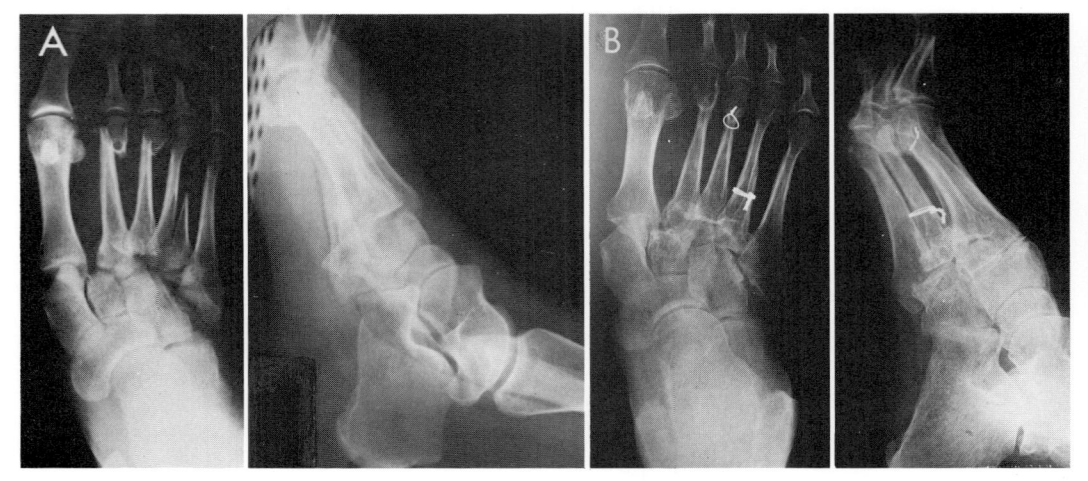

Fig. 33-23.—**A,** anteroposterior and lateral views of tarsometatarsal dislocation sustained in an automobile accident. There were fractures of the second, third, fourth and fifth metatarsals, of the second and third cuneiform and of the cuboid. Treatment by open reduction and wire fixation and a plaster boot. Patient returned to her job as secretary 8 weeks after operation. **B,** 9 months postoperative; satisfactory result.

PHALANGEAL FRACTURES

Phalangeal fractures may be caused by objects falling on the toes or by the stubbing of toes while walking barefoot. Diagnosis and treatment usually are easy.

If only a single phalanx is fractured, normally there is no disability. If the fifth toe is fractured, it may be wise to strap this toe to the adjacent one in order to

Fig. 33-24.—**Left,** open fracture dislocation of second and third toes. Treatment by amputation, followed by plastic surgery. **Right,** 7 months after injury.

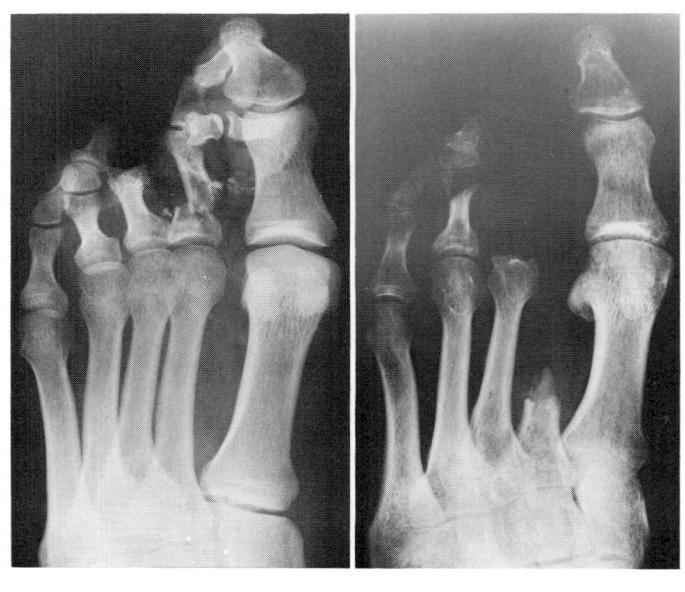

prevent continual displacement at night and during bathing, when the shoe is removed. Usually the wearing of the stocking and shoe provides adequate protection. A Jones bar, 1/2 inch wide and 1/4 inch high, placed diagonally across the sole of the shoe just proximal to the metatarsal heads, or a steel plate inserted between the layers of leather in the sole, effectively prevents painful motion of the toes during walking. Phalangeal fractures usually are asymptomatic after 6 weeks, but the fracture line may be clearly visible in x-ray films for 6 months to a year.

Simple fracture of the phalanges may be quite disabling when multiple, but if the toes are carefully protected by bits of foam rubber or felt on the plantar surface, and strapped one to the other with cotton or gauze between them to prevent maceration, no disability need be expected. Treatment should be directed toward avoiding hammer-toe deformity, rotation deformity or lateral deviation. The sooner a shoe can be worn the quicker the bones will be molded to a functional position. If one of the lesser toes is fractured, disability lasts for 2–3 weeks; in the case of the great toe, 4–5 weeks.

Severe injuries to the great toe usually demand individual consideration, as, for example, the following case of a 14-year-old girl who sustained a comminuted fracture of the two phalanges of her left great toe. The injury occurred in the playroom of her home, where she accidentally kicked a wall.

Five days after injury, open reduction under general anesthesia was carried out as follows: An Esmarch ankle tourniquet was applied. A linear incision was made on the tibial side of both phalanges, exposing the comminuted fracture of the proximal phalanx and the single fracture of the distal phalanx. Care was taken to wash out the blood and minute bone fragments from the interphalangeal joint.

A towel clip was placed on the tip of the toe for traction and the fragments in the proximal phalanx were manipulated into position and held in place by another towel clip. Then, using an electric drill, a small threaded Kirschner wire was placed through the small fragment on the tibial side of the toe and the larger frag-

Fig. 33-25. — Anteroposterior and lateral views of comminuted fracture of the proximal and distal phalanges of the left great toe.

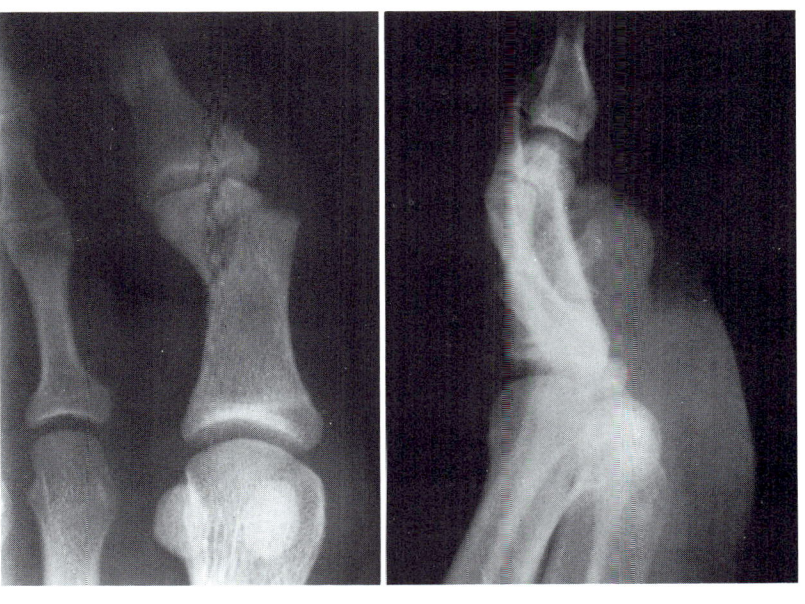

858 / Robert J. Joplin

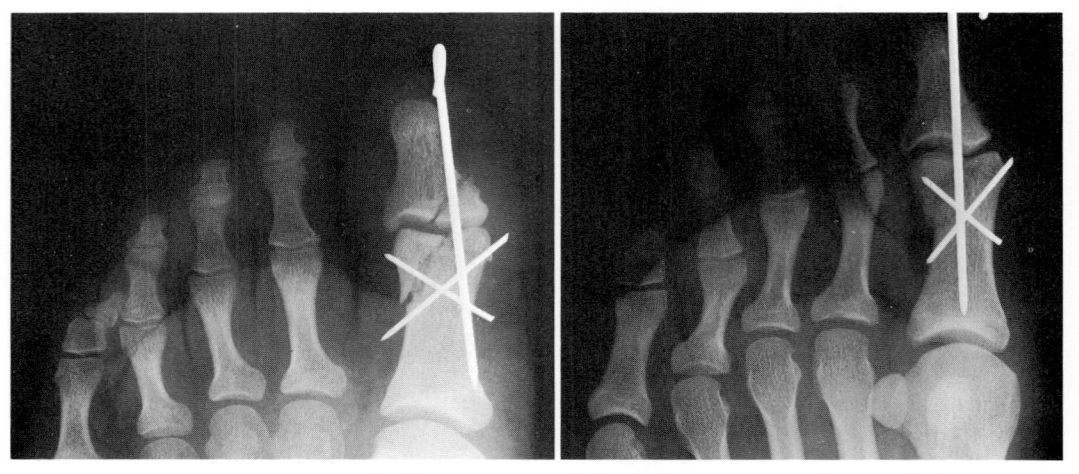

Fig. 33-26.—Anteroposterior and oblique views of the left great toe with threaded Kirschner wires impaling the fragments of the proximal phalanx and the smooth, heavier Kirschner wire holding the distal phalangeal fragments as well as the alignment of both phalanges.

ment was transfixed, approximating it from the tibial side.

Finally, a larger smooth Kirschner wire was passed through the distal phalanx along the underside of the proximal phalanx to avoid displacing the threaded wires and to hold the two phalanges in alignment.

After the application of the wires, the fragments appeared to be in excellent alignment by direct inspection.

X-ray films taken 3 days later showed less than a perfect hairline reduction, but the alignment of the fragments that formed the joint was excellent.

Films taken 1 month postoperatively showed that healing was progressing normally. The smooth Kirschner wire was removed in the office and the patient was admitted to the hospital 2 weeks later for removal of the threaded wires. This was done under sodium pentothal anesthesia.

X-ray films taken 2 months later

Fig. 33-27.—Showing the maintenance of position and the progress in healing of the fragments (3 weeks later) by comparison with Figures 33-25 and 33-26.

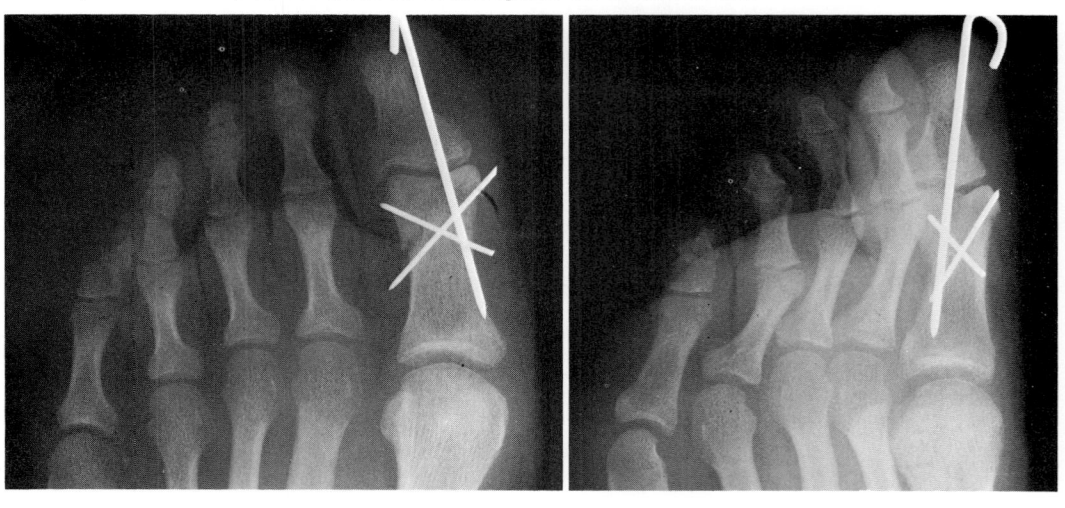

Chapter 33: INJURIES OF THE FOOT / 859

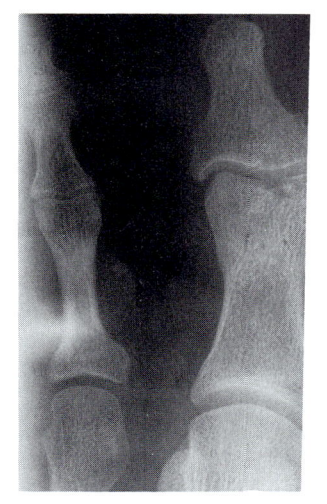

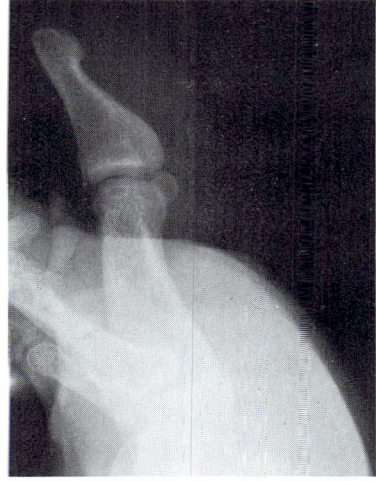

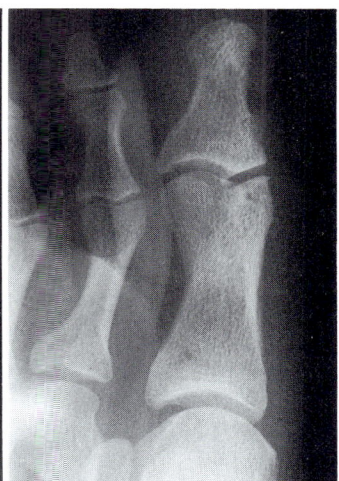

Fig. 33-28.—Anteroposterior, lateral and oblique views showing healing of the fractures in both phalanges approximately 4½ months after injury.

showed an excellent result. On examination 8 months following removal of the wires, the patient reported that she was able to participate in all school activities. Photographs of the two toes showed no differences between them. There was limited flexion in the interphalangeal joint, which, according to the patient, caused no difficulty. It is anticipated that flexion will improve in time, since the articular cartilage space is only slightly diminished.

Open fractures of toes require debridement, tetanus antitoxin, chemotherapy and repair of tendons. If the blood supply of the toe is imperiled, amputation may be necessary. Deformity may be prevented by skeletal traction, using a needle in the terminal phalanx (not in the soft tissue), or by a threaded Kirschner wire longitudinally through the phalanges.

Caution must be exercised in cases of open fracture. At the Fracture Clinic of

Fig. 33-29.—Photograph of both feet to show by comparison excellent cosmetic result at follow-up about 10 months later. It is too early for final result.

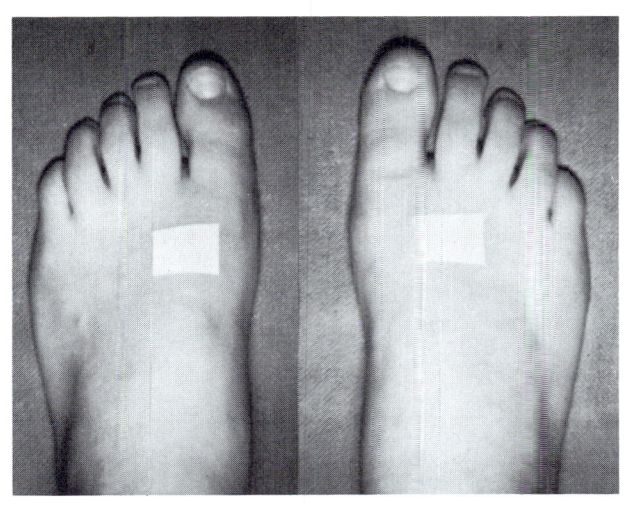

Massachusetts General Hospital, 2 cases of fracture of the foot, each produced by an ax cutting through the shoe into the great toe, resulted in tetanus, with 1 patient succumbing.

In a review of a series of phalangeal fractures, end results were available in only 16 cases. In 11 of these 16 (almost 70%), the results were excellent ($E_4F_4A_4$).

TREATMENT OF INJURIES OF SOME LESSER BONES OF THE FOOT

Some of the most annoying problems occur in isolated fractures of single bones of the foot. Their seeming insignificance may delay diagnosis and treatment. Sudden, exquisite, localized pain should indicate trouble to the patient, but many simply limp along, hoping that the pain will go away. This may lead to postponement of diagnosis until valuable time is lost and the patient has undergone unnecessary suffering.

Some examples of these fractures are: Freiberg's infraction of a metatarsal head; fractured sesamoid; fractured accessory scaphoid; fractured tarsal navicula.

FREIBERG'S INFRACTION OF A METATARSAL HEAD. — While bathing, a 15-year-old girl stepped on a sea urchin. One of its spines stuck in the sole of her foot and penetrated the head of the fourth metatarsal. She immediately withdrew her foot, but a portion of the spine broke off and remained in her foot. On her return home in the fall she had a protective limp on the right side. Eventually, the family had her consult a physician, who took x-rays. The films demonstrated a Freiberg's infraction of the head of the fourth metatarsal of her right foot.

She has procrastinated about suggested treatment and deformity has persisted. Although she is not completely disabled, she may be prevented from enjoying normal function of her foot in athletics, dancing, etc., indefinitely.

A similar diagnosis was made on a girl of 13 years who denied any history of injury, but limped and suffered a persist-

Figs. 33-30 and 33-31.—Typical examples of Freiberg's infraction.

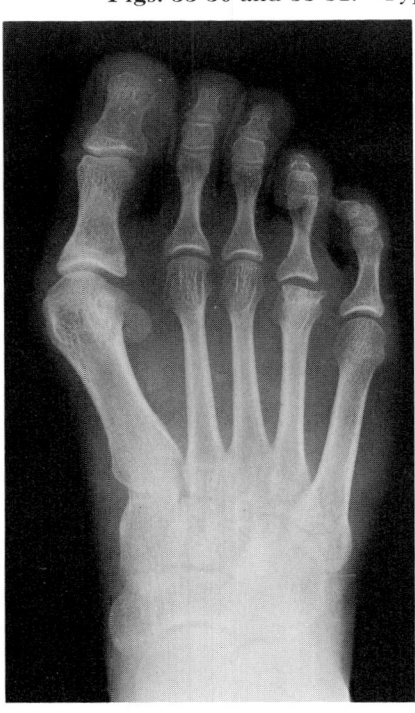

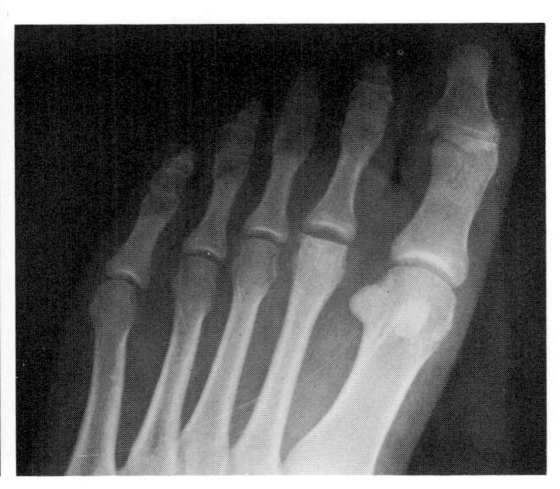

Chapter 33: INJURIES OF THE FOOT / **861**

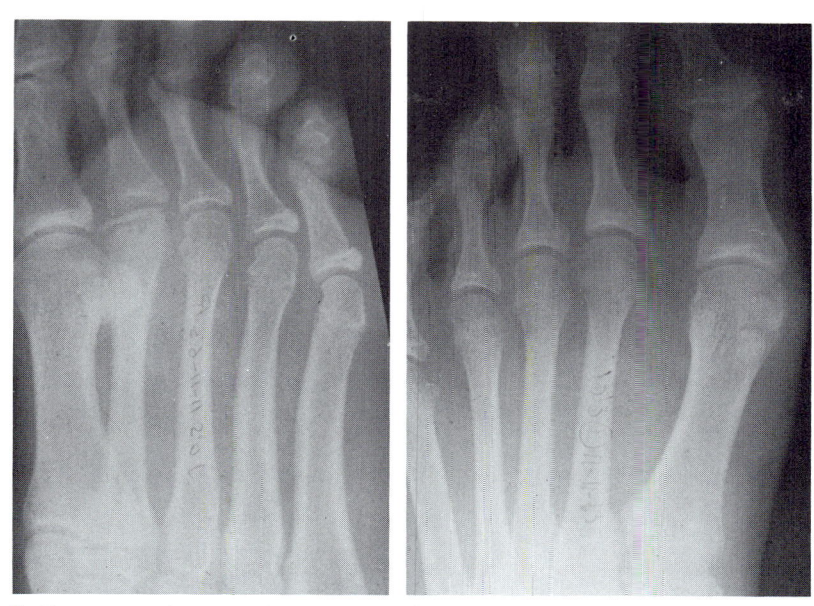

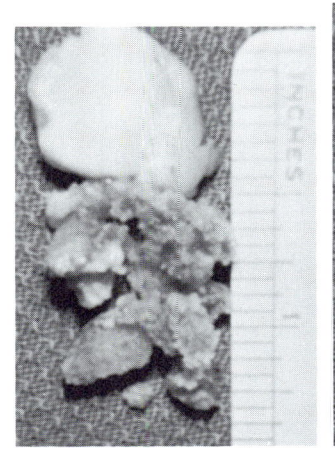

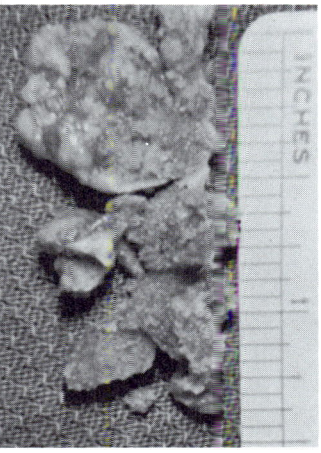

Fig. 33-32 (left). — Typical view of Freiberg's infraction of head and neck of second metatarsal of right foot. The shortening of the shaft in comparison with the left, or normal, side, the increased size and flattening of the articular surface are characteristic findings.

Fig. 33-33 (right). — The normal left foot with longer second metatarsal shaft, normal head and round head are quite noticeably different from the one on the injured right foot shown in Figure 33-32.

ent, annoying pain in the second metatarsal of her left foot. She first noticed this 5 months prior to her initial visit to my office. X-ray films taken at the time of her visit demonstrated the lesion, but she, too, has procrastinated about definitive treatment.

Definitive treatment can be achieved, however, as was demonstrated in the following case.

Fig. 33-34 (left). — Articular surface of the excised head of second metatarsal and fragments of bone comprising both head and neck of the portion removed.

Fig. 33-35 (right). — Other side of the portions of the head and neck removed, showing the degree of necrosis present approximately 6 months after injury.

862 / *Robert J. Joplin*

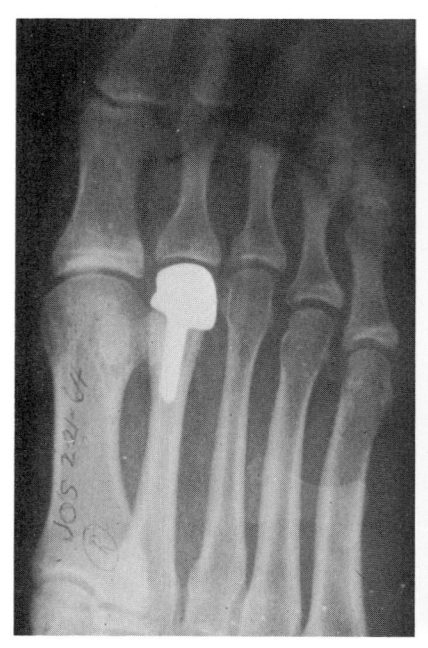

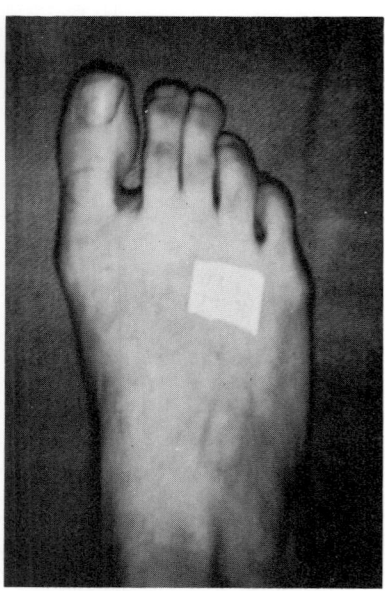

Fig. 33-36 (left).—The Vitallium stem prosthesis after insertion into shaft of second metatarsal of right foot.
Fig. 33-37 (right).—Photograph of patient's injured foot at follow-up visit 7 years after surgery shows an essentially normal extremity. The final result was rated $A_4E_4F_4$.

Fig. 33-38 (left).—Follow-up x-ray film 8 years after surgery. Note the small fragment of bone on the fibular side of the prosthesis. She has lost no time from her work and skis frequently.
Fig. 33-39 (right).—Appearance of both feet 8 years after surgery. (Photograph taken on same date as x-ray film shown in Fig. 33-38.)

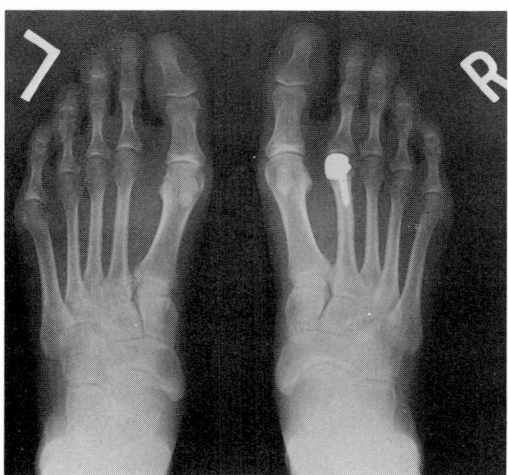

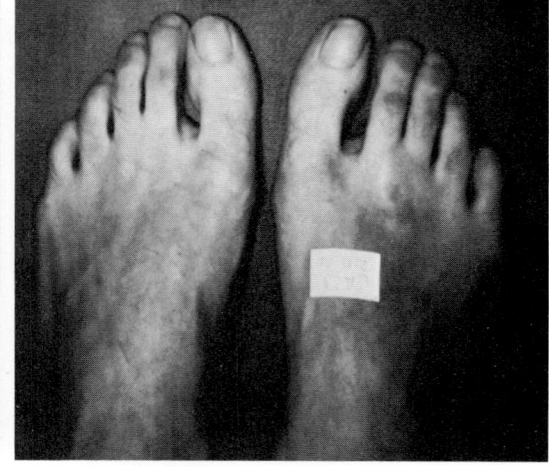

Chapter 33: INJURIES OF THE FOOT / 863

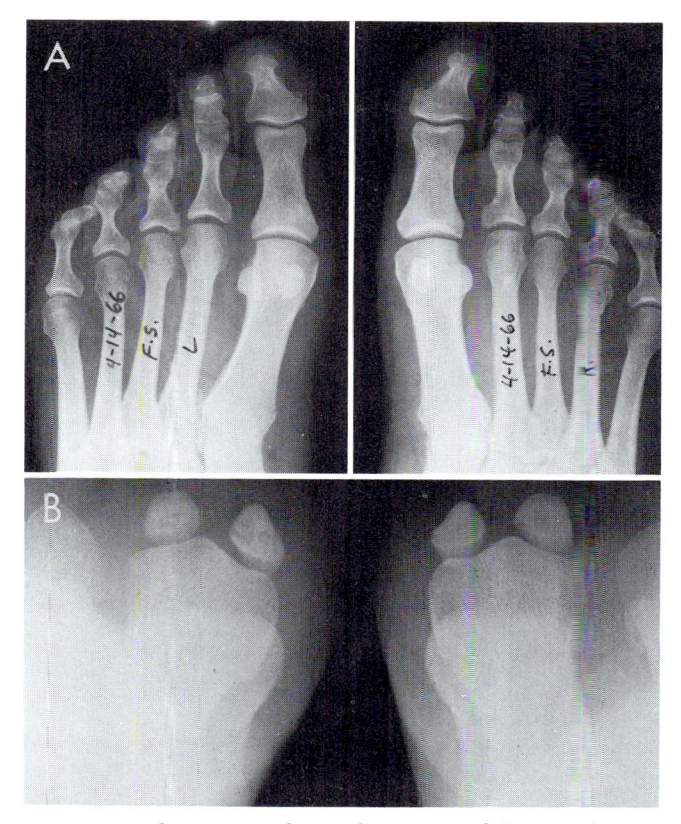

Fig. 33-40. — Demonstrating a faint, irregular, rather serrated fracture line running transversely across the tibial sesamoid in both the anteroposterior (**A**) and sesamoid (**B**) views of the left foot.

Fig. 33-41. — Showing the sesamoid bone just after removal in the operating room before (**A**) and after (**B**) pulling the fragments apart to demonstrate the fracture line and callus within.

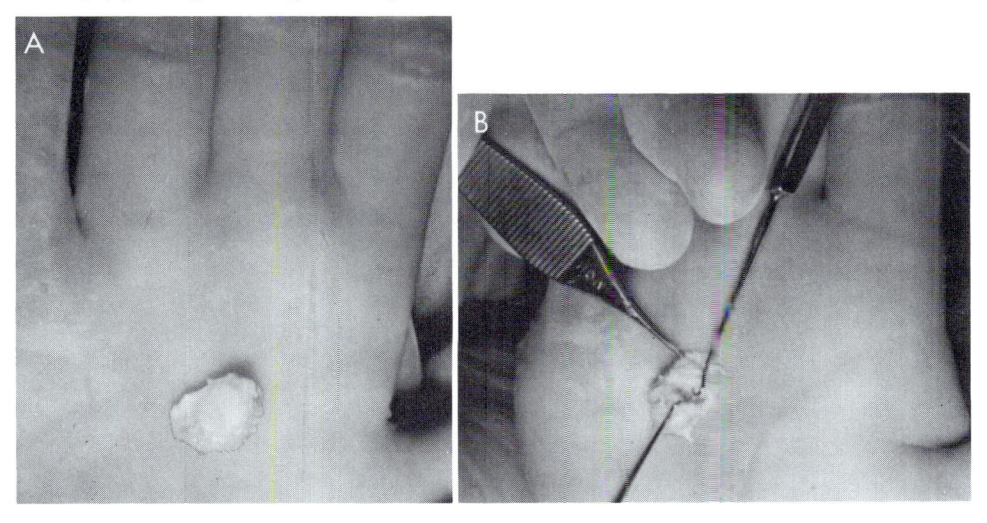

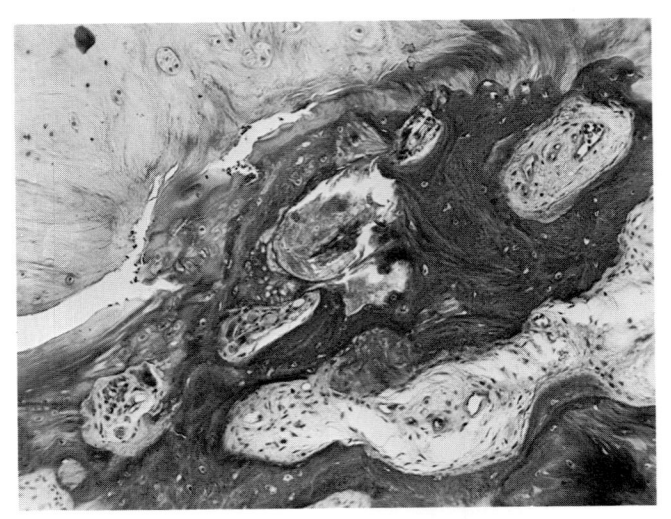

Fig. 33-42.—Microfracture of the sesamoid bone involving articular cartilage and underlying bone. There is fibrous union.

FREIBERG'S INFRACTION: A NEW WAY OF TREATMENT.—A 14-year-old girl stubbed the toes of her right foot on a step. The next day she was able to walk, but the lesser toes were swollen. She was able to run, but there was tenderness of the heads of the metatarsals of the second and third toes, with pain radiating to the second and third toes.

Examination revealed localized swelling of the second metatarsophalangeal joint, with some tenderness on palpation in this area.

Freiberg's infraction was suspected and confirmed on x-ray films.

The young lady was purported to be the fastest runner in her school and was anxious to compete in that sport the following spring. In order to ready her for this, and with the approval of her referring physician, it was decided to place a Vitallium prosthesis on the shaft of the

Fig. 33-43.—Revealing traumatic changes of the proper digital nerve (**A**) and a neuroma (**B**) in continuity with its localized enlargement.

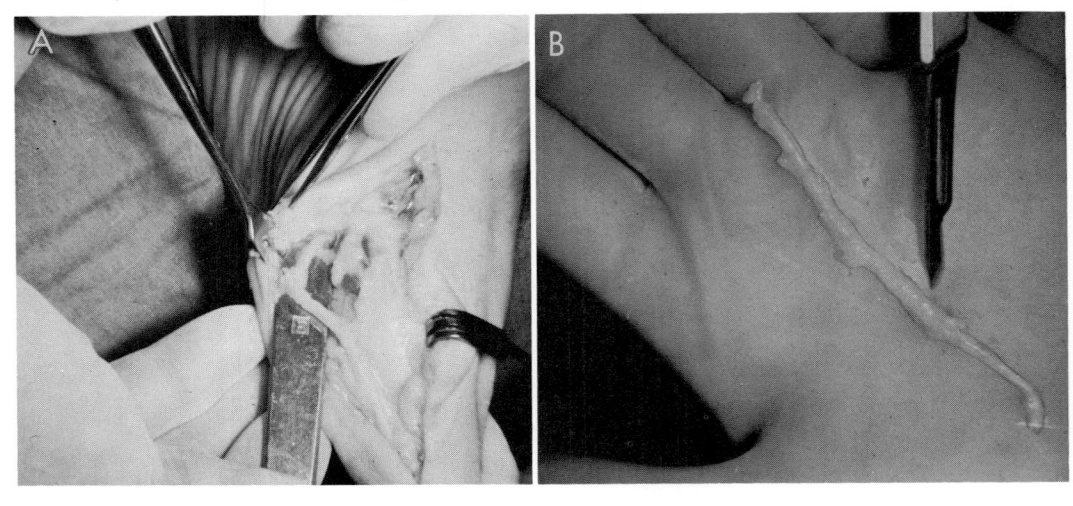

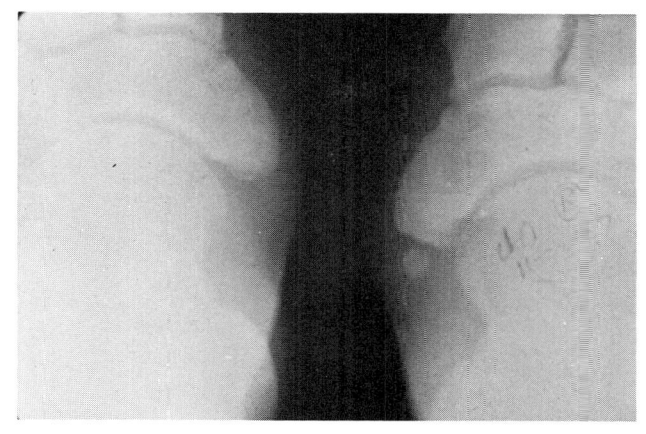

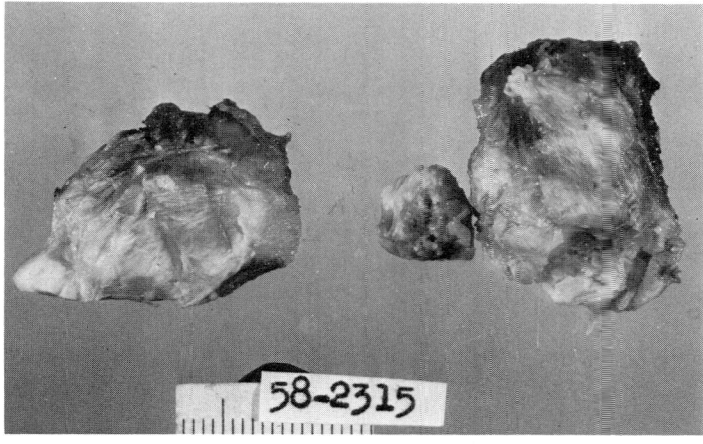

Fig. 33-44 (top).—Anteroposterior view of both right and left feet to show the intact accessory scaphoid on the left and the recently separated (fractured) one on the right.

Fig. 33-45 (bottom).—Photograph of the gross specimens removed. The recently separated fragment can be seen on the specimen at the right.

second metatarsal. X-ray films of the opposite foot were sent to the Austenal Company for the manufacture of a Vitallium prosthesis the size of the head of the second toe. On arrival of the prosthesis in February of the following year, operation was carried out as follows: An incision was made over the dorsal surface of the second metatarsal. The head of the second metatarsal was excised; the articular surface came off quite easily and appeared necrotic beneath the glistening cartilage, which was slightly yellow in its center. A Vitallium stem prosthesis was inserted, with the base of the prosthesis snug on the amputated neck. Sterile dressings were applied. Pathologic examination of the specimen confirmed the diagnosis.

Convalescence was uneventful, with partial weight bearing allowed 10 days after operation and full weight bearing by 3 weeks. A photograph taken 7 years after operation and x-ray films and a photograph taken 1 year later show a satisfactory result. The patient was working as a hostess and dental hygienist, standing on her feet most of the day without pain.

FRACTURED SESAMOID.—Strange as it may seem, the smallest bone in the foot can be not only most annoying, painful

866 / Robert J. Joplin

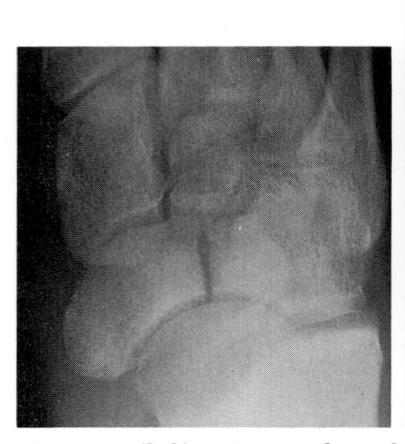

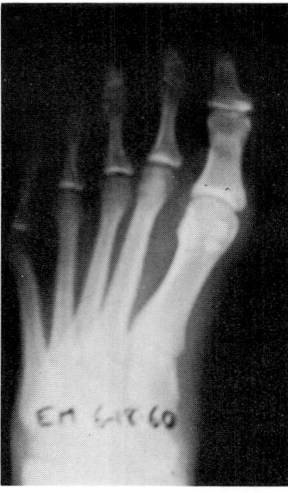

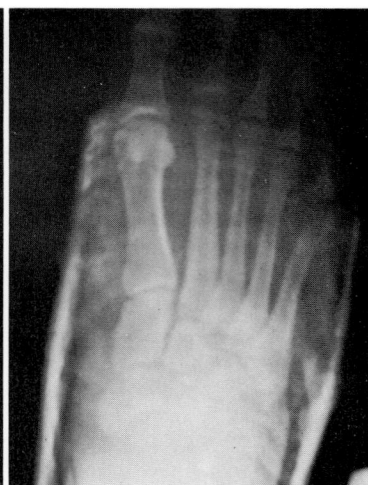

Fig. 33-46 (left).—Fractured tarsal navicula. This is a vertical fracture through the tarsal navicular that divides the bone into a lateral third and medial two-thirds. The fragments are separated about 2 mm but otherwise are in good alignment.

Fig. 33-47 (right).—Anteroposterior view of right foot in plaster-of-Paris boot, revealing good position of fragments. X-ray film of left foot was taken to eliminate possibility of a bipartite navicula. The fracture was due to acute injury.

and disabling but may be the most controversial when a positive diagnosis is required.

A 42-year-old female sustained marked pronation weight-bearing stress of the foot with exquisite pain localized beneath her first metatarsophalangeal joint. Pain persisted on weight bearing.

When seen 1 month following injury, the swelling had subsided somewhat, but localized tenderness beneath the head of the first metatarsal was present. The diagnosis of fractured sesamoid was confirmed on x-ray, which showed a faint, somewhat serrated line transversely across the sesamoid. Due to continuing pain and disability, the sesamoid was excised. Pathologic study revealed "fracture and early callus formation."

An incidental finding was a traumatized proper digital nerve on the inferior tibial aspect of the ball of the foot. Be-

Fig. 33-48 (left).—Anteroposterior and oblique views after removal of the plaster boot, demonstrating that there was no fracture of any other tarsal bones.

Fig. 33-49 (right).—X-ray film approximately 9 months after injury, revealing bone atrophy and evidence suggestive of bridging of bone across the fracture line.

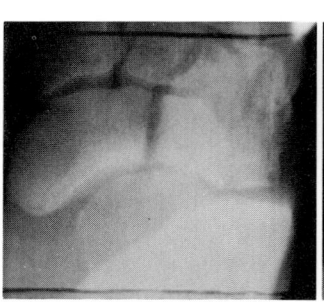

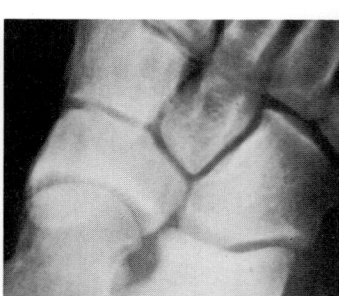

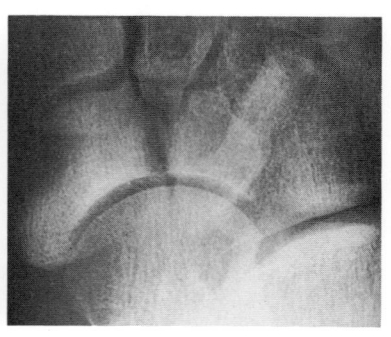

Chapter 33: INJURIES OF THE FOOT / 867

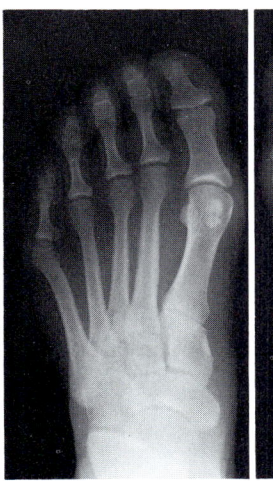

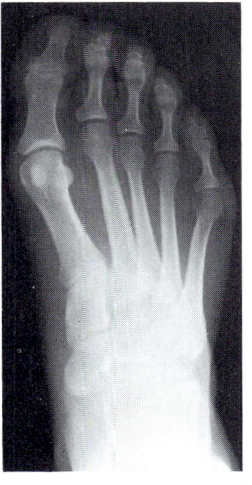

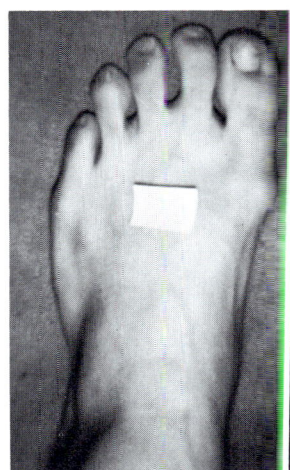

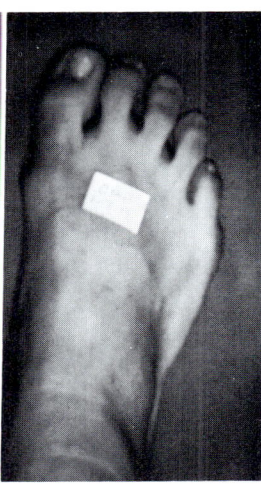

Fig. 33-50 (left).—Anteroposterior view of both feet approximately 19 months after injury, showing only faint signs of old fracture of right tarsal navicular.

Fig. 33-51 (right).—Photograph of both feet, taken at same time as x-ray film in Figure 33-50, indicating essentially normal feet. The final result was rated excellent ($A_4E_4F_4$).

cause this nerve was enlarged and demonstrated signs of localized trauma, a diagnosis of perineural fibrosis of the proper digital nerve was made and the damaged nerve was excised. Postoperatively there was complete relief from discomfort.

FRACTURED ACCESSORY SCAPHOID.—One is likely to underestimate the disability from a fractured accessory tarsal scaphoid.

An 18-year-old soccer player was kicked on the inner side of the foot, sustaining a separation of the tarsal accessory scaphoid on the right, confirmed on x-ray films. Conservative therapy, including rest, strapping and heat failed to relieve a painful snapping on the inner side of the right foot with each step. A diagnosis of a fractured or detached accessory scaphoid was made and excision of the fractured tarsal scaphoid was carried out.

No gross evidence of fracture could be detected. Convalescence was uneventful, with relief from pain postoperatively. Examination of the excised specimen showed an infraction with healing.

FRACTURED TARSAL NAVICULA.—A 16-year-old girl developed pain in the foot after running. X-ray films revealed a vertical fracture through the narrow portion of the tarsal navicula opposite the middle of the second cuneiform. A plaster boot was applied.

After removal of the cast, a circumferential 2-inch gauze bandage was applied around the tarsal area of the right foot and the patient began a non-weight-bearing crutch gait.

The patient was seen again the following autumn. She had discarded crutches but was wearing the circumferential gauze bandage and was bearing weight. X-ray films 6 months later revealed considerable bone atrophy generally but evidence of bridging of bone across the gap, which indicated healing.

Later x-ray films after injury revealed healing of the fractured tarsal navicula with only faint signs of the old fracture. The patient had no symptoms.

BIBLIOGRAPHY

1. Allan, J. H.: Trauma to the foot and ankle, Surg. Clin. North Am. 27:1505, 1947.
2. Bertelsen, A., and Hasner, E.: Primary results of treatment of fracture of the os calcis by "foot-free walking bandage" and early movement, Acta Orthop. Scand. 21:140, 1951.
3. Blair, H. C.: Comminuted fractures and fracture dislocations of the body of the astragalus, Am. J. Surg. 59:37, 1943.

4. Böhler, L.: Diagnosis, pathology and treatment of fracture of the os calcis, J. Bone Joint Surg. 13:75, 1931.
5. Boyd, H. B., and Knight, R. A.: Fractures of the astragalus, South. Med. J. 2:160, 1942.
6. Bradford, C., and Larsen, I.: Sprain fractures of the anterior process of the os calcis, N. Engl. J. Med. 244:970, 1951.
7. Christopher, F.: Fractures of the anterior process of the calcaneus, J. Bone Joint Surg. 13:877, 1931.
8. Conn, H. R.: The treatment of fractures of the os calcis, J. Bone Joint Surg. 17A:392, 1953.
9. Conwell, H. E., and Alldredge, R. H.: Complete compound comminuted fracture dislocation of the astragalus, Surgery 1:222, 1937.
10. Cotton, F. J.: Os calcis fractures, Trans. Am. Surg. Assoc. 34:404, 1916.
11. Cotton, F. J., and Henderson, F. F.: Results of fractures of the os calcis, Am. J. Orthop. Surg. 14:290, 1916.
12. Cotton, F. J., and Wilson, L. F.: Fractures of the os calcis, Boston M. & S. J. 159:559, 1908.
13. Dachtler, H. W.: Fractures of the anterior superior portion of the os calcis due to indirect violence, Am. J. Roentgenol. 25:629, 1931.
14. Essex-Lopresti, P.: The mechanism, reduction technique and results of fractures of the os calcis, Br. J. Surg. 39:395, 1952.
15. Gallie, W. E.: Subastragalar arthrodesis in fractures of the os calcis, J. Bone Joint Surg. 25:731, 1943.
16. Geckeler, E. O.: Comminuted fractures of the os calcis, Arch. Surg. 61:469, 1950.
17. Gellman, M.: Fractures of the anterior process of calcaneum, J. Bone Joint Surg. 33-A:382, 1951.
18. Gibson, A., and Inkster, R. C.: Fractures of the talus, Can. Med. Assoc. J. 31:357, 1934.
19. Harris, R. I.: Fractures of the os calcis: Their treatment by triradiate traction and subastragalar fusion, Ann. Surg. 124:1082, 1946.
20. Harris, R. I.: Fracture of the os calcis, Surg. Gynecol. Obstet. 84:374, 1947.
21. Hermann, O. J.: Conservative therapy in fractures of the os calcis, J. Bone Joint Surg. 19:709, 1937.
22. Lipscomb, P. R., and Ghormley, R. K.: Old and new fractures and fracture-dislocations of the astragalus, Surg. Clin. North Am. 23:995, 1943.
23. McKeever, F. M.: Fracture of the neck of the astragalus, Arch. Surg. 46:720, 1943.
24. McKeever, F. M.: Fractures of tarsal and metatarsal bones, Surg. Gynecol. Obstet. 90:375, 1950.
25. Palmer, I.: The mechanism and treatment of fractures of the calcaneus; open reduction with the use of cancellous graft, J. Bone Joint Surg. 30-A:1, 1948.
26. Pridie, K. H.: A new method of treatment for severe fractures of the os calcis, Surg. Gynecol. Obstet. 82:671, 1946.
27. Schrock, R. D., Johnson, H. F., and Walters, C. H., Jr.: Fractures and fracture-dislocations of the astragalus (talus), J. Bone Joint Surg. 24:560, 1942.
28. Taylor, R. G.: The treatment of claw toes by multiple transfers of flexor into extensor tendons, J. Bone Joint Surg. 33-B:539, 1951.

34 | Epiphyseal Injuries
CLEMENT B. SLEDGE

THE WEAKEST LINK in the articulated skeleton of a growing child is the epiphyseal growth plate. Its strength varies with growth rate, sex and hormonal status,[21] but, as a rough approximation, it is 20–50% as strong as adjacent bone and ligaments.[17] Injuries that produce ligamentous tears, fractures or dislocations in adults often will produce injuries of the growth plate in children, and radiographic examination of such "sprains" and "torn ligaments" is mandatory to assess the true nature of such injuries. Of all injuries of the long bones during childhood, approximately 15% involve the epiphyseal plate[10,26] and about one-third will produce some disturbance in longitudinal growth. In 10% of injuries of the epiphyseal plate, the growth abnormality will be significant.[25] The incidence of significant deformity can be reduced by recognition of the injury and rational treatment, based on an understanding of the anatomy and physiology of the epiphyseal growth apparatus.

HISTORICAL NOTE

Epiphyseal separations were suspected long before the discovery of x-rays by Röntgen in 1895, but only those associated with gross deformity could be recognized; these were in the distal femur, proximal humerus, distal humerus and distal radius in that order of frequency.[22] In 1898, John Polland published the first treatise on epiphyseal injuries, in which he discussed their anatomy and radiographic features and outlined methods of treatment. Since that time, numerous articles have appeared discussing these important injuries and their incidence, outlining plans of treatment and suggesting factors that influence subsequent growth at the injured plate. Most important among these is the excellent paper by Salter and Harris,[26] which provides the commonly used scheme of classification followed in this chapter. Our understanding of epiphyseal growth and the contribution of the various epiphyseal plates to skeletal growth is largely due to the work of Blount[5,6] and Green and Anderson.[14]

EPIDEMIOLOGY

A recent analysis of 330 epiphyseal injuries from the Mayo Clinic,[22] excluding injuries from birth to 12 months, revealed an overwhelming predominance of injuries to the distal radius (Table 34-1). Distal epiphyses were injured more frequently than proximal in all long bones except the humerus; boys were injured more frequently than girls in a ratio of 2:1; 62% of the injuries involved the upper extremity and the peak ages of incidence were 11–12 in females and 13–14 in males. The injuries of the distal humerus had earlier peak incidence — 4–5 for girls and 5–8 for boys. The increased incidence in males may be explained by their greater exposure to trauma and by the weaker epiphyseal plates in males.[21] The greater susceptibility of

TABLE 34-1.—INCIDENCE OF INJURY
TO THE VARIOUS EPIPHYSES[22]

LOCATION	FREQUENCY (%)
Distal radius	29.6
Distal tibia	17.8
Phalanges	12.1
Proximal humerus	6.7
Distal fibula	6.3
Distal humerus	6.0
Distal femur	5.4
Distal ulna	3.6
Phalanges (toes)	3.3
Metacarpals	3.0
Proximal femur	2.1
Proximal tibia	1.8
Metatarsals	1.8
Proximal radius	0.3

the plate during growth spurts produces an earlier age of peak incidence in females.

Larson and McMahan[20] reported that 6% of 371 athletic injuries in patients 15 years of age or younger were epiphyseal injuries and that the obese "Fröhlich type" and the tall lanky individual with ligamentous laxity and poor muscle development were particularly susceptible.

In addition to frank fractures through the epiphyseal plate seen in athletic injuries, Little League pitchers develop chronic affections of the epiphyseal plates around the elbow. Adams[1] reported that 80 Little League pitchers, age 9–14, whom he examined all had some degree of epiphysitis, osteochondritis, accelerated growth or separation of the medial humeral condyle. There also were some with osteochondritic lesions of the capitellum or radial head. He suggested that pitchers with open epiphyseal plates in the elbow be limited to 2 innings of pitching and that the throwing of curve balls be prohibited in this age group.

Another injury seen with increased frequency in the child athlete is the deceleration injury of the proximal tibial epiphyseal plate seen in broad jumpers and baseball players sliding into base.

ANATOMY AND PHYSIOLOGY OF THE EPIPHYSEAL PLATE[23]

Longitudinal growth of the skeleton occurs at the epiphyseal plates by the sequential and orderly replication of chondrocytes and their subsequent elaboration of a hyaline matrix composed of collagen and protein-polysaccharide. The cells become hypertrophic and partially degrade the surrounding matrix, which then is calcified, invaded by blood vessels and replaced by bone.[27] Since this sequence is dependent on proliferation of chondrocytes, it is the viability of these cells that will determine if an injury to the plate will produce abnormalities of growth. The germinal zone lies adjacent to the true epiphysis of the bone and receives its nutrition from vessels that penetrate the secondary center of ossification in the epiphysis. After formation of the secondary center (epiphyseal ossification center), a bony plate overlies the germinal zone. Vessels enter the epiphysis, branch and divide to form an arborizing network above the bone plate, which they then penetrate at numerous intervals as terminal arterioles (see Fig. 34-2, C). Each of these terminal branches supplies 4–10 cell columns of the plate but does not penetrate the columns themselves.[28] The blood supply to these crucial germinal cells thus is of a terminal nature and is susceptible to injury in two places —as it enters the epiphysis and as it arborizes through the subepiphyseal bone plate.

Just as the proliferation of chondrocytes in the germinal zone is dependent on the epiphyseal vessels, the progressive alteration of the plate (hypertrophy of cells, degradation of matrix with calcification and replacement by bone) is brought about by invasion of the plate by the metaphyseal vessels. Four-fifths of the vessels penetrating the metaphyseal side of the plate are terminal branches of the nutrient artery and supply the central portion of the plate. The peripheral one-

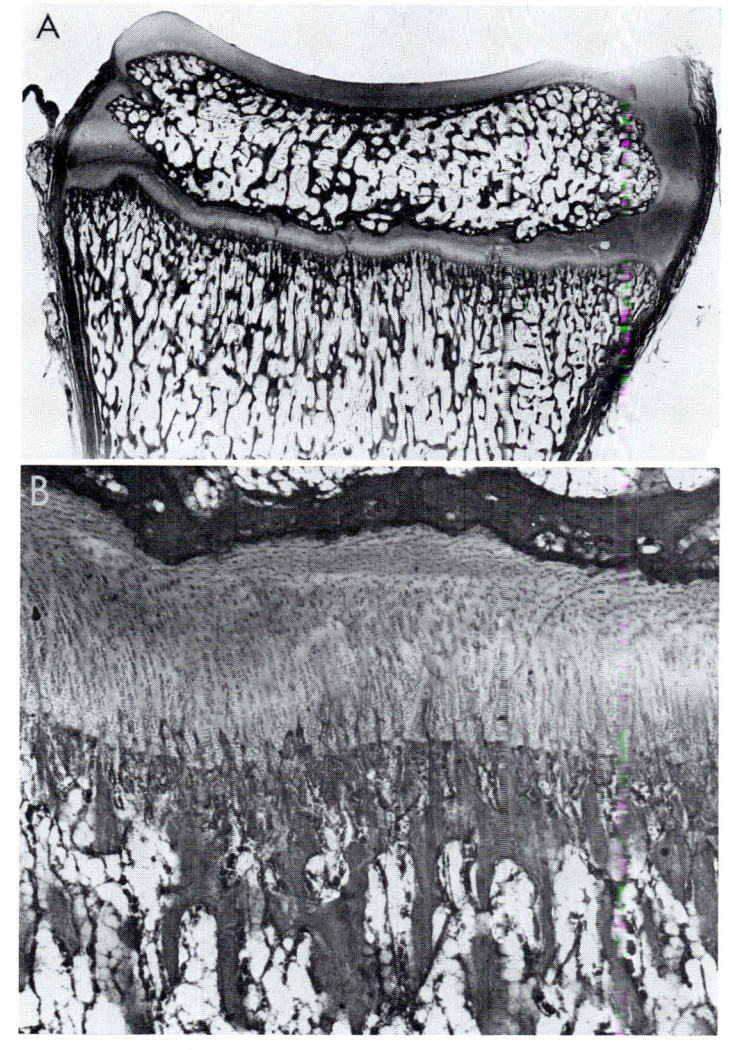

Fig. 34-1.—**A,** cross section of the proximal tibial epiphysis of a 12-year-old child. **B,** high-power photomicrograph of the epiphyseal plate with the various zones apparent. See Figure 34-2, *C* for diagrammatic representation.

fifth of the plate is supplied by vessels that penetrate the metaphysis from the surrounding soft tissues.

Trueta[28] has clearly demonstrated the dual nature of the blood supply of the epiphyseal plate and the results of interruption of either component. Transient ischemia to the germinal zone by interruption of the epiphyseal vessels leads to death of those cells and failure of growth. Since the metaphyseal vessels are responsible only for removal of the cartilaginous plate, their interruption leads to an increased thickness of the plate as chondrocytes pile up. On re-establishment of the metaphyseal blood supply, vascular invasion of the thickened plate rapidly results in restoration of a normal

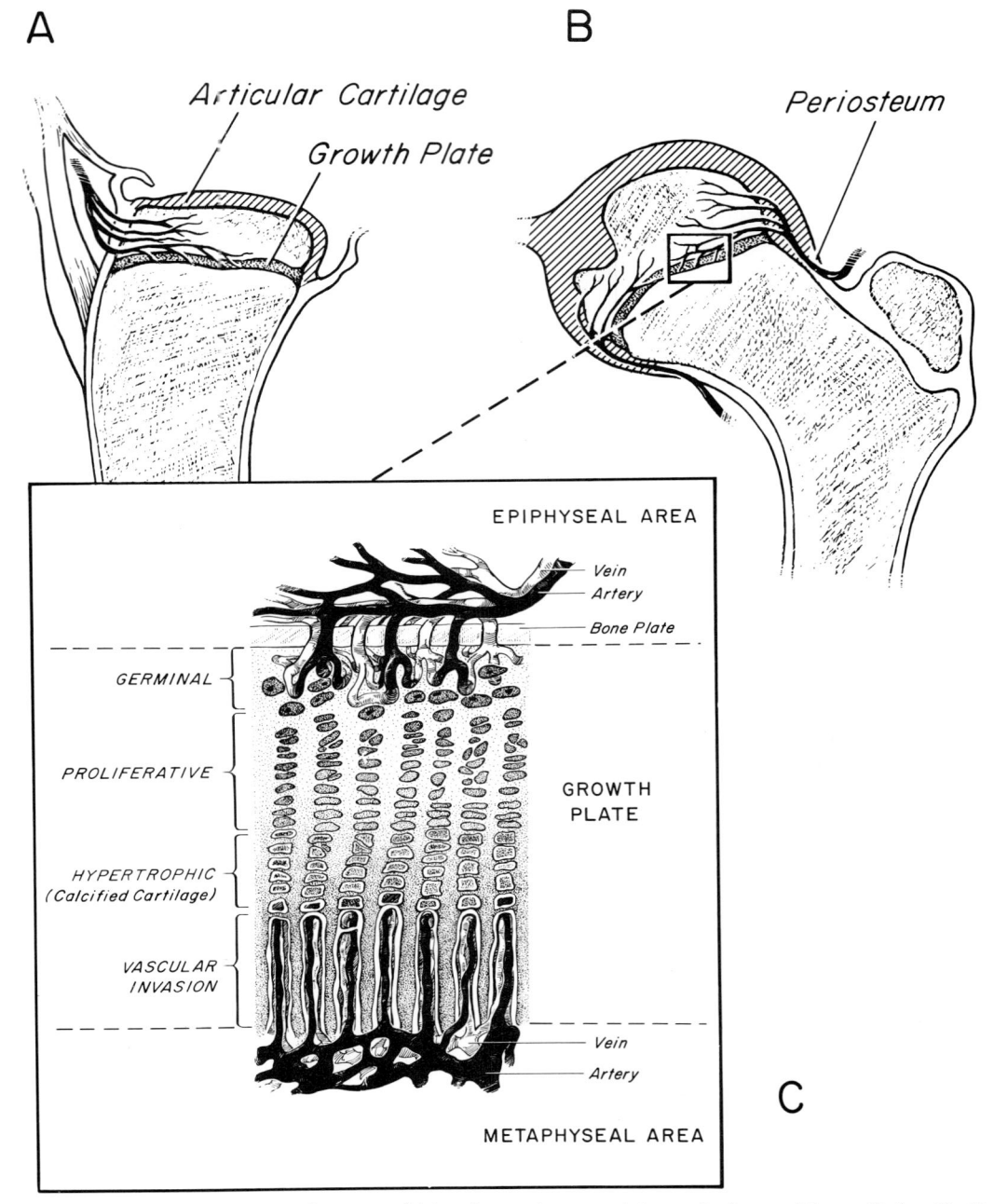

Fig. 34-2.—The two general types of blood supply to epiphyseal plates. (From Dale, G. G., and Harris, W. R.: Prognosis of epiphyseal separation, J. Bone Joint Surg. 40-B:116, 1958.) **A**, the more common type of blood supply through abundant peripheral soft tissue attachments to the secondary center. **B**, the less common type of blood supply, in which the course of the artery traversing the rim of the epiphyseal plate renders it liable to injury. **C**, diagrammatic representation of the blood supply to the germinal zone of an epiphyseal plate. Blood vessels enter the secondary center of ossification, perforate the bony plate overlying the germinal zone and arborize to supply the columns of proliferating cells. The vessel is vulnerable as it enters the ossification center and again as it divides into terminal arterioles and penetrates the bony plate.

thickness without alteration of growth.

In addition to this all-or-none response of the germinal layer of the epiphyseal plate to interruption of its blood supply, the plate apparatus is responsible for the plasticity of growing bone and its responsiveness to pressure.[29] In 1862, Hueter and Volkmann separately stated what has since been known as the law of Hueter and Volkmann that "pressure parallel to the axis of epiphyseal growth affects the rate of such growth and that increased pressure inhibits growth and decreased pressure favors growth."[15] This rule of epiphyseal growth is used widely in the correction of deformities in the growing child, ranging from plaster correction of clubfoot and correction of tibial torsion with night splints to correction of angular deformities by the use of staples. Experimental work leading to the development of epiphyseal stapling as a clinically useful procedure demonstrated that the forces of growth in the child can break staples that are able to withstand 900 pounds of distraction in tests.[5] It also was demonstrated that minor degrees of pressure can slow growth without stopping it entirely.[4, 6] Since stapling of the epiphyseal plate does not damage the epiphyseal blood supply, one may leave staples in situ with the expectation that growth will continue after the removal of the staples. Staples have been safely left in place for up to 2 years. The mechanism by which pressure affects the rate of growth of the epiphyseal plate is not known. It appears to be a biologic expression of the physical-chemical principle of Le Châtelier, which states that pressure on a chemical equilibrium will result in a shift of that equilibrium in the direction that relieves that pressure. Since the growing epiphyseal plate exerts considerable pressure, pressure applied to the plate will result in diminution of the growth rate. Ehrlich, Mankin and Treadwell[13] recently have demonstrated that the first change seen in the epiphyseal plate after stapling is a decrease in the rate of DNA synthesis in the proliferating cells, followed by a decrease in the cellular content of degradative enzymes and a loss of polysaccharide content.

Given the fact that the ultimate outcome of a fracture through the epiphyseal plate depends on the integrity of the blood supply to the germinal cells, it is apparent that a knowledge of the blood supply to each epiphysis and the pathway of the fracture line would be necessary to predict the outcome of an epiphyseal fracture. Fortunately, these anatomic variables are limited and only a few basic concepts are necessary.

BLOOD SUPPLY TO THE EPIPHYSIS

Two types of epiphyseal blood supply can be identified. The most common type exists in epiphyses that have periosteal or ligamentous attachments at their margins (Fig. 34-2, A). Fractures through this type of plate are less likely to damage the epiphyseal blood supply because of this arrangement. The less common type of blood supply exists in epiphyses that are entirely intra-articular, such as the proximal femoral and proximal radial epiphyses. In this situation, epiphyseal vessels traverse the margins of the plate, closely attached to the plate by the perichondral rim (Fig. 34-2, B). These vessels are extremely susceptible to injury. The fracture line emerging from the plate is quite likely to rupture such vessels, leading to avascular necrosis of part or all of the secondary center of ossification and death of the subjacent germinal zone of the plate. Fortunately, this vascular arrangement exists in only these two epiphyses, neither of which is particularly prone to injury because of its anatomic location and wide range of motion.

COURSE OF THE FRACTURE LINE
(Fig. 34-3)

The partial loss of matrix that accompanies hypertrophy of epiphyseal chondrocytes plus the Swiss cheese configuration of the hypertrophic zone produces an

TYPE	INCIDENCE (%)	USUAL SITE	PROGNOSIS-GROWTH
I	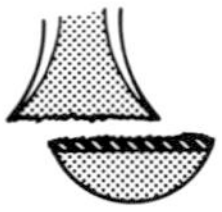 6	Proximal Femur Distal Femur (Young) Proximal Humerus (Young)	Poor * Fair † Good
II	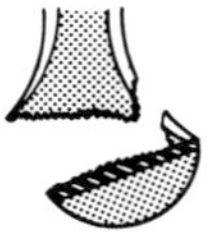 75	Distal Radius Proximal Radius Proximal Humerus (Older) Distal Femur (Older)	Incomplete → Good with accurate reduction Complete → Poor * Good Fair †
III	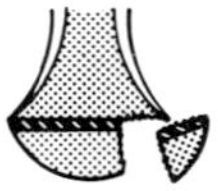 8	Distal Tibia Phalanges	Fair ‡ Good
IV	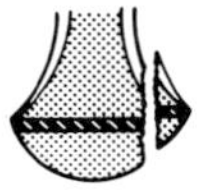 10	Humerus – lateral condyle	Good ‡
V	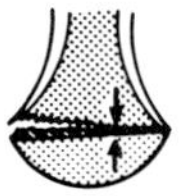 1	Distal Tibia Proximal Tibia	Poor Poor

Fig. 34-3.—Classification of epiphyseal injuries. The classification is based on the course of the fracture line through or across the plate, and its prognostic value relates to the potential for vascular damage. *—The blood supply of totally intra-articular epiphyses (proximal femur and proximal radius) is precarious. Avascular necrosis of the secondary center of ossification and growth arrest, therefore, are frequent complications of epiphyseal separations in these locations. †—The irregular plane of the distal femoral epiphyseal plate, producing a central "break," may result in damage to the central germinal layer and growth retardation. ‡—Types III and IV require exact reduction because of their involvement of the articular surface. In Type IV, the possibility of cross-bridging between metaphysis and epiphysis also demands exact reduction.

area of weakness. The deposition of mineral salts in the zone of provisional calcification reinforces the plate, leaving the hypertrophic zone just adjacent to the calcified zone as a localized zone of weakness that offers little resistance to shearing or tensile forces. The fracture begins on the side subjected to tension and propagates through the hypertrophic zone.[16] If the apparent force is purely shear, a linear fracture through the hypertrophic zone results (Type I). Combinations of shear with tension and compression are more common, however, and the fracture line, after traversing most of the width of the plate in the hypertrophic zone, veers off into the cancellous metaphysis, then out through the cortex, leaving a triangular fragment of metaphysis attached to the epiphysis and epiphyseal plate on the compression side (Type II). Tension from attached ligaments or muscle origins may produce avulsions of a portion of the epiphysis (Type III), seen commonly in the phalanges, distal tibia and around the elbow. Since the fragment usually is pulled off with some tissue attachments intact, the growth prognosis is excellent and treatment should be directed toward producing a smooth articular surface. The same considerations apply to Type IV fractures, produced by compression or tension, except that imperfect reduction may leave metaphyseal cancellous bone contiguous with cancellous bone of the secondary center of ossification in the epiphysis, and healing of these two structures will produce a bony bridge that will terminate growth on that side of the plate, producing an angular deformity if the fracture is peripheral and growth potential remains, and closure of the plate if the fracture is in the central portion. Epiphyses held rigidly in a mortise by bone or ligamentous structures and adjacent to uniaxial joints are susceptible to Type V injuries, which carry the poorest prognosis. In these, the cribriform subepiphyseal bone plate is crushed, damaging the vessels supplying the germinal zone. Growth abnormalities uniformly result. The proximal and distal tibial epiphyses are examples of such susceptible structures. Angular forces applied at a right angle to the plane of joint motion produce crushing on the compression side. It is paradoxic that the radiologically most innocuous lesion, therefore, carries the worst prognosis.

The prognostic variables are simple to state: anatomic arrangement of blood supply (Type A or B), pathway of the fracture line (Types I, II, III or IV) and the presence or absence of compression damage to the subepiphyseal bone plate. The severity of deformity is related, of course, to the growth contribution of the individual epiphyseal plate (Table 34-2). Some element of compression often accompanies "typical" epiphyseal fractures, and vascular damage may not be suspected on initial assessment of the injury. Therefore, it is suggested that all epiphyseal injuries be assessed radiographically for at least 1 year following injury or until the age of usual closure of that plate (Table 34-3).

TABLE 34-2.—RELATIVE CONTRIBUTION TO OVER-ALL LENGTH BY INDIVIDUAL EPIPHYSEAL PLATES

Humerus:	proximal—80% distal—20%	Femur:	proximal—30% distal—70%
Radius:	proximal—25% distal—75%	Tibia:	proximal—55% distal—45%

TABLE 34-3.—TIME OF APPEARANCE AND OF OSSIFICATION OF EPIPHYSES*

EPIPHYSIS	APPEARANCE	AGE AT COMPLETE OSSIFICATION
Upper humerus	At 7 weeks	19–20 years
Internal epicondyle of humerus	As early as 7 years; not constantly present until 11 years	15–17 years
External epicondyle of humerus	Not ordinarily as separate epiphysis	15–17 years
Capitellum	At 17 months	15–17 years
Trochlea humeri	As early as 8 years; not constantly present until 11 years	15–17 years
Head of radius	Occasionally at 5 years; constant at 7 years	13–14 years
Olecranon	At 8 years	14 years
Distal radius	At 6 months	20–21 years
Distal ulna	At 6–7 years	20–21 years
Head of femur	At 7–12 months	15–16 years
Greater trochanter	At 5 years	15–16 years
Lesser trochanter	At 9–11 years	15–16 years
Distal femur	Present at birth	19 years
Proximal tibia	Present at birth	19 years
Distal tibia	At 5 months	18 years
Proximal fibula	At about 5 years	15–18 years
Distal fibula	At 13 months	18 years

*From Cohn, I.: Normal Bones and Joints (New York: Paul B. Hoeber, Inc., 1924).

GENERAL NOTES ON EPIPHYSEAL SEPARATIONS

Since the crux of the problem is not the mechanical damage of the plate but whether the separation interferes with the blood supply of the epiphysis, treatment of these injuries should be designed carefully to avoid further injury to the epiphyseal blood supply. This relates not only to closed manipulative treatment but also to open surgical treatment. Excessively strenuous attempts at closed reduction, particularly if treatment is delayed beyond 10 days and healing has already begun, may easily produce vascular damage. In Types III and IV, where restoration of a smooth articular surface is the paramount aim of treatment (along with prevention of cross-union in Type IV), it often is necessary to use internal fixation that traverses the epiphyseal plate. Campbell et al.[9] have clearly shown the innocuous nature of small smooth wires or threaded wires and screws removed in a few weeks. The diameter of such defects in the plate is critical, because such defects will be filled in by cancellous bone, which, if sufficiently strong, will produce an epiphysiodesis. Small cancellous bridges seemingly are unable to withstand the considerable pressures developed by the remaining epiphyseal growth apparatus and will not produce permanent growth retardation.

Since periosteum is intact on one side of Types I and II injuries, it may be used as a hinge to effect anatomic reduction. In the event that anatomic reduction is not obtained easily, residual angular deformities may be tolerated because of the tendency of subsequent growth to correct such angular deformities, particularly in the young child and particularly if the deformity is in the direction of motion of the adjacent joint. Often it is better to accept residual angulation than to risk further damage to the plate by repeated manipulation. Healing of such separations is rapid, and immobilization usually is not necessary for longer than 4-6 weeks, depending on the size of the bone and whether it is exposed to repeated angular stress if unprotected. Type III injuries often will require open reduction and internal fixation but they also heal rapidly. Type IV injuries almost always require open reduction and internal fixation, and rapid healing can be expected.

The importance of x-ray examination in all injuries suspected of producing damage to the epiphysis has already been stressed. Two views at right angles constitute the minimal examination and if questions still exist, oblique views and comparable views of the opposite extremities should be obtained. The metaphyseal fragment associated with the Type II injury has been referred to radiographically as Thurston Holland's sign[18] and often is the only evidence that a Type II injury has been sustained and reduced spontaneously. It also indicates the side of the intact periosteal hinge, useful in carrying out manipulative reduction. A smaller fragment of metaphyseal bone often is pulled off the tension side of a Type I or II injury and is known as the "lamella sign."[25] A history of the mechanism of injury often is the only indication that a Type V injury may have been sustained.

MANAGEMENT OF INJURIES

DISTAL RADIAL EPIPHYSIS.—This injury is analogous to a Colles fracture in adults and the treatment is essentially the same. Reduction usually is quite simple, utilizing the intact dorsal periosteum. Immobilization with the forearm in pronation, the elbow at a right angle and the wrist somewhat volarly flexed for 3 weeks usually is adequate (Fig. 34-4).

PROXIMAL RADIAL EPIPHYSIS.—Injury here fortunately is quite rare, since it is of the Type II variety. The susceptibility of the blood supply of this epiphysis has already been stressed and gentle, accurate reduction should be attempted by

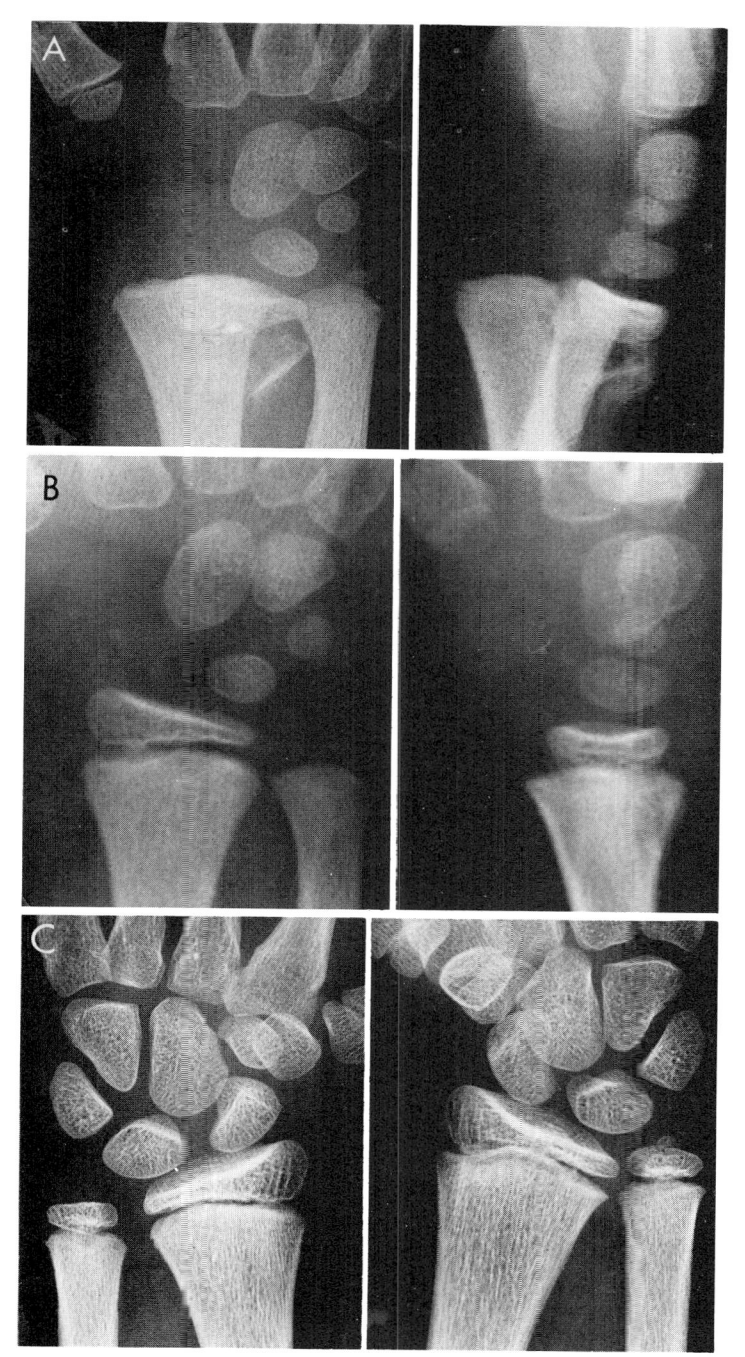

Fig. 34-4.—**A,** anteroposterior and lateral views of separation of the distal radial epiphysis in a 6-year-old boy. Note the sizable metaphyseal fragment on the ulnar side. **B,** immediately after closed reduction with an excellent anatomic restoration except for persistence of slight dorsal displacement. **C,** anteroposterior views of both wrists 4 years later. Minimal growth retardation resulted in the right distal radius.

direct pressure on the radial head with the elbow joint opened by varus stress. Pronation and supination carried out in this position with direct pressure on the epiphysis usually will result in satisfactory reduction (Fig. 34-5). If more than 15 degrees of residual angulation remains, limitation of pronation is to be expected and open reduction should be carried out. Great care should be exercised to preserve all soft tissue attachments to the epiphysis and thereby minimize the extent of the almost inevitable avascular necrosis of the epiphysis. The functional limitation secondary to premature closure is less than the limitation due to malposition of the epiphysis. Of 15 separations of the proximal radial epiphysis, 7 fused completely and 2 fused partially. All of these had an increase in the carrying angle and no patient had a perfect end result. Eighty per cent had reduction of pronation secondary to angulation of the radial head. Treatment of this injury should be directed toward restoration of the position of the proximal radial epiphysis to provide a normal range of pronation and supination.

PROXIMAL HUMERUS. — The mechanism of this injury usually is described as a fall on the extended, adducted arm. The patient falls backward, extends the arm to break the fall and lands with the hand under the buttocks. The injuries are either Type I (10%) or Type II (90%).[12] The separated epiphysis assumes a position of flexion, abduction and slight external rotation (Fig. 34-6). Reduction can be obtained by traction with the arm in the overhead position, followed by plaster immobilization in the "salute" position for 3 or 4 weeks. Up to 20 degrees of residual angular deformity and 50% contact can be accepted with the expectation that remodeling and the wide range of motion of the glenohumeral joint will produce a good functional result. Approximately 30% of these injuries will have some growth disturbance and in half of these it will be greater than ½ inch but rarely of any functional significance.

Fig. 34-5. — **A,** anteroposterior and lateral views of a fracture of the radial head in a 12-year-old boy. There is marked displacement of the proximal radial epiphysis. **B,** after reduction. **C,** 4 years after injury with uninjured side for comparison. Some deformity of the radial head and slight shortening of the radial shaft can be seen. The carrying angle was normal; flexion 140 degrees; fixed flexion 10 degrees; pronation 45 degrees; supination 85 degrees.

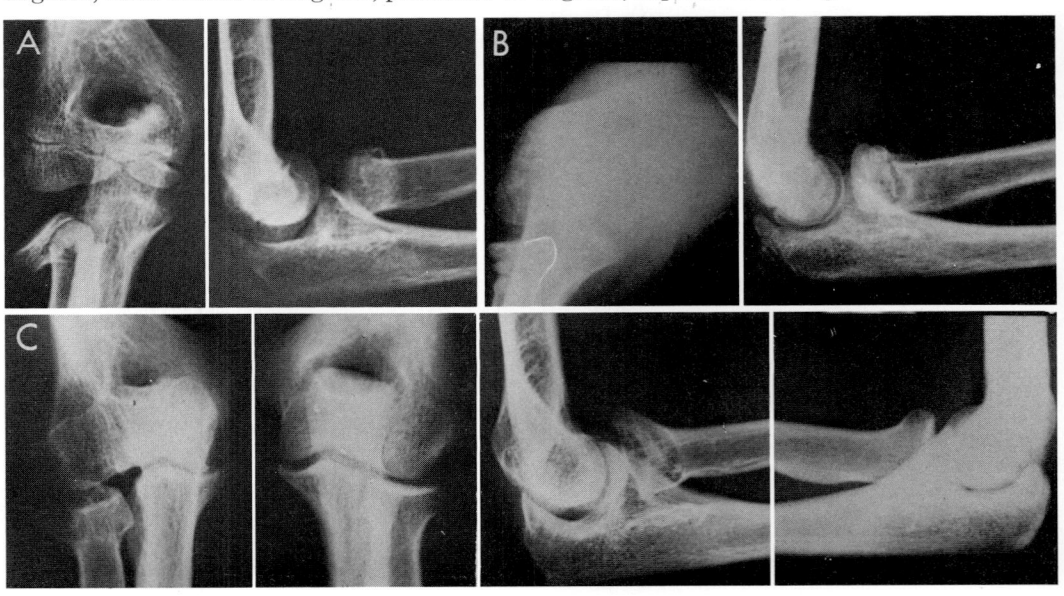

Chapter 34: EPIPHYSEAL INJURIES / 879

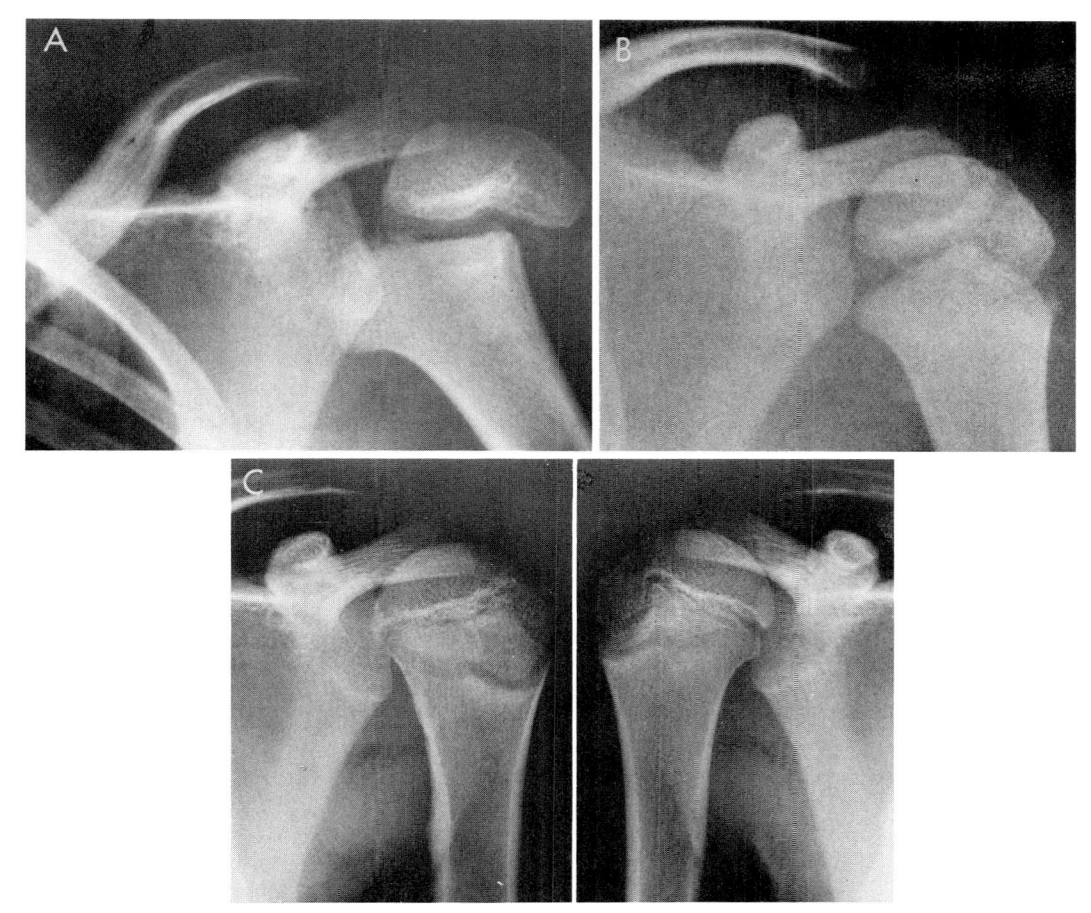

Fig. 34-6.—**A**, anteroposterior view of left shoulder of 6-year-old boy showing moderate displacement of the proximal humeral epiphysis. **B**, postreduction view. **C**, 4 years later, left and right proximal humeral epiphyses, showing minimal growth disturbance.

DISTAL HUMERUS.—Epiphyseal separations of the distal humerus are rare but it is important to distinguish between this lesion, which should be treated by a closed reduction and managed in a fashion similar to that of a supracondylar fracture, and a Type IV injury of the lateral humeral condyle.[19] If displaced, such an injury of the lateral condyle should be treated by open reduction and internal fixation to restore a smooth joint surface and to realign the epiphyseal plate. Internal fixation may be obtained either by sutures in the periosteum, Kirschner wires or by a nail. The elbow should be immobilized for 3 weeks at 90 degrees and if the fixation device traverses the epiphyseal plate, it should be removed. The prognosis from this injury, handled properly, is excellent. Inadequate reduction will result in a valgus deformity of the elbow and delayed ulnar nerve paralysis.

PROXIMAL FEMORAL EPIPHYSIS.—This injury, fortunately, is rare, since almost inevitably it leads to loss of blood supply of the proximal femoral epiphysis with consequences of both avascular necrosis of the femoral head and premature fusion

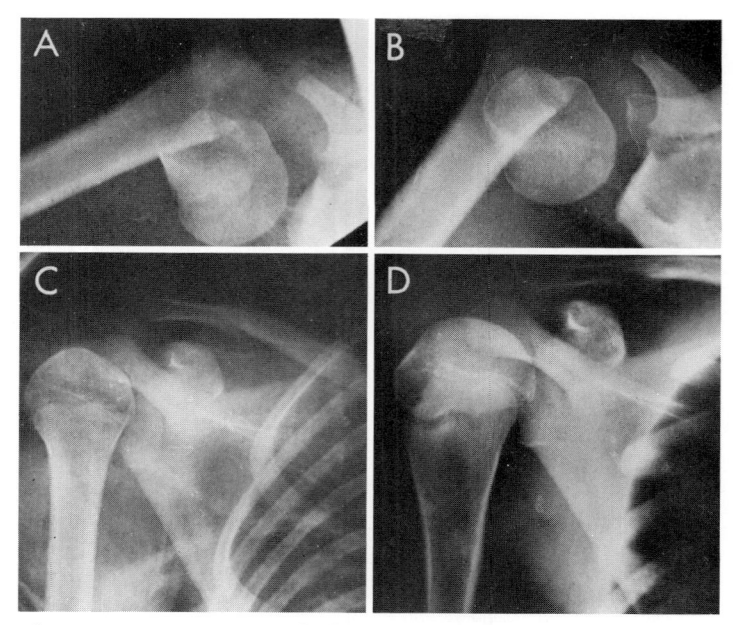

Fig. 34-7.—**A** and **B**, anteroposterior and oblique views showing separation of the proximal humeral epiphysis with severe displacement of the proximal fragment. **C**, anteroposterior view immediately after reduction by closed manipulation in the overhead position. **D**, end result showing complete correction and normal growth.

of the epiphyseal plate. Most reported cases have been of Type I, although there have been rare reports of Type II injuries to this epiphysis. Occasionally it is difficult to distinguish between a traumatic separation and a chronic slipped epiphysis, particularly in the adolescent. Helpful features are the history of the injury, the age of the child and the radiographic appearance, which may demonstrate some early remodeling in the case of the chronic slip (Table 34-4). In a recent series reported by Ratliff,[24] 13 such injuries were identified. Premature fusion of the epiphyseal plate occurred in 8 of the 13 and avascular necrosis of the secondary center of ossification in 7 of the 13. Premature fusion and avascular necrosis or nonunion individually or together occurred in 11 of the 13 patients. In general, patients who escaped the complication of avascular necrosis were under the age of 5. The age-related patterns of blood supply to the proximal femoral epiphysis have been well described by Trueta,[28] and it is possible in certain age groups to have injury to the blood supply of the epiphyseal plate without injuring the blood supply to the ossification center through the ligamentum teres. The reverse also is possible, producing avascular necrosis without premature fusion.

DISTAL FEMUR.—The injuries usually are Type II with a metaphyseal fragment and theoretically should have a good prognosis. However, the anatomy of the

TABLE 34-4.—DISTINCTION BETWEEN TRAUMATIC SEPARATIONS AND SLIPPED CAPITAL FEMORAL EPIPHYSES[24]

CHARACTERISTIC	TRAUMATIC SEPARATION	SCFE
Age	9 years	11–16 years
Onset	Sudden	Gradual
Mechanism	Severe violence	No injury or minor
Endocrine defect	None	Often

distal femoral epiphyseal plate is somewhat unusual in that its central portion has a large proximal peak. The fracture line traversing the hypertrophic zone may cut across the base of this peak, damaging the blood supply to the germinal cells in the central portion and resulting in premature closure of this central portion. Another mechanism has been proposed by Brashear,[7,8] who suggests that this peak or apex of the distal femoral epiphyseal plate may be crushed during the process of dislocation of the epiphysis, thereby damaging the germinal cells in the central portion. The presence of a metaphyseal fragment seems to offer some protection to the epiphyseal cartilage adjacent to it, whereas the epiphyseal cartilage not protected by a metaphyseal fragment frequently shows evidence of significant crush injury.

The distal femur represents a departure from the usual rather innocuous Type I and Type II injuries in that "it would thus appear that some degree of shortening due either to premature ossification or retardation of growth occurs quite frequently following fractures involving the distal femoral epiphyseal cartilaginous plate."[3]

A particularly serious injury involving the lower femoral epiphysis is that produced by hyperextension (Fig. 34-8). The posterior aspect of the metaphysis, displaced into the popliteal space, may damage the popliteal vessels. Reduction, therefore, should be obtained as gently and speedily as possible, and if there is any question as to the integrity of the popliteal circulation, surgical exploration is indicated. Salter and Harris[26] have pointed out that reduction is accomplished most easily by placing the patient face down, applying traction on the bent

Fig. 34-8.—**A,** lateral view of distal femoral epiphysis in a 7-year-old boy who was struck by an automobile. The proximal metaphysis is displaced posteriorly into the popliteal space. Treatment consisted of traction and flexion of the knee with pressure over the distal shaft posteriorly. **B,** anteroposterior and lateral views 5 years later showing the absence of deformity and continued growth at epiphyseal plate.

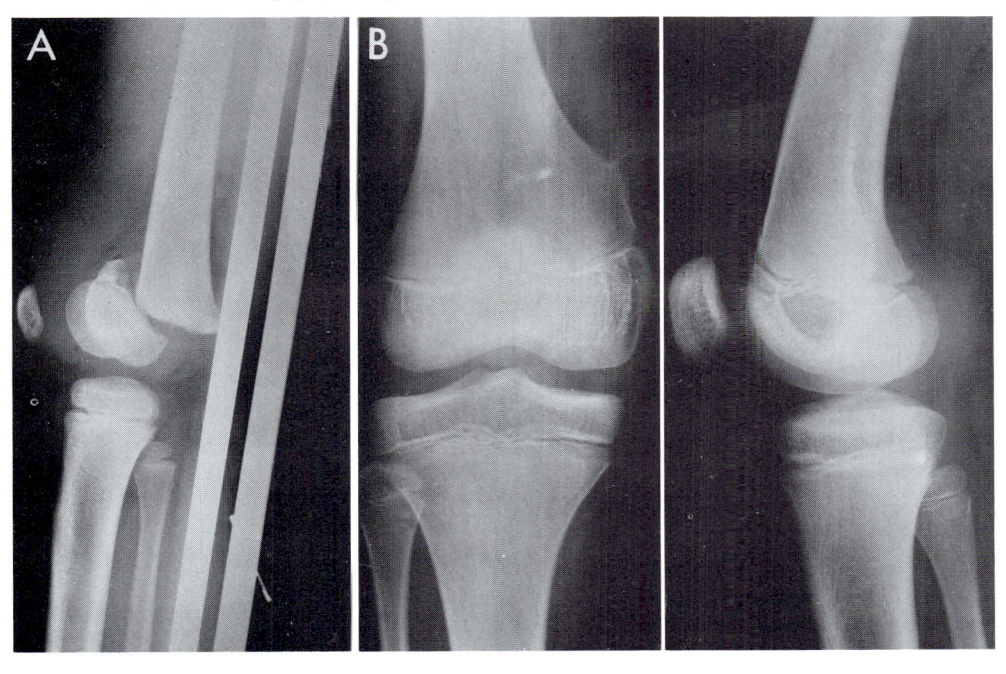

knee while pushing the proximal fragment anteriorly. Reduction is stable with the knee flexed to 90 degrees with careful observation of the circulation. The amount of flexion may be reduced after 10 days and total immobilization does not need to exceed 3 weeks.

PROXIMAL TIBIA.—The proximal tibial epiphyseal plate is somewhat protected from injury by the long anterior lip at the insertion of the patellar tendon. Epiphyseal separations and dislocations therefore are quite rare but may be sustained by athletic activity such as broad jumping and base sliding (Fig. 34-9). The recurvatum deformity resulting from premature closure of the anterior lip of the epiphysis produces a hyperextension deformity requiring osteotomy for correction. The

Fig. 34-9.—**A,** lateral and anteroposterior views of a fracture through the proximal epiphysis of the tibia in a 9-year-old boy who was struck by an automobile. **B,** a Kirschner wire was inserted in the femur, following which closed reduction was carried out and excellent position was obtained. **C,** x-ray films taken 3 months after injury revealing satisfactory healing.

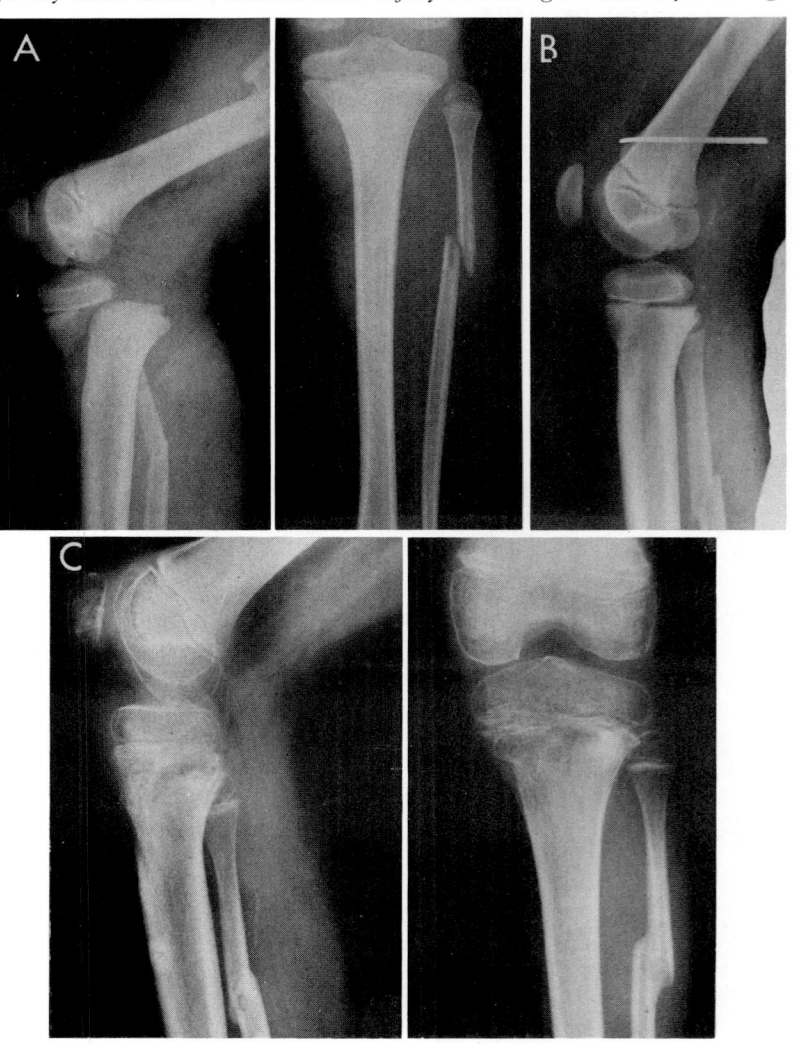

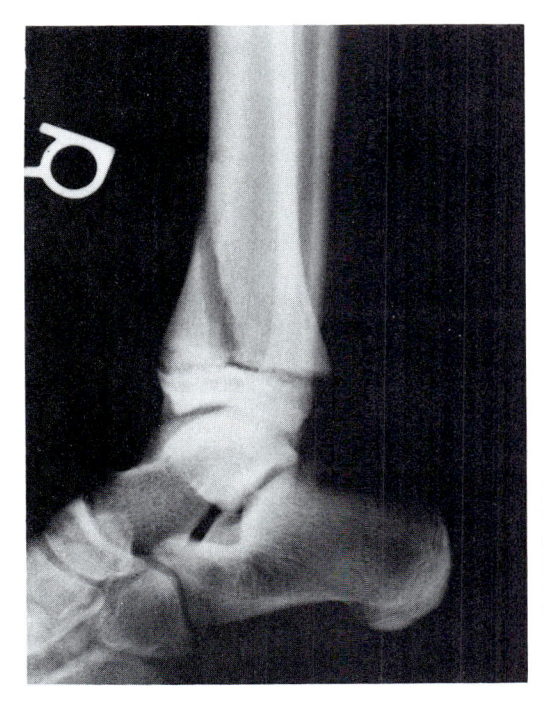

Fig. 34-10.—Type I injury to the distal tibial epiphysis sustained in a skiing accident. This injury results from falling forward over a high rigid boot with failure of heel release. The prognosis is excellent following closed manipulative reduction.

Fig. 34-11.—**Left,** anteroposterior view of the distal end of the right tibia of a 14-year-old girl who sustained a Type III injury in a fall. **Right,** anteroposterior view 15 months after injury showing satisfactory healing with an excellent articular surface and no growth abnormality.

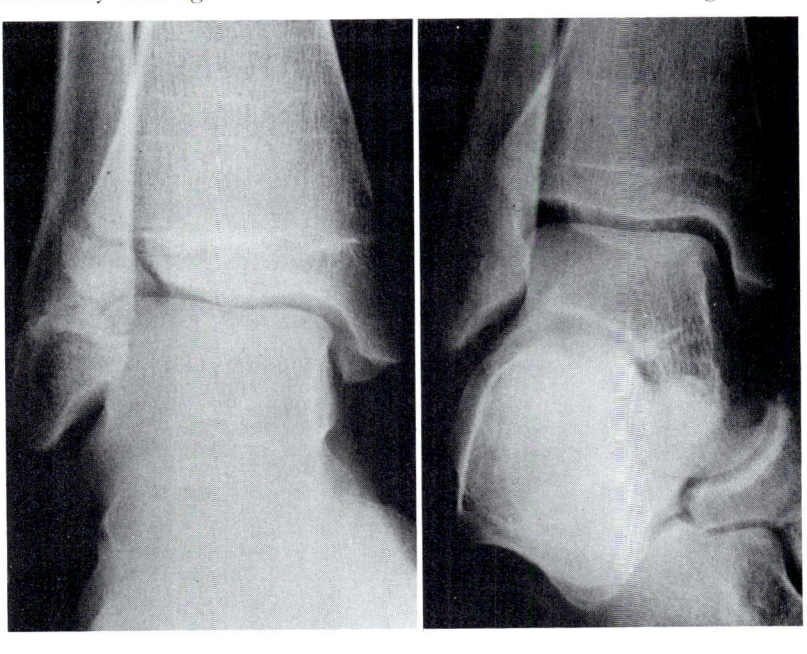

injury carries with it the same danger to the popliteal vessels described under hyperextension injuries to the distal femur.

Stress in the coronal plane may produce a Type V crush injury of the proximal tibial plate with its development of angular deformity following premature closure on the compressed side.[2]

DISTAL TIBIA.—Since the distal tibial epiphysis is adjacent to a joint that moves in only one plane and is enclosed by strong unyielding lateral ligaments, a variety of injuries may be sustained by this epiphyseal plate. Forces in the sagittal plane, seen particularly in skiing, usually will produce Type II injuries and may have a long metaphyseal fragment (Fig. 34-10). These usually are managed adequately by closed reduction. Forces acting in the coronal plane usually will produce a Type III injury (Figs. 34-11 and 34-12) and anatomic reduction is necessary to restore a smooth joint surface. This reduction usually can be accomplished by closed means but occasionally open reduction and internal fixation will be necessary. Forces in the coronal plane, if severe enough, may produce Type V crushing injuries and, indeed, this epiphyseal plate is the most common location of this ominous injury. Repeated corrective osteotomies may be necessary to maintain alignment of the ankle joint during growth. Since it is quite common for the undamaged portion of the plate to continue to grow for some time, the correction obtained by one osteotomy usually is not sufficient and will have to be repeated until growth in the uninjured portion ceases spontaneously.

Fig. 34-12.—Anteroposterior view of the left thumb showing a Type III injury to the epiphysis of the proximal phalanx. This injury was sustained in a skiing accident by the same mechanism that produces a "gamekeeper's thumb" in adults. The thumb was forced into radial deviation; the collateral ligaments held and avulsed the ulnar half of the epiphysis. Closed manipulation to restore articular congruity and maintenance of reduction for 3 weeks led to a satisfactory result.

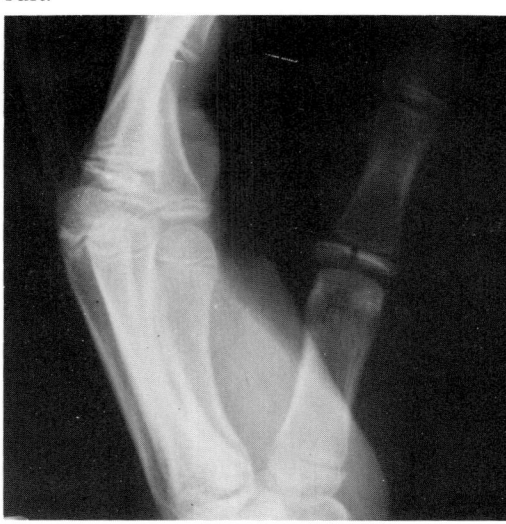

BIBLIOGRAPHY

1. Adams, J. E.: Injury to the throwing arm: A study of traumatic changes in the elbow joints of boy baseball players, Calif. Med. 102:127, 1965.
2. Aitken, A. P.: Fractures of the proximal tibial epiphyseal cartilage, Clin. Orthop. 41:92, 1965.
3. Aitken, A. P., and Magill, H. K.: Fractures involving the distal femoral epiphyseal cartilage, J. Bone Joint Surg. 34-A:96, 1952.
4. Arkin, A. M., and Katz, J. F.: The effects of pressure on epiphyseal growth: The mechanism of plasticity of growing bone, J. Bone Joint Surg. 38-A:1056, 1956.
5. Blount, W. P., and Clark, G. R.: Control of bone growth by epiphyseal stapling, J. Bone Joint Surg. 31-A:464, 1949.
6. Blount, W. P., and Zeier, F.: Control of bone length, JAMA 148:451, 1952.
7. Brashear, H. R.: Epiphyseal fractures of the lower extremity, South. Med. J. 51:845, 1958.
8. Brashear, H. R.: Epiphyseal fractures: A microscopic study of the healing process in rats, J. Bone Joint Surg. 41-A:1055, 1959.
9. Campbell, C. J., Grisolia, A., and Zanconato, G.: The effects produced in the cartilaginous epiphyseal plate of immature dogs by experimental traumata, J. Bone Joint Surg. 41-A:1221, 1959.
10. Compere, E. L.: Growth arrest in long bones as a result of fractures that include the epiphysis, JAMA 105:2140, 1935.
11. Dale, G. G., and Harris, W. R.: Prognosis of epiphyseal separations, J. Bone Joint Surg. 40-B:116, 1958.
12. Dameron, T. B., and Reibel, D. B.: Fractures involving the proximal humeral epiphyseal plate, J. Bone Joint Surg. 51-A:289, 1969.
13. Ehrlich, M. G., Mankin, H. J., and Treadwell, B. V.: Biochemical and physiological events during closure of the stapled distal femoral

epiphyseal plate in rats, J. Bone Joint Surg. 54-A:309, 1972.
14. Green, W. T., and Anderson, M.: Experiences with epiphyseal arrest in correcting discrepancies in length of the lower extremities in infantile paralysis: A method of predicting the effect, J. Bone Joint Surg. 29:659, 1947.
15. Haas, S. L.: The changes produced in the growing bone after injury to the epiphyseal cartilage plate, J. Orth. Surg. 1:67, 166 and 226, 1919.
16. Harris, W. R., and Hobson, K. W.: Histological changes in experimentally displaced upper femoral epiphyses in rabbits, J. Bone Joint Surg. 38-B:914, 1956.
17. Harsha, W. N.: Effects of trauma upon epiphyses, Clin. Orthop. 10:140, 1957.
18. Holland, T. C.: A radiological note on injuries to distal epiphyses of the radius and ulna, Proc. R. Soc. Med. 22:23, 1929.
19. Kaplan, S. S., and Reckling, F. W.: Fracture separation of the lower humeral epiphysis with medial displacement, J. Bone Joint Surg. 53-A:1105, 1971.
20. Larson, R. L., and McMahan, R. O.: The epiphyses and the childhood athlete, JAMA 196:607, 1966.
21. Morscher E.: *Strength and Morphology of Growth Cartilage under Hormonal Influence of Puberty* (Basel and New York: S. Karger, 1968).
22. Peterson, C. A., and Peterson, H. A.: Analysis of the incidence of injuries to the epiphyseal growth plate, J. Trauma 12:275, 1972.
23. Rang, M.: *The Growth Plate and Its Disorders* (Baltimore: The Williams & Wilkins Company, 1969).
24. Ratliff, A. H. C.: Traumatic separation of the upper femoral epiphysis in young children, J. Bone Joint Surg. 5-B:757, 1968.
25. Rogers, L.: The radiography of epiphyseal injuries, Radiology 96:289, 1970.
26. Salter, R. B., and Harris, W. R.: Injuries involving the epiphyseal plate, J. Bone Joint Surg. 45-A:587, 1963.
27. Sledge, C. B.: Biochemical events in the epiphyseal plate and their physiological control, Clin. Orthop. 61:37, 1968.
28. Trueta, J.: *Studies of the Development and Decay of the Human Frame* (Philadelphia: W. B. Saunders Company, 1968).
29. Trueta, J., and Tres, A.: The effect of pressure upon the epiphyseal cartilage of the rabbit, J. Bone Joint Surg. 43-B:800, 1961.

35 | Operative Treatment of Fractures

EDWIN F. CAVE, ROBERT J. BOYD
and JAMES G. HUDDLESTON

AS THE YEARS PASS, the operative treatment of fractures is gradually finding its proper place in fracture management. Whereas 2 or 3 decades ago the open treatment of fractures in many clinics, and in the United States especially, without question was overdone, we believe that presently over the country there is a swing back, at least to some degree, to the more conservative approach and that open reduction and internal fixation as a form of treatment is leveling off. As this has happened in the United States, however, certain clinics in Europe, having developed effective forms of material for openly stabilizing fractures, have done an excessive number of open reductions on long bones and often without good reason.

As has been emphasized elsewhere (see Chapter 5), the fundamental principles of bone healing do not change and it must be realized that the vast majority of long-bone fractures will heal with reasonable reduction and alignment and sufficiently prolonged external fixation.

When the over-all results of the operative treatment of fractures are contemplated, it is most difficult to determine whether the advantages of operative treatment outweigh the disadvantages, considering the disasters that sometimes follow the open reduction of long-bone fractures. One case of osteomyelitis following an elective operation on a closed fracture will not soon be forgotten by the operating surgeon. The surgeon must repeatedly ask himself: "Will the fracture heal in a reasonable time with nonoperative methods?" Or "Do I have the experience and training, the tools and the surroundings to ensure a better result in a shorter period by operating on the fracture at hand?"

The success or failure of the operation will depend largely on the surgeon. Therefore, the student must be inculcated with fundamental surgical principles and taught to realize the importance of proper training and of postgraduate study, and must develop careful judgment in the selection of cases for operation. Improper operative interference is the most common cause of delayed union or nonunion of fractures.

K. W. Starr[21] wisely stated: "If the dread of bone infection following operation on fractures remains like the sword of Damocles over our therapeutic head during the next decade, surgical training, not the pathology of bone, is at fault."

The operative management of fractures received its greatest stimulus from the work of Sir Arbuthnot Lane at Guy's Hospital in London in the latter part of the nineteenth century. In 1912, Sherman of Pittsburgh also advocated early operative reduction of long-bone fractures. The metals used by these two surgeons caused tissue reactions and frequently had to be removed. (Sherman later abandoned his "vanadium steel" in favor of 18-8 SMo stainless steel). Venable and Stuck, in their excellent monograph *The Internal Fixation of Fractures*, point out that in 1922 C. M. Johnson of Pittsburgh secured patents for a chrome-nickel stainless steel that contained 10–20% chromium and 9–25% nickel and was characterized by the presence of about 2% silicon; later studies caused the proportions to be altered to 18% chromium and 8% nickel with a substantial proportion of silicon; this latter proportion is used basically in all the present-day "18-8 stainless steels." In 1946, Key[6] observed the deleterious effects of electrolytic reaction in body fluids between the different types of stainless steels. Moreover, he found that the stainless steels vary enormously in their resistance to corrosion and that mixing of stainless steels in the same patient produces destruction of bone. By present standards, 18-8 SMo stainless steel (Table 35-1) can be used in the body without danger. Even so, there still is some slight disintegration of the metal, which can be demonstrated by analyzing tissue around the metal; however, the corrosion of the metal is minimal and the interference with healing of the soft tissue is slight. Although reaction in the tissue occurs rarely after using 18-8 SMo stainless steel, breakage is by no means uncommon. We do not, as yet, have the ideal stainless steel for internal fixation of fractures.

In 1929, Venable and Stuck advocated the use of Vitallium, an alloy of cobalt, chromium and molybdenum with small amounts of manganese, silicon and carbon. Vitallium is used extensively in the manufacture of plates, screws, nails, molds for arthroplasty, prostheses, etc. It is a very hard alloy that is less malleable than most and hence cannot be machined. Therefore, appliances made of Vitallium must be cast in molds. Vitallium as now manufactured (Table 35-2) can be bent to conform to the part if necessary.

TABLE 35-1. — SPECIFICATIONS OF STAINLESS STEEL 18-8 SMo

Chromium	17–20%
Nickel	10–14%
Molybdenum	2–4%
Manganese	2% maximum
Carbon	0.08% maximum
Silicon	0.75% maximum
Phosphorus	0.03% maximum
Sulfur	0.03% maximum
Iron	Remainder
Rockwell hardness	30–35° C

TABLE 35-2. — SPECIFICATIONS OF VITALLIUM

Cobalt	65%
Chromium	30%
Molybdenum	3%
Manganese, Silicon, Carbon	Remainder

TRAINING OF THE FRACTURE SURGEON

The surgeon operating on a fracture must not only have perfected his skill in operative techniques but must be grounded in sound surgical principles as to the over-all management of the entire patient and be able to treat soft tissues as well as bone; he must also be able to anticipate the possible complications of surgery. He must have sufficient knowledge to deal with them should they develop. He must be more than a "carpenter." He must treat the entire patient and not just the x-ray film and the local injury. Specialization may mitigate against such broad experience and therefore it is up to the various qualifying boards in American surgery to make certain that the surgeon who operates on a fracture is surgically trained in all aspects and in fundamentals. He must have sufficient knowledge and judgment to select the fracture that is to be treated by closed means and to choose properly the case to be operated on.

Selection of Cases for Operation

The following fractures, in most cases, should be treated primarily by operation:

Chapter 35: OPERATIVE TREATMENT OF FRACTURES / 889

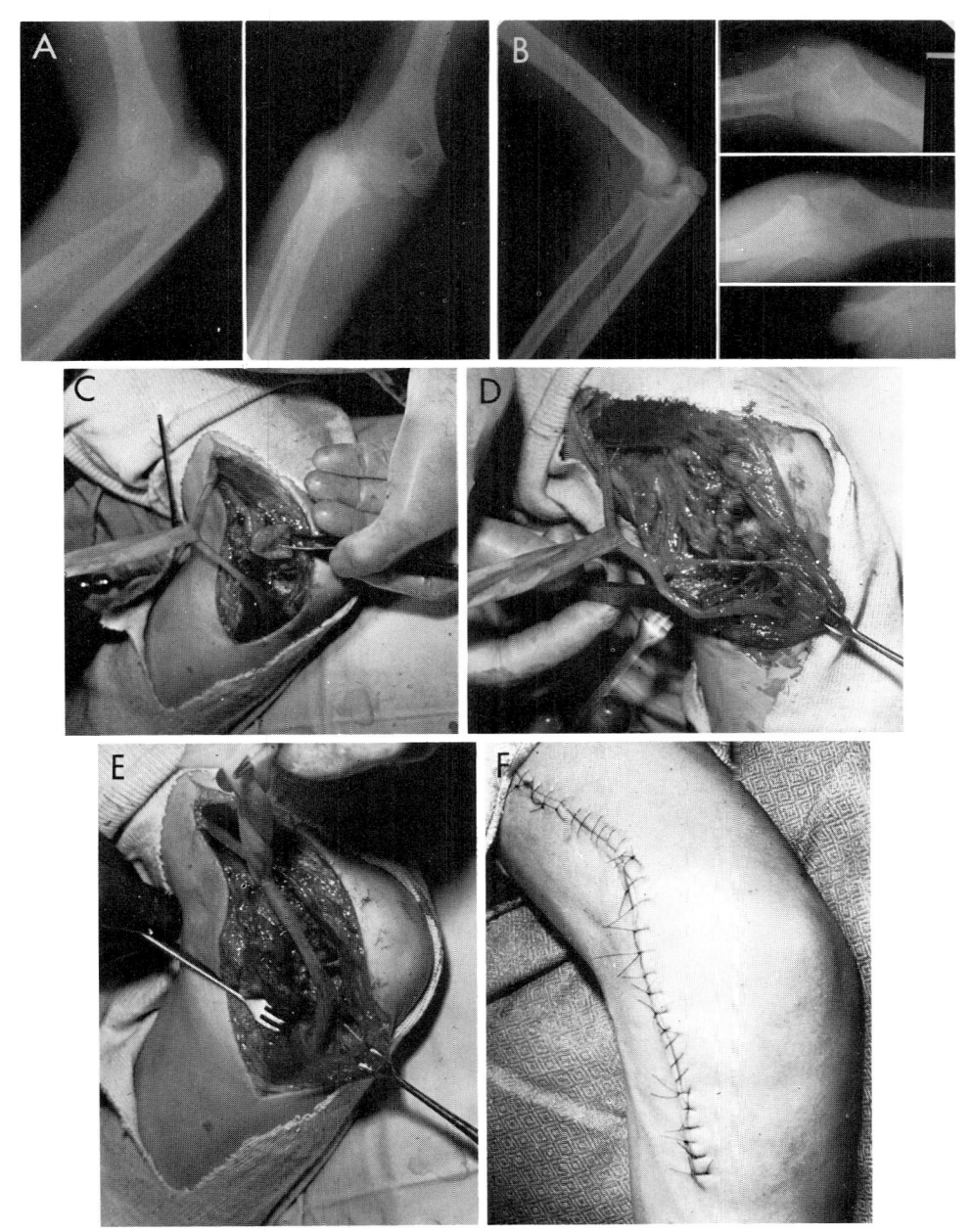

Fig. 35-1.—**A**, posterolateral dislocation of the elbow with fracture of the mesial humeral epicondyle, which was pulled into the elbow joint by the attached flexor muscles. **B**, the dislocation was reduced but the fractured fragment remained within the joint, later requiring removal of the loose fragment and transplantation of the ulnar nerve. **C** reveals the fragment and retraction of the ulnar nerve at the time of exposure at operation. **D**, mobilization of the ulnar nerve. **E**, transplantation of the ulnar nerve at the time of exposure at operation. **F** shows the incision. Note that the operation was done with the patient in a prone position. (From Cave, E. F.: Sir Robert Jones Lecture, Bull. Hosp. Joint Dis. 26:127, 1965.)

1. Fractures of the olecranon with separation of fragments.
2. Fractures of the lateral condyle of the humerus with marked rotation in children or in adults.
3. Displaced fractures of the femoral neck.
4. Patellar fractures with separation of the fragments and laceration of the quadriceps expansion.
5. Major vascular injury associated with fracture.
6. Displaced fractures of the spine with progressive neurologic deficit.

There is a group of fractures in which open reduction and internal fixation usually are contraindicated:

1. Essentially all fractures in children under the age of 12, except fractures of the lateral humeral condyle.
2. Impacted fractures of the surgical neck of the humerus.
3. Impacted fractures of the femoral neck in valgus.

PREPARATION OF THE PATIENT

Once operation is decided on, certain fundamental rules must be followed in the preparation of the patient. The usual principles, applicable in any major operation, must be observed. Operation should be carried out as soon as the patient is in the optimal condition that can be obtained.

Stabilization of the fracture will help materially to reduce the shock that accompanies injury. The only reason for delay is an unfavorable condition of the local tissue or of the patient. Although the surgeon cannot plan every detail of his operation beforehand, he should have in mind a general scheme as to his method of reduction and fixation of the fracture. He should look over his instruments before the operation and be certain that the necessary tools are on the "sterile table." Nothing is more frustrating than not to have the proper size of drill, screws, plates, etc., at hand the moment they are needed.

For local management, the following should be observed:

1. One careful preparation of the extremity is sufficient.
2. It probably is better to do the local preparation in the operating room under anesthesia. This requires: (a) sufficient help in handling the injured extremity to prevent additional trauma; (b) cutting of toenails and fingernails; (c) careful shaving; (d) gentle scrubbing with gauze immersed in liquid soap and water; (e) the application of an antiseptic solution of the surgeon's choice.
3. Positioning of the patient. The posi-

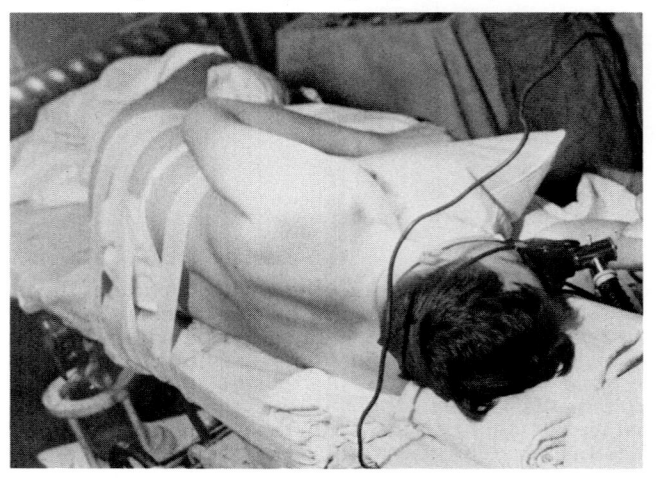

Fig. 35-2.—Position of patient for exposing superior aspect of the shoulder joint.

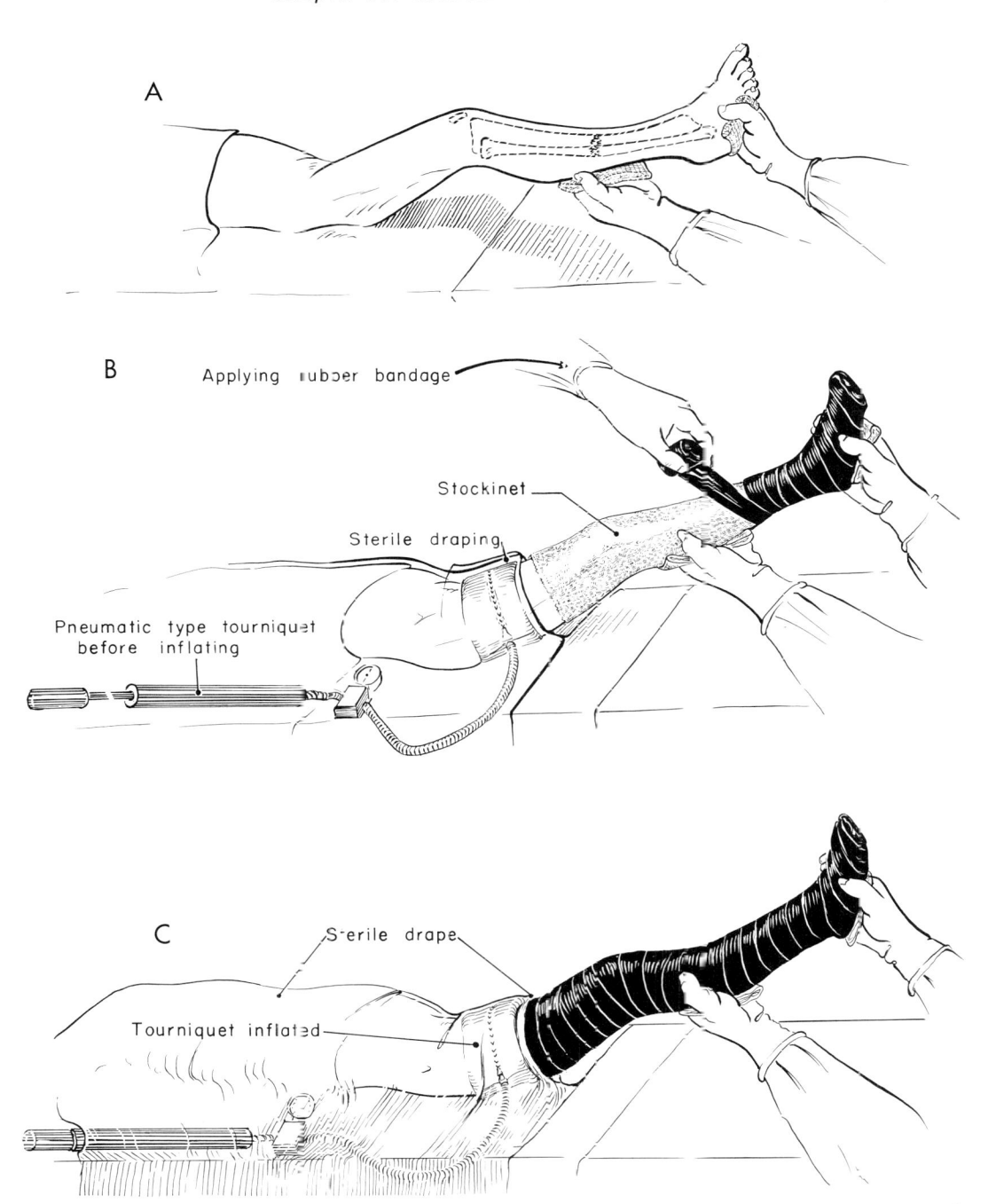

Fig. 35-3.—Preparation of patient for surgery for fracture. The extremity must be supported adequately; if a tourniquet is used, it should be the pneumatic type. **A**, preparation of skin. **B** and **C**, draping of extremity and application of tourniquet. Before the tourniquet is inflated, a rubber Esmarch bandage should be used to deplete the extremity of blood. The tourniquet then is inflated and the Esmarch bandage removed.

tion of the patient can add to the ease with which the operation is accomplished or it can produce insurmountable difficulties. For instance, most operations on the elbow should be done with the patient in a prone position. When exposing the superior aspect of the shoulder joint, the operative side of the patient should be well elevated at an angle of at least 45 degrees or more. An arthrodesis of the tarsus is performed more easily with the patient lying on the opposite side, even though two incisions, both mesial and lateral, may be necessary.

4. The extremity should be draped carefully.

5. The use of a tourniquet is optional. If a tourniquet is used, the pneumatic type should be applied before the extremity is prepared. After the usual draping and before inflation of the tourniquet, a rubber Esmarch bandage should be applied from below upward over stockinet covering the extremity. After the bandage is applied, the tourniquet should be inflated to the degree desired. The Esmarch bandage then is removed.

OPERATIVE TECHNIQUES

Various parts of the skeleton, if operated on, call for different forms of internal fixation. Often it is a matter of choice of the individual surgeon. For instance, some surgeons prefer to stabilize a long bone with plates and screws whereas others like the medullary nail. Therefore, the surgeon undertaking the task at hand should use the apparatus that in his opinion is the most suitable to the occasion and that can be applied more effectively by him. The most common long bone subjected to open reduction and internal fixation is the tibia.

The operative approach and fixation of a forearm fracture are diagrammed in Figure 35-4. The skin incision must be adequate to allow subperiosteal exposure of the fragments without undue tension on the skin edges. Superficial sensory nerves must be avoided. Various materials have been used to cover the skin and prevent possible contamination of the deep tissues. Such materials are stockinet, held by metal clips, or one of the more recently utilized plastic materials, through which skin incisions can be made. Where possible, the incision should follow muscle planes down to bone. The periosteum and muscles are carefully and sufficiently reflected, in one layer from the ends of the broken bones, to allow gentle manipulation and reduction of the fragments with bone clamps. All major fragments are brought into line and fitted as accurately as possible to their normal position. When this is done, the surgeon decides what type of internal fixation to use. He has a choice of screws, a plate and screws, bands, circular wires or medullary nails. Rarely will suture material such as silk or catgut give stability to any fracture.

During the past few years, the "compression plate" has been advocated and popularized, especially by the Swiss surgeons, Müller, Allgöwer and Willenegger. The principle of compression is not new, nor is the controversy concerning this principle. Eggers et al.[4] discussed the problem in 1949, after having applied compression forces to the bones of an animal's skull. Albert Key[6] also wrote rather extensively on the problem and advocated compression, especially for the arthrodesis of joints. Charnley went even further and devised an effective apparatus for carrying out stabilization of a joint that had been subjected to a fusion operation.

In the early 1930s, Clay Murray of New York City was a firm believer in "rigid fixation" and employed a transfixation screw or screws, placed at a right angle to the plate and screws.

However, credit must be given to Müller, Allgöwer and Willenegger for developing a mechanically sound combination of plate and screws for compressing a long-bone fracture. Presently in our clinic we believe that the compression plate is of value in the management of

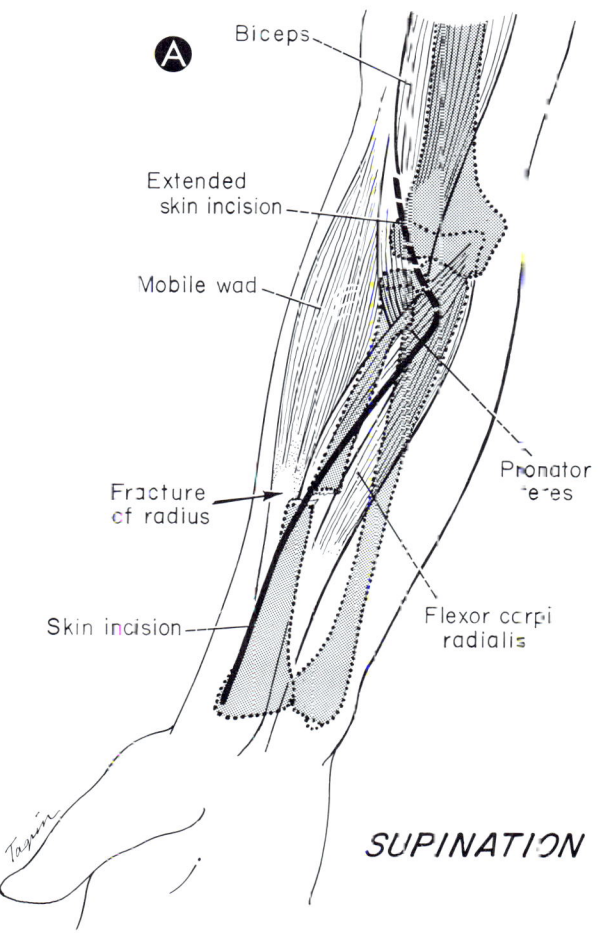

Fig. 35-4. — Operative approach and fixation of a long-bone fracture. (**Continued.**)

adult fractures of the forearm, which cannot be reduced and held by external fixation. Occasionally it is indicated in humeral shaft fractures, which require rigid fixation because of associated nerve and vascular injuries. It is less often necessary in lower-shaft fractures of the femur with soft tissue problems. The compression plate rarely is indicated in the management of fresh fractures of the tibia, but in the minds of some surgeons it may be the method of choice in the treatment of nonunion of the radius, ulna, humerus, femur and tibia, although many in our clinic still prefer the medullary nail for the management of nonunion of a fracture of the femoral shaft.

Whether the compression factor is of real advantage in making fractures unite promptly is debatable. C. Andrew Bassett[1] of New York has written as follows:

". . . the rigidity of internal fixation is increased by *properly* applied compression. Furthermore, the applied compression *does not* lead to resorption of bone and only slowly diminishes over a period of months as the fracture repair is proceeding. The pattern of repair is modified in that very little or no internal and exter-

PRONATION

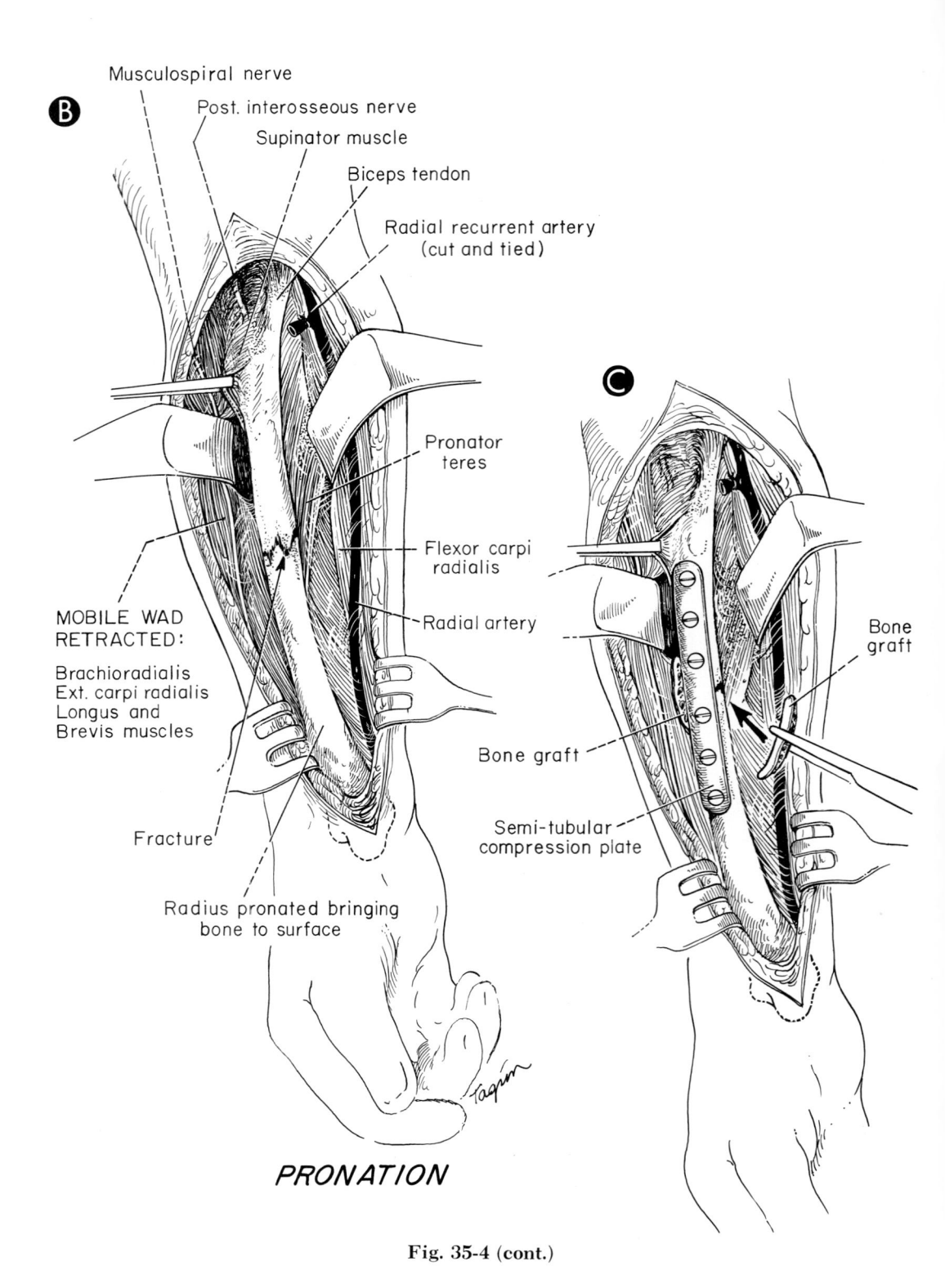

Fig. 35-4 (cont.)

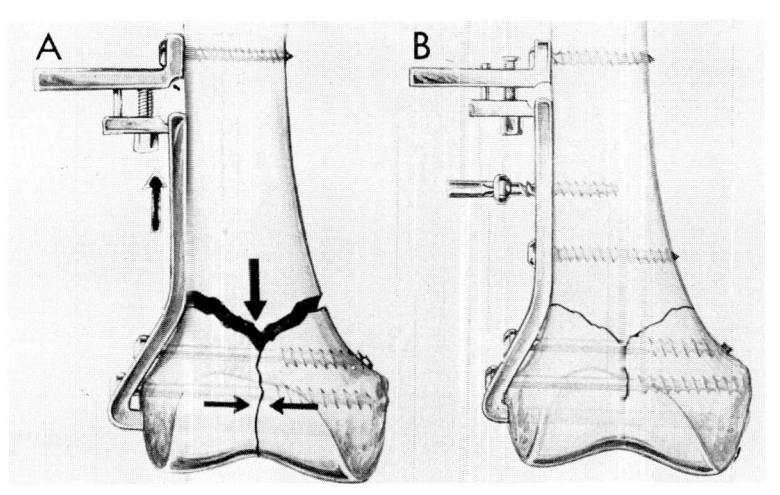

Fig. 35-5.—Compression of fractured bone surfaces is advocated by some authorities to promote rapid healing of bone. The "compression" plate as demonstrated here is used to approximate and stabilize a fracture of the lower end of the femoral bone. A, internal fixation of the condyles and thereafter compression toward the shaft of the femur. B, fixation of the plate with screws to the shaft. (From Müller, M. E., Allgöwer, M., and Willenegger, H.: *Technique of Internal Fixation of Fractures* [Springer-Verlag New York, 1965].)

nal callus appears in the rigidly fixed, compressed fracture and healing is per primum. By this I mean that the zone of cortical osseous necrosis is diminished and osteogenesis springs from regenerating vascular and cellular elements within the haversian canals. If apposition of contiguous fragments is absolute, there is a longitudinal repair process, oriented parallel to the axis of the bone. Proliferating-migrating vessels and perivascular cells bridge the discontinuity from both fragments and set the stage for 'creeping substitution' of the dead osteons on either side. In this way, the fracture is slowly 'reworked' or rewoven. The process requires about 12–18 months to be completed.

"As with most things in life, we never 'get something for nothing' and a price is paid for this pattern of osseous union. First, since the plate is rigid, the supported fragments have some of the mechanical 'signals' modified; and porosis in the underlying bone results. In addition, since there is little or no external or internal callus, premature removal of the plate leaves an unsupported repair region which may be significantly weaker.

"Despite these negative factors, I believe that compression, properly used, has increased the expectation of union and permits earlier function than with most methods of internal fixation. The technique has not changed my indications for operation on a fracture, but if the fracture is opened, compression seems to be one of the best methods for repair."

At present, we believe that the objections to the ASIF plate and screws are as follows:

1. The plate is very large and its presence directly under skin, as in the case of the tibia, is undesirable.

2. In a number of cases, the metal thus far used has caused reaction in tissue and often has had to be removed.

3. We think that without question the plate frequently has been used without proper indication. For instance, it is unnecessary to apply any form of internal fixation to an oblique fracture of the tibia with the fibula intact, unless there is marked angulation, which cannot be corrected by manipulation and external fixation. Many of the illustrations in *Technique of Internal Fixation of Fractures* by Müller and his colleagues[15] suggest

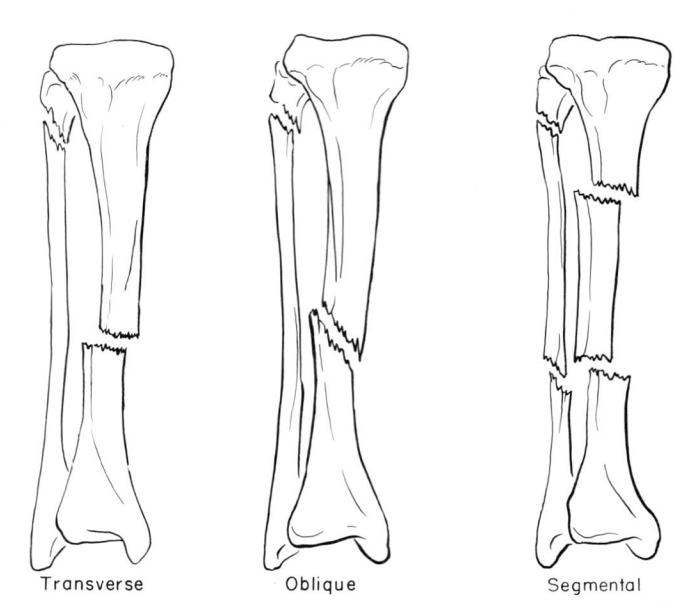

Fig. 35-6.—Types of long-bone fractures. Any of the three types may be comminuted.

that the plate and screws have been used unnecessarily.

4. Compression plating makes evaluation of fracture healing difficult. The plates should be left in at least 12–18 months before considering removal, unless by chance they cause reaction in soft tissue, in which case earlier removal will be indicated and further external protection of the fracture carried out.

Fig. 35-7.—Types of long-bone fractures with appropriate internal fixation. **A,** plate and screw fixation for transverse comminuted closed or open fractures. **B,** screw fixation for spiral oblique fracture. **C,** medullary nail for segmental fracture.

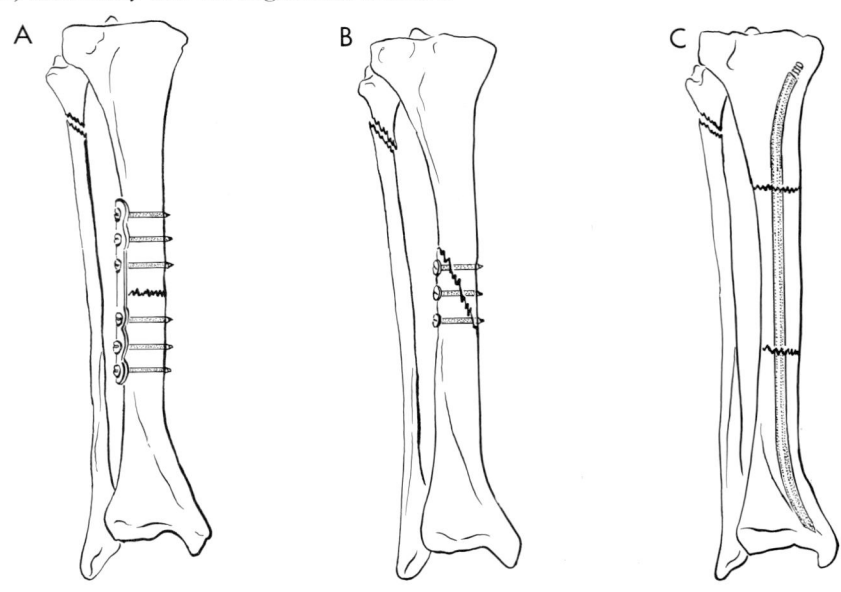

5. Wide exposure is necessary to apply the compression plate, as presently it is designed with at least 2 and preferably 3 screws on either side of the fracture margins. Dr. Louis Anderson, with extensive experience in the use of this technique, suggests that the plates be applied over periosteum. We see no advantage to this technique and believe that it is just as destructive to periosteum as would be the routine periosteal reflection.

In general, there are three types of long-bone fractures: (1) transverse, (2) oblique and (3) segmental. Any of the three may be comminuted. And, in general, the methods of internal fixation vary as follows: (1) plate and screws for the transverse or short oblique fracture, (2) screws only for the long oblique fracture and (3) a medullary nail for the segmental fracture. A combination of a plate and/or screws may be used for the comminuted fracture.

Technique of Applying Plates and Screws

The technique of fixation of bone by plates and screws used by L. T. Peterson[16] is an excellent one. The plate should conform to the shape of the bone and any inequality should be adjusted by accurate shaping of the plate before it is fixed. It is not good technique for the screws to bend the plate to fit the bone, since, in so doing, a spring action results and the screw is immediately subjected to a strong pulling-out force. The screw should fit in the center of the hole in the plate so that the head of the screw will have uniform contact and pressure on the plate. If the screw is not centered properly as it is tightened, the countersink in the plate will tend to force it to one side, thereby damaging the good threads already cut in the bone and producing a strain that probably will lead to necrosis and early loosening of the screw.

In order to have uniform contact between plate and screws, it is important to drill vertically to the plate as well as in the center of the hole. A drill guide will aid in determining this direction. The drill point should be turned without describing an arc, which tends to enlarge the hole. A motor-driven drill possesses certain advantages over the hand drill because it is mechanically powered and the operator can devote his attention to direction. If the drill is thrust through the bone at high speed, it will burn the bone and produce necrosis. Therefore, a slow rate of speed is desired; this not only avoids unnecessary bone damage but it is safer for the patient and the operator. The drill must be sharp and of proper size, and it should be just slightly smaller than the screw that is to be used. The screw should pass through both cortices of bone. A screw with a pilot point is desirable because the point of the screw will "find" the hole in the opposite cortex. The point of the screw should project through the length of the pilot point. Sometimes it is necessary to insert screws at an angle in order to engage some of the bone fragments. It is best to use a separate screw for this purpose, since angular screws give poor contact with the plate. In fixing a bone graft, a flat-headed screw may be desirable because a tapered screw head tends to split the bone. This hazard can be eliminated, however, by the use of a countersink, which will serve to make the screw head less prominent. The countersink is also useful where fragments are secured by screws without the use of plates.

THE SLOTTED PLATE. — The idea behind the slotted plate was that after its application muscle contraction was believed to cause impaction of the fracture. In clinical experience, such has not been proved true, and in most clinics the "slotted plate" has been abandoned.

The Addition of Bone

The addition of bone at the time of open reduction and internal fixation frequently is indicated. Many surgeons prefer to add bone, particularly if delay in open reduction has been necessary. The

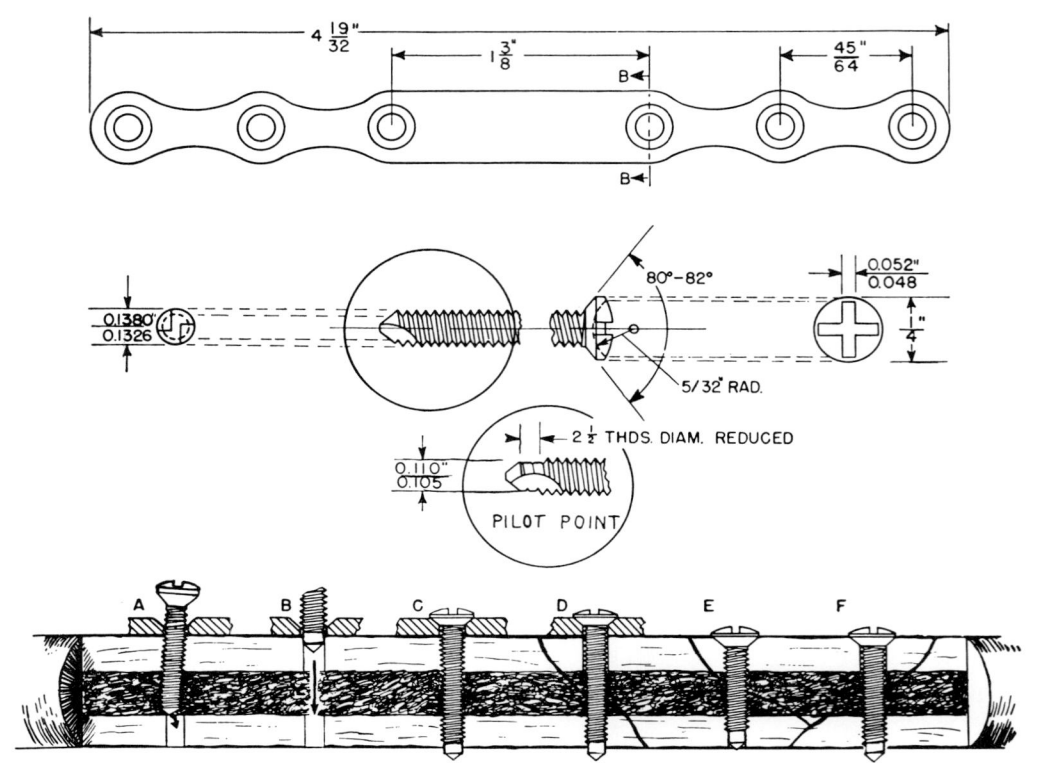

Fig. 35-8. — Details of construction of plates and screws (18-8 SMo stainless steel). Inset shows the cruciate head, the cutting flutes and the pilot point of the screw. The lower drawing shows the technique in plate and screw fixation.

A, a long screw without pilot point inserted at slight angle in relation to the drill hole. This procedure is common in actual practice. The point may completely miss the hole or it may hit the hole eccentrically. Then, as the point is forced into line, it will tend to strip the threads already cut in the proximal cortex.

B, a screw with a pilot point. The tip accurately fits the drill hole and tends to direct the screw properly. Furthermore, the pilot point holds the screw, so that the screw may be controlled more easily without the use of a screw-holding device on the screwdriver. A longer pilot point would be more effective for both purposes, but this portion of the screw does not engage the bone.

C, a long pilot-point screw, properly centered and of optimal length.

D, enlarging the hole in the proximal cortex. After both cortices have been drilled with a no. 35 drill, the hole in the proximal cortex is enlarged by a no. 27 drill (0.144 inch) so that the threads engage only the distal cortex. The whole screw acts as a pilot point. This method makes possible the impaction of fragments when the screw is tightened.

E, two fragments of bone, fixed with a screw without use of a plate. The hole in the proximal cortex has been countersunk. This avoids the tendency for the tapered head to split the bone; it also makes the head less prominent.

F, the proximal hole enlarged as in **D**, and countersunk as in **E**, permitting impaction of the fragments. Methods **E** and **F** are applicable in fixation of fragments and of onlay bone grafts.

(From Peterson, L. T.: Fixation of bones by plates and screws, J. Bone Joint Surg. 29:335, 1947.)

Chapter 35: OPERATIVE TREATMENT OF FRACTURES

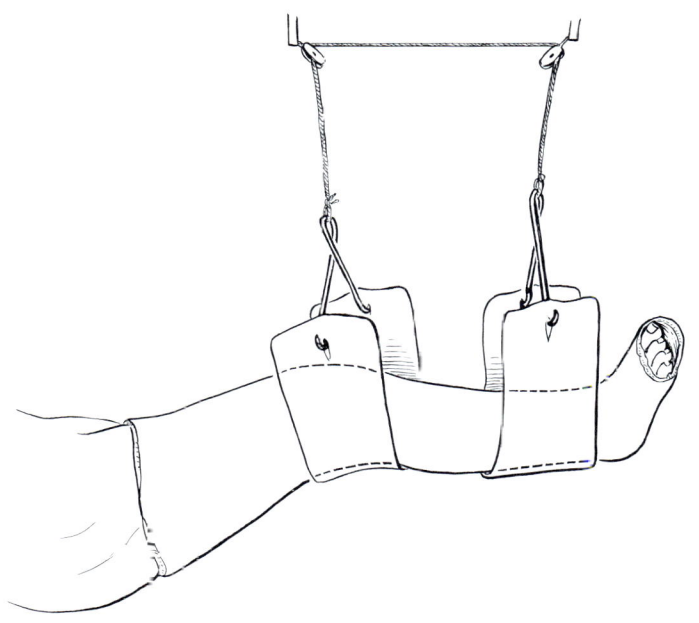

Fig. 35-9. — Elevation of the extremity after injury or after operation will eliminate swelling and encourage wound healing.

bone can be an osteoperiosteal graft from the surface of one fragment or it may be taken from the ilium. It should be placed subperiosteally, preferably where muscle will cover the graft.

Closure of the Wound

If a tourniquet is used, it is released before the wound is closed. An attempt is made to repair the periosteum with fine suture material. Subcutaneous tissues are carefully repaired and the skin is closed without tension, using relaxing incisions, if necessary.

Usually some form of external fixation or traction is necessary after open reduction and internal fixation. Plaster of Paris still is the most reliable material in most hands. When used, it should include the joints above and below the region of fracture.

Postoperative Elevation

After operation, the extremity is suspended for a period of 10 days to prevent congestion of the wound, since congestion predisposes to infection. Whether the plaster casing should be split must be determined by the individual surgeon. If the plaster has been applied properly with adequate padding, there is, as a rule, no need to split the casing; but when there is doubt concerning its suitability, not only the plaster casing but also the padding underneath the plaster should be divided and separated in order to prevent circulatory or nerve damage.

The First Dressing

Generally speaking, it is not necessary to inspect the wound before the time to renew the plaster casing at the end of 10 days or 2 weeks, provided that there is no undue swelling of the extermity, the temperature remains normal, pain diminishes steadily and the blood count remains within normal limits. When the plaster casing is changed, the stitches can be removed and new plaster applied with little padding. This will ensure a more accurate fit of the plaster.

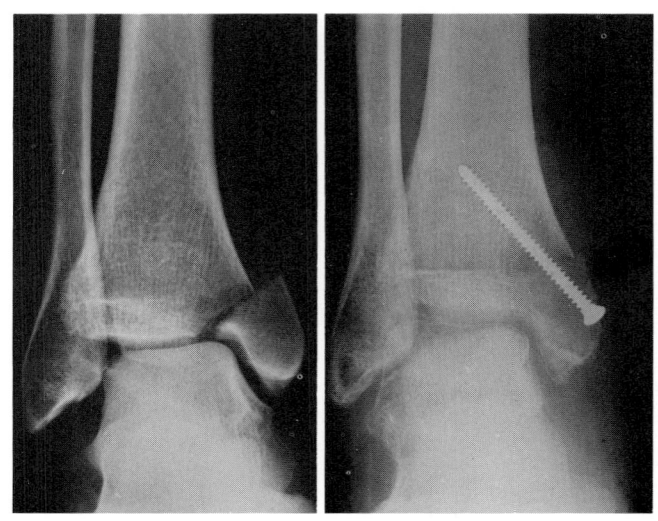

Fig. 35-10.—Use of a single screw for fixation of internal malleolus. **Left,** displaced fracture of internal malleolus. **Right,** reduction and bone union of fracture.

Other Forms of Internal Fixation

USE OF SCREWS ALONE.—A single screw is useful in securing a condylar fragment or a malleolus. Many oblique and some comminuted fractures, particularly those with large butterfly fragments, can be secured with screws alone and without the use of a plate. In other words, a large third fragment can be used for stabilizing

Fig. 35-11.—Use of screws alone for stabilizing long oblique fracture. **A,** torsional fractures of tibia and fibula secondary to skiing injury. **B,** end result 1 year later; complete bone union.

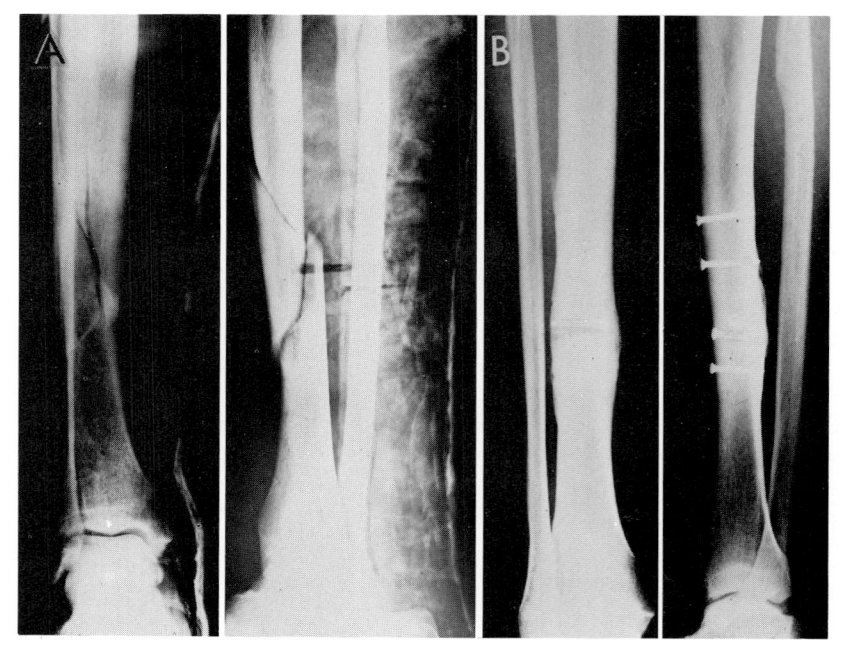

Chapter 35: OPERATIVE TREATMENT OF FRACTURES / 901

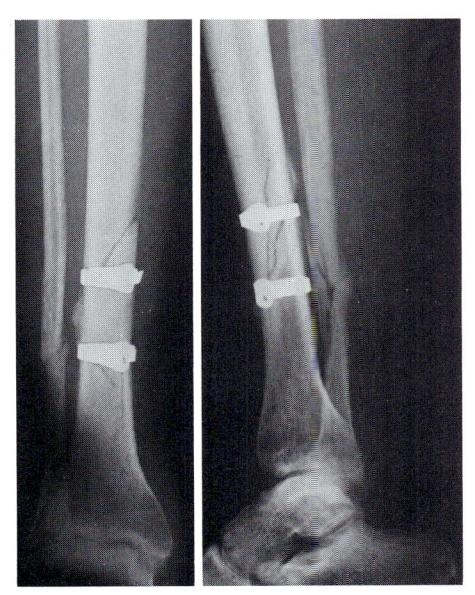

Fig. 35-12.—Parham bands applied for oblique fracture of lower end of tibia.

the main fragments, just as a plate would be employed. A good rule to follow in the management of any fracture is: "The less hardware the better"; but sufficient metal must be applied to give stability to the fracture.

PARHAM BANDS.—Some surgeons find Parham bands very useful, particularly in the management of oblique fractures of the femur, humerus and tibia. These bands are applied easily, but they must be removed, especially from the tibia, at the end of 6 or 8 weeks because, as new bone is formed, the band is covered, and eventually it tends to cut through the shaft of the bone, thus predisposing to refracture. After removal of the bands from the tibia, plaster must be reapplied until union is firm. The bands are made of stainless steel and require special instruments for their application. They may be indicated when it is not possible to apply screws. They may also be used in conjunction with the medullary nail in the femur or tibia to secure comminuted fragments.

Treatment of Long-Bone Fractures by Medullary Nailing

The treatment of long-bone fractures has been greatly enhanced during the past 20 years by intramedullary fixation with metallic nails, pins or rods. This form of treatment was used in ancient times in severe open fractures. In 1897, Nicolaysen proposed such a form of treatment and in 1921 Groves advocated the use of a "long steel strut" in badly comminuted fractures. However, because of the poor quality of metal available, the method was abandoned until 1940, when Küntscher showed that the method was sound and that the medullary canal could tolerate a large cylinder of steel, occupying nearly its entire diameter, and still allow the fracture to heal.

Medullary nailing has, with considerable justification, replaced plate and screw fixation in many long-bone fractures, particularly those of the femur. The ulna, fibula, tibia, humerus and radius have been so treated less frequently. Nails of various types have been devised: the original Küntscher (the "cloverleaf"), the diamond-shaped nail of Hansen and Street, the Rush nail and the Lottes nail for use in the tibia.

Medullary Nailing of the Femur

So-called blind nailing of femoral fractures, where the nail is introduced at the trochanteric level and driven down the canal across the fracture line into the distal fragment without exposing the fracture, has considerable merit if the surgeon has the tools and the ability to direct the nail properly. The technique of inserting the medullary nail without exposure of the fracture, used rather extensively in some European clinics, has been greatly aided by the employment of the image intensifier and a television screen. This technique can be used for a long-bone fracture in good alignment and is especially useful in the management of pathologic fracture of the femur without

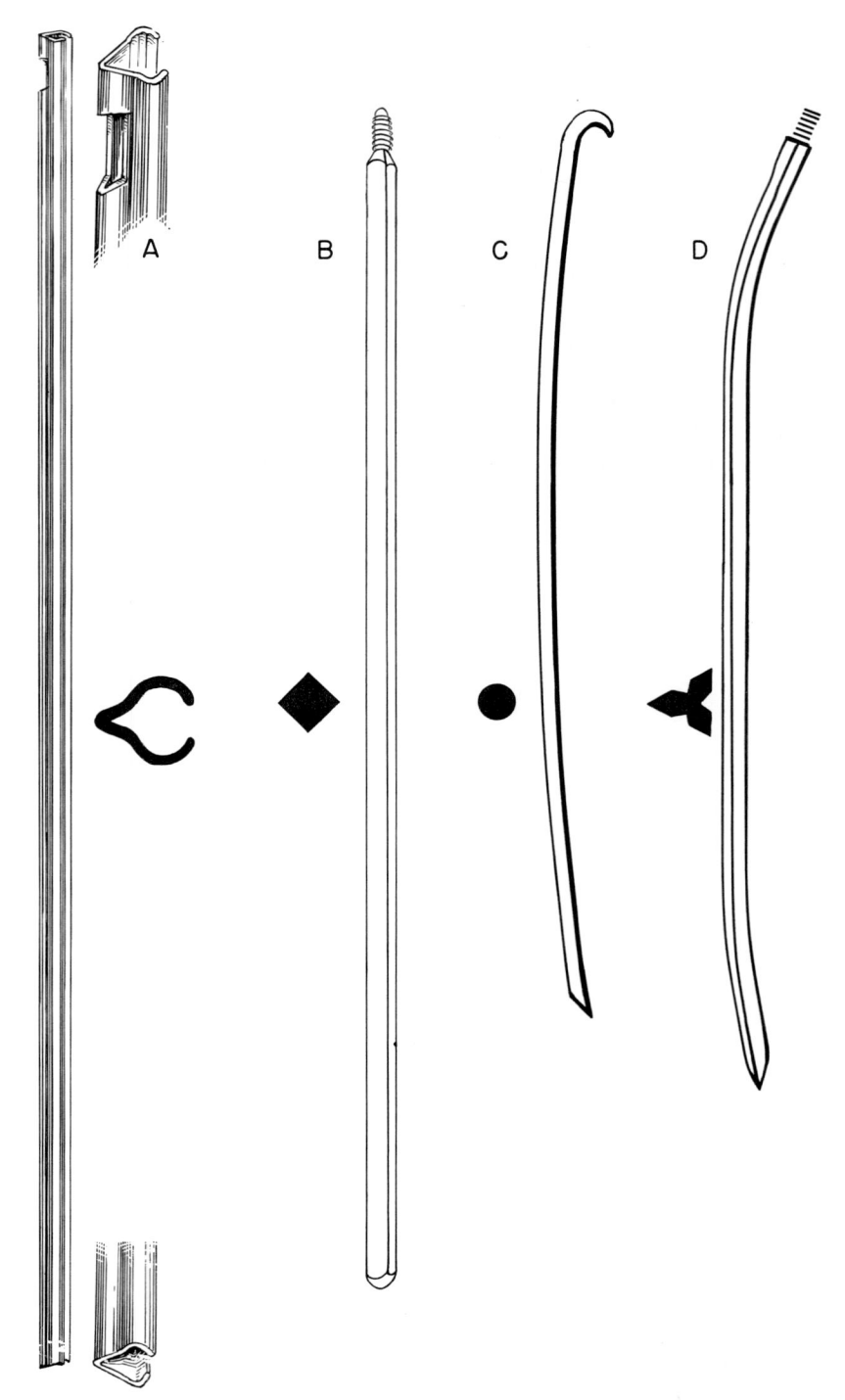

Fig. 35-13.—Types of medullary nails, longitudinal and cross-section views. **A**, cloverleaf (Küntscher) nail. **B**, Hansen-Street nail. **C**, Rush nail. **D**, Lottes nail.

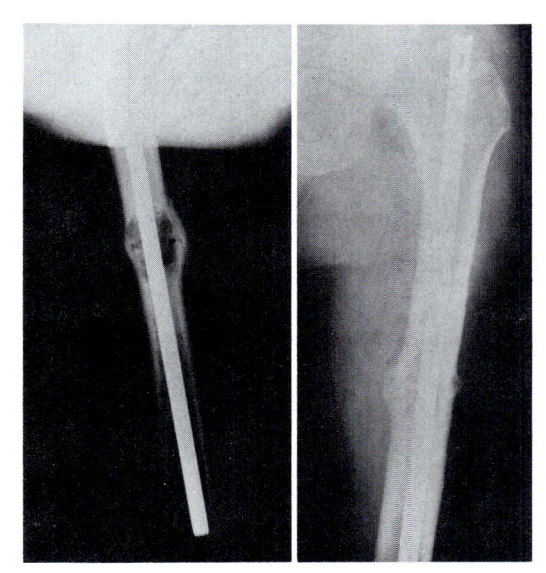

Fig. 35-14. — Postoperative biopsy of metastatic tumor and insertion of Küntscher nail for stabilization of pathologic fracture of left femur. (From Cave, E. F.: Complications of Orthopedic Surgery, in *Traumatic Medicine and Surgery for the Attorney* [Washington, D. C.: Butterworths, 1966].)

displacement. For the ordinary fracture of the femur, however, most frequently the fracture is exposed, the size of the canal measured, the fracture reduced and the nail driven either retrograde or directly down the canal.

INDICATIONS FOR NAILING. — The indications for medullary nailing of the femur are broad or narrow, depending on the skill and experience of the surgeon with this technique and the facilities at hand. Many surgeons will continue to use traction or plaster fixation, or both, and, at times, open reduction with plate and screw stabilization; but in the hands of the skilled bone and joint surgeon who is familiar with the technique, medullary nailing may be the method of choice.

Medullary nailing is not indicated in recent fractures in young children; otherwise, age is not a factor. This method is not necessarily the most desirable form of treatment for fresh femoral fractures, but in delayed union or nonunion and in pathologic fractures many believe that it is the best means of treatment available. The use of the medullary nail in open fractures is a reasonable procedure if adequate debridement can be carried out prior to insertion of the nail. There is no question that stabilization of any fracture tends to diminish the risk of infection and promote healing of soft tissue. If adequate debridement cannot be done, a soft tissue wound can be left open for a few days and closed secondarily. Medullary nailing can be used in femoral shortening or for correction of rotation or angulation deformity. It is a tremendous aid in the management of the patient with associated severe abdominal and chest wounds or with extensive burns where external fixation is not possible, provided, of course, that the patient can tolerate the major operation required for insertion of the nail. Thus, the method may well play an important role in war or disaster surgery.

THE CLOVERLEAF NAIL. — This nail is manufactured of 18-8 SMo (see Fig. 35-13, A) stainless steel or Vitallium in diameters of 7–12 mm and in lengths of 14–17 inches. It is cloverleaf shaped when viewed in cross section and it is hollow, so that is may be driven over a guide rod. It has torsional strength produced by curves in both sides of a U design. The nail apex has a well-rounded curve to induce strength, and the "eye" for extraction should be at least the diameter of the nail from the end.

The use of this nail requires direct exposure of the fracture. With the patient lying on the side opposite that of the injury, the fracture is exposed by means of an anterolateral incision (preferred for the lower half of the femur), a posterolateral incision (preferred for the upper third of the femur) or a directly lateral incision.

The fragments are mobilized. The proximal fragment is brought up into the wound and the size of the canal estimat-

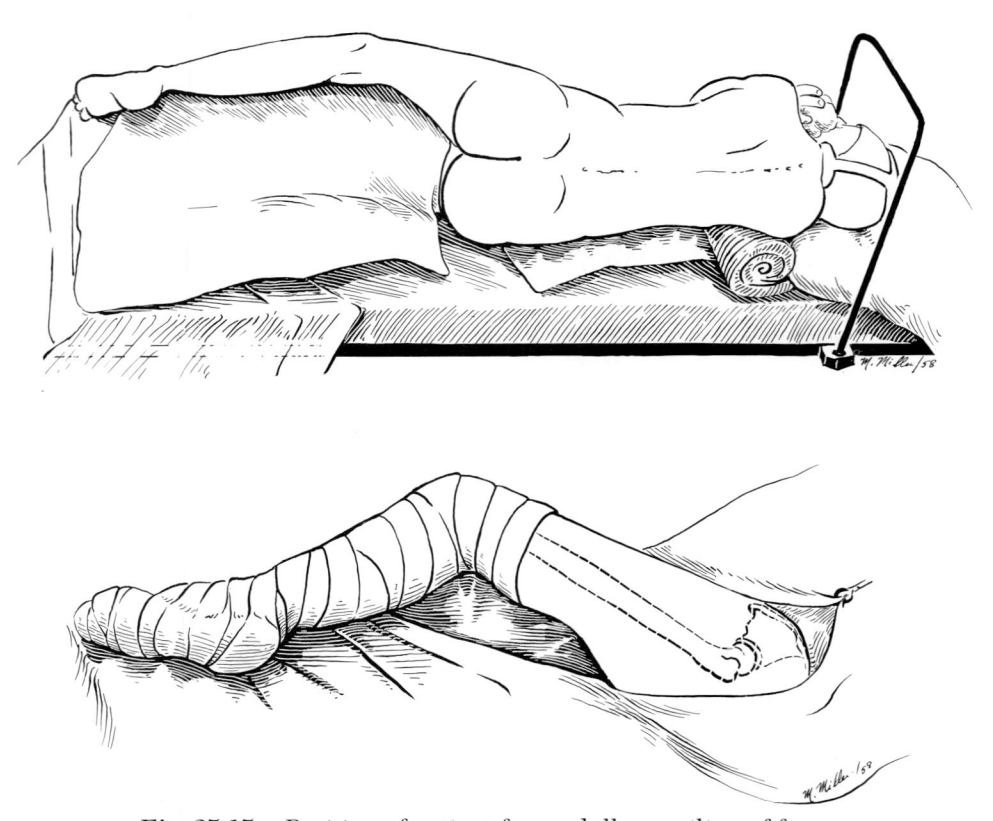

Fig. 35-15.—Position of patient for medullary nailing of femur.

ed by gently inserting a medullary nail of known diameter. The nail must fit the narrowest part of the medullary canal, which is in the upper portion of the shaft. On the other hand, if the canal is unusually large, as may be true in osteoporosis, two "nested" Küntscher nails may be required to give stability to the fracture. The usual diameter selected is 10, 11 or 12 mm. If the fracture is an old one and the bone is sclerosed and the canal narrow at the fracture site, the medullary canal must be enlarged with a reamer to accommodate the proper size nail. However, extensive reaming of the femoral shaft should be discouraged.

A guide rod of known length then is inserted in the proximal fragment and tapped gently upward through the greater trochanter, where it makes its exit and becomes subcutaneous as it is driven farther upward. A stab incision then is made over the guide-rod point. A nail of chosen diameter is inserted over the guide rod and driven about 1 inch into the cortical bone at the level of the greater trochanter. The guide rod is withdrawn and inserted into the hollow nail above and driven down to the fracture site. The hollow nail is temporarily removed. The fracture then is reduced and the guide rod driven well into the distal fragment, down to the level of the adductor tubercle. Portable x-ray films, which include the knee and the fracture site, then are taken in anteroposterior and lateral views and the amount of guide rod projecting above the trochanter is measured. This amount is subtracted from the known length of the guide rod, which gives the

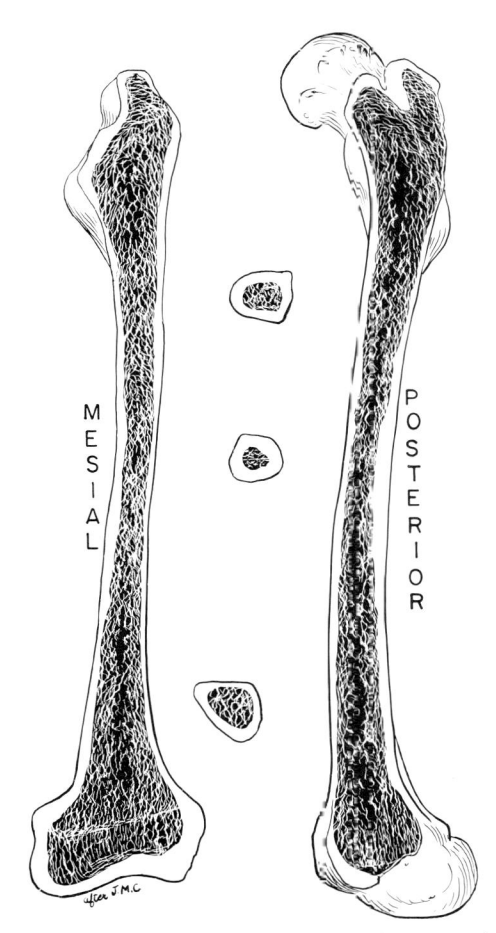

Fig. 35-16.—Cross section of femur. The normal curve of the femoral shaft is anterior and the narrowest part of the canal is in the upper portion of the shaft of the bone. (From Sofield, H. A.: Anatomy of medullary canals, Am. Acad. Orthop. Surgeons Lect., Vol. VIII, 1951.)

exact length of nail desired. The average femur in the adult will require a nail 16 or 16½ inches in length and from 10 to 12 mm in diameter. While reduction of the fracture is maintained by a bone clamp, the hollow nail is inserted over the upper end of the guide rod and driven over the guide rod, down across the fracture line. After the nail is well across the fracture line, the guide rod may be withdrawn and the nail further inserted to the level of the adductor tubercle. As the nail is driven in, the femur must be straightened to accommodate the straight nail. The anterior bow of the femur must be eliminated; otherwise, the nail will impinge against the anterior cortex. The nail should be tapped gently. If it is driven forcibly, it may become impinged and extraction and reinsertion may be extremely difficult or impossible, or it may be forced through the cortex or into the knee. It should project no more than ½ inch above the greater trochanter.

If there are large fragments in addition to the two main fragments, it may be necessary to use supplementary fixation—either short screws through one cortex, circular wires or Parham bands—to maintain stability of these fragments. The incision is closed in layers, dressing applied and the leg bandaged from toes to groin. The leg is suspended in a Hodgen splint. Active muscle-setting exercises for the foot, leg and thigh are begun as soon as wound soreness subsides. After wound healing, normally within a week or 10 days, the leg is removed from the splint and active knee motion is encouraged. During the next few days, sufficient muscle strength and joint mobility will be recovered to allow walking with crutches. The patient's weight should be distributed equally between the injured leg and the crutches. The use of crutches is required until solid bone union is evident by x-ray films. This will require from 6 to 12 months in most cases.

Removal of the nail.—The only reasons for removal of the nail are: (1) pain over the upper end of the nail, which may occur if the nail projects more than about ½ inch above the greater trochanter, (2) a bent nail and (3) a broken nail.

Complications of Medullary Nailing

The medullary nail can be the most efficient form of internal fixation of fractures or its use may be accompanied by many technical difficulties—and, at times, disaster. Possible complications are:

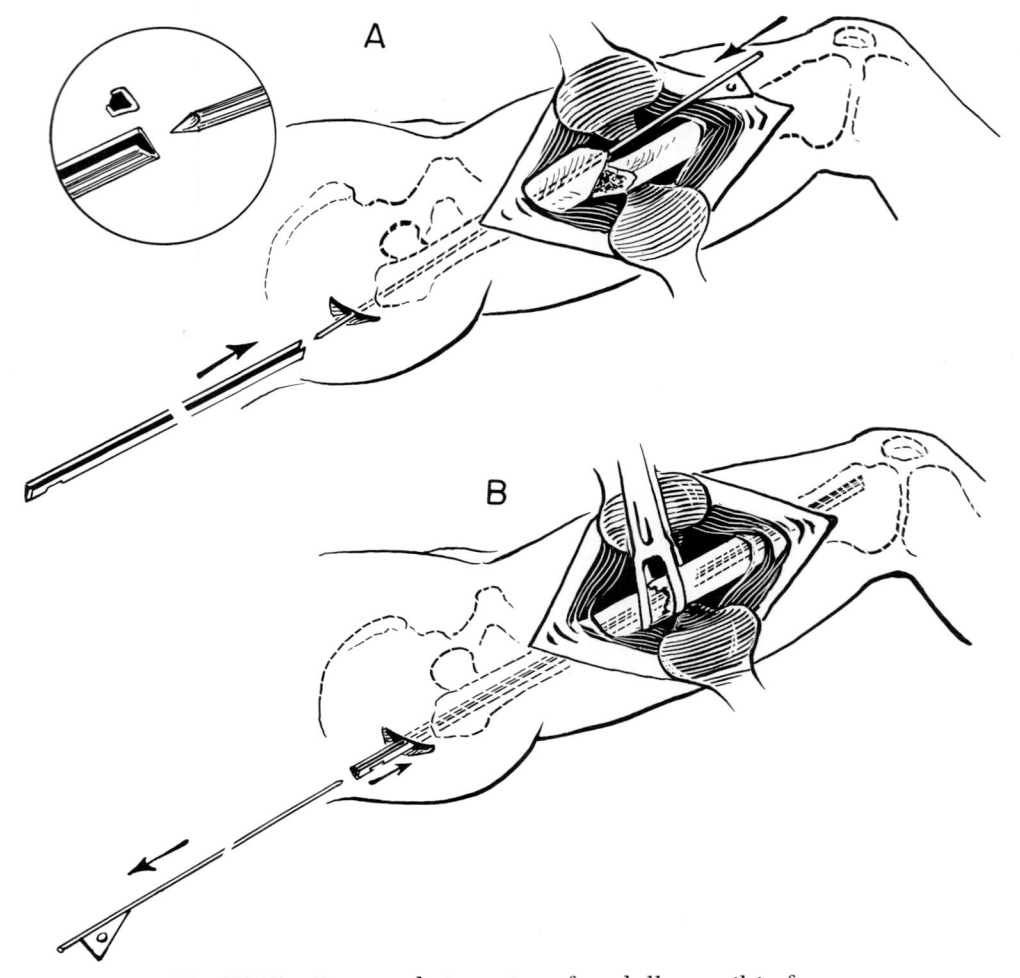

Fig. 35-17.—Retrograde insertion of medullary nail in femur.

1. Infection.
2. Hemorrhage and shock.
3. Impingement of the nail against the cortex, making insertion or removal difficult.
4. Comminution of the fracture.
5. Driving the nail too far into an adjacent joint, particularly in osteoporotic bone.
6. Failure of the nail to fit, with resultant rotation at the fracture site.
7. Too much projection of the nail above the greater trochanter.
8. Bending of the nail.
9. Breaking of the nail.
10. Fat embolism—reported surprisingly rarely.

BENDING OR BREAKING OF THE NAIL.—This complication occurs occasionally and is due to excessive stress on the nail before bone union has progressed sufficiently to contribute some strength to the fracture site. A fall, a misstep or too early full weight bearing, particularly if there is delayed union, usually is responsible for this mishap. Nails of small diameter, i.e., 9 mm or less, are more likely to fail.

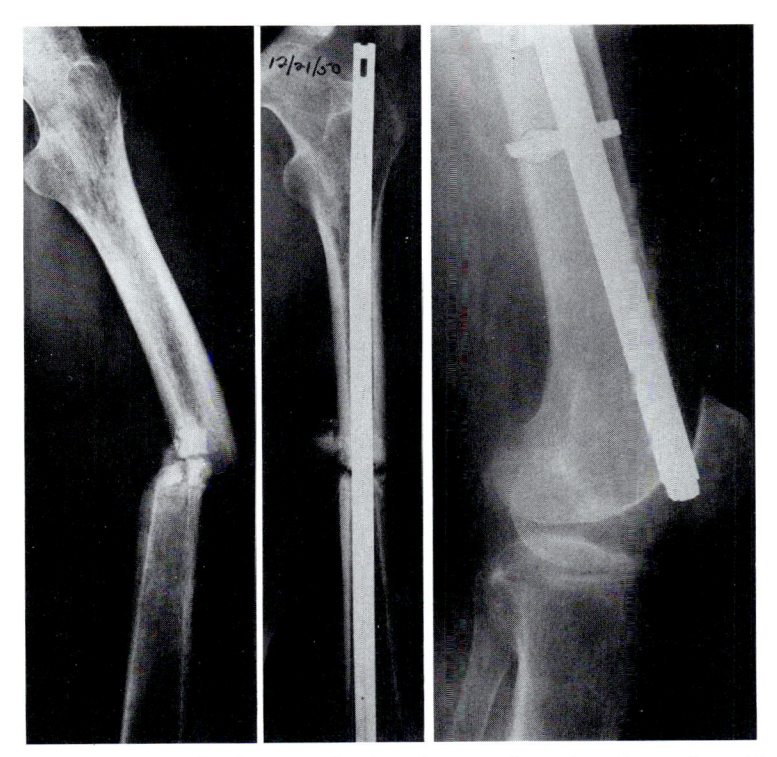

Fig. 35-18 (left). — The cloverleaf (Küntscher) nail, extending distally to the adductor tubercle and projecting proximally the width of the "eye" of the nail. The anterior bow of the femur is eliminated to conform to the straight nail.

Fig. 35-19 (right). — Example of a technical error in inserting the femoral medullary nail. With porotic bone, the nail is easily driven through the cortex or into the knee joint. Portable x-ray films taken during the operation will prevent this error.

To prevent this complication, the patient should walk with crutches and guarded weight bearing until union has progressed satisfactorily.

Once a nail has bent, it should be straightened and replaced by another, preferably a larger one. The Hansen-Street nail will not lose much strength if bending does not exceed 30 degrees. In the case of the Küntscher nail, however, any deformation of the nail at the point of bending results in marked loss of rigidity. Except in rare instances, a bent nail of any type should be considered defective and replaced by a new one. Ordinarily, the nail can be straightened by manipulation of the leg under anesthesia and then replaced during the same procedure through a trochanteric incision without exposing the fracture site.

If the nail breaks, the fracture site must be exposed and the proximal fragment either extracted through this incision or driven out through the trochanter, using another nail as a driver. Removal of the portion of the nail in the distal fragment may prove difficult. If the nail cannot be grasped with pliers or clamps and extracted, a hole may be drilled in the exposed end, using a motor-driven, high-speed steel drill. This portion of the nail then can be removed with an extractor or suitable hook. For a Küntscher nail, a screw extractor or "easy out" may be used. Once the old nail has been removed, the fracture should be treated like any other

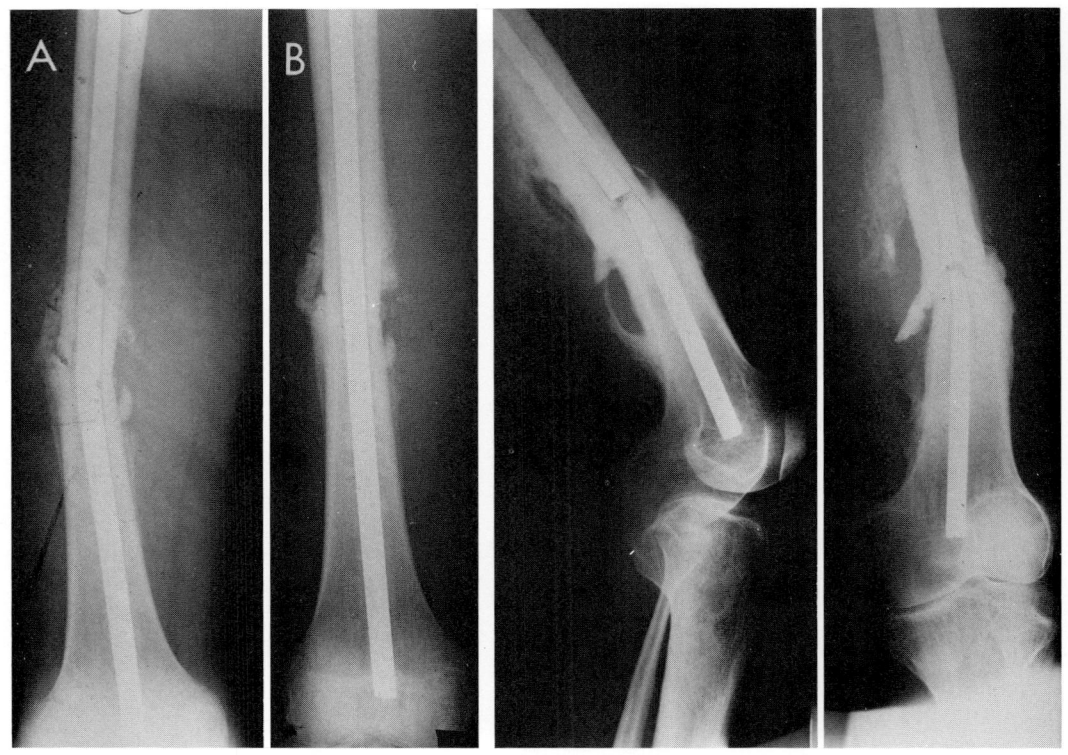

Fig. 35-20 (left).—**A,** bent medullary nail, the result of discarding crutches too soon. Under anesthesia, the nail and the femur were straightened manually. The nail was removed without exposing the fracture site and a new nail (**B**) was inserted.

Fig. 35-21 (right).—Lateral and anteroposterior views of a broken medullary nail, which resulted from discarding crutches too soon. Both fragments of the nail were removed and another nail was inserted. In addition, a walking plaster spica was applied for 4 months. Bone union resulted.

Fig. 35-22.—The pull-out screw extractor devised by Cherry and supplemented by Southwick and Austin's vise-grip pliers. This device is effective for removing broken cloverleaf medullary nails. Note that the base of the extractor (*B*) is larger than the apex (*A*), so that with each blow the grasp on the nail is made more secure. (From Southwick, W. O., and Austin, G. N.: A practical method for extracting impacted intramedullary nails, J. Bone Joint Surg. 38-A:226, 1956.)

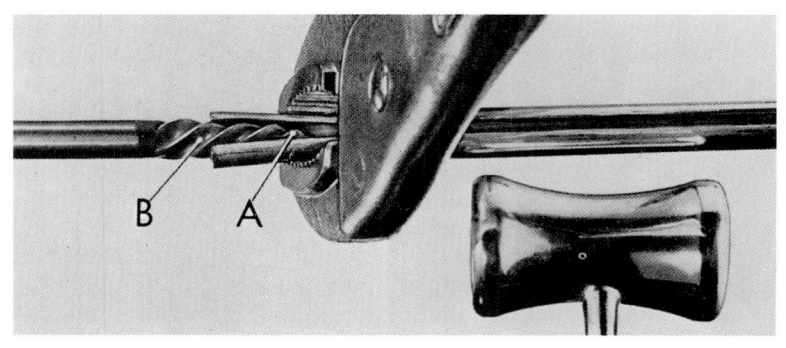

nonunion—by fixation with a new nail and iliac grafts.

SEPSIS FOLLOWING INTRAMEDULLARY FIXATION.—In the event of wound sepsis following open reduction and intramedullary fixation, adequate dependent drainage should be established and appropriate chemotherapy instituted. Reports in the literature and experience at Massachusetts General Hospital indicate that the nail should not be removed until the fracture has healed (see Fig. 5-14, p. 130). Adequate drainage and excision of scar and of sequestra should be carried out as the need arises while the fracture is healing. When solid healing has occurred, the nail may be removed. Although sepsis along the nail tract may occur even with drainage through the trochanteric wound, the nail is, as a rule, well tolerated.

Other Types of Medullary Fixation

THE RUSH NAIL.—This nail is made of 18-8 SMo stainless steel, Type 316. The content of this steel is given in Table 35-3.

The Rush nail is solid, cylindrical in shape and flexible; it is manufactured in various lengths and diameters and is suitable for use in all long bones. The principle of its medullary fixation is that of three-point pressure. This type of nail is extremely useful in stabilizing fractures of the ulna and fibula but is applied less easily to the radius. For femoral or humeral fractures, two of the nails may be required.

When inserting the Rush nail, it usually is advisable to expose and reduce the fracture and then make a small drill hole in either the distal or proximal end of the broken bone. The nail then can be gently tapped into the shaft to the fracture site, the fracture reduced and held with a bone clamp and the nail further gently tapped or guided with strong pliers into the other fragment. If impingement is encountered, the nail should be rotated back and forth as it is inserted into the canal. It should be driven well into the bore so that the hook on the proximal end can be locked into cortical bone.

THE LOTTES TIBIA NAIL.—Another type of nail, designed by Lottes of St. Louis, is used for tibial fractures. It is made of 18-8 SMo stainless steel, is triflanged and is curved to allow its insertion at the level of the tibial tubercle. It has a diameter of $3/8$ inch and is available in lengths of $9\frac{1}{2}$–14 inches, the lengths varying by $\frac{1}{2}$ inch.

Lottes usually avoids exposing the fracture by carrying out a closed reduction; then, with the patient's knee flexed over the end of the operating table, he drives the nail across the fracture line well into the distal fragment. The nail can be used

TABLE 35-3.—SPECIFICATIONS OF THE RUSH NAIL

Chromium	17.54%
Nickel	12.89%
Molybdenum	2.27%
Manganese	1.67%
Carbon	0.059%
Silicon	0.50%
Phosphorus	0.024%
Sulfur	0.020%

Fig. 35-23.—Use of the Rush nail for intramedullary nailing of fracture of upper end of the ulna.

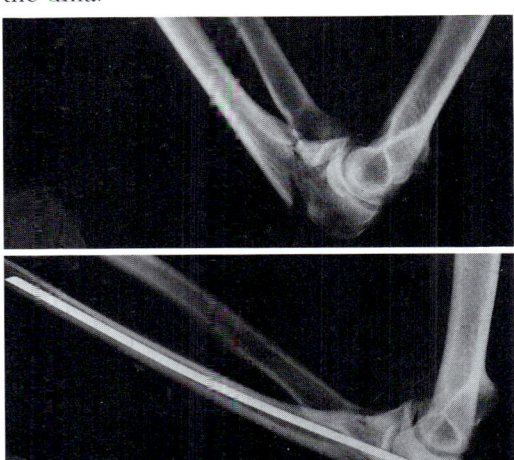

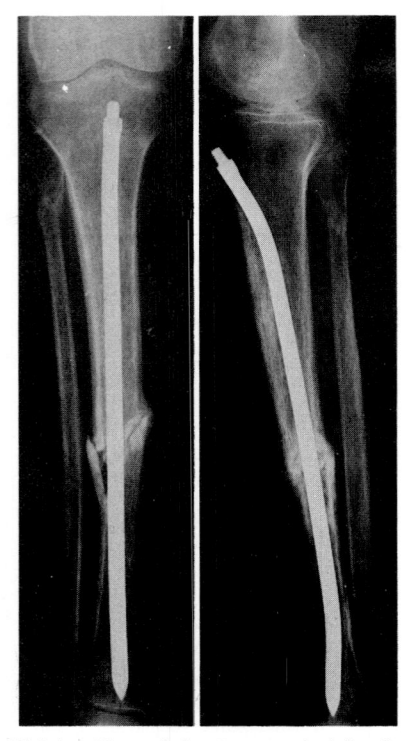

Fig. 35-24.—Use of the Lottes nail for fixation of tibial fracture.

for "any fracture in the middle one-third or upper portion of the tibia and for multiple segmental fractures" (see Chapter 31). It has also been employed in selected open fractures and in cases of delayed union or nonunion of the tibia.

In cases of nonunion of long bones in proximity to joints, the form of treatment used occasionally at Massachusetts General Hospital has been to introduce a medullary nail through the adjacent joint. This treatment has been used in fractures of the humerus, when a Rush nail has been driven down through the humeral head. In 6 cases of prolonged nonunion of the tibia, a Küntscher nail was introduced through the knee. This procedure was used only in extreme cases when no other form of internal fixation would suffice (see Chapter 5).

Fractures Treated by Excision of Fragments

The patella and the olecranon perform similar functions in the knee and elbow, respectively. When they are fractured, they may, at times, be treated similarly — that is, by excision (see Chapters 19 and 30). The severely comminuted patellar

Fig. 35-25.—Restoration of elbow motion after olecranon excision following old fracture. **A,** olecranon fracture that had been treated by catgut suture 18 months previously. Motions were: 15 degrees fixed flexion to 60 degrees further flexion. **B,** 2 months after olecranon excision. Motions were: 5 degrees fixed flexion; further flexion, 145 degrees — essentially normal. **C,** the excised olecranon.

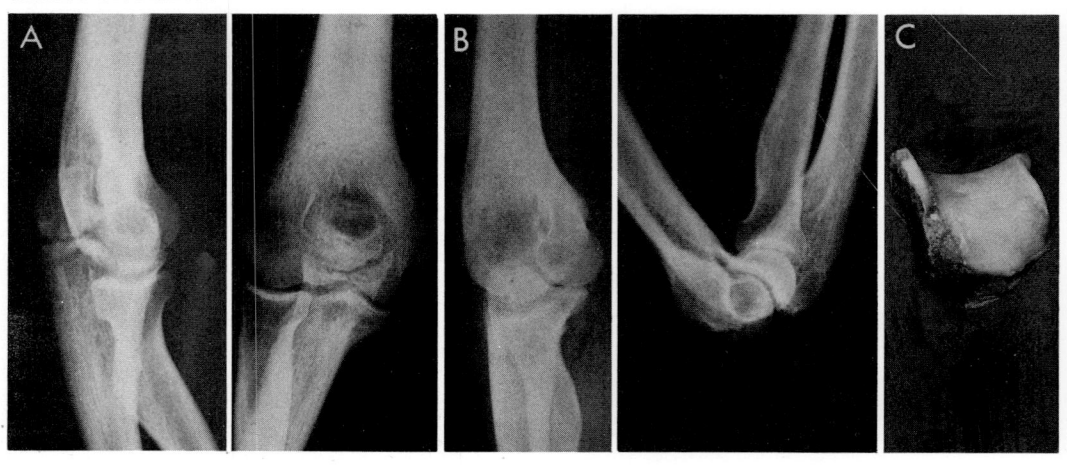

fracture is managed best by excision of all fragments and suture of the quadriceps and patellar tendons. When there is a transverse fracture, the surgeon may elect to excise the smaller fragment and suture the tendon to the remaining larger fragment.

Olecranon fractures, particularly in older adults, are managed effectively by excision of the fragment and suture of the triceps tendon to the ulna if, at the time of operation, passive displacement of the joint is not possible. Excision of the olecranon is followed by early use of the elbow and a good return of function. Treatment by excision may also be used for the following: the internal humeral epicondyle that has been pulled into the elbow joint; old displacements of the outer or inner end of the clavicle, if painful; the ununited spinous process of a vertebra; an ununited neck or base of the fifth metatarsal.

Much has happened as a result of the operative treatment of fractures in this century to condemn the procedure in many instances. The unsatisfactory outcomes have largely been due to lack of fundamental training and judgment on the part of the surgeon, resulting in poor selection of cases and faulty operative technique. If the surgeon is trained properly and exercises careful judgment in the selection of cases, this form of fracture management has much to recommend it. However, no surgeon should operate on a fracture unless: he and his assistants are trained properly, the proper instruments are available, the operating room is adequate, sterilization is trustworthy and the patient's general condition is satisfactory.

BIBLIOGRAPHY

1. Bassett, C. A.: Personal communication.
2. Brav, E.: Personal communication.
3. Cherry, H. L.: Simple effective extractor, J. Bone Joint Surg. 36-A:400, 1954.
4. Eggers, G. W. N., Shindler, T. O., and Pomerat, C. M.: The influence of the contact-compression factor on osteogenesis in surgical fractures, J. Bone Joint Surg. 31-A:693, 1949.
5. Groves, E. W. H. *On Modern Methods of Treating Fractures* (Bristol, England: John Wright & Sons, Ltd., 1916).
6. Key, J. A.: Electrolytic absorption of bone due to the use of stainless steels of different composition for internal fixation, Surg. Gynecol. Obstet. 83:319, 1946.
7. Küntscher, G.: Die Marknagelung von Knochenbruchen, Arch. Klin. Chir. 200:443, 1940.
8. Lane, W. A.: *The Operative Treatment of Fractures* (London: Medical Publishing Co., 1914).
9. Lane, W. A.: The operative treatment of single fractures, Surg. Gynecol. Obstet. 8:344, 1909.
10. Lottes, J. O.: Blind nailing technique for insertion of the triflange medullary nail, JAMA 155:1039, 1954.
11. Luck, V. J.: Medullary fixation of the femur, Am. Acad. Orthop. Surgeons Lect. 8:2, 1951.
12. Lund, F. B.: The Parham and Martin band in oblique fractures, Surg. Gynecol. Obstet. 23:545, 1916.
13. Müller, M. E., Allgöwer, M., and Willenegger, H.: *Technique of Internal Fixation of Fractures* (New York: Springer-Verlag, 1965).
14. Nicolaysen, J.: Lidt om diagnosen og behandlingen fr. colli femoris, Nord. med. Ark. N.F. 7:1, 1897.
15. Parham, F. W.: A new device for treatment of fractures, New Orleans M. & S. J. 66:451, 1913–14.
16. Peterson, L. T.: Fixation of bones by plates and screws, J. Bone Joint Surg. 29:335, 1947.
17. Rush, L. V., and Rush, J. L.: Fixation of fractures by longitudinal pin, Am. J. Surg. 78:324, 1949.
18. Rush, L. V., and Rush, J. L.: Technique for longitudinal pin fixation of certain fractures of the ulna and femur, J. Bone Joint Surg. 21:619, 1939.
19. Sherman, M. S., and Phemister, D. B.: Pathology of ununited fractures of neck of femur, J. Bone Joint Surg. 29:19, 1947.
20. Southwick, W. O., and Austin, G. N.: A practical method for extracting impacted intramedullary nails, J. Bone Joint Surg. 38-A:266, 1956.
21. Starr, K. W.: *The Causation and Treatment of Delayed Union in Fractures of the Long Bone* (St. Louis: The C. V. Mosby Company, 1947).
22. Street, D. M., Hansen, J. J., and Brewer, B. J.: Medullary nail: Presentation of new type and report of cases, Arch. Surg. 55:423, 1947.
23. Venable, C. S., and Stuck, W. G.: *The Internal Fixation of Fractures* (Springfield, Ill.: Charles C Thomas, Publisher, 1947).
24. Winant, E. M.: Personal communication.

36 | Use and Abuse of Metal Implants

JONATHAN COHEN and THORNTON BROWN

THE USE of internally implanted devices for the fixation of fractures is becoming increasingly common. More and more devices are being developed for the treatment of fractures. In this chapter we will consider some of the characteristics of these devices, which we will call bone fasteners. This term is used to distinguish them from other devices, such as endoprostheses and nonorthopedic implants. It is not our purpose to discuss specific uses of different bone fasteners, including their indications or contraindications. Rather, we will first summarize the current status of the metallurgy of these devices, particularly with reference to recognizing the ways in which they can fail and the reasons for failure. We will then review some of the biologic and mechanical interactions between the devices and the host that may influence the results of treatment.

METALLURGY

For a metal to be suitable for use in bone fasteners, it must be well tolerated in the tissues. Tolerance, of course, involves both the tissues and the metal. When a metal is not tolerated by tissues, not only are the tissues inflamed but the metal also is affected and shows signs of having reacted. We will consider first the reaction in the metal, i.e., corrosion.

Corrosion

The discussion of corrosion will be confined to situations in which *modern* surgical metals are used in fracture fixation. These modern metals include 3 groups of alloys that have been singled out for these applications: (1) the stainless steels of the 316 and 317 classes; (2) the cobalt chromium alloys (stellites) and (3) titanium and its alloys.*

STAINLESS STEELS.—The 2 classes of stainless steel used for surgical implants are characterized by a content of about 3% molybdenum, which accounts for the occasional designation of some steels in this group as SMO. The general class is known as 18-8 because all the steels in this group have about 18% chromium and 8% nickel. The word "stainless," by definition, means that there is at least 11% chromium in the formulation. There are hundreds of varieties of stainless steel that do not have the 18-8 chromium-nickel ratio, and only a few that do. Nearly all the latter have been tried out for surgical implant applications, and the 316 and 317 types have been found to be most corrosion resistant in tissues. One variety in particular, 316-L, the L desig-

---

*The American Society for Testing and Materials has elaborated standard specifications for these 3 metals (ASTM Annual Standards, Part 7, pp. 1004–16, 1971, 1916 Race Street, Philadelphia).

913

nating a low-carbon formulation, is the most popular today.

It should be noted that, in different countries, analogous alloys may have slighty different specifications as to chemical composition and, of course, different designations. The AISI system of nomenclature (American Iron and Steel Institute) is the most well known here and abroad, but devices of foreign origin may not meet the accepted chemical compositions and specifications of this system.

The chemical compositions of stainless steels developed for different purposes vary widely because varying amounts of different elements are introduced to provide desired characteristics. Thus, changes in carbon content on the order of tenths or even hundredths of 1% strongly affect the hardness of the product and other physical properties which are of vital concern to those who manufacture the finished item. Similarly, other elements—for instance, chromium, nickel and molybdenum—have a significant but lesser effect on the physical properties, but a great influence on corrosion resistance. Still other elements (e.g., sulfur and phosphorus) may be residuals from the original ore and may constitute undesirable inclusions. The problems of specifications and the responsibilities of various organizations to have meaningful specifications, and to adhere to them, are particularly difficult when imported devices are in question. These devices often will have compositions that do not meet U.S. formulations. Surgeons and patients should be aware of these differences and their implications, if such devices are used.

COBALT CHROMIUM ALLOYS.—The cobalt chromium alloys were invented in 1907 by Haynes, who later formed the Haynes Stellite Company. Hence the designation of the most commonly used alloys in this group as stellites (HS with a number indicating the specific formulation). Each one of this class of alloys contains more than 50% cobalt and about 20–30% chromium. The 2 most popular of the surgical stellite alloys are marketed as Vitallium, but other proprietary names are also used (Vinertia, Zimaloy). It should be appreciated that there is a significant difference in the chemical composition of the 2 stellites marketed as Vitallium. One, "cast" Vitallium, has about 27% chromium and no tungsten. The other, "wrought" Vitallium, has 19% chromium and 14% tungsten. The words "cast" and "wrought" are generally omitted from labels and markings.

TITANIUM AND ITS ALLOYS.—The relatively recent development of these metals, primarily for aerospace application, followed the discovery that these metals can be quite strong and quite resistant to corrosion, yet are much lighter than either the stellites or the stainless steels. Titanium and its alloys have only recently been given wide application in surgical implants, now that the techniques of fabrication have been worked out for aerospace purposes. These techniques are much more difficult than those used for the better known alloys. It has not yet been established to what extent the titanium alloys are superior in corrosion resistance to the other alloys mentioned, if indeed they are. Long-term studies on toxicity are not yet available. Similarly, no thorough evaluation has been made of the many titanium alloys which may be superior to the ones now in use. The ones in use are primarily 99% titanium (unalloyed) and Ti 6Al4V (6% aluminum and 4% vanadium).

The 3 classes of metals just described have been singled out because of their resistance to corrosion in chloride-containing fluid, an attribute which makes them suitable for marine and industrial applications. It is for this reason that they have been and continue to be studied intensively. Since the tissue environment resembles sea water so far as corrosion testing and marine experience are concerned, the results of this research can be applied to the use of metals for bone fasteners. However, only in the last 3 years or so have any attempts been made to formulate specifically for surgical implants metals that will have more resistance to corrosion in chloride-containing fluids than the metals currently in use. Although these attempts have been encouraging, they have not yet dealt with the question of whether tissue and tissue fluids differ significantly from sea water in relation to corrosion. Not even the first step has been taken in the attack on this problem, despite the obvious need to explore the potential capacity of several of the components of the tissues and tissue fluids (such as the phosphates, protein complexes and even enzymes) to influence corrosion.

TYPES AND RATE OF CORROSION. — Corrosion of bone fasteners must be reviewed in the light of how long the fastener must remain in contact with tissue and how long it must provide the mechanical function for which it was implanted. In other words, the time scale of the corrosion process in relation to the particular fracture situation must be appreciated before one can judge how well a metal meets the minimal need for corrosion resistance. On the surface of all the metals listed, all selected because of their resistivity, extensive but superficial corrosion occurs rather quickly, as it does on all metal objects, in the form of tarnish or rusting. However, this corrosion does not become significant, provided each metal is properly prepared and cleaned prior to use. In addition to this immediate surface reaction, however, are 3 other, significant kinds of corrosion that affect these classes of metals. How significant each one is depends mostly on the rate and duration of the corrosion process. Other important factors determining the significance of corrosion are the volume of metal involved and the exact location of the deteriorative process as well as its mechanical and biologic consequences. The 3 important types of corrosion are (1) crevice corrosion, (2) pit corrosion and (3) fretting corrosion (Fig. 36-1).

Unfortunately, the available methods to measure the amount and rate of these 3 types of corrosion are not standardized. The usual measurements of weight loss of standard metal coupons under standard experimental conditions (in milligrams per kilogram per year), or of penetration, as in pitting (in micrometers per year measured at the deepest point in a pit) are obviously not adequate measurements, although the orders of magnitude of corrosion may be characterized by these means.

In general, the rates of corrosion for the 3 classes of metals under discussion are somewhat as follows:

1. Stainless steels kept in salt solutions will show grossly evident pits on the surfaces after some months, whereas in crevices they will show corrosion in a few weeks. Using stronger corrodents and specially designed crevices, stainless steels will show gross evidence of corrosion within days. If fretting is added to the aforementioned conditions, extensive corrosion will develop in a few weeks even with milder corrodents.

2. The cobalt chromium alloys, particularly the wrought Vitallium formulation, are also susceptible to pitting under the same conditions but the pits are smaller and less undercut than those in the stainless steels and take longer to develop. A similar difference is noted with crevice and fretting corrosion. Because stellites ordinarily are harder (more wear resistant) than steel, particularly the cast formulations, they resist the fretting corrosion process to a much greater degree. Nevertheless, observations of a great many standard clinical situations (several screw-plate interfaces per case) have revealed that fretting corrosion either of the underside of screw heads or of the mating surface of countersink holes in the plate is a common occurrence, even after a few weeks or months of implant residence in a patient.

3. Titanium is held to be much more

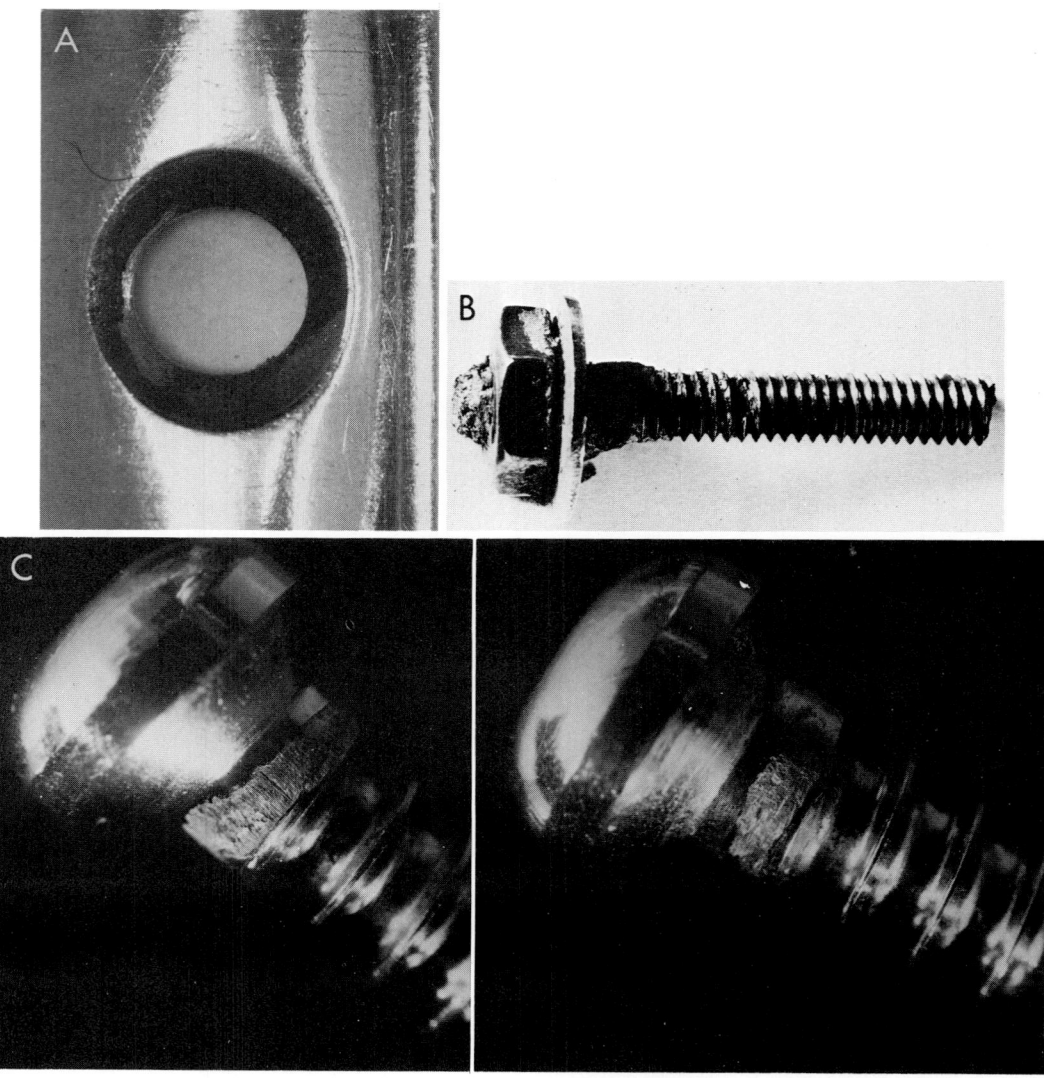

Fig. 36-1—**A**, screw hole in a bone plate that had remained in a patient for 1 year. Fretting corrosion is evident in the 3 irregular gray areas on the countersink. The largest area *(right lower)* is nearly diagonally oriented to the thinner area to the left, the 1 being on the outer part of the countersink, the other on the inner part, indicating the direction of rocking motion of the screw. **B**, broken bolt, with nut and washer, has pitting corrosion sufficient to reduce the profile of the threads *(center)* and weaken the bolt so that it broke *(right)*. There is also crevice corrosion between nut and washer. This is a large crevice. The smaller the crevice, the greater the likelihood of crevice corrosion. **C**, heads of 2 screws (from a compression plating); corrosion is evident on the neck, where compression force narrowed the crevice, and on the chamfer (underhead).

resistant to corrosion in chloride solutions than either of the other 2 classes of alloys. It owes its resistance to the rapid formation of a thin layer of oxide on its surface, which then protects the surface against further reaction. Despite the resistance of the titanium alloys to pit and crevice corrosion, titanium implants produce high concentrations of titanium in the nearby tissue, showing that loss of metal from the implants has occurred. Furthermore, if there is fretting, titanium is especially vulnerable because of its poor resistance to wear. Well-documented clinical examples of corrosion of titanium, however, have not yet been reported. There are, however, reports of blackening of tissues in contact with titanium devices after only a few months of implantation.

From the foregoing, it is evident that all 3 groups of metals are corrodible in tissues to some degree and that the amount of corrosion varies for the different metals and in particular situations. However, each of these metals is currently in widespread use — a fact that must indicate that each is sufficiently corrosion-resistant to warrant clinical application.

Tissue Reaction

The tissue's reaction to the metal of the fastener, the other side of the 2-way street, is inflammation. This always occurs to some degree, as in response to any foreign material. When the reaction is severe enough to cause significant symptoms, the tissue intolerance to the metal is considered a metal failure. How failure of treatment is related to metal failure will be taken up later.

The inflammation related to a metal implant must be evaluated with respect to its degree and with respect to the possibility of another cause. Frank suppurative infection, with bacteria demonstrated in the exudate, need hardly be mentioned, except for the possibility that the pre-existent, lesser degree of chronic inflammation due to the metal and the tissue necrosis around the fastener as a result of insertional trauma (or the fracture itself) may constitute a *locus minoris resistentiae*. Here blood-borne, or locally implanted, bacteria may thrive.

Purulent inflammation, severe in degree, hardly ever occurs about a metal in the absence of bacterial infection. Although corrosion products may elicit this kind of inflammatory reaction, experience has shown that it happens rarely and then only in relation to metals which are not acceptable for surgical implantation today. We refer to the cases, which still crop up occasionally, in which fasteners of vanadium steel, of stainless steels of types other than those already described or of other unacceptable metals (including welds) have been used. Most of these implants date back several decades, when metals and manufacturing processes of types now unacceptable were still being used. But even at present, there is the rare instance in which a wrong metal will be discovered to be the basis of tissue reaction and corrosion. These instances, past and present, will be easily recognized by the surgeon, because the inflammation caused by the corrosion products is accompanied by severe gross staining of the tissues by these products and because, histologically, the presence of large amounts of rust extracellularly and in histiocytes is pathognomonic.

Setting aside these cases of severe inflammation, there is the much more common moderate degree of inflammation (Fig. 36-2) and scarring around the fastener made of acceptable metal. In this situation, several clinical aspects other than infection and corrosion must be considered. Persistent mechanical instability of the fracture, in the presence of an ineffective bone fastener, in itself can give rise to chronic inflammation and scarring. If nonunion persists for several weeks or months, the slight cyclic bending of a bone plate or rod may first evoke significant tissue reaction and then may cause

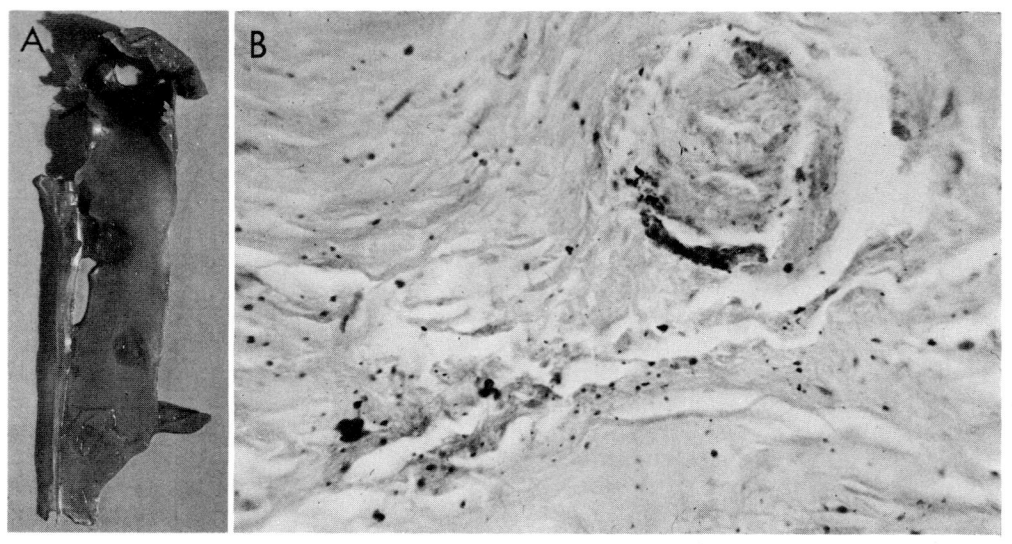

Fig. 36-2.—A, strip of tissue removed from a patient who had a Smith-Petersen nail and Thornton plate in situ for 3 years. The metal was type 316-L stainless steel. The hole in the tissue *(arrow)* was where the nail penetrated into the femoral neck. The smaller holes below are where screws penetrated the femoral shaft. Each hole is surrounded by a dark discoloration (brownish at operation), indicating corrosion products. B, photomicrograph of part of wall of the fibrous capsule. This part showed no discoloration, yet rust particles are numerous, intracellularly and extracellularly, amid the fibrous tissue of the scar.

the fastener to break. The cyclic bending at the fracture site is then augmented, intensifying the scarring. Histologic and bacteriologic study of the tissue removed in these cases may contribute the important information that corrosion products are present in significant amounts, but it is more usual to find no demonstrable cause of the inflammation in the tissue. The clinical aspects of the case, therefore, which must be coordinated with the tissue findings to determine the cause for the corrosion and tissue reaction, would be: (1) the extent of necrosis from the original fracture and operative trauma; (2) the mechanical stability achieved after reduction and maintained thereafter; (3) the time intervals between the original injury and the original operation and between the original and the secondary operation, when the tissue was obtained; (4) the time when the fastener showed signs of corrosion and/or breakage, and (5) the metallurgical findings on examination of the fastener after removal. The complexity of this analysis varies in each case, but enough has been said to provide a general view of the problems.

Corrosion of Metal Implants

Further discussion of corrosion would lead us into aspects of the corrosion problem that are not strictly germane to the fixation of fractures. We will limit further consideration of corrosion to a series of the most frequently asked questions and try to provide answers that are up-to-date.

Question: If 1 alloy is better than the others with respect to corrosion resistance, why not use it exclusively?

Answer: Each of the alloys has attributes that make it preferable in certain ways. One of these attributes is ease of manufacturing. The methods of manufacture using steel are more advanced, more adaptable and cheaper than those available for either cobalt chromium or titanium. Good grades of type 316 and 317 stainless steel are readily available at relatively low cost from several steel manufacturers. By good grades, we mean steels relatively free of dirt (inclusions) and conforming not only in their composition to standards, but also furnished in the specific state of hardness required for the particular processes to be used in manufacture. The fact that stainless steel can be hardened or softened to some degree by physical manipulations also allows the manufacturer to regulate somewhat the physical properties of the steel not only during manufacture but also in the end product.

The alloy HS 21, the most corrosion-resistant cobalt chromium alloy under consideration here, is several times more expensive than steel. Devices manufactured of this alloy are usually cast, because the techniques of machining and of reducing the large ingots to bar or wire dimensions are difficult, due mostly to the fact that the alloy work-hardens so quickly. Although methods of extruding HS 21 (and thus avoiding the casting process) are now being developed, they are expensive and not yet generally available. As a consequence, devices made from this alloy are manufactured by special casting methods, the first of which was devised as recently as 1929, by Prangle and co-workers. Casting as a manufacturing method introduces the possibility that the end product may contain small voids and concentrations of inclusions. With casting there is also less firm control over the dimensions of the end product. To avoid these defects, there must be much stricter attention to the details of manufacture than is necessary in the fabrication of steel products.

The manufacturing process for devices made of wrought cobalt chromium alloys is also more difficult and expensive than that of steel devices. The very limited and diminishing use of wrought alloys, compared with the use of HS 21, despite the somewhat better physical properties of the wrought alloy, is explained by its lesser corrosion resistance.

Titanium and its alloys also are difficult and expensive to manufacture and, at present, the more complicated designs of bone fasteners are not being made from titanium. Difficulties are also being encountered in quality control of both the dimensions and the worked surfaces of titanium devices, notably those of screw threads. Since titanium and its alloys are so difficult to use in the manufacture of implants, it is understandable that only a relatively few manufacturers are marketing products made of this metal. From the point of view of the user, titanium products must be examined carefully with respect to quality control. The user should also be certain that the products come from a reliable source. Nevertheless, the excellent corrosion resistance of titanium should be reason enough to continue to use this material in the manufacture of surgical implants, at least until better metals are obtainable.

Question: If corrosion is so important and occurs with all metals, why can so many surgical implants remain in situ for years without causing trouble?

Answer: There is no doubt that thousands of devices, after holding the bone fragments together for the few weeks or months required for union of a fracture, thereafter cause no symptoms or significant changes visible on x-rays. However, it is rare indeed that the reactive tissue (Fig. 36-3) that encapsulates a metal implant remains thin and uninflamed after it has been in situ for several years. The usual picture is that of a thickened capsule of fibrous tissue in which there are chronic inflammatory changes. On occasion, after as long as 10 or even 20 years, this capsule breaks down and inflammation of a more acute type is seen in the surrounding tissue. However, the relationship between the production of corrosion products and the development of fibrous tissue is by no means a proportional one. The exact mechanisms by which corrosion products cause irritation in the tissue are not known. There is ample evidence, however, that corrosion products are irritative. First, the pH within a crevice where corrosion is occurring can be depressed to as low as 2. Second,

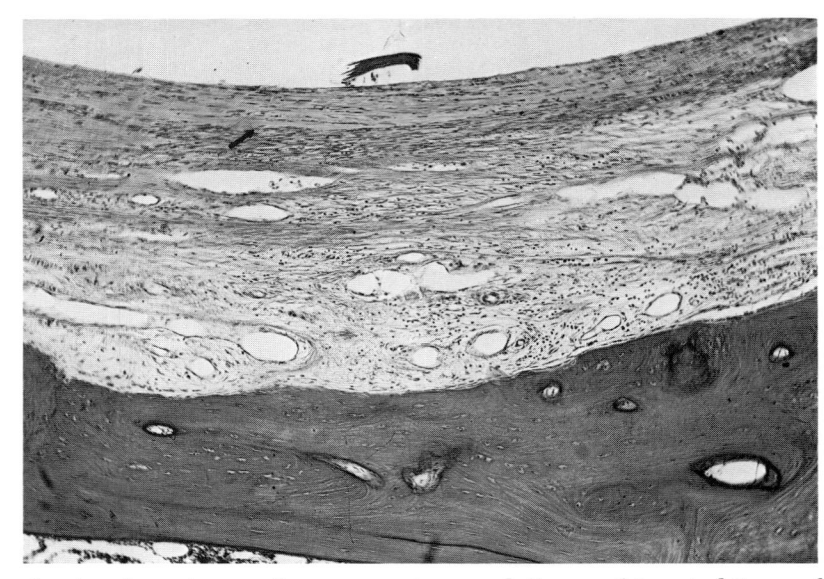

Fig. 36-3.—Section from tissue adjacent to an intramedullary nail inserted 3 years before. The fibrous reaction *(arrow)*, the particles of metal or metal corrosion product *(right, on surface)* and the subjacent mild chronic inflammation are the principal features. Sclerosis of bone is not seen.

corrosion products can be seen regularly in phagocytic cells (Fig. 36-4) near the sites of conversion of metal into corrosion products. Third, in prospective studies to determine whether residual symptoms occur with metal implants, the experience has been that such symptomatology may be expected in more than half the cases.

Question: If corrosion is a continuing

Fig. 36-4.—Foci of cells showing accumulation of particles of metal or metal products. These were black on the sections, whereas nuclear fragments were blue. Cells morphologically identical with fibrocytes and fibroblasts contained the particles, as well as histiocytes. Some of these "fibrocytes" had particles in their cytoplasm strung out in a line with the nucleus *(arrow)*.

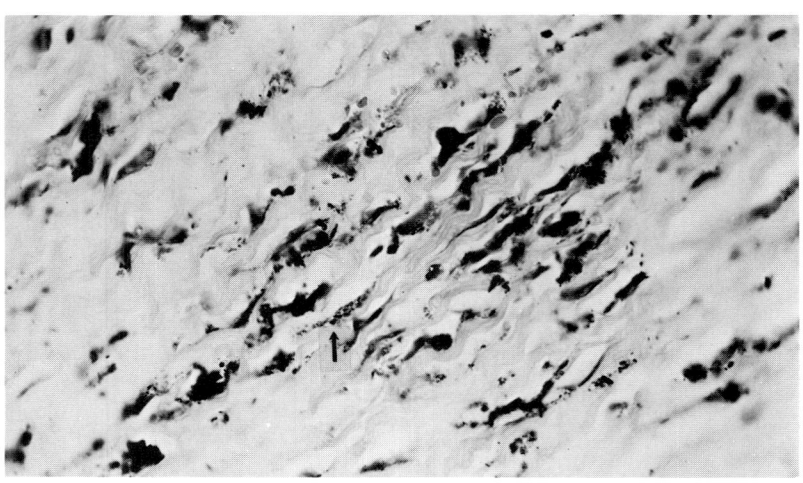

process, would it not be good policy to remove all metal implants, if possible, after they have accomplished their purposes?

Answer: Many factors must be weighed in the answer to this question. Our own judgment is that in all young people, i.e., under 30 years of age, removal of the appliance is warranted because the long-term effects of implanted metal are not known. Short-term study of corrosion processes rarely permits conclusions that will be pertinent after 30 or 40 years of exposure of an implant to the corrodent. Long-term toxicity studies are lacking and are not likely to be accomplished. It is easy to decide to remove a surgical device if it has accomplished its purpose and has begun to cause symptoms of pain or inflammation. It is in the borderline case, in which symptoms are minimal, the operative risk is considerable or difficulties in removing the device are anticipated that expert judgment is required.

Question: Since experience has shown that corrosion is only important in a minority of cases, are there any special circumstances in which corrosion is more apt to occur?

Answer: The more metal items implanted in a given patient, the greater the likelihood of significant corrosion. The greater the opportunity for fretting to occur between 2 pieces of metal within the same patient, the greater the opportunity for corrosion. If the design of a device is such that there are many crevices and if there is a good chance for motion between components of the fastener (Fig. 36-5), a corrosion-prone situation exists.

Question: Is a mixture of metals to be avoided categorically?

Answer: It is true that the more diverse 2 metals are, particularly if they are in contact, the greater the chance that a corrosion cell will be formed. However, a large experience with mixtures of different stainless steel components has not

Fig. 36-5. — Plate and screws used in internal fixation of a fracture of the tibia. Note the fretting corrosion at the countersink of most of the screw holes and on the chamfer (underhead) of most of the screws. In this site crevice corrosion is prone to occur and the fretting motion of metal on metal continually exposes new surfaces for reaction by breaking through the protective layer of oxides (corrosion products). The underside of the plate, next to the bone, also shows areas of crevice corrosion, the crevice being between bone and plate.

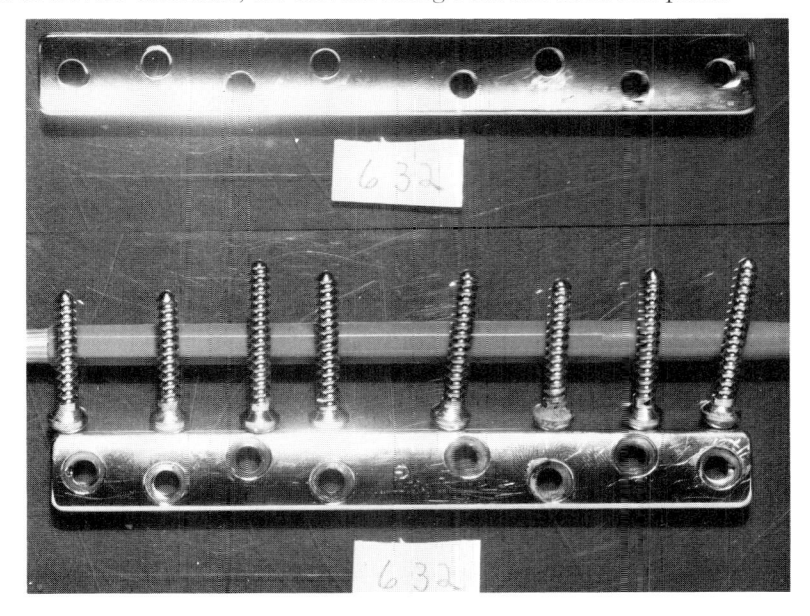

shown a much greater potentiality for corrosion with such mixtures than with components made of metal of the same formulation. We therefore cannot, purely on the basis of experience, advocate that all stainless steel items be purchased from the same manufacturer, nor can we state without reservation that a mixture of steels from different manufacturers is bad practice.

By the same token, experience with mixtures of Vitallium and steel implants in the same patient seems to be comparable, i.e., there does not seem to be a significantly greater tendency for corrosion when these metals are mixed. There has not been sufficient clinical experience in which titanium and cobalt chromium or titanium and stainless steel objects have been used together in the same patient to make any statement about these mixtures (Fig. 36-6).

These statements, however, should not be taken as assurances that all the presently accepted surgical metals can be used together indiscriminately. From the statistical and metallurgical points of view it seems likely that pure metal of any 1 type in all components of a device would be preferable in the long run to multiple metals in the different components.

Question: What physical properties of the different alloys relate to the choice of 1 alloy over the others?

Answer: Some of the physical properties which are the result of methods of manufacture, e.g., casting, have already been discussed. All the metals mentioned have ultimate tensile strengths a good deal greater than 50,000 psi and often approaching 100,000 psi (greater by far than the tensile strength of bone). Although the ultimate tensile strength is an indicator of the resistance of the material to breakage, a more important indicator is the yield strength. This, in general, is a measure of the tensile strength and the

Fig. 36-6.—Part of a cobalt chromium plate and 3 type 316 steel screws removed after 24 months because of pain. Note the collection of dark powder at periphery of the screw holes (some of it has been scraped off the center one for analysis). Corrosion products are also evident on the middle screw. Color photographs of this specimen showed 2 rings of the colors of the rainbow on the plate concentric with the middle hole. Analysis of the powder by spectrography revealed both iron and cobalt, iron being in greater amount. The tissues showed mild chronic inflammation with blackish discoloration.

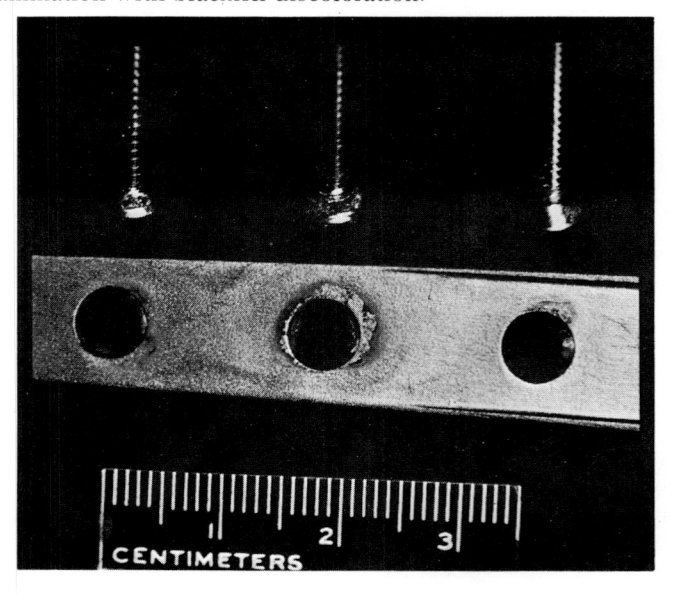

degree of elasticity of the material. A still more important property from the point of view of the manufacturer, is ductility. If a metal is not sufficiently ductile to permit the usual machining manipulations, the process of manufacture is very expensive and exacting.

All these considerations guide the fabricator of surgical implants in seeing that the end product is strong enough (high tensile strength) for its intended usage, yet flexible enough (adequate elastic modulus) so that brittle failure with slight bending or impact stress does not occur. Specifications for these properties are now available for a variety of bone fasteners, thanks to the efforts of the F-4 Committee of the ASTM. However, it is impossible for the surgeon, at the operating table or during gross inspection of his material before operation, to be sure that these specifications have been met. At present, the reliability of the fabricator of the fastener is the only assurance a surgeon has that the fastener has the required physical properties.

Question: The transfer of bits of metal from instruments, such as screw drivers or clamps, to the device being implanted has been proposed as 1 method whereby corroding metals may be introduced into the tissues. The implication is that the instruments should be made of metal with corrosion resistance equal to that of the implant. How important is this, practically?

Answer: All the evidence indicates that, although such transfer occurs regularly, it has no clinical significance. Examination of thousands of screws that have been removed has shown that the site of corrosion, if there is any, practically never involves the slot (Fig. 36-2, A) and that no preferential localization of inflammation in the tissue in juxtaposition to the slot has been evident. Since the screw slot always is the site of some metal transfer, it would seem that this process is not the determining one, at least with respect to tissue reaction.

Question: Are there any methods of treating the metals now in use to make them more corrosion resistant?

Answer: The practicalities of any surgical operation are such that no type of plating, cladding or surface treatment of metals would be adequate; since scratching of the surface-protective layer would lay bare the material that is to be protected. The same difficulty would be present in any composite, e.g., metal-reinforced polymers, that might be thought applicable by providing 1 component for strength and another for corrosion resistance. The metal to be used therefore has to have "self-healing" properties as regards resistance

Question: What improvements can we expect in the near future with respect to bone fasteners?

Answer: The manufacturers of bone fasteners are in fairly lively competition and quality control in the production of standard fasteners will probably improve in due course. Manufacturers are also continuing to standardize dimensions, so that components made by 1 company will be more likely to fit those of others. The ASTM is acting as the principal agency for developing standards. It is a nongovernmental organization that includes representatives of the consumers as well as the producers. The Food and Drug Administration, as the protector of the public's interest in this field, is also exerting efforts to upgrade the quality of existing devices. Research is being done to improve the metals and their fabrication. We believe that in a few years new metals and new ways to fabricate them will supplant those in use today.

FAILURE

When a bone fastener is used in the treatment of a fracture, failure may occur, due either to failure of the device or to clinical failure. Failure of the device, i.e., a metal failure, may be either a mechanical or a corrosion failure. Clinical failure, i.e., a bad result, may be due to infection or other complication or to problems related to the presence of the implant in the tissues. These general types of failure — device failure and clinical failure — may occur singly or in combination. Thus, the device may fail but the clinical result be entirely satisfactory. Or the device may perform well but the fracture fail to unite. Or the device may fail and there may also be nonunion. The most common situation is clinical failure without evidence of failure of the device. When both types of failure occur, it is important to show what relationship exists between them.

Pure corrosion failure, which causes clinical failure, is epitomized by the patient whose fracture heals after fixation with a plate and screws, but who, after months or years, has pain at the fracture site. If the surgeon removes the metal and examines it adequately, he finds some elements showing corrosion. He also finds evidence of inflammation in the tissue near 1 or more of the screws and adjoining portions of the plate. He may discern discoloration of the tissues caused by corrosion products. Biopsies of these tissues then show scar and active chronic inflammation. If the correct tissue specimens are properly processed, corrosion products will be visible in histiocytes and perhaps also in the fibrocytes (Fig. 36-4), even at some distance from the site of the device.

Despite these changes, the clinical result almost always is successful, since removal of the offending, corroding material relieves the symptoms. Metal from such a failure is illustrated in Figure 36-7.

It should be noted, however, that the same evidence of corrosion and the same type of inflammation and scar tissue formation but to a lesser degree may be present without accompanying symptoms. Are we to call such evidence of corrosion metal *failure*, in the face of obvious clinical success? Perhaps a specific amount or rate of corrosion and scarring, which is tolerable, must be exceeded if symptoms are to develop. Perhaps individuals differ in their tolerance for local tissue irritation. Again, perhaps local anatomic factors, such as the proximity of sensory nerves, as well as the irritation of moving structures, such as muscles or synovial membranes in proximity to the inflamed area, are auxiliary factors that produce symptoms. These possibilities have yet to be properly assessed.

If the objective of internal fixation of fractures is that during the lifetime of the patient the fastener will reside in this tissue without corrosion, then by definition the presence of any corrosion must be considered a failure. Unfortunately, it is impossible to quantitate corrosion in vivo

Fig. 36-7.—Screw removed from patient having clinical failure. There is pitting corrosion in the screw threads sufficient in degree to weaken the screw and cause it to break. In this patient the corrosion products were voluminous and sufficiently irritative to cause a sterile inflammation, which ultimately was drained before removal of the metal. (From Cohen, J., and Hammond, G.: Corrosion in a device for fracture fixation, J. Bone Joint Surg. 41-A:524, 1959.)

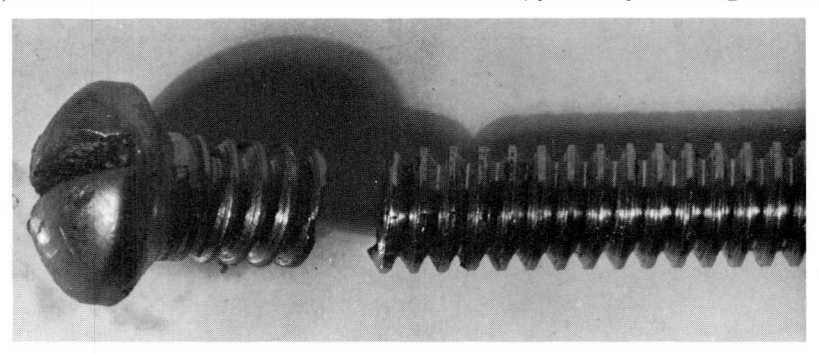

with sufficient accuracy to establish a definable line between metal success and metal failure, at least in the present state of the art.

Corrosion, by itself, rarely if ever is a cause of nonunion of a fracture. The rate of corrosion of modern surgical metals in vivo is too slow to compromise the strength of a device to the extent that it breaks before the fracture has had a chance to heal. However, cases have been reported in which corrosion was responsible for breakage of the fasteners. In such cases there usually is not extensive destruction of metal, but rather formation of points of weakness (stress raisers) where the fracture of the appliance is instigated. In other words, the break in the metal starts at a point where stress has been concentrated because of a corrosion pit (Fig. 36-7). In most of these cases, the process known as corrosion fatigue has been evident. Under these circumstances, sufficient stress has been applied to the device to weaken it, and the break then occurs at a point where plastic deformation of grains and grain boundaries (Fig. 36-8) in the metal has been potentiated by the corrosion discontinuity.

Failure of a metal device in an obvious way, such as breaking, bending or the components coming apart, would not seem to deserve much discussion. Yet individual situations may not always be simple, and the medicolegal importance of the proper assignment of blame, if there is blame, justifies some discussion. It seems platitudinous to state that designation of the failure of a device as mechanical is a judgment, based on what was expected of the device. If a screw breaks under an inordinate load, the blame for the break should fall on the one who allowed the inordinate load to be applied. If the load was not inordinate, and the defect was in composition, design, fabrication or application, the appropriate assignment of blame can be made on the evidence (Fig. 36-9).

However, we must recognize how difficult it is to define what an inordinate load is. Even under the best of circumstances a strict definition is impossible. Whether or not the hardware is appropriate depends on an accumulation of experience and judgment, as is evident in the following example. A subtrochanteric, essentially transverse, uncomminuted fracture of the femur can be fixed by sev-

Fig. 36-8.—**A,** part of roentgenogram showing a broken screw. The radiolucent interval between the plate and bone (femur) indicates loosening, and the relative motion has permitted the screw head to be well displaced from its original position. Displacement occurred long after the fracture had healed, since radiographs 1 year after fracture did not show the screw to be broken. **B,** low-power metallograph of the screw shows pitting on the left. **C** and **D,** in slightly higher power, the transgranular and intergranular corrosive process is seen.

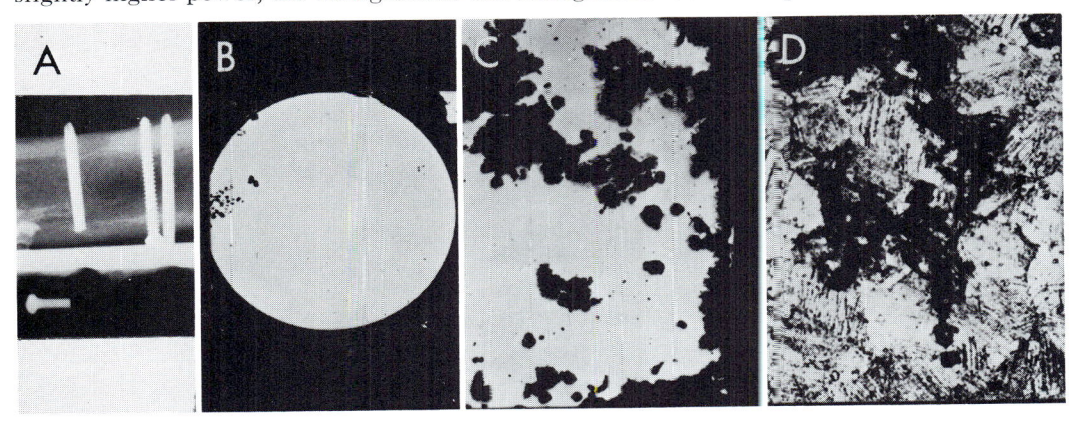

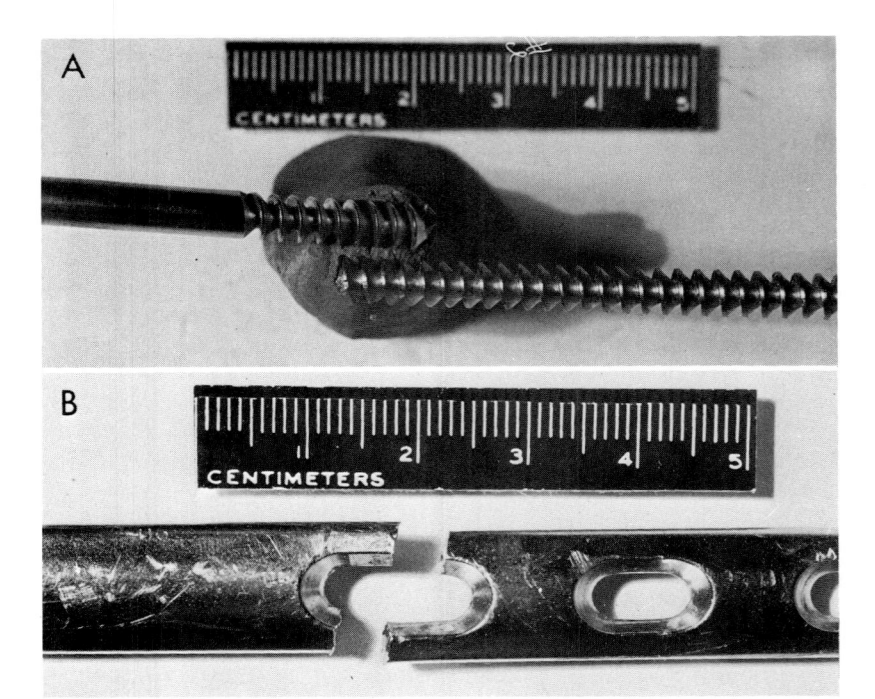

Fig. 36-9.—Two examples of defects in design (or application). **A**, broken olecranon screw, used for fixation of an ulnar fracture from the olecranon. The annealed condition of the screw and its thin core diameter were not satisfactory for the use to which it was put. The screw should have been harder and thicker. **B**, slotted plate with sharp edges at the holes—stress-raising features which predispose to breakage. Fracture surfaces of the metal on metallography indicated recurrent, cyclic stresses with work hardening and gradual deformation and breakage. The amounts of stress and cycles of stressing, although not matters which can be estimated except through detailed clinical history and educated speculation, were excessive. Either they should have been minimized or the design features altered so that the device can withstand greater and more protracted stressing.

eral devices available to the surgeon. However, the load applied to the device postoperatively may vary widely. If the surfaces of the fracture are jagged and the 2 fragments interlock well at the time the device is inserted, and if postoperatively the patient engages in minimal activity and does not bear weight on the extremity, we have a situation in which the loading is kept to a minimum. If the device fails, especially if failure occurs during the first few weeks after operation, one may well suspect some defect in its design, fabrication or application. Such a situation would warrant full examination of the appliance itself and of its past history.

On the other hand, let us suppose that during application of the device used for fixation of the aforementioned subtrochanteric fracture, some distraction of the fracture surfaces occurred and 1 screw was inserted into the fracture site where it did not get a good grip on the bone. The obvious consequences of this situation would be a much greater load on a localized segment of the device, fracture healing that would be delayed or prevented by the distraction, and a less efficient attachment of the plate to the femoral shaft. The result might well be that the device would come apart or pull away from the bone or that 1 of its components would break, even if the patient were as inactive as in the previous situation.

The assignment of blame for failure of the device in the second case would rest on a consideration of all the evidence and a judgment of the relative importance of the individual bits of evidence. If the fracture had been fixed as described and the plate broke despite minimal activity, whether 1 day, 6 months or 2 years after operation, the blame would fall on the mistake in operative technique. The accumulation of metallurgical data on possible defects in the device would be beside the point. Any device will break if badly applied or if loaded beyond its designed capacity. The fact that it breaks at a demonstrated point of weakness is irrelevant.

However, if the device was applied properly and if the point of weakness where failure occurred was indicative of a defect in design (such as a thin flange on a Thornton plate to support the attachment of the Smith-Petersen nail — Fig. 36-10) or if there was a defect in fabrication (such as a casting void), these features would obviously be relevant.

There is no easy way to explain all or even the largest number of the observed failures. Each situation must be considered in detail and attention given to the kind of fracture, the likelihood of healing with the type of treatment administered (clinical judgment), all the details of treatment, including the minutiae of the operative situation and the day-by-day or week-by-week conduct of after-care, and finally the clinical and metallurgical evidence accumulated once failure is encountered. The best prophylaxis against failure is proper clinical judgment in the selection of the device and meticulous technique in its application. It goes without saying that devices of the best design for the fractures to be treated must be available and that the reliability of any device in large measure is assured by the reliability of the manufacturer.

Fig. 36-10. — Break in Thornton plate removed 3 months after implanting for treatment of intertrochanteric fracture. No metallurgical defects at break surface were grossly demonstrable, but corrosion on bolt, washer and plate-hole periphery is easily seen. Metallography (not done) could have shown the presence or absence of stress corrosion. Design of plate obviously reveals inadequate strength at break site in view of forces to be expected. Did patient bear full weight? Was appliance tight at all times? Did bone absorption allow loosening of appliance? All of these factors may have had a part in causing breakage.

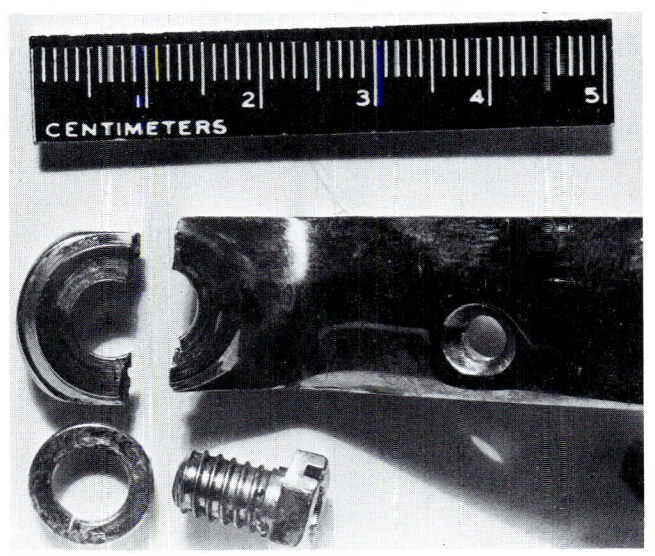

MECHANICAL AND BIOLOGIC INTERACTIONS OF HOST AND IMPLANT

Up to this point we have considered metallurgical, biologic and mechanical factors that may influence what happens after a bone fastener has been inserted. These factors, of course, include design and fabrication of the implant, chemical interaction between the tissues and the metal, mechanisms of mechanical and clinical failure and like factors that become operative once the fastener is in situ. Other more general biologic and mechanical aspects of fracture treatment may be important considerations in determining whether a metal implant is used or abused. These considerations vary with specific fracture situations, but a few general remarks would seem appropriate.

Mechanical Interactions

An important mechanical consideration is the rigidity of fixation needed and obtainable in a given situation. Such rigidity depends on many factors, including the stresses to which the particular fracture site will be subjected (muscle forces, as well as those applied externally), the strength of available fasteners, the location and plane of the fracture, the degree of comminution and the interlocking of the fracture surfaces. If the surgeon concludes that anatomic reduction is needed but rigid internal fixation cannot be achieved, he may elect to use a metal implant and supplement this fixation with a plaster cast or traction. Or, if during the procedure it becomes apparent that rigid internal fixation, orginally thought to be obtainable has in fact not been achieved, the surgeon may resort to supplemental external fixation. However, as a general principle, use of a metal implant should have as its goal an anatomic reduction and fixation sufficiently rigid to permit early motion. The implantation of metal to achieve a lesser goal is likely to be considered abuse.

Modern implants and techniques, such as those developed by the AO group, have made it possible to achieve adequate fixation of some fractures which formerly could not be treated with implanted fasteners. However, there remain situations in which, for a variety of reasons, the use of metal fasteners is impractical or inadvisable. These reasons include the small size of the comminuted fragments, the severity of the osteoporosis, the amount of disruption of a joint surface and the lack of experience of the surgeon with the particular fracture problem. It scarcely seems necessary to remark that an unsuccessful attempt at open reduction and internal fixation may in itself be a cause of nonunion even when there is no complication, such as postoperative infection, foreign body reaction, or the like.

The thickness and mobility of the surrounding soft tissues as opposed to the bulk of the implant are also mechanical features the surgeon must consider if he is to avoid abuse of metal. A bone fastener can be applied to the surface of a bone with safety only when the wound can be closed without tension and when there is sufficient, adequately vascularized soft tissue overlying the implant to minimize the risk of soft tissue necrosis and loss of skin. The volume of the implant required indeed may be a crucial consideration. Another is the position the implant must occupy with respect to moving parts, such as tendons and ligaments. If, once it is in situ, the fastener will limit excursion or otherwise impair function of these structures, internal fixation may jeopardize function of the part.

Still other mechanical factors which relate to the proper use of metallic devices for internal fixation lie in the realm of technique and judgment. Although these factors are discussed in connection with specific fractures elsewhere in this book, no consideration of the use and abuse of metals would be complete without some reference to the importance of preoperative planning and technique in the successful application of metal fasteners.

Once the decision to use internal fixation has been made, the surgeon must select the device with design features that make it suitable for the job to be accomplished. He must also be sure that the instruments and assistance necessary to apply the device in an optimal fashion will be available. Alternative devices should be on hand in the event that the procedure planned proves not to be feasible. Success can only be achieved if the device is adequate and is applied so that it can function in the way for which it was designed. Thus, a femoral intramedullary rod must be of sufficient length and diameter to provide the needed strength and stability. The screw holes drilled in bone for plate fixation must be accurately placed and tapped to provide maximal strength of fixation. If a plate must be bent to fit the bone fragments, the bending should be done carefully with a proper bending device to avoid undue weakening. The plate must also be sufficiently ductile to allow mechanical bending, and examination of its surface after bending should reveal no fissuring or crazing indicative of inordinate weakening. The fracture surfaces and fragments should be accurately fitted together to ensure maximal surface contact and stability. In this connection it should be kept in mind that, with rare exceptions, the goal of internal fixation is to establish conditions under which the bone fastener holds the fracture fragments in position so that they resist the deforming forces. Rarely will a fastener by itself withstand these forces long enough for union to occur.

Biologic Interactions

The biologic interactions of the metals with the tissue are related primarily to the effects that the process of insertion and the presence of the fastener in the tissues have on vascularity, resistance to infection and healing potential of the bone and soft tissues. When the risks entailed in the use of a metal fastener are considered, it should be obvious that even the gentlest of surgical exposures may be the final, slight, but determinate additional trauma that makes it impossible for the severely traumatized skin and soft tissue to recover. By the same token, scarred, adherent avascular skin and soft tissues cannot be incised, reflected, retracted and sutured and still continue their precarious existence. If the tissues are in this precarious state, as they so often are over an ununited fracture of the tibia, a metallic implant may be contraindicated, at least until adequate soft tissue coverage has been restored by a pedicle graft. Possible exceptions are insertion of an intramedullary rod without exposing the fracture site and implantation of a compression plate through a posterior incision.

Similarly, the extent of damage to the 2 blood supplies of a bone—the endosteal and periosteal—may vary. The fastener selected and the site of application, so far as possible, should preserve the existing blood supply. To apply double plates to an ununited fracture previously fixed with an intramedullary rod may destroy virtually all the blood supply to the bone ends throughout the extent of the bone exposed subperiosteally for the application of the plates.

Another biologic consideration is the effect of a bone fastener on the resistance of the tissues to infection and on the growth of bacterial contaminants within the wound. The factors related to decrease of resistance include the introduction of a foreign body, the additional trauma to tissues consequent to the surgical approach, and the exposure of more tissue to contamination. On the other hand, the immobilization of the bone fragments and surrounding tissues made possible by internal fixation may enable the local tissues to combat bacterial contamination, thereby preventing bacterial growth and clinical infection. Also, rigid internal fixation often permits fracture healing even in the presence of an established infection; after healing, the infection can be controlled by the removal of the implant, wound debridement and appropriate antibiotics. The often difficult decision relative to the insertion and removal of the bone fasteners in contaminated or infected fractures must be based on expert clinical judgment.

A final biologic consideration relates to the patient as a whole. When use of a metallic fastener is contemplated, one must not lose sight of the patient's total problem, especially when there are multiple injuries. Will the gains to be derived from successful internal fixation be negated by the effects of other injuries? For example, the patient with fractures of both upper extremities cannot use crutches. He therefore may have nothing to gain from an open reduction of a fracture of the femoral shaft already adequately aligned in traction, and he may have everything to lose from a postoperative infection and chronic osteomyelitis of the femur.

The aforementioned rather general statements about the mechanical and biologic factors that may determine whether metal is used or abused may have more meaning if specific situations are considered.

CASE 1.—A closed transverse fracture of the midshaft of the femur of a young man with no other injuries.

A variety of treatment regimens may be used in this situation. Common to all methods of internal fixation is a reduction in the amount of displacement of the fragments, so that less callus is needed to bridge the fracture gap. When the various available types of internal fixation are considered, certain mechanical and biologic consequences should come to mind.

Fixation by a long plate with screws, though technically relatively easy, provides less stability than other methods. This is true primarily because the very firm callus needed to unite the fragments of a femur in adults takes many weeks or even many months to develop. During this interval, absorption of bone around the screws may diminish the stability, or fatigue failure of the plate or screws may result in loss of all fixation.

Double plating, of course, provides more stability, but the large exposure required, the technical difficulties of the procedure and the need to remove the plates in separate procedures to reduce the risk of refracture are distinct drawbacks. Compression plating no doubt produces more rigid fixation and closer contact of the fracture surfaces but has similar disadvantages. All types of plating require rather widespread stripping of the periosteum, hence loss of periosteal circulation. This loss may be of considerable significance if the endosteal circulation has been destroyed. The major blood supply to the cortex comes through the endosteal circulation, which is fed by the nutrient vessels. The principal nutrient artery to the femur enters near the lesser trochanter; other, smaller arteries are located near the distal end. In the fracture of the midshaft, therefore, vascular impairment would not be an important objection to use of a plate, since the endosteal circulation would probably not have been seriously impaired.

Perhaps the major objection to plating of the femoral fracture considered here is the extent of the surgical exposure. There would be wide opening of tissue planes, the inevitable operative trauma to soft tissues and the attendant risk of a disastrous postoperative infection in a young man who physiologically could tolerate closed treatment with every expectation of a satisfactory result.

The remaining method of internal fixation applicable to this fracture is intramedullary nailing. The significant design features of intramedullary rods pertain to length and strength sufficient to provide stability. Whether the cloverleaf nail of Küntscher or another type, including the various self-broaching devices, is used is largely a matter of personal preference. The procedure may be done either with or without exposing the fracture site when facilities for blind nailing are available. To expose the fracture site in order to align the fragments under direct vision, a relatively small incision will suffice. This reduces the surgical insult to the blood supply and soft tissues considerably. However, any exposure of the fracture site, no matter how small, is not to be taken lightly. It carries all the risks of full exposure although to a lesser degree. Thus, blind nailing without exposure of the fracture clearly has advantages, although these are offset to a considerable degree by the technical difficulties. Moreover, blind nailing is feasible only if the necessary special equipment is available, and it is mandatory that the surgeon and operating room personnel have had the necessary experience with this equipment.

Unlike plates and screws which mostly damage the periosteal circulation, intramedullary rods will damage only the endosteal circulation. The damage will vary, perhaps with the type of rod used, and certainly with the extent of reaming of the medullary cavity. The significance of this damage, in the patient under consideration, would be minimal, since the periosteal circulation has not been seriously impaired. The success of the method of Küntscher with the extensive reaming that it entails emphasizes that loss of endosteal circulation is usually a small price to pay for stability of fixation.

For the fracture in Case 1 we may therefore conclude that the use of metal should be avoided if satisfactory position of the fragments can be achieved by closed methods. If metal is used, intramedullary nailing must be placed high on the list of choices for mechanical and biologic reasons. It should be emphasized that intramedullary nailing especially by the blind technique, is fraught with pitfalls. If they are not avoided, disaster may follow.

CASE 2.—A closed transverse fracture of the tibia just below its midpoint in a man, 45 years old.

For such a fracture there is much evidence that closed treatment using a total-contact cast and early weight bearing is the safest and most reliable method. One may make a strong case for the view that internal fixation in the treatment of most fractures of this type is indeed "abuse of metal." However, for purposes of this discussion, let us assume there are compelling reasons to achieve rigid internal fixation, complete restoration of normal anatomic relationship and the earliest possible return of normal function. To achieve these goals a compression plate is probably the method of choice, although an intramedullary rod inserted blindly under x-ray control might be expected to be satisfactory. Devices producing less stable fixation would not be appropriate.

Let us therefore review some of the principles of design, fabrication and application of a compression plate. Compared to bone plates in the generic sense, a compression plate must be much thicker. The usual coaptation plate is designed only to control forces that may cause displacement or disalignment of the bone fragments. The compression plate must also withstand a compression force applied to the screw heads. The force is maintained by means of the apposition of the countersinks in the screw holes against the undersurfaces (chamfers) of the screw heads. Mechanical considerations thus require a greater depth of the countersink and chamfer to allow the application and maintenance of the required force. Moreover, the effective application of this force to the bone fragments also requires better holding power of the bone on the screws than would be needed for a coaptation plate. Thus, there is a need for a technique more precise than that employed in ordinary plating. Self-tapping screws should not be used; rather, the cortical bone should be meticulously tapped before each screw is inserted.

Since the compression plate must be thicker than a coaptation plate and hence must have a larger cross-sectional area, one may well ask, "Could the design be altered without loss of needed strength, thereby reducing the tensile strength specification slightly for ease of machining during fabrication?" Better corrosion resistance may then be possible (if the plate is to be made of steel). Some designs of commercially available steel compression plates show that these considerations have been operative, and in these devices the steel is softer than in coaptation plates. This softening is achieved either by annealing or by altering the specifications for the actual chemical composition of the steel.

The mechanical interaction of a screw with the bone is much influenced by the great difference in modulus of elasticity between bone and metal. Because of this difference, it is desirable to keep the width of the crevice between the threads of the screw and the bone to a minimum. Therefore, all bone dust from drilling and tapping should be removed from the hole before each screw is inserted, and only drills and taps with appropriate dimensions and cutting specifications suitable for a mineral (noncompliant) material should be used. In this way, insertion of the screw will not cause microscopic crushdown of bone substance because of too tight a fit. Similarly, the final turn of the screw must not be so forceful that the bone threads are crushed or stripped. Improper fit of a screw, whether too tight or too loose, reduces the effectiveness of the compression.

The character of the tibial bone in which the screw holes are drilled and tapped also influences the holding power and maintenance of compression force in this situation. The compact bone of the young athlete obviously is less porous, thicker and more suitable for the application of a compression plate than the bone of an older individual with osteoporosis. The physical character of the bone material may be an overriding reason, in some cases, to avoid the use of a compression technique altogether. It also should be evident that during fracture healing the bone becomes more porous than it was prior to fracture. It is thus more prone to resorption, with resultant loosening of the screws—an instance of the interaction of the biologic and mechanical factors affecting the quality of the fixation.

The condition of the fracture surfaces, of course, is a mechanical factor that influences compression fixation. The fracture in Case 2 is transverse and noncomminuted, an ideal situation for rigid compression fixation. However, even in this situation there is comminution at a microscopic order of magnitude. When the 2 main fragments are fitted together, they can never be so disposed that the whole area of their fracture surfaces is in immediate contact. Some tissue elements always will intervene. At the minimum, those elements are a thin film of blood, or exudate, and microscopic bits of bone, or marrow. What is considered a hairline reduction therefore means some interposition of tissue elements.

The thickness of the interposed tissue at the least is on the order of hundreds of microns (human hair may be $100-300\mu$ thick). While the grossly apparent, jagged projections on the surface of 1 fragment may fit well into corresponding recesses in the other, at the level of the haversian systems, there is not a tight fit. When a fracture occurs, whether created by a torsional, shear or traction force, individual haversian systems break and tend to pull out of 1 fragment or the other, leaving interstitial lamellae behind. These small $(200-300\mu)$ projections may well abut 1 against the other when the fracture is reduced and maintain the fracture gap. The following mechanical situation would then obtain: Asperities of bone would be in contact, between which there would be gaps containing blood, exudate, etc. Application of the compression force would distribute that force in the bone substance of the asperities, compressing them to the point of their maximal compressibility. Then, if further force is applied, some asperities would be crushed, thus subjecting a larger number (and cross section) of them to the load. Equilibrium would be reached when there is sufficient bony contact to carry the load. At that point there still would be soft tissue and spaces between the 2 major fracture fragments, and during healing blood vessels would grow into these spaces and callus would be formed within them. Compression fixation therefore reduces but does not eliminate the fracture gap.

In considering the use of metal in Case 2 as in Case 1, the same considerations with respect to the periosteal and endosteal circulation of the bone fragments apply. However, here there is the additional factor of the thin layer of soft tissue covering the tibia. Necrosis of this skin and subcutaneous tissue is a hazard that must be added to the risk of infection and impaired bone healing secondary to avascularity of the bone fragments. The advantages of compression plate fixation (restoration of normal anatomic relationship, stability and earlier restoration of function) are attractive but may not be worth the risk. In the case under consideration, a total-contact cast with early weight bearing could be expected to give an excellent result with minimal risk.

This chapter has touched on many aspects of fracture treatment using metal bone fasteners. It should be obvious that use of metal implants in the treatment of fractures can benefit the patient immeasurably. However, there are many problems related to this use: metallurgical, mechanical, bacteriologic and biologic. Many of these problems are being solved or at least show promise of being solved. At the same time, recent experience with early weight bearing and cast bracing has convincingly demonstrated the safety, convenience and excellent results of treatment without implanted metal. It behooves the surgeon to remember that it may be easy to use metal, but it is also all too easy to abuse it.

37 | Treatment of Open Fractures

THOMAS VANDER SALM and EDWIN F. CAVE

THE TREATMENT of open fractures historically has improved in response to the demands created by battlefield wounds. Churchill, quoting Allbutt, reminds us "again how large and various was the experience of the battlefield, and how fertile the blood of warriors in rearing good surgeons."[5] Although such a statement falls harshly on us in these times, it is no less true. Most of our present principles of trauma surgery in general and of treatment of open fractures in particular have been born of the necessity created by war.[1, 2, 5, 7-9, 12-14] These principles will be discussed in this chapter.

GENERAL PRINCIPLES IN THE APPROACH TO THE PATIENT

Of a patient's several injuries, the open fracture is often the most obvious, although it may be the least threatening. Therefore, the orthopedic surgeon will frequently be the first physician to evaluate a patient who has injuries of a life-threatening but extraorthopedic nature. He would be well advised to be accomplished in the general approach to, and initial management of, trauma in general.

One of the few mnemonics worth remembering is an excellent aid to the logical approach to the trauma patient. The letters in CRASH PLAN represent: Cardio-Respiratory, Abdomen, Spine, Head, Pelvis, Limbs, Arteries and Nerves in decreasing order of urgency.

The orthopedic surgeon by his training will be intimately familiar with the PLAN but can well use the CRASH to help organize his thoughts on the initial investigation and management of a seriously wounded patient. The particulars of this management are detailed in other chapters and will not be pursued here.

PRINCIPLES OF FRACTURE HANDLING

In the Emergency Room

As the patient is quickly evaluated, his orthopedic care can be divided into general and local therapy.

GENERAL MEASURES. — An intravenous needle must be inserted, and blood should be drawn simultaneously for hematocrit, white cell and differential counts, for other tests appropriate to the patient and, most important, for typing and cross matching of blood. Resuscitation, if necessary, may be initiated with use of lactated Ringer's solution and colloid replacement until blood of the specific type is available.

Tetanus toxoid should be administered if it has not been received in the past year. If the immunization history is uncertain or if the wound is exceptionally dirty and devitalized, human hyperimmune globulin should be used.

Antibiotics should be given. We usually use a synthetic penicillin together with a drug active against gram-negative organisms for 5 days.

LOCAL THERAPY.—The wound should be inspected briefly and with sterile precautions; it should not be probed. It is then covered with a sterile dressing and the fracture appropriately splinted. For lower leg fractures, a pillow splint is often the easiest and best (Fig. 37-1). A Thomas splint is appropriate for the femur.

Standard x-rays should then be obtained, if possible. Suspected fractures of the skull or spine cannot be properly evaluated on portable x-ray film; however, with present day techniques and improved x-ray machines, most fractures of the extremities can be successfully defined with portable x-ray films. The less the patient is moved the better, and

Fig. 37-1.—Emergency room treatment. **A,** emergency care. The condition of the patient should be evaluated and the following done: The leg should be supported by pillows; bleeders ligated; sterile gauze placed in wound; needle placed in vein for blood for typing and for intravenous administration of fluids and medication. **B,** patient prepared for transportation from emergency room to x-ray department or operating table.

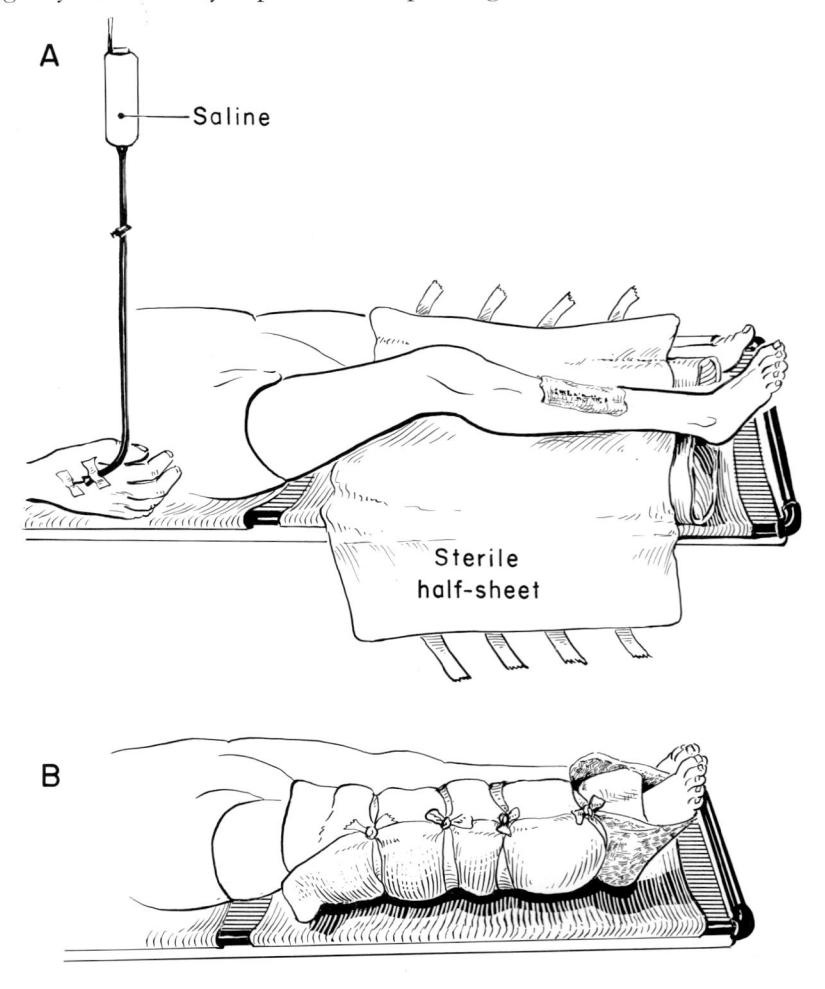

it may be advisable to bypass x-ray on the way to the operating room and obtain films once there.

Delay must be avoided, and prompt transfer to the operating room is essential after completing initial evaluation and necessary emergency room treatment.

Operative Management

It is here that we rely so heavily on the lessons learned from war experience. The *sine qua non* of management in open fractures is good debridement. This cannot be overemphasized.

PREPARATION.—The skin should be carefully prepared (Fig. 37-2). It is wise to protect the wound itself from the irritating preparation agents with a succession of dry sponges. During these procedures, it may be expeditious to stabilize the fracture with Kirschner wire traction placed in a bone distal to the fractured bone. The area prepared should be adequate to

Fig. 37-2.—Operating room treatment. **A,** skin preparation. To protect wound from solutions, sterile gauze should be placed in the wound. **B,** sharp debridement, accompanied by saline irrigation, to remove nonviable tissue and foreign material. Fracture reduction and fixation are then carried out, followed by external fixation or traction. Delayed primary wound closure is preferred (see text).

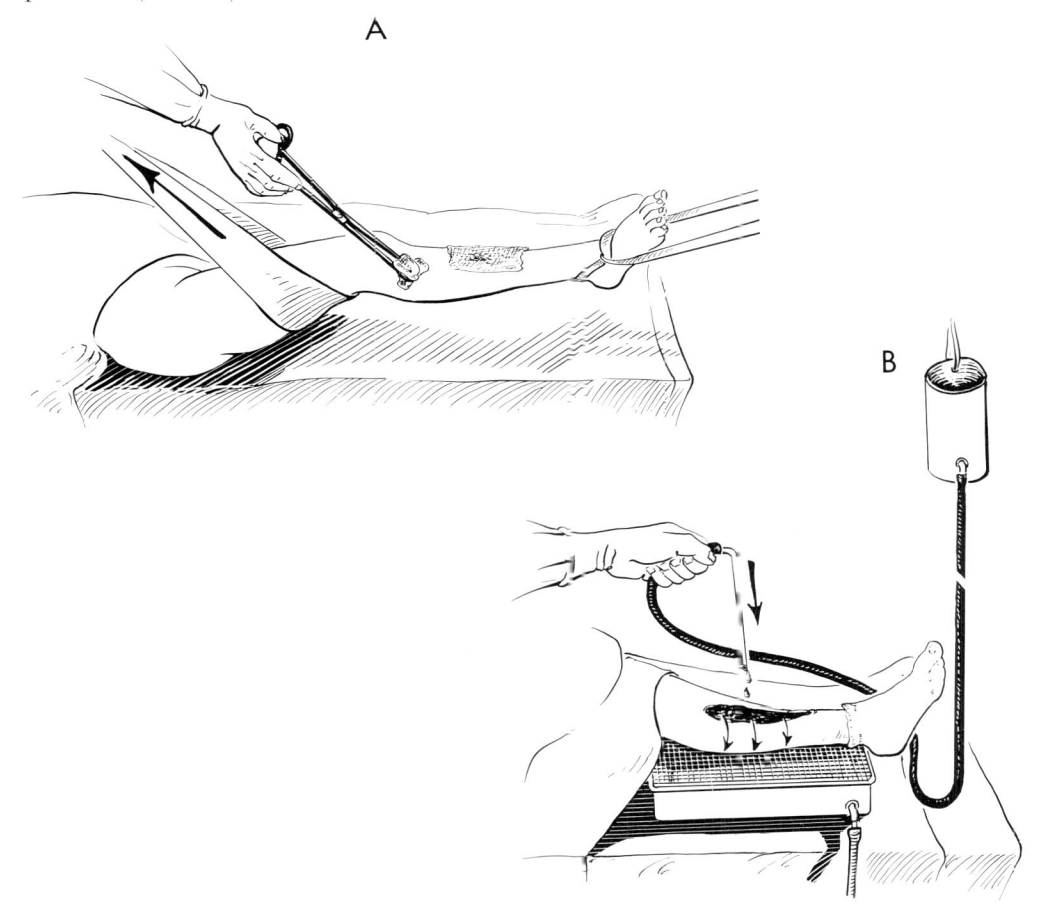

encompass easily all possible incisions necessary in the debridement.

DEBRIDEMENT.—This all important step is carried out meticulously in layers, from superficial to deep, using sharp dissection. Gentle handling of soft tissues cannot be overemphasized. Copious saline irrigation is usually helpful in further cleansing the wound.

1. *Skin.*—Often the edges of the skin will require excision to insure removal of contused, dirty areas of questionable viability. This is performed sharply and completely, even though it is realized that there may be inadequate skin to close later. Extension of the laceration may be required to obtain adequate exposure; this should be done without hesitation (Fig. 37-3). The laceration can often be converted into a standard incision for the specific exposure desired.

2. *Fascia.*—This should be meticulously debrided where necessary.

3. *Muscle.*—Debridement of muscle is of paramount importance. It must be absolutely complete and yet must be carefully done. Muscle of questionable viability should be sacrificed. The local anatomy must be known and respect given to vital structures. Bleeding is controlled.

4. *Bone.*—Dirty bone should be cleaned as well as possible. The periosteum should not be stripped if healthy, and free bone fragments in general should be retained as they act as bone grafts.

5. The wound should be thoroughly irrigated with physiologic electrolyte solution.

6. If a fasciotomy is necessary, it may be done either through the same incision or through separate incisions where more convenient.

To re-emphasize: The attainment of a clean, fresh wound is the factor. Without this, the probable result will be sepsis.

SKIN CLOSURE.—Whether or not to close the skin primarily will depend on the contamination of the wound and the adequacy of debridement. If both conditions are optimal, a primary closure may be effected. This may be either with primary suture, with split-thickness graft or with relaxing incisions and complementary split-thickness graft. The guiding principle is that the wound must not be closed under tension.

If, however, there is any question about the adequacy of debridement, or if more than 4–6 hours have elapsed from the time of injury, delayed primary closure is preferable. To this truth many papers attest.[3-6, 8, 9, 12] This method is at all times the safest and, even in rather minor, clean injuries, often the best.

The technique is simple. After thorough debridement, the wound is layered with compress gauze and on this gauze sponges are loosely packed. A sterile dressing is then applied to the entire wound; the dressing should not be taken down until from 3 to 6 days postinjury. The dressing is removed under completely sterile conditions in the operating room and the wound, if it appears clean grossly, is closed with sutures.[3, 8, 12]

Peacetime wounds are usually far less severe than war wounds and the surgeon is thus afforded the opportunity to close them primarily more often. But in so doing he should realize that his transgression of the sound principle of using delayed primary or secondary closure is possible only because the otherwise healthy patient can usually handle small amounts of enclosed contamination. To re-emphasize, when there is doubt, it is safer not to close the wound primarily.

The question of closure over exposed bones and joints must be considered, and the same basic principles apply. If the tissues extending down to bone are dirty and/or of questionable viability, they should be packed open down to bone, with plans for delayed primary closure. Conversely, if the bone is clean and immediately supra-adjacent tissues are healthy, the bone should be covered even if the more superficial wound is left open.

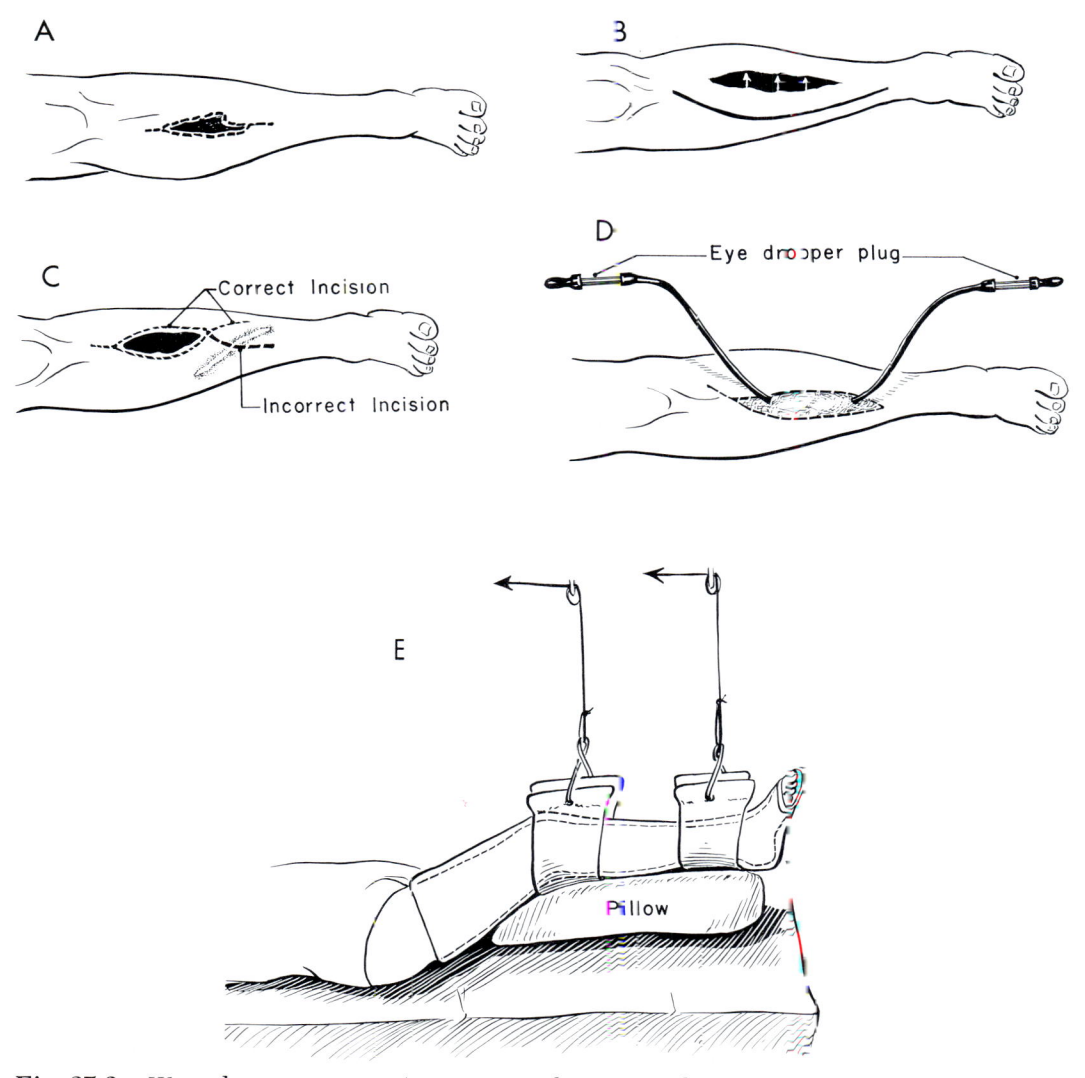

Fig. 37-3.—Wound management. **A,** preparing for surgery by enlarging wound in line of extremity and excising the edges of the skin. **B,** tension avoided by using relaxing incision when necessary. **C,** crossing of old scars avoided. **D,** wound left open and lightly packed with saline gauze fluff when viability of tissues is in doubt. **E,** immediate postoperative elevation to eliminate congestion and lessen pain.

For joints the established teaching is that complete closure should always be carried out after adequate irrigation and careful debridement. But even joints have been shown to heal well if initially left open for 1–2 days following injury.[2] For dirty joints, therefore, a sterile dressing should be applied following debridement and irrigation and closure undertaken in the operating room 1–2 days later.

FRACTURE FIXATION.—Fracture immobilization may be effected with either internal or external fixation. This is discussed after the operative care of the open fracture because we believe that, when possible, external fixation is preferable. There are, of course, cases in which internal fixation is necessary; some forearm fractures are examples. But even in these, unless the open wound is minimal and the tissues healthy, consideration should be given to debriding the wound and obtaining soft tissue healing first. Then, as a secondary procedure, the fracture can be internally fixed by an appropriate method.

In the majority of open fractures, and in tibial fractures specifically, internal fixation is not indicated.[1] After the wound is closed and dressed, the fracture is held reduced and a circular cast (bivalved if indicated) is applied. The cast may be removed and reapplied or windowed to change the dressing or complete a delayed primary closure. Otherwise it need not be removed except for signs of sepsis or as dictated by the fracture per se. Open femoral fractures are best treated with balanced suspension and Kirschner wire traction through the tibial tuberosity (in adults), unless internal fixation is opted for, after soft tissue healing has occurred. The length of treatment and the timing of weight bearing are determined as for simple fractures.

COMPLICATIONS AND TREATMENT

Nonunion

In our series, nonunion was slightly more prevalent with internal than external fixation, occurring in 18% of 44 patients with, and in 12% of 68 patients without, internal fixation. Nonunion is defined arbitrarily as healing delayed beyond 18 months or incomplete healing interrupted by operative intervention at a shorter interval.

The clinical findings are tenderness and pain at the fracture site, increased local skin temperature and x-ray appearance of nonhealing. There is usually instability and often progressive deformity at the fracture site. In our experience, nonunion has, as a rule, been associated with infection. When it is not, treatment consists of autogenous bone grafting, followed by internal and/or external fixation. Cases associated with sepsis are discussed below.

Sepsis

As can be seen in Table 37-1, the incidence of sepsis seems unchanged from the preantibiotic era in a review of open fractures from 1930 to 1965. The incidence of severe complications, such as gas gangrene or amputation secondary to sepsis, and death due to sepsis have been greatly reduced in the antibiotic era. This same review pointed out the expected relation between severity of injury and incidence of infection, and between severity of injury and severity of sepsis (Fig. 37-4). The criteria used for grading wounds are shown in Table 37-2.

The prevention of sepsis in open fractures of any type is dependent on the adequacy of the surgical procedure. Of paramount importance is thorough debridement. When adequacy of debridement is questionable, the wound must not be closed primarily. When the wound can be primarily closed, it must not be closed under tension.

The contribution of ancillary measures is difficult to assess. Antibiotic use is especially open to question on an empiric basis, but on the theoretical ground that all wounds are contaminated, antibiotic therapy would seem helpful when used for short periods. In any case, without proper care in the operating room the ancillary measures are for naught.

TYPES OF INFECTIONS. — Numerous studies have shown that all these wounds are bacterially contaminated within as little as one-half hour after injury,[13, 14] and it is reasonable to assume that most are contaminated at the moment of injury. The organisms cultured are the skin organisms, plus those exogenous organisms present in the dirt locally. The common

TABLE 37-1.—INCIDENCE OF SEPSIS IN 407 OPEN FRACTURES, 1930–65*
(FROM FOLLOW-UP STUDIES)

	1930–45 (132 CASES)	1945–55 (130 CASES)	1955–65 (145 CASES)	TOTAL (407 CASES)
Upper extremity	9% (5/54)	0% (0/37)	19% (7/37)	9% (12/128)
Lower extremity	32% (25/78)	13% (12/93)	24% (26/108)	23% (63/279)
Total incidence	23% (30/132)	9% (12/130)	23% (33/145)	18% (75/407)
Gas gangrene	2.3% (3/132)	0% (0/130)	0% (0/145)	0.7% (3/407)
Amputation due to sepsis	5.3% (7/132)	1.5% (2/130)	3.4% (5/145)	3.4% (14/407)
Death due to sepsis	1.5% (2/132)	0% (0/130)	0% (0/145)	0.5% (2/407)

*Because of a recoding of hospital records, charts were not available for review for 1960–61 and were only partially available for 1959 and 1962.

bacteria recovered in the study by Pulaski, Meleney and Spaeth were *Staphylococcus aureus, Staph. albus*, hemolytic streptococcus, enterobacilli and clostridia, the clostridium usually being *C. welchii*.

Superficial infection, if treated properly, usually has few adverse consequences. Local debridement and/or wet dressings should be sufficient. Deep infection requires formal drainage and appropriate antibiotic therapy. All necrotic

Fig. 37-4.—Degree of sepsis in relation to severity of open fractures (in 431 open fractures).

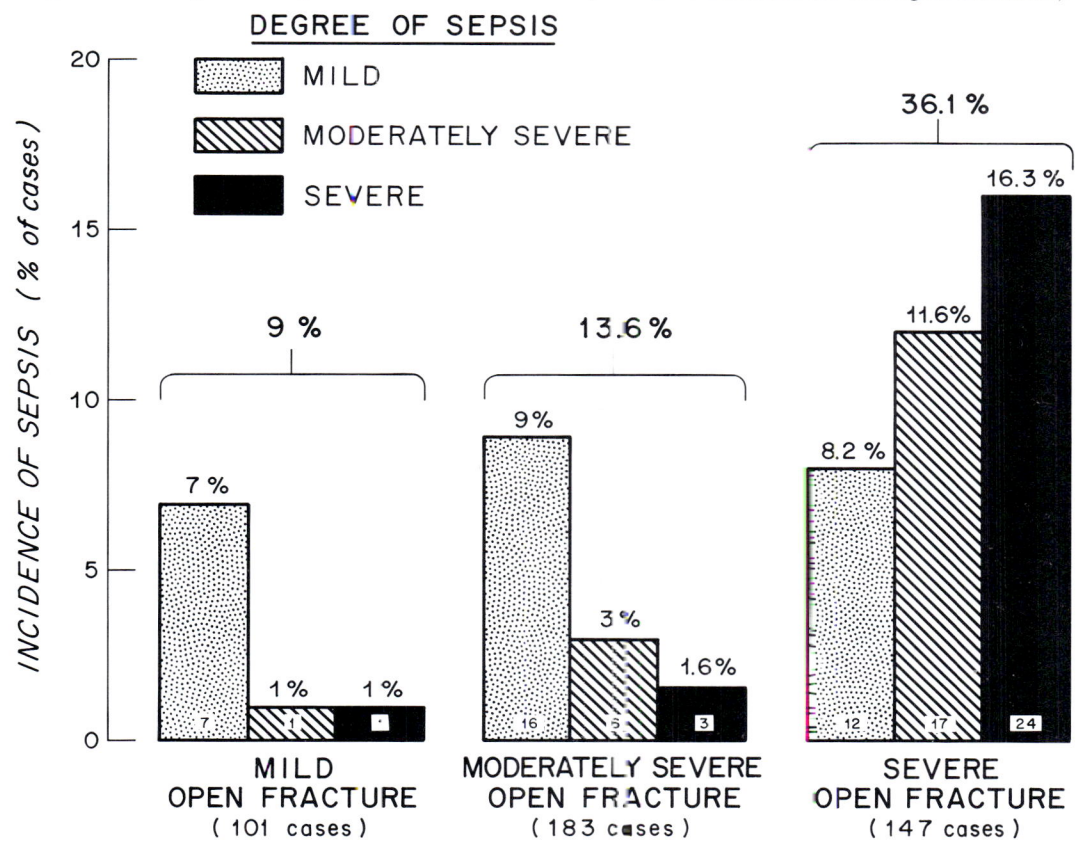

TABLE 37-2.—CRITERIA FOR
GRADING WOUNDS

NONINFECTED WOUNDS
Mild—puncture wound at the fracture site, clean
Moderate—larger wound with appreciable exposure of fracture site but with soft tissues in good condition and the degree of wound soiling not extensive
Severe—wound with soft tissue necrosis and with dirt and foreign material embedded in the soft tissues or bone fragments

SEPTIC WOUNDS
Mild—superficial wound slough or abscess down to the muscle layer, which healed within a relatively short time
Moderate—wound in which fracture site was involved by infection and which required opening but healed without complication of long-term osteomyelitis or invasive sepsis
Severe—wound with osteomyelitis requiring further treatment, invasive sepsis, gangrene, amputation or death due to sepsis from the fracture

tissue must be removed, the debridement followed by secondary closure or healing by granulation. The treatment and diagnosis of specific types of sepsis—clostridial myositis and fasciitis, necrotizing fasciitis, Meleney's synergistic gangrene, streptococcal myositis and gangrene and tetanus—are well described by Patman.[10] (See Chapter 38 for further discussion of sepsis.)

Far less dramatic than these infections, but often more devastating in terms of disability, is the infection that goes on to chronic osteomyelitis. This is generally associated with nonunion, and treatment is exasperating at best. The sepsis on the one hand and the nonunion on the other seem to perpetuate one another and therapy must be aimed at both. The bastions of therapy are excision of the draining wound, localization and excision of the sequestrum, thorough curettage of dead bone and, finally, bone grafting at a later date. The grafting should be carried out through a separate incision and in uncontaminated tissue. Using this approach, it is often possible to obtain stability before the infection is eradicated. Indeed, stability may be a prerequisite to eradication of the osteomyelitis. The details of this therapy are given in Chapter 38.

SUMMARY

The hallmark of good treatment of open fractures is thorough, careful debridement. Although primary closure of the skin is often possible in open fractures in civilians, the most universally applicable method is that of delayed primary closure. Immobilization in most cases should be with external fixation or traction.

BIBLIOGRAPHY

1. Brown, P. W., and Urban, J. G.: Early weight-bearing treatment of open fractures of the tibia, J. Bone Joint Surg. 51-A:59, 1969.
2. Burkhalter, W. D.: Four lessons from war, Emergency Med., p. 95, March, 1970.
3. Cannon, B., and Constable, J. D.: Reconstructive Plastic Surgery of the Lower Extremity, in Converse, J. M. (ed.), *Reconstructive Plastic Surgery* (Philadelphia: W. B. Saunders Company, 1964), Vol. 4, p. 1811.
4. Cannon, B.: Plastic surgery skin transplantation, N. Engl. J. Med. 239:435, 1948.
5. Churchill, E. D.: The surgical management of the wounded in the Mediterranean Theater at the time of the fall of Rome, Ann. Surg. 120:268, 1944.
6. Cleveland, M.: The emergency treatment of bone and joint casualties, J. Bone Joint Surg. 32-A:235, 1950.
7. Converse, J. M.: Early skin grafting in war wounds of the extremities, Ann. Surg. 115:321, 1942.
8. Key, J. A.: Treatment of compound fractures in the antibiotic age, JAMA 146:1091, 1951.
9. Lowry, K. F., and Curtis, G. M.: Delayed suture in management of wounds, Am. J. Surg. 80:280, 1950.
10. Patman, R. D.: Surgical Infections—Prophylaxis—Relation to Trauma, in Shires, G. T. (ed.), *Care of the Trauma Patient*. (New York: McGraw-Hill Book Company, Inc., 1966).
11. Peebles, T. C., Levine, L., Eldred, M. C., and Edsall, G.: Tetanus-toxoid emergency boosters, N. Engl. J. Med. 280:575, 1969.
12. Pool, E. H.: War wounds: Primary and secondary suture, JAMA 73:383, 1919.
13. Pulaski, E. J., Meleney, F. L., and Spaeth, W. L. C.: Bacterial flora of acute traumatic wounds, Surg. Gynec. Obstet. 72:982, 1941.
14. Rustigan, R., and Cipriani, A.: Bacteriology of open wounds, JAMA 33:224, 1947.
15. Schmeisser, G.: A syllabus on musculoskeletal trauma from lectures given at Johns Hopkins Medical School, 1965.
16. Urist, M. R., and Quigley, T. B.: Use of skeletal traction for mass treatment of compound fractures, AMA Arch. Surg. 67:834, 1951.

38 | Sepsis Following Trauma: Prevention and Control

JOHN F. BURKE

GENERAL PRINCIPLES

THE RATE OF DEATH or serious functional loss as a direct result of trauma has markedly decreased over the past few years, primarily because of the development of effective methods for dealing with massive injury to the cardiovascular-respiratory system and because of more efficient triage at the time of injury. Unfortunately, as the number of deaths related directly to trauma decrease, there have been an increase in mortality and a striking increase in numbers of patients with a severe functional loss due to a septic process developing in the period following resuscitation and primary repair. It is now clear that to ensure a long-term satisfactory outcome in the patient whose life is saved through accurate treatment in the emergency ward and operating room, the patient must be kept free of sepsis during the period of recovery and healing.

The management of trauma rests on an accurate understanding of the anatomic and physiologic disturbances caused by injury, and their early repair. It must, however, be recognized that repair from the patient's point of view includes healing and return to function. Repair, then, not only involves the restoration of anatomic continuity and alignment of soft tissue or fracture but equally rests on the prevention or early obliteration of sepsis while healing takes place. In fact, the major impediment to accurate healing and return to normal function is sepsis. Although the important advances in physiologic knowledge and their application to the trauma patient have greatly increased his chance for immediate survival, the later development of sepsis, particularly that which occurs in the injured tissues themselves, will at least impair the functional result and could cost the patient his life.

The successful management of trauma therefore depends not only on the timely repair of physiologic and anatomic injuries but also on the prevention or successful management of septic sequelae. In an attempt to outline the logical approach to the problem of postinjury sepsis, this discussion will be divided into 2 parts. The first will discuss the clinical information and techniques useful in preventing infection; the second will discuss the clinical information and techniques important in the treatment of established sepsis.

MEASURES IMPORTANT IN PREVENTING SEPSIS

It is almost always easier to prevent sepsis than to treat a bacterial infection once established. Further, the patient who heals without bacterial complication is far more likely to have a satisfactory functional result than the patient who experiences a septic episode, no matter

943

how effective the treatment. In the seriously injured patient, the direct injuries to tissue and the subsequent anesthetic and surgical maneuvers required for their repair in themselves seriously decrease the patient's usual high resistance to bacterial infection. This loss of normal host resistance is particularly prominent locally in the injured tissues. Areas of hematoma, relative ischemia, post-traumatic swelling and direct soft tissue damage all combine with the physiologic derangement of circulation and respiration to make the seriously injured patient an easy mark for infection. This defect in the patient's ability to defend himself against bacteria begins immediately after injury and is perhaps at its lowest level immediately before resuscitation in the emergency ward. In fact, in the physiologically unstable patient, anesthesia and operation, if carried out before adequate resuscitation, may seriously further decrease the patient's ability to withstand bacterial invasion. If the natural mechanisms are not at least partly operational, there is no possibility of preventing sepsis.

With these concepts in mind, it follows that, to prevent sepsis, measures aimed at repairing defects in host resistance and supplementing the natural resistance must begin as shortly after injury as possible. These preventive measures can be divided into several areas for the purpose of discussion. For clarity, each concept will be discussed separately. It is important, however, to realize that in practice they should be carried out not sequentially but simultaneously and as early as possible after injury. The areas are: (1) restoration of normal physiology; (2) removal of lethally injured tissue and the accompanying bacterial contamination produced at the time of injury; (3) avoidance of further bacterial contamination of tissue, and (4) *preventive antibiotics*.

Restoration of Normal Physiology

The comprehensive treatment of an injured patient must include measures designed to prevent infection. Of these, the immediate application of effective maneuvers that bring the patient back to a condition of near normal physiology provides the basis on which all other sepsis preventive and therapeutic activity rests. Not immediate anatomic repair of vascular occlusion, or early and accurate debridement, or the most extensive use of antibiotics will prevent infection unless there are simultaneous repair of circulatory volume and respiratory exchange and the return to normal of cardiovascular-respiratory function. For example, low cardiac output, in addition to seriously compromising the functions of the brain, the kidney and the heart, produces peripheral underperfusion. This hypoperfusion of skin, subcutaneous tissue and muscle greatly reduces tissue resistance to bacteria, particularly in the contaminated traumatic wound itself. This effect of cardiovascular inadequacy is more subtle but is nonetheless as potentially damaging as renal failure or cardiac arrest. Immediate correction of circulatory failure is universally recognized as essential to prevent death from central nervous system or cardiac failure. However, it is not widely recognized that immediate correction of circulatory failure is also essential to prevent a decrease in host resistance that would allow contaminating bacteria to invade traumatized or partially ischemic tissue and threaten the patient's life through sepsis.

These effects of peripheral underperfusion on the ability to defend against bacterial invasion have been well documented.[12, 13] In short, the immediate and long-term recovery of the injured patient, especially the patient with a large, contused open wound, gut injuries or open fracture, depends on the early re-establishment of adequate central as well as peripheral circulation.

In the long run, then, it is not sufficient merely to prevent the patient's death from shock in the immediate postinjury period. The trauma surgeon must also prevent the development of sepsis. Although infection may not be obvious for several days or weeks following trauma, the bacterial contamination causing infection often occurs at the time of, or closely following, the injury. Infection is inevitable in contaminated tissue if the natural mechanisms of host resistance cannot function. Since a major portion of these mechanisms are intimately associated with, and dependent on, the circulation, treatment must include repair of defects in host resistance to bacteria along with the maintenance of central nervous system, cardiac and renal function in the over-all plan to return the injured patient to society. In this regard, the peripheral arteriospasm produced by vasoconstrictive agents, which are occasionally suggested as a means of increasing the level of central arterial pressure, should be avoided in the treatment of traumatic shock.

The exact ways in which circulatory volume and near normal peripheral, as well as central, circulation can be most effectively repaired have been given in the chapter on shock (Chapter 11). It must be kept in mind, however, that the physiologic defects caused by red cell loss are, at least at this time, most effectively repaired by red cell replacement.

Although the intimate relationship between effective host resistance and tissue perfusion gives high priority to the repair of defects in circulatory volume, cardiac output and level of tissue perfusion, other systemic abnormalities must be corrected before adequate antibacterial defenses can be expected. Respiratory function and efficient gas exchange are vital. Electrolyte concentration, acid-base equilibrium and hydration are also crucial areas. Pre-existing disease states, such as chronic renal disease, malnutrition and diabetes, must be carefully controlled.

None of the above maneuvers is new or even unusual in any sensible plan for the resuscitation of the seriously injured patient. What is perhaps not widely recognized is that although brain, heart and kidney function can be maintained with the maintenance of central perfusion in the face of severe peripheral hypoperfusion, host resistance to bacteria, particularly in the area of open contaminated wounds, cannot. Resuscitation, then, must include not only central but also the peripheral aspects of normal physiology.

Removal of Lethally Injured Tissue and Contaminating Bacteria

Following close behind in importance in the prevention of post-traumatic sepsis are the measures which eliminate devitalized tissue, foreign bodies and contaminating bacteria from the patient's wounds at the time of initial medical care. The techniques worked out to accomplish this, particularly in military surgery, have been collected into a system called "Debridement and Initial Wound Repair." In the years since World War I, simple and clear cut concepts have been developed, In actual clinical application, however, these concepts are apt to present considerable technical and judgment difficulties. Debridement includes the removal of all devitalized tissue and foreign bodies with their burden of bacteria from the wound as early as possible following trauma. Although the idea of removing dead tissue or foreign bodies is simple enough, the problems faced by the surgeon in carrying this out may be extremely difficult. The difficulties involve 2 problems: first, actually telling injured tissue destined to die from injured tissue destined to recover; second, the reticence of the surgeon to sacrifice muscle, tendon or skin, which he cannot be positive will die, when its removal would produce a nonrepairable loss of function. Debridement is, therefore, often incomplete. Devitalized tissue, bacteria and occasionally small foreign bodies may go unrecognized and remain in the wound, leading to a high probability of disastrous suppuration. Experience has, therefore, instructed that following debridement of a traumatic wound, unless the surgeon can be absolutely certain of removal of all dead or potentially devitalized tissue, the wound must be allowed to remain open, to be closed from 3 to 7 days later. This maneuver, known as *delayed primary closure* or *secondary closure*, provides reliable drainage of the entire wound and also provides an opportunity for accurate and repeated inspection, allowing for the immediate debridement of further tissue if necessary. Both are important in preventing the development of sepsis which would be all but inevitable in a closed contaminated wound containing necrotic tissue. The combination of early excision of dead tissue, removal of dirt and bacteria, thorough and careful irrigation of the wound with saline, gentle tissue handling, accurate hemostasis and delayed primary closure has greatly reduced the risk of infection and subsequent loss of function that follows destruction of additional tissue through suppuration.

In the classic method of delayed primary closure, the edges of the debrided wound are held apart by a thin layer of fine mesh gauze and the entire wound is covered by an occlusive dressing to prevent further bacterial contamination. The area of the wound is splinted in a position of rest to prevent strain and motion. In the next few days, if exudate, local pain, developing cellulitis or systemic reactions indicate, the wound can be examined without difficulty and further debridement carried out if necessary. If in 3 days there is no sign of suppuration or devitalized tissue on inspection, the wound is definitively closed, usually on the ward, using local anesthesia. If suppuration is present, the wound is again debrided, the gauze replaced and further delay undertaken before final closure.

The thin layer of gauze allows the wound to be examined on clinical demand without seriously delaying the process of healing. The classic method of delayed primary closure has the disadvantages of (1) loss of considerable fluid, electrolyte and protein from the wound surface and (2) an increase in scar tissue formation generated by the foreign body effect of the gauze, which is allowed to remain in contact with the wound for a matter of days. Recently, split-thickness cadaver skin allografts have been substituted for the gauze layer holding the wound edges apart.[9] The cadaver skin provides physiologic closure of the wound while maintaining all the advantages of classic delayed primary closure. Fluid, electrolyte and protein loss are reduced to near zero, and scar tissue formation is not greater than that seen in primarily closed wounds. The technique of delayed primary closure and the use of split-thickness skin grafts as temporary primary closure are demonstrated in Figure 38-1.

On occasion, it may be impossible to close soft tissue wounds primarily because of post-traumatic swelling, even if no tissue is lost. This may happen because of the size of the wound or because of the inherent immobility of skin, such as that found in the lower third of the leg. These wounds cannot be closed primarily without tension unless plastic surgical procedures, such as the swinging of a flap or the harvesting and transfer of split-thickness autograft, are used. In an emergency operation, these additional plastic procedures greatly complicate the technical operative problems and considerably prolong the operative and anesthesia time. Again, the temporary use of previously harvested split-thickness cadaver skin allografts may be employed.[9] The skin allograft supplies all the benefits of primary closure without the additional operative time and surgical trauma required to harvest an autograft. The method has also proved far superior to the use of occlusive dressings in the management of large, open wounds, open fractures or open reduction of fractures of the lower third of the tibia and fibula, where soft tissue protection of underlying bone is impossible to achieve by primary closure.

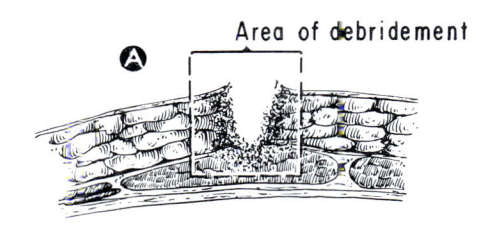

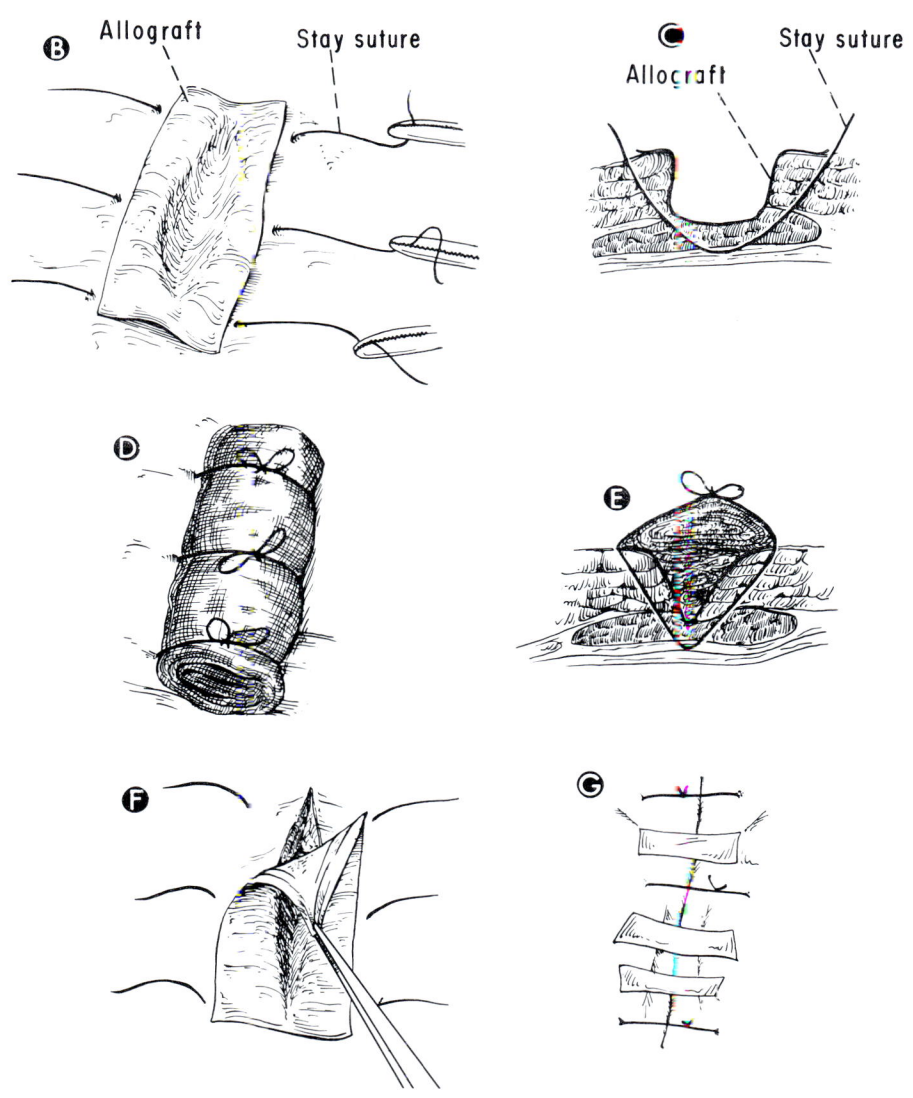

Fig. 38-1.—Technique of allografting followed by delayed closure. **A,** area to be debrided. **B,** allograft placed as the usual split-thickness skin graft. **C,** relation of debrided area to allografted surface and to stay suture tract. **D** and **E,** stent holds allograft in place on debrided surface. **F,** removal of allograft at time of definitive closure. **G,** appearance of wound following closure.

Avoidance of Further Bacterial Contamination

For practical purposes, although the major contamination of an open wound occurs at the time of injury, it is well to remember that bacterial contamination continues until the wound is closed or otherwise protected through medical intervention. In this regard, the nature of the bacterial contamination produced within the hospital itself is of particular importance to the patient, for it differs markedly from that at the place of injury. The species of bacteria likely to enter a wound at the time of injury are usually sensitive to available antibiotic substances. The hospital strains of bacteria may be more virulent and, even more important, much more apt to be resistant to antibiotic substances. As a result, infection caused by contamination of a traumatic wound at a place of work or on the roadside almost always responds to vigorous antibiotic treatment. Infection produced by hospital strains of bacteria is much more difficult to treat. In order to lower the risk of sepsis in the trauma patient, therefore, further bacterial contamination must be avoided, including that occurring in the hospital.

The measures used to protect a patient from continuing bacterial contamination do not differ from those involved in accurate aseptic technique and prevention of cross infection and are well known to the surgeon. Preventive measures themselves can be divided into 2 broad categories. The first contains those measures aimed at preventing further contamination of a traumatic open wound itself and the second includes those measures designed to protect the patient's blood stream and respiratory or urinary tract from bacteria. Both, however, rest on the same foundation. It is beyond the scope of this chapter to give a detailed description of the techniques required to protect the injured patient's respiratory tree following intubation, or his blood stream following intravenous or intra-arterial cannulation, but it is well to emphasize that there must be exact attention to detail if success is to be achieved.

The problem of preventing contamination in the hospital is greatly complicated by the confusion generated by a medical emergency. Inadvertently, many injured patients are heavily contaminated by bacteria in the emergency room when the details of sterile techniques are temporarily lost sight of because of the urgent requirements of cardiovascular collapse, massive hemorrhage or respiratory insufficiency. Occasionally, tracheostomy tubes, Foley or intravenous catheters, surgical instruments or dressing sponges are contaminated in the rush and confusion of emergency resuscitation of a dying patient. Unfortunately, the life saved by this emergency resuscitation may later be lost as a result of sepsis generated by bacterial contamination during the period of resuscitation. This sequence of events can only be halted if further bacterial contamination is prevented.

As in the restoration of normal physiology, protection of the patient from further contamination must begin as soon as possible following injury. Although the handling of the patient at the scene of the accident, his transportation and his treatment in the emergency ward are crucial steps in the progress toward resuscitation, it is well to remember that the patient continues at risk until the wound is closed and all catheters, tubes and drains have been removed.

Needless to say, it is essential to employ impeccable surgical and aseptic technique throughout the patient's operative and postoperative periods. In surgical procedures, the use of a foreign body should, if possible, be avoided. An accurate hemostasis, gentle tissue handling and precise anatomic reconstruction using accurately placed sutures without tension will provide the best long-term result.

Preventive Antibiotics

The return to a near normal physiologic state and the cleansing of the wound by removal of contaminating bacteria, foreign bodies and dead tissue, followed by physiologic primary closure, make up the most important parts of the treatment regime leading to timely healing without infection. Unhappily, it is not always possible to achieve completely these goals, and in such clinical situations it is to the patient's advantage to supplement his ability to defend himself against bacteria with an antibiotic. The term "preventive antibiotics" most accurately describes this form of antibiotic use, for the antibiotic, to be effective, must be delivered before infection begins. The concept behind this use of antibiotic substances is the prevention of a bacterial lesion,[5] not treatment.

There is now considerable experimental and clinical evidence documenting the effectiveness of preventive antibiotics in both elective[4, 7] and emergency surgery.[8, 10] In these studies, a number of points important in the prevention of sepsis following serious injury have been demonstrated. First, preventive antibiotics can markedly decrease the risk of postoperative or post-trauma infection if given at a time they can supplement the natural antibacterial activity of the patient's tissues. Second, preventive antibiotics have a diminishing effect with time following bacterial contamination. They are most effective when the antibiotic substance is in the tissue before bacteria arrive. If the antibiotic substance arrives in the tissue following the bacteria, its preventive effect is progressively less.

To be as effective as possible, then, an antibiotic substance must be given to the injured patient as soon after injury as possible. In fact, whenever there is risk of infection in trauma, the antibiotic should be given with the initial fluid replacement, along with the treatment for shock or acidosis. Preventive measures cannot wait until the more dramatic activities related to the repair of massive blood loss or respiratory insufficiency are carried out. They must be among the initial therapeutic activities in the resuscitation of the seriously injured patient.

The selection of antibiotic and its optimal dose level cannot be easily regimented for preventive antibiotic usage. The ever-present danger of less than normal perfusion of traumatized areas prompts the use of a daily dose of antibiotic toward the upper end of the recommended dose level. The intravenous route of administration is perhaps the most useful, because of the frequent abnormalities of gastrointestinal tract function and the unreliability of intermuscular absorption in the seriously injured patient. Since it is urgently necessary to deliver antibiotic substances to the injured tissue as soon as possible if infection is to be prevented, the intravenous route has proved to be not only the most reliable but also the fastest.

The exact choice of antibiotic must rest with the clinical judgment and experience of the surgeon. Usually, a single antibiotic with minimal toxicity and wide spectrum in regard to gram-positive bacteria should be chosen. Multiple antibiotics should be used only when the probability of life-threatening infection is high. Oxacillin, cephalothin, ampicillin and tetracycline have all been used with success as preventive antibiotics. The combinations of penicillin and tetracycline or kanamycin and oxacillin have also been used.

CONTROL OF ESTABLISHED INFECTION

General Principles

Before effective treatment of an infection in a traumatic wound can begin, the diagnosis of the infection itself must be established. The earlier this can be accomplished, the less likely infection is to become generalized and the smaller the tissue damage and eventual secondary functional loss due to local bacterial invasion. The final level of performance of an extremity or joint may well depend on the prompt recognition and immediate treatment of a beginning infection in a traumatic wound. In smaller superficial wounds the early appearance of the cardinal signs of inflammation—pain, heat, redness and swelling—make diagnosis easy. The early diagnosis of deep sepsis complicating extensive trauma, when wounds may extend into body cavities or deeply into intramuscular spaces, is far more difficult. The patient may complain of tightness in the region of the wound or local pain or tenderness. These signs are not always present. Systemic signs of infection, such as spiking fever, leukocytosis, malaise and ileus (and in overwhelming sepsis, shock) are clinical indicators which must be carefully evaluated. Early signs, such as a rapidly spreading cellulitis that often indicates a beta-hemolytic streptococcal infection, or the presence of crepitus in the tissue telling of infection caused by gas-forming organisms, may be the first indication of serious infection.

As soon as the diagnosis of infection is made, treatment must begin in order to confine the bacterial spread to as small an area of tissue as possible.

The over-all principles regarding treatment of established infections in traumatic wounds are the same for small wounds in which treatment is on an outpatient basis and for life-threatening infections in massive wounds. These principles are (1) the prevention of closed-space, expanding infection by establishing and maintaining drainage of loculated purulent material; (2) the debridement of tissue devitalized by trauma, foreign body or septic process; (3) an antibiotic supplement to host resistance if bacterial invasion of tissue surrounding the wound is present; (4) general systemic support as required.

The exact techniques chosen for debridement and for drainage and its maintenance (it must be kept in mind that drainage of a closed-space infection accomplishes little over the long term if the space is allowed to seal again shortly after drainage), the mechanisms of systemic support, and the decision to use or not to use antibiotics depend on the extent of the wound, its anatomic location, the general condition of the patient and the invasive nature of the bacteria. These clinical decisions are of first-order importance and must vary with the clinical problems presented. For example, wound infections involving the brain or the thoracic or abdominal cavity cannot be dealt with in the same manner as sepsis following an open fracture of the femur or a small superficial soft tissue wound of the forearm.

Although treatment of infection in the anatomic or physiologic special areas of the body is detailed elsewhere, there are several general principles worth emphasizing. As noted before, the ease or difficulty encountered in bringing a post-traumatic wound infection under control is, at least in part, related to the possibility or impossibility of (1) wide debridement of bacterially involved tissue and (2) establishment of efficient, open, continuous drainage of the affected site. In a soft tissue wound of an extremity, it is physiologically and functionally reasonable to open an infected area widely, thus providing adequate drainage, and to maintain this drainage by packing the wound open until the infection has cleared. In this type of wound, the sacrifice of skin, subcutaneous tissue and muscle is not limited by a devastating loss of function. On the other hand, for physiologic reasons, it is difficult to establish and impossible to maintain open drainage of an infection of the peritoneum or pleural cavities. Similarly, because of devastating loss of function, it is impossible to debride large areas of the brain in order to remove all bacteria-containing tissue. These special cases must be recognized and adequate alternative methods employed.

Treatment of Specific Bacterial Infection

Despite the similarity in the over-all philosophy of treatment of bacterial infection in traumatic wounds, there are important differences in the metabolic behavior of certain bacteria which lead to differences in the pathophysiologic evolution of infection caused by these bacteria. Perhaps the most important difference is the variation in susceptibility or insusceptibility of bacterial species to antibiotic substances. The general principles outlined in the foregoing section are applicable in an over-all sense to all pyogenic infection. In this section we will consider (1) the specific antibiotic sensitivities of the various clinically important bacterial species which may be used as a guide to specific therapy and (2) several clinical syndromes caused by specific bacterial species that are different enough from the usual pyogenic infection to require special treatment. As a general rule, in all cases of sepsis requiring medical treatment, culture identification of bacteria and their antibiotic sensitivities should be carried out as an initial step in management.

The common bacterial species found in clinical medicine and especially following trauma are outlined in Table 38-1. The suggested antibiotic for a specific infection, the dose and route of administration are to be used as guidelines only. The exact clinical situation, the patient's allergic or sensitivity history and hospital epidemiologic considerations must be carefully considered before an antibiotic is chosen for therapeutic use.

Infections caused by the beta-hemolytic streptococcus, *Clostridium tetani*, and *Cl. welchii* are life-threatening processes, differing from the usual pyogenic infection because of invasive characteristics or toxin formation. A brief description of each clinical syndrome, its prevention and treatment is given here.

BETA-HEMOLYTIC STREPTOCOCCAL INFECTIONS.—These are notable because of their early onset, rapid spread through the tissue and early and frequent life-threatening invasion of the blood stream. The old-fashioned term "blood poisoning" was usually applied to a beta-hemolytic streptococcal septicemia. This streptococcus commonly produces a rapidly evolving, bright red cellulitis (erysipelas) or lymphagitis (red streak) which may begin hours after traumatic contamination of a wound and progress to a fatal septicemia in 48 hours. Fortunately, the organism is sensitive to antibiotic therapy, particularly with penicillin, and clinically has not presented problems related to development of antibiotic resistance. The sensitivity and lack of development of resistance to penicillin provide a basis for the prevention of this infection by early use of preventive antibiotics. Preventive penicillin therapy has proved particularly effective in burn patients. In addition, if a beta-hemolytic streptococcal infection develops, it is easily eliminated by the use of therapeutic antibiotics given early. The life-threatening quality of this infection lies in its ability to produce a rapidly evolving systemic infection, creating the possibility of extensive bacterial invasion before diagnosis and treatment can be instituted.

TETANUS.—Tetanus (lockjaw)[1, 14] is a clinical syndrome caused by the spore-forming, strictly anaerobic, gram-positive bacillus *Cl. tetani*. The bacteria do not produce disease by direct invasion but by the elaboration of a toxin, so that even the most minute wounds can initiate clinical tetanus. *Clostridium tetani* is found widely distributed in nature, being a common inhabitant of the gastrointestinal tract of domestic animals, and is widely distributed in soil. Because the

TABLE 38-1.—Antibiotic Therapy in Surgical Infections

Surgical Infection Caused by	Drug of Choice and Dosage	Alternative Drugs
Gram-positive cocci		
Staphylococcus aureus (non-penicillinase producing)	Penicillin G $1-5 \times 10^6$ units q 4–6 hr (parenteral) Penicillin V 0.25–1 gm q 6 hr (oral)	Cephalothin, vancomycin, erythromycin, lincomycin
Staph. aureus (penicillinase producing)	Oxacillin or Cloxacillin 0.5–1 gm q 4–6 hr (parenteral) 0.25–1 gm q 6 hr (oral) Nafcillin 0.5–1 gm q 4–6 hr (parenteral) 0.25–1 gm q 6 hr (oral) Dicloxacillin 0.25–1 gm q 6 hr (oral)	Cephalosporin, methicillin, lincomycin, erythromycin
Gram-positive bacilli		
Clostridium tetani	Penicillin G 10×10^6 units daily (parenteral)	Cephalosporin, tetracycline
Cl. welchii (gas gangrene)	Penicillin G 10×10^6 units daily (parenteral)	Cephalosporin, tetracycline
Bacillus anthracis	Penicillin G $1-5 \times 10^6$ units q 4–6 hr (parenteral)	Erythromycin, tetracycline
Gram-negative bacilli		
Escherichia coli	Ampicillin 0.5–1 gm q 4–6 hr (parenteral)	Gentamicin, kanamycin, tetracycline, polymyxin
Aerobacter	Kanamycin 15 mg/kg/day in 2 doses (parenteral)	Gentamicin, tetracycline, polymyxin, carbenicillin
Klebsiella pneumoniae	Cephaloridine 0.25–1 gm q 4–6 hr (parenteral)	Kanamycin, chloramphenicol, polymyxin
Proteus mirabilis	Ampicillin 0.25–1 gm q 4–6 hr (parenteral)	Gentamicin, kanamycin, cephalosporin
Other *Proteus sp.*	Gentamicin 1–3 mg/kg/day q 4–6 hr (parenteral)	Kanamycin, chloramphenicol, tetracycline c̄, streptomycin, cephalosporin
Providencia	Carbenicillin 2–4 gm/day q 4–6 hr (parenteral)	Gentamicin
Pseudomonas aeruginosa	Gentamicin 1–3 mg/kg/day q 4–6 hr (parenteral)	Carbenicillin, polymyxin
Bacteroides	Tetracycline 0.25 mg q 6 hr (parenteral or oral)	Erythromycin, chloramphenicol, lincomycin
Actinomyces	Penicillin G $1-5 \times 10^6$ units q 4–6 hr (parenteral)	Tetracycline, sulfonamide
Candida albicans	Amphotericin B	

tetanus bacillus produces disease by toxin formation, which diffuses throughout the tissue, devastating or even lethal tetanus can be caused by bacterial growth which produces no clinically detectable inflammation in the most minor wounds. In addition, natural tissue resistance to the tetanus bacillus is high, so that under usual circumstances contamination with the bacteria or its spores does not produce bacterial invasion or infection. However, if the natural host resistance is diminished by devitalized tissue or foreign bodies and anaerobic conditions are produced, a tetanus infection may be established.

Prophylaxis. — In the area of preventive medicine, tetanus is theoretically 1 of the easiest diseases to prevent. As in betahemolytic streptococcal infection the tetanus infection is amenable to prevention using antibiotics. Even more important, the disease can be completely prevented by antitetanus toxin immunization using tetanus toxoid. Unhappily, the civilian public health measures attempting to produce a uniformly immunized population have fallen far short of the goal. Many patients come to the emergency ward following trauma without adequate tetanus immunization. Even though the clinical disease of tetanus is rare today, it is seen sporadically throughout the country. Therefore, its occurrence must be considered and preventive measures taken as a routine part of any emergency treatment of a traumatic wound.

In the prevention of clinical tetanus, 2 factors are important: the treatment of a traumatic wound so that bacterial growth does not develop and the insuring of an adequate level of circulating antitetanus antibody in the injured patient. The treatment of wounds and use of preventive antibiotics are the same as described for other bacterial infections. However, in the present context, the treatment of puncture wounds[2] is particularly important, because the depth of the wound and the narrowness of the opening to the skin surface prevent efficient cleansing of the wound. Foreign bodies, such as rust, dirt or bits of cloth inserted at the time of injury, may remain unnoticed. Further, purulent exudates resulting from infection deep in a puncture wound tend to pocket, since the external opening of the wound is soon sealed by a protein coagulart, and a closed-space infection is produced. In the emergency treatment of puncture wounds, therefore, special attention should be paid to establishing a widely opened egress to the depth of the wound to secure adequate cleansing, debridement and continuing drainage.

An adequate amount of antitetanus antibody should be insured. This can be accomplished actively or passively. Active immunization is carried out by immunization with adsorbed tetanus toxoid in 3 separate injections of 0.5 ml each. The second injection is given 4–6 weeks after the first and the third injection is given 6 months to 1 year after the second. A booster dose of adsorbed tetanus toxoid is indicated in 6–10 years following the third injection. Passive immunization is carried out with human tetanus immune globulin given as soon after injury as possible.

The general principles of tetanus prophylaxis in traumatic wounds can be briefly outlined as follows:

1. The surgeon must determine what is required for adequate prophylaxis against tetanus for each patient with an open wound.

2. All patients, regardless of immunization status, must undergo meticulous debridement for removal of all dead tissues and foreign bodies.

3. All patients who have traumatic wounds should receive adsorbed tetanus toxoid intramuscularly at the time of injury unless they have had a booster dose or have completed their initial immunization series within 5 years of injury.

4. The decision to use passive immunization with human tetanus immune globulin must rest on the character of the wound, the conditions under which it was created, previous treatment, the age

of the wound, and the tetanus immunization status of the patient.

5. All patients treated should be given an accurate record of the tetanus immunization provided, as well as instructions for completing active immunization, if necessary.

The specific measures indicated for patients with traumatic wounds may be divided into 2 broad categories: the measures indicated for patients previously immunized and the measures required for patients not previously immunized.

If the patient has been immunized within the past 6–10 years but has not had a booster dose within the past 5 years, a single booster dose of adsorbed tetanus toxoid should be given. In severe, neglected or heavily contaminated wounds, a dose of adsorbed tetanus toxoid should be given unless it is certain the patient has had a booster dose within the previous year. Most of the patients who have been actively immunized more than 6 years before the injury will be satisfactorily treated with a single injection. In the tetanus-prone wounds, the patient should be given, in addition to the single dose of tetanus toxoid, 250 units of human tetanus immune globulin. Penicillin or oxytetracycline[11] therapy should also be considered.

In patients suffering from traumatic wounds who have not been previously immunized but who have clean, sharply inflicted wounds in which tetanus is unlikely, an initial immunizing dose of 0.5 ml of adsorbed tetanus toxoid is indicated at the time of injury. Completion of the full immunization regime should follow. For all other wounds except the minor wounds, adsorbed tetanus toxoid should be given as an initial immunizing dose and, in addition, 250–500 units of human tetanus immune globulin should be given. Again, penicillin or oxytetracycline therapy should be given.

Treatment.—In clinical medicine, the diagnosis of tetanus may be suspected in a patient who suffers irritability, insomnia, tremor, rigidity or spasm of muscles, particularly those muscles adjacent to the wound. The incubation of the disease varies from 4 to 21 days, but clinically the disease is usually seen between 7 and 10 days after injury. The mortality and severity of the clinical disease are inversely proportional to the length of incubation. The cases of tetanus with short incubation periods have a serious prognosis.

The treatment of tetanus embodies 3 main objectives: the removal of the source of tetanus toxin production, the neutralization of circulating toxin already produced and the symptomatic treatment of the patient's muscle spasms. Removal of the source of tetanus toxin production is accomplished by thoroughly debriding the wound containing tetanus bacilli by wide excision. Recurrent anaerobic conditions must be prevented at all costs, so the wound is left open following debridement unless specific conditions demand its closure. The destruction of circulating tetanus toxin is accomplished by administering human tetanus immune globulin daily for about 10 days. Antibiotics,[1] usually penicillin, cephalosporin or oxytetracycline, are usually given to the patient in order to prevent further bacterial growth.

Because the main symptom of tetanus is muscle spasm, sedation and a quiet, dark environment are essential. Valium has proved useful for sedation. In the severely ill patient with pharyngeal spasm, tracheostomy should be performed and muscle relaxants used as necessary to assure adequate respiration with a respirator. Nutrition may be maintained with a nasogastric tube, and constant, expert nursing care is essential.

Patients being treated for tetanus should have immunization begun, using tetanus toxoid. The clinical disease does not uniformly confer immunity.

GAS GANGRENE (CLOSTRIDIAL MYOSITIS).—Gas gangrene[3] is a life-threatening bacterial infection involving destruction of muscle and must be clinically separated from gas-forming infections which do not carry the grim prognosis of clostridial myositis. Gas gangrene usually develops early following muscle injury, often within 12 hours. It is characterized by a rapid pulse, restlessness, severe pain, a thin, brownish discharge from the area of the wound and profound toxemia. Swelling and edema are prominent in the affected tissue, and crepitus may be present in the area of swelling. Bubbles are occasionally seen in the discharging serosanguineous exudate.

Treatment of gas gangrene must be immediate and thorough if success is to be achieved. Prompt excision of the entire involved muscle mass should be carried out. If the wound involves an extremity, immediate amputation may be necessary. Antibiotics are useful in controlling bacterial growth and should be given intravenously in large doses. Penicillin or tetracycline have proved effective. The clinical use of gas gangrene antitoxin is not clearly established. If used, it should be administered as early in the clinical disease as possible in doses consisting of 10,000–15,000 units per kilogram of body weight. The treatment of gas gangrene with hyperbaric oxygen has, in some instances, proved useful.[5] In weighing the use of hyperbaric oxygen treatment, consideration must be given to the hazards of transporting critically ill patients over long distances and of delaying surgical intervention while arrangements and transportation to hyperbaric facilities are carried out.

BIBLIOGRAPHY

1. American College of Surgeons: A guide to prophylaxis against tetanus in wound management, Bull. Am. Col. Surg. 57:10, 1972.
2. American College of Surgeons Committee on Trauma: Prophylaxis against Tetanus, in *The Management of Fractures and Soft Tissue Injuries* (2d ed.; Philadelphia: W. B. Saunders Company, 1965).
3. Altemeier, W. A., and Furste, W. L.: Collective review—gas gangrene, Surg. Gynecol. Obstet. 84:507, 1947.
4. Bernard, H. R., and Cole, W. R.: The prophylaxis of surgical infection: The effect of prophylactic antimicrobial drugs on the incidence of infection following potentially contaminated operations, Surgery 56:151, 1964.
5. Boerema, I.: An operating room with high atmospheric pressure, Surgery 49:291, 1961.
6. Burke, J. F.: The effective period of preventive antibiotic action in experimental incisions and dermal lesions, Surgery 50:161, 1961.
7. Burke, J. F.: Preoperative antibiotics, Surg. Clin. North Am. 43:665, 1963.
8. Burke, J. F.: The significance of time between injury and treatment, Conn. Med. 29:110, 1965.
9. Burke, J. F., and Bondoc, C. C.: A method of secondary closure of heavily contaminated wounds providing "physiologic primary closure," J. Trauma 8:228, 1968.
10. Fullen, W. D., Hunt, J. L., and Altemeier, W. A.: The time factor in antibiotic prophylaxis of penetrating wounds of the abdomen, Surg. Forum 22:58, 1971.
11. Goodman, L. S., and Gilman, A.: *Pharmacological Basis of Therapeutics* (4th ed.; New York: The Macmillan Company, 1970).
12. Miles, A. A.: Nonspecific defense reactions in bacterial infections, Ann. NY Acad. Sci. 66:356, 1956.
13. Miles, A. A., Miles, E. M., and Burke, J. F.: The value and duration of defense reactions of the skin to the primary lodgement of bacteria, Br. J. Exp. Pathol. 38:1, 1957.
14. Robles, N. L., et al.: Tetanus prophylaxis and therapy, Surg. Clin. North Am. 48:799, 1968.

39 | Injuries to Major Tendons*

EDWIN F. CAVE and ROBERT J. BOYD

ANATOMY

A TENDON IS a strong arrangement of fibrous tissue in which the fibers of a muscle end and which serves as a bridge for attaching the muscle to a bone or other structure. Tendons vary in size from that of the quadriceps muscle to the diameter of the extensor digiti minimi of the fifth finger of the hand. They have little, if any, elasticity, and they are nourished by an inefficient blood supply. Nerves supplying tendons end in what is known as "neurotendinous spindles." Tendons vary in length from a maximum of approximately 8 in. for the plantaris tendon to only a few millimeters.

MECHANISM OF INJURY

Tendons may be injured by 1 of 3 methods: a direct blow by a blunt object, which may severely bruise or lacerate the tendon; a blow by a sharp instrument, which divides the skin and tendon underneath; or an indirect pull, such as that sustained by the Achilles tendon when the calf muscles are suddenly contracted with the foot fixed to the floor. The more frequent type of injury is that due to a sudden indirect muscle contraction which pulls the tendon apart.

PATHOLOGIC PROCESS

The tendon may rupture at 1 of 3 points: its musculotendinous junction; the central portion of the tendon; or its bony attachment (Fig. 39-1). When the

Fig 39-1.—Common sites of tear of Achilles tendon: *1*, at musculotendinous junction; *2*, in the central portion of tendon; *3*, at its bony attachment. (From Lawrence, G. H., Cave, E. F., and O'Connor, H.: Injury to the Achilles tendon: Experience at the Massachusetts General Hospital 1900–1954, Am. J. Surg. 89:795, 1955.)

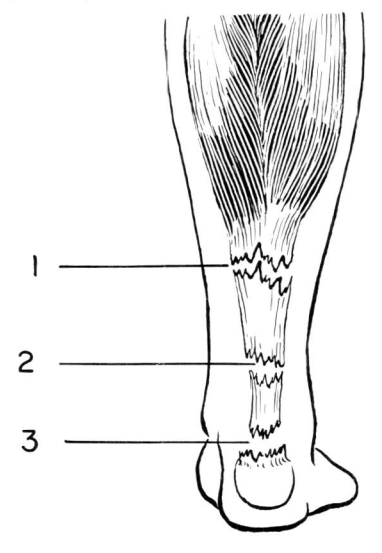

---

*[Although injuries to major tendons are discussed elsewhere in this volume with particular reference to various individual joints, it seems worthwhile to include a separate chapter on the general subject of trauma to major tendons.—Ed.]

separation occurs at the musculotendinous junction or in the central portion, the result is a fraying out of the tendon. If the tendon ruptures from its bony attachment, the rupture is apt to be more of a transverse tear, and there is less fraying out of the tendon fibers.

SYMPTOMS AND SIGNS

The sudden rupture of the tendon by an indirect means may be accompanied by a loud snap, as in rupture of the plantaris tendon. The first symptom is that of weakness. Pain in the injured part is not a consistent symptom, but there will be inability to flex or extend the part unless accessory muscles can be brought into play. In rupture of the Achilles tendon, plantar flexion of the foot can often be carried out by the intact flexors of the toes and the posterior tibial tendon. However, with a baseball finger, where the extensor tendon is ruptured and no accessory muscle can be utilized, there will be no ability to extend the distal phalanx of the finger.

If the tendon is superficial, an actual defect in its contour may be palpated. This is frequently possible in Achilles tendon ruptures or when the quadriceps is separated from its patellar attachment. Immediate weakness and pain are followed by a moderate amount of swelling and perhaps by some discoloration.

TREATMENT

Except in rare instances, most tendon injuries require surgical repair to restore function. Those that do not necessarily demand operative treatment are injuries to the extensor tendon of the finger (baseball finger) or to the plantaris tendon, which is not essential for good function of the calf muscle group. However, the Achilles tendon, the quadriceps tendon, the long head of the biceps, the distal end of the biceps, the patellar tendon, the extensor of the thumb, the flexor hallucis longus, and the anterior tibial and posterior tibial tendons usually require surgical repair.

Achilles Tendon

In a review of tendon injuries treated at Massachusetts General Hospital over 50 years, injuries to Achilles tendon comprised one-fifth of all large tendon injuries. During this period, 31 patients were treated for injuries to the Achilles tendon; 23 of these were followed for a sufficient time to permit adequate evaluation of the type of treatment carried out. Five patients received delayed treatment and had surgical repair of the ruptured Achilles tendon from 2 to 14 months following injury. The group followed consisted of 4 women and 19 men, ranging in age from 17 to 71 years. The injury was not bilateral in any of these cases.

The predominant symptom was pain; weakness in plantar flexion was the most common sign. On examination, a palpable gap in the continuity of the tendon was present in all patients.

The test for Achilles tendon continuity described by Thompson and Doherty[7] has proved to be very helpful. With the patient prone and the ankle free, a firm squeezing of the sole of the foot will cause definite plantar flexion of the foot if there is continuity of the tendon.

The dehiscence of the tendon was complete in 16 patients, with the plantaris tendon remaining intact in 6 of these complete ruptures. The separation occurred at the musculotendinous junction in 8, in the tendon itself in 14, and at its insertion into the os calcis in 1. The findings at operation were usually those of hemorrhage and a markedly frayed tendon.

Following exposure of the tendon, suturing was done in all patients in this series (Fig. 39-2). With 1 exception, all patients were immobilized for a period of 3–4 weeks in toe-to-groin plaster to hold the knee in flexion and the foot in slight equinus position. After a variable period of protected weight bearing, all the pa-

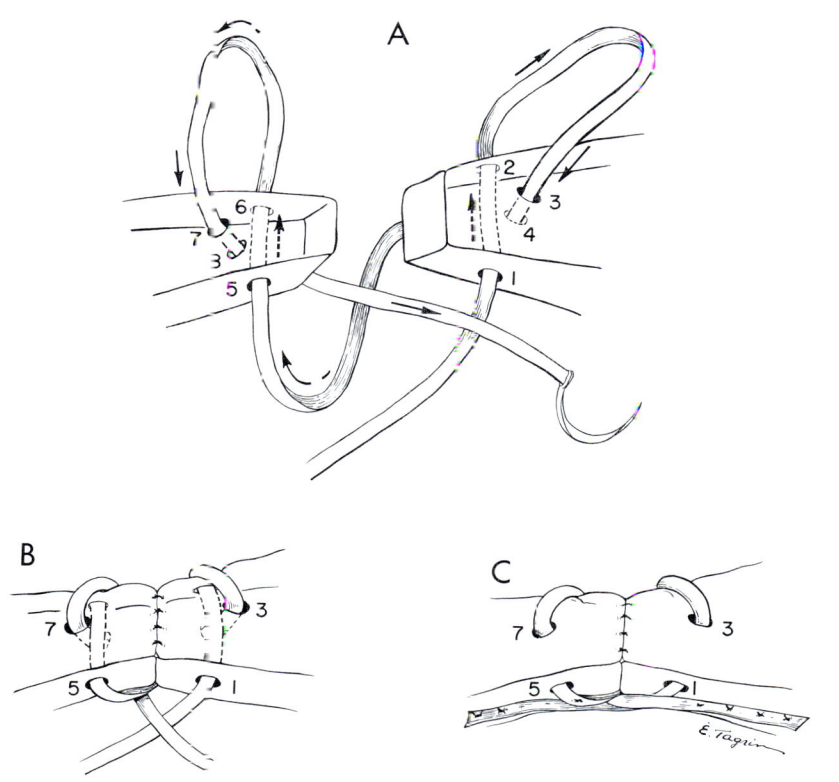

Fig. 39-2.—Diagrammatic sketches showing technique of approximating divided Achilles tendon. **A,** placing the suture. The 2 ends of the tendon are mobilized and brought up into the wound. A mattress suture of fascia ⅜ in. wide and 8 in. long (taken with a fascial stripper) is used to approximate the separated tendon. **B,** approximating the divided tendon and tightening the fascial strip. A reinforcing layer of silk is used to suture the tendon edges. **C,** suture of ends of fascial strip to side of tendon. (From Lawrence, G. H., Cave, E. F., and O'Connor, H.: Injury to the Achilles tendon: Experience at the Massachusetts General Hospital, 1900–1954, Am. J. Surg. 89:795, 1955.)

tients were able to return to work or resume previous activity in 3–5 months and to walk with no limp and with normal ankle motion.

Following operation, all 23 patients obtained good functional results. All were able to stand on tiptoe on the injured side and had forcible plantar flexion and dorsiflexion of the foot through a full range of motion. It may therefore be concluded that, regardless of the method of suture, careful repair of the tendon followed by 4–6 weeks of plaster immobilization will give a good result.

Recent reports of the nonoperative treatment of Achilles tendon rupture[2] suggest that acceptable results can be obtained by this method, although further experience and careful comparison of similar cases will be required before final assessment can be made. Our own experience with simple cast immobilization for these injuries is limited. Our current practice is to repair the ruptured tendon except in those patients whose age, level of activity or medical condition precludes surgical treatment.

Quadriceps Tendon

A rupture of the quadriceps tendon occurs at its bony attachment to the patella. Characteristically, such a rupture occurs in middle-aged or older adults and is practically always sustained when there is a sudden contracture of the quadriceps muscle as the knee is flexed from 30 to 60 degrees, thereby pulling the quadriceps tendon from its patellar attachment. The tear is usually complete. Immediate pain and inability to extend the knee against gravity are signs. Palpation will reveal a defect between the patella and the quadriceps tendon. Complete laceration of the tendon from its bony attachment frequently occurs, and surgical repair is always required.

X-ray films of the knee should be made to determine whether there is a fracture of the patella or a simple separation of the quadriceps tendon from its bony attachment.

Operation should be carried out as soon as possible. A parapatellar incision, a straight longitudinal incision or a transverse incision may be used. A transverse incision which adequately exposes the point of injury is preferred. The blood clot is removed from between the patella and the torn quadriceps; the knee is exposed in order to remove cartilaginous or bone fragments. Repair is carried out using silk to suture the lateral expansions and using fascia as a mattress suture through the tendon and through drill holes in the patella (Fig. 39-3).

Postoperative immobilization in a plaster cylinder is utilized until the wound is healed. Quadriceps-setting exercises are started on the first day after operation and are continued for an indefinite period. As soon as the wound is satisfactorily

Fig. 39-3.—Repair of quadriceps tendon by fascial strip removed from same thigh. **A,** placing mattress suture of fascia. **B,** horizontal view of same. **C,** approximation of tendon to patella by tightening fascial strip. A reinforcing layer of silk suture is added.

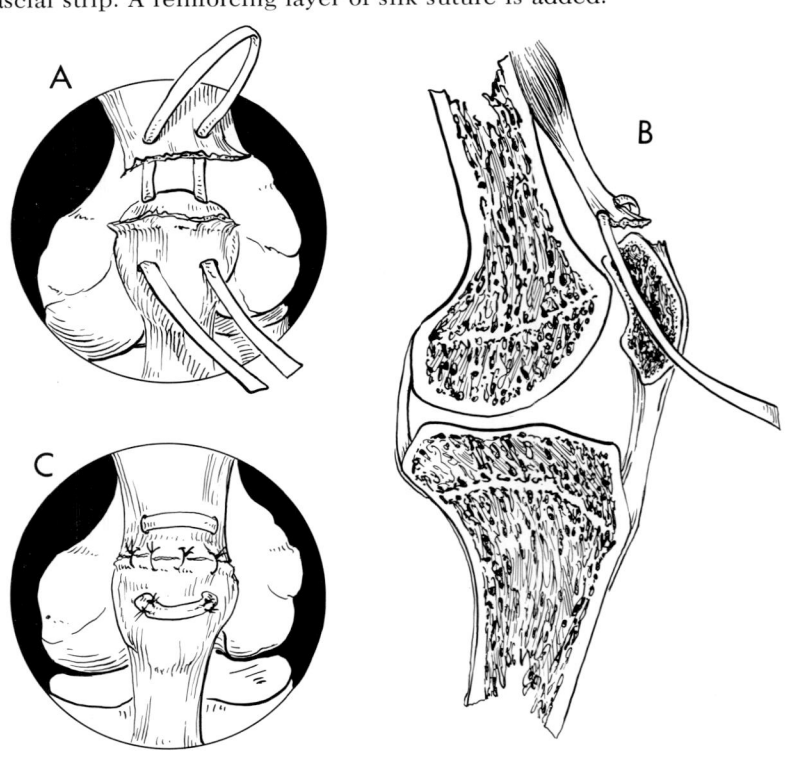

healed, gentle active flexion of the knee is encouraged. The patient is kept in bed until he can lift the leg against gravity with the knee fully extended and until he has from 70 to 90 degrees of active flexion of the knee. Such restoration of flexion indicates flexibility of the quadriceps muscle. This places less strain on the line of suture as flexion of the knee is carried out. Careful instruction in crutch walking is essential. Full weight may be borne, but precaution must be taken to avoid sudden flexion of the knee. The patient must guard against catching the heel or toes of the foot as he walks with crutches. Crutches are continued for 5–6 weeks. During this period, an essentially normal motion of the knee is restored.

Long Head of the Biceps Tendon

Rupture of the long head of the biceps tendon is usually produced by a sudden lifting motion with the elbow flexed. There may be only slight pain and disability at onset; frequently such an injury goes unrecognized for a few days, when there is noticeable bulging of the biceps muscle belly. This calls the patient's attention to the disability, and frequently he seeks medical advice too late to effect adequate attachment of the biceps tendon. Usually the injury causes so little disability that the patient is reluctant to have surgical repair carried out.

However, if the patient is seen within a matter of days, it is possible to expose the long head of the biceps tendon and suture it to the upper shaft of the humerus. The tear generally occurs at the glenoid attachment or at the level of the surgical neck of the humerus, and repositioning of the tendon is usually not possible.

The ruptured tendon is exposed through the deltopectoral approach, reflecting the deltoid from its attachment to the clavicle. The interval between the deltoid and the pectoralis major muscles is located. The cephalic vein is retracted or ligated and the deltoid muscle retracted laterally. The ruptured tendon is usually found lying anterior to the subscapu-

Fig. 39-4.—Repair of rupture of long head of biceps tendon. **A,** rupture possible at glenoid attachment *(1)* or at level of surgical neck of humerus *(2)*. Suture at the glenoid is usually not possible. Consequently, the distal fragment is sutured to the upper end of the humeral shaft under a flap of bone (**B** and **C**). (See text.)

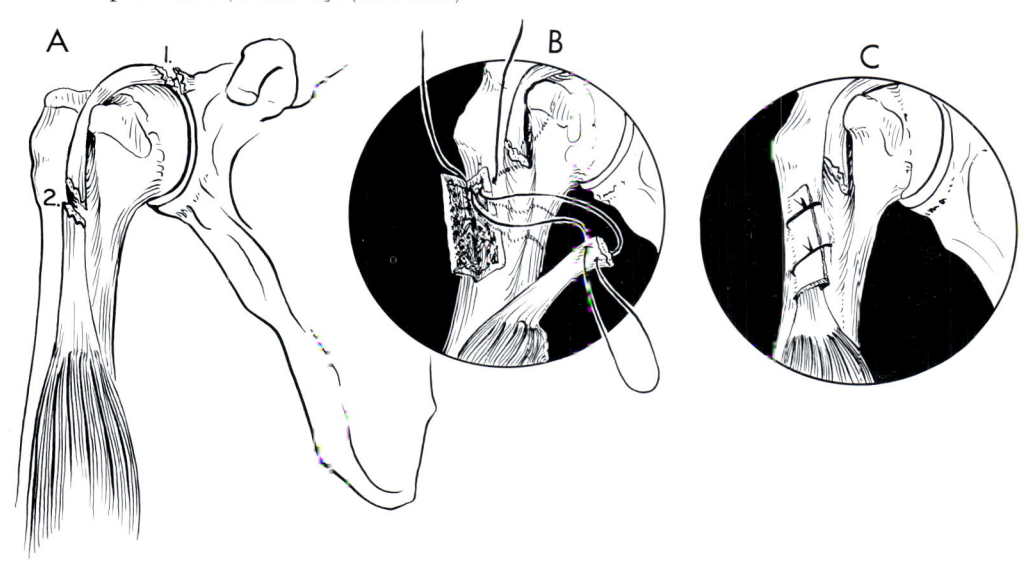

laris tendon, though occasionally it may be necessary to detach the upper portion of the pectoralis major insertion into the humerus to locate the end of the ruptured tendon. The tendon is pulled upward and sutured to the upper end of the humeral shaft (Fig. 39-4). Braided silk is passed through the tendon into 2 drill holes in the upper humeral shaft, firmly reattaching the tendon.

Postoperatively, the arm is immobilized for 3–4 weeks in a light hanging cast, with the elbow at 90 degrees, permitting use of the hand. At the end of this period of immobilization, gentle active flexion and extension of the elbow are encouraged until a full range of elbow motion is obtained. The patient should be cautioned to avoid sudden forceful contracture of the biceps muscle and to avoid lifting heavy objects for a period of 6 weeks following tendon repair, so that the tendon may become firmly reattached.

Distal Biceps Tendon

Rupture of the distal biceps tendon from its radial attachment is rare. It occurs when lifting a heavy object with the elbow flexed; with a sudden contracture of the biceps muscle the tendon is pulled from its attachment to the biceps tubercle at the upper end of the radius. Usually there is immediate pain and some limitation of motion of the elbow. However, flexion of the elbow can frequently be carried out by the supinator muscle, which acts as a substitute. There is immediate swelling. Careful palpation in the anterior aspect of the arm may reveal a defect between the muscle and the upper end of the radius.

Surgical repair (Figs. 39-5 and 39-6) should be carried out as soon as possible after injury and before contracture of the biceps muscle shortens the tendon. If operation is done within a few days, the tendon can be reattached to the radius by placing a drill hole through the upper end of the radius and suturing the tendon to bone with silk. If operation is delayed, fascia lata repair of the tendon may be used to bridge the gap between the contracted tendon and the biceps tubercle of the radius. After operation, the elbow should be kept in a flexed position of about 90 degrees for 4 weeks. Active use

Fig. 39-5.—Repair of rupture of distal biceps tendon. Although rarely separated, this tendon can usually be sutured to its radial attachment if the elbow is flexed. The tendon is sutured to bone under a flap of bone and periosteum at the level of the bicipital tubercle.

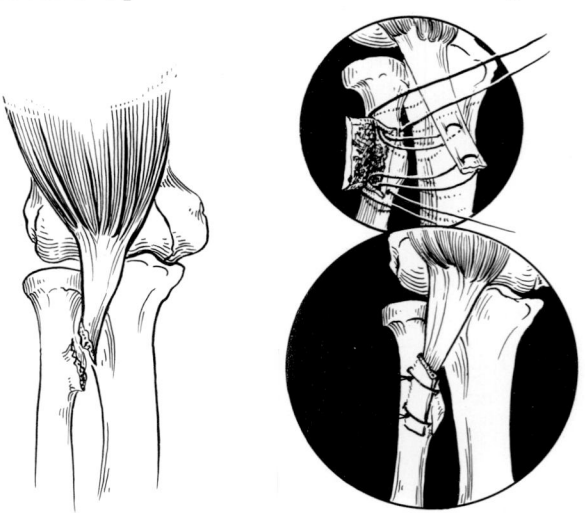

Chapter 39: INJURIES TO MAJOR TENDONS / 963

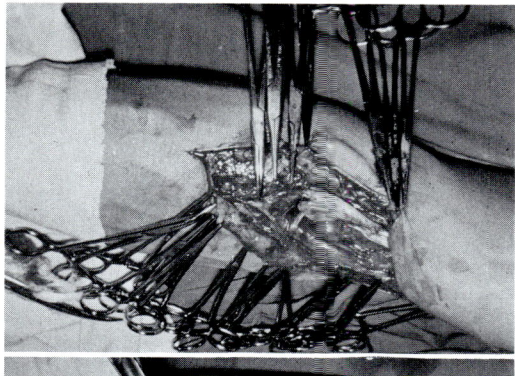

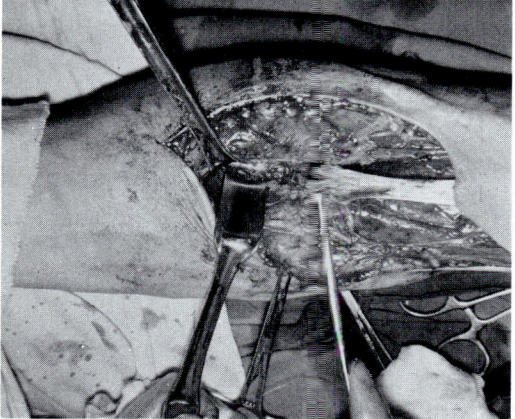

Fig. 39-6.—Complete rupture of the attachment of the distal biceps tendon. There was complete separation from the radius, secondary to heavy lifting. Through a "hockey-stick" incision, the distal biceps tendon was reattached to the upper end of the radius (see Fig. 39-5).

of the elbow should then be encouraged. If repair is carried out early, a good functional result should be obtained.

Extensor Tendon of the Thumb

Characteristically, rupture of the extensor pollicis longus tendon occurs at the level of the radial styloid. Vigorous attempts at reduction of Colles' fractures with traction exerted on the thumb and the wrist in ulnar deviation will cause a rupture of this tendon (Fig. 39-7). The tendon is stretched over the broken fragments of the radius, producing a laceration at this level.

Many instances of late rupture of this tendon are reported in the literature. The rupture occurs after prolonged wear and tear on the tendon as it moves to and fro over the roughened or ragged dorsal surface of the fractured radius. Pain at the site of rupture and inability to extend fully the distal phalanx of the thumb are the usual signs.

Immediate surgical repair is indicated. The tendon is approached through a longitudinal incision beginning at the wrist and extending proximally along the dorsum of the radius to the junction of the middle and lower third of this bone. If contracture of the extensor pollicis longus muscle has taken place so as to prevent primary suture of the proximal end to the distal end, then a tendon transfer procedure is indicated to restore functional extension to the distal phalanx of the thumb. A free tendon graft, using the palmaris longus tendon, may be utilized to bridge the gap between the severed tendon ends. However, a more satisfactory procedure is to use the extensor indicis proprius tendon, which is divided just distal to the dorsal carpal ligament and is relocated through the tunnel of the extensor pollicis longus tendon and sutured to the distal fragment of this tendon. The pull-out wire technique is recommended as the method of suture when approximating the severed tendon ends and when a tendon transfer procedure is performed (see Chapter 23).

Postoperatively, the extremity is immobilized in plaster for 3 weeks, maintaining the thumb in its functionally opposed position with the distal phalanx in maximal extension. The wrist is held in approximately 15 degrees of extension. At the end of 3 weeks, the plaster is removed for brief periods during the day, and the patient is given exercises to restore flexibility to the wrist and thumb. Caution must be exercised for an additional 3 weeks to avoid sudden full flexion and opposition of the thumb and palmar flexion of the wrist; otherwise, too much tension may be placed on the su-

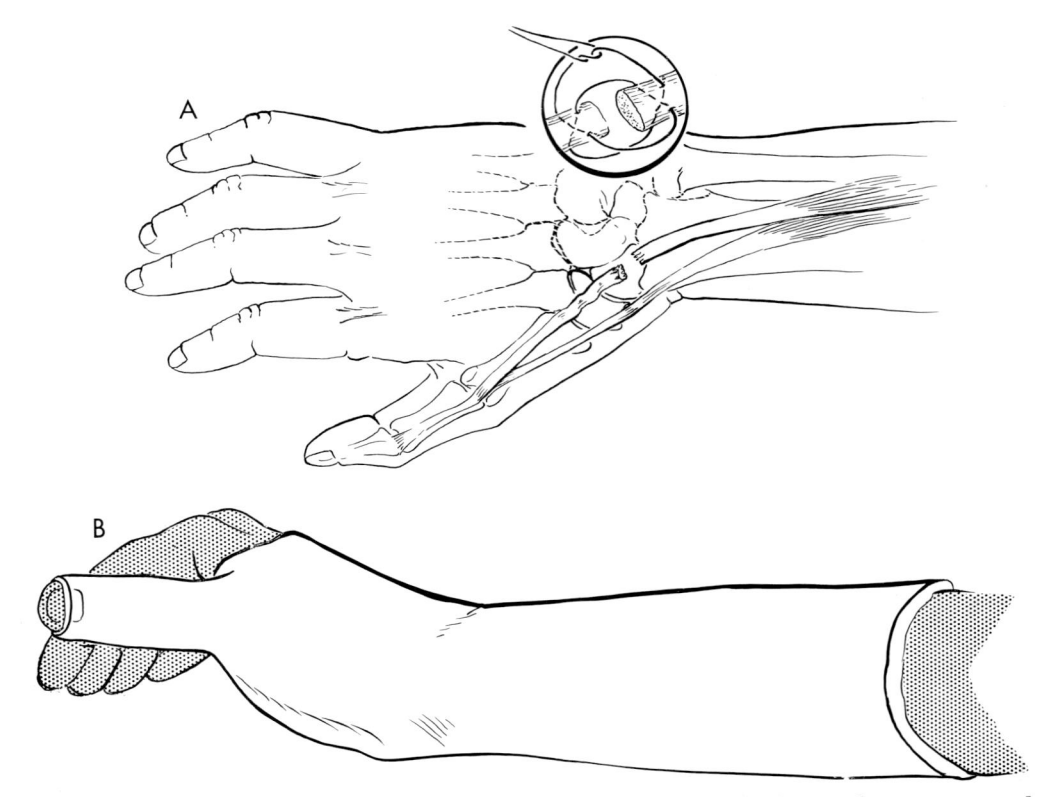

Fig. 39-7.—Repair of extensor pollicis longus tendon. Occasionally this tendon is separated in Colles' fracture, or it may be pulled apart by manipulation of the fracture. **A**, the tear is usually at the level of the radial styloid. Direct suture of the tendon *(inset)* is indicated as soon as possible, to prevent contracture of the proximal portion. If it is not possible to suture the tendon under the transverse carpal ligament, the subcutaneous positioning of the sutured tendon will suffice, or the distal end of divided tendon may be sutured to the extensor indicis proprius tendon (see text). **B**, plaster immobilization after tendon repair.

ture line in the tendon, causing it to break. An adequate temporary plaster splint for the thumb and wrist is used during this 3-week period. Six weeks after tendon suture the patient may begin to regain full function of both the wrist and thumb.

Direct trauma with a blunt or sharp instrument may divide this tendon. If the wound is dirty or if there is a delay greater than 4–6 hours between the time of injury and the time repair is contemplated, debridement and primary suture of the skin laceration should be performed. Repair of the tendon should be postponed until the laceration has completely healed and the danger of wound infection has passed.

Additional discussion of this problem is found in Chapter 23.

Extensor Tendon of the Finger (Baseball Finger)

Rupture of the extensor tendon of the finger is very common and usually results from a direct blow on the distal end of the extended finger. Such an injury produces a transverse separation of the extensor tendon from the dorsum of the distal phalanx of the finger. As a rule, the lateral expansions of the tendon remain intact. Therefore, if prompt application of a splint with the distal interphalangeal joint in hyperextension and the proximal interphalangeal joint in 30 degrees of flexion is carried out, good function and ability to hyperextend the finger will be restored. The splint should be worn for a period of 6 weeks. Even if treatment is delayed, complete restoration of function is possible by the use of a splint for at least 6 weeks. Many authorities recommend primary operative repair of the tendon (Chapter 23), although in our experience splinting has proved very satisfactory. An acceptable alternative to plaster or metal splinting is taping as illustrated in Figure 23-8.

Not infrequently in such an injury, a fragment of the dorsum of the proximal portion of the phalanx will be pulled off. If the fracture is old, surgery is performed (Fig. 39-8), removing the bone fragment and suturing the tendon to the phalanx with fine silk. Postoperatively, the finger must be immobilized in a splint that holds the distal interphalangeal joint in hyperextension and the proximal interphalangeal joint in 30 degrees of flexion for at least 6 weeks. At the end of 6 weeks, exercises to restore full function to the finger are encouraged.

Patellar Tendon

Rupture of the patellar tendon is rare. It is not infrequent in Paget's disease of the tibia, when the tendon actually separates from its bony attachment at the tibial tubercle. Symptoms are comparable to those experienced when the quadriceps is lacerated, and there is inability to extend the knee. X-ray films of the knee in this type of injury may reveal actual separation of a portion of the tibial tubercle. If in good position, this fragment may reattach itself if the leg is immobilized in plaster with the knee in complete extension for a period of 6–8 weeks. If there is wide separation of the fragment or if the injury is confined to the tendon attachment, surgical repair is indicated. Direct exposure of the tendon and suture of the tendon to the tibial tubercle with heavy silk will effect a good result, provided plaster immobilization follows repair for a period of 6 weeks.

If the patellar tendon ruptures through its midportion or at its inferior patellar attachment, surgical repair is indicated, using silk or fascial sutures.

Fig. 39-8. — Repair (as sometimes indicated) in old case of separation of extensor tendon from distal phalanx. **A**, mattress suture of fine silk or wire is passed through the tendon. One end of the suture is first passed through a small drill hole in the base of the phalanx from right to left, while the other end of the suture is passed through from left to right. **B**, the 2 ends are brought back through the tendon and tied. **C**, a postoperative splint is worn for about 6 weeks.

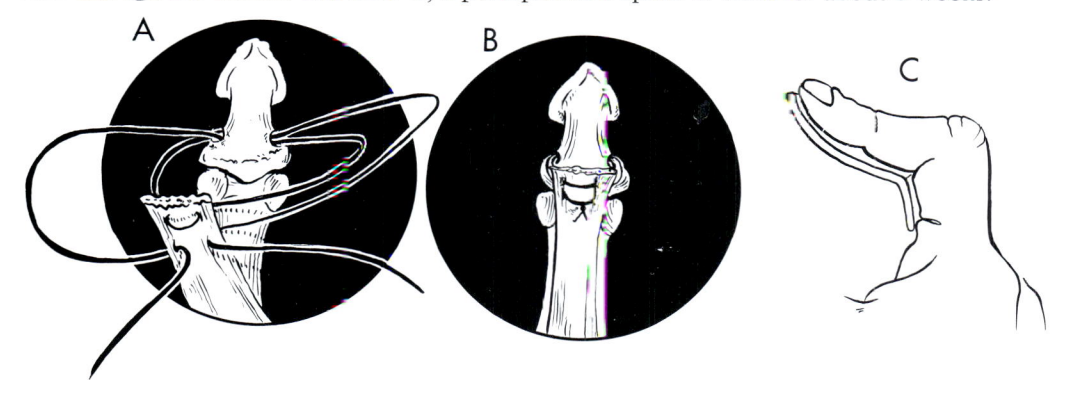

Anterior and Posterior Tibial Tendons

Division of the anterior and posterior tibial tendons is rarely due to a sudden contracture of the muscles; rather, it is usually caused by a direct blow or laceration. Unfortunately, the injury frequently goes unrecognized because functions of these 2 tendons can be taken over by associated muscles.

Spontaneous rupture of the posterior tibial tendon is an exceptionally rare injury. Only 1 case of a spontaneous partial rupture is reported in the literature. This occurred in a 65-year-old steamfitter, who slipped while carrying lead pipes downstairs and jumped down 4 steps, landing on his foot and twisting the ankle. Pain and swelling over the medial aspect of the ankle were not noted until 10 days after the injury, and this disability persisted until 6 months after injury, when the posterior tibial tendon was explored and found to be partially lacerated. After repair of the tendon the patient returned to work, with only occasional discomfort in the region of the ankle.

A similar injury was repaired in our fracture clinic. The patient, a 57-year-old woman, complained of recurrent ankle sprains and for 3 months had increasing pain and swelling over the posteromesial aspect of the left ankle. The preoperative diagnosis was "ganglion" or possibly "synovioma." At operation a complete laceration and fraying out of the posterior tibial tendon was found at the level of the internal malleolus (Fig. 39-9). Repair was carried out by bringing the 2 frayed ends together and suturing them with silk. A plaster boot was worn for 6 weeks.

The following are illustrative cases of traumatic lacerations of the posterior and anterior tibial tendons.

CASE 1.—A boy, 10, sustained a laceration over the medial malleolar region of the left ankle while swinging an ax. The skin laceration was sutured. Eighteen months after the injury he complained that he did not walk properly and that the left foot was more pronated than the right. Examination disclosed a well-healed scar just behind the medial malleolus and a posterior tibial tendon that was not functioning.

The posterior tibial tendon was explored and found to be completely divided; there was a 3-in. gap between the divided ends. Repair of the tendon was carried out, using as a graft a third of the Achilles tendon, 4 in. long. The tendon graft was sutured to the proximal stump of the tendon, passed through a drill hole in the tarsal navicular bone and then sutured to the distal stump of the posterior tibial tendon.

Following operation, the leg was immobilized in a toe-to-groin plaster for 6 weeks with the foot in inversion and dorsiflexion and the knee flexed at 45 degrees. Good function of the posterior tibial tendon was restored.

CASE 2.—A 15-year-old schoolboy sustained a laceration over the anterior tibial tendon just above the ankle while chopping wood. The skin wound was sutured on the day of the injury, but the anterior tibial tendon was not inspected. Four days following repair of the laceration the boy noticed that he could only weakly dorsiflex and invert the foot. Examination showed that the anterior tibial tendon was not functioning and that he could not walk on the heel of the foot.

The anterior tibial tendon was explored through an incision incorporating the old scar and was found to be divided across half its diameter. A repair of the tendon was carried out, using silk sutures, and a short leg plaster casing was applied, with the foot in inversion and dorsiflexion. The plaster was removed in 6 weeks. Seven months following repair of the lacerated tendon the boy was engaged in normal activities. The tendon was functioning normally.

CASE 3.—A similar, late end-to-end repair of the extensor hallucis longus above the ankle in a housewife, 42, was carried out 6 weeks after laceration by a small glass fragment from an exploding bottle. Excellent restoration of extension of the great toe was achieved.

The original wound should have been carefully explored before closure so that

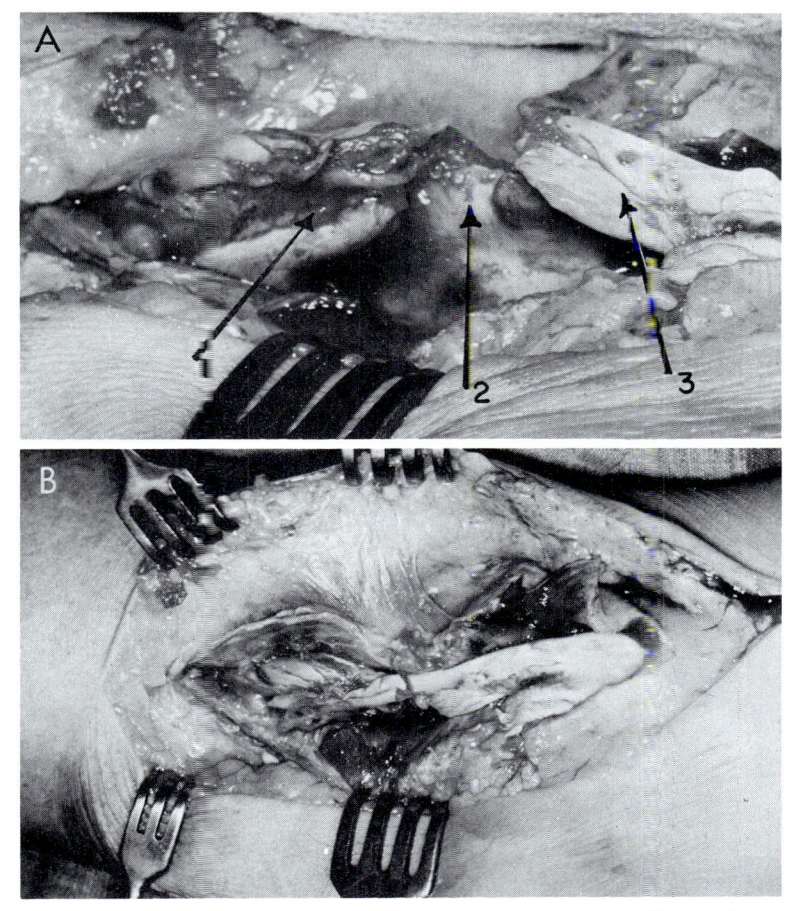

Fig. 39-9.—A, complete rupture of posterior tibial tendon at level of left ankle, a rare injury. *1*, proximal end of tendon; *2*, internal malleolus; *3*, distal end of tendon. B, tendon repair. Two ends of tendon were brought together and sutured with silk. Plaster immobilization was used for 6 weeks. At end of 5 months patient was symptom-free; tendon function was normal.

the tendon laceration would not have been missed.

The surgeon must carefully consider the possibility of a divided anterior or posterior tibial tendon if there has been a laceration around the ankle on the anterior or posteromedial aspect. When injury is suspected, the tendon should be explored before the subcutaneous tissue and skin are sutured. Prolonged disability may be prevented and earlier complete function restored to the lower extremity by immediate tendon repair.

Flexor Hallucis Longus Tendon

Separation of the flexor hallucis longus tendon from the distal phalanx of the great toe is rare, only 1 case has been seen at the fracture clinic of Massachusetts General Hospital. This injury occurred to a boy who was running upstairs and whose weight was suddenly borne fully on the distal portion of the great toe. The tendon was separated from its bony attachment. In such a case, surgical repair is indicated.

BIBLIOGRAPHY

1. Cronkite, A. E.: The tensile strength of human tendons, Anat. Rec. 64:173, 1935.
2. Gillies, H., and Chalmers, J.: The management of fresh ruptures of the tendo Achillis, J. Bone Joint Surg. 52-A:337, 1970.
3. Lawrence, G. H., Cave, E. F., and O'Connor, H.: Injury to the Achilles tendon: Experience at the Massachusetts General Hospital, 1900–1954, Am. J. Surg. 89:795, 1955.
4. Lea, R. B., and Smith, L.: Nonsurgical treatment of tendo Achillis rupture, J. Bone Joint Surg. 54-A:1398, 1972.
5. McLaughlin, H. L.: Repair of major tendon ruptures by buried removable sutures, Am. J. Surg. 74:758, 1947.
6. McMaster, P. E.: Late ruptures of extensor and flexor pollicis longus tendons following Colles' fracture, J. Bone Joint Surg. 14:93, 1932.
7. Thompson, T. C., and Doherty, J. H.: Spontaneous rupture of tendon of Achilles: A new clinical diagnostic test, J. Trauma 2:126, 1962.

40 | Soft Tissue Repairs

BRADFORD CANNON and JOHN REMENSNYDER, JR.

SOFT TISSUE INJURY is, to a greater or lesser degree, the inevitable accompaniment of a fracture. In most fractures the amount of soft tissue injury is fortunately not so severe or extensive that the final result is jeopardized. But the surgeon treating a fracture should be prepared to choose an appropriate method of dealing with soft tissues and to use the method effectively in the face of any difficulties. The concept that deep healing can be no better than the surface closure is perhaps nowhere better exemplified than in the management of trauma.

Difficulties of wound closure arise not only in severe open injuries with obvious soft tissue loss; they may also complicate open reduction of a closed fracture (Fig. 40-1) or the ill-advised use of a plaster casing or splint. Restoration of the skin covering at the time of reduction and fixation of the fracture is desirable to prevent further external contamination, to reduce the hazards of infection and to minimize fibrosis and interference with local blood supply. Thus, wound closure as an essential part of the definitive treatment of any fracture which is operated on cannot be disregarded for considerations of exposure of the fracture site or anatomic reduction of the bone. But closure must be carried out with thoughtful concern for skin circulation, avoidance of tension in the suture line and resort to delayed primary closure or other methods if immediate suture is hazardous or impossible.

In any active fracture service there will be wounds which break open because of deep infection or failure of the suture line to heal; there will be areas of ischemic necrosis of the skin; there will be avulsion or losses of skin arising from the trauma itself, and there will be deep wounds associated with fractures. The purpose of this chapter is to recount some of the soft tissue complications that have been observed and to call attention to possible ways in which these complications can be treated.

Skin, the barrier between external and internal milieus and thus the key to every wound closure, is nourished by a plexus of blood vessels that course immediately beneath the dermis, sending branches into the skin papillae. These in turn are supplied by larger vessels in the subcutaneous fat superficial to the deep fascia. The pattern of the deeper vascular channels is governed by the even larger vessels lying deep to the fascial layer. Thus, the blood supply of the skin over the perforating branches of the internal mammary vessels, or along the course of the thoracoepigastric vessels, or around the knee where the multiple geniculate branches are given off by the popliteal artery, follows an established pattern. These patterns are useful in the planning of repairs.

The arrangement of vessels in the skin and in most other areas of the body, with the exception of the long axis of an ex-

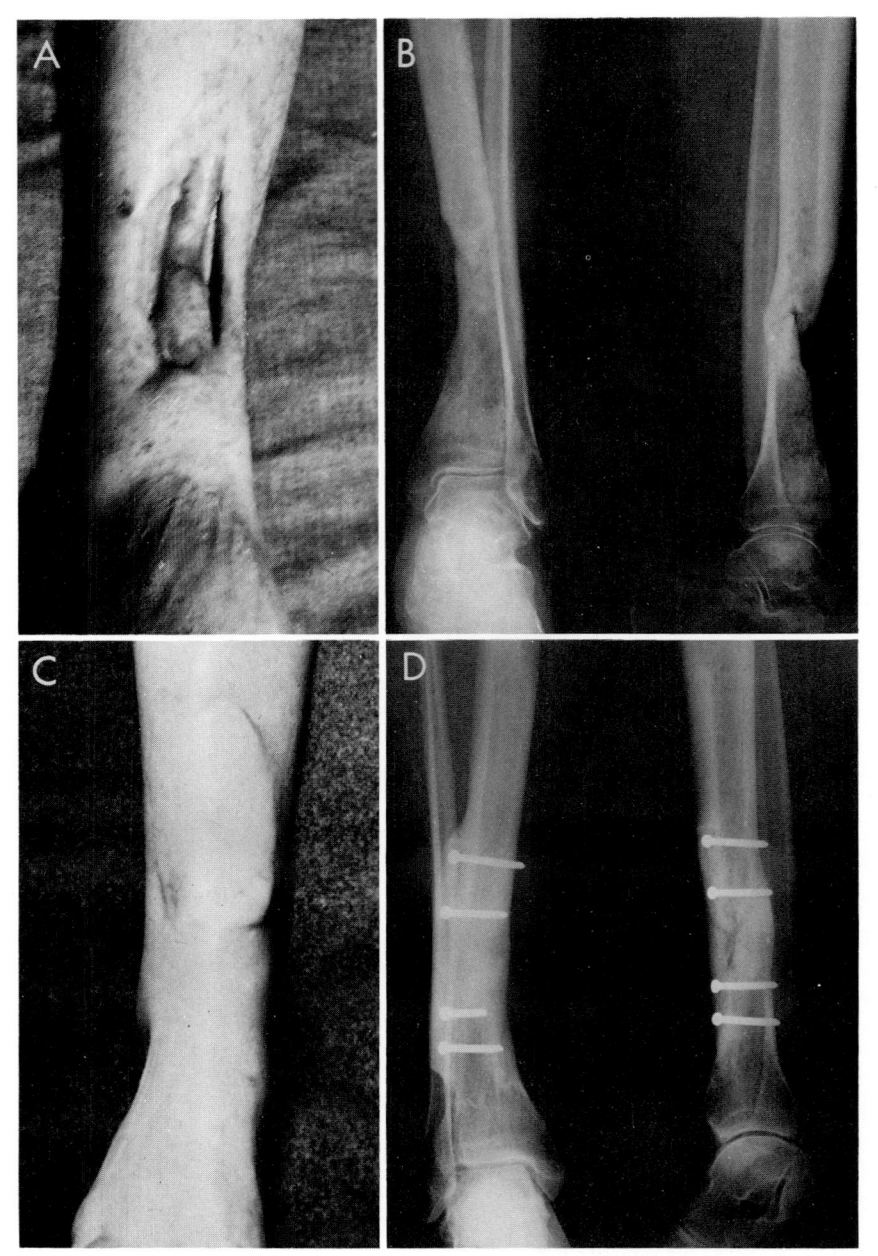

Fig. 40-1.—Closed comminuted spiral fracture of the tibia treated by open reduction and plating. **A,** when the wound broke open, there was considerable necrosis of skin, sequestration of much of the anterior tibia and serious infection in the local tissues. The granulating areas surrounding the exposed bone were closed promptly by skin grafts; after the sequestra were removed, the viable bone was also covered with skin grafts. **B,** with elimination of infection by wound closure, bone union progressed to a solid but weak bone bridge in the tibia. **C,** a direct flap from the opposite thigh was used to replace the skin grafts and provide a well-vascularized and flexible cover of normal skin over the damaged tibia. **D,** finally, the tibia was strengthened by a bone graft inserted beneath the flap.

tremity, does not follow a linear course. Vascular anastomoses across the midline of the trunk are said to be fewer than in the adjacent subcutaneous tissues. And the skin of the lower leg, especially the anterior surface where there is minimal subcutaneous tissue, is notoriously susceptible to ischemia and necrosis. When trauma is encountered or repairs contemplated in these areas of random circulation, special attention must be given to judging the condition of the skin. Care must be exercised in the manipulation of the skin to avoid closure under tension and to avoid marginal necrosis by constricting sutures.

METHODS OF WOUND CLOSURE

The surgeon has the choice of 4 methods of wound closure: linear closure, closure with a free skin graft, closure with a local flap and closure with a remote flap. Familiarity with the advantages and disadvantages, and the indications and limitations of each method will simplify the selection of the most suitable.

Linear Closure

The normal method of wound closure is by approximation of the edges. The wound may be an incised wound, in which the edges are smooth and undamaged, or it may be an open wound, with ragged crushed edges that must be excised before closure can be safely carried out. Suture must be without undue tension and with carefully placed stitches. The edema of the tissues at the fracture site may be great enough to prevent closure without tension despite the absence of skin loss. The so-called fracture blister is merely an evidence of the impaired circulation associated with acute edema. Compromise of the local blood supply by tight sutures may result in necrosis at the margins where the sutures are constricting, or it may produce enough regional ischemia to cause wider destruction of skin. Exposure of subcutaneous tissues or bone, serious infection in the devitalized tissues and long delays in healing of all tissues will result. Blanching of the skin, an evidence that blood is being expressed from the tiny vessels of the skin, is the best warning of impaired circulation. Delayed primary closure so well demonstrated in World War II and used routinely in some fracture services today should always be kept in mind in fractures of the distal extremities (lower leg and forearm). In these areas with a limited skin envelope, the deep swelling that accompanies the acute injury is more likely to produce wound complications in an open injury or following an open reduction. Edema following trauma uncomplicated by infection slowly subsides in a few days. In the meantime, the precursors of the healing process are gathering in the injured area so that closure at or about the seventh day progresses without delay.

The distribution of the blood supply to the skin and subcutaneous tissues described previously calls for suturing with a minimal number of skin stitches. Skin approximation can perhaps best be secured by sutures buried in the fatty subcutaneous tissue and by subcuticular stitches of fine suture material. Loose closure of the deep inelastic fascia will suffice with adequate skin covering. If direct closure cannot be carried out, some alternative method, such as a free skin graft or a local flap, must be used.

Closure by Skin Transplantation

Skin may be transplanted in 2 ways: (1) free transplantation or skin grafting, which means that the skin is completely detached from the body in its transfer, and (2) transplantation as a flap, which means that at all times the skin and subcutaneous tissues remain attached to the body and receive blood supply through this attachment or pedicle. The free skin graft must be thin, without any subcutaneous tissue to survive and grow after transfer, whereas the flap must retain the subcutaneous tissues in which its nutrient vessels course.

Skin Grafting

Free split-skin grafting is 1 of the most useful techniques available to the surgeon dealing with trauma. Unfortunately, use of these grafts is too frequently overlooked. There are few traumatic wounds with skin loss that cannot be closed by a skin graft, applied either on a raw surface of subcutaneous tissue or on muscle, or even on cancellous bone. In most acute wounds, the direct application of a skin graft is possible. Only if hemostasis is a problem is there reason to postpone the application of a graft, and in that situation the graft should certainly be applied before 4–5 days have passed. Whether the skin graft will provide the definitive covering or not is immaterial. Its immediate function is to convert the open wound into a closed one, so that deep healing can progress. Final evaluation of the stability of the skin graft can be made at a later date.

A properly prepared, clean, granulating wound—following failure of primary wound closure, infection or ischemic necrosis of skin—can be closed by a skin graft. Both the general condition of the patient and the local condition of the wound will improve as the total area of raw surface is reduced. Even the granulating wound surrounding exposed tendon or bone should be promptly closed with a graft. The drainage will diminish, the care of the wound is made easier, and the necrotic tissue will sequester with less reaction. Not infrequently, what appears to be devitalized bone or nonviable tendon will begin to show evidence of recovery when no longer bathed in purulent exudate. Blood vessels appear on the surface and epithelium spreads rapidly from the surrounding grafted skin (Fig. 40-2).

SECURING THE SKIN GRAFT.—The split-skin graft, as the name implies, is cut at approximately the midthickness of the dermis. The cut is considerably deeper than the rete pegs and germinal layer that form the base of the normal epidermis. Skin grafts thus consist of the normal epidermis and variable thicknesses of the dermal layer, determined by the depth of the cut. The roots of the hair follicles and the sebaceous and sweat glands, which lie in the depths of the dermis, are the only epithelial elements that remain. These specialized structures are developmental offshoots of ectodermal tissue. From the transected openings of these structures pour out the cells that re-establish the epidermal layer. The term "dedifferentiate" has been used to define the reversion of the function of the cells lining these special structures to that of the more simple squamous epithelial type. Spontaneous healing of the donor site, which is usually complete in 12–14 days, is marked by the restoration of an intact impervious outer layer of skin. The dressing on the donor site should be left undisturbed until healing is complete lest the delicate new epidermis be traumatized and the healing time prolonged.

The graft may be cut with a razor, with a special thin-bladed knife or with 1 of several machines termed "dermatomes." For any wound with impaired blood supply or with chronic low-grade sepsis, it is desirable to obtain a thin sheet of skin because a thinner sheet of skin is more apt to survive. To survive, the graft must be transplanted either to a freshly prepared raw surface or to a granulating surface free from active infection. At first the graft is nourished by osmotic interchange with the underlying tissues, but within 2–3 days there is abundant evidence of active circulation and revascularization of the skin. If nutrition of the skin graft is inadequate because of an unhealthy local wound or general malnutrition of the patient, the graft may be overwhelmed by sepsis or autolysis and fail to survive.

The skin graft has a high resistance to infection. Its successful "take" is associ-

Chapter 40: SOFT TISSUE REPAIRS / 973

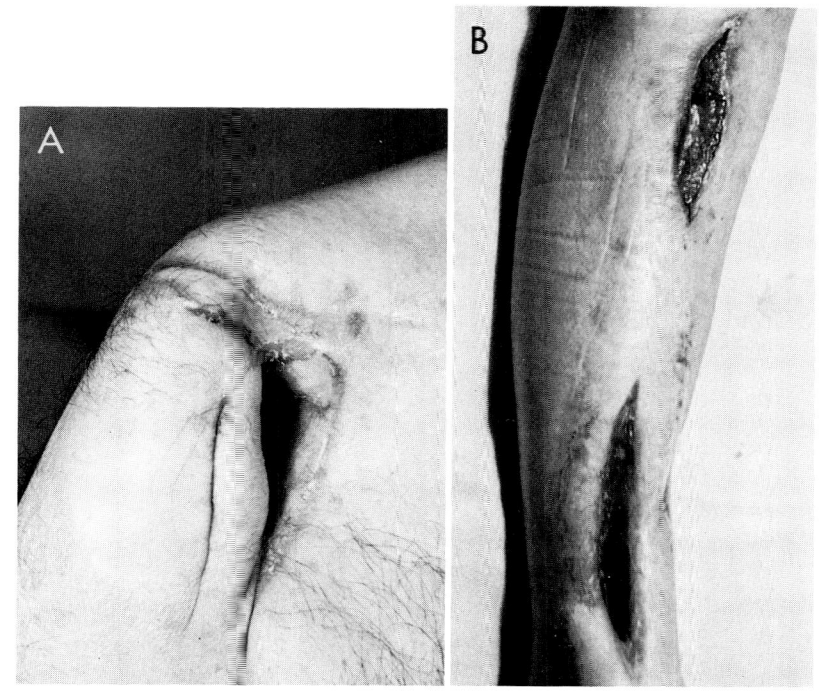

Fig. 40-2. — Granulating bone defects closed with skin grafts. Localized osteomyelitis was controlled by wound closure. **A**, necrosis and infection of head of humerus following open reduction; removal of the head was necessary. After the deep concavity was lined with the skin grafts, infection in the bone subsided and the remaining raw surface healed spontaneously. Repair with a flap was contemplated later. **B**, infection of tibial shaft following intramedullary nailing. Decortication of the bone was necessary for adequate drainage, after which both upper and lower cavities were lined successfully with skin grafts. Photograph shows condition of upper cavity at time of skin grafting and healed distal cavity.

ated with a rapid reduction in the bacterial content of the underlying wound. Well-documented evidence is reported of a 71% decrease in the bacterial count of a granulating surface in 2 hours after grafting. Success is influenced by the condition of the wound, the thickness of the graft, the temperature of the skin surface, and the intangibles — the surgeon's judgment and skill. Although a thin skin graft is more likely to succeed on a wound of doubtful condition, a thicker split-skin graft will shrink less and will provide a smoother, more stable surface. Thin grafts cut with a dermatome are difficult to unglue from the drum or adhesive-strip backing and often may tear when removed. Therefore a thin graft can perhaps be best cut with a knife or its equivalent.

The dermis is what provides elasticity, texture and toughness of the skin, as well as anchorage and stability for the epidermis. It does not regenerate. When destroyed, it is replaced by scar tissue, which lacks the elastic fibers and consequently the resiliency that characterizes the dermis. Spontaneous epithelial spread across a granulating surface will provide a protective layer of "scar epithelium," but this thin sheet may be unstable and ulcerate repeatedly without the anchorage and cushioning support of the underlying dermis. Epidermoid carcinoma may develop in such scars if they are allowed to become the site of recurrent or chronic ulceration or irritation.

Transfer of a Flap

The flap method of transplanting skin differs from the free skin graft since the flap remains attached at all times to the body by a pedicle. The flap consists of not only the full thickness of the skin but also the underlying subcutaneous fat, in which the nutrient vessels of the skin lie. It may be transplanted in 2 principal ways: as a direct flap or as a delayed flap.

Transfer of a *direct flap* is possible when sufficient blood supply through the attachment or pedicle can be insured, either because recognized major blood vessels are present in the pedicle or because the attachment is sufficiently broad to contain enough nutrient blood vessels. The statement has been made that no flap should be more than twice as long as the width of its attachment or pedicle. If this rule is followed to the letter, there will be instances of necrosis of the distal end of the flap because of inadequate blood supply. It is preferable, if possible, that the direct flap from local or remote sources be no more than half again as long as the width of the attachment. This places limitations on the availability of direct flaps for major repairs. However, it is usually feasible to use a direct flap from the trunk for any part of the upper extremity, and most repairs of the lower extremity can be carried out with a direct flap from the opposite leg.

By the *delayed transfer* of a flap is meant the gradual cutting of the major blood vessels entering a flap on 3 sides, leaving intact the blood vessels at the base or pedicle of the flap as the sole blood supply when the flap is finally moved. By this method, longer and narrower flaps can be safely transferred to an adjacent local area or to a more remote part of the body. It should be emphasized that the delay of a flap is a multiple-stage procedure. After the pattern of the flap has been outlined on the skin, incisions are made on either side of the long axis of the flap. These are carried down to the deep fascia. Both the small subdermal vessels and the deeply lying, larger vessels in the subcutaneous fat are interrupted by this cut. At this primary procedure, unless the flap is more than 3–4 times the length of its base or pedicle, the flap may be completely undermined, thereby interrupting the vessels which emerge through openings in the deep fascia. The flap is sutured back in place after ligation of all active bleeding points, or it may be formed into a rope or tube by suturing the skin edges of the flap together. Sometimes the skin defect can be closed beneath a tubed flap, but more often a free skin graft is necessary for closure.

Tubing a flap allows multistage transfer of a flap from 1 area to another without an exposed raw surface. The disadvantages of tubing are several: the width of the flap is limited by the mechanics of tubing, some circumferential shrinkage of the tube cannot be prevented, formation of a tube in an obese person is hazardous because of poor skin healing, and adjusting the flap at the final step may be awkward because of its rounded form. The advantage of transfer without an exposed raw surface usually outweighs these disadvantages.

After the first step in the preparation of the flap is completed, major blood vessels at the distal end of the flap still remain. These must be severed before the final transfer can be safely accomplished. Thus, the final step in preparation requires the making of an incision across the end of the flap down to the deep fascia. It will not be necessary to undermine the flap at this operation because the vessels on its undersurface should have been cut and tied at an earlier procedure. However, in a large flap, i.e., 1 with a length greater than 3–4 times the width of its base or pedicle, several preliminary delaying procedures are almost invariably necessary. Sometimes four or more such procedures are expedient to interrupt the blood supply gradually and to insure the viability of the skin and subcutaneous layer of the flap.

Occasionally, small hematomas or

areas of induration may occur in a flap during its preparation. Accumulations of blood should be evacuated and areas of induration watched until they have completely subsided. Transfer of a flap in the presence of local or diffuse induration, localized infection or accumulations of blood is foolhardy and can result only in disastrous partial or complete tissue loss.

TYPES OF FLAPS.—A local skin flap may be taken from an adjacent untraumatized area and shifted into the defect left by the trauma (Fig. 40-3). It is unwise to use a local flap if the site from which the flap is to be secured is one that is subject to trauma or weight bearing (Fig. 40-4). Such areas include the skin overlying the malleoli or other prominences (Fig.

Fig. 40-3.—**A,** ulceration over the lateral aspect of the knee, with proved connections to the joint, which was closed successfully after preliminary debridement and preparation of the wound. **B,** repair by local single-pedicled flap, which rotated forward to cover the defect, and by skin graft covering the donor area.

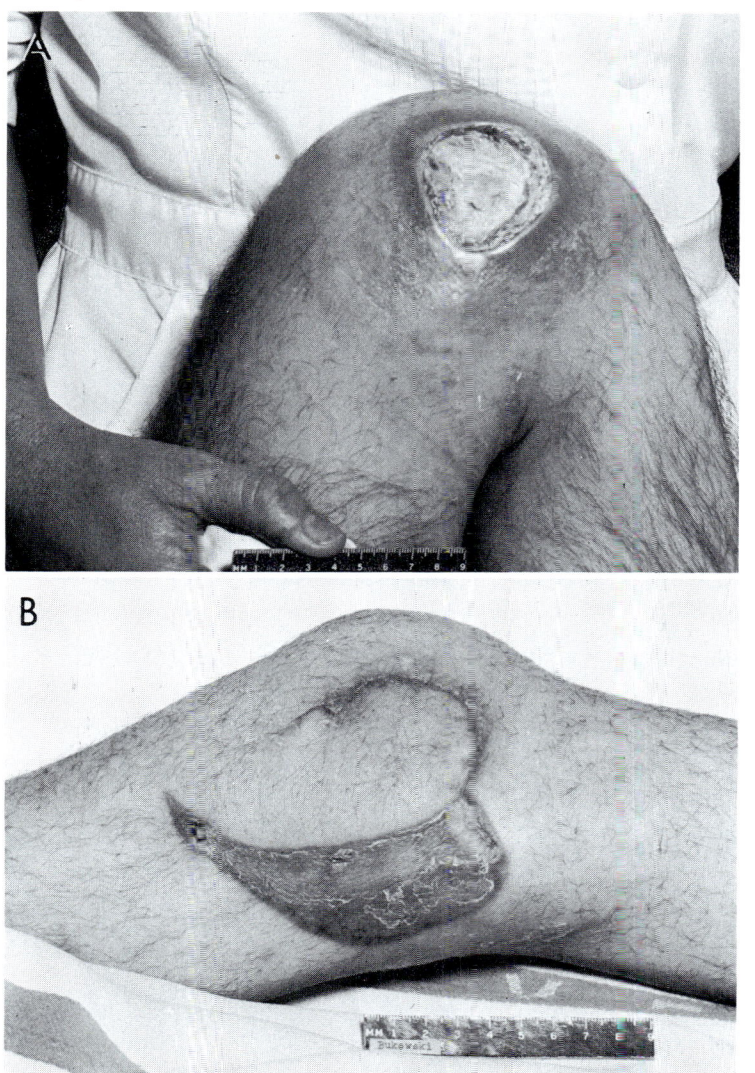

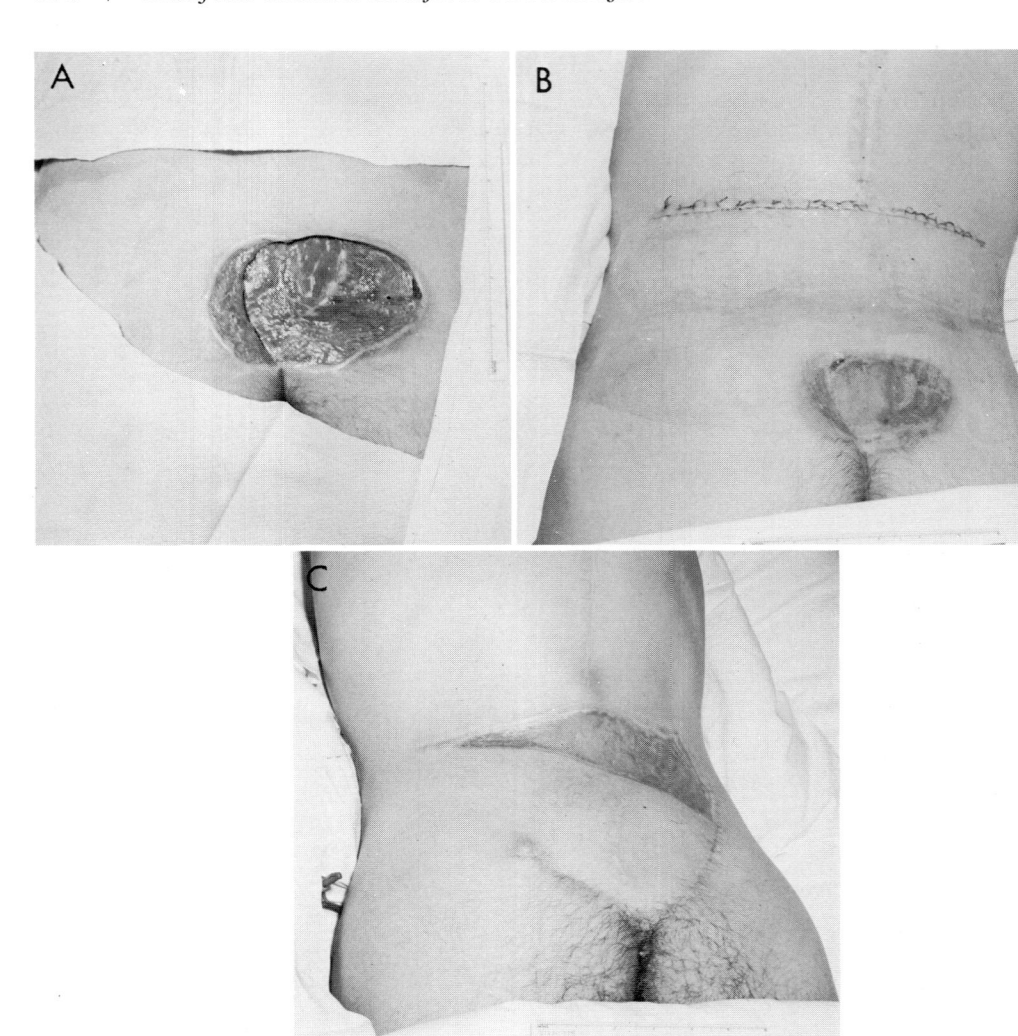

Fig. 40-4.—**A,** sacral pressure ulcer in a paraplegic. **B,** ulcer was closed primarily with a skin graft at the time of the first-stage delay of a flap in the lumbar region, a non-weight-bearing area. At operation the skin of the flap was completely undermined, all bleeding carefully controlled, and the wound closed. At a second operation the end of the flap was cut and sutured. **C,** in the final operation, the skin graft was removed and the flap shifted over the sacrum. The donor site of the flap was closed with a skin graft. (From Cannon, B., O'Leary, J. J., O'Neil, J. W., and Steinsieck, R.: An approach to the treatment of pressure sores, Ann. Surg. 132:760, 1950.)

40-5), the weight-bearing areas of the sole of the foot (Fig. 40-6) and the tactile areas of the hands.

If there is not sufficient tissue available locally to form a flap or if the defect is too large to cover with local tissue, a flap from another part of the body may be necessary. In the upper extremities the skin of the trunk can be utilized as a direct flap, prepared and applied either at the time of the debridement or at the time of excision of the scar tissue. These flaps can be measured to fit the defect exactly. They should have a broad base of attachment to serve as a source of blood supply and a well-vascularized layer of

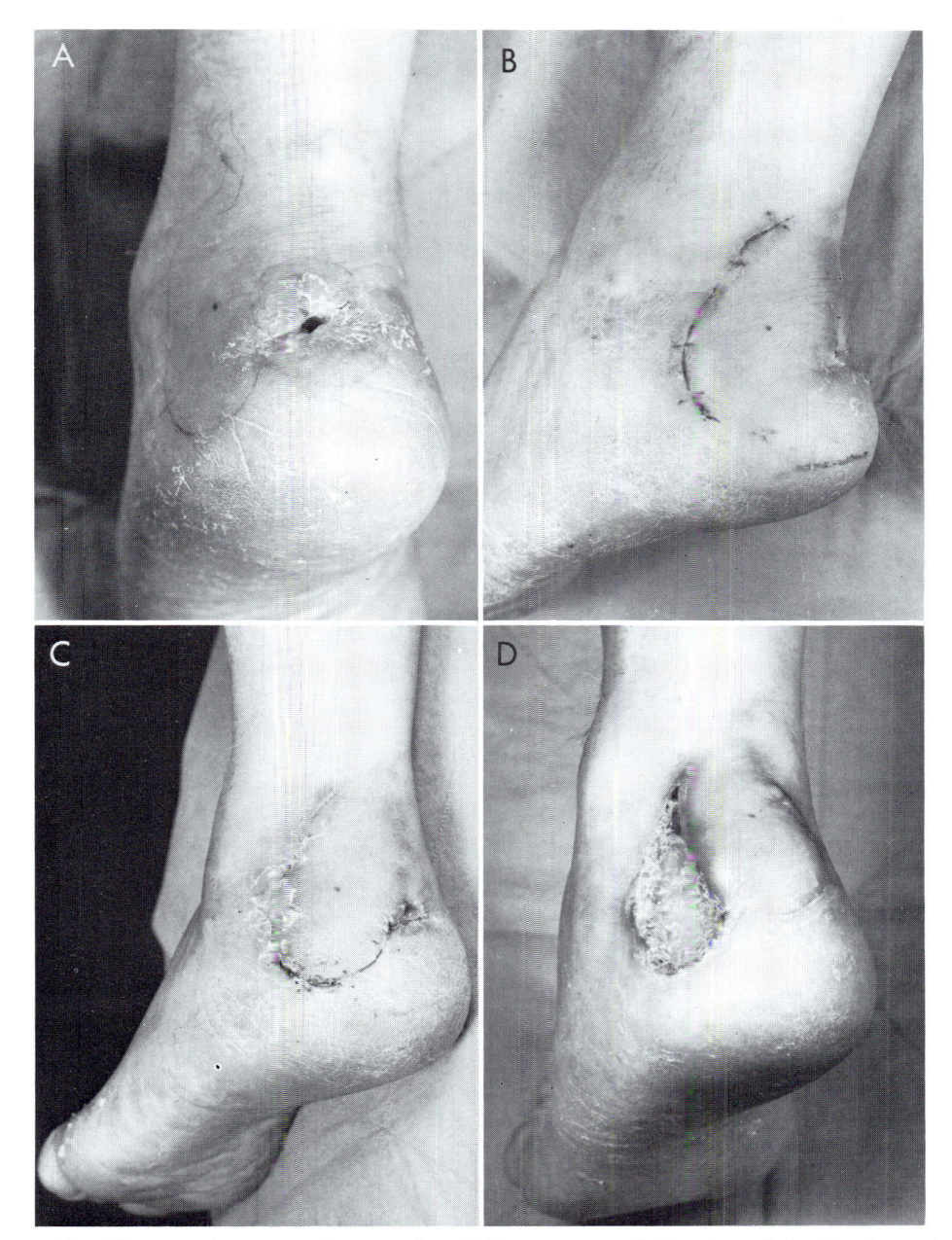

Fig. 40-5.—Chronic ulcer over the os calcis following immobilization of the leg in a plaster cast. Repair in 3 stages with a local flap has proved the most expeditious and permanently stable method of repair in all but very large defects. **A,** the lesion with the flap outlined on the lateral side. **B,** at the first step, 1 border of the flap is incised and the area completely undermined. **C,** the second operation consists in incising the distal margin of the flap. The junction of the flap with the scar is not cut because no major vessels could remain in the scar. **D,** final transfer of the flap, which is now elevated completely for the first time. The ulcer and surrounding scar tissue are excised. The donor area of the flap is closed with a skin graft. (From Cannon, B., and Constable, J. D.: Reconstructive Plastic Surgery of the Lower Extremity, in Converse, J. M. (ed.), *Reconstructive Plastic Surgery* [Philadelphia: W. B. Saunders Company, 1964].)

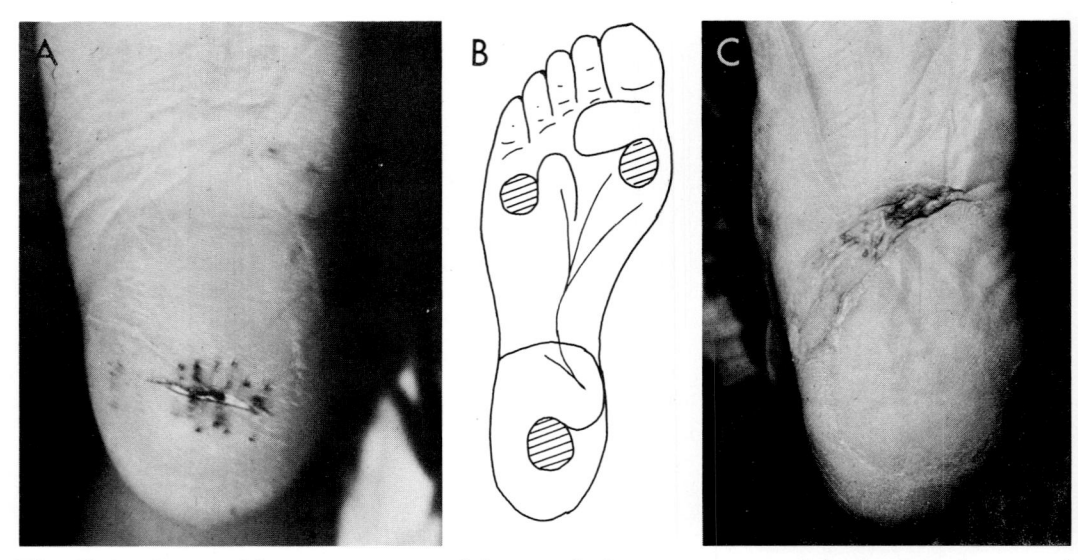

Fig. 40-6.—**A**, unstable scar in center of the weight-bearing portion of the heel. **B**, diagram of non-weight-bearing donor sites appropriate for plantar flaps. **C**, scar was excised and the defect repaired by a local single-pedicled flap from the plantar arch. The donor site of the flap was covered by a graft which is wrinkled but has good stability.

subcutaneous fat to provide a cushion between the skin and the deeper tissue (see Fig. 40-15).

In the lower extremities the problem is more difficult, and the transfer of a flap from 1 leg to another requires stoicism on the part of the patient, and forethought, planning and care on the part of the surgeon. Many flaps can be transferred directly, such as those about the knee, where there is abundant blood supply, as previously noted. Covering the front of the tibia often requires a retrograde flap in the opposite thigh. Such a flap can usually be transferred without the need of a delaying procedure. A flap from the medial aspect of the opposite calf is often the best source of skin for the sole of the foot (see Fig. 40-11). The calf may also be the source of covering for repairs either in front or in back of the opposite knee.

Defects of large areas of the lower extremity are the kind that require the greatest planning and skill, because remote flaps from the abdominal wall or elsewhere must often be transferred by means of an intermediate carrier, such as the forearm or hand. In preparing the original flap, sufficient tissue must be projected to insure complete coverage of the damaged area. Not only must the quantity be adequate but the method of transfer must be forecast. For example, an abdominal tubed flap to cover the tibial crest must be attached appropriately to its intermediate carrier, the forearm or hand, so that it will lie comfortably in the long axis of the lower leg, not at right angles to it. Such simple concepts are often overlooked. The surgeon will be enlightened by practicing these inelegant positions on himself (see Fig. 40-14).

CARE OF THE OPEN WOUND

There is no substitute for diligence in the care of the chronic open wound. No topical or parenteral medication has yet replaced faithful mechanical cleansing, careful daily debridement and frequent changes of dressing. The skin surrounding the wound, as well as the wound itself, must be kept scrupulously clean. Hair should be shaved off and all local epithelial debris washed vigorously away. Exposed bone need not be trimmed away, but loose sequestra should be lifted from the wound. A single layer of fine gauze (44-mesh), moistened to increase its capillarity and held firmly against the granulating surface, has the advantage of minimal adherence to the wound itself without obstructing the wound drainage. Bits of necrotic tissue will adhere to the gauze and come away when the dressing is changed. Contact of the gauze with the whole wound surface is necessary. In any concave wound or in one with a deep pocket the gauze should be packed loosely into the cavity to eliminate all "dead space" in which exudate may accumulate and provide a local medium for infection. Preventing accumulations of exudate in such cavities is important in the care of a wound.

DELAYED PRIMARY CLOSURE

Delayed primary closure finds its greatest usefulness following acute trauma. After the wound has been appropriately debrided, the fracture reduced and the bones immobilized, an attempt at closure can be made. If, because of edema or skin loss, there is any significant degree of tension in suturing the skin, a minimum of approximation is done (Fig. 40-7). Even bare bone can be left uncovered by soft tissue. A dry dressing is loosely packed into the uneven contours of the unclosed wound. Under no circumstances should this dressing be changed until the patient is appropriately anesthetized in the operating room 5–7 days later. The healing stimulus defined recently by a number of investigators is then at its maximum. No "prep" of the wound is needed or desirable—in fact, it is harmful. If the dressing is removed and replaced or if the operative closure is delayed, the condition of the wound will deteriorate, bacteria will gain a foothold, and it will become an infected wound. At 5–7 days no attempt should be made to carry out a layer closure, because the tissues will seldom accept a series of buried sutures. It is better to use loose stay sutures, which will engage all layers of the wound, collapse any dead spaces and allow surface drainage through the gaps in the skin edges between the sutures.

SKIN GRAFTING

A wound that cannot be sutured within the prescribed several days after injury, or one that has opened spontaneously because of tension, sepsis or necrosis of skin, is best converted from an open into a closed wound by a free skin graft. It should always be recognized that the prime function of the graft is to close the wound. Healing of the deeper tissues (skin, muscle, etc.) can then progress without the delays that accompany infection, fibrosis and diminished blood supply. If the location of a graft or the condition of the deeper tissues requires later replacement of the graft with a flap, the graft will still have served the important emergency function of protecting the wound.

On a freshly dissected surface the skin graft had best be sutured, but on a granulating surface it is seldom necessary or wise to suture a graft, especially on an extremity where effective "snubbing" of the graft in place with a circular bandage is possible. Usually the graft will adhere promptly to a clean granulating surface, probably by the interaction of plasma ingredients both on the undersurface of the graft and on the granulating surface. A single sheet of skin is preferable to scraps of skin, but wounds with many uneven contours may require the fitting of several pieces of graft to the complex surface. Trimming the skin graft to leave a narrow margin of raw surface between the edge of the graft and the normal surrounding skin is desirable. If an overlap is left, the graft adheres to the skin; and any exudate at the junction will be forced beneath the graft and may destroy it. The unnourished graft over avascular tissues invites infection which can cause de-

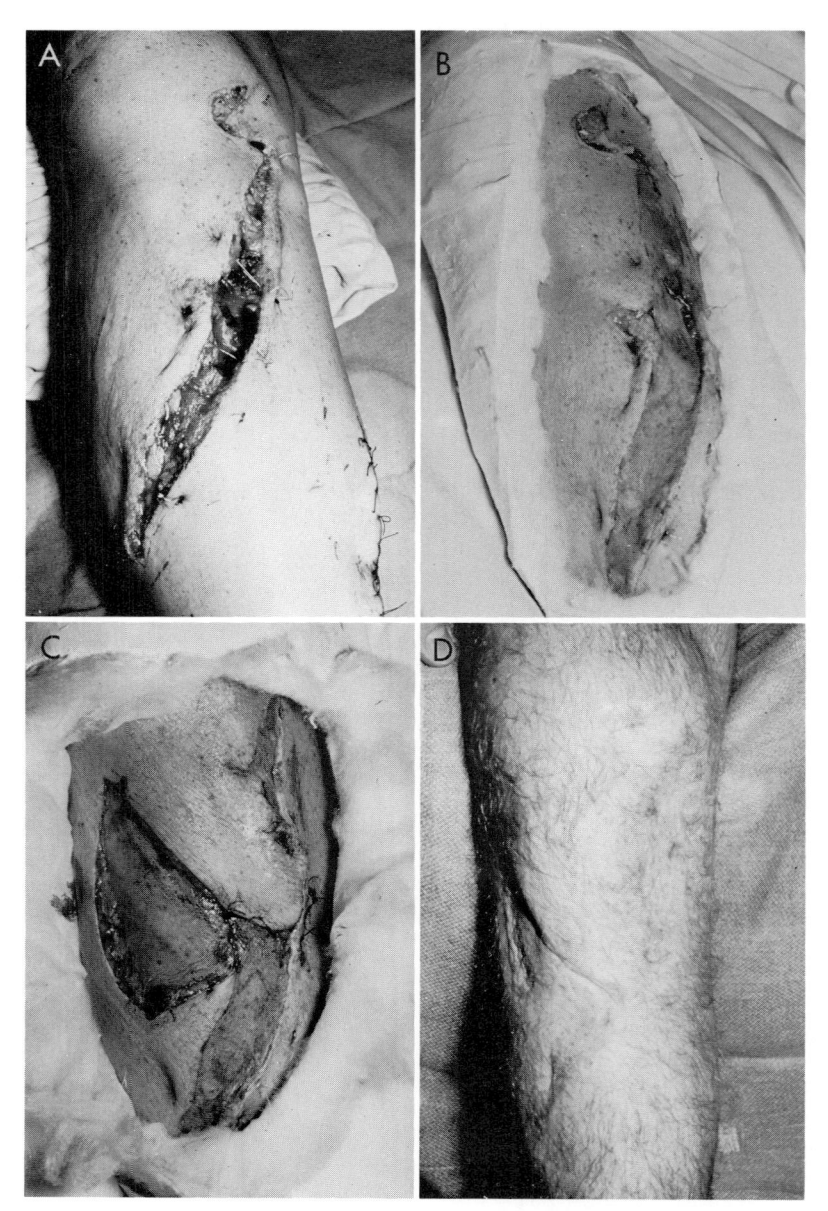

Fig. 40-7.—Serious compound injury of the lower leg. **A,** after the fracture had been reduced and the bone stabilized, wound closure was attempted, but the edema already present in the leg caused tension on the suture line sufficient to impair the skin circulation. Therefore, loose closure was done, leaving a gap of approximately 2 cm in the widest part, unfortunately immediately overlying the fracture line. **B,** the skin graft on the raw surface over the fracture had insufficient nutrition to survive in this critical area. **C,** a direct, local, single-pedicled flap was rotated over this area to provide protection for the healing bone and to avoid a suture line immediately over the fracture. Operation was performed through the window in the plaster cast without disturbing the fracture fixation. **D,** primary healing of the bone was secured without any local suppuration. Full weight bearing was begun within a few months. (From Cannon, B., and Constable, J. D.: Reconstructive Plastic Surgery of the Lower Extremity, in Converse, J. M. (ed.), *Reconstructive Plastic Surgery* [Philadelphia: W. B. Saunders Company, 1964].)

struction of viable skin. Neither a deep sinus from which there is drainage nor a small bleeding vessel is a contraindication to grafting. The skin graft should be perforated, allowing the drainage or the blood to escape into the dressing. Holes in the skin graft should likewise be made over exposed bone, tendon or islands of epithelium if the area is larger than 5–10 mm.

Immobilization of the graft and support with moderate compression by a protective dressing is desirable. The dressing for a concavity or a deep pocket must be fitted accurately to the space in order to fulfill its function of holding the graft in place. Likewise, if the part is oval in shape, as for the forearm and hand, the dressing must be higher on the volar and dorsal surfaces than on the lateral surface, in order to secure uniform circumferential compression.

There is evidence that grafts may do better if maintained at normal skin temperature. Occasionally, therefore, in areas where the problem of immobilization is slight or where the graft is glued firmly to the raw surface, dressings may be omitted. It is essential to check the wound daily in order to empty any accumulations of exudate beneath the graft and to remove the crusts that form at the graft margin. The exudate would, of course, normally be absorbed into a dressing if one were used, but without a dressing, the exudate dries and may act as a barrier to drainage. A cradle or other protection is desirable to prevent contact of the graft with the bedclothing, which could dislodge it. The successful graft will be well vascularized and adequately secure in position to resume wet dressings in 4–5 days. The resumption of wet dressings will simplify the care by eliminating the crusting. The dressing also acts as a splint to on-growing epithelium and protects the skin graft itself when the sheltering cradle is removed.

Cultures are desirable in determining the bacterial flora in the wound and in selecting the antibiotics for preventing invasive infection. A valuable clue to the condition of the wound, other than observation, is the pH. The more alkaline the pH (7.2 or above), the higher the percentage of successful skin grafts.

The drilling of holes in the bony cortex devoid of periosteum, or in eburnated bone at the fracture site, in order to establish vascular connections between the marrow cavity and the overlying soft tissues, is a useful adjunct to the attachment of a skin flap or preparation for the application of a free skin graft. Vascular channels between the marrow cavity and the outer surface of the cortex serve as anchorage for the otherwise easily dislodged soft tissue. Nothing is gained by drilling necrotic bone, which must be completely resected before a wound can be closed.

Postoperative Care of Grafts and Flaps

There is no hard-and-fast rule about the time for the first change of dressing of a skin graft. Observation of the graft daily, if no dressing is used, will allow the most careful check of the progress of healing. If a dressing is used, daily inspection in the first few days after operation is risky because removal of the dressing may dislodge the graft. If the dressing, serving the important function of immobilizing the graft, must be removed and replaced, the surgeon should weigh his ability to restore as good a dressing as that originally applied against the risks involved in postponing the removal of the dressing until the graft is more firmly healed in place.

The following routines have generally been followed. Grafts without dressings are observed daily. Grafts on small granulating surfaces where a good dressing can be reapplied are examined on the third or fourth day. Larger grafts or grafts applied at the donor site of a flap are examined between the fifth and seventh days.

Dressings are applied to all flaps postoperatively. Moderate resilient compression (cotton waste) is maintained on the end of the flap with minimal compression on the pedicle. The end of the flap is usually inspected within the first few hours after operation. Cyanosis of the skin is considered a serious prognostic sign because it means that venous return from the flap is inadequate. This may result from kinking of the pedicle, too great pressure on the pedicle or improper preparation of the flap. When cyanosis is present, the flap should be completely exposed, the pedicle examined, and efforts made to change the position so that the circulation will be improved. If the congestion persists for more than 24 hours, it is seldom possible to salvage the congested part of the flap.

A complete change of the dressing on a flap is usually done by the fifth or sixth day. This is repeated daily or every second day thereafter. In complex flaps from the trunk to the arm, or from 1 leg to the other, there may be small raw surfaces that could not be closed with a skin graft at the time the flap was transferred. These are often not easily accessible and must be carefully watched and kept scrupulously clean. Invasive infection from these surfaces can produce thromboses in the pedicle and loss of the flap.

The pedicle of most flaps can be severed in 18–21 days. Earlier separation of the pedicle is possible, but premature cutting involves risks that can be minimized by maintaining the attachment for a few more days. Several tests (histamine flare, saline wheal, fluorescein or simply temporary compression of the pedicle) can be used to judge the circulation. Even after 3 weeks, these observations may make *staged* cutting of the pedicle desirable. Final separation will be postponed until circulation between the flap and the recipient surface is assured. Staged cutting across the pedicle can require 2 or more operations.

INDICATIONS FOR AND USES OF FLAPS

Since serious soft tissue damage is a common accompaniment of lower leg fractures, these injuries have often been the reason for combined efforts by the hospital fracture and plastic services. The leg is subject to direct trauma from the automobile bumper, from heavy industrial materials, from power equipment and from logging operations, and to indirect trauma from falls with twisting of the tibia while the ankle or knee is fixed. Compound injuries, avulsions of skin and detachment of comminuted bone fragments occur because the thick cushion of flexible soft tissue which overlies most other long bones is lacking over the tibial tubercle, the tibial crest and the malleoli. The small tight muscular compartments of the lower leg pose additional considerations in the management of the traumatized soft tissues (see Fig. 40-12).

The timing of treatment of any fracture of the lower leg may well be determined by the condition of the soft tissues. Delay in treatment of the simple fracture should always be considered when there is extreme swelling with or without blistering of the skin (an indication of locally impaired circulation). It is difficult, however, to postpone attack on a displaced or open fracture. Open reduction of the closed fracture before organization and resorption of the hematoma have begun is less complex because the parts are more easily identified and mobilized. The risk in operative treatment of closed fractures is one of imperfect wound healing, which can prolong recovery for years if wound disruption, infection and bone necrosis develop. Perhaps the pendulum has swung too far in the direction of operative interference for lower leg fractures.

Two types of open wound are common in the tibial crest. One is the jagged, roughly circular, open wound which must be debrided and may be extended upward and downward to expose and stabilize the fracture. The other is the elliptical wound that either evolves from the first as edema of the soft tissues increases or results from tissue loss in the long axis of the tibia.

The incision above and below the circular defect may be sutured unless edema is great, but the defect itself cannot be sutured without tension and must therefore be closed with a rotation flap of adjacent tissue. A single-pedicled flap, half again as large as the circular defect, can be raised from the lateral surface of the leg with the pedicle lying proximally. The flap is rotated medially to cover the exposed fracture line, and the donor surface closed with a skin graft (Fig. 40-8).

An unstable scar or ulceration on the back of the heel is a not uncommon complication of fracture immobilization. Resurfacing with a rotation flap is indicated. Delay of the flap is advisable in the area of random circulation (see Fig. 40-5).

The second type of wound, because the defect is elliptical in shape rather than circular, is best closed with a double-pedicled flap, also from the lateral surface of the leg. This flap can be very

Fig. 40-8. — Open fracture of right tibia through which an open reduction was carried out. **A**, the wound broke down, exposing the metal plate (*arrow*). Intensive daily local care and general antibiotic therapy improved the condition of the wound sufficiently to permit direct closure. **B** and **C**, single-pedicled local flap was used because of the circular shape of the wound and because the condition of the lateral tissues was too uncertain to tolerate elevation of a double-pedicled flap. The bone plate was removed at the time of closure and a skin graft was used to close the donor area of the flap. **D**, the dimensions of a single-pedicled flap must be measured as indicated in the diagram, insuring that the radius or length of the flap will reach the limits of the defect.

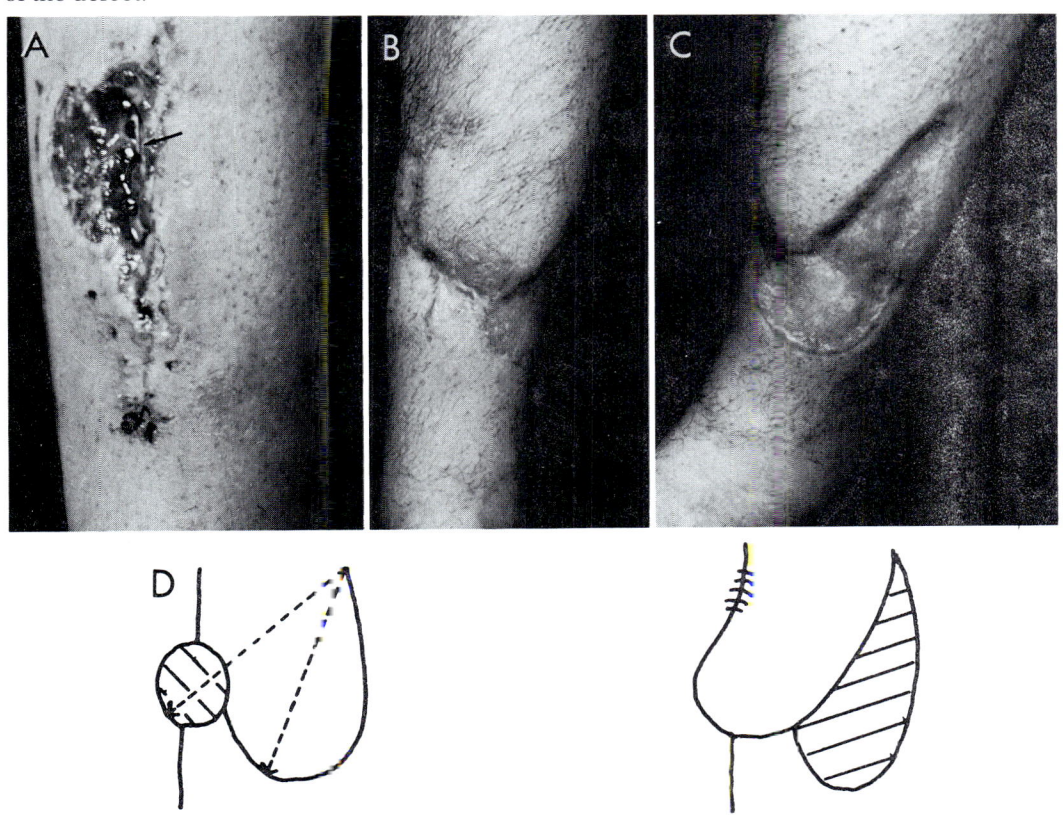

SINGLE PEDICLED FLAP

accurately measured in its preparation. Its width should be *half the length* of the primary wound, and the lateral incision which permits its mobilization should be parallel to the margin of the wound and *twice as long* as the length of the wound. These measurements will insure free mobilization of the flap when it is completely undermined and will also insure an adequate blood supply. The flap that is too narrow may not survive and the flap that is too wide may not be easily moved into place over the tibia. This donor surface is also closed with a skin graft (Fig. 40-9).

More complex but equally effective methods of treatment are required for larger defects or for those in which local

Fig. 40-9.—Open fracture of tibia treated by plating. **A**, the wound broke open, exposing the fracture line and the metal plate. Although infected, the condition of the wound was so much improved by intensive local care (gentle debridement, daily wet dressings and carefully placed gauze packing) that direct closure after removal of the metal plate was successful. **B** and **C**, result of closure with a local, double-pedicled flap of adjacent skin and use of a free graft on the donor site. **D**, dimensions of the flap: the relaxing incision of the flap is twice as long as the primary scar and the width of the flap is more than half the length of the primary scar.

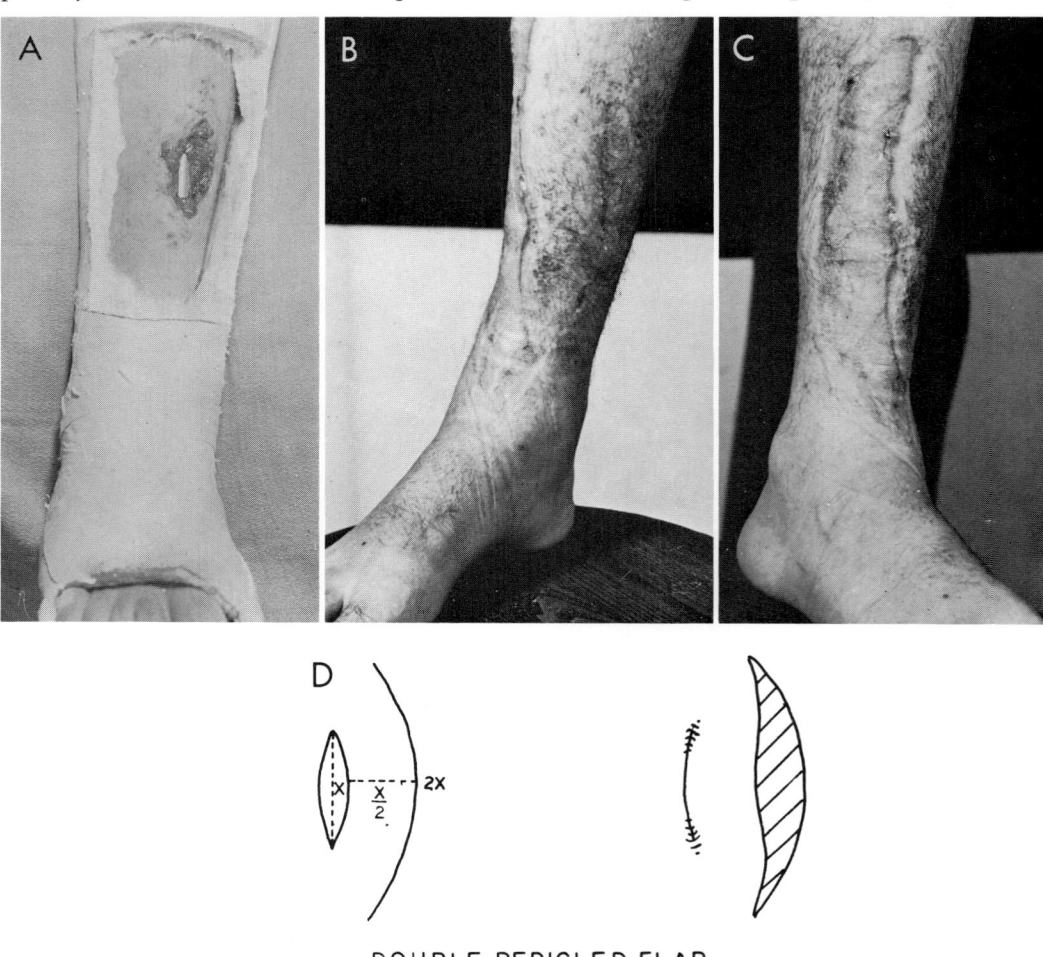

DOUBLE PEDICLED FLAP

Chapter 40: SOFT TISSUE REPAIRS / 985

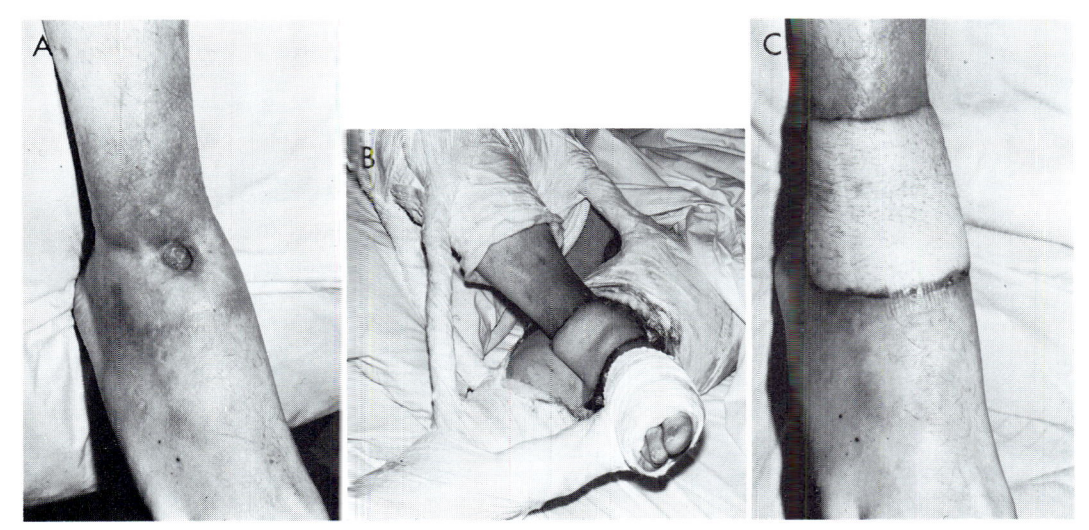

Fig. 40-10. – Open fracture of ankle with infection, spontaneous fusion of the ankle joint and a draining sinus from which sequestra have been removed. **A**, the sinus is now lined by healthy granulation tissue and has minimal drainage. The surrounding scar tissue was excised, the bone pocket saucerized and the surface repaired with a direct flap from the opposite thigh (**B**). "Cross-leg" position was maintained for 18 days. **C**, final result.

Fig. 40-11. – Repair of avulsion of anterior sole of foot that included all skin and subcutaneous tissues. **A**, primary wound was closed with a skin graft. **B**, definitive covering was provided by a direct flap from the opposite calf, which replaced the skin graft. Each leg was wrapped in a cast and the casts joined by plaster struts. **C**, at follow-up 8 years later, well-cushioned skin flap was still stable. (From Cannon, B., and Trott, A. W.: Expeditious use of direct flaps in extremity repairs, Plast. Reconstr. Surg. 4:415, 1949.)

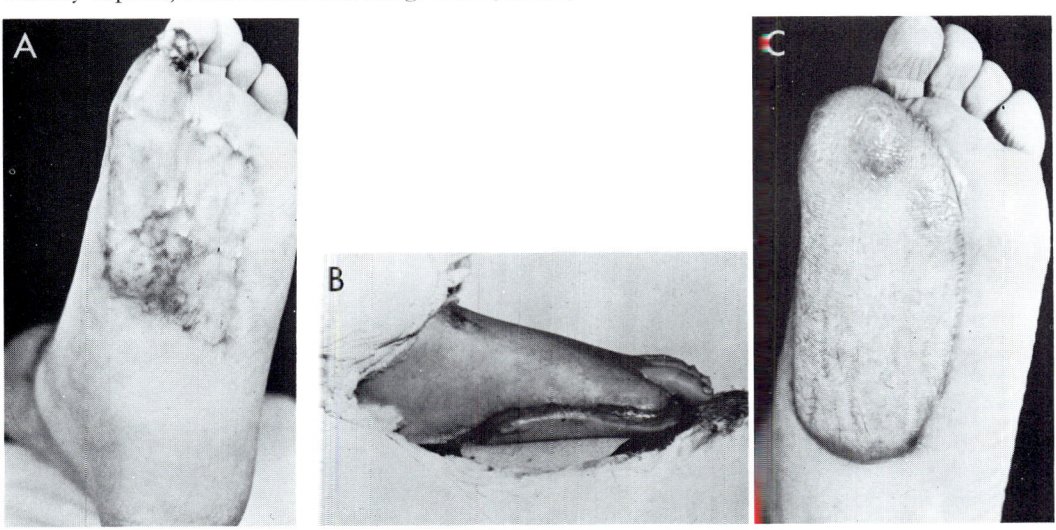

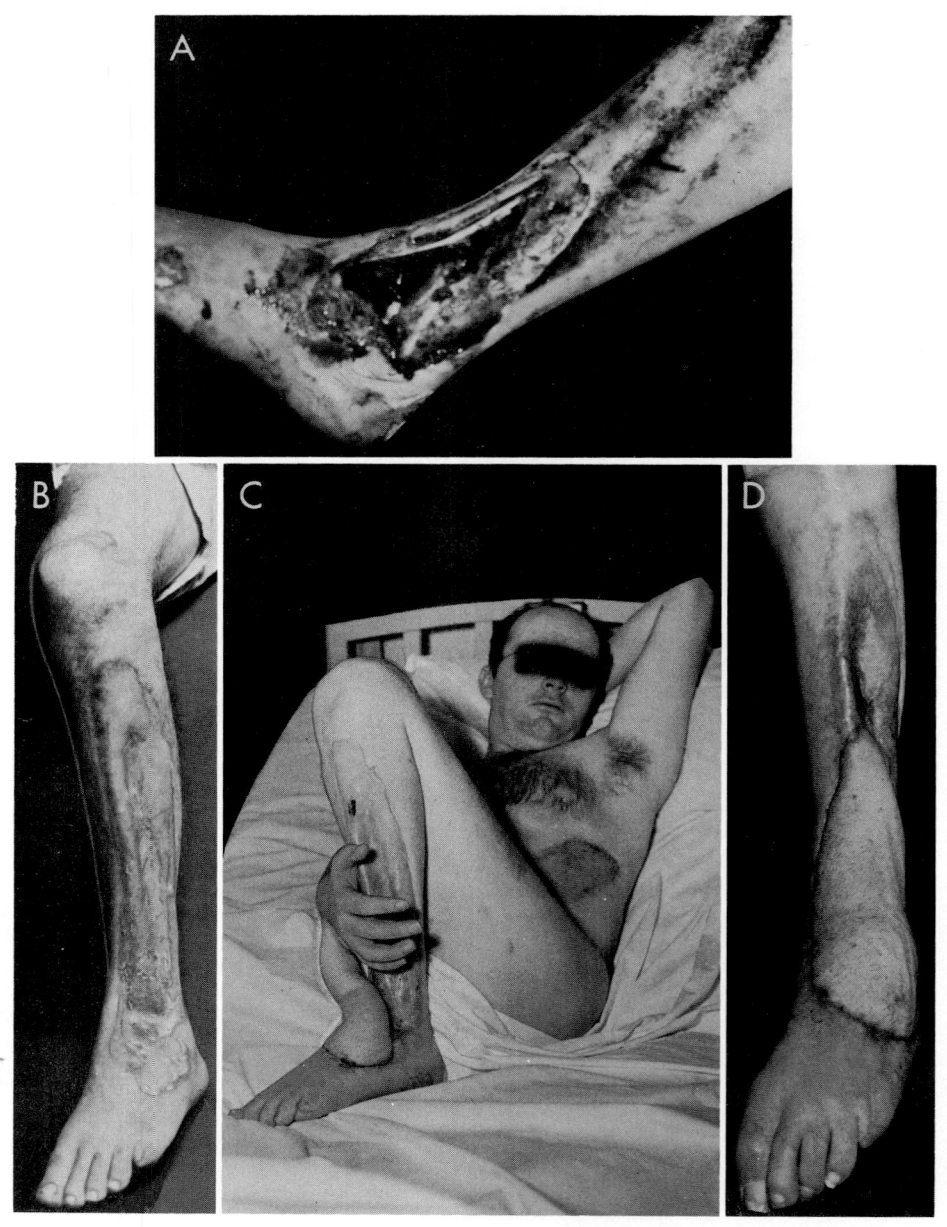

Fig. 40-12.—**A,** severe crushing injury with necrosis of skin and destruction of contents of anterior compartment of the lower leg. Operative debridement of all devitalized tissue was carried out within 24 hours and the wound closed immediately with a free skin graft from the opposite thigh (**B**). The skin graft proved stable except over the ankle joint, where it lay directly on the joint surfaces. **C and D,** a tubed flap from the abdominal wall, with the wrist as the intermediate carrier, was transferred in multiple stages to replace the skin graft in the lower half of the leg and to provide a cushion over the ankle joint. When the patient began to move the ankle, the flap separated from the bone at this level. Better anchorage for the flap was secured by drilling multiple holes in the thick bony cortex of the tibia and the talus.

tissue is unsuitable because uncovering vulnerable weight-bearing areas or bony prominences is undesirable. The direct "cross-leg" flap may be transferred from the opposite normal thigh or even the calf to the injured foot or leg (Figs. 40-10 and 40-11). Multistage delaying of the flap is seldom necessary, but a delaying procedure ensures less risk of complications. The position and direction of the scars at the junction of the flap and the normal skin must be carefully planned. A scar

Fig. 40-13. — The complex problem that can follow open reduction of the tibia if primary healing does not occur. Previous attempts at bone grafting of the ununited tibia failed because of insufficient skin covering and inadequate blood supply. These can be provided only by a flap when bone is exposed, as in **A**, **B**, the wound was finally closed by a skin graft which provided a source of spreading epithelium for the several small areas of exposed bone. **C–F**, the multistage transfer of a tubed flap from the abdominal wall with the hand as an intermediate carrier was then begun. The tubed flap was chosen in order to fill the large concave defect in the tibia with well-vascularized fatty tissue to eliminate "dead space" and provide improved blood supply to the surrounding bone (G). The skin margins of the tube are reflected and the central core of the tube fills the bony defect. The tubed flap is ideal for these purposes but requires many stages and awkward positioning for its accomplishment. (From Cannon, B., and Constable, J. D.: Reconstructive Plastic Surgery of the Lower Extremity, in Converse, J. M. (ed.), *Reconstructive Plastic Surgery* [Philadelphia: W. B. Saunders Company, 1964].)

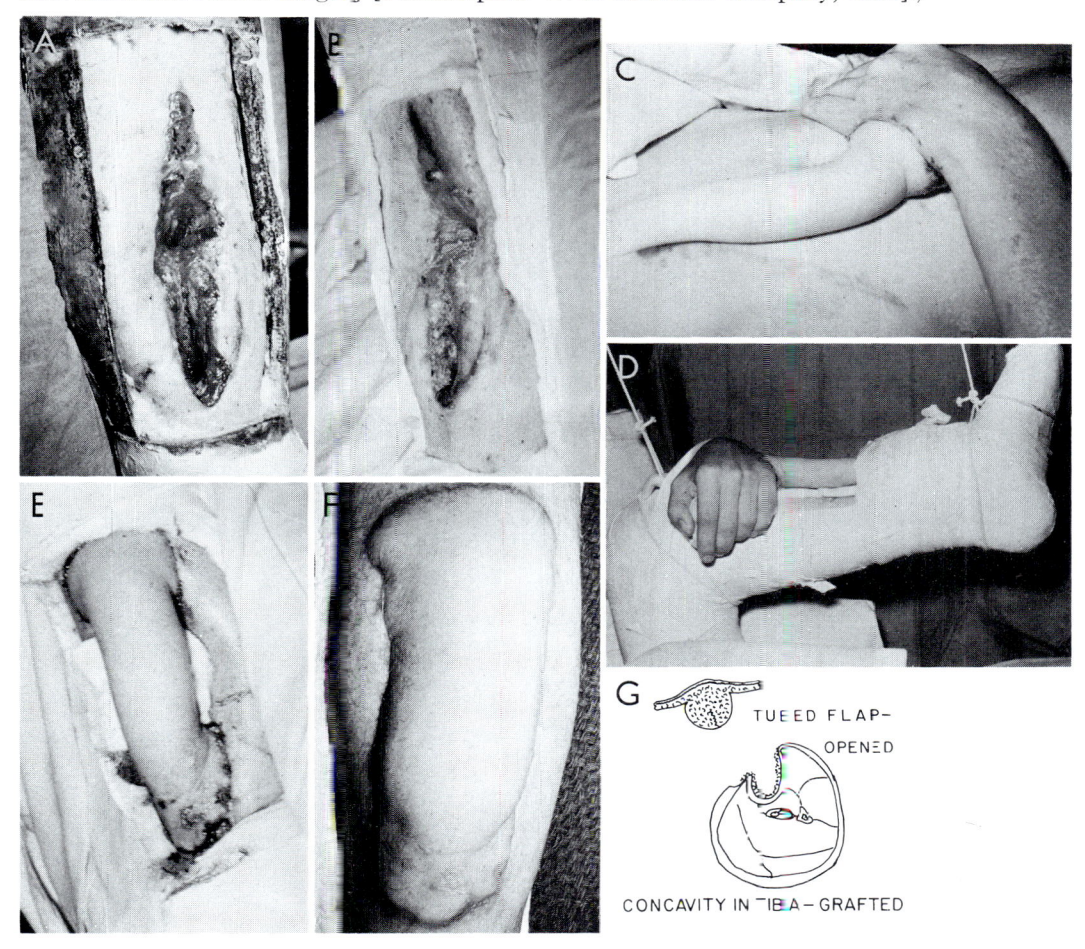

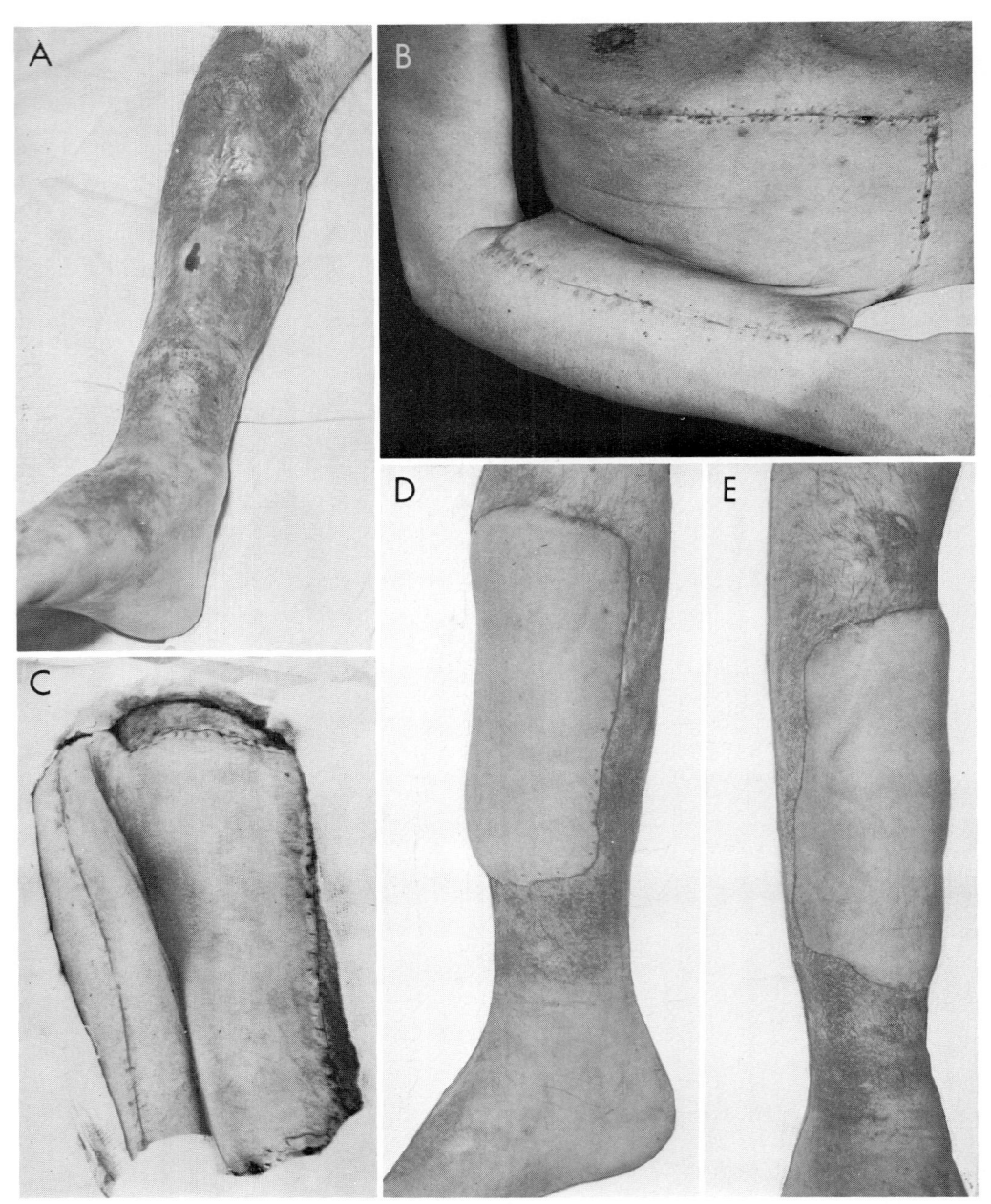

Fig. 40-14.—**A**, extensive loss of skin on the leg requiring resurfacing of the whole front of the lower leg and covering of the tibia by an open jump flap from the abdominal wall. **B** and **C**, 7 operations, in 12 weeks, were required to complete the procedure, using the forearm as a direct intermediate carrier. **D** and **E**, final appearance. (From Cannon, B., Lischer, C. E., and Brown, J. B.: Open jump flap repairs of the lower extremity, Surgery 22:335, 1947.)

Chapter 40: SOFT TISSUE REPAIRS / 989

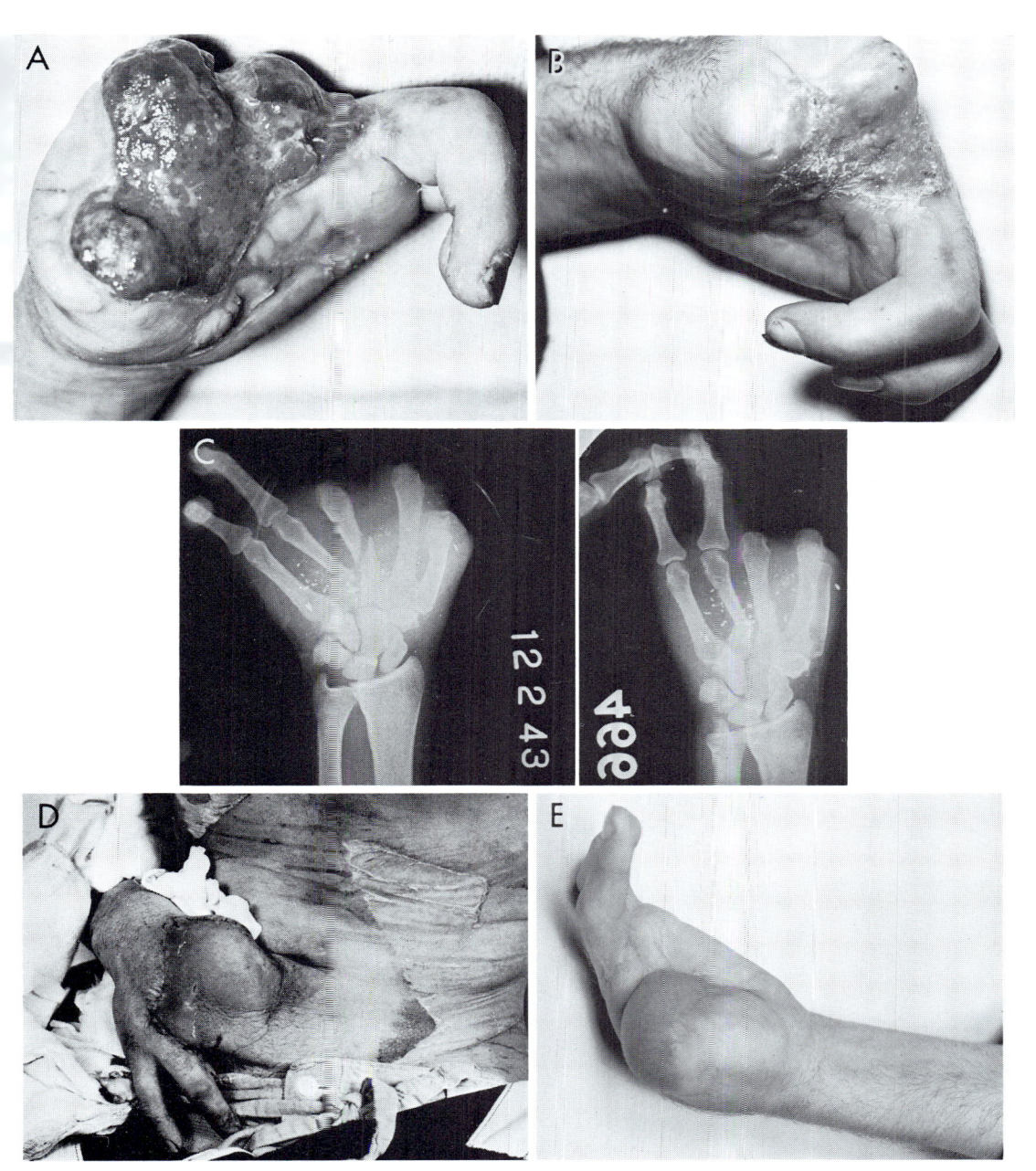

Fig. 40-15.—A, an explosion caused loss of thumb and 2 digits, leaving open stump. B, prompt skin grafting of the raw surface hastened reduction of edema. C, in addition, the position of the fractured metacarpals was improved. D, definitive repair was done electively with replacement of the graft by an abdominal flap. E, functional result proved satisfactory with return of sensation to the skin flap and a sufficiently bulky thenar eminence against which the remaining digits opposed.

over a malleolus or in the middle of a weight-bearing area will not be as stable as undamaged skin (see Fig. 40-6). Scars across a flexion crease are undesirable because tension associated with constant motion may produce hypertrophy of the scar. Thus, sacrifice of normal skin may be necessary for proper placement of marginal scars.

The donor site of the flap and as much as possible of the pedicle of the flap that bridges the gap between the legs should be closed with a skin graft. The legs must be supported comfortably and maintained accurately in position throughout the estimated 3 weeks during which the flap is growing to the opposite leg. Plaster casts are wrapped on each leg at operation and attached to each other by struts (Fig. 40-11). Care must be taken to avoid compression or kinking of the pedicle of the flap by the overlying leg when a cross-leg position is necessary. Also to be avoided is pressure on the tissues of the underlying donor leg even if the pedicle of the flap does not lie beneath it. The transfer of a flap from 1 leg to another is at best an uncomfortable experience, and in older patients alternative but more time-consuming methods may be preferable.

Very large defects or long and broad defects of the lower leg may require the transfer of larger flaps from the abdominal wall. Either tubed flaps attached to the wrist or hand as the intermediate carrier (Figs. 40-12 and 40-13) or open jump flaps with a broad attachment to the long axis of the forearm (Fig. 40-14) may be used. Both of these are multistage procedures and require even more cumbersome and uncomfortable positions for the patient. Despite the drawbacks, these large flaps have proved most effective in furnishing good covering for the injured area and have made salvage of the leg possible.

The methods and techniques that have been described are equally applicable to other parts of the body: forearm and hand (Fig. 40-15), head and neck, upper arm and trunk (Fig. 40-16). Less tissue is available for local flap repairs in the hand and forearm but flaps from the anterior trunk or groin can be transferred by a 2-

Fig. 40-16. — **A**, soft tissue loss on the lateral surface of the upper arm with interruption of continuity of the humerus. Function of the forearm and hand was unimpaired. **B** and **C**, direct flap from the chest wall was used to provide covering preliminary to successful bone grafting of the humerus. (From Cannon, B.: Some recent developments in plastic surgery, Surg. Clin. North Am. 27:1106, 1947.)

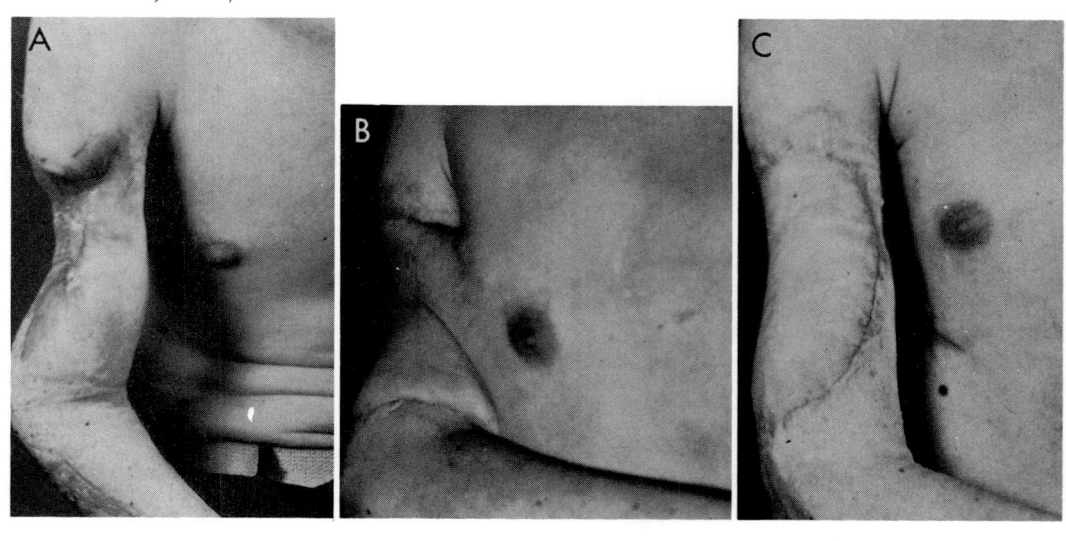

stage procedure. For the volar surface of the hand or forearm the pedicle is usually upward toward the chest, and for the dorsal surface it is usually downward toward the groin. Fixation for almost all upper extremity flaps from the abdominal or chest walls can be secured adequately with adhesive strapping.

The flap itself is protected and supported by a firm resilient dressing so arranged that the pedicle is not compressed and the flap can be easily inspected at intervals in the immediate postoperative period. Such an inspection will often reveal alterations in the normal circulation to the flap—alterations that are still correctable. Cotton waste is an ideal medium for the dressing because it provides resiliency and can be teased aside to permit the inspections without disturbing the dressing as a whole. Interpretation of the color of the flap is most important. Seldom does a flap fail because of inadequate arterial supply. The normal arterial pressure is usually sufficient to pump blood into a flap, but if the pedicle is kinked or inadequate, the venous outflow at a much lower pressure may be impeded. Persistent bluish discoloration of a flap, due to venous congestion, is often a grave sign of impending necrosis.

Flaps, particularly from the abdominal wall, may need to be thinned after the deep surgery is completed. The fat provides a good gliding medium for the repaired or adherent tendons and a good blood supply for bone grafts or nerve suture. Sensation returns to flaps in a matter of months if the local nerve supply is intact; but if the regional nerve is destroyed, anesthesia will persist. Until sensation returns, the patient must be warned to avoid injury or trauma to the anesthetic skin.

SUMMARY

In evaluating the best method for any extremity surface repair, the sequence of choices usually is: (1) excision of the scar and closure; (2) resurfacing with a free skin graft if the underlying tissue is sufficiently vascular to accept the graft; (3) shifting of a single- or double-pedicled local flap as either a direct or delayed flap, and (4) transfer of remote flaps. The skin graft is most useful for primary or early wound closure at the time of initial debridement, for the covering of ulcerations in the chronic wound or reducing its size, and for repair of the donor area of a flap. In the majority of extensive repairs, necessitated by previous major deep trauma, the use of a remote flap may prove the most rapid and effective method of securing a satisfactory result. The prime indication for the use of a flap is to replace superficial and deep scars with normal skin and subcutaneous tissue. Such replacement is of the greatest importance for better protection over bony prominences, for replacement of unstable scar tissue and for securing healthy tissue through which definitive deep repairs to bone, tendon and nerve may be carried out. The practice of delayed primary closure will often preclude grave wound complications that can prolong healing for months or years.

BIBLIOGRAPHY

Barsky, A. J.: *Principles and Practice of Plastic Surgery* (Baltimore: Williams & Wilkins Company, 1950).

Brown, J. B.: Closure of surface defects with free skin grafts and pedicle flaps, Surg. Gynecol. Obstet. 84:862, 1947.

Brown, J. B., and Cannon, B.: The repair of surface defects of the foot, Ann. Surg. 120:417, 1944.

Brown, J. B., Fryer, M. P., and McDowell, F.: Permanent pedicle blood-carrying flaps for repairing defects in avascular areas, Ann. Surg. 134:486, 1951.

Brown, J. B., et al.: Direct flap repair of defects of the arm and hand, Ann. Surg. 122:706, 1945.

Cannon, B.: Plastic surgery: Skin transplantation, N. Engl. J. Med. 239:435, 1948.

Cannon, B.: Open grafting of raw surfaces, N. Engl. J. Med. 256:672, 1957.

Cannon, B.: Plastic surgery of the extremities, Am. Acad. Orthop. Surg. Instructional Course Lectures, XVIII, p. 258, 1961.

Cannon, B., Graham, W. C., and Brown, J. B.: Restoration of grasping function following loss of all 5 digits, Surgery 25:420, 1949.

Cannon, B., Lischer, C. E., and Brown, J. B.: Open jump flap repairs of the lower extremity, Surgery 22:335, 1947.

Cannon, B., O'Leary, J. J., O'Neil, J. W., and Steinsieck, R.: An approach to the treatment of pressure sores, Ann. Surg. 132:760, 1950.

Cannon, B., and Trott, A. W.: Expeditious use of direct flaps in extremity repairs, Plast. Reconstr. Surg. 4:415, 1949.

Churchill, E. D.: Surgical management of wounded in Mediterranean theater at time of fall of Rome, Ann. Surg. 120:268, 1944.

Coakley, W. A., McCoy, S. M., and Kelleher, J. C.: The use of direct forearm flaps in resurfacing defects of the soft tissues of the lower extremities, Plast. Reconstr. Surg. 6:413, 1950.

Connelly, J. R.: Pedicle coverage in nonunion of fractures, Plast. Reconstr. Surg. 3:727, 1948.

Converse, J. M.: Early skin grafting in war wounds of the extremities, Ann. Surg. 115:321, 1942.

Converse, J. M.: Plastic repair of the extremities of non-tubulated pedicle skin flaps, J. Bone Joint Surg. 30-A:163, 1948.

Conway, H., Stark, R. B., and Joslin, D.: Cutaneous histamine resection of a test of circulatory deficiency of tubed pedicles and flaps, Surg. Gynecol. Obstet. 93:185, 1951.

Dunphy, J. E., and Udupa, K. N.: Chemical and histochemical sequences in the normal healing of wounds, N. Engl. J. Med. 253:847, 1955.

Eades, C. C., Bass, S. A., Lewis, S. R., and Blocker, T. G., Jr.: Bacterial studies of the burn wound in relation to therapy and skin grafting procedures, Surg. Forum 9:805, 1959.

Kelly, R. P., Rosatio, L. M., and Murray, R. A.: Traumatic osteomyelitis: Use of skin grafts; technic and results, Ann. Surg. 122:1, 1945. II. Subsequent treatment, ibid. 123:688, 1946.

Knight, M. P., and Wood, G. O.: Surgical obliteration of bone cavities following traumatic osteomyelitis, J. Bone Joint Surg. 27:547, 1945.

Macomber, W. B., and Patton, H. S.: Split-thickness graft—useful adjunct in tube pedicle preparation, Surg. Gynecol. Obstet. 84:97, 1947.

Mason, M. L.: Wound healing, Surg. Gynecol. Obstet. 69:303, 1939.

Robinson, D. W.: Problems in fractures of the tibia, AMA Arch. Surg. 63:53, 1957.

Stark, R. B.: The cross-leg flap procedure, Plast. Reconstr. Surg. 9:173, 1952.

Webster, J. P.: Thoraco-epigastric tubed pedicles, Surg. Clin. North Am. 17:145, 1937.

41 Chest Injuries: Chest Wall, Lung, Esophagus and Pleural Spaces

ASHBY C. MONCURE and
J. GORDON SCANNELL

THERE ARE THREE primary considerations in the management of severe chest injuries—two immediate and one late. These are: (1) immediate and often profound disturbances of cardiorespiratory function, (2) hemorrhage and (3) the late complications of infection damaged lung and crippled thoracic cage. The management of the bony injury is secondary to these important considerations.

The immediate goals in management of the patient who has suffered a severe chest injury are as follows: (1) Resuscitation has been carried out to the extent that significant circulatory disturbances and asphyxia are relieved. (2) Bleeding has been controlled. (3) The chest wall is stable and cough and breathing are painless enough to be effective. If positive-pressure ventilation has been necessary, the patient is successfully relieved of this need. (4) The respiratory passages are cleared of secretions. (5) The pleural cavities are free from significant amounts of blood and air, so that both lungs are expanded or expanding. (6) External wounds have been debrided and dressed satisfactorily. (7) Traumatic rupture of great vessels, bronchus, esophagus and diaphragm have been excluded or dealt with.

With these objectives in mind, it is possible to construct a clinically useful outline of the management of chest injury. Each item will be considered, first in terms of disturbance of function and second in terms of practical management of that disturbance. It is recognized that such separation is an artificial device, easier to accomplish on paper than when confronted with a severely injured patient.

RESUSCITATION

It is clear that accurate diagnosis is of paramount importance in the treatment of shock associated with serious chest injury. The state of shock, usually a consequence of failure of the heart as a pump or a volume deficit of the fluid that is pumped, may, in the setting of acute chest injury, result from a mechanical cause, such as a positive-pressure pneumothorax or cardiac tamponade. On the other hand, blood loss may be concealed, and exsanguination into a pleural cavity may occur without great embarrassment to respiration. Concurrent intra-abdominal hemorrhage from an injured viscus may go unappreciated in the events surrounding resuscitation of a lethargic, hypoxic patient.

The ultimate effectiveness of resuscitative measures in large part is dependent on the promptness of their institution. First priority is the establishment of an adequate airway and effective gas exchange. This is accomplished by examination of the upper airway; clearing of the oro- and hypopharynx; inspection and palpation of the entire chest wall for evidence of an open wound, instability and the presence of crepitus. By auscultation and prompt radiologic examination, the presence of fluid and/or air within the pleural space can be ascertained.

In the patient with severe maxillofacial injury or overt cervical spine injury, tracheostomy is mandatory if oro- or nasotracheal intubation is impossible. In the patient who shows evidence of inadequate ventilation (roughly a respiratory rate of greater than 35 per minute or the demonstration of arterial blood PCO_2 of greater than 60 mm Hg), prompt airway control and mechanical ventilation with high concentration of O_2 are made possible by orotracheal intubation with a 38-mm-diameter cuffed tube in the adult male and a 36- or 34-mm cuffed tube in the adult female. An open wound of the pleural space requires an initial sterile dressing and prompt operative attention. An unstable chest wall may require prolonged positive-pressure ventilation. Pleural blood or air makes necessary the placement of intercostal catheters for its evacuation and subsequent expansion of the lung.

Once adequate ventilation has been established, the management of shock will depend on the cause or causes of the shock state, with particular attention to cardiogenic and hypovolemic factors.

The most urgent cardiogenic problem is, of course, cardiac arrest. Treatment of this requires prompt external massage, with use of an unyielding surface under the thorax, and adequate endotracheal ventilation from the start. Attention should be placed on proper application of pressure over the heart, avoiding excessive force and pressure over the rib joints and xiphoid process, with frequent evalu-

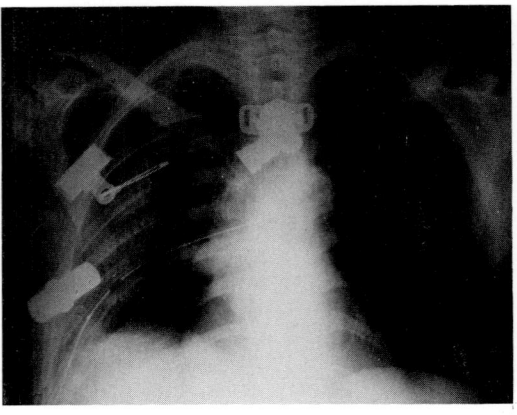

Fig. 41-1.—Chest plate of a 50-year-old man with a right lateral chest wall flail segment, requiring endotracheal intubation and subsequent tracheostomy with intermittent positive-pressure ventilation, after progressive deterioration of respiratory function. Note indwelling intercostal catheter in this setting.

ation of the efforts by return of a palpable pulse and blood pressure. Early correction of metabolic acidosis, universally present following cardiac arrest, requires adequate amounts of sodium bicarbonate administered through a large functional intravenous line. A monitoring electrocardiogram should be available to establish the presence of ventricular fibrillation or cardiac standstill and enable those directing treatment to evaluate the need for countershock for reversion of ventricular fibrillation plus the effect of adjunctive drugs to maintain cardiac activity and blood pressure.

The agents most useful as adjuncts in cardiac resuscitation are: (1) myocardial stimulants, epinephrine or isoproterenol; (2) antiarrhythmic agents, lidocaine, procaine amide; (3) calcium; (4) corticosteroids. Myocardial stimulants are indicated to stimulate a ventricular response in asystole or to coarsen the amplitude of ventricular fibrillation prior to countershock. They are contraindicated in the patient who can be reverted to an organized rhythm and maintain an effective beat. Antiarrhythmic agents are most useful when the heart can be shocked into an organized rhythm but are contraindicated in asystole and low-amplitude fibrillation. Calcium is useful for its direct stimulant effect on myocardial contractility after ventricular fibrillation has been corrected. Corticosteroids may have some benefit for their vasodilating effects. It should be re-emphasized that sodium bicarbonate should be given promptly and repeatedly during resuscitative efforts to reverse the metabolic acidosis (presumably from poor tissue perfusion) that universally accompanies cardiac arrest.

The hypovolemic state suggested by peripheral vasoconstriction and evidence of blood loss, documented by low hematocrit and low central venous pressure (below 5 cm saline while not being ventilated by positive pressure) is corrected initially by intravenous administration of buffered salt solution, low molecular weight dextran, plasma and type-specific blood as each becomes available in turn. The use of a blood-warming device has been found helpful in avoiding the precipitous drop in body temperature associated with rapid administration of large amounts of bank blood. If operation is contemplated, attention to monitoring of body temperature and avoidance of hypothermia with a heating blanket should be considered.

Ongoing moment-to-moment monitoring of the recently resuscitated patient is made possible by an indwelling arterial line, most conveniently placed percutaneously in the radial artery at the hyperextended wrist to allow continuous determination of PO_2, PCO_2 and pH. A central venous pressure radiopaque line, generally placed in an arm vein percutaneously and threaded into a mediastinal great vein, permits sequential determination of central venous pressure. Its position should be confirmed by a chest film. When used in association with other information, it reflects hypovolemia when low (under 5 cm saline) or overhydration, congestive heart failure or cardiac tamponade when high (over 12 cm saline). Measurement should be made while the patient is not being ventilated and fluctuations are present in the saline column. Determination of urine output each hour by use of an indwelling catheter reflects the state of tissue perfusion. Under 40 ml per hour is inadequate in the adult. A continuous visual pattern of the electrical activity of the heart is accomplished by placement of chest leads led to a standard monitor.

Above all, successful management of the severely injured patient requires frequent objective examination by the surgeon in charge. He must be aware that valid clinical judgment requires accurate information and that incomplete information can be disastrously misleading. He must also be ever alert to the possibility of multiple, covert, treatable organ system injury in the setting of major trauma, either civilian or military.

CONTROL OF BLEEDING

Control of bleeding is axiomatic in the management of any severe injury. The problem in chest injury is to identify the scource of the bleeding and to decide whether it is continuing.

Arterial bleeding into the chest may be from two sources: low-pressure bleeding from the pulmonary circuit or high-pressure bleeding from a systemic artery, usually an intercostal. In addition, there may be troublesome and dangerous hemorrhage from a systemic vein held open by bone injury and bleeding into an enormous body cavity.

Bleeding from the lung is of the low-pressure variety, and, when stopped, is not prone to begin again. Such bleeding is not likely to be affected by re-expansion of the lung. Systemic bleeding is high-pressure, is largely independent of the state of the lung and is poorly tamponaded by massive hemothorax. Aspiration of the hemothorax, therefore, is logical and advisable as a means of both re-expanding the lung and determining the status of bleeding. Ordinarily, the detection of blood in the pleural space is not difficult, particularly if only the simplest of x-ray facilities are available. Aspiration should be carried out with a wide-bore needle (no. 18 gauge usually will suffice). If blood is found, a large intercostal catheter (no. 24 F or no. 28 F) should be placed through a low interspace, usually in the area between the anterior and posterior axillary line, and connected to gentle suction. Evidence of continuing hemorrhage after initial evacuation of blood from the pleural space (greater than 150 ml per hour for several hours) demands prompt thoracotomy through a posterolateral approach, which allows flexibility in dealing with any intrathoracic problem.

Thoracotomy in the presence of severe chest injury, particularly damage to the lung, may present a serious problem if an open and functioning indwelling pleural catheter is not present, for the respiratory effort attendant on the induction of anesthesia and insertion of an endotracheal tube, in addition to the maintenance of positive-pressure breathing, may lead to the rapid accumulation of air under pressure in the pleural space.

STABILIZATION OF THE CHEST WALL

To be effective, a chest wall must be not only relatively rigid but also painless enough to permit cough and ventilation.

Certain rigidity of the chest wall is essential; otherwise, paradoxical motion of the chest occurs. Under the latter circumstances, the chest wall is drawn in on inspiration and bulges out on expiration. As a result, the bellows-like action of the thorax is abolished and the underlying lung is not ventilated. In extreme cases, the lung on the affected side may become the air space from which the contralateral lung is ventilated. This, the phenomenon of "pendulum air," is illustrated in Figure 41-2. Whatever its practical importance, the concept of pendulum air serves to emphasize the dangers of the "stove-in" or "flail" chest. Paradoxical motion of an injured chest usually presupposes that the rib cage has been broken anteriorly and posteriorly. Ribs 3 through 10 are fractured most commonly, since they are exposed and have the least muscle protection. Posterior fractures usually are apparent in the roentgenogram, whereas anterior fractures frequently can be ascertained only by physical examination. A special situation may occur in the case of impact injury to the sternum (the common steering-post injury), in which bilateral anterior fractures are present.

Lesser degrees of paradoxical motion may be controlled by supporting bandages, light shot bags and similar splinting as long as total immobilization of the thorax is avoided. Severe crushing injuries, in the face of inadequate ventilation, are managed best by endotracheal intubation and subsequent tracheostomy, allowing intermittent positive-pressure ventilation to be instituted. Intermittent positive-pressure therapy restores thoracic cage stability and intrathoracic volume, improves alveolar ventilation, decreases the work of breathing and also relieves anxiety and pain. It also allows effective administration of oxygen, to overcome the effect of shunting frequently found in this setting, secondary to atelectasis and pulmonary contusion. Presumably the latter is in large part due to the compression-decompression phenomenon that occurs with blunt trauma and produces the morphologic picture of diffuse, disseminated, congestive and hemorrhagic atelectasis. High inspired oxygen pressures have been shown to be associated with pulmonary damage. There is an early exudative phase characterized by alveolar edema and congestion, intra-alveolar hemorrhage and a fibrin exudate with formation of prominent hyaline membranes without an associated inflammatory component. There is also a late proliferative phase characterized by pronounced alveolar and interalveolar septal edema, fibroblastic proliferation with early fibrosis and prominent hyperplasia of the alveolar lining cells.

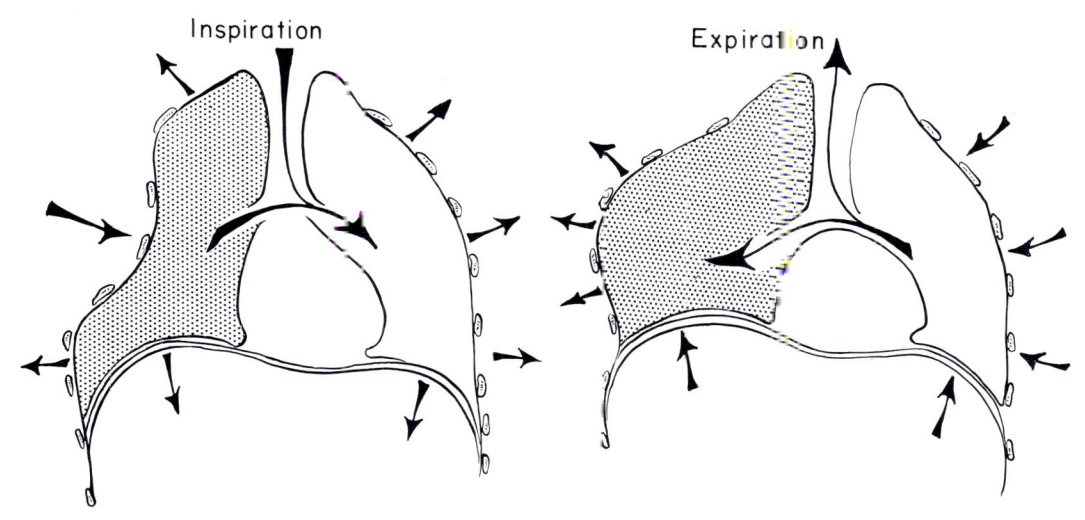

Fig. 41-2. — Diagram illustrating the hazards of paradoxical motion of the chest wall. Volume of the involved side is *reduced* on inspiration, and ventilation of the uninjured side may be to and from the injured side — i.e., "pendulum air."

However, to withhold oxygen for fear of oxygen damage when the patient is hypoxemic may result in serious and fatal complications from hypoxemia before the signs of oxygen toxicity become apparent. Thus, oxygen is administered in a concentration required to maintain an arterial PO_2 of 100 mm Hg. Severely injured patients, those receiving numerous blood transfusions and those receiving prolonged artificial ventilation not infrequently exhibit radiographic changes suggestive of pulmonary edema, physiologically manifested by deteriorating blood-gas exchange. As a rule, diuretic therapy and severe fluid restriction will lead to clinical improvement. At the same time, they pose the puzzling dilemma of balancing overhydration against systemic hypovolemia from continuing blood loss. The determination of whether intermittent positive-pressure ventilation should be continued depends entirely on arterial blood-gas determinations, the length of time being quite variable, depending on the severity of the injury the presence of other complications, such as lung contusion, and the presence of extrathoracic considerations, such as concomitant head injury. If intermittent positive-pressure ventilation is necessary in the management of chest wall instability, a period of at least 10 days is to be expected before chest wall stability is gained to the extent necessary to permit effective spontaneous ventilation. A prolonged period of progressive "weaning" from artificial ventilation is not unusual. The avoidance of post-tracheostomy tracheomalacia, thought to be usually due to excessive pressure from the tracheostomy tube's expanded cuff, should be attempted by assiduous attention to the type of cuff and the amount and duration of pressure within it.

The nutrition of the ventilated patient should not be neglected, and if effective alimentation by the oral route is not possible, the placement of a gastrostomy tube for tube feedings or a mediastinal great vein catheter for administration of a high-glucose protein "hyperalimentation" solution should be considered.

In lesser degrees of chest injury, distressing pleuritic pain should be treated by intercostal block, repeated if necessary. An effective combination of drugs has been the use of 2% lidocaine

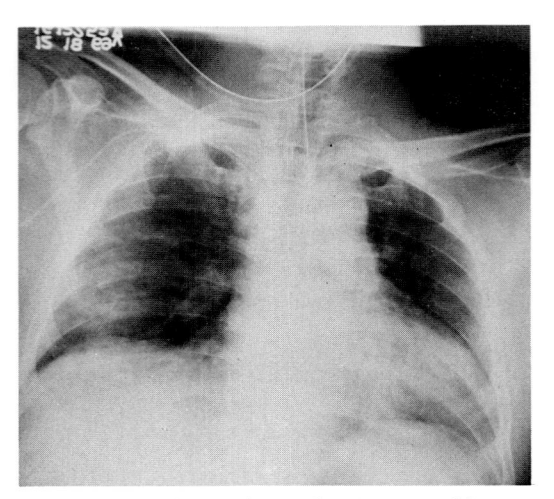

Fig. 41-3.—Chest plate of a 50-year-old man with a right lateral chest wall flail segment managed successfully with multiple intercostal nerve blocks, aggressive pulmonary physiotherapy and mask oxygen, with careful monitoring by sequential arterial blood gas determinations.

(Xylocaine) with epinephrine, together with tetracaine (Pontocaine) 1 mg added per ml of lidocaine solution. The maximal allowable dose of Xylocaine is 500 mg in a 70-kg man. When used, this ordinarily produces anesthesia for at least 6 hours before additional administration is necessary.

The technique of intercostal block is simple. Skin wheals are raised posterior to the angle of the ribs to be blocked, usually 2 or 3 ribs above and below the level of pain. Through the skin wheal, a 1-inch no. 22 needle is inserted down to the underlying rib, and the angle then is shifted so that the needle tip slides a few millimeters below the lower border of the rib. Aspiration at this point will determine that the needle does not lie within an intercostal vessel or within the pleural space. After this check, 3–5 ml of the aforementioned solution is injected. It is important to remember that this maneuver is not infrequently followed by pneumothorax—if this did not already exist as a result of the original injury. Such a pneumothorax is not a serious complication if recognized and treated properly. When the block is carried out close to the neck of rib, it is in reality a paravertebral block. Under these circumstances, great care must be exercised not to introduce the anesthetic agent intraspinally along a dorsal nerve root.

Tight adhesive strapping has little place in the treatment of fractured ribs, although light support with an elastic adhesive bandage may provide symptomatic relief.

MAINTENANCE OF A CLEAR AIRWAY

In the preceding section, the importance of ensuring an effective cough was emphasized. By coughing, the patient manages to keep his tracheobronchial tree clear of secretions. To administer oxygen to a patient who is drowning in his own secretions is remarkably futile. Furthermore, the accumulation of tenacious secretions in the smaller branches of the bronchial tree leads to atelectasis and presumably facilitates the development of bronchopneumonia. If the patient is unable to keep the airway clear, active steps must be taken to help him. In order of simplicity, these are: (1) tracheal aspiration by catheter, (2) bronchoscopic aspiration, (3) oro- or nasotracheal intubation, (4) tracheostomy.

The proper use of tracheal aspiration is so important that a few words concerning technique are in order. It is best to use a relatively firm catheter—for example, a new red-rubber 16 F. Fairly strong suction is required, and this is applied to the catheter by a Y or T tube so that intermittent suction can be obtained by occluding and releasing the side-arm vent. To minimize the gag reflex, topical anesthesia of the pharynx with 4% cocaine or a similar agent may be used. If the patient can cooperate, he is given a gauze sponge and is instructed to pull his tongue outward, thereby tilting the epiglottis forward. The operator then inserts the lightly lubricated tube into the patient's nostril. If it is advanced only during inspiration—particularly inspiration that immediately follows a forced cough—the catheter will enter the trachea. The patient must be urged not to swallow; otherwise, the tube will almost certainly enter the esophagus. The entrance of the catheter into the trachea is heralded by pronounced coughing. The catheter then is advanced first into one major bronchus, then into the other, suction being applied intermittently. If the patient's head is turned to the left, the catheter will enter the right main bronchus, and vice versa. Tracheal suction, although not pleasant, should not be an excessively uncomfortable procedure. Its immediate effect often is dramatic.

Tracheal aspiration is helpful in association with other techniques of pulmonary physiotherapy, such as rapid sequential percussion with a cupped hand over the atelectatic and consolidated segments of lung, followed by compression of the rib cage with both hands in association with postural drainage. Administered oxygen should be warmed and humidified. The atelectatic or consolidated area of the lung should be kept upright as much as possible to facilitate drainage. Occasionally, bronchoscopy is necessary to clear the tracheobronchial tree.

Tracheostomy often is lifesaving in the management of secretions when there is associated severe head injury, but its use should not be reserved for such extreme cases. Tracheostomy makes it possible to keep the airway clear at all times with a minimum of disturbance to the patient.

Vigilance must be exercised in detecting the development of pulmonary sepsis, the identification of the responsible organism and its drug susceptibility. The evolution of drug-resistant infecting organisms is common, and appropriate alteration of antibiotic therapy frequently is necessary during the course of hospitalization. Bronchopneumonia may produce remarkable alveolar-arterial oxygen gradients, and must be differentiated from pulmonary contusion, congestive heart failure, fluid overload, fat emboli and multiple pulmonary emboli. Each of these entities responds to different therapy; therefore, proper identification of the responsible pulmonary process is most important.

MANAGEMENT OF BLOOD AND AIR IN THE PLEURAL SPACE

One of the primary objectives of treatment in chest injuries is to expand the lung on the involved side and to restore the normal intrathoracic dynamics as soon as possible. This is most obvious when a positive-pressure pneumothorax is present.

A positive-pressure or tension pneumothorax is the result of a valvar leak into an otherwise closed pleural space. With a closed injury, this injury usually is from the parenchyma of the lung, although it may be from a major bronchus, the trachea or, on rare occasions, from the esophagus. Very often, as the lung collapses, a tear in its surface will seal; if it does not, a dangerous degree of positive intrapleural pressure may develop, which, by displacing the mediastinum away from the injured side, may encroach on the other, presumably uninjured, lung. In addition to producing a respiratory embarrassment, positive intrathoracic pressure may seriously interfere with venous inflow into the chest and therefore into the heart, with a result of lowering of cardiac output to dangerous levels. The treatment is to create a valvar leak out from the pleural space.

The diagnosis of a tension pneumothorax may be confirmed by a chest film, but the latter is not needed to make the diagnosis. Respiratory embarrassment, tracheal shift away from the injured side, absent breath sounds and particularly subcutaneous emphysema following injury confirm the diagnosis and demand prompt action. The first step is needle aspiration, done most easily in the second or third interspace anteriorly, about 2 inches lateral to the border of the sternum so as to avoid injury to the internal mammary vessels. This is an emergency procedure. Usually it is wise, in civilian hospital practice, to institute prompt closed drainage by intercostal catheter in every traumatic pneumothorax that initially is at positive pressure, which reaccumulates after one aspiration or where the patient will require intermittent positive-pressure ventilation.

For closed drainage, a 20 F catheter is inserted either by clamp technique or by means of a trocar through the second or third intercostal space anteriorly or the fifth or sixth laterally. The catheter then is connected to three-bottle suction (Fig. 41-4) or to water-seal drainage (Fig. 41-5). Used intelligently, either form of drainage is satisfactory. When available, three-bottle suction is preferable, since it ensures a continuous "negative" pressure of a known degree. The danger of reopening a leak in an injured lung by suction is more fancied than real.

Ordinarily, 48 hours of closed drainage is adequate. After that time, the danger of introducing infection along the tube is increased, partly related to the difficulty of maintaining an airtight closure of the chest wall around the catheter. Usually, after 48 hours the leak in the lung is sealed and the lung itself is expanded or is expanding satisfactorily. To demonstrate the presence of a continuing air leak if three-bottle suction has been used, one can convert to water-seal drainage or modify the original system by leading the tube from the patient to a water seal in the first bottle.

The management of blood in the pleural space may present greater practical difficulties than the management of air. There are many compelling reasons for aspirating a hemothorax of significant

Fig. 41-4.—Diagram of a satisfactory method of chest suction. The center bottle serves as a safety valve to prevent the suction in the system from reaching unphysiologic levels. The first bottle is merely a trap. The third bottle acts as a water-seal valve in case the suction tubing is disconnected from its source.

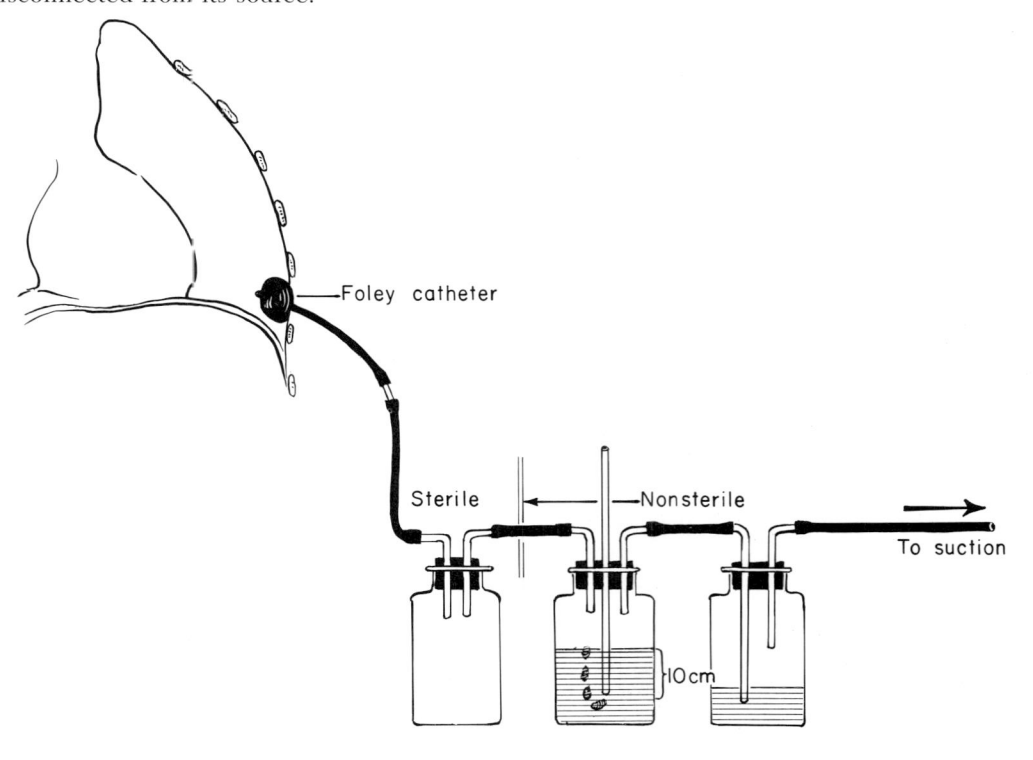

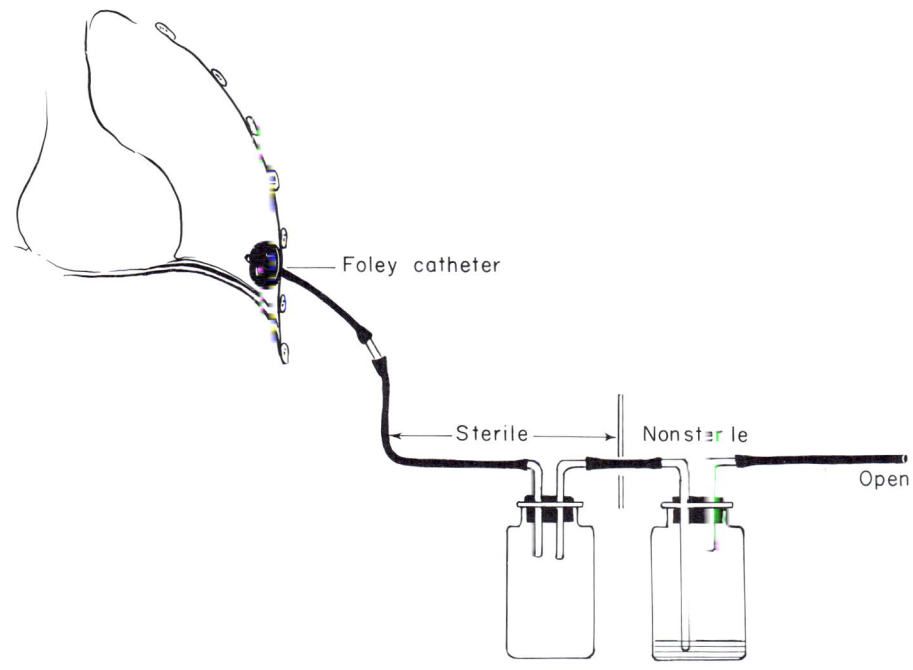

Fig. 41-5.—Diagram of water-seal drainage. The sterile bottle acts as a trap and prevents siphonage of water into the chest if the apparatus should be lifted above the level of the patient's chest.

amount. In the first place, it is important to relieve, so far as possible, any encroachment on the lung. Second, as already stated, it is essential to determine the source and status of intrathoracic bleeding. The third reason is the avoidance of the late crippling effects of fibrothorax.

Obviously it is important to define "significant" hemothorax. Certainly this term includes any hemothorax detectable by physical examination. It also includes one that produces 25% collapse of the underlying lung, or which may be estimated, by x-ray examination, to exceed 500 ml. It includes any hemothorax that increases to an appreciable extent while under careful observation.

MANAGEMENT OF THE EXTERNAL WOUND

The care of the external chest wound involves the principles that apply to wounds of the soft parts in general, in addition to the problem of the external wound that communicates with the pleural space—the so-called sucking wound. Prompt closure is mandatory, but certain precautions are necessary in order to ensure that there is no underlying wound of the lung that may lead to a pressure pneumothorax when the external wound is closed. The principle here is to close the external wound but to provide, at the same time, for closed pleural drainage by way of an intercostal catheter.

The method of closure of the chest wound depends on the exigencies of the situation and the facilities available. Under emergency conditions, a voluminous gauze dressing, applied firmly, provides adequate occlusion. Subsequently, this dressing may be removed, the wound debrided and an anatomic layer closure of the chest wall carried out. At the time of definitive closure, associated injuries to the lung and thoracic contents may be dealt with. If the latter are extensive, a separate incision may be necessary for adequate exposure. The surgeon should not feel compelled to limit his choice of incision to the one that an unkind fate has provided.

The important practical point to remember is that the emergency dressing should not be applied so tightly as to prevent the escape of air should a positive-pressure pneumothorax develop. The dressing should function as an effective flap valve.

SPECIAL CONSIDERATIONS

No discussion of chest trauma would be complete without some mention of cardiac tamponade, direct cardiac injury and injury to the great vessels, which may be the result of the most common form of severe injury today—the automobile accident. The classic situation is the steering-post injury with a depressed fracture of the sternum or anterior chest wall. The underlying pathophysiology and treatment necessary are dealt with in Chapter 43.

The esophagus, tucked away in the depths of the mediastinum, rarely is injured in chest injuries. When seen, the injury usually is a tear, which frequently is at the level of the tracheal bifurcation and manifested either by cervical subcutaneous emphysema or by hydrothorax. Prompt exploration and repair is needed, after confirmation by contrast study and esophagoscopy.

Traumatic rupture of the tracheobronchial tree is not common. When present, it occurs to either main stem bronchus. The diagnosis is suggested by the presence of pneumomediastinum and subcutaneous emphysema extending up into the neck. This diagnosis also should be entertained when there is continued massive escape of air through an intercostal catheter. Laminagraphy and bronchoscopy are used to document its presence, and prompt operative repair is indicated.

Most traumatic ruptures of the diaphragm occur on the left and generally are posterocentral in position. The traumatic opening may be quite large, permitting intrathoracic displacement of abdominal contents. The diagnosis may be delayed, revealed only by serial films showing migration of abdominal viscera into the hemithorax. Operative repair should be undertaken as promptly as the circumstances dictate or permit.

SUMMARY

An effort has been made to present a clinically useful outline with a brief discussion of each of the major disturbances of function encountered in chest injury, as well as practical suggestions on how to manage each aspect. Obviously, each surgeon may argue his own personal preferences, but there should be fundamental agreement on the objectives of treatment. In summary, these are:

1. Prompt resuscitation.
2. Control of serious hemorrhage.
3. Restoration of a stable and painless chest wall.
4. Maintenance of a clear airway.
5. Removal of blood and air from the pleural space.
6. Satisfactory closure of the external wounds.
7. Anatomic repair of seriously injured intrathoracic contents.

BIBLIOGRAPHY

Avery, E. E., Mörch, E. T., and Benson, D. W.: Critically crushed chests, J. Thoracic Surg. 32:291, 1956.

Bendixen, H. H., Egbert, L. D., Hedley-White, J., Pontoppidan, H., and Laver, M. B.: *Respiratory Care* (St. Louis: The C. V. Mosby Company, 1965).

Blair, E., Topuzlu, C., and Deane, R. S.: Major Blunt Chest Trauma, in *Current Problems in Surgery* (Chicago: Year Book Medical Publishers, Inc., May, 1969).

Churchill, E. D.: Trends and practices in thoracic surgery in Mediterranean theatre, J. Thoracic Surg. 13:307, 1944.

Gianelly, R. E., and Harrison, D. C.: Drugs Used in the Treatment of Cardiac Arrhythmias, in *Disease-a-Month* (Chicago: Year Book Medical Publishers, Inc., January, 1969).

Moore, F. D., Lyons, J. H., Pierce, E. C., Morgan, A. P., Drinker, P. A., MacArthur, J. D., and Dammin, G. J.: *Post-traumatic Pulmonary Insufficiency* (Philadelphia: W. B. Saunders Company, 1969).

Pontoppidan, H., Laver, M. B., and Geffin, B.: Acute Respiratory Failure in the Surgical Patient, in Welch, C. E. (ed.), *Advances in Surgery* (Chicago: Year Book Medical Publishers Inc., 1970), Vol. 4, pp. 163–254.

Shires, G. T., Carrico, C. J., Baxter, C. R., Giesecke, A. H., Jr., and Jenkins, M. T.: Principles in Treatment of Severely Injured Patients, in Welch, C. E. (ed.), *Advances in Surgery* (Chicago: Year Book Medical Publishers, Inc., 1970), Vol. 4, pp. 255–324.

Wise, A., Topuzlu, C., Mills, E. L., Page, H. G., and Blair, E.: The importance of serial blood gas determinations in blunt chest trauma, J. Thorac. Cardiovasc. Surg. 56:520, 1968.

42 | Cardiac Trauma: Heart and Great Vessels

WILLARD M. DAGGETT, ELDRED D. MUNDTH,
MORTIMER J. BUCKLEY and
W. GERALD AUSTEN

ALTHOUGH THE OCCURRENCE of major injury to the heart or great vessels results in a high mortality rate,[1,2] the excellent survival rates achieved for patients who reach the hospital after major cardiovascular injury[9-12, 16-18] emphasize the importance of this type of injury in the over-all management of the traumatized patient. Trauma to the heart and great vessels may result from either blunt or penetrating injury. Blunt trauma most commonly derives either from compression injury (for example, compression of the sternum against the steering wheel in an automobile accident) or from shear stress injury as the result of the deceleration forces operative in an automobile collision.[18] Penetrating injury may result from a stab wound with a knife, ice pick or stiletto or from a gunshot wound that may be associated with a retained intracardiac or intravascular missile. Even blunt trauma may result in secondary penetrating injury to the heart or great vessels from the sharp end of an associated fractured rib or clavicle. The mechanism of injury to the heart or great vessels is of more than academic interest, as management of the patient may be influenced substantially by the causal factors involved in a given injury.

MANAGEMENT OF THE PATIENT IN THE EMERGENCY ROOM IN RELATION TO CARDIOVASCULAR TRAUMA

Any discussion of specific problems related to trauma to the heart and great vessels must begin with a consideration of the patient as he presents in the emergency room. Immediate establishment of an adequate airway is of primary importance, as in all cases of major trauma. Hypoxia resulting from an occluded or damaged airway may significantly influence the outcome of treatment of major cardiac injury and may specifically impair the function of an already damaged heart. The immediate insertion of large-bore intravenous cannulas and a central venous pressure cannula should coincide with the prompt processing of blood for transfusion. Patients with major cardiovascular injury who arrive in the emergency room usually require intravascular volume expansion before cross-matched blood is available. This immediate goal can be accomplished with albumin-containing solutions and plasma. Arterial blood gas determinations should be carried out promptly to correct, if present, either hypoxia or acidosis resulting from inadequate cardiac output. Similarly, serum electrolytes and, in particular, serum potassium should be assessed immediately, as hyperkalemia resulting from massive trauma or inadequate cardiac output may result in fatal arrhythmias in an already damaged heart. In the absence of evidence of urethral injury, insertion of a Foley catheter will facilitate the measurement of hourly urinary output as an important sign of adequate perfusion. Equipment should be immediately available for electric defibrillation, electrocardiographic monitoring and pericardicentesis, as required. Definitive treatment of patients with major trauma to the heart and great vessels in many instances requires the availability of cardiopulmonary bypass.

BLUNT TRAUMA TO THE HEART AND GREAT VESSELS

BLUNT CARDIAC TRAUMA. — Blunt trauma to the myocardium is a frequent occurrence after compression injury of the sternum against the steering wheel in an automobile accident. The appreciation of sternal fracture or disruption of costochondral cartilages on admission of the patient to the emergency room will heighten the surgeon's suspicion of the possibility of underlying myocardial trauma. The evaluation of the patient's condition should include an immediate electrocardiogram and, most important, serial electrocardiograms thereafter for evidence of evolving myocardial injury as a result of myocardial contusion.[4] Ordinarily, treatment for myocardial contusion is nonoperative and is identical to that for acute myocardial infarction. Contusions of the ventricle occur more frequently on the right than on the left. This type of injury often is associated with arrhythmias. The occurrence of atrial fibrillation or ventricular premature beats should lead the surgeon to suspect underlying myocardial contusion. Often the injury is unsuspected, and sudden ventricular fibrillation may be the first sign of a serious underlying myocardial contusion. The importance of immediate and serial electrocardiograms after sternal compression injury cannot be overemphasized. Similarly, determinations of cardiac enzyme levels should be undertaken, but the interpretation thereof may be complicated by either skeletal muscle or hepatic injury. Although myocardial contusion often has been thought to be benign in nature, a number of deaths from arrhythmias, cardiac failure or rupture of the ventricle have been reported.[6] Immediate recognition of the possibility of myocardial contusion and institution of appropriate antiarrhythmic therapy may significantly influence the outcome.

In addition to the myocardial contusion, compression injury to the heart may result in other intracardiac injuries, such as traumatic ventricular septal defect and, less commonly, traumatic atrial septal defect, aortic valvar insufficiency or rupture of the papillary muscles or chordae tendineae, leading to tricuspid or mitral valve regurgitation.[1] Ventricular aneurysms as a late sequel to myocardial contusion have been treated successfully by surgical excision.[15]

Apart from arrhythmias, the most important accompaniment of myocardial contusion from the standpoint of immediate management may be the occurrence of hemopericardium and cardiac tamponade. The clinical signs of cardiac tamponade include elevated central venous pressure in the presence of arterial hypotension, narrow pulse pressure, pulsus paradoxus and a widened cardiac shadow on roentgenogram. However, the roentgenogram frequently may be difficult to interpret unless a very large effusion is present. A relatively small amount of blood, that is, 150 ml, may cause significant cardiac restriction in a pericardial cavity of normal size. Although the clinical signs of cardiac tamponade are well known, the rate of development of such

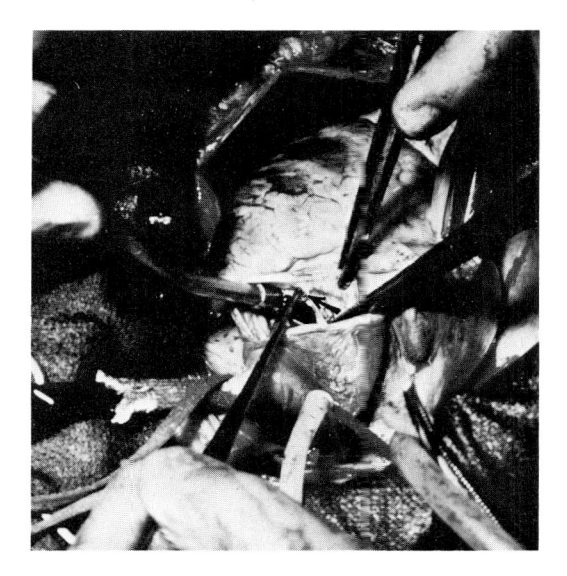

Fig. 42-1.—Operative view of traumatic aortic regurgitation in a 43-year-old male without previous history of heart disease; arrow indicates torn leaflet of aortic valve. The patient had sustained a steering wheel injury in an automobile accident 3 months earlier, after which clinical signs of aortic valve regurgitation developed. Prosthetic replacement of the torn aortic valve was followed by an uneventful recovery.

signs is critical to successful management of the patient. Slowly developing tamponade from a superficial myocardial injury or from pericardial vessels may be relieved adequately by pericardicentesis with appropriate direct electrocardiographic monitoring. On the other hand, rapidly developing signs of tamponade or the recurrence of tamponade following an initial pericardicentesis should lead to immediate operative intervention for control of bleeding vessels and adequate assessment of the extent of cardiac injury. Standby cardiopulmonary bypass should be available during the operation whenever possible. Argument continues to rage concerning closed pericardicentesis) versus open operative treatment of the patient with signs of traumatic cardiac tamponade; however, the selection of the appropriate surgical approach will depend largely on the nature of the injury, the rapidity of development of signs of cardiac restriction and the extent of continuing blood loss

BLUNT TRAUMA TO THE GREAT VESSELS. — Blunt trauma to the pulmonary artery or its branches may result from direct compression due to an automobile accident, a fall or a blow from a falling object. Patients with injuries of this type most often will present with shock, respiratory distress and clinical and roentgenographic evidence of hemothorax. Associated rib fractures almost always are observed, except in children, in whom the compressive forces often are transmitted through the elastic chest wall to the underlying thoracic viscera. The mechanism of injury is of great importance in dictating the early phases of treatment. History of compression injury to a hemithorax with the accumulation of blood in the pleural space requires the insertion of a chest tube for evacuation of the blood and reexpansion of the lung. Many such injuries result from a contusion or superficial tear of the lung or laceration of a vessel in the chest wall. Continued bleeding through the chest tube and shock that is unresponsive to blood replacement make open thoracotomy necessary for control of major pulmonary arterial or intercostal arterial bleeding. Brisk hemorrhage of dark blood from the right hemithorax may also result from tears of either the vena cava or the right atrium.

Probably the most important type of blunt trauma to the great vessels to be considered here is traumatic disruption of the thoracic aorta.[14] This injury has gained increasing attention because of its highly lethal nature and because of the development of techniques that make possible the successful treatment of this otherwise highly fatal injury. Traumatic rupture or dissection of the aorta almost invariably results from shear stress injury caused by the deceleration forces operative on a person in an automobile acci-

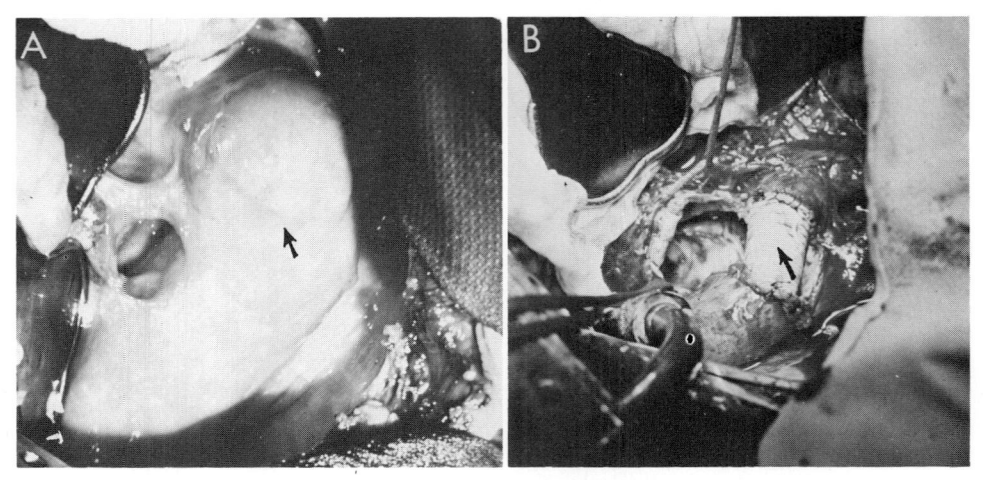

Fig. 42-2.—**A**, arrow indicates traumatic false aortic aneurysm at the aortic isthmus as a late sequel to an automobile accident of 20 years earlier. The aneurysm had shown recent increase in size with associated chest pain, making operation advisable. Pathologic examination revealed a false aneurysm of traumatic origin. **B**, arrow indicates tightly woven Teflon graft bridging the space previously occupied by the traumatic aortic aneurysm. The medial wall of the aneurysm, which was firmly adherent to trachea and esophagus, was left in place and excluded by the graft.

dent at the moment of impact. The vast majority of traumatic aortic ruptures occur at the aortic isthmus, where the aorta is fixed by the ligamentum arteriosus, intercostal vessels and left subclavian artery. The lower part of the thoracic aorta and the ascending aorta are less common sites of traumatic disruption. Occasionally cases involving rupture of the innominate artery or carotid arteries have been reported. In autopsy series of patients who died from injuries received in automobile accidents, traumatic rupture of the aorta is a frequent finding. Although approximately 80% of patients sustaining this type of injury die before reaching the hospital,[19] conversely, 20% do reach the hospital alive and can be saved if the injury is recognized immediately and emergency surgery is undertaken. One of the major difficulties in the treatment of traumatic aortic rupture is recognition of this injury within the limited time available for definitive surgical treatment to be applied successfully. Although reports have appeared of successful operations performed up to 1 month

Fig. 42-3.—Angiographic illustration of traumatic disruption of the aortic isthmus with associated dissection indicating "pseudo-coarctation." This 20-year-old male, a passenger in an automobile accident, displayed upper-extremity hypertension, barely palpable femoral pulses and a loud systolic murmur over the chest, as well as dysphagia caused by esophageal compression from the expanding hematoma.

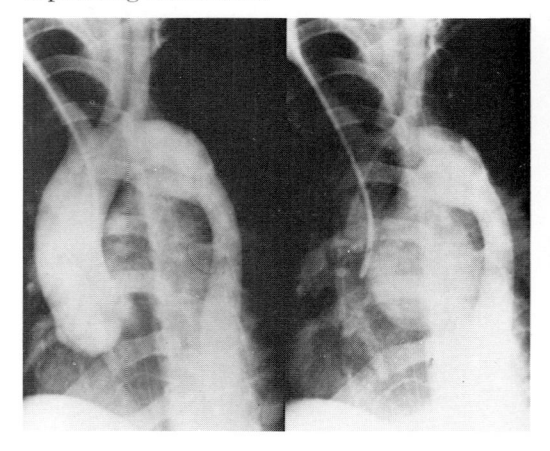

after injury, it has been estimated that a patient with traumatic disruption of the aorta probably has no more than a 50% chance of surviving 48 hours after reaching the hospital. Reports occasionally appear of successful treatment of late-developing traumatic aneurysms of the thoracic aorta. On the other hand, successful treatment of any significant number of patients with traumatic rupture of the aorta requires immediate recognition of the injury, its delineation by angiography and emergency surgical repair utilizing extracorporeal circulation.

The patient with traumatic rupture of the aorta resulting from deceleration injury usually presents in hemorrhagic shock; hemothorax, usually left-sided, often is present. Occasionally such patients will exhibit proximal (upper extremity) hypertension and may present the picture of "pseudocoarctation" with diminished femoral pulses and a systolic murmur. An expanding hematoma may cause dysphagia and hoarseness.

Associated injuries, including fractures, head injuries and internal abdominal injuries, are common and may divert attention from the aortic injury.

A widened mediastinum demonstrated on plain chest roentgenogram in a patient following an automobile accident is an indication for immediate aortography. Although anteroposterior portable views of the chest commonly employed in traumatized patients may exaggerate the width of the mediastinum, assessment of this radiologic sign clearly is of value in selecting management. In some patients, the hematoma around the aorta may be visible in a lateral view of the chest when the anteroposterior view appears unremarkable. Attar et al.[2] have reported 24 patients with observed widening of the

Fig. 42-4 (left).—Plain anteroposterior chest roentgenogram in an 8-year-old male 6 hours after an automobile accident in which the patient was the driver. The upper mediastinum, as indicated by the white arrows, was typically widened and dictated angiography, which was diagnostic of a tear in the aortic isthmus. The black arrow points to a left-sided pleural effusion, which often attends this type of injury and which was shown to be frank blood by thoracentesis. The aortic disruption was treated successfully by resection and grafting.
Fig. 42-5 (right).—Anteroposterior chest roentgenogram in a 22-year-old male who was a passenger in an automobile involved in a high-speed collision 12 hours earlier. As indicated by the white arrows, the mediastinum is widened. The black arrow indicates a gas bubble in the stomach, which has herniated into the left chest through a ruptured left hemidiaphragm. This patient underwent immediate aortography documenting an aortic isthmus tear. Surgical correction of the injuries included resection and grafting of the ruptured aortic isthmus, removal of a lacerated spleen and repair of the torn left hemidiaphragm. The patient recovered uneventfully.

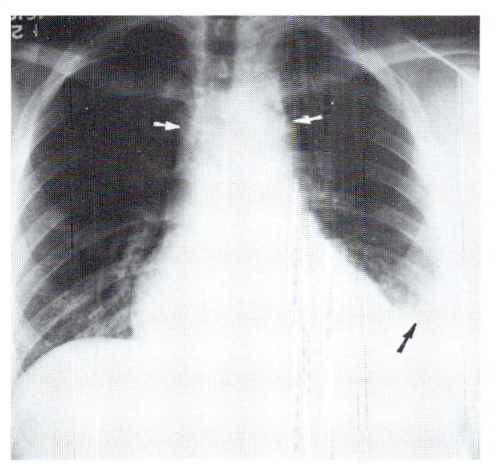

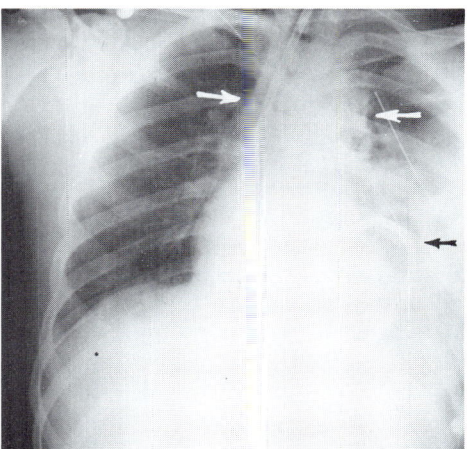

mediastinum following trauma, of whom 7 were shown to have a ruptured thoracic aorta. Aortography can be accomplished at low risk even in the presence of other injuries. Because of the lethal nature of traumatic aortic rupture and because of the success of operative therapy when it is instituted promptly, aortography is mandatory in all patients with a widened mediastinum after trauma from an automobile accident. A widened mediastinum may also be caused by mediastinal hematoma from torn small vessels in the mediastinum. Injuries of this type usually are self-limited and can be managed conservatively. Diagnostic techniques, on the other hand, should be directed toward injuries of the major vessels.

The angiographic documentation of rupture of the descending thoracic aorta should lead to immediate left thoracotomy, resection of the traumatized aorta and replacement with a graft. We favor a tightly woven Teflon graft to prevent bleeding through the graft in association with the required heparinization.[5] This type of repair is carried out with either left heart bypass (that is, pumping oxygenated blood from the left atrium into the femoral artery), partial femoral vein to femoral artery cardiopulmonary bypass with an oxygenator or a combination of both. Our preference for surgical repair of rupture of the aortic isthmus has been a combination of femoral vein to femoral artery bypass and left heart bypass. This method has evolved from our experience with dissecting aortic aneurysms and appears to offer significant advantages over either technique used alone. In this method, the left femoral vein is cannulated for drainage of the inferior vena cava. The venous blood is passed through a bubble oxygenator and pumped back into the femoral artery. Similarly, a cannula is placed in the left atrium through the appendage to facilitate maintenance of low left atrial pressures during aortic cross-clamping. The use of either method alone during aortic cross-clamping may result in left ventricular stretch, high left-sided filling pressures and postoperative pulmonary edema and left ventricular failure. In this type of surgery, adequate perfusion pressure and flow to the lower half of the body still may be accompanied by postoperative acute renal failure as a consequence of left ventricular failure if left heart decompression is not adequate during the period of aortic cross-clamping. An additional technique that has facilitated this type of surgery is the use of a Carlens double-lumen endotracheal tube, which permits complete deflation of the left lung during the rapid and often difficult exposure of the ruptured thoracic aorta. Another distinct advantage of this technique is the prevention of undue trauma to the left lung with the patient heparinized and with the vigorous retraction required on the inflated lung in order to gain adequate exposure. With the

Fig. 42-6.—Aortic angiogram in the patient whose chest x-ray is displayed in Figure 42-5. The white arrow shows an acute false aneurysm at the aortic isthmus, which resulted from a circumferential aortic intimal tear.

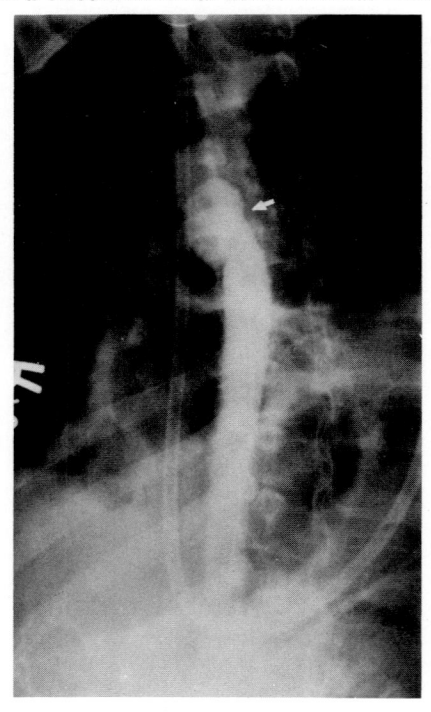

approach described, we recently have achieved survival in 13 of 18 patients operated on in an acute condition after traumatic rupture of the aorta.

Occasionally, a patient may survive the acute injury and show different clinical signs that still may lead to an accurate diagnosis and successful treatment. Patients with a partial tear of the aortic isthmus and a developing adjacent mediastinal hematoma may complain of hoarseness resulting from compressive paralysis or tearing of the left recurrent laryngeal nerve, dysphagia from esophageal compression and hemoptysis or dyspnea from compression of the left bronchus. The appreciation of these signs and symptoms should lead to the proper diagnosis by aortography and successful treatment in the patient who is first seen days to weeks after the acute injury.

Rarely, the rupture occurs in the ascending aorta; total cardiopulmonary bypass is required to repair the aorta in this location.

PENETRATING TRAUMA TO THE HEART AND GREAT VESSELS

STAB WOUNDS OF THE HEART.—Stab wounds of the heart with stilettos, kitchen knives and even ice picks have been observed, and knowledge of the nature of the injuring weapon may be of some value in the early stages of management of the patient. The patient with a stab wound of the heart usually exhibits the clinical signs of shock and pericardial tamponade. As Naclerio[2] has pointed out, the initial appearance of the patient on entry to the emergency room may be extremely deceptive. Patients who are unconscious and from whom a blood pressure reading cannot be obtained may be resuscitated quickly by pericardicentesis or rapid open thoracotomy to relieve critical pericardial tamponade from a relatively minor cardiac injury. On the other hand, the condition of a patient with relatively good hemodynamics after a stab wound of the heart may deteriorate rapidly and he may die before definitive surgery can be undertaken. The arguments mentioned previously concerning closed (pericardicentesis) versus open surgical treatment of patients with penetrating wounds of the heart may be confusing and misleading to the surgeon who encounters this type of injury only occasionally. Many series have been reported documenting low mortality rates with both management approaches.[9, 12] The type of treatment selected, however, appears to be less important in these reported series than the nature of the injury and the rapidity with which circulatory collapse develops. Patients who are first seen several hours after a stiletto or ice pick stab wound of the heart may be selectively relieved of moderate cardiac tamponade by pericardicentesis. Such patients observed closely in an intensive care setting with electrocardiographic, arterial and venous pressure monitoring frequently can be managed conservatively, with surgical intervention available for the occasional patient whose condition shows late deterioration.

On the other hand, the patient arriving in the emergency room in circulatory collapse as a result of a stab wound of the heart should be treated on the spot by left anterolateral thoracotomy in the fourth interspace, open evacuation of the blood-filled pericardium and cardiorraphy of the stab wound. This classic emergency method of dealing with stab wounds of the heart has yielded an impressive number of survivors, in whom any delay of definitive therapy would have resulted in death.[12] In certain hospitals, an intermediate group of patients with moderately well-maintained hemodynamics may be brought directly from the emergency room to the prepared operating theater for a more controlled open procedure under optimal operating conditions; initial pericardicentesis in the emergency room may be helpful. The exact mode of treatment must be dictated by the nature of the injury and the timing of physiologic events that may either permit or preclude a more deliberate approach to management.

Of particular importance in the hemodynamic management of pericardial tamponade is the recognition that cardiac output is reduced by restriction of stroke volume. Thus, during the rapid preparation for definitive relief from tamponade, adequate cardiac output may be temporarily maintained for perfusion of the brain and other vital organs by transiently increasing cardiac filling pressures to high levels with intravascular volume expansion with plasma or albumin. The appreciation of this hemodynamic principle is important and may avoid the occasional tragedy of a patient who emerges from the operating room with a live heart but a dead brain

MISSILE WOUNDS OF THE HEART.—Gunshot wounds of the heart and other missile wounds as may result from exploding stoves or gas tanks usually are fatal immediately because of the extent of injury deriving from the energy imparted to the missile. The classic work of Harken[8] in World War II clearly established that patients reaching a major medical facility have a significant chance for survival if immediate surgical treatment is instituted. Only rarely will the condition of such patients allow conservative treatment; the availability of cardiopulmonary bypass for treatment of this type of injury is essential. The myocardial injury should be repaired and the foreign body removed. Migration of retained missiles to and from the heart has been well documented[3] and offers an indication for their removal, if possible, even in the occasional patient who survives the immediate injury.

PENETRATING WOUNDS OF THE GREAT VESSELS[13].—Stab wounds or gunshot wounds of the lung and branches of the pulmonary artery frequently can be managed conservatively. Continued bleeding into the chest is an indication for operation, but more often the indication for surgery is related to bronchial damage with continuing air leak.

Penetrating wounds of the thoracic aor-

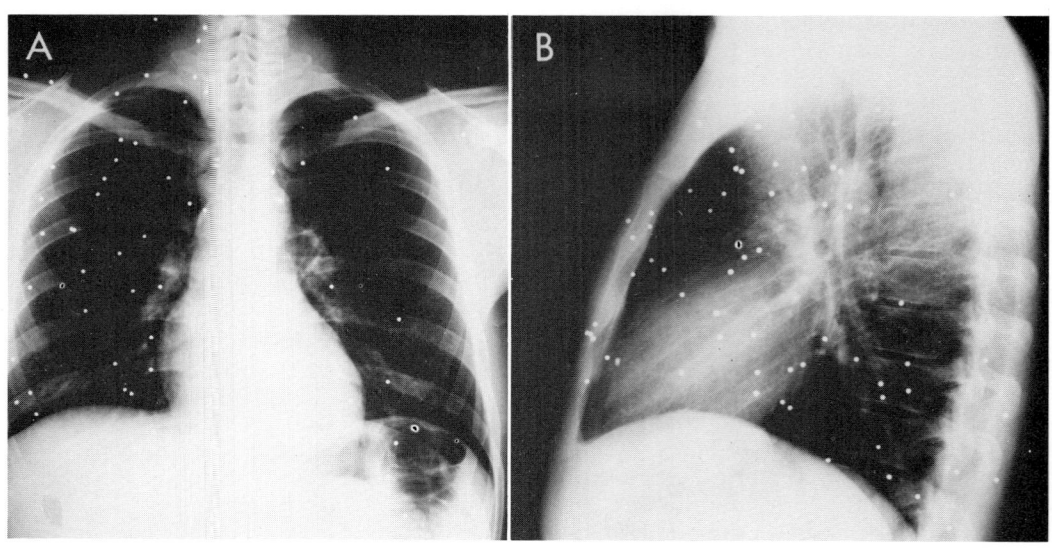

Fig. 42-7.—Anteroposterior (A) and lateral (B) views of the chest taken in a 12-year-old boy who sustained a shotgun wound of the heart and lungs during a riot. Angiography and fluoroscopy showed that the two pellets were lodged in the right ventricular myocardium. The patient was treated nonoperatively and recovery was uneventful.

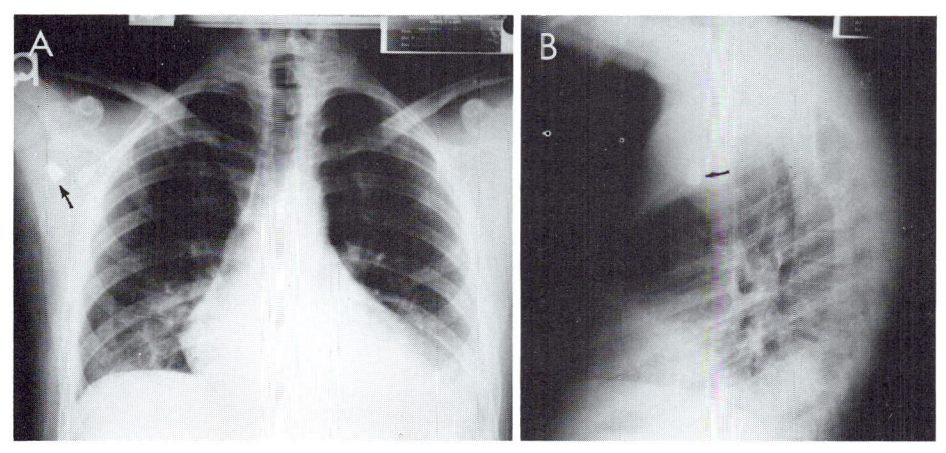

Chapter 42: CARDIAC TRAUMA: HEART AND GREAT VESSELS / 1013

Fig. 42-8.—Anteroposterior (A) and lateral (B) chest roentgenograms taken in a 24-year-old male who sustained a gunshot wound of the heart from a 32-caliber pistol. The bullet, which initially entered the chest through the left axilla, came to lie outside the chest wall in the right pectoral area and is indicated by the arrow. This patient initially was treated conservatively with bilateral chest tube drainage for hemothoraces. Four days later the patient developed a continuous murmur over the precordium that was shown angiographically to result from a fistula between the left anterior descending coronary artery and the right ventricle. Because of continuing electrocardiographic signs of anterolateral ischemia, the patient underwent closure of the fistula and saphenous vein aortocoronary bypass grafting to the left anterior descending coronary artery. The patient's subsequent recovery was uneventful.

ta, by stabbing or gunshot, are relatively uncommon. Symbas and Sehdeva,[20] in reporting their experience with 6 such patients in 1969, found a total of 43 reported cases of penetrating wounds of the aorta in the world literature. Stab wounds or gunshot wounds of the thoracic aorta invariably require open surgical treatment. Ordinarily, extracorporeal circulation is required, as with nonpenetrating traumatic disruption of the thoracic aorta. Because of the urgency of required treatment of this type of injury, an aorta-to-aorta silastic bypass shunt[20] may provide a satisfactory alternative to extracorporeal circulation.

BIBLIOGRAPHY

1. Aleksandrow, D., Wysznacka, W., Szczerban, J., and Krus, S.: Traumatic rupture of the right papillary muscle in a patient with congenital atrial septal defect, Am. Heart J. 69:686, 1964.
2. Attar, S., Ayella, R. J., and McLaughlin, J. S.: The widened mediastinum in trauma, Ann. Thorac. Surg. 13:435, 1972.
3. Bland, E. F., and Beebe, G. W.: Missiles in the heart. A twenty-year follow-up report of World War II cases, N. Engl. J. Med. 274:1039, 1966.
4. Brooks, S. H., Nahum, A. M., and Siegel, A. W.: Causes of injury in motor vehicle accidents, Surg. Gynecol. Obstet. 131:185, 1970.
5. Daggett, W. M., and Austen, W. G.: Biomedical engineering applications to cardiovascular surgery, Am. J. Surg. 114:139, 1967.
6. DeMuth, W. E., Jr., and Zinsser, H. F., Jr.: Myocardial contusion, Arch. Intern. Med. 115:434, 1965.
7. Fromm, S. H., Carrasquilla, C., and Lucas, C.: The management of gunshot wounds of the aorta. The use of Dacron grafts to replace the injured aorta, Arch. Surg. 101:388, 1970.
8. Harken, D. E.: Foreign bodies in, and in relation to, thoracic blood vessels and heart; techniques for approaching and removing foreign bodies from chambers of heart, Surg. Gynecol. Obstet. 83:117, 1946.
9. Isaacs, J. P.: Sixty penetrating wounds of the heart: Clinical and experimental observations, Surgery 45:696, 1959.
10. Maynard, A. L., Brooks, H. A., and Froix, C. J. L.: Penetrating wounds of the heart, Arch. Surg. 90:680, 1965.
11. Mulder, D. G., and Grollman, J. H., Jr.: Traumatic disruption of the thoracic aorta, Am. J. Surg. 118:311, 1969.
12. Naclerio, E. A.: Penetrating wounds of the heart, Dis. Chest 46:1, 1964.
13. Parmley, L. F., Mattingly, T. W., and Manion, W. C.: Penetrating wounds of the heart and aorta, Circulation 17:953, 1958.
14. Parmley, L. F., Mattingly, T. W., Manion, W. C., and Jahnke, E. J., Jr.: Nonpenetrating traumatic injury of the aorta, Circulation 17:1086, 1958.

15. Pupello, D. F., Daily, P. O., Stinson, E. B., and Shumway, N. E.: Successful repair of left ventricular aneurysm due to trauma, JAMA 211:826, 1970.
16. Rittenhouse, E. A., Dillard, D. H., Winterscheid, L. C., and Merendino, K. A.: Traumatic rupture of the thoracic aorta: A review of the literature and a report of five cases with attention to special problems in early surgical management, Ann. Sur. 170:87, 1969.
17. Smyth, N. P. D., Hirsch, E. F., and Santos, D. S.: Penetrating wounds of the heart, Dis. Chest 49:538, 1966.
18. Spencer, F. C., Guerin, P. F., Blake, M. A., and Bahnson, H. T.: Report of fifteen patients with traumatic rupture of thoracic aorta, J. Thorac. Cardiovasc. Surg. 41:1, 1961.
19. Strassmann, G.: Traumatic rupture of aorta, Am. Heart J. 33:508, 1947.
20. Symbas, P. N., and Sehdeva, J. S.: Penetrating wounds of the thoracic aorta, Ann. Surg. 171:441, 1970.

43 | Management of Respiratory Failure Associated with Chest Trauma

KENNETH W. TRAVIS, HENRIK H. BENDIXEN and BENNIE GEFFIN

AMONG CIVILIANS in the United States, accidental death due to chest injury occurs every 40 minutes.[7] The increasing epidemiologic importance of chest trauma is emphasized further by the fact that in the United States, in 1968, an estimated 55,000 persons died in motor vehicle accidents. Chest injury accounts for 15–25% of such automotive fatalities.[11, 25] In one small survey of 28 traffic victims with otherwise minor injuries, 84% died as a result of chest and upper-airway injury.[18]

Many factors influence the mortality of chest trauma. Seventy per cent of vehicular deaths occur in rural areas, away from emergency care facilities and with less than optimal first-aid and transportation available.[18] In addition to the extent of thoracic and pulmonary injury, survival was influenced by shock, associated injuries and delayed diagnosis of the chest injury.[7, 16] Over-all mortality from isolated thoracic injuries ranges from 7.2% to 13%.[6, 7] With associated injuries, mortality is nearer 25–40%.[33]

WHAT IS TRAUMATIZED

THE CHEST. — Direct injury to the chest may result from penetrating wounds or blunt trauma. In each category, rib fracture, pneumothorax, hemothorax or laceration and contusion of lung parenchyma, conducting airways, esophagus and great vessel or cardiac injury can occur. Flail chest refers to an unstable chest wall segment caused by multiple rib or sternal fractures or by costochondral dislocations. The paradoxical movement of the flail segment, appearing as a collapse of the chest during inspiration and expansion, compromises ventilation, tends to decrease lung volume and severely hinders coughing.

In children, severe lung contusion may be present with little external evidence of trauma[28] whereas in adults, extensive rib fractures frequently are indicative of severe pulmonary injury. Pathologically, the pulmonary contusion is characterized by endobronchial edema, retained secretions, patchy or confluent areas of parenchymal edema, alveolar rupture and blood-stained intra-alveolar exudates.

Lung contusion becomes evident by chest film in 2–24 hours,[2] but it may be suspected earlier by falling oxygen tension and the appearance of blood in the sputum. Lung rupture can result from penetration by fractured rib fragments. Bronchial tears, lacerations of great vessels or the thoracic duct, pericardial tamponade, myocardial contusion and ruptured hemidiaphragm with intrathoracic herniation of abdominal contents have also been reported.[11, 27, 29]

ASSOCIATED INJURIES

Head injury, extremity or pelvic fractures and intra-abdominal or retroperitoneal injuries frequently and seriously complicate chest trauma. These associated injuries may direct attention away from the subtle chest insult, and simultaneous heavy administration of narcotics for pain aggravates hypoventilation. Aspiration of gastric contents is a continuing threat. When fire accompanies the accident, inhalation of noxious gases can produce chemical pneumonitis, and concurrent methemoglobin or carboxyhemoglobin lowers the oxygen-carrying capacity of blood. Circulatory compensation for hypoxemia can be reduced further by hypovolemia, myocardial contusion, pericardial tamponade, acidosis or pre-existing heart disease.

EARLY MANIFESTATIONS

Early clinical signs and symptoms of serious chest injury include pain, apprehension, dyspnea, tachypnea, tachycardia and limitation of chest movement. Cyanosis invariably is a sign of serious pulmonary pathology.

DIAGNOSIS

The diagnosis of pulmonary injury is made on clincial, radiologic and laboratory grounds. Initially, flail may be concealed by muscle spasm or voluntary splinting. Tachycardia, tachypnea, mild hypertension, sweating and cyanosis suggest hypoxemia or hypercapnia. However, this is assessed best by arterial blood gas analysis. Hypotension and shock accompany severe injuries in the young and moderate or severe injuries in the elderly or debilitated. To supplement the physical examination, an upright chest film is valuable in demonstrating intrapleural air or fluid.

FUNCTIONAL DISTURBANCE

In addition to the extent of anatomic derangement, one must carefully evaluate the resulting or evolving functional disturbance, keeping in mind certain salient physiologic principles.

Figure 43-1 depicts lung volumes and capacities. Each tidal volume (VT) is composed of air that participates in gas exchange (alveolar ventilation, or VA) and air that does not (dead space ventilation, or VD). Thus: VT = VD − VA (equation 1).*

Gas filling the conducting airways occupies anatomic dead space (VD anatomic); normally, this quantity is about 1 cc per pound of body weight.[36] Whenever an area of the lung is overventilated in relation to perfusion, an alveolar dead space (VD alveolar) is present. Thus: VD physiologic = VD anatomic + VD alveolar (equation 2). One of the most useful indices of ventilatory efficiency is the ratio of dead space ventilation to the tidal volume (VD/VT).

Normally, in the 70-kg adult,
VT = VD + VA (equation 3)
450 = 150 + 300
VD/VT = 0.33

By collecting expired gas, determining the partial pressure of CO_2 and relating that value to the simultaneously drawn arterial Pa_{CO_2}, one can calculate VD/VT using the Enghoff modification of the Bohr equation as follows:

$$VD/VT = \frac{Pa_{CO_2} - Pe_{CO_2}}{Pa_{CO_2}}$$

(equation 4)

The clinical application of the VD/VT ratio is described in Figure 43-2.

Normally, vital capacity is 70 cc/kg, 70–80% of which can be exhaled in the

---
*Equations are grouped at the end of the chapter.

Chapter 43: MANAGEMENT OF RESPIRATORY FAILURE WITH CHEST TRAUMA / 1017

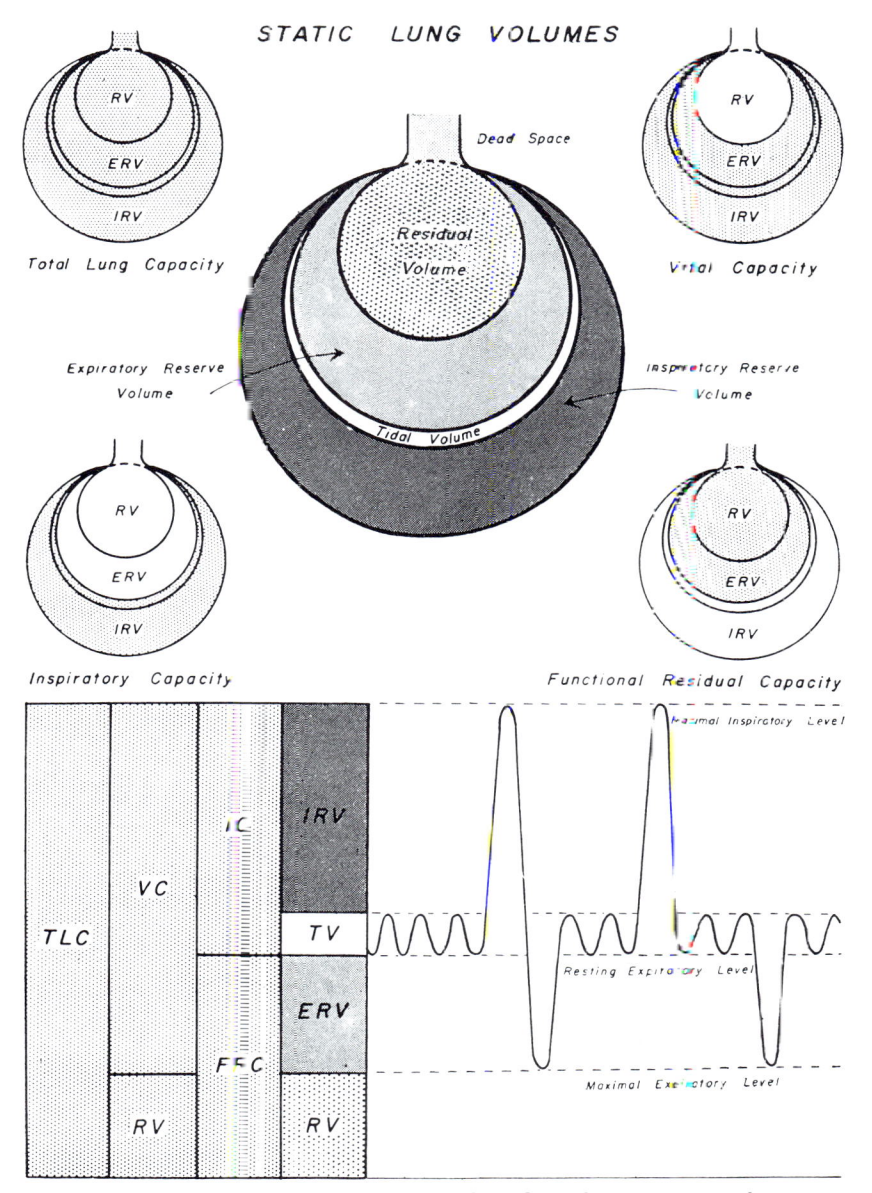

Fig. 43-1.—Lung volumes and capacities. (Reproduced, with permission, from Comroe, J. H., Jr., et al.: *The Lung* [2d ed.; Chicago: Year Book Medical Publishers, Inc., 1962].)

first second. The second vital capacity (FEV_1) is reduced when airway resistance is increased by acute or chronic reduction in airway caliber or secretions. Bedside measurement of vital capacity provides an index to the patient's ability to cough or re-expand collapsing lung segments.[35] Following trauma, both the total and timed vital capacities may be reduced.

That quantity of gas remaining in the lung at the end of a normal exhalation is

Fig. 43-2.—Pulmonary effects of nonthoracic trauma. Beyond a VD/VT of 0.6, minute ventilation must increase greatly to present progressive carbon dioxide retention. (Reproduced, with permission, from Pontoppidan, H.: Treatment of respiratory failure in nonthoracic trauma, J. Trauma 8:941, 1968.)

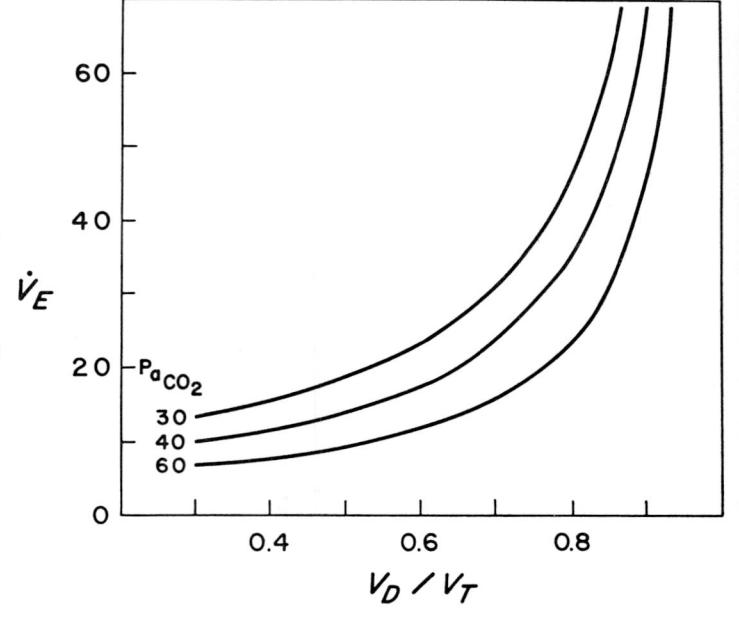

the functional residual capacity (FRC). Normally, FRC constitutes approximately 50% of total lung capacity[13] and is defined as that point at which the differing relaxation pressure-volume curves of the chest wall and lung are equal and opposite.[3] FRC constitutes one of the body's few oxygen reservoirs.[9] It is reduced normally in the supine position and may be reduced greatly after chest trauma.[23, 34]

Ventilation is the movement of gases against tissue and airway resistances. It is expressed as volume per unit time. Total

Fig. 43-3.—Work of breathing—normal work diagram. The area enclosed by the ellipse represents work done to overcome resistance. The area A-B-C-D-A represents the energy cost of stretching the lungs. The total energy cost of a breath equals area A-B-C-D-A plus the area to the right of the line B-C. (Modified, with permission, from Peters, R. M.: The work of breathing following trauma, J. Trauma 8:916, 1968.)

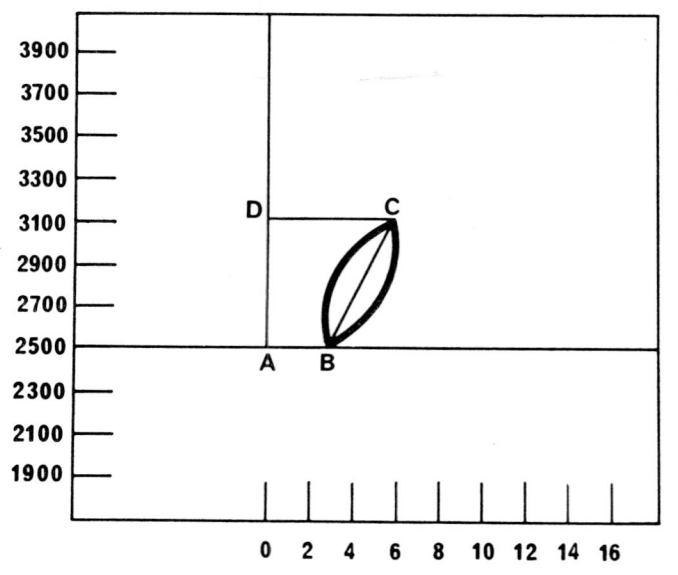

Chapter 43: MANAGEMENT OF RESPIRATORY FAILURE WITH CHEST TRAUMA / 1019

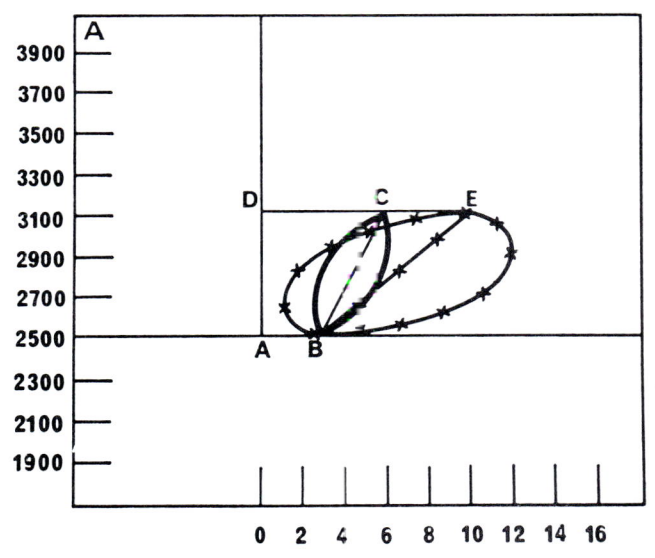

Fig. 43-4.—Work of breathing. The effect of both increased resistance and compliance. The total area A-B-E-C-D-A, including the area enclosed by the loop, is greatly increased. (Modified, with permission, from Peters, R. M.: The work of breathing following trauma, J. Trauma 8:920, 1968.)

compliance is a static volume-pressure measurement (V/P) that reflects the elastic properties of the lung and chest wall. Airway resistance is a dynamic measurement expressed in cm H_2O/liter/sec. Poiseuille's equation demonstrates the critical role of airway caliber in determining airway resistance and flow.[14]

$$\dot{V} = \Delta P \times \frac{\pi}{8l} \times \frac{R^4}{\eta}$$

where $\dot{V}$ = flow, ΔP = pressure difference, r = radius of lumen, l = length and η = viscosity of the gas. Work of breathing may be represented conceptually as overcoming compliance and resistance forces and graphically by pressure-volume loops.

Exhalation is accomplished normally with little energy expenditure. One merely reclaims potential energy imparted to the lung and chest during inspiration (see Fig. 43-2). Figure 43-3 represents the traumatized patient with reduced compliance and increased airway resistance whose work of breathing is increased.

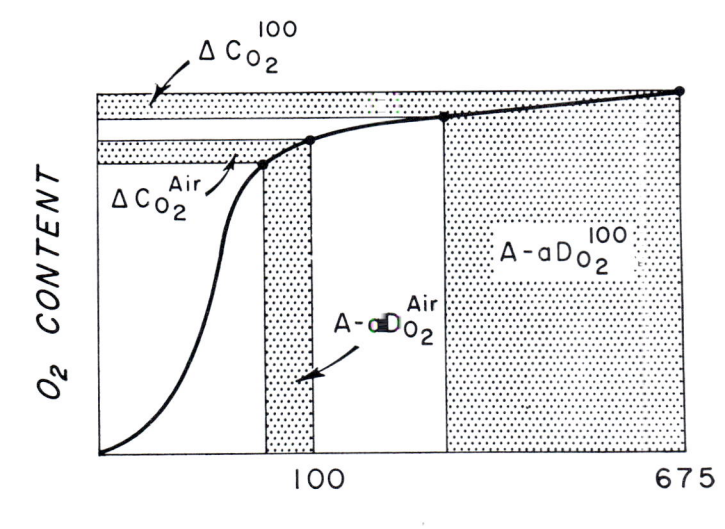

Fig. 43-5.—When high concentrations of oxygen are breathed, a given fall in oxygen content will correspond to a larger fall in Pa_{O_2} than when the same degree of content fall occurs on the steeper portion of the oxyhemoglobin dissociation curve. (Reproduced, with permission, from Pontoppidan, H.: Treatment of respiratory failure in nonthoracic trauma, J. Trauma 8:940, 1968.)

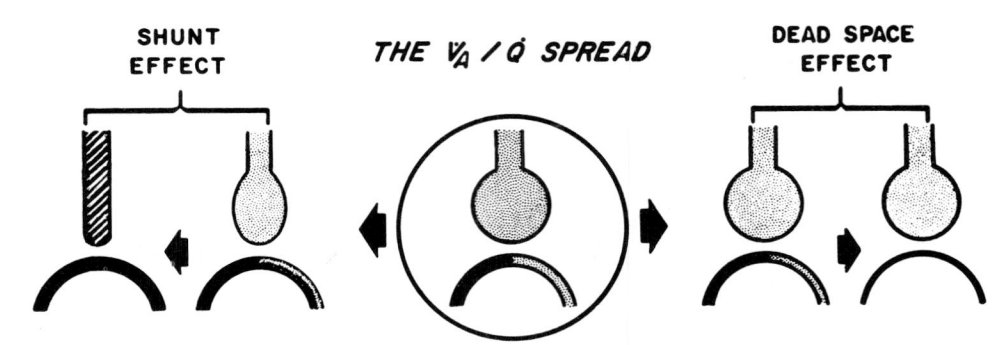

Fig. 43-6.—The VA/Q spread takes off in either direction from the normal ratio of VA and Q for the individual gas exchange unit. When ventilation diminishes and ceases while perfusion remains constant, a *shunt effect* is present. When perfusion diminishes and ceases while ventilation remains constant, a *dead-space effect* is present. (Reproduced, with permission, from Holiday, D.: *Clinical Anesthesia* [Philadelphia: F. A. Davis Company, 1967].)

At rest, 4 liters per minute of alveolar ventilation (VA) is matched by 5 liters per minute of blood (Q).[13] As long as this VA/Q ratio of 0.8 exists, as long as the distribution of VA/Q ratio across the lungs is normal and as long as the oxygen concentration and quantities of gas and of blood are sufficient, normal blood gases result. Two to 4% of the cardiac output normally bypasses ventilated alveoli via anatomic channels, such as thebesian vessels or bronchial communications, resulting in slight venous admixture in arterial blood. Abnormal shunting refers to the continued perfusion of collapsed, filled or otherwise nonfunctioning alveoli, which further increases venous admixture and is reflected in the increased alveolar to arterial oxygen difference (A-aDO$_2$) and falling Po$_2$. Measurement of the A-aDO$_2$ on 100% oxygen provides a sensitive index of shunting, as explained in Figure 43-5.

TABLE 43-1.—CAUSES OF HYPOXEMIA

1. Collapse—compression, atelectasis
2. Pneumonic
   a) Consolidation
3. Contusion
4. Infarction and emboli
5. Pulmonary edema
6. Hypoventilation

TABLE 43-2.—CAUSES OF INCREASED DEAD SPACE

1. Hypotension
2. Hypovolemia
3. Emboli
4. Air trapping
5. Dead space effect of shunting
6. Redistribution of tidal volume from collapsed, perfused lung areas (as with atelectasis, pneumonia or congestion)

The ventilation-perfusion (V/Q) spectrum is represented in Figure 43-6.

Events contributing to increased shunting are listed in Table 43-1 and those causing increased physiologic dead space are listed in Table 43-2.

PATHOPHYSIOLOGY

In crushing injuries of the chest, the inward movement of the flailing segment during inspiration disallows expansion of the underlying lung, and atelectasis results. Further collapse and retention of secretions occur as a result of pain, muscle spasm, increased secretions, shallow breathing and an inefficient cough mechanism. The pleural spaces may also contain air, blood or herniated abdominal viscera. Bronchiolar obstruction and alveolar edema caused by lung contusion

Chapter 43: MANAGEMENT OF RESPIRATORY FAILURE WITH CHEST TRAUMA

reduce compliance, increase airway resistance and intensify hypoxemia still further. Blood loss aggravates tissue hypoxemia, increases dead space and both respiratory and metabolic acidosis evolve.

WET LUNG SYNDROME

The wet lung syndrome is characterized by acute infiltrative changes affecting one or both lungs, impaired gas exchange, reduced lung compliance, increased airway resistance and increased extravascular pulmonary water and blood.

Clinically, this syndrome presents with respiratory difficulty of varying degrees, arterial desaturation, high P_{CO_2} and increased secretions. In its most severe form, it is clinically identical to the pulmonary edema of acute left ventricular failure. (Pulmonary wedge pressure determinations will help in the differential diagnosis.) A great diversity of conditions can lead to this pathophysiologic state. In all cases, however, interstitial edema is present. In patients who have been subjected to chest trauma, it may follow contusion of the lungs, particularly if

Fig. 43-7. — Vital capacity, compliance, oxygenation and weaning efforts improve with reversal of positive fluid balance. M = mercuhydrin 2 ml IM. V/P = volume/pressure = effective compliance on the ventilator. (Courtesy of H. Pontoppidan.)

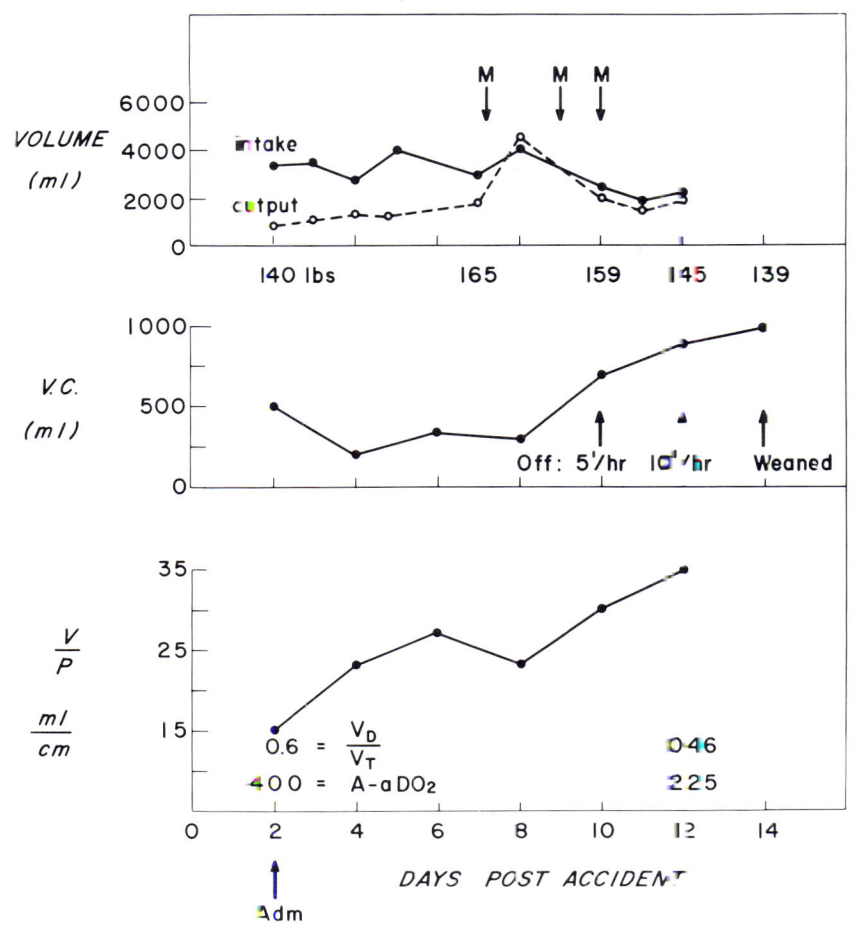

TABLE 43-3. — NONTHORACIC CAUSES OF PULMONARY INSUFFICIENCY*

1. Craniocerebral trauma
2. Hypotension — low pulmonary perfusion
3. Acidosis
4. Fat emboli
5. Microthrombosis, particulate microemboli
6. Fluid overload
7. Bacteremia
8. Graft vs. host rejection
9. Hypoxemia
10. Oxygen toxicity
11. Toxin
12. Circulating vasoactive substances

*Modified from Pomerantz, M., and Eiseman, B.: Experimental shock lung model, J. Trauma 8:650, 1968, and Aviado, D., Adenosine diphosphate and vasoactive substances, J. Trauma 8:880, 1968.

TABLE 43-4. — CLINICAL INDICATIONS FOR IMMEDIATE INTUBATION AFTER TRAUMA

1. Cardiac arrest
2. Upper airway obstruction
3. Cervical fracture with resulting intercostal paralysis
4. Overt, symptomatic flail chest
5. Coma

an excess of solute has been administered. Microemboli or small-vessel coagulation or sludging have been invoked as causes. It has also been described as a complication of artificial ventilation in association with water retention.[39] Because of the inefficiency of gas exchange in these patients, ventilatory requirements are increased. Fluid restriction, diuretics and the maintenance of normal levels of serum albumin, however, often will lead to marked improvement.[1, 10, 12, 38, 39] Figure 43-7 depicts the clinical course of a patient with chest trauma in whom relative fluid overload was reversed with diuretics.

Other factors that additionally contribute to lung injury in trauma are listed in Table 43-3.

EARLY TREATMENT

At the scene of the accident or in the emergency room, management consists first of resuscitation. A clear airway, stabilization of the chest wall by positive-pressure manual ventilation with a "bag and mask" or endotracheal tube and oxygenation are first-order requirements. Adequate ventilation thus is ensured and paradoxical breathing eliminated. Evacuation of blood and air from the pleural cavities and restoration of circulating blood volume with correction of acid-base parameters are accomplished virtually simultaneously.

Continued bleeding into the trachea from a ruptured bronchus requires placement of an endobronchial tube or blocker to prevent drowning of the uninjured lung. Indications for immediate intubation appear in Table 43-4. Once physiologically stable, the patient may be transported. Figure 43-8 shows a ventilator used to control ventilation during transfer.

Later manifestations of trauma may include the development of tension pneumothorax, intra-abdominal bleeding from hepatic or splenic rupture or cerebral and pulmonary deterioration from fat emboli.

Continuous monitoring of arterial blood gases and vital capacity measurements are mandatory, for they assist greatly with the early diagnosis of respiratory failure. General indications for respiratory support appear in Table 43-5.

MAINTENANCE OF RESPIRATORY CARE

In 1956, Avery, Mörch and Benson[5] reported the use of a volume-limited ventilator to treat a crushing chest injury. "Internal pneumatic stabilization" (ibid.) sustains alveolar patency until the chest wall no longer moves paradoxically and has generally supplanted various external fixation techniques. (In selected cases, combined operative and internal stabilization may reduce the total time necessary for artificial ventilation.)

In general, intervention with intuba-

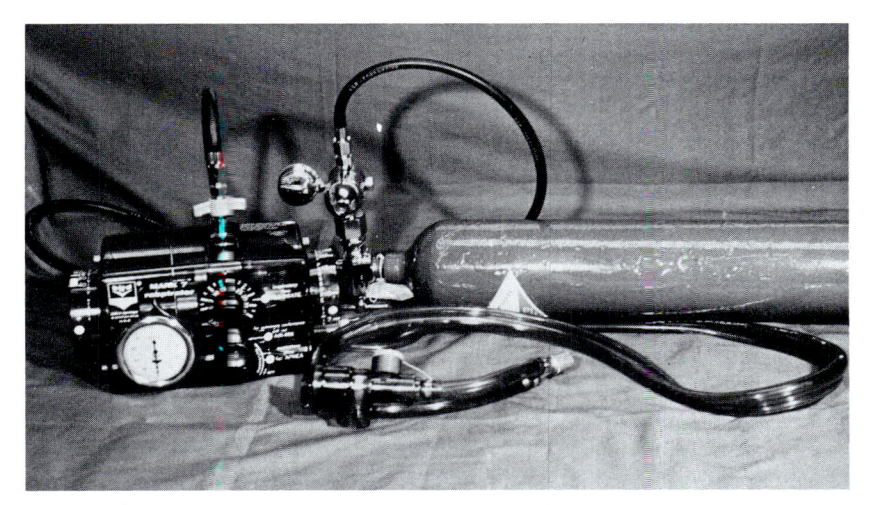

Fig. 43-8.—A Bird Mark 8 respirator powered by an "E" cylinder oxygen tank facilitates transportation of the patient who requires mechanical ventilation.

tion and mechanical ventilation should be early. Delay allows for the development of disturbances in gas exchange, shunting and inefficient CO_2 elimination. High airway pressures and high oxygen concentrations then are required[7, 35]; thus, a new set of hazards is introduced. A polyvinyl chloride (Portex) nasotracheal tube with a prestretched, high-volume, low-tension cuff[27] is readily inserted under topical anesthesia and may be used initially for artificial ventilation. Once circulatory stability has been established, tracheostomy through the second tracheal ring[26] should be performed and a tracheostomy tube with a low-tension cuff used.

Synchronizing the patient with the ventilator is of special importance and can be facilitated by appropriate individualization of flow settings, mild hyperventilation[5] and narcotics such as morphine (2–10 mg intravenously as needed). Sedatives such as diazepam or barbiturates can be used when pain is not present. Muscle relaxants such as succinylcholine, curare or gallamine are employed when the above measures fail,

TABLE 43-5.—INDICATIONS FOR RESPIRATORY SUPPORT*

		ACCEPTABLE RANGE	CHEST PHYSICAL THERAPY, OXYGEN, CLOSE MONITORING	INTUBATION TRACHEOSTOMY VENTILATION
Mechanics	Respiratory rate	12–25	25–35	>35
	Vital capacity, ml/kg	70–30	30–15	<15
	Inspiratory force, cm H_2O	100–50	50–25	<25
Oxygenation	A-aDO_2, mm Hg	50–200	200–350	>350
	Pa_{O_2}, mm Hg	100–75 (air)	200–70 (on mask O_2)	<70 (on mask O_2)
Ventilation	V_D/V_T	0.3–0.4	0.4–0.6	>0.6
	Pa_{CO_2}, mm Hg	35–45	45–60	>60

*Reproduced, with permission, from Pontoppidan, H.: Treatment of respiratory failure in nonthoracic trauma, J. Trauma 8:940, 1968.

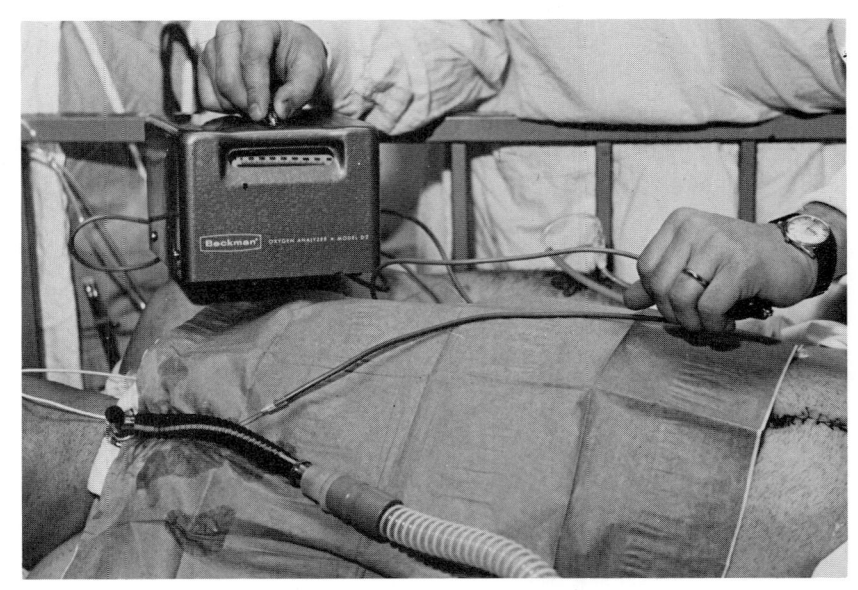

Fig. 43-9.—A Beckman paramagnetic oxygen analyzer allows monitoring of inspired oxygen concentrations.

particularly in the marginally oxygenated, agitated patient in whom perfect ventilator-patient synchrony and reduced oxygen consumption are crucial.[37] Once pulmonary compliance and resistance have been affected favorably, the need for such pharmacologic adjuncts lessens.

Setting the Ventilator

Tidal volumes of 10–15 ml/kg with an inspiratory to expiratory time ratio not exceeding 1:1 (generally 1:2) and a frequency of 8–12 breaths per minute provide good ventilation and adequately

Fig. 43-10.—An endotracheal tube adapter (15 mm) of internal diameter 3, 4 or 5 mm is placed on the exhalation port of an Emerson Postoperative Ventilator to serve as an exhalational retard. (We now prefer to place a tubing from the exhalation port 5–10 cm under water, thus avoiding air trapping, which can occur if the patient coughs or gets out of phase with the ventilator, which has a fixed flow retard.)

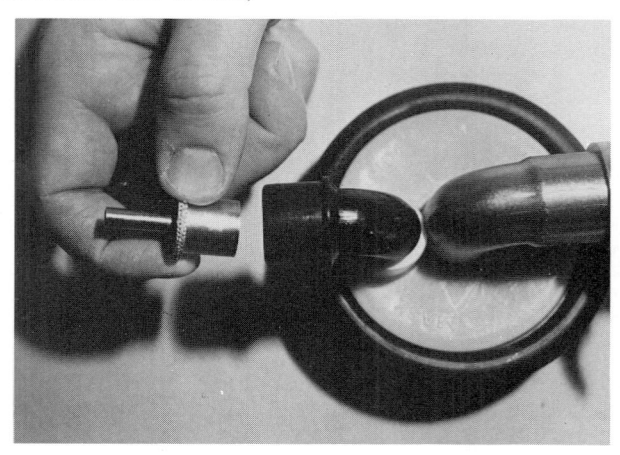

Chapter 43: MANAGEMENT OF RESPIRATORY FAILURE WITH CHEST TRAUMA / 1025

stabilize any flail segment.[24] Inspired oxygen is adjusted (Fig. 43-9) to achieve an arterial oxygen tension of 70–90 mm Hg. The Pa_{CO_2} should be kept between 30 and 40 mm Hg.* This may require the addition of mechanical dead space and reduction of the respirator rate.

When the $A-aDO_2$ is large, an expiratory retard that produces an end-expiratory pressure of 5–10 cm H_2O may improve oxygenation.[4]

Figure 43-10 shows an Emerson ventilator with a #4 endotracheal tube adapter fitted to the exhalation port. This constriction serves as an expiratory retard. Its effect on lung volume is shown in Figure 43-11. Cardiac output may be depressed by this maneuver[20] and, if so, can be treated with the transfusion of colloid.

GENERAL CARE

Figure 43-12 is a nursing care sheet used in the Respiratory Care Unit of the University of California at San Diego.

Physician's orders read as follows:

A. Ventilator: indicate time on or off; per cent oxygen, volume settings, degree of expiratory retard.

B. Tracheobronchial care:

1. Turn side-back-side every hour in supine and semi-Fowler's position. (Include trunk-down [5–10°] position twice daily unless medically or surgically contraindicated.)

2. Suction: Sterile, gloved endotracheal suction hourly or as needed. Precede with 6–8 chest hyperinflations, chest physiotherapy and instillation of 2–4 ml of normal saline. Take no more than 15 seconds for suctioning.† Follow with 6–8 chest hyperinflations. (NOTE:

---

*Except in patients having chronic hypercapnia. PCO_2 should be regulated to maintain pH values of between 7.35 and 7.45. Dosages: succinylcholine: 20–100 mg as bolus or 1 gm in 500 ml as concentrated infusion; gallamine: 20–60 mg IV every hour as needed; curare: 3–12 mg in increments every hour as needed.

†In severely affected patients, special precautions should be taken during endotracheal suctioning, as the PO_2 may fall precipitously.

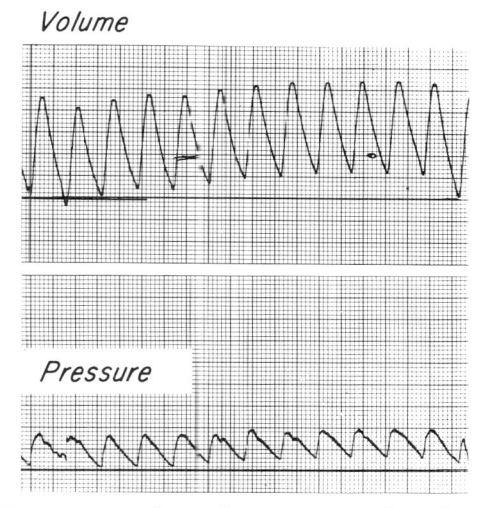

Fig. 43-11.—The volume stepup from baseline as end-expiratory pressure increases indicates an increment in FRC. Exhalational retard and end-expiratory pressures frequently will raise the Pa_{O_2} in acute trauma.

Most self-inflating bags give 50% oxygen; when the patient requires greater concentrations, an oxygen reservoir must be constructed [Fig. 43-13].) Chest physiotherapy in the postural drainage position facilitates removal of secretions. Differential endobronchial suction should be performed. If secretions are exceptionally tenacious, agents such as N-acetylcysteine may be helpful. Bronchodilators, intermittent ultrasonic nebulizations and antibiotics may be needed.

3. Sputum cultures twice weekly.

4. Deflation of the tracheostomy cuff is performed every 2–4 hours for $1/2$–2 minutes as tolerated, always with the patient in the head-down position. Prior to deflation, the mouth should be cleared of secretions and pressure should be applied with the ventilator or self-inflating bag as the cuff is deflated slowly. The cuff should be reinflated carefully just to the point of minimal leak during positive pressure. Overinflation of the cuff may damage or obstruct the trachea.

General measures include:

1. Weight daily: adult patients receiving only intravenous fluids lose 500 gm

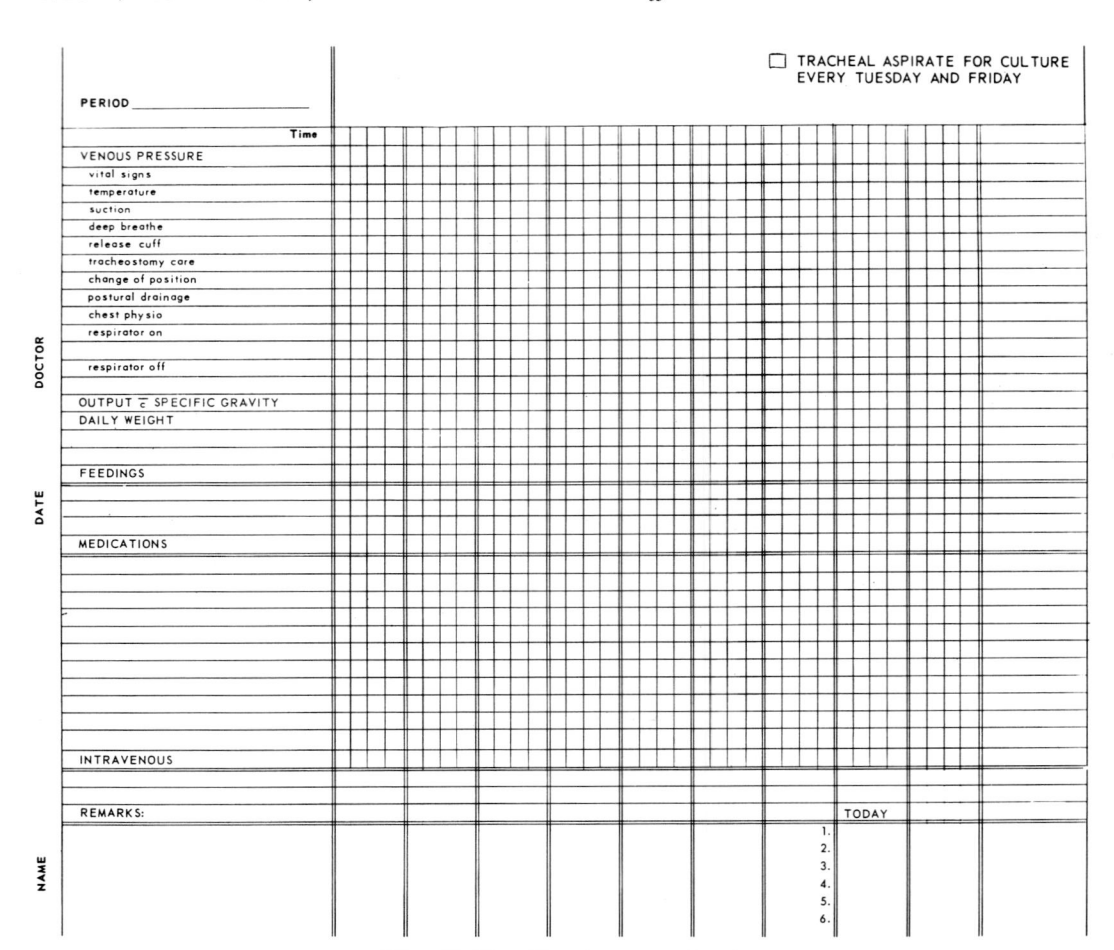

Fig. 43-12.—Nursing care sheet.

Fig. 43-13.—The large-bore corrugated tubing serves as an oxygen reservoir, allowing concentrations of oxygen nearer to 100% to be delivered by this self-inflating bag.

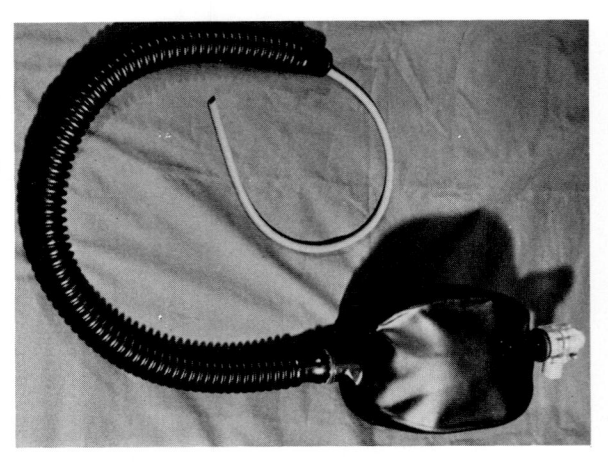

per day. A stable weight may indicate fluid retention.[39]

2. Periodic electrolyte, hematologic and hepatic function tests

3. Check all stool or gastric aspirate for blood.

4. Active and passive physical therapy exercises with special exercises to strengthen accessory muscles of respiration.

5. Nutrition

  a) Intravenous fluids are satisfactory for several days in most patients.

  b) Intravenous hyperalimentation may be useful when the gastrointestinal tract is defunctional.[15] Care must be taken, however, to avoid over-hydration.

  c) Oral alimentation can be accomplished in patients with tracheostomy or nasotracheal tubes. Before feeding with the cuff deflated, one can document protective laryngeal reflexes or a competent swallowing mechanism by having the patient drink a dilute methylene blue solution.[8] If none appears in the tracheal aspirate, proceed with feeding.

  d) If there is repeated aspiration with the cuff deflated and the patient has difficulty in swallowing with the cuff inflated, a soft Penrose feeding tube will allow feeding and minimize the hazard of tracheo-esophageal fistula.

6. Shivering in the hypoxic patient can be stopped by Thorazine or one of the muscle relaxants. Central venous and arterial pressure monitoring facilitates adjustment of intramuscular volume or vasopressor needs when these agents are used.

7. Digitalis and diuretics frequently are required by patients receiving respiratory care.

PHYSIOLOGIC ASSESSMENT OF RESPIRATORY FUNCTIONS

Daily measurements include:
1. Determination of alveolar to arterial oxygen gradient A-aDO$_2$ on 100% oxygen with simultaneous collection of expired gas for calculation of the VD/VT ratio.

2. Vital capacity and inspiratory force.
3. Periodic tests include:

  a) Fluoroscopy, if weaning is unexplainably prolonged and one suspects diaphragmatic fixation or paralysis.

  b) Tests not readily available but which are helpful include:
   i. Cardiac output determination.
   ii. Functional residual capacity measurements.
   iii. Flow-volume tracings.
   iv. Pulmonary artery and wedge pressures.

COMPLICATIONS OF MECHANICAL VENTILATION

The most serious problems are listed in Table 43-6. Other more minor practical problems, however, may also occur and, if not dealt with adequately, can seriously hamper the efficiency of the artificial ventilation.

1. Fighting the ventilator. Optimal efficiency of artificial ventilation requires that the patient and the machine operate synchronously. When "fighting" of the ventilator occurs, ventilation often is reduced and inspired oxygen concentrations are altered. The high airway pressures generated lead to depression of the circulation; in addition, the danger of a pneumothorax occurring increases.

Hypoxia or hypercapnia always must be considered as a possible cause, as these states stimulate respiratory drive. At times, the arterial blood gases may be normal, and the increased respiratory drive may be caused by CSF acidosis; e.g., caused by CSF hemorrhage.[19] Usually, however, this asynchrony is the result of an inappropriate ventilatory pattern with normal blood gases. Ensuring that tidal volumes are large (10–15 ml/kg) and that the PCO$_2$ is between 30 and 35 corrects the problem in most cases. Sudden alteration in pulmonary mechanics, however, may also affect the patient's comfort. This may occur when secretions have been retained, when a pneumothorax occurs or when the airway

TABLE 43-6.—COMPLICATIONS OF
MECHANICAL VENTILATION*

A. *Physiologic Effects*
 1. Cardiovascular system
  a) Reduced cardiac output when automatic function is impaired
 2. Respiratory system
  a) Artificial airway results in:
   i. Reduced bacterial defenses
   ii. Bypass of nasal filter and humidification
   iii. Less effective cough
  b) Improved V/Q from improved ventilatory pattern
  c) Reduced compliance
 3. CNS
  a) Increased venous pressure
  b) Reduced cerebral blood flow with overventilation
 4. Metabolism
  a) ? Reduced work of breathing
  b) Hormonal elaboration
   ? ADH, aldosterone with altered water metabolism
B. *Pathologic Developments*
 1. Pulmonary infections, atelectasis, sepsis. These can be avoided with chest physiotherapy, regular position change and suctioning
 2. Pneumothorax or subcutaneous emphysema†
 3. Wet lung
 4. GI bleeding
 5. Oxygen toxicity
 6. Tracheal damage: malacia or stenosis
 7. Ventilatory discoordination-diaphragmatic paralysis
 8. Psychosis

*Modified from Geffin, B.: Complications Associated with Ventilator Therapy, 1969. Annual Refresher Course Lectures, Annual Meeting of American Society of Anesthesiologists, October 25–29, 1969.
†Subcutaneous emphysema developing during mechanical ventilation may be caused by pneumothorax, malpositioned thoracostomy tube, subpleural alveolar rupture, carinal tear, mediastinal placement of tracheostomy tube or gas exiting at the tracheal stoma during continuous positive-pressure breathing.

becomes partly occluded for some other reason. Apprehension and pain aggravate the problem.

2. Development of an air leak from sudden rupture of cuff. This can cause a sudden reduction in alveolar ventilation and may require urgent remedy. Compression of the submental region causes the base of the tongue and epiglottis to compress the glottis and re-establish a leak-free system. Usually, however, it is more practical to increase the tidal volume delivered by the ventilator in order to compensate for the leak that is occurring.

3. Accidental decannulation. Failing successful recannulation, artificial ventilation must be resumed either with a tight-fitting anesthesia mask, 100% oxygen and a sponge occluding the leaking tracheal stoma or with mouth-to-mouth resuscitation. In the interim, preparations should be made for an endotracheal intubation.

4. Respiratory obstruction. Endotracheal tubes, being long, narrow and often difficult to keep clear with suction catheter, not infrequently develop occluding concretions from sputum unless humidity is carefully maintained. Nasotracheal tubes, although well tolerated, increase the airway resistance and work of breathing still further because of their increased length and tortuous route. In addition, nasal swelling and kinking can aggravate the situation further. Despite these problems, endotracheal intubation is the method of choice in all emergencies in preparation for tracheostomy and when an artificial airway is required for only a few days. It is a simple procedure, can be accomplished speedily and offers an efficient direct route to the patient's respiratory tree. Tracheostomy thus can be performed with the ensurance of adequate ventilation. Other airway problems that might occur are illustrated in Figures 43-14 and 43-15.

STABILIZATION OF THE FLAIL CHEST

Stabilization of a flail chest usually takes up to 3 weeks to occur; stabilization precedes complete healing.[1, 11, 16] Among 27 patients with flail chest treated in the Respiratory Care Unit of Massachusetts General Hospital, the interval for chest

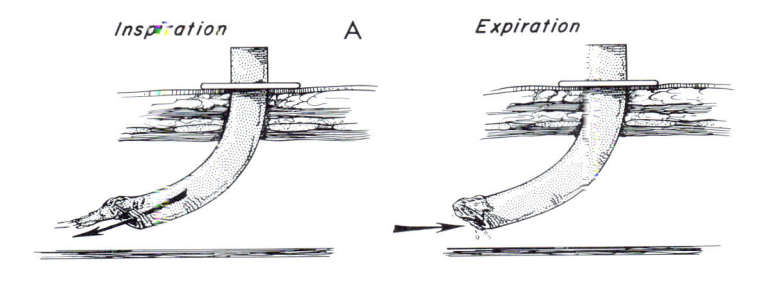

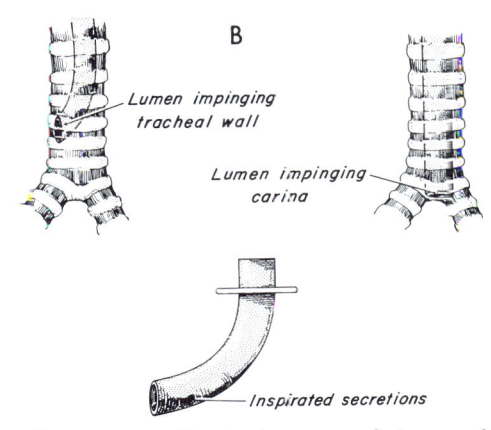

Fig. 43-14. — Common mechanical causes of airway obstruction.

stabilization was 2–42 days. Eighty-five per cent of these were stable within 20 days (mean 13 days). Mechanical ventilation usually was required for longer (3–61 days, mean 17 days) because of concomitant injuries and pulmonary damage. Efforts to wean before stability has been re-established causes the return of paradox and may delay the healing process.

WEANING FROM THE VENTILATOR

Weaning from ventilatory support begins when the following criteria for stability and over-all lung function are met:
1. Absence of gross paradox in a conscious, cooperative patient.
2. Vital capacity of 15 ml/kg or greater.
3. Effective cough mechanism.
4. Inspiratory force of −20 or greater.
5. A-aDO$_2$ on 100% oxygen less than 350 mm Hg.
6. VD/VT ratio of <0.6.

Frequently, the A-aDO$_2$ rises with spontaneous ventilation. Oxygen concentrations, therefore, need to be increased at this time and weaning periods increased as tolerated. The ability to breathe spontaneously during meals and throughout the night generally represents a rapidly declining need for artificial ventilation

EXTUBATION

Criteria for extubation include:
1. Successful weaning from the ventilator for at least 24 hours. This is associ-

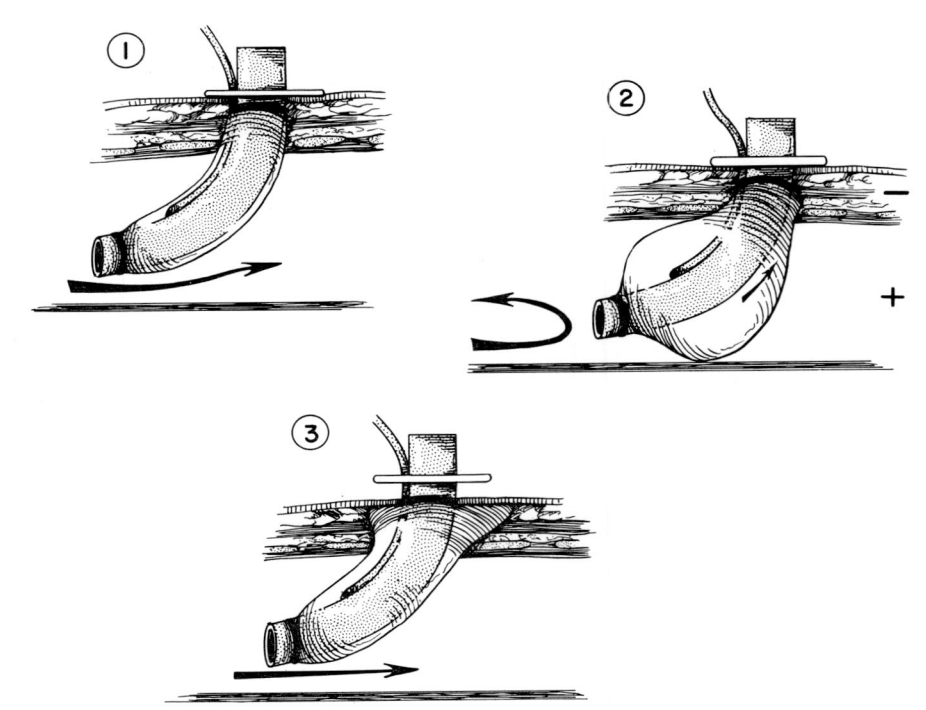

Fig. 43-15.—Migratory tracheostomy tube. Outward migration of the tube can occur if the cuff, which lies partly outside the trachea, is progressively inflated.

ated with an adequate vital capacity, inspiratory force and acceptable A-aDO$_2$ and VD/VT ratio.

2. An intact swallowing mechanism, protecting against aspiration.

3. An ability to cooperate for such supportive measures as IPPB, wearing of mask or nasal oxygen or taking deep breaths on command.

One may temporize by inserting a fenestrated tracheostomy tube,[8] tracheal button or small tracheostomy tube for 24 hours prior to extubation. This is acceptable particularly in patients with neuromuscular diseases, pre-existing pulmonary disease, or in those in whom reintubation or opening of the tracheostomy would be exceptionally difficult. In many younger, more vigorous patients, extubation may be accomplished directly without this intermediate step. Most patients need supplemental oxygen and supportive measures for several days after decannulation.

CONCLUSION

In this chapter the problems of acute respiratory insufficiency in relation to chest injuries have been described. These principles, however, apply generally to the management of all patients requiring artificial ventilation. A controlled respiratory care environment, close physiologic monitoring, meticulous attention to detail and the coordinated professional efforts of many individuals are essential for success.

EQUATIONS

1. Alveolar-arterial oxygen difference (A-aDO$_2$). To find alveolar oxygen tension:

$PA_{O_2} = Pb - Pa_{H_2O} - PA_{CO_2}$
(when breathing 100% O_2 for 15 minutes)
Pa_{O_2} = arterial oxygen tension
where PA_{O_2} = alveolar O_2
Pb = barometric pressure
PA_{H_2O} = 47 mm Hg at 37°
$PA_{CO_2} = Pa_{CO_2}$ = usually 40 mm Hg

E.g.: In a healthy young adult breathing 100% O_2:
A = 760 − 47 − 40
A = 673
Arterial blood values: Pa_{O_2} 573, Pa_{CO_2} 40, pH 7.40
∴ A-aDO_2 = 673 − 573
A-aDO_2 = 100 mm Hg

2. Dead space to tidal volume ratio
$$VD/VT = \frac{Pa_{CO_2} - PE_{CO_2}}{Pa_{CO_2}}$$
where VD = physiologic dead space
VT = tidal volume
Pa_{CO_2} = arterial carbon dioxide tension
PE_{CO_2} = mixed expired carbon dioxide tension

3. VD/VT − corrected for compressible volume
$$VD/VT^{corr} = \frac{Pa_{CO_2} - PE_{CO_2}{}^{corr}}{Pa_{CO_2}}$$

4. $PA_{O_2} = FI_{O_2}(Pb - P_{H_2O}) - Pa_{CO_2}$
$$\therefore FI_{O_2} = \frac{Pa_{O_2} + Pa_{CO_2}}{Pb - P_{H_2O}}$$

E.g.: A-aDO_2 = 400; desired Pa_{O_2} = 80
P_{CO_2} = 40
Pb = 760
$$FI_{O_2} = \frac{480 + 40}{760 - 47}$$
= 0.73 or 73%

BIBLIOGRAPHY

1. Abrams, L. D., and Clarke, D. B.: The management of thoracic injuries, Postgrad. Med. J. 43:639, 1967.
2. Alfano, S. S., and Hale, H. W.: Pulmonary contusion, J. Trauma 5:647, 1965.
3. Angostini, E., and Mead, J.: Statics of the Respiratory System, in Fenn, W. O., and Rahn, H. (eds.), Handbook of Physiology, Sec. 3, Respiration (Washington, D. C.: American Physiological Society, 1964, Vol. I, Chap. 13, pp. 387–407.
4. Ashbaugh, D. G., Petty, T. L., Bigelow, D. B., and Harris, T.M.: Continuous positive-pressure breathing (CPPB) in the adult respiratory distress syndrome, J Thorac. Cardiovasc. Surg. 57:31, 1969.
5. Avery, E. A., Mörch, E. T., and Benson, D. W.: Critically crushed chests, J. Thorac. Surg. 32: 291, 1956.
6. Baragh, W., Greths, H. W. C., and Slawson, K. B.: Crush injuries of the chest, Br. Med. J. 2:131, 1967.
7. Bassett, J. S.: Blunt injuries to the chest, J. Trauma 8:418, 1968.
8. Bendixen, H. H., Egbert, L. D., Hedley-Whyte, J., Laver, M. B., and Pontoppidan, H.: Respiratory Care (St. Louis: The C. V. Mosby Company, 1965), Chap. 15.
9. Bendixen, H., and Laver, M. B.: Hypoxia in anesthesia: A review, Clin. Pharmacol. Ther. 6: 510, 1965.
10. Brewer, L. A., Burbank, B., Samson, P. C., and Schiff, C. A.: The "wet lung" in war casualties, Ann. Surg. 123:343, 1946.
11. Brewer, L. A., and Steiner, L. C.: The management of crushing injuries of the chest, Surg. Clin. North Am. 48:1279, 1968.
12. Chinard, F. P.: The Permeability Characteristics of the Pulmonary Blood-Gas Barrier, in Caro, C. (ed.), Advances in Respiratory Physiology (Baltimore: The Williams & Wilkins Company, 1966) pp. 106–144.
13. Comroe, J., et al.: The Lung (2d ed.; Chicago: Year Book Medical Publishers, Inc., 1962).
14. Cooper, J. D., and Grillo, H. C.: The evolution of tracheal injury due to ventilatory assistance through cuffed tubes: A pathologic study, Ann. Surg. 169:334, 1969.
15. Dudrick, S. J., Wilmore, D. W., and Vars, H. M.: Long-term total parenteral nutrition with growth, development and positive nitrogen balance, Surgery 64:134, 1968.
16. Duff, J. H.: Flail chest: A clinical and physiological study, J. Trauma 8:63, 1968.
17. Fatal Motor Vehicular Accidents. Stat. Bull. Metropol. Life Ins Co. 50:7, 1969.
18. Frey, C. F., Huelke, D. F., and Gikas, P. W.: Resuscitation and survival in motor vehicular accidents, J. Trauma 9:292, 1969.
19. Froman, C., and Crampton-Smith, A.: Hyperventilation associated with low pH of cerebrospinal fluid after intracranial haemorrhage, Lancet 1:780, 1955.
20. Geffin, B.: Personal communication.
21. Geffin, B., and Pontoppidan, H.: Reduction of tracheal damage by the prestretching of inflatable cuffs, Anesthesiology 31:162, 1969.
22. Grillo, H. C.: The management of tracheal stenosis following assisted respiration, J. Thorac. Cardiovasc. Surg. 57:52, 1969.
23. Hedley-Whyte, J.: Personal communication.
24. Hedley-Whyte, J., Pontoppidan, H., and Morris, M. J.: The response of patients with respiratory failure and cardiopulmonary disease to different levels of constant volume ventilation, J. Clin. Invest. 45:1543, 1966.
25. Hughes, R. K.: Thoracic trauma, Surg. Clin. North Am. 48:789 1968.
26. Jackson, C., and Jackson, C. L.: Tracheotomy, Am. J. Surg. 46:519, 1939.

27. Jackson, F. R.: Traumatic aortic rupture after blunt trauma, Dis. Chest 53:577, 1968.
28. Kilman, J. W., and Charnock, E.: Thoracic trauma in infancy and childhood, J. Trauma 9:863, 1969.
29. McGrath, J. P.: Burst trachea, Br. J. Surg. 55:77, 1968.
30. Mulder, D. S., and Rubush, J. L.: Complications of tracheostomy: Relationship to long-term ventilatory assistance, J. Trauma 9:389, 1969.
31. Murphy, D. A., MacLean, L. D., and Dobell, A. R. C.: Tracheal stenosis as a complication of tracheostomy, Ann. Thorac. Surg. 2:44, 1966.
32. Nadel, J. W., Wolfe, W. G., Graf, P. D., Youker, N., Zamel, G. H., Austin, J. H. M., Hinchcliffe, W. A., Greenspan, R. H., and Wright, R. R.: Powdered tantalum for roentgenographic examination of human airways, N. Engl. J. Med. 283:281, 1970.
33. Perry, J. F., and Galway, C. F.: Chest injuries due to blunt trauma, J. Thorac. Cardiovasc. Surg. 49:684, 1965.
34. Pontoppidan, H.: Personal communication.
35. Pontoppidan, H.: Bedside pulmonary function tests and their interpretation. Fourth Annual Symposium on Acute Medicine, Respiratory Intensive Care. University of Pittsburgh, Pittsburgh, Pennsylvania, May 14–16, 1970.
36. Radford, E. P.: Ventilation standards for use in artificial respiration, J. Appl. Physiol. 7:451, 1955.
37. Safar, P., and Kinkel, H. G.: *Prolonged Artificial Ventilation in Clinical Anesthesia/Respiratory Therapy* (Philadelphia: F. A. Davis Company, 1965), p. 132.
38. Skillman, J. J., Parikh, B. M., and Tanenbaum, B. J.: Pulmonary arteriovenous admixture, improvement with albumin and diuresis, Am. J. Surg. 119:440, 1970.
39. Sladen, A., Laver, M. B., and Pontoppidan, H.: Pulmonary complications associated with water retention during prolonged mechanical ventilation, N. Engl. J. Med. 279:448, 1968.
40. Suwa, K., and Bendixen, H. H.: Change in Pa_{CO_2} with mechanical dead space during artificial ventilation, J. Appl. Physiol. 24:556, 1968.
41. Wylie, W. D., and Churchill-Davidson, H. C.: *A Practice of Anaesthesia* (Chicago: Year Book Medical Publishers, Inc., 1960), p. 598.
42. Wylie, W. D., and Churchill-Davidson, H. C.: *A Practice of Anaesthesia* (Chicago: Year Book Medical Publishers, Inc., 1960), p. 584.

44 | Management of Abdominal Injuries

GRANT V. RODKEY and CLAUDE E. WELCH

IN THIS CHAPTER, consideration will be limited to those types of abdominal visceral injuries inflicted by external trauma. Iatrogenic or "spontaneous" visceral injuries will be deliberately excluded. Since wounds of the liver and extrahepatic biliary system are described in a separate chapter, they will be omitted from this discussion.

GENERAL CONSIDERATIONS

Abdominal injuries are relatively frequent in both military and civilian experience. In the former, most such wounds are the result of penetrating missiles or metallic fragments whereas the majority of civilian cases result from nonpenetrating or blunt trauma. Nevertheless, blast injuries and other mechanisms contribute significant numbers of blunt abdominal injuries to military experience, and an increasing incidence of penetrating abdominal wounds is seen in civilian hospitals as a consequence of the rising frequency of violent crimes in urban areas. In either situation, the difficulties of diagnosis and treatment may be enhanced significantly by pre-existing disease, by drug or alcohol usage and especially by multiple systems injuries, often including brain damage.

Penetrating abdominal wounds in civilian practice are not usually associated with injuries to other systems and permit prompt diagnosis and treatment with low mortality rates. If the fact of visceral injury is not immediately apparent on admission, x-ray examination of the wound tract and attentive observation of the patient's progress may, in some cases, eliminate the need for laparotomy. Increased severity of wounding and the lack of facilities for close observation make nonoperative treatment of penetrating abdominal injuries impractical among military casualties

On the other hand, blunt abdominal injuries often do not immediately declare the need for surgical repair and frequently are associated with injuries to other organ systems that may mask the diagnosis and complicate the treatment. Thus, it is among this group of patients that mortality and morbidity following abdominal trauma are greatest.

DIAGNOSIS OF ABDOMINAL VISCERAL INJURY

Penetrating abdominal wounds may produce evident injury to abdominal organs, as manifested by severe pain, shock, increasing abdominal girth or partial evisceration If such signs are absent, plain and upright or lateral decubitus x-ray examination may demonstrate free gas beneath the diaphragm if a hollow viscus has been penetrated. If the diagnosis remains in doubt, injection of the sinus tract with Hypaque may establish whether the peritoneal cavity has been entered. If the diagnosis of visceral injury still remains in doubt, repeated examinations to elicit evidence of pain, tenderness, spasm, shock or sepsis should be carried out. Finally, one always should suspect abdominal injury in the presence of penetrating wounds of the chest, back, buttocks or thigh.

Blunt abdominal trauma is associated with much greater difficulty in the diagnosis of visceral injury. Furthermore, such injuries commonly are associated with head injuries, thoracic injuries, fractures, extensive soft tissue damage and shock, so that immediate appropriate treatment must be instituted if the patient is to be saved. Thus, in many cases, diagnosis and treatment must proceed simultaneously and proper management may require immediate transfer of the patient to the operating room.

Symptoms

If the patient is conscious, symptoms of abdominal injury include pain, nausea, vomiting, hematemesis, hematuria, anxiety, thirst and air hunger. Of these, the most constant is pain, which may vary from mild to severe, may be localized or generalized over the abdomen or may be referred to the back or to the shoulders as a manifestation of diaphragmatic irritation.

Physical Signs

Local physical signs that may indicate underlying visceral injury include evidence of a wound tract, severe contusion or ecchymosis, fractures of lower ribs on either side or of the pelvis, tenderness, spasm, absence of liver dullness, diminished or absent peristaltic sounds, shifting dullness and increasing abdominal girth. Digital rectal examination should not be omitted, and if blood is encountered, sigmoidoscopy should be included in the examination. Urine should be examined promptly for evidence of gross and microscopic hematuria. In all cases of severe trauma, a Foley catheter should be inserted into the bladder and placed on gravity drainage. A nasogastric tube should be passed and the gastric aspirate should be examined for gross or occult blood. This tube should be left in place and allowed to drain.

Systemic signs of visceral injury include rapid respiratory rate, rising pulse rate and falling blood pressure. Every severely injured patient should have vital signs monitored and charted at intervals not greater than 15–30 minutes over the first few hours of observation. During the first few hours after wounding, the development of shock without external blood loss should be assumed to be due to interstitial or intracavitary hemorrhage; later, sepsis and peritonitis may contribute to the severity of the signs. In this regard, it should be remembered that head injuries rarely cause shock, although they may be associated with bradycardia and widened pulse pressure.

Diagnostic Paracentesis

Almost to be considered as an extension of the physical examination is the use of abdominal paracentesis to identify intraperitoneal hemorrhage. There are several acceptable techniques for this, but a very satisfactory method is to insert a large-bore Intracath well out in each flank directed into the peritoneal cavity. This can be accomplished painlessly with local anesthesia, and if no fluid is encountered, the plastic tubes may be left for later aspiration. If initial paracentesis is negative, it should be repeated at subsequent intervals if signs of intraabdominal injury persist. An alternative method is to perform the paracentesis with a peritoneal dialysis set, infuse Ringer's lactate into the peritoneal cavity and then allow the infusate to siphon off to be examined for evidence of blood.

Although the paracentesis should be positive in more than 50% of cases of abdominal visceral injury, failure to obtain blood or fluid on repeated aspirations does not exclude such injuries. Finally, if aspirate is obtained, it should be examined for amylase content as a clue to pancreatic injury.

X-ray Examination

The early use of x-ray examination as an adjunct to the diagnosis of abdominal visceral injury is advisable. Plain and erect or lateral decubitus films of the abdomen may reveal foreign bodies, enlargement or loss of detailed outlines of liver or spleen, obliteration of the psoas shadows, free gas in the peritoneal cavity or retroperitoneal planes, serrated filling defects along the greater curvature of the stomach or evidence of separation of bowel loops by intraperitoneal fluid. The finding of fractures in the lower thoracic cage on either side, fractures of the bodies or transverse processes of the spine or fractures of the pelvis may give further clues as to the possible nature of underlying visceral injury. Fractures of the left lower ribs often are associated with damage to the spleen and fractures of the right lower ribs are associated with damage to the liver. Fractured transverse processes of vertebrae D8–L2 often are accompanied by injuries to the kidney. Fractures of the pelvis may cause tears of the urethra or bladder and may be associated with severe retroperitoneal hemorrhage from extensive bone injury or tears of the iliac veins and their tributaries.

If more than a few red cells are found on urinalysis, an intravenous or infusion pyelogram should be done as soon as feasible, in order to discover whether one or two kidneys are present and to assess the degree of renal damage. Even in an unprepared patient, this study will demonstrate the presence or absence of gross damage to the kidneys.

Selective angiography recently has become an important adjunct in the evaluation of the injured patient (see Chapter 10). If intravenous pyelograms do not clearly define the extent of renal injury, selective angiography should be performed. This examination may be extremely helpful in the acutely injured patient in cases of suspected aortic intimal dissection and thrombosis and in cases of severe hemorrhage associated with extensive fractures of the pelvic girdle. Among patients in whom delayed splenic rupture is questioned, and in those who may exhibit hematobilia as a late manifestation after trauma, selective angiography may be of critical importance.

Radiographic study of a wound tract may be quite informative in cases in which doubt exists as to whether the peritoneal cavity has been entered. The examination must be performed with attention to detail – particularly in prevention of backflow of the contrast medium from the external opening of the wound tract. Interpretation is not always easy and errors have included both false negative and false positive readings. Even with this aid, the surgeon who delays exploring a penetrating abdominal wound assumes a heavy responsibility.

In cases of pelvic injury, cystograms with anteroposterior and oblique views may reveal the presence of retroperitoneal pelvic hematomas as well as information regarding the integrity of the bladder.

Finally, in some cases, instillation of opaque contrast material into the gastrointestinal tract may give valuable information. Barium should be avoided, but Gastrografin or Hypaque may be injected safely through a Levin tube and may reveal ruptures of stomach, duodenum or jejunum. In cases of intramural hematoma of these organs, this maneuver has been especially informative.

GENERAL TREATMENT

Resuscitation and Early Supportive Therapy

In the patient with multiple severe injuries, physical examination and diagnostic procedures must be integrated with urgently required therapy for life support. The immediate requirement in every case is adequate respiratory exchange. Usually, in an unconscious patient or one with severe trauma to head, neck or thorax, this is accomplished most expeditiously by tracheal intubation with a cuffed endotracheal tube. The cuff is inflated and respirations are controlled manually if respiratory failure is noted.

The second step in priority is control of external blood loss. Local compression or clamping exposed bleeding vessels should accomplish this within moments of the patient's admission. Rarely, a tourniquet may be required.

Restoration of circulating blood volume is the third objective of resuscitation. To be accomplished rapidly, this requires a large intravenous conduit, which always must be located above the diaphragm. If the veins in the arms are collapsed and inaccessible, the external jugular or subclavian veins may be cannulated swiftly. Failing this, an antecubital cutdown should be carried out immediately. In either case, a long plastic cannula should be used to permit monitoring of the central venous pressure (CVP) and a large blood sample should be drawn. Part of the sample should be dispatched by messenger to the blood bank; the remainder should be sent to the laboratory for appropriate examinations. These should include hemogram and amylase. Pending the receipt of crossmatched whole blood, circulatory support should be accomplished by rapid infusion of crystalloid solutions, plasma, dextran, albumin or universal donor blood (Type O Rh D negative) as the requirements indicate.

Finally, whenever indicated by the severity and location of the injuries, an antigravity suit may be used to help stabilize the patient's circulatory function. This may be especially helpful in cases of pelvic fracture with massive retroperitoneal hemorrhage.

Antibiotics

Patients with suspected abdominal visceral injuries should be given broad-spectrum antibiotic therapy. In patients who have not been sensitized previously, intravenous penicillin in dosages of 2.5 million units every 6 hours may be combined with streptomycin, 0.5 gm intramuscularly every 12 hours. Alternatively, ampicillin in dosages of 2.0 gm every 6 hours or tetracycline in amounts of 0.5 gm every 6 hours may be given intravenously. Wounds should be cultured and antibiotic therapy should be tailored to demonstrated bacterial sensitivities.

Gastric Aspiration

The importance of gastric aspiration as a diagnostic aid has been noted. A Levin tube left in the stomach will reduce the danger of aspiration of gastric contents during operation, reduce the hazard of peritoneal contamination in cases of injury to hollow viscera and aid in prevention of postoperative distention and wound dehiscence. At times, however, a Levin tube will not collapse the stomach completely, particularly if a large meal had been ingested shortly before injury. The stomach then should be emptied by insertion of a large-bore tube and gastric lavage before induction of anesthesia.

Urinary Drainage

A Foley catheter should be inserted into every severely wounded patient and placed on gravity drainage. It gives immediate evidence of continuing or delayed hematuria and also provides an accurate index of urine output. Usually, an amount of 50 ml/hour of urine indicates satisfactory circulatory and renal function. When used in conjunction with CVP monitoring, the rate of urine output provides a sensitive indication of the patient's response to restorative treatment.

Laparotomy

As soon as the diagnosis of abdominal visceral injury has become reasonably certain, the patient should be explored at the earliest moment consistent with his adequate response to resuscitative measures. In a few instances, continued intraabdominal hemorrhage will be so furious that laparotomy and control of hemorrhage must be included among the immediate lifesaving requirements. In less urgent cases, early laparotomy permits control of continued peritoneal bacterial soiling and enzymatic digestion as well as persistent hemorrhage.

In general, laparotomy will be required in all penetrating wounds, in all patients with rupture of the urethra or bladder, all patients with extensive disruption of the kidney, patients with x-ray evidence of free gas in the peritoneal cavity and those patients who yield free blood on peritoneal tap or lavage. Those cases of blunt abdominal trauma that do not present clear-cut evidence of underlying visceral injury pose a difficult dilemma: Is it more dangerous to delay or to operate? Such instances require skillful, individualized surgical judgment, which must also take into consideration such matters as age of the patient, obesity, extent of associated injuries and available resources for treatment. Occasional instances of negative exploration inevitably result from erroneous evaluation; this may be preferable to sustaining increased mortality by delaying or withholding laparotomy in such doubtful situations.

In some cases of severe, multiple injuries, laparotomy should be carried out simultaneously with operations by other operating teams (neurosurgical, orthopedic). Such patients usually are received in severe shock, and a high proportion of them fall in the group who respond poorly to resuscitative treatment. Mortality rates in treatment of such desperate injuries will be expected to exceed 60%.

Anesthesia

In cases of suspected abdominal injury, general anesthesia that permits delivery of oxygen in high concentration through a cuffed, inflated endotracheal tube and complete muscle relaxation is a basic requirement. Rapid induction and placement of the endotracheal tube are particularly important to avoid regurgitation and aspiration in patients who have ingested food shortly prior to wounding.

Patients who have sustained combined abdominal and thoracic injuries present special anesthesia problems, which may include instability of the chest wall, compression of lungs by air, blood or abdominal viscera, pulmonary contusion or laceration, bronchial rupture, cardiac contusion and hemopericardium. Accurate preoperative assessment of these problems is essential. Rarely, thoracotomy must take precedence over laparotomy in resuscitative treatment in these complicated cases.

Incisions

Placement of abdominal incisions will depend on the location of wounds, if any. Wound tracts should be avoided and debrided only after completion of laparotomy and suture of the incision. Paramedian incisions offer maximal flexibility in respect to length and exposure and permit strong closure. Figure-of-eight sutures of #34-gauge monofilament stainless steel wire to the rectus fascia combined with frequently placed retention sutures to include the deep fascia will give excellent support to these incisions.

In the instances in which thoracoabdominal incisions may be required, the upper end of the paramedian incision may be extended obliquely across the costal margin at the appropriate level. Stabilization of these wounds may be enhanced by a figure-of-eight wire suture to reapproximate the costal margin. In many cases of combined abdominothoracic trauma, separate abdominal and thoracic incisions may be preferable for security of wound closure. Enterostomies and drains, if required, should be brought out through separate incisions from the primary laparotomy.

Control of Hemorrhage

In cases of visceral injury accompanied by massive intraperitoneal hemorrhage, release of intra-abdominal pressure by opening the peritoneum may be accompanied by a precipitous fall in blood pressure and cardiac arrest. This should be anticipated by having large-bore intravenous conduits with transfusions running in each arm and preparations to hasten the infusions by pressure if necessary. A minimum of 8–10 units of whole blood should be immediately at hand in the operating room at the commencement of the incision. Entry through the abdominal wall should be swift, and there should be an adequate number of operative assistants to permit manual compression with gauze packs placed over organs that are the sites of major hemorrhage. In children and young adults who have sustained extreme blood loss, consideration should be given to cross-clamping the abdominal aorta to divert all the available blood volume to the vital organs. If there is massive bleeding from a burst liver, primary manual compression must be supplemented by cross-clamping the portal triad and perhaps by obstructing backflow through the hepatic veins as described in Chapter 45. Tears in the vena cava or aorta may bleed freely into the peritoneal cavity and should be compressed manually while dissection is carried out to obtain proximal and distal control; appropriate repair of the defect then should be accomplished at once.

Hemorrhage from ruptured spleen or from mesenteric tears may also be massive. Such bleeding should be controlled manually or by clamping identified points of arterial hemorrhage pending definitive treatment of the problem, as described in later sections.

Retroperitoneal hemorrhage may be present with or without free intraperitoneal bleeding. Injuries to the great vessels, mesenteric tears, lacerations of renal vessels or kidneys or pelvic fractures with sacroiliac separations are the chief sources of such hematomas. Unless they are found coincidentally with large intraperitoneal bleeding, they are not likely to cause profound shock as an immediate consequence to laparotomy.

Fortunately, many cases of abdominal injury will not present such massive bleeding. In any event, control of hemorrhage remains the first priority after the initial incision.

Control of Fecal Contamination

Disruption of the hollow viscera contributes fecal and bacterial contamination, which should be controlled as soon as hemorrhage has been stanched. Wounds of the right colon permitting escape of liquid feces with a high concentration of mixed bacterial flora are most serious in this respect. Initial study for colonic tears should begin at the cecum and progress distalward to the rectum. Defects discovered should be closed temporarily with noncrushing clamps until evaluation of the entire enteric tract has been completed.

On completion of inspection of the colon, the terminal ileum should be identified, and examination cephalward on the bowel should be continued to the ligament of Treitz.

Inspection of the duodenum should be accompanied by incision of its lateral peritoneal attachments and reflection forward of the second portion if any evidence of duodenal injury is noted. Wounds of the third and fourth portions of the duodenum may be exposed by reflecting the right colon and its mesentery and incising the ligament of Treitz.

If there is evidence of gastric injury,

the gastrocolic omentum should be divided to allow access to the lesser omental bursa and inspection of the posterior gastric wall.

During the entire exploratory phase of the operation, each defect should be temporarily occluded; no attempt at specific treatment is indicated until the extent of injuries has been defined.

TREATMENT OF SPECIFIC INJURIES

Spleen

Ruptures of the spleen usually are readily apparent on exploration. Less evident are contusions or subcapsular hematomas. All splenic injuries should be managed by splenectomy to avoid the hazard of delayed rupture of this organ—an event occurring in most instances within 2 weeks of wounding but rarely as late as 2 years postinjury.

Certain technical features are important in splenectomy (Fig. 44-1). First, the spleen is mobilized from its bed by gentle manual dissection, bringing it forward so that the pedicle can be visualized accurately. This is facilitated by packing a large gauze sponge into the former splenic bed during the remainder of the operation. Careful attention must be given to gastric decompression to avoid aspiration secondary to pressure on the stomach during the manipulations and to avoid inadvertent gastric injury during the procedure. Unless care is exercised, injury to the tail of the pancreas may occur when the splenic pedicle is clamped. Whenever possible, the splenic artery and vein should be ligated separately—each with a ligature of #0 chromic catgut and a stitch ligature of nonabsorbable suture material. Throughout the procedure, vigilance should be exercised to avoid injury to the adjacent splenic flexure of the colon.

In some cases, hemorrhage in the hilum of the spleen may make identification of the vessels quite difficult. In such an event, splenic artery and vein may be dissected through the lesser omental bursa along the superior border of the pancreas.

If the splenic injury is associated with fragmentation of the organ, an attempt should be made to remove all the tissue debris to prevent the late complication of splenosis.

Pancreas

Due perhaps to its rather inaccessible and protected location, injuries to the pancreas are sustained infrequently and recognized less often. Pancreatic injury should be suspected particularly in all direct blows to the upper abdomen, penetrating wounds of the upper abdomen and upper lumbar region and in injuries marked by transmission of great force to the torso. Clues to the presence of pancreatic disruption may be elevated amylase levels in the blood or peritoneal aspirate and, in severe cases, decreased concentration of blood calcium. With or without such indications, every laparotomy for abdominal trauma should include careful examination of the pancreas. In thin patients, division of the gastrohepatic omentum gives good access to the body and tail of the pancreas; in other cases, it may be necessary to expose the organ by division of the gastrocolic omentum. Evidence of pancreatic injury may include blood-stained fluid, edema, retroperitoneal hematoma, fat necrosis, contusion or transection of the pancreas. Associated injuries to the duodenum, extrahepatic bile ducts, stomach and transverse colon should be carefully excluded.

The surgical management of pancreatic injuries is controversial and must be adapted to each case, with attention to associated injuries and the general condition of the patient. It is generally agreed that accurate hemostasis and sump drainage is mandatory. With respect to the treatment of severe contusions or transections of the pancreas there is less una-

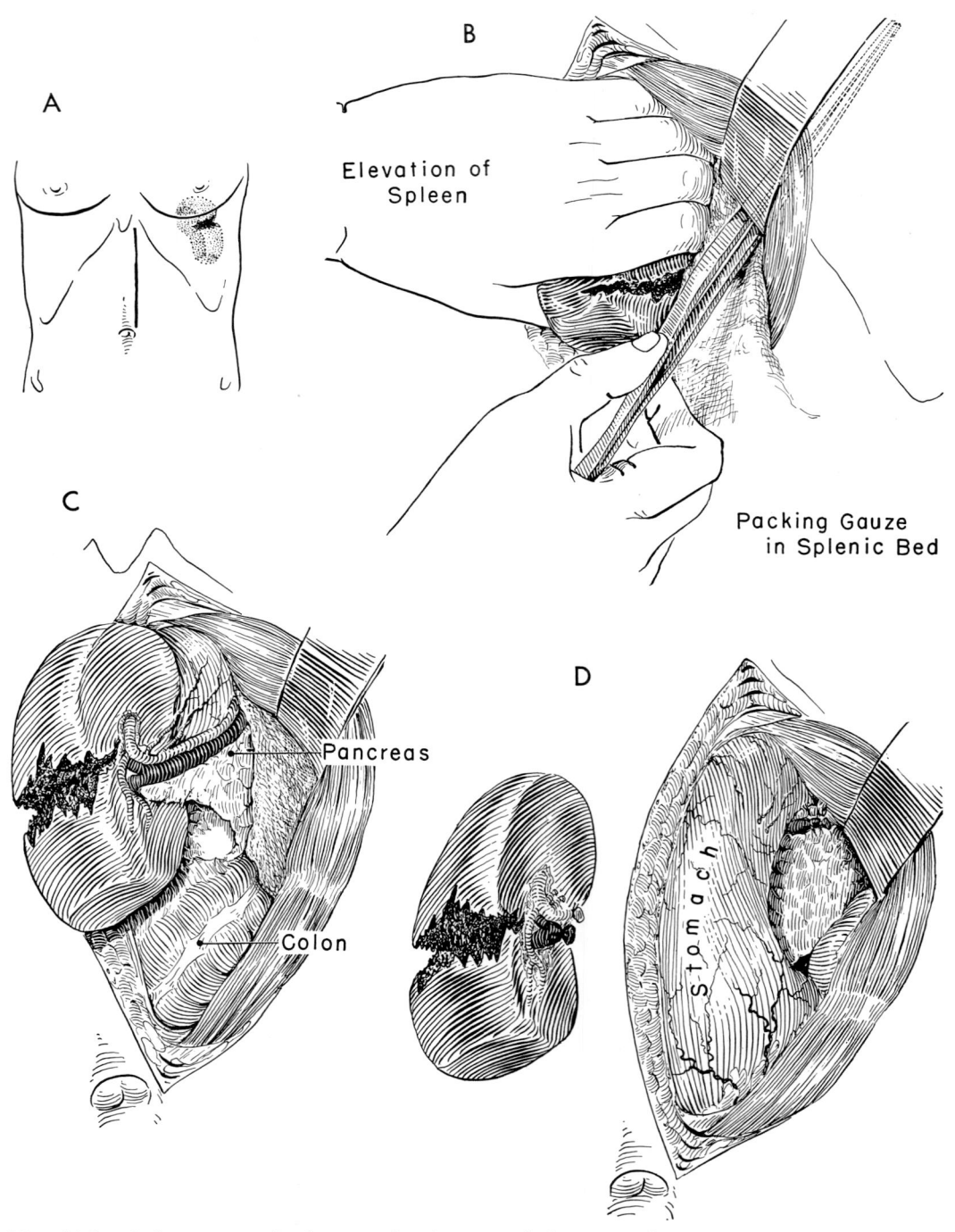

Fig. 44-1.—Splenectomy for lacerated spleen. **A,** left paramedian incision. **B,** elevation of spleen by packing gauze against diaphragm. **C,** showing intimate relationship of pancreas, stomach and colon. **D,** appearance after individual ligation of splenic vessels.

nimity of opinion. In general, when the circumstances of injury and the condition of the patient permit extended operating time, it is advisable to attempt preservation of pancreatic tissue by bringing up a loop of jejunum Roux en Y for reconstruction. In other situations, resection of the damaged distal pancreas should be performed (Fig. 44-2). Complications are frequent and may include hemorrhage, abscess, pseudocyst and external fistula. Decompression of the biliary tract by cholecystostomy or T-tube choledochostomy should be considered in cases of extensive pancreatic injury.

Stomach

Injuries to the stomach are relatively infrequent, usually are due to penetrating wounds and often are associated with injuries to surrounding viscera. Blunt injuries to the stomach may follow direct, high-velocity blows to a localized area in the epigastrium and may vary in severity from laceration to complete transection of the body of the stomach, the pylorus or the cardia.

At exploration, adequate exposure of both anterior and posterior walls of the stomach has been emphasized. Wounds should be debrided, converted to linear configuration by traction sutures and closed by suture. In most instances, continuous suture with #2-0 chromic catgut through all layers as the first row is desirable for accurate hemostasis; in addition, specific arteries in the gastric wall should be ligated individually. An outer row of interrupted nonabsorbable sutures to the seromuscular layer completes the repair. Postoperative decompression by Levin tube or gastrostomy should be routine. Rarely, extensive gastric injuries may require repair by bringing up a loop of jejunum and suturing it to the stomach. In rare instances, partial gastric resection and Billroth II reconstruction may be indicated. In cases of transection of the cardia or lower esophagus, interposition of a segment of jejunum or colon may be required.

Duodenum

Wounds of the duodenum occur in approximately 5% of abdominal visceral injuries, more commonly due to penetrating than to blunt trauma. In either case, there is a high incidence of associated injuries to surrounding organs. Penetrating injuries may vary from simple lacerations to those with extensive destruction of the duodenal wall — as from the blast of a shotgun or missile. Typically, nonpenetrating injuries result from sharp blows to the epigastrium and do not cause extensive destruction of the duodenum. A small proportion of these are located in the retroperitoneal portion of the duodenum — a situation that may obscure and delay the diagnosis. Contusion of the duodenum may result in formation of an intramural hematoma, which may either subside spontaneously or result in obstruction, delayed necrosis and disruption of the duodenal wall.

At exploration, disruption of the duodenum may be evident immediately or, in case of retroperitoneal tears, may be indicated by surrounding hematoma with varying degrees of black or green discoloration secondary to leakage of duodenal contents. If any evidence of duodenal injury is noted, complete exposure of the organ is mandatory. All surrounding organs must be subjected to the most careful scrutiny to detect associated injuries. Specifically, stomach, pancreas, liver, extrahepatic biliary tract, jejunum, transverse colon and right kidney should be included in this study.

There is no general pattern of surgical repair to fit the variety of injuries that occur in this area, but some universal principles apply. These include accurate hemostasis, debridement of necrotic tissue, restoration of integrity of the gastrointestinal tract and its tributary biliary and pancreatic ducts, conservation of all

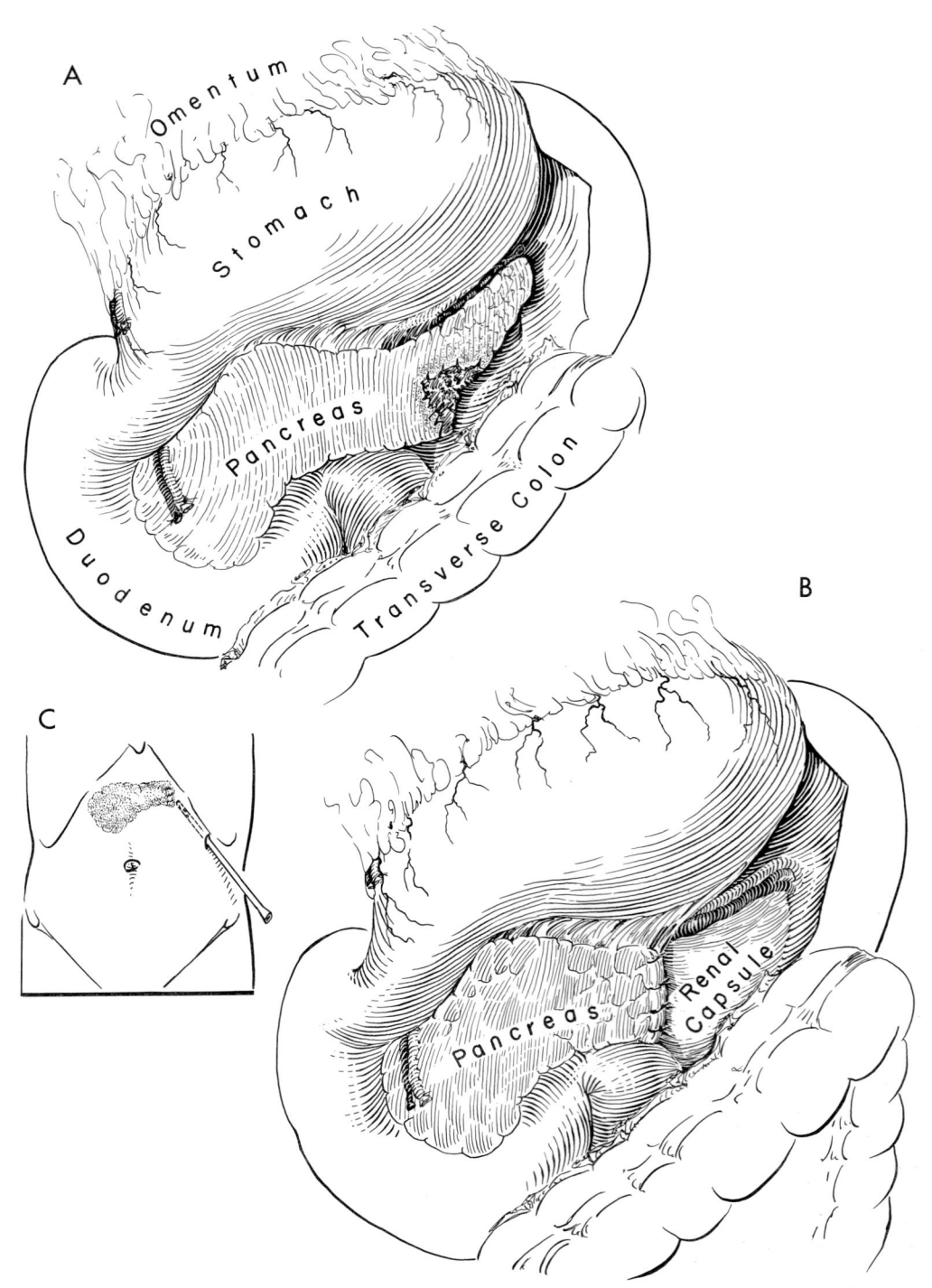

Fig. 44-2.—Repair of contusion of tail of pancreas. **A,** pancreas exposed through the gastrocolic omentum. **B,** resection of tail. **C,** drainage instituted through left flank.

nontraumatized tissue, adequate drainage, postoperative gastric decompression by Levin tube or gastrostomy and, in selected cases, T-tube drainage of the common bile duct. Wounds without extensive tissue destruction may be treated by debridement and two-layer suture or by direct anastomosis (Fig. 44-3). Patients with more extensive loss of duodenal wall may be patched by bringing up a loop of jejunum and suturing it over the defect. Other maneuvers that may be useful in these complicated cases include the bringing up of a loop of jejunum Roux en Y for jejunoplasty, duodenojejunostomy (side-to-side or end-to-side), gastroduodenostomy, partial gastrectomy with Billroth II anastomosis (perhaps with vagotomy) and pancreaticoduodenectomy. Unfortunately, escalation of the magnitude of the operative procedure in such cases all too frequently is bal-

Fig. 44-3.—Repair of laceration of posterior surface of duodenum. **A**, mobilization of duodenum by cutting the lateral peritoneal attachments and reflecting the right colon downward. **B**, closure of duodenum by two layers of sutures.

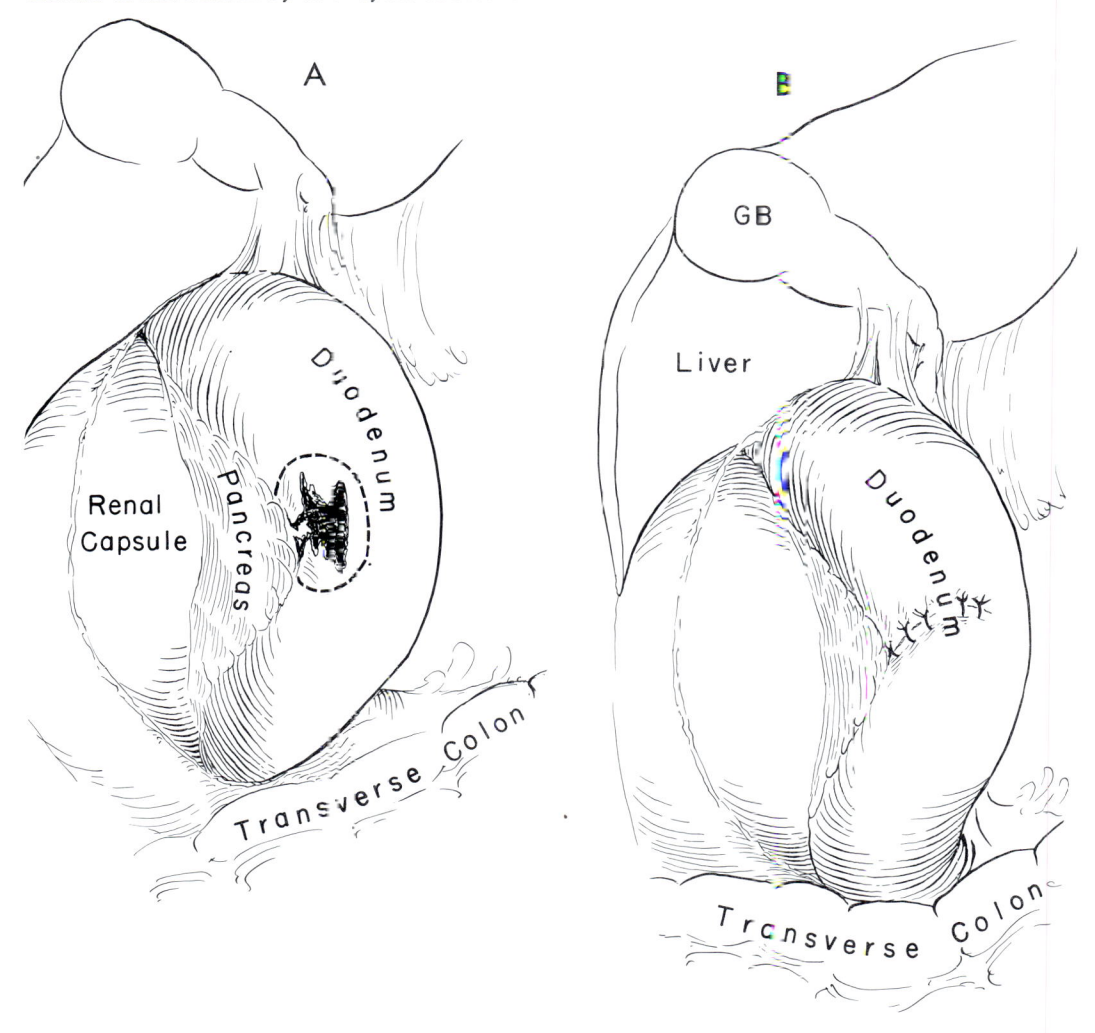

anced by a declining operative survival rate.

Intramural hematomas of the duodenum, in some instances, will respond to treatment by nasogastric decompression and parenteral fluids. However, if the symptoms develop rapidly and are associated with elevated blood amylase levels, early exploration is advisable. In such circumstances there is a frequent association of retroperitoneal rupture of the duodenum or pancreatic injury. If the lesion is found to be only hematoma of the duodenum, drainage of the hematoma by incision of the seromuscular layer with supplementary gastrostomy and jejunostomy is the preferred treatment.

Complications following surgical repair of duodenal injuries are frequent and severe. They include early duodenal obstruction, hemorrhage, fistula, pancreatitis, peritonitis, subphrenic abscess and late duodenal stenosis.

Small Bowel and Mesentery

Penetrating wounds of the small bowel and its mesentery are relatively common and tend to be multiple. Ordinarily, they are not associated with extensive destruction of tissue, but location of several perforations in adjacent portions of bowel may make segmental resection preferable to individual repair of each lesion. On the other hand, when the wounds are few or widely spaced, simple closure by two-layer suture transversely to the long axis of the bowel is optimal (Fig. 44-4).

Avulsion of the mesentery from a segment of intestine greater than 2.5 cm in length or combined injury of bowel and adjacent mesentery should be treated by resection of the bowel and its subtended mesentery to normal tissue with end-to-end two-layer anastomosis (Fig. 44-5).

Blunt injuries to the small bowel often result in a single disruption fairly close to one of the fixed points (ligament of Treitz, ileocecal junction). Depending on the extent of injury, they should be treated by simple transverse repair or by resection and anastomosis.

Mesenteric injuries frequently are obscured by hematoma formation. The hematomas should be evacuated and accurate hemostasis accomplished by ligation of injured arteries and veins. Any portion of bowel found to be devascularized thereafter should be resected.

Rarely, the superior mesenteric artery may be lacerated or avulsed. In such a situation, an attempt should be made to insert a graft from the aorta to restore mesenteric flow.

Colon and Rectum

Wounds of the colon present such a variety in location and extent that their proper management requires a high de-

Fig. 44-4.—Closure of minor injuries to small intestines. **Left,** a smooth defect (a short, sharp incision), which may be closed by two layers of sutures. **Right,** plastic closure completed by second layer of interrupted sutures.

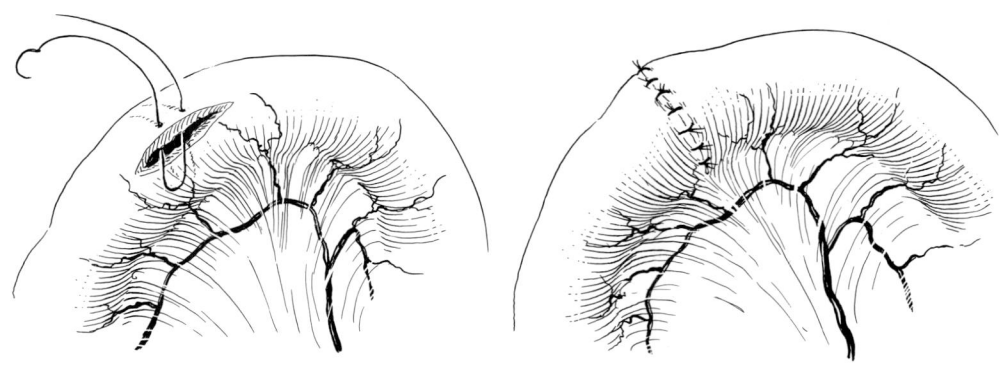

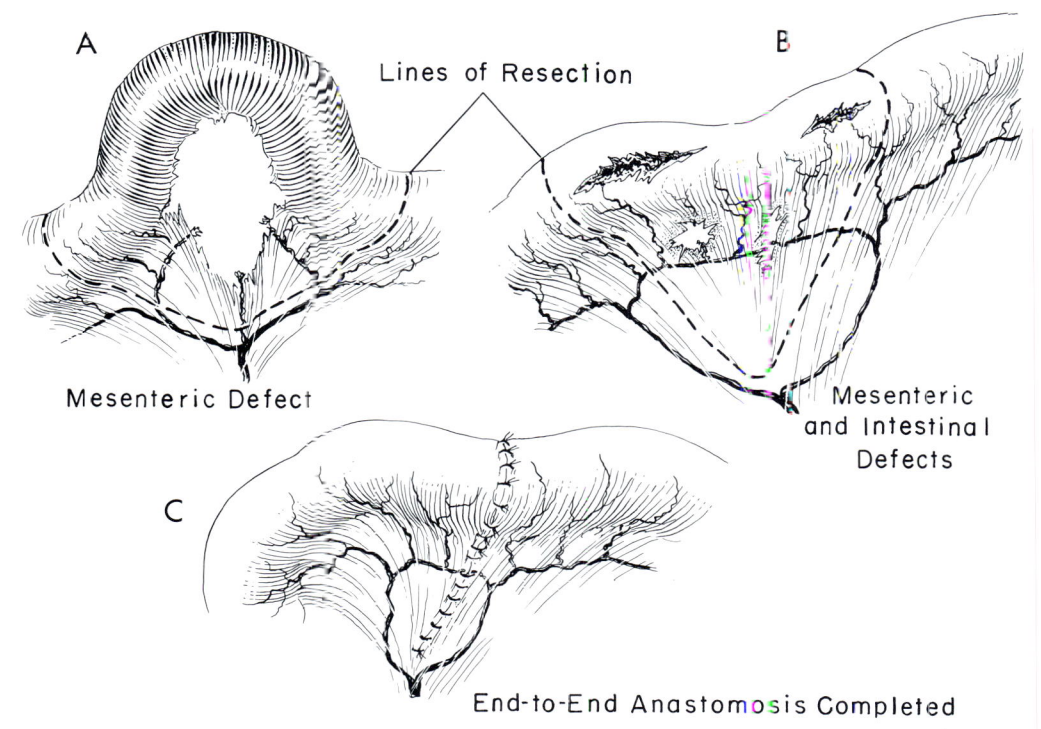

Fig. 44-5. — Injuries of small intestine treated by resection. **A**, resection for avulsion of mesentery. **B**, resection for long ragged defects. **C**, completion of an open end-to-end anastomosis.

gree of surgical sophistication. The difficulties of the surgeon and the hazards for the patient are compounded when, as frequently is the case, they occur concomitantly with other visceral injuries.

Military experience in World War II demonstrated clear-cut improvement in mortality rates when all colonic wounds were treated by exteriorization (Fig. 44-6) or by suture and proximal colostomy (Fig. 44-7). During the Korean War, application of the same principles in treatment led to a further reduction in mortality rate from about 37% to 15%. Mortality rates due to the required subsequent colostomy closure were shown to be approximately 0.5%. Thus, this method of treatment is broadly applicable to colonic injuries, relatively safe and particularly useful in patients with severe or multiple injuries because of the minimal dissection and operating time required. The rather prolonged periods of morbidity and disability entailed are of secondary importance.

In civilian practice, colonic injuries often are less extensive and may be operated on more quickly after wounding than in military experience. This has led to the primary suture of colonic wounds that are not associated with extensive injury to the colon, gross fecal contamination or wounds of other viscera (Fig. 44-8). However, there is a heavy responsibility on the surgeon who elects this course, and the patient's postoperative care must be especially monitored.

Wounds of the cecum and ascending colon require mobilization of these structures by incision of the peritoneum in the lateral gutter to permit inspection of retroperitoneal surfaces. Simple wounds of the cecum may be treated by tube cecostomy that is brought out through an

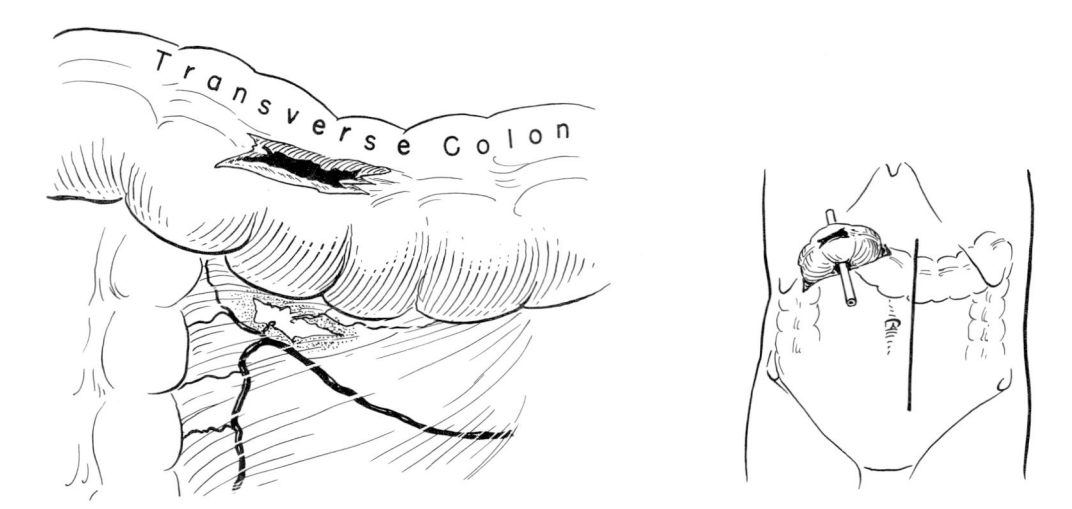

Fig. 44-6.—Repair of extensive ragged defects of colon. **Left,** damage to bowel and to mesentery. **Right,** exteriorization of wound through separate incision.

incision in the right lower quadrant (Fig. 44-9).

More extensive wounds of the right colon with minimal fecal soilage and a short interval from wounding may be treated by right colectomy and ileotransverse colostomy (Fig. 44-10). If conditions are less favorable, resection of the damaged bowel, ileostomy and transverse colostomy with drainage of the right gutter and pelvis is much safer than attempted anastomosis.

Wounds of the transverse and descending portions of the colon are readily treated by exteriorization of the injured segment, and the mobility of the mesentery in these regions makes this procedure quite simple. Release of attachments of the flexures and incision of the lateral reflection of peritoneum of the descending colon are important points of technique in avoiding tension on the colostomy.

Lower sigmoid and rectal wounds cannot be exteriorized. They should be sutured and drained with concomitant

Fig. 44-7.—Repair of wound of low sigmoid or rectum by a completely defunctioning transverse colostomy, made after suture of the sigmoid laceration.

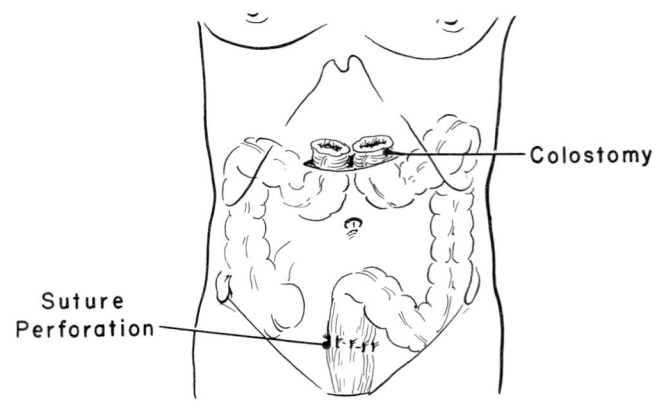

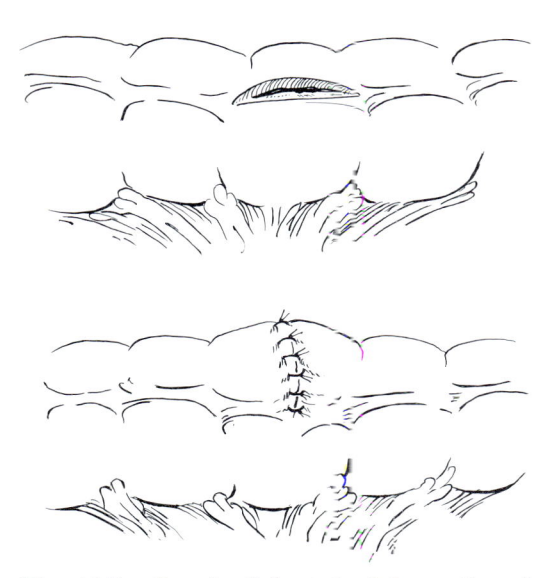

Fig. 44-8.—Repair of short, fresh laceration of colon. **Top,** stab wound. **Bottom,** transverse closure by primary suture.

completely defunctioning transverse colostomy.

Wounds of the rectum that can be exposed by incising the peritoneal floor should be repaired transabdominally with drains brought out in the left lower quadrant or through the perineum with an incision placed lateral to the coccyx. Lower wounds of the rectum should be repaired through a postanal perineal incision with appropriate drainage. In either case, defunctioning transverse colostomy should be done as a final step in the operation.

Peritoneal toilet following repair of colonic injury should be meticulous. If fecal soilage has been extensive, irrigation of the peritoneal cavity with a kanamycin-bacitracin solution may be advantageous.

Complications following repair of colonic injury are relatively common and may include leakage of suture lines, fistula, pelvic and subphrenic abscesses, wound abscess and intestinal obstruction.

Anal Sphincter

Lacerations of the anal sphincter should be repaired primarily and require a defunctioning transverse colostomy. Local repair should be accomplished through a curving incision placed well

Fig. 44-9.—Repair of single laceration of cecum. **Left,** laceration. **Right,** closure of laceration around a large rubber tube.

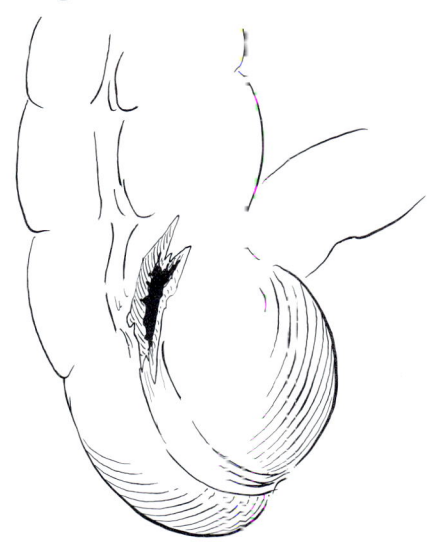

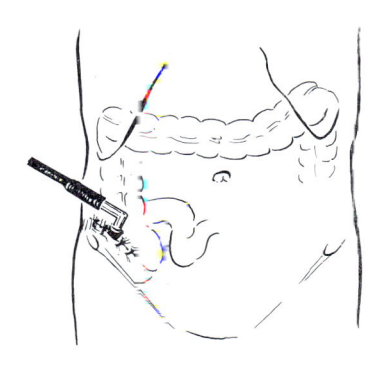

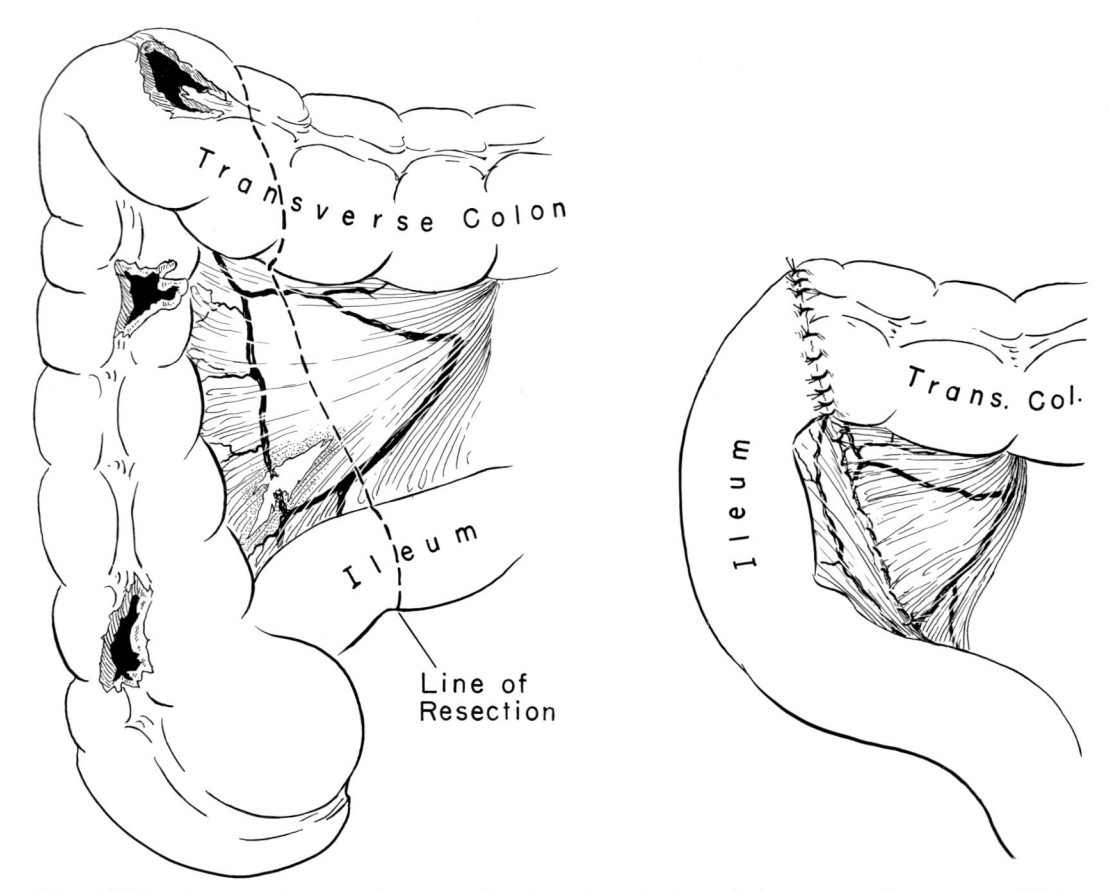

Fig. 44-10.—Repair of severe injuries of right colon. **Left,** mobilization and resection. **Right,** end-to-end ileocolostomy.

away from the anal verge. Edges of the defect in the sphincter muscle should be approximated by mattress sutures of #34-gauge stainless steel wire, which are tied over buttons on the perineum to permit later removal. Additional sutures of fine catgut may be placed as necessary to maintain anatomic repair of the muscle. Accurate healing, function of the sphincter and any required dilatation of the anal ring should be prerequisites to closure of the colostomy.

Retroperitoneal Hematomas

Reference to retroperitoneal hematomas has already been made in the section on Control of Hemorrhage. Large hematomas in this location usually are secondary to fractures of the kidney, tears of the renal vessels, injuries to aorta or inferior vena cava, mesenteric injury or extensive fractures of the pelvis — often with sacroiliac dislocation. Although not all such hematomas will require exploration, if they are large or expanding, usually they should be explored and treated appropriately. Before incising the retroperitoneal planes, one should have several units of whole blood on hand in the operating room, since from 2,500 to 5,000 ml of blood may be shed very rapidly during the initial phase of the exploration.

Extensive renal fractures may require nephrectomy, but if a portion of the kidney retains its blood supply and drainage system, this renal tissue should be preserved. Injuries to the renal artery and vein should be repaired whenever feasible.

Wounds of the aorta and inferior vena cava should be sutured after suitable exposure and control of blood flow proximal and distal to the injury. Occasionally, ligation of the inferior vena cava may be required, but this is less ideal in terms of both immediate and late sequelae.

The management of mesenteric hematomas has been discussed in the section on Small Bowel and Mesentery and will not be reviewed here.

Retroperitoneal hematomas secondary to severe pelvic fractures are increasing in frequency and often are noted among pedestrians who have been struck by automobiles. Sacroiliac disarticulation is observed frequently in these cases, and autopsy studies indicate that tears of the iliac veins may be present. The combination of large hematoma accumulation, large areas of raw fractured bone and tears of the large pelvic veins or their tributaries makes this a most formidable surgical challenge. Recently, selective angiographic studies have helped to demonstrate the specific site of hemorrhage and to control hemorrhage by pharmacologic or mechanical means. If one is forced to intervene surgically, bilateral hypogastric artery ligation in continuity may be effective if one has been unable to define the precise site of hemorrhage preoperatively. Mortality rates indicate that these extensive shattering injuries to the pelvic girdle are among the most serious abdominal wounds.

Finally, severe retroperitoneal injuries may involve the adrenal glands. The surgeon should be alert to the possibility of hemorrhagic shock compounded by acute adrenal insufficiency.

Urogenital Tract

Of all abdominal organs, the kidney is injured most frequently in blunt trauma. Most of these wounds are minor contusions and heal with supportive treatment. As has already been noted, rupture of the kidney may require partial or complete nephrectomy, and trauma to the renal pedicle occasionally may be irreparable.

If nephrectomy is contemplated, either an oblique flank incision or the thoracoabdominal approach may be employed. The advantage of better visualization of the renal pedicle afforded by the latter approach is somewhat offset by the increased hazard of opening the chest cavity in patients sustaining multiple injuries. The ureter should be doubly ligated, with one of the ties being a suture ligature of nonabsorbable material. Nephrectomy wounds should be drained, since urinary drainage, secondary hemorrhage, sepsis and urinary fistula may occur as complications.

Injuries that cause ureteral injury require exposure, visualization and repair of this structure to avoid serious retroperitoneal urinary extravasation. Trivial ureteral injuries may be repaired by simple suture, but more extensive injuries require excision of damaged tissue and reanastomosis. Low ureteral injuries may be managed most effectively by reimplantation into the bladder. In either case, a T-tube may be employed as a stent, with the side arm of the tube being brought out through a stab wound away from the ureteral anastomosis. Drainage of the retroperitoneal space is mandatory.

Rupture of the bladder may be suspected when insertion of a catheter fails to produce appreciable amounts of urine. This observation should be checked by instilling Hypaque into the bladder and obtaining frontal and oblique x-ray films. Wounds of the bladder are treated by suture and suprapubic cystostomy. The latter procedure is also required in severe cases of injury to the posterior urethra. Sometimes it is possible to catheterize the urethra through the bladder; at other times, primary repair of the bladder neck is required.

Injuries of the internal genital organs in the female are rare. Occasionally, the gravid uterus may be lacerated by gunshot or stab wounds. Blunt injuries may rupture the uterus, particularly during the last trimester of pregnancy. Treatment in each case must be particularized, but transabdominal emptying and repair of the uterus will be required in most instances.

Diaphragm and Abdominal Wall

Traumatic rupture of the diaphragm occurs occasionally as a manifestation of severe injury to the torso. This occurs much more frequently on the left than on the right, is associated often with other abdominal visceral wounds and pelvic fractures and dislocation of abdominal organs into the chest. Signs of this injury include prominence and immobility of the left chest wall, absence of breath sounds on that side, bowel sounds over the left lower thorax, shifting of the heart to the right, tympanites of the left chest on percussion and elevation of the left diaphragm noted on chest x-ray examination.

Because of the association with other abdominal injuries, the acutely ruptured diaphragm should be repaired transabdominally by interrupted nonabsorbable sutures. Accurate hemostasis should be ensured by suture ligatures wherever necessary.

Rarely, blunt injuries to the abdomen may cause subcutaneous rupture of the abdominal wall. These cases will have a high incidence of associated visceral injury, and laparotomy usually will be required. Repair of the abdominal wall should be carried out at the time of initial operation, but a high incidence of late hernias in such wounds should be anticipated. Marlex mesh is a satisfactory adjunct to the repair of such defects, but its use should be reserved for a secondary operation.

POSTOPERATIVE CARE

The postoperative management of patients with abdominal injuries requires meticulous care. Associated injuries must not be neglected. Continued use of oxygen, antibiotics, gastrointestinal decompression and whole blood, as required, should be the universal rule. Parenteral fluids and electrolytes should be administered as needed. Except in the presence of severe cardiovascular disease or marked oliguria, it usually is adequate to plan on a daily quota of 2,000 ml of 5% dextrose in water, 500 ml of 5% dextrose in saline and 40 milliequivalents of potassium. Additional increments of water, sodium chloride and potassium are added to cover all extrarenal losses, as from gastric suction, fistulas or other drainage tubes. Frequent determinations of the hemoglobin and of blood electrolytes are made during the first few postoperative days to ensure accurate replacement therapy. When peristaltic activity is restored, as judged by the passage of flatus, the nasogastric tube is removed and gradual resumption of oral nutrition is begun. Drains are mobilized on the seventh postoperative day and removed a day or two later if no excessive exudate is observed. Sutures are removed no earlier than the tenth postoperative day; they may be left much longer if the circumstances of nutrition, distention or local wound healing require such delay.

Common complications encountered after repair of abdominal injuries include peritonitis, intra-abdominal abscess, small bowel obstruction, wound abscesses and wound dehiscence. Abscesses occur most commonly in the wound, the pelvis and the subphrenic space. They also may be formed in the peritoneal cavity between adjacent loops of bowel or mesentery and the omentum. Wound abscesses should be treated by opening the involved area widely. Abscesses within the peritoneal cavity should be drained by an incision through the abdominal wall directly over the presenting mass, whereas pelvic abscesses may be drained through the vagina or rectum. Subphrenic abscesses are drained by resecting the twelfth rib on the affected side and evacuating the pus through the

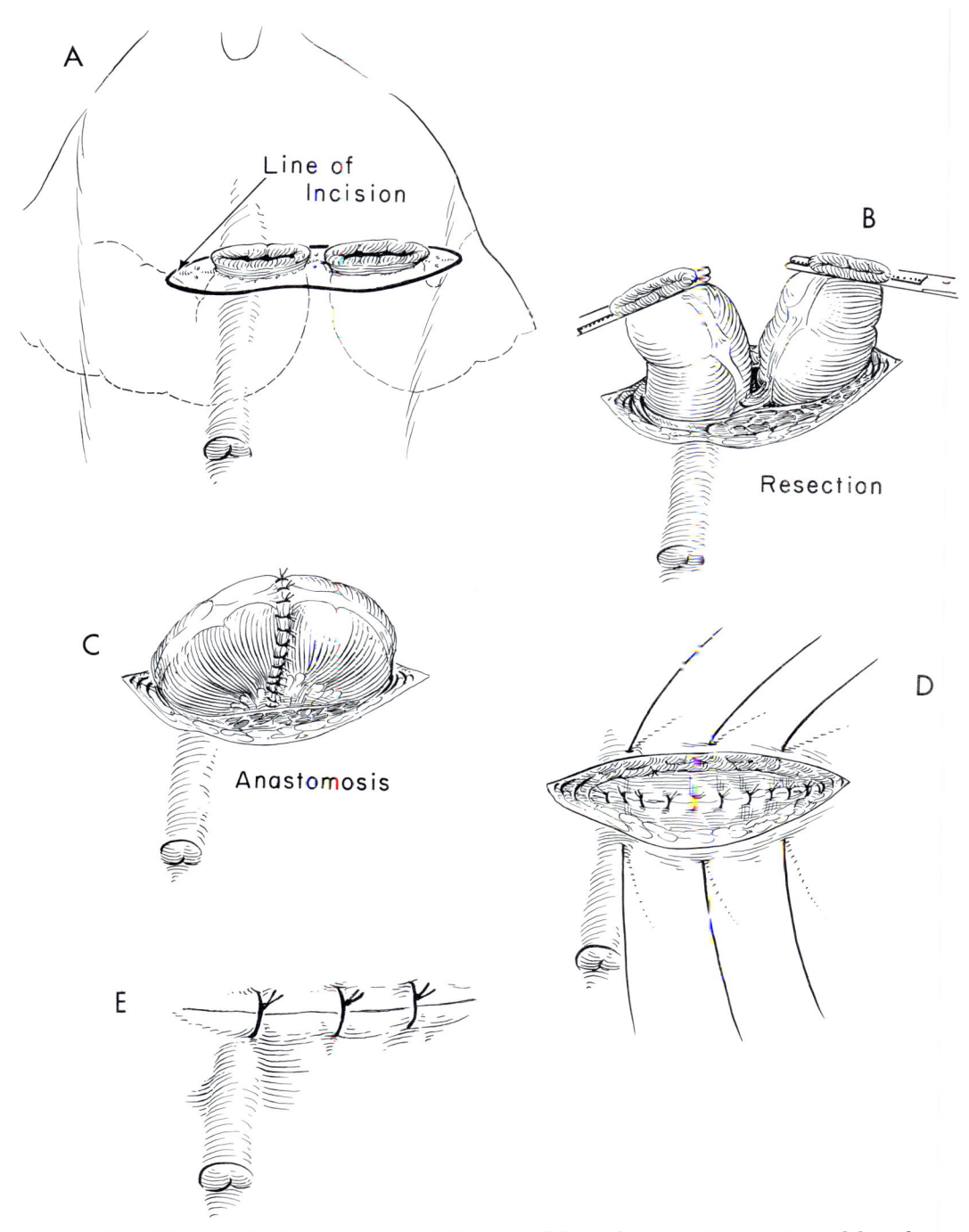

Chapter 44: MANAGEMENT OF ABDOMINAL INJURIES / 1051

Fig. 44-11.—Closure of colostomy. **A,** mobilization of the colostomy. **B,** resection of the edematous stomas. **C,** open end-to-end, two-layer anastomosis. **D,** preparation for delayed primary closure; subcutaneous tissue and fat held open by gauze pack for 48 hours. **E,** appearance after delayed primary closure.

rib bed. Cigarette drains should be left in all abscess cavities and withdrawn gradually as the cavities are obliterated. Wound dehiscence should be repaired by closely placed wire sutures that extend through all layers of the abdominal wall. Small bowel obstruction may be decompressed temporarily by the use of long intestinal tubes, but often will require lysis of adhesions or the use of bypassing anastomoses. Thromboembolism always is a threat, particularly among older civilian patients, and prophylaxis should include elastic bandaging of the legs, active exercises and early ambulation. Carefully monitored Coumadin prophylaxis may be used in patients whose convalescence requires prolonged immobilization. Established thrombophlebitis is definitively treated by anticoagulants when there is no special reason to expect intra-abdominal or gastrointestinal hemorrhage. In those cases unsuitable for anticoagulant therapy, bilateral superficial femoral vein ligation or application of a Teflon clip to the inferior vena cava are alternative methods of treatment.

Pulmonary complications contribute significantly to mortality in patients with severe abdominal trauma, operation and massive blood replacement. These include shunting, atelectasis, aspiration pneumonia, emboli and pulmonary edema. The pathogenesis and treatment of these conditions have been reviewed recently by Webb.

Colostomy Closure

No set time can be fixed for the closure of a defunctioning colostomy. In general, one should wait until the edema and inflammatory reaction in the wound have subsided. In most cases, a delay of 2–3 weeks will be adequate, but under military conditions a longer period may be more desirable. It is wise to demonstrate the integrity of the defunctioned bowel by barium enema before closure of the colostomy is performed. Although extraperitoneal closure of colostomies and Mikulicz resection with crushing of the spur have been recommended by some, modern techniques make intraperitoneal closure (Fig. 44-11) much safer and far more satisfactory. Stronger wound repair and better function of the anastomosed bowel are to be expected from intraperitoneal closure. It is wise to prepare the bowel preoperatively by 48 hours of liquid diet combined with vigorous mechanical cleansing of the gut. This should include castor oil 2 days preoperatively and enemas on the evening preceding anticipated colostomy closure. The colostomy stomas and intervening skin are excised and discarded and an open, end-to-end anastomosis is performed. The repaired bowel then is dropped back into the peritoneal cavity and peritoneum and deep fascia are sutured in separate layers. Healing of these wounds without sepsis is promoted if the procedure of delayed closure of fat and skin, as recommended by Coller and Volk, is used.

MORTALITY

The over-all mortality rates in treatment of abdominal injuries are complex data that may not be strictly comparable in different series. Factors that have been shown to decrease the probability of survival after wounding include advanced age, pre-existing disease, multiple organ and systems injuries, increased time interval from wounding to surgical treatment and profound shock secondary to massive blood loss. Among any large series of traumatized patients is a group who survive long enough to be admitted to the emergency service and expire before any effective therapy can be administered. There is also another group whose injuries are so severe that they do not live to be transported to the hospital. Thus, in a study of traffic victims in Birmingham, England, each patient was found to have more than three injuries, two-thirds had head injuries, one-third had chest injuries and one-half had serious hemorrhage. One-third of the victims were killed outright and one-half of the remainder died within 12 hours.

The mortality rate for all abdominal injuries treated by the Second Auxiliary Surgical Group during World War II was 24%. Aalpoel reported a mortality rate of 8.9% in cases treated during the Korean War. Results among casualties in the Vietnam War are not yet clarified; however, among patients evacuated postoperatively to Clark Air Base Hospital, Whelan and his associates found the over-all mortality rate to be 6.2%. Of those patients requiring reoperation, 15.4% died. The special hazards of dehiscence secondary to infection and the stress of air evacuation with intestinal gas expansion has prompted these authors to emphasize again the importance of layer closure of the abdominal wounds with closely spaced through-and-through retention sutures.

Experience in civilian hospitals generally indicates that mortality rates from blunt abdominal injuries range between 10% and 15%; penetrating injuries are associated with somewhat lower mortality rates.

It is evident that figures for comparison of mortality rates have limited usefulness. If we are to improve our results in the therapy of abdominal injuries, we must concentrate our efforts on salvaging those patients presenting multiple severe organ and multiple systems injuries. This will require attention along the entire chain of treatment—including improved first-aid; better transport to hospitals, organization of emergency ward teams with general, orthopedic and neurosurgeons and immediate standby support from anesthesiologists, radiologists, clinical laboratories, blood banks and operating rooms. Present mortality rates in excess of 50% for injuries of this type should provide ample stimulus for educational and organizational adaptation.

BIBLIOGRAPHY

Aalpoel, J. A.: Abdominal wounds in Korea, Ann. Surg. 140:850, 1954.

Allen, R. E., Eastman, B. A., Halter, B. L., and Connolly, W. B.: Retroperitoneal hemorrhage secondary to blunt trauma, Am. J. Surg. 118:558, 1969.

Artz, C. P., Bronwell, A. W., and Sako, Y.: Experiences in the management of abdominal and thoraco-abdominal injuries in Korea, Am. J. Surg. 89:773, 1955.

Beebe, G. W., and De Bakey, M: *Battle Casualties: Incidence, Mortality, and Logistic Considerations* (Springfield, Il: Charles C Thomas, Publisher, 1952).

Berger, W. J., Jr.: Evaluation of "Intracath" method of abdominal paracentesis, Am. Surg. 35:23, 1969.

Biggs, T. M., Beall, A. C., Jr., Gordon, W. B., Morris, G. C., Jr., and De Bakey, M.: Surgical management of civilian colon injuries, J. Trauma 3:484, 1963.

Braunstein, P. W., Skudder, P. A., McCarroll, J. R., Musolino, A., and Wade, P. A.: Concealed hemorrhage due to pelvic fracture, J. Trauma 4:832, 1964.

Carter, J. W., and Sawyers, J. L.: Pitfalls in diagnosis of abdominal stab wounds by contrast media injections, Am. Surg. 35:107, 1969.

Charron, J. W., and Brault, J. P.: Recognition and early management of injuries to the urinary tract, J. Trauma 4:702, 1964.

Cleveland, H. C., and Waddell, W. R.: Retroperitoneal rupture of the duodenum due to non-penetrating trauma, Surg. Clin. North Am. 43:413, 1963.

Coller, F., and Volk, N.: The delayed closure of contaminated wounds. Trans. South. Surg. Gynecol. Assoc. 52:449, 1939.

Cornell, W. P., Ebert, E. A., and Zuidema, G. D.: X-ray diagnosis of penetrating wounds of the abdomen, J. Surg. Res. 5:142, 1965.

DiVincenti, F. C., Rives, J. D., Laboude, E. J., Fleming, I. D., and Cohn, I., Jr.: Blunt abdominal trauma, J. Trauma 8:1004, 1968.

Foley, W. J., Gaines, R. D., and Fry, W. J.: Pancreato-duodenectomy for severe trauma to the head of the pancreas and the associated structures: Report of 3 cases, Ann. Surg. 170:759, 1969.

Frey, C. F., Hullke, D. F., and Gikas, P. W.: Resuscitation and survival in motor vehicle accidents, J. Trauma 9:292, 1969.

Friedmann, P.: Selective management of stab wounds of the Abdomen, Arch. Surg. 96:292, 1968.

German, J. D., and Davis, W. C.: Peritoneal splenosis following traumatic rupture of the spleen, Am. Surg. 32:329, 1966.

Gissane, W., and Bull, J.: A study of 183 road deaths in and around Birmingham in 1960, Br. Med. J. 1:1716, 1961.

Guerrier, K., Albert, D. J., Mahoney, S. A., Izant, R. J., and Persky, L.: Delayed nephrectomy after trauma, J. Trauma 9:455, 1969.

Hauser, C. W., and Perry, J. F., Jr.: Control of massive hemorrhage from pelvic fractures by hypogastric artery ligation, Surg. Gynecol. Obstet. 121:313, 1965.

Hill, M. C.: Roentgen diagnosis of duodenal injuries, Am. J. Roentgenol. 94:356, 1965.

Izant, R. J., Jr., and Drucker, W. R.: Duodenal obstruction due to intramural hematoma in children, J. Trauma 4:797, 1964.

Jones, E. L., Peters, A. F., and Gasior, R. M.: Early management of battle casualties in Vietnam, Arch. Surg. 97:1, 1968.

Khauna, H. L., Hayes, B. R., and McKeown, K. C.: Delayed rupture of the spleen, Ann. Surg. 165:477, 1967.

Ludewig, R. M., and Wangensteen, S. L.: Aortic bleeding and the effect of external counterpressure, Surg. Gynecol. Obstet. 128:252, 1969.

MacLean, L. D.: The traumatic rupture of the diaphragm, Postgrad. Med. 29:383, 1961.

Martin, L. W., Henderson, B. M., and Walsh, N.: Disruption of the head of the pancreas caused by blunt trauma in children: A report of 2 cases treated with primary repair of the pancreatic duct, Surgery 63:697, 1968.

Mathewson, C., Jr., and Morgan, R.: Intramural hematoma of the duodenum, Am. J. Surg. 112:299, 1966.

McCarroll, J. R., Braunstein, P. W., Weinberg, S. B., Seremetis, M. G., and Cooper, M.: The pathology of pedestrian automotive accident victims, J. Trauma 5:421, 1965.

McIndoe, A. H.: Delayed hemorrhage following traumatic rupture of the spleen; Br. J. Surg. 20:249, 1932.

Medical Dept., United States Army: *Surgery in World War II*, Vol. II. Office of the Surgeon General, Dept. of the Army, Washington, D. C., 1955: Giddings, W. P., and Wolff, L. H.: Factors of Mortality, pp. 213-221. Giddings, W. P., and McDaniel, J. R.: Wounds of the Jejunum and Ileum, pp. 241-254. Chun, C. F., and Hauver, R. V.: Wounds of the Colon and Rectum, pp. 255-274.

Miller, D. R.: Transection of the esophagus at the esophago-gastric junction by blunt trauma, J. Trauma 8:1105, 1968.

Mills, M.: The management of thoraco-abdominal wounds, Milit. Med. 132:602, 1967.

Morehous, D. D., and MacKinnon, K. J.: Urological injuries associated with pelvic fractures, J. Trauma 9:479, 1969.

Morse, T. S.: Infusion pyelogram in the evaluation of renal injuries in children, J. Trauma 6:693, 1966.

Morton, J. R., and Jordan, G. L.: Traumatic duodenal injuries: Review of 131 cases, J. Trauma 8:127, 1968.

Motsay, G. J., Manlove, C., and Perry, J. F.: Major venous injury with pelvic fracture, J. Trauma 9:343, 1969.

Mule, J. E. and Adaniel, M.: The management of trauma to the pancreas, Surgery 65:423, 1969.

Nance, F. C. and Cohn, I., Jr.; Surgical judgment in the management of stab wounds of the abdomen; Ann. Surg., 170:569-577, 1969.

Nelson, J. B., Jr., Zipperman, H. H., Christensen, N. M., and Mathewson, C. Jr.: Diaphragmatic injuries and post-traumatic hernia, J. Trauma 2:36, 1962.

Nick, W. V., Zollinger, R. W., and Pace, W. G.: Retroperitoneal hemorrhage after blunt abdominal trauma, J. Trauma 7:652, 1967.

Nick, W. V., Zollinger, R. W., and Williams, R. D.: The diagnosis of traumatic pancreatitis with blunt abdominal injuries, J. Trauma 5:495, 1965.

Noon, G. P., Beall, A. C., Jr., and De Bakey, M.: Surgical management of traumatic rupture of the diaphragm, J. Trauma 6:344, 1966.

Oglesby, J. E., Smith, D. E., Mahoney, W. D., and Baugh, J. H.: Complete duodenal transection in blunt trauma, Am. J. Surg. 116:914, 1968.

Olsen, W. R.: The emergency department and the critically injured patient, Surg. Gynecol. Obstet. 129:113, 1969.

Parkinson, E. B.: Perinatal loss due to external trauma to the uterus, Am. J. Obstet. Gynecol. 90:30, 1964.

Parrish, R. A., Edmondson, H. T., and Moretz, W. H.: Duodenal and biliary obstruction secondary to intramural hematoma, Am. J. Surg. 108:428, 1964.

Perry, J. F., Jr.: A five-year survey of 152 acute abdominal injuries, J. Trauma 5:53, 1965.

Perry, J. F., Jr., and McClellan, R. J.: Autopsy findings in 127 patients following fatal traffic accidents, Surg. Gynecol. Obstet. 119:586, 1964.

Poer, D. H.: Evaluation of colostomy for present-day surgery, Arch. Surg. 61:1058, 1950.

Pridgen, J. E., Herff, A. F., Jr., Watkins, H. O., Halbert, D. S., Avila, R. D., Crouch, D. M., and Prud'homme, J. L.: Penetrating wounds of the abdomen: Analysis of 776 operative cases, Ann. Surg. 165:901, 1967.

Printen, K. J., Freeark, R. J., and Shoemaker, W. C.: Conservative management of penetrating abdominal stab wounds, Arch. Surg. 96:899, 1968.

Redman, H. C., Renter, S. R., and Bookstein, J. J.: Angiography in abdominal trauma, Ann. Surg. 169:57, 1969.

Resnicoff, S. A., and Morton, J. H.: Changing concepts concerning duodenal hematomas, J. Trauma 9:559, 1969.

Rooney, J. A., and Pesek, J. G.: Transection of the stomach due to blunt abdominal trauma: Review of previous reports and presentation of 2 new cases, J. Trauma 8:487, 1968.

Root, H. D., Hauser, C. W., McKinley, C. R., LaFave, J. W., and Mendiola, R. P., Jr.: Diagnostic peritoneal lavage, Surgery 57:633, 1965.

Root, H. D., Keizer, P. J., and Perry, J. F.: Peritoneal trauma, experimental and clinical studies, Surgery 62:679, 1967.

Sargent, F. T., and Williams, R. D.: The effects of explosive decompression on the gastro-intestinal tract: A preliminary report, J. Trauma 4:618, 1964.

Schmitt, H. J., Jr., Patterson, L. T., and Armstrong, R. G.: Reoperative surgery of abdominal war wounds, Ann. Surg. 165:173, 1967.

Seavers, R., Lynch, J., Ballard, R., Jernigan, S., and Johnson, J.: Hypogastric artery ligation for uncontrollable hemorrhage in acute pelvic trauma, Surgery 55:516, 1964.

Shirkey, A. L., Quast, D. C., and Jordan, G. L.: Superior mesenteric artery division and intestinal function, J. Trauma 7:7, 1967.

Slate, R. W., Gatzen, L. C., and Laning, R. C.: One hundred cases of traumatic rupture of the spleen, Arch. Surg. 99:498, 1969.

Stahl, W. M.: Resuscitation in trauma; the value of central venous pressure monitoring, J. Trauma 5:200, 1965.

Steichen, F. M., Dargan, E. L., Pearlman, D. M.,

and Weil, P. H.: The management of retroperitoneal hematoma secondary to penetrating injuries, Surg. Gynecol. Obstet. 123:581, 1966.

Storstren, K. A., and ReMine, W. H.: Rupture of the spleen with splenic implants: Splenosis, Ann. Surg. 137:551, 1953.

Sturim, H S.: The surgical management of pancreatic injuries, J. Trauma 5:693, 1965.

Sullivan, M. B., Jr., Morgan, J. M., and Murdaugh, H. V., Jr.: Management of the post-traumatic oliguric state, J. Trauma 3:268, 1963.

Tank, E. S., Eraklis, A. J., and Gross, R. E.: Blunt abdominal trauma in infancy and childhood, J. Trauma 8:439, 1968.

Taylor, F. A., Morgan, W. W., Jr., Lucero, J. I., and Owen, J. C.: Abdominal trauma from seat belts, Am. Surg. 35:313, 1969.

Teschan, P. E.: Management of patients with post-traumatic renal insufficiency, J. Trauma 3:181, 1963.

Thompson, D. P., Schulta, E., and Benfield, J. R.: Celiac angiography in the management of splenic trauma, Arch. Surg. 99:494, 1961.

Vannix, R. S., Carter, R., Henshaw, D. B., and Joergenson, E. J.: Surgical management of colon trauma in civilian practice, Am. J. Surg. 106:364, 1963.

Webb, A. J., and Taylor, J. J.: Traumatic intramural hematoma of the duodenum, Br. J. Surg. 54:50, 1967.

Webb, W. R.: Pulmonary complication of non-thoracic trauma: Summary of the National Research Council Conference, J. Trauma 9:700, 1969.

Weckesser, E. C., and Putnam, T. C.: Perforating injuries of the rectum and sigmoid colon, J. Trauma 2:474, 1962.

Weinstein, E. C., and Pallais, V.: Rupture of the pregnant uterus from blunt trauma, J. Trauma 8:1-11, 1968.

Whelan, T. J., Jr., Burkhalter, W. E., and Gomez, A.: Management of War Wounds, in Welch, C. E. (ed.), *Advances in Surgery* (Chicago: Year Book Medical Publishers Inc., 1968), Vol. 3, pp. 227-350.

Williams, R. D., and Sargent, F. T.: The mechanism of intestinal injury in trauma, J. Trauma 3:288, 1963.

Wilson, R. F., Taggett, J. P., Pucelik, J. P., and Walt, A. J.: Pancreatic trauma, J. Trauma 7:643, 1967.

Wise, R. A., Chutrapakul, S., and Balankura, O.: Adrenal gland injury in blunt abdominal trauma, Am. Surg. 160:97., 1964.

Witte, C. L.: Mesentery and bowel injury from automotive seat belts, Ann Surg. 167:486, 1968.

Wren, H. B., Texada, F. J., Krementz, E. T., and Creech, O., Jr.: Traumatic rupture of the diaphragm, J. Trauma 2:147, 1962.

45 | Liver and Extrahepatic Biliary System

RONALD A. MALT

LIVER

THREE PRINCIPLES should guide the surgeon who operates to remedy the consequences of hepatic trauma:

1. Since tissue distal to a complete transection of the major inflow vessels will die as a result of inadequate collateral circulation, it should be removed.
2. Undrained collections of bile or blood probably will become infected. Their formation should be deterred by scrupulous ligation of open vessels and ducts and by continuous aspiration of any fluid.
3. Resections along anatomic planes are practical when formal lobectomy actually is necessary, but it rarely is.

In putting these principles into action, knowledge of the detailed anatomy of the liver is almost excess baggage. The surgeon is well equipped if he knows the following facts:

1. A plane passing between the gallbladder fossa and the inferior vena cava marks the division between the right and left hepatic lobes.[30]
2. The right and left branches of the portal vein and the hepatic artery supply these lobes.
3. A major division of the right hepatic artery and a branch of the portal vein define the anterior and posterior segments of the right lobe. A division of the vessels on the left defines medial and lateral segments.
4. Venous drainage from the extremities of the liver is through the right and left hepatic veins, but much of the central part of the liver is drained by the middle hepatic vein.
5. The three hepatic veins tend to enter the vena cava at a common point only 4–5 cm below the diaphragm.

Types of Injury

A *subcapsular hematoma* of the liver often results from diffuse shearing of superficial parenchymal vessels or from localized trauma, as from a retractor squeezing the liver during an operation in the right upper quadrant. If several liters of blood are deposited under the capsule, there may be early signs of hypovolemia and later, perhaps, indications of free rupture of the blood into the liver substance or into the peritoneal cavity. This problem usually is dealt with by opening the capsule, ligating any points still bleeding and, perhaps, transposing the free surface of the greater omentum to the site of the injury. Sump drains are placed as in any other injury to the liver.

Both blunt trauma and penetrating wounds can produce *capsular tears*, and, in a good many of these, hemostasis will be spontaneous by the time of operation. These injuries are either repaired with mattress sutures of 0 chromic catgut or are left open with sumps or drains placed

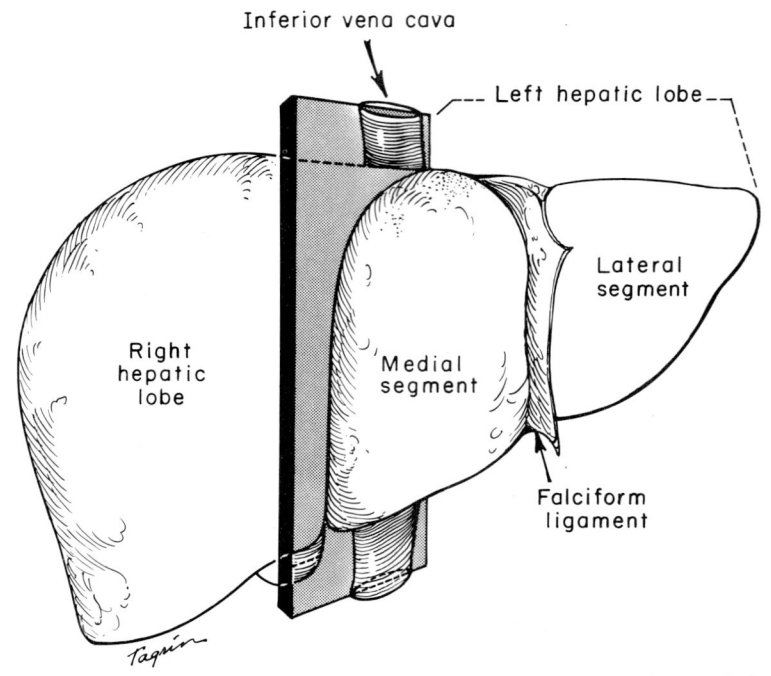

Fig. 45-1.—The anatomic right and left lobes of the liver. The plane of division passes through the fossa of the gallbladder.

nearby, provided that there is no leakage of blood or bile.

The deeper *penetrating wound,* typically a stab or bullet wound, should be closed only if there is no leakage from open vessels or ducts. Otherwise, accumulation of blood and bile within the liver can form the medium for development of an intrahepatic abscess. Such wounds are better left open, to be aspirated by a sump drain; they may need to be opened further, in fact, to permit ligation of vessels and ducts.

The management of major *avulsing lacerations,* whether from penetrating or blunt injury, and of bursting injuries of the liver[27] will be the concern of the rest of this chapter. This is the kind of trauma that causes major segments of liver to be irremediably separated from their blood supply and biliary drainage. Sometimes the injury is also associated with injury to the vena cava itself.

Diagnosis

Every injured patient showing signs of shock or low blood volume in the absence of external bleeding should be at once suspected of harboring a torn liver. The distinction between injuries to the liver and to the spleen or the aorta, for example, is not always clear but often can be sharpened merely by observation of the external signs of trauma and the location of any fractured ribs. In every injury to the liver, the possibility of damage to the right colon, duodenum, kidney, pancreas, vena cava and aorta should be entertained, as well as the chance of remote injuries.

Routine laboratory tests, except for serial determination of hematocrits, usually are of little help, but special examinations are of considerably more value. Although failure of a diagnostic paracentesis to yield blood must be discounted,

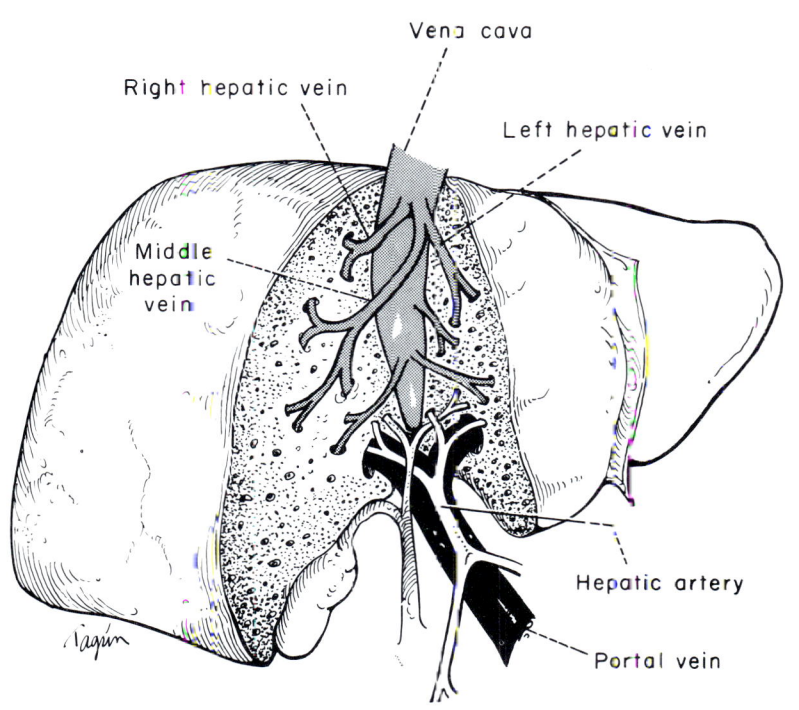

Fig. 45-2.—The major venous drainage of the liver is through the right, middle and left hepatic veins. Numerous smaller veins also enter the cava.

aspiration of blood may be possible in 80–95% of patients with major liver injuries.[28] In those patients, the roentgenographic examination may also show the virtually diagnostic picture of haziness or an enlarged liver in the right upper quadrant, a high diaphragm, widening of the flank stripe and a fractured right costal margin.[33] Lack of response to a rapid infusion of 500–1,000 ml of Ringer's solution has also been said to have diagnostic value[23] but cannot, of course, differentiate between rupture of the liver and other major vascular damage.

Seldom is there time for more complicated studies. When they are possible, hepatic angiography for assessment of the integrity of deep structures in the liver is a valuable guide to strategy.[1] Angiography can also alert the surgeon to the possibility that the right hepatic artery originates from the superior mesenteric artery ("replaced" right hepatic artery) or that the left hepatic artery originates from the left gastric artery ("replaced" left gastric artery). If either of these anomalies is present (about 20% of patients inclusive), cross-clamping of the portal triad will not occlude the vascular inflow to the liver, and accidental injury to the hepatic arteries is possible. Accessory hepatic arteries are other causes of mystifying hemorrhage (see Fig. 45-9).

Preoperative Preparation

When injury to the liver is massive, attempts to restore homeostasis before surgery usually are fruitless. The best that can be hoped for is the insertion of a #15-gauge catheter into each upper extremity or into a subclavian vein followed by rapid infusion of blood, dextran or saline

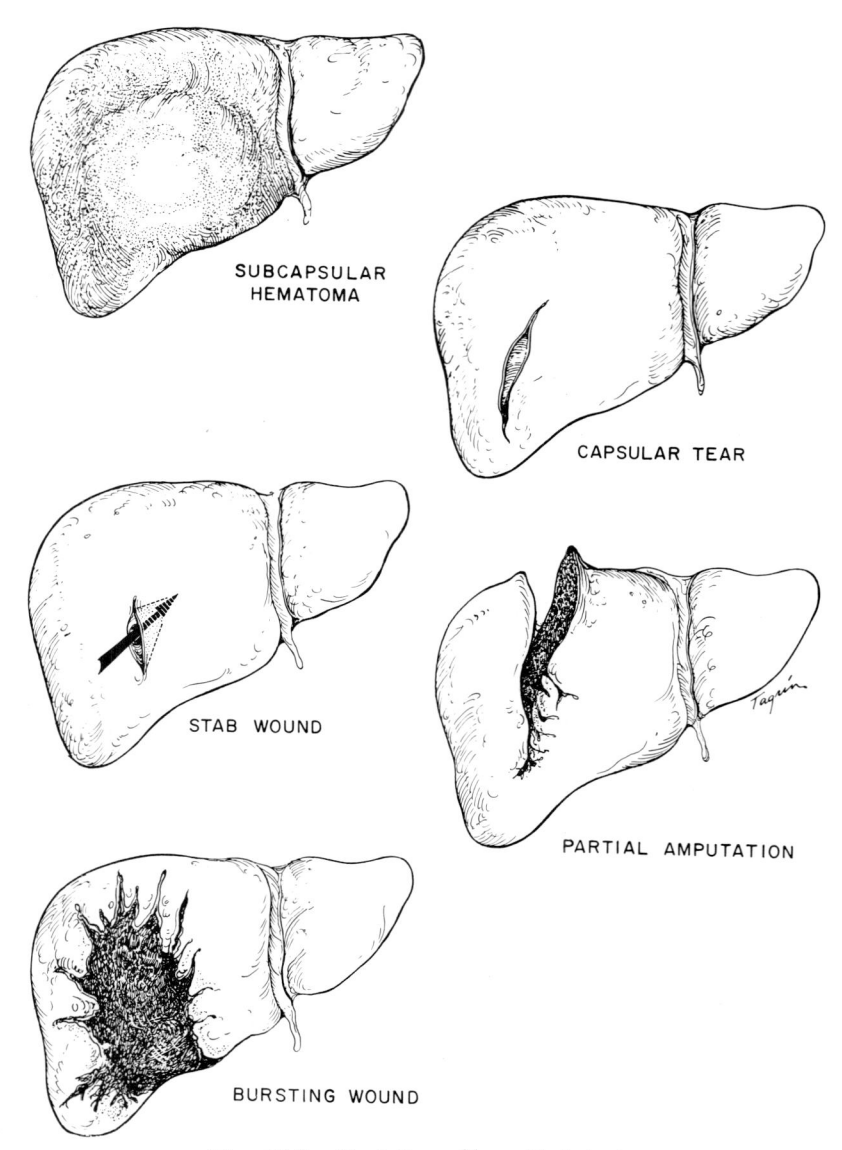

Fig. 45-3.—Varieties of hepatic injuries.

solution. Since absence of a normal splanchnic reservoir makes the vasomotor stability of these patients precarious,[41] a central venous pressure cannula should be placed as a guide to adequacy of replacement. Inasmuch as the inferior vena cava may have to be cross-clamped during surgery, fluids preferably should not be administered through veins in the lower extremities. The value of an inflated antigravity suit to diminish sequestration of blood in the extremities and to counteract the lost tamponading effect of intra-abdominal pressure after anesthesia

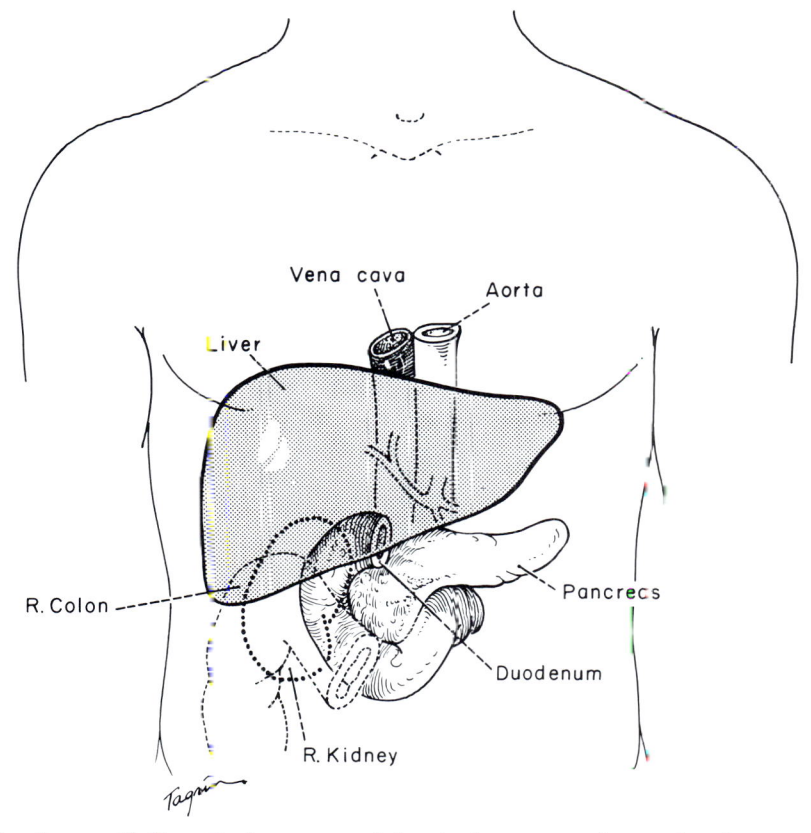

Fig. 45-4.—Susceptibility of other upper abdominal organs to forces that damage the liver.

is induced remains to be explored; it seems to have value in maintaining intravascular volume until blood transfusions are available.

Bloods to be cross-matched for transfusion should be as fresh as possible. Although a customary allotment is 1 unit of fresh blood (less than 24 hours old) for every 4 units of older blood, a special attempt should be made in dealing with hepatic trauma to have at least half the transfusions from recent blood collections and to call in donors for really fresh blood. Since coagulation factors produced by the liver will be deficient if a massive liver resection is necessary, the freshest blood and fresh-frozen plasma should be withheld until hemostasis is virtually complete. Serum fibrinogen concentrations and fibrinolytic activity should be measured so that fibrinogen and epsilon-aminocaproic acid (EACA) can be given if necessary.

Heat exchangers to warm the transfusions[36] and thermal blankets to regulate the patient's temperature are valuable. During the early stages of the operation, deliberate moderate hypothermia produced by cold transfusions is desirable to permit prolongation of the safe period for occluding all hepatic blood flow, but regulation should be controllable to prevent profound hypothermia.

When time permits, several feet of soft polyvinyl tubing (about ⅝ in. internal diameter) and a #34 F cuffed endotra-

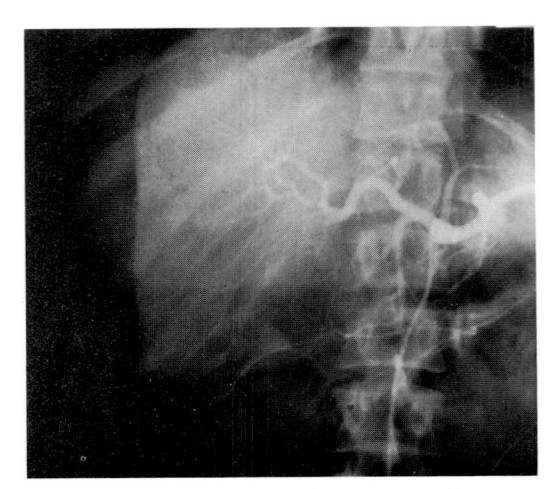

Fig. 45-5.—Angiogram showing a subcapsular hematoma resulting from a kick in the chest. The liver is separated from the rib cage by the hematoma. (Figs. 45-5–45-8 were kindly provided by Dr. Donald J. Fleischli.)

cheal tube should be sterilized for use as internal vascular shunts.[2, 10, 39]

Operation

CONTROL OF BLEEDING.—In the treatment of massive liver injury, whether associated or not with damage to surrounding organs or blood vessels, the most useful initial approach is a long right paramedian incision. A copious supply of gauze packs should be at hand, because shoveling with them is the only way to evacuate the abdomen expeditiously. As soon as the basic landmarks are apparent, pads are pressed against the shattered liver substance and held by an assistant while the surgeon manually identifies the portal triad and compresses it with fingers of one hand or with a Crafoord clamp. Continued bright bleeding from the parenchyma thereafter is a signal to search for the nonoccluded replaced right or left hepatic arteries already described. Massive bleeding from an inapparent source is a signal to inspect especially the right posterior-superior part of the liver under the diaphragm[21]

and to convert the original incision for exploration of the abdomen into a thoracoabdominal incision, as will be discussed below.

Peripheral lobar lacerations are readily handled with encircling fingers, with a large springy clamp or with a choker tourniquet.[13] However, in major central lacerations of the liver, two potentially lethal problems may yet remain: (1) exsanguination from associated tears of the vena cava or of the major hepatic veins and (2) air embolism through these rents during an inspiratory phase. To ameliorate at least one part of this situation, although it may play havoc with venous return, the anesthetist should have the patient in a reverse Trendelenburg position and should try to maintain a positive pressure within the airway from the time the cava is uncovered until control of it is achieved. The patient may be tilted to the left if air embolism is inevitable.

Sometimes exposure through a right

Fig. 45-6.—Extravasation of contrast substance through ruptured arteries *(arrows)*. Other roentgenograms showed adjacent fractured ribs. The celiac axis is filled by collaterals from injection of the superior mesenteric artery but not by direct celiac injection; this finding is consistent with stenosis of the celiac axis.

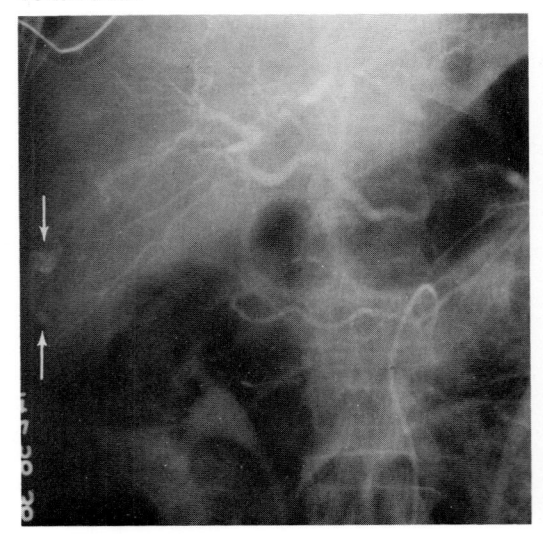

paramedian incision is sufficient enough that caval injuries can be controlled with application of either a sidewall clamp or with several Allis forceps, particularly if all of the ligamentous attachments of the liver are divided. On occasion in major vascular injuries, complete control of the infrahepatic and suprahepatic vena cava by cross-clamping is necessary.[2, 42] In this event, simultaneous occlusions of the aorta will minimize pooling of blood in the lower extremities.[22] Nonetheless, if the cava has to be cross-clamped, other adjuncts to permit control without obstructing venous return must be applied soon.

One of the most useful is to open immediately into the left hemithorax through the seventh or eighth intercostal space without dividing the costal margin. As soon as a hand can be inserted, the index and middle fingers can compress the supradiaphragmatic vena cava, oc-

Fig. 45-7.—Intravascular shunt proposed for controlling tears in the vena cava or hepatic veins.

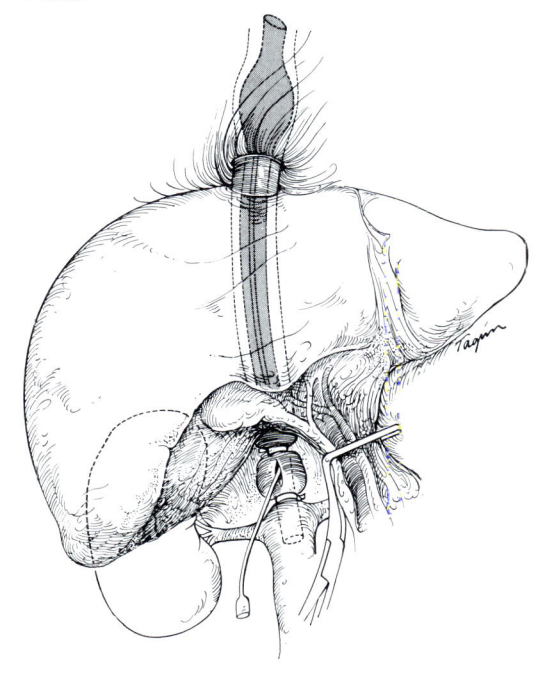

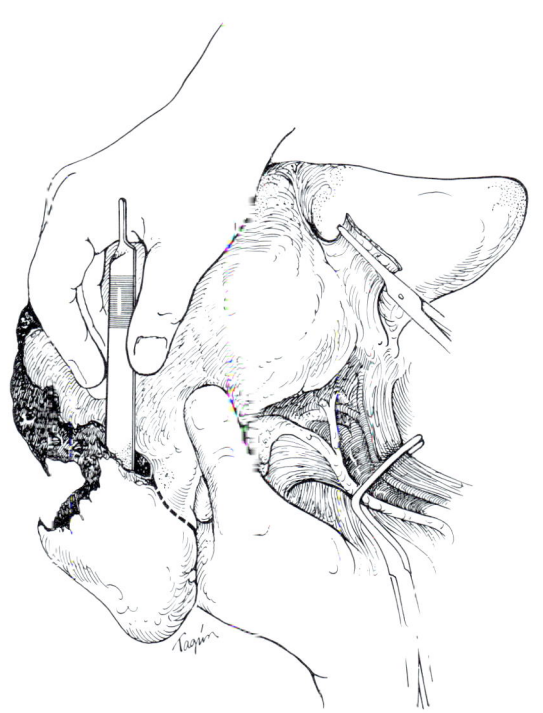

Fig. 45-8.—Guillotine removal of functionally complete sublobar lacerations. Bile ducts and blood vessels are ligated individually. Mattress sutures may be used to control ooze from the rest of the parenchyma.

clude it and push the infradiaphragmatic vena cava and liver toward the surface of the abdominal incision. With this exposure, which incidentally eliminates the effect of negative intrathoracic pressure in predisposing to air embolism, and with the added view provided by removing any clamp between the liver and the diaphragm, lacerations sometimes become visible and thus amenable to direct control by clamping and then undersewing the clamps. On occasion, this maneuver may also permit repair of injury in the left hepatic lobe, even near the midline, without the necessity of a formal thoracoabdominal incision. Division of the falciform ligament permits retraction on its hepatic end, the better to expose the suprahepatic vena cava for cross-clamping.

If control of bleeding is not instant and the surgeon is not able to mobilize all of the ligamentous attachments of the liver, the incision must be deepened radially through the diaphragm at once to permit the liver to fall into the thorax and thus expose its root. As this incision is made, thought should be given to avoiding the phrenic nerve and the inferior phrenic blood vessels. Severed vessels should be methodically sought after vascular compensation is restored.

Since failure to control bleeding promptly usually spells death, an attempt at placing an internal vascular shunt should be considered if the simpler means of controlling hemorrhage from the vena cava and hepatic veins fail. One approach to the problem involves passing a long polyvinyl tube distal through the right atrium and drawing the inferior vena cava above and below the tear snug around it.[39] The upper end of the tube may be permitted to protrude through a purse-string suture in the atrium, but obviously should have a sidewall hole in its intra-atrial portion, about 20 cm from the end in the inferior vena cava, to permit caval blood to enter the heart. Another approach also appears practical.[2, 10] A standard cuffed endotracheal tube, preferably silastic or polyethylene, is passed via a venotomy through the tear and is seated above the diaphragm by inflation of the cuff. Encircling tapes above and below the point of insertion complete the vascular control. When all else fails, the only recourse may be compression of the cava and liver with packs until anatomic removal of the injured segments is carried out.

CHOICE OF RESECTION. — The direct approach is best. After the suspensory ligaments are divided, as may be required, fractures of the periphery of either the right or left lobe should be completed as guillotine amputations.[15, 25, 31] Attempts to convert them into formal lobectomies or segmentectomies are meddlesome and unnecessary. Because major lacerations more central in the right lobe nearly always enter through both anterior and posterior segments, they should be handled by total right lobectomy if they involve the vena cava. When they do not involve the cava, guillotine amputations are usually possible.

Deep lacerations in the medial segment of the left lobe are controlled more easily by total left lobectomy than by ill-advised attempts to resect the medial segment and to preserve the left lateral segment. Only when the injury is in the left lateral segment, in essence, the tissue to the left of the falciform ligament, should formal segmental resections be entertained in major liver trauma, but the guillotine technique usually is possible here also. Such a resection is easily performed through an abdominal incision alone and is quickly compensated for by the body.[9]

The extraordinary situation of a major shattering injury to both lobes probably is managed best by excision of as much devitalized tissue as possible combined with mattress sutures placed deep in the tissue to remain.[25] Ligation of one or both of the branches of the hepatic artery ought to be considered,[5, 27] but for this desperate prescription to have any chance of success, particular attention must be paid to maintaining the blood pressure and to preventing infection in the postoperative period.[8]

In the uncommon event that a formal lobectomy is necessary because of massive injury or because of damage to the cava or hepatic veins, the plane of resection ought to avoid the true anatomic division (the gallbladder fossa) in order to reduce the possibility of a longitudinal incision through the middle hepatic vein, which courses in an anteroposterior direction in the gallbladder fossa. The easier planes are, for a right lobectomy, from 2 cm to the right of the gallbladder fossa to 2 cm to the right of the vena cava and, for a left lobectomy, from 2 cm to the left of the fossa to 2 cm to the left of the vena cava.[26] These planes will provide

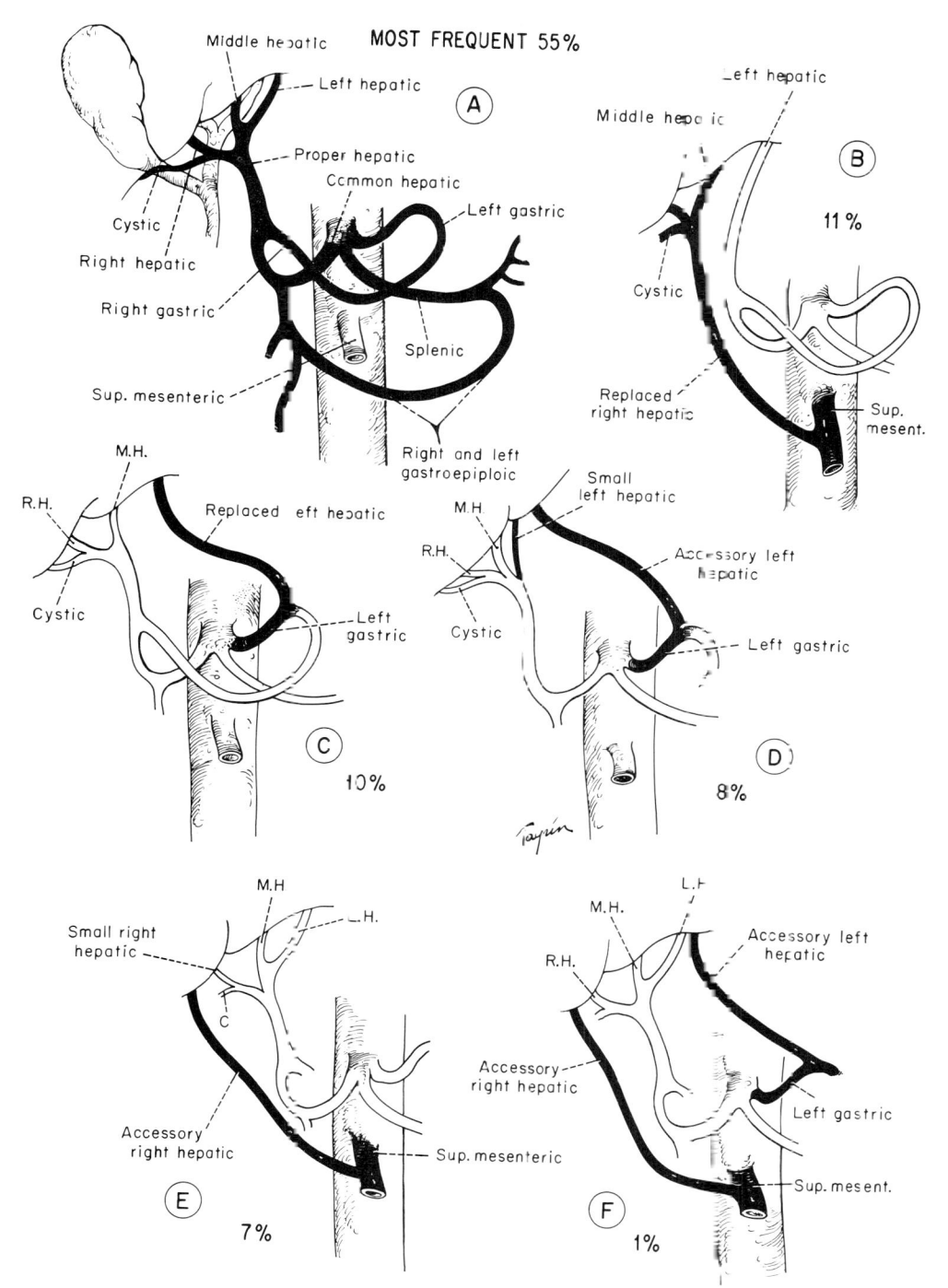

Fig. 45-9.—Major anatomic variations of the hepatic arterial supply to the liver. **A,** normal. **B,** replaced right hepatic artery arising from the superior mesenteric artery. **C,** replaced left hepatic artery arising from the left gastric artery. **D,** accessory left hepatic artery. **E,** accessory right hepatic artery. **F,** accessory left and right hepatic arteries.

stumps of suitable length for the hepatic veins and a cushion of liver around the cava to hold stitch ligatures.

Resections of the left lateral segment should avoid the plane of the falciform ligament to prevent cutting through the branch of the left portal vein running in a posteroanterior direction at this point. The preferred plane of resection, therefore, is 2–3 cm to the right or left of the falciform ligament.

TECHNIQUE OF RESECTION. — All anatomic resections of the liver begin with division of the falciform ligament, ligamentum teres and suspensory ligaments.[1, 5, 6, 12, 18, 21, 26, 29, 33-35] The clamp attached to the round ligament becomes a handle to move the liver up and down or sideways as the need for exposure demands.

Although the safe period of total occlusion of the total hepatic inflow at normothermic temperatures before a period of unclamping and transient perfusion is said to be 20 minutes, seldom is there any difficulty with 30 minutes of total local circulatory arrest in the normally hypothermic victim of massive trauma given many transfusions of cool blood. Nonetheless, arterial inflow should be restored early to the undamaged liver tissue. Both major hepatic lobectomies and left lateral segmentectomy should begin with identification and occlusion of the ipsilateral hepatic artery high in the gastrohepatic omentum. A prudent gesture at this point is to insert a firm rubber catheter through the common hepatic duct into the division of the hepatic duct to be spared. The branch of the portal vein on the side of the trauma then is identified and occluded; in about a quarter of cases, the bifurcation of the portal vein will be intrahepatic. In lobectomies, division and ligation of these vessels — or of the replaced and accessory right and left hepatic arteries described earlier — completes securing of the vascular inflow. The ipsilateral hepatic duct becomes readily accessible and the lobe to be removed becomes visibly demarcated from the lobe that is to stay. The common variations in anatomy in the area in which all these strictures bifurcate is shown in Figure 45-9.

In performance of a left lateral segmentectomy it is easier to maintain occlusion of the whole left hepatic artery and left branch of the portal vein than to attempt to identify the segmental vessels near the hilum. Identification of the appropriate vessels to the lateral segment often is simpler after the parenchyma has been divided to the depths.

Following mobilization of the appropriate suspensory ligaments, the liver substance in the proper plane is split with the handle of a scalpel or by finger fracture to prevent retraction of severed vessels cut with a sharp blade. All tubular structures, irrespective of size, are individually divided between hemostatic clamps and secured with fine silk or clips. The dissection is carried back to the root of the liver, where the appropriate major hepatic vein is identified and divided; minor veins are tied individually.

In the absence of a cross-clamped vena cava or a cava threaded with an internal shunt, unexpected massive bleeding may be precipitated at two points in the resection. If bleeding is encountered when a good deal of parenchyma has yet to be divided, almost certainly the middle hepatic vein has been sliced longitudinally during a dissection too close to the anatomic midline; either the vein can be repaired or a more extended hepatectomy done. More frequently, hemorrhage occurs when only a minute, and apparently inconsequential, amount of tissue far to the posterior end of the liver remains to be divided. In this instance, a bold last swipe may transect or avulse the ipsilateral vein or, on the left, may divide a middle hepatic vein that empties into the left hepatic vein rather than into the cava. Compression and elevation of the supradiaphragmatic cava with fingers as has already been described may well be lifesaving. Intermittent constriction of the intrapericardial superior vena cava by an encircling tape may engorge the smaller branches of the hepatic vein enough to make their identification and control easier.[19]

TERMINAL HEMOSTASIS.— If all vessels and ducts have been secured as encountered, the amount of ooze from the raw surface after either formal lobectomy or guillotine removal of lesser segments usually will be minimal. No further hemostatic measures are necessary in this event. A test for unsuspected bile leakage is carried out easily by injecting saline solution into the common hepatic or bile duct and searching for its appearance at the plane of resection[14]; using methylene blue for this purpose unnecessarily obscures the issue.

Should troublesome oozing persist, either a series of 0 chromic catgut mattress sutures may be placed over buttresses of omentum and tied firm or interlocking catgut sutures may be employed. The use of hemostatic, supposedly absorbable, sponges is to be condemned, for they may persist for many months as foreign bodies and foci of sepsis.

After hemostasis is complete, there is no reason that the raw surface cannot be allowed to remain that way, except that the unfinished surface is alien to the surgeon's eye. If omentum or the flap of falciform ligament is brought up to shield this area or to help in final hemostasis, the tissue cover should be made loose rather than watertight, so that exudate will not be trapped.

The essential final step is the placement of large sump drains plus Penrose drains to provide evacuation of the subphrenic and infrahepatic regions and the cut section of the liver. Two or three sumps usually are required and are left in place for as long as they evacuate liquid.

Argument no longer exists about whether the common bile duct should be vented. Although greater likelihood of survival has been attributed to relief from pressure surges within the biliary system[35] and to the removal of the fibrinolytic action of bile,[43] controlled studies show twice the mortality when T-tubes are used.[24] T-tubes should not be used unless the common bile duct as well as the liver is injured.

Postoperative Course

The central venous pressure catheter is valuable since the capacity of intravascular volume in patients with hepatic resections seems brittle—easily overloaded, provoking pulmonary edema or easily under-replaced, precipitating vasomotor collapse. To avoid thrombophlebitis, the usual hastily placed central venous pressure catheter must not be allowed to remain in situ more than 48 hours.

Besides the potential need for replacement of whole blood, there always is a requirement for plasma after hepatectomy. As an estimate, if the normal catabolism of albumin at 10.9 gm/day in the average man[37] is increased one-third by the metabolic demands of convalescence and even as little as 2 liters of high-protein exudate are lost into the peritoneal cavity, one-third of the total exchangeable albumin will be depleted in a single day; the intravascular volume accordingly will be quite depleted. Because the regenerating liver is not well enough redifferentiated during this time to make much of a contribution to replacement, transfusion of 175 gm of albumin, or more, may be required during this period.[29]

Although hypoglycemia, resulting from lack of glycogen stores, is infrequent, a drip of 10% glucose ought to be running from the beginning of surgery until homeostasis is adequate several days later. Placing a gastrostomy is wise.[29]

Vitamin K may be required to support prothrombin function at levels compatible with the surgeon's ease, but only infrequently is it truly needed to counteract a frank bleeding diathesis attributable to lack of prothrombin. Administration of EACA and transfusions of fibrinogen or of fresh whole blood or fresh plasma sometimes will rectify other less-well-defined problems of coagulation.[20]

Complications

The early difficulties relate to maintenance of vascular volume and local bleeding. The later difficulties relate to bleeding, sepsis and the hepatorenal syndrome. Since support of the intravascular volume has already been discussed, and since the thing to do about intra-abdominal bleeding is to stop it, the major residual difficulty is infection, which is more easily prevented by adequate sump drainage than treated with antibiotics and incision after it occurs. The best prophylaxis against hepatorenal syndrome seems to be maintenance of blood pressure at all times, removal of devitalized tissue and, perhaps, use of mannitol during the operation.

If persistent gastrointestinal bleeding occurs following injury to the liver, hepatic angiography should be given preference to roentgenograms of the gastrointestinal tract in order to identify the site of bleeding and to avoid obscuring the view with barium. Post-traumatic hemobilia sometimes may subside, giving an opportunity to defer its correction until the patient is somewhat better, but the trouble often will persist or recur. Under the circumstances, control occasionally will be possible by unroofing a cavity and tying the vessel responsible. Often, a resection will be necessary if the bleeding vessel is clearly limited to a lobe or to a segment.[44] If resection is not feasible, sometimes ligation of the common hepatic artery proximal to the gastroduodenal artery will suffice.[45] Although ligation of the proper hepatic artery itself or of the right or left hepatic arteries is more to be feared in these potentially hypotensive and infected patients than in otherwise normal people undergoing laparotomy,[3, 8] these possibilities should be kept in active reserve.

Stress ulcers[18] and fatty metamorphosis of the liver are handled according to usual principles. The rare post-traumatic cysts usually can be evacuated and drained and fistulas repaired by standard methods. Complications of the wound, the perihepatic spaces, the lungs and other viscera[4, 40] are virtually the same as after any major injury in which an abdominal or thoracoabdominal operation has been necessary. However, the lungs seem to be especially vulnerable after hepatic trauma, sometimes showing widespread infiltration and abnormalities in diffusion. Overtransfusion may be an etiologic factor.

EXTRAHEPATIC BILIARY SYSTEM

In contrast to bursting injuries of the liver that become surgical emergencies because of acute blood loss, injuries of the extrahepatic biliary system make themselves known by causing pain—pain, abdominal tenderness and shock—which usually is said to clear within a day or two, before returning after another few days transformed into signs of localized fluid collection, jaundice and choluria.[26] Victims of transection of the portal vein or hepatic artery probably die of these or of other injuries before they reach a hospital. In complete transection of the extrahepatic biliary ducts, stools may be acholic.

Except for transections of the intrahepatic portions of the bile ducts, liver injury and biliary injury rarely seem to coexist. The absence of liver injury is not assurance that a blow to the right upper quadrant has not transected the extrahepatic biliary system—quite the contrary. Transection of the ducts probably requires a direct and localized injury undiffused by rupture of other organs and severe enough to shear fixed portions of the ducts against unyielding posterior structures or away from fixed points. For these reasons, the usual sites of injury are in the free portion of the common duct as it traverses the spine and the terminal portion behind the pancreas; however, they may be anywhere—and of any size, from pinpoint to complete transections.[11, 17, 38] The rarity of ruptures of the hepatic artery and portal vein, even in medicolegal cases, suggests that the elasticity, distensibility or location of these vessels usually protects them from isolated trauma.

Even when injury is restricted to the gallbladder, the biliary system will be harder to repair and the patient will be sicker when the injury has been unattended for days; it therefore follows that repair is best done at the time of injury. Cholecystectomy takes care of injuries to the gallbladder. The principles for reconstruction of other injuries are the same as for repair of operative injuries of the duct, and the results may be inferred to be about the same. Although no one has had enough experience with this uncommon problem to have an authoritative opinion, end-to-end anastomosis of the duct probably is best, followed in preference by choledochojejunostomy or cholecystojejunostomy into a Roux en Y loop or choledochoduodenostomy. Obviously, an undamaged gallbladder and cystic duct should not be removed despite an apparently successful union on common duct and bowel. Late strictures may occur, and the availability of the gallbladder may provide the way out of a difficult situation. Drainage of the peritoneal cavity is indispensable. Complications are handled as with injuries to the liver.

BIBLIOGRAPHY

1. Ackroyd, F. W., Pollard, J., and McDermott, W. V.: Massive hepatic resection in the treatment of severe liver trauma, Am. J. Surg. 117:442, 1969.
2. Albo, D., Christensen, C., Rasmussen, B. L., and King, T. C.: Massive liver trauma involving the suprarenal vena cava, Am. J. Surg. 118:960, 1969.
3. Almersjö, O., Bengmark, S., Engevik, L., Hafström, L. O., Loughridge, B. P., and Nilsson, L. A.: Serum enzyme changes after hepatic dearterialization in man, Ann. Surg. 167:9, 1968.
4. Amerson, J. R., and Stone, H. E.: Experiences in the management of hepatic trauma, Arch. Surg. 100:150, 1970.
5. Aronsen, K. F., Bengmark, S., Dahlgren, S., Engevik, L., Ericsson, B., and Theren, L.: Liver resection in the treatment of blunt injuries to the liver, Surgery 63:236, 1968.
6. Baker, R. J., Taxman, P., and Freeark, R. J.: An assessment of the management of non-penetrating liver injuries, Arch. Surg. 93:84, 1966.
7. Balasegaram, M.: Blunt injuries to the liver: Problems and management, Ann. Surg. 169:544, 1969.
8. Brittain, R. S., Marchioro, T. L., Hermann, G., Waddell, W. R., and Starzl, T. E.: Accidental hepatic artery ligation in humans, Am. J. Surg. 107:822, 1964.
9. Bucher, N. L. R., and Malt, R. A.: *Regeneration of Liver and Kidney* (Boston: Little, Brown & Company, 1970).
10. Chávez-Peón, F., Gonzalez, E., and Malt, R. A.: Vena cava catheter for asanguineous liver resection, Surgery 67:694, 1970
11. Dobbie, R. P., and Stormo, A. C.: Complete transection of the common bile duct, the sole sequela of blunt abdominal trauma, J. Trauma 8:9, 1968.
12. Donovan, A. J., Turrill, F. L., and Facey, F. L.: Hepatic trauma, Surg. Clin. North Am. 48:1313, 1968.
13. Doty, D. B., Kugler, H. W., and Moseley, R. V.: Control of the hepatic parenchyma by direct compression: A new instrument, Surgery 67:720, 1970.
14. Dow, R., and Thompson, N.: Bile stasis after hepatic resection, Surg. Gynecol. Obstet. 127:1075, 1968.
15. Fischer, R. P., Stremple, J. F., MacNamara, J. J., and Guernsey, C. J.: The rapid right hepatectomy, J. Trauma 11:742, 1971.
16. Fish, J. C., and Nippert, R. H.: Traumatic hemobilia: The dilemma of delay, J. Trauma 9:546, 1969.
17. Fletcher, W. S., Mahnke, D. E., and Dunphy, J. E.: Complete division of the common bile duct due to blunt trauma. Report of a case and review of the literature, J. Trauma 1:87, 1961.
18. Foster, J. H., Lawler, M. R., Welborn, M. B., Holcomb, G. W., and Sawyers, J. L.: Recent experience with major hepatic resection, Ann. Surg. 167:651, 1968.
19. Gentile, J. M., and MacLean, L. D.: Improved technique for human hepatic resection, Am. J. Surg. 117:424, 1969.
20. Groth, C. G.: Changes in Coagulation, in Starzl, T. E., *Experience in Hepatic Transplantation* (Philadelphia: W. B. Saunders Company, 1969), pp. 159–175.
21. Hardy, K. J.: Liver trauma: Royal Melbourne Hospital experience, 1956 to 1969, Med. J. Aust. 1:929, 1970.
22. Heany, J. P., Stanson, W. K., Halbert, D. S., Swidel, J., and Vice, T.: An improved technique for vascular isolation of the liver. Experimental study and case reports, Ann. Surg. 163:237, 1966.
23. Lane, T. C., Johnson, H. C., and Walker, H. S. J.: Extrahepatic biliary decompression in traumatized canine livers, Surgery 62:1039, 1967.
24. Lucas, C. E., and Ledgerwood, A. M.: Controlled biliary drainage for large injuries of the liver, Surg. Gynecol. Obstet. 137:585, 1973.
25. Lucas, C. E., and Walt, A. J.: Critical decisions

in liver trauma: Experience based on 604 cases, Arch. Surg. 101:277, 1970.
26. Madding, G. F., and Kennedy, P. A.: *Trauma to the Liver* (2nd ed.; Philadelphia: W. B. Saunders Company, 1971).
27. Mays, E. T., and Wheeler, C. S.: Demonstration of collateral arterial flow after interruption of hepatic arteries in man, N. Engl. J. Med. 290:993, 1974.
28. McClelland, R., Shires, T., and Poulos, E.: Hepatic resection for massive trauma, J. Trauma 4:282, 1964.
29. McDermott, W. V., and Ottinger, L. W.: Elective hepatic resection, Am. J. Surg. 112:376, 1966.
30. Michels, N. A.: Newer anatomy of the liver and its variant blood supply and collateral circulation, Am. J. Surg. 112:337, 1966.
31. Morton, J. R., Roys, G., and Brecker, D. L.: A review of 1,068 cases of civilian liver injury, Surg. Gynecol. Obstet. 134:298, 1972.
32. Moyle, W. D., and Karl, R. C.: Rupture of the extrahepatic biliary ducts by external blunt trauma, J. Trauma 9:623, 1969.
33. Nemhauser, G. M., Cleveland, R. J., Benfield, J. R., and Thompson, J. C.: Resectional therapy in massive liver injury, J. Trauma 9:537, 1969.
34. Payne, W. D., Terz, J. J., and Lawrence, W.: Major hepatic resection for trauma, Ann. Surg. 170:929, 1969.
35. Perry, J. F., Root, H. D., Hauser, C. W., and Keizer, P. J.: Treatment of hepatic injuries, Surgery 62:853, 1967.
36. Pilcher, D. B.: Penetrating injuries of the liver in Vietnam, Ann. Surg. 170:793, 1969.
37. Rossing, N.: The normal metabolism of ^{131}I-labeled albumin in man, Clin. Sci. 33:593, 1967.
38. Rydell, W. B.: Complete transection of the common bile duct due to blunt abdominal trauma, Arch. Surg. 100:724, 1970.
39. Schrock, T., Blaisdell, F. W., and Mathewson, C.: Management of blunt trauma to the liver and hepatic veins, Arch. Surg. 96:698, 1968.
40. Solhein, K., and Aune, S.: Traumatic liver rupture, Injury 1:39, 1969.
41. Stone, H. H., Long, W. D., Smith, R. B., and Haynes, C. D.: Physiologic considerations in major hepatic resections, Am. J. Surg. 117:78, 1969.
42. Waltuck, T. L., Crow, R. W., Humphrey, L. J., and Kauffman, H. M.: Avulsion injuries of the vena cava following blunt abdominal trauma, Ann. Surg. 171:67, 1970.
43. Wasowski, J. R.: Drainage of the common bile duct in experimental injury to the liver, Am. J. Surg. 115:787, 1968.
44. Whelan, T. J., and Gillespie, J. T.: Treatment of traumatic hemobilia, Ann. Surg. 162:920, 1965.
45. Wilkinson, G. M., Mikkelsen, W. P., and Berne, C. J.: The treatment of post-traumatic hemobilia by ligation of the common hepatic artery, Surg. Clin. North Am. 48:1337, 1968.

46 | Injuries to the Genitourinary Tract

WALTER S. KERR, JR.

KIDNEY

ETIOLOGY.—Renal trauma occurs most frequently in young males. It can be conveniently divided into 2 categories, nonpenetrating and penetrating.

Nonpenetrating trauma.—The most common cause is an accident, occurring in traffic, in athletics, at work or at home. The mechanisms of injury (Fig. 46-1) are (1) a direct or transmitted force to the kidney through the rib cage or through the abdomen and (2) an indirect force (contrecoup injuries). The former is the most common. In the latter, the body is abruptly stopped, as in a fall or an automobile accident, and the kidney continues to move, causing separation of, or damage to, the renal pedicle.

Penetrating trauma.—The second category of renal injury consists of penetrating wounds caused by knives or missiles. These accidents are becoming more common in some strife-torn cities. High-velocity missile injuries that occur in combat result in shattered kidneys and usually are associated with severe injuries to adjacent structures.

PATHOLOGY.—Early pathologic findings range from (1) simple contusion to (2) mild or severe parenchymal fractures with disruption of the capsule and/or collecting system to (3) fragmented kidneys and (4) damaged or separated renal pedicles (Fig. 46-1, C). Late pathology includes scarring, varying degrees of atrophy, cyst formation and calcification. Extravasation of urine may lead to scarring around the ureter, with ureteral obstruction and hydronephrosis and possibly pyonephrosis; or scarring around the renal artery, with resulting atrophy of the kidney and occasionally hypertension.

COMMON SYMPTOMS AND SIGNS.—The common complaints include varying degrees of pain and tenderness in the flank and adjacent areas. If clots are formed and obstruct the ureter, typical renal colic may be present. When there is severe hemorrhage from the kidney, evidence of hematoma in the flank with an expanding mass will be found and a state of shock will develop.

Hematuria may be either microscopic or gross. Commonly, bleeding may last a short time, and thus, in suspected trauma, microscopic examination of the urine should be done early.

Diagnosis

A careful history is taken, if possible, to determine the type of injury and the direction of the blow. Knowledge of previous kidney pathology and results of previous intravenous urograms should be recorded.

A thorough, careful examination of the flank and abdomen for tenderness, mass and rigidity are essential. In penetrating

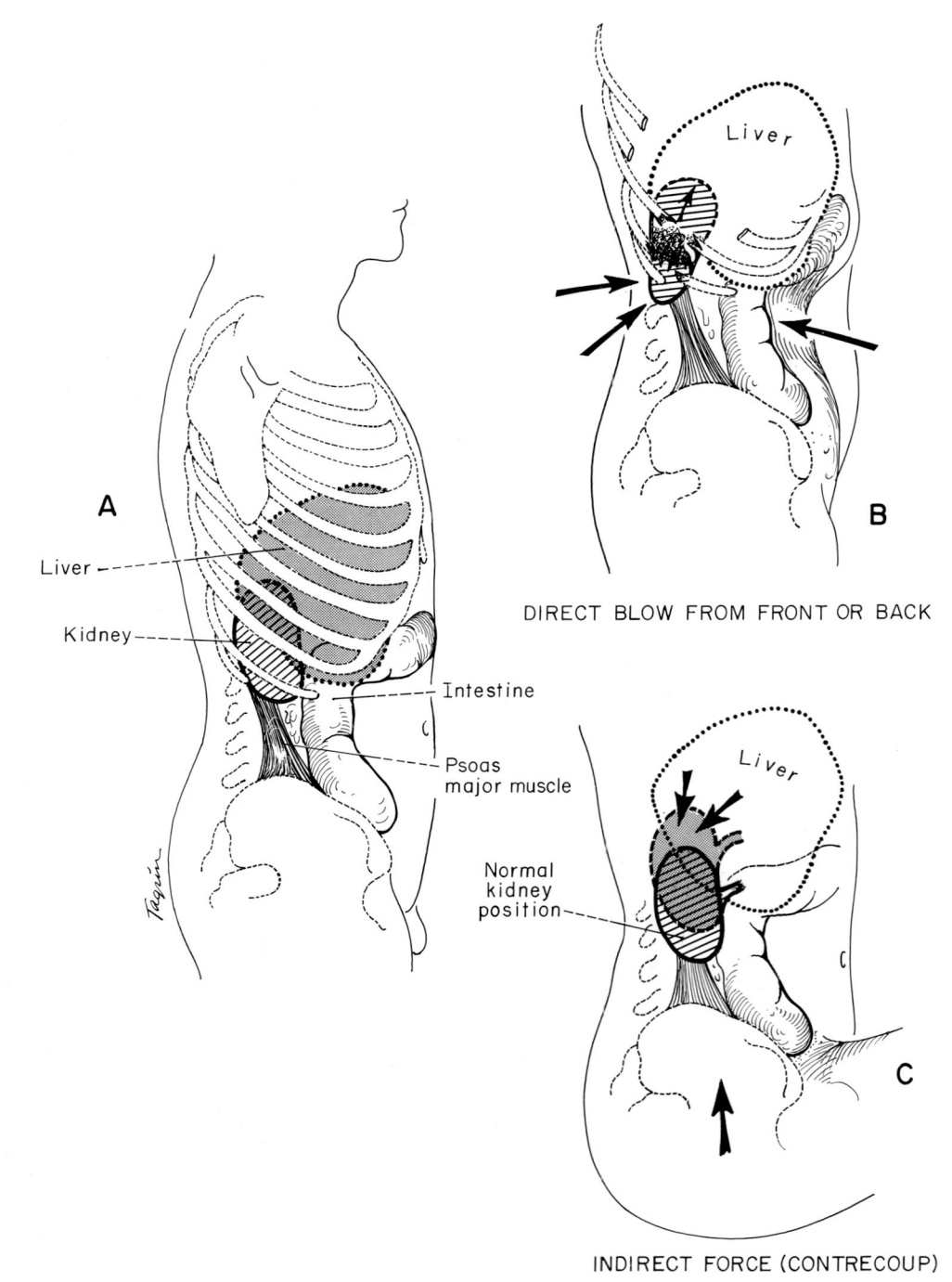

Fig. 46-1.—Mechanisms of injury. **A,** normal anatomic relationships. **B,** direct or transmitted force. **C,** indirect force.

wounds, both the entry and exit wounds should be identified. If rupture of an intraperitoneal viscus is suspected, 4 quadrant taps or peritoneal lavage are indicated. One must look for evidence of bone fractures in adjacent ribs or vertebrae. If a hematoma or mass is present, outline it with a marking pencil so that changes in size can be recognized.

ROENTGENOGRAPHY.—In renal trauma the following studies should be considered.
KUB
Infusion IV urography with nephrotomography
Retrograde pyelography
Renal angiography
Renal venography
Renal scan

KUB.—The KUB films should be carefully inspected for: (1) asymmetry or loss of renal outline; (2) fractures, especially of adjacent ribs and vertebrae; (3) blurring or obliteration of the psoas shadow; (4) signs of peritoneal irritation; (5) elevation of the diaphragm or atelectasis.

Infusion intravenous urography with nephrotomography.—Hypaque sodium 25% in a 300-ml bottle is available and allows an infusion intravenous urography to be easily done. The 300 ml of fluid is run in at body temperature in 3–10 minutes. When combined with nephrotomography it is the most useful, simple study one can obtain in patients with renal trauma. In addition to giving vital information regarding the kidneys, it outlines the ureters and bladder. It can be done without bowel preparation in nonfasting, hydrated patients with excellent results.

In such a study the films should be checked for: (1) the state of the other kidney; (2) evidence of segmental decreased or absent function; (3) evidence of extravasation of dye; (4) separation of a pole of the kidney; (5) no function. If a kidney is not visualized, it could be due to an absent kidney, an ectopic kidney, a nonfunctioning kidney due to pre-existing disease, a fragmented kidney or injury to the renal pedicle.

Retrograde pyelography.—Indications for this technique include: (1) history of severe allergy to iodine; (2) nonfunctioning of the kidneys, thought to be due to chronic infection or suspected congenital abnormalities (20% of Persky and Forsythe's series[8]); (3) suspected ectopic kidneys; (4) other cases of unsatisfactory urograms when renal angiograms are not available.

Renal angiography.—Emergency renal angiograms now are easily obtainable in many community hospitals as well as in large centers. Angiography gives the most detailed information of both the parenchyma and the vascular system and should be done in patients with suspected injury to the renal blood supply and when visualization of the parenchyma is inadequate.

Renal venography.—Renal venography is helpful if renal vein thrombosis is suspected. It can be done at the same time that selective angiography is performed.

Renal scan.—This is recommended by Kazmin el al.[6] in identifying areas of parenchymal damage. If facilities and enthusiastic personnel are available, renal scan should be considered.

Grades of Injury Judged Radiologically

Grading the injuries radiologically provides guidelines for treatment.[13]

Grade I.—Simple contusion of the kidney. The IV urogram is normal in all respects. There is no evidence of a collecting system defect and no obliteration of caliceal systems.

Grade II.—Parenchymal damage without evidence of lacerated capsule or collecting system. An intravenous urogram may show displacement or spreading of the caliceal pattern, due to bleeding within the parenchyma.

Grade III.—Lacerated capsule and parenchyma with intact collecting system. The KUB will show a blurred kidney shadow and obliteration of the psoas muscles and possibly displacement of the kidney as a result of bleeding from the parenchyma or capsular vessels.

Grade IV.—Severe injury to the parenchyma, capsule and/or collecting system. This group includes fragmented kidneys. The KUB will again show loss of renal shadow, possible loss of psoas shadow and possible displacement of the kidney. The intravenous urogram shows extravasation of urine outside of the kidney if the kidney is still functioning. If the kidney is badly fragmented, there will be little or no function.

Grade V.—Injury to the renal pedicle is most often seen after a contrecoup injury. Injuries to the renal pedicle include laceration or separation of 1 or both renal vessels, thrombosis of the renal vessels and spasm of the renal artery. The intravenous pyelogram shows no function if the renal artery is partially or completely separated. There would be evidence of extrarenal hemorrhage on that side. If there is only spasm or thrombosis of 1 of the vessels, the renal outline should be normal, without evidence of perirenal bleeding. A renal angiogram should be made.

Treatment

All patients with grade I and grade II injuries will respond to conservative treatment. They should remain at bedrest until the urine is free from evidence of bleeding for 24 hours. All patients with

Fig. 46-2.—A bulldog clamp has been placed on the right renal artery before opening Gerota's fascia and exposing the right kidney.

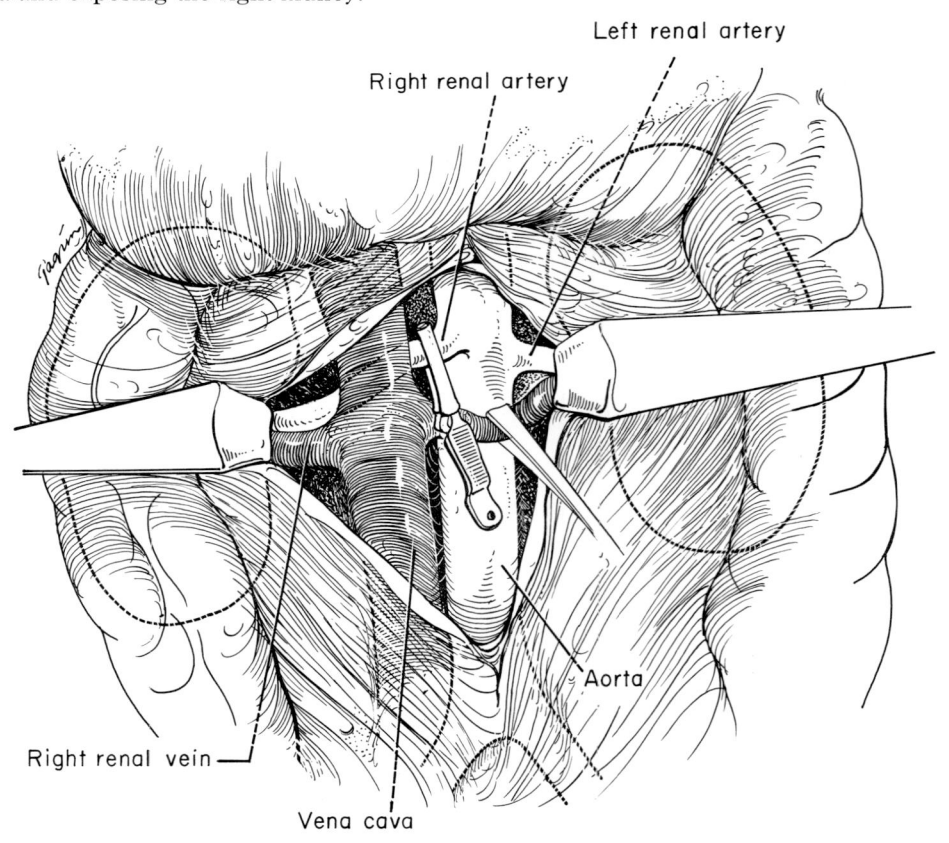

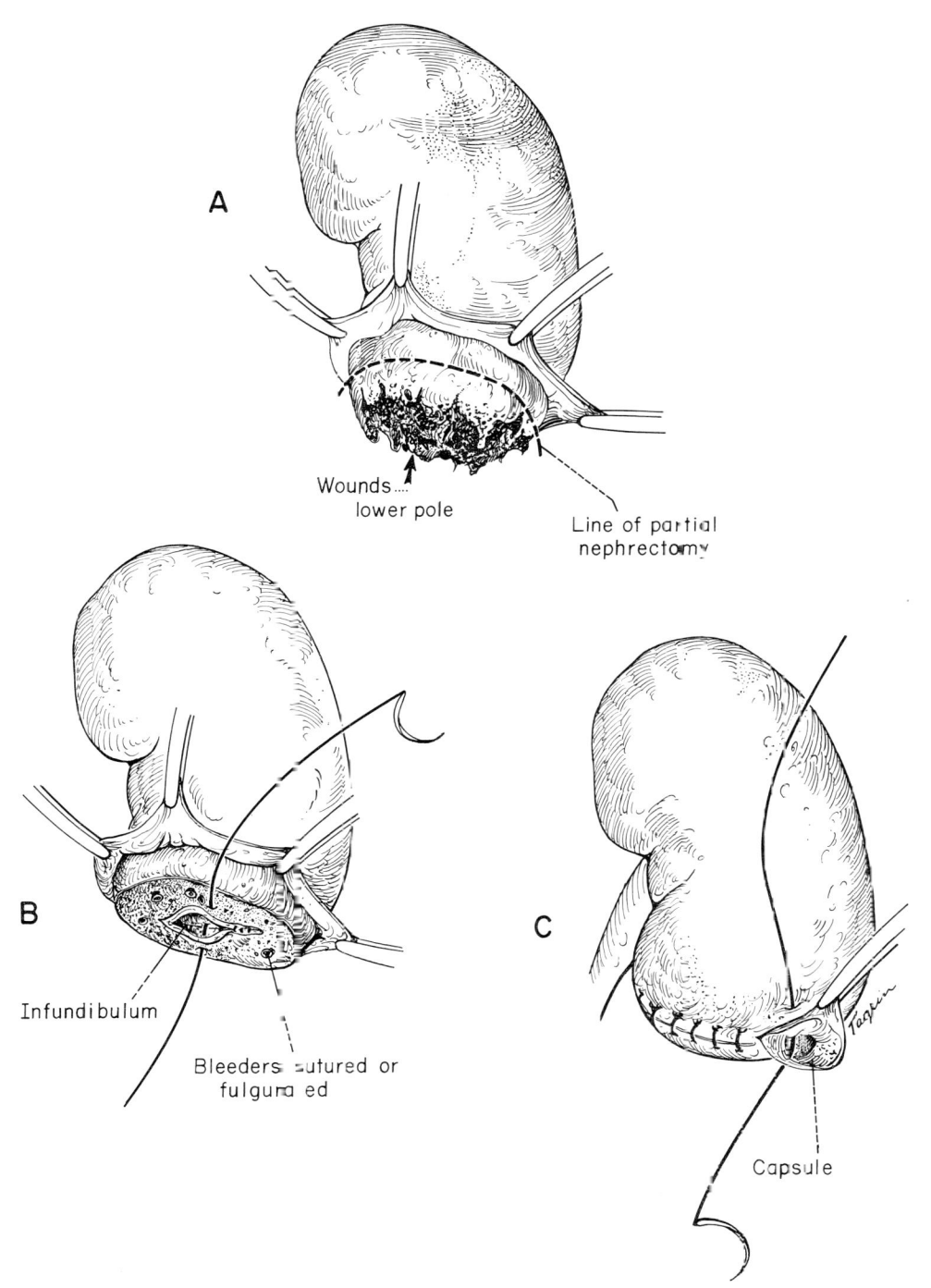

Chapter 46: INJURIES TO THE GENITOURINARY TRACT / 1075

Fig. 46-3.—Kidney repair. A, devascularized tissue is excised. B and C, bleeders are fulgurated or sutured, the calix or infundibulum closed and the capsule repaired.

grade V and some with grade IV lesions must be operated on. In grade V lesions operation should be done as soon as the diagnosis is made and the patient's general condition permits.

Patients with grades III and IV lesions who do not respond to treatment of shock, or who have associated intra-abdominal injuries, should be operated on promptly. All mild or moderate injuries heal, and only a few complications develop, such as hydronephrosis or infection, that necessitate secondary operation.

SURGICAL TREATMENT.—Surgical treatment should be directed to the conservation of renal tissue whenever possible. If exploration becomes necessary because of continued bleeding, reconstruction of the kidney with removal of as little of the kidney as possible should be the goal. Scott and associates[11] have emphasized the advisability of exploring such kidneys through an abdominal incision, so that control of the renal vessels may be obtained before opening Gerota's fascia (Fig. 46-2). Opening of Gerota's fascia first results in loss of a tamponading effect, and bleeding may be so brisk and uncontrollable that a kidney otherwise salvageable may have to be removed to control the bleeding. Devascularized kidney tissue should be removed, with hemostasis obtained by either coagulating the renal arterials or using fine stitch-ligatures.

When a partial nephrectomy is done, the capsule should be approximated with catgut sutures, if possible (Fig. 46-3). If there is insufficient capsule to do this, a patch of peritoneum or fascia may be used. A nephrostomy or pyelostomy may be indicated. Drainage of the area through a retroperitoneal stab wound is advisable when there is evidence of infection or continued bleeding from surrounding tissues.

If infection of a hematoma or extravasated urine occurs in patients treated conservatively, incision and drainage will be indicated.

Secondary hemorrhage may occur between the seventh and fourteenth day and necessitate exploration. This is an excellent reason to keep the patients quiet and resting and under close supervision for this period. Perirenal cysts developing as a result of perirenal hemorrhage sometimes become large and need to be drained.

URETER

Ureteral injuries from nonsurgical causes are uncommon.[14] Damage by knife or bullet wounds are the most common. Occasionally, blunt trauma may avulse the ureter, or the ureter may be damaged by fractures of the pelvis or vertebrae. Since these ureteral injuries are so rare, the possibility is usually not considered until complications or urinary extravasation occur.

Diagnosis

Unless the possibility is suspected, diagnosis is difficult, for often there are no symptoms or signs, and accompanying injuries are obvious and sufficient to explain the clinical condition. Hematuria may be noted. Its absence is easy to understand, because it is easier for blood from the ureteral vessels to extravasate, rather than to find its way into a contracted and at times retracted ureteral opening. An intravenous urogram may demonstrate a damaged ureter or extravasation of dye if the defect is large enough.[3] A retrograde urogram will provide the most definitive study. Indigo carmine given intravenously at the time of abdominal exploration will help discover injured ureters since the dye will stain the surrounding area blue.

Complications of a leaking ureter may be (1) retroperitoneal or intraperitoneal sepsis or (2) an expanding mass with or without evidence of sepsis or leakage of urine via the drain site. Again, suspicion is of the greatest help.

Chapter 46: INJURIES TO THE GENITOURINARY TRACT / 1077

Treatment

Conservation of kidney tissue is the prime consideration. Early diagnosis and surgical correction of the defect will give the best result. An oblique, end-to-end anastomosis, using fine #5 chromic sutures, gives excellent results (Fig. 46-4). Carleton and Scott[3] report no complications in 25 patients having primary closure with either interrupted or interlocking sutures. The wound should be drained.

If the injury is close to the bladder,

Fig. 46-4.—Surgical correction of ureteral injury. **A** and **B**, the ureter is debrided and the ends fishmouthed. **C** and **D**, meticulous approximation is done with fine #5 chromic catgut interrupted or locking sutures.

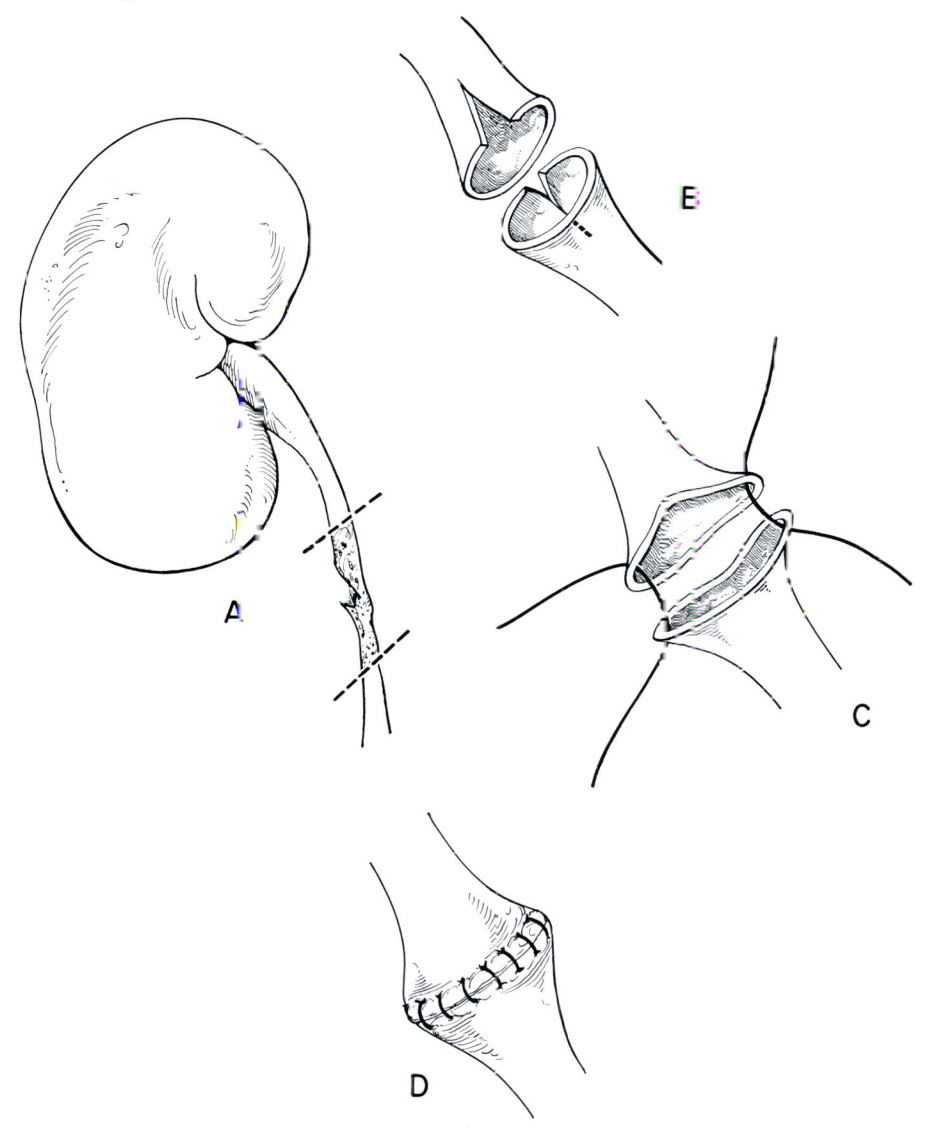

reimplantation into the bladder or into a flap of bladder can be done. A ureteroureterostomy may be indicated in some situations.

If the ureter cannot be satisfactorily approximated because of the patient's poor condition, nephrostomy will preserve the kidney until reconstruction can be carried out.

BLADDER

TYPES OF INJURY.—Bladder injuries should be suspected and investigated whenever there is trauma to the abdomen and pelvis. The types of injury include simple contusion, intraperitoneal rupture, extraperitoneal rupture and combined intra- and extraperitoneal rupture.

Simple contusion is the most common injury. Intraperitoneal rupture often occurs when the patient sustains abdominal injury when the bladder is full. The distended bladder and overlying peritoneum split posteriorly, with leakage into the peritoneal cavity.

Retroperitoneal ruptures are seen with fractures of the pubic rami. The lacerations are commonly located on the anterior and lateral portions of the bladder, close to the pubis. Urine extravasates extraperitoneally, extending around the bladder and rectum in severe cases. Prather and Keiser[10] in 1951 found approximately 10% of a total of 1,798 cases of fractured pelvis had associated rupture of the bladder. In 82% the bladder ruptures were extraperitoneal.

Combined intraperitoneal and extraperitoneal ruptures are usually associated with perforating injuries.

SYMPTOMS AND SIGNS.—The symptoms and signs will depend on the severity and location of the injury. A contused bladder may bleed microscopically or grossly. Extravasation of urine causes lower abdominal pain and tenderness. Shoulder pain will be noted as urine reaches the diaphragm. A suprapubic mass may develop. Extravasated, infected urine will result in signs of toxicity.

Diagnosis

A description of the accident will be helpful. A history of a large intake of fluid prior to the abdominal trauma, such as a steering wheel injury, would suggest the possibility of intraperitoneal rupture. The physical findings described above should be kept in mind.

A KUB film showing a pelvic fracture, especially of the pubic bones, would make one suspicious of either an extraperitoneal laceration of the bladder or damage to the membranous urethra. Diagnosis of a ruptured bladder is made definite by obtaining a cystogram. If possible, especially in pelvic fractures where the membranous urethra may be injured, a urethrogram should be obtained as the initial step. After the urethrogram has been obtained, a Foley catheter is passed into the bladder and the amount of urine present is recorded. The sediment should be examined for red cells and white cells. If white cells are present, a gram stain should be done and a specimen for culture and sensitivities sent to the laboratory.

CYSTOGRAPHY.—An ampule of Hypaque or Urokon and 250 ml of saline are instilled into the bladder gently. Anteroposterior, right and left oblique films are obtained. A delayed anteroposterior film taken 10 minutes or so after the first may reveal leakage not seen on the original x-ray. The bladder should be drained, the amount recorded and another film taken. Extravasation, obscured by the full bladder, may be visible on this last film (Figs. 46-5 and 46-6). A cystogram with negative findings in the presence of clinical evidence of extravasation should be ignored, because the laceration may have been small and sealed over by the time the cystogram was obtained. Cystoscopy is not a reliable method of demonstrating laceration.

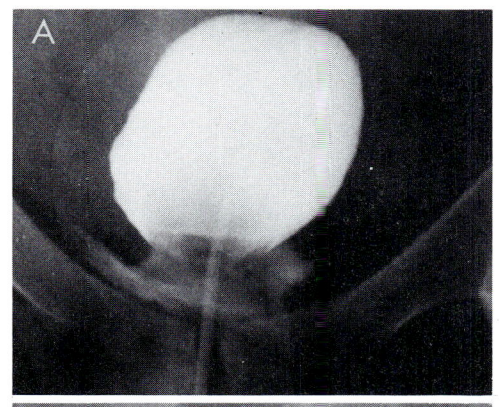

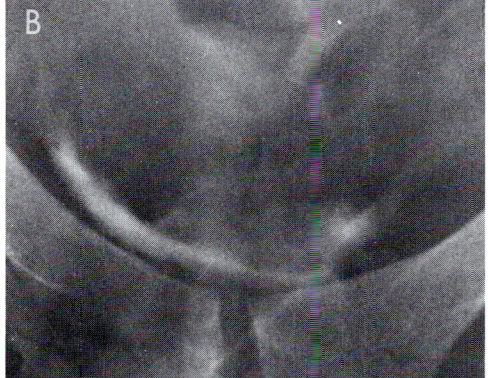

Chapter 46: INJURIES TO THE GENITOURINARY TRACT / 1079

Fig. 46-5.—A, cystogram showing extravasation of dye. B, delayed film after emptying bladder demonstrates more extensive extravasation.

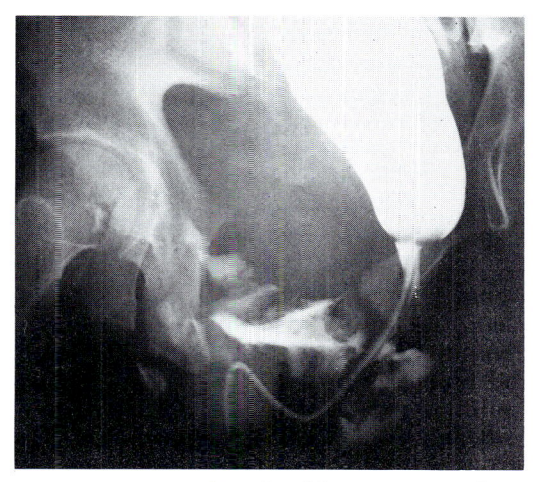

Fig 46-6.—Teardrop bladder, resulting from extensive retroperitoneal hemorrhage from badly fractured pelvis.

Treatment

CONTUSION.—The bleeding from a contused bladder will usually stop with Foley catheter drainage.

INTRAPERITONEAL RUPTURES.—The peritoneum and bladder should be opened through a midline incision. Bleeding must be controlled. Adjacent organs should be inspected for injury. The bladder defect or defects should be carefully closed with 00 or 000 chromic catgut continuous sutures in 2 layers. The bladder should be drained with the urethral catheter and a suprapubic catheter, size 26 or 28 Fr. The wound should be adequately drained with Penrose drains brought out through a stab wound. The suprapubic tube should be removed as soon as the urine is clear. The Foley catheter should be left in at least a week.

EXTRAPERITONEAL EXTRAVASATION.—Small lacerations that are associated with sterile urine respond to Foley catheter drainage in most instances. Larger lacerations with continued bleeding should be managed surgically. The bladder is exposed suprapubically and the laceration closed. Drainage of the bladder by the suprapubic tube and drainage of the retroperitoneal space are carried out.

Pelvic hematomas that become infected should be explored suprapubically, with insertion of the suprapubic tube in the bladder and adequate drainage. Free bone fragments should be removed. Kanamycin, 500 mg intramuscularly every 12 hours, in the presence of good kidney function is very effective against most gram-negative organisms. Keflin intravenously and gentamicin intramuscularly are an excellent combination which cover all gram-negative bacteria, including pseudomonas and *Staphylococcus aureus*.

URETHRA

The male urethra is divided into the anterior urethra and the posterior urethra. In the anterior urethra, the portion distal to the fixed triangular ligament, the penile portion is mobile, the bulbous portion fixed. The posterior urethra consists of the membranous urethra, located within the triangular ligament, and the prostatic urethra.

ETIOLOGY.—Anterior urethral injuries result from external or internal (instrumentation) trauma. Injuries to the pendulous portion are relatively rare because of the mobility of the penis. The bulbous portion (between the suspensory and triangular ligaments) is fixed and easily contused or lacerated by falling astride an object.

Posterior urethral injuries are caused by pelvic fractures, penetrating wounds or instrumentation.

PATHOLOGY.—Minor trauma to the urethra may cause bleeding that usually stops by itself. Moderate trauma will cause more bleeding into the urethral lumen, the wall of the urethra and periurethral tissues, and spasm of the urethra resulting in obstruction and inability to void.

Severe trauma may cause destruction

Fig. 46-7.—Leakage from urethra below the triangular ligament (urogenital diaphragm) results in extravasation in scrotum, perineum, penis and lower abdominal wall. Separation of the membranous urethra results in extravasation in the periprostatic, the retropubic and occasionally the perirectal area.

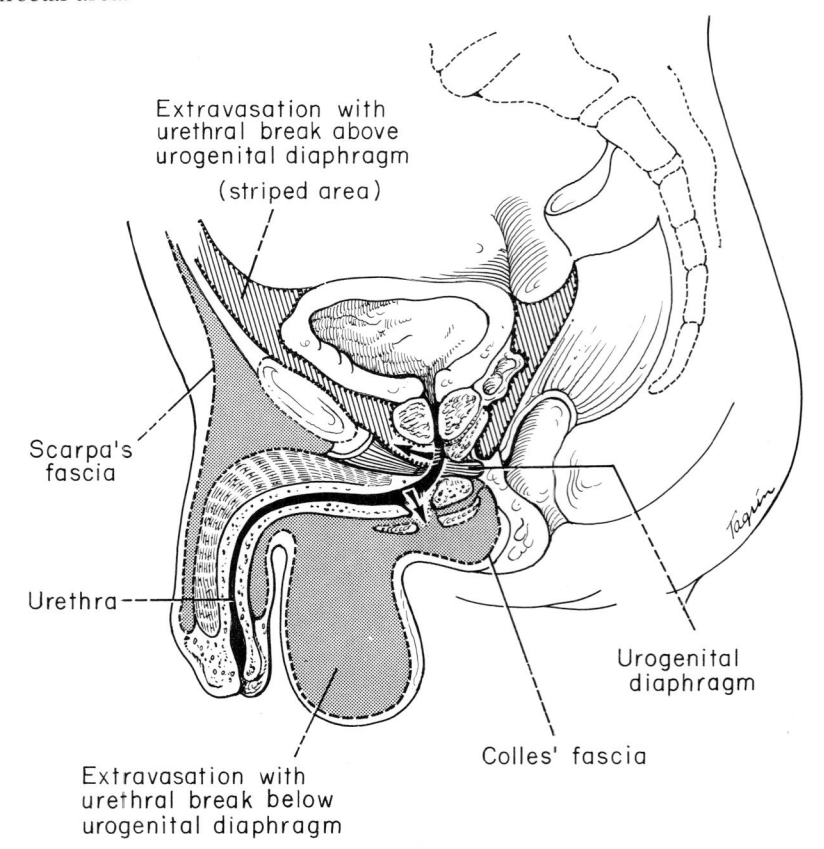

of the injured portion or separation of the urethra, with the formation of hematoma and with extravasation of urine. Lacerations of the anterior urethra result in extravasation within Colles' fascia and possible extension beneath Scarpa's fascia. Extravasation would thus be in the perineum, scrotum, penis and lower abdominal wall (Fig. 46-7). Laceration or separation of the membranous urethra results in extravasation in the retropubic (extraperitoneal), periprostatic and perirectal areas.

Urethral strictures may occur even after the mildest injuries, are very common and are often difficult to repair.

CLINICAL FINDINGS. — Clinical findings include bleeding from the urethral meatus, external evidence of bleeding along the penis or in the perineum and the inability to void, due to obstruction, separation or spasm of the urethra.

Diagnosis

The site of injury in the urethra as well as the extent of injury should be determined in all but the simplest injuries. This can easily and quietly be done in most cases by urethrography. A #10 Foley catheter is inserted so that the balloon can be inflated with 3 ml fluid just inside the penis (fossa navicularis). The patient is placed in an oblique position and the urethra is gently filled with a water-soluble iodine solution. The urethrogram should be obtained while instilling the dye. Exerting too much pressure with the syringe will, if there is an obstruction, cause extravasation of dye into penile blood vessels and lymphatics, resulting in a confusing picture. Exerting such pressure should be avoided.

Panendoscopy provides additional information regarding site and extent of injury. Examination of the anterior urethra by this method should be painless and can be done with the patient supine. The diagnosis of complete separation of the membranous urethra is easy to make. The urethrogram demonstrates dye in the retropubic (extraperitoneal) space (Fig. 46-8). On rectal examination, the prostate moves away from the examining finger from its usual fixed position (Fig. 46-9). A catheter will not pass into the bladder. Frequently, in the excitement of the activity on the emergency ward, a catheter is passed into the bladder before obtaining a urethrogram. In such cases, a small plastic feeding tube can be passed along the Foley catheter and approximately 10 ml of iodine dye introduced, with the Foley catheter on traction to prevent the dye from escaping into the bladder. This method will give an excellent urethrogram and demonstrate partial separation of the urethra. This is very useful and necessary information in cases of partial separation of the membranous urethra in patients with extensive pelvic hematomas and infected urine. This technique was introduced by McLaughlin at Massachusetts General Hospital.[13]

Treatment

Minor anterior urethral injuries causing only minimal bleeding, no interference with voiding and no lacerations need no specific treatment.

Fig. 46-8. — Urethrogram in case of complete transection of membranous urethra, showing extravasation of dye in retroperitoneum.

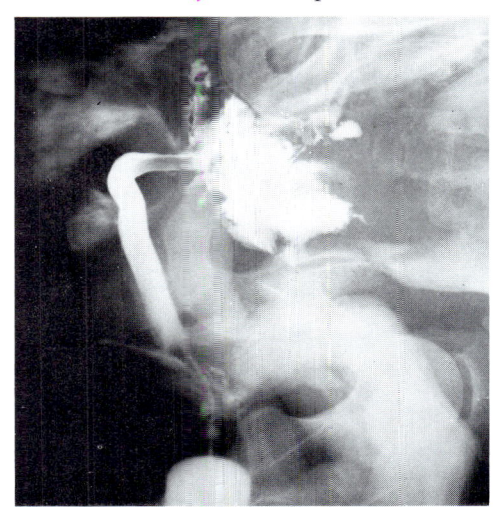

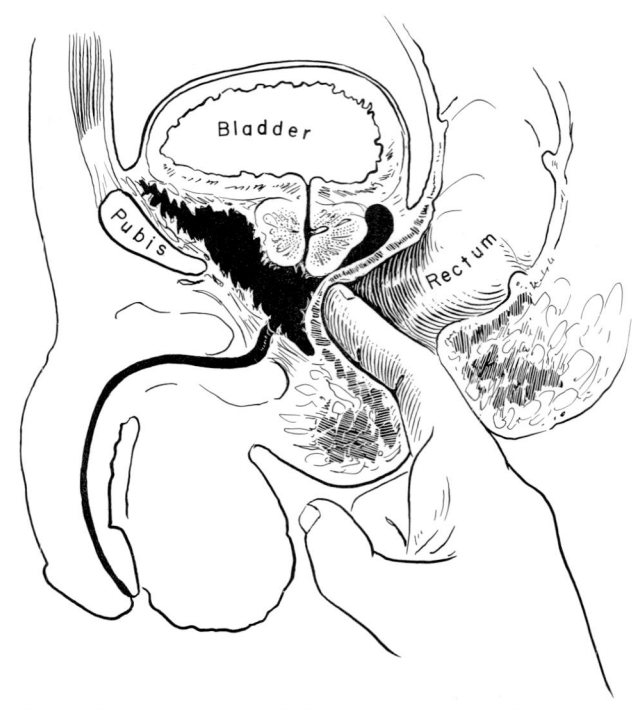

Fig. 46-9.—Unusual mobility of the apex of the prostate is found in complete transection of the urethra.

In more severe injuries, with persistent bleeding but no evidence of extravasation on the urethrogram, catheter drainage for a few days and antibiotic coverage should be instituted. The catheter will control the bleeding and help heal a small, undetected laceration. If periurethral bleeding does not stop with catheter drainage and external pressure, the site should be opened, the hematoma evacuated and bleeding controlled.

Severe anterior urethral injuries, with urethrographic or external evidence of separation of the urethra, should be exposed and debrided and the hemorrhage stopped. The ends of the urethra should be obliquely cut and approximated with interrupted #4 catgut sutures over a suitable size catheter, e.g., a #20 in an adult. Careful closure of overlying layers in staggered fashion, so suture lines are not above one another, is ideal. Additional urethral length to insure reapproximation without tension can be obtained by freeing the urethra in 1 or both directions.[2] A suprapubic cystotomy is advisable in most cases. The urethral catheter should be left in 10 days.

All patients with urethral injury from the mildest to the most complicated should be checked for stricture formation over a period of 6 months.

The treatment of posterior urethral injuries is frequently difficult. Incomplete lacerations of the membranous urethra should be treated with catheter drainage for 3 weeks, plus antibiotic and supportive therapy. If evidence of an infection in the retropubic area occurs, drainage should be provided and any devitalized bone fragments removed.

The ideal treatment for complete separation of the membranous urethra is anastomosis of the separated urethra. Unfortunately, rarely is this possible, because these patients are often verging on a state

Chapter 46: INJURIES TO THE GENITOURINARY TRACT / 1083

of shock from pelvic fractures and associated injuries of abdomen, head and extremities. Thus, the treatment of separated urethra is dictated by the general condition of the patient (see Chapter 25). Placement of a suprapubic tube in the bladder is the simplest and safest maneuver for patients in a critical condition. If the general condition can be improved and maintained, the next goal would be to place a urethral catheter in the bladder, inflate the Foley balloon and put the

Fig. 46-10. — Banks' method of using interlocking sounds in complete transection of the membranous urethra. **A**, male sound has been passed through the urethra and is interlocked with the female sound passed through the bladder and prostatic urethra. (**Continued**.)

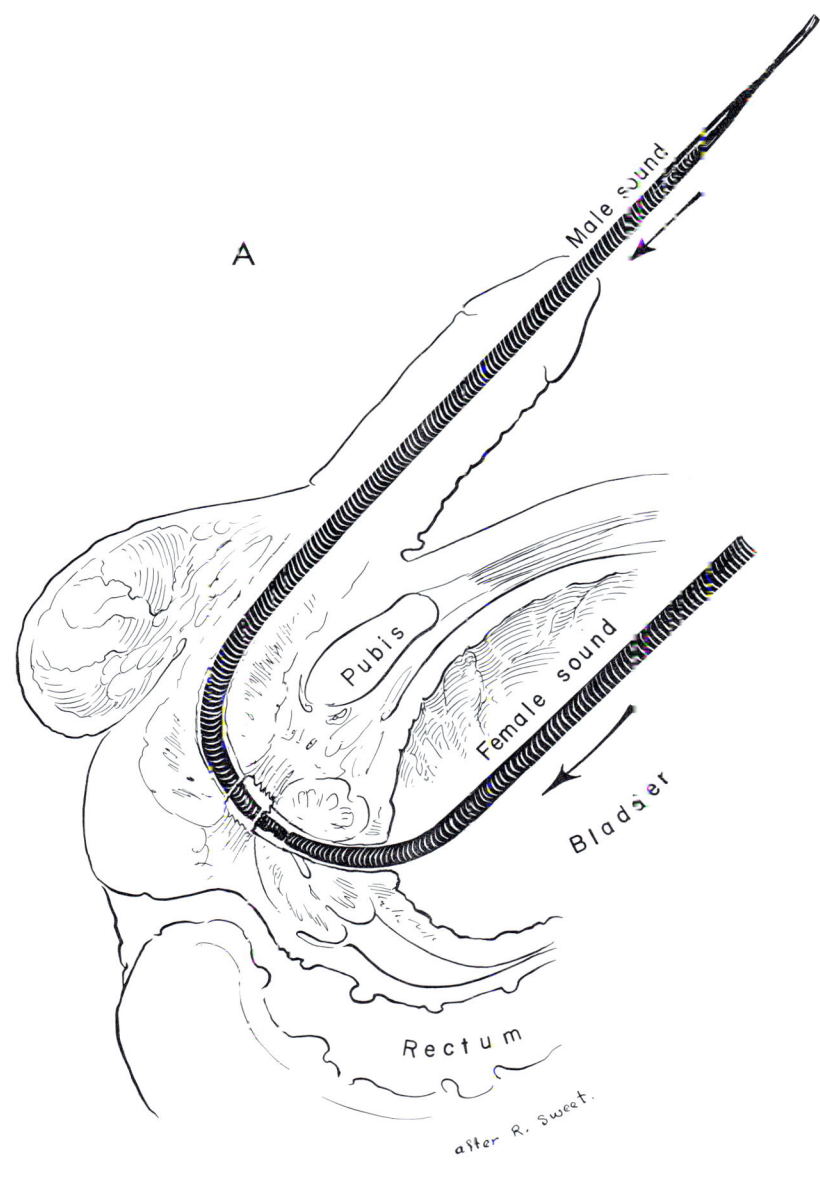

balloon on 1½ lb of tension. The Banks method[1] of using interlocking sounds is used to introduce a #22, 30-ml Foley catheter into the bladder. (Figs. 46-10, A–C). A heavy silk suture at the end of the Foley catheter is brought out through the suprapubic cystotomy. This silk suture allows reintroduction of a Foley catheter if the bag of the original one deflates and the catheter is pulled out. A #24 mushroom catheter should be left in the suprapubic cystotomy. The Foley catheter should be kept on tension at a 45-degree angle for 6 weeks by a pulley suspended over the abdomen. This will avoid pressure and fistula formation of the penile urethra which sometimes occurs when the traction is over the foot of the bed.

DeWeerd of the Mayo Clinic reported on 24 patients treated in this manner. In 22 healing took place without troublesome stricture formation.[4] Seitzman[12] reported being able to perform the ideal procedure—primary anastomosis of the urethra—in selected cases. Again, all patients should be informed of the possible long-term complication of stricture and

Fig. 46-10 (cont.). — **B,** male sound is introduced into the bladder and will be used to guide the attached soft rubber catheter through the urethra. (**Continued.**)

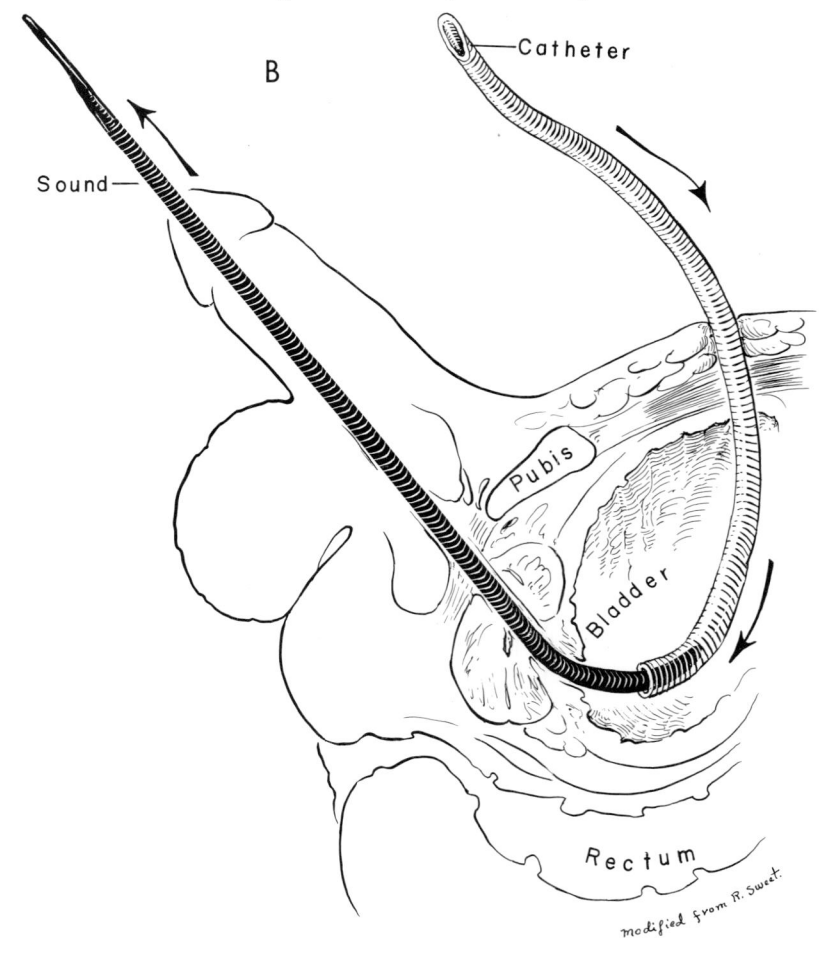

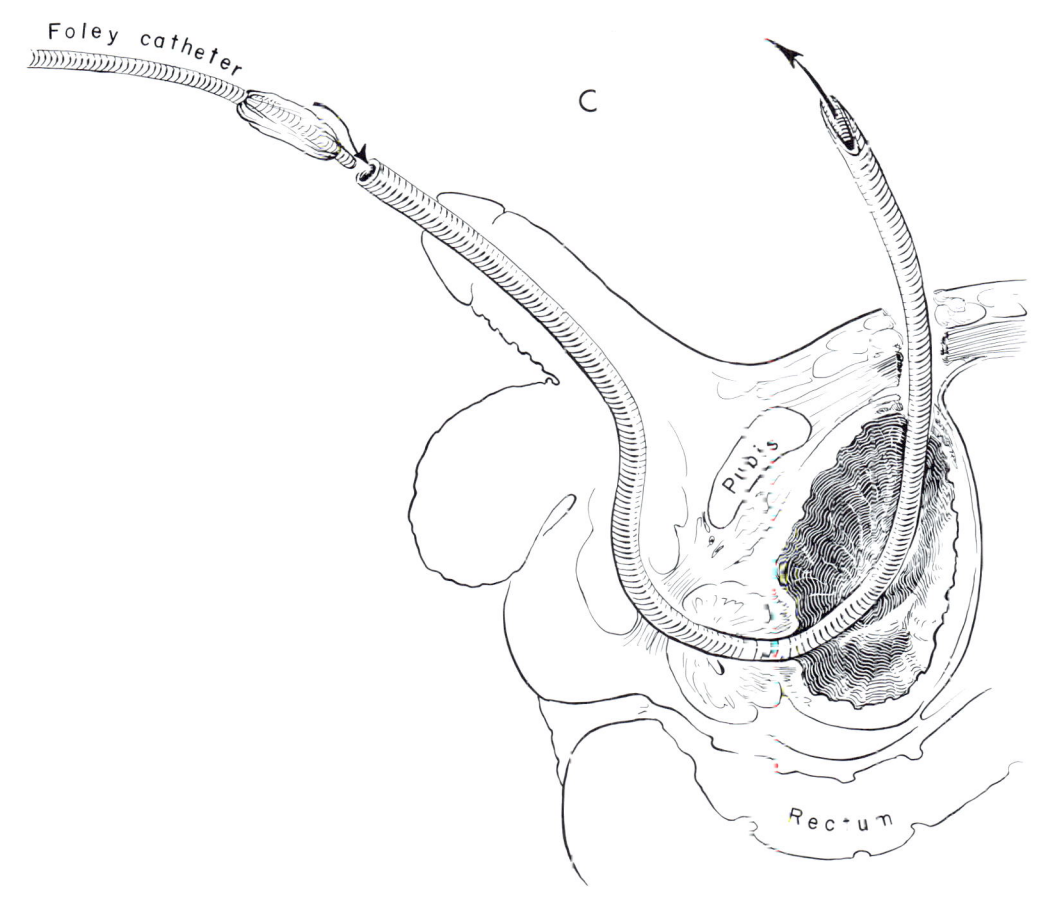

Fig. 46-10 (cont.).—C, a #22, 30-ml Foley catheter is sewn to the soft rubber catheter and will be drawn into the bladder, and the bag inflated. A heavy silk suture sewn in the end of the Foley will be brought out through the cystotomy.

the necessity for careful follow-up and possible plastic correction.

PENIS

The penis may be contused, lacerated or amputated. Avulsion of the skin of the penis and scrotum is not uncommon in industrial and farm machinery accidents. Avulsion of the penile skin is best treated by debridement and immediate skin grafting.

Lacerations should be carefully debrided. Arterial and venous bleeding must be carefully controlled with ligatures. If the urethra is lacerated, it should be approximated with interrupted #4 chromic catgut sutures over a #18 Foley catheter. The catheter should be left in place for 7 days. Lacerations should be closed carefully in layers with fine #4 chromic catgut sutures.

Amputation should be treated by debridement and control of bleeding. The tunica albuginea should be closed with #3 chromic catgut suture and the urethra should be sutured to the skin with 6 or 8 sutures of #4 chromic catgut. A Foley catheter should be left in place for 7 days.

SCROTUM AND TESTES

Avulsion of the scrotum in industrial accidents is not uncommon. The scrotum has great regenerative powers, and often simple closure is all that is necessary. If the scrotum has been extensively avulsed and there is not room to replace the testes within the scrotum, the testes may have to be placed subcutaneously for the time being.

Testicular injuries are not common. If the tunica albuginea is lacerated, bleeding should be controlled and the tunica closed with interrupted fine catgut sutures. If the spermatic cord is severed but the vas deferens is intact, an effort should be made to save the testis, for often the artery coming along the vas deferens will be sufficient to keep the testis from atrophying.

BIBLIOGRAPHY

1. Banks, H.: Ruptured urethra: A new method of treatment, Br. J. Surg. 15:262, 1927.
2. Blumberg, N.: Anterior urethral injuries, J. Urol. 102:210, 1969.
3. Carleton, C. E., Jr., and Scott, R., Jr.: Initial management of ureteral injuries: Report of 78 cases, J. Urol. 105:335, 1971.
4. DeWeerd, J.: Paper presented before Association of Genito-Urinary Surgeons, Chicago, May 12, 1971.
5. Evans, A., and Mogg, R. A.: Renal artery thrombosis due to closed trauma, J. Urol. 105:330, 1971.
6. Kazmin, M. H., Swanson, L. F., and Cockett, A. T. K.: Renal scan: The test of choice in renal trauma, J. Urol. 97:189, 1967.
7. McLaughlin, A. P.: Personal communication.
8. Persky, L., and Forsythe, W. E.: Renal trauma in childhood, JAMA 182:709, 1962.
9. Pollard, J. J., and Nebesar, R. A.: Abdominal angiography; N. Engl. J. Med. 279:1035, 1968.
10. Prather, G. C., and Keiser, T. F.: The bladder and fracture of the bony pelvis: The significance of a "tear drop" bladder as shown by cystogram, J. Urol. 63:1021, 1950.
11. Scott, R., Carleton, C. E., and Goldman, M.: Penetrating injuries of the kidney: An analysis of 181 patients, J. Urol. 101:247, 1969.
12. Seitzman, D. M.: Repair of the severed membranous urethra by the combined approach, J. Urol. 89:433, 1963.
13. Vermillion, C. D., McLaughlin, A. P., III, and Pfister, R. C.: Management of blunt renal trauma, J. Urol. 106:478, 1971.
14. Walker, J. A.: Injuries of the ureter due to external violence, J. Urol. 102:410, 1969.
15. Waterhouse, K., and Gross, M.: Trauma to the genitourinary tract: A 5-year experience with 251 cases, J. Urol. 101:241, 1969.

47 | Peripheral Nerve Injuries
RAYMOND N. KJELLBERG and JAMES C. WHITE

INJURIES TO PERIPHERAL NERVES can be repaired by careful surgeons with thoughtful preparation and straightforward techniques. Because of the variable frequency with which these are encountered in civilian practice, operators are encouraged to utilize the lessons derived from military casualties which have been systematically appraised in our own and other countries.[27] The complexity and variability of these injuries can lead an individual surgeon to false security when based upon "clinical impression" alone. The cost to the patients and society of unnecessarily prolonged disability becomes an increasingly important consideration.

ANATOMIC STRUCTURE

The spinal nerves arise from the cord at each segment of the neuraxis as a posterior (sensory) and an anterior (motor) root. These roots join together in the intervertebral foramen and form a single nerve; this is covered by a fibrous tissue sheath, the epineurium, which is in continuity with the dura mater. Within this sheath the nerve is divided by fibrous connective tissue septa into bundles of fibers, or funiculi, each of which has a fibrous covering known as the perineurium. Each funiculus, in turn, contains numerous nerve fibers. A nerve fiber consists of a central axon surrounded by myelin, a complex substance containing proteins and lipids, which forms a sheath of variable thickness around the axon. Surrounding the myelin sheath is the neurilemma or sheath of Schwann; this in turn is surrounded by a thin layer of collagen and fibrous connective tissue, the endoneurium, which is the inward extension of the perineurium. The myelin sheath is interrupted periodically by constrictions, the nodes of Ranvier. The larger, more heavily myelinated fibers, which conduct with the greatest velocity, transmit skeletal motor impulses or tactile and postural sensation. The smaller, lightly myelinated and nonmyelinated fibers carry impulses to the blood vessels, sweat glands and arrectores pilorum muscles in addition to the greater portion of the impulses transmitting pain, the rate of conduction in these is slow.

Each large peripheral nerve is made up of a number of fascicles, or funiculi. After each branch enters a nerve, its fibers, as Sunderland and Ray[22] have found, ascend for a short distance within a single funiculus. At a higher level in the nerve, the funiculus loses its identity because its fibers intermingle with those of other funiculi. In the course of nerve regeneration after division and suture, it is manifestly impossible to secure anything like nearly perfect regeneration. Not only is it impossible for individual sensory, motor or autonomic fibers to find their original distal Schwann tubes, but even the gross funicular pattern can never be accurately reapposed (Fig. 47-1). Nevertheless, provided a sufficient number of motor and sensory axons reach corresponding end-organs, the motor and sensory areas of the

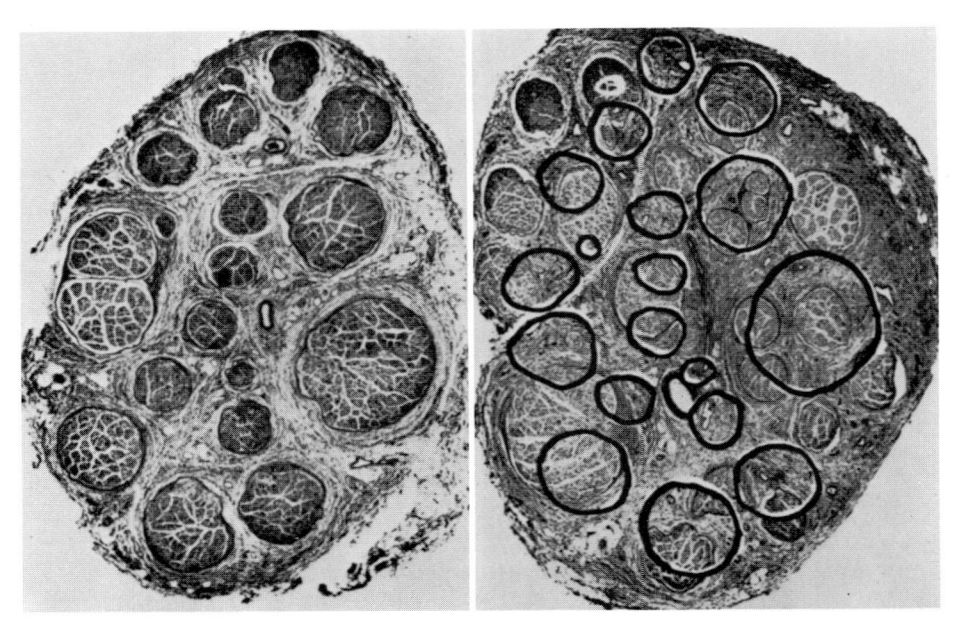

Fig. 47-1.—Following resection of a segment of nerve with a neuroma. **Left,** a pattern of fiber arrangement in the proximal segment. **Right,** the funicular pattern of the proximal section traced upon the distal section indicates the imperfect alignment of fiber bundles. (From Woodhall, B., and Beebe, G. W.: *Peripheral Nerve Regeneration: A Follow-Up Study of 3,656 World War II Injuries,* VA Medical Monograph [Washington, D. C.: Government Printing Office, 1956].)

cerebral cortex can soon readjust to restore useful function.

METABOLIC DETERMINANTS IN NERVE REPAIR

A cut axon proceeds through a metabolic sequence (chromatolysis). The cell body, the nutrition factory, is optimally suited for recovery between 19 and 21 days following injury. The distal axon simply dies. In a divided peripheral nerve, many factors, frequently indeterminate or unalterable, contribute to the recovery. Delays beyond the initial 19–21-day waiting period are accompanied by a 1% reduction in motor recovery for every 6 days of postponement of the definitive neurorrhaphy. For moderate-sized nerves, such as the median, ulnar, radial, peroneal and tibial, these guidelines hold true. For large nerve trunks, such as the sciatic nerve or brachial plexus, regardless of the timing of a repair, the outlook for recovery in digital motor function remains poor. For smaller digital nerves, any delay appears unnecessary, and the prognosis after repair is generally very good.

The metabolic response to trauma and regeneration concerns 3 different cellular levels.

1. The spinal cord, particularly the anterior horn cells and the less thoroughly studied sensory cells in the ganglia of the posterior spinal roots.

2. The proximal nerve stump.

3. The distal severed and separated part of the peripheral nerve and its associated end-organs.

Within the spinal cord, the motor cell bodies whose axons have been severed (Fig. 47-2) progressively enlarge for approximately 10–20 days, remain swollen while there is active regeneration, and thereafter, with maturation, return slowly

Chapter 47: PERIPHERAL NERVE INJURIES / 1089

A   Phase of Neuronal Survival

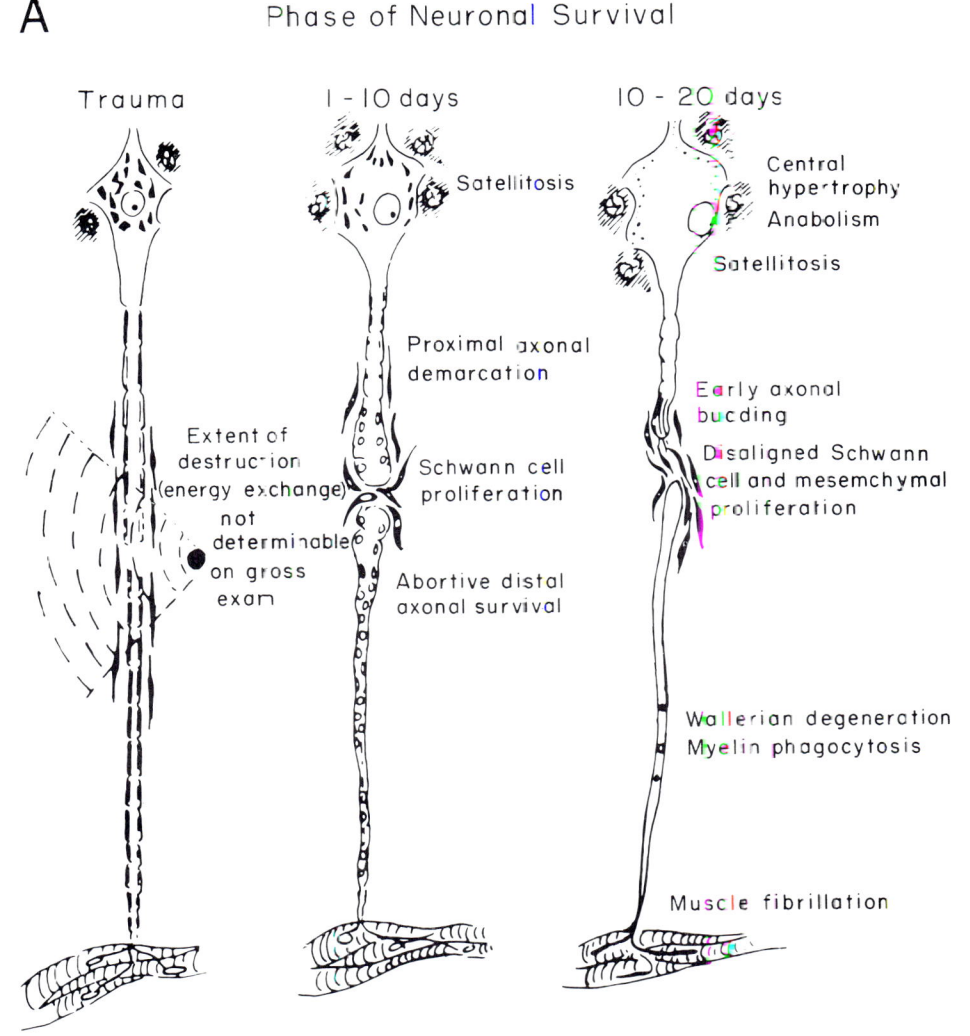

Trauma   *1 - 10 days*   *10 - 20 days*

- Satellitosis
- Extent of destruction (energy exchange) not determinable on gross exam
- Proximal axonal demarcation
- Schwann cell proliferation
- Abortive distal axonal survival
- Central hypertrophy
- Anabolism
- Satellitosis
- Early axonal budding
- Disaligned Schwann cell and mesemchymal proliferation
- Wallerian degeneration
- Myelin phagocytosis
- Muscle fibrillation

Fig. 47-2.—Composite drawing outlining the metabolic phase in nerve repair and illustrating the multiple processes which take place simultaneously. **A**, phase of neuronal survival. **(Continued.)**

to normal size. The biochemical phenomena have been studied by Ducker et al.[4]

Ribonucleic acids in the cytoplasm and in the Nissl substances migrate peripherally and break up into smaller particles. The amount of ribonucleic acid (RNA) aggregations from large particles to submicroscopic particles gives the picture of "chromatolysis" and represents a transformation of RNA into a more active form. Increases in enzymatic activity and in the incorporation of amino acids point to increased metabolism. The anabolic proteosynthesis evidently is required for maintenance of neuronal survival and cellular function after trauma and for regeneration of a new distal axon.

When a nerve lesion is close to the cell

B   Phase of Repair

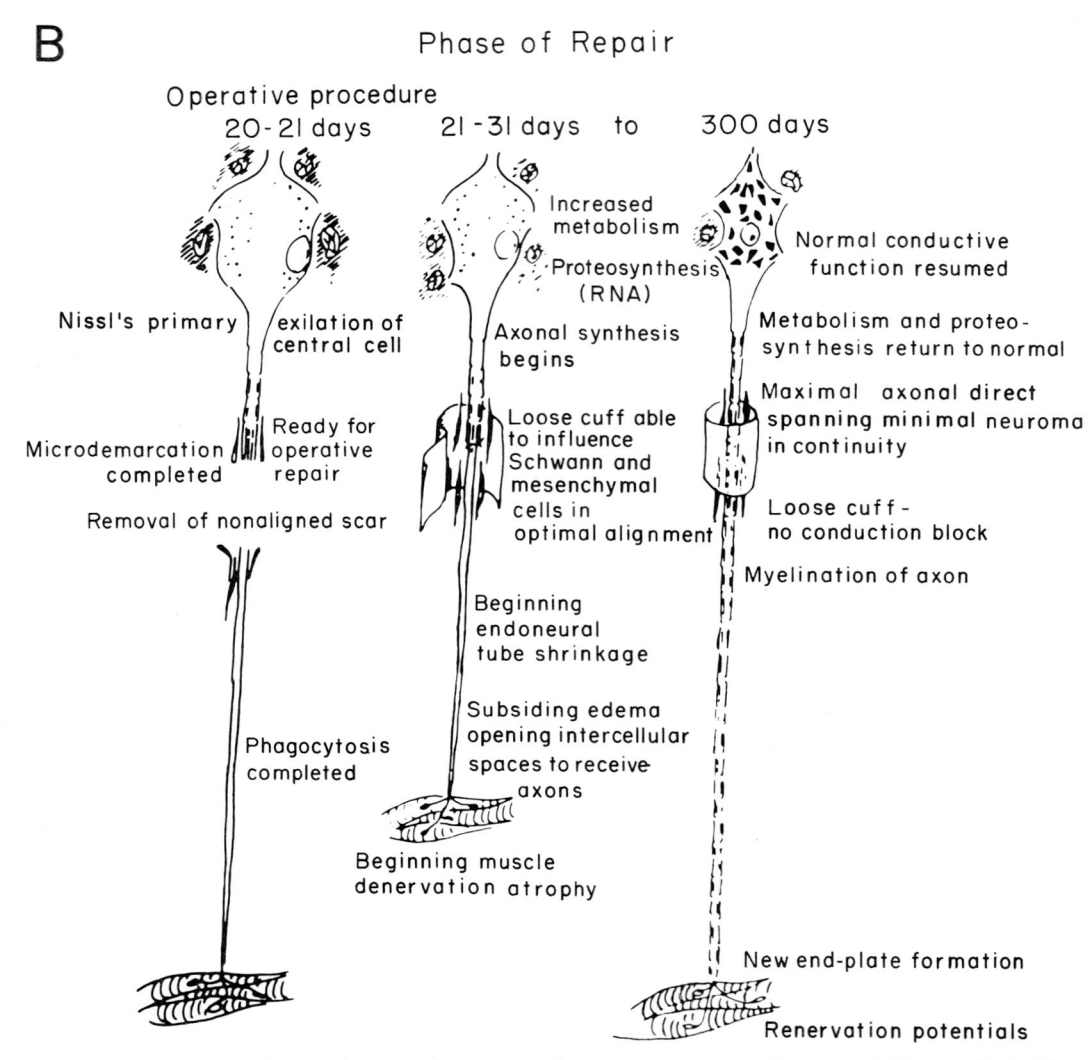

Operative procedure
20-21 days   21-31 days   to   300 days

- Nissl's primary
- exilation of central cell
- Microdemarcation completed
- Ready for operative repair
- Removal of nonaligned scar
- Phagocytosis completed

- Increased metabolism
- Proteosynthesis (RNA)
- Axonal synthesis begins
- Loose cuff able to influence Schwann and mesenchymal cells in optimal alignment
- Beginning endoneural tube shrinkage
- Subsiding edema opening intercellular spaces to receive axons
- Beginning muscle denervation atrophy

- Normal conductive function resumed
- Metabolism and proteosynthesis return to normal
- Maximal axonal direct spanning minimal neuroma in continuity
- Loose cuff – no conduction block
- Myelination of axon
- New end-plate formation
- Renervation potentials

Fig. 47-2 (cont.) – **B**, phase of repair. (From Ducker, T. B., Kempe, L. G., and Hayes, G. J.: The metabolic background for peripheral nerve surgery, J. Neurosurg. 30:270, 1969.)

body, a large percentage of cell mass is lost. Such changes of the cell body in the cord may take up to 2 years in rats and many years in man. The amount of distal axon to be replaced may exceed the metabolic capability of the cell. The nerve cell during successful regeneration replaces 50–100 times the organic material contained in the cell body. In unsuccessful nerve repairs, regeneration into the peripheral endoneural tubes may begin, but the central cell may not maintain its hypertrophic anabolic state for the extended period of months required to complete the resynthesizing process, as in cases of high transection. Also, during this period, shrinkage occurs in the distal endoneural tubes with fibrosis and atrophy of the distal muscles, further downgrading the prognosis.

The changes in the central body of the anterior horn cells are less marked in more peripheral lesions where the neuronal disruption is minimal. The phase of neuronal survival is shortened to less than 2 weeks and the phase of repair to 2–3 months. If the extent of destruction of the peripheral stump at the time of original trauma is minimal, the definitive operative repair may be safely carried out earlier than usual. The prognosis is good since the regeneration requirements are small.

The clinical experience of World War II provided statistically significant proof that, in general, a delay in definitive neurorrhaphy up to 19 days had no harmful effect. In fact, in over one-half the patients who had suture repair less than 2 weeks after injury resuture was required because of excessive mesenchymal tissue build-up within the anastomosis. One of us (J.C.W.) has learned that appraisal of clinical material from the Vietnam conflict favors delay of suture repair to 6 weeks after injury. Only after the neuron has shown the chromatolytic hypertrophic alterations, which, depending on the level of the lesion, take from several days to 2 weeks to develop fully, is its axon capable of regenerating peripherally. Operative intervention at this time alters the appearance of the cell within the spinal cord minimally, and the neuron continues a pattern of changes nearly identical to that of a crush lesion where surgical repair was not required. The hypertrophic cell with its increased proteosynthesis acts as if it were metabolically primed for a delayed repair (Fig. 47-2).

Following recovery from the initial trauma, the percentage of the remaining intact cell that is lost after a delayed suture in which the axon is cut back to healthy fascicles is very small. Excessive mesenchymal tissue build-up at the anastomosis becomes much less of a problem, in that the regenerating neuron begins to penetrate the repair site immediately before a heavy scar forms and solidifies.

Long delays in operative repair may be harmful to the cell within the spinal cord. After some 2–3 months proteosynthesis decreases, and the nerve cell morphologically begins to disintegrate. A late surgical repair with the necessary cutting back into normal nerve from the region of neuroma will initiate again the metabolic cycle, with cellular hypertrophy, etc. Although the changes in this cell are less, the neuron cannot respond a second time with maximal metabolic effort.

The glial cells that surround the neuron within the central nervous system also undergo morphologic, biochemical and histochemical changes. The simultaneous neuronal and perineuronal glial reaction strongly suggests a close interaction between nerve cell and glial cell.

Within 1 hour of cutting a peripheral nerve, there is marked swelling from the point of severance that extends about 0.5–1 cm both proximally and distally. This extends a greater distance after the nerve has suffered additional contusion. The amount of swelling is greater than previously realized, for the cross-sectional area of the nerve gradually increases 3–4 times. The swelling consists of both intra- and extracellular edema, mostly a gel-like amorphous substance containing a large quantity of acid mucopolysaccharide. It persists for a week or more and subsides slowly thereafter.

Within 2 or 3 days after transection of a nerve, there is a cellular proliferation in both stumps composed chiefly of Schwann cells which initially outnumber the mesenchymal cells of endoneural, perineural and vascular origin. In man, when a nerve is lacerated distally with a sharp object, the retrograde destructive changes may be minimal and axon sprouting may begin at 4 days. However, in peripheral nerve injuries due to contusion, especially the blast wave of a high-velocity missile, such a situation rarely occurs. The typical trauma involving a nerve is extensive, with distal and proximal fascicular disruption extending several centimeters. An accurate demarcation of the retrograde destruction cannot be made for many days after injury. During this period, the surviving Schwann cells proliferate; this may even occur within a normal intact epineurium. At the time of a 3-week-delayed operative repair, it is necessary to cut back proximally and distally for a considerable distance to identify a normal fascicular pattern. The mesenchymal scar is for the most part not longitudinally aligned, so that any early axonal regeneration becomes entangled and in time forms a neuroma. These supportive elements dominate the dynamic action in the early post-traumatic period, and one sees only the earliest signs of axonal regeneration.

The direction of the regenerating axons starts as an ameboid extension and is dependent on "contact guidance" of the existing supportive element. The orientation of the mesenchymal and ectodermal elements appears dependent on the state of the wound and physical influences rather than chemotaxis. Accordingly, the best longitudinal alignment of the supportive structures is brought about by cuffing the anastomotic site. Recent studies of Ducker et al.[4,5] indicate that a pliable, elastic, short, thin tube of silicone rubber possesses physical properties that encase and support the mesenchymal proliferation, force longitudinal alignment and yet do not constrict the nerve. Consequently, maximal direct spanning takes place when the axonal bulb pushes across a structured anastomosis. Silastic cuffs are preferred over the tantalum cuffs used previously because of the tendency of the latter to fragment. Ducker[6] has recently found significantly improved results in 50 Vietnam cases that were compared at the end of a year with results in a corresponding number of uncuffed cases.

If the mesenchymal tissue buildup has not been structured and consequently has become disoriented, the regenerating axon may twist and turn and, at times, turn back on itself. With primary nonstructured repair in higher primates and in man, the gross and histologic appearance of the nerve repair is a neuroma-in-continuity.

With primary repair, it is nearly 4 weeks before the axons cross the anastomosis and 6 weeks before there is a sizable number in the distal segment.

If repair of a proximally severed nerve is carried out 3 weeks after injury, the axon sprouts from the now metabolically active cell and pushes buds into the anastomotic site almost immediately. The edema begins to subside, and the intercellular spaces open to allow the swollen axonal bud to pass through. The long-term appearance is a healthier anastomosis with only a minimal neuroma-in-continuity.

As in the proximal stump, the early changes in the distal stump are reactive swelling plus proliferation of connective tissue and Schwann cells. The sequence and timing are very similar; however, only the supporting structures contain intact cells with stepped-up metabolism. At an anastomosis, half or more than half of the supportive structures seen in the various stages of repair come from the distal stump. Increase in deoxyribonucleic (DNA) and RNA in the peripheral stump occur in these neurolemmal cells. These active, metabolic, multiplying cells should also be structured to provide a longitudinal alignment for the downgrowing axons. Proximally, the same phenomenon occurs with the additional progressive enlargement from ingrowing neurons and is called a "neuroma." At a repair, unless the entire area of disruption has been trimmed back, regenerating axons become entangled in a bed of connective tissues and collagen and develop into a neuroma-in-continuity.

When a nerve has been only partly severed, a lateral neuroma will form by sprouting of axon tips and Schwann cells through the disrupted funiculi and epineuron. The degree of spontaneous recovery will depend on the number of severed funiculi and the degree of injury to the axis cylinders within the remaining intact, but more or less contused, part of the nerve.

The peripheral stump reaction differs from the proximal one chiefly in the absence of neural elements. The distal axon undergoes a series of changes which end in wallerian degeneration. Electrical excitability disappears after a few hours. At the margin of transection, axon thickenings can be seen with the light microscope as early as 24–48 hours after injury. Enzymes, like diphosphopyridine nucleotide diaphorase in the neuron and acid phosphatase in the surrounding myelin, will increase transiently.

A delay of 3 weeks in repair allows this cellular debris of myelin and degenerated axons to be phagocytosed by macrophages. It appears that the regrowing axons are less impeded when advancing into clean endoneural tubes. With the passage of time, the empty endoneural sheaths of the peripheral segment shrink, eventually to one-tenth their original diameter. The intersheath perineural tissue also shrinks. The preservation of these mesenchymal elements is dependent on the presence of the nerve fiber to maintain an anatomic, metabolic and functional relationship. Without the nerve fibers, this shrinkage becomes irreversible and downgrades further the prognosis of an unduly postponed nerve repair. Even with optimal axonal regeneration and blood supply, the endoneural tubes contract and re-expand to only 60–80% of their normal cross-sectional areas.

Not only the peripheral axon but also the muscle is metabolically dependent on the nerve cell body. After sectioning of a nerve, muscle fibers shrink, endomysium and perimysium thicken and muscle spindles atrophy. After several months or years, the muscle fiber may fragment and disintegrate.

Even as the muscle is being surrounded by fibrous tissue, it may survive 10 years with active fibrillations. However, any denervation atrophy of muscles is harmful to reinnervation because the thickening of the muscle sheath hinders end-plate formation. The sensory end-organs are less dependent for survival on being reinnervated. The World War II study yielded no evidence that the time from injury to repair influenced sensory recovery in any way. Admittedly, we know little about the response to trauma and wound healing of sensory nerve injuries. Golubov[7] has shown that retrograde changes in the cells of the posterior spinal root ganglia are similar to those described in the anterior horn of gray matter in the spinal cord. Since many of the same histometabolic and pathologic changes occur, the timing of the repair of a sensory nerve is probably dependent on the same principles.

DEGREES OF INJURY

The proportion of the whole cross section of the injured nerve, the length involved and the distance from the cell body (above) are critical in determining the time and nature of operative repair. The varying types of trauma alter the appraisal of injury: (1) sharp clean division, (2) pressure (3) traction, (4) contusion, or shock-wave injury, as in high-velocity missile wounds. In any case, the number or proportion of fibers temporarily or definitively interrupted constitutes the primary basis for classifying degrees of injury. The classical monograph of Haymaker and Woodhall[8] provides such a clear and authoritative basis for such classification that their examples are reproduced here.

First degree.—Concussion or compression of fibers is present without degeneration. Recovery may begin in a period of minutes and is always complete within a month, since few, if any, fibers degenerate (Fig. 47-3).

Second degree.—The axons are destroyed, but their Schwann sheaths remain intact. Therefore wallerian degeneration follows, but each axon regener-

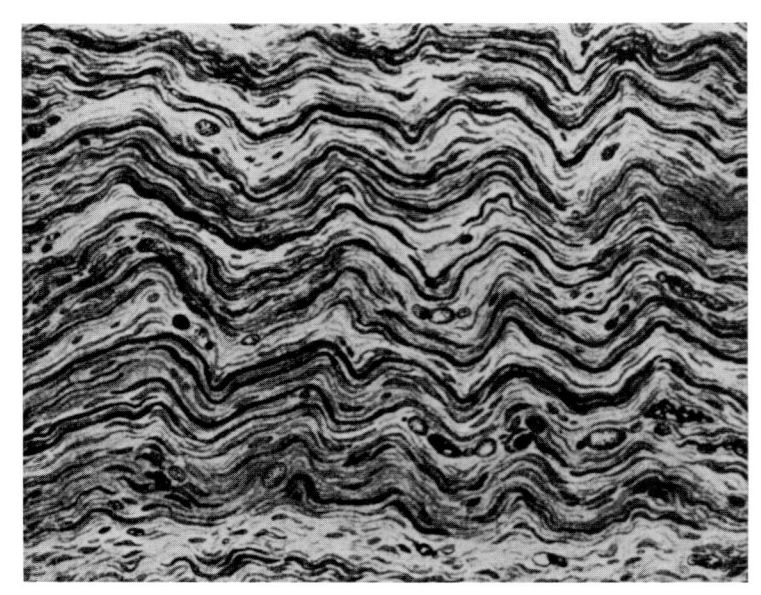

Fig. 47-3.—First-degree injury. This section of the sciatic nerve was stained to bring out myelin sheaths. A number of myelin sheaths have disappeared or have degenerated, indicated by their greyness. The ringlets are evidence of wallerian degeneration. Time interval from injury to operation is not known. (From Spielmeyer, W.: *Zur Klinik und Anatomie der Nervenschussverletzungen* [Berlin: Springer-Verlag, 1915].)

ates within its endoneurial tubule and eventually reaches its original end-organ.

Third degree.—Here there is a more serious injury in continuity, with the epineurium preserved but with disorganization of many of the funiculi and endoneurial tubules (Fig. 47-4). There is usually some intrafunicular hemorrhage and resultant fibrosis.

Fourth degree.—With more serious injury in continuity, there is disruption of all the funiculi and individual nerve fibers. This results in severe endoneurial scarring and a dense neuroma-in-conti-

Fig. 47-4.—Third-degree injury. Rifle bullet wound of right forearm, with comminuted fracture of radius and paralysis of median nerve. The small fascicle in the upper part of the nerve passes through the region of injury without interruption. The larger fascicle expands to form a fairly symmetrical neuroma. (WR-184; from Lyons, W. R., and Woodhall, B.: *Atlas of Peripheral Nerve Injuries* [Philadelphia: W. B. Saunders Company, 1949].)

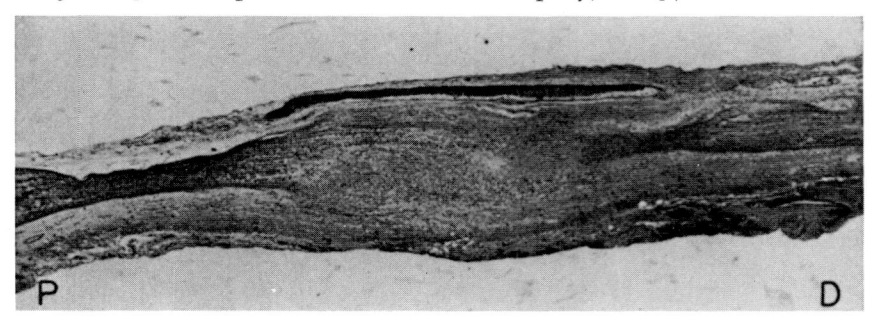

Chapter 47: PERIPHERAL NERVE INJURIES / 1095

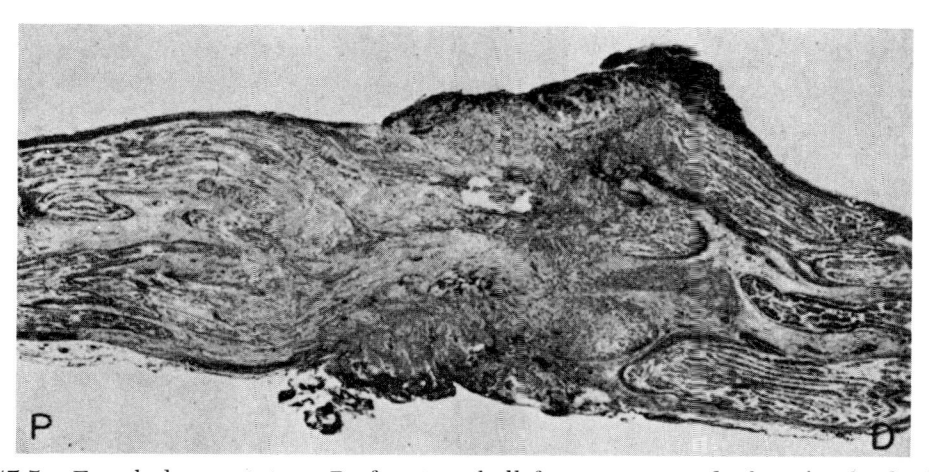

Fig. 47-5.—Fourth-degree injury. Perforating shell fragment wound of upper third of arm, with immediate median nerve paralysis. No spontaneous improvement occurred. Resection of neuroma-in-continuity with end-to-end suture was carried out 3 months later. Specimen shows the proximal nerve segment *(P)* with small proximal neuroma fused to distal nerve segment *(D)* by mass of scar tissue involving all components of nerve structure and thus completely interrupting the nerve. (VA-67C; from Haymaker, W., and Woodhall, B.: *Peripheral Nerve Injuries* [Philadelphia: W. B. Saunders Company, 1953].)

Fig. 47-6.—Partial fourth-degree injury. Shell fragment wound of left posterior thigh, with partial sciatic nerve division. Resection of neuroma-in-continuity and end-to-end anastomosis were done 3 months later. Specimen is that of a neuroma-in-continuity in which about four-fifths of the nerve segment has been transformed into a lateral neuroma *(N)*, with one-fifth of the fibers remaining intact. The epineurium adjacent to the normal fibers is not disrupted. (VA-12C. from Haymaker, W., and Woodhall, B.: *Peripheral Nerve Injuries* [Philadelphia: W. B. Saunders Company, 1953].)

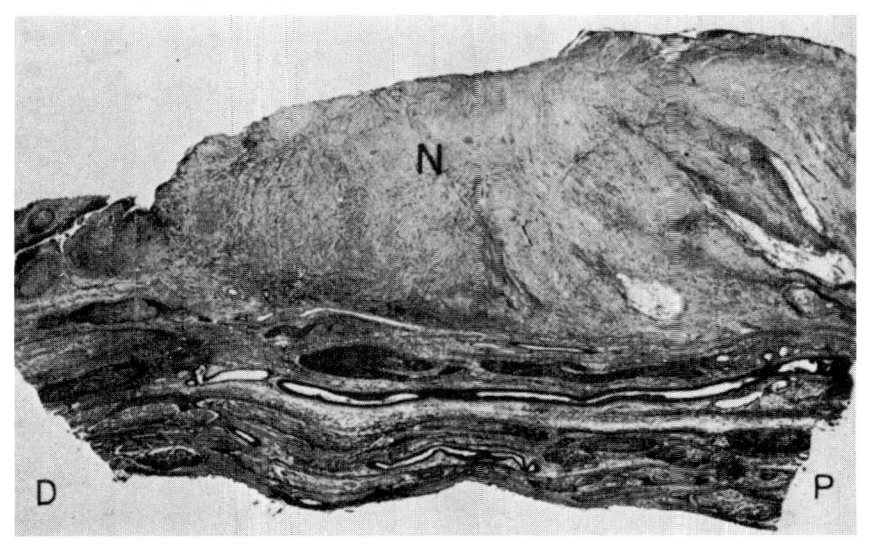

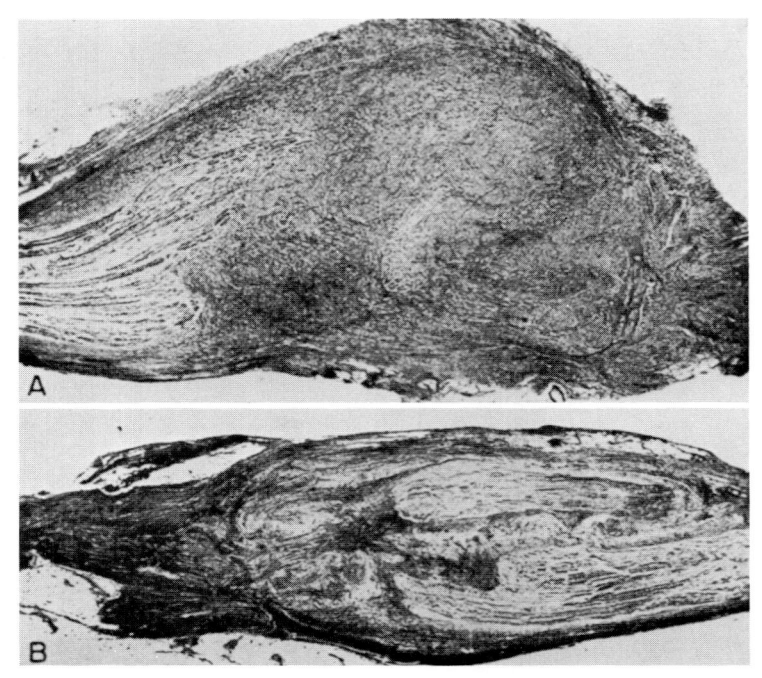

Fig. 47-7.—Fifth-degree injury. Mortar shell fragment wound of ulnar nerve with complete disruption of nerve segment. End-to-end suture was performed 8 months after injury. **A,** proximal nerve segment, characterized by fascicles fanning out to form a typical swollen, neuromatous bulb, surrounded by fragments of scar tissue (proximal neuroma). **B,** distal glioma of the same specimen. The distal fascicles are embedded in firm scar tissue and the tip of the glioma is covered by adhesions. (HG-195; from Lyons, W. R., and Woodhall, B.: *Atlas of Peripheral Nerve Injuries* [Philadelphia: W. B. Saunders Company, 1949].)

nuity (Figs. 47-5 and 47-6). No useful regeneration can bridge the barrier of scar tissue, and so the scar tissue must be excised and the healthy ends of the nerves sutured.

Fifth degree.—The nerve trunk is severed, with retraction of its ends and the formation of a proximal neuroma and distal glioma (Fig. 47-7).

After complete severance or intraneuronal destruction, there is immediate and total paralysis of all forms of sensation, muscular movement and vasomotor and sudomotor activity. The ability of the distal segment to conduct an electrical stimulus is lost within a few hours. Chronaxy rises, and the paralyzed muscle fibers begin to fibrillate. By the end of 2–3 weeks, the electrical reaction of degeneration is complete, with well-advanced fragmentation of the axons and disintegration of their surrounding myelin. Muscular atrophy becomes noticeable within a month.

With the lesser second- and third-degree injuries, there is usually some preservation of sensation and sweating because the small, unmyelinated fibers that mediate deep pain and sympathetic activity may be in part preserved. A Tinel paresthesia (a tingling sensation on tapping over the nerve) can soon be elicited over the site of injury and later at the level of advance of regenerating nerve fiber tips.

TYPES OF INJURY

Seddon[16] has divided nerve injuries into 3 categories: neurapraxia, axonotmesis and neurotmesis.

Neurapraxia.—In neurapraxia there is

concussion with brief physiologic loss of function and return to normal conduction within a period ranging from minutes to a few weeks. There is no axonal degeneration.

Axonotmesis.—This is also an injury in continuity, but with more severe contusion and wallerian degeneration of the axons within their Schwann sheaths. Since the latter remain intact, regeneration will ultimately be complete or nearly so.

Neurotmesis.—In neurotmesis there is complete severance of a nerve trunk or some of its funiculi.

DIAGNOSIS OF INJURY

The diagnosis of injury to a peripheral nerve is not difficult; it is only missed if the surgeon fails to look for it when he is confronted with a wound involving blood vessels and tendons or with a difficult fracture. The characteristic loss of sensation that follow interruption of the common nerves to the extremities is illustrated in many texts and in great detail in the excellent plates in Pollock and Davis' *Peripheral Nerve Injuries*.[14] The skin is tested by pricking with a pin, remembering that absence of sensibility may be limited to the autonomous zone shown in Figures 47-8 and 47-9.

The total area of innervation of any cutaneous nerve tends to shrink with time—to the tips of the second and third digits in the case of injury to the median nerve and to the little finger when the ulnar nerve has been severed. In the case of the radial nerve, overlap from the median and ulnar nerves may be so extensive that no numbness can be detected on

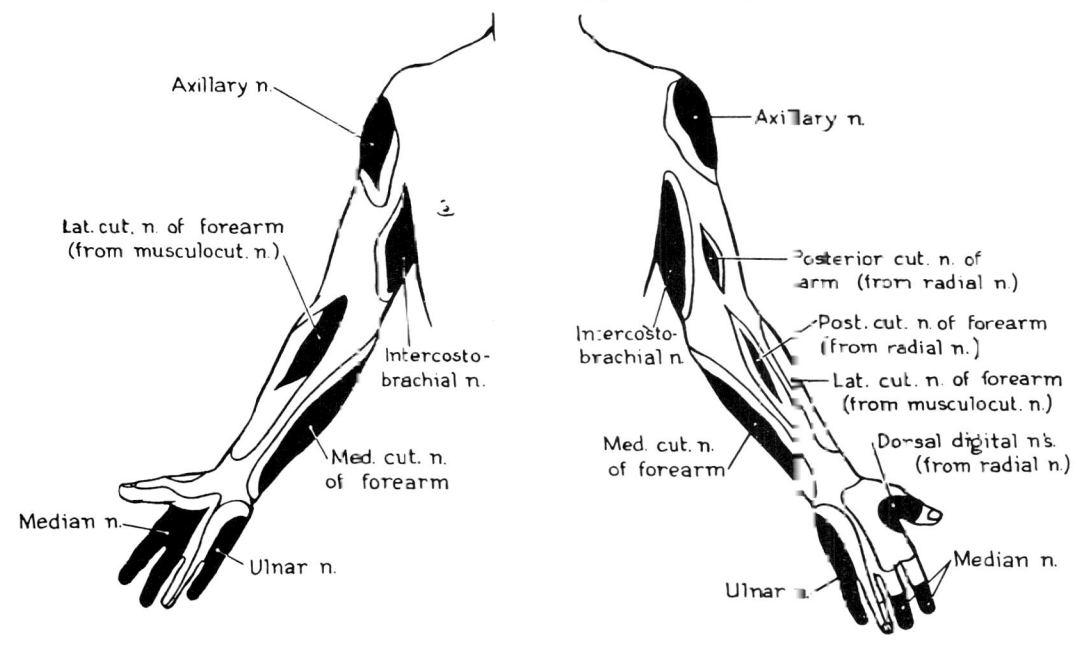

Fig. 47-8.—Sensory deficit following interruption of individual nerve trunks of the upper limb. The black areas represent the autonomous zones and the surrounding lines indicate the approximate border of tactile anesthesia and thermoanesthesia. The cutaneous area between the autonomous zone and the encircling border of retained pain sensibility is referred to as the "intermediate zone." The autonomous zones represent the smallest encountered in the hundreds of cases studied from this standpoint. (Figs. 47-8 and 47-9 from Foerster, O.: Die Symptomatologie der peripheren Nerven, in Lewandowsky, M. H.: *Handbuch der Neurologie* [Berlin: J. Springer, 1929], Erganzungsbd. 2. Teil, pp. 975–1508.)

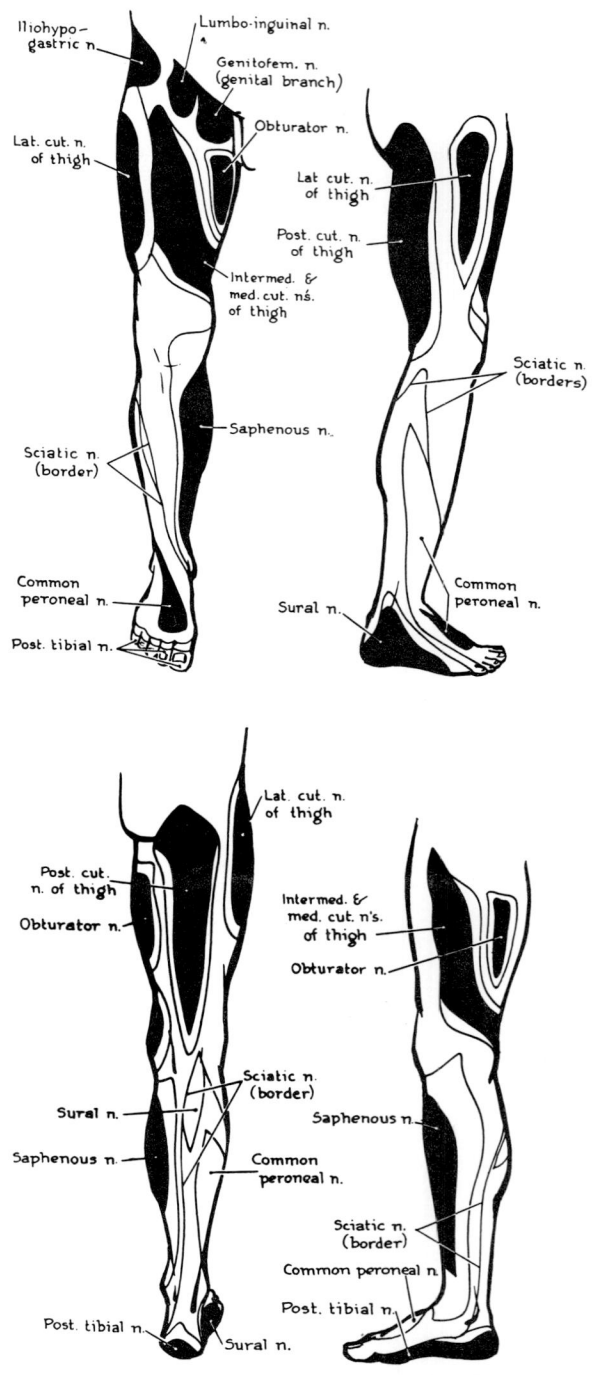

Fig. 47-9.—Sensory deficit following interruption of individual nerve trunks of the lower limb. The pattern is the same as that in Figure 47-8.

the dorsum of the hand. Usually, cutaneous sensory loss is limited to a small area at the base of the thumb and index finger. When a physician is in doubt as to whether the contraction of sensory loss is caused by regeneration or overlap, he can easily determine the cause by blocking neighboring nerves with procaine. Loss of sweating and elevated skin resistance follow a very similar pattern. The interpretation of paralysis requires a knowledge of motor innervation and of how to test the individual muscles. The muscles supplied by the peripheral nerves are shown in Tables 47-1 and 47-2. Methods of testing the activity of the muscles are

TABLE 47-1.—SPINAL AND PERIPHERAL INNERVATION OF MAJOR MUSCLES OF ARM AND HAND*

	UPPER ARM		FOREARM		HAND	
Musculocutaneous: C5–7	Coraco-brachialis Biceps Brachialis	C6, 7 C5, 6 C5, 6				
Axillary: C5–6	Deltoid	C5, 6				
Radial: C5–8	Triceps Brachioradialis	C7, 8 C5, 6	Extensor carpi radialis Supinator Extensor digitorum Extensor digiti minimi Extensor carpi ulnaris Abductor pollicis longus Extensor pollicis longus and brevis Extensor indicis	C6, 7, 8 C5, 6 C7, 8 C7, 8 C7, 8 C7, 8 C7, 8 C7, 8		
Median: C6–7 Lateral head mainly to forearm muscles C8, T1 Medial head mainly to intrinsic muscles of hand			Pronator teres Flexor carpi radialis Palmaris longus Flexor digitorum sublimis Flexor digitorum profundus (F2, 3) Flexor pollicis longus Pronator quadratus	C6, 7 C6, 7, 8 C7, 8, T1 C7, 8, T1 C7, 8, T1 C8, T1 C7, 8, T1	Abductor pollicis brevis Opponens pollicis Flexor pollicis brevis First and second lumbricals	C8, T1 C8, T1 C8, T1 C7, 8
Ulnar: C8, T1			Flexor carpi ulnaris Flexor digitorum profundus (F4, 5)	C8, T1 C8, T1	Abductor digiti minimi Opponens digiti minimi Third and fourth lumbricals Interossei Adductor pollicis Flexor pollicis brevis	C8, T1 C8, T1 C8, T1 C8, T1 C8, T1 C8, T1

*The muscles are listed in the order of origin of their motor branches from the main nerve trunks, from above downward. With this knowledge it is possible to figure the level at which any major nerve is transected, and likewise to follow the rate of motor reinnervation after repair or spontaneous regeneration.

TABLE 47-2.—SPINAL AND PERIPHERAL INNERVATION OF MAJOR MUSCLES OF LEG AND FOOT*

	THIGH			
Femoral: L2–4	Rectus femoris	L2–4		
	Vastus lateralis	L2–4		
	Sartorius	L2–4		
	Vastus intermedius and medialis	L2–4		
Obturator: L2–4	Adductor magnus	L2–4		
	Adductor longus and brevis	L2–4		
	Gracilis	L2–4		
Sciatic: L4–S3	Adductor magnus	L5–S1		
	Semimembranosus and semitendinosus	L4–S2		
	Biceps femoris	L5–S2		
	POSTERIOR CALF			FOOT
Tibial: L4–S3	Gastrocnemius	S1, 2	Intrinsic plantar muscles, which are difficult to test	L5–S2
	Soleus	L5–S2		
	Tibialis	L5–S2		
	Flexor digitorum longus	L5–S2		
	Flexor hallucis longus	L5–S2		
Peroneal: L4–S2	Superior branch:		Extensor digitorum brevis	S1, 2
	Peroneus longus and brevis	L5–S2		
	Deep branch:			
	Tibialis anterior	L4, 5		
	Extensor digitorum longus	L4–S2		
	Extensor hallucis longus	L5–S2		

*The muscles are listed in the order of origin of their motor branches from the main nerve trunks, from above downward. With this knowledge it is possible to figure the level at which any major nerve is transected, and likewise to follow the rate of motor reinnervation after repair or spontaneous regeneration.

clearly illustrated in Haymaker and Woodhall's *Peripheral Nerve Injuries: Principles of Diagnosis*[8] and in the British Medical Research Council monograph entitled *Peripheral Nerve Injuries*, edited by Seddon.[12]

It is important for the examiner to be aware of the possibility of abnormalities in motor innervation; e.g., the first dorsal interosseus is often supplied by the median, rather than the ulnar, nerve. It is also important not to be misled by the common "trick movements" that can be performed by other nerves; e.g., the elbow can be flexed by the brachioradialis muscle (supplied by the radial nerve) when the musculocutaneous nerve has been injured and the biceps paralyzed. When dealing with an uncooperative individual or a patient with suspected hysterical paralysis, infallible evidence can always be obtained by intraneuronal stimulation of the nerve or electromyographic testing of the muscles[8, 11] or by the absence of sweating and elevated skin resistance.[15] The latter follow the pattern of the cutaneous sensory supply.

A more difficult matter of diagnosis is the pathologic extent of nerve injury. First-, second- and third-degree injuries (neurapraxia, axonotmesis and even a partial intraneuronal disruption) will make a worthwhile or even a perfect recovery if left alone, or they can best be treated by a delayed neurolysis at a subsequent date. If there is an open wound that requires closure, the state of the underlying nerves can usually be observed at the time of debridement of the wound. At the same time, severed ends should be anchored as close together as possible with single sutures to prevent further retraction. When there has been a closed fracture, dislocation of a joint or compression of the extremity, the surgeon must wait and observe the course of events. The nerve often will need to be explored 19–21 days after the injury if progress is inadequate by clinical and electrodiagnostic criteria. The charts of the levels of origin of the muscular rami from the major nerves given in Haymaker and Woodhall's monograph and summarized in Tables 47-1 and 47-2 are most useful in following the progress of motor reinnervation. Tinel's sign is rarely reliable evidence of worthwhile regeneration, but the physician can observe the progressive innervation of muscles charted in the Tables 47–1 and 47–2 and obtain electrical evidence of their reinnervation by the reduction in chronaxy and the cessation of fibrillation, together with the appearance of voluntary contraction potentials in the electromyogram.

NERVE REPAIR

Timing of Operation

A digital nerve may be sutured immediately. Immediate suture may also be performed in occasional instances of distal injury to larger nerves if the wound is free from serious contamination and the nerve has been severed by a knife or penetrating glass fragments. Instances in which uncertainty exists should have operation deferred to 19–21 days following injury. Longer periods of delay are advisable after severe contusions. The policy in Vietnam was to wait up to 6 weeks in gunshot wounds.[3]

After suitable delay, inspection and palpation of nerves permit more satisfactory appraisal of the condition of the nerve ends and adjacent portions of the nerve trunk. This is especially important in a bullet or other high-velocity missile injury, the shock-wave impact of which always produces damage beyond the immediate point of impact. Postponement of nerve repair in other wounds compounded with bone and blood vessel injury or widespread crush of tissue also allows better appraisal of the linear extent of injury. Furthermore, immediate suture in these circumstances is inadvisable because wide dissection to obtain slack carries the risk of spreading infection, there is insufficient time to use the operating room microscope, and there is the danger of separation of the sutures in the softened epineurium. However, delays beyond 3–6 weeks should be strenuously avoided because the prospect of recovery of motor function begins to decrease at this time. There is a 1% loss of function for each 6 days thereafter.

It is more judicious with brachial plexus injuries to allow 3 months to elapse to define the prognosis for recovery of hand function. A fairly clear indication of spontaneous recovery ordinarily exists by this time. Since suture repair of the lower brachial plexus rarely results in recovery of useful hand function, this therapeutic goal can be excluded from consideration. In contrast, however, suture repair of the upper brachial plexus carries good expectation for recovery of the supraspinatus, deltoid and biceps. Reasonable recovery of the forearm flexors, triceps and sometimes the wrist extensors may occur. Further gains may be realized by later tendon transfers. The outlook for recovery of sensation to the fingertips tends to be discouraging.

It is unclear from the data whether neurolysis will alter the prognosis favorably, although some workers favor it. Traumatic aneurysms of the axillary artery may be discovered by exploration but can normally be diagnosed by palpation, auscultation and angiography. In any case, it is unwise to resect any nerve lesion unless the complete disruption of neural elements is perfectly clear by inspection and electrical testing. Avulsion of nerve roots can normally be confirmed by a cervical myelogram which demonstrates extravasation of dye into extraspinal pockets and does not require exploration.

Lesions of the lumbar and sacral plexuses are so rare that published experience provides little useful guidance.

Intraoperative Examination

With the point of injury clearly exposed, the course to follow will be governed by the type of wound (Fig. 47-10). When there is a neuroma in continuity, it is important to decide whether an adequate number of fibers can grow down through the zone of endoneurial scarring. A fairly accurate assessment can be made by 1 of the following methods.

METHOD 1.—Palpation of the segment of nerve injured in order to detect the presence of a constrictive scar.

METHOD 2.—Electrical stimulation by means of an alternating current transformer producing 60-cycle sine waves or a condenser discharge giving square-topped waves of 1 millisecond duration. If 1 of these stimulators is not available, a faradic current of the type supplied by the Harvard inductorium will do.

Sensory.—Can the patient feel a stimulus applied to the distal end of the neuroma?

Motor.—Does a stimulus of 10–15 volts above the neuroma produce any contraction of the muscles below? This test will be painful unless the nerve is blocked by injecting local anesthetic solution into its trunk a few centimeters above.

METHOD 3.—Infiltration of sterile saline solution, checking to see if the solution passes areas of suspected fibrosis.

Technique of Nerve Suture

We favor the use of an operating microscope for nerve suture. In addition to the obvious advantages of magnification to 6 or 10 power, the brilliance of the illumination of the operative field enhances the detail and promotes gentleness of manipulation. Efforts at aligning perineural blood vessels and major funiculi are facilitated. Magnifying lenses or loupes offer an alternative when a microscope is not available.

1. Suture must be performed at a level of healthy epineurium with preservation of the nerve vuniculi and relative freedom from scar.

Fig. 47-10.—Gunshot wound of median nerve in midforearm. Surgical exposure, several months after injury, shows wide retraction of end-bulbs *(B)* with intervening scar *(S)*. The proximal neuroma lies to right, with the nerve *(N)* above emerging from under the superficial head of the pronator teres muscle *(P)*.

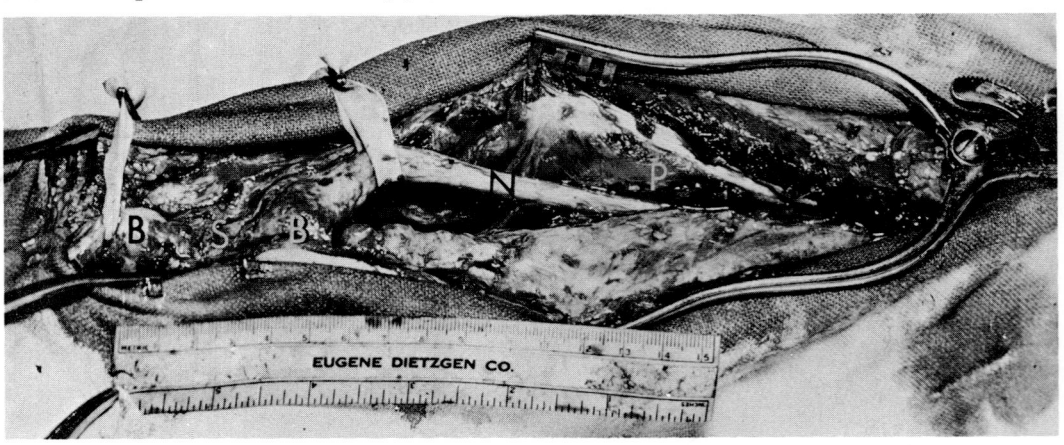

2. The suture should be made with very fine, nonabsorbable stitches and accurate apposition of the epineurium.

3. There should be as little rotation of the nerve ends as possible.

4. The completed suture must not be under tension.

5. The sutured nerve should be placed in as healthy a bed of tissue as circumstances permit.

6. The suture must be protected from disruption by immobilizing the contiguous joints.

Except in the case of a fresh laceration, exploration of an injured nerve should be carried out under local anesthesia. This is best done by infiltrating the tissues in the line of incision with procaine or longer lasting Xylocaine with added epinephrine. Care should be taken not to infiltrate the nerve itself, because its function must be tested electrically in case a neuroma-in-continuity is found. (A tourniquet cannot be used if local anesthesia is employed because of the resultant painful ischemia.)

Long incisions should be planned with care to permit satisfactory exposure and to avoid linear contracting scars across the joints. When the position of the retracted end-bulbs is uncertain, these can be located most easily by exposing the nerve above and below in healthy tissue. It is always advisable to free up a considerable length, in order to gain slack. This is quite harmless (except in the leg), provided care is taken not to injure any important branches. Fortunately, nerves have an extensive longitudinal blood supply, so that their lateral vascular supply can be sacrificed over many inches without risk of ischemic necrosis.

When there is no chance of effective regeneration through a neuroma-in-continuity, or when there has been separation of the nerve ends, as in Figure 47-10, it is necessary to resect the scarred portion back to healthy tissue. This is best done by making serial sections with a safety-razor blade held in a hemostat until the separate fascicles can be seen under the operating microscope. The zone of scar tissue in a neuroma has the pale, uniform texture of "fish flesh." In striking contrast is the characteristic appearance of the cross section of healthy nerve, in which the individual fascicles stand out as multiple small projections. Before resection of any neuroma-in-continuity, a marker suture should be placed at corresponding points in the epineurium above and below the area to be resected, so that the free ends can be sutured afterward with a minimum of rotation.

For suturing it is best to use either very fine (6-0) black silk or 3-mil tantalum wire. Metallic stitches have the feature that they can be seen in x-ray films, and subsequent separation of the suture line can thus be detected.

Clinical and experimental evidence favors use of a cuff at the suture line. Silastic is currently considered superior to tantalum[5] because it is soft and less likely to be painful or to fracture, and it provokes even less glioma-neuroma formation proximal and distal to the tube itself. Experience with war wounds[6] does not favor use of a cuff with the radial or perineal nerve. If placed at joints—elbow or wrist—cuffs should be removed after a few weeks.

The tubes should be 3 times larger in cross section than the nerve. For example, a 1-mm nerve requires a cuff 1.7 mm in diameter; a 3-mm nerve requires a cuff 5.2 mm in diameter; a 10-mm nerve requries one 17.4 mm in diameter. Smaller tubes constrict the repair site. The large tubes allow for swelling in the immediate postoperative period and force longitudinal alignment of the rapidly proliferating supportive structures during this critical period. Consequently, there is more direct axonal spanning, which in turn improves function.

When the 2 ends of healthy nerve are ready for approximation, stay sutures should be placed in the epineurium 180 degrees apart, tied and held taut at either side by fine hemostats. Individual stitches are then placed and tied 1 or 2 mm apart on the anterior exposed half of the circumferences, taking care to include only the firm, thick epineurial sheath and to tie each suture snugly (Fig. 47-11). When this row has been completed, there should be an accurate approximation of the outer sheath of the nerve with no protrusion of its contents. One of the original stay sutures is then passed beneath and the nerve trunk rotated 180 degrees to expose its posterior wall for suture. After the suture has been completed all the way around, the repaired nerve is dropped back into a bed of healthy muscle or adipose tissue.

In addition to accurate approximation, it is of vital importance that the suture be free from any tension. Sometimes it is necessary to compromise by not carrying the resection all the way back to entirely normal tissue. Generally, however, and particularly in civilian type injuries, adequate slack can be gained by 1 of the following methods.

Achieve adequate extent of neurolysis.—This may include, if necessary, the entire length of the forearm, upper arm,

Fig. 47-11.—Technique of neurorrhaphy. Prior to suture, the end-bulbs were cut back to healthy nerve structure free from scar. (Procedures described in the text have also been utilized to permit approximation and suture free from tension and with minimal rotation.) **A,** stay sutures *(1 and 2)* placed on opposite sides to approximate severed ends of nerve with minimal rotation. Epineurial suture *(3)* is started. **B,** epineurial suture on anterior surface completed. The long end of stay suture *2* is passed beneath the nerve, while suture *1* is drawn across its surface in the opposite direction. **C,** method of rotating nerve. Traction on stay sutures will now present its posterior aspect. **D,** epineurial suture completed.

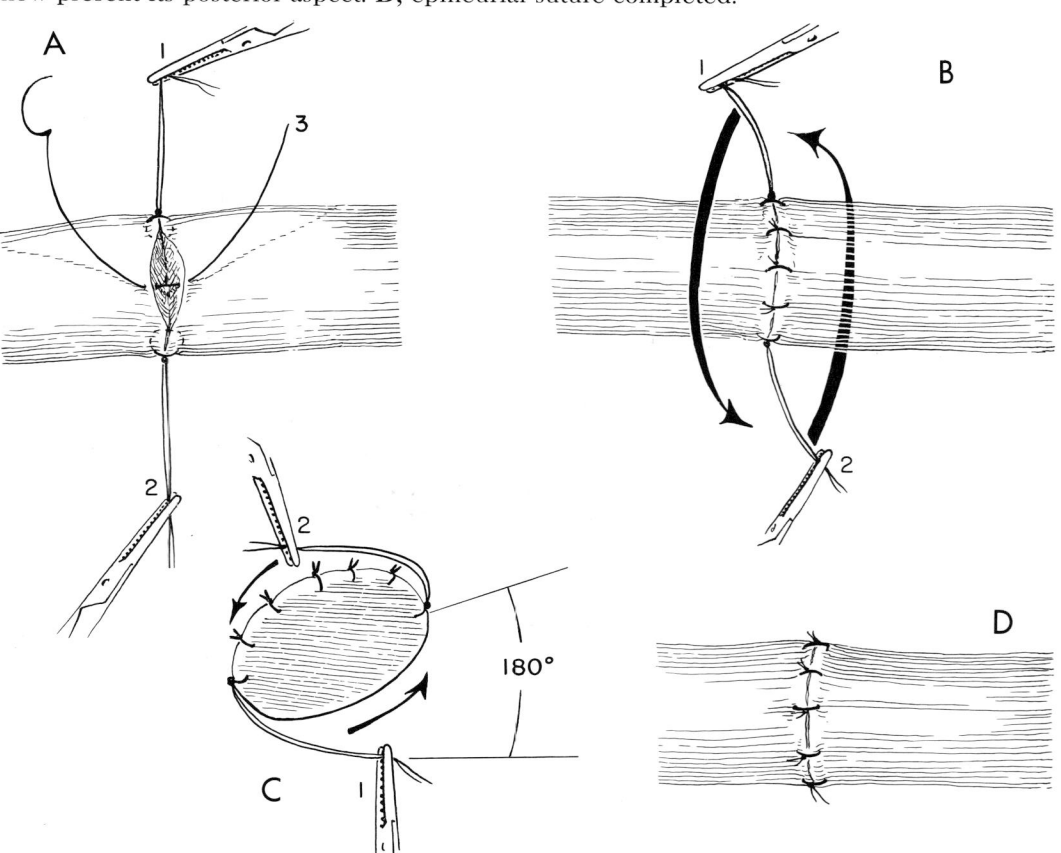

thigh and lower leg. The extent of neurolysis, however, should not be carried any farther than necessary. In wartime experience, sciatic and tibial sutures seemed to do poorly when the nerve was freed up over the greater part of the leg.

Position joints to shorten course of nerve.—In injuries to the brachial nerves, the elbow and wrist are flexed. The hip is extended and the knee flexed after a sciatic suture.

Transpose or reroute nerve.—A standard procedure in ulnar nerve sutures is to shift the nerve from its epicondylar groove to a position in front of the elbow. As Learmonth[9] first recommended, it is advisable to cut the flexor muscles a few millimeters from their insertion in the medial condyle, to lay the ulnar nerve alongside the median and then to resuture the muscle attachments (Fig. 47-12). In treating old fractures of the internal condyle with injury to the nerve in the epicondylar groove, the orthopedic surgeons at Massachusetts General Hospital often resect a portion of the condyle in addition to transposing the ulnar nerve.

Other maneuvers of similar type are: (1) transposing the median nerve into a more superficial position by cutting the superficial head of the pronator radii teres muscle and resuturing it behind the nerve; (2) passing the radial nerve in front of the humerus so that, after suture, it passes in a straighter course through a tunnel beneath the biceps muscle (this step gains only 3–4 cm of length); (3) resection of the parotid gland in difficult sutures of the facial nerve, as recommended by White.[24] The third procedure gains 1 or 2 cm of added slack and permits a far better exposure for deep sutures between the ramus of the mandible and the stylomastoid foramen.

Grafts for Excessive Defects in Peripheral Nerves

Use of pedicle grafts has been more successful than any other method of bridging excessive defects in peripheral nerves. These grafts can be utilized only with the sacrifice of a contiguous large nerve. In Selverstone's case,[18] in which there was an extensive gap in both the median and ulnar nerves at the elbow, the proximal end of the median nerve was sutured to the nearby ulnar nerve, which was then divided above in the axilla. As a result, axons and longitudinal blood vessels from the median nerve grew into the upper decentralized segment of the ulnar nerve, which was still supplied by its lateral vascular branches. After several months, when Tinel's sign showed regeneration of median axons throughout the upper ulnar segment, this pedicle, now supplied by newly formed longitudinal blood vessels, was turned down and sutured to the lower end of the median nerve. The patient thereby regained good function of the more important median innervation of the forearm and hand. A number of other successful examples of this ingenious procedure have been reported.

Free autografts must never be longer than 4 cm to have reasonable hope of success. The sural nerve is a favorite donor site for such grafts. The relatively small caliber of the sural nerve is not a limitation. In the case of a large-caliber nerve, several smaller nerves laid side by side (the cable graft of Tarlov[23]) have a better prospect of success than a free homograft of large caliber.

Homografts are a choice of last resort. To be used at all, these grafts should be fresh frozen and irradiated with 2 million rads. The gamut of problems of autoimmunity and tissue rejection are shared by nerve homografts and their use should be considered quasi-experimental.

The whole subject of nerve grafting is ably reviewed in the Medical Research Council monograph, *Peripheral Nerve Injuries*, edited by Seddon.[12] Seddon reports many successes with cable grafts in bridging large defects in major nerves, and even a few successes with main trunk autografts, provided the gap to be bridged does not exceed a few centimeters in length.

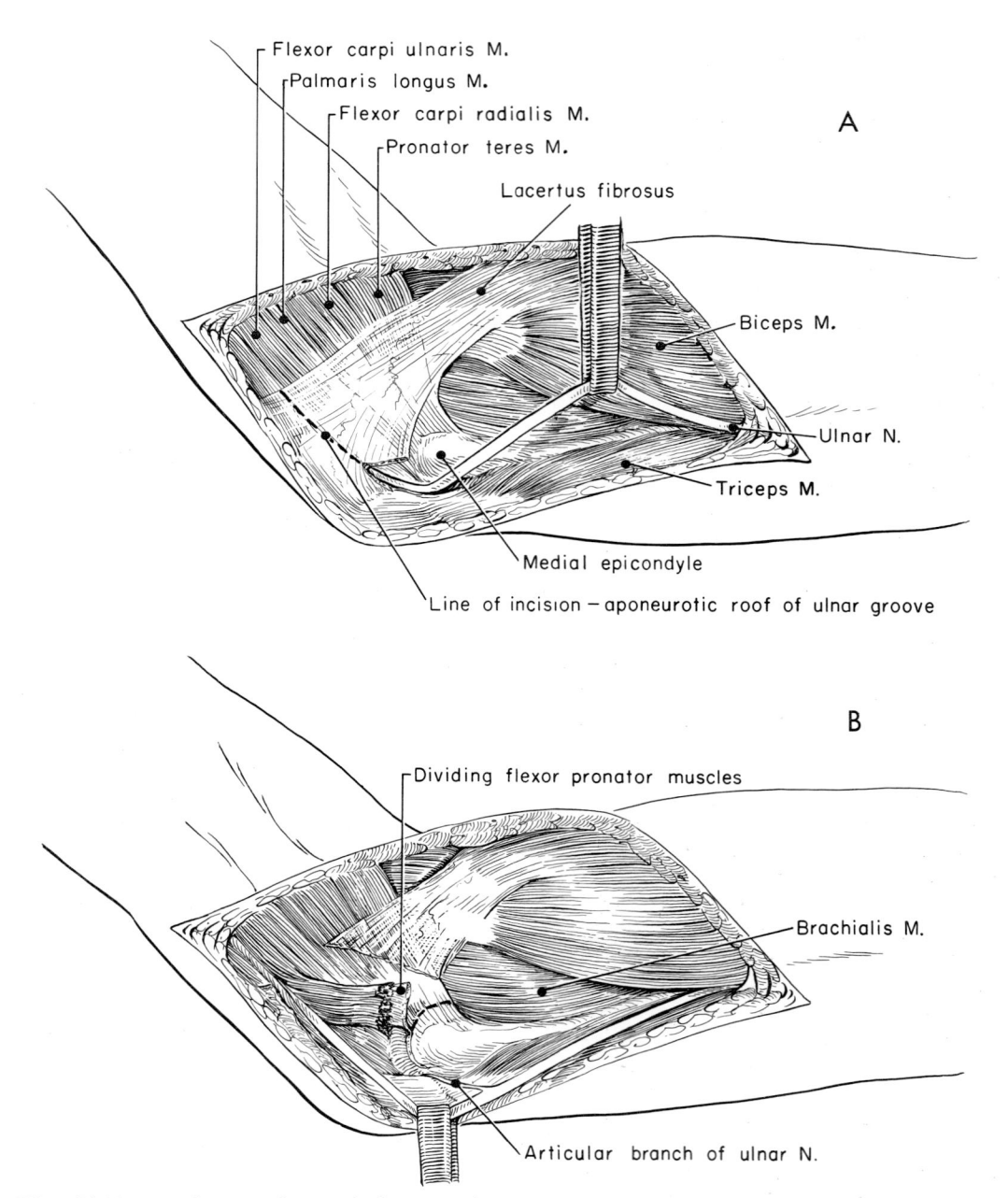

Fig. 47-12.—Technique for transplanting ulnar nerve. **A,** nerve exposed above the epicondylar groove by division of intermuscular septum between biceps and triceps muscles. The lacertus fibrosus fascia and aponeurotic roof of the epicondylar groove are next divided. **B,** ulnar nerve elevated and freed below by separating the 2 heads of the flexor carpi ulnaris and retracting the forearm flexor muscles medially. The attachment of the flexor pronator muscle heads to the medial condyle of the humerus is then cut. It is often necessary to sacrifice the branch to the elbow. The flexor pronator muscles are turned back, exposing the median nerve. **(Continued.)**

Chapter 47: PERIPHERAL NERVE INJURIES / 1107

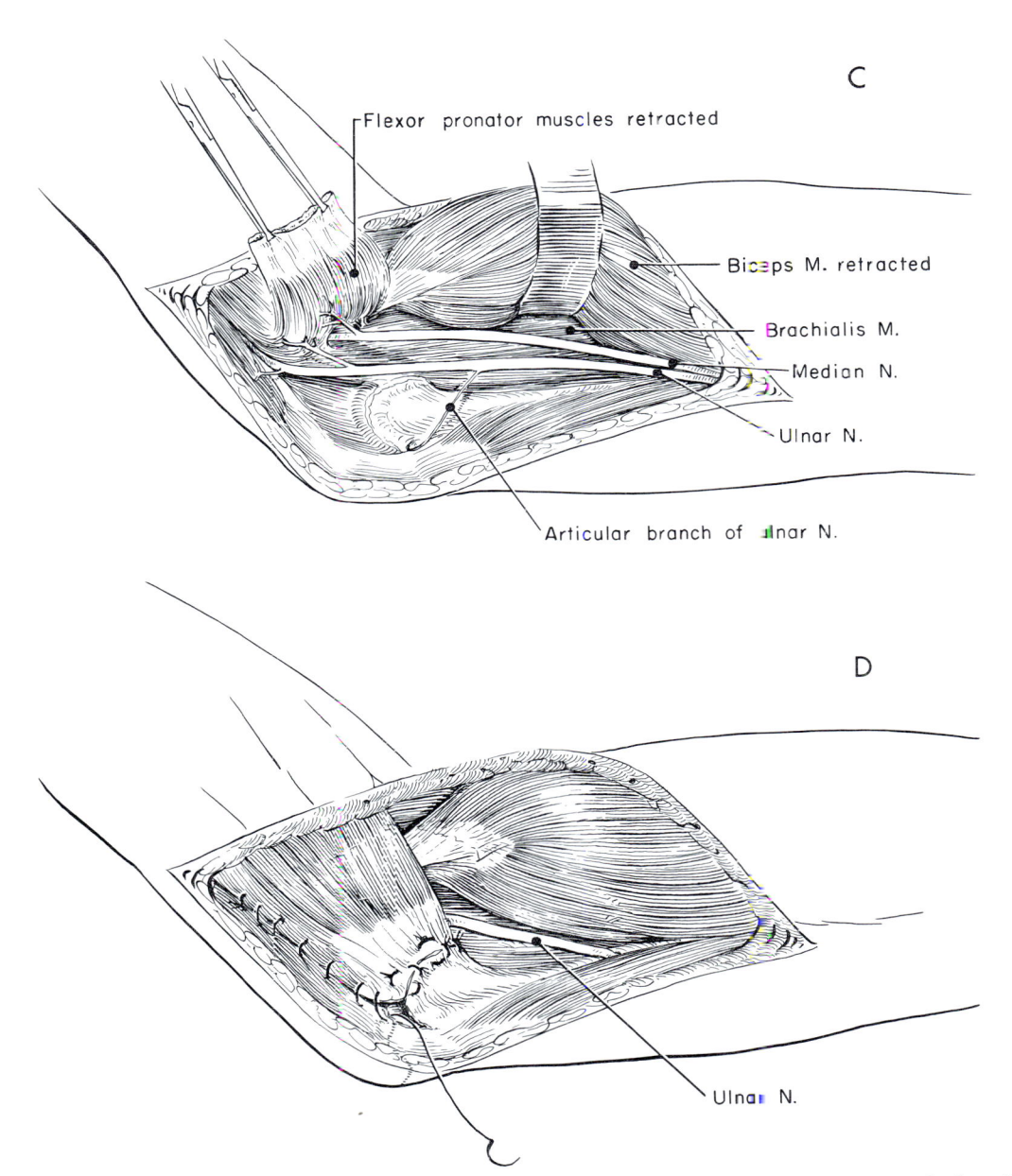

Fig. 47-12 (cont.). — **C,** ulnar nerve transposed in front of the humeral condyle and placed alongside the median nerve. **D,** severed muscle attachments are sutured with fine silk or stainless-steel wire. (Modified from Learmonth, J. R.: A technique for transplanting the ulnar nerve, Surg. Gynecol. Obstet. 75:792, 1942.)

Bone Shortening

As proposed by Dandy,[3] shortening of the humerus or femur is a logical step in cases of ununited fractures. The clavicle also can be shortened or excised and the shoulder moved inward in difficult repairs of plexus injuries.

POSTOPERATIVE CARE

After neurorrhapy, tension and disruption of the suture must be prevented by immobilization of neighboring joints in flexion, but splints must be applied with extreme caution and only for the shortest possible period. In a high sciatic suture, it is essential to apply a plaster spica to maintain extension of the hip as well as flexion of the knee. Regeneration of severed nerves is of little value if a useful range of joint movement is sacrificed by overprolonged splinting. Splinting of the wrist, elbow or knee in acute flexion need never be maintained for more than 3 weeks. At the end of this period, the joint can gradually be extended and the splint removed daily for passive flexion and massage. Physiotherapy and full range of joint movement should be started within a month. By this time, tissue regeneration should safeguard the suture against disruption.

After the initial splint necessary to prevent disruption of the sutures is no longer required, special splints are useful to maintain the paralyzed extremity in a functional position. These permit use of the intact muscles and prevent stretching of those that are paralyzed during the long period of motor recovery. These include: a wrist cock-up, elastic finger-extension splint for radial palsies; the so-called knuckle-bender splint to prevent clawing of the fingers in lumbrical paralysis (this holds the metacarpophalangeal joints in flexion and the proximal interphalangeal joints in partial extension); the lower leg spring brace that holds the shoe in neutral position to prevent foot drop after peroneal injuries.

During the prolonged course of reinnervation, the patient must be taught to exercise the normal muscles and joints of the extremity as actively as possible. Galvanic stimulation of paralyzed muscles will also do much to maintain muscle tone until voluntary movement returns, provided facilities are at hand for daily application. Every possible means must be employed to maintain good function of joints and soft parts in order to have a useful extremity when nerve regeneration is completed.

RECOVERY AFTER NERVE SUTURE

The course of reinnervation can be followed by downward extension of Tinel's sign, the gradual return of sensation, and muscular contraction. Shortening of chronaxy, electromyographic evidence of loss of paralytic fibrillation and the disappearance of the reaction of degeneration will all precede the return of active movement. Full recovery will require about 6 months when nerve suture is at the wrist or ankle, 1 year at the level of the elbow or knee, and 18 months to 2 years when the suture is in the axilla or upper thigh.

Action potentials may be seen as early as 17 days following experimental nerve crush but is more usual after 6 weeks. The conduction velocity reaches 75% of normal in 12 months and remains at this level up to the succeeding year. Conduction of a regenerating nerve occurs when larger axons develop and does not occur when only smaller axons are present. The further conduction is enhanced, the greater the degree of myelinization. By 12 weeks, action potentials are found up to 18 cm from the crush, and at increasing amplitude the more proximal to the crush. The increased amplitude reflects the greater population of axons. The electromyogram shows a decrease in number of fibrillations and denervation potentials and the appearance of motor units.

Tables 47-3 and 47-4 from Woodhall and Beebe's *Peripheral Nerve Regenera-*

TABLE 47–3.—MEAN POWER OF AFFECTED MUSCLES FOLLOWING COMPLETE SUTURE*

NERVE AND MUSCLE	NO. CASES	MEAN POWER AS % OF NORMAL — ALL CASES	CASES WITH MOVEMENT AGAINST RESISTANCE
Median			
Flexor carpi radialis	141	55.99	†
Flexor pollicis longus	103	33.16	46.78
Flexor digitorum profundus 2	155	31.13	45.95
Opponens	187	23.69	†
Abductor pollicis brevis	124	13.67	33.24
Ulnar			
Flexor carpi ulnaris	253	59.57	†
Flexor digitorum profundus 4 & 5	304	33.92	44.07
Abductor digiti V	425	9.63	24.81
Adductor pollicis	393	23.66	†
1st dorsal interosseous	305	10.90	28.42
Radial			
Triceps	39	57.05	†
Brachioradialis	111	48.56	†
Extensor carpi radialis	175	41.26	49.12
Extensor digitorum	167	28.08	44.66
Extensor carpi ulnaris	177	36.07	†
Abductor pollicis longus	113	14.69	†
Extensor pollicis longus	169	19.14	36.76
Tibial			
Gastrocnemius and soleus	32	55.94	63.93
Tibialis posterior	37	35.68	†
Flexor digitorum longus	53	10.09	35.67
Flexor hallucis longus	54	9.44	34.00
Interosseous	76	3.36	†
Sciatic-tibial			
Gastrocnemius and soleus	125	46.08	58.77
Tibialis posterior	129	18.72	†
Flexor digitorum longus	133	3.31	36.67
Flexor hallucis longus	133	2.82	31.25
Interosseous	120	.42	†
Peroneal			
Tibialis anterior	128	17.38	46.35
Extensor digitorum longus	137	8.61	31.89
Extensor hallucis longus	134	6.68	35.80
Peroneus longus	135	17.00	42.50
Sciatic-peroneal			
Tibialis anterior	166	5.91	31.65
Extensor digitorum longus	167	2.25	23.50
Extensor hallucis longus	165	2.36	27.79
Peroneus longus	168	4.26	26.52

*Tables 47–3 to 47–6 from Woodhall, B., and Beebe, G. W.: *Peripheral Nerve Regeneration: A Follow-up Study of 3,656 World War II Injuries* (Washington, D. C.: Government Printing Office, 1956).
†Not calculated.

TABLE 47-4.—PERCENTAGE OF AFFECTED MUSCLES CONTRACTING AND MEAN POWER FOLLOWING COMPLETE SUTURE

NERVE AND MUSCLE	HIGH LESIONS				LOW LESIONS				STATISTICAL TESTS†
	N*	% CONTRACTING	MEAN POWER ALL CASES	MEAN POWER CASES MOVING AGAINST RESISTANCE	N*	% CONTRACTING	MEAN POWER ALL CASES	MEAN POWER CASES MOVING AGAINST RESISTANCE	
Median									
Flexor carpi radialis	103	96.52	51.99	60.17	38	92.31	66.84	74.71	°
Flexor pollicis longus	70	88.46	27.93	41.60	33	91.43	44.24	56.15	°
Flexor digitorum profundus 2	106	87.72	22.26	36.88	49	94.12	50.31	60.12	°°
Opponens	96	75.75	18.44	34.04	91	91.75	29.23	45.08	°°
Abductor pollicis brevis	63	78.12	12.38	35.45	61	82.81	15.00	31.55	NS
Ulnar									
Flexor carpi ulnaris	178	96.14	56.63	66.32	75	97.44	66.53	72.32	°
Flexor digitorum profundus 4 & 5	206	93.69	31.67	41.82	98	95.05	38.65	48.56	NS
Abductor digiti V	232	84.87	7.20	21.14	193	90.40	12.55	28.16	°°
Adductor pollicis	217	84.85	18.94	33.69	176	92.51	29.49	40.23	°°
1st dorsal interosseous	164	78.41	8.96	25.77	141	86.84	13.16	30.93	°
Tibial									
Gastrocnemius and soleus	125	94.16	46.08	58.77	32	94.29	55.94	63.93	NS
Tibialis posterior	129	68.66	18.72	53.67	37	85.00	35.68	60.00	°°
Flexor digitorum longus	133	27.61	3.31	36.67	53	65.52	10.09	35.67	°
Flexor hallucis longus	133	28.36	2.82	31.25	54	67.24	9.44	34.00	°
Interosseous	120	14.05	.42	50.00	76	51.81	3.36	31.92	°
Peroneal									
Tibialis anterior	166	58.93	5.91	31.65	128	75.19	17.38	46.35	°°
Extensor digitorum longus	167	42.94	2.25	23.50	137	65.94	8.61	31.89	°°
Extensor hallucis longus	165	35.33	2.36	27.79	134	54.41	6.68	35.80	°
Peroneus longus	168	55.29	4.26	26.52	135	71.01	17.00	42.50	°°

*Number of muscles studied.
†Probability that observed difference between means for all muscles, or a larger difference, might arise by chance. Results are abbreviated as follows: NS = Not significant ° = Significant at .05 level °° = Significant at .01 level.

tion[26] show the over-all degree of recovery of motor power after military wounds in World War II. Current civilian nerve injuries could be expected to have a better prognosis than these, since the former include many high-velocity missile wounds and in many instances suture was done after several months rather than in the optimal interval of 19–21 days. Technical features, microsurgical technique and silicon cuffing could also improve the outcome.

In general, several patterns of motor recovery are evident. Lesions below the elbow may realize a better recovery of power by a factor of 2 than those in the upper arm. Recovery of extrinsic musculature of the hand is about twice as satisfactory as that of intrinsic muscles. The recovery of tibial innervation is better than peroneal and, so far as the muscles of the calf are concerned, compares with the median and ulnar innervation. The intrinsic muscles of the foot rarely recover. Peroneal sutures give only a 17% chance of recovery from foot drop.

The use of a cuff about a nerve suture was considered to promote a 20–25% better motor recovery than not using a cuff in World War II patients, but the cuff fractured and produced marked reactions years later. The value of the newer Silastic cuffs that have been used in some of the recent war injuries from Vietnam has not yet been accurately assessed. In 50 cases re-examined after a year, Ducker (reported at the Congress of Neurological Surgeons in Toronto, 1968) found the early end results slightly superior to those with the tantalum cuffs. Tantalum wire appears to slightly aid motor recovery, but the difference is not statistically significant. Delay of suture past 19–21 days impairs motor recovery 1% for each 6 days of delay. A gap bridged by autogenous graft loses 6% in motor recovery for each centimeter of gap.

Preadolescents are noted to have qualitatively far better recoveries than adults. In a 9-year-old girl whose median and ulnar nerves had been severed in the axilla, functional recovery has been nearly perfect. Nine years later, she has no noticeable handicap in playing the piano, typing or distinguishing coins with her eyes closed. In a boy, 12, who had replantation of an arm cut off below the shoulder by the wheels of a train, it was possible to suture the median, ulnar and musculocutaneous nerves 4 months after injury. Six years later he was working as an automobile mechanic.

Sensory recovery in the World War II cases is summarized for pain and touch thresholds in Tables 47-5 and 47-6. No recovery of pain sensibility occurred

TABLE 47–5.—DEEP-PRESSURE PAIN RESPONSE AND SUPERFICIAL PAIN THRESHOLD FOR COMPLETELY SUTURED LESIONS, BY NERVE, AUTONOMOUS ZONE ONLY

THRESHOLD°	MEDIAN %	ULNAR %	RADIAL %	TIBIAL %	PERONEAL %	SCIATIC-PERONEAL %	SCIATIC-TIBIAL %
No sensation of pain	8.5	11.9	5.8	19.0	15.5	22.7	23.3
Deep-pressure pain only	13.6	18.1	14.9	23.2	15.5	27.6	35.7
Superficial pain, 40 gm	14.5	16.2	15.9	15.4	17.0	17.0	12.8
Superficial pain, 30 gm	8.0	8.2	6.2	5.6	4.3	4.4	3.4
Superficial pain, 20 gm	11.7	12.1	6.2	6.9	9.4	2.9	4.3
Superficial pain, 10 gm	17.3	17.5	22.1	16.8	11.9	11.8	11.9
Superficial pain, 6 gm	10.8	6.2	10.7	2.7	10.2	3.7	2.5
Superficial pain, <6 gm	15.7	9.8	18.1	10.5	16.2	9.8	6.2
Total	100.1	100.0	99.9	100.1	100.0	99.9	100.1
No. of lesions	236	430	188	95	142	163	129

°About 6% of all cases were classified as "hypalgesia, unmeasured," and distributed proportionately over the frequencies for thresholds from 40 gm to 6 gm.

TABLE 47-6.—DEEP-PRESSURE AND SUPERFICIAL TOUCH RESPONSES FOR COMPLETELY SUTURED LESIONS, BY NERVE, AUTONOMOUS ZONE ONLY

THRESHOLD*	M, %	U, %	R, %	P, %	T, %	SP, %	ST, %
No sensation, or threshold >50 gm	18.3	24.5	11.8	29.4	34.8	47.2	49.7
Deep pressure felt with 50 gm / Deep pressure felt with 35 gm	4.6	4.9	4.4	3.1	8.0	6.6	6.3
Deep pressure felt with 25 gm	5.4	7.9	6.7	15.9	8.1	6.6	4.7
Superficial pressure felt with 16 gm	23.2	27.7	21.1	14.3	22.8	9.9	21.3
Superficial pressure felt with 5 gm	21.8	16.6	20.0	13.5	10.7	8.6	9.4
Superficial pressure felt with 3 gm	11.4	9.6	17.8	11.1	4.0	5.3	5.5
Superficial pressure felt with <3 gm	15.3	8.8	18.2	12.6	11.6	15.5	3.1
Total	100.0	100.0	100.0	99.9	100.0	99.7	100.0
No. of lesions	241	433	187	143	95	163	129

*About 5% of all cases were classified as "hypesthesia, unmeasured," and distributed proportionately over the frequencies for thresholds from 50 gm to 3 gm.

in the vicinity of 10% in the median, ulnar and radial distributions. On the other hand, recovery to essentially normal pain detection occurred in 10-20% in median, ulnar, radial, tibial and peroneal lesions, but in less than 10% in sciatic lesions. Varying degrees of hypalgesia were distributed between these extremes.

Fewer factors appear to contribute to the degree of sensory recovery. In particular, the time of suture does not affect the quality of recovery. Cuffs about the suture may aid recovery, and suturing with silk is just barely better than suturing with tantalum wire.

Lesions of the brachial plexus yield relatively poor motor or sensory recovery in the digits. Suture repair yields about 80% "useful" recovery of flexion of the elbow; abduction of shoulder and triceps responds less well. However, wrist movement and sensation are rated at only 15-20%, finger flexion at 6%, and extension or intrinsic control of the muscles of the hand at essentially 0. Exploration and lysis, if done to establish prognosis, should be performed between 3 and 6 months after injury.

ORTHOPEDIC MEASURES TO CORRECT PERSISTENT PARALYSIS

When a useful degree of motor recovery fails to take place, the function of a paralyzed extremity can be improved greatly by a number of orthopedic procedures. These are well described by Campbell[2] and by Bunnell.[1] Excellent functional results after irreparable radial nerve injury may be obtained by transferring wrist flexor tendons to the long extensors of the fingers and thumb.

Irreparable ulnar nerve injuries may require no reconstructive surgery if the functional disability is mild. The clawhand deformity which may occur can be improved by transfer of the flexor sublimis tendons to the lateral bands of the dorsal aponeurosis of the proximal interphalangeal joints of the fourth and fifth fingers, as described by Bunnell.[1]

For irreparable median nerve injuries, function may be improved by transplanting the extensor carpi radialis brevis muscle to the flexor pollicis longus. Flexion of the index and the middle fingers may be improved by attaching their flexor profundus tendons to the functioning flexor profundus tendons of the ring and little fingers. The flexor carpi ulnaris may be used to produce opposition of the thumb. Its detached tendon is sutured to that of the extensor pollicis brevis after it has been run obliquely across the palm and through a fascial loop attached to the hamate bone. There is no truly satisfactory reconstructive surgery for combined complete ulnar and median lesions.

Deltoid paralysis due to axillary nerve injury produces inability to abduct the arm. Transplants of the trapezius muscle (Mayer) or of the triceps and short head of the biceps (Ober), as described in Campbell,[2] can improve function in these cases.

Irreparable injury to the musculocutaneous nerve results in inability to flex the elbow. Advancing the origin of the forearm flexor muscles on the humerus (Steindler) is of benefit.

In the lower extremity, injury of the femoral nerve results in paralysis of the quadriceps femoris muscle. Despite such paralysis, patients can learn to walk without apparatus (or with a cane at most) with an excellent gait. Transplant of a number of muscles in various combinations (biceps femoris, semitendinosus, sartorius and tensor fascia femoris) to the patella may improve extensor power and lessen the tendency for the knee to "give way."

Complete lesions of the sciatic nerve produce so much sensory deficit in the foot that amputation is often necessary eventually because of trophic ulceration. Foot drop due to irreparable peroneal nerve palsy produces a steppage type of gait that may be corrected by wearing a short foot-drop brace. Stabilization of the foot by ankle fusion, by triple arthrodesis or by transplant of the functioning posterior tibial tendon anteriorly through the interosseous membrane may enable the patient with foot drop to discard his brace with improvement in function of the extremity.

PAINFUL SYNDROMES AFTER NERVE INJURY

A final complication of nerve injury that deserves mention is persistent pain. In lateral neuromas from penetrating wounds, the burning discomfort of causalgia may become a source of intense suffering within a few hours or days. This syndrome, so well described by Weir Mitchell,[13] is characterized by diffuse burning pain and trophic disturbances with glossy skin and tapering fingers. The pain is distinctly related to emotional disturbances; the victim prefers to remain alone in a quiet closed room with the extremity protected by a moist towel against changes in temperature and even drafts of air. Experience has taught that neither resection of the neuroma nor any other operation on the injured nerve can be counted on to give effective relief. If the pain is relieved temporarily by stellate or lumbar sympathetic block, an appropriate sympathectomy will give permanent relief White, Heroy and Goodman[25] and Shumacker[19]). In a review of results in 32 veterans of World War II 2–7 years after injury, it was found that a properly performed sympathectomy almost always relieved true causalgic pain. In high sciatic injury, it is important to carry the resection of the sympathetic chain upward to include the first lumbar and the twelfth thoracic ganglia. Failures occurred consistently after incomplete sympathetic denervation or periarterial stripping and in many instances when the neuroma was resected and the nerve sutured. The British, however, claimed quite a number of successes prior to the advent of sympathectomy.

Other types of pain and discomfort are common after nerve injury when there is lasting paralysis or when there is partial recovery after neurolysis or suture. Usually the discomfort consists only of minor complaints—a feeling of coldness, paresthesia or spontaneous twinges of pain—and these are not a serious problem. On the other hand, a few unfortunate individuals have a permanent state of sensitivity in the partially reinnervated skin, which is best described as "over response." This is particularly incapacitating after injury to the median or tibial nerves, when the sufferer is unable to grasp firmly with his hand or bear full weight in walking. Occasionally, the condition has improved after a secondary suture with better sensory recovery, but often there is no solution except by recourse to anterolateral cordotomy or dorsal rhizotomy. Cutting the pain fibers in the dorsal root, when done by an expert. offers a good chance of success with little risk of serious complications in the case of sciatic and tibial injuries.

BIBLIOGRAPHY

1. Bunnell, S.: *Surgery of the Hand* (2d ed.; Philadelphia: J. B. Lippincott Company, 1948).
2. Campbell, W. C., in Speed, J. S., and Knight, R. A. (eds.): *Operative Orthopedics* (3d ed.; St. Louis: C. V. Mosby Company, 1956).
3. Dandy, W. E.: A method of restoring nerves requiring resection, JAMA 122:35, 1943.
4. Ducker, T. B., Kempe, L. G., and Hayes, G. J.: The metabolic background for peripheral nerve surgery, J. Neurosurg. 30:270, 1969.
5. Ducker, T. B., and Hayes, G. J.: Experimental improvements in the use of silastic cuff for peripheral nerve repair, J. Neurosurg. 28:582, 1968.
6. Ducker, T. D.: Personal communication.
7. Golubov, G.: Changes in the spinal cord and spinal ganglia from traumas of the peripheral nerves and their connections with regeneration of the nerve and gravity of the trauma, Izv. Inst. Mortol. 4:109, 1961.
8. Haymaker, W., and Woodhall, B.: *Peripheral Nerve Injuries: Principles of Diagnosis* (2d ed.; Philadelphia: W. B. Saunders Company, 1953).
9. Learmonth, J. R.: A technique for transplanting the ulnar nerve, Surg. Gynecol. Obstet. 75:792, 1942.
10. Malt, R. A.: Replantation of Severed Arms, in Egdahl, R. H., and Mannick, J. A. (eds.): *Modern Surgery* (New York: Grune & Stratton, Inc., 1970).
11. Marinacci, A. A.: Electromyography as an adjunct in neurological diagnosis, Bull. Los Angeles Neurol. Soc. 18:25, 1953.
12. Medical Research Council, Nerve Injuries Committee, in Seddon, H. J., ed.: *Peripheral Nerve Injuries* (London: Her Majesty's Stationery Office, 1954).
13. Mitchell, S. W.: *Injuries of Nerves and Their Consequences* (Philadelphia: J. B. Lippincott Company, 1872).
14. Pollock, L. J., and Davis, L.: *Peripheral Nerve Injuries* (New York: Paul B. Hoeber, Inc., 1933).
15. Richter, C. P., and Katz, D. T.: Peripheral nerve injuries determined by the electrical skin resistance method: I. Ulnar nerve, JAMA 122: 648, 1943.
16. Seddon, H. J.: Three types of nerve injury, Brain 66:237, 1943.
17. Seddon, H. J.: War injuries of peripheral nerves, Br. J. Surg. (War Surgery, supp. 2) 36: 325, 1949.
18. Selverstone, B.: The pedicle principle in nerve grafting, Bull. Am. Coll. Surg. 32:226, 1947.
19. Shumacker, H. B.: Causalgia: III. A general discussion, Surgery 24:485, 1948.
20. Sunderland, S.: Factors influencing the course of regeneration and the quality of the recovery after nerve suture, Brain 75:19, 1952.
21. Sunderland, S.: Rate of regeneration in human peripheral nerves: Analysis of the interval between injury and onset of recovery, Arch. Neurol. 58:251, 1947.
22. Sunderland, S.: and Ray, L. J.: The intraneural topography of the sciatic nerve and its popliteal divisions in man, Brain 71:242, 1948.
23. Tarlov, I. M.: *Plasma Clot Suture of Peripheral Nerves and Nerve Roots: Rationale and Technique* (Springfield, Ill.: Charles C Thomas, Publisher, 1950).
24. White, J. C.: Suture of facial nerve after injury at base of skull: Method of gaining exposure and slack by resection of parotid gland; J. Neurosurg. 5:284, 1948.
25. White, J. C., Heroy, W. W., and Goodman, E. N.: Causalgia following gunshot injuries of nerves: Role of emotional stimuli and surgical cure through interruption of diencephalic efferent discharge by sympathectomy, Ann. Surg. 128: 161, 1948.
26. Woodhall, B., and Beebe, G. W.: *Peripheral Nerve Regeneration: A Follow-up Study of 3,656 World War II Injuries*, VA Medical Monograph (Washington, D.C.: Government Printing Office, 1956.)

48 | Peripheral Vascular Injuries

ASHBY C. MONCURE and R. CLEMENT DARLING

ARTERIAL INJURY

MAJOR ARTERIAL injury accompanying fracture may be manifested by immediate hemorrhage or by arterial insufficiency and eventual loss of function or limb. Arterial hemorrhage announces itself stridently and forces prompt and specific action on the part of the surgeon. Traumatic arterial insufficiency may be more subtle and may be unrecognized by the inattentive or uninformed physician.

This chapter is designed as a guide to recognition, understanding and treatment of vascular injuries. The discussion is based on the thesis that the therapeutic ideal of restoration of normal anatomy and function should be applied just as vigorously in the treatment of major arterial injury as in the treatment of fractures.

Natural History of Acute Arterial Occlusion

An understanding of the mechanisms and sequelae of acute arterial insufficiency is necessary for its intelligent treatment. After traumatic interruption of the major arterial supply to an extremity, a predictable sequence of events takes place: vasoconstriction, vasodilation and the development of collateral circulation. These 3 phases will be discussed in sequence.

VASOCONSTRICTION. – The body first responds with a spasm of the vessels of the affected part. This may be considered a protective mechanism against further hemorrhage. It is partially a reflex constriction, mediated through the sympathetic nervous system, and partly a traumatic arteriospasm intrinsic to the artery. During this phase of vasoconstriction the circulation of the extremities is most strikingly diminished.

VASODILATION. – After several hours, the second phase, vasodilation, takes place. This condition represents an effort on the part of the organism to increase the circulation to the part. The point of occlusion in the main artery is bypassed by means of flow through the maximally dilated collateral channels.

Nonoperative therapy in the early phases of acute arterial occlusion is directed at minimizing the duration of the vasoconstriction and encouraging the dilation of the collateral vessels. Hemorrhagic shock, pain and cold are all strong stimuli to vasoconstriction. Therefore, adequate blood replacement, comfort and warmth are important to the early termination of the constrictive phase. Sympathetic blocks will diminish the reflex component of the vasospasm but will not affect traumatic arteriospasm.

During the very unstable period of the circulatory readjustment, thrombosis is taking place in the occluded artery. If the patient is fortunate, this thrombosis will extend from the point of occlusion proximally and distally to the first significant branch of the artery. If he is unfortunate, the thrombus will extend farther, usually in a distal direction; it may occlude the major arterial tree to the part. The latter sequence will interrupt inflowing collateral branches and thwart the efforts of the body to restore circulation. The mobilization and reinforcement of blood-clotting mechanisms accompanying trauma encourage the thrombosis. Good collateral flow tends to limit it. The 2 factors of greatest practical consideration in the development of extending thrombus are slow blood flow and passage of time. These are within the control of the surgeon.

Surgical procedures performed on extremities with precarious circulation tend to reinaugurate the "spastic" phase and interfere with circulation. If the surgical procedure will, of itself, improve circulation, this disadvantage is overcome. Ill-considered operations may reverse the vasodilation and decrease collateral flow, resulting in further extension of thrombus.

DEVELOPMENT OF COLLATERAL CIRCULATION.—The third phase of gradual collateral hypertrophy begins following stabilization of thrombosis and vasodilation. The process takes place rapidly over a period of 4–6 months and then more slowly over a period of years. Collateral arteries parallel to the occlusion grow in response to the need for blood in the part and may, especially in the young patient, restore the circulation almost to normal. Usually this collateral circulation never develops a capacity for flow possessed by the original vessel. Residual arterial insufficiency may be apparent as easy fatigue, intermittent claudication, cold intolerance or greater susceptibility to the circulatory complications of old age and atherosclerosis.

Sequelae of Ischemia

When the initial ischemia is not too severe and distal thrombosis has not been extensive, the extremity survives the acute occlusion with only the functional impairments mentioned. Circulation may, however, be sufficiently impaired to result in ischemic death of tissue and gangrene. The likelihood of gangrene depends on the site of arterial occlusion. Table 48-1 correlates amputation with site of arterial trauma in battle injuries and emphasizes the importance of restoring arterial continuity in injuries of such major arteries as the common femoral and popliteal, especially when their bifurcations have been destroyed. Other factors, such as associated injury in the area of impaired circulation and associated arteriosclerosis, will affect limb survival in any given case.

The previously described sequence of vascular responses continues in the presence of gangrene. Dilatation of collateral circulation in this instance will reinforce doubtful circulation near the line of demarcation between the dead and living tissue. The adverse effect of early amputation on unstable circulation at the site of amputation must be kept in mind.

TABLE 48–1.—CORRELATION OF SITE OF INJURED VESSEL AND SUBSEQUENT ISCHEMIC LIMB LOSSES*

INJURED ARTERY	NO. CASES	AMPUTATION, %
Subclavian	21	28.6
Axillary	74	43.2
Brachial		
Above profunda	97	55.7
Below profunda	209	25.8
Radial	99	5.1
Ulnar	69	1.5
Radial and ulnar	28	39.3
Common iliac	13	53.8
External iliac	30	46.7
Internal iliac	1	0.0
Common femoral	106	81.1
Superficial femoral	177	54.8
Deep femoral	27	0.0
Popliteal	502	72.5
Anterior tibial	129	8.5
Posterior tibial	265	13.6
Anterior and posterior tibial	91	69.2

*Modified from DeBakey, M. E., and Simeone, F. A.: Battle injuries of the arteries in World War II, Ann. Surg. 123:534, 1946.

The level of skin demarcation and the level of muscle demarcation may be quite different. The nutrient arteries to muscle are frequently end-arteries, so occlusion may result in death of the entire muscle. Thus, at midthigh amputation after thrombosis of common and superficial femoral arteries, the entire anterior thigh musculature may be found necrotic beneath viable skin and subcutaneous tissue.

In certain instances ischemia may not be severe enough to cause massive death of all tissues but may just affect the more vulnerable tissues, such as nerve and muscle. In a similar manner, temporary circulatory arrest will injure the more vulnerable tissues. Muscle will suffer necrosis after 6–8 hours of arrested circulation. When necrosis is not extensive, patchy scarring with little interference with function will result. With extensive necrosis, a heavy dense contracting fibrous replacement of the muscle ensues. Death of peripheral nerve will occur after 12–24 hours of ischemia. Both sensory and motor deficits result. Regeneration of both of these components is likely to be incomplete. This combination of muscle necrosis and peripheral nerve injury may be seen in patients having surgical restoration of circulation after long periods of arrest secondary to trauma or embolus, or having circulation drastically reduced for long periods by tight plaster or displaced bone. Severe degrees of this injury are recognized as Volkmann's contracture (see Chapter 49).

Recognition of Major Arterial Injury

Prompt recognition of major vascular injury is essential to its successful treatment. Delay allows irreversible ischemic injury to take place and also encourages the propagation of intravascular thrombus. Loss of limb because of improper treatment is seen too frequently, and delay because of failure to determine the state of the arterial circulation is the most common fault.

It is easy to miss major vascular injury if the physician is not constantly alert to its possibility. Major degrees of extremity ischemia may be concealed by a general picture of shock and vasoconstriction. Extremities hidden in plaster casings and bandages may suffer serious circulatory impairment that will be missed by the incurious. It is, therefore, important to assess vascular injury in the initial examination of the patient and to continue to check circulation particularly through the early mobile phases of body readjustment to trauma.

Major arteries may suffer lacerations which demand repair but still may not have interruption of arterial flow or show evidence of arterial insufficiency. Such injuries are not always made apparent by hemorrhage. Thus, a penetrating injury of the popliteal space with laceration of the popliteal artery may bring the patient to the hospital in shock but produce no hematoma, loss of peripheral pulses or active bleeding at the time of admission. The nature of the injury should be suspected from the location of the wound and the evidence of past major blood loss and will be confirmed by exploration of the wound or hemorrhage on recovery from shock.

A closed fracture requiring a disproportionate amount of blood for correction of shock and showing excessive hematoma should be suspected of being associated with injury to a major blood vessel even if there is no loss of distal circulation. One can usually reconstruct the mechanism of injury to a major artery when the injury is from displaced bone ends or from the original trauma. Excessive bleeding from a fracture site is occasionally a manifestation of a specific blood dyscrasia. Therefore, bleeding time, clotting time, blood smear, prothrombin time, observation of clot for fibrinolytic activity and partial thromboplastin time should be a part of the work-up in such cases. When a bleeding defect is not present, prompt surgical exploration and repair of the vessel should be performed. Procrastination in these cases not only results in excessive blood loss and cumbersome hematoma but may lead to the development of false aneurysms or arteriovenous fistulas that will require surgery at a later date and under less favorable circumstances, owing to scarring and fibrosis. Restoration of normal arterial anatomy, either by suture repair or by arterial graft, should be the objective of surgery in false aneurysm or arteriovenous fistula, even when operation is carried out late.

Acute arterial insufficiency is seen after supracondylar elbow fractures, fractures and dislocations of the knee and femoral shaft fractures and secondary to swelling within tight circular casings on the extremities. It may, of course, accompany any injury to a major artery. When arterial insufficiency appears in a traumatized extremity, therapy should be active rather than expectant. The possibility of an external cause, such as a tight dressing of plaster or displaced bone, must first be ruled out or, if present, corrected. If circulation is not restored by these measures, obstruction of a major artery within the limb is likely and surgical exploration with correction of the defect is indicated. Such surgery is urgent and should not be deferred. Expectant therapy is allowable only when the insufficiency is very mild and when the injured vessel is small and so situated that it can be expected to have a good collateral circulation.

It is important to localize the point of obstruction well. There is danger of operating on the peripheral manifestation of a more proximal occlusion. More than 1 fruitless fasciotomy has been performed in a calf when the primary disorder was femoral artery occlusion from a fractured femoral shaft. The point of obstruction can usually be located by determining the level at which peripheral pulses disappear. Care must be taken to be sure the palpated pulse is synchronous with the patient's radial pulse; the examiner may be confused by feeling his own finger pulse. This should be checked by the use of an oscillometer. The most readily available is an aneroid blood-pressure manometer. The cuff is inflated to a point just below systolic pressure at various levels on the extremity to determine the presence or absence of a pulse. Arteriography by percutaneous injection of dye, such as Renografin, is easily done and frequently successful in delineating the point of arterial occlusion.

Exposing the vessel at the point of occlusion may reveal any 1 of a number of causes for the obstruction. It is most gratifying to find that, after correction for a tense hematoma in the fascial compartment of the artery or other extra-arterial pathology, good arterial flow is resumed. The surgeon may, however, find a segment of artery where pulsations stop or are greatly diminished. This may be reversible segmental arteriospasm without thrombosis, but it should be looked on with the greatest suspicion. More likely there is subintimal hematoma, thrombosis or other anatomic reason for the occlusion. If caused by arteriospasm, the occlusion will disappear with the external application of papaverine to the vessel. The commercially available 1-ml ampule containing 30 mg papaverine may be used. The wound must not be closed in the hope that the "spasm" will go away. Rather, a persistent lesion should be explored by arteriotomy and mobilization with primary repair or a graft should be carried out if the artery is injured and thrombosed.

There may be an obviously contused or lacerated segment. The contused vessel must be excised at least 1 cm beyond obvious contusion, because to leave traumatized endothelium is to invite thrombosis.

A lacerated artery may be repaired by careful suture, provided the laceration is a sharp one without associated contusion. This is unusual in civilian practice except in the instance of a knife wound, and the surgeon should never hesitate to resect questionable vessels and insert an appropriate graft.

Every fracture of an extremity should

be considered to have an associated vascular injury until proved otherwise. When the attending physician is in doubt, competent consultation must be sought promptly and without hesitation, before loss of the limb becomes inevitable. If adequate facilities for reconstructive surgery are not available or if the surgeon is inexperienced, it is preferable to ligate and divide an injured artery than to attempt repair or to put in an unsatisfactory graft. The patient should then be transferred to a hospital where adequate facilities and competent vascular surgeons are available.

Operative Techniques

Major arterial injury is an indication for surgical exploration. Again, it is essential that the surgeon be prepared to do reconstructive surgery. The goal is re-establishment of normal vascular anatomy.

A few technical considerations are important.

EXPOSURE.—Reconstructive vascular surgery is impossible without wide exposure of the injured vessels. Good exposure is obtained through conventional longitudinal incisions running parallel to the vessel and allowing extension for exposure of additional artery, if need be. These incisions should be made initially, without wasting time trying to work through the primary wound.

CONTROL OF BLEEDING.—With good exposure, control of vessels proximal and distal to the injury is easy. Bad exposure, however, creates conditions incompatible with good technique. Pressure applied by the assistant, both proximal and distal to the source of bleeding, will allow the surgeon to expose blood vessels calmly and adequately, instead of blindly clamping at the bleeding source, which may do serious damage both to the artery and to the concomitant vein.

Care must be taken in temporarily occluding vessels not to injure them. Arteriosclerotic vessels are particularly vulnerable because the fragile atheromatous layer is easily split. Serrated clamps, good for normal vessels, may damage heavy atheromatous vessels. Bulldog clamps with weak springs will not injure such vessels. A modified Bethune lung tourniquet clamp or a Crafoord clamp is good for control of very large vessels, such as the aorta. Special instruments are not essential, however. Excellent atraumatic control can be secured by means of a tape that is passed beneath the vessel, drawn tight and clamped (Fig. 48-1).

BLOOD VESSEL SUTURE.—Two general principles are of great importance in blood vessel suture.

1. Intact, uninjured endothelium must be presented to the blood stream to avoid thrombosis. Injured tissue in contact with the blood stream will cause the formation of thrombus. For this reason, great care should be taken not to abrade or pinch the endothelium with forceps during blood vessel suture. Cut edges of the blood vessel must be everted to keep the injured tissue from the blood stream.

2. The suture line must not compromise the lumen of the artery, since this will slow the flow of blood, which in turn encourages thrombosis. To avoid such damage requires the careful placement of fine stitches not more than 1 mm from the edge of the vessel and the use of atraumatic needles and fine suture material, 5-0 to 6-0. Care must be taken in the placement and tying of sutures so as to avoid "puckering up" of a vessel on the suture, thus narrowing it.

Contrary to previous teachings, extensive excision of adventitia at the site of a vascular suture line is unnecessary and actually injurious because it seriously disturbs the circulation of the vessel wall. This is especially true with sclerotic vessels, where the adventitia is important to the vessel strength. Rupture of the artery formerly was a common complication of periarterial sympathectomy when adventitia was extensively excised.

If major vessels must be divided, clo-

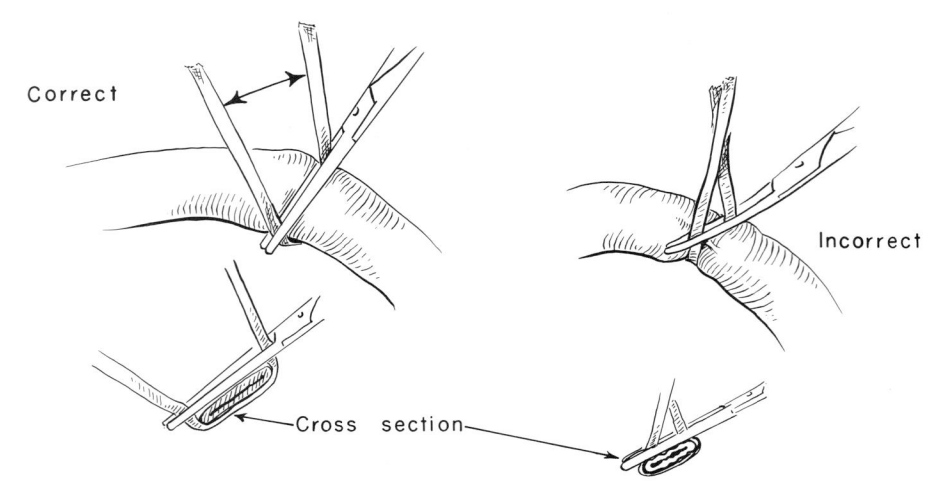

Fig. 48-1.—Atraumatic control of major artery without the use of special instruments; a shoelace and a hemostat are shown here.

sure by suturing the ends is preferable to use of a ligature, (1) because suturing does not require the generous cuff that ligation does, and consequently is not so wasteful of important vessel length and collateral branches, and (2) because this more secure method avoids the possibility of secondary hemorrhage due to slough of the vessel at the site of ligature or cutting through or breakage of a ligature. Suture closure of an artery should be performed next to a branch (Fig. 48-2). An arterial laceration is closed with a running everting suture through the full thickness of the vessel wall.

In a normal elastic artery, anastomosis can be performed by a modification of the original Carrel technique. Everting mattress stay sutures are placed first. Traction is maintained on the stay sutures to stretch the margin of the vessel during the placement of the running suture between them in order to keep them from narrowing the lumen. The running suture can be an over-and-over Carrel stitch or a running everting mattress suture, depending on the preference of the surgeon and the ease with which the vessel edges evert. Rigid atheromatous arteries smaller than the common iliac are best anastomosed with interrupted everting mattress sutures (Fig. 48-3). The more difficult sutures in the atheroma are placed first.

Fig. 48-2.—Suture closure of a major artery next to a branch avoids possible necrosis distal to a ligature and formation of a thrombus in the blind segment.

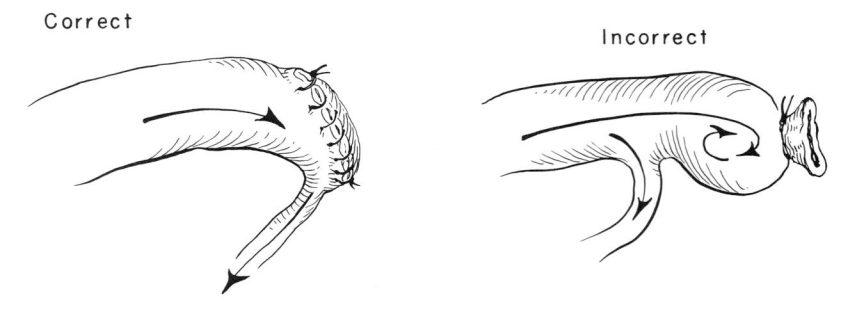

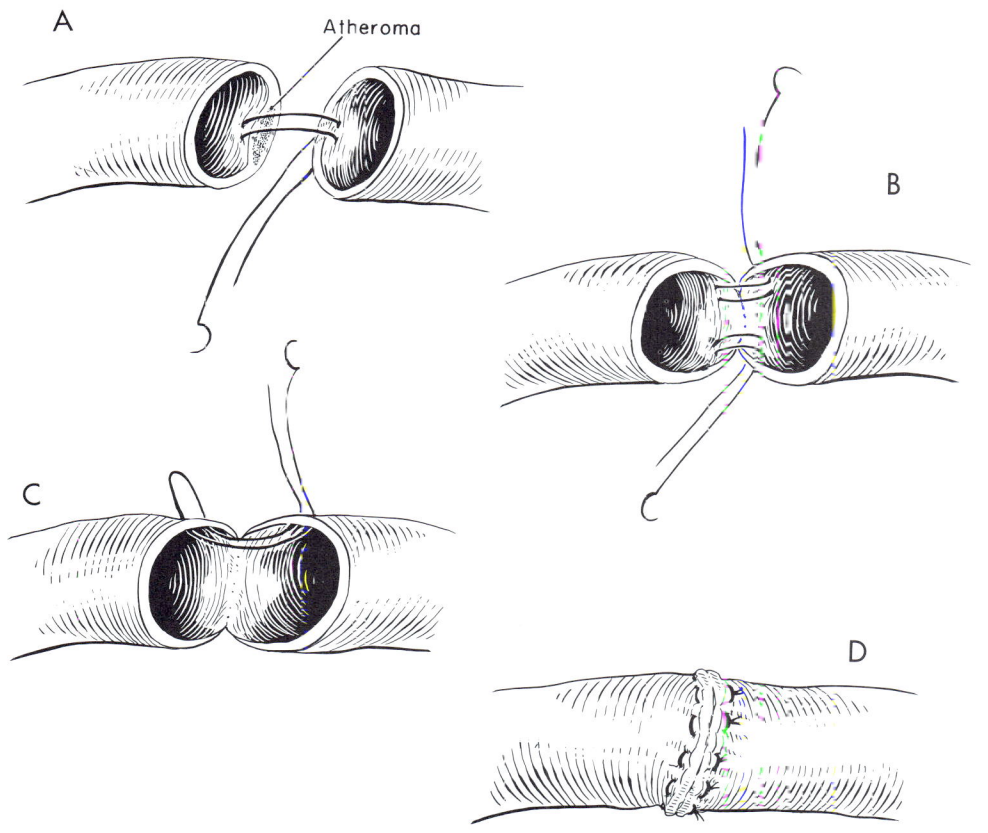

Fig. 48-3.—End-to-end anastomosis in a rigid arteriosclerotic vessel is accomplished with interrupted everting mattress sutures, placed first in the more rigid portions of the vessel.

In small arteries, when there is sufficient length, as in some simple transections and in all grafts, an oblique anastomosis (Fig. 48-4) is preferable to the standard end-to-end suture. This is a quick and simple method and avoids constriction of the suture line that is the primary reason for failure.

A gentle and meticulous technique with complete control of all bleeding points is necessary for good results. Hematomas favor sepsis and also result in necrosis of the grafts.

GRAFTS.—Within the past 15 years reconstructive arterial surgery has come of age with the development of durable suture materials, the construction of porous prosthetic tubes with materials that will allow tissue ingrowth (thus obviating the problems of procurement, sterilization, preservation and late failures formerly present with the use of arterial homografts) and the realization that autografts, such as the reversed saphenous vein, can be used with a high degree of success in small vessel defects and in areas traversing natural creases. With adequate inflow and an open distal arterial tree, demonstrated by brisk back-bleeding or by direct assessment by backing out an inflated embolectomy balloon catheter (after Fogarty), technical errors at the proximal and distal anastomotic sites would seem to be the most frequent cause of graft failure from thrombosis.

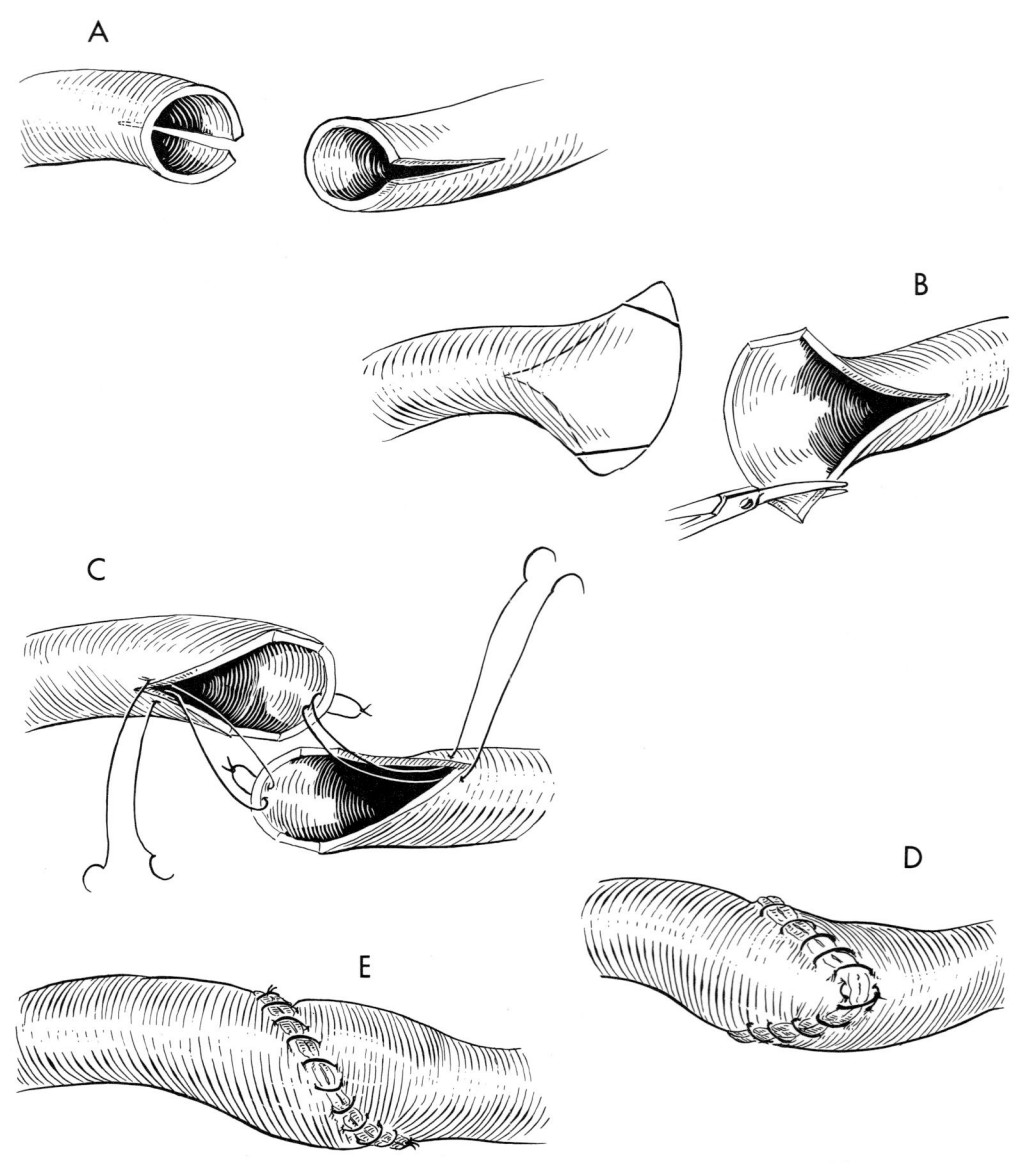

Fig. 48-4.—When there is sufficient vessel length, as with a graft, the oblique anastomosis shown here is preferred.

The reversed saphenous vein, when interposed as a substitute in arterial defects, has the advantages that viable autogenous tissue should have over prosthetic materials, i.e., relative resistance to sepsis and the ability to angulate at body creases without compromise of the lumen by kinking. Thus, use of the saphenous vein, in the setting of trauma, should be considered when a deficit in arterial length cannot be overcome by isolating the dividing tethering branches proximally and distally. Including the groin and the upper thigh in the sterile field will facilitate its harvest. On delivery of the saphenous vein from the leg, it should be inflated with heparin-saline solution and all side branches securely ligated with fine nonabsorbable suture material. The distal end should be marked to allow the surgeon to determine accurately at any time the positioning of the vein in the reversed state. A longitudinal marking suture should be run through the adventitia the length of the vein to obviate twisting the graft when the proximal anastomosis is carried out. Anastomosis should be accomplished meticulously, with fine, permanent suture materials. The cut edges of the graft and artery are everted and the suture interrupted at several points to avoiding a pursestring effect. Points of temporary occlusion with vascular clamps immediately proximal and distal to anastomoses should be probed before completion of the suture line to be sure the vessel has not been crushed or constricted by the clamp.

If a suitable saphenous vein is not available, the use of ultralight-weight, knitted Dacron grafts should be considered, taking care to "preclot" the prosthetic tube before its placement.

Administration of antibiotics having a bactericidal effect against both gram-positive and gram-negative organisms should supplement debridement of nonviable tissue and meticulous hemostasis to aid in preventing infections. Adequately reconstructed vessels should not require the use of anticoagulants postoperatively to maintain their patency, but dilute heparin (1,000 units/100 ml saline solution) should be injected intra-arterially beyond each of the controlling clamps during the procedure in order to avoid thrombosis and air embolus.

In the situation in which tissue injury is of such magnitude or contamination of such degree that sepsis is quite likely, a vein autograft or prosthetic graft may be brought through a clean area and anastomosed proximally and distally to normal vessel, thereby bypassing the suspect area. This tactic may allow restoration of vascular continuity in that special circumstance in which direct primary repair or graft interposition will lie in a less than optimal bed of tissue.

DISTAL THROMBOSIS. — As the interval between the initial arterial occlusion and operation approaches 12 hours, clot propagation down the vessel becomes an increasingly serious problem. After this period of time, some degree of distal thrombosis is the rule. Distal thrombosis probably accounts for the majority of failures in arterial embolectomy and is most familiar to surgeons in this connection.

Removal of a distal thrombus is essential to the success of any procedure to reestablish arterial flow, since distal obstruction to flow would result in rapid thrombosis at the site of a proximal repair, arteriotomy or graft. It is possible to remove even an extensive distal thrombus and every effort should be made to do so.

The Fogarty embolectomy catheter of appropriate size should be passed gently proximally and distally through the arteriotomy (Fig. 48-5). When it can be advanced no further the balloon should be inflated with sterile injectable saline until slight resistance is met when withdrawing the catheter. This tension forcing the balloon against arterial wall should be maintained by adjusting the volume of saline in the balloon as the catheter is withdrawn, thus extricating the thrombus. This maneuver should be repeated until the surgeon is reasonably certain the arterial tree is cleared of thrombus and brisk back-bleeding is restored. Inspection of extricated thrombus may reveal a cast of the distal arterial tree and allow the surgeon to assess the success of the maneuver.

If the catheter cannot be passed beyond the distal bifurcation of the vessel, such as the popliteal or brachial bifurcation, a separate incision should be made at this level and the vessel isolated just above its bifurcation. Thereafter, a trans-

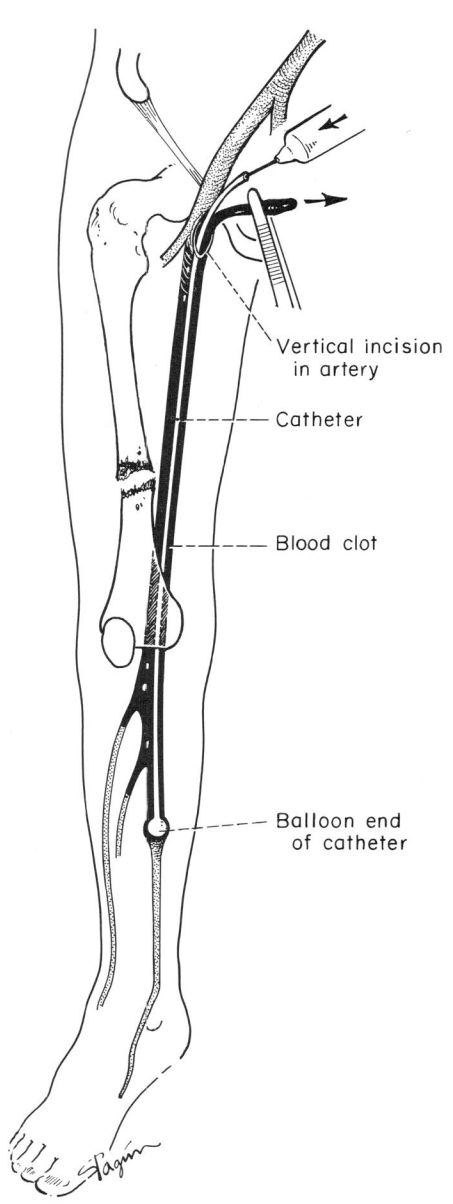

Fig. 48-5.—Thrombectomy, accomplished by backing out an inflated Fogarty embolectomy catheter, is mandatory on exploration of an artery when back-bleeding is not brisk.

verse arteriotomy with passage of the embolectomy catheter down either distal vessel may be carried out. Arteriograms subsequently may show profound spasm of the arterial tree, and restoration of the distal pulses may only be appreciated some hours after thrombectomy.

SEPSIS AND SECONDARY HEMORRHAGE.—Sepsis involving the ligature of a major vessel was a familiar and much feared complication of amputation in the days before asepsis, but for a long time it has been so uncommon in civilian surgery as to be almost forgotten. With the great increase in the number of operations involving arterial grafts, sepsis and major secondary hemorrhage have again become, on occasion, a matter of great concern.

Tissue devoid of circulation is helpless in the presence of infection. Once a graft is infected, rupture and hemorrhage from the suture line are almost inevitable. Such weakness is intrinsic in a vascular graft, a fact which stresses the importance of rigid aseptic technique.

Certain avoidable practices weaken the resistance of a vessel to infection and may increase the likelihood of secondary hemorrhage if sepsis should occur. The arterial ligature devascularizes tissue beyond the tie. Stripping adventitia destroys the vasa vasorum. An arterial suture line placed too tightly compromises the circulation of the vessel wall and major hemorrhage may result.

Secondary hemorrhage usually occurs from 1 ro 2 weeks postoperatively. Control of major secondary hemorrhage poses a formidable problem. The surest method of control is proximal ligation of the artery through a new incision and a clean field, with division of the artery at the point of ligation. Thereafter, a vein autograft or prosthetic graft may be brought through a clean area and anastomosed proximally and distally to normal vessel, thereby bypassing the area of hemorrhage. If this is not possible or if the patient is not in a condition to tolerate it, control of the hemorrhage at the source may be attempted. If control is attempted through the septic field at the site of the hemorrhage, any involved graft must be excised and the artery must be closed with fine sutures placed with minimal tension and great care so as not to strangulate tissue. When secondary hemorrhage occurs from the side wall of the artery, the vessel should be divided and the ends sutured. This arterial suture line should be isolated from the body of the wound by covering it with a flap of well-vascularized tissue, and the body of the wound should be drained. Appropriate antibiotics, confirmed by sensitivity testing, should be used.

ANTICOAGULANTS.—At the time of surgery, after wound hemostasis has been secured, local intravascular injection of dilute heparin solution, as described above, is useful. Systemic use of anticoagulants in the postoperative period, however, is contraindicated because of the frequency of major hemorrhagic complications. If good flow is obtained through vessels properly sutured and untraumatized, thrombosis will not occur. If there is poor flow through an improperly performed anastomosis or a traumatized vessel, thrombosis will be inevitable—whether or not anticoagulants are used.

SYMPATHETIC BLOCKS.—Paravertebral sympathetic blocks with procaine or similar drugs may be used in the therapy of acute ischemia, but should never be persisted in as a definitive treatment. Blocks should always be considered ancillary to restoration of normal vascular anatomy.

VENOUS INJURY

Although restoration of arterial function is a primary concern after trauma to an extremity, the consequences of venous injury, direct or indirect, must not be overlooked. The effect may be due to local damage, or it may be of a more general nature, as a result of the hypotension accompanying the shock of injury.

In general, local repair of the lacerated vein should not be attempted, because thrombosis at the site of the injury is likely to develop. The vena cava and the larger vessels of the neck, axilla and pelvis provide an exception to this principle, because in these areas the channel is large and blood flow from divergent

Fig. 48-6.—Method of application of a serrated vena caval clip immediately below the renal veins. Excellent exposure is provided by approaching the vessel retoperitoneally through the bed of the resected right twelfth rib.

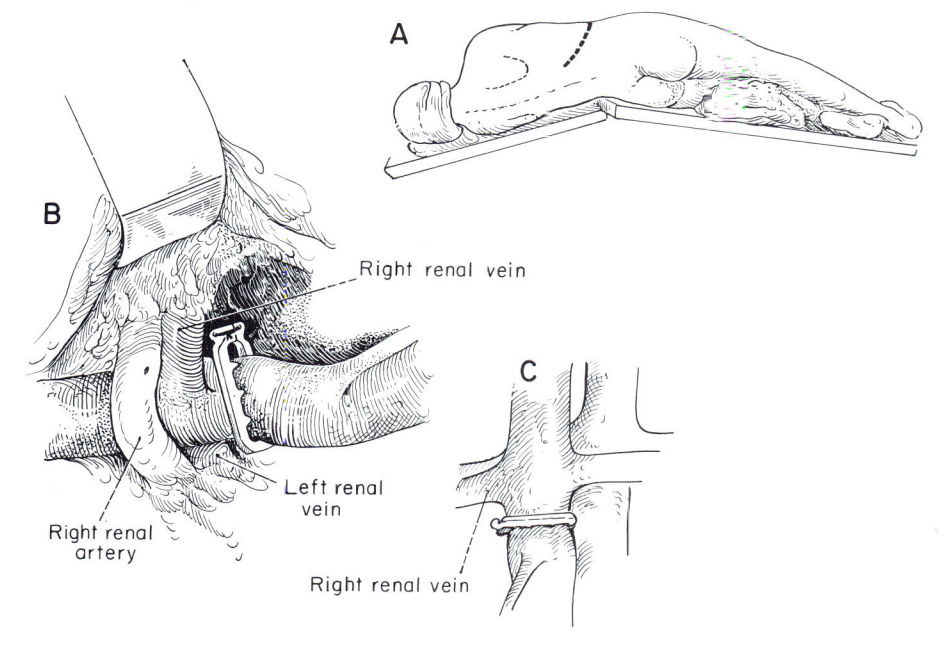

sources is present. The increased likelihood of thrombosis in a vein requires that the repair be performed with scrupulous attention to the previously mentioned principles of blood vessel suture. All the smaller veins of the extremities themselves can be ligated with little serious disturbance of limb circulation, and even the inferior vena cava below the renal veins can be interrupted if its repair is impossible. Distal venous stasis and edema secondary to interruption can be controlled by elevation and elastic support.

By far the most important venous disorder associated with trauma is venous thrombosis with secondary embolism. Most injuries of any degree provide 2 of the prime prerequisites for thrombus formation—slowing of the blood flow, and roughening of an area of venous intima somewhere in the body. Although many emboli find their origin from venous thrombi at the site of injury itself, it has been well demonstrated that thrombi may develop in veins distant from the site of trauma. The most common location for such spontaneous venous thrombosis is in the deep veins of the legs, where it may produce the familiar clinical entity of thrombophlebitis. Not infrequently it occurs also in the veins of the pelvis, in which case clinical signs are absent.

Fig. 48-7.—In established thromboembolic disease, when systemic anticoagulation is contraindicated and inferior vena caval interruption cannot be safely accomplished, bilateral interruption of the common femoral veins below the saphenofemoral junction should be carried out.

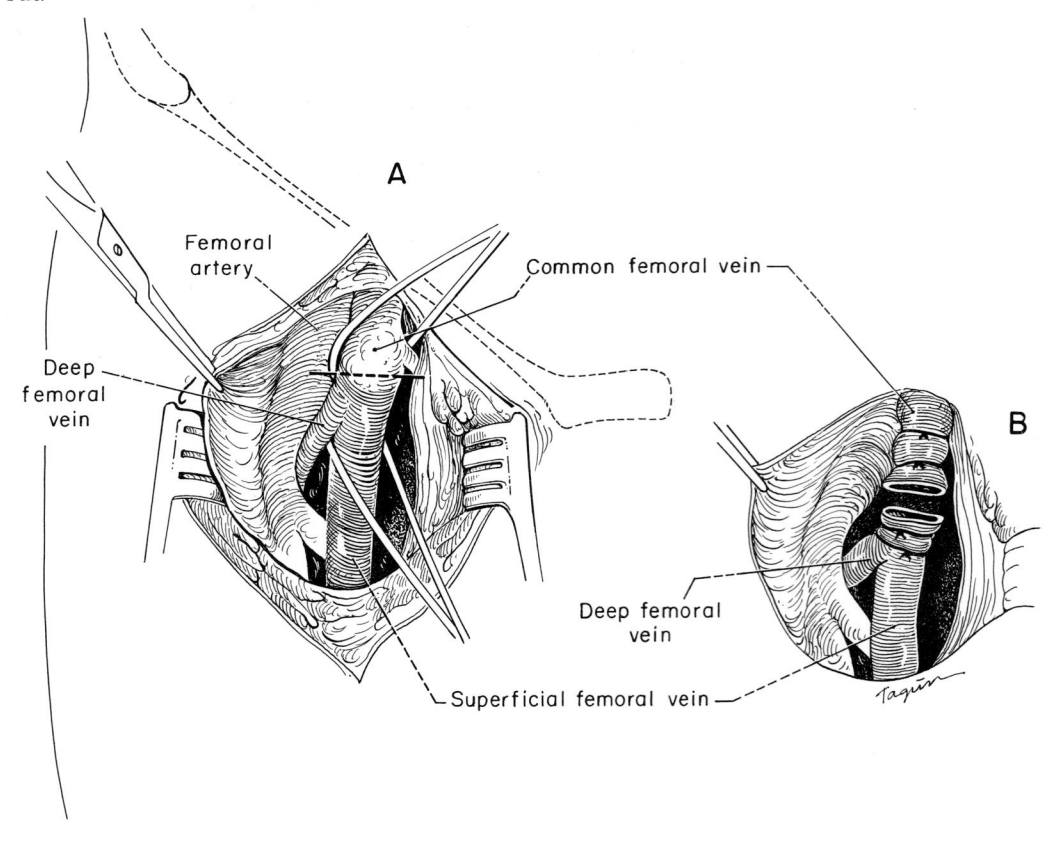

The diagnosis of deep vein thrombosis and pulmonary embolism in the injured is often difficult. Local signs may be lacking or may be obscured by casts, traction or other forms of therapy to the injured part. Pleuritic pain or hemoptysis is most difficult to assess in the presence of a chest wall or lung injury. In the elderly immobilized patient particularly, venous thrombosis must ever be suspected, and any patient exhibiting an unexplained simultaneous elevation in temperature pulse and respiratory rate should be regarded with concern.

It becomes obvious that measures aimed at preventing peripheral thrombosis are of special value in the injured. Restoration of blood volume and blood pressure by proper replacement is a first essential. Movement in bed, both active and passive, should be encouraged. Patients should become ambulatory as soon as possible. Compression support to the lower extremities may be of value. Prophylactic anticoagulants may be helpful, but in traumatic injuries are frequently contraindicated for obvious reasons.

In the event of a recognizable thrombophlebitis or a sublethal pulmonary embolus, systemic anticoagulation should be initiated with heparin, if not contraindicated, and the activity of the heparin should be monitored with sequential determination of partial thromboplastin time. In the event that anticoagulation is contraindicated for major reasons and the presence of pulmonary embolus is unequivocally documented by pulmonary angiogram, interruption of the inferior vena cava just below the renal veins

Fig. 48-8.—Iliofemoral venous thrombotic occlusion is best managed by evacuation of the proximal venous system with an embolectomy catheter and interruption of the common femoral vein.

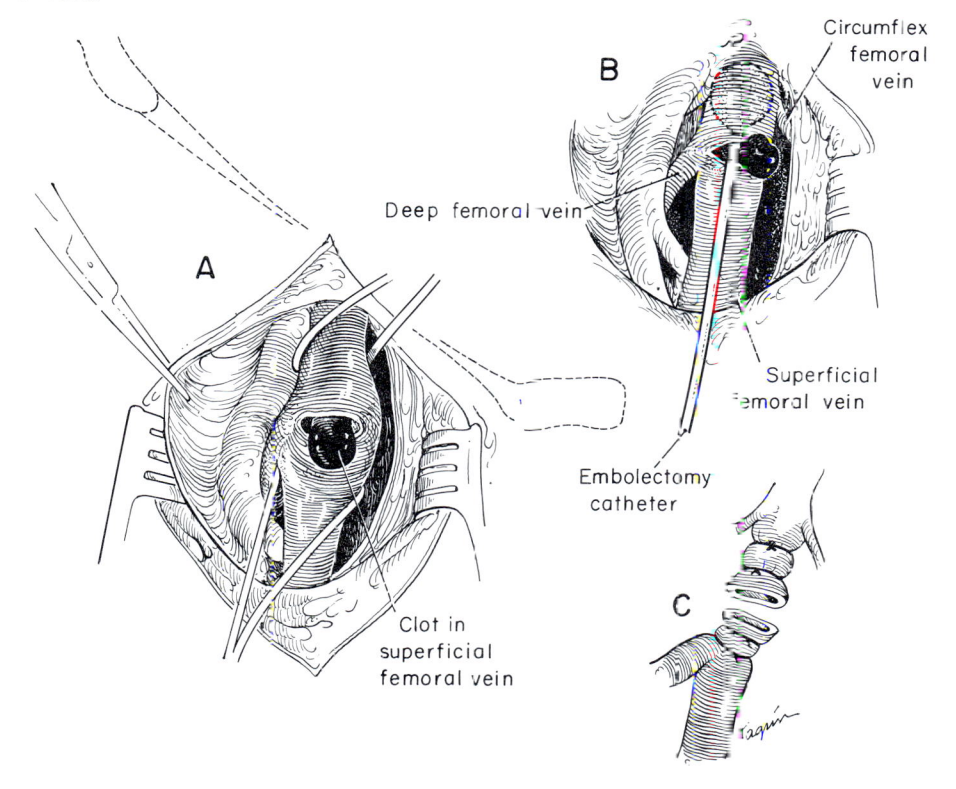

should be undertaken (Fig. 48-6). If it is felt that the patient cannot tolerate this procedure, interruption of the common femoral vein bilaterally in the groin under local anesthesia should be carried out (Fig. 48-7). The common femoral vein should be interrupted flush with a major branch proximally and should be interrupted below the saphenofemoral junction.

The patient with phlebitis and edema rising above the knee can be presumed to have iliac vein thrombosis. If seen within 48 hours of the beginning of thigh and groin edema, the iliac venous system may be evacuated with the use of a Fogarty embolectomy catheter, and common femoral vein interruption performed (Fig. 48-8). After this period, the thrombus becomes too adherent to remove and systemic anticoagulation with heparin, if not contraindicated, should be initiated.

In summary, traumatic arterial injury will be manifested by either bleeding or arterial insufficiency. Prompt recognition and treatment are essential in both conditions. Modern techniques of vascular surgery allow the primary mechanical defect to be corrected in almost all cases. The goal of therapy should always be the restoration of normal vascular anatomy.

Clean lacerations of the great veins may be repaired. In general, injuries to veins of the extremities should be treated by ligation next to a major branch because of the danger of thrombosis and embolization. Systemic anticoagulation is the initial treatment of choice in established thromboembolic disease unless specifically contraindicated. In the latter instance, or where failure has been documented by pulmonary angiography, interruption of the inferior vena cava or, if not possible, of the common femoral veins bilaterally, should be carried out.

BIBLIOGRAPHY

Darling, R. C.: Peripheral arterial surgery, N. Engl. J. Med. 280:26, 84, 141, 1969.

Hershey, F. B., and Calman, C. H.: *Atlas of Vascular Surgery* (2d ed.; St. Louis: C. V. Mosby Company, 1967).

Levin, P. M., Rich, N. M., and Hulton, J. E.: Collateral circulation in arterial injuries, Arch. Surg. 102:392, 1971.

Strandness, D. E.: *Collateral Circulation in Clinical Surgery* (Philadelphia: W. B. Saunders Company, 1969).

49 | Volkmann's Contracture
WILLIAM C. QUINBY, JR.

VOLKMANN'S CONTRACTURE of muscle is a clinical tragedy. No matter how expertly a fracture is treated, the beneficial effects are nullified if muscle contracture develops. The preceding chapter gives detailed consideration to the management of blood vessel injuries, which frequently are the basis for muscle ischemia. It is fitting to add a clinical consideration of Volkmann's syndrome and a review of our present knowledge of the processes that produce it.

NATURE OF THE PROCESS

Classic Volkmann's ischemic contracture is the result of infarction of the muscles of the forearm subsequent to fractures of the elbow, humerus or forearm bones. The major involvement is of the flexor muscles. It has become a vanishing clinical entity since Volkmann[39] and Leser[26] emphasized its relationship to impaired circulation. The fundamentally ischemic cause of the process is now accepted, and the histologic picture of muscle infarction has been established as the ultimate criterion for diagnosis. A similar process has been shown to involve the leg muscles subsequent to injuries of the femur, knee or tibia; and ischemic changes of the intrinsic muscles of the hand have been described.

Evidence of damage to nerves of the extremities is frequently part of Volkmann's syndrome — so much so, that the muscular changes were originally thought to be secondary to denervation alone. Three lines of observation, however, have shown that denervation is not the cause: (1) histologically the degeneration of muscle which follows denervation is a diffuse fibrosis rather than an infarction; (2) Volkmann's contracture may occur without demonstrable damage to nerves; and (3) characteristic lesions of nerves are produced by the same ischemic processes that cause muscle infarction. The current concept, then, is that ischemia is the cause of the lesions of muscle and nerve and that such ischemia is not sufficiently complete to cause gangrene of all tissues but selectively affects those having a special structure and metabolism most sensitive to circulatory impairment.

The infarcted muscle usually becomes a sterile sequestrum surrounded by fibrous tissue that cannot be penetrated by peripheral regenerating muscle fibers. The sequestrum may ultimately calcify or become infected, but most commonly it is slowly replaced by dense scar, with fibrotic atrophy and complete fixation of the forearm structures contiguous to it. The characteristic clawhand, with stiffening of the small joints, is due partly to contracture in the forearm and partly to disuse. When nerves are also damaged, the sensory loss and further degenerative processes of muscle render the extremity painful and useless

It has been difficult to produce the Volkmann process in experimental animals. The laboratory evidence which exists, however, forms the basis for preventive treatment.

MECHANISMS OF ISCHEMIA

EDEMA.—On theoretical grounds, ischemia of tissue cells occurs whenever stasis sufficient to interfere with exchange of oxygen and cellular metabolites is found. It follows that edema and extravasation of blood *in a confined space* will produce a progressive ischemia with impairment of capillary, venous and arterial circulations as pressure increases. The tissue ischemia of edema is illustrated clinically in instances of tight bandages, casings or splints applied to extremities. The pressure that may exist in a confined space following injury is obvious when the fascia is split over such spaces as the flexor muscle compartment of the forearm or the anterior tibial or gastrocnemius compartments of the leg. The fascial confinement of muscle is favorable to the production of ischemia of edematous origin.

VENOUS AND LYMPHATIC OBSTRUCTION.—Acute venous obstruction causes a transient ischemia by blocking the outflow of blood from an extremity. By rapid dilatation, the collateral venous pathways are sufficient to provide adequate flow centrally unless most of the major veins are obstructed completely and simultaneously. However, before the collateral channels can dilate effectively, sudden extensive venous obstruction may cause an ischemia sufficient to damage muscle. Lymphatic obstruction has a similar effect, but to a milder degree. When venous and lymphatic obstruction occur together, the edema is intensified and the degree of ischemia is augmented. It is often difficult to distinguish between the 2 components, but there is much evidence that acute venous obstruction by this mechanism may be a significant factor in the development of Volkmann's contracture.

The acute mechanism is distinguished from chronic or partial venous or lymphatic obstruction, wherein the effects of stasis are greatest in the skin and subcutaneous tissues and only manifested as cramps and fatigue by the muscles.

ARTERIAL OBSTRUCTION.—As stated in Chapter 48, the susceptibility of tissues to infarction appears to depend on the pattern of arterial supply and on the metabolic demands of the specific tissue. Anatomic studies of the forearm and lower leg muscles show that such areas are susceptible to infarction in the event of damage to a single major artery. However, experimentally it is difficult to produce a pure muscle infarct by isolated arterial ligation. The results are either (1) transient, with rapid recovery, or (2) total, producing gangrene of all tissues distal to the ligation. Concomitant tourniquets and muscle incisions bear little relationship to the clinical Volkmann's syndrome, but Brooks[5] produced infarction and contracture in dogs by venous ligation in conjunction with arterial obstruction of varying duration. Indeed, his work threw the weight of conviction toward venous obstruction as the special determining feature of Volkmann's contracture.

TRAUMATIC VASOSPASM.—Recent understanding of the physiologic behavior of arteries has emphasized that arterior vasospasm which involves the major artery *and its collaterals* is an outstanding component of the initial phase of most ischemic contractures. The 2 vasospastic patterns which have been demonstrated are discussed in the preceding chapter. Resection of a segment of damaged artery will interrupt the starting point of either mechanism, whereas procaine injections of the sympathetic nerves will affect the spinal reflex mechanism alone. There is little doubt that reflex or intrinsic arterial vasospasm is the chief determinant of the varied circumstances under which Volkmann's contracture develops. Awareness of occult mechanisms such as intramural arterial hematoma or perivascular processes that cause spasm will display a proximate cause for muscle ischemia in most cases.

THROMBOSIS.—Thrombosis of arteries or veins with propagation of the clot is not a conspicuous feature of Volkmann's syndrome in the acute phase. Extensive thrombosis is more commonly associated with frank gangrene. Histologic study of the small vessels has shown some stasis and clumping of cells in the venules but no widespread thrombosis. However, in any vascular injury the possibility of thrombosis as an exceptional factor must not be neglected.

ALTERED MUSCLE METABOLISM.—The usual greenish color of the muscle infarct and the sterile inflammatory process that accompanies it have stimulated a review of studies on muscle regeneration and the chemical changes that follow ischemia. After simple injury, new muscle buds from each side of the damaged area show strong tendencies to bridge small gaps and to re-establish continuity of the fiber. The success of regeneration appears to depend on the viability of the sarcolemmal sheath and nuclei. By contrast, the muscle infarct contains no viable cells and incites a peripheral inflammatory and fibrous reaction which cannot be penetrated by new muscle buds. In mild forms the infarctions may be spotty through a muscle belly, with sufficient viable areas between to permit recovery of function; but the massive infarct is surrounded by an inflammatory and fibrous reaction before muscle regeneration becomes active. Although chemical studies of normal muscle metabolism and changes following ischemia have been reported, there is little information regarding the constitution of infarcted muscle. The irritative feature, the hardness of the muscle and the rapid contracture have been compared to rigor mortis and contrasted with the flaccidity of muscle in a gangrenous extremity. There is a need for greater understanding of the chemical processes involved.

RECOGNITION OF IMPENDING VOLKMANN'S CONTRACTURE

Although current knowledge may be incomplete, it is advisable to place the preventive management of impending Volkmann's contracture within the reach of all surgeons. Constant suspicion, early recognition and active therapy directed against the mechanisms outlined in the preceding section form the basis for successful care.

Clinical Features

Volkmann's contracture most frequently follows supracondylar fracture of the humerus in children. The characteristic displacement of bone angulates the brachial artery against the upper fragment and may damage the artery's wall. The artery may be caught between the fragments or ruptured. The fascia of the biceps muscle spreads to form a tight roof to the antecubital space, and most of the venous and lymphatic channels of the forearm cross the space anteriorly. After reduction, the position of fragments is best maintained by flexion of the elbow and plaster splints. All of the initiating components of ischemia are present in some degree: arterial injury with diffuse reflex vasospasm, venous obstruction and local swelling in a confined space, further confined by the position of flexion and by pressure externally applied.

The earliest clinical signs of impending Volkmann's contracture in the hand are those of impaired circulation. There is pallor, coldness and evidence of ischemia beneath the fingernails, followed by swelling. The radial pulse is usually absent, although a pulse has been demonstrable in a few patients in whom the contracture developed later. The clinical signs are rapidly progressive. Muscle ischemia first becomes apparent by an inability to extend the fingers actively and by resistance to passive extension. Severe pain usually accompanies the syndrome, particularly if the muscles are put under tension. If there is also damage to the nerves, however, pain may be virtually absent. With some exceptions, the quartet of "pain, pallor, pulselessness and paralysis" are cardinal signs of trouble, and perhaps "pressure" within the tissues should be added. When neglected, the process runs an increasingly severe course for a few days, after which there may be some return of the radial pulse and apparent improvement in the circulatory status of the hand. But the damage to muscles has been done, and the progressive fixation and contracture continue. Ultimately the fingers can only be extended when the wrist is flexed, the forearm tissues are hard and wasted, and the skin of the hand is thin and atrophic. There may eventually be almost complete regeneration of nerves, but paresthesias and hypersensitivity often persist.

Volkmann's contracture also occurs following fractures of both bones of the forearm or around the elbow joint. The clinical features are the same. It is worth remembering that external injury in the absence of fracture has caused some cases and that *any* series of events which sets off the mechanisms of ischemia is essentially dangerous.

The same sequence of events applies to the lower leg. The femoral and popliteal arteries are even more essential to the viability of the lower leg than the brachial artery is to the arm. Injury to the anterior tibial artery may produce selective necrosis of the muscles of the anterior tibial compartment, and contractures that involve the gastrocnemius and produce a clawfoot are more disabling. In fracture of the femur, the site of arterial injury may be in the thigh and the signs of ischemia may be evident only in the calf. Contractures are reported less frequently in the leg than in the arm, either because total ischemia with gangrene is more prevalent or because the ultimate disability is not so dramatic. Reports of ischemic necrosis of the flexor sublimis following injury to the hand without fracture demonstrate the occult nature of the rare case.

Minor degrees of ischemia probably occur more often than is recognized. There is no certain way to determine the degree of ischemia compatible with recovery of function. Onset may be during manipulative reduction rather than at the time of fracture or may be a few days after injury. Experienced surgeons have had the process develop under their eyes when they thought the danger period had passed. Injured patients, particularly children, are unable to give adequate subjective warning through their symptoms. The physician must make the observations and act on them with conviction if tragedy is to be avoided.

Identification of Impending Contracture

Suspicion that ischemic contracture may develop is based on repeated clinical examinations. The initial examination is the most important and must include evaluation of the following.

1. The over-all circulatory status of the patient.
2. The type of injury to the extremity, using roentgenograms when appropriate.
3. The circulatory status of the injured extremity compared with that of the contralateral one.
4. The presence or absence of accompanying neurologic deficit.

The color, temperature, nailbed circulation, edema, venous engorgement, sensation and active and passive motion of the fingers or toes must be observed and recorded. The radial and ulnar pulses must be palpated and compared. Oscillometry may be useful. The same examinations should be made after each manipulation or change in position of the extremity, and frequent (at least hourly) recording of finger-tip color and function and of the radial pulse should be made for 48 hours after definitive therapy of the injury. The state of the peripheral circulation is more significant than the presence or absence of a palpable radial pulse. Pain in the extremity out of proportion to that reasonably attributable to the injury is an important sign.

Angiography is generally avoided, since added vasospasm may accompany its use and the results may tend to confuse decisions.

MANAGEMENT OF IMPENDING CONTRACTURE

REDUCTION OF THE FRACTURE. — If the foregoing signs of ischemia are noted and if the bone is broken, the fracture should be reduced by manipulation. Griffiths[16] states that many contractures follow manipulative reduction; however, others believe that reduction often releases an artery that is impinged by one of the fragments. In either case, if ischemia begins or persists, all external pressure is removed and the extremity is placed in a position of partial extension and elevation. Repeated manipulations are inadvisable if the first one is thorough.

NONOPERATIVE MEASURES AGAINST VASOSPASM. — Papaverine is used to relax the spastic muscle of the arterial wall. It may be administered intravenously, but it does not appear to have more than temporary value. Procaine block of the sympathetic ganglia has occasionally relieved the ischemia, but this also must be repeated for sustained effect. Both types of treatment often have temporary and confusing effects. Their danger is that more active treatment will be unduly postponed. Unless the return of a good circulation is prompt, unequivocal and sustained through 48 hours, operation should be undertaken directly. Severe ischemia has produced irreversible necrosis of muscle in 6–8 hours. Although operations done at longer intervals have been followed by good recovery, procrastination is unsafe.

Operative Management

The aims of operation are to release pressure in confined tissue compartments, to relieve venous obstruction, to relieve arterial obstruction and vasospasm and to identify gross injury to nerves.

Efforts to obtain accurate reduction of the fracture are of secondary importance and must be limited to those which clearly help the circulatory status. Since it is imperative to preserve all collateral circulation, internal fixation of the fracture must not entail additional dissection and generally should be avoided.

Past experience has shown that extensive splitting of the fascia over the muscle bellies and antecubital or popliteal spaces often relieves the ischemia. This maneuver releases pressure and minimizes the harmful effects of edema and venous obstruction. It is obvious that attempts to close such a wound primarily will reproduce pressure and ischemia. The deep fascia must not be closed and skin closure should be done only if there is no tension. In a few days, when the swelling has subsided, secondary skin closure may be done by grafting or in accordance with the principles of wound management developed in World War II.

Although the circulation may improve after splitting the fascia, the integrity of the arterial flow must be assured. In the preceding chapter the recognition and management of arterial injury and vasospasm are treated in detail, and the reader should study that material carefully. It is worth repeating that the arterial injury may be hard to find, that the surgeon must not rest until a good peripheral circulation is obtained and that present methods of direct repair or grafting are effective.

In the arm, recovery of the circulation after resection of the grossly damaged segment of the brachial artery has been good. When no gross arterial lesion is seen and no improvement follows exposure of the artery and application of heat or procaine, resection of the area where spasm begins has also proved successful. In the lower extremity, the use of an arterial graft should be considered much more seriously. Articles which deal specifically with impending Volkmann's syndrome do not include considerations of grafting or primary repair, but experience with war wounds and other forms of arterial insufficiency indicates that grafting is advisable after resection of a damaged segment in the lower extremity unless the peripheral circulation is excellent.

If gross damage to major nerves is identified, primary repair should not be attempted, since it is difficult to determine the extent of the injury. Three or 4 weeks later there will be accurate demarcation, and a complete resection with suture of all damaged nerves can be done. Ischemic lesions of nerves are not grossly identifiable, and they show a high degree of ultimate recovery. If careful study shows no evidence of regeneration after a month, exploration of the nerves should be done.

MANAGEMENT OF ESTABLISHED MUSCLE ISCHEMIA

Every doctor is concerned with the prevention of Volkmann's contracture. Unfortunately, recognition and therapy have occasionally been so delayed that large clinics continue to report established cases.

Established Case Seen Early

There is no way to determine accurately how much damage is done in the early stages of any given case. Therefore, even though pain, a swollen hard forearm, nerve deficit and inflexibility of the hand predict that muscle necrosis has occurred, it is best to operate up to 48 hours after onset. Experience with wounds and peripheral vascular disease indicates that unanticipated recovery of muscle may occur if good blood flow is re-established in the major arteries. Operation may be harmful in cases of mild ischemia, but in the severe extensive case, there is little to be lost and possibly much to be gained.

Operations done 3 days or more after onset have not been successful. Because an extensive infarct ultimately fixes the adjacent tissues together, it is tempting to excise in order to reduce the eventual restricting scar to a minimum.

There is no rule that applies universally. It is difficult to gauge the extent of necrosis and to predict the ultimate regeneration with accuracy, and the dangers of introduction of infection or reinauguration of ischemic mechanisms are real. Unless nerve involvement is progressive, it is probably best to use measures designed to minimize contracture and maintain maximal function of joints. Such measures consist of exercises, physiotherapy, external splints and traction devices.

Mild Established Case

Ischemic changes may be so mild and spotty through the muscle bellies that evidence of contracture is not clear until the fracture has healed and the slow restriction of finger motion arouses suspicion of trouble. In such instances, it has been customary to use physiotherapy and finger traction to regain range of motion. Any reduction in the vigor of treatment may be followed by recurrence of the hand's contraction. In this event, after long trial with such treatment, it may be wise to liberate the muscles from scar at operation or to lengthen the flexor tendons in order to regain function.

Severe Established Case

If established contracture is neglected, the effects of disuse are added to those of the basic process. They are atrophy of the joints, contraction of joint capsules, vasomotor instability, hyperesthesia and loss of mass of normal muscles. Nerve deficit is quite variable. Complete evaluation of the problem requires repeated examination during the course of intensive physiotherapy; exercises; appropriate splinting; and constant gentle finger traction which is designed to overcome, insofar as possible, the effects of disuse. Former teaching indicated that maximal improvement must be gained from such measures before corrective or reconstructive operations are considered. These measures may require months of faithful work. Repeated electromyographic records, studies of muscle response to electrical stimulation, and detailed neurologic evaluations should be made in order to assess the potential function available in the damaged muscles and nerves. The continued growth of bones in children effectively increases the deformity. In recent years a more active surgical approach directed toward release of nerves has been favored, and experience with detachment of involved muscles from their origins on the medial condyle, with the advancement of entire groups distalward, has produced better results than have combinations of procedures that basically work around the dense infarct, such as muscle or tendon lengthening and tendon transplantation. When nerve deficit persists, neurolysis or repair of nerves imbedded in dense scar is beneficial. The operations on bone are designed to provide the most favorable structural basis for the action of those muscles shown to have a useful degree of contractility. Resection of carpal bones, arthrodesis, removal of epiphyses and osteotomy are among the operations used. Capsulotomy may improve neglected joints. The results of each operation must be fully developed before another is undertaken.

Seddon[32] has described the repair of ischemic nerve lesions and excision of the muscle infarct 3–6 months after onset in patients who have a respectable amount of functional muscle. The removal of the binding necrotic mass permits greater benefit to be gained from reconstructive procedures. Whether excision of the infarct is preferable to muscle-slide operations is not determinable because each case presents such an individual problem.

The reconstructive problem is a challenge to surgical ingenuity. Essential hand functions, such as the ability to pinch and grasp, take precedence over less important ones. Throughout a course of management, which may last for years, it is imperative to have the full confidence and cooperation of the patient and to continue physiotherapy and exercises. At best, results are often imperfect.

SUMMARY

Volkmann's ischemic contracture in classic form is seen with decreasing frequency and appears almost totally preventable if suspicion, intensive observation and active operative therapy are employed. Vascular and trauma surgery have broadened experience so that, in many areas of the distal extremities, varying degrees of muscle ischemia from a wide variety of causes are recognized as essentially the same process as Volkmann[39] and Leser[26] described. In most cases direct injury to, or reflex or traumatic vasospasm of, the arterial side of the circulation is responsible for muscle ischemia sufficient to produce spotty or solid infarction. The sterile inflammatory reaction and swelling that rapidly follow intensify the arterial insufficiency in anatomically confined compartments. Either preventive or active therapy directed at these mechanisms is the more successful the earlier it is used. There is no place for the "wait and see" management the moment symptoms or signs appear.

In established contracture seen early or late there is a trend toward earlier and broader operation, provided care is taken not to augment the original ischemic damage. Whether this approach will improve functional results is not entirely clear but is promising.

BIBLIOGRAPHY

1. Adams, R. D., Denny-Brown, D., and Pearson, C. M.: *Diseases of Muscle* (New York: Paul B. Hoeber, Inc., 1953.
2. Albert, M., and Mitchell, W. R. D.: Volkmann's ischemia of the leg Lancet 1:519, 1943.
3. Barns, J. M., and Trueta, J.: "Arterial spasm": An experimental study, Br. J. Surg. 30 74, 1942.
4. Blount, W.: Volkmann's ischemic contracture (Editorial), Surg. Gynecol. Obstet. 90:244, 1950.

5. Brooks, B.: Pathologic changes in muscle as a result of disturbance of circulation: An experimental study of Volkmann's ischemic paralysis, Arch. Surg. 5:188, 1922.
6. Bunnell, S.: Ischemic contracture, local, in the hand, J. Bone Joint Surg. 35-A:88, 1953.
7. Campbell, J., and Pennyfeather, C. M.: The blood supply of muscles, with special reference to war surgery, Lancet 1:294, 1919.
8. Clark, L., and Blomfield, L. B.: Efficiency of intramuscular anastomoses, with observations on regenerating muscle, J. Anat. 79:15, 1945.
9. Clark, L., and Blomfield, L. B.: An experimental study of the regeneration of mammalian striped muscle, J. Anat. 80:24, 1946.
10. DeBakey, M., and Simeone, F. A.: Battle injuries of the arteries in World War II, Ann. Surg. 123:534, 1946.
11. Eichler, G. F., and Lipscomb, P. R.: The changing therapy of Volkmann's contracture plan 1955-1965 at the Mayo Clinic, Clin. Orthop. 50:215, 1967.
12. Foisie, P. S.: Volkmann's ischemic contracture: An analysis of its proximate mechanism, N. Engl. J. Med. 226:671, 1942.
13. Gardner, R. C.: Impending Volkmann's contracture following minor trauma to palm of the hand, Clin. Orthop. 72:261, 1970.
14. Gay, A. J., and Hunt, T. E.: Reuniting of skeletal muscles after transsection, Anat. Rec. 120:853, 1955.
15. Griffiths, D. L.: Volkmann's ischemic contracture, Br. J. Surg. 28:239, 1940.
16. Griffiths, D. L.: The management of acute circulatory failure in an injured limb, J. Bone Joint Surg. 30-B:280, 1948.
17. Harmon, J. W.: A histological study of skeletal muscle in acute ischemia, Am. J. Pathol. 23:551, 1947.
18. Harmon, J. W., and Gwynn, R. P.: The recovery of skeletal muscle fibers from acute ischemia as determined by histologic and chemical methods, Am. J. Pathol. 25:741, 1949.
19. Holmes, W., Highet, W. B., and Seddon, H. J.: Ischemic nerve lesions occurring in Volkmann's contracture, Br. J. Surg. 32:259, 1945.
20. Homans, J.: Vasomotor and other reactions to injuries and venous thrombosis, Am. J. Med. Sci. 205:313, 1943.
21. Hughes, C. W., Lineberger, E. C., and Bowers, W. F.: Anterior tibial compartment syndrome: A plea for early surgical treatment, Milit. Med. 126:124, 1961.
22. Hughes, J. R.: Ischemic necrosis of the anterior tibial muscles due to fatigue, J. Bone Joint Surg. 30-B:581, 1948.
23. Jones, S. G.: Volkmann's contracture, J. Bone Joint Surg. 17:649, 1935.
24. Jones, S. G., and Cotton, F. J.: Ischemic paralysis of the leg simulating Volkmann's ischemic contracture, J. Bone Joint Surg. 17:659, 1935.
25. Leriche, R., and Fontaine, R.: Experimental and clinical contribution to the question of the innervation of the vessels, Surg. Gynecol. Obstet. 47:631, 1928.
26. Leser, E.: Untersuchungen über Ischämischen Muskellahmungen und Muskelkontrakturen, Sammlung klin. Vortrage 249:287, 1884.
27. Lipscomb, P. R.: The etiology and prevention of Volkmann's ischemic contracture, Surg. Gynecol. Obstet. 103:353, 1956.
28. Lipscomb, P. R., and Burleson, R. J.: Vascular and neural complications in supracondylar fractures of the humerus in children, J. Bone Joint Surg. 37-A:487, 1955.
29. MacFarlane, M. G., and Spooner, S. J. L.: Chemical changes in muscle during and after ischemia, Br. J. Exp. Pathol. 27:339, 1946.
30. Murphy, J. B.: Myositis, JAMA 63:1249, 1914.
31. Parkes, A. R.: Traumatic ischemia of peripheral nerves, Br. J. Surg. 32:403, 1944-45.
32. Seddon, H. J.: Volkmann's contracture: Treatment by excision of the infarct, J. Bone Joint Surg. 38-B: 153, 1956.
33. Seddon, H. J.: Volkmann's ischemia in the lower limb, J. Bone Joint Surg. 48-B:627, 1966.
34. Seddon, H. J.: War injuries of peripheral nerves, Br. J. Surg. (War Surgery, supp. 2) 35:151, 1946–47.
35. Shaw, R. S.: A more aggressive approach toward the restoration of blood flow in acute arterial insufficiency, Surg. Gynecol. Obstet. 103:279, 1956.
36. Thomas, J. J.: Nerve involvement in the ischemic paralysis and contracture of Volkmann, Ann. Surg. 49:330, 1909.
37. Thompson, S. A., and Mahoney, L. S.: Volkmann's ischemic contracture and its relationship to fracture of the femur, J. Bone Joint Surg. 33-B:336, 1951.
38. Volkmann, R. von: Krankheiten der Bewegungsorgane, in Pitha and Brillroth (eds.): *Chirurgie* (Erlangen, Germany, 1869), Vol. 2, p. 846.
39. Volkmann, R. von: Die Ischämischen Muskellahmungen und Kontrakturen, Zentralbl. Chir. 8:801, 1881.

50 | Treatment of Burns

WILLIAM C. QUINBY, JR., and JOHN F. BURKE

THE MANAGEMENT of burns has kept pace with the advances in surgery. It has both borrowed from and contributed to the body of pathophysiologic knowledge that introduces quantitative data as a replacement for clinical dogma. The alterations in organ function that follow an extensive burn are being deciphered, their interrelationships made more clear and the direction and timing of treatment based on more solid ground.

As each advance has reduced some dangers to the patient, others equally threatening come to the surface. Perhaps nowhere in surgery is the patient's life at risk from so many disorders of function for so long as in the case of a deep, extensive burn. Surely nowhere are pain and physical and emotional suffering any greater. Even if life is saved, the prevention and correction of deformity are tremendous tasks, and the ultimate restoration of function is imperfect at best.

The experience of the past 20 years reinforces the conviction that the survival of the severely burned patient depends on the maintenance of the integrity of unburned organs. This in turn depends on the interval of time between the burn and the complete and permanent closure of the wound. The same objective applies to prevention of suffering, deformity and loss of function of lesser burns. Although personnel, equipment and expertise necessary to the survival of a severely burned patient have called forth special burn units and hospitals, moderate and minor burns are the province of all surgeons. Here attention to the principles and details of management are equally important.

The history of burn management is replete with the endless search for remedies, patent medicines and miracles which will turn abject failure into success. It is difficult to discuss the pros and cons of all the methods of treatment in current practice. Therefore, the emphasis here is on our present understanding of pathophysiology of the various organ systems encountered in burn care. The principles and aims of specific management rather than the details are accentuated, with discussion limited to those that apply to the point in consideration.

The major considerations are with scald burns, flame burns and flash burns, since they are most frequently seen. Brief consideration is given wounds of special types, but the material in other chapters on shock, respiratory physiology, metabolic response to trauma and infection is only reiterated here as it applies to burn trauma.

BURN SHOCK

The impact of traumatic wounds on circulating blood volume in the absence of overt hemorrhage was recognized 50 years ago. Studies by Underhill and associates[17] and by Blalock[3] established the concept of leakage from damaged capillaries and put wound shock, burn shock and tourniquet shock on a comprehensible basis. Increasingly sophisticat-

1137

ed research techniques over the years have shown that the circulatory effects that attend a burn wound are exceedingly complex.

Losses from Circulatory Blood

In the acute burn wound, the graded destruction of capillaries and small vessels by heat causes them to leak a protein-rich filtrate of the circulating plasma. Circulating red cells are damaged or destroyed as well. In addition the concept that a "toxin" or "kinin" elaborated from the burned tissue increases the general endothelial permeability and causes unburned capillaries at a distance also to "leak" a fluid similar in composition to interstitial fluid is supported by study and clinical experience. Thus, a vigorous dynamic state exists both in the burned area and in the neighboring undamaged tissues.

Movement of water, electrolytes and colloidal substances across capillary membranes may occur in a more complex way than according to Starling's law. The studies of Guyton and Coleman[9] on tissue pressures may clarify what does, in fact, occur. The adrenocortical alarm reaction, the cardiac output, the pH, oxygenation and viscosity of the blood, the microcirculation and direct or evaporative losses through damaged skin are but a few of the factors that influence what will be lost from the circulating blood after a burn injury. Losses begin immediately, are of major proportions in the first 8–10 hours, reach an equilibrium after 48–72 hours and are followed by a return of extravascular fluid to the circulation from the third to the seventh day after injury. The type and depth of burn cause variations in the timing of these events.

As coagulation seals the capillaries at the interface of the burn, overt leakage is superseded by an inflammatory process. Loss of water through burned skin continues, while the exudate of inflammation or infection causes additional loss of body fluids and protein. This continues as long as the wound remains unhealed. Most of the surface losses decrease abruptly on epithelialization of the wound or on closing it with skin grafts. Thus, although the initial management of burn shock is of critical importance, the wound makes constant demands on the body to maintain nutrition because of large losses of protein, water and energy from an inflammatory reaction that persists for weeks. Metabolic balance studies, both in the patient and the laboratory, have established some generalizations that direct management.[5]

1. The quantity of fluid rendered ineffective for the circulation immediately after the burn is directly proportional to the area of body surface burned.

2. While damaged vessels exude a plasma filtrate of high protein content, a large volumetric component whose composition is similar to interstitial fluid and contains sodium and water is also lost.[2, 11]

3. In deep and extensive burns, there is an initial destruction or impairment of red cells that rarely exceeds 10% of the total red cell mass.[10, 12, 14]

4. The exchanges of fluid between the circulating blood and the tissues is governed by the size of the extravascular space and by tissue pressures, so that the direct relationship between body surface area (BSA) burned and predicted losses from the blood does not constantly hold in a burn over 50% of BSA.

5. The nature and rates of metabolic change within the wound may be strongly affected by renal, cardiac, pulmonary and neuroendocrine function.

6. The inflammatory response evoked by the burn wound makes extraordinary demands on all functions of the body which are greatly intensified by the invasion of bacteria.[6]

7. Although it has been suggested that "neurogenic" shock and fat embolism play a role in initial burn shock, it is difficult to decipher such components in the presence of rapid changes that occur soon after the burn.

Treatment

Aims

It is a reasonable therapeutic objective to maintain the volume and composition of the circulating blood within the normal range throughout the course of the burned patient. With limited or superficial burns, losses are small and can be replenished by oral intake alone. Burns up to 10% of BSA in children and 15% in adults usually do not require intravenous support, although exceptions must be made in the very young, the aged, the infirm and under other special circumstances. With extensive burns, losses are so great that unless anticipated in the plan of therapy there is rapid blood volume depletion. Burn formulas for fluid replacement have been developed that equate the BSA burn with total surface area or the patient's weight as volumetric guidelines for therapy in the acute phase of the burn.

Two decades ago, blister fluid was used as a model for the losses through burned capillaries. Consequently, replacement for wound losses was considered to be best if its protein content was at least 4 gm/100 ml. An additional allotment of dextrose and water was given to replace urinary and insensible water loss. With recognition of the large expansion of the interstitial space and sodium losses, the emphasis has shifted to crystalloid solutions of isotonic sodium content with buffering substances added. Lactated Ringer's solution is currently in vogue.

Experience has shown that crystalloid solutions administered intravenously pass through damaged capillaries more easily than do solutions containing colloids. If blood volume is to be maintained by crystalloid alone, significantly larger quantities are needed, and the patient's interstitial space is expanded to a greater extent than with added colloid. After the capillaries have sealed, the sequestered interstitial fluid of crystalloid therapy returns to the circulation more rapidly than does the fluid lost when colloid is given with lactated Ringer's. Therefore, the total volume required for resuscitation varies with the type of fluid administered.[7]

In patients with cerebral injury from anoxia or with pulmonary injury at the time of burn, fluid therapy aims to minimize brain swelling or interstitial pulmonary edema while maintaining adequate blood volume. Since treatment with crystalloid alone often results in serum protein concentrations as low as 3 gm/100 ml during the acute phase of fluid losses, it is reasonable to increase the proportion of colloid given when these dangers are suspected.

The fluid which acutely expands the interstitial space returns to the circulating blood in about a week, but a protein-rich fluid is permanently lost in blisters or in coagulation around eschar. In addition, red cell destruction by the initial burn is reflected in low hemoglobin or hematocrit values. Therefore, a further objective of therapy during the first week is to replace the protein that is irretrievable and the red cells that have been destroyed.

Replacement Formulas

Early studies by Cope and Moore[5] formed the basis of a plan of therapy in which 75 ml of plasma and 75 ml of crystalloid were administered for each percent of BSA burned: to this was added 2,000–3,000 ml of dextrose and water to replenish insensible and urinary losses. These figures applied to the average 70-kg patient. The rate of administration was adjusted to maintain urine output between 50 and 200 ml an hour. A "water tolerance test," consisting of rapid infusion of 1,500 ml of dextrose or dextrose and saline solution, was employed to distinguish the anuria of inadequate blood volume from that of renal shutdown in patients whose output was not maintained on this regimen. In the aged and in patients with pulmonary burns, experience showed these quantities to be excessive. Other adjustments were made for body size based on a normogram which converted weight and height into square meters of body surface. These refinements resulted in a formula in which 75 ml of colloid and 15 ml of crystalloid/% BSA burned/sq m of total BSA was administered for burn wound losses, with dextrose and water (1,500 ml/sq m BSA) supplied for insensible losses.[4] The total volume estimate was for the first 24 hours after the burn.

At the other extreme, Moyer and associates[11] and Baxter and Shires[2] have emphasized sodium loss of interstitial fluid and showed that in extensive burn patients resuscitation can be successful with the use of crystalloid solution alone. Clinical experience here showed that 3.5–4.5 ml of lactated Ringer's solution/% BSA burned/kg body weight sustained urine flow, normal blood gases and normal central venous pressure in a series of patients and in experimental animals.

An early formula proposed by Evans et al.[8] advocated 1 ml of colloid and 1 ml of crystalloid/% BSA burned/kg body weight with an added 2,000 ml of dextrose and water for insensible and urinary losses per 24 hours following the burn. At the Brooke Army Medical Center these quantities have been modified to call for 0.5 ml of colloid plus 1.5 ml of crystalloid/% BSA burned/kg, with the added 2,000 ml of dextrose and water per 24 hours.[15] Extensive experience with both of these formulas has authenticated their effectiveness.

Evidence of initial hemolysis and studies that show significantly diminished life span of red cells following a severe burn have prompted resuscitation with whole blood combined with crystalloid solutions.[1] It is significant that 60% or more of a whole blood transfusion is composed of plasma with anticoagulant and that this therapy results in an increasing hematocrit and blood viscosity during the first 48 hours after a burn.[13]

In search for an inexpensive and available colloidal substance devoid of the dangers of hepatitis that may accompany plasma, low-molecular-weight dextran solutions have been tried and will indeed act effectively as colloid.[16] Although coagulation defects may limit their use and protein deficits will occur, the dextrans are important in the event of mass casualty.

Many resuscitation programs have advocated oral fluids in the form of liquids containing sodium, potassium or sodium bicarbonate. Allowance for the quantity of these fluids ingested and retained has been made in all formulas.

If attention is directed to the composition of the circulating blood after reabsorption of edema fluid a week after burn, there may be no detectable abnormality in burns up to 25% of BSA, because red cell and plasma losses usually are small enough to be compensated for by the body. In extensive burns, however, it is common to find the hematocrit and serum protein levels abnormally low at this time if crystalloid alone or crystalloid and plasma according to the Brooke formula have been used as resuscitative fluids. Although proof is lacking, it is a clinical impression that more red cells and more albumin or plasma are needed to return blood values to normal if this therapeutic effort is begun at 7–10 days following the burn than if these substances are incorporated in the initial plan of resuscitative therapy.

Monitoring during Therapy

The management of a healthy young adult who sustains a flash or flame burn of up to 20% of body surface can be conducted successfully in the community hospital. Adequate therapy of early fluid losses is determined by urine output and hematocrit levels. These 2 time-honored indexes can be supplemented by serum electrolytes and osmolality determinations. Necessary replacements for deficits are usually at hand.

The presence of smoke inhalation, cerebral anoxia, a questionable laryngeal burn or serious concomitant disease of age greatly compounds the problem of fluid therapy. Here the distinction between burn shock and organ dysfunction from some other cause requires personnel and monitoring which postulate intensive care. Infants and small children require pediatric intensive care. Deep burns of more than 30% of the body represent a statistically serious hazard to life at any age.

The essential feature of all fluid resuscitation is an accurate monitoring of intake and output. In an extensive burn, oral fluids are frequently sequestered in the stomach or vomited and thus invalidate total intake measurements. The stomach should be emptied with a tube and kept empty.

A central venous pressure catheter line is placed in all extensive burns and in those with a cerebral, cardiac or pulmonary component. It can also be used for fluid administration or drawing of blood samples. Since, in many patients, the tip of the line may not be truly "central," a change in the venous pressure measurement is more significant than its absolute reading.

Urine specific gravity, osmolality and volume are sensitive indexes of blood volume and composition and should be monitored hourly in severe burns. This requires an inlying bladder catheter. Unless severe dehydration and acidosis have occurred because of delay in restoring renal perfusion and blood volume, acute tubular necrosis of the kidney is a rarity. It can be identified by examination of the urinary sediment for casts in the presence of high sodium concentration and low urine osmolality.

Because topical applications of 0.5% silver nitrate dressings or Sulfamylon have metabolic effects on the serum sodium and blood pH, respectively, careful monitoring of these values is required. If blood samples are hard to obtain, the urinary sodium concentration is a reasonable reflection of the serum sodium and is best kept between 20 and 80 mEq/L.

Cardiac monitoring is appropriate, where indicated, and evidences of respiratory inadequacy must be followed carefully. An initial evaluation of the blood gas values and pH together with serum electrolytes, serves as a base line of tissue oxygenation and should be repeated every 8 hours for the first 3 days. Chest x-ray, repeated at appropriate intervals, may identify atelectasis, pulmonary injury or pulmonary edema in the first few days after burn.

Implementation

Assessment of the burn is of primary importance in the decisions as to intensity of the monitoring and type of therapy required. Obviously, burns of minor extent or depth do not require hospital care or elaborate treatment. If need for intravenous supplements or laboratory data is deemed likely, the patient should enter a hospital until the requirements are clear. Babies, the elderly and patients with pre-existing cardiac or pulmonary injury must be carefully evaluated even though the burn is not large.

It is clear that a variety of solutions can be used successfully in the resuscitative phase of acute burn shock.[2, 4, 5, 7] The essential feature is to restore an effective circulating blood volume as quickly as possible after the burn. Since reabsorption of burn edema fluid after 48 hours may be quite rapid, it is equally important to decrease the rate of administration as soon as diuresis becomes evident to avoid volumetric overload of the circulation. All formulas emphasize that half the first day's complement be given in the first 8 hours following the burn and that the second day's volume need only be about half that calculated for the first 24 hours.

In the modern day it is rare to lose a patient in the early shock phase of even very extensive burns if volume replacement is administered promptly. Formulas serve only as predictions. They must be modified by the evidence of adequacy or excess in accordance with the patient's response as determined by repeated measurements. The hematocrit and hourly urine output are the simplest reliable indexes of adequate blood volume, whereas central venous pressure, dyspnea, auscultation, chest x-ray and blood gas values identify circulatory overload.

It is difficult to maintain a normal composition of the circulating blood during the acute phase of fluid shifts. In most burn centers it is agreed that plasma or albumin should be given if the serum protein concentration falls to less than 3 gm/100 ml and that blood transfusion is indicated if the hematocrit falls below 30% in the first 48 hours after the burn. During the phase of reabsorption of fluid from the interstitial space, however, such value changes often reflect dilution that subsides with normal diuresis.

Since urine output is so significant, the integrity of renal function must be established quickly. If an initial acidosis due to dehydration is recognized, it should be corrected at once with intravenous administration of sodium bicarbonate, 0.5 mM/kg. If scant, dark-red urine indicates hemoglobinuria, both mannitol and sodium bicarbonate protect the renal tubular function if given early with the initial volume replacement.

Intensive monitoring can be tapered off after 5–7 days, but nutritional losses are insidious, and later effects of sepsis may be rapid and severe. If organs are to function at their best, it is essential to identify anemia, hypoproteinemia, electrolyte imbalance, metabolic acidosis or alkalosis and respiratory insufficiency by regular testing and to correct them promptly.

INFECTION

Sources and Types of Organisms

It is reasonable to assume that the heat of a burning agent sufficient to destroy skin will also destroy most of the bacteria on it. Although cultures of fresh burns support this assumption, they frequently show that materials applied to the wound before arrival at a hospital have contaminated the surface. The hospital environment provides opportunities for cross infection, whether airborne or by contact with the apparatus or personnel necessary to patient care. Even the most elaborate techniques may fail to prevent wound contamination in the burned patient.

Autogenous contamination of burn wounds may arise from bacteria in hair follicles or sweat glands of the patient's skin; these are predominantly staphylococci. The frequent finding of contamination of burns of the upper thighs and buttocks with gram-negative organisms supports the place of fecal organisms in autocontamination, whereas the patient's nose, throat and skin often harbor beta-hemolytic streptococcus.

Although mixtures of organisms may be present at any time in the burn wound, swab cultures generally show that the beta-hemolytic streptococcus is an early contaminant, to be accompanied or followed by staphylococcus, and within days or weeks by gram-negative organisms, such as pseudomonas, klebsiella, aerobacter, enterobacter and those of the coliform group.[28] Clostridia also present a constant hazard wherever there is burned tissue.[31] Quantitative studies show that about 10^2 or 10^3 organisms/gm tissue are found on contaminated wounds. When colonization occurs, the numbers rise to $10^4 - 10^6$ bacteria/gm tissue. Invasion of surrounding tissues usually predicts 10^8 or more organisms. *Pseudomonas aeruginosa*, the verdoglobin of which fluoresces under ultraviolet light, can be identified when the wound population exceeds 10^6 bacteria/gm tissue, and green fluorescence can also be seen in the urine.[34, 37]

Although bacteria differ in their virulence, invasive qualities and local destructive effects, their presence inevitably deepens the burn wound. In a first-degree burn, little dead pabulum for multiplication of bacteria exists, but the fluid of unruptured blisters may become infected and result in tissue destruction, more violent inflammatory reaction and enlargement of the wound. Formerly it was held that the eschar of full-thickness burns (or eschar produced by topical application of tannic acid, gentian violet or other protein coagulants) formed a protective covering relatively impermeable to bacteria and to the loss of body fluids. Cannon and Cope[23] showed that these escharotics merely deepen the burn. Colonization of tissues below an eschar inevitably occurs, and the septic process progresses at a deeper level. The inflammatory response and its metabolic demands are intensified, and the multiplication and invasion of bacteria into contiguous tissues and the blood stream are favored because the eschar prevents the escape of septic exudate, as in an undrained abscess.

It also was thought that the granulation tissue bed that develops after the eschar has separated from a full-thickness burn is "healthy" and relatively free from bacteria. Although this may be true at times, it is clear that chronic granulation tissue harbors large numbers of bacteria, quickly becomes edematous and produces an inflammatory exudate that can demolish epithelium or a superimposed skin graft. With such infected granulation tissue there is a constant danger of deeper invasion and blood stream contamination.

In the past 15 years, death from gram-negative septicemia has superseded death from shock or renal failure in patients with deep or extensive burns because the patients have lived long enough for the full range of septic processes to develop. Bacteremia is identified on blood cultures which may be contaminated from intravenous lines or bacteria in the wound close to the venipuncture. A diagnosis of septicemia is authenticated by positive results of blood cultures, but in practice represents a composite of clinical findings that reflect organ dysfunction. Hyper- or hypothermia, cerebral obtundation, tachycardia and septic shock, hypoxia, ileus and oliguria are all attendant features. Unless repeated blood stream invasion can be controlled by elimination of the source of organisms, the clinical picture of septicemia may come on at any time from a few days to a few weeks after a severe burn. Ultimately, microabscesses develop in many tissues and rapidly lead to organ failure.[38]

Measures for Control

LOCAL AND ENVIRONMENTAL. — Since infection in the burn wound has such serious consequences, many efforts to control it have been made. Prevention of contamination is successful in superficial burns if the wound is thoroughly cleaned and protected from the environment by occlusive dressings. Since deeper wounds cannot be as effectively cleaned, colonization occurs from skin glands and residual bacteria when there is significant devitalized tissue. Because coagulated plasma in the form of a scab is nature's dressing and because the exudate at the surface saturates dressings and permits further bacterial multiplication, the "exposure method" of treating a burn wound has had success in shallow burns but not in deeper burns. Contamination and colonization inevitably occur after 8–12 days in deeper burns, whether exposed or dressed. It is of primary importance repeatedly to assess the progress of the wound by clinical and bacteriologic observations because extensive epithelialization will occur from viable skin glands if bacterial action can be minimized.

Prevention of contamination by isolation, gown, gloves and hand washing is directed toward cross infection, and strict aseptic surgical techniques are used in wound care to minimize autogenous infection. The more rigidly adhered to, the more effective are such control measures. Recently, significant improvement has attended the development of a totally enclosed unit that surrounds the bed. Here the environmental bacterial population is markedly reduced by a constant downward laminar flow of filtered air from the ceiling. Temperature and humidity can be adjusted, an effective barrier to cross infection is produced, and autogenous bacteria are wafted downward away from the wounds through exit grilles in the floor. Other strict patient isolation units, such as the "life island" have also been on trial. Virtually all nursing and active therapy can be carried on without entering these units. Clinical results and bacteriologic studies support the effectiveness of such special environmental control.

TOPICAL AGENTS. — In 1963 there was a revival of effective topical agents when Moyer and associates[33] introduced 0.5% silver nitrate wet dressings and when use of 10% Sulfamylon ointment, originally developed for wounds during World War II, was revived.[29, 32] Both 0.1% gentamicin cream[37] and 1% silver sulfadiazine ointment[26] also have shown significant effectiveness. Betadyne ointment, silver nitrate gel and local applications of multiple antibiotics are included among agents used topically. Each has its good points and its shortcomings,[22, 29] but there is no question that a significant degree of control over colonization and subsequent invasive infection has attended their use. Sulfamylon cream has had a wide application because it penetrates the depth of an eschar. Direct injection of antibiotics beneath full-thickness eschar has also been tried with benefit.

As control of wound bacteria becomes more effective, the separation of eschar is retarded because bacterial action promotes its autolysis and digestion. In deep burns without infection, the unresolved wound may persist for weeks unless debrided. Manipulation of a septic wound, however, is accompanied by showers of bacteria in the blood stream and may be followed promptly by septicemia. Surgeons often hesitate to upset the balance between patient and organisms by anything more than gentle debridement of eschar. The improved control of wound bacteria by topical agents has reduced this danger and greatly prolonged the interval after the burn during which surgical manipulation of the wound can be conducted safely. None of the agents "sterilizes" the burn wound nor holds bacterial proliferation in control indefinitely,[27] but by inhibition of destructive bacterial action for a significant period they permit shallowly burned areas to heal spontaneously and active surgical procedures to be done on deep burns. The institution of effective topical therapy is an outstanding advance in burn therapy of the past decade.

SYSTEMIC ANTIBIOTICS. — The same principles apply to the use of antibiotics in burns as to their use in other areas of trauma, but a complicating factor is the span of time from injury to closure of the wound.[24] The beta-hemolytic streptococcus does not become resistant to penicillin and is also controlled by kanamycin or erythromycin in penicillin-sensitive patients. Oxacillin is effective against penicillin-resistant staphylococci. Most of the gram-negative pathogens are controlled by gentamicin — although pseudomonas organisms may develop resistance rapidly — and carbenicillin is also effective. Predominant organisms cultured from the sputum, urine, the wound or blood may show good sensitivity to other specific antibiotics, which then become the preferable ones in therapy. Prolonged treatment or use of multiple antibiotics leads to the development of resistant strains and superinfection with candida or other fungi. Indeed, long-term suppression of bacteria by topical agents alone favors the emergence of candida in the wound. If candida septicemia truly occurs, amphotericin B is an effective although highly nephrotoxic agent.

Because of the dangers of superinfection and resistance, the indications for antibiotic therapy must be clear. They are grouped as preventive, empirical or specific. Preventive penicillin therapy has had a long clinical trial directed against early wound contamination by the beta-hemolytic streptococcus and toward protection of injured air passages from airborne organisms. Its effectiveness is suggested because minor superficial burns may become infected with streptococcus when it is not used and because it is rare to culture these organisms from the wounds of patients who have received penicillin. Similar findings in throat, sputum or tracheal cultures support the clinical habit of administering penicillin for 5 days after a burn in which respiratory tract damage is suspected.

Organisms may be disseminated locally and into the blood stream by manipulation of a colonized burn wound. To minimize these dangers, antibiotics should be given before, during and for 24–48 hours after surgical debridement or excision of contaminated wounds. Protection against both gram-negative and gram-positive organisms is confirmed by the low incidence of septicemias following aggressive surgery of wounds when preventive antibiotic therapy has been employed. The appropriate antibiotics may be determined according to the predominant organisms cultured from the wound. Penicillin or oxacillin with gentamicin are effective agents in most cases.

In patients with critical burns it may be necessary to institute antibiotic therapy when the clinical diagnosis of septicemia, spreading pneumonitis or uncontrolled infection is secure but a specific causative organism has not been isolated. During the time necessary for bacteriologic identification the patient's condition may deteriorate seriously, and the empirical use of agents against staphylococci or gram-negative organisms is justified. Here the needs are desperate, and the effectiveness of such choice only authenticated by blood cultures which ultimately grow out positive or by marked clinical improvement of the patient. On occasion, with a sick patient, smears of urine or tracheal aspirates will show abundant organisms and provide indications for empirical therapy pending culture reports.

Specific therapy is indicated when tracheal, urine or blood cultures give positive results, but treatment aimed at organisms cultured from the wound is rendered ineffective by the presence of necrotic tissue. The diagnosis of invasive infection is difficult because hypermetabolism and the inflammatory reaction of large wounds make fever and leukocytosis common features of most major burns. Efforts to suppress bacteria in colonized wounds for long periods by antibiotics lead only to drug resistance and failure ultimately to avoid invasive sepsis.

IMMUNOLOGY. — In most burn centers wide differences are found in the clinical response of patients to burns of similar severity and bacterial population in the wound. Studies have been directed along 3 lines. One concept is that denatured protein of burned skin may elaborate substances which are toxic to general cell metabolism, particularly in the first hours or few days after the injury. Other investigations are concerned with immunoglobulin titers of the patient as an index of innate resistance to infection or wound bacteria.[20, 36] Finally, the emergence of pseudomonas sepsis as a major factor in modern burn mortality has led to clinical trial of active or passive immunization of patients, using pseudomonas polyvalent vaccine or hyperimmune polyvalent antiserum.[25]

To date, specific toxic substances have not been identified clearly enough to merit clinical concern. Suggestive evidence of a "burn toxin," operative in the early phases after injury, is only borne out in laboratory animals.

Although a pattern of decreased IgA and IgM titers in the first postburn week is followed by a marked increase that persists after the wound is closed, there is inconsistent correlation of such findings with burn morbidity or mortality.

Early results suggested that there was benefit to patients treated with a polyvalent pseudomonas vaccine at the time of injury. However, a month is required to produce high titers by active immunization, and correlation with wound flora is inconsistent. Hyperimmune pseudomonas antiserum has been used clinically but not widely enough for evaluation. Volunteer donors are required, and at least 3 major groups of pseudomonas organisms must be included in the immunization process. Thus, protection against pseudomonas infection by immunologic measures is not yet established clinically and has not been applied to other serious burn infections with klebsiella or staphylococci.

There has been considerable study of the cellular responses of the reticuloendothelial system, of lymphocytes and of polymorphonuclear leukocytes in burned patients.[19, 35] The correlation of bacterial density in the wound with the clinical course of the patient has been made on the natural assumption that phagocytic mechanisms against bacteria are strong determinants of what develops in the wound and in the patient. A somewhat cyclic neutrophil activity has been identified. Lymphocytic activity has been used as a reflection of the immune reactions of the body, as recognized in transplantation work. The reticuloendothelial function is less specific and requires greater understanding. This important area of investigation is in its infancy and as yet has limited therapeutic application or use in predicting the course of a burn.

ALLOGRAFTS AND HETEROGRAFTS.—For many years allografts have been used in burn therapy when autogenous skin was insufficient to cover extensive burn wounds or when the patient could not tolerate anesthesia or the added hazard of donor site wounds. Since a successful "take" of allografts closes the wound for 2–3 weeks before there is rejection by the host, nutritional losses and colonization of the portion of the wound covered by allografts is prevented.[30] With the process of rejection, however, open wounds again occur, and infection as well. Successful allografts become vascularized and intimately incorporated with the host after 3–4 days, in the same manner as an autograft. At a week from grafting they are so adherent that it is difficult to remove them.

Bacterial counts of granulating burn wounds have shown a marked reduction within hours of application of skin grafts to the surface, provided most of the devitalized tissue has previously been removed. This bacteriostatic effect favors the epithelialization of partial-thickness burns from hair follicles and skin glands. Allografts applied to uncontaminated partial-thickness burns may adhere and vascularize in some areas. They are gradually lifted off as the host epithelium regenerates beneath them. Further refinements have led to the use of allografts as a biologic dressing that is unfavorable to bacterial growth. In infected wounds, the expectation is not that they will vascularize and "take." Instead, they must be removed and be freshly applied every day or whenever septic wound exudates appear beneath them—a nicety of technique in judgment of wound care.

Heterografts of pigskin underwent empirical clinical trial as much as 60 years ago. Currently their availability commercially has resulted in extensive trial as a primary burn dressing or as a substitute for human allografts on open burn wounds when allografts are not available. True take and vascularization are not seen, but heterografts are protective against contamination of a fresh wound and aid in the reduction of bacteria in an infected or granulating one.

CLOSTRIDIAL INFECTION.—Active immunization against tetanus has been accomplished so thoroughly in early childhood, the school years or during military service that clinical tetanus is a rarity in the United States, although its incidence in patients with burn injury is occasionally reported.[31] The sensitivity of the organism to penicillin, the development of human tetanus immune globulin and laboratory evidence that Sulfamylon inhibits clostridial growth further reduce the incidence of overt clinical tetanus. Nonetheless, the deep burn wound provides all the requirements for growth of the organism. A booster dose of 0.5 ml of tetanus toxoid provides adequate protection in patients who have been fully immunized as long as 10 years prior to injury. When such a record is uncertain, or when no previous immunization can be documented, 500 units of human tetanus globulin is administered at once and active immunization with tetanus toxoid begun. Second and third doses of toxoid should follow at monthly intervals.

Since common burns involve the skin and rarely destroy muscle, the occurrence of myositis of gas gangrene is limited to unusual circumstances, such as electrical burns or instances in which occlusion of arterial supply results in ischemia or gangrene of deep tissues. Here no positive form of immunization or antiserum is readily available, although penicillin or tetracycline afford significant protection. The elimination of the site of clinical gas gangrene by wise excision or, in extreme circumstances, by amputation, is essential to management.

BURN WOUND

Evolution

The agent that produces a burn damages or destroys cells by denaturation and coagulation of protein. The extent of damage is a function of the intensity and duration of the heat. The earliest reaction to injury is one of capillary dilatation and increased blood flow to the area. The swelling which rapidly follows reflects leakage of components of the circulating blood from injured and adjacent capillaries and expansion of the interstitial space.

The redness of sunburn reflects capillary dilatation. If the burn is deeper, blisters form, representing intradermal collections of a dilute plasma. If the entire thickness of the skin is heat coagulated, it is not perfused and will not swell, but the same processes go on at the interface between damaged and undamaged tissues whatever the depth of the destruction. Burn wounds are traditionally classified as first second and third degree, according to whether the response indicates superficial, partial-thickness or full-thickness destruction of the skin. Most flame burns encountered are a mixture of the 3 "degrees," whereas hot water rarely burns deeply except in the very young or very old. Burns from chemical agents, electricity and inflammable liquids may extend into the fat, deep fascia, joint capsules or muscles and represent a fourth "degree" which has significant clinical implications.

The burn wound undergoes a dynamic sequence in which initial tissue swelling causes further ischemia and loss of some cells not originally destroyed by heat, so that the full extent and depth of injury may not be clear for 3 or 4 days. By this time damaged capillaries have thrombosed or sealed, wound edema begins to be absorbed, and local circulation is adequate to support those cells which will ultimately survive. There is no conclusive evidence that this sequence can be altered by applications of ice water or external pressure dressings designed to limit edema.

The progress of the uninfected burn wound after the first 3 or 4 days is characterized by an inflammatory process which varies among individuals but follows the pattern of demarcation, autolysis, phagocytosis and a cellular and metabolic inflammatory response that occurs whenever destroyed tissue has to be dealt with by the body. In shallow burns the superficial layer is cast off as the epidermis regenerates beneath it. In deep dermal burns the separation is slow because the dense collagenous dermal layer of the skin resists autolytic digestion. In full-thickness burns new capillary buds form the basis of a vascular granulation tissue as the dead skin separates at a level below the deep dermal pegs.

If bacterial contamination can be prevented, a deep second-degree burn re-epithelializes from a few residual skin glands over a period of weeks, but the quality of the healed surface is poor because of excessive fibrosis and loss of the reticular structure of the dermal layers of connective tissue. After the eschar of full-thickness burns has separated, granulation tissue continues to be formed, to exude protein from the exposed capillary buds at the surface and to harbor a significant inflammatory reaction, the maturation of which results in fibrosis of the deeper layers and edematous granulations superficially. Wound contraction slowly follows, and epithelial spread in a thin layer from the periphery closes the wound. Here the quality of the closure is poor, due to dense fibrosis and the fragile nature of the epithelial covering.

Even after closure by epithelium or graft the process of rearrangement of the wound continues. It is poorly understood. Simultaneously more connective tissue is formed than is desirable (the so-called hypertrophic scar), while contractures of the new fibrous tissue develop. The former process produces raised, reddened, bulky, inelastic and disorganized fibrous tissue covered by epithelium at the borders of the wound, edges of skin grafts and even areas of partial-thickness skin loss. The latter foreshortens the distance between any 2 points in the wound and forms bands which may be kept in a constant "live" or active state if overstretching of inelastic scar fractures capillaries, reactivates the inflammatory process and retards the resolution of fibrous tissue. After a year or more, hypertrophic scar settles down and flattens out. The process of wound contracture relaxes moderately for 3-6 months after the wound has healed but ultimately becomes dense, unyielding and relatively avascular.

Much investigation is in progress to clarify the dynamics of contraction in an open wound. The origin and nature of collagen, which is a major component of wound closure, the balance between collagen formation, rearrangement and absorption, the nature of granulation tissue and the nature and mediation of hypertrophic scar are under study.

Most important is a better understanding of the biologic processes at work before and after a skin graft is applied to an open wound; for, although mechanisms are poorly understood, the healing of a burn wound is subject to the same deterrents of devitalized tissue, hematomas, dead space, excessive motion, ischemia, trauma, malnutrition and bacterial infection that apply to all soft tissue wounds. There is little evidence that any substance applied to the wound "stimulates" healing. After devitalized tissue has been removed, closure of the wound with a skin graft promptly effects a barrier against bacteria and promotes destruction of contaminants in the wound. Water and nutritional components are retained in the body, and the inflammatory reaction subsides.

Studies of autograft "take" describe the processes of vascularization, revitalization and spread of epithelium from transplanted skin. The process of rejection of allografts has clarified the immune responses of the recipient. Many studies have shown that any factor which interferes with normal healing also reduces the "take" of grafts. Whereas the spread of epithelium from the wound edges or the periphery of a graft has received appropriate emphasis as an essential feature of wound closure, the effects of the dermal layers of grafts on collagen formation and fibrosis deserve more study.

Management

Management of the burn wound is determined by accurate appraisal of its severity, its location, the presence or absence of sepsis, its observed or predictable progress and the impact on the patient. What is done or not done in the earliest stages dictates what may occur weeks later. Time is of the essence. In all cases the therapeutic result is directly proportional to the intensity of wound care. The prime objective of earliest possible wound closure must govern management. The nicety of judgment concerns whether or not the body will spontaneously heal the wound more quickly than this can be accomplished by surgical manipulations. Temporary control of wound infection by topical agents has greatly increased the interval of time during which active surgical maneuvers can be carried out safely. This time is precious and must be used to maximal advantage.

APPRAISAL.—Most burns are of uneven depth and distribution. Scald burns are rarely deep; flaming clothing usually produces full-thickness destruction in most areas; the hot smoke of a house fire may cause a severe baking type of injury, and chemicals or electricity may produce profound destruction that is not apparent at the surface. The presence of blisters, the sensitivity to touch or pinprick, the blanching response of capillaries to pressure, and the consistency of the injured areas contribute to the evaluation. With extensive burns, it is often crucial to distinguish moderate depth, partial-thickness from full-thickness injury. Difficulty is encountered when broken blisters expose a bright red, inflamed base that must be distinguished from the redness produced by hemoglobin fixed in the capillaries by heat that predicts a full-thickness injury. Thrombosis of intradermal veins always designates third-degree burn. A technique of intravenous injection of patent blue dye which accentuates hyperemic partial-thickness burn and does not stain full-thickness areas is helpful in determination of depth[7] but is hazardous to the patient, which precludes its use. The profuse blood supply to the face and genitalia protects against invasive infection, and regeneration of epithelium is also favored because of plentiful hair follicles. The prediction of ultimate tissue loss is difficult, and spontaneous repair is often suprisingly good with facial and genital burns.

As time passes, shallow burns can be observed to heal from the edges, whereas full-thickness eschar remains stiff, develops cracks which admit infection, and ultimately shows fluctuation or gradual separation of connective tissue pegs, depending on the degree of bacterial action. Intermediate between these extremes are second-degree burns which have a variable course, depending on depth and activity of infection. The simultaneous processes of separation of eschar and epithelial regeneration in the deep dermis often present as a whitish base mixed with punctate red spots and some dried eschar. The appearance and appraisal vary according to the moisture in dressings and the quantity of exudate. A gluey, soft, connective tissue eschar adheres to viable dermal pegs in the skin despite dressing changes or efforts to speed the separation by active debridement. It is common for such separation to persist for weeks before the area will either show spontaneous healing or accept a skin graft.

Treatment of the Clean Wound

Superficial burns should be cleaned and protected from further bacterial contamination. A neutral soap or pHisoderm is adequate if rinsed with saline. Hexachlorophene is absorbed from extensive raw areas with serious systemic effects and should be avoided. A moderately wide-meshed gauze is used to cover the wound and is kept in place by an occlusive dressing. Motion is limited by splinting or by adding sufficient bulk to the dressing so that external motion is not transmitted to the wound surface. Impregnation of the gauze with substances designed to prevent adherence to the wound should not interfere with its ability to transmit wound exudates to the surrounding dressing. The dressing should remain in place for 5 days unless fever or increased pain indicate infection. Revaluation will authenticate the estimate of the depth of the burn and determine whether or not to alter treatment. Protection is provided until epithelialization is complete.

Second-degree burns should receive the same primary treatment, except that use of topical ointments may be indicated. A decision as to ultimate depth and preferential management should be made within 7 or 8 days. When observations indicate destruction at the deep dermal level, strong consideration should be given to active surgical debridement or excision and graft of such areas. Although uninfected deep dermal burns will eventually heal and displace the eschar, the process may be slow and the resulting deformities severe. A more active program of management frequently is advisable.

Over the years a number of clinical trials of enzymic debriding agents have been made. Proteolytic enzymes derived from papaya or figs and collagenases produced by bacteria have been the chief sources of such substances. The problems have been to limit the debriding effects to dead tissue, so that the wound is not enlarged, and to maintain the concentration within the appropriate range of pH. Although investigation continues, at present no enzyme preparation has yet attained the position of preferred clinical treatment.

Full-thickness burns of limited extent should be primarily excised and autografted. Exceptions occur in burns of the face and genitalia or when the condition of the patient precludes general anesthesia. Since even with modern topical agents bacteria ultimately invade the wound and reduce the chances of successful take of grafts, excision must be undertaken early when graft take of 95–100% is the rule and the ravages of sepsis, pain and prolonged hospital care are avoided.[42] In most patients primary excision can be safely carried out within 12–14 days of injury, although the decision is influenced by the appearance of the wound and the organisms cultured.

Extensive full-thickness burn injury presents the problem of a lack of donor site skin sufficient to close a large area of excision. Yet here it becomes even more important to excise and close as much of the burn as possible, since ultimate mortality is directly proportional to the area of the wound and the infection attendant thereto. Thus, repeated "primary partial excision" of full-thickness areas is established as a critically important extension of the principle of removal of dead tissue.[43, 45] Since repeated harvest of autogenous skin from limited donor sites can usually be made at intervals of 10–14 days, a significant percentage of the entire burn can often be excised and closed before serious wound colonization occurs. Allografts may be used to close excised areas temporarily and are replaced with autografts as they become available.[40] Although severe problems attendant on blood loss and the trauma of operation impose a stringent protocol on this therapeutic attitude, the alternative of extensive infected sloughing wounds which will inevitably occur justifies such risks. There is growing clinical experience that supports such aggressive management.

Excision of burned areas aims to remove all of the tissue that is destroyed and no normal tissue. In practice it is difficult to realize this ideal. On the one hand, the entire purpose of excision is defeated if damaged cells which will not support a graft or resist infection are left in the wound; on the other hand, the tangential excision of progressively deeper slices of eschar until a healthy tissue bed is reached is attended by serious loss of blood.[48] Excision can be done more easily with less hemorrhage if it is carried out at the level of muscle fascia.[55] The deformity that results from absence of subcutaneous fat is significant but there is gradual improvement through fat regeneration over the years. Burns of extremities should be excised under tourniquet control to limit blood loss.

The technical features of skin grafting are treated in many texts. Suffice it to say that failure of grafts to take is a serious occurrence. Motion of the graft on the tissues beneath, exudate or hematomas which lift it from its bed and infection at its periphery are the major causes of failure. Although compromises which entail mesh-grafting[53] or other techniques may be dictated by the circumstances of each patient, meticulous care must be taken to close the excised wound completely.

Nowhere is the importance of such principles more forcefully demonstrated than in the burned hand, which presents intricate problems of judgment and care.[50, 51] The palm rarely suffers full-thickness flame burn, but the relatively thin and elastic skin of the dorsum is essential to normal function and is frequently burned most deeply over the extensor surface of the joints. If the burn is distinctly a partial-thickness injury and shows good sensitivity to pinprick for the first 5 days, spontaneous healing should occur if infection is controlled. Topical agents and allografts provide this protection and assurance. During the period of healing, elevation, careful splinting and supervised periods of active and passive motion produce the best results.

Full-thickness burns of the hands too often are combined with similar wounds of the upper extremity or generalized body burns that assume priority in treatment so that life may be saved. The circulation to the hand is severely compromised by circumferential burns of the extremity. The damage caused by ischemia in the first few hours is frequently reflected in ultimate necrosis of the distal fingers and inordinate fibrosis of the intrinsic muscles of the hand. Escharotomy of all constricting mechanisms must be done early and be reviewed repeatedly to determine adequacy. In the hand, incisions may need to be extended along the lateral sides of the fingers and include fasciotomy of thenar or hypothenar muscles.

Excision and graft of the dorsum in full-thickness burns of the hand are strongly indicated as soon as the condition of the patient will permit. The best results are obtained when the graft is fairly thick and large enough to cover most of the dorsum. The junctions of grafts should not be placed over a joint area. Because pain, prolonged immobilization and an unhealed wound cause such severe joint stiffness and later contracture, it appears preferable to perform primary excision on some hand burns that are of deep second-degree depth. The decision must be made within the first 3–4 days, however, if good results are to be obtained.

Treatment of the Infected Wound

Even superficial burns become infected. To prevent deepening of the wound, frequent dressings with saline and topical agents are indicated. Cultures must be taken to guide specificity of treatment. With early recognition and appropriate attention such wounds heal rapidly.

There are more exudate, dead tissue and infected blister fluid in shallow, partial-thickness wounds. Topical agents are effective in limiting the growth of existing organisms, and the debriding effect of "wet to dry" saline or 0.5% silver nitrate dressings is beneficial in extensive burns in the hospital. If beta-hemolytic streptococcus is cultured, penicillin therapy is indicated for 10 days even though culture results may turn negative. Otherwise, antibiotics should be withheld unless clear evidence is found of local or bloodstream invasion with a specific organism. Allografts or heterografts that are changed every 8–12 hours also limit the destructiveness of large areas of infected burn.[41, 49]

Deep partial-thickness infected burns present problems of judgment, in that the quantity of dead tissue for bacterial multiplication is significant, and the organisms involve the deeper layers. These areas are often mixed with full-thickness burn areas, and the patient may be quite toxic from invasive infection. It becomes imperative to use all methods to limit bacterial growth, including active wound debridement, topical antibacterial agents and systemic antibiotics appropriate to the organisms cultured. Vigorous wound manipulation may cause septicemia, but repeated, frequent dressings and tedious removal of all dead tissue that will come away without bleeding is beneficial. The objectives are to control invasive infection with systemic antibiotic therapy and to eliminate the septic source as rapidly as possible. In rare instances wound excision must be undertaken despite its hazards. Allografts and heterografts are beneficial to areas that are not grossly purulent or do not contain large amounts of dead tissue.[46]

The full-thickness infected burn from which the eschar has not separated often harbors gross pus in the subcutaneous fat. A careful search for areas of fluctuation and excision of overlying eschar can be done with each dressing. In critical cases it is mandatory to excise or to drain the source of general septicemia by unroofing it. On occasion, salvage of a patient who is clearly in gram-negative septicemic shock can be accomplished by radical debridement and excision of infected tissue. The specific wound management is dictated by the patient's condition. The principles and objectives remain the same.

The infected, granulating full-thickness burn that contains unseparated tissue and heavy wound exudate harboring large numbers of bacteria may be the result of prolonged hypermetabolism, weight loss, inadequate nutrition and inability to close the wounds because grafts will not take. Such patients are at extreme risk. Attempts to close the wounds with autografts are unsuccessful and often produce a larger wound in the unhealing donor site. Quantitative studies of such wounds show large numbers of bacteria. Septicemia and generalized infection become common, with bacterial counts of 10^7 and 10^9/gm tissue. In addition to judicious removal of all eschar or dead tissue, the problem becomes that of restoring the patient's nutritional status and reducing the size of the wound. Severe anemia and hypoproteinemia are the rule, so that large quantities of intravenous fluid replacement are mandatory. Heterografts and allografts are effective in wound care both because they reduce the bacteria in the wound and limit the loss of protein from the edematous granulating surface.[39, 41] Modern intravenous hyperalimentation may salvage the patient who cannot accept sufficient calories by mouth, and the danger of introducing infection via intravenous central lines must be taken. Antibiotics are strongly indicated on an empirical basis, to be made more specific as culture results are reported. If infection can be controlled and nutrition improved, the "take" of an allograft becomes an excellent index of whether the patient's own skin will take in the same area.[56]

It is worth emphasis that such heavily contaminated wounds may kill the patient even though they do not represent a large percentage of the body surface. Attention to every detail of metabolic and nutritional balance is necessary for success. Even if the patient improves significantly, it may be found that grafts will not adhere unless the exuberant, edematous granulation tissue is first removed. This often can be done with minimal trauma to the deep tissues and presents an excellent bed more favorable to success of grafting.

Chemical Burns

A large number of dilute acid or alkaline agents are common to everyday life, while stronger ones are used extensively in industry or laboratories. Burns from vesicant gases and incendiary agents, such as white phosphorus, are part of the misfortunes of war. As with thermal burns, the basic process of destruction of tissue is through coagulation of protein. Some evidence exists that protein neutralizes acids more quickly than alkalies, so that caustic action of strong bases continues longer, and therefore more deeply, than acids of equivalent chemical strength. White phosphorous particles produce a thermal burn that is lessened by exclusion of oxygen, since particles spontaneously reignite in air at temperatures above 90 F.

Fortunately, most common injurious chemical substances are water soluble or can be washed off the surface of the body. Although it is conceptually attractive to neutralize acute acid burns with weak alkaline solutions, and vice versa, appropriate materials are rarely at hand. The most practical therapy is to dilute the chemical agent at once with copious amounts of water to reduce its potency and damaging effects. It is necessary to pick white phosphorous particles out of the tissues, and a 1% solution of copper sulfate has been found to stain them so that they can be identified. Since copper is toxic, it should not be used for extensive initial irrigation. The involved area should be kept soaking wet with saline prior to debridement at operation

When the destructive agent has been eliminated, the management of the chemical burn wound does not differ in practice from thermal burns. Since the chemical burn is usually not extensive, the principle of primary excision of areas of full-thickness skin destruction should be followed, although a conservative approach is indicated with facial or genital involvement. Since strong chemicals penetrate deeply, excision of all destroyed tissue may require judgment as to whether or not tendons, muscle and other important structures will be viable. In this event the wound should be covered with a sterile dressing and reviewed within 48–72 hours, at which time demarcation of nonviable tissue may indicate further excision. Tendon and periarticular structures will be protected from the added damage of drying if allografts are used to cover the wound after a primary excision of uncertain completeness. On a rare occasion a limited burn of deep structures vital to function may be closed with a full-thickness pedicle flap. In most cases, early aggressive wound care produces the best results.

Electrical Burns

The basic mechanism of electrical injury is most likely thermal. Clinical experience shows that a significant difference exists in the injuries produced by low voltage and high voltage currents.[44, 52] The short circuit and electrical spark that occurs on contact with house currents up to 220 volts usually produces a localized thermal injury, best exemplified when an infant puts the end of a home electrical outlet cord in its mouth. The wet tissues are highly conductive, and local tissue destruction is deep.

Flash burns from proximity to high-tension arcs of intense but brief heat also produce a thermal burn of the skin. However, if contact is made with a single high-tension source carrying thousands of volts, the body then becomes the most accessible pathway to the current for grounding, and wounds both of entrance and of exit of the current are produced. The part of the body closest to any grounding mechanism represents the path of least resistance. An example is the boy who stands on a metal fence as he grasps a high-tension wire and sustains obvious entrance and exit wounds, which may appear quite localized. The course taken by the current through the tissues of the body may be diffuse and shows unpredictable variations. The pathways of maximal conductivity are demonstrated by clinical experience that shows extensive damage across flexor surfaces of joints and deep destruction of muscle and fascia along the course of major blood vessels, even though the overlying skin usually gives no early sign of the destruction beneath. Finally whether thermal in origin or through other mechanisms, the blood vessel walls sustain primary injury, the extent of which becomes apparent only as thrombosis occurs during the subsequent 10 days. Therefore, the initial manifestations of electrical injury resemble the crush syndrome with extensive occult destruction of muscle which releases hemoglobin, requires large blood volume replacement and is highly susceptible to infection by pyogenic and clostridial bacteria. Progressive thrombosis of injured arteries is followed by further tissue necrosis, so that detection of the extent of the wounds and the dangers of sepsis are unresolved for many days.

The management of the low-voltage electrical injury is guided by the principles of excision and debridement of destroyed tissue in 1 or more stages as the extent of damage becomes defined.[54] The same treatment applies to the entrance and exit wounds of high-tension burns, although here it is common to discover localized deep destruction which may even necrose bone. In many patients the involvement is most severe near points of entry or where current has arced across the flexion creases of joints. Operation discloses progressively less severe effects on muscle and fascia as exploration proceeds centrally; it is as if the current had gradually become dissipated as it flowed up an arm or leg.

After resuscitation it is essential to determine where necrosis from direct contact or arterial thrombosis has occurred. This can only be done at operation and may require exploratory incisions through normal skin or as extensions of areas of cutaneous burn. Obviously damaged muscle is purple and soft, but fibers which will ultimately necrose are only slightly pale, of normal texture and may even bleed. It is a universal experience that the initial excision which has apparently been carried to margins of bleeding viable tissue is rarely adequate. Since vascular thrombosis is progressive, repeated explorations, enlargement of wounds and debridement are required to discover and excise further devitalized tissue. Amputation is frequently necessary, although every effort should be made to retain what initially appears to be a useless extremity unless severe infection supervenes. Since secondary major arterial hemorrhage is a constant hazard, points of arterial ligation should be buried in normal tissue, if possible.

Surgical therapy of high-tension electrical burns resembles that of war wounds. After each debridement the wound is gently packed open, until ultimately the findings of healthy granulating tissues give evidence that the process of arterial thrombosis has reached its limit and no devitalized tissue remains. Only then is it clear that the dangers of infection have passed and that measures to close the wound can be undertaken.

FUNCTION OF SYSTEMS AND ORGANS

Respiratory Impairment

DIRECT CAUSES. — Primary injury to the respiratory tract from heat, smoke and fumes accompanies many burns and is an outstanding cause of death in the early postburn days or weeks.[69] The pattern of injury reflects the circumstances at the time of the burn. In the experimental animal, hot air rarely causes injury distal to the carina. Steam produces airway damage farther distally, the hot carbon particulate matter of smoke carries the heat deeper into the lung, and gases or fumes given off by some combustible materials enter and damage alveoli. Manifestly, the respiratory injury may reflect any or all such mechanisms.[74]

Laryngeal or tracheal edema follows the pattern of a cutaneous burn and results in early upper airway obstruction. Similarly, injury from the tracheal through the bronchiolar level causes swelling, exudate and denudation of epithelium with diffuse obstructive effects and atelectasis. Combustion products such as sulfur and nitric oxide gases resemble phosgene war gas and cause a rapid alveolar pulmonary edema.

It is rarely clinically possible to identify these mechanisms individually, since all are seen as obvious respiratory distress from hypoxia, and, except for the stridor of laryngeal edema, physical and x-ray signs are usually normal. Furthermore, the hypoxic evidences of a "pulmonary burn" may not become detectable until the third day after injury, and evidence of hypervolemic pulmonary edema, atelectasis or early pulmonary infection may be absent. The only clinical manifestations may be an increasing respiratory rate, with initial lowering of blood P_{CO_2} values followed by increasing restlessness and falling blood P_{O_2} values.[63]

The dangers of tracheal intubation or ventilatory support for patients with respiratory involvement are greatly compounded by the susceptibility of the injured airways to infection. Whereas early tracheostomy was formerly advocated on suspicion of damage to the airways, the almost inevitable sequelae of sepsis, tracheitis and pneumonitis are strong arguments for a conservative approach. This is only safe if intensive observation, pulmonary physiotherapy and monitoring of blood gases are available.[70] The details of respiratory management[65] are given in Chapter 43. Suffice it to say that any direct manipulation of the burned airway should be grounded on strong positive indications and that all inlying tracheal tubes should be removed promptly when respiratory function shows they are not absolutely necessary.[61]

When primary respiratory injury is suspected, it is reasonable to use a large dose of corticosteroids designed to diminish the inflammatory response and its secondary effects on aeration. To be effective, this must be begun as early as possible after the burn and continued for 3-4 days. It is clinically difficult to assess the value of steroids in any way other than empirical use in a large number of cases. There appear to be few ill effects, however. The same reasoning applies to the use of antibiotics for the first 5 days after injury. Penicillin is favored, but results of tracheal cultures should guide therapy. Scrupulous aseptic technique in aspirations or tracheostomy care are mandatory. Two weeks are required for the burned tracheal or bronchial epithelium to separate and heal and twice that time for the cilia which protect the lung against sepsis to regenerate.

INDIRECT MECHANISMS.—Severe anoxia at the time of the burn may damage the brain and cause central respiratory mechanisms to be lost. Resuscitation usually requires tracheal intubation and respiratory assistance until the brain recovers. Experience shows that full return of cerebral function should be anticipated in most instances, particularly in children.

Circumferential involvement of the thorax and upper abdomen by full-thickness burns causes a restriction of thoracic excursion. Although the degree to which this mechanism impairs normal respiration is difficult to measure, the restriction is clinically obvious, and the release of thoracic confinement by escharotomy is often dramatic.

Defects of 3 mechanisms involving oxygen transport by red cells are recognized in burn care. Carbon monoxide poisoning at the time of the burn can be measured and is treated by high concentrations of inhaled oxygen and maintenance of normal blood pH. A rare instance of methemoglobinuria is encountered when 0.5% silver nitrate dressings are used and organisms capable of converting nitrates to nitrites are present in the wound.[72] Methemoglobin levels as high as 3 gm/100 ml have been identified; these rapidly return to normal when use of silver nitrate is discontinued. Finally, since stored bank blood is often low in content of the 2,3-diphosphoglycerate enzyme responsible for release of oxygen from red cells at the tissue level, extensive transfusion therapy should include a significant portion of fresh blood.

As with general trauma and infection, the burned patient demonstrates a very high metabolic rate, cardiac output and oxygen requirement. It is not surprising occasionally to find a syndrome of high-output respiratory failure, identified by tachypnea and deteriorating blood gas values, when extensive sepsis and chronically unhealed wounds exist. If severe malnutrition and hypoproteinemia have also been present, autopsy shows diffuse pulmonary interstitial edema, hyaline membranes and alveolar thickening, which support the clinical impression that oxygenation of the blood is impaired at the alveolar level. Combinations of these mechanisms produce a type of respiratory failure that requires immediate respiratory assistance, vigorous correction of anemia and hypoproteinemia and the administration of furosemide to prevent hypervolemia. Control of sepsis in the burn wound and its closure prevent recurrence, but until that time it is important to recognize that oxygen requirements in the presence of open wounds and hypermetabolism approach the limits of the body's respiratory mechanisms of supply and that minimal added demands from whatever cause result in critical tissue hypoxia. Respiratory assistance and rapid correction of basic causes alone may save the patient.

Renal Impairment

The power of adjustment of normal kidneys is so great that nearly 80% of maximal renal function can be lost before the kidneys fail to accomplish the demands of the body. This vast reserve may be reduced by a general hypoxia at the time of the burn and is further impaired when diminished renal perfusion occurs because vascular volume is not reconstituted quickly. The destruction of red cells with extensive or deep burns adds free hemoglobin to the renal load, which appears as acid hematin owing to the acidity of the urine. With an electrical burn, muscle damage may release myoglobin as well. The presence of these substances with hypoperfusion results in obstruction of renal tubules. This mechanism of renal shutdown is the one most familiar to early burn therapy and is greatly compounded in patients with pre-existing renal disease. Other forms of renal impairment include a specific interstitial nephritis secondary to administration of kanamycin, gentamicin, polymyxin or oxacillin and, rarely, a true renal cortical necrosis. Hypoperfusion from gram-negative septicemia is reflected in low renal output, and specific renal abscesses with parenchymal invasion often is a terminal occurrence in patients who die of uncontrolled sepsis.

Since acute tubular necrosis may be accompanied by polyuria rather than oliguria,[60] it is important to identify it by examination of the urinary sediment and osmolarity of the urine. In acute burns, oliguria usually reflects inadequate blood volume replacement. Damage is minimized by establishing urine flow with mannitol and alkalinizing the urine with sodium bicarbonate, 0.5 mm/kg. Repair of renal tubular damage is usually substantial within 12–14 days if further damage can be avoided. Rarely, full renal failure may require dialysis and the intricate metabolic management that it entails.

Cardiac Function

Studies of burn toxins in patients with acute burns suggest that an early depressive effect on myocardial function may occur.[59, 66] It is more certain that the marked hypermetabolism and increased cardiac output of large infected burns impose severe demands on the myocardium. At autopsy, degenerative changes in the muscle fibers have been described, while embolic abscesses, valvulitis and endocarditis may occur as part of an overwhelming septicemia.

Pre-existing disease will determine the bounds within which the myocardium can meet the metabolic or volumetric demands. There is nothing peculiar to burns about identification of right or left heart failure, or treatment of arrhythmias. A constant area of debate is whether or not digitalis should be used. Because major changes in electrolyte concentrations are expected early in burn therapy, there is some hazard of inducing arrhythmia. In critical cases of sepsis with requirement for large volume replacement, the empirical use of digitalis may be justified. In general, it should be used only on specific indication, as is true also of inotropic agents or specific medications to control arrhythmias.

Cerebral Function

Fires in a closed space may consume most of the available oxygen and produce high concentrations of carbon monoxide. Victims often become unconscious, fail to escape and sustain severe body burns as a result. The sensitivity of the brain to anoxia may be manifested as a "watershed" syndrome wherein hypovolemia and decrease in arterial oxygen combine to cause maximal cerebral damage to the portions of the cerebral cortex farthest from the midline and with the least vigorous perfusion.[57] Such patients require early resuscitation and maximal oxygen concentrations in the circulating blood. Anoxic cerebral injury is followed by cerebral edema, so that general therapy must be designed to anticipate it. Early replacement fluid should contain adequate colloid with volume kept to a minimum. Respiratory assistance and anticonvulsants may be necessary. Unless the electroencephalogram shows no cortical activity for at least 3 days, "brain death" cannot be assumed, and dramatic recovery frequently follows a program of consistent support.

Hypoproteinemia, excessive fluid volume, high fever and electrolyte imbalance are reflected in the appearance of cerebral symptoms.[57] Throughout the course of therapy it is necessary to avoid water intoxication and to maintain homeostasis for maximal cerebral function.

Gastrointestinal Function

The gastrointestinal tract quickly reflects all major disturbances of hypoxia, hypoperfusion, electrolyte balance, sepsis, anemia and hypoproteinemia by reduction in peristaltic activity. This ileus is seen immediately after a severe burn and results in gastric retention, so that vomiting with associated dangers of aspiration becomes an important hazard to the patient. The stomach should be emptied and kept empty until ileus subsides.

Acute gastric or duodenal ulceration has been recognized as a concomitant of severe burns for many years.[67] Although Curling's ulcer is classically duodenal and is interpreted as a response to stress, similar to ulcers from steroid administration, gastric ulcerations are also common in prolonged burn treatment, and diffuse superficial gastric erosions may follow gastric distention or an episode of hypoxia and hypoperfusion. Whether or not the same mechanisms cause such varied types of ulceration is unclear, but all respond best to measures designed to combat gastric hyperacidity or retention. Both treatment and prevention involve frequent intake of milk or antacids given by nasogastric tube, if necessary. When prevention is begun in the early phases of injury, the incidence of gastrointestinal hemorrhage or proved peptic ulcer is markedly reduced. Rarely, uncontrolled hemorrhage requires operation, and this must be undertaken even though the incision is made through cutaneous burn.

Efforts to maximize oral caloric intake may result in diarrhea because of a heavy osmolar load or because the component of dietary protein exceeds the abilities of the patient to break it down completely for resynthesis. Here there is no alternative but to cut back sharply on intake until the symptoms subside. Opiates in small doses are helpful.

Edema from hypoproteinemia is quickly reflected as intestinal hypomotility, with probable impairment of absorption. Syndromes such as partial obstruction at the level of the superior mesenteric artery are probably based on such circumstances. Finally, it is clearly recognized that 1 of the earliest signs of invasive sepsis and septicemia is ileus. In all cases, correction of the cause is more effective than specific gastrointestinal treatment.

Metabolic and Nutritional Responses

Acutely burned patients are subject to the neuroendocrine mechanisms that have been dissected in the laboratory over the past 25 years and others which collectively make up the metabolic response to trauma. The early shock phase of burn injury presents a particularly severe interval, in which tissue necrosis, fluid and electrolyte shifts, alterations in the body's fluid compartments and impairments of organ function from toxins, anoxia or hypoperfusion are most active.[62] The persistence and ultimate infection of a large burn wound cause a prolongation of the mechanisms of injury and a sustained hypermetabolic response, in the course of which it is difficult to study the individual components that contribute to the over-all metabolic derangements. To the original concept of an alarm reaction in which the hypophyseal-adrenocortical axis was emphasized, there have been added studies of serum cortisol levels, implication of a renin-angiotensin-spironolactone mechanism, more detailed examination of thyroid function and investigation of calcium metabolism. From the therapeutic standpoint, understanding has not advanced far enough to support specific endocrine manipulation during the course of a burn. Deficits in electrolyte balance, protein, red cell mass and volume of circulating plasma are corrected as they occur, however.

The persistence of the burn wound not only is the stimulus for a marked hypermetabolism from evaporative water loss and energy expenditure but also is a cause for continuous nutritional depletion from wound exudates. Measurements show cardiac outputs up to 5 times normal, with corresponding caloric requirements. It is not suprising that the body reflects these metabolic demands in an elevated temperature, which must be distinguished from fever caused by extensive sepsis. Shivering can be controlled by chlorpromazine and fever by antipyretics, whereas invasive sepsis requires specific antibiotics. It is important to recognize that moderate fever is a concomitant of large burn wounds. It most often reflects hypermetabolism and not sepsis amenable to antibiotic treatment.

Since protein metabolism is so central to the burned patient's nutrition, nitrogen balance studies that include measurement of wound exudates have been accentuated in metabolic studies. The results demonstrate a negative nitrogen balance which persists even after the wounds are closed. The deficit often exceeds the bounds of tolerable protein intake by mouth, and forced feeding results in diarrhea which defeats its purpose. Many dietary supplements of simplified protein constituents help to overcome problems of intake, and recent refinements have also produced oral fat supplements for incorporation into the diet or tube feedings. Maximal intake of carbohydrate is essential to all high-caloric dietary regimens, and regular vitamin supplements are given orally or intravenously.

Patients do best if high-calorie foods are offered frequently throughout the 24 hours. If anorexia or vomiting occurs, tube feedings can be used. Gastric distention can be avoided by preliminary aspiration followed by slow administration of a blenderized feeding. There is no dietary supplement as effective as oral foods that are palatable to the patient and none simpler than milk and its products.

In recent years the improvements in

intravenous hyperalimentation give promise of significant support in solving the over-all problems of nutrition. This route can supply 3,000 calories a day. Since severely burned adults may require almost twice that quantity to avoid malnutrition, the necessity for oral feedings remains. Also, there have been promising improvements in fat solutions that can be administered through peripheral veins. The essential feature of all intravenous nutrition is that administration can be continuous rather than sporadic. A heavy hyperosmolar carbohydrate load not only places volumetric demands on the circulation but also taxes the insulin-producing power of the pancreas. It is important to prevent contamination in the centrally placed intravenous catheters required to administer hyperosmolar fluids. Only meticulous care of apparatus and solutions guards against septicemia, which is the direct result of infection in the lines and is difficult to identify in patients who have many potential mechanisms of bloodstream contamination. Prompt removal of central lines is the first step if the patient shows signs of septicemia.

Musculoskeletal Function

Since most burns do not extend to muscles, joints or bones, the major therapeutic consideration concerns maintenance of function and protection against joint stiffness and the crippling deformities of contracture. With minor burns limited to flat surfaces or those where immobilization is essential to the care of grafted areas, splints and bulky dressings afford the physiologic rest necessary to wound care during the relatively short period required for healing. Deep burns that cross joints demand aggressive treatment designed to close the wound with viable skin as quickly as possible. In this manner the underlying joint is protected against infection and excessive periarticular fibrosis, and active efforts to maintain full ranges of motion can be instituted early after healing.

Whether or not early operation is indicated for any part of the body, it is essential that all joints near burned areas be splinted to prevent contracture and that general measures of physiotherapy be applied daily or more often to retain joint function.[73] These measures are particularly important in burns of the hands, where contractures, the boutonniere deformity or stiffness may cause permanent crippling.

Extensive experience has shown that use of skeletal traction permits elevation of burned extremities, facilitates dressings, minimizes edema, improves the success of grafting procedures and prevents or overcomes late wound contractures and joint deformity. This is now well established in burn care.[64] Although sepsis may occur around the tract of a pin and rarely a sequestrum may develop, skeletal suspension and traction should be used confidently when they serve a definite function, and pins should be removed if they become loose or as soon as they are no longer useful.

Weight loss, debility and pain limit the patient's motion in bed. Prevention of pressure sores over the heels, sacrum, scapulae or spine demands excellent nursing care. Despite extensive dressings and inlying tubes or lines, a burned patient should be gotten out of bed whenever possible

Pain and Suffering

Pain is a constant feature of burn injury. Even with trivial burns it is annoying. In care and therapy of major burns there is a constant concern with control of pain without adding drug dependency to the list of the patient's problems. Another essential factor of management is to provide adequate sleep for patients whose metabolic rate is high, whose active care runs around the clock and who are virtually never comfortable. Much of the basal need is satisfied by tranquilizing and sedative drugs, such as diazepam, meprobamate and chlorpromazine, instead of specific analgesics, narcotics or barbiturates that may require escalation of dosage to remain effective. It is essential that combinations of drugs be minimized and that control of pain be as specific as possible.

Although full-thickness burn areas are relatively intensitive from the time of injury, other areas are not, and the changing of dressings often is so uncomfortable as to represent a terrifying daily experience. Minor debridement can be done and skin grafts applied to wounds without anesthesia. Tranquilizers, with or without minimal narcotic dosage, are preferred to control anxiety and pain. Various short-acting inhalation anesthetics to cover the pain of major dressings are effective but hazardous if given at the bedside. Ketamine given intravenously represents a great advance despite a tendency to unpleasant hallucinatory aftereffects. In general, patients can be treated humanely and effectively with appropriately gentle dressing techniques and with ketamine anesthesia for more significant manipulations. The periods of withdrawal of oral intake which general anesthesia necessitates must be minimal.

Although adjustment of the patient and family to the devastating effects of a burn is commonly consigned to the rehabilitation phase of the injury, there is ample evidence that early and constant support is essential to the ultimate salvage of the patient as a human being. Conversely, when such supportive measures are not utilized from the start, patients may lose heart and fail to participate actively in treatment and the physical and emotional processes so necessary for nutrition, maintenance of physical functions and cosmetic or functional reconstructive measures. The burn need not be large for such crippling emotional effects to occur, although usually it is deep enough to leave a scar. The full tragedy of facial or hand burns is realized slowly as the patient recovers and the disappointments and limitations of reconstructive surgery become apparent. Unhappily no society has developed the universal ability to accept such visible deformities with compassion rather than revulsion or staring.

The most beneficial surgical treatment available is rapid wound closure. Here, as in all features of burn care, constant attention, companionship and support must be provided by doctors and nurses. Since their clinical duties unavoidably add to a patient's discomfort, even the most dramatic results may be nullified unless other benevolent forces are brought to bear. This involves family and personnel skilled in psychologic and sociologic disciplines, which may include psychiatry and religion.[71] These persons form the bridge between the patient and a future worthwhile existence and are essential to the ultimate success of all treatment.

BIBLIOGRAPHY

Shock

1. Abbott, W. E., Pilling, M. S., Griffin, G. L., Hirshfeld, J. W., and Meyer, F. L.: Metabolic alterations following thermal burns: V. The use of whole blood and an electrolyte solution in the treatment of the burned patient, Ann. Surg. 122:678, 1945.
2. Baxter, C. R., and Shires, T.: Physiological response to crystalloid resuscitation of severe burns, Ann. NY Acad. Sci. 150:874, 1968.
3. Blalock, A.: Disorders of the Circulatory System: Shock or Peripheral Circulatory Failure, in *Principles of Surgical Care* (St. Louis: C. V. Mosby Company, 1940).
4. Burke, J. F., and Constable, J. D.: Systemic changes in replacement therapy in burns, J. Trauma 5:242, 1965.
5. Cope, O., and Moore, F. D.: The redistribution of body water and the fluid therapy of the burned patient, Ann. Surg. 126:1010, 1947.
6. Cotran, R. S.: The delayed and prolonged vascular leakage in inflammation, Am. J. Pathol. 46:589, 1965.
7. Davies, J. W. L., Jackson, D. M., and Cason, J. S.: A comparison of the efficacy of plasma and sodium salts, Ann. NY Acad. Sci. 150:852, 1968.
8. Evans, E. I., Purnell, O. J., Robinett, P. W., Batchelor, A., and Martin, M.: Fluid and electrolyte requirements in severe burns, Ann. Surg. 135:804, 1952.
9. Guyton, A. C., and Coleman, T. G.: Regulation of interstitial fluid volume and pressure, Ann. NY Acad. Sci. 150:537, 1968.
10. Moore, F. D., Peacock, W., Blakely, E., and Cope, O.: The anemia of thermal burns, Ann. Surg. 124:811, 1946.
11. Moyer, C. A., Margraf, H. W., and Monafo, W. W., Jr.: Burn shock in association with extravascular sodium deficiency: A report on

the treatment with Ringer's solution with lactate, Arch. Surg. 90:799, 1965.
12. Muir, I. F. K.: Red cell destruction in burns with particular reference to the shock period, Br. J. Plast. Surg. 14:273, 1961.
13. Quinby, W. C., and Cope, O.: Blood viscosity and the whole blood therapy of burns, Surgery 32:316, 1952.
14. Raker, J. W., and Rovit, R. L.: Acute red blood cell destruction following severe thermal trauma in dogs, Surg. Gynecol. Obstet. 98:169, 1954.
15. Reiss, E., Artz, C. P., Davis, J. H., and Amspacher, W. H.: Fluid and electrolyte balance in burns, JAMA 152:1309, 1953.
16. Sorensen, B., Sejresen, P., and Thomsen, M.: Dextran solutions in the treatment of burn shock, Scand. J. Plast. Reconstr. Surg. 1:68, 1967.
17. Underhill, F. P., Kapsinow, R., and Fish, M. E.: Studies on water exchange in animal organism, Am. J. Physiol. 95:302, 1930.

Infection

18. Alexander, J. W., Brown, W., Mason, A. D., Jr., and Moncrief, J. A.: The influence of infection on serum protein changes in severe burns, J. Trauma 6:780, 1966.
19. Alexander, J. W., Dionigi, R. and Meakins, R. L.: Periodic variation in the antibacterial function of human neutrophils and its relationship to sepsis, Ann. Surg. 173:206, 1971.
20. Arturson, G., Hogman, C. F., Johansson, S. G. O., and Killander, J.: Changes in immunoglobulin levels in severely burned patients, Lancet 1:546, 1969.
21. Burke, J. F.: Isolation Techniques and Their Effectiveness, in Polk, H. C., and Stone, H. H., (eds.): *Contemporary Burn Management* (Boston: Little, Brown & Company, 1971), p. 141.
22. Burke, J. F., Bondoc, C. C., and Morris, P. J.: Metabolic effects of topical silver nitrate therapy in burns covering more than 15% of the body surface, Ann. NY Acad. Sci. 150:674, 1968.
23. Cannon, B., and Cope, O.: Rate of epithelial regeneration: A clinical method of testing various agents recommended in the treatment of burns, Ann. Surg. 117:85, 1943.
24. Collentine, G. E., Jr., Waisbren, B. A., and Mellender, J. W.: Treatment of burns with intensive antibiotic therapy and exposure, JAMA 200:939, 1967.
25. Feller, I., Vial, B., Collahen, W. S., and Waldyke, J.: Use of vaccine and hyperimmune serum for protection against Pseudomonas septicemia, J. Trauma 4:451, 1964.
26. Fox, C. L., Jr.: Control of pseudomonas infection in burns by silver sulfadiazine, Surg. Gynecol. Obstet. 128:1021, 1969.
27. Hummel, R. P., Rivera, J. A., and Artz, C. P.: Evaluation of several antibiotics used locally on granulating wounds caused by thermal injury, Ann. Surg. 146:808, 1957.
28. Langohr, J. L., Owen, C. R., and Cope, O.: Bacteriologic study of burn wounds, Ann. Surg. 125:452, 1947.
29. Lindberg, R. B., Moncrief, J. A., and Mason, A. D., Jr.: Control of experimental and clinical burn wound sepsis by topical application of sulfamylon compounds, Ann. NY Acad. Sci. 150:950, 1968.
30. MacMillan, B. G., and Altemeier, W. A.: Homograft skin: A valuable adjunct to the treatment of thermal burns, J. Trauma 2:130, 1962.
31. Monafo, W. W., Brentano, L., et al.: Gas gangrene and mixed clostridial infections of muscle complicating deep thermal burns, Arch. Surg. 92:212, 1966.
32. Moncrief, J. A., Jr., Lindberg, R. B., Switzer, W. E., and Pruitt, B. A., Jr.: Use of topical antibacterial therapy in the treatment of the burn wound, Arch. Surg. 92:558, 1966.
33. Moyer, C. A., Brentano, L., Gravens, D. L., Margraf, H. W., and Monafo, W. W.: Treatment of large human burns with 0.5% silver nitrate solution, Arch. Surg. 90:812, 1965.
34. Polk, H. C., Jr., Ward, C. G., Clarkson, J. G., and Taplin, D.: Early detection of pseudomonas burn infection: Clinical experience with Wood's light fluorescence, Arch. Surg. 98:292, 1969.
35. Rittenbury, M. S., and Hanback, L. D.: Phagocytic depression in thermal injuries, J. Trauma 7:523, 1967.
36. Ritzman, S. E., Larson, D. L., McClung, C., Abston, S., Falls, D., and Goldman, A. S.: Immunoglobulin levels in burned patients, Lancet 1:1152, 1969.
37. Stone, H. H.: Review of pseudomonas sepsis in thermal burns: Verdoglobin determination and gentamicin therapy, Ann. Surg. 163:297, 1966.
38. Teplitz, C.: Pathogenesis of pseudomonas vasculitis and septic lesions, Arch. Pathol. 80:297, 1965.

Wound

39. Artz, C. P., Becker, J. M., Sako, Y., and Bronwell, A. W.: Postmortem skin homografts in the treatment of extensive burns, Arch. Surg. 71:682, 1955.
40. Bondoc, C. C., and Burke, J. F.: Clinical experience with viable frozen human skin and a frozen skin bank, Ann. Surg. 174:371, 1971.
41. Brown, J. B., Fryer, M. P., Randall, P., and Lus, M.: Postmortem homografts as biological dressings for extensive burns and denuded areas: Immediate and preserved homografts as life-saving procedures, Ann. Surg. 138:618, 1953.
42. Cope, O., Langohr, J. L., Moore, F. D., and Webster, R. G., Jr.: Expeditious care of full-thickness burn wounds by surgical excision and grafting, Ann. Surg. 125:1, 1947.
43. Cramer, L. M., McCormack, R. M., and Carrol, D. B.: Progressive partial excision and early grafting in lethal burns, Plast. Reconstr. Surg. 30:595, 1962.
44. DiVincenti, G. S., Moncrief, J. A., and Pruitt, B. A.: Electrical injuries: A review of 65 cases, J. Trauma 9:497, 1969.
45. Jendren, W. H., Constable, J. D., and Zawacki, B. E.: Early partial excision of major burns in children, J. Pediatr. Surg. 3:445, 1968.
46. Jackson, D.: A clinical study of the use of skin homografts for burns, Br. J. Plast. Surg. 7:26, 1954.
47. Leape, L. L., and Randolph, J. G.: The early

surgical treatment of burns: II. Clinical application of intravenous vital dye (patent blue V) in the differentiation of partial and full-thickness burns, Surgery 57:886, 1965.
48. Meeker, I. A., Jr., and Snyder, W. H., Jr.: Dermatome debridement and early grafting of extensive third degree burns in children, Surg. Gynecol Obstet. 103:527, 1956.
49. Miller, T. A., Switzer, W. E., Foley, F. D., and Moncrief, J. A.: Early homografting of second degree burns, Plast. Reconstr. Surg. 40:117, 1967.
50. Moncrief, J. A., Switzer, W. E., and Rose, L. R.: Primary excision and grafting in the treatment of third degree burns of the dorsum of the hand, Plast. Reconstr. Surg. 33:305, 1964.
51. Peacock, E. E., Jr., Madden, J. W., and Trier, W. C.: Some studies on the treatment of burned hands, Ann. Surg. 171:903, 1970.
52. Robinson, D. W., Masters, F. W., and Forrest, W. J.: Electrical burns: A review and analysis of 33 cases, Surgery 57:385, 1965.
53. Tanner, J. C., Jr., Vandeput, J., and Olley, J. F.: The mesh skin grafts, Plast. Reconstr. Surg. 34:287, 1964.
54. Wells, D. B.: The treatment of electric burns by immediate resection and skin graft, Ann. Surg. 90:1069, 1929.
55. Whittaker, A. H.: Treatment of burns by excision and immediate grafting, Am. J. Surg. 85:411, 1953.
56. Zarkoff, L. I., Mills, W., Sr., Duckett, S. W., Jr., Switzer, W. E., and Moncrief, J. A.: Multiple uses of viable cutaneous homografts in the burned patient, Surgery 59:368, 1966.

Systems and organs

57. Antoon, A. Y., Volpe, J. J., and Crawford, J. D.: Burns encephalopathy, Pediatrics 50:609, 1972.
58. Barr, P. O., Burke, G., Liljedahl, S. O., and Plantin, L. O.: Oxygen consumption and water loss during treatment of burns with warm dry air, Lancet 1:164, 1968.
59. Baxter, C. R., Cook, W. A., and Shires, G. T.: Serum myocardial depressant factor of burn shock, Surg. Forum 17:1, 1966.
60. Baxter, C. R., Zedlitz, W. H., and Shires, G. T.: High output acute renal failure complicating traumatic injury, J. Trauma 4:567, 1964.
61. Cooper, J. D., and Grillo, H. C.: The evolution of tracheal injury due to ventilatory assistance through cuffed tubes: A pathologic study, Ann. Surg. 169:334, 1969.
62. Davies, J. W. L., and Liljedahl, S. O.: Metabolic Consequences of an Extensive Burn, in Polk, H. C., and Stone, H. H. (eds.): *Contemporary Burn Management* (Boston: Little, Brown & Company, 1971), p. 151.
63. Harrison, H. N.: Respiratory tract injury, pathophysiology and response to therapy among burned patients, Ann. NY Acad. Sci. 150:627, 1968.
64. Larson, D. L., Evans, E. B., Abston, S., and Lewis, S. R.: Skeletal suspension and traction in the treatment of burns, Ann. Surg. 168:981, 1968.
65. Lee, A. B., and Kinney, J. M.: Ventilatory management of the pulmonary burn, Ann. NY Acad. Sci. 150:738, 1968.
66. Merriman, J. W., Jr., and Jackson, R.: Myocardial function following thermal injury, Circ. Res. 11:669, 1962.
67. Moncrief, J. A., Switzer, W. E., and Teplitz, C.: Curling's ulcer, J. Trauma 4:481, 1964.
68. Mulder, D. S., and Rubush, J.: Complications of tracheostomy: Relativity to long term ventilatory assistance, J. Trauma 9:389, 1969.
69. Phillips, A. W., Tanner, J. W., and Cope, O.: Burn therapy: IV. Respiratory tract damage and the meaning of restlessness, Ann. Surg. 158:799, 1963.
70. Pontoppidan, H., Laver, M. B., and Geffin, B.: Acute Respiratory Failure in the Surgical Patient, in C. E. Welch (ed.): *Advances in Surgery* (Chicago: Year Book Medical Publishers, Inc., 1970), Vol. 4, p. 163.
71. Quinby, S. V. C., and Bernstein, N. R.: How children live after disfiguring burns, Psychiatry Med. 2:146, 1971.
72. Ternberg, J. L., and Luce, E.: Methemoglobinemia: A complication of the silver nitrate treatment of burns, Surgery 63:328, 1968.
73. Willis, B.: The use of orthoplast isoprene splints in the treatment of the acutely burned child: Further report, Am. J. Occup. Ther. 24:1, 1970.
74. Zirka, B. A., Sturner, W. Q., Astarjian, N. K., Fox, C. L., Jr., and Fener, J. M., Jr.: Respiratory tract damage in burn: Pathophysiology and treatment, Ann. NY Acad. Sci. 150:618, 1968.

51 | Injuries Due to Cold

FRANK C. WHEELOCK, JR., and LESLIE W. OTTINGER

ALTHOUGH it is true that in civilian life injuries due to cold are relatively uncommon, they can and do occur sufficiently often to deserve our consideration. In this chapter we will describe the important pathologic and physiologic factors and outline appropriate treatment. Since frostbite is the most serious cold injury, most of our discussion will center on this. The less common and less serious injuries—trench foot, immersion foot and chilblain—will be discussed at the end of the chapter.

HISTORICAL CONSIDERATIONS

Frostbite has been a major consideration in military campaigns for centuries—perhaps most familiar to us from the history of the American Revolution and the Napoleonic Wars. More recently, it is of record that there were 115,361 cases of frostbite or trench foot in the British forces in World War I and 46,000 cold injuries among United States troops in World War II. The latter group averaged 50 days of hospitalization. That it was a serious problem in this war is further supported by the fact that cold injury caused more casualties to the British Air Force than did enemy fire from 1942 to 1944.[4] Even more recently, many cold injuries from the Korean War have been reported.[9]

Other dramatic reports of cold injury are to be found in the annals of various mountain-climbing expeditions and in tales of shipwrecks. In many cases, a lack of fundamental knowledge of prevention and treatment is obvious in these reports—a situation that has caused needless damage to those involved.

DEFINITIONS AND FACTORS PRODUCING INJURY DUE TO COLD

Frostbite is a term applied when a part is cooled enough to solidify—that is, to the point of actually freezing. Trench foot and immersion foot are cold injuries from lesser temperatures, usually requiring prolonged exposure in the presence of moisture. Freezing does not occur.

The production of frostbite depends on local conditions of the exposed part and on the general condition of the person involved. Air is a poor conductor of heat whereas metal is an excellent conductor, so that touching very cold metal is indeed dangerous. Moving air will produce frostbite much more effectively than quiet air. As an example, Washburn[11] points out that a thermometer reading of 20° F with a 45-mph wind is equivalent to −40° F with a wind of 2 mph. The duration of the exposure obviously is of great importance also.

The patient's general condition plays a major role. If one is generally cold, blood is shunted away from surface areas to keep the vital organs warm enough to function. In this event, peripheral frostbite can occur more easily. Lack of oxygen or inadequate food intake curtails activity that would generate heat and help prevent frostbite. On the other hand, excessive activity is dangerous in that too much heat can be lost via the lungs and by evaporation of sweat. Injury, fear, panic, exhaustion, habitual smoking and advanced age increase the occurrence and extent of injuries due to cold. Alcohol is the most common predisposing factor in civilian practice, being noted in 65% of our cases at Massachusetts General Hospital. It is generally accepted that racial background is of importance in that Negroes tolerate cold poorly[6] whereas Eskimos and certain South American Indians have great resistance to cold. Yet another obvious factor may be the presence of occlusive arterial disease, which allows tissues to be injured more easily.

Prevention consists fundamentally of wearing adequate clothing and avoiding the generally predisposing factors. If a part shows signs of early frostbite, it should be warmed rapidly. Outside, this is done best by placing it next to some part of one's own or someone else's body. If feet are frostbitten seriously and the victim must climb or walk to get to safety, it is best to walk on the frozen foot. Once thawed, the foot may be too painful to use and the victim must be carried.

PATHOLOGY AND PHYSIOLOGY

Two important physiologic changes are involved in frostbite. First there is the tissue injury from the actual freezing and, second, there are vascular changes that cause further damage later on. Years ago it was thought that ice crystals formed within the cells and broke the cell membranes. Now, due to the work of Meryman,[7] it has been shown that the ice crystals — except in terribly rapid freezing at very low temperatures — are extracellular. As these crystals form and grow, the cells are dehydrated and eventually may be destroyed by the effect of dehydration on enzyme action. That skin can recover from a frozen state has been shown experimentally by Weatherley-White et al.,[12] who grafted frozen and thawed skin to a new site with a successful take. Normal skin, grafted to a previously frozen bed, did not survive, indicating that vascular changes had occurred.

The second major effect of frostbite is on the vascular supply in the involved area. With exposure to cold, the blood supply to the area is reduced by vasospasm to the point that even before freezing occurs flow may be almost nonexistent — a situation that pertains until the part is thawed. An important series of vascular changes following rewarming have been demonstrated by Bellman and Adams-Ray.[1] They noted that blood flow was present immediately after thawing but decreased after a few minutes. Within a day, new vessels appeared at the margins of the injury and, eventually, revascularization of the entire area could occur. They also noted spasm of the small arteries and veins in the early stages and, later on, permanent narrowings and irregularities of these vessels. In addition, Knoze et al.[3] have shown that injury to the vessel wall can alter the endothelium in such a way that platelets stick and produce thrombi. This, plus increased blood viscosity due to loss of albumin by capillary leakage, can lead to thrombosis of small vessels. Edema forms and further impedes the flow of blood through the previously frozen areas.

If this injury has been severe enough, blisters may form in the viable areas during the phase of capillary leakage. If the distal tissue is dead, vesicles will be found at the proximal margin of injury only. Later there is bleeding into the blisters, so they become black, usually by the fifth day, a condition that does not mean that the whole area is to be lost. After many weeks, these black areas of skin may desquamate and an entire cast of the part may come off, revealing new thin skin underneath. Nerve damage by frostbite may produce a combination of pain and varying degrees of diminished sensation.

Later on, after healing, an increase in collagen in the subcutaneous area is present. Excessive sweating and sensitivity to cold are frequent long-term sequelae, with an increase in susceptibility to recurrent frostbite.

CLINICAL FINDINGS

In civilian practice, we seldom see a patient with frostbite still in the frozen stage; that is to say, with the injured part hard, white and numb. Usually the police or rescue party have thawed the area. Following the rewarming, the tissue softens, may become red and pain starts. Later, edema develops and blisters may form within 24 hours if the injury has been sufficient. When very deep damage has occurred, there will be blister formation only at the proximal margin. Later — in about 5 days — bleeding into the blistered area will result in the development of black areas.

Demarcation between viable and necrotic tissue is very slow to occur, so any decision regarding amputation is best deferred for 60–90 days. During this time, the injured area and nearby parts may sweat excessively and be unusually cold.

EARLY TREATMENT

We have discussed the two major causes of damage from frostbite — namely, the actual freezing and the secondary vascular changes. Treatment, therefore, is directed at the correction of these problems. The actual freezing should be corrected by rapid rewarming. The old teaching of slow rewarming — even with rubbing, which compounds the trouble by adding physical trauma — has long since been shown to be the worst possible thing to do. This method is less painful, which probably is the reason it has been favored for so many years. Rapid rewarming is accomplished by immersion of the part in water at 108–112° F (42–44° C) for 20 minutes. Dry heat is not desirable, as the temperature cannot be well controlled. Meanwhile, the patient's body in general should also be warmed appropriately. Pain of moderate severity will ensue and should be treated by medication.

The injured part should be treated very gently — not cleaned roughly — and either dressed very lightly or left between sterile sheets. If the room is cool, exposure will result in some undesirable further vasospasm, so such exposure is to be avoided. Elevation might reduce blood flow and dependency might increase edema, so a neutral position seems best. Since secondary infection may increase the damage, the use of prophylactic antibiotics in some of the more severe cases is indicated. Obviously, aseptic technique is to be used in the care of the infected areas. Blisters should not be opened unless one is convinced that they have already become infected. Later on — some days later, when the blisters have broken — gentle debridement by instruments or by whirlpool baths may help clean up the involved areas. At this point, exercises should be started to maintain motion in the joints.

Treatment of the vascular component of the injury must be considered early. Heparin and cortisone have been found to be of little help.[3] Low molecular weight dextran will reduce platelet adhesiveness and therefore should be used unless there is a contraindication (as there might be in a patient with significant cardiac impairment). Another agent — not widely tested yet — that may prove useful in the prevention of thrombosis is the surface-active agent Pluronic F 86 (poloxalkol).

The use of Priscoline (tolazoline), given in a proximal artery or by mouth, has been mentioned as helpful in the early stages. A more definitive approach is an early sympathectomy, as advised by Martinez et al.,[5] Shumacker and Kilma[10] and others. In a good-risk patient who is going to have significant tissue loss, this is advisable. The operation will obviate vasospasm, lessen pain, encourage revascularization, lessen edema, conserve tissue, hasten demarcation and reduce late hyperhidrosis. Recently, an interesting "controlled" evaluation of this was observed at our hospital. A 34-year-old alcoholic male came in with frostbitten feet. It was elected to sympathectomize the more involved side. Ultimately, this foot required a transmetatarsal amputation and the side that originally looked favorable ended with a below-knee amputation. Despite our prejudice against such anecdotal reporting, this patient seemed of special interest.

LATE TREATMENT

The decision as to the timing and extent of amputation can be difficult and is best deferred for more than 2 months. As judged by the Korean War experience as reported by Edwards and Leeper,[2] 10% of the victims will require some form of amputation of a digit or more. Sixty-three of the 71 patients in this group returned to duty after hospital stays of 44–165 days. In civilian practice, dealing with older patients, the amputation rate might be higher.

An example of the difficulties encountered in making accurate prognoses and of the long hospitalizations that may be needed was a Massachusetts General Hospital patient. He was a 14-year-old boy who sustained frostbite of both feet when he ran away from home. On admission, it was estimated that there would be no tissue loss. This was far from accurate, as eventually he had bilateral transmetatarsal amputations and a hospital stay of 143 days.

During this long period of recovery from serious frostbite damage, the lesion is not very painful, and, for obvious reasons, narcotics should be avoided. Weight bearing is not permitted when the lower extremity is involved. When the blebs have ruptured spontaneously, gentle debridement is indicated—often done best by whirlpool baths using hexachlorophene (pHisoHex) as recommended by Mills et al.[8] Sterile fluffy dressings keeping the toes separated may be desirable. When it is clear that a digit or more must be amputated, the incision should be right at the margin of living tissue—allowing the stump end to heal by secondary intention in many cases. This conserves tissue and is far from the principles and techniques employed in patients with vascular disease.

If uncontrolled sepsis develops and a foot must be removed, a guillotine type of amputation as low as possible is in order, with later appropriate plastic closure.

Summary of Treatment

Frostbite is treated best by rapid rewarming in a bath at 108–112° F for 20 minutes. Care is taken to warm the patient in general at the same time. A suitable soft dressing or sterile sheets should be used to protect the area against infection. Prophylactic broad-spectrum antibiotics are given. The vascular injury is treated by the use of dextran initially. If major damage is suspected and if the patient's general condition permits, sympathectomy is carried out.

When there is deep injury, the long-term treatment is conservative until it is quite certain that amputation is indeed required. This then is done very close to the line of demarcation—using secondary skin grafting if indicated.

OTHER FORMS OF COLD INJURY

Prolonged and repeated exposure to temperatures near but above freezing, especially in the presence of moisture, can produce several different lesions or syndromes. All reflect local tissue injury, may be associated with tissue loss and may be quite disabling, depending on the severity. It is thought that the damage is due to anoxia caused by increased viscosity of the blood and due to stasis.

Trench Foot

Trench foot, which rarely may involve the hands as well, seldom is seen in civilian practice but has long been a common problem in cold-weather military campaigns. Usually three factors are contributory in its development. These are prolonged exposure to cold, wetness and immobilization of the extremity, both by inactivity and by tight shoes or bindings. The typical victim has been pinned down in a wet trench or foxhole for several days without the opportunity to dry or exercise his feet. Initially, a numb, white extremity is produced. With warming, it becomes erythematous, edematous and painful. These three findings are, in fact, typical of all cold injuries unless actual freezing has occurred. Blisters often form, with the subsequent development of black eschars. These eventually peel off to reveal thin atrophic epithelium or shallow ulcers. Loss of digits is not common but may be seen. Often it is as long as 3 months before the patient is able to ambulate without discomfort. The general principles of conservative management described for frostbite should be applied. Immersion foot is a similar lesion, produced by long exposure to water, and is seen commonly in mariners. Its evolution and treatment are the same.

Chilblain

Chilblain is a lesion usually found on the extensor surface of the fingers over the phalanges. It is thought to be the result of repeated episodes of cold exposure. Although relatively common in England and Scotland, it is quite rare in the United States. Red, itchy nodules first form. These then become painful, may ulcerate and are slow to disappear. They tend to recur seasonally in the same area. Therapy consists of eliminating, insofar as possible, further exposure to cold.

Erythrocyanosis

Erythrocyanosis tends to involve the skin over the lower tibia, again in response to repeated exposure to cold. Since trousers eliminate this exposure, it almost never occurs in males. The lesion is similar to chilblain but is more extensive. Its evolution is the same and, again, prevention of further exposure of the area is the only effective treatment.

BIBLIOGRAPHY

1. Bellman, S., and Adams-Ray, J.: Vascular reactions after experimental cold injury, Angiology 17:339, 1956.
2. Edwards, A. E. and Leeper, R. W.: Frostbite: An analysis of seventy-one cases, JAMA 149:1199, 1952.
3. Knoze, D. M., et al.: The use of autosludging agents in experimental cold injuries, Surg. Gynecol. Obstet. 129:1019, 1969.
4. Lewis, R. B.: The Wellcome Prize Essay 1951, Local cold injury—frostbite, Milit. Surg. 110:25, 1951.
5. Martinez, A., et al.: The specific arterial lesions in mild and severe frostbite: Effect of sympathectomy, J. Cardiovasc. Surg. 7:495, 1966.
6. Meehan, J. P.: Individual and racial variations in vascular response to a cold stimulus, Milit. Med. 116:330, 1955.
7. Meryman, H. T.: Mechanics of freezing in living cells and tissues, Science 124:515, 1956.
8. Mills, W. J., et al.: Frostbite: Experience with rapid rewarming and ultrasonic therapy, Alaska Med. 3:28, 1961.
9. Orr, K. D., et al.: Cold injuries in Korean surgery, Medicine 31:177, 1952.
10. Schumacher, H. B, and Kilma, J. W.: Sympathectomy in the treatment of frostbite, Arch. Surg. 89:575, 1964.
11. Washburn, B.: Frostbite: What it is—How to prevent it—Emergency treatment, N. Engl. J. Med. 266:974, 1962.
12. Weatherley-White, R C., et al.: Experimental studies in cold injury, J. Surg. Res. 4:17, 1964.

52 | Rehabilitation Medicine

DONALD S. PIERCE

REHABILITATION of a patient following fracture or other orthopedic injury entails both the proper support of the injured member and, at the same time, the re-strengthening to a normal level of musculature that has undergone atrophy because of either disuse secondary to cast immobilization or transient neurologic deficit. It may also entail the re-education of muscles in which function has been changed by tendon transfer following neurologic injury secondary to fracture or dislocation particularly in the upper extremity or the cervical spine.

To this end, rehabilitation of the orthopedic patient suffering from fracture or other injury makes use of the services of highly trained allied health personnel — the physical therapist and the occupational therapist. Broadly speaking, the physical therapist is trained in the application of exercise and physical modalities in disorders of the back, neck and extremities. The occupational therapist's skills lie in the area of functional rehabilitation, often with more specific concentration on the upper extremity. This may include the re-education of the patient in the use of his hands following fracture, burns or other trauma to the hand or upper extremity, or may involve hand splinting, manual dexterity training and prevocational evaluation and testing. The concept of the occupational therapist as a person carrying out a project with the patient to keep him amused or to train him in some activity for which he might be suited after his period of hospitalization is, in the former instance, no longer true of the profession and, in the latter instance, only a small part of the work done by the occupational therapist with modern training.

Immobilization of nearly all patients with fractures or joint dislocations for a varying period leads to atrophy of the musculature in the extremity or extremities involved. At the same time, secondary to immobilization for prolonged periods in plaster, there may be fibrosis around a joint or joints and shortening of the musculature of the extremity, known as myostatic contracture. It is the purpose of the rehabilitative process, therefore, to restore the normal strength of the musculature under consideration and to reduce the fibrosis and concurrent limitation of joint motion to a minimum in a way that is as free from pain as possible to the patient and brings about the most normal possible function of the extremity following fracture or other neuromusculoskeletal injury.

Although there is no known modality that will reliably cause the dissolution of scar tissue or intramuscular fibrosis, the application of heat by a variety of methods, and sometimes of cold through the use of ice packs, has been found to reduce muscle spasm and thereby to allow increased passive and active range of joint motion early in the treatment of the postfracture patient. The ability of the physical therapist to passively stretch muscles that have been kept at a finite length by plaster immobilization, by reducing muscle spasms through the application of heat or by icing, will result in a more rapid increase in joint motion, which can be taken over by the patient actively as he regains muscle power from his exercise program. A reduction of pain, secondary to the reduction of muscle spasm by heating or icing, will also allow a more rapid progress of muscle strengthening and bring about the total rehabilitation of the affected extremity or extremities more rapidly.

In addition to a decreased range of motion, the afflicted joints may have intra-articular pathology present, and may simply show a reactive synovitis secondary to beginning of motion after prolonged immobilization. In the stretching of muscles shortened by myostatic contracture, it may be necessary for the physical therapist or the occupational therapist to apply a brace or splint to the leg or hand under consideration, which will produce a constant dynamic pull or guard a joint from motion in an undesirable direction or overstretching of the joint capsule and associated ligamentous structures.

In the rehabilitation of the upper-extremity fracture patient, particularly in fractures of the hands or in fractures in which immobilization of the hands has been necessary, the occupational therapist may have to construct from a temporary material, such as Orthoplast or Prenyl, a mold for the hand to rest on or a dynamic splint, in which outriggers are attached to a plastic base, strapped to the arm with Velcro, and slings placed around the fingers, in order to place a dynamic pull on the flexor tendons and flexor musculature. Alternatively, in hands in which extension contractures exist following fracture, glove traction splints or other types of dynamic splints to produce metacarpophalangeal joint flexion and a steady traction pull on a shortened extensor mechanism may also require construction by the occupational therapist. Under her guidance, an expert orthotist may be asked to construct metallic splints to carry out the same functions over longer periods. With the help of such a team, it may be possible for the orthopedic surgeon to discontinue plaster immobilization of an upper-extremity fracture earlier and to begin a program of active rehabilitation at an earlier date than otherwise could be done. The occupational therapist will also concurrently teach the patient the reuse of his upper extremity for normal activities of daily living and, if required, for activities in his previous occupation or in a new occupation. In the area of the lower extremity, it usually is the province of the orthopedic surgeon to prescribe a brace, after discussion of the patient's exercise program with the physical therapist, to guard against overuse of a particular joint and overstretching of contracted muscles and tendons. In this situation, the skills of a certified orthotist will be of paramount importance in the rehabilitative process.

The second area in which the physical therapist will act as a member of the health care team in rehabilitating the orthopedic patient is in a retraining in gait, following the removal of immobilization devices after healing of lower-extremity fractures. The physical therapist may begin treatment by having the patient stand between parallel bars, ambulating with the support of the parallel bars; then, as the patient's strength increases from his exercise program and his balance and the ability to handle himself improves, he is progressed to a four-legged walker or moved directly to a pair of axillary crutches. If a proper relationship exists between the orthopedic surgeon and the physical therapist, the measuring for crutches, selection of crutches and training in their use generally will fall in the province of the physical therapist.

It is important that the orthopedic surgeon or other physician treating the fracture patient be familiar with the skills and training of both the physical therapist and the occupational therapist and that he be well acquainted with the uses of all types of assistive devices — devices for ambulation, braces and splints and the common modalities used by the physical therapist and the occupational therapist in reduction of muscle spasm and pain and the promotion of joint motion and muscle strength. In prescribing physical or occupational therapy, the surgeon should lay down broad guidelines for the physical therapist or the occupational therapist. He should specify what the limits of exercise should be, both from the patient's general physical condition and from the degree of healing of the fracture or joint injury, how far the joint may be moved safely, how far muscles may be stretched, how much pressure may be applied across the fracture site and what angular moment can be applied at the fracture site with safety. He should include in his prescription any contraindications to certain exercises, ranges of motion or modalities. He should not, however, if he knows the capabilities of his physical therapist, attempt to limit or specifically and exactly prescribe what exercises or what modalities should be used in any stage of the physical therapy or occupational therapy program, but should give the therapist a broad latitude in putting together the best possible program for the individual patient, and develop a relationship with the therapist such that she will refer to the surgeon and consult with him frequently on the patient's treatment. Thus, both surgeon and therapist are aware of the patient's progress and the methods being used to achieve it. Such a working relationship will produce the most rapid rehabilitation for the orthopedic patient.

CRUTCH WALKING

Many patients with fractures of the lower extremity require the use of crutches at some time during their convalescence. Accordingly, it is essential that these patients be equipped with the proper size of crutches and that they receive instructions in their use.

SELECTION OF CRUTCHES. — Most patients have a single fracture or fractures of only one lower extremity, and the choice of crutches presents no particular problem. The crutch can be either a standard double upright underarm type or, as may be preferred, an adjustable underarm crutch (see Fig. 52-1, A). The crutch should be provided with a suction tip and very often with an underarm axillary pad. For the patient having good triceps power, an aluminum crutch with a forearm loop (see Fig. 52-1, C) may be used. The aluminum crutch may be used in place of a cane when the patient requires more stability than is provided by a cane alone. It is also preferred by patients who are required to use crutches for an extended period. There is a certain convenience in using this type of crutch, since the patient is able to release his grasp from the handle while the crutch remains supported on the forearm. Special arm and hand supports may be utilized in particular cases in which there are complications of arthritis or muscle weakness.

MEASURING FOR CRUTCHES. — To measure a patient for crutches, the height of the crutches — or their length — and the level of the handpiece are the points of consideration. The length of the crutches is important, because if they are too long there will be pressure in the axilla and against the radial nerve, causing a crutch paralysis or radial nerve palsy. If the crutches are too short, improper stance will result. The hand level is important. It should be such that an angle of 30 degrees of flexion is present at the elbow joint.

One method of measuring is to have the patient lie straight in bed and to measure from the anterior fold of the axilla to a point 6 inches from the level of the bottom of the foot — that is, 6 inches out from the side of the level of the bottom of the foot. An alternative method is to

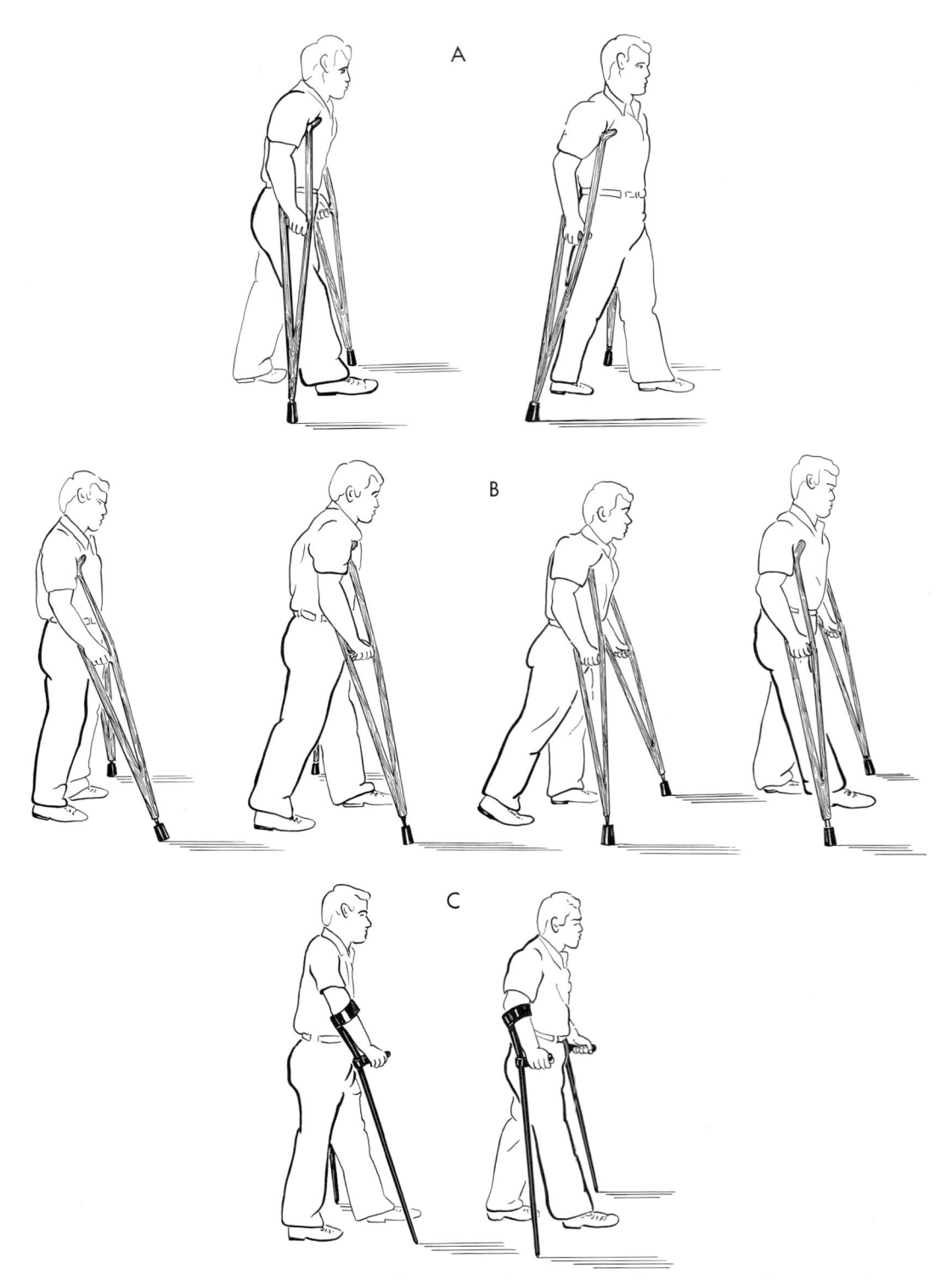

Fig. 52-1.—**A**, three-point gait. **B**, four-point alternate gait. **C**, two-point alternate gait.

measure from the anterior point of the axilla to the foot and add 2 inches. In many instances, it is best to utilize adjustable crutches so that the length and the level of the hand grasp are finally decided when the patient is up.

ACCESSORIES.—Rubber covers for the shoulderpiece are helpful to prevent undue pressure, and a large suction tip, 1½ or 2 inches in length, is helpful also. Small round tips are not safe because they do not hold well at all angles with the ground.

THREE-POINT CRUTCH GAIT.—For patients with fractures of one lower extremity, the usual gait prescribed is the three-point gait (Fig. 52-1, A). This gait is used to avoid full weight bearing on the affected extremity. The crutch sequence is: (1) both crutches and the weaker lower extremity; then (2) the stronger lower extremity. In this way, the two crutches and weaker limb are placed simultaneously, and then the stronger limb, supporting the whole body weight, is advanced.

FOUR-POINT ALTERNATE CRUTCH GAIT.— This gait (Fig. 52-1, B) is used for bilateral involvement and is the most elementary gait. It is a safe gait because there are three points of support on the floor, but it is slow because the weight must be shifted constantly. The sequence is as follows: (1) right crutch, (2) left foot, (3) left crutch, (4) right foot.

TWO-POINT ALTERNATE CRUTCH GAIT.— For a patient who has mastered the four-point alternate crutch gait, the two-point alternate crutch gait (Fig. 52-1, C) may be taught, since the latter increases speed. Actually, it can be as fast as the walk of the average normal person. This gait requires more balance control because only two points are supporting the body at one time. Crutch sequence: (1) right crutch and left foot simultaneously, (2) left crutch and right foot simultaneously.

EXERCISE

It has been noted that virtually every patient who has had immobilization of an extremity, cervical spine or trunk for fracture or dislocation, or both, will have undergone a variable degree of disuse atrophy and/or neurogenic atrophy of muscle, and if the joints involved are to be supported properly and normal activity again engaged in, it is necessary to attain normal muscle strength and full range of motion in all joints as rapidly as possible and as painlessly as possible. A prescription of an exercise program should stipulate the limitations of range of motion, so that the physical therapist may safely guide the patient. Where indicated, the positioning of the part to the extremity and the support in certain areas should be stipulated. Whether range of motion of the affected joint is to be active or passive, or both, or whether it is to be active with assistance by the therapist should be stated. Customarily, exercises are divided into passive, active and resistive. It should be emphasized that passive stretching to obtain motion in the early after-care of fractures usually is contraindicated, as there may be a reactive synovitis created in the joint, which will both diminish the effect of the exercise program and decrease the range of motion rather than increase it. Active motion or active assisted motion, with the patient doing most of the moving, should be the order of activity in early fracture rehabilitation. Pain and muscle spasm produced by the exercise signal that the limits of exercise have been reached, or exceeded, and the therapist should take steps to see that pain, or fear of it, does not lessen the patient's willingness to participate in his rehabilitation program. The physiologic effects of active exercise are well known. It is this type of exercise that is most effective in bringing about hypertrophy of muscles, increasing muscle fiber diameter. At the same time, exercise increases both arterial and venous circulation, leading to a decrease in swelling. As an end result there is greater muscle power, increased range of motion in the joints and increased nutrition and circulation for the affected area. One technique that warrants special discussion is that of progressive resistance exercise. When strong bony union has been secured in fractures, particularly of the weight-bearing bones, the individual may not be able to resume full activity because of muscle weakness. This is particularly true if long immobilization without joint range of motion or any exercise has resulted from plaster immobilization. The progressive resistance exercise technique is aimed at quickly developing muscle power by applying near-maximal resistance and a low repetition rate of exercise. An excellent example is that of knee extension exercise, used in the case of fractured femurs (Fig. 52-2). Applications have also been developed for the hip, back and leg musculature (Fig. 52-3). Special equipment is available for use in hospital departments, but for quadriceps, an aluminum boot or shoe that straps onto the patient's foot, with a bar for weights, may be supplied for home use.

A newer technique that has great merit, especially in the area of early fracture rehabilitation before bony union is strong enough to withstand independent and entirely unguarded motion, particularly in areas where joints have been injured, is the technique of proprioceptive neuromuscular facilitation, originated by Kabat, Kaiser and Knott.[3] Although somewhat complicated from the point of view of the physiology on which it is based, this concept may be summarized by pointing out that it does not require a joint to go through a full range of motion, or more than 10–15 degrees of joint motion, in order to exercise all of the muscles of an extremity. The principle is based on placement of the patient's extremity in such a position by the therapist that as the therapist resists the rotational efforts on a patient's part in a static position, he is required to use all of the muscles of an extremity to maximal ability in order to attempt to derotate in a functional pattern the extremity that the therapist is placing under rotational stress (Fig. 52–4). As muscle strength develops and bony strength and joint range allow, the pattern of motion may be increased in joint range to what is called rhythmic stabilization of a joint or joint complex, such that the joint may be allowed to move through a partial or full range of motion with rotatory resistance to derotational force being applied by the therapist in a pattern that is normal for that extremity in actual functional use. In a period of 10–20 minutes, an extremity can be exercised to the point at which the muscles are warm and have been put through a substantial period of isometric contraction, which is known to be the most effective method of building muscle strength in hypertrophying muscle fibers.

This newer technique has considerable advantages over the older progressive resistance exercise technique, in

Fig. 52-2.—Technique of progressive resistance exercise for developing strength of knee extensors.

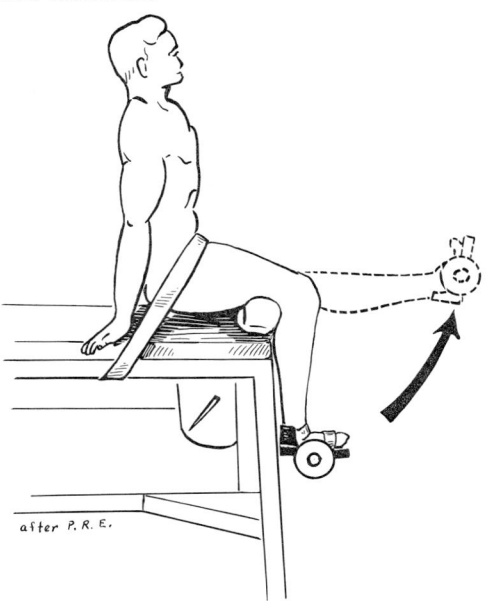

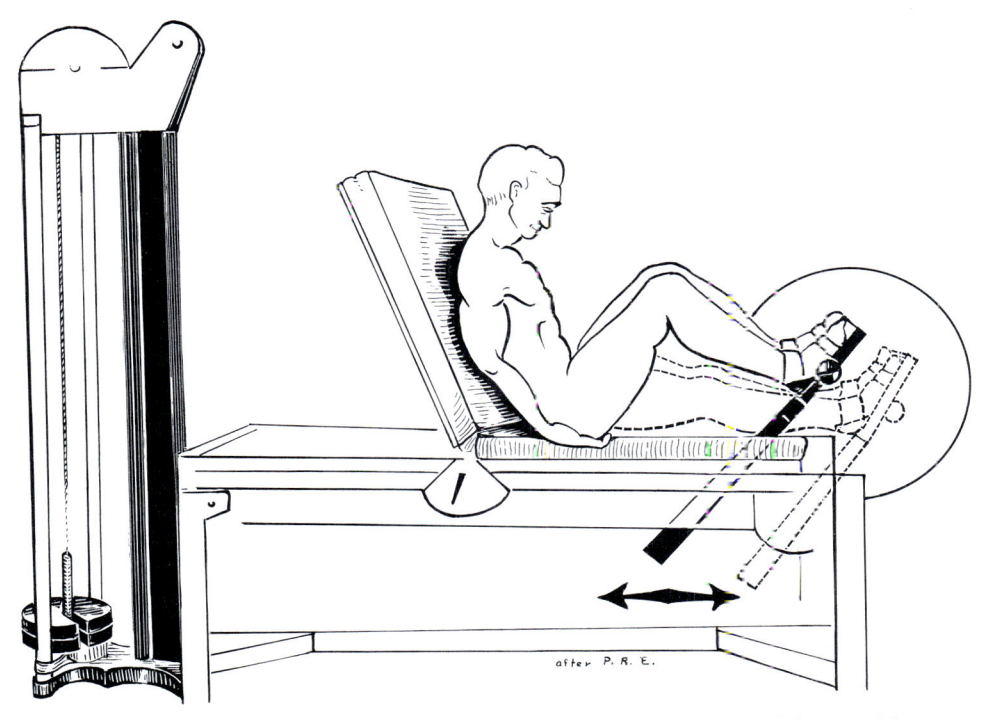

Fig. 52-3.—Technique of progressive resistance exercise for combined hip and knee extension.

that it does not require a full range of motion and in the case of the knee does not require that the patella be pulled across the underlying femoral cartilage surface under load. The drawback to this technique is, of course, that in its initial stages it must be carried out by a trained physical therapist familiar with the method. A good therapist can teach the technique, within limits, to a member of the family, to be carried out at home later in the physical therapy program. The program should be checked by the therapist once a week.

The use of heat and ice has been mentioned in the reduction of muscle spasm and pain as an adjunct to programs of joint ranging and exercise. The application of ice to the muscles in question is simply carried out by placing ice cubes in a plastic bag, wrapping them in several layers of toweling and placing them on the muscle so as not to injure the skin. It should be noted here that great care must be taken to be certain that no damage occurs to injured tissue and that where impaired sensation exists, the therapist should be very careful not to allow too much cold to affect the skin.

HEAT

Heat as a modality in rehabilitation can be produced in a number of ways. All methods have in common the production of heat within the tissues at a variable rate. It should be noted that these are adjuncts to a proper exercise program and that they are not treatments within themselves, although they may greatly enhance the exercise program and make the patient a great deal more comfortable. One additional safeguard should be pointed out. Prolonged use of ultrasound and diathermy is contraindicated and probably should be stopped after 6 treat-

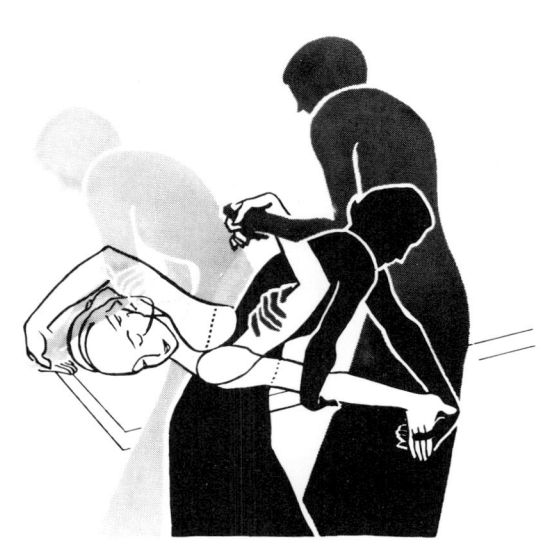

Fig. 52-4.—Proprioceptive neuromuscular facilitation technique for upper extremity with elbow flexion. (Reproduced, with permission, from Knott, M., and Voss, D. E.: *Proprioceptive Neuromuscular Facilitation. Patterns and Techniques* [2d ed.; New York: Hoeber Medical Division, Harper & Row, Publishers, 1968].)

ments, as there is mounting evidence that the continued use of diathermy, and possibly ultrasound, may have deleterious effects on body tissues and may even be capable of denaturing proteins and causing fibrosis on extended use. The possible connection between the use of diathermy on cervical musculature over a prolonged period and radiation type of cataracts is being studied by the United States Public Health Service.

Among the known physiologic effects of heat is sedative action for relief from pain. Although a slight raising of tissue temperature elevates the pain threshold, it seems likely that the most important mechanism for relief from pain is through reduction of muscle spasm. The primary local response to heat, however, is change in circulation. An increased arterial flow is produced, resulting in a dilated capillary bed and increased blood supply. This increased blood supply, however, is not without an undesirable effect; namely, increased swelling. In most traumatized areas there is some injury to the lymphatic and venous drainage, and excessive heating may cause increased swelling and pain, with loss of motion. For this reason, the use of heat alone is deprecated, whereas heat may be quite beneficial when followed by proper massage and exercises, including attention to positioning during both heat application and later exercises.

There are a great many methods for applying heat. In general, those that are applied most easily, may be repeated as often as needed and are least costly are the most desirable.

CONDUCTIVE HEATING.—Perhaps the simplest forms of heating are conductive. This includes the use of warm-water soaks, hot packs and heating pads.

Hot-water soaks can also be given in the form of whirlpool baths. Here, the agitation of the water is thought to have an additional stimulative effect on the cutaneous circulation and in the relief from muscle spasm, together with certain psychologic therapeutic actions. The whirlpool bath has the disadvantage of requiring dependency of the part immersed. This works against venous return and, in the presence of edema, may not be as effective as other agents that can be given with the part horizontal or elevated.

One of the most effective methods of conductive heating is a hot moist pack known commercially as the Hydrocollator. This consists of a ribbed canvas pack containing a gelatinous material that has a high absorptive power for water, so that, after the pack is saturated with water and heated, it may be held up with only a few drops falling out, thus obviating the need for wringing. After the heat is given off in the form of vapor, the pack remains dry instead of cold and wet. The pack is wrapped in five or six thicknesses of turkish toweling, adjusted to comfortable warmth and the toweling reduced as cooling occurs. This pack is suitable for home use. It is safe to heat the water to as high as 170° or 180° F, or slightly below boiling. The safe temperature of the water baths, on the other hand, ranges between 104° and 110° F.

Another form of conductive heating often of value, particularly for the hand, is the paraffin bath. Proper mixtures of paraffin wax and oil (usually 7:1) are used so that the melting point is between 125° and 130° F. By repeated immersions, a layer of wax solidifies like a glove. The injured part then may be either left in the melted paraffin or wrapped in towels for the desired length of time.

It has been found that adequate local heating can be obtained in about 30 minutes by the conductive methods described.

RADIANT HEATING. — Another relatively simple method of heating utilizes radiant energy, which is absorbed by the tissues and converted to heat. The energy source is infrared radiation, which may be obtained from the usual tungsten-filament light bulbs of sufficient wattage, nonluminous infrared coils or carborundum elements. The larger the area to be treated the greater the wattage needed, the range being from 250 to 1,500 watts. Heat lamps safe for home use are available, including lamps with Pyrex bulbs and inside reflective coating and lamps with metallic reflectors properly insulated to prevent overheating. One necessary precaution is that the source of heat be so angled that in case of breakage of the bulb, hot parts will not fall onto the skin. The heating source is set at a comfortable distance; this will vary between 15 and 30 inches on the average, depending on the wattage of the bulb or element. Adequate rise in temperature usually can be obtained by infrared radiation in 30 minutes.

CONVERSIVE HEATING. — The conversive method of heating employs the principle of converting high-frequency electromagnetic energy into heat in the tissues. This is known as "diathermy" and, depending on the frequency, is either shortwave or microwave. So far as is known, diathermy has no proved effect on tissues other than that resulting from increased temperature. Because of the ability of high-frequency electrical energy to penetrate tissues, deep heating effects are obtainable in less time than with other methods of applying heat. It is, therefore, possible to obtain adequate heating in 20 minutes by the use of diathermy. Most of this electrical energy is absorbed by the blood in the tissues and is an effective stimulus to circulation. It is not generally accepted that diathermy has a specific beneficial effect on a formation of callus; in fact, some evidence indicates that excessive heating by diathermy possibly may cause osteoporosis or decalcification of bone by increasing circulation. Because of the large amounts of energy that are delivered to the tissues, it is especially important that there be normal sensation if diathermy is to be used, as is necessary with all forms of heat application. The use of diathermy over growing epiphyses is contraindicated. The correct technique of application of diathermy is dependent on knowledge of its physics and training in methods of operation. The technical details are beyond the scope of this discussion. In the after-care of fractures, the prolonged use of diathermy without exercise therapy is contraindicated.

ULTRASOUND. — Presently, the newest method for the application of heat involves the use of high-frequency vibratory energy in the form of ultrasound waves. The vibrations are too rapid to be heard by the human ear (700,000–1,000,000 per second). Ultrasound generators now available are effective in producing local heat. This can be done in 5–10 minutes by direct application of the sound applicator to the skin through a proper coupling medium, such as mineral oil or a water bath. So far as is known, the fundamental effects of ultrasound application result from the increase in temperature produced when the mechanical energy is converted to heat in the body. Although consideration of the physics involved shows that the ultrasonic energy, when applied to a limb, may selectively increase bone temperature, it has not yet been demonstrated that this is a desirable method of treatment for fractures and so it is not recommended for this purpose.

MASSAGE

The beneficial effects of massage as part of the rehabilitation program are dependent on the type of movement and the dosage. In the early treatment of fractures, superficial stroking may have a sedative effect, with relief from pain and muscle spasm. Deeper massage, when permissible, is a greater stimulus to circulation. The greatest effect, however, is on the venous return, which is facilitated both reflexly and mechanically. In view of this, properly executed massage may lead to some decrease in swelling. For all practical purposes, however, massage is of benefit only in the most skilled hands and under the expert guidance of the physician or surgeon. Because of the danger from massage in inexpert hands and without proper medical supervision, it is best to omit this aspect of the treatment if there is any doubt in the surgeon's mind.

ELECTRODIAGNOSIS

Whenever there is a suspicion of nerve lesion, electrodiagnostic tests are of utmost importance. Electrodiagnostic tests include direct muscle stimulation for the determination of electrical excitability, the determination of a response to galvanic stimulation, with a measurement of chronaxy and/or complete strength-duration curve, and, most important, electromyography and nerve conduction studies.

Electromyography consists of the measurement of the electrical potentials from resting and actively contracting muscle in which, 21 days or more after injury to the peripheral nerve innervating the muscle, there will be definite changes connoting denervation and a gradual change with reinnervation. It is possible to tell with considerable accuracy whether the nerve to the muscle has been totally lost and, later on, whether there is nerve regeneration. Visual and audio records are produced, using a cathode-ray oscilloscope and a loudspeaker. If the physician observes denervation potentials, indicating fibrillation of denervated muscle fibers, a nerve injury undoubtedly is present. As the nerve regenerates, or if the muscle is not totally denervated, action potentials will be seen representing normal motor-unit activity, indicating that the nerve has not been completely severed or is not totally lacking in conduction.

Nerve conduction studies are carried out by stimulating the nerve above the suspected level of injury, placing a surface electrode over the muscle innervated by the nerve or over the path of the nerve below it, picking up the impulse and measuring the time taken for the stimulus to reach the point of pickup. The period of conduction, if conduction occurs, is compared with a table of normal conductions for that particular nerve and the degree of impairment noted.

ELECTROTHERAPY

Normally innervated skeletal muscle that has become weak or atrophied from disuse or immobilization may be made to contract by appropriate electrical stimulation. The currents used for this purpose must have certain physical characteristics for optimal effect. The current must have sufficient intensity to overcome the threshold of excitability, each individual impulse must have sufficient duration to overcome the time factor of excitability and the waveform of the individual impulse must have an abrupt rise, so that the threshold is not raised by the process of accommodation. There must be an adequate frequency of individual impulse to produce a sustained smooth tetanic muscle contraction. Every well-equipped hospital physical therapy department should have a variety of commercially available stimulators that can be used for this purpose.

Some generators are quite elaborate, having mechanical means of surging the current on and off gradually; others have a manual control by which the therapist can make and break the current. From the point of view of comfort, the individual impulse of short duration with high voltage and minimal amperage produces the least sensory stimulation or pain. The current used for the greatest number of years is that produced by an induction coil or faradic current, although at present this current is less popular than that produced by various oscillating-tube circuits. A general rule to follow is to have the electrical stimulation produce an individual impulse, usually of about a millisecond duration. The frequency should be between 50 and 200 per second, and the intensity should be easily controlled by an appropriate potentiometer. If the current is unidirectional, the cathode, or negative pole, usually is applied at the motor point of the muscle. One of the most comfortable currents producing a strong contraction is similar to a static machine, in that a high-voltage discharge in a vacuum tube is produced and enters the muscle through glass and air spacing. Such a generator is commercially available.*

Although a number of stimulators are available, their value in therapy is not well established, with certain exceptions. It is generally accepted that a voluntary contraction is the most effective way of getting back power of normally innervated muscle. However, in some cases of prolonged immobilization, a patient may seem to forget how to contract a muscle, and electrical stimulations of the muscle may help in muscle re-education. This use of electrotherapy seems to be the most logical, from our present knowledge.

In the presence of a nerve injury, completely denervated muscles may also be made to contract by appropriate electrical currents. Because denervated muscle has specific characteristics of electrical excitability, the selection of currents must be in keeping with this excitability. Intensities are in the same range as those for innervated muscle but the time characteristic of excitability is quite different. Stimuli of longer duration must be used, in keeping with the increased chronaxy, or time threshold of excitability. The average duration of a rectangular waveform stimulus for denervated muscle is 50 milliseconds. The frequency of stimulation needed to produce the sustained contraction is also different, and for denervated muscle the frequency need only be approximately 10 per second. Therefore, a current of adequate intensity with impulses of 50 milliseconds duration and with a frequency of 10 per second can be used satisfactorily to stimulate denervated muscle. Again, the current may be turned on mechanically slowly in a surge wave and similarly turned off, by sharp make and break, with a manual switch. It has been shown that the atrophy of denervation cannot be prevented by electrical stimulation, nor does this stimulation have an effect on the regeneration of the nerves. Experimental work suggests that only stimulation at least twice a day every day for 5–10 minutes at a time per individual muscle, and with maximal contraction, has any physiologic effect. Consequently, electrical stimulation of denervated muscle is, in most instances, confined to testing purposes.

INSTRUCTION OF PATIENT IN HOME CARE

The importance of the active cooperation of the patient in securing a good end

---

*Produced by the Batrow Laboratories, Inc., Branford, Connecticut.

result has been stressed. It rarely is possible to provide enough supervised physical and occupational therapy to make sure that the patient has sufficient active use of the involved part to secure return of function. Therefore, it is necessary to instruct the patient and instill in him the desire to improve results through his own efforts. Accordingly, it is good practice to teach the patient to use simple methods of heat application and, in particular, to encourage him to do exercises at home that he can repeat many times a day without any elaborate apparatus.

In more difficult cases, especially those that require the regaining of a particular skill, occupational therapy may provide a home program of activity that the patient may practice for many hours on his own, with only the necessary checks of progress and supervision of exercises or other therapy activities whenever seen by the physician. Years of experience have shown that in perhaps the majority of uncomplicated fractures adequate advice from the surgeon regarding a home exercise program, including, if indicated, application of heat of a simpler type, may be sufficient to secure good return of function. Individuals vary greatly, however, in their ability to learn how to exercise properly, and it may be a time-consuming procedure to supervise patients in a home exercise program to make sure that it is done effectively. For some individuals, a few supervised treatment sessions in physical therapy may be of immeasurable value in teaching them how to carry out an effective home program.

PROBLEMS IN REHABILITATION

Rehabilitation medicine procedures, applied adequately, are successful in rehabilitating most patients with uncomplicated fractures. However, a sizable number of patients have complications and more serious injuries, particularly of weight-bearing joints, that require procedures beyond those available in the usual physical and occupational therapy departments. These patients usually present long-term problems of after-care because of the severe trauma and the long period of disability, and other factors become important in management.

Prolonged periods of immobilization in the hospital or at home may lead to considerable psychologic, as well as physiologic, disability simply from inactivity and boredom. Some of the physiologic effects are, of course, to a large extent obviated by instructing and interesting the patient in an active exercise program for the uninvolved muscles of the body, since such exercises tend to maintain a more normal metabolism. Other adverse effects of immobilization and inactivity may also be in part prevented by occupational therapy to provide an interest in an activity within his reach while immobilized. In addition, it is important to consider the objectives and problems of economic rehabilitation and return to employment.

The importance of an over-all approach to rehabilitation of the seriously injured patient cannot be overemphasized. This has been manifested again and again by those caring for patients who have been involved in industrial accidents. It is generally believed—and there are statistics to bear out the belief—that if the disability is unnecessarily prolonged for months or years, the chances for successful rehabilitation, even with the best facilities, are greatly hampered by delay in making the facilities available to the patient.

It is, of course, obvious that no amount of expert rehabilitation can make up for a lack of proper fracture reduction and good anatomic realignment of all functioning parts.

A review of the fracture patients referred to the Bay State Medical Rehabilitation Clinic at Massachusetts General Hospital in its first 3-year period showed that about 30% of the new patients each year were referred for treatment of fractures. About 25% of these had upper-extremity fractures, usually with such complications as severe limitation of adjacent joint motion, and tendon or nerve injuries. The largest percentage of patients (75%) had involvement of the weight-bearing joints of the lower extremities that incapacitated them for months or years.

The procedures usually included at this stage of rehabilitation should begin with an evaluation of patient motivation. It should be emphasized, however, that proper motivation cannot be expected to be automatic, since it is dependent on orientation as to what end result is to be expected in the particular case. Realistic goals must be established in the event of permanent residual disability, and provision made for guidance and necessary training in the learning of new skills. In some cases, of course, lack of function can be explained not on organic disability or on lack of motivation but on a deep-seated emotional reaction to the disability. This usually is treated with guidance or with the active therapeutic participation of a psychiatrist. In this series at the Rehabilitation Clinic, there were no patients with frank psychiatric disorders related to their trauma.

Experience has shown that an all-inclusive rehabilitation program may be of definite value in the most difficult cases. Such a program may include graduated physical activity under supervision and often group activities correlated with occupational therapy procedures to improve work tolerance and to stimulate interest in productive activity. Social service workers are helpful in orienting the patient to the program and helping with economic and social problems related to his injury, as well as in securing help for him in such matters as compensation and transportation and in explaining his disability to other members of the family. In a large general hospital it may be possible to utilize the hospital industries in a therapeutic manner. For example, patients often can be stimulated to work in the hospital carpentry shop or plumbing shop, in the dietetic department, in bookkeeping, accounting or printing or in the almost endless occupations that are part of any hospital administration and are similar to those in which the patient was employed previously or in which he may seek to be employed in the future. In a sheltered, protective environment, associated with the rehabilitation clinic, the patient may be encouraged to increase his work activity and to develop the self-assurance so important in rehabilitation. The ability to work in a group with other people is an aspect of treatment not to be neglected in a complicated case.

The rehabilitation of patients with permanent disabilities includes proper vocational testing, guidance and, when indicated, retraining in another type of employment. Retraining can be accomplished only through knowledge and understanding of the agencies available for this purpose and by work with these agencies in providing an evaluation of the particular patient and his physical and intellectual capabilities and interests. The United States Government has provided, through the departments of vocational rehabilitation in all states, facilities for this type of counseling and for the necessary vocational training. It is urged that the physician caring for seriously injured patients be aware of all the available rehabilitation procedures and refer the patient to appropriate agencies for necessary occupational and physical therapy.

BIBLIOGRAPHY

1. DeLorme, T. L., and Watkins, A. L.: *Progressive Resistance Exercise* (New York: Appleton-Century-Crofts, Inc., 1951).
2. DeLorme, T. L., West, F. E., and Shriber, W. J.: Influence of progressive-resistance exercises on knee function following femoral fractures, J. Bone Joint Surg. 32-A:910 1950.
3. Knott, M., and Voss, D. E.: *Proprioceptive Neuromuscular Facilitation. Patterns and Techniques* (2d ed.; New York: Hoeber Medical Division, Harper & Row, Publishers, 1968).

53 Replanting Amputated Arms

RONALD A. MALT and WILLIAM H. HARRIS

THE CIRCUMSTANCES that combine to call for replanting a severed limb are rare, indeed. Nonetheless, several dozen successful replantations during the past decade testify to the utility of the operation when it is indicated.[4, 8, 14, 18, 25] A well-executed operation in the proper patient can give him an arm far better than any prosthesis now available—or likely to be available in the near future.

To have any semantic justification, replantation* must be defined as the reuniting of a part completely separated from the body, except, perhaps, for a strand of skin and areolar tissue. Only by adhering to this definition can the aspects of the operation that distinguish it from repair of traumatized limbs in general be made clear. Only to the extent that the unique problems of preservation of the amputated part, provision of lymphatic and venous drainage and re-establishment of neural function are noteworthy does replantation deserve being treated as a separate entity.

The essence of the operation is for the surgeon to maintain the faculty of balanced judgment and to integrate into one large operation the individual procedures that would repair separately each of the injured structures. This chapter will consider these factors only as they relate to reuniting parts of arms, inasmuch as a lower extremity is almost never suitable for replantation.

EMERGENCY CARE

First priority obviously must be given to relieving any abnormalities in the respiratory, vascular and nervous systems that compromise survival of the patient. Only then should attention be diverted to the possibility of electively replacing an amputated limb.

Intrinsic hemostatic mechanisms often will spontaneously stop hemorrhage from the completely severed vessels in the proximal amputation stump. Elastic fibers removed from stretch contract the lumen, which, during the inevitable phase of hypotension, becomes occluded with a platelet and fibrin plug. Seldom is there major bleeding. For this reason, there rarely is need to put a tourniquet on the stump, especially as the time of its removal will be uncertain. The major vessels should be tied or clamped and venous oozing controlled with a firm elastic bandage; damage produced by a tourniquet should not be added to the burdens of the traumatized stump. Not only is direct destruction of tissue possible but thrombogenic mechanisms conceivably could be activated after release of a tourniquet that has been in place for some time. Naturally, antitetanus and

---

*The preferred word is *replantation*, "a planting again," not *reimplantation*, which means "The (re-) uniting of structures by suturing one inside the other" or "(to) set (again) securely or deeply."— Webster's New International Dictionary, 2d ed.

antibiotic therapy should be instituted as in any major injury of this kind.

To lower its metabolic requirements, the amputated part should be immersed in ice as soon as possible. Freezing will not occur; the slowed metabolism will deter autolysis—for how long, no one knows. Six to 8 hours is a reasonable guess for amputations in the upper forearm or arm—longer for more distal amputations, which consist mainly of metabolically sluggish tendons and bone. Recent observations suggest that one way of estimating viability of muscle masses is to measure pH at the surface.[2] Acidotic muscle appears to have the potentiality of being revitalized if the blood flow can be restored, but alkalotic muscle seems to be irreversibly damaged.

There may also be merit in flushing the vascular system via a readily accessible artery, not only to speed cooling of the core of the severed part further but to remove sludged and altered blood. By inserting a large-bore plastic cannula into the artery and compressing the vessel around it with the fingers, direct mechanical damage to the artery can be minimized; by restricting the pressure of perfusion to that obtainable from an intravenous drip hanging not more than 6 feet above the limb, mechanical disruption of the capillary bed can be limited.

The chemical composition of the ideal

Fig. 53-1.—Possible reasons for occlusion of small blood vessels (modified from Strock and Majno,[22] with permission). The ideal perfusate for a severed limb, besides preserving the part, would block all the deleterious responses, which are: (1) arteriolar spasm, (2) microemboli, (3) anoxic swelling of leukocytes, (4) sticky endothelium, (5) direct endothelial injury, (6) compression by interstitial edema, (7) compression by perivascular cells, (8) endothelial swelling, (9) constriction by collagen fibers, (10) formation of intravascular blebs, (11) histamine leaks, (12) platelet thrombosis, (13) intravascular clotting. (Courtesy of P. E. Strock and G. Majno.)

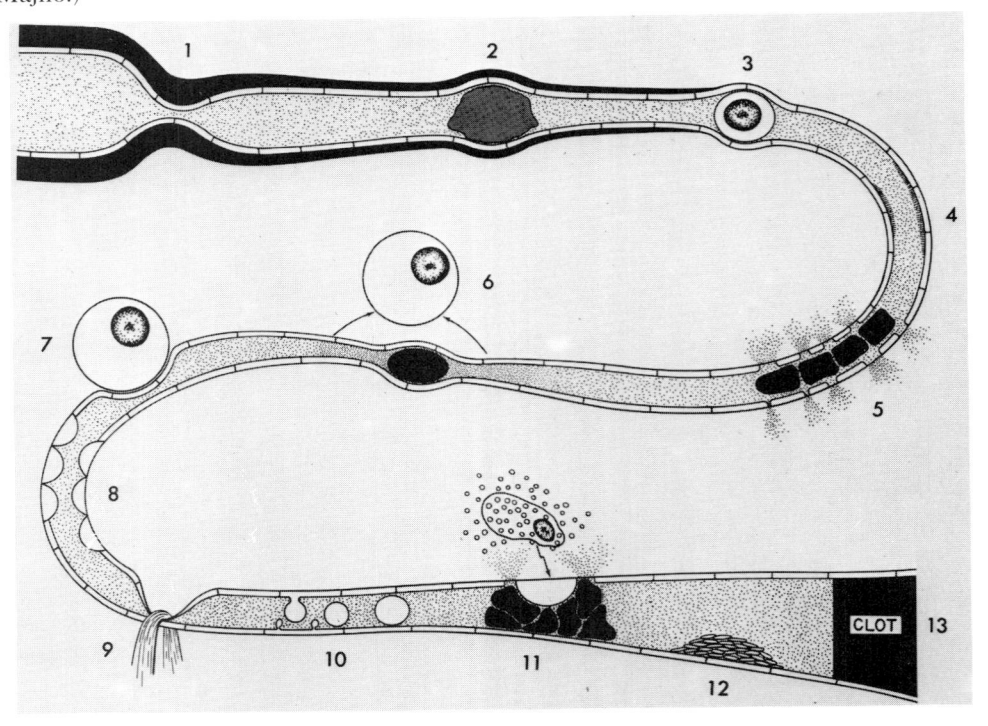

perfusate for this purpose has not been settled. Theoretically, the perfusate should block all 13 of the mechanisms that may impair vascular flow even after restoration of the vascular system[22] (Fig. 53-1). For these purposes, saline solution or lactated Ringer's solution may be as good as anything else now available,[16] but if the experience of perfusion for organ transplantation can be transposed, the ideal perfusate should have a composition similar to that of the intracellular environment. The addition of heparin (5,000 units/500 ml) or of dextran to the perfusate probably is worthwhile.

JUDGMENT

Once the bleeding is controlled and the amputated part is preserved, there is a hiatus during which the possibility of a replantation can be weighed calmly. The decision is made in two steps: (1) Can it be done? and (2) Should it be done? The major consideration in the first question is whether the patient has any serious visceral injuries or any damage that could become functionally severe if left unattended during the time necessary to perform a replantation. If the amputation was the result of a single slice or blow to an extremity, these are not serious issues, but if the damage was a consequence of trauma to the whole body, they are. Assessment of the integrity of the amputated part and of the stump, by both direct examination and roentgenography, needless to say, are also essential elements in deciding whether the replantation can be performed.

The prime factors in determining whether the replantation should be done are the site of amputation, the age and the aspirations of the patient and the resources of the surgical team. Replantation of the upper extremity should receive careful consideration because the arm has a reasonable potentiality for nerve regeneration, shortening is of little consequence and even the best prostheses cannot replace the function of the hand. By contrast, amputations of the lower extremity rarely should be considered. The chances of reinnervation are poor, the hazards of an anesthetic foot are great, shortening of the limb in comparison with the other is a definite handicap and prostheses are far more satisfactory. In essence, the hand is complex, prehensile and should be restored to as near that state as is possible; the functions of the lower extremity in support and locomotion often are well served by a substitute. Every now and again, however, a case might be made for performing a usually questionable replantation if the sole object is to get a longer stump for a better prosthesis, as in the difference between amputation at the shoulder and one at the elbow.

On the other hand, not all amputations of an upper extremity are ideal. Avulsing injuries, which tear the arm from the body, may well also avulse the spinal roots of the nerves so that no return of function will be possible; a cervical myelogram may disclose characteristic diverticula of the dura in these situations. In crushing injuries, so much nerve or muscle tissue may be lacking that return of function will be unlikely. At the other end of the arm, replantation of any single digit except the thumb rarely would seem to be worthwhile.

The more distal the amputation the better the prognosis, because misalignment of nerve fibers as they grow across an anastomosis is less of a problem. Patients over 40 years of age with high amputations have a poor prognosis for anything but limited return of feeling and crude flexion. The younger the patient the better, because his chances both for neural regeneration and for relearning new pathways of response are great compared with those of older people.[12]

Even if both anatomy and physiology seem ideal for a reunion, one further facet of the patient needs to be evaluated— his psychologic state. This is a complex issue and, obviously, a complete assessment cannot be made, but nevertheless a good many inferences can be made by a perceptive surgeon. On the one hand, the dependent, timid person or the one with an irregular work record or with a regularly posted hospital chart probably will do badly no matter how skillful the operation. The patient who wants to support his family, who perhaps works hard doing so and who appears to have stoicism and spunk even while in the emergency ward can virtually be counted on to be a strong ally during rehabilitation. On the other hand, the vigorous person will also adapt better to a prosthesis, and perhaps a timid person will use his own imperfect limb better than a prosthesis. No easy formula can substitute for clinical judgment in predicting how the patient himself will influence the result.

Finally, the surgeon must make a realistic appraisal of resources available for the whole effort at replantation—the skill, the personnel and the facilities required for the task. The technical capacity to restore an arm does not constitute an indication to carry out the operation.

OPERATION

Once the feasibility of replantation has been decided, the principles are to remove foreign matter scrupulously, to stabilize the fracture, to repair the vessels, to approximate the nerves and to close the soft tissues.

PRELIMINARY DEBRIDEMENT.—In a good many amputations there are grease and foreign bodies ground into the wound. Since sepsis is the major cause of late failure of initially successful replantations, removal of these substances should be meticulous and thorough right from the start, because they will never be accessible again. Nonviable tissue must be removed without compromise. Yet, at the same time, debridement of the amputated part should be limited to the tissue that is clearly destroyed. Final debridement has to wait until blood flow is restored, for only then will the borders between dead and living tissue be declared.

FRACTURE.—Paradoxically, the initial event of the replantation itself is not restoration of circulation. Primary attention is given to the skeleton, because osseous stability is necessary to permit and to maintain effective vascular restoration.

The basic rules in restoration of bony continuity are:

1. Shorten the limb generously.
2. Use internal fixation.
3. Give precedence to osseous stability over attempts to gain union.

Since a discrepancy in length of one upper extremity compared with the other is of little consequence, shortening may be liberal, for it affords important advantages. It allows better bony contact and alignment and, hence, stability. It permits vascular repair without tension and perhaps without grafting. It immediately eases the burden of closing the soft tissues and helps in nerve repair later (Fig. 53-2).

The individual measures most applicable to each amputation will depend on the exact location and type of fracture. Because the limb will be anesthetized and may be swollen after the operation, reliance on plaster fixation alone is unwise. For this reason and also because of the need for osseous stability to facilitate the vascular repair, immediate internal fixation is required. Intramedullary fixation or plate-and-screw fixation are preferable because they add little bulk to the extremity and usually can be applied without adding much additional soft tissue and circulatory injury.

Replantation proximal to the shoulder rarely is feasible. For division through the surgical neck of the humerus, the best device to provide fixation is the AO Y-plate on the proximal humerus.[17] It provides control of the proximal fragment through cancellous screws into the humeral head and controls the distal fragment through cortical screws into the diaphysis. In most fractures, the com-

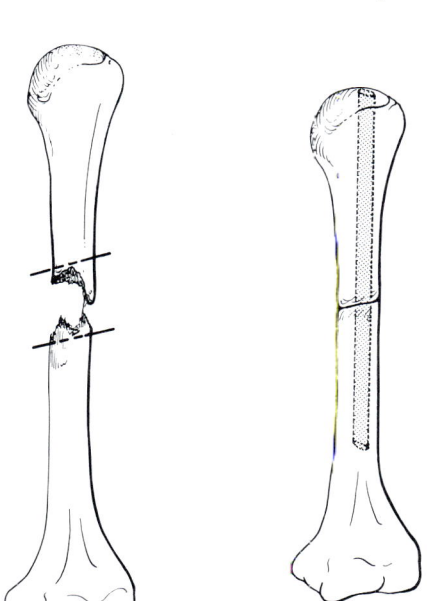

Fig. 53-2.—Fashioning the osseous framework. Bones should be shortened for ease in uniting other structures in the arm and should be contoured for maximal stability and cortical contact.

pression afforded by this plate across the fracture site will be a great asset in obtaining stability. Humeral diaphyseal fractures are best repaired using either a Küntscher rod or a heavy compression plate.

The anatomic complexities around the elbow mean that considerable ingenuity may be required in stabilizing an amputation in this region. Some distal humeral fractures can be fixed with an inverted Y-plate, but most will require crossed Kirschner wires from behind the flexed elbow through the humerus, across the elbow joint and down the medullary cavity of the radius or, conversely, across the ulna and up the humerus.

In the forearm, control of rotation is the special problem and is managed best by the use of fixation with plates. This method, especially with AO plates, usually is far preferable to intramedullary fixation in this region. The AO tubular forearm plates are of particular value.

At the wrist, as at the elbow, the crossed, buried Kirschner-wire fixation provides the adaptability required. If the carpus has received significant damage, primary fusion of the wrist is indicated. Shaping the radius for fusion will permit both improvement of the contact with the remaining carpus or metacarpal bases and shortening of the limb.

Fixation can be achieved by passing a Kirschner wire longitudinally down the medullary cavity of the second or third metacarpal, through the base of the metacarpal into the radius and then locking it in place by dorsiflexing the wrist.[13] Excellent stability is ensured when a second wire is passed through the base of the fifth metacarpal diagonally into the radius (Fig. 53-3). Kirschner wires are best for the fixation of metacarpal and thumb amputations also. Indications for replantation of a single digit other than the thumb must be rare.

Devices such as the Charnley compression clamp and Roger Anderson pins should be avoided because they provide an avenue for infection to enter the anesthetic limb.

Because the immediate needs for skeletal restoration are solely those of stability, bone grafting should not be done at the time of replantation. It adds time to the operation, trauma to the patient and bulk to the tissue mass without relieving the immediate problem. The graft will be unable to contribute to stability for many weeks until it is united. Usually the necessity for grafting can be obviated by shortening the limb, but if grafting is needed, it should be done later as an elective procedure.

BLOOD VESSELS.—In a field in which few things are complicated, arguments can begin over trivia. The two points of view concerning vascular repair in replantation are, on the one hand, that the veins should be repaired first and the other, that the arteries should have preference. In favor of giving priority to the veins is the scarcely debatable fact that if the surgeon restores flow in the arteries with no

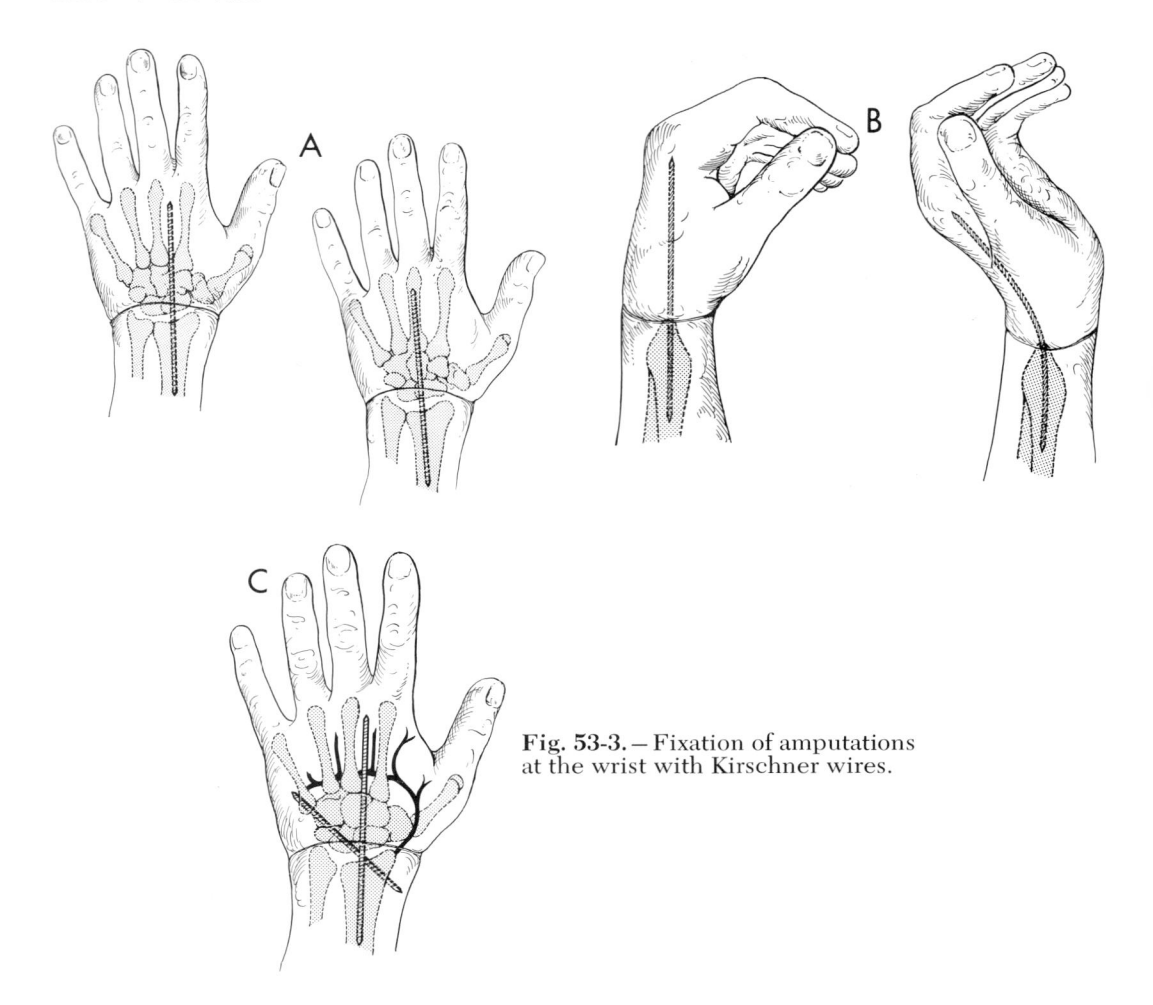

Fig. 53-3.—Fixation of amputations at the wrist with Kirschner wires.

place for the blood to go, he is in the uncomfortable situation of having to allow hemorrhage from the cut ends of the veins or else to clamp many of them and thus to provoke venous stasis and hypertension. Even in repairs at the wrist, arteriovenous anastomoses are open wide enough that the loss of blood can be brisk. In favor of the primacy of arterial repair is the unarguable point that the sooner arterial circulation is restored the better.

The resolution is simple. If the veins are of good size and easily accessible, at least one of them should be reconstituted as the first step in vascular repair; this short delay in restoring arterial flow will not harm the limb. If the veins are flimsy or difficult to locate, an arterial anastomosis should be done first; perhaps the bloody efflux will even help in identifying the veins.

Above the elbow there scarcely are any problems in vascular repair, as the vessels are large and strong. The veins are joined by over-and-over stitches of 5-0 Teflon-impregnated Dacron between triangulating stay sutures 120° apart. Practically the only caution is to avoid purse-stringing the anastomosis by being sure that the stay sutures are pulled wide apart and by placing the intervening su-

Chapter 53: REPLANTING AMPUTATED ARMS / 1189

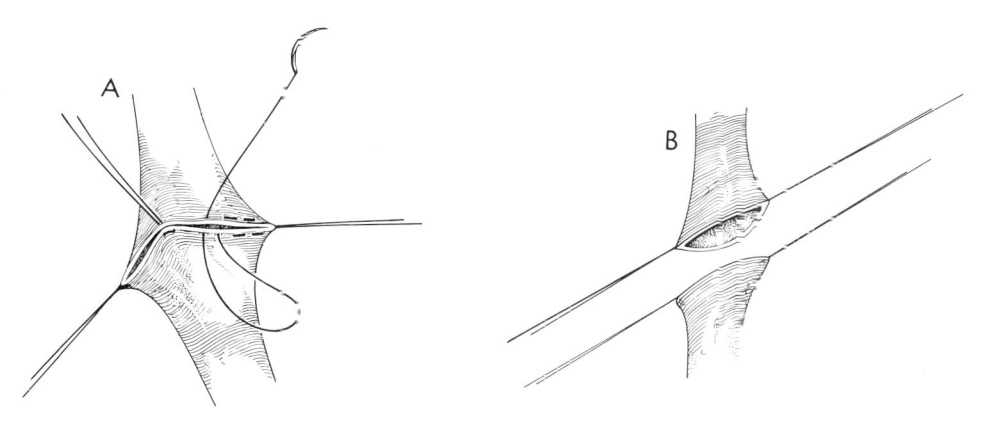

Fig. 53-4.—Anastomoses of large veins (**A**) and arteries (**B**).

tures with just enough tightness to coapt the walls of the vessels (Fig. 53-4, *A*). Since the deep veins of the upper arm entwine in a plexus around the artery, it may be necessary to join two veins side to side to get a vessel suitable for anastomosis. If a path for venous return cannot be established by these methods, an arthrodesis of the next proximal joint might be considered in an effort to utilize the intramedullary route for venous drainage.[11]

The arterial repair is simpler—over-and-over stitches between guy sutures 180° apart (Fig. 53-4, *B*). As a rule, it is well to divulse the ends of the artery with a smooth clamp or with hydrostatic pressure to achieve a lumen considerably larger than was present at the start.[21]

Below the elbow, the situation presents greater difficulties. In the first place, there are two arteries, and both of them ought to be repaired to avoid a fibrosis of intrinsic musculature of the hand that sometimes follows repair of one when the collateral circulation is inadequate. In the second place, everything about the vessels is smaller.

To facilitate repair, a few mechanical aids are helpful. A lowpower magnifying loupe with a long focal distance provides enlargement but does not constantly require reaccommodation of the eyes from near to far vision (Optivisor, Donegan Optical Co., Kansas City 1.5–2.5×; 30–20 cm focal length). A straight Barraquer's ophthalmic needle holder (Dixey Instruments, London) is a sturdy and responsive instrument lacking the annoying click-lock that dislodges a needle when it is opened.[5] Jewelers' forceps and a Jacobson fork for counterpressure against the intima (V. Mueller Co., Chicago) are indispensable. Buncke clamps are handy for hemostasis.[4] With these instruments, particularly if reinforced by practice with an operating microscope, anastomosis of vessels in adults as far distal as the palmar arch is not terribly difficult, provided that all vessels are well divulsed (Fig. 53-5).

The venous union at this level is carried out as with the larger veins except that interrupted sutures are used between the stay sutures and that the suture

Fig. 53-5.—Microsurgical anastomoses of arteries. Small tubes tied gently around the vessels provide hemostasis during surgery.

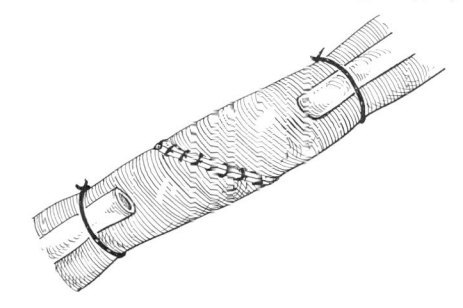

material is 7-0. Using the same material and interrupted sutures, the only difference in the arterial anastomosis is that the two stay sutures are placed 120° apart on top of the artery. This maneuver permits the back side to balloon out and helps to prevent sewing the walls together.

Another useful trick for insurance is to pass a polyethylene catheter through an arteriotomy some distance proximal to the proposed anastomosis. The catheter should be of large enough size just to be short of distending the distal artery. The repair then can be carried out over this strut, the catheter withdrawn and the proximal arteriotomy closed.

In all likelihood, if vessels in an adult are so small that they cannot be joined with these methods, the replantation is not worth doing. The sole exception may be replantation of a digit, which would require true microsurgery. The applications for microsurgery in children naturally are more extensive.

A frequently asked question concerns the use of systemic anticoagulants. They do have a role in preventing clotting from stagnant flow during the time that circulation is occluded before the vascular anastomoses are done. A single intravenous injection of perhaps 4,000 units of heparin is given; following that, anticoagulants should not be used. They do not prevent plugging of an imperfect anastomosis[19] but they do predispose to bleeding, which next to sepsis is the greatest cause of late failure of replantations.

DEFINITIVE DEBRIDEMENT. — After the circulation of blood is restored, a moment of triumph is appropriate. That moment will be brief, indeed, if attention is not soon turned to the problem of debridement. For the reasons stated earlier, every last bit of nonvital tissue must be removed at this point in an effort to prevent sepsis. Furthermore, wide areas of coapted soft tissues are necessary for adequate lymphatic regeneration and drainage.

NERVES. — Since the preponderance of amputating injuries are the result of blunt or shearing trauma with diffuse injury to nerves, and since the effects of anoxia on the capacity of the nerves to regenerate has not been explored, the repair of the nerves almost always should be delayed in performing a replantation. The patient will be in better condition at a later time, the surgeon will be fresher, distinction between injured and unharmed nerves will be more precise, the perineurium will hold stitches better and, if grafts are required, a less hurried job can be done. Therefore, at the initial operation, nerve ends should merely be brought end to end to prevent retraction and to aid later identification.[1, 20, 23, 24] The optimal time for the delayed repair seems to be after 3 weeks.[6] The tissues still will be soft at that time and the nerves will be biologically ready to regrow.

Primary repair of nerves should be undertaken only when the injury is sharp and when the period of ischemia is brief. These conditions will be met infrequently.

SOFT TISSUE CLOSURE. — The objectives are to surround the bone with its associated hardware and the vascular anastomoses each with a layer of well-vascularized tissue and to provide a broad union of muscle. Although some shifting of the soft tissues may be necessary to accomplish these goals, these rearrangements should be carried out freely, without concern for the functional or cosmetic handicaps that they may present later. Coverage of the site of replantation is essential; difficulties so produced can be repaired at another time.

If good coverage with muscle is possible, surfacing of the defect with skin is not essential at this time. There are, in fact, advantages to reinspecting the wound after 4–5 days and in applying split-thickness grafts at that time.

If good coverage is not possible, consideration should again be directed to whether the effort is worthwhile. Perhaps the patient would be far better off with one operation, a prosthesis and vocational rehabilitation than with a tenuous replantation, multiple operations and the possibility of developing detrimental personality traits during the prolonged rehabilitation. If a replantation is desirable notwithstanding these hazards, the details of cutting well-vascularized remote soft tissue flaps will, of course, depend on the relation of the defect to appropriate donor tissue.

POSTOPERATIVE CARE

Once a carefully padded cast is applied to the anesthetic limb and the limb is elevated, there ought to be scarcely any special needs after surgery. We have seen little lymphedema in these cases and think that it will not be much of a problem if venous drainage is good and if clean soft tissue planes are approximated over a broad area. If it occurs, the two approaches to its remedy are to perform prompt and generous fasciotomies and to consider shunting blood from blocked veins through silicon rubber tubing to patent veins in the other arm until the time that the drainage channels through small veins become adequate,[9] if they will. Fasciotomy has well-recognized benefits when muscle subjected to profound ischemia swells following revascularization. Benefits from a shunt have yet to be established, but looked promising in one case. An arthrodesis to facilitate venous return, as mentioned earlier, would seem to be practical only during the effort at replantation itself.

Although vascular occlusion can, in theory, be coped with according to standard surgical methods, in actuality few, if any, replantations have been rescued once an occlusion has developed following the operation. Thrombosis in the operating room likewise is ominous unless some major and totally correctable technical error is the cause. Cyanosis of the nail beds is such a bad sign that a case for reamputation can almost be made as soon as it is recognized, whether during the operation or afterward.

If collected experience is any criterion, infection makes the situation just about as grim as vascular occlusion. Prevention is more worthwhile than treatment. Aside from knowing the usual principles for correction of wound infection, physicians who do not often deal with infections in the presence of fractures stabilized by internal fixation should realize that these are instances in which the usual truism of removing hardware from a wound does not prevail. Maintenance of stability with metal fixation actually is paramount to the control of infection, if the limb still can be saved.

REAMPUTATION. — Almost as much of a challenge for every surgeon who attempts a replantation as the operation itself is his capacity for facing failure realistically. He must be objective about assessing the condition of the limb and act with dispatch when there is no reasonable chance for success. Although the commitment of the surgeon, the patient and the family toward a successful result can create an atmosphere promoting and sustaining false hope, no surgeon should undertake a replantation unless he is fully prepared to reamputate swiftly if the course of events is bad. The harm that may result from delay and procrastination is real, particularly in regard to sepsis.

PRESERVATION OF MOVEMENT. — During the period between the reattachment and the resumption of sensation and of volitional movement, the mobility of all joints and muscles must be maintained, within limits set by proper care of the fracture. A full range of passive motion should be carried out several times a day beginning in the first week following operation. Although preservation of muscle bulk is more of an unsolved problem, there is an indication that galvanic stimulation of the intrinsic musculature several times a day will help to maintain function.[10] As for the sensory receptors, there is no evidence that denervation of any duration will rob them of their receptivity.

NERVE REPAIR. — Providing useful sensation in an upper extremity is the main goal of replantation. Even if the hand is seriously compromised and the wrist joint is barely movable, fingers with feeling are valuable.

Since the end-receptors do not atrophy, repeated attempts at neurolysis in restoring sensation are worthwhile. To maintain the best muscle function, re-exploration should be entertained as soon as signs of neural regeneration fail to match the usual rate of about an inch a month. Electromyograms are valuable documentations of progress—or lack of it. One of the dangers of primary nerve repair is that the surgeon may be satisfied with a modicum of recovery and never know how much more might have been possible had he done an ideal job at another operating session.

The principles of neural repair are to arrange tissues so that an anastomosis without tension can be made, to resect the end-neuromas serially and squarely with a sharp blade until a maximal number of fresh fasicles are visible, to make the repair with fine, nonreactive perineural stitches and to splint the extremity for at least 3 weeks in an effort to remove distracting forces.[7] Of the several devices for facilitating squared cuts of the nerve, the most generally useful probably is a strip of heavy brown paper or Webril wrapped snugly around the nerve to hold it compressed in preparation for a single accurate division with a razor blade. Sutures of Teflon-impregnated Dacron, sizes 5-0 to 7-0, are good for the interrupted perineural stitches, reinforced in some instances by a single "tension" stitch of heavier material.

Although the use of adjuncts to nerve repair remains unsettled, one or all of them certainly should be tried before giving up on the hope of nerve repair. A thin silastic sheath to guide the regrowing fibers and to limit the anastomotic neuroma is the simplest prosthesis and the one least likely to cause trouble. Autografts from the sural, lateral femoral cutaneous and brachial cutaneous nerves are distinctly worth employing to bridge a gap, despite the markedly poorer results than when direct nerve unions are possible. As a last hope, irradiated nerve allografts can be attempted, with the anastomoses protected with silastic and the immune response diminished with azathioprine.

REHABILITATION. — While reinnervation is taking place, physical therapy several times daily must be maintained if joints are to be limber and the muscles are to remain capable of responding. Early vocational rehabilitation and return to work are desirable.

Function will continue to return over a period of several years. Restoration of active motor power will depend not only on the extent of motor activity present from those muscles innervated above the amputation and those restored to function by the nerve repair but on the imaginative use of tendon transfers and successful education of the patient to use them well. An example of an especially useful tendon transfer is the reversal of the extensor carpi radialis longus to restore elbow flexion, leaving its origin attached at the elbow and activating the tendon in the axilla through attachment to the pectoralis major muscle.

In this final phase of treatment, as in the ones before it, indispensable ingredients to success are a knowledgeable and enthusiastic physician to integrate the plan of treatment and a stable, highly motivated patient capable of readjusting his self-image and his goals.

BIBLIOGRAPHY

1. Bateman, J. E.: *Trauma to Nerves in Limbs* (Philadelphia: W. B. Saunders Company, 1962).
2. Berman, I. R., Leimieux, M. D., and Aaby, G. V.: Responses of skeletal muscle pH to injury: A new technique for determination of tissue viability, Surgery 67:507, 1970.
3. Buncke, H. J., Cobbett, J. R., Smith, J. W., and Tamai, S.: *Techniques of Microsurgery* (Somerville, N. J.: Ethicon, Inc.).

4. Chase, R. A.: The severely injured upper limb. To amputate or reconstruct: that is the question, Arch. Surg. 100:382, 1970.
5. Cobbett, J. R.: Microvascular surgery, Surg. Clin. North Am. 47:521, 1967.
6. Ducker, T. B., Kempe, L. G., and Hayes, G. J.: The metabolic background for peripheral nerve surgery, J. Neurosurg. 30:270, 1969.
7. Edshage, S.: Peripheral nerve suture. A technique for improved intraneural topography: Evaluation of some suture materials. Acta Chir. Scand. Supp. 331, 1964.
8. Engber, W. D., and Hardin, C. A.: Replantation of extremities, Surg. Gynecol. Obstet. 132:901, 1971.
9. Halmagyi, A. F., Baker, C. E., Campbell, H. H., Evans, J. G., and Mahoney, L. J.: Replantation of a completely severed arm followed by reamputation because of failure of innervation, Can. J. Surg. 12:222, 1969.
10. Jackson, E. C. S., and Sedcon, H. J.: Influence of galvanic stimulation on muscle atrophy resulting from denervation, Br. Med. J. 2:485, 1945.
11. Lemperg, R. D., and Arnoldi, C. C.: Intramedullary blood flow through arthrodesis-treated joints: An experimental study in rabbits, Angiology 21:368, 1970.
12. Lindsay, W. K., Walker, F. G., and Farmer, A. W.: Traumatic peripheral nerve injuries in children: Results of repair, Plast. Reconstr. Surg. 30:462, 1962.
13. Malt, R. A., and Harris, W. H.: *Replantation of Limbs* (Somerville, N. J.: Ethicon, Inc., 1965).
14. Malt, R. A., and McKhann, C. F.: Replantation of severed arms, JAMA 189 716, 1964.
15. McNeil, I. F., and Wilson, J. S. P.: The problems of limb replacement, Br. J. Surg. 57:365, 1970.
16. Mehl, R. L., Faul, H. A., Shorey, W. D., Schneewind, J. E., and Beattie, E. J.: Patency of the microcirculation in the traumatically amputated limbs—a comparison of common perfusates, J. Trauma 4 495, 1964.
17. Müller, M. E., Allgower, M., and Willenegger, H.: *The Technique of Internal Fixation of Fractures* (Berlin: Springer-Verlag. 1965).
18. Rosenkrantz, J. G., Sullivan, R. C., Welch, K., Miles, J. S., Sadler, K. M., and Paton, B. C.: Replantation of an infant's arm, N. Engl. J. Med. 276:609, 1967.
19. Salzman, E. W.: The limitations of heparin therapy after arterial reconstruction, Surgery 57:131, 1965.
20. Seddon, H. J.: *Peripheral Nerve Injuries*. Medical Research Council Special Report, Series 282 (London: H. M. Stationery Office, 1954).
21. Shaw, R. S.: Treatment of the extremity suffering near or total severance with special consideration of the vascular problem, Clin. Orthop. 29:56, 1963.
22. Strock, P. E., and Majno, G.: Microvascular changes in acutely ischemic rat muscle, Surg. Gynecol. Obstet. 129:1213, 1969.
23. Sunderland, S.: *Nerves and Nerve Injuries* (Edinburgh: E. & S. Livingstone, Ltd., 1968).
24. White, J. C.: Nerve regeneration after replantation of severed arms, Ann. Surg. 170:715, 1969.
25. Williams, G. R.: Replantation of amputated extremities, Monogr. Surg. Sci. 3:53, 1966.

54 | Fat Embolism

JAMES H. HERNDON

As Dr. Oliver Cope has stated, "From time to time, patients with fractures of a major bone, particularly the femur, die in shock; and the striking finding of postmortem examination is capillaries of the lung and brain filled with fat."[3] This clinical syndrome was first described by Zenker in 1862, and since, with the experience offered by several major wars, fat embolism has become a definite clinical entity that can be seen on any active fracture service. Its incidence varies from 10% to 65% (clinical syndrome),[7,10] depending on the series reported, with autopsy evidence that it is even more common (in the range of 80–100%).[9] A significant mortality of between 5% and 15% has been reported.[4]

PATHOGENESIS

The source of the fat still is the subject of considerable controversy. In all likelihood, each of the two main theories proposed has some validity. In 1924, Gauss[5] believed that the fat was released from the marrow of the fractured bone into the venous circulation. In 1951, evidence to support this theory was offered by Armin and Grant,[2] who demonstrated bone marrow emboli in lung capillaries after fractures of long bones in experimental animals.

The second, or physiochemical, theory, proposed by Lehman and Moore,[6] is more intriguing. It states that trauma in some way leads to a disturbance of normal blood fat emulsion, with formation of large fat globules. Evidence for this theory is only indirect, but, interestingly, the syndrome of fat embolism has been reported in other conditions, such as sickle cell crisis, poisoning, childbirth, severe burns, alcoholism, use of the pump oxygenator, following renal transplantation, after external cardiac massage, in patients with steroid-induced fatty liver and in simulated high-altitude flights.

Recently, a complicated, poorly understood relationship between lipid emulsion and blood cells and coagulation factors has been the subject of many investigations. Platelet adhesiveness and red blood cell aggregation increase with hyperlipemia. Fibrin thrombosis and an intravascular coagulopathy have also been implicated as possible mechanisms.

PATHOPHYSIOLOGY

Sevitt[9] reported that the major insult to the body by embolic fat was in the central nervous system. However, we agree with Peltier[8] that the major site of injury is in the lung. At Massachusetts General Hospital we have recently reported 17 cases of severe fat embolism and in each the clinical course was one of severe pulmonary insufficiency, and death from hypoxemia appeared to be the most immediate danger.

Regardless of the mechanism of formation, fat globules lodge in pulmonary arterioles and capillaries. They are coated with adhering platelets and are acted on by lipase hydrolyzing the neutral fats to free fatty acids. Thus, because of the mechanical blockage of arterioles, AV shunting is increased and, as Peltier[8] has demonstrated, the free fatty acids are toxic to lung parenchymal cells, leading to disruption of the capillary-alveolar membrane and curtailing of pulmonary surfactant activity. Pulmonary edema, hemorrhage and alveolar collapse develop. Also, serotonin is released from the large number of platelets present, leading to further vasoconstriction and bronchoconstriction. A severe respiratory insufficiency results, which requires prompt, correct treatment for survival of the patient.

CLINICAL MANIFESTATIONS

The appearance of the clinical syndrome occurs anywhere from 12 hours to 4 days after injury.[9] Classically, the patient develops a tachycardia, tachypnea and a fever up to 103 degrees (Fig. 54-1). Dyspnea may become prominent, with evidence of increasing respiratory insufficiency, although cyanosis is not a common finding.

With systemic emboli, petechiae have been reported in as high as 50% of cases. Usual distribution includes the anterior chest wall, axillary folds, neck, fundi and conjunctivae. With emboli to the brain, symptoms vary from headache to irritability and may progress to delirium or coma. Involvement of other major organs has been noted but not reported.

DIAGNOSIS

The diagnosis of fat embolism is largely clinical. There are, however, ancillary diagnostic aids. Fluffy densities in both lung fields, often similar to pulmonary edema, have been reported as high as 36% with chest roentgenograms (Fig. 54-2). Electrocardiograms show variable nondiagnostic abnormalities. Adler and Peltier[1] have shown the serum lipase to be elevated in 50% of cases. These results are similar to those in our series (Fig. 54-3).

We have found the presence of fat in the urine to be reliable and it can be found in up to 57% of cases. Fat globules

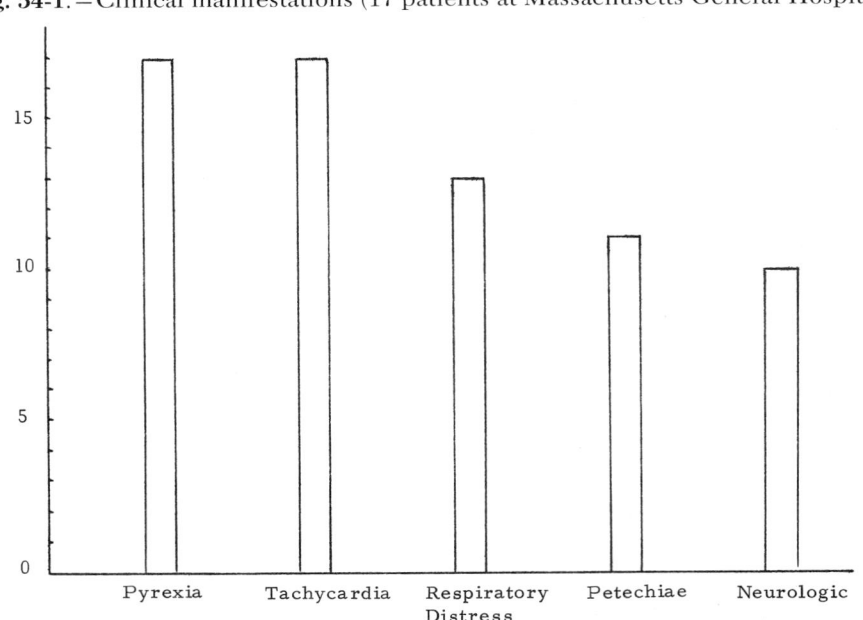

Fig. 54-1.—Clinical manifestations (17 patients at Massachusetts General Hospital).

Chapter 54: FAT EMBOLISM / 1197

in the sputum or cerebrospinal fluid are of little value.

Within 24 hours, hemoglobin values decrease as much as 4–5 grams. The reason for this is obscure. Some investigators have believed that it was secondary to pulmonary hemorrhage. In a few of our cases, hemolysis appeared to play a significant role, with the appearance of methemalbumin.

The most important laboratory test, and one that is essential for management of the patient, is arterial blood gases. In our series, the arterial P_{O_2} often was as low as 40 mm Hg. Often there was a slight increase in pH, with hyperventilation occurring in response to hypoxia.

None of these tests nor numerous others reported are consistently diagnostic of fat embolism. Further study of the reliability and usefulness of these laboratory tests is needed to aid the clinician.

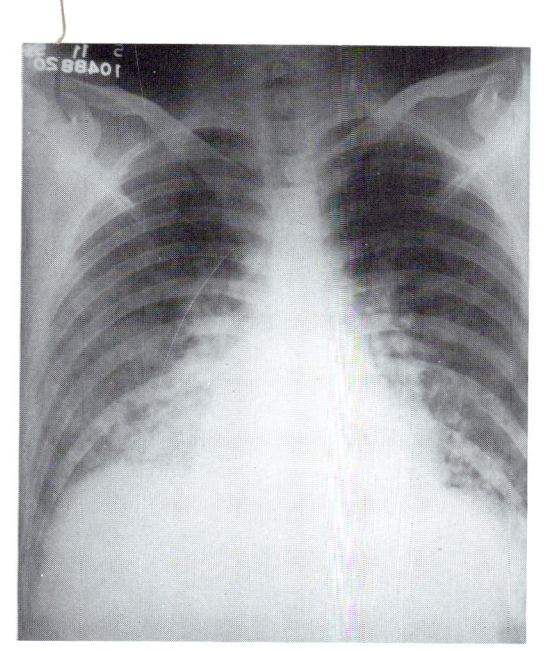

Fig. 54-2.—Chest roentgenogram demonstrating the usual fluffy "snowstorm" infiltrate characteristic of fat embolism.

TREATMENT

Because of the poor understanding of the pathophysiology of fat embolism, a

Fig. 54-3.—Laboratory data (17 patients at Massachusetts General Hospital).

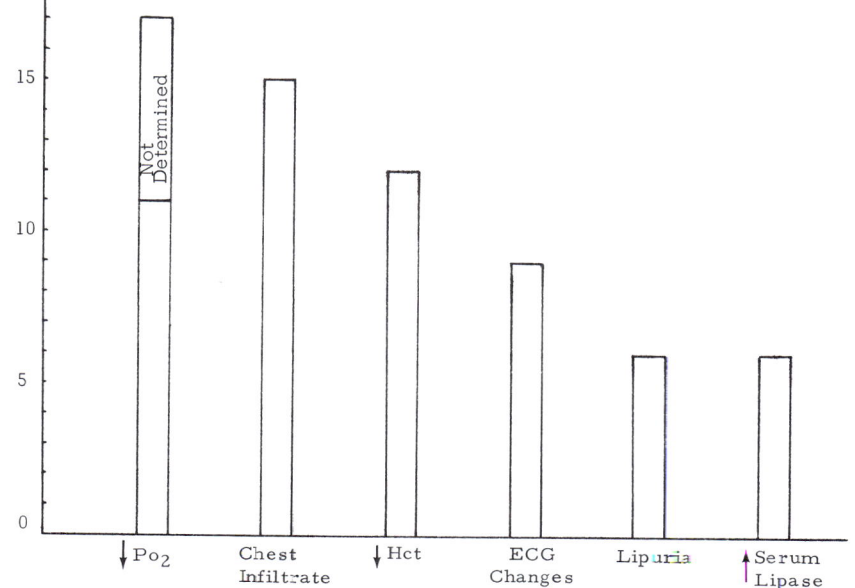

wide range of treatments has been proposed. We divide therapy into two components—supportive and specific. Supportive therapy includes immobilization of the fracture, no unnecessary manipulation and treatment of the respiratory distress with oxygen, digitalis for heart failure, aminophylline for bronchospasm, maintenance of an adequate airway and respirators if necessary.

Specific therapy, such as heparin, intravenous alcohol, low molecular weight dextran, detergents, emulsifying agents and others, has been advocated, but, in our experience, these add little to the treatment of the patient.

We have used corticosteroids in large doses (similar to that required in septic shock), with dramatic response in the recovery of the patients from a severe pulmonary insufficiency (Table 54-1). We believe that it is an essential treatment for severe fat embolism and rely on it solely, with only additional supportive care.

TABLE 54-1.—IMPROVEMENT FOLLOWING CORTICOSTEROID THERAPY (13 PATIENTS AT MASSACHUSETTS GENERAL HOSPITAL)

Pulse	12–48 hours
PO_2	12–24 hours
Compliance	48–72 hours
Chest x-ray	12–48 hours
Neurologic status	36–72 hours

BIBLIOGRAPHY

1. Adler, F., and Peltier, L. F.: The laboratory diagnosis of fat embolism, Clin. Orthop. 21: 226, 1961.
2. Armin, J., and Grant, R. F.: Observations on gross pulmonary fat embolism in man and in the rabbit, Clin. Sci. 10:441, 1951.
3. Cope, O.: In Cave, E. F. (ed.), *Fractures and Other Injuries* (Chicago: Year Book Medical Publishers, Inc., 1958), p. 121.
4. Fuchsig, P., Brucke, P., Blumel, G., and Gottlub, R.: A new clinical and experimental concept of fat emboli, N. Engl. J. Med. 276: 1192, 1967.
5. Gauss, H.: The pathology of fat embolism, Arch. Surg. 9:593, 1924.
6. Lehman, E. P., and Moore, R. M.: Fat embolism, including experimental production without trauma, Arch. Surg. 14:621, 1927.
7. Mallory, J. B., Sullivan, E. R., Burnett, C. H., Simeone, F. A., Shapiro, S. L., and Beecher, H. K.: The general pathology of traumatic shock, Surgery 27:629, 1950.
8. Peltier, L. F.: Fat embolism: A current concept, Clin. Orthop. 66:241, 1969.
9. Sevitt, S.: *Fat Embolism* (London: Butterworths, 1962).
10. Sutton, G. E.: Pulmonary fat embolism and its relation to traumatic shock, Br. Med. J. 2:368, 1918.

Index

A

ABDOMEN, 1033–1055
  angiography, 198–206
  injuries, 1033–1055
    anesthesia in, 1037
    antibiotics in, 1036
    diagnosis, 1033–1035
    fecal contamination in, 1038–1039
    gastric aspiration in, 1036
    general considerations, 1033
    hemorrhage control in, 1038
    incisions, 1037–1038
    laparotomy in, 1037
    liver injuries and, 1061
    management, 1033–1055
    mortality in, 1052–1053
    paracentesis in, 1034–1035
    postoperative care, 1050–1052
    radiography of, 1035
    resuscitation and, 1035–1036
    signs, physical, 1034
    symptoms, 1034
    treatment, 1035–1050
    treatment, early supportive, 1035–1036
    treatment, general, 1035–1039
    urinary drainage in, 1036
  in physical examination, 185
  wall
    lower, extravasation due to urethral leakage, 1080
    treatment, 1050
ABDUCTION
  fingers, 17
  foot, 35
  hip, 30
  shoulder, 18–19
  thumb, 13, 15
  toes, 36
ACE SPLINTS: for clavicle fractures, in children, 413

ACETABULUM
  divisions of, primary, 692
  fracture (see Fractures, acetabulum)
  fracture-dislocation of, 697
  hip capsule and ligament attachments to, 699
  lip disruption, 712
  rim, radiography of, 688
  wall of, 693
    disruption of, 713
ACETAMINOPHEN: temperature control by, 312
ACHILLES TENDON (see Tendons, Achilles)
ACID-BASE DISORDERS, 53–54
ACIDOSIS, 53
  lactic, treatment, 54
  metabolic
    shock and, sodium bicarbonate in, 220
    shock and, treatment of, 220
    treatment, 54, 220
  respiratory, treatment, 54
  sodium bicarbonate and, 53, 220
ACOUSTIC NERVE, 293
ACROMIOCLAVICULAR
  dislocations (see Dislocations, acromioclavicular)
  pin-screws, Simmons-Martin, 407
  separation
    Kirschner pin in, 406
    reduction, open, 406–407
    sling for, 405
  trauma, 404–409
    complications, 409
    diagnosis, 404–405
    incidence of, 404
    inspection, 404
    mechanism, 404
    palpation, 404–405
    treatment, 405–409
    treatment, after-treatment, 408–409
    treatment, operative, 405–408
    types of, 404
    x-rays in, 405
ACROMION FRACTURES, 416
ACTH: and 17-hydroxycorticosteroid secretion, 45, 47
ADDUCTION
  in acetabular fracture, 701
  fingers, 17
  foot, 35
  hip, 30
  shoulder, 18–19
  thumb, 13
  toes, 36
ADH: secretion, 41
ADHESIVE CAPSULITIS: and shoulder dislocations, 440
ADOLESCENCE: epiphysitis during, 381
ADRENAL
  insufficiency
    cortisol in, 47
    desoxycorticosterone acetate in, 47
    hydrocortisone in, 47
    prednisolone in, 47
    prednisone in, 47
  response to stress, 47
ADRENOCORTICOTROPIC HORMONE: and 17-hydroxycorticosteroid secretion, 45, 47
AGE
  forearm fractures and, 499
  shoulder dislocations and, recurrent, 417, 440
AGED: shoulder fracture dislocation in, 445
AIR
  in orbit, 257
  "pendulum," 997
  in pleural space, management, 999–1001
AIRPLANE SPLINT: in humeral neck fracture, 444
AIRWAY, 178–180
  clear, maintenance of, 998–

1200 / INDEX

AIRWAY (cont.)
　999
　in face trauma, 244
　in head trauma, 270
　obstruction
　　common mechanical
　　　causes, 1029
　in shock, hypoxic, 225
ALBUMIN: serum, 49
ALCOHOL
　head trauma and, 283
　-induced coma, 283
ALDOSTERONE
　response, sensitivity of, 41
　secretion, 41–43
ALIGNMENT: in tibial and
　fibular fractures, 799
ALKALOSIS, metabolic, 53
　treatment, 54
ALLEN, A. W., 4
ALLISON, N., 2
ALLOGRAFTS (see Grafts)
AMNESIA
　anterograde, 279–280
　retrograde, 279
AMPHOTERICIN B: in surgical
　infections, 952
AMPICILLIN: in surgical
　infections, 952
AMPUTATION
　arm
　　reamputation after
　　　replantation failure, 1191
　　replanting (see
　　　Replantation of arms)
　of extremities, ischemic, and
　　vascular injuries, 1116
　after fibular fracture, 807
　finger, index, painful stump,
　　576
　after tibial fracture, 807
　in toe fracture-dislocations,
　　856
　wrist, fixation in, 1188
ANAL SPHINCTER: treatment,
　　1047–1048
ANASTOMOSIS
　of arteries
　　large, 1189
　　microsurgical, 1189
　end-to-end, for
　　arteriosclerotic vessel,
　　1121
　tendon to terminal phalanx,
　　566
　vascular, with graft, 1122
　of veins, large, 1189
ANESTHESIA
　(See also Anesthetist)
　in abdominal injuries, 1037
　in face trauma, 248–249
　in femoral neck fracture,

　　displaced, 633–634
　in forearm fractures, 500
　in hand soft tissue injuries,
　　556–557
　induction of, and anesthetist,
　　238–239
　problems associated with,
　　237
　shock and, 213–239
　spinal, and cortisol excretion,
　　44
ANESTHETIST, 235–242
　(See also Anesthesia)
　anesthesia induction and,
　　238–239
　cardiac massage and, 235–
　　236
　cardiovascular system and,
　　unstable, 238
　ear trauma and, 240–241
　eye trauma and, 240–241
　full stomach and, 239
　maxillofacial trauma and,
　　240–241
　neurologic trauma and, 239–
　　240
　pain and, 242
　patient evaluation and, 236–
　　237
　physiologic problems and,
　　241–242
　problems for, 237
　resuscitation and, 235–236
　shock and, 238
ANEURYSM: aortic, traumatic
　false, 1008
ANGIOGRAPHY, 197–211
　abdomen, 198–206
　aorta
　　intimal tear, 199
　　isthmus, tear of, 1009
　　isthmus, traumatic
　　　disruption, 1008
　　rupture, 199
　catheter approach, 197
　cerebral, 278
　chest, 198, 199
　after disk surgery, 206–210
　extremities, 206
　femoral artery tear, 205
　fistula, arteriovenous, 205,
　　206
　hematoma
　　extradural, 298
　　hepatic, 1062
　　renal, 203–204
　　spleen, 201
　　subdural, 279
　after hip surgery, 206–210
　kidney, 202–203, 205, 1073
　　hematoma, 203–204
　　rupture, 204

　liver, 198–200
　　hematoma, subcapsular,
　　　1062
　　indications for, 198
　　rupture, 200
　　method, 197
　in multiple trauma, 209, 210
　of myocardial shotgun
　　wound, 1012
　pancreas, 202
　　pseudocyst, 202
　pelvic hemorrhage, 207
　　with fractures, 208, 210
　retroperitoneal hemorrhage,
　　207
　spleen, 194, 200–202
　　hematoma, 201
　　rupture, 201
　vessels, great, 198
ANKLE, 809–836
　anatomy
　　of clinical significance,
　　　813–815
　　of surgical importance, 816
　arthritis of, 138
　articulation
　　at distal end of fibula, 813
　　at distal end of tibia, 813
　bone injuries, 823–836
　　surgery, indications for,
　　　829–830
　　types of, 823–824
　dislocation, 821, 833
　extension, 32
　flexion, 32
　fracture (see Fracture, ankle)
　fracture-dislocation (see
　　Fracture, -dislocation,
　　ankle)
　joint
　　fusion of, 852
　　medial capsule, transverse
　　　fiber of, 821
　ligaments of, 815, 820–823
　　anatomy, 818–819
　　deltoid, tear of, 830
　　lateral, rupture of, 822
　　medial, rupture of, 823
　　medial, tear of, 821, 829
　manipulation of, 811
　motion, 32, 817–820
　muscles of, 815–817
　radiography of, 811–813
　　positions for, 812
　reduction of, 811
　rotation, external, leverage
　　forces in, 810
　tendons of, 815–817
　　Achilles (see Tendons,
　　　Achilles)
　　flexor hallucis longus, 817
　　peroneal, 815

INDEX / 1201

posterior tibial, 815–817
trauma, 809–836
treatment, emergency, 809–811
twisted, 820, 822
ANKYLOSIS, 37
  of cervical spine, fracture in, 375
ANOMALIES (see Deformity)
ANTIBIOTICS
  in abdominal injuries, 1036
  in burn infections, 1144–1145
  in face trauma, 249
  in hand soft tissue injuries, 561–562
  for sepsis prevention, 944, 949
  in shock, 230
  in surgical infections, 952
ANTICOAGULANTS: and arterial injuries, 1125
ANTICONVULSANTS: in head trauma, 311–312
ANTIDIURETIC HORMONE: secretion, 41
AO COMPRESSION PLATES: in tibial and fibular fractures, 804
AORTA
  aneurysm, traumatic false, 1008
  angiography (see Angiography, aorta)
  intra-aortic balloon assist, in cardiogenic shock, 224–225
  isthmus
    rupture, angiography, 199
    tear, angiography of, 1009
    tear, aortography of, 1009
    traumatic disruption, 1008
AORTIC VALVE REGURGITATION: traumatic, 1007
AORTOGRAPHY, 198
  of aortic isthmus tear, 1009
  intravenous, 198
ARM
  (See also Forearm)
  innervation of, 1099
  replanting (see Replantation of arms)
  sensory deficit after nerve trunk interruption in, 1097
  upper, flaps for, 990
ARTERIES, 1115–1125
  anastomoses of, 1189
    microsurgical, 1189
  cerebral, extracranial occlusion, 284
  femoral, tear, angiography of,

205
  grafts for, 1121–1123
  hemorrhage control, 1119
  hepatic, anatomic variations in, 1065
  injuries, 1115–1125
    anticoagulants and, 1125
    blocks and, sympathetic, 1125
    hemorrhage and, secondary, 1124–1125
    major, atraumatic control of, 1120
    major, recognition of, 1117–1119
    sepsis and, 1124–1125
  ischemia, sequelae of, 1116–1117
  obstruction, in Volkmann's contracture, 1130
  occlusion, natural history of, 1115–1116
  pressure, measurement of, 216
  spinal, 321
  surgery, 1119–1125
    exposure, 1119
    techniques, 1119–1125
  suturing of, 1119–1121
  thrombosis, distal, 1123–1124
  vasoconstriction, 1115
  vasodilation, 1115–1116
ARTERIOSCLEROSIS: vascular, anastomosis for, 1121
ARTERIOVENOUS FISTULA: angiography, 205, 206
ARTHRITIS
  ankle, 138
  septic, after hip nailing, 650
ARTHROPLASTY: primary cup, 714
ASIF PLATE AND SCREWS: discussion, 895–896
ASPIRATION
  gastric, 186–187
  of hemarthrosis, in radius head fracture, 492–493
ASPIRIN: temperature control by, 312
ATLAS
  dislocation, 351, 377–379
    anterior, 359
  fracture, bursting, 368–369
ATROPHY: and forearm fractures, 501
AUFRANC, O. E., 6
AUSTIN'S VISE-GRIP PLIERS, 908
AVASCULAR NECROSIS (see Necrosis, avascular)
AVULSION
  in ankle fractures, 824

of calcaneus, 841
of elbow
  epicondyle, and dislocation, 475–477
  epiphysis, 494
of finger, due to ring, 577
of foot, 985
in hand injuries, 573
of knee posterior cruciate ligament, 761
  treatment, 761
of ligamentum patellae, 767
  treatment, 767
of liver, 1058
of radius, 141
of scalp, treatment, 265
of spine, 613
  anterior, 756
  cord fracture, 335
in tibial fracture, 758–760
of tibial tubercle, 767
  treatment, 767
AXONOTMESIS, 1097

B

BACK: physical examination, 185–186
BACTEREMIC SHOCK: treatment of, 229–230
BALLOON: intra-aortic balloon assist in cardiogenic shock, 224–225
BAND (see Parham bands)
BANDAGE: Esmarch, 891
BANKART LESION, 424
BANKART PROCEDURE IN RECURRENT ANTERIOR SHOULDER DISLOCATIONS, 425–432
  after-treatment, 431–432
  modified
    instruments for, 431
    steps in, 428–430
  objective, 425
  position of patient, 425, 426
  shoulder exposure, 426–431
  skin incision in, 425–426, 427
BANKS METHOD: in complete urethral transection, 1083–1085
BÉNARD'S OPERATION: in navicular nonunion, 534
BARTON TONGS: and spinal cord trauma, 330, 332
BARTON'S FRACTURE, 525
BASAL METABOLIC RATE, 56–57
BASEBALL FINGER, 569
  treatment, 964–965
BATTLE'S SIGN, 275

1202 / INDEX

BECKMAN PARAMAGNETIC
  OXYGEN ANALYZER, 1024
BELT
  pubic, 614
  sacroiliac, 612
BEND: lateral, cervical spine,
  22
BENNETT FRACTURE-
  DISLOCATION: of thumb,
  592
BICEPS
  muscle, in humeral shaft
    fracture, 462
  tendon (see Tendons, biceps)
BIGELOW'S METHOD: for
  posterior hip dislocation,
  687
BILIARY SYSTEM: extrahepatic,
  1068–1069
BIRD MARK 8 RESPIRATOR,
  1023
BIRTH: symphysis pubis tear
  during, 613–614
BLADDER, 1078–1079
  contusion, 1079
  cord, 383
  cystography, 1078
    in extravasation, 1079
  extravasation
    cystography of, 1079
    extraperitoneal, 1079
  function loss after spinal cord
    contusion, 334
  injuries, 1078–1079
    diagnosis, 1078
    signs, 1078
    symptoms, 1078
    treatment, 1079
    types of, 1078–1079
  laceration, 608
  rupture, intraperitoneal, 1079
  teardrop, 1079
BLEEDING (see Hemorrhage)
"BLIND" TECHNIQUE: Rush
  nails in humerus shaft
  transverse fracture, 464
BLOCK
  brachial plexus, in forearm
    fracture, 500
  in hand soft tissue injuries,
    557
  myelographic, and vertebral
    fracture, 383
  nerve (see Nerve, block)
  spinal subarachnoid space,
    329
  sympathetic, and arterial
    injuries, 1125
BLOCKING AGENTS: in shock,
  229
BLOOD
  ACD, and acidosis, 53

losses, in burns, 1138
plasma (see Plasma)
in pleural space,
  management, 999–1001
pressure, arterial,
  measurement of, 216
studies, 186
supply
  to carpal bones, 528
  to epiphysis, 872, 873
  to epiphysis, plate, 872
  to shoulder, 399
  to spinal cord, in fetus, 321
  tibial, 120
transfusions (see Transfusions)
"BLOWOUT" FRACTURES: of
  orbit, 256–257
BÖHLER-BRAUN FRAME: in
  femoral supracondylar
  fracture, 778
BÖHLER CLAMP: for foot, 842
BOLSTER METHOD: in
  acetabular fractures, 701
BOLT
  corrosion of, 916
  transfixion, in humeral
    fractures, 489
BONE
  ankle (see Ankle, bone
    injuries)
  callus, 96
  carpal (see Carpal bones)
  cyst, causing humeral
    fracture, 169
  in debridement of open
    fractures, 938
  defects, granulating, skin
    grafts in, 973
  deformity, correction of, 149
  facial, damage to, 266
  foot (see Foot, injuries, bone)
  formation, in immobilized
    patient, 61
  grafts (see Grafts, bone)
  healing
    (See also repair below)
    necrotic compact, 83–87,
      88
    necrotic compact,
      differentiation in, 83–86
    necrotic compact,
      inflammatory response
      in, 83
    necrotic compact, necrosis
      in, 83
    necrotic compact,
      remodeling in, 86–87
    necrotic compact,
      revascularization in, 83–
      84
    primary, 104–106
    primary (in dog), 105

small hole in bone, 87–91
innominate, disruption, 714
long
  fractures (see Fractures,
    long-bone)
  malunion of, 115–166
  nonunion of, 115–158
loss, and nonunion, 122
navicular (see Navicular
  bone)
repair, 71–113
  (See also healing above)
  dead course cancellous, 73–
    82
  dead course cancellous,
    cytodifferentiation in,
    79–81
  dead course cancellous,
    inflammatory response
    in, 75, 78
  dead course cancellous,
    necrosis in, 73–75
  dead course cancellous,
    revascularization in, 78,
    80
  general considerations, 73
  remodeling in, 82
resorption, in immobilized
  patient, 61
sclerosis of, 121
-seeking radioisotopes, 61
shortening, 122–123
  in peripheral nerve
    injuries, 1108
  producing union, 126
shoulder, 400
slabs, iliac, in tibia
  nonunion, 123
spicules, rotating femoral
  head fragment, 637
temporal, fracture, 293
toleration of metal, 116
BOOT: plaster-of-Paris, for foot,
  866
"BOOT-TOP" FRACTURES, 132
"BOUTONNIERE" DEFORMITY,
  570
BOWEL
  small, treatment, 1044
  after spinal trauma, 395
  function loss after cord
    contusion, 334
BRACE
  cast (see Fractures, femur,
    shaft, brace, cast)
  for clavicle fracture, 147
  halo, 360
BRACHIAL PLEXUS BLOCK: in
  forearm fracture
  treatment, 500
BRACHIALIS MUSCLE: in
  humeral fracture, 462

BRADYARRHYTHMIAS: in shock control of, 220
BRAIN
  contusion
    contrecoup, 282
    coup, 280
    stem, decerebrate rigidity due to, 275
  coverings, trauma, 286–291
  death, and irreversible coma 313–314
  scanning, radioisotope, 278–279
  trauma
    coverings of brain, 286–291
    gunshot causing, 307
    intrinsic, 279–283
    penetrating, 306–308
    primary, 276, 281
    secondary, 276
BREAST CARCINOMA, metastatic
  femoral fractures and, 172, 174
  hip fractures and, pathologic, 676
BREATHING
  (See also Respiration, Respiratory)
  high oxygen concentrations, 1019
  intermittent positive-pressure, 994
  work of
    compliance increase and, 1019
    normal work diagram, 1013
    resistance increase and, 1019
BROWN-SÉQUARD SYNDROME: and spinal cord trauma, 336
BRYANT TRACTION: in femoral shaft fractures, 731, 732–733
BULLDOG CLAMP: in kidney surgery, 1074
BULLET WOUND (see Gunshot wounds)
BUNNELL METHOD, 566
BUR-HOLE EXPLORATION, 278
BURN(S), 1137–1162
  basal metabolic rate and, 57
  cardiac function in, 1156–1157
  cerebral function in, 1157
  chemical, 1152–1153
  electrical, 1153–1154
  forearm, 579
  gastrointestinal function in, 1157–1158
  grafts in, 1146
  hand, 579
  infections, 1142–1147
    antibiotics in, systemic, 1144–1145
    clostridial, 1146–1147
    control measures, 1143–1147
    control measures, environmental, 1143–1144
    control measures, local, 1143–1144
    immunology in, 1145–1146
    organisms, sources of, 1142–1143
    organisms, types of, 1142–1143
    topical agents in, 1144
    treatment, 1151–1152
  metabolic responses in, 1158–1159
  musculoskeletal function in, 1159
  nutritional responses in, 1158–1159
  pain of, 1159–1160
  renal impairment in, 1156
  respiratory impairment in, 1154–1156
    direct causes, 1154–1155
    indirect mechanisms, 1155–1156
  shock, 1137–1142
    blood losses in, 1138
  shock, treatment, 1139–1142
    aims, 1139
    implementation, 1141–1142
    monitoring during, 1140–1141
    replacement formulas, 1139–1140
  ulcers and, gastrointestinal, 56
  wound, 1147–1154
    appraisal, 1149
    clean, treatment, 1149–1151
    evolution, 1147–1148
    infected, treatment, 1151–1152
    management, 1148–1152

C

CALCANEUS: avulsion of, 841
CALCIFICATION: of thoracic vertebra, 347
CALCIUM: for hyperalimentation, 65
CALLUS
  bone, 96
  periosteal, 100
  requirement increase with malposition, 119
CALORIC BALANCE: by IV feeding, 65
CAMBIUM, 91
CAPITATE (see Dislocations, capitate)
CAPITELLUM
  epiphyseal displacement, 485
  elbow cubitus valgus deformity after, 494
  fractures (see Fractures, capitellum)
CAPSULITIS: adhesive, and shoulder dislocations, 440
CARBENICILLIN: in surgical infections, 952
CARBOHYDRATE METABOLISM, 47–48
CARCINOMA (see Breast carcinoma)
CARDIAC (see Heart)
CARDIOGENIC SHOCK (see Shock, cardiogenic)
CARDIOPULMONARY BYPASS UNITS, 223
CARDIOVASCULAR (see Heart, Vessels)
CARE
  after abdominal surgery, 1050–1052
  after acetabular fracture, 701
  after ankle fracture reduction, 825–829
  of chest injuries, general, 1025–1027
  emergency, in replantation of arm, 1183–1185
  emergency room, of open fractures, 935–937
  after femoral fracture
    neck, 646–647
    supracondylar, 779–782
  of flaps, 981–982
  of grafts, 981–982
  in hand soft tissue injuries (see Hand, soft tissue injuries, care)
  home, patient instruction for, 1179–1180
  of knee
    after dislocation, 785
    meniscus, 764
  after nerve surgery, 1108
  nursing
    care sheet in chest injuries, 1026

CARE (cont.)
    after spinal cord trauma,
        339–340
    after patellar fracture
        surgery, 772
    respiratory, maintenance of,
        1022–1025
    of soft tissue open wounds,
        978–979
    after tibial fracture reduction,
        787, 789
CAROTID
    angiography in extradural
        hematoma, 298
    -cavernous fistula and skull
        fracture, 291–292
CARPAL BONES, 527–553
    anatomy, 528–529
        skeletal, 528
    blood supply of, 528
    development of, 527–528
    dorsal approach to, 538
    radiography of, 529–531
    trauma, 527–553
        severe, 544
        treatment, 531–553
        types of, 527
CARPOMETACARPAL JOINT
    dislocations (see
        Dislocations,
        carpometacarpal joint)
    flexion, 14
    fracture-dislocation, 592
CARTILAGE
    hip, destruction after trauma,
        716–717
    knee, semilunar, 762–764
CAST
    brace (see Fractures, femur,
        shaft, brace, cast)
    in forearm fractures, 501
    hanging, in humeral shaft
        fracture, 458–460, 465
    immobilization fracture
        healing, diaphysis, 91–
        98
    spica (see Spica)
    total contact, in tibial and
        fibular fractures, 797
CAT SCANNING, 279
CATHETER
    Fogarty embolectomy, 1124
    Swan-Ganz, 217
CAUDA EQUINA, 317–341
    anatomy, 317–324
    fractures, 333–336
    trauma, 317–341
CAVE, E. F., 5
CECUM: laceration, repair, 1047
CELIAC AXIS: stenosis of, 1062
CELLS
    source of, 73

types of, 73
CEPHALOHEMATOMA, 287
CEPHALORIDINE: in surgical
    infections, 952
CEPHALOTHIN: in bacteremic
    shock, 230
CEREBRAL
    angiography, 278
    artery occlusion, extracranial,
        284
    concussion, 279–280
    contusion, 280–283
    edema (see Edema, cerebral)
    fat embolism, 284–286
    function, in burns, 1157
    laceration, 280–283
    palsy, and hip fracture, 653
CEREBROSPINAL FLUID
    otorrhea, and skull fracture,
        293–295
    rhinorrhea, and skull
        fracture, 293–295
CEREBRUM (see Cerebral)
CERVICAL SPINE (see Spine,
    cervical)
CHEEK LACERATIONS:
    treatment, 265
CHEMICAL BURNS, 1152–1153
CHERRY SCREW EXTRACTOR,
    908
CHEST, 993–1003
    angiography, 198, 199
    flail
        segment, 994, 998
        stabilization of, 1028–1029
    injuries, 993–1003
        associated injuries, 1016
        bleeding in, control of,
            995–996
        care, general, 1025–1027
        diagnosis, 1016
        discussion of, 1015–1016
        early manifestations, 1016
        external wound,
            management, 1001–1002
        functional disturbances
            and, 1016–1020
        nursing care sheet, 1026
        pathophysiology, 1020–
            1021
        respiratory failure and,
            1015–1032
        special considerations in,
            1002
        treatment, early, 1022
        motor function chart and,
            328
        physical examination, 185
        plate, 994, 998
        suction, method, 1000
    wall
        flail segment, lateral, 998

        flail segment, right, 994
        paradoxical motion,
            hazards of, 997
        stabilization of, 996–998
CHILBLAIN, 1167
CHILDBIRTH: symphysis pubis
    tear during, 613–614
CHILDREN
    capitellar epiphysis fracture
        with rotational
        displacement, 485
    clavicular fractures, splints
        for, 412, 413
    fibular fractures, healing of,
        795–796
    forearm fractures, 509, 510–
        512
    hip fractures, 675–677
    humerus supracondylar
        fractures in, prognosis,
        482
    infant (see Infants)
    mandibular fractures, 263
    olecranon fractures, 491–492
    radiation damage to
        epiphysis, 192
    radius
        epiphyseal separation,
            493–494
        head dislocation, 473–474
    tibial fractures, healing of,
        795–796
CHIP FRACTURE: of capitellum,
    484–485
CHLORIDE: for
    hyperalimentation, 65
CHLORPROMAZINE: in
    hypovolemic shock, 229
CHROMIUM COBALT ALLOYS:
    corrosion of, 914
CINERADIOGRAPHY: in cervical
    spine surgery, 362
CIRCULATION
    assisted, in shock, 222–225
    collateral, development of,
        1116
    interruption in navicular
        fractures, 532
    support of, 40–43
        homeostatic mechanisms
            of, 43
CITRIC ACID CYCLE, 52
CLAMP
    Böhler, for foot, 842
    bulldog, in kidney surgery,
        1074
CLAMPING: of vessels, in face
    trauma, 243–244
CLAVICLE
    acromioclavicular (see
        Acromioclavicular)
    anatomic considerations, 404

cross section of, 404
dislocation, treatment, 405
fractures (see Fractures, clavicle)
nonunion, 130, 147–148
resection of distal end of, 408
sternoclavicular (see Dislocations, sternoclavicular)
CLEANSING: of facial wounds, 249
CLIP: vena caval, below renal veins, 1125
CLOSTRIDIAL
infection, in burns, 1146–1147
myositis, 954–955
CLOVERLEAF
nail (see Nails, Küntscher)
rods, 503
CLOXACILLIN: in surgical infections, 952
COAGULATION, 49–50
hypercoagulation, 49–50
hypocoagulation, 50
COAGULOPATHY: consumption, 49
COAPTATION SPLINT: for humerus shaft fractures, 460
COBALT CHROMIUM ALLOYS: corrosion of, 914, 922
COCAINE
in face trauma, 248
in nasal fractures, 251
COLD INJURIES, 1163–1167
clinical findings in, 1165
definitions concerning, 1163–1164
factors producing, 1163–1164
historical considerations, 1163
pathology, 1164–1165
physiology, 1164–1165
treatment
early, 1165–1166
late, 1166
summary of, 1166
COLISTIN: in bacteremic shock, 230
COLLAR SLING (see Sling, collar and cuff)
COLLES' FRACTURE (see Fractures, Colles')
COLON
laceration, repair, 1047
ragged defects, repair, 1046
severe injuries, repair, 1048
stab wound, 1047
treatment, 1044–1047
COLOSTOMY

closure
diagram, 1051
discussion, 1052
ileocolostomy, end-to-end, 1048
transverse, completely defunctioning, 1046
COMA
alcohol-induced, 283
irreversible, and brain death, 313–314
patients, transportation of, 271
position, 271
postictal, 284
COMPACTION: definition of, 107
COMPOSITIONAL CHANGES, 61–64
COMPRESSION: of fractures, 895
COMPRESSION PLATE, 895
AO, in tibial and fibular fractures, 804
in clavicle nonunion, 148
in femur nonunion, 150
fracture healing and, 104–106
rigid fixation with, 503
in tibia fracture, 140, 804
COMPUTERIZED AXIAL TOMOGRAPHY, 279
CONTRACTURE
muscle, after nerve suture, 1110
Volkmann's (see Volkmann's contracture)
CONVALESCENCE
fat mobilization during, 48–49
gastrointestinal symptoms during, 56
metabolic response and, 56–64
oxygen consumption during, 56
stool tests during, 56
CORD BLADDER, 383
CORONOID PROCESS FRACTURE: and elbow dislocation, 474
CORROSION (see Metal implants, corrosion)
CORTICOSTEROIDS: in fat embolism, 1193
CORTISOL
actions of, 45–46
in adrenal insufficiency, 47
conditioning role of, 46
excretion, 43–47
COTTON FRACTURES of malleolus, 832
COUNTERPULSATION, 223
CRANIAL

intracranial see Intracranial)
nerve trauma, and skull fracture, 292–293
wires, for traction after spinal cord trauma, 331
CRANIOTOMY, 302
bifrontal, 303
CRIBRIFORM PLATE FRACTURES, 293
CROSSUNION: of forearm bones, 509
"CRUSH SYNDROME," 56
CRUTCHES, 1171–1173
measuring for, 1171, 1173
selection of, 1171
walking with, 1171–1173
walking with, gaits, 1172, 1173
four-point alternate, 1172, 1173
three-point, 1172, 1173
two-point alternate, 1172, 1173
CUBITUS
valgus (see Valgus, cubitus)
varus, after humeral fracture, 483
CUFF
rotator (see Rotator cuff)
sling (see Sling, collar and cuff)
"CUSHINGOID," 60
CYCLOPROPANE, 240
CYLINDERIZATION, 108
CYST
bone, causing humeral fracture, 169
pancreas pseudocyst, angiography, 202
CYSTOGRAPHY OF BLADDER, 1078
in extravasation, 1079
CYTODIFFERENTIATION: in bone repair, 79–81
CYTOPLASM, 79

D

DAVIS SKID, 539
DEAD SPACE
increase, causes of, 1020
to tidal volume ratio, 1031
DEATH
abdominal injuries, mortality in, 1052–1053
brain, and irreversible coma, 313–314
DEBRIDEMENT
face, 249
fractures, open, 938
bone in, 938
fascia in, 938

1206 / INDEX

DEBRIDEMENT (cont.)
  muscle in, 938
  preparation for, 937–938
  skin in, 938
  in replantation of arms, 1186
    definitive, 1190
    preliminary, 1186
DECEREBRATE RIGIDITY: due to brainstem contusion, 275
DECOMPRESSION: in spinal cord trauma, 338
DEFORMITY
  bone, correction of, 149
  Madelung's, 493
  at wrist, 474
  trap door flap, 267
  varus, after femoral fracture, 656, 658
DELIVERY: symphysis pubis tear during, 613–614
DELTOID-SPLITTING INCISION: to shoulder, 450
DERMATITIS: radiation, 193
DERMATOMAL MAP: of body, 324
DESOXYCORTICOSTERONE: in adrenal insufficiency, 47
DEXAMETHASONE: in head trauma, 310
DIABETES INSIPIDUS: and head trauma, 312
DIAMOND-SHAPED RODS, 503
DIAPHRAGM: treatment, 1050
DIAPHYSIS
  angulation, correction of, 198
  displacement, correction of, 108
  fracture healing, 101–104
    after cast immobilization, 91–98
DIAZEPAM
  in head trauma, 312
  in status epilepticus, 312
DICLOXACILLIN: in surgical infections, 952
DIGIT(S) (see Fingers, Toes)
DIGITALIZATION: in shock, 219
DIGOXIN: in shock, 219
DIPHENYLHYDANTOIN: in head trauma, 311–312
DISK SURGERY: angiography after, 206–210
DISLOCATIONS
  acromioclavicular, 407–408
    acute complete, 408
    chronic, 407–408
  ankle, 821, 833
  atlas, 351, 377–379
    anterior, 359
  capitate, 542–549
    diagnosis, 546
    mechanism of, 544–546
    old, 546–549
    radiography of, 548
    treatment, 546–549
  carpometacarpal joint, 593–594
    dorsal, 592
    volar, 592
  clavicle, treatment, 405
  elbow, 469–495
    anterior, 472–473
    anterior, myositis ossificans after, 473
    anterior, olecranon fracture and, 475
    differentiated from humeral fractures, 469
    lateral 473
    lateral, epicondylar avulsion and, 475–477
    posterior, 469–472
    posterior, collar and cuff sling in, 471
    posterior, condylar fracture and, 475
    posterior, coronoid process fracture and, 474
    posterior, diagnosis, 469
    posterior, radial fracture and, 474–475
    posterior, reduction in, 470–472
    posterior, x-rays in, 469–470
    posterolateral, 889
  fibula, proximal, 786
    treatment, 786
  fractures and (see Fracture, -dislocation)
  hand, 591–594
  hip, 681–692
    anterior (see hip, anterior below)
    associated fractures, 704
    complications, 704
    follow-up study, 704
    incidence by type, 685, 687
    intra-articular changes after, 704
    manipulation of, closed, 687–688
    necrosis after, avascular, 715
    posterior (see hip, posterior below)
    prognosis, 701–703
    prognosis, complicated cases, 701–703
    prognosis, femoral head injury and, 703
    prognosis, uncomplicated cases, 701
    recurrent, 692
    sciatic nerve injury and, 704
    vascular injuries and, 704
  hip, anterior, 682–683
    diagnosis, 682
    mechanism of, 681, 682
    radiography of, 682
    reduction, closed, 682–683
    treatment, 682–683
    typical deformity in, 682
  hip, posterior, 683–692
    Bigelow's method in, 687–688
    dashboard injury, 686
    diagnosis, 683–687
    by direct blow to knee, 685
    femoral shaft fracture and, 688–690
    mechanism of, 683
    prognosis, 691–692
    prone method in, 688
    radiography of, 685–687
    reduction, open, 690–691
    reduction, prone technique, 690
    Stimson's method in, 688
    treatment, after-care, 691
    typical deformity in, 686
    unfavorable signs, 691–692
  interphalangeal joint, 591–593
  knee, 784–785
    posterior, 785
    rotary, 785
    treatment, 785
    treatment, care after, 785
  lunate, 537–539
    Kienböck's disease after, 540
    late effects of, 539
    old, treatment of, 538–539
  metacarpal, 551
  metacarpophalangeal joint, 592, 593
  nose, 250–251
  patella, traumatic, 767–768
    treatment, 768
  radius head, 473–474
    diagnosis, 473–474
    reduction in, 474
    ulna fracture and (see Monteggia's fracture)
  sacroiliac joint, 610, 614–617
  shoulder, 417–441
    anterior (see shoulder, anterior below)
    atraumatic, 417
    atraumatic, recurrent, 439–440

chronic, 418
exercises and, 422–423
incidence of, 417
number and distribution of, 403
posterior (see shoulder, posterior below)
recurrent, age and, 417
recurrent, incidence of, 417
transient, 418
traumatic (see shoulder, traumatic below)
types of, 417–418
unreduced, 418
voluntary, 417
shoulder, anterior, 418–436
acute, 418
appearance of, 418
diagnosis, 418
immobilization in, 422
recurrent (see shoulder, anterior, recurrent below)
reduction (see shoulder, anterior, reduction below)
x-rays in, 418, 419
shoulder, anterior, recurrent, 423–436
Bankart procedure in (see Bankart procedure)
Gallie-LeMesurier procedure in (see Gallie-LeMesurier procedure)
Hybbinette-Eden procedure in (see Hybbinette-Eden procedure)
Magnuson-Stack procedure in (see Magnuson-Stack procedure)
Nicola procedure in (see Nicola procedure)
pathologic factors, 423–424
Putti-Platt procedure in (see Putti-Platt procedure)
Rowley Bristow procedure in, Heflet modification, 435–436
surgical procedures, 424–436
shoulder, anterior, reduction 418–421
after-care, 422–423
elevation method, 420
Kocher method, 420–421
steps in, 419–420
Stimson method, 420
shoulder, posterior, 417–418,
436, 437
diagnosis, 436, 437
primary traumatic, 437, 439
recurrent, 437
recurrent, voluntary, 440
reduction, 422
reduction, after-care, 422–423
unrecognized, 436
x-rays in, 436, 437
shoulder, traumatic, 417
capsulitis and, adhesive, 440
complications of, 440–441
nerve injuries and, 440
shoulder, traumatic, old unreduced, 437–439
manipulation in, 437
open reduction in, 437–439
shoulder, traumatic, recurrent, 440–441
age and, 440
constitutional factors, 441
degree of injury and, 440–441
humeral head defects and, 441
shoulder, traumatic, rotator cuff injury and, 440
spinal cord, 353
atlantoaxial, 335
atlantooccipital, 335
cervical, 353
sternoclavicular, 409–411
diagnosis, 409
palpation, 409
reduction in, closed, 409
reduction in, open, 409–411
treatment, 409–411
x-rays in, 409
talus, 848–850
posterior, 850
tarsometatarsal, 852–855
radiography of, 856
ulna (see Galeazzi's fracture)
vertebra, 344
anterior, 349, 371–373, 374
anterior, halter traction in, 352
posterior, 375–376
posterior, healed 376
unilateral rotary 349, 370–371
DIURETICS: in shock, 222
2,3-DPG, 55
DRAINAGE
urinary, in abdominal injuries, 1036
water-seal, 1001
"DRAWER" SIGN: for knee

cruciate ligament rupture, 759
DRESSINGS
face, 267
after fracture surgery, 899
DRILL HOLE: in bone, healing of, 89
DRUGS: pressor, 41
DUNLOP'S TRACTION: in humeral fracture, 480–481
DUODENUM
posterior laceration, repair, 1043
treatment, 1041–1044
ulcers, 56
DURA
hematoma (see under Hematoma)
watertight closure of, 307

E

EAR TRAUMA: and anesthetist, 240–241
EDEMA
cerebral
fluids in, 311
glucose in, 311
intracranial pressure and, management, 308
elevation after fracture to prevent, 899
of hand, 564
in soft tissue injuries, 555
in Volkmann's contracture, 1130
ELASTIC BANDAGE: with sponge rubber, for knee, 754
ELBOW
anatomy of, 470
cubitus valgus deformity after capitellar epiphyseal displacement, 494
dislocation (see Dislocations, elbow)
epicondyle
avulsion and dislocation, 475–477
displacement, degrees of, 476
operative view of, 476
extension, 10
flexion, 10
proprioceptive neuromuscular facilitation technique for, 1176
fracture, 469–495
external condyle, and

1208 / INDEX

Elbow (cont.)
　　dislocation, 475
　　fracture-dislocations, 474–478
　　hyperextension, 10
　　motion of, 10
　　　restoration by olecranon excision, 910
　　"nursemaid's" (see Dislocations, radius head)
　　"pulled," 473–474
　　in shoulder trauma examination, 403
Electrical burns, 1153–1154
Electrocardiogram monitor, 216
Electrodiagnosis: in rehabilitation, 1178
Electrotherapy: in rehabilitation, 1178–1179
Elevation
　　after fracture, 899
　　method, in shoulder dislocation reduction, 420
Embolectomy: Fogarty catheter in, 1124
Embolism
　　fat (see Fat embolism)
　　after femoral shaft fracture, 747
　　thromboembolism, femoral vein interruption in, 1126
Emerson Postoperative ventilator, 1024
Endocrine functions, 64
Endotracheal
　　intubation, 994
　　tube adapter, 1024
Energy
　　balance after surgical procedure, 58
　　expenditures, 56–58
　　requirements, 56–58
Epicondyle (see Elbow, epicondyle)
Epinephrine, 40–41
　　contraindicated in hand soft tissue injuries, 556
　　in shock, 219
Epiphysis, 869–885
　　appearance time of, 875
　　blood supply to, 872, 873
　　capitellum, displacement, 485
　　　elbow cubitus valgus deformity after, 494
　　elbow

　　　avulsion of, 494
　　　external condylar, displacement of, 494–495
　　femoral (see Femur, epiphysis)
　　fracture line course, 873–875
　　humeral (see Humerus, epiphysis)
　　injuries, 493–494, 869–885
　　　classification, 874
　　　epidemiology, 869–870
　　　historical notes, 869
　　　incidence, 870
　　　management, 876–884
　　ossification of, 875
　　plate
　　　anatomy of, 870–873
　　　angulation, correction of, 109
　　　blood supply to, 872
　　　contribution to over-all length by individual plates, 875
　　　photomicrograph of, 871
　　　physiology of, 870–873
　　radial (see Radius, epiphysis)
　　radiation damage, in growing child, 192
　　separation, general notes, 876
　　thumb, type III injury, 884
　　tibial (see Tibia, epiphysis)
Epiphysitis: in adolescence, 381
Equations: relating to respiration, 1030–1031
Erythrocyanosis, 1167
Esmarch bandage, 891
Ethacrynic acid: in cardiogenic shock, 222
Eversion (see Foot, eversion)
Examination, 177–189
　　face, 244–248
　　laboratory, 186–187
　　patient, 184–186
　　　history, 184
　　　physical, 184–186
　　　　abdomen, 185
　　　　back, 185–186
　　　　external signs, 184
　　　　extremities, 184
　　　　head, 184–185
　　　　in humeral shaft fractures, 457
　　　　neck, 184–185
　　　　pelvis, 185–186
　　　　thorax, 185
　　　　vital signs, 184
　　x-ray, 187
Exchange transfusion: and sodium excretion rates in

　　urine, 42
Exercise, 1173–1175
　　after humeral fracture shaft, 466
　　　supracondylar, 482
　　of knee (see Knee, exercise of)
　　in rehabilitation, 1173–1175
　　resistance, progressive, technique
　　　for hip extension, 1175
　　　for knee extension, 1174, 1175
　　shoulder (see Shoulder, exercises)
Extension
　　ankle, 32
　　elbow, 10
　　fingers, 17
　　hip, 28
　　knee, 31
　　shoulder, backward, 18–19
　　spine, 25
　　　cervical, 22
　　toes, 36
　　wrist, 12
Extensor tendons (see Tendons, extensor)
Extremities
　　(See also specific sites)
　　amputations, ischemia and vessel injury, 1116
　　angiography, 206
　　lower, motor function chart for, 328–329
　　in physical examination, 184
　　upper
　　　motor function chart and, 326–327
　　　proprioceptive neuromuscular facilitation technique for, 1176
Extubation, 1029–1030
Eye trauma: and anesthetist, 240–241
Eyelid lacerations: treatment, 265

F

Face
　　bony damage to, 266
　　fractures (see Fractures, face)
　　lacerations, treatment, 265
　　maxillofacial trauma and anesthesia, 240–241
　　nerve, 293
　　trauma, 243–268
　　　anesthesia and, 248–249
　　　antibiotics in, 249
　　　dressings for, 267

emergency care, 243–244
examination, 244–248
hemorrhage and, 240–241
management, general considerations in, 248–249
nerve, 293
postoperative care, 267–268
soft tissue, management of, 264–267
soft tissue, shotgun blast causing, 266
transportation of patients, 243–244
vessel clamping in, 243–244
wound preparation, 249
x-rays, positions for, 246, 247
FARADIC STIMULATION: of flexor muscle belly, 475
FASCIA
in debridement of open fractures, 938
lata repair in acromioclavicular separation, 406
strip, in quadriceps tendon repair, 960
FAT EMBOLISM, 1195–1198
cerebral, 284–286
hypoxia and, 286
clinical manifestations, 1196
corticosteroids in, 1198
diagnosis, 1196–1197
laboratory data in, 1197
pathogenesis, 1195
pathophysiology, 1195–1196
radiography of, showing "snowstorm" infiltrate, 1197
treatment, 1197–1198
FAT METABOLISM, 48–49
FAT MOBILIZATION: during convalescence, 48–49
FAT, orbital: prolapse, 256
FECES
contamination in abdominal injuries, 1038–1039
stool tests during convalescence, 56
FEEDING
(See also Nutritional) IV
caloric balance by, 65
nutritional balance by, 65
FEET (see Foot)
FEMORAL
artery, tear, angiography of, 205
vein

iliofemoral, occlusion, 1127
interruption in thromboembolism, 1126
FEMUR
distal, management, 880–882
epiphysis
capital, separation and slipping, 880
distal, displacement, 881
distal, displacement, posterior, 775
distal, separation of, traumatic, 774–776
distal, separation of, traumatic, treatment, 774–776
proximal, management, 879–880
fractures (see Fractures, femur)
head
anatomic relationship to neck, 629–630
fragment, spicules of bone rotating, 637
in hip dislocation prognosis, 703
molding after acetabular fracture, 695
necrosis, avascular, origin, recognition and prevention, 650
positions of, anatomic and valgus, 643
stabilization by Ray trochanteric screw, 691
neck
anatomic relationship to head, 629–630
internal architecture, 642
normal, cross section of, 905
shaft, 719–751
anatomy, 719–722
nailing hip to avoid splitting shaft, 641
nailing in femoral neck fracture and, 640
FETUS
radiation hazards, 192
spinal cord blood supply in, 321
FEVER (see Temperature)
FIBRINOGEN, 49
FIBRINOLYSIN, 49
FIBROBLASTS: and metal implants, 920
FIBROCYTES: and metal implants, 920
FIBULA
dislocation, proximal, 786
treatment, 786
fixation to tibia, rigid, 817

fractures (see Fractures, fibula)
hypertrophy, 155
pseudarthrosis, 138
strut graft, in cervical spine surgery, 366
transplant, for radius fracture and avulsion, 141
FICK DETERMINATION: of cardiac output, 217
FINGERS
abduction, 17
adduction, 17
avulsion due to ring, 577
baseball, 569
treatment, 964–965
exercises, after humeral fracture, 482
extension, 17
extensor tendon
separation repair, 965
treatment of, 964–965
hyperextension, 17
index
amputation, painful stump, 576
loss of radial aspect, 574
metacarpophalangeal joint dislocation, 592
loss of, treatment, 989
mallet, 569
motion of, 16–17
radiography in hand fractures, 594
tip, clean slicing injury, 574
FISTULA
arteriovenous, angiography, 205, 206
carotid-cavernous, and skull fracture, 291–292
FIXATION
in femoral fracture, extracapsular, 657
failure of fixation, 671
of fibula to tibia, rigid, 817
of fibular fracture, with intramedullary nail, 828
of hip fractures (see Fractures, hip, fixation devices)
in humerus neck surgical fractures, 447
internal
in Colles' fracture, 519
in femoral neck fracture, complication of, 649
of long-bone fractures, 896
shoulder fracture-dislocation, 445–446
of trimalleolar fracture, 835
intramedullary
clavicle fractures, 414

1210 / INDEX

FIXATION (cont.)
  forearm fractures, 502
  in osteotomy, complete, healing of, 98–101
  sepsis after, 909
  lag-screw, in displaced humeral neck fracture, 446
  in long-bone fractures, 893–894
  of malleolus fracture, with screws, 900
  of navicular fracture, 545
  nonrigid, in forearm fractures, 505
  in open fractures, 939–940
  plate, in humeral shaft fracture, 463
  prophylactic, in metastatic fractures, 174
  rigid, with compression plates, 503
  screw (see Screws)
  teeth in occlusion, 260
  of tibia to fibula, rigid, 817
  in wrist amputations, 1188
FLAIL CHEST (see Chest, flail)
FLAP (see Grafts, flap)
FLEXION
  ankle, 32
  carpometacarpal joint, 14
  elbow, 10
  hip, 27
  interphalangeal joint, 14
  knee, 31
  metacarpophalangeal joint, 14
  shoulder (see Shoulder, flexion)
  spine
    cervical, 22
    dorsal, 23–24
    lumbar, 23–24
  thumb, 15
  toes, 36
  wrist, 12
FLUID(S)
  in cerebral edema, 311
  requirements and intracranial pressure, 311
  therapy, 43
FLUOROSCOPY
  proper use of, 193–194
  risks of, 192
FOGARTY EMBOLECTOMY CATHETER, 1124
FOOT, 837–868
  abduction, 35
  adduction, 35
  anatomy of, 838
  avulsion, 985
  Böhler clamp for, 842

eversion
  active, 34
  hind part, 33
fractures of phalanges, 856–860
injuries, 837–868
  bone, treatment, 860–867
  bone, Vitallium prosthesis in, 862
innervation of, 1100
inversion
  active, 34
  calcaneus avulsion causing, 841
  hind part, 33
ligaments, anatomy of, 818–819
motion, 33–35
  hind part, 33
  after os calcis excision, 848
  in plaster-of-Paris boot, 866
  radiography, positions for, 812
soft tissue injuries, 837–839
trench, 1167
tuber joint angle, normal, 843
FOREARM
  (See also Arm)
  anatomy of, 497–499
  bow, in children, 510
  burns, 579
  fractures (see Fractures, forearm)
  loss of, major, 579–580
  motion of, 11
  muscles, rotatory pull of, 498
  nerves, gunshot wound of, 1102
  nonunion (see Nonunion, forearm)
  pronation, 11
  supination, 11
  support, in humeral shaft fractures, 459
FORMULAS: replacement, in burn shock, 1139–1140
FOSSA
  glenoid, fracture, 416–417
  posterior, hematoma, 305–306
FRACTURE(S)
  acetabulum, 692–704
    associated fractures, 704
    bursting (see acetabulum, bursting below)
    central, 694
    complications, 704
    decisions concerning, 693
    incidence by type, 685, 687
    inner wall, 693–694
    inner wall, molding to

femoral head after, 695
inner wall, treatment, 693–694
intra-articular changes after, 704
investigation of, 693
management guidelines, 692
posterior, 695–698
posterior, dislocation in, 697
posterior, radiography of, 696
posterior, treatment, 695–696
prognosis, 703–704
sciatic nerve injuries and, 704
stabilization of, 693
superior dome, 697, 698
superior dome, reduction failure in, 699
superior dome, vertical cleft, 698
treatment, after-care, 696–698
treatment, emergency, 692
types of, 692–693
vascular injuries and, 704
acetabulum, bursting, 698–701
  adduction in, 701
  Bolster method in, 701
  Kilfoyle's method in, 701
  manipulative techniques, 701, 702
  Ray's screw method in, 701
  Rowe's method in, 701
  severe, 700
  treatment, follow-up care, 701
  treatment, initial, 699–701
acromion, 416
ankle
  associated open wounds, 824
  avulsion, 824
  causes of, 809
  classification of, 823–824
  explosion, 833
  immobilization, 825
  immobolization, length of, 834–835
  management after plaster cast removal, 835–836
  manipulations, closed 824–825
  manipulations, general principles of, 825
  mechanism of, 809
  open, 834
  open, infection and, 985

INDEX / 1211

reduction, 826–827
reduction, care after, 825–829
reduction, open, 833
atlas, bursting, 368–369
Barton's, 525
bone addition in, 897–899
"boot-top," 132
capitellum, 484–486
  chip, 484–485
  epiphysis, with rotational displacement, in children, 485
  hemicapitellum, 484, 485–486
  hemicapitellum, treatment, 486
  treatment, 486
  types of, 484
cauda equina, 333–336
clavicle, 411–416
  closed manipulation, unsuccessful, 415
  comminuted, 411
  deformity of, 411
  diagnosis, 411–412
  fixation in, intramedullary, 414, 415
  immobilization in, 412, 413
  Kirschner pin in, 414, 415
  mechanism of injury, 411
  palpation, 411
  reduction in, open, 414
  splints for, 412, 413
  transverse, 411
  treatment, 412–416
  treatment, duration of, 412
  treatment, operative, 412, 414–416
  x-rays in, 412
Clinic of Massachusetts General Hospital, history of, 1–7
closure, delayed primary, and sepsis, 946
Colles'
  comminuted, 515
    Kirschner wire in, 519
  malunited, 523–524
  reduction of, 518
  splints for, plaster, 519
  traction, thumb, 518, 519
compression of, 895
coronoid process, and elbow dislocation, 474
cotton, of malleolus, 832
cribriform plate, 293
diaphysis, healing, 101–104
  after cast immobilization, 91–98
-dislocation
  acetabulum, 697

ankle, 823, 829, 833
ankle, reduction, open, 831
ankle, rotary, severe, 830
Bennett, of thumb, 592
bimalleolar, unstable, 834
carpometacarpal joint, 592
elbow, 474–478
hip, 712, 713, 715
humerus, Rush nail in, 446
shoulder, fixation, internal, 445–446, 447, 448, 449
shoulder, manipulation, closed, 442–443
shoulder, reduction, open, 443–455
shoulder, treatment, 442–446
shoulder, types of, 441
spinal cord, 333–334
talus, 849
toes, 856
vertebra, 344, 369
vertebra, anterior, 350, 373–375
vertebra, lumbar, 387–390
vertebra, lumbar, articular processes in, 389
vertebra, lumbar, extension and, 388
vertebra, lumbar, reduction, 388–390
vertebra, lumbar, reduction, table position for, 389
vertebra, posterior, 377
vertebra, thoracic, 381–384
wrist, 547
dressing after surgery, 899
elbow, 469–495
  condyle, external, and elbow dislocation, 475
elevation after, 899
epiphysis, fracture line course, 873–875
excision of fragments, 910–911
face, 261
  indicators of, 249–250
  malocclusion of teeth in, 260
  management of, 249–264
femur
  compositional data after, 63
  condyle, lateral, 784
  extracapsular (see femur, extracapsular below)
  head, 712
  head, anatomic relationship to neck, 629–630
  head, bone spicules rotating fragment, 637

intracapsular (see femur, intracapsular below)
Küntscher nail for, 907
lower end (see femur, supracondylar below)
metabolic data after, 62
metastatic, 172–174
nailing, medullary, 901–905
nailing, medullary, insertion error, 907
nailing, medullary, insertion, retrograde, 906
nailing, medullary, patient position for, 904
neck (see femur, neck below)
nonunion (see Nonunion, femur fractures)
pathologic, Küntscher nail in, 903
pathologic, from osteogenesis imperfecta, 168
screw for, break due to corrosion, 925
shaft (see femur, shaft below)
supracondylar (see femur, supracondylar below)
trochanteric (see femur, extracapsular below)
femur, extracapsular, 654–673
  comminuted, 658
  comminuted, 4-part, anatomy of, 662
  comminuted, with large fragment, 665
  comminuted, severe, 658
  comminuted, unstable, 659, 665
  comminuted, unstable, 4-part, 669
  comminuted, varus deformity and, 658
  complications, 668–673
  complications, structural failures causing, 668
  complications, technique errors causing, 668–669
  external rotation of lower fragment, 656
  fixation devices, 657
  fixation, failure of, 671
  linear, without displacement, 656
  nonunion, 669–673
  nonunion, management, 672
  Paget's disease and, 660
  postoperative management,

FRACTURE(S) *(cont.)*
  668
  stable, 662
  surgery, 657–668
  surgery, after-treatment, 668
  surgery, technique, 657–658
  traction in, Russell, 655
  transportation in, 654–657
  treatment, 657–668
  treatment, emergency, 654–657
  types of, 657
  unstable, 670–671
  unstable, comminuted, 659, 666
  unstable, comminuted, 4-part, 669
  unstable, heart disease and, 664
  unstable, management of, 663
  unstable, trochanteric and subtrochanteric combination, 667
  varus deformity and, 656
femur, intracapsular, 625–654
  anatomic considerations, 627–629
  anatomic deformity, 625–626
  cerebral palsy and, 653
  radiography of, 626–627
  treatment, emergency, 626
femur, neck
  anatomic relationship to femoral head, 629–630
  complications, 648–652
  complications, treatment, 652
  displaced, 632–646
  displaced, anesthesia in, 633–634
  displaced, as emergency, 632–633
  displaced, mechanism of displacement, 628
  fixation, internal, complication of, 649
  impacted, 629–632
  impacted, conservative management, 630–631
  impacted, favorable, 632
  impacted, positions favoring union and function, 631
  impacted, radiography of, 633
  impacted, unfavorable, 634, 635
  internal architecture of neck, 642
  management, summary of, 652–654
  nailing (*see* Nailing, of femoral neck fractures)
  prognosis, 647–648
  range of fracture lines, 627
  reduction, anatomic guides in, 638
  reduction, closed, difficult cases, 646
  reduction, principles of, 635–639
  spicules of bone rotating head fragment, 637
  surgical after-care, 646–647
  tissue reactions to metal implants, 918
  Vitallium prosthesis for, 116
  wire migration in, 649
femur, shaft, 719–751
  anatomic considerations, 719–722
  brace, cast, 738–743
  brace, cast, completed, front and side views, 743
  brace, cast, indications, 738
  brace, cast, technique, 738–743
  comminuted, of mid-distal shaft, 739
  comminuted, severe, 721
  complications, 747–749
  delayed union in, 747–749
  embolism after, 747
  first aid, 722–724
  hip dislocations and, posterior, 688–690
  immobilization, duration of, 736–738
  immobilization, improvised, 724
  infection after medullary nailing, 130
  infection, and thigh drainage, 130
  isolated closed transverse, 740
  knee function impairment after, 749
  nonunion, 747–749
  oblique, of midshaft, 720
  open, 727, 746
  in Paget's disease, 745
  pathologic, 745, 746–747
  polycentric hinged knee joints used, 742
  reduction, closed, 736–738
  reduction, open, 743–746
  sepsis and, 747
  signs of, 722
  spiral, of midshaft with "butterfly" fragment, 725
  splints for, 723
  splints for, Keller-Blake, 723
  symptoms of, 722
  traction, 728–738
  traction, Bryant, 731, 732–733
  traction, 90-90-90, 734–736
  traction, pillow and sling, 734
  traction, Rowe method, 734
  traction, Russell, 732, 733
  traction, skeletal, 730–736
  traction, skin, 728–730
  traction, straps, types of, 729
  traction, suspension, 733–734, 735
  traction, through tibial tubercle, 733
  transverse, Küntscher rod used, 748
  treatment, 722–747
  treatment, definitive, 724–728
  vascular injury in, 722
  wires for, Kirschner, 730, 733
femur, supracondylar, 776–784
  Böhler-Braun frame for, 778
  comminuted, 780
  comminuted, T, 783
  conservative treatment, 779–782
  conservative treatment, technique, 779
  diagram of, 777
  Hodgen splint with Pearson attachment for, 778
  postreduction care, 779–782
  surgery, 782–784
  surgery, technique, 782–784
  T, 779
  T, comminuted, 783
  T, screws for, 784
fibula, 793–808
  alignment in, 799
  AO compression plates for, 805
  cast for, total contact, 797
  closed, comminuted, severe, 800
  comminuted, 800, 801

comminuted, delayed healing causing amputation, 807
comminuted, open, 805, 806
comminuted, after unnecessary open reduction and internal fixation, 139
delayed union, 805–808
displacement in, 799, 831
evaluation, initial, 793–795
fixation, with intramedullary nail, 823
grafts in, bone, 155
healing, in children, 795–796
healing in shortened position, 828
healing times, 795–796
Lottes nail for, 804
mechanism of, 793
midshaft, 823
nonunion (*see* Nonunion, fibula fractures)
open, 801–805
open, bone grafting in, 151
open, comminuted, 805, 806
open, skin grafting in, 151
Parham bands for, 804
proximal, 786
proximal, treatment, 786
radiography of, 793–795, 829
reduction, closed, 796–802
reduction, closed, contact and, 799
reduction, closed, length and, 799–800
reduction, closed, plaster roll for unstable fracture, 802
reduction, open, 803–805, 831
rotation deformity in, 799
screws for, 900
stable, 794
treatment, 796–808
type of, 793
unstable, 794, 800–801
unstable, reduction of, 802
fixation (*see* Fixation)
of foot phalanges, 856–860
forearm, 497–512
age and, 499
anesthesia, 500
cast in, 501
in children, 509, 510–512
contour restoration in, in children, 509
fixation, intramedullary, 502
fixation, nonrigid, 505
greenstick type, in children, 510–512
gross motion after fall, 505
iliac bone graft in, 505
incidence of, 499
mechanism of injury, 499
nonunion (*see* Nonunion, forearm)
open, 504–505, 506–509
operative techniques, 502–506
pins in, Sage, 502
plates in, 4-hole semitubular, 504
pronation fractures, 511
reduction in, closed, by manipulation, 500–501
reduction in, open, 501–506
refracture, 512
resorption at fracture line, 504
sex and, 499
supination fractures, 511
traction in, 500
treatment, 500–506
x-rays in, 499–500
x-rays in, positioning for, 499
Galeazzi's (*see* Galeazzi's fracture)
glenoid fossa, 416–417
greenstick (*see* Greenstick fracture)
hand, 594–602
classification, 595–602
intra-articular, 597–602
open, 600, 602
radiography of, 594–595
stable, 595–596
unstable, 596–597, 598
unstable, immobilization in, 596–597
unstable, skeletal traction in, 597
hangman's, of spinal cord, 335
head
depressed, x-ray studies, 277
linear, x-ray studies, 277
healing, 71–113
angulated fractures, 109–110
biology of, 92
compression plate and, 104–106
diaphysis, 101–104
diaphysis, after external cast immobilization, 91–98
displaced fractures, 107–110
elevation and, 899
features of, 106–110
hematoma in, 98
osteoporosis and, 106
pathologic, 167
remodeling in, 106–107
rotation and, 110
variation in, 106
hemicapitellum, 484, 485–486
treatment, 486
hip, 619–680
(*See also* femur *above*)
in children, 675–677
complications, clinical 673–675
epidemiology, 624–625
fixation devices, complications of, 651–652
fixation devices, design for, 623–624
fixation devices, materials for, 623–624
historical considerations concerning, 620–623
ipsilateral, and cerebral palsy, 653
Pare's description of, 621
pathologic, 675
pathologic, breast carcinoma and, 676
Smith-Petersen nail for, 622
humerus
condyle, external, 486–487
condyle, external stable type, 487
condyle, external, unstable type, 487
dicondylar, 484
epicondyle, mesial, 889
head (*see* humerus head *below*)
intercondylar, greenstick type, 484
Lottes nail in, 143, 144
neck (*see* humerus neck *below*)
nonunion (*see* Nonunion, humerus fractures)
Parham bands in, 145
pathologic, and bone cyst, 159
Rush pin in, 146
shaft (*see* humerus shaft *below*)
supracondylar (*see*

1214 / INDEX

FRACTURE(S) *(cont.)*
  humerus, supracondylar
    below)
    T fractures, 487–490
    T fractures, open
      reduction, function after,
      488
    T fractures, reduction
      technique, 489
    T fractures, treatment,
      487–490
    transcondylar, 484
    tuberosity, displaced
      fracture, 442
    Y fractures, 487–490
    Y fractures, reduction
      technique, 489
    Y fractures, treatment,
      487–490
  humerus head, 441–446
    bursting, 441
    diagnosis, 441–442
    shattered, Laurence Jones
      technique, 448
    shattered, Neer
      replacement prosthesis,
      449
    treatment, 442–446
    x-rays in, 441–442
  humerus neck, 441–446
    diagnosis, 441–442
    displaced, lag-screw
      fixation, 446
    impacted, treatment, 442
    splint in, abduction, 444
    splint in, airplane, 444
    surgical fixation of, 447
    treatment, 442–446
    x-rays in, 441–442
  humerus shaft, 455–467
    anatomic considerations,
      455–457
    cast in, hanging, 458–460
    complications of, 464, 466
    etiology of, 457
    exercises and, 466
    oblique, long spiral open
      reduction, 463
    physical examination, 457
    radial nerve injuries and,
      466–467
    reduction in, open, 461–
      464
    reduction in, open, utility
      incision in, 462
    segmental, open reduction,
      463
    spica in, plaster of Paris,
      460
    splint in, coaptation, 460
    traction in, axial, skin-
      adhesive technique, 461

    traction in, skeletal, 460–
      461
    transverse, cast in,
      hanging, 465
    transverse, grafts in,
      fibular, 465
    transverse, grafts in, iliac,
      465
    transverse, grafts in,
      osteoperiosteal tibial,
      465
    transverse, olecranon wire
      traction in, 465
    transverse, Rush nails in,
      "blind" technique, 464
    transverse, spica in, 465
    transverse, Vitallium plate
      in, 465
    treatment of, 457–464
    treatment of, general
      considerations, 457–458
    types of, 457
  humerus, supracondylar,
    478–483
    differentiated from elbow
      dislocation, 469
    extension type, 479–482
    extension type, after-
      treatment, 481–482
    extension type,
      complications of, 482
    extension type, exercises
      after, 482
    extension type, traction in,
      Dunlop's, 480–481
    extension type, traction in,
      skeletal, 481
    extension type, treatment,
      479–481
    extension type, vessels in,
      480
    flexion type, 482–483
    flexion type, treatment,
      482–483
    malunited, 483
    osteotomy in, 483
    prognosis, 482
  ilium, 610, 611
    comminuted, 612
  immobilization, discussion
    of, 117
  jaw, 261
  Jefferson's, 368–369
  knee, posterior cruciate
    ligament, 761
    treatment, 761
  LeFort, 258
  long-bone
    fixation, internal, 896
    fixation and operative
      approach, 893–894
    nailing, medullary, 901–

      909
    types of, 896
  malleolus
    bimalleolar, 831
    classification of, 823–824
    cotton, 832
    fixation with screw, 900
    grafts, in, slotted, 166
    medial, 830–831
    medial, diagram of, 832
    Potts, 831
    trimalleolar, 832
    trimalleolar, lag screws in,
      835
  mandible, 263–264
    at angles, 262, 264
    neck of condyle, in
      children, 263
    sites of, 247
  maxilla, 258, 259–263
    varieties of, 258
  metacarpals
    grafts in, 989
    second, 551
  metastatic, 171–175
    femur fractures, 172–174
  metatarsal, 851–855
    complete transverse
      comminuted, 855
    fifth, proximal end of, 855
    radiography of, 856
    tarsometatarsal dislocations
      and, 853–855
  Monteggia's *(see* Monteggia's
    fracture)
  navicular, 542–549
    circulation interruption in,
      532
    delayed union in, 533
    diagnosis, 546
    fixation by graft, 545
    fresh, 531–532
    immobilization in, plaster,
      532
    mechanism of, 544–546
    nonunion *(see* Navicular
      bone, nonunion)
    reduction, open, 545
    treatment, 546–549
  nonunion *(see* Nonunion)
  nose, 250–252
    cartilage in, 244–245
    examination, 244–245
    reduction methods, 251
    splints in, metal, 252
    types of, 250
  odontoid process, 346, 377–
    379, 380
    at base, 378
    nonunion in, 352, 359
    radiography of, 351
  olecranon, 490–492

INDEX / 1215

comminuted, 490–491
elbow dislocation and, anterior, 475
excision to restore elbow motion in, 910
simple, 490
treatment, in adult, 490–491
treatment, in children, 491–492
open, 935–942
  approach to patient, principles, 935
  complications, 940–942
  debridement (see Debridement, fractures, open)
  emergency room care, 935–937
  emergency room, general measures, 935–936
  emergency room, local therapy, 936–937
  fixation, 939–940
  grading wounds, criteria for, 942
  infections after, types of, 940–942
  nonunion, 940
  principles for handling, 935–940
  sepsis and, 940–942
  sepsis degree and fracture severity, 941
  skin closure, 938–939
  surgery, 937–940
  surgery, preparation for, 937–938
  transportation and, 936
  treatment, 935–942
operative treatment (see Surgery of fractures)
orbit
  "blowout," 256–257
  examination, 245
os calcis, 839–848
  anterior process, 842
  anterior process, technique for diagnosis, 841
  bone graft in, 844
  bone graft in, for deformities, 845
  comminuted, with displacement, 843
  conservative treatment, 844–847
  "duckbill" type, 840
  functional progress by type of treatment, 847
  incidence of, 839
  mechanism of, 844
  Palmer technique in, 844

radiography of, 843
surgery, 847–848
types of, 839–844
patella, 768–774
  comminuted, 771, 773
  lateral plateau, 768
  marginal 773–774
  marginal, treatment, 774
  osteochondral, 774
  osteochondral, treatment, 774
  polar, comminuted, 773
  polar, treatment, 772–773
  with separation, 770
patella, transverse, 769, 771–772
  conservative treatment, 771–772
  postoperative care, 772
  surgery, 772
  surgery, technique, 772
pathologic, 167–175
  classification of, 167
  definition of, 167
  femur, Küntscher nail in, 903
  femur, metastatic, 172–174
  femur, from osteogenesis imperfecta, 168
  femur, shaft, 745, 746–747
  healing times, 167
  hip, 675
  hip, and breast carcinoma, 676
  humerus, and bone cyst, 169
  humerus, and giant-cell tumors, 170
  metastatic, 171–175
  in Paget's disease, 169, 745
  spine, and steroids for pemphigus, 168
  treatment, 170–171
  treatment, of underlying condition, 170
  types of, 167, 170
  vertebral compression, 168
pelvis, 605–617
  associated injuries, 605–607
  avulsion, 613
  hemorrhage and, angiography, 208, 210
  isolated, 609–613
  mechanism of, 608–609
  posterior arch distortion and, 614–617
  stress, 613
  teardrop bladder after, 1079
  treatment, 609–617
  treatment, results of, 617

Potts, 851
radius
  closed, Rush rods in, 503
  distal end (see radius, distal end below)
  head (see radius head below)
  healing time, 508
  nonunion (see Nonunion, radius fractures)
  open, 141
  ulna dislocation and, distal (see Galeazzi's fracture)
radius, distal end, 513–525
  associated injuries, 516
  Colles' (see Fractures, Colles' above)
  complications, 522–524
  mechanism of injury, 513–515
  prognosis, 521–522
  radiography of, 516
  reduction by manual method, 517
  splints for, plaster, 517
  surgery of, 518–521
  traction, 518
  treatment, 516–521
radius head, 878
  in adult, 492–493
  in adult, treatment, 492–493
  comminuted, in adult, 492
  elbow dislocation and, posterior, 474–475
reduction of (see Reduction)
replantation of arms and, 1186–1187
result rating scheme from Massachusetts General Hospital, 846
sacro iliac joint, 611
sacrum, 612
scaphoid, 865
  accessory, 867
scapula, 416–417
  of body, 416
  complications of, 416
  diagnosis, 416
  incidence of, 416
  neck of, 416–417
  spine of, 416
  treatment, 416–417
  x-rays in, 416
sesamoid, 865–867
  microfracture, 864
shoulder
  number and distribution of, 403
  shattered, 444
skull
  basilar, and

1216 / INDEX

FRACTURE(S) (cont.)
  hemotympanum, 295
  complications of, 291–295
  cranial nerve trauma and, 292–293
  depressed (see skull, depressed below)
  fistula and, carotid-cavernous, 291–292
  "growing," 289
  hematoma and, extradural, 295
  linear, 287–289
  linear, diagnosis, 289
  otorrhea and, cerebrospinal fluid, 293–295
  rhinorrhea and, cerebrospinal fluid, 293–295
  skull, depressed, 289–291
    closed, 290
    comminution, 289
    compound, 290
    compound, treatment, 290–291
    elevation of, 291
    in infants, 290
    "ping-pong ball" variety, 290
  Smith's, 525
  spinal cord, 333–336, 353
    (See also spine below)
    bilateral avulsion, through arch of axis, 335
    cervical, 353
    compression, 334
    compression, hyperflexion causing, 335
    hangman's, 335
    linear, 335
    Meurig-Williams plates in, 334
    myelography in, 334
    paraparesis, bowel, bladder and sexual function loss after, 334
    teardrop, 335–336
  spine
    (See also spinal cord above)
    cervical, ankylosed, 375
    cervical, essential points in, 379–381
    compression, and steroids for pemphigus, 168
    transverse processes, 391–393
    transverse processes, multiple, 393
  splints for (see Splints)
  surgeon, training of, 888–890
  surgery of (see Surgery of fractures)
  talus, 848–850
    functional progress by type of treatment, 848
    necrosis after, avascular, 851
    open, comminuted, 853
  tarsal navicular, 850–851, 866, 867
    compression, 854
  temporal bone, 293
  tibia, 793–808
    alignment in, 799
    anterior margin, 832
    avulsion, 758–760
    avulsion, conservative treatment, 760
    avulsion, radiography of, 760
    avulsion, repair of, 761
    avulsion, surgery of, 760
    cast for, total contact, 797
    comminuted (see tibia, comminuted below)
    delayed union, 805–808
    dicondylar, 789–790
    dicondylar, conservative treatment, 789–790
    dicondylar, surgery, 790
    displacement in, 799
    epiphysis, proximal, 882
    evaluation, initial, 793–795
    grafts in, bone, 155, 156
    healing, in children, 795–796
    healing times, 795–796
    Kirschner wire in, 882
    lateral plateau, 787, 789
    lateral plateau, bolt, nut and washer used, 789
    lateral plateau, treatment technique, 787
    Lottes nail for, 804, 910
    mechanism of, 793
    medial condyle, 787
    medial plateau, 787
    medial plateau, surgery, 789
    nonunion (see Nonunion, tibia fractures)
    open, 140, 801–805
    open, bone grafting in, 151
    open, comminuted, 805, 806
    open, skin grafting in, 151, 152
    Parham bands for, 804, 901
    plate for, 970, 984
    plate for, AO compression, 804
    plate for, corrosion of, 921
    plateau, comminuted, 787–789, 790
    plateau, comminuted, conservative treatment, 788
    plateau, comminuted, postoperative care, 789
    plateau, comminuted, surgery, 788–789
    plateau, comminuted, surgery, technique, 788–789
    proximal, 786–787
    proximal, conservative treatment, 787
    proximal, with displaced fragment, 787
    proximal, postreduction care, 787
    radiography of, 793–795
    reduction, closed, 796–801
    reduction, closed, contact and, 799
    reduction, closed, length and, 799–800
    reduction, closed, plaster roll for unstable fracture, 802
    reduction, open, 140, 803–805, 983, 987
    reduction, open, and plating, 970
    rotation deformity in, 799
    screws for, 900
    screws for, corrosion of, 921
    spiral, 970
    stable, 794
    treatment, 796–808
    type of, 793
    unstable, 794, 800–801
    unstable, reduction of, 802
    weight-bearing surface, 824
  tibia, comminuted, 800, 801
    closed, 800, 970
    delayed healing causing amputation, 807
    open, 805, 806
    plateau (see Fractures, tibia, plateau, comminuted above)
    after unnecessary open reduction and internal fixation, 139
  toes
    great, 857
    Kirschner wires for, 858
  trochanteric, nonunion, 669–673
    management, 672
  ulna

INDEX / 1217

closed, Rush rods in, 503
healing time, 508
nonunion, 142
radial head dislocation and
  (see Monteggia's
  fracture)
Rush nail for, 909
screw for, complications
  with, 926
vertebra
  body, 345, 390–391
  body, bursting, 369–370
  body, wedge-compression,
    374
  bursting, 348
  compression, and
    osteoporosis, 168
  first cervical, bursting,
    368–369
  lumbar, bursting, 390–391
  lumbar, bursting,
    compression in, 392
  lumbar, wedge-
    compression, 384–387
  lumbar, wedge-
    compression, treatment
    386–387
  thoracic, compression, 383
  thoracic, wedge-
    compression, 381
  wedge-compression, 348,
    367
Volkmann's contracture after,
  1133
wrist, 551
zygoma, 253–259
  approach to, intraoral, 254
  arch, depressed fracture,
    253
  arch, depressed fracture,
    Gillies method, 253
  arch, wiring in, 254
  examination, 245
  unstable, Kirschner wire
    in, 255
FREIBERG'S INFARCTION, 860–
  865
  examples of, typical, 860
  of metatarsal head, 860–863
  new treatment method, 864–
    865
  radiography of, 861
FROSTBITE, 1163
  (See also Cold injuries)
FUROSEMIDE: in cardiogenic
  shock, 222

G

GAITS (see Crutches, walking
  with, gaits)
GALEAZZI'S FRACTURE, 506

onlay iliac graft in, 506
reduction in, closed, 500
treatment, 506
GALLIE-LEMESURIER
  PROCEDURE, 432–433
  after-treatment, 433
  approach, 433
  object, 433
  repair, 433
GAMMA GLOBULINS, 49
GANGLION: gasserian, 293
GANGRENE: gas, 954–955
GAS GANGRENE, 954–955
GASSERIAN GANGLION, 293
GASTRIC (see Stomach)
GASTROINTESTINAL (see
  Intestine, Stomach)
GENETIC EFFECTS: of
  radiation, 192–193
GENITAL TRACT
  injuries, 1071–1086
  treatment, 1049–1050
GENTAMICIN
  in shock, bacteremic, 230
  in surgical infections, 952
GILLIES METHOD: for elevation
  of depressed zygomatic
  arch fractures, 253
GLENOHUMERAL JOINT
  motion, of shoulder, 21
  muscles, and exercise, 423
GLENOID
  fossa, fracture, 416–417
  pincers, 431
GLOBULINS: gamma, 49
GLUCOCORTICOIDS: in head
  trauma, 309–310
GLUCOSE
  in cerebral edema, 311
  for hyperalimentation, 65
  metabolism, 48
GLYCEROL: in head trauma,
  309
GONADOTROPINS: secretion, 64
GONIOMETER, 10
GRAFTS
  allografting and sepsis, 947
  arterial, 1121–1123
  bone
    autogenous, fresh, 163,
      165–166
    bank, 163
    dowel, 163, 165
    in fibula fracture, 155
    in fibula fracture, open,
      151
    heterogenous, 163, 165–
      166
    homogenous, 163, 165–166
    iliac (see Ilium, grafts)
    inlay, 162
    inlay, sliding, 159

in navicular bone
  nonunion, 534–536
in navicular bone
  nonunion, technique,
    534–536
onlay, 159–162
onlay, double, 162
onlay, from ilium, 161
onlay, in tibia nonunion,
  121
onlay, tibial, for humerus
  fracture, 146
onlay, "twin," 162
in os calcis fractures, 844
in os calcis fractures, for
  deformities, 845
osteoperiosteal
  "neighborhood," 163,
    164
in pathologic fracture from
  giant-cell tumor, 170
in radius nonunion, 157
rejection of, 163, 165
slotted, 163, 165
slotted, in united malleolus
  fracture, 166
in spinal surgery, cervical,
  365
technique, 159–166
in tibia fracture, 155, 156
in tibia fracture, open, 151
tibial (see tibial below)
in burns, 1146
of forearm and hand, 579
fibular
  in humerus shaft fracture,
    465
  strut, in cervical spine
    surgery, 366
flap, 974–978
  for ankle fracture with
    infection, 985
  for arm, upper, 990
  in burns of forearm and
    hand, 579
  direct 974
  in finger loss, 989
  for foot avulsion, 985
  for heel scar, unstable, 978
  indications for, 982–991
  for leg, 988
  in leg crushing injury, 986
  length of, 984
  neurovascular island,
    techniques of, 576
  pedicle, for scalp, 388
  postoperative care, 981–
    982
  scalp, pedicled, 388
  for soft tissue closure,
    974–978
  in thumb loss, 989

GRAFTS (*cont.*)
   for tibial fracture, 938, 984, 987
   transfer of, 974–978
   transfer of, delayed, 974
   types of, 975–978
   for ulcer, knee, 975
   for ulcer, os calcis, 977
   for ulcer, sacral pressure, in paraplegia, 976
   uses of, 982–991
   iliac (*see* Ilium, grafts)
   in navicular fracture, 545
   for nerves, peripheral, 1105–1107
   onlay, saw removal, 160
   sepsis and, 947
   skin, 979–991
     in bone defects, granulating, 973
     in fibula fracture, open, 151
     in finger loss, 989
     in foot avulsion, 985
     in leg crushing injury, 986
     for leg, lower, 980
     postoperative care, 981–982
     in soft tissue closure, 972–974
     in soft tissue closure, securing graft, 972–974
     in thumb loss, 989
     in tibia fracture, 151, 987
     in tibia fracture, open, 152
   Teflon, and aortic aneurysm, 1008
   tibial
     in forearm nonunion, 508
     in navicular fracture nonunion, 533
     osteoperiosteal, in humeral shaft fracture, 465
     in wrist fracture, 551
   vascular, in anastomosis, 1122
GREENSTICK FRACTURE
   forearm, in children, 510–512
   humerus intercondylar, 484
GROWTH HORMONE, 64
GUILLOTINE REMOVAL: of hepatic sublobar lacerations, 1063
GUNSHOT WOUNDS
   brain, 307
   face, 266
   femur fractures and, 124, 126
   flank, hematuria after, 203–204
   hand, 578
   humerus fracture and, 146

   spinal cord causing quadriplegia, 337

H

HALO
   brace, 360
   in spinal trauma, cervical, 355
HALTER TRACTION: in vertebral dislocation, 352
HAND
   burns, 579
   dislocations, 591–594
   edema of, 564
   fractures (*see* Fractures, hand)
   function after forearm fracture treatment, 507
   innervation of, 1099
   joints, anatomy of, 583–584
   lacerations, 564
   ligament injuries, 583–603
     collateral, 585–589
     collateral, anatomy, 584
     collateral, old injuries, 585
     collateral, recent injuries, 585
     collateral, rupture, with early repair, 588
     incomplete, 586
     rupture, complete, 586
     sprain, 586
   loss of, major, 579–580
   shotgun injury of, 578
   in shoulder trauma examination, 403
   skeletal injuries, 583–603
   soft tissue injuries, 555–581
     acceptance of injury by patient, 563
     anesthesia for, 556–557
     anger of patient after, 562
     antibiotics in, 561–562
     bag for elevation after surgery, 561
     block used, axillary, 557
     care of, follow-up, 562
     care of, intraoperative, 559–560
     care of, postoperative, 560–561
     care of, preoperative, 558–559
     denial by patient after, 562
     edema only, 555
     equipment for, 557–558
     history, 556
     incised wounds, 555
     malingering after, 563
     multiple, complicated, 601
     nature of, 555–556

     neurosis after, compensation, 563
     neurosis after, patterns of, 563
     open wounds, 555–556
     physical examination in, 556
     psychologic patterns after, 562–564
     repair principles, 556–564
     repair principles, general, 556
     severe crushing with avulsion, 573
     severe flaying injury, 572
     simple, 564–572
     tissue loss, 555, 572–579
   tendons of, injuries, 564–572
     extensor, 568–572
     extensor communis, 570
     flexor, 565–568
     flexor, areas of injuries, 566
     flexor, divided, 565
     flexor, silicone rod used, 567
HANGING CAST: in humeral shaft fracture, 458–460, 465
HANGMAN'S FRACTURE: of spinal cord, 335
HANSEN-STREET NAIL, 902
"HATCHET" DEFECT: in humeral head, 425
HAVERSIAN SYSTEMS: mature, 87
HEAD
   fractures (*see* Fractures, head)
   jerking backward causing atlantoaxial dislocations, 335
   physical examination, 184–185
   trauma
     airway in, 270
     alcohol and, 283
     anticonvulsants in, 311–312
     dexamethasone in, 310
     diabetes insipidus and, 312
     diagnosis, 269–315
     diagnosis, conditions complicating, 283–286
     diphenylhydantoin in, 311–312
     evaluation of, 272–279
     first aid for, 270–272
     glucocorticoids in, 309–310
     glycerol in, 309
     hyperosmolar agents in, 309

hyperventilation and,
  management, 308–309
laboratory studies, 276–279
lumbar puncture in, 278
management, nonsurgical
  adjuncts to, 308–313
mannitol in, 309
methylprednisolone in, 310
nervous system disorders
  and, 283–284
pharmacologic agents in,
  309
phenobarbital in, 311–312
problem of, 269–270
pupils in, dilated, 274
shock and, 272
steroids in, 310
temperature control and,
  312
transportation, 270–272
treatment of, 269–315
x-ray studies, 276–279
HEADACHE: in subdural
  hematoma, 303
HEALING
bone (see Bone, healing)
fracture (see Fracture,
  healing)
osteotomy, complete, treated
  by intramedullary
  fixation, 98–101
HEART, 1005–1014
arrest, treatment of, 183
disease, and femoral fracture,
  extracapsular, 664
function, in burns, 1156–1157
insufficiency, 50
massage, 222
  anesthetist and, 235–236
missile wounds of, 1012
monitoring, in shock, 216
output
  Fick determination of, 217
  hypoxia and, 50
  oxygen and, 52
rate control, in shock, 220–221
shotgun wound of, 1012,
  1013
stab wounds of, 1011–1012
trauma, 1005–1014
  blunt, 1006–1007
  emergency room
    management, 1005–1006
  penetrating, 1011–1013
unstable system, and
  anesthetist, 238
HEAT IN REHABILITATION,
  1175–1178
conductive, 1176–1177

conversive, 1177
radiant, 1177
ultrasound, 1177–1178
HEEL
cord, 815
unstable scar of, 978
HEFLET MODIFICATION: of
  Rowley Bristow
  procedure, 435–436
HEMARTHROSIS
of knee, traumatic, 755
in radius head fracture,
  aspiration of, 492–493
HEMATOCRIT
changes after hemorrhage, 44
oxygen and, 52
HEMATOMA
cephalohematoma, 287
extradural
  acute, 295–300
  acute, bur holes, 299
  acute, pressure-cone
    formation, mechanism of,
    297
  angiography in, 298
  diagnosis, 296
  removal, 297–298
  skull fracture and, 295
fossa, posterior, 305–306
in fracture healing, 98
intracranial, 295–308
kidney, angiography of, 203–204
liver, subcapsular, 1057
  angiography of, 1062
retroperitoneal, treatment,
  1048–1049
spleen, angiography, 201
subdural, 281
  acute, 300–302
  acute, bifrontal craniotomy
    in, 303
  angiography, 279
  chronic, 302–305
  chronic, removal of, 305
HEMATURIA: after bullet
  wound of flank, 203–204
HEMIANOPIA, 284
HEMICAPITELLAR FRACTURE,
  484, 485–486
HEMIDIAPHRAGM: tear of,
  repair, 1009
HEMIPARESIS, 284
detection of, 274
HEMIPELVIS ROTATION, 608
counterclockwise, 611
HEMORRHAGE
in abdominal injuries,
  control, 1038
arterial, control of, 1119
in chest injuries, control of,
  995–996

external, control of, 180–181
in face trauma, 240–241
  vessel clamping in, 243–244
  hematocrit changes after,
    44
in hypovolemic shock, 227
internal, control of, 181
in liver injuries, control,
  1062–1064
pelvic, angiography, 207, 208
plasma volume changes after,
  44
preretinal, 284
retroperitoneal, angiography,
  207
secondary, and arterial
  injury, 1124–1125
sodium excretion rates in
  urine and, 42
subarachnoid, 284
HEMOSTASIS: terminal, and
  liver injuries, 1067
HEMOTHORAX, 236
HEMOTYMPANUM: and basilar
  skull fracture, 295
HENRY'S INCISION, 144
HEPATIC (see Liver)
HETEROGRAFTS (see Grafts)
HILL-SACKS LESION, 424
HIP
adduction, 30
anatomy, 620
capsule, attachment to
  acetabulum, 699
cartilage destruction in, 716–717
dislocations (see
  Dislocations, hip)
extension, 28
flexion, 27
fracture (see Fractures, hip)
fracture-dislocation, 712, 713,
  716
girdle, and motor function
  chart, 328–329
ligaments, attachment to
  acetabulum, 699
motion, 27–30
nailing to avoid femoral shaft
  splitting, 641
necrosis of, avascular, 712–716
protrusion, intrapelvic, and
  acetabular fracture, 694
reconstruction, 711–717
  early, 711–712
  late, 712–717
replacement, total, 714
rotation, 29
sepsis and, 717
surgery, angiography after,

HIP (cont.)
    206-210
    surgical approaches to, 704-710
        anterior, anatomy and, 706
        anterior, technique, 704-709
        lateral, diagrams, 708
        lateral, incisions for, 707
        lateral, patient position for, 707
        lateral, technique, 709-710
        lateral, technique, intertrochanteric line presentation, 708
        posterior, to expose external rotators, 709
        posterior, to expose sciatic nerve, 709
        posterior, incisions for, 707
        posterior, patient position for, 707
        posterior, technique, 710
    trauma, 619-680
HISTIOCYTES: and metal implants, 920
HISTORY: of Fracture Clinic of Massachusetts General Hospital, 1-7
HODGEN SPLINT: for femoral supracondylar fracture, 778
HOME CARE: patient instruction for, 1179-1180
HORMONES
    adrenocorticotropic, and 17-hydroxycorticosteroid secretion, 45, 47
    antidiuretic, secretion, 41
    growth, 64
HOSPITAL PERSONNEL: radiation hazards, 193
HUMERUS
    distal, management, 879
    epiphysis
        displacement, proximal, 879
        displacement and separation, 880
    fractures (see Fractures, humerus)
    head
        defects, "hatchet," 425
        defects, in recurrent shoulder dislocations, 441
        displacement, 441
        fracture-dislocation, Rush nail in, 446
        retractor, 431
    interruption of, flaps in, 990

proximal, management, 878
shaft
    displacement, 441
    exposure of, 462
    tumors, giant-cell, and pathologic fracture, 170
HYBBINETTE-EDEN PROCEDURE, 433-434
    after-treatment, 434
    approach, 433
    object, 433
    repair, 433-434
HYDROCORTISONE (see Cortisol)
17-HYDROXYCORTICOSTEROID SECRETION RATES
    ACTH administration and, 45, 47
    surgery and, 45, 47
HYPERALIMENTATION: nutrients and minerals for, 65
HYPERCALCIURIA: after immobilization, 61
HYPERCOAGULATION, 49-50
HYPEREXTENSION
    elbow, 10
    fingers, 17
    knee, 31
    of spine
        cervical, 376-377
        cord, 336
HYPERFLEXION: causing compression spinal cord fractures, 335
HYPEROSMOLAR AGENTS: in head trauma, 309
HYPERTROPHY: of fibula, 155
HYPERVENTILATION: and head trauma management, 308-309
HYPOCOAGULATION, 50
HYPONATREMIA: treatment, 47
HYPOTHALAMUS: and temperature, 312
HYPOTHERMIA
    renal, in hypovolemic shock, 228
    spinal cord, 339
HYPOVOLEMIA
    pressor response to, 41
    shock in (see Shock, hypovolemic)
HYPOXEMIA: causes of, 1020
HYPOXIA, 50-53
    cerebral fat embolism and, 286
    in shock (see Shock, hypoxic)

I

ILEAL LOOP: problems with, after spinal trauma, 394-395
ILEOCOLOSTOMY: end-to-end, 1048
ILIAC (see Ilium)
ILIOFEMORAL VEIN: occlusion, 1127
ILIUM
    bone slabs, in tibia nonunion, 121
    fractures, 610, 611
        comminuted, 612
    grafts
        in capitellar epiphyseal separation, 494
        in clavicle nonunion, 147
        in forearm fractures, 505
        in humeral shaft fractures, 465
        massive, 161
        onlay, 161
        onlay, in Galeazzi's fracture, 506
        removal technique, 162
        subperiosteal, 162-163
        in tibial fracture, 140
    rotation, 611
IMMOBILIZATION
    of fractures, 117
    clavicle, 412, 413
    hypercalciuria after, 61
    metabolic response to, 60-61
    osteoporosis, in fracture healing, 106
    plaster, in navicular fracture, 532
    in shoulder dislocations, anterior, 422
    in spinal trauma
        cervical, 357-360
        cord, 330-333
    urinary tract infection after, 61
IMMUNOLOGY: and burn infections, 1145-1146
IMPLANTS
    (See also Replantation)
    metal (see Metal implants)
INFANTS
    clavicular fractures, splints for, 412, 413
    skull fractures in, depressed, 290
INFARCTION (see Freiberg's infarction)
INFECTIONS
    after burns (see Burn, infections)
    after nailing, medullary, 129
        femoral shaft fracture, 130
    nonunion and (see Nonunion, infection and)
INFLAMMATION IN BONE

HEALING
  dead course cancellous, 75–78
  necrotic compact, 83
INNERVATION (see Nerves)
INNOMINATE BONE: disruption of, 714
INOTROPIC AGENTS: in shock, 218–219
INSPIRATORY FORCE METER, 240
INTERMITTENT POSITIVE-PRESSURE VENTILATION, 994
INTERPHALANGEAL JOINT
  collateral ligament anatomy of, 584
  dislocations, 591–593
  flexion, 14
  proximal, injuries of, 585
  volar plate, 590
INTESTINE
  function, in burns, 1157–1158
  small
    closure of minor injuries, 1044
    resection of, 1045
  ulcer, 56
INTRACRANIAL
  hematomas, 295–308
  pressure
    cerebral edema and, management, 308
    fluid requirements and, 311
INTRAMEDULLARY
  fixation (see Fixation, intramedullary)
  nails (see Nails, intramedullary)
INTUBATION
  endotracheal, 994
  immediate, clinical indications for, 1022
  nasal, 248
  tracheal, 236
INVERSION OF FOOT
  active, 34
  hind part, 33
IPPB, 994
IRRADIATION (see Radiation)
ISCHEMIA
  arterial, sequelae of, 1116–1117
  extremity losses and vascular injuries, 1116
  muscle, in Volkmann's contracture, management, 1134–1135
  in Volkmann's contracture, 1130–1131, 1134–1135
ISOPROTERENOL, 41

in shock, 219
hypovolemic, 229
ISOTOPE (see Radioisotope)

J

JAW: fractures, 261
JEFFERSON'S FRACTURE, 368–369
JEWETT NAIL (see Nails, Jewett)
JIG
  in femoral shaft fracture, 742
  for Jewett nail, 661
JOINT(S)
  (See also specific sites)
  acromioclavicular (see Acromioclavicular)
  ankle (see Ankle)
  carpometacarpal (see Carpometacarpal joint)
  glenohumeral (see Glenohumeral joint)
  of hand, anatomy of, 583–584
  interphalangeal (see Interphalangeal joint)
  knee (see Knee)
  malalignment, correction of, 109
  metacarpophalangeal (see Metacarpophalangeal joint)
  motion, 9–37
    measurement of, 9–37
    recording of, 9–37
  positioning in nerve suturing, 1105
  sacroiliac (see Sacroiliac joint)
  sternoclavicular (see Dislocations, sternoclavicular)
  talofibular, separation of, 823
JONES, D.F., 2

K

KANAMYCIN
  in shock, bacteremic, 230
  in surgical infections, 952
KARYOLYSIS, 79
KELLER-BLAKE SPLINT: for femoral shaft fracture, 723
KIDNEY, 1071–1076
  angiography (see Angiography, kidney)
  contusion, 612
  failure, "crush syndrome," 56
  hypothermia, in hypovolemic shock, 228
  impairment in burns, 1156

injuries, 1071–1076
  diagnosis, 1071–1073
  etiology, 1071
  grade I, 1073
  grade II, 1073
  grade III, 1073–1074
  grade IV, 1074
  grade V, 1074
  mechanisms of, 1072
  nonpenetrating, 1071
  pathology, 1071
  penetrating, 1071
  radiography of, 1073
  repair, 1075
  signs, common, 1071
  surgery, 1076
  symptoms, common, 1071
  treatment, 1074–1076
ischemic syndrome, 55
nephrotomography of, 1073
pyelography of, 1073
scars of, 1073
in shock, 228
surgery, 1076
  exposure technique, 1074
urography of, 1073
veins, vena caval clip below, 1125
venography of, 1073
KIENBÖCK'S DISEASE, 539–542, 543
  diagnosis, 542
  etiology, 539–541
  after lunate dislocation, 540
  pathology, 541
  radiography of, 541–542
  signs of, 542
  symptoms, 542
  treatment, 542
KILFOYLE'S METHOD: in acetabular fracture, 701
KIRSCHNER PIN
  in acromioclavicular separation, 406
  in clavicle fractures, 414, 415
  in clavicle nonunion, 147
  in Colles' fracture, 519
  in femoral shaft fractures, 730, 733
  in thumb carpometacarpal joint fracture-dislocation, 592
  in tibial fracture, 882
  in toe fractures, 858
  in wrist amputations, 1188
  in zygoma fracture, 255
KNEE
  cartilage, semilunar, 762–764
  contusions, 755
  dislocations (see Dislocations, knee)
  elastic bandage over sponge

1222 / INDEX

KNEE (cont.)
  rubber for, 754
  exercise of, 754–755
    convalescent phase, 755
    early phase, 755
      late phase, 755
      techniques, 754–755
  extension, 31
  extensor apparatus, 765–767
    common injuries of, 765
    muscle ruptures, 766
    muscle ruptures, treatment, 766
  flexion, 31
  fracture, of posterior cruciate ligament, 761
    treatment, 761
  function impairment after femoral shaft fracture, 749
  hemarthrosis, traumatic, 755
  hyperextension, 31
  immobilization, motion after, 755
  instability, rotary, test for, 758
  ligaments, 756–762
    collateral, external, 758
    collateral, internal (see ligaments, collateral, internal below)
    collateral, medial, tears of, 756
    cruciate (see ligaments, cruciate below)
    trauma of, 756–762
  ligaments, collateral, internal, 756–758
    conservative treatment, 757
    diagnosis, clinical, 756
    meniscus lesions associated with, 764–765
    surgery, 757–758
    surgery, technique, 757–758
  ligaments, cruciate
    anterior, 758–760
    anterior, meniscus lesions associated with, 764–765
    posterior, 761
    posterior, avulsion fracture of, 761
    posterior, avulsion fracture, treatment, 761
    rupture, "drawer" sign for, 759
    sketch demonstrating, 759
  meniscus, lateral, 764
    treatment of, 764
  meniscus, medial, 762–764
    conservative treatment, 763
    displacement of, 756

    ligament lesions associated with, 764–765
    postoperative care of, 764
    surgery of, 763–764
    surgery of, technique, 764
  motion, 31
    after immobilization, 755
  polycentric hinged joints, in femoral shaft fracture, 742
  quadriceps tendon rupture, 766–767
    treatment, 767
  soft tissue injuries, 755–756
    treatment, 756
  synovitis and, traumatic, 755–756
  trauma, 753–791
    general considerations, 753–755
    rest and, 753–754
  ulcer, 975
KOCHER METHOD: reduction of anterior dislocated shoulder, 420–421
KREBS CYCLE, 52
KÜNTSCHER
  nails (see Nails, Küntscher)
  rod, in femoral shaft fracture, 748

L

LABORATORY
  examination, 186–187
  studies, in head trauma, 276–279
LACERATIONS
  cerebral, 280–283
  cheek, treatment, 275
  eyelids, treatment, 265
  face, treatment, 265
  hand, 564
  lip, scar after, 267
  trachea, and anesthetist, 241
LACTIC ACID, 52–53
LACTIC ACIDOSIS: treatment, 54
LAG SCREWS (see Screws, lag)
LAPAROTOMY: in abdominal injuries, 1037
LAURENCE JONES TECHNIQUE, 448
LEAN TISSUE: metabolic response of, 58–60
LE FORT FRACTURES, 258
LEG
  crushing injury, grafts in, 986
  flaps for, 988
  innervation of, 1100
  lower, skin graft for, 980
  sensory deficit after nerve trunk interruption in,

1098
  straight leg raising test, 26
LEGAL PROBLEMS: with x-ray, 191–192
LIGAMENTS
  ankle (see Ankle, ligaments of)
  foot, anatomy, 818–819
  of hand (see Hand, ligament injuries)
  of hip, attachment to acetabulum, 699
  of knee (see Knee, ligaments)
  shoulder, 399, 400
LIGAMENTUM PATELLAE, avulsion of, 767
  treatment, 767
LIMBS (see Extremities)
LIP LACERATIONS: scars after, 267
LIVER, 1057–1068
  anatomy, 1058
  angiography (see Angiography, liver)
  arteries, anatomic variations in, 1065
  capsular tears, 1057–1058
  hematoma, subcapsular, 1057
    angiography of, 1062
  injuries, 1057–1068
    abdominal injuries and, 1061
    complications, 1068
    diagnosis, 1058–1059
    hemorrhage control in, 1062–1064
    hemostasis, terminal, 1067
    postoperative course in, 1067–1068
    preoperative preparation in, 1059–1062
    resection, choice of, 1064–1066
    resection, technique of, 1066–1067
    surgery, 1062–1067
    types of, 1057–1058, 1060
  lacerations
    avulsing, 1058
    sublobar, guillotine removal of, 1063
  penetrating wounds, 1058
  veins of, 1059
  tears, shunt for, 1063
LOCKJAW (see Tetanus)
LOTTES NAIL (see Nails, Lottes)
LYMPHATIC OBSTRUCTION: in Volkmann's contracture, 1130
LYMPHOMA: metastases causing femoral fracture, 173

INDEX / 1223

LUMBAR
  spine (*see* Spine, lumbar)
  vertebra, 384–391
    bony anatomy of, 320
LUNATE
  dislocations (*see* Dislocations, lunate)
  Kienböck's disease of (*see* Kienböck's disease)
  reduction of
    closed, 537, 538
    closed, method, 538
    open, through dorsal incision, 539
LUNG
  capacities, 1017
  compliance, 1021
  congestion, 50
  effects of nonthoracic trauma on, 1018
  function disturbances, 1013–1020
  insufficiency, 50
  nonthoracic causes, 1022
  shotgun wound, 1012
  volumes, 1017
    effects of respirator on, 1025
  wet lung syndrome, 1021–1022

M

MADELUNG'S DEFORMITY, 496
  at wrist, 474
MAGNESIUM: for hyperalimentation, 65
MAGNUSON-STACK PROCEDURE, recurrent shoulder dislocations, 434
  after-treatment, 434
  approach, 434
  exposure, 434
  object, 434
  repair, 434
MALFORMATIONS (*see* Deformity)
MALINGERING: after hand soft tissue injuries, 563
MALLEOLUS
  "buttonholing" of, 821
  fracture (*see* Fractures, malleolus)
  fracture-dislocation, unstable, 834
  tendon pulley forces on, 827
MALLET FINGER, 569
MALOCCLUSION OF TEETH: and face fracture, 260
MALPOSITION: callus requirement increase

with, 119
MALUNION
  Colles' fracture, 523–524
  femur fractures, 150
  forearm, 508–509
  humeral fractures, supracondylar, 483
  long bones, 115–158
MANDIBLE
  fractures (*see* Fractures, mandible)
  x-rays of, positions for, 247
MANIPULATION
  forearm fractures, 500–501
  of shoulder
    in dislocations, old unreduced traumatic, 437
    in fracture-dislocations, 442–443
MANNITOL
  in cardiogenic shock, 222
  in head trauma, 309
MAP: dermatomal, of body, 324
MARBLE, H.C., 3
MASSACHUSETTS GENERAL HOSPITAL FRACTURE CLINIC: history of, 1–7
MASSAGE: in rehabilitation, 1178
MAXILLA
  fractures, 258, 259–263
  varieties of, 258
  floating, direct wiring to orbital rim, 259
MAXILLOFACIAL TRAUMA: and anesthesia, 240–241
MEDIASTINUM: widening due to trauma, 1009
MEDICAL PERSONNEL: radiation hazards, 193
MEDICINE, REHABILITATION (*see* Rehabilitation)
MEDULLARY
  nail (*see* Nail, medullary)
  nailing (*see* Nailing, medullary)
MENISCUS (*see* Knee, meniscus)
MESENCHYMAL TISSUE, 80
MESENTERY: treatment, 1044
METABOLIC ACIDOSIS: treatment, 54
METABOLIC ALKALOSIS: treatment, 54
METABOLIC RESPONSE TO TRAUMA, 39–69
  acute, 40–50
  complications and, 50–56
  convalescence and, 56–64
  features of, 64
  therapy and, 50–56

METACARPAL
  first, dislocation, 551
  fractures (*see* Fractures, metacarpals)
METACARPOPHALANGEAL JOINT
  collateral ligament anatomy of, 584
  dislocations, 592, 593
  flexion, 14
  thumb (*see* Thumb, metacarpophalangeal joint)
METAL
  bone toleration of, 116
  harmful use of, 131
  implants (*see* Metal implants *below*)
  splints, in nose fractures, 252
  unnecessary use of, 131
METAL IMPLANTS, 913–933
  application defects, 926
  biologic interactions with host, 929–933
    cases illustrating, 930–932
  corrosion, 913–917, 918–923
    of bolts, 916
    discussion of, 918–923
    questions and answers concerning, 918–923
    rate of, 915–917
    of screws, 916, 924, 925
    types of, 915–917
  design defects, 926
  failures, 923–927
  fibroblasts and, 920
  fibrocytes and, 920
  histocytes and, 920
  mechanical interactions with host, 928–929
  metallurgy, 913–923
  tissue reaction to, 917–918, 920
METALLURGY: and metal implants, 913–923
METASTASES
  in breast carcinoma (*see* Breast carcinoma, metastatic)
  fractures due to, 171–175
    of femur, 172–174
METATARSAL
  fractures (*see* Fractures, metatarsal)
  head, Freiberg's infarction of, 860–863
METHOHEXITAL, 240
METHYLMETHACRYLATE REINFORCEMENT: in myeloma microfractures, 173

1224 / INDEX

METHYLPREDNISOLONE
  in head trauma, 310
  in shock, hypovolemic, 228
MEURIG-WILLIAMS PLATES: in spinal cord fractures, 334
MICROFRACTURE: of sesamoid, 864
MICROSURGICAL ANASTOMOSES: of arteries, 1189
MINERALS: for hyperalimentation, 65
MONITORING
  ECG, 216
  oxygen concentrations, 1024
  shock, 216–218
    burn, during treatment, 1140–1141
MONTEGGIA'S FRACTURE, 477–478
  anterior, 477
  posterior, 478
MORPHINE
  ADH activity and, 41
  in shock, hypovolemic, 229
MORTALITY (see Death)
MOTION
  ankle, 32
  elbow, 10
  fingers, 16–17
  foot, 33–35
  hind part, 33
  forearm, 11
  hip, 27–30
  joint (see Joint, motion)
  knee, 31
  shoulder (see Shoulder, motion)
  spine, 25–26
    cervical, 22
    lumbar, 23–24
  thumb, 13–15
  toes, 36
  wrist, 12
MOTOR
  function chart, 326–329
  impulses, 320
  neuron lesions, lower, 395
MUSCLES
  of ankle, 815–817
  biceps, in humerus shaft fractures, 462
  brachialis, in humerus shaft fractures, 462
  contracture after nerve suture, 1110
  in debridement of open fractures, 938
  forearm, rotatory pull of, 498
  function, in burns, 1159
  glenohumeral joint, and exercise, 423
  ischemia in Volkmann's contracture, management, 1134–1135
  of knee extensor apparatus, ruptures, 766
    treatment, 766
  metabolism in Volkmann's contracture, 1131
  power after nerve suture, 1109–1110
  proprioceptive neuromuscular facilitation technique, 1176
  shoulder, 399, 401
  trauma, 55–56
MYELOGRAPHY
  block in, and vertebral fracture, 383
  in spinal cord fracture, 334
  of subarachnoid space, 329
MYELOMA: metastases causing fractures, 173
MYOCARDIUM: shotgun wound of, 1012
MYOGLOBIN, 55
MYOSITIS
  clostridial, 954–955
  ossificans, 717
    after elbow dislocation, 473

N

NAFCILLIN: in surgical infections, 952
NAIL(S)
  (see also Nailing)
  cloverleaf (see Küntscher below)
  Hansen-Street, 902
  intramedullary
    in fibular fracture, 828
    in humerus shaft fractures, 465
    tissue reaction to, 920
  Jewett
    in femoral fracture, extracapsular, 661
    jig for, 661
  Küntscher
    diagram of, 902
    discussion of, 903–905
    in femoral fracture, 174, 907
    in femoral fracture, pathologic, 903
    in femoral fracture, pathologic, due to lymphoma, 173
    in pathologic fracture in Paget's disease, 169
    removal of, 905, 908
  Lottes, 902
    discussion, 909–910
    in fibular fracture, 804
    in humeral fracture, 143, 144
    in tibial fracture, 804, 910
  medullary
    in ankle fracture-dislocation, 830
    in femur fracture, ununited infected, 124
    types of, 902
  Rush, 902
    discussion of, 909
    for forearm fractures, 507
    for humeral head fracture-dislocation, 446
    for humeral shaft fracture, "blind" technique, 464
    specifications, 909
    for ulnar fracture, 909
  sliding, in femoral fracture due to breast carcinoma, 174
  Smith-Petersen, 622
  tissue reaction to, 918
NAILING
  (See also Nail)
  of femoral neck fractures
    anatomic guides in, 638
    arthritis after, septic, 650
    femur head positions in, anatomic and valgus, 643
    importance of impacting in, 644
    lead markers for angle of nail, 639
    nail length determination method, 644
    nailing hip to avoid femoral shaft splitting, 641
    placement of nail, 639–646
    poor positions of fragments after, 648
    position of nail, 642–646
    radiography as guide in, 645
    usual angle of nail with femoral shaft, 640
  medullary
    bending of nail, 906–909
    breaking of nail, 906–909
    complications of, 905–909
    of femur, 901–905
    of femur, insertion error, 907
    of femur, patient position for, 904
    of femur, retrograde insertion, 906

indications for, 903
infection after, 129
infection after, femoral shaft fracture, 130
of long-bone fractures, 901–909
sepsis after, 909
tissue reaction to, 920
NARCOTICS, 240
NASAL (see Nose)
NAVICULAR BONE
 fractures (see Fractures, navicular)
 nonunion, 533–536
  Barnard's operation in, 534
  drilling, 534
  graft for, bone, 534–536
  graft for, bone, technique, 534–536
  spatula used in, 535
 radial approach to, 535
 rotation, in capitate dislocation, 545
 subluxation, 542–549
  diagnosis, 546
  mechanism of, 544–546
  rotation, 548
  treatment, 546–549
 tarsal, fracture, 850–851, 866, 867
  compression, 854
NECK
 jerking backward causing atlantoaxial dislocations, 335
 in physical examination, 184–185
NECROSIS
 aseptic, in capitellar epiphyseal fracture, 485
 avascular
  of femoral head, 650
  of hip, 712–716
  after talar fracture, 851
 in bone healing, necrotic compact, 83
 in bone repair, dead course cancellous, 73–75
 radiation, 193
 tubular, acute, 55–56
NEER REPLACEMENT PROSTHESIS: in shattered humeral head, 449
NEPHROTOMOGRAPHY: of kidney, 1073
NERVES
 acoustic, 293
 of arm, 1099, 1190, 1192
  gunshot wound of, 1102
 block
  in face trauma, 248
  intercostal, 998

cranial, trauma, and skull fracture, 292–293
digital, traumatic changes in, 864
in elbow dislocations, posterior, 471
facial, 293
of foot, 1100
of hand, 1099
of leg, 1100
olfactory, 292
optic, 292
peripheral, 1087–1114
 anatomic structure, 1087–1088
 grafts for, 1105–1107
 injuries (see peripheral, injuries below)
 repair, 1101–1108
 repair, metabolic determinants in, 1088–1093
 repair, metabolic determinants in, composite drawing outlining, 1089–1090
 rerouting, 1105
 resection, for neuroma, 1088
 surgery (see peripheral, surgery below)
 suturing (see peripheral, suturing below)
 transposing, 1105
 trunk interruption, sensory deficit after, in arm, 1097
 trunk interruption, sensory deficit after, in leg, 1098
peripheral, injuries, 1087–1114
 bone shortening and, 1108
 diagnosis, 1097–1101
 fifth degree, 1096
 first degree, 1093, 1094
 fourth degree, 1094–1096
 fourth degree, partial, 1095
 painful syndromes after, 1113–1114
 paralysis after, orthopedic measures in, 1112–1113
 second degree, 1093–1094
 third degree, 1094
 types of, 1096–1097
peripheral, surgery, 1101–1114
 examinations during, 1102
 examinations during, methods, 1102
 examinations during, motor, 1102
 examinations during, sensory, 1102

postoperative care, 1108
 timing of, 1101–1102
peripheral, suturing
 joint positioning in, 1105
 muscle contracture after, 1110
 muscle power after, 1109–1110
 neurolysis and, 1104
 pain after, 1111
 recovery after, 1108–1112
 technique, 1102–1105
 touch response after, 1112
proprioceptive neuromuscular facilitation technique, 1176
radial injury, in humeral shaft fracture, 466–467
in replantation of arms, 1190
 nerve repair, 1192
sciatic
 exposure of, in hip surgery, 709
 in hip dislocations and acetabular fractures, 704
shoulder, 399
in shoulder dislocations, 440
trigeminal, 293
ulnar, transplantation technique, 1106–1107
wrist, median
 approach to, 549
 sensory changes after trauma, 548
 traumatic neuritis of, 549–550
NERVOUS SYSTEM DISORDERS: and head trauma, 283–284
NEURAPRAXIA, 1096–1097
NEURITIS: traumatic, of wrist median nerve, 549–550
NEUROGENIC SHOCK: treatment of, 230–231
NEUROLOGIC
 examination, in shoulder trauma, 403
 syndromes, and spinal cord trauma, 336
 trauma, and anesthesia, 239–240
NEUROLYSIS: and nerve suturing, 1104
NEUROMA
 digital nerve and, 864
 of peripheral nerves, resection in, 1088
NEURONS: lower motor neuron lesion, 395
NEURORRHAPHY: technique, 1104

1226 / INDEX

NEUROSIS AFTER HAND SOFT TISSUE INJURIES
  compensation, 563
  patterns of, 563
NEUROTMESIS, 1097
NEUROVASCULAR ISLAND FLAP:
  techniques of, 576
NICOLA PROCEDURE, 434-435
  after-treatment, 435
  approach, 435
  exposure, 435
  object, 434
  repair, 435
NICOTINAMIDE ADENINE DINUCLEOTIDE, 52
90-90-90 TRACTION: in femoral shaft fracture, 734-736
NITROGEN: excretion, 59
NITROUS OXIDE, 240
NONUNION
  "boot-top" fracture, 133
  capitellar epiphyseal displacement, 494
  causes of, local, 116
  clavicle, 130, 147-148
    compression plate in, 148
  clinical findings, 120
  closed fractures, causes of, 117, 119
  femur fractures, 123-127
    closed, treatment of, 123-127
    comminuted, 127
    compression plate in, 150
    infected, 142
    infected, medullary nail in, 124
    open, treatment of, 127
    shaft, 747-749
    "walking" plaster spica for, 128
  fibula fractures, 138, 805-808
    closed, 127-128
    displaced, 148
    infection and, 136-137
    Parham bands causing, 131
    Rush pin causing, 131
    secondary to open fractures, 128
    segmental, 135
    treatment, 151
  forearm fractures, 128-129, 506-508
    causes of, 508
    grafts in, dual tibial onlay, 508
    infection and, 144
  humerus fractures, 144, 145
    comminuted, 143, 146
    infection and, 142-144
    shaft, 129-130, 466

  infection and, 115-158
  femur fractures, 124, 142
  fibula fracture, 136-137
  forearm fractures, 144
  humerus fractures, 142-144
  tibia fracture, open, 136-137
  long bones, 115-158
  in navicular fracture (see Navicular bone, nonunion)
  in odontoid process fracture, 352, 359
  of open fractures, 940
    causes of, 119
  radius fractures, 142
    grafts in, bone, 157
    "wire loop," causing, 157
  roentgenography, 120-121
  tibia fractures, 138, 805-808
    closed, 127-128
    displaced, 148
    faulty application of plate and screws causing, 123
    grafts in, onlay, 121
    iliac bone slabs in, 121, 123
    infection and, 136-137
    Parham bands causing, 131
    Rush pin causing, 131
    secondary to open fractures, 128
    segmental, 135
    treatment, 125, 151, 156
  of trochanteric fractures, 669-673
    management, 672
  ulna fractures, 142
NOREPINEPHRINE, 40-41
  in shock, 219
  dislocations, 250-251
  fractures (see Fractures, nose)
  intubation, 248
NUCLEAR CLUMPING, 79
"NURSEMAID'S ELBOW," 473-474
NURSING CARE (see Care, nursing)
NUTRIENTS: for hyperalimentation, 65
NUTRITIONAL
  (See also Feeding)
  balance, by IV feeding, 65
  responses, in burns, 1158-1159

O

OCCLUSION
  cerebral arteries, extracranial,

  284
  teeth, fixation methods of, 260
ODONTOID PROCESS (see Fractures, odontoid process)
OLECRANON
  excision to restore elbow motion, 910
  fracture (see Fractures, olecranon)
  screw for, broken, 926
  wire traction in humerus shaft fractures, 465
OLFACTORY NERVE: trauma, 292
OPERATIVE TREATMENT OF FRACTURES (see Surgery of fractures)
OPTIC NERVE, 292
ORBIT
  air in, 257
  fat, prolapsed, 256
  fractures (see Fractures, orbit)
  rim, floating maxilla wired to, 259
  trauma, 254
ORGAN TRANSPLANTATION, 314
OS CALCIS
  excision, foot after, 848
  fractures (see Fractures, os calcis)
  ulcer, 977
OSSIFICATION
  endochondral, 96
  epiphyseal, 875
OSTEOBLASTS, 72
OSTEOCLASTS, 72, 76, 77
OSTEOCYTIC OSTEOLYSIS, 72
OSTEOGENESIS IMPERFECTA, 168
OSTEOLYSIS: osteocytic, 72
OSTEOMYELITIS: bone defects and skin grafts, 973
OSTEONS, 77, 87
OSTEOPERIOSTEAL GRAFT
  "neighborhood," 163
  tibial, in humeral shaft fracture, 465
OSTEOPOROSIS, 61
  in fracture healing, 106
  nonunion and, 122
  vertebral compression fracture and, 168
OSTEOTOMY
  complete, treated by intramedullary fixation, healing of, 98-101
  in humerus supracondylar fracture, 483
  scapular neck, wedge, 439

INDEX / 1227

OTORRHEA: cerebrospinal fluid, and skull fracture, 293–295
OXACILLIN
  in shock, bacteremic, 230
  in surgical infections, 952
OXYGEN
  alveolar-arterial oxygen difference, 1030–1031
  analyzer, Beckman paramagnetic, 1024
  breathing high concentrations of, 1019
  cardiac output and, 52
  concentrations, monitoring of, 1024
  comsumption, 51
    during convalescence, 53
  hematocrit and, 52
  reservoir, self-inflating bag for, 1026
  tank, 1023
  therapy in shock, 221–222
OXYGENATION, 1021
OXYHEMOGLOBIN DISSOCIATION CURVE
  in acidosis, 53–54
  in alkalosis, 53–54

P

PAGET'S DISEASE, fractures in, 169
  femoral
    extracapsular, 660
    shaft pathologic, 745
PAIN
  anesthetist and, 242
  of burns, 1159–1160
  after nerve suture, 1111
  spinothalamic tracts and, 323
  syndromes after peripheral nerve injury, 1113–1114
PALMER TECHNIQUE: in os calcis fracture, 844
PA_{O_2}, 1031
PALPATION
  acromioclavicular joint, 404–405
  clavicle, 411
  shoulder, 403
  sternoclavicular, 409
PALSY
  cerebral, and hip fracture, 653
  Todd's, 284
PANCREAS
  angiography, 202
  contusion of tail, repair, 1042
  pseudocyst, angiography, 202
  treatment of, 1039–1041
PAPILLEDEMA, 284

PARACENTESIS
  in abdominal injuries, 1034–1035
  diagnostic, 186
PARALYSIS
  after nerve injuries, peripheral, orthopedic measures in, 1112–1113
  radial nerve, and humerus shaft fractures, 466
PARAPARESIS: after spinal cord contusion, 334
PARAPLEGIA
  spinal cord and, 317
  spinal stab wound causing, 337
  transient, 339
  ulcer in, sacral pressure, 976
PARATHYROID: function changes, 64
PARÉ'S DESCRIPTION: of hip fracture, 621
PARHAM BANDS, 129
  discussion, 901
  in fibular fractures, 804
  in humerus fractures, 145
  infection after, 155
  nonunion due to, 131
  in tibial fractures, 804
PATELLA
  bilateral tripartite, 771
  dislocations, traumatic, 767–768
    treatment, 768
  fractures (see Fractures, patella)
  ligamentum patellae avulsion, 767
    treatment, 767
  tendon, treatment of, 965
PATELLECTOMY
  postoperative care, 773
  technique, 773
PATHOLOGIC FRACTURES (see Fractures, pathologic)
PATIENT EVALUATION: and anesthetist, 236–237
PEARSON ATTACHMENT: and Hodgen splint for femoral supracondylar fracture, 778
PEDICLE FLAP: scalp, 288
PELVIC SLING, 616
PELVIS, 605–617
  anatomy, 607
  collapse of, inward, 609
  fractures (see Fractures, pelvic)
  hemipelvis rotation, 608
    counterclockwise, 611
  hemorrhage, angiography, 207, 208

  in physical examination, 185–186
  rotation, counterclockwise, 610
  trauma, 605–617
    distortion of posterior arch and, 614–617
PEMPHIGUS: steroids for, and spinal fracture, 168
"PENDULUM AIR," 997
PENICILLIN
  in bacteremic shock, 230
  in surgical infections, 952
PENIS
  extravasation due to urethral leakage, 1080
  injuries, 1085
PERINEUM: extravasation due to urethral leakage, 1080
PERIOSTEUM
  callus, 100
  long bone, normal (in rabbit), 91
PERITONEUM: retroperitoneal hematoma, treatment, 1048–1049
PERSONNEL: radiation hazards, 193
PHALANGES
  (See also Fingers, Toes)
  of foot, fractures of, 856–860
  terminal, anastomosing tendon to, 566
PHARMACOLOGIC AGENTS: in head trauma, 309
PHENOBARBITAL: in head trauma, 311–312
PHENOXYBENZAMINE: in hypovolemic shock, 229
PHENYLEPHRINE: in neurogenic shock, 231
PHOSPHORUS: for hyperalimentation, 65
PHOTOMICROGRAPH: of epiphyseal plate, 871
PHYSICAL EXAMINATION (see Examination, physical)
PHYSICAL THERAPY: after spinal trauma, 395–396
PHYSIOLOGIC PROBLEMS: and anesthetist, 241–242
PILOT POINT SCREWS: discussion, 898
PIN
  Kirschner (see Kirschner pin)
  Rush (see Rush pin)
  Sage, in forearm fractures, 502
  -screws, Simmons-Martin acromioclavicular, 407
PINCERS, 431
  glenoid, 431

PINEAL GLAND: as radiographic indicator, 278
PLASMA
  loss in hypovolemic shock, 227
  volume changes after hemorrhage, 44
PLASTER
  immobilization in navicular fracture, 532
  of Paris
    boot, for foot, 866
    slab, in humeral fracture, 481
    spica (see Spica, plaster of Paris)
    splints (see Splints, plaster)
PLATE(S)
  application techniques, 897
  ASIF, discussion, 895–896
  chest, 994, 998
  cobalt chromium, corrosion of, 922
  compression (see Compression plate)
  construction of, 898
  corrosion of, 921, 922
  epiphysis (see Epiphysis, plate)
  4-hole semitubular, in forearm fractures, 504
  in humeral shaft fracture, 463, 465
  Meurig-Williams, in spinal cord fracture, 334
  6-hole, 505
  slotted, 897
    complications with, 926
    improper application and delayed union, 118
  stainless steel, in T and Y fractures of humerus, 489
  Thornton
    break in, 927
    tissue reaction to, 918
    in tibial fracture, 970, 984
    nonunion due to faulty application, 123
  Vitallium, in humeral shaft fracture, 465
PLATELET: count, 49
PLEURAL
  effusion, 1009
  space, management of blood and air in, 999–1001
PLIERS: Austin's vise-grip, 908
PNEUMATIC TOURNIQUET, 891
PNEUMOCEPHALUS, 293
PNEUMOTHORAX, 236
  tension, 236
POTASSIUM: for hyperalimentation, 65

POTTS FRACTURE, 831
PREDNISOLONE: in adrenal insufficiency, 47
PREDNISONE: in adrenal insufficiency, 47
PRESSOR DRUGS, 41
PRESSURE
  arterial, measurement of, 216
  intracranial (see Intracranial, pressure)
PROCAINE: in face trauma, 248
PROPRIOCEPTIVE NEUROMUSCULAR FACILITATION TECHNIQUE, 1176
PROSTATE: mobility in complete urethral transection, 1082
PROSTHESIS
  Neer replacement, in shattered humeral head, 449
  Vitallium (see Vitallium prosthesis)
PROTEIN
  for hyperalimentation, 65
  serum, 49
PROTHROMBIN TIME, 49
PSEUDARTHROSIS, 103
  fibula, 138
  tibia, 138
"PSEUDOCOARCTATION," 1008
PSEUDOCYST: pancreas, angiography, 202
PUBIC BELT, 614
"PULLED ELBOW" (see Dislocations, radius head)
PUPILS: dilated, in head trauma, 274
PUTTI-PLATT PROCEDURE, 432
  after-treatment, 432
  approach, 432
  objective, 432
  repair, 432
  subscapularis tendon division in, 432
PYELOGRAPHY: of kidney, 1073
PYKNOSIS, 79
PYRUVATE, 52

Q

QUADRICEPS TENDON (see Tendons, quadriceps)
QUADRIPLEGIA
  spinal cord bullet wound causing, 337
  spinal cord teardrop fracture causing, 335

R

RACCOON SIGN, 275
RADIAL DEVIATION: wrist, 12
RADIAL NERVE INJURY: in humeral shaft fracture, 466–467
RADIATION
  abuse of, 191–195
  dermatitis, 193
  diagnostic, 187
    of abdominal injuries, 1035
    of acetabulum, fracture, posterior, 696
    of acetabulum, rim, 688
    in acromioclavicular trauma, 405
    of ankle, 811–813
    of ankle, positions for, 812
    of atlas dislocation, 351
    of capitate dislocation, 548
    of carpal bones, 528, 529–531, 550
    cineradiography in cervical spine surgery, 362
    in clavicle fractures, 412
    of elbow dislocation, 469–470
    in embolism, fat, 1197
    face, positions for, 246, 247
    in femoral fracture, impacted, 633
    in femoral fracture, intracapsular, 626–627
    in femoral fracture, neck, as nailing guide, 645
    of fibular fractures, 793–795, 829
    of foot, positions for, 812
    of forearm fracture, 499–500
    of forearm fracture, positioning for, 499
    of Freiberg's infarction, 861
    general principles in, 194–195
    of hand fractures, 594–595
    head trauma, 276–279
    of hip dislocation, anterior, 682
    of hip dislocation, posterior, 685–687
    of humeral fractures, 441–442
    of kidney injuries, 1073
    of Kienböck's disease, 541–542
    KUB films, 1073
    mandible, positions for, 47
    of metatarsal fractures, 856
    nonunion, 120–121

of odontoid process
  fracture, 351
of odontoid process
  fracture, follow-up, 346
of os calcis fractures, 843
radius fractures, distal end,
  516
in scapula fractures, 416
in shoulder dislocations,
  anterior, 418, 419
in shoulder dislocations,
  posterior, 436, 437
in spinal cord trauma, 325,
  329
in sternoclavicular
  dislocations, 409
of tarsometatarsal
  dislocations, 856
of tibial fracture, 793–795
of tibial fracture, avulsion,
  760
of vertebra, thoracic
  decalcified, 347
of wrist joint, 550
hazards, 192–193
  to medical personnel, 193
historical background, 191
legal problems, 191–192
necrosis, 193
use of, 191–195
RADIOGRAPHY (see Radiation,
  diagnostic)
RADIOISOTOPE(S)
bone-seeking, 61
brain scanning, 278–279
RADIUS
anatomy, 513
avulsion, 141
bow, 503
curves of, 498
dislocations (see
  Dislocations, radius)
epiphysis
  distal, management, 876
  distal, separation, 877
  of head, 475
  proximal, displacement,
    878
  proximal, management, 876
  separation, in children,
    493–494
fractures (see Fractures,
  radius)
head
  epiphysis, 475
  fractures (see Fractures,
    radius head)
  "silver-fork" deformity, 513–
    515
RAY'S SCREWS (see Screws,
  Ray's)

RECALCIFICATION TIME, 49
RECONSTRUCTION (see Hip,
  reconstruction)
RECTUM
  repair, 1046
  treatment, 1044–1047
REDUCTION
  of acetabular fracture,
    reduction failure in, 699
  of ankle, 811
    fracture, 826–827, 833
    fracture-dislocation, 831
  closed
    of capitate, 545
    in fibular fractures (see
      Fractures, fibula,
      reduction, closed)
    in forearm fractures, 500–
      501
    of hip dislocations, 682–
      683
    of lunate, 537, 538
    of lunate, method, 538
    sternoclavicular
      dislocations, 409
    in tibial fractures (see
      Fractures, tibia,
      reduction, closed)
  of Colles' fracture, 518, 519
    malunited, 523–524
  of elbow dislocations,
    posterior, 470–472
  of femoral fractures
    neck, anatomic guides in,
      638
    neck, difficult cases, 646
    neck, reduction principles,
      635–639
    shaft, 736–737, 743–746
  humerus fractures
    shaft, 461–464
    T fractures, 488, 489
    Y fractures, 489
  nose fractures, 251
  odontoid process fracture,
    352, 359
  open
    acromioclavicular
      separation, 405–407
    in clavicle fractures, 414
    fibular fractures, 803–805,
      831
    in forearm fractures, 501–
      506
    in hip dislocations,
      posterior, 690–691
    of lunate, through dorsal
      incision, 539
    of navicular fracture, 545
    in sternoclavicular
      dislocations, 409–411

tibia fractures, 140, 803–
  805, 983, 987
tibia fractures, and plating,
  979
unnecessary, disaster after,
  152–154
of wrist fracture, 551
prone technique, in posterior
  hip dislocation, 690
of radius
  fracture of distal end,
    manual method, 517
  head dislocation, 474
shoulder dislocations
  anterior (see Dislocations,
    shoulder, anterior,
    reduction of)
  old unreduced, 437, 439
  posterior, 422
shoulder fracture-dislocations,
  443–445
of spinal cord fracture-
  dislocation, 353
of trimalleolar fracture, 835
vertebra
  fracture, 351
  fracture-dislocation,
    lumbar, 388–390
zygoma fractures, temporal
  approach, 253
REFRACTURE: forearm bones,
  502
REGURGITATION: of aortic
  valve, traumatic, 1007
REHABILITATION, 1169–1181
  crutches in (see Crutches)
  electrodiagnosis in, 1178
  electrotherapy in, 1178–1179
  exercise in (see Exercise)
  heat in (see Heat in
    rehabilitation)
  home care, patient
    instruction for, 1179–
    1180
  massage in, 1178
  problems in, 1180–1181
  after replantation of arms,
    1192
  ultrasound in, 1177–1178
REMODELING
  bone, clinical implications,
    72–73
  in bone healing, necrotic
    compact, 86–87
  in bone repair, 82
  in fracture healing, 106–107
  internal, 107
RENAL (see Kidney)
REPLANTATION OF ARMS,
  1183–1193
  debridement (see

1230 / INDEX

REPLANTATION OF ARMS (cont.)
Debridement, in replantation of arm)
emergency care, 1183–1185
failure causing reamputation, 1191
fashioning the osseous framework, 1187
fractures and, 1186–1187
judgment in, 1185–1186
movement preservation, 1191–1192
nerves in, 1190
repair of, 1192
postoperative care, 1191–1192
rehabilitation after, 1192
soft tissue closure in, 1190–1191
surgery, 1186–1191
vessels in, 1187–1190
RESPIRATION
(See also Breathing)
equations relating to, 1030–1031
in hypoxic shock, 225
mechanical ventilation, 1023
complications of, 1027–1028
RESPIRATOR
Bird Mark 8, 1023
effects on lung volume, 1025
Emerson Postoperative, 1024
setting of, 1024–1025
weaning from, 1029
RESPIRATORY
acidosis, treatment, 54
care, maintenance of, 1022–1025
embarrassment, causes of, 178
failure, 1015–1032
management, 1015–1032
functions, physiologic assessment, 1027
impairment in burns, 1154–1156
direct causes, 1154–1155
indirect mechanisms, 1155–1156
support, indications for, 1023
REST: and knee trauma, 753–754
RESUSCITATION, 993–995
in abdominal injuries, 1035–1036
anesthetist and, 235–236
RETICULOSPINAL TRACTS: and spinal cord trauma, 323
RETINA: preretinal hemorrhage, 284
RETRACTOR: humeral head, 431

RETROPERITONEAL
hematoma, treatment, 1048–1049
hemorrhage, angiography, 207
REVASCULARIZATION: in bone repair, 78, 80
RHINORRHEA: cerebrospinal fluid, and skull fracture, 293–295
RIGIDITY: decerebrate, due to brainstem contusion, 275
RING AVULSION: of finger, 577
RODS
cloverleaf, 503
diamond-shaped, 503
Küntscher, in femoral shaft fracture, 748
Rush (see Rush rods)
types of, 503
ROENTGENOLOGY (see Radiation)
ROGERS FRAME: after spinal cord trauma, 332
ROTATION
defects and fracture healing, 110
hip, 29
scapula, 402
shoulder, 20
spine, 26
cervical, 22
thumb, 15
ROTATOR CUFF TRAUMA, 446–450
diagnosis, 447–448
shoulder dislocation and, 440
treatment, 448–450
ROWE METHOD IN FRACTURES
acetabular, 701
femoral shaft, 734
ROWLEY BRISTOW PROCEDURE: Heflet modification, 435–436
RUBBER: sponge, with elastic bandage, for knee, 754
"RUM FITS," 283
RUPTURE
of ankle ligament
lateral, 822
medial, 823
of aorta
isthmus, angiography of, 199
thoracic, angiography of, 199
of biceps tendon
distal, 962
distal, complete, 963
long head of, 961
of bladder, intraperitoneal, 1079
of hand ligaments
collateral, with early repair, 588
complete, 586
of kidney, angiography of, 204
of knee cruciate ligament, "drawer" sign for, 759
of knee extensor apparatus muscles, 766
treatment, 766
of knee quadriceps tendon, 766–767
treatment, 767
of liver, angiography of, 200
spleen, angiography, 201
of tibial tendons, posterior, repair, 967
RUSH
nail (see Nail, Rush)
pin
in humeral fracture, 146
nonunion due to, 131
rods
in radius fractures, closed, 503
in ulnar fractures, closed, 503
RUSSELL TRACTION (see Traction, Russell)

S

SACROILIAC BELT, 612
SACROILIAC JOINT
dislocations, 610, 614–617
fracture, 611
lacerations, 608, 609
SACRUM
fracture, 612
ulcer due to pressure, in paraplegia, 976
SAGE PIN: in forearm fracture, 502
SCALP
avulsion, treatment of, 265
sutures, 287
trauma, 286–287
flaps in, bridging, 288
flaps in, pedicle, 288
flaps in, sliding, 288
repair of, 284
SCANNING
brain, 278–279
CAT, 279
of kidney, 1073
SCAPHOID FRACTURES, 865
accessory, 867
SCAPULA
fractures (see Fractures, scapula)

neck, wedge osteotomy, 439
  rotation, 402
SCAPULOTHORACIC MOTION: of
    shoulder, 21
SCAR
  after laceration below lip,
    267
  unstable, of heel, 978
SCIATIC NERVE (see Nerves,
    sciatic)
SCLEROSIS: bone, 121
SCREWS, 900–901
  application
    faulty, causing tibia
      nonunion, 123
    techniques, 897
  ASIF, discussion, 895–896
  in capitellar epiphyseal
    separation, 494
  construction of, 898
  corrosion of, 916, 921, 922,
    924, 925
  extractor, Cherry and
    Southwick, 908
  in femoral fracture,
    supracondylar T, 784
  in fibular fracture, 900
  in humeral fractures
    neck surgical, 447
    shaft, 465
    shaft segmental, 463
  infection after, 155
  lag
    in humeral neck fracture,
      displaced, 446
    in trimalleolar fracture, 835
  long, discussion, 898
  in malleolus fracture fixation,
    900
  for olecranon, broken, 926
  pilot point, discussion, 898
  pin-screws, Simmons-Martin
    acromioclavicular, 407
  Ray's
    in acetabular fractures, 701
    trochanteric, 691
  in tibial fracture, 900
  in wrist fracture, 551
SCROTUM
  extravasation due to urethral
    leakage, 1080
  injuries, 1086
SCUDDER, C.L., 1
SEPSIS, 943–955
  allografting and, 947
  ankle fracture and, 985
  antibiotics in
    preventive, 944, 949
    surgical infections, 952
  arterial injury and, 1124–
    1125
  avoidance of further bacterial
    contamination, 948
  bacterial infections, specific,
    treatment, 951–955
  closure and
    delayed primary, 946
    secondary, 946
  controlling established
    infection, 949–955
    principles, general, 949–
      951
  femoral shaft fractures and,
    747
  after fixation, intramedullary,
    909
  hip and, 717
  host resistance to bacteria
    and hypoperfusion, 945
  open fractures and, 940–942
    grading wounds, criteria
      for, 942
    incidence, 941
    sepsis degree and fracture
      severity, 941
  prevention, important
    measures in, 943–949
    antibiotics, 944
  principles concerning,
    general, 943
  removal of contaminated
    bacteria and, 945–947
  removal of injured tissue
    and, 945–947
  restoration of normal
    physiology and, 944–945
SEPTIC ARTHRITIS: after hip
  nailing, 650
SEQUESTRECTOMY, 152
SESAMOID FRACTURES, 865–
    867
  microfracture, 864
SEX: and forearm fractures, 499
SEXUAL FUNCTION: loss after
  spinal cord contusion,
    334
SHOCK, 213–234
  acidosis and, metabolic
    sodium bicarbonate in, 220
    treatment, 220
  anesthesia and, 238–239
  anesthetist and, 238
  antibiotics in, 230
  bacteremic, treatment of,
    229–230
  blocking agents in, 229
  bradyarrhythmias in, control
    of, 220
  burn (see Burn, shock)
  cardiogenic
    counterpulsation in, 223
    ethacrynic acid in, 222
    furosemide in, 222
    intra-aortic balloon assist
      in, 224–225
    mannitol in, 222
    treatment, 218
  circulation and, assisted,
    222–225
  definition of, 213–214
  digitalization, 219
  digoxin in, 219
  diuretics in, 222
  epinephrine in, 219
  general measures, 230–231
  head trauma and, 272
  heart rate control in, 220–
    221
  hypovolemic
    chlorpromazine in, 229
    hemorrhage control in, 227
    isoproterenol in, 229
    methylprednisolone in, 228
    morphine in, 229
    phenoxybenzamine in, 229
    plasma loss control in, 227
    renal hypothermia in, 228
    treatment of, 226–227
  hypoxic
    airway obstruction in, 225
    respiration in, 225
    treatment of, 225–226
    ventilation in, 225
  inotropic agents in, 218–219
  isoproterenol in, 219
  kidney in, 228
  monitoring systems, 216–218
  neurogenic, treatment of,
    230–231
  norepinephrine in, 219
  oxygen therapy in, 221–222
  pathologic physiology, 214–
    216
  steroids in, 228–229
  tachyarrhythmias in, control
    of, 221
  tachycardia in, ventricular,
    221
  treatment of, 181–183, 218–
    231
  vasopressors in, 229
  volume expansion in, 220
  volume replacement in,
    227–228
  volume therapy, 230
SHOTGUN WOUND (see Gunshot
    wounds)
SHOULDER
  abduction, 18–19
  adduction, 18–19
  anatomy, 399–403
  blood supply, 399
  bones, 400
  dislocations (see
    Dislocations, shoulder)
  exercises, 450–452

1232 / INDEX

SHOULDER (cont.)
  in dislocation, 422–423
    early pendulum, 450–452
    in humerus supracondylar fracture, 482
    resistive, 451, 452
    stretching, 451, 452
  exposure
    posterior, 438
    superior, 438
  extension, backward, 18–19
  flexion
    forward, 18–19
    horizontal, 18–19
  fracture (see Fractures, shoulder)
  fracture-dislocation (see Fracture, -dislocation, shoulder)
  function, 399–403
  girdle, and motor function chart, 326–327
  joint exposure, patient position for, 890
  ligaments, 399, 400
  motion, 18–21, 399–400, 402–403
    clinical examination, 403
    glenohumeral, 21
    scapulothoracic, 21
  muscles, 399, 401
  nerves, 399
  palpation, 403
  rotation, 20
  slings (see Sling, shoulder)
  subluxation, transient recurrent anterior, 436
  surgical approaches to, 450
    anterior, 450
    deltoid-splitting incision, 450
    posterior, 450
    utility incision, 450
  trauma, 399–453
    clinical examination, 403
    incidence of, 403
    neurologic examination, 403
SHUNT
  for hepatic vein care, 1063
  for vena caval tear, 1063
SIGMOID: low, repair of, 1046
SIGMOIDOSCOPY, 186
SILICONE ROD: after flexor tendon removal, 567
"SILVER-FORK" DEFORMITY, 513, 515
SIMMONS-MARTIN ACROMIOCLAVICULAR PIN-SCREWS, 407
SKELETAL TRACTION (see Traction, skeletal)

SKELETON
  of hand, 583–603
  musculoskeletal function in burns, 1159
SKIN
  -adhesive technique, axial traction in recumbency, for humeral shaft fractures, 461
  closure in open fractures, 938–939
  in debridement of open fractures, 938
  grafts (see Grafts, skin)
  traction, in femoral shaft fractures, 728–730
  transplant, in soft tissue closure, 971–978
SKULL
  fractures (see Fractures, skull)
  traction (see Traction, skull)
SLING
  in acromioclavicular separation, 405
  collar and cuff
    in elbow dislocation, 471
    in humerus fractures, 481
  in humerus shaft fractures, long spiral oblique, 463
  pelvic, 616
  shoulder
    double sling, 421
    sling-and-swathe, 421
    wraparound, 421
  in traction for femoral shaft fracture, 734
SLOTTED PLATE (see Plate, slotted)
SMITH-PETERSEN, M.N., 5
SMITH-PETERSEN NAIL, 622
  tissue reaction to, 918
SMITH'S FRACTURE, 525
SODIUM
  bicarbonate
    in acidosis, 53
    in acidosis, metabolic, and shock, 220
  chloride in metabolic alkalosis, 54
  excretion rates in urine hemorrhage and, 42
  transfusion and, exchange, 42
  for hyperalimentation, 65
SOFT TISSUE, 969–992
  care of open wounds, 978–979
  closure, 971–978
    delayed primary, 979
    flap for (see Grafts, flap)
    linear, 971

methods, of, 971–978
  in replantation of arms, 1190–1191
  skin grafts in (see Grafts, skin)
  by skin transplant, 971–978
face trauma
  management of, 264–267
  shotgun blast causing, 266
in foot injuries, 837–839
in forearm fractures, 507
in hand injuries (see Hand, soft tissue injuries)
in knee injuries, 755–756
  treatment, 756
repairs, 969–992
SOUTHWICK SCREW EXTRACTOR, 908
SPHINCTER: anal, treatment, 1047–1048
SPHYGMOMANOMETRIC SYSTEM, 216
SPICA
  in humerus shaft fractures, 460, 465
  plaster of Paris
    in humerus shaft fractures, 460
  "walking," in ununited femur fracture, 128
SPICULES: of bone rotating femoral head fragment, 637
SPINE
  anesthesia, and cortisol excretion, 44
  arteries of, 321
  avulsion, 613, 756
  cervical, 345–381
    bend, lateral, 22
    decompression of, 366
    dislocations, essential points in, 379–381
    extension, 22
    flexion, 22
    fracture, ankylosis and, 375
    fracture, essential points in, 379–381
    graft for, fibular strut, 366
    hyperextension of, 376–377
    immobilization of, 357–360
    motion, 22
    neurologic symptoms, onset of, 345
    rotation, 22
    in shoulder examination, 403
    surgery (see cervical, surgery below)

traction and, 357–360
trauma, 345–381
trauma, common types, 366–379
trauma, dangerous to cord, 345–353
trauma, distribution of types, 358
treatment, definitive methods, 355–357
treatment, emergency, 353–354
treatment, halo and frame used, 355
treatment, initial evaluation and, 354–355
cervical, surgery
  anterior operation, 363–366
  anterior operation, technique, 363–366
  bone graft in, 365
  cineradiography in, 362
  posterior operation, 360–363
  posterior operation, technique, 361–363
cord, 317–341
  anatomy, 317–324
  Barton tongs and, 330, 332
  blood supply, in fetus, 321
  bullet wound of, causing quadriplegia, 337
  cervical, cross section of 323
  cervical spine injury dangerous to, 345–353
  concussion, 336
  contusion, 336
  diagram of, 318
  dislocations (see Dislocations, spinal cord)
  evaluation, basic, 324–330
  evaluation, clinical, 324–325
  fracture (see Fractures, spinal cord)
  fracture-dislocation, 333–334
  function, interruption of, complete, 372
  function, interruption of, partial, 373
  hypothermia, 339
  immobilization, 330–333
  laboratory studies, 325–330
  motor function chart and, 326–329
  motor impulses and, 320
  relationship to root level and vertebral body level, 322
  Rogers frame and, 332
  traction and, cervical, 330–331
  traction and, cervical, by cranial wires, 331
  transverse section through, 319
cord, trauma, 317–341, 343–345
  anterior, 336
  Brown-Séquard syndrome and, 336
  care after, medical and nursing, 339–340
  central cervical, 336
  decompression in, emergency, 338
  equipment needs in, 356
  functional goals in, 356
  immediate therapy with medical adjuvants, 325
  neurologic syndromes and, 336
  radiography of, 325, 329
  reticulospinal tracts and, 323
  surgery of, indications for, 336–339
  surgery of, late considerations, 339
  transportation after, 325
  visceral activity and, 323
dorsal
  flexion, 23–24
  motion, 23–24
extension, 25
flexion, causing disengagement of articular processes, 382
fractures (see Fractures, spine)
lumbar, 384–391
  flexion, 23–24
  motion, 23–24
  puncture, 186
  puncture, in head trauma, 278
motion, 25–26
neurologic considerations, 343–397
rotation, 26
stab wound causing paraplegia, 337
subarachnoid space block, 329
thoracic, 381–384
transverse processes, fractures of, 391–393
  multiple, 393
trauma, 343–397
  bowel and, 395
  cervical spine (see cervical, trauma *above*)
  to cord (see cord, trauma *above*)
  physical therapy after, 395–396
  team approach to, 396
  urinary tract and, 393–395
  upper, 381–384
SPINOTHALAMIC TRACTS: pain and temperature, 323
SPLEEN
  angiography (see Angiography, spleen)
  lacerated, splenectomy for, 1040
  treatment of, 1039
SPLENECTOMY: for lacerated spleen, 1040
SPLINTS, 183–184
  abduction, in humeral neck fracture, 444
  airplane, in humeral neck fracture, 444
  in clavicle fractures, 412, 413
  coaptation, for humerus shaft fractures, 460
  in femoral shaft fracture, 723
  Hogden, for femoral supracondylar fracture, 778
  Keller-Blake, for femoral shaft fracture, 723
  metal, in nose fractures, 252
  plaster
    in clavicle fracture, 413
    in Colles' fracture, 519
    in forearm fracture, 501
    in radius fracture, distal end, 517
  Velpeau, in clavicle fracture, in children, 413
  wool, in clavicle fracture, in infant, 413
SPONDYLOSIS: cervical, and spinal cord trauma, 336
SPONGE RUBBER: with elastic bandage, for knee, 754
SPRAIN: of hand ligaments, 586
STAB WOUND: of spine, causing paraplegia, 337
STAINLESS STEEL (see Steel, stainless)
STATUS EPILEPTICUS: diazepam in, 312
STEEL, STAINLESS
  corrosion of, 913–914
  18-8 SMo
    for plates and screws, 898
    specifications, 888
  plates, in humerus fractures, 439

STEEL, STAINLESS (cont.)
  316, corrosion of screws
      using, 922
  316-L, tissue reaction to, 918
STENOSIS: of celiac axis, 1062
STERNOCLAVICULAR
      DISLOCATIONS (see
      Dislocations,
      sternoclavicular)
STEROIDS
  in head trauma, 310
  for pemphigus, and multiple
      compression fractures of
      spine, 168
  in shock, 228–229
STIMSON METHOD
  in hip dislocation, posterior,
      688
  in shoulder dislocation,
      reduction, anterior, 420
STOMACH
  aspiration, 186–187, 1036
  emptying, artificial, 239
  full, and anesthetist, 239
  function, in burns, 1157–
      1158
  treatment, 1041
  ulcer, 56
STOOLS (see Feces)
STRAIGHT LEG RAISING TEST,
      26
STREPTOCOCCAL INFECTIONS:
      beta-hemolytic, 951
STRESS: adrenal response to,
      47
SUBARACHNOID HEMORRHAGE,
      284
SUBARACHNOID SPACE
  block, spinal, 329
  myelography of, 329
SUBDURAL HEMATOMA (see
      Hematoma, subdural)
SUBSCAPULARIS TENDON
      DIVISION: in Putti-Platt
      procedure, 432
SUFFERING (see Pain)
SUPINATION: forearm, 11
SURGEON: fracture, training of,
      888–890
SURGERY OF FRACTURES, 887–
      911
  bone addition, 897–899
  closure of wound, 899
  dressing, first, 899
  elevation, postoperative, 899
  Esmarch bandage in, 891
  excision of fragments, 910–
      911
  long-bone, operative
      approach and fixation,
      893–894
  preparation of patient, 890–
      892
  selection of cases, 888–890
  shoulder joint exposure,
      patient position for, 890
  techniques, 892–911
  tourniquet for, pneumatic,
      891
  training of fracture surgeon,
      888–890
SURGERY: general, priority of,
      188–189
SUTURE(S)
  mattress, interrupted
      everting, for
      arteriosclerotic vessel,
      1121
  scalp, 287
SUTURING
  nerves (see Nerves,
      peripheral, suturing)
  of vessels, 1119–1121
SWAN-GANZ CATHETER, 217
SWAN NECK DEFORMITY, 590
SWATHE: in humerus shaft
      fractures, 463
SWELLING (see Edema)
SYMPATHETIC BLOCKS: and
      arterial injuries, 1125
SYMPHYSIS PUBIS
  tear during childbirth, 613–
      614
  widening after trauma, 608
SYNOVITIS: of knee, traumatic,
      755–756
SYNOVIUM TEARS: and patellar
      fracture, 770

T

TACHYARRHYTHMIAS: in shock,
      control of, 221
TACHYCARDIA: ventricular, in
      shock, 221
TALOFIBULAR JOINT:
      separation of, 823
TALUS, 813
  dislocations, 848–850
      posterior, 850
  fracture (see Fractures, talus)
  fracture-dislocation, 849
  instability of, 822
  mechanical features of, 814
TARSAL NAVICULAR FRACTURE,
      850–851, 866, 867
  compression, 854
TARSOMETATARSAL
      DISLOCATIONS, 853–855
  radiography of, 856
TEAM APPROACH: after spinal
      trauma, 396
TEARDROP BLADDER, 1079
TEARDROP FRACTURES: of
      spinal cord, 335–336
TEETH
  malocclusion, and facial
      fractures, 260
  occlusion, fixation methods
      of, 260
TEFLON GRAFT: and aortic
      aneurysm, 1008
TEMPERATURE
  control and head trauma, 312
  spinothalamic tracts and, 323
TEMPORAL BONE: fractures,
      293
TENDONS, 957–968
  Achilles, 815
    divided, technique of
      approximating, 959
    lengthening in Volkmann's
      contracture, 149
    tears of, common sites, 957
    treatment of, 958–959
  anatomy of, 957
  of ankle (see Ankle, tendons
      of)
  biceps
    distal, rupture, complete,
      963
    distal, rupture, repair, 962
    distal, treatment, 962–963
    long head, rupture repair,
      961
    long head, treatment, 961–
      962
    in shoulder fracture-
      dislocation, 443
  extensor
    of finger (see Finger,
      extensor tendon)
    pollicis longus, repair, 964
    of thumb, treatment, 963–
      964
  flexor hallucis longus,
      treatment, 967
  of hand (see Hand, tendons
      of)
  injuries, 957–968
    mechanism of, 957
    signs of, 958
    symptoms of, 158
  knee quadriceps, rupture of,
      766–767
    treatment, 767
  major, 957–968
  patellar, treatment, 965
  pathologic processes in,
      957–958
  pulley forces on malleoli,
      827
  quadriceps
    repair by fascial strip, 960
    treatment of, 959–961
  reflexes, deep, examination

in head trauma, 275
subscapularis, division, in Putti-Platt procedure, 432
tibial
  posterior and anterior, treatment, 966–967
  posterior, rupture repair, 967
  treatment of, 958–967
TESTES: injuries, 1086
TETANUS, 951–954
  prophylaxis, 953–954
  treatment, 954
TETRACYCLINE
  in bacteremic shock, 230
  in surgical infections, 952
THERAPY, 177–189
  immediate, 187–188
THIGH DRAINAGE: in infection of femoral shaft fracture, 130
THORACIC SPINE, 381–384
THORACIC VERTEBRA (see Vertebra, thoracic)
THORAX (see Chest)
THORNTON PLATE
  break in, 927
  tissue reaction to, 918
THROMBECTOMY, 1124
THROMBOEMBOLISM: femoral vein interruption in, 1126
THROMBOPLASTIN TIME: partial, 49
THROMBOSIS, 49
  arterial, distal, 1123–1124
  in Volkmann's contracture, 1131
THUMB
  abduction, 13, 15
  adduction, 13
  carpometacarpal joint fracture-dislocation, 592
  epiphysis, type III injury, 884
  extensor tendon, treatment of, 963–964
  flexion, 15
  ligament injuries, collateral, pathology, 587
  loss of, treatment, 989
  metacarpophalangeal joint dislocation, 592
    ligament rupture, 586
    volar plate injury, 589
  motion, 13–15
  rotation, 15
  traction in Colles' fracture, 518, 519
THYROID: function changes, 64
TIBIA

approach to
  lateral, 122
  posterior, 154
blood supply, 120
distal, management, 884
epiphysis
  distal, type II injury, 883
  distal, type III injury, 883
  proximal, cross section, 871
  proximal, fracture, 882
fixation to fibula, rigid, 817
fractures (see Fractures, tibia)
grafts (see Grafts, tibial)
proximal, management, 882–884
pseudarthrosis, 138
tubercle
  avulsion from, 767
  avulsion from, treatment, 767
  traction through, in femoral shaft fracture, 733
TIBIAL TENDONS (see Tendons, tibial)
TIDAL VOLUME: dead space to tidal volume ratio, 1031
TISSUE
  lean, metabolic response of, 58–60
  mesenchymal, 80
  reactions to metal implants, 917–918
  soft (see Soft tissue)
TITANIUM: corrosion of, 914–915
TODD'S PALSY, 284
TOES
  abduction, 36
  adduction, 36
  extension, 36
  flexion, 36
  fracture (see Fractures, toes)
  fracture-dislocation, 856
  great
    fractures of, 857
    Kirschner wires used for, 858
  motion, 36
TOMOGRAPHY: Computerized Axial, 279
TOUCH
  response after nerve suture, 1112
  sensibility, 323
TOURNIQUET: pneumatic, 891
TRACHEA
  intubation, 236
  laceration, and anesthetist, 241
TRACHEOSTOMY, 994
  emergency, 179
  in face trauma, 248–249

tube, migratory, 1030
TRACTION
  axial, in humerus shaft fractures, 461
  Bryant, in femoral shaft fractures, 731, 732–733
  cervical, after spinal cord trauma, 330–331
  Dunlop's, in humerus supracondylar fracture, 480–481
  in femoral shaft fractures (see Fractures, femur, shaft, traction)
  in forearm fractures, 500
  halter, in vertebral dislocation, 352
  90-90-90, in femoral shaft fracture, 734–736
  olecranon wire, in humerus shaft fractures, 465
  in radius fractures, distal end, 518
  Russell, in femoral fracture extracapsular, 655
    shaft, 732, 733
  skeletal
    in femoral fractures, shaft, 730–736
    in hand fractures, unstable, 597
    in humerus shaft fractures, 460–461
    overhead, in humerus supracondylar fracture, 481
  skin, in femoral shaft fractures, 728–730
  skull
    in dislocation of cervical spinal cord, 353
    in fracture of cervical spinal cord, 353
    in odontoid process fracture, 352, 359
    in vertebral fracture, 351
  spinal trauma and, cervical, 357–360
  straps, types of, 729
  suspension, in femoral shaft fracture, 733–734, 735
  thumb, in Colles' fracture, 518, 519
TRAINING: of fracture surgeon, 888–890
TRANSFIXION BOLT: in humerus fractures, T and Y, 489
TRANSFUSIONS
  exchange, and sodium excretion rates, 42
  multiple, 54–55

1236 / INDEX

TRANSPLANTATION
  fibula, for radius fracture and avulsion, 141
  nerve, ulnar, technique, 1106–1107
  organ, 314
  skin, in soft tissue closure, 971–978
TRANSPORTATION
  coma patients, 271
  face trauma patients, 243–244
  in femoral fractures, extracapsular, 654–657
  head trauma patients, 270–272
  in open fractures, 936
  after spinal cord trauma, 325
TRAP DOOR FLAP DEFORMITY, 267
TREATMENT (see Therapy)
TRENCH FOOT, 1167
TRIGEMINAL NERVE, 293
TROCHANTERIC FRACTURE NONUNION, 669–673
  management, 672
TUMORS: humerus giant cell, and pathologic fracture, 170

U

ULCER
  gastrointestinal, 56
  knee, 975
  os calcis, 977
  sacral pressure, in paraplegia, 976
ULNA
  dislocations (see Dislocations, ulna)
  fractures (see Fractures, ulna)
ULNAR DEVIATION: wrist, 12
ULNAR NERVE: transplantation technique, 1106–1107
ULTRASOUND: in rehabilitation, 1177–1178
UNION
  by bone shortening, 126
  delayed, 115–158
    causes of, local, 116
    clavicle fractures, 415
    early weight bearing and, 134
    "hardware" and, 134
    humerus shaft fractures, 465, 466
    improperly applied slotted plate causing, 118
    unnecessary surgery causing, 134
  forearm, cross union, 509

UREA: in head trauma, 309
URECOLINE: in urinary complications after spinal trauma, 394
URETER INJURIES, 1076–1078
  diagnosis, 1076
  surgery, 1077
  treatment, 1077–1078
URETHRA, 1080–1085
  injuries, 1080–1085
    diagnosis, 1081
    etiology, 1080
    findings in, clinical, 1081
    pathology, 1080–1081
    treatment, 1081–1085
  laceration, 608
  leakage from, causing extravasation, 1080
  transection, complete
    Banks' method in, 1083–1085
    mobility of prostate in, 1082
    urethrography in, 1081
URETHROGRAPHY: in complete urethral transection, 1081
URINARY TRACT
  infection, after immobilization, 61
  injuries, 1071–1086
  spinal trauma and, 393–395
  treatment, 1049–1050
URINE
  drainage, in abdominal injuries, 1036
  studies, 186
UROGRAPHY: of kidney, 1073

V

VALGUS, CUBITUS
  after elbow displacement, 494
  after humeral fracture, 483
VALVES: aortic, traumatic regurgitation, 1007
VAN GORDER, C. W., 4
VA/Q SPREAD, 1020
VARUS
  cubitus, after humeral fracture, 483
  deformity, after femoral fracture, 656, 658
VASCULAR (see Vessels)
VASOCONSTRICTION, 1115
VASODILATION, 1115–1116
VASOPRESSORS: in shock, 229
VASOSPASM
  prevention in impending Volkmann's contracture, 1133
  traumatic, in Volkmann's

contracture, 1130–1131
VD/VT, 1031
VEINS, 1125–1128
  anastomoses of, 1189
  arteriovenous fistula, angiography of, 205, 206
  central venous pressure, 237
  femoral, interruption in thromboembolism, 1126
  iliofemoral, occlusion, 1127
  injuries, 1125–1128
  of liver, 1059
  tears, shunt for, 1063
  obstruction, in Volkmann's contracture, 1130
  renal, vena caval clip below, 1125
VELCRO STRAP: in femoral shaft fracture, 742
VENA CAVA
  clip, below renal veins, 1125
  tears, shunt for, 1063
VENOGRAPHY: of kidney, 1073
VENTILATION (see Respiration, Respiratory)
VENTILATOR (see Respirator)
VENTRICULAR TACHYCARDIA: in shock, 221
VERTEBRA
  body level, relationship to spinal cord and exciting root level, 322
  dislocation (see Dislocation, vertebra)
  fracture (see Fractures, vertebra)
  fracture-dislocation (see Fracture, -dislocation, vertebra)
  lumbar, 384–391
  anatomy, bony, 320
  thoracic, 381–384
  thoracic, decalcified, 347
  radiography of specimen, 347
  sagittal section of, 347
  thoracic, transverse section through, 319
"VERTICAL SECTOR:" principle of, 458
VESSELS, 1005–1014
  after acetabular fractures, 704
  arteriosclerotic, anastomosis for, 1121
  clamping, in face trauma, 243–244
  in elbow dislocations, 471
  in femoral shaft fracture, 722
  grafts for, with anastomosis, 1122
  great, 1005–1014
  great, angiography, 198

great, trauma, 1005–1014
  blunt, 1007–1011
  emergency room
    management, 1005–1006
  penetrating, 1011–1013
after hip dislocations, 704
insufficiency, 50
peripheral, 1115–1128
  injuries, 1115–1128
  injuries, ischemic
    extremity losses and,
    1116
  in replantation of arms,
    1187–1190
  revascularization in bone
    repair, 78, 80
  small, occlusion, reasons for,
    1184
  in supracondylar humerus
    fracture, 480
  suturing of, 1119–1121
  unstable system, and
    anesthetist, 238
VIBRATION SENSIBILITY, 323
VISCERAL ACTIVITY: and spinal
  cord trauma, 323
VITAL CAPACITY, 1021
VITAL SIGNS: in examination,
  184
VITALLIUM
  plate, in humerus shaft
    fracture, 465
  prosthesis
    in femur neck fractures,
    116
    for lesser bones of foot,
    862
  specifications, 888
VOLAR PLATE INJURY, 589–591
  swan neck deformity and,
    590
  thumb metacarpophalangeal
    joint, 589
VOLKMANN'S CONTRACTURE,
  1129–1136
  Achilles tendon lengthening
    in, 149
  arterial obstruction in, 1130
  edema in, 1130
  after humerus supracondylar
    fracture, 479, 481
  impending

clinical features, 1131–
  1132
fracture reduction and,
  1133
initial examination in, 1132
management, 1133–1134
recognition of, 1131–1133
surgery, 1133–1134
vasospasm prevention in,
  1133
ischemia in, mechanisms of,
  1130–1131
lymphatic obstruction in,
  1130
muscle ischemia in,
  management, 1134–1135
muscle metabolism in, 1131
nature of process, 1129–1130
thrombosis in, 1131
vasospasm in, traumatic,
  1130–1131
venous obstruction in, 1130
VOLUME
  expansion in shock, 220
  replacement in shock, 227–
    228
  therapy in shock, 230

W

WALKING (see Crutches,
  walking with)
WATER-SEAL DRAINAGE, 1001
WATERS POSITION, 246
WEANING: from ventilator,
  1029
WEBBING AND RING SPLINTS:
  for clavicle fractures, 413
WEBRIL SPLINTS: for clavicle
  fractures, in children,
  413
WET LUNG SYNDROME, 1021–
  1022
WILSON, P.D., 3
WIRE(S)
  buttons, in fixation of teeth in
    occlusion, 260
  cranial, for traction after
    spinal cord trauma, 331
  in femoral fracture,
    extracapsular, with
    Jewett nail, 661

in fixation of teeth in
  occlusion, 260
Kirschner (see Kirschner
  wire)
loop in radius nonunion, 157
migration in femoral neck
  fractures, 649
olecranon wire traction in
  humerus shaft fractures,
  465
WIRING
  fixing maxilla to orbital
    rim, 259
  in zygoma fracture, 254
WOOL SPLINTS: in clavicular
  fracture, in infant, 413
WORK OF BREATHING (see
  Breathing, work of)
WRIST
  amputations, fixation in, 1188
  anatomy, diagrams, 514
  combined injuries of, 550–
    552
  extension, 12
  flexion, 12
  fracture of, 551
  fracture-dislocation of, 547
  Madelungs deformity at, 474
  motion, 12
  nerve, median
    approach to, 549
    sensory changes after
      trauma, 548
    traumatic neuritis of, 549–
      550
  radial deviation, 12
  in shoulder examination, 403
  trauma, 520
  ulnar deviation, 12

X

X-RAY (see Radiation)
XYLOCAINE: in face trauma,
  248

Z

ZYGOMA
  displacement, 254
  fractures (see Fractures,
    zygoma)

← PZ